The Adult Spine

Principles and Practice

Second Edition

The Adult Spine

Principles and Practice

Second Edition

Editor-in-Chief

JOHN W. FRYMOYER, M.D.

Dean, College of Medicine
Professor of Orthopaedics
Department of Orthopaedics and Rehabilitation
University of Vermont
Burlington, Vermont

Associate Editors

THOMAS B. DUCKER, M.D.

Professor of Surgery
Department of Neurosurgery
The Johns Hopkins University School of Medicine
Baltimore, Maryland

NORTIN M. HADLER, M.D.

Professor of Medicine and Microbiology/Immunology
School of Medicine
University of North Carolina at Chapel Hill
and Attending Rheumatologist
University of North Carolina Hospitals
Chapel Hill, North Carolina

JOHN P. KOSTUIK, M.D.

Professor
Department of Orthopaedic Surgery
The Johns Hopkins University School of Medicine
Baltimore, Maryland

JAMES N. WEINSTEIN, D.O., M.S.

Division of Orthopedics and Neurosurgery
Senior Faculty Member
Center for Clinical Evaluative Sciences
Dartmouth Medical School
Dartmouth Hitchcock Medical Center
Hanover, New Hampshire

THOMAS S. WHITECLOUD III, M.D.

Ray J. Haddard, Jr. Professor and Chairman
Department of Orthopaedic Surgery
Tulane University School of Medicine
New Orleans, Louisiana

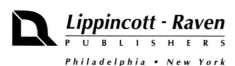 **Lippincott - Raven**
P U B L I S H E R S
Philadelphia • New York

© 1997, Lippincott-Raven Publishers. All rights reserved. This book is protected by copyright. No part of it may be reproduced, stored in a retrieval system, or transmitted, in any form or by any means—electronic, mechanical, photocopy, recording, or otherwise—without the prior written consent of the publisher, except for brief quotations embodied in critical articles and reviews. For information write
Lippincott–Raven Publishers, 227 East Washington Square, Philadelphia, PA 19106-3780.

Materials appearing in this book prepared by individuals as part of their official duties as U.S. Government employees are not covered by the above-mentioned copyright.

Printed in the United States of America

9 8 7 6 5 4 3 2 1

Library of Congress Cataloging-in-Publication Data

The adult spine: principles and practice/editor-in-chief, John W. Frymoyer; associate editors, Thomas B. Ducker . . .[et al.]—2nd ed.
    p. cm.
   Includes bibliographical references and index.
   ISBN 0-7817-0329-8
   1. Spine—Abnormalities.   2. Spine—Wounds and injuries.
  3. Spine—Diseases—Treatment.   4. Spine—Surgery.
   I. Frymoyer, John W. [DNLM: 1. Spinal Diseases. 2. Spine.
  WE 725 A244 1996]
  RD768.A32   1997
  617.5′6—dc20
  DNLM/DLC
  for Library of Congress   95-23863

Care has been taken to confirm the accuracy of the information presented and to describe generally accepted practices. However, the authors, editors, and publisher are not responsible for errors or omissions or for any consequences from application of the information in this book and make no warranty, express or implied, with respect to the contents of the puplication.

The authors, editors, and publisher have exerted every effort to ensure that drug selection and dosage set forth in this text are in accordance with current recommendations and practice at the time of publication. However, in view of ongoing research, changes in government regulations, and the constant flow of information relating to drug therapy and drug reactions, the reader is urged to check the package insert for each drug for any change in indications and dosage and for added warning and precautions. This is particularly important when the recommended agent is a new or infrequently employed drug.

Some drugs and medical devices presented in this publication have Food and Drug Administration (FDA) clearance for limited use in restricted research settings. It is the responsibility of the health care provider to ascertain the FDA status of each drug or device planned for use in their clinical practice.

The First Edition of *The Adult Spine* was dedicated to our teachers, many of whom were the pioneers who shaped the entire field of spinal diagnosis and management. The list was extensive and included F.P. Dewar, John Hall, Edgar Kahn, Ludwig Kempe, William Kirkaldy-Willis, Stephen Krane, Henry Metzger, Alf Nachmenson, Richard Schneider, Edwards Simmonds, Henk Verbiest, Partick Wall, and Leon Wiltse.

In addition, two particular great people who influenced the thinking about spinal disorders died after publication of the First Edition. Ian Macnab and Harry Farfan, as much as any two individuals, shaped our thinking of spinal stability and instability, and how we can think about, diagnose, and treat elusive causes of low back pain. It is to their memory that we pay particular tribute.

Finally, the job of an Editor-in-Chief is to keep the multiple authors working in harmony and toward a common purpose. In the case of *The Adult Spine* this job has been made easier because of the focus and good will of the Associate Editors. In addition, the environment in which we work must support the effort. For that reason, this Edition is dedicated to Lois and Warren McClure, whose establishment of a Musculoskeletal Research Center has provided a focus for scholarly activity at the University of Vermont. More important, their dedication to many causes, through giving with "warm hands," has been an inspiration to all of us fortunate enough to be associated with them.

Contents

Volume 1

PART I: EPIDEMIOLOGY, DISABILITY, AND SOCIETAL IMPACT
Editor: Nortin M. Hadler

PART II: GENERAL ISSUES OF SPINAL DISORDERS
Editor: James N. Weinstein

Diagnostic Studies

General Operative Considerations

General and Degenerative Conditions

Metabolic Disease

Inflammatory Disorders

Degenerative Conditions of the Cervical Spine

Volume 2

PART IV: THORACIC AND THORACOLUMBAR SPINE
Editor: John P. Kostuik

Trauma to the Thoracolumbar Spine

Adult Spine Deformities

PART V: LUMBAR SPINE AND SACRUM
Editor: John W. Frymoyer

Low Back Disorders: Diagnosis and Conservative Treatment

Physical Therapy and Education

Congenital Abnormalities

Degenerative Conditions and Disc Herniation: Diagnosis and Treatment

Stenosis/Neurogenic Claudication

Segmental Instability

PART VI: SACRUM AND COCCYX
Editor: John W. Frymoyer

Subject Index follows Chapter 112

Contributors

Rodney H. Adkins, Ph.D.   *Spinal Cord Injury Project, Rancho Los Amigos Medical Center, 7601 East Imperial Highway, Downey, California 90242*

Pieter F. van Akkerveeken, M.D., Ph.D.   *Orthopedic Surgeon, Director, Rugadviescentra Nederland, Utrechtseweg 92, 3702 AD Zeist, The Netherlands*

David B. Allan, M.B., Ch.B., F.R.C.S.   *Consultant Orthopaedic Surgeon, Queen Elizabeth National Spinal Injury Unit, Southern General Hospital, Govan Road, Glasgow G51 4TF, Scotland*

Paul A. Anderson, M.D.   *Clinical Associate Professor, Department of Orthopaedic Surgery, University of Washington, Orthopaedics International, Suite 400, 1600 East Jefferson Street, Seattle, Washington 98122*

Gunnar B. J. Andersson, M.D., Ph.D.   *Professor and Chairman, Department of Orthopedic Surgery, Rush-Presbyterian-St. Luke's Medical Center, 1653 West Congress Parkway, 1471 Jelke, Chicago, Illinois 60612*

Charles Neuville Aprill III, M.D.   *Spine Radiologist, Magnolia Diagnostic, 4303 Magnolia Street, New Orleans, Louisiana 70115*

Steven J. Atlas, M.D., M.P.H.   *Instructor in Medicine, Harvard Medical School, Department of Medicine, Massachusetts General Hospital, 50 Staniford Street, 9th floor, Boston, Massachusetts 02114*

Michele Crites Battié, Ph.D.   *Professor and Chair, Department of Physical Therapy, University of Alberta, 2-50 Corbett Hall, Edmonton, Canada T6G 2G4*

Ulrich Batzdorf, M.D.   *Professor of Neurosurgery, Department of Surgery/Neurosurgery, University of California, Los Angeles, Box 956901, Los Angeles, California 90095-6901*

Jean C. Beckham, Ph.D.   *Assistant Professor, Department of Psychiatry and Behavioral Sciences, Duke University Medical Center, Box 2969, Durham, North Carolina 27710*

Daniel R. Benson, M.D.   *Professor of Orthopaedic Surgery, Department of Orthopaedics, University of California, Davis, 2230 Stockton Boulevard, Sacramento, California 95817*

Thomas N. Bernard, Jr., M.D.   *Clinical Assistant Professor, Department of Orthopaedics, Tulane University School of Medicine, New Orleans, Louisiana, and Anderson Orthopaedic Clinic, 500 North Fant Street, Anderson, South Carolina 29621*

Louis Bessette, M.D., F.R.C.P.(C.), M.S.   *Department of Medicine, Laval University, Le Centre Hospitalier de l'Université, 2705 Boul. Lavrier, Ste-Foy, Quebec, GIV 4G2, Canada, current address: Brigham and Women's Hospital, 75 Francis Street, Boston, Massachusetts 02115*

Stanley J. Bigos, M.D.   *Professor of Orthopaedics and Environmental Health, Department of Orthopaedics, University of Washington, 1959 Pacific Avenue N.E., Box 356500, Seattle, Washington 98195*

Jane F. Bleasel, M.B.B.S., F.R.A.C.P.   *Department of Rheumatology, Rachel Forster Hospital, 150 Pitt Street Redfern, Sydney, New South Wales 2065, Australia*

Scott D. Boden, M.D.   *Associate Professor of Orthopaedic Surgery, Director, The Emory Spine Center, Emory University School of Medicine, 2165 North Decatur Road, Decatur, Georgia 30033*

Henry H. Bohlman, M.D.   *Professor, Department of Orthopaedic Surgery, Case Western Reserve University, Director, Reconstructive and Traumatic Spine Surgery Center, University Hospitals of Cleveland, 11100 Eucllid Avenue, Cleveland, Ohio 44106*

Michael J. Bolesta, M.D.   *Assistant Professor of Orthopaedic Surgery, Department of Orthopaedic Surgery, The University of Texas Southwestern Medical School, 5323 Harry Hines Boulevard, Dallas, Texas 75235-8883*

Stefano Boriani, M.D.   *Modulo di Chirurgia Vertebrale della 5ᵃ Divisione, Rizzoli Institute, Via G.C. Pupilli 1, Bologna 40137, Italy*

Deke J. Botsford, M.D.   *Resident, Faculty of Medicine, Department of Surgery, University of Toronto, 1 King's College Circle, Toronto, Ontario, Canada M5S 1A8*

Eric A. Brandser, M.D.   *Assistant Professor, Department of Radiology, University of Iowa Colege of Medicine, University of Iowa Hospitals and Clinic, 200 Hawkins Drive, Iowa City, Iowa 52242*

Antonio Briccoli, M.D.   *Associate Professor, Department of General Surgery, University of Moderna, Modena, Italy*

Mark R. Brinker, M.D.   *Clinical Associate Professor of Orthopaedic Surgery, Tulane University School of Medicine and, Director of Orthopaedic Research, St. Luke's Medical Center, Department of Orthopaedic Surgery and, Residency Program, Cleveland, Ohio and, Texas Orthopedic Hopital, Fondren Orthopedic Group, L.L.P., 7401 S. Main, Houston, Texas 77030*

James C. Butler, M.D.   *Associate Professor, Department of Orthopaedic Surgery, Tulane University School of Medicine, 1430 Tulane Avenue, New Orleans, Louisiana 70112*

James N. Campbell, M.D.   *Professor of Neurosurgery, Department of Neurosurgery, The Johns Hopkins University School of Medicine, 600 North Wolfe Street, Meyer 5-109, Baltimore, Maryland 21287-7509*

Laura C. Campanacci, M.D.   *Orthopaedic Consultant, Department of Orthopaedics, Rizzoli Institute, via Pupilli 1, Bologna 40137, Italy*

Rodolfo Capanna, M.D.   *Chairman, Orthopaedic Department, Centro Ortopedico Traumatologico, Policlinico Careggi, University of Florence, L. Palagi 1, Florence 50100, Italy*

Timothy S. Carey, M.D., M.P.H.   *Associate Professor, Department of Medicine, University of North Carolina at Chapel Hill, The Sheps Center for Health Services Research, Suite 210, Chapel Hill, North Carolina 27599-7110*

J. David Cassidy, D.C., Ph.D., F.C.C.S.(C.)   *Director of Research, Department of Orthopaedics, Royal University Hospital, 103 Hospital Drive, Saskatoon, Saskatchewan, S7N OW8, Canada*

John R. Cassidy, M.D.   *Suite 610, 1921 Waldemere Street, Sarasota, Florida 34239*

Jens R. Chapman, M.D.   *Assistant Professor, Chief of Orthopaedic Spine Service, Department of Orthopaedic Surgery, Harborview Medical Center, University of Washington, 325 Ninth Avenue, Seattle, Washington 98104*

Charles R. Clark, M.D.   *Professor, Department of Orthopaedic Surgery, University of Iowa College of Medicine, 200 Hawkins Drive, Iowa City, Iowa 52242*

Andrew H. Cragg, M.D.   *Attending Radiologist, Department of Interventional Vascular Medicine, Fairview Riverside Medical Center, 2450 Riverside Avenue, Minneapolis, Minnesota 55454*

Mark K. Crawford, M.D.   *Assistant Professor, Chief, Division of Spine Surgery, Department of Orthopaedics, University of New Mexico Health Sciences Center, Albuquerque, New Mexico 87131-5296*

Gregory R. Criscuolo, M.D.   *Assistant Professor of Neurosurgery, Division of Neurological Surgery, Yale University School of Medicine, 333 Cedar Street, New Haven, Connecticut 06520-8039*

Stephen L. Curtin, M.D.   *Tucson Orthopaedic Institute, P.C., Suite 200, 2424 N. Wyatt Drive, Tucson, Arizona 85712*

Stephen M. David, M.D.   *Resident, Department of Orthopaedic Surgery, Carolinas Medical Center, 1000 Blythe Boulevard, P.O. Box 32861, Charlotte, North Carolina 28232*

Richard B. Delamarter, M.D.   *Associate Clinical Professor, Division of Orthopaedic Surgery, University of California, Los Angeles Medical Center, 100 UCLA Medical Plaza, Suite 755, Los Angeles, California 90024*

Richard A. Deyo, M.D., M.P.H.   *Professor, Departments of Medicine and Health Services, Back Pain Outcome Assessment Team, University of Washington, 1107-NE 45th Street, Suite 427, Seattle, Washington 98105-4631*

Elizabeth A. Dienes, M.D.   *Medical Director, MRI, Venice Hospital, 540 The Rialto, Venice, Florida 34285*

John F. Ditunno, Jr., M.D. *Professor, Department of Rehabilitation Medicine, Jefferson Medical College of Thomas Jefferson University, 111 South 11th Street, Suite 9410, Gibbon Building, Philadelphia, Pennsylvania 19107-5098*

Ronald G. Donelson, M.D. *Assistant Professor, Department of Orthopedics, SUNY-HSC at Syracuse, 550 Harrison Center, Suite 130, Syracuse, New York 13202*

Craig A. Dopf, M.D. *Department of Orthopedics, Meriter Park Hospital, 202 S. Park Street, Madison, Wisconsin 53715*

Thomas B. Ducker, M.D. *Professor of Surgery, Department of Neurosurgery, The Johns Hopkins University School of Medicine, 600 North Wolfe Street, Baltimore, Maryland 21205*

Ann-Christine Duhaime, M.D. *Associate Neurosurgeon, Children's Hospital of Philadelphia, University of Pennsylvania School of Medicine, 34th and Civic Center Boulevard, Philadelphia, Pennsylvania 19104*

Carol L. Durett, M.B.A. *Clinical Instructor, Biomedical Technologies, University of Vermont and, Financial Services Specialist, Fletcher Allen Health Care, 111 Colchester Avenue, Burlington, Vermont 05401*

Jiri Dvořák, M.D. *Spine Unit, Department of Neurology, Schulthess Hospital, Lengghalde 2, 8008 Zürich, Switzerland*

Thomas A. Einhorn, M.D. *Professor, Department of Orthopaedics, Mount Sinai Medical Center, One Gustave L. Levy Place, New York, New York 10029-6574*

Stephen M. Eisenstein, Ph.D., F.R.C.S.(Ed.) *Director, Center for Spine Studies, The Robert Jones & Agnes Hunt Orthopaedic Hospital, Keele University, Oswestry, Shropshire SY10 7AG, United Kingdom*

Georges Y. El-Khoury, M.D. *Professor of Radiology and Orthopaedic Surgery, Department of Radiology, The University of Iowa College of Medicine, University of Iowa/Hospitals and Clinics, 200 Hawkins Drive, Iowa City, Iowa 52242-1077*

Beth A. Elliott, M.D. *Assistant Professor of Anesthesiology, Mayo Medical School, Department of Anesthesiology, Mayo Clinic, 200 First Street SW, Rochester, Minnesota 55905*

Joseph E. Epstein, M.D., F.A.C.S. *Clinical Professor of Neurological Surgery, Department of Neurosurgery, Albert Einstein College of Medicine, Bronx, New York and, Long Island Neurosurgery Association, 410 Lakeville Road, Suite 204, New Hyde Park, New York 11042*

Nancy E. Epstein, M.D., F.A.C.S. *Clinical Associate Professor, Department of Neurosurgery, Cornell University Medical College and, North Shore University Hospital, Manhasset, New York 11030, Long Island Neurosurgery Assoc., Suite 204, 410 Lakeville Road, New Hyde Park, New York 11042*

Thomas J. Errico, M.D. *Associate Professor of Clinical Orthopedics and Neurosurgery, Department of Orthopedics, New York University Medical Center, Suite 84, 530 First Avenue, New York, New York 10016*

Stephen I. Esses, M.D., F.R.C.S.(C.), F.A.C.S. *Professor, Department of Orthopedic Surgery, Baylor College of Medicine, 6550 Fannin, Suite 2526, Houston, Texas 77030*

David F. Fardon, M.D. *Clinical Associate Professor of Orthopedic Surgery, University of Tennessee, Knoxville Orthopaedic Clinic, 1128 Weisbarger Road, Knoxville, Tennessee 37909*

Roger B. Fillingim, Ph.D. *Research Assistant Professor, Department of Dental Ecology, University of North Carolina at Chapel Hill, CB 7455, Chapel Hill, North Carolina 27599-7455*

Christopher S. Formal, M.D. *Associate Professor, Department of Rehabilitation Medicine, Magee Rehabilitation Hospital, 6 Franklin Plaza, Philadelphia, Pennsylvania 19102*

Robert D. Fraser, M.B.B.S., M.D., F.R.A.C.S. *Head, Spinal Unit, Clinical Professor, Department of Orthopaedics & Trauma, Royal Adelaide Hospital, North Terrace, Adelaide, 5000 South Australia*

Bruce E. Fredricksen, M.D. *Professor of Orthopedic and Neurologic Surgery, Department of Orthopedic Surgery, SUNY Health Science Center, 550 Harrison Center, Suite 100, Syracuse, New York 13202*

Gary E. Friedlaender, M.D. *Professor and Chairman, Department of Orthopaedics and Rehabilitation, Yale University School of Medicine, P.O. Box 20871, 333 Cedar Street, New Haven, Connecticut 06520-8071*

John W. Frymoyer, M.D.   *Dean, College of Medicine, Professor of Orthopaedics, Director, McClure Musculoskeletal Research Center, Department of Orthopaedics and Rehabilitation, University of Vermont, E109 Given Building, Burlington, Vermont 05405*

Francis W. Gamache, Jr., M.D.   *Associate Professor, Department of Surgery, The New York Hospital-Cornell Medical Center, 525 East 68th Street, New York, New York 10021*

Steven R. Garfin, M.D.   *Professor of Orthopaedic Surgery, Department of Orthopaedics, University of California, San Diego, 200 W. Arbor Drive, San Diego, California 92103-8894*

Alessandro Gasbarrini, M.D.   *Orthopaedic Consultant, Department of Orthopaedics, Rizzoli Institute, via Pupilli 1, Bologna 40137, Italy*

Kevin Gill, M.D.   *Clinical Associate Professor, Department of Orthopedics, University of Texas Southwestern Medical Center, Dallas, Texas 75235 and, Southwest Orthopedic Institute, Suite 560, 5920 Forest Park Road, Dallas, Texas 75235*

Russell H. Glantz, M.D.   *Associate Professor of Neurology, Department of Neurological Sciences, Rush-Presbyterian-St. Luke's Medical Center, 1725 West Harrison Street, Chicago, Illinois 60612*

Vijay K. Goel, Ph.D.   *Professor and Chairman, Department of Biomedical Engineering, University of Iowa, College of Engineering, EB1202, Iowa City, Iowa 52242*

Leon J. Grobler, M.B., Ch.B., M.Med., F.C.S.   *Associate Professor of Surgery, Department of Orthopaedic Surgery, Bowman Gray School of Medicine, Wake Forest University, Medical Center Boulevard, Winston-Salem, North Carolina 27157-1070*

Nortin M. Hadler, M.D.   *Professor of Medicine and Microbiology/Immunology, School of Medicine, University of North Carolina at Chapel Hill and, Attending Rheumatologist, University of North Carolina Hospitals, 3330 Thurston Building, Campus Box 7280, Chapel Hill, North Carolina 27599-7280*

Scott Haldeman, D.C., M.D., Ph.D., F.R.C.P.   *Associate Clinical Professor, Department of Neurology, University of California, Irvine, Adjunct Professor, Los Angeles College of Chiropractic, 16200 East Amber Valley Drive, Whittier, California 90609-1166*

Jerome C. Hall, M.D.   *Resident in Orthopedics, Department of Orthopedics, Mount Sinai Medical Center, One Gustave L. Levy Place, New York, NY 10029-6574*

Manny (Nachman) Halpern, M.A., C.P.E.   *Occupational and Industrial Orthopaedic Center, New York University Medical Center, Hospital for Joint Diseases, 63 Downing Street, New York, New York 10014*

Edward N. Hanley, Jr., M.D.   *Chairman, Department of Orthopaedic Surgery, Carolinas Medical Center, Clinical Professor, Department of Surgery, School of Medicine, University of North Carolina at Chapel Hill, 1000 Blythe Boulevard, P.O. Box 32861, Charlotte, North Carolina 28232*

Russell W. Hardy, Jr., M.D.   *Professor, Department of Neurosurgery, University Hospitals of Cleveland, 11100 Euclid Avenue, Cleveland, Ohio 44106-4915*

Mitsuo Hasue, M.D.   *Department of Orthopaedic Surgery, Japanese Red Cross Medical Center, 4-1-22 Hiroo, Shibuya-ku, Tokyo, Japan 150*

Rowland G. Hazard, M.D.   *Associate Professor, Department of Orthopaedics and Rehabilitation, University of Vermont, Burlington, Vermont 05405*

Michael H. Heggeness, M.D., Ph.D.   *Associate Professor, Department of Orthopedic Surgery, Baylor College of Medicine, Suite 2501, 60 Fannin Street, Houston, Texas 77030*

Kenneth B. Heithoff, M.D.   *Medical Director and Chairman, Department of Radiology, Center for Diagnostic Imaging, Suite 190, 5775 Wayzata Boulevard, St. Louis Park, Minnesota 55416*

John G. Heller, M.D.   *Associate Professor of Orthopaedic Surgery, Department of Orthopaedic Surgery, Emory University Hospital/School of Medicine, 2165 N. Decatur Road, Decatur, Georgia 30033*

Richard J. Herzog, M.D.   *Medical Director, San Francisco Neuro Skeletal Imaging, Suite 100, and San Francisco Spine Institute, Suite 140, 1850 Sullivan Avenue South, Daly City, California 94015*

Richard T. Holt, M.D.   *Clinical Associate Professor, Department of Orthopaedic Surgery, Tulane University School of Medicine, and Assistant Professor, Volunteer Faculty, University of Kentucky, 210 E. Gray Street #601, Louisville, Kentucky 40202*

Paul D. Hooper, D.C.   *Professor, Co-Chair, Department of Principles and Practice, Los Angeles College of Chiropractic, 16200 East Amber Valley Drive, Whittier, California 90609-1166*

Terese T. Horlocker, M.D.   *Assistant Professor, Department of Anesthesiology, Mayo Clinic, 200 First Street SW, Rochester, Minnesota 55905*

Serena S. Hu, M.D.   *Assistant Professor of Orthopedics, University of California, San Francisco, 533 Parnassus Avenue, U471, San Francisco, California 94143-0728*

Robert Huler, M.D.   *Assistant Professor, Department of Orthopaedic Surgery, Indiana University Medical Center, 541 Clinical Drive #600, Indianapolis, Indiana 46202-5111*

Michael H. Huo, M.D., M.S.   *Assistant Professor, Department of Orthopaedic Surgery, The Johns Hopkins University School of Medicine, Bayview Medical Center, 4940 Eastern Avenue, Baltimore, Maryland 21224*

Jorge E. Isaza, M.D.   *Clinical Assistant Professor, Department of Orthopaedic Surgery, Tulane University School of Medicine, 1430 Tulane Avenue, New Orleans, Louisiana and, Spine Surgery PSC, Suite 601, 210 East Cray Street, Louisville, Kentucky 40202*

Malcolm I. V. Jayson, M.D., F.R.C.P.   *Professor of Rheumatology, University of Manchester, Rheumatic Diseases Centre, Clinical Sciences Building, Hope Hospital, Eccles Old Road, Salford M6 8HD, United Kingdom*

Parviz Kambin, M.D.   *Clinical Associate Professor, Department of Orthopaedics, University of Pennsylvania School of Medicine, The Graduate Hospital, Medical Institute for Orthopaedic and Spine Surgery, 1125 Lancaster Avenue, Berwyn, Pennsylvania 19312*

Jeffrey N. Katz, M.D., M.S.   *Assistant Professor of Medicine, Harvard Medical School, Division of Rheumatology/Immunology, Brigham and Women's Hospital, 75 Francis Street, Boston, Massachusetts 02115*

Francis J. Keefe, Ph.D.   *Professor of Medical Psychiatry, Department of Psychology, Duke University Medical Center, Pain Management Program, Durham, North Carolina 27710*

Timothy L. Keenen, M.D.   *Associate Professor, Department of Orthopaedics, Oregon Health Science University, 3181 SW Sam Jackson Park Road, Portland, Oregon 97201*

Lee A. Kelley, M.D.   *2001 Peachtree Road, N.E., Atlanta, Georgia 30309*

Robert B. Keller, M.D.   *Adjunct Professor, Department of Family and Community Medicine and Surgery, Dartmouth Medical School and, Maine Medical Assessment Foundation, P.O. Box 4682, 18 Spruce Street, Augusta, Maine 04330-1682*

Shinichi Kikuchi, M.D.   *Professor, Department of Orthopaedic Surgery, Fukushima Medical College, 1 Hikarigaoka, Fukushima, Japan 960-12*

Jeffrey D. Klein, M.D.   *Clinical Assistant, New York University School of Medicine, Attending Medicine Spine Physician, Hospital of Joint Diseases and, 109 Park Avenue, New York, New York 10028*

John P. Kostuik, M.D., F.R.C.S.(C.)   *Professor, Department of Orthopaedic Surgery, The Johns Hopkins University School of Medicine, 600 North Wolfe Street, Baltimore, Maryland 21287-0882*

Martin H. Krag, M.D.   *McClure Center for Musculoskeletal Research, Department of Orthopaedics and Rehabilitation and Vermont Rehabilitation Engineering Center for Low Back Pain, University of Vermont, Burlington, Vermont 05405-0084*

Thomas K. Kristiansen, M.D.   *Associate Professor, Department of Orthopaedics and Rehabilitation, University of Vermont, Staffold Hall, Room 430, Burlington, Vermont 05405-0084*

Noshir A. Langrana, Ph.D.   *Professor, Department of Mechanical and Aerospace Engineering, Rutgers University, Brett and Bower Roads, Piscataway, New Jersey 08855-0909*

Henry LaRocca, M.D. *(deceased)*   *Clinical Professor, Department of Orthopaedic Surgery, Tulane University School of Medicine, New Orleans, Louisiana 70112*

Steven A. Lavender, Ph.D. *Assistant Professor, Department of Orthopedic Surgery, Rush-Presbyterian St. Luke's Medical Center, 1653 West Congress Parkway, Chicago, Illinois 60612*

Casey K. Lee, M.D. *Professor, Department of Orthopaedics, University of Medicine and Dentistry of New Jersey, New Jersey Medical School, 185 South Orange Avenue, Newark, New Jersey 07103*

Roland R. Lee, M.D. *Assistant Professor, Department of Radiology, The Johns Hopkins University School of Medicine, 600 N. Wolfe Street, Baltimore, Maryland 21287*

Matthew H. Liang, M.D., M.P.H. *Professor of Medicine, Professor of Health Policy and Management, Harvard Medical School, Multipurpose Arthritis Center, Brigham and Women's Hospital, 75 Francis Street, Tower 16B, Boston, Massachusetts 02115*

Donlin M. Long, M.D., Ph.D. *Professor and Director, Department of Neurosurgery, The Johns Hopkins University School of Medicine, 600 North Wolfe Street, Baltimore, Maryland 21287-7709*

Mark A. Lorenz, M.D. *Associate Professor, Department of Orthopedics, Loyola University Medical Center, 550 West Ogden Avenue, Hinsdale, Illinois 60525*

Marianne L. Magnusson, Dr.Med.Sc. *Assistant Professor, Department of Orthopaedic Surgery, The University of Iowa Hospitals and Clinics, 200 Hawkins Drive, Iowa City, Iowa 52242-1088*

Leonard N. Matheson, Ph.D. *Assistant Professor, Department of Occupational Therapy, Washington University School of Medicine, St. Louis, Missouri and, Director, ERIC Human Performance Laboratory, Employment and Rehabilitation Institute of California, 600 South Grand Avenue, Suite 106, Santa Ana, California 92705*

John A. McCulloch, M.D., F.R.C.S.C. *Professor, Department of Orthopaedics, Northeastern Ohio Universities College of Medicine, Summa Health Systems, 444 North Main Street, Akron, Ohio 44310*

Robin A. McKenzie, O.B.E., F.C.S.P., F.N.Z.S.P.(Hon.), Dip.M.T. *President, The McKenzie Institute International, P.O. Box 93, 8 Parata Street, Waikanae, New Zealand*

Robert F. McLain, M.D. *Associate Professor of Orthopaedic Surgery, Department of Orthopaedics, University of California, Davis, 2230 Stockton Boulevard, Sacramento, California 95817*

Robert A. McNutt, M.D. *Professor, Department of Medicine, University of Wisconsin Medical School, Milwaukee Clinical Campus, Sinai Samaritan Medical Center, 945 North Twelfth Street, P.O. Box 342, Milwaukee, Wisconsin 53233*

Arnold H. Menezes, M.D. *Professor and Vice Chairman, Division of Neurosurgery, Department of Surgery, University of Iowa Hospitals and Clinics, 200 Hawkins Drive, Iowa City, Iowa 52242*

Vert Mooney, M.D. *Professor of Orthopaedic Surgery, Department of Orthopaedics, University of California, San Diego, La Jolla, California 92037*

Roland W. Moskowitz, M.D. *Professor of Medicine, Case Western Reserve University School of Medicine, Director, Division of Rheumatic Diseases, University Hospitals of Cleveland, 11100 Euclid Avenue, Cleveland, Ohio 44106*

Mary Newton, M.Ed., M.C.S.P. *Superintendent Physiotherapist, Department of Physiotherapy, Clydebank Health Center, Kilbonie Road, Clydebank G81, Scotland*

Eugene J. Nordby, M.D. *Associate Clinical Professor, Department of Orthopaedics, University of Wisconsin Medical School, 6234 S. Highlands, Madison, Wisconsin 53705-1115*

Margareta Nordin, R.P.T., Dr.Sci. *Adjunct Associate Professor, New York University School of Medicine, Director, Occupational and Industrial Orthopaedic Center, New York University Medical Center, Hospital for Joint Diseases, 63 Downing Street, New York, New York 10014*

Richard B. North, M.D. *Associate Professor, Department of Neurosurgery, The Johns Hopkins University School of Medicine, Meyer 7-113, 600 North Wolfe Street, Baltimore, Maryland 21287-7710*

J. Desmond O'Duffy, M.B. *Professor, Department of Medicine, Mayo Medical School, Consultant in Medicine, Mayo Clinic, 220 First Street, SW, Rochester, Minnesota 55905*

Jeffrey H. Owen, Ph.D. *Associate Professor, Department of Neurology, The Johns Hopkins University School of Medicine, Carnegie 2-24, 600 North Wolfe Street, Baltimore, Maryland 21287*

Marco Pappagallo, M.D. *Assistant Professor, Departments of Neurology, Neurosurgery, and Anesthesiology/Critical Care, The Johns Hopkins University School of Medicine, 601 N. Carolina Street, 5066A, Baltimore, Maryland 21287*

J. Russell Parsons, Ph.D. *Associate Professor, Department of Orthopaedics, University of Medicine and Dentistry of New Jersey, New Jersey Medical School, 185 South Orange Avenue, Newark, New Jersey 07103*

Reed B. Phillips, D.C., D.A.C.B.R., Ph.D. *President, Los Angeles College of Chiropractic, 16200 East Amber Valley Drive, Whittier, California 90609-1166*

Dennis A. Plante, M.D. *Associate Professor, Department of Medicine, University of Vermont, 2 Blair Park, Williston, Vermont 05495*

Malcolm H. Pope, Dr. Med. Sc., Ph.D. *University of Iowa Foundation Distinguished, Professor, Department of Orthopaedics and Preventive Medicine, University of Iowa Hospitals and Clinics, Iowa Spine Research Center, 1 Hawkins Drive, Iowa City, Iowa 52242*

John A. Prodoehl, M.D. *Resident in Orthopaedics, Department of Orthopaedic Surgery, The Medical College of Pennsylvania, 3300 Henry Avenue, Philadelphia, Pennsylvania 19129*

Kevin A. Rahn, M.D. *Ft. Wayne Orthopaedics, 7601 West Jefferson, Ft. Wayne, Indiana 46804*

Wolfgang Rauschning, M.D., Ph.D. *Professor of Clinical Anatomy, Department of Orthopaedic Surgery, Uppsala University, Academic University Hospital, S-751 85 Uppsala, Sweden*

John J. Regan, M.D. *Associate Clinical Professor, Department of Orthopedic Surgery, University of Texas Southwestern Medical Center, Texas Back Institute, 6500 W. Parker, Plano, Texas 75093*

Steven H. Rose, M.D. *Assistant Professor, Mayo Medical School, Department of Anesthesiology, Mayo Clinic, 200 First Street, SW, Rochester, Minnesota 55905*

David Rothbart, M.D. *Chief Resident, Section of Neurosurgery, Yale University School of Medicine, 333 Cedar Street, New Haven, Connecticut 06405*

Marilyn G. Rothwell, R.N.C. *Clinical Assistant Professor, Department of Medicine, University of Vermont, Given Health Care Center, 1 South Prospect Street, Burlington, Vermont 05401*

Joel S. Saal, M.D. *Clinical Instructor, Functional Restoration, Stanford University, Suite 110, 2884 Sand Hill Road, Menlo Park, California 94025*

Jeffrey A. Saal, M.D. *SOAR-The Physiatry Group, Suite 110, 2884 Sand Hill Road, Menlo Park, California 94025*

Aaron Sandler, B.S. *Spine Unit, Schulthess Clinic, Lengghalde 2, 8008 Zurich, Switzerland*

Mark T. Scarborough, M.D. *Associate Professor, Department of Orthopaedics, University of Florida, P.O. Box 100246, Gainesville, Florida 32610*

John G. Scaringe, D.C., D.A.C.B.R. *Associate Professor, Co-Chair, Department of Principles and Practice, Los Angeles College of Chiropractic, 16200 East Amber Valley Drive, Whittier, California 90609-1166*

John D. Schlegel, M.D. *Associate Professor, Department of Orthopedic Surgery, University of Utah School of Medicine, 50 North Medical Drive, Salt Lake City, Utah 84132*

Luis Schut, M.D. *Professor of Neurosurgery and Pediatrics, Departments of Surgery and Pediatrics, University of Pennsylvania, 34th and Civic Center Boulevard, Philadelphia, Pennsylvania 19106*

Henry H. Sherk, M.D. *Professor, Department of Orthopedic Surgery, The Medical College of Pennsylvania, 3300 Henry Avenue, Philadelphia, Pennsylvania 19129*

Ien H. Sie, M.S., P.T. *Spinal Cord Injury Project, Rancho Los Amigos Medical Center, 7601 East Imperial Highway, HB-206, Downey, California 90242*

D. Hal Silcox III, M.D. *Assistant Professor, Department of Orthopaedic Surgery, Emory University, 2165 North Decatur Road, Decatur, Georgia 30033*

James W. Simmons, M.D. *Alamo Bone and Joint Clinic, Suite 1200, 8122 Datapoint Drive, San Antonio, Texas 78229-3364*

Tony P. Smith, M.D. *Professor, Department of Radiology, Duke University Medical Center, Erwin Road, Durham, North Carolina 27710*

Brett R. Stacey, M.D. *Assistant Professor, Department of Anesthesiology, University of Pittsburgh School of Medicine, 4601 Baum Boulevard, Pittsburgh, Pennsylvania 15213*

Steven Stecker, M.D. *Department of Orthopedics, New York University Medical Center, 530 First Avenue 8U, New York, New York 10016*

John C. Steinmann, D.O. *Clinical Professor, Department of Orthopedic Surgery, Loma Linda University, 11234 Anderson Street, Loma Linda, California 92354*

Leslie N. Sutton, M.D. *Professor, Department of Neurosurgery, University of Pennsylvania, Children's Hospital of Philadelphia, 34 Street and Civic Boulevard, Philadelphia, Pennsylvania 19104*

Tetsuya Tamaki, M.D., Ph.D. *Professor and Chairman, Department of Orthopaedic Surgery, Wakayama Medical College, 27-7 Bancho, Wakayama, Japan 641*

Tom Arild Torstensen, B.Sc.(Hones) *Project Leader, Specialist in Manual Therapy MNFF, Centre for Physiotherapy Research and Development, PB 7009 Majorstuen, 0306 Oslo, Norway*

Alfred B. Traina, D.C., F.A.C.O. *Professor, Director, Clinical Science Division, Los Angeles College of Chiropractic, 16200 East Amber Valley Drive, Whittier, California 90609-1166*

Nobuyuki Tsuzuki, M.D. *Professor, Department of Orthopaedic Surgery, Saitama Medical Center, Saitama Medical School, 1981, Tsujido, Kamoda, Kawagoe, Saitama 350, Japan*

Henry M. Tufo, M.D. *Professor of Medicine, University of Vermont College of Medicine, Fletcher Allen Health Care, Colchester Avenue, Burlington, Vermont 05401*

Dennis C. Turk, Ph.D. *Professor, Department of Psychiatry, Anesthesiology, and Behavioral Science, University of Pittsburgh School of Medicine, Pain Evaluation and Treatment Institute, 4601 Baum Boulevard, Pittsburgh, Pennsylvania 15213*

Gordon Waddell, D.Sc., M.D., F.R.C.S. *Professor, Department of Orthopaedic Surgery, Western Infirmary, Glasgow G11 6NT, Scotland*

Robert L. Waters, M.D. *Clinical Professor, Department of Orthopedic Surgery, University of Southern California, Rancho Los Amigos Medical Center, Harriman Building, Room 117, 7601 East Imperial Highway, Downey, California 90242*

Steven H. Weeden, M.D. *Resident in Orthopaedic Surgery, The University of Texas-Houston Medical School, Scott and White Memorial Hospital, Scott, Sherwood, and Brinkley Foundation, Texas A&M University Health Science Center, College of Medicine, Temple, Texas 76508*

James N. Weinstein, D.O., M.S. *Division of Orthopedics and Neurosurgery, Senior Faculty Member, Professor, Center for Evaluative Clinical Sciences, Dartmouth Medical School, Dartmouth Hitchcock Medical Center, Hanover, New Hampshire 03755*

Sherri R. Weiser, Ph.D. *Occupational and Industrial Orthopaedic Center, New York University Medical Center, Hospital for Joint Diseases, 63 Downing Street, New York, New York 10014*

Joseph G. Werner, Jr., M.D. *Orthopedic Surgeon, Browne & Reichard, P.S.C., Suite 100, Baptist East Office Park, 4001 Kresge Way, Louisville, Kentucky 40207*

Thomas S. Whitecloud III, M.D. *Ray J. Haddard, Jr. Professor and Chairman, Department of Orthopaedic Surgery, Tulane University School of Medicine, 1430 Tulane Avenue, New Orleans, Louisiana 70112*

David G. Wilder, Ph.D. *Visiting Associate Professor and Senior Scientist, Department of Biomedical Engineering, University of Iowa, Iowa Spine Research Center, 200 Hawkins Drive, Iowa City, Iowa 52242*

Leon L. Wiltse, M.D. *Clinical Professor, Department of Orthopaedic Surgery, University of California at Irvine, and Long Beach Memorial Hospital, 2888 Atlantic Avenue, Long Beach, California 90806-1553*

David Wright, M.B., Ch.B., B.Med.Sci., M.D., M.R.C.P. *Senior Registrar in Rheumatology and Rehabilitation, Musculoskeletal Unit, Freeman Road Hospital, Freeman Road, Newcastle Upon Tyne NE7 7DN, United Kingdom, and Hunters Moor Rehabilitation Centre, Hunters Road, Newcastle Upon Tyne, United Kingdom*

Joy S. Yakura, M.S., P.T. *Spinal Cord Injury Project, Rancho Los Amigos Medical Center, 7601 East Imperial Highway, Downey, California 90242*

Hansen A. Yuan, M.D. *Professor, Departments of Orthopaedic and Neurological Surgery, State University of New York Health Science Center, at Syracuse, Syracuse, New York 13202*

Thomas A. Zdeblick, M.D. *Associate Professor of Orthopaedic Surgery, Department of Surgery, University of Wisconsin Hospital and Clinics, 600 Highland Avenue, G5/314, Madison, Wisconsin 53792-3228*

Seth M. Zeidman, M.D. *Clinical Instructor, The Johns Hopkins University School of Medicine, Assistant Professor, The Uniformed Services University of the Health Sciences, Staff Neurosurgeon, Division of Neurosurgery, Department of Surgery, Walter Reed Army Medical Center, Building II, Room 5C09, Washington, D.C. 20307*

Mark C. Zimmerman, Ph.D. *Associate Professor of Orthopaedics, Co-Director, Laboratories for Orthopaedic Research, Department of Orthopaedics, University of Medicine and Dentistry of New Jersey, New Jersey Medical School, 185 South Orange Avenue, Newark, New Jersey 07103-2714*

Michael R. Zindrick, M.D. *Clinical Associate Professor, Department of Orthopedic Surgery, Loyola University Medical Center, Maywood, Illinois 60153 and, Hinsdale Orthopedics Assoc., S.C., 550 West Ogden Avenue, Hinsdale, Illinois 60521*

S. James Zinreich, M.D. *Associate Professor of Radiology, Department of Radiology/ Neuroradiology, The Johns Hopkins University School of Medicine, 600 N. Wolfe Street, Baltimore, Maryland 21205-0810*

Preface to the First Edition

Two decades ago a small handful of books and no journals were available to physicians and surgeons who daily encountered spinal disorders. Today, multiple journals and texts are devoted to this topic; yet a comprehensive text has been unavailable to bring together the epidemiology and socioeconomic consequences of spinal disease, its causation and diagnosis, its prevention, and the myriad of non-operative and operative approaches that are used with varying degrees of success.

The editors and publisher of *The Adult Spine* identified this important need two years ago. Our overall goal was simple: create a book that would serve as *the* reference text for every physician treating adult spine disorders. Our approach was somewhat more complex: Identify all of the important topics in spinal disorders from the foramen magnum to the coccyx, and get the recognized authorities to produce chapters that give the reader the most up-to-date information on those topics. Write chapters that can stand alone so that the reader can find the needed information, illustrated with original drawings and radiographs, and supported by a complete bibliography. At the same time, our editorial group was charged with the important task of making the individual chapters form a comprehensive whole.

The task has been complex. The effort has been monumental to produce a two-volume text comprising 104 chapters, over 400 original illustrations and 2,000 images, and a bibliography of nearly 9,000 references. To complete such a project in two years and thus keep the text at the "cutting edge" has required remarkable devotion from the editors, publisher, illustrators, and librarians.

All of us associated with this project are proud of the final product. We hope you, who read this text, will find it contains all of the important, timely information you need to understand and treat your patients with spinal disorders. If you and they benefit, then our efforts will have been well worth it.

John W. Frymoyer
Thomas B. Ducker
Nortin M. Hadler
John P. Kostuik
James N. Weinstein
Thomas S. Whitecloud III

Preface

Seven years ago our editorial group, and the publisher, then Raven Press, concluded there was an international need for a comprehensive treatise on disorders of the adult spine. We stated a simple goal, "Create a book that would serve as the reference text for every physician treating adult spine disorders." The key to whatever successes the First Edition had was the dedication of a group of expert authors who had the ability to synthesize the extensive and diverse literature, such that those who treat spinal disorders can do their work more effectively. Based on extensive reviews, and other information, the editors were heartened by the success of the First Edition.

Since the publication of the First Edition, we have watched the continued progress in the understanding of spinal disorders, and concluded it was now time for a new edition. While planning, we recognized some topics had changed little, for example, the history of spinal disorders. At the same time we were anxious to include all new information, as well as being responsive to suggestions for improvement made by reviewers, and by our readers. As this work progressed, it became apparent there are many changes. In the First Edition, we speculated on the impact of "health reform." Today, health reform and managed care dominate much of the United States press. In virtually all other industrialized nations health reform of one or another variety is taking place. In the quest to improve health care, there has been major advances in clinical outcomes research and the management of quality, and these form new and important foci for the first section. Similarly, there has been major advances in our understanding of many of the pathologic bases of symptoms, signs, and disease. Thus, the Second Edition updates our understanding about the mechanisms of disease, pain, and its pathophysiologic basis, as well as our insights into the mechanisms of actions of commonly used drugs. In each of the sections devoted to anatomic areas of the spine new chapters written by authors who bring their expert opinion about what constitutes optimum diagnosis and treatment are found. As the expertise to manage more complex disorders has increased, there has been a reappraisal, and in some instances a basic reformulation of how this new technology should be used.

Readers will find this Second Edition continues to contribute to the betterment of the care our patients receive, and will find it useful in their practice.

Acknowledgments

The editors and publisher of the Second Edition of *The Adult Spine* continue the commitment made in the First Edition. We wanted a book that is comprehensive, contains the latest information, stimulates the reader and contributes to the understanding that there are diverse opinions surrounding all aspects of the diagnosis and treatment of spinal disorders. Although this edition builds on the First Edition, the task put to the authors remained monumental. Almost 50% of the new edition represents new authors and new material. The chapters, with very few exceptions, have undergone major revision and refocusing based on the advances that occurred in the past five years.

Particular tribute goes to our secretarial staff, Deborah A. Logsdon and Peggy Stover, as well as to the editors' spouses, who have again survived their husbands' dedication and time to this project.

This continued updating of *The Adult Spine* will again give you, the reader, a vital source of new and timely information to guide the diagnosis and treatment of your patients. Its usefulness to you will make the effort involved in preparing a book of this scope well worthwhile for all of us involved in the Second Edition of *The Adult Spine.*

The Adult Spine

Principles and Practice

Second Edition

The Adult Spine: Principles and Practice,
2nd edition, J.W. Frymoyer, Editor-in-Chief.
Lippincott-Raven Publishers, Philadelphia © 1997.

CHAPTER 1

Introduction

John W. Frymoyer, Thomas B. Ducker, Nortin M. Hadler, John P. Kostuik, James N. Weinstein, and Thomas S. Whitecloud III

It is much more important to know what sort of patient has a disease, than what sort of disease a patient has.
—WILLIAM OSLER

Five years ago the editors of the first edition of *The Adult Spine* defined an editorial mission. We saw the need for a comprehensive volume devoted to the adult spine with the breadth and depth that did justice to the information accumulated over the prior 60 years. We observed that prior to 1930 spinal disorders scarcely warranted a literature, that tuberculosis, spinal deformities, and the sequelae of poliomyelitis occupied the vast majority of the limited publications. Further, we noted that prior to 1950 spinal disorders had minimal socioeconomic impact.

As we structured the first edition our challenge was to present science and research intertwined with the art of medical care in the context of a complex socioeconomic

J. W. Frymoyer, M.D.: Dean, College of Medicine, Professor, Department of Orthopaedics and Rehabilitation, University of Vermont, Burlington, Vermont 05405.

T. B. Ducker, M.D.: Professor of Surgery, Department of Neurosurgery, Johns Hopkins Medical Institutions, Baltimore, Maryland 21205.

N. M. Hadler, M.D.: Professor of Medicine and Microbiology/Immunology, University of North Carolina at Chapel Hill; Attending Rheumatologist, University of North Carolina Hospitals, Chapel Hill, North Carolina 27599-7280.

J. P. Kostuik, M.D., F.R.C.S.(C.): Professor, Department of Orthopaedic Surgery, Johns Hopkins Medical Institutions, Baltimore, Maryland 21287-0882.

J. N. Weinstein, D.O., M.S.: Division of Orthopedics and Neurosurgery, Senior Faculty Member, Center for Clinical Evaluative Sciences, Dartmouth Medical School, Dartmouth Hitchcock Medical Center, Hanover, NH 03755.

T. S. Whitecloud III, M.D.: Professor and Chairman, Department of Orthopaedic Surgery, Tulane University School of Medicine, New Orleans, Louisiana 70112.

and social climate in which spinal disorders occur and in which care is rendered.

In the ensuing five years we have been gratified by the response to the first edition as reflected in both its content and technical quality. We learned a great deal about technical quality when the first edition was awarded one of three prizes from the American Medical Writers Association. We learned a great deal about the quality of the content from the many reviews. The overwhelming response was praise; however, we found that some topics should be expanded or refocused. Starting from this foundation, we now present the second edition.

This new edition is structured along the same lines of the first edition. We start in Part I with the major economic, social, industrial, and disability issues posed by spinal disorders. We have expanded upon this area by including greater focus on the new science of outcome measurements and quality improvement as well as more emphasis on the array of approaches used to improve the function of people with chronic disabilities.

Part II is the broad outlines of the biologic basis of spinal disorders. It cannot be emphasized strongly enough that a basic premise of this book is that clinical diagnosis is based on a well conceived hypothesis derived from the history and physical examination. The utilization of sophisticated technology is only as appropriate as it confirms the clinical hypothesis.

Part III is again familiar territory and deals with the pathophysiologic basis of those few causes of spinal disorders that are well understood and for which specific medical or surgical treatments can be directed.

The last four sections of the book are related to the four anatomic areas comprising the spine. You will find the full gamut of disorders, their diagnosis, conservative and operative management, as well as the specific operative approaches, and the use of complex and simple devices. Reconceptualization of older techniques, such as correction of deformities, is juxtaposed to the latest technology such as thoracoscopy, fixation devices, and laser technology. At the same time we make the reader aware of the very latest development, we also want your awareness heightened about the devices, techniques, and treatments for which there is well established scientific evidence and for those whose efficacy is yet proven. We also have asked the authors to be clear about the risks and complications. As the reader looks at the alternatives, the balance of risk, and benefit, particularly when benefit is yet to be fully established, is of critical importance.

Finally, a comprehensive book such as this can only have it's greatest value when the reader is stimulated to continuously ask questions. Not all the answers will be found here, and indeed for some topics legitimate controversy can and should be identified. For example, is lumbar disc excision best accomplished by standard techniques, or is their a growing role for a variety of percutaneous techniques. Has laser discectomy reached a level of development where it can and should be recommended for treatment? And in 1996 do we have sufficient evidence to decide who should receive any surgical treatment, when non-operative therapy would suffice. You as readers can draw your own conclusions, and we the editors hope this book will serve as a useful means of improving the care received by your patients.

The Adult Spine: Principles and Practice,
2nd edition, J.W. Frymoyer, Editor-in-Chief.
Lippincott-Raven Publishers, Philadelphia © 1997.

CHAPTER 2

The History of Spinal Disorders

Leon L. Wiltse

   L. L. Wiltse, M.D.: Clinical Professor, Department of Orthopaedic Surgery, University of California at Irvine; and Long Beach Memorial Hospital, Long Beach, California 90806.

Is there a thing of which it is said,
"See, this is new"
It has been already,
In the ages before us.

—ECCLESIASTES 1:10

While reviewing for this chapter, I was again struck by how dependent our research and treatment is on the work of those who came before us. Mixter (192) stated this eloquently when describing his dependence on the work of Bell (21,22), Middleton and Teacher (188), Kocher (157), Elsberg (85–87), and Dandy (71), which led to his and Barr's description of the ruptured intervertebral disc. In 1949 he stated, "Had it not been for the reports of the various workers in neurosurgery, in pathology, in neurology, and in orthopedics, the focusing of attention on rupture of the intervertebral disc and its importance as a clinical entity would have been impossible."

Even the remarkable discoveries of Louis Pasteur (217) and Joseph Lister (167) came only after painfully slow lesser advances by their predecessors. Only rarely has medical knowledge made a great leap forward based on a single individual's sudden and dramatic insights. Notable exceptions are Conrad Roentgen's (237) discovery of the x-ray and Alexander Fleming's (90) serendipitous recognition of the antimicrobial properties of penicillin. Even these discoveries might have easily gone unpursued had not the scientists recognized the importance of their chance observations and pursued them.

This may well be the *sine qua non* for making advances; that is, the psychological make up (call it energy, insight, brilliance, or what you will) that causes one to pursue a chance observation or a chance thought. Most "flashes of insight" never get beyond just that. There can be little doubt that there is many a "mute inglorious Milton" (285) among us who had a good idea upon which he never acted.

This chapter is intended to give an overview of the history of spinal disorders, rather than a detailed account of every significant event. My task is made easier by other contributors to this volume as they describe the more specific history as it relates to their particular topics. Nevertheless, there are bound to be omissions, particularly of the contributions made from other countries with whose language and literature I may be unfamiliar. For these omissions, I apologize at the outset.

I have organized this chapter to cover first the major advances in medicine that made our present level of spine care possible, and subsequently to discuss some historical aspects of the treatment of spinal cord injuries, spinal deformities (especially scoliosis), cervical spine disorders, and disorders of the lumbar spine, in that order.

GENERAL HISTORY OF SPINAL DISORDERS

Imhotep, 2686–2613 B.C.

In looking back through the history of the treatment of spine disorders, it is noted that Imhotep, the Vizier of Djoser (37), the second Pharaoh of the Third Dynasty, was an astronomer, magician, priest, and physician, as well as the architect for the step pyramid at Sakkarah. This structure remained the largest building ever built until the pyramids of Giza.

Imhotep probably wrote the first treatises on surgery, which much later came into the possession of Edwin Smith (37) and are known as the Edwin Smith Papyrus. Imhotep remains much better known than the Pharaoh he served. The papyrus was found in the tomb at Thebes, was sold to Edwin Smith in 1862, and later translated by Breasted in 1930 (37). The papyrus describes 48 mainly osseous lesions, some of which involve the spine. This can be considered the first orthopedic paper ever produced. Considering this was written about 4,630 years ago, the accuracy of Imhotep's observations is incredible. He identified sprains, vertebral subluxations, and dislocations. He also differentiated upper cord injuries that caused quadriplegia from those injuries of the middle regions of the body that caused paraplegia of the lower extremities. He realized that paralysis resulted from severing the spinal cord, but he did not understand why.

Hippocrates, 1460–1375 B.C.

Early writings, particularly those of the Greeks, are steeped in mythology. These were largely done by members of the cult of Aesculapius, to which Hippocrates (233) (Fig. 1) apparently belonged. Although he belonged to this cult, by the time he did his writing, mythology had largely given way to more scientific medicine. There almost certainly was a man named Hippocrates who was born in about 460 B.C. on the island of Cos during the Age of Pericles. His grandfather was a physician, as was his father, whose name was Heraclides.

Hippocrates is credited with being instrumental in separating medicine from mythology. The philosophy of rationalism that he promoted led to an environment that has been characterized as one of the most memorable epochs in the intellectual development of the human race. The material attributed to him is regarded more as a compilation of many people's thoughts than the work of one man. This so-called hippocratic collection was put together by an Egyptian scholar appointed by the king Ptolemy Soter (37) (323–285 B.C.). This scholar and his group assembled all the writings of that epoch that seemed to have even a hippocratic flavor and called them

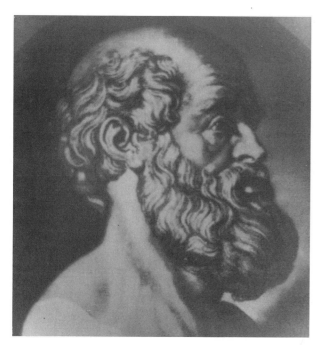

FIG. 1. Hippocrates (1460–1375 B.C.).

the work of Hippocrates. One of the likely genuine contributions of Hippocrates is his "bench" for reduction of fractures and fracture dislocations. This device was actually a traction table and is surprisingly similar to the tables in use today (Fig. 2).

We can say that hippocratic medicine was rational but still quite removed from the scientific reasoning of today. Some have used the term "prescientific." This should not be considered a reproach to the physicians of the

time. They brilliantly constructed an enviable stage of medicine.

Even if we do not know with certainty exactly what part of the collection Hippocrates wrote, we should nevertheless consider him the pre-eminent representative of a significant stage of medicine, the stage in which war was waged on all magico-religious medical practices and in which medicine consciously sought to become fully scientific and at least succeeded in becoming partially rational. To go further in one's praise of him is to fall into hagiography; we must marvel at the enormity of the task that the people who assembled his works assumed. The proof of their success lies in the fact that for two millennia, no better work was accomplished. Hippocratic medicine traversed the centuries somewhat like Aristotelian logic; and if since the nineteenth century the errors of the physicians of that era have been seen to be more profound than those of the logician, it is because the domain that the physician explored was much more complex.

Galen, 130–200 A.D.

Galen (51) (Fig. 3) was born in Greece but later moved to Rome and became the physician to the emperor, Marcus Aurelius. During his stay in Rome he made accurate and extensive anatomic dissections. Galen may be re-

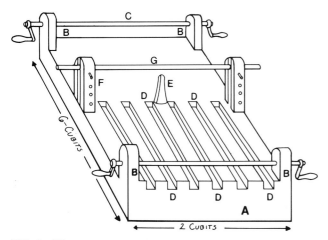

FIG. 2. Hippocrates's traction table. A cubit was the distance from the tip of the olecranon to the tip of the middle finger on an ancient king (about 18 inches). **A:** Main board, about 9 feet by 3 feet. **B:** Feet for the axles. **C:** Axle tree. **D:** Grooves, 3 inches by 3 inches. **E:** Peroneal post. **F:** Pillars to support cross-beam (bar). **G:** Cross-bar or beam. This cross bar can be placed at different heights in the pillars that support it.

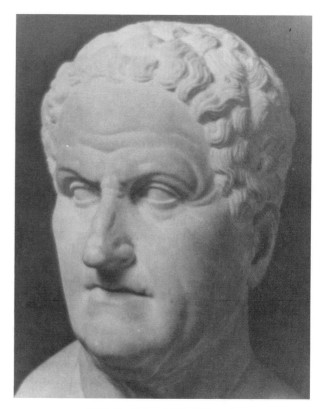

FIG. 3. Galen (130–200 A.D.).

garded as the founder of experimental physiology and embryology as well as, next to Hippocrates, the greatest physician of antiquity. He described the muscular system as a "unified but complex organ of locomotion" and demonstrated the physiological relationship between nervous and muscular systems. He also recognized and named various muscles and showed that vessels contained blood that they carried to and from the tissues. Although his work describes the capillary system, Galen never did completely visualize the circulatory system. This remained for Harvey.

Galen named some deformities of the spine, such as lordosis, kyphosis, and scoliosis, and was the first person to attempt active correction of such deformities. His complete works were based to a large extent on the writings of Hippocrates, and for several centuries were the outstanding treatises on medicine. Galen has been whimsically called "the first sports medicine specialist" because he was appointed and served as the official doctor for the gladiators of the amphitheater. This position provided him with material for his anatomic and neurophysiological research. He confirmed Imhotep's and Hippocrates's observations that injuries to the cervical cord caused a certain level of loss of sensation and motor function while injuries in lower areas caused a different level of paralysis. He assigned to the brain the role of presiding over sensation and voluntary motion and noted that hemisections paralyze the ipsilateral parts below the brain. Galen's accomplishments are even more remarkable when one considers that because of laws forbidding human dissection, except for accidental observations, his studies were done on Barbary apes and Rhesus monkeys.

Oribasius, 325–400 A.D.

The next important contributor was another Greek physician, named Oribasius (213), who moved to Rome at the invitation of the Emperor Julian. He improved on Hippocrates's "bench" by adding a cross bar, which could be used as a lever for the treatment of fracture dislocations. By means of this bar, forward pressure could be made on a gibbus to reduce the deformity while at the same time, by turning the various cranks, strong traction could be maintained on the torso and on the legs.

Paulus of Aegina, 625–690 A.D.

Paul of Aegina (41) was another Greek physician and is notable because he was the last of the Greek physicians who helped preserve the medical writings that had been compiled over the previous 1,000 years. His compendium of medicine was the most important of the era and was done about the time of the fall of Rome. The idea of using splints after reduction of spine fractures is ascribed

to him. He seems also to have performed the first laminectomies in cases where the posterior elements were fractured and pushed into the cord. Unfortunately, many of the skills of this ancient era were lost during the Dark Ages. The magnitude of this loss is underscored by the fact that the next successful laminectomy was not done until 1828, by Alban Smith (263) of Danville, Kentucky.

Dark Ages

After the fall of Rome, the Dark Ages settled like a black cloud over Europe. During this era, no great new contributions were made. Instead, the physicians of the time simply improved on hippocratic methods. As far as the spine was concerned, most of their efforts were directed toward the treatment of fracture dislocations. Treatment of scoliosis was deemed nearly hopeless, as was the gibbus of tuberculosis. They, of course, did not recognize that the "hump" was caused by tuberculosis and that it was due to the same disease that affected the lung. Although great surgeons and great teachers of medicine did exist during the Dark Ages, there were few basic contributions to the development of spine care. With the decline of the civilizations of Alexandria and Rome, there arose a mysticism at least as unscientific as that which existed before Hippocrates. This mysticism, combined with the appalling illiteracy of the period, virtually abolished medical progress.

In 1210, however, Roland (41) of Parma did write his famous Chirurgica. He discarded Hippocrates's "bench" and recommended only manual manipulation of fractures and dislocations of the spine. He did use traction bands around the torso and pelvis but these were pulled on by hand rather than by the type of windlass seen in the hippocratic bench.

RENAISSANCE OF MEDICINE

Andreas Vesalius, 1514–1564

Vesalius (17) (Fig. 4) was born in Brussels but worked largely in Padua, Italy. He occupies one of the foremost places in the history of medicine. Not only was he the inaugurator of the real science of anatomy, but he was the founder of modern medical science as we now understand it. It is of interest to note that his epic-making *De Humani Corporis Fabrica Liberi Septum,* published in 1543, immediately aroused violent opposition. This book, with its magnificent engravings by Jan Stephan Van Calcar, slowly but surely reached a most eminent position from which it has never been displaced. Even today, it stands as a valuable and practical anatomic text. It also possesses the distinction of being the masterpiece

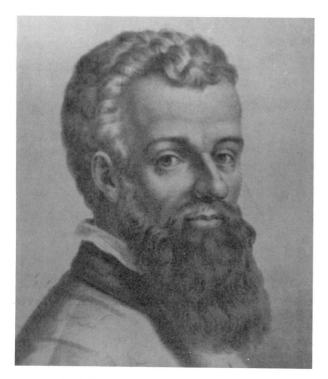

FIG. 4. Andreas Vesalius (1514–1564).

of a great pioneer. This work by Vesalius and his engraver, Jan Calcar, "set the standard for that naturalness of form, that suggestion of texture and depth, which is still known as the anatomical norm." Jan Calcar's engravings set a standard that all subsequent medical artists must emulate.

Vesalius's other great contribution, aside from correcting some of Galen's errors, was his assertion that anatomy must be learned from dissections with one's own hands, not just from books. He also established the concept "that to know the body, the doctor must know its anatomy." His teachings seem even more relevant today, when physicians treating spinal disorders often fail to look systematically for the anatomic cause of spinal pain.

Ambrose Paré, 1510–1590

Although Vesalius was a brilliant anatomist, Paré (214) (Fig. 5) was by far the outstanding surgeon of the Renaissance. He was born into a poor family in Laval, in northern France. His family was too humble to afford the fee for the license that was needed to practice. At that time, there was a rigid caste system in medicine. Physicians were the ruling hierarchy, then came the surgeons, and last the barber surgeons who basically were tradesmen. Paré was forced to belong to this last group. Despite his barber surgeon status, Paré eventually attained an official position as "Premier Surgeon and Counselor" of France. His great treatise, *Dix Liv de la Chirurgie*, has

been translated into all major languages and remains today one of the classics of medical literature.

His contributions include the introduction of the practice of ligaturing the great vessels after amputations instead of cauterizing them with boiling oil. He inaugurated the idea of gentle treatment of wounds. His most famous apothegm was, "I dressed him and God healed him." The discovery that wounds heal better with simple dressings than with cauterization with boiling oil stands as an everlasting monument to him. This last discovery was Paré's greatest contribution and was totally accidental. He was a military surgeon and on the day of a great battle, the oil supply ran out. He applied a "digestive" that was really a mild poultice of egg yolk, vegetable oil, and turpentine. He could not sleep that night, expecting to find his patients who did not get the boiling oil to be seriously infected or dead. To his surprise and delight, they were quite pain free and generally recovering better than those treated early in the day with the hot oil. Of this experience he said, "Then I resolved never again so cruelly to burn the poor victims of gunfire."

Antony Van Leeuwenhoek, 1632–1723

The discovery of microbes is one of the landmark scientific discoveries of medicine and can be largely attrib-

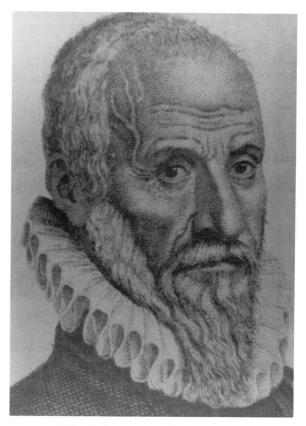

FIG. 5. Ambrose Paré (1510–1590).

uted to the work of a single person, Van Leeuwenhoek (286) (Fig. 6). Van Leeuwenhoek worked alone. His discovery was unanticipated because it was not a natural outgrowth of previous biological knowledge, or others' research.

Antony Van Leeuwenhoek was born in 1632 in Delft, Holland. He came from a middle class family, and for most of his adult life held a minor post as a civil servant in the town government. Like many Europeans with this type of job, he had lots of free time, so he took up "microscopy" as a hobby. Although he had no formal training, he learned to grind lenses and made by far the best lens of that time. One of these surviving lenses has a magnification power of ×270, and some of his lenses that have been lost were even more powerful. He was a patient, careful worker. One day, he looked through his microscope and saw an unsuspected new world teaming with life. He knew he had made a profound discovery. Although he surmised that these animated particles were important, the discovery that they could cause disease had to await Louis Pasteur of France, 200 years later.

The dignitaries of the world beat a path to Van Leeuwenhoek's door. The Czar of Russia and the Queen of England both visited him and looked through his microscopes. He died at the age of 90 in his home town of Delft.

Nicholas Andry, 1658–1742

The eighteenth century is of special importance to orthopedic surgery. It was during this time that Nicholas Andry (244) (Fig. 7) published the first book on the musculoskeletal system, entitled *L'Orthopedie.* It is a classic in orthopedic literature. During this time orthopedics itself became a specialty, the first orthopedic hospital was established, and orthopedic literature became organized

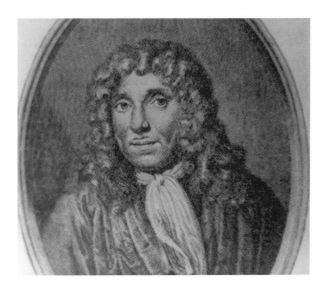

FIG. 6. Antony Van Leeuwenhoek (1632–1723).

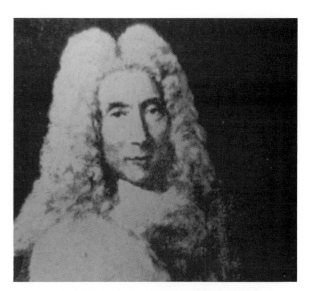

FIG. 7. Nicholas Andry (1658–1742).

and widely available. Nicholas Andry was the guiding force behind many of these accomplishments and is considered by many to be the father of orthopedic surgery. He wrote extensively on curvature of the spine with a special reference to the effects of bad posture and the value of postural training. He considered muscle imbalance to be of prime importance in skeletal deformities and used graded exercises, rest, and supportive apparatus for its treatment.

Andry was more a teacher and writer than an innovator. His classic drawing of the crooked tree bound to the straight stake has been used as a logo by dozens of orthopedic clubs and societies in the years since Andry's time.

Percivel Pott, 1717–1788

Percivel Pott of London (223–225) is important to those who treat spinal disorders for his classic description in 1769 of the deformity and sequelae of tuberculosis of the spine. The importance of his contribution is recognized by the eponym, "Pott's disease." Although the tuberculous nature of spinal deformity had been surmised by Hippocrates and confirmed by Galen, it was Pott's classic description that finally brought the condition to clarity for the practitioner.

Louis Pasteur, 1823–1895

Born the son of a tanner in the town of Dole in eastern France, Pasteur (217) (Fig. 8) was trained as a chemist. His "great observation," which he made about 1857, was that micro-organisms in the air produce fermentation, and that without micro-organisms fermentation or putrefaction cannot occur. He found that by boiling wine or broth, all organisms were killed. He even found that

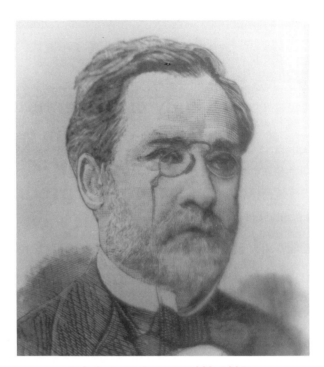

FIG. 8. Louis Pasteur (1823–1895).

exposing the broth to temperatures well below boiling for a longer period of time would sterilize it. Thus, pasteurization was born. His observations paved the way for the work of Lister, Koch, and later for the principles of aseptic surgery.

Although Pasteur was not the first person to suggest the germ theory of disease, his persistent championship of this theory greatly influenced the scientific community's eventual acceptance of it.

Pasteur is listed number 12 in Hart's *The 100 Most Influential Persons of History* (122). Interestingly, during his student days, his chief professor rated him as only "mediocre" in chemistry, which was his major.

Ignas Phillip Semmelweis, 1818–1865

Ignas Semmelweis (256) was born in 1818. He was assigned to the obstetrical wards of Vienna Allgemeines Krankenhaus, where women entering the obstetrical wards were assigned either to section 1 or section 2, according to the day of admission. Section 1 was staffed by the professor and medical students and section 2 by midwives. The medical students examined all patients with great care. They also performed autopsies, attempting to determine the cause of fatal puerperal fever. The midwives didn't go to the ward, examine patients, or perform autopsies. The incidence of death from puerperal fever was over 10% in section 1, whereas in section 2, where the midwives worked, the incidence was 1%. This observation led Semmelweis to believe that the medical students and the professors did something to

cause the infections, and suspected it was related to their dissections in the morgue or the examinations of patients predelivery. He decided it was their dirty hands that was causing the infection. He admonished everyone to wash their hands before touching patients. His teaching was met with nothing but resistance, and even outright hostility. His chief, Professor Klein, was especially hostile to him.

Semmelweiss made a second profound observation when one of the professors was nicked by a scalpel while in the morgue. The professor died of septicemia within a few days, leading Semmelweis to conclude that whatever was causing the infections could be transferred by an instrument from a person who had died of infection to a well person. Later, an infected patient was admitted to a ward where the new healthy patients awaited delivery. A pelvic examination was done on the infected patient, followed by a pelvic examination on the other ten healthy patients in the ward. All ten healthy patients died of puerperal fever. Thus, Semmelweis drew the third conclusion. Whatever it was that was causing infection could be transferred from one living person to another. He surmised that by simple cleanliness, transfer of the infective substance might be prevented. Washing of the hands seemed to be a logical solution. Even though he was able to prove his belief, his teachings were blocked for years. This resistance is all the more difficult to understand when it is remembered that Greek physicians 2,000 years earlier had insisted on cleanliness between physicians and their patients.

Part of the reason for the resistance was Dr. Semmelweis's personality. He was described as extremely high-strung and somewhat arrogant, but at the same time shy. In his later years, he suffered from a progressive organic brain syndrome. He would stand at church doors, and when newly married couples came out, he would admonish them to be delivered at home and especially not to go near the public obstetrical facility. Finally, he was taken to an insane asylum. Two weeks later, on August 14, 1865, he died at the age of 47, perhaps from beatings by attendants attempting to subdue him in the asylum (208).

It is interesting to note that at least 4 years before Semmelweis made his observations, Oliver Wendell Holmes (136), the physician-poet of Boston, published a remarkable original paper on the subject of puerperal fever. Here are some excerpts of that paper:

> A physician holding himself in readiness to attend cases of midwifery, should never take any active part in the post-mortem examination of cases of puerperal fever.
>
> If a physician is present at such autopsies, he should use thorough ablution, change every article of dress, and allow 24 hours or more to elapse before attending to any case of midwifery. It may be well to extend the same caution to cases of simple peritonitis.
>
> Similar precautions should be taken after the autopsy or surgical treatment of cases of erysipelas, if the phy-

sician is obliged to unite such offices with his obstetrical duties.

On the occurrence of a single case of puerperal fever in his practice, the physician is bound to consider the next female he attends in labor, unless some weeks, at least, have elapsed, as in danger of being infected by him and it is his duty to take every precaution to diminish her risk of disease and death.

Although Holmes's paper never received much attention, there is solid evidence that Semmelweis had read it.

It is interesting to contemplate the reason these two men were treated as they were by the profession. Holmes was born in 1809 at Cambridge, Massachusetts, one of the "Brahman caste of New England." He worked at prestigious Boston hospitals. Yet, despite these sterling credentials, his views brought bitter personal abuse on him (116). Semmelweiss, too, was violently opposed by the obstetrical hierarchy. Perhaps it was Semmelweis's near insane dedication, his fighting with his professor, Klein, and his firing from the Vienna Krankenhaus that cast so strong a spotlight on him that his ideas were finally accepted. Eventually, both Holmes and Semmelweiss were given the honor due them.

Discovery of Anesthesia

No one person can be credited with the discovery of anesthesia. Sir Humphrey Davy (74,215), Dr. Crawford Long (168), Dr. Horace Wells (299), and Dr. William T.G. Morton (201) all contributed to this monumental discovery.

Sir Humphrey Davy (112,215), an English chemist, on April 9, 1799, discovered that pure nitrous oxide was perfectly respirable. He tried it out on himself and found it "intoxicated" him. His continued experiments were reported in a paper published in 1800, in which he stated, "Nitrous oxide appears capable of destroying physical pain. It may probably be used to advantage during surgical anesthesia." People discovered its intoxicating properties and called it "laughing gas." Its frivolous use at parties may have held up its acceptance as an anesthetic, because it was not taken seriously.

Ether had been synthesized in 1835 by the famous French chemist Jean Baptiste Dumas (242). Dr. Crawford Long, a country practitioner in Jefferson, Georgia, appears to have been the first to use ether as an anesthetic. It, too, was used as an intoxicant at parties. Dr. Long noticed at one of these parties that after ether inhalation, even severe injuries caused no pain. In 1842, only 7 years after ether's discovery, he began using it in his patients.

Dr. Horace Wells, a dentist in Hartford, Connecticut, probably deserves the most credit for bringing the possibilities of anesthesia to the attention of the world, but his task was not without difficulties. When he made a demonstration at the Massachusetts General Hospital in late January of 1845, with Dr. John Warren, a surgeon (201), the anesthesia failed to work and Dr. Wells was laughed out of the amphitheater with cries of "Humbug!" from the students.

It was William T.G. Morton (201), an ex-partner in practice with Horace Wells, who finally established anesthesia in its rightful place. On October 16, 1846, in the operating room at the Massachusetts General Hospital, William Morton served as anesthesiologist while John C. Warren removed a fairly large tumor from the neck of a patient named Gilbert Abbott. The students were all prepared to shout "Humbug!" as they had at Dr. Wells. This time the anesthesia proved completely effective, the demonstration was an overwhelming success, and anesthesia was forever established.

John C. Warren (297) was probably the most prestigious surgeon in America at that time. Personally, he was a cold, sarcastic man with a sort of mocking manner (perhaps he needed such a personality to spend so much time doing major surgery without anesthesia). It is said that this emotionless man was moved to tears by Dr. Morton's demonstration and at the conclusion of the operation uttered the now-famous words, "Gentlemen, this is no humbug."

The ability to put an end to the pain of major surgery is certainly one of the greatest inventions in all human history. Few inventions are so highly valued by individual human beings, and few have made such a profound difference in the human condition. The grimness of surgery in the days when the patient had to be awake while the surgeon sawed through his bones is so frightful as to be almost beyond contemplation. Consider that in the same operating room, only a few months before Morton made his famous demonstration, a surgeon was to operate on a woman with a severe cancer of the tongue. When the surgeon put the white hot iron in her mouth to fulgurate the cancer, she died of sheer pain and fright (201).

Joseph Lister, 1827–1912

Joseph Lister (167) (Fig. 9) was born in Upton, England, in 1827. His great contribution to medicine was his promulgation of antiseptic surgery, which was accomplished with the use of wound irrigations and carbolic acid spray. It was Lister's dogged persistence that persuaded the world that antisepsis was beneficial. This task was not easy and took him years.

Lister was of small build. His face was not the face of a fighter but had, rather, the benign cast of a good Quaker. He was a poor public speaker, almost painfully shy, and had a mild stammer. Although he was blessed with few other natural gifts, he did have a faculty for diligence, tenacity, and absolute consistency in thought and action. He had one more asset: luck in choosing the right wife. He married Agnes Syme, daughter of the famous Scot-

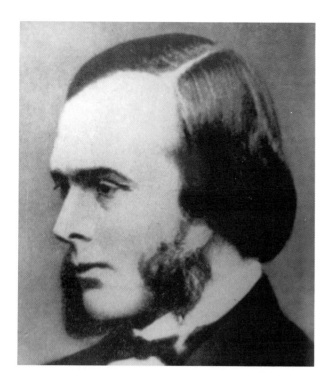

FIG. 9. Joseph Lister (1827–1912).

tish surgeon James Syme. She was his constant supporter through all his tribulations. Having a famous surgeon for a father-in-law likely did him no harm.

Lister believed that infection descended from the air, when in fact most of the things in the air were harmless yeasts and molds. He did not realize that infection is generally transmitted from one person to another or from one site in the body to another. He bathed wounds in a weak solution of carbolic acid solution and wrapped the wounds in dressings soaked with carbolic acid, a process called "carbolization." He even sprayed the room with this solution. Toward the end of his career, he was swinging strongly toward the idea of aseptic surgery. He was still soaking his instruments and wounds in carbolic acid solution and was still admonishing hospital personnel to keep everything as clean as possible, especially their hands.

Robert Koch, 1843–1910

Robert Koch (156) was born in Klausthal, Germany, the son of a miner. He began his medical practice as a civil servant doing county practice in the town of Wollstein, Germany. He did his experiments in a small, make-shift laboratory divided from his consultation room by a screen. By 1880 he was able to prove beyond question that infectious disease and wound suppuration were caused by micro-organisms. He proved that specific infections were caused by the anthrax bacillus and also by the tuberculosis bacillus. Of greatest importance to

orthopedic surgeons, however, was his discovery of Staphylococcus. He enunciated the four postulates that bear his name:

Organisms must be found in all cases of a given disease.
They must be isolated and grown in pure culture.
They must reproduce the original disease when introduced into a suitable host.
They must be found in the host so infected.

Koch's work irrevocably proved the germ theory of disease for all time and filled in the final gaps in the road toward aseptic surgery.

William S. Halstead, 1852–1922

The introduction of the rubber glove by Halstead (286) (Fig. 10) in 1890 was a great step forward for aseptic surgery.

William Stewart Halstead was Professor of Surgery at Johns Hopkins University. In the spring of 1889, he became enamored with Miss Caroline Hampton, a nurse, who had just completed her training in New York and had come to Baltimore. She rose rapidly in the nursing hierarchy at Johns Hopkins Hospital and soon became Operating Room Supervisor. In the winter of 1889–1890, she began to develop such severe skin irritation from the constant exposure to bichloride of mercury that she was prepared to quit and leave the hospital with intentions of going back to New York. Since "necessity is the mother of invention," Halstead must have considered her a "necessity," so he developed the rubber surgical glove. Miss Hampton continued to work as Operating Room Supervisor for a while but was lost to the

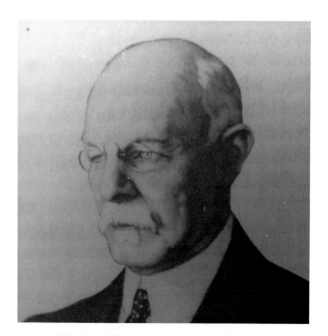

FIG. 10. William S. Halstead (1852–1922).

operating room when in the spring of 1890 she married Dr. Halstead.

Halstead is also famous for his meticulous handling of tissues, evidenced by his tiny hemostats.

William Halstead was born into a wealthy and socially prominent New York family. He first went into practice in New York City and developed a very busy, lucrative practice. He left New York in 1886 at age 34 to get over his cocaine addiction. Six years later, in 1892, he was called to the chair of surgery at Johns Hopkins. He was then 40 years old.

His personal idiosyncrasies were many. He was at once shy, aloof, aristocratic, witty, sarcastic, demanding, and brilliant. He was the only person in Baltimore who wore a top hat in summer. He personally picked over his coffee beans, discarding any not properly roasted. When he and his wife gave a dinner party, he would go to the store and select the wood for the fireplace. Yet, incongruously, he loved to go to prize fights and would watch for hours while the combatants beat each other to insensibility, wearing the scanty boxing gloves of the day. He must have been a most difficult man to live with; yet in my research, I found no evidence of complaint from Caroline.

Aseptic Surgery

In the 1880s a German doctor by the name of Curt Schimmelbusch (250) discovered that exposing instruments, bandages, and linens to live steam would kill all microbes, including spores. He carried his idea into practice. During the 1880s he and the French scientist Terrier (286) popularized steam sterilization. Steam killed everything that grew. Thus was ushered in the era of aseptic surgery.

Alexander Fleming, 1881–1955

Alexander Fleming (90) (Fig. 11) was born in Lochfield, Scotland. He became a bacteriologist. In 1928, he made his epochal discovery of the antibacterial powers of the mold from which penicillin is derived. This chance observation has been cited as a "triumph of accident and shrewd observation." Mold had accidentally developed on a Staphylococcus plate. Fleming discovered that the mold had created a bacteria-free circle around itself. Experimenting further, he found that a liquid mold culture prevented growth of Staphylococci, even when the mold was diluted 800 times. He named this substance "penicillin" and reported his work in 1929, but his report didn't attract much notice until the late 1930s when two British medical researchers, Howard Florey and Ernst Chain, repeated his work and verified his results. They purified the penicillin and tested the substance first on

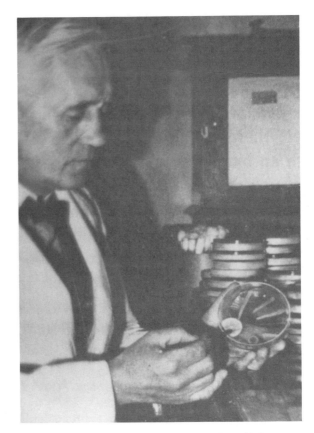

FIG. 11. Alexander Fleming (1881–1955).

laboratory animals and then on humans. Fleming, Florey, and Chain shared the Nobel prize in 1945.

In the ensuing 40 years since Fleming made his famous observation, there has been remarkable progress in general medicine and surgery, affecting the safety and efficacy of spinal surgery. Such advances as our ability to type and cross-match blood, the safe and efficient use of anesthesia, innovations in cardiac care, discovery of better antibiotics, and developments in fluid and electrolyte balance have made surgery safe for all ages, from the premature infant to the centenarian.

DIAGNOSTIC TECHNIQUES

William Conrad Roentgen, 1845–1923

Toward the end of the nineteenth century a discovery was made of such magnitude that the practice of spine surgery became forever different. Conrad Roentgen (237) (Fig. 12), a physicist of German ancestry who was born in Holland, discovered the x-ray while he was working at the University of Wurzberg. On Friday, November 8, 1895, he was experimenting with a Hittoff-Crookes tube. He had covered the tube with black paper, so no light could possibly get out, but he noticed that a fluorescent screen lying nearby glowed when the electric cur-

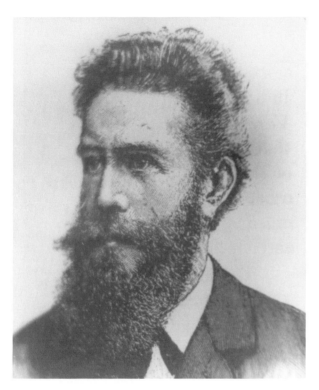

FIG. 12. William Conrad Roentgen (1845–1923).

rent was turned on. He became so fascinated with it that his wife barely got him to come to dinner that night. During the next few days, he put wire and also his own thumb in the x-ray beam, making pictures of each one. He persuaded Frau Roentgen to hold her hand in the beam for 15 minutes, and a good reproduction of the bones of her hand was made on a photographic plate. Two rings on her fingers also showed clearly. This is probably the most famous roentgenogram in the world. It has been reproduced thousands of times and is remarkably good. Frau Roentgen was actually shocked and worried at seeing a picture of her bones. It seemed to her to portend death. Roentgen immediately recognized the implications of his discovery, and before the end of the next year x-ray machines could be found in physicians' offices in many places in the United States and Europe. Roentgen, true to the high scientific tradition of the day, refused to accept monetary gain from his momentous discovery. He did receive a Nobel prize and thus was compensated in the best way a true scientist could be.

Myelography

Air myelography was introduced by Dandy (71) in 1918. This procedure never worked well in the spine but was a valuable procedure for the diagnosis of lesions in the brain.

In the years following World War I, Sicard (260), a neurosurgeon in Paris, was using injections of Lipiodol as a treatment for painful conditions in the lower back. In 1920, his assistant (it may have been Forestier) injected a patient's back with 8 or 10 cc of Lipiodol. After the injection he drew the plunger back and to his horror, noted what was obviously spinal fluid. He went to his professor, Sicard, in great agitation. Sicard said, "Is the patient all right?" The assistant answered that the patient had suffered no ill effects. They then put the patient under the fluoroscope and to everyone's surprise, a fine myelogram was seen. This was the birth of Lipiodol for myelography (Fig. 13).

Lipiodol was never a good material for this purpose. It tended to form globules and also was found later to produce arachnoiditis far too frequently.

In 1941, Strain and co-workers (272) introduced pantopaque, another oil-based material. This remained the contrast of choice in the United States until metrizamide was introduced.

The disadvantages of an oil-based myelogram and the

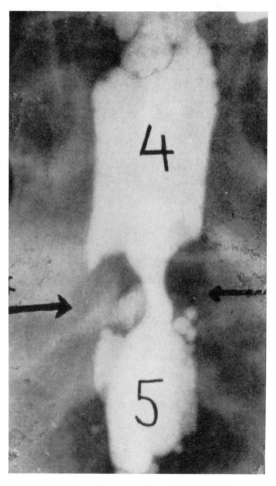

FIG. 13. Lipiodol myelogram, about 1932. This is an extraordinarily good myelogram of a case of degenerative spondylolisthesis at L4-5. Lipiodol had a tendency to break up into globules, which made accurate interpretation impossible.

advantages of one based on water were realized early on. In 1931, Arnell and Lidstrom of Sweden (12) recommended a water-soluble contrast, skiodan (Abradil). This material was used for many years but never became popular because it could be used only in the lumbar area and required the use of general anesthesia. There followed a succession of water-soluble materials, including Thorotrast, Conray, Dimeray, Dimerex, and finally, in the 1970s, metrizamide. Metrizamide has largely given way to iohexol and iopamidol, which are now being used extensively.

Discography

Discography was first reported by Lindblom (165) in 1948. After his report, the procedure was used by a few people but never gained much popularity until the last few years. It still remains controversial despite widespread use.

Computed Tomography and Magnetic Resonance Imaging

The development of the computed tomography (CT) scan and magnetic resonance imaging (MRI) are also interesting stories. In each case, there was a step-by-step advance, each forward step being totally dependent on a previous discovery.

In the development of the CT scan, Radon (229) in 1917 made a mathematical calculation that could have permitted the reconstruction of CT images. However, because the computer was not yet developed, nothing came of it. Then 40 years later, one evening William Oldendorf (211) (Fig. 14), a neurologist at UCLA, was at a cocktail party at which some engineers were discussing an experimental x-ray machine that might be used by orange growers to detect dehydrated areas in oranges. Dr. Oldendorf believed that a similar system might show tumors in the brain and published his work in 1961 (211), which showed drawings of the basic apparatus for CT. This report remains a classic.

Like Radon in 1917, R.N. Bracewell (34), an Australian radio astronomer between 1956 and 1979, made the necessary calculations for CT reconstruction, but again his work was not fully appreciated.

In 1963, A.M. Cormak (60), an American physicist, described the mathematics related to Bracewell's lines but added an important link by showing how such a reconstruction could be applied to tomography. During this same time an English engineer and computer expert, G.N. Houndsfield (137), began working in the central laboratories of EMI, Ltd. In 1967, he was able to develop a functional scanner. By this time he had the good fortune that computer technology had evolved to a level of sophistication necessary for his elaborate calculations.

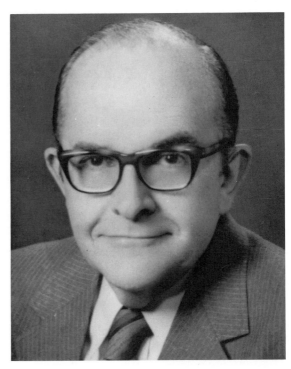

FIG. 14. William Oldendorf (born 1925), Professor of Neurology and Psychiatry, University of California at Los Angeles.

The first good brain image was made in 1972. Houndsfield's final breakthrough represents a fortunate confluence of engineering excellence, ingenuity, persistence, computer excellence, and the excellent facilities of the EMI laboratory. In 1979 Houndsfield and Cormack shared the Nobel prize in medicine. Many believe that Oldendorf should have been included.

The history of the development of MRI is also fascinating (286), again demonstrating that the development of most advanced techniques is a matter of inching forward, with many different scientists contributing important building blocks of knowledge. In 1869, Mendeleev (211), a Russian, and Meyer (221), a German, within a few months of each other classified the 60 known elements into the periodic table. In about 1895, Rutherford (245), a New Zealander working at Cambridge University, discovered alpha, beta, and gamma radiation. He was the first to show that the atom had a nucleus that contained all its positive charges. In 1913, Niels Bohr (264), also working at Cambridge University, postulated that each atom had a number of electrons equal to the number of positive charges in the nucleus, which proved to be correct.

In 1952, Bloch (25), at Stanford, and Purcell (227), at Harvard, shared a Nobel prize for the discovery of the nuclear magnetic resonance (NMR) phenomenon.

In 1972, Damadian (70), an American, patented an imaging device using the principles of magnetic resonance. Others gradually pushed MRI to the point of medical usefulness. Moore and Hinshaw (199), physicists at Nottingham, England, in particular, are to be credited because on May 18, 1979, they constructed an imaging unit that produced the first head scan using MRI. Soon thereafter, a group at Aberdeen, Scotland, headed by Reid (232), developed a unit that gave fairly clear and sharp images of the thorax and abdomen.

Electromyography

Using a string galvanometer (221), Piper recorded voluntary contractions in the forearm flexors of a man in 1907. He found distinctive rhythms for each muscle, which he thought indicated the degree of innervation received from the central nervous system. Buchanan (44) and Wertheim-Salomonson (301) confirmed the findings of Piper. Soon thereafter (1928), tracings of paralyzed peripheral nerves were produced by Proebster (226). He is most often credited with beginning clinical human electromyography.

In 1935, Lindsley (166) made the first tracings of a patient with myasthenia gravis, and Denny-Brown (75), using a bipolar needle electrode, was able to differentiate between fasciculations and fibrillations.

In 1948, Hodes and Larrabee (133) of Germany reported nerve conduction velocities, but this technique became popular in the United States only in the late 1960s.

Somatosensory Evoked Potentials

The first use of somatosensory evoked potentials was reported by a Japanese, Professor Tamaki (276). The technique was initially invasive and required an operation to place the electrodes. Then in the late 1970s, noninvasive placement of electrodes was developed by Richard Brown (43), an electrical engineer, and Clyde Lester Nash (204), an orthopedic surgeon at Case Western Reserve in Cleveland. Dr. Betty Grundy (113), an anesthesiologist, showed how anesthesia can affect evoked potentials. This led to spinal cord monitoring. This modality has improved but still, as of this writing, is not established in what many believe to be its rightful place. It does appear that these techniques hold great promise, and most believe they will be useful in the future.

HISTORY OF TREATMENT OF SPINAL CORD INJURY

The history of medicine is, in fact, the history of humanity itself.
—FIELDING H. GARRISON, 1870–1935 (102)

The history of spinal injury is intimately involved with the history of treatment of the spine. Most of the discussions of treatment of the spine in the Edwin Smith Papy-

rus (37), the hippocratic collection (4), and in other writings up to the 1800s had to do with spinal injury.

During the nineteenth century great advances were made in other areas of medicine, which made effective treatment of spinal cord injury possible. Louis Pasteur opened the new science of bacteriology. Lister created a system of antiseptic surgery. Anesthesia was developed. Semmelweis showed the mode of transmission of disease. Koch discovered and isolated pathogens and, with his four postulates, further explained their mode of transmission. Schimmelbusch (250) and Terrier introduced gas sterilization, and thus aseptic surgery was ushered in. Halstead (286) introduced rubber gloves, and caps, masks, and gowns were worn. Better surgical instruments were developed. Electricity was harnessed, which brought brighter, more versatile lighting and, later, power tools. Near the close of the century, in 1895, Roentgen discovered the x-ray.

The most widely discussed topic concerning the treatment of spinal cord injury during the nineteenth century was the laminectomy. This operation, as previously mentioned, was performed by Paul of Aegina (3) in the seventh century A.D. After that time it was described by almost all the great surgeons, but these reports fail to describe actual cases attempted. Antoine Louis used this principle in 1762 for the successful removal of a bullet lodged in the spinal column. The first real laminectomy was done in 1814 by a London surgeon, Henry Cline. Although Cline's patient died in 9 days, the whole medical profession became interested in the possibilities of this operation. Probably more physicians condemned it than approved of it, and heated arguments over its efficacy were published. The most notable adversaries were Sir Astley Cooper (58,59) (in favor of) and Sir Charles Bell (21,22) (against).

In 1829, Alban Smith (263) of Danville, Kentucky, appears to have been the first since Paul of Aegina to perform a laminectomy successfully.

Malgaigne (178) in 1847 was the first since Hippocrates to use hyperextension for the treatment of spinal dislocations. Hippocrates had tried it and failed.

Most of the real advances in specific treatment of spinal injury have been in the twentieth century. In 1911, Albee (6) and Hibbs (127) described methods of fusing the spine. This was a landmark advance. Crutchfield (69) developed his famous tongs in the early 1930s. But the discovery of penicillin by Fleming (90) in 1929, ushering in the era of antibiotics, was one of the greater moments in the treatment of the spinal cord–injured patient, and proved to be as much benefit for these people as any other discovery in history. Without antibiotics, the treatment of paraplegia as we know it would not be possible. The Stryker turning frame developed in the late 1930s by Homer Stryker (273) of Kalamazoo, Michigan, allowed better care of the paraplegic patient.

Harrington (120) instrumentation made it possible to

surgically reduce and hold spinal fractures. Thus began the era of early stabilization of spine fractures. The halo, developed by Nickel (224) and his group at Rancho Los Amigos Hospital in Downey, California, represents an important advance in the treatment of cervical fractures. It makes early mobilization and ambulation possible. Of interest is that Dr. F.A. Bloom (207), an orthodontist, described in a personal communication with Dr. Nickel the use of the halo. This gave Nickel the idea that it might be used in cervical fractures.

The concept of intermittent catheterization alone, popularized by Sir Ludwick Guttman (210), changed the life expectancy of a paraplegic from a few years to a near normal lifespan.

Pedicle screws with plates or rods, first used in the spine by Roy-Camille (241,242) of France, make it possible to hold a spine fracture with a short segment fusion. In this day, when paraplegics are becoming more active, participating in athletics, and doing most things a noninjured person does, the short fusion is immensely valuable, as it makes spine motion possible and often makes the difference between whether a handicapped person can compete or not.

HISTORY OF SCOLIOSIS AND OTHER SPINAL DEFORMITIES

Only the man who is familiar with the art and science of the past is competent to aid in its progress in the future.
—THEODOR BILLROTH, 1829–1894, Zurich

Scoliosis is derived from the Greek word meaning curvature, but is used to describe only lateral deviations, often associated with rotation, rather than abnormalities in the sagittal plane.

Spinal deformities have been recognized since ancient times. In "De Articulationes" of the Corpus Hippocraticum (4), there is a description of normal and abnormal spinal curves. One passage states, "There are many varieties of curvature of the spine even in persons who are in good health, for it takes place from natural conformation and from habit, and the spine is liable to be bent from old age and from pains." The possible relationship between spinal deformity and pulmonary disease was also mentioned, and it is just possible tuberculous kyphosis was recognized.

Hippocrates noted, "When a gibbosity seizes persons who have already attained their full growth, it usually occasions a crisis of the then existing disease." We do not know what the "existing disease" might have been, but clearly tuberculosis was one possible explanation.

Treatment was considered to be difficult and ineffective. The poor prognosis in patients with early onset of spine deformity was described. No clear distinction was made between the deformity of tuberculosis and that of true scoliosis. Treatment of spine deformities was by forcible traction, both horizontal and with underarm and leg distraction in suspension (see Fig. 2).

Galen coined the word "scoliosis" (51), but he made little new contribution to its treatment and basically followed Hippocrates's teaching.

From the fifth to the fifteenth centuries, little progress was made in treatment of spine deformities. However, Paul of Aegina (3) did write a treatise of Seven Books, which was a bright light in a dark period, and does describe some aspects of spine deformity.

Ambrose Paré (214) thought that poor posture was a probable cause of scoliosis. He described congenital scoliosis and recognized cord compression from the curvature as a cause of paraplegia. His treatment of scoliosis adhered closely to the hippocratic method, but he added a steel corset made by armorers, thus antedating by several hundred years the development of bracing in western Europe and in the United States.

Andry (10), who was the first to use the word "orthopedia" in 1741, wrote about spine curvatures, giving special attention to postural and sitting habits as a preventive measure and to corsets and exercise as methods of treatment.

The "jury mast" for sustained head traction during ambulation was developed by Levacher in 1764 (164). Myotomies were advocated by Guerin in 1839 (114). Volkmann resected protruding ribs in 1889 (294). Royle (243) in 1928 reported on resection of hemivertebrae.

Throughout the nineteenth century, postural habits continued to be considered the cause of most spinal deformities, including scoliosis. Exercises and body bracing were the recommended treatment, and distraction in bed or on a frame was used for attempted correction.

Ingenious vertical distraction frames with corrective pressure pads appeared under the name of Hoffa (135) and others in Germany. Louis Sayre (249) applied plaster torso casts in vertical suspension. Bracket and Bradford (36) in 1895 devised a horizontal distraction frame with a "localizer" attachment, very similar to that later used by Risser in 1952 (234) (Fig. 15). As treatment evolved, the etiologic factors involved in scoliosis became increasingly evident, and surgical treatment emerged. Although Calot (47,48) performed a fusion for tuberculosis of the spine before Hibbs (127), he abandoned the procedure as unsuccessful. The successful surgical treatment of scoliosis can be attributed to Hibbs (127). His original method of spine fusion was developed in 1911 for tuberculosis of the spine. In this article he suggested the possible use of the procedure for scoliosis, and later (in 1914) performed the first fusion for that condition. With Risser and Fergusson, he published an end result study of 360 fusions for scoliosis (234). In this same article, the use of the turnbuckle corrective cast was described, to which the name Risser cast (256) is commonly attached.

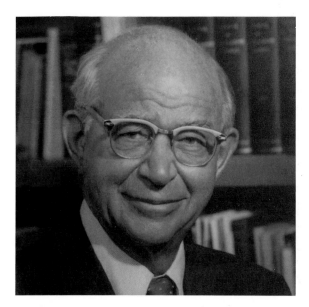

FIG. 15. Joseph Risser (1892–1982), Los Angeles.

During the decade of 1930 to 1940, treatment of scoliosis by fusion fell into disrepute because of the poor results. Steindler's (269) fusion results were so poor that he gave up the idea entirely and again resorted to exercises, bracing, and attempts to establish better compensation and balance.

In 1941, a group of 425 cases of idiopathic scoliosis was studied by a committee of the American Orthopaedic Association (7). They made a dismal report, giving the following conclusions: 60% of cases treated by exercise and braces but no fusion progressed and 40% were unchanged. Correction and fusion in a group of 180 cases studied specifically for rate of fusion showed pseudarthrosis in 54 of 214 patients treated by fusion; 29% lost all correction. Of the entire group, 69% had an end result rated poor or fair and 31% good or excellent.

Fusion with preoperative cast correction provided fairly good results in the hands of the few orthopedic surgeons who chose to study the problem thoroughly, paying meticulous attention to details of cast application, technique of fusion, and protection of the fusion by external support until graft maturation. Through the efforts of Goldstein (107,108), Risser (234), Cobb (56), and a very few others, surgical treatment of scoliosis slowly began to regain its proper status. In 1946, Blount and Schmidt (26,27) devised a distraction brace, combined with lateral pressure pads. This early Milwaukee brace was at first used only in the preoperative treatment of scoliosis. Its success in curvature correction led to improvement in fit and construction and to increasing enthusiasm for its use. Such changes led to greater correction of the curvature and ultimately to use of the appliance as an ambulatory brace in the non-operative treatment of lesser curves. It has proved fairly successful in a high percentage of properly selected patients.

The advent of Harrington instrumentation (119) (Fig. 16) marked the next milestone in the surgical treatment of the scoliotic spine. The early use of this device was not successful because many inexperienced orthopedic surgeons considered it the answer to all scoliosis problems and used it as a substitute for meticulous fusion and cast techniques. Widespread experience with several hundred scoliotic spines treated by fusion proved of great benefit when Harrington instrumentation was added to cast correction and meticulous fusion (118).

Like other innovators before him, Harrington had difficulty getting his technique accepted. He was severely criticized at first as being too radical and of performing too dangerous an operation where simpler safer methods would suffice. His system won the day, however, and became for many years the gold standard for surgical treatment of scoliosis.

In 1965, Hodgson (134) described his method of anterior opening wedge osteotomy for congenital kyphosis. The results were satisfactory with up to 25° of final correction. Since that time, the anterior approach for spine deformities has become increasingly recognized as a necessary procedure for most patients with a sharply angulated kyphosis or kyphoscoliosis and for the release of cord impingement in paraplegia. The work of Moe (195–197), Winter (195), Hall (195), Leatherman (195), Simmons (261), and others has established this anterior approach as a vital and necessary addition to the surgical treatment of spinal deformities.

The use of the halo for distraction of the spinal column was developed at Rancho Los Amigos Hospital in Dow-

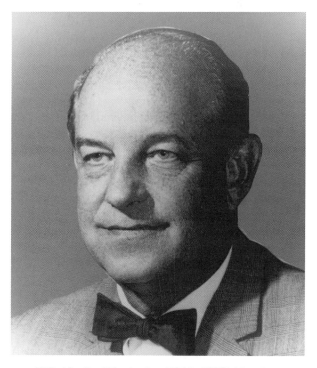

FIG. 16. Paul Harrington (1911–1980), Houston.

ney, California, by Nickel, Perry, and Garrett (207), and provided yet another means for curve correction in difficult cases. The halo was originally connected to a body cast to provide stable spine distraction in paralytic spines. With a tracheostomy and mechanical breathing assistance, surgical fusion of the collapsing spine became a relatively safe procedure in patients with severe respiratory depletion. Later, at some scoliosis services, femoral traction was added, which became a fairly common method of correcting severe forms of scoliosis (159).

The halopelvic hoop was developed by Dewald (77) in Chicago. It was popularized in Hong Kong by Hodgson, Yau, and O'Brien (209), and has become yet another accepted form of correction in certain severe spine deformities (209).

In 1969, A.F. Dwyer (81) of Australia reported a new method of correcting lateral curvatures of the spine by anterior disc excision combined with the insertion of special screws and compression of the vertebral bodies with a fixed cable. Excellent correction was obtained and, with that advance, anterior instrumentation has gained wide acceptance for use in selected cases of severe deformity. Improvements have been made using modifications of Dwyer's instrumentation.

The founding of the Scoliosis Research Society at the University of Minnesota in 1966 must be considered an important milestone in progress of scoliosis treatment. For the first time, a large group of enthusiastic orthopedic surgeons came together in the United States and Canada for the express purpose of standardizing scoliosis treatment and solving the many problems brought about by divergent opinions. No organization has created such worldwide stimulation toward progress in scoliosis treatment.

In 1982, Eduardo Luque (171) of Mexico City published reports of the use of his system for treating scoliosis. This was a very real addition to the scoliosis surgeon's armamentarium, because it allowed segmental stabilization and the avoidance of postoperative casts.

Because of some problems associated with getting the wires around the laminae, Drummond (80) in Wisconsin developed a system whereby the wire could be attached to the bases of the spinous processes. Although this technique is not as biomechanically efficient as the sublaminar wires, it is much safer.

In 1984, Yves Cotrel and J. Dubousset (63) of Paris presented their technique using a system of pedicle screws, rods, cross links, and hooks. This system basically rotates rather than distracts. This instrumentation represents a great improvement over previous systems.

From all these advances, treatment of scoliosis has come of age and is no longer haphazard. Centers for the study of and treatment of scoliosis are being formed in increasing numbers. Scoliosis research societies are being organized all over the world, and information of value is being given international attention. Highly motivated

orthopedic surgeons, whose main interest is scoliosis, are freely exchanging opinions with their fellows. Their motive is the development of the best possible treatment of scoliosis.

HISTORY OF DISORDERS OF THE CERVICAL SPINE

To understand a science it is necessary to know its history.
—AUGUSTE COMPTE, 1798–1857 (I) (57)

When the early clinicians wrote about the cervical spine, they were almost totally concerned with injuries rather than acquired nontraumatic disc disease. The following case report is from the Edwin Smith Papyrus written 5,000 years ago (37). It contains a description of an acute neck injury. Here is an erom Case 31:

If thou examines a man having a dislocation in a vertebra of his neck, shouldst thou find him numb in his two arms [and] two legs on account of it, while his phallus is erected on account of it [and] urine drops from his member without him being aware of it, his flesh has received wound, both his eyes are bloodshot, it is a dislocation of a vertebra of his neck, extending to his backbone [lower cervical], which causes him to lack feeling in both his arms and legs. If, however, the middle vertebra of his neck is dislocated, it is an [emissio seminis] which befalls his phallus. Diagnosis: thou shouldst say concerning him, one having a dislocation of his neck while he is not conscious of his two legs and his two arms and his urine dribbles. This is an ailment not to be treated.

Between the ancient Egyptian and the Greek period the medical literature is sparse. In Homer's *Odyssey,* we find the description of one of Odysseus's aides, who fell off a roof after drinking heavily the night before, sustaining acute quadriplegia, and soon afterward, "his soul went down to Hades. . . ."

In I Samuel 4:18, we find the description of a neck injury:

And it came to pass, when he [the messenger] made mention of [the loss of] the ark of God, that he [Eli] fell from off the seat backward by the side of the gate and his neck brake, and he died; for he was an old man and heavy. And he had judged Israel forty years.

Hippocrates (32,86) wrote of cervical injuries in his book, *On the Articulations.* In general he was pessimistic about the value of treatment. An interesting excerpt from the same work attributed to Hippocrates is as follows: "No head injury, however trivial, should be taken lightly," indicating that even at that time doctors were acutely aware of the dangers associated with head trauma. It seems likely Hippocrates was referring to intracranial injury and did not realize that a good share of the danger from head injury was associated cervical damage. Even today the incidence of cervical spine injury associated with head injury in accidental death is not fully appreciated by most doctors, since postmortem examinations of individuals dead on arrival at hospitals do not always include the cervical spine, especially the craniovertebral area. This principle has recently been confirmed by Bohlman (29).

The principle of traction to the cervical spine was well appreciated by Hippocrates, but the only way he knew of applying head traction in his time was with swaths and bandages. In fact, the use of traction for neck injuries was reported by Bontecou (31) only in 1887. He placed adhesive tape on a patient's face and attached 20 pounds of traction to reduce a fracture. In 1929, Taylor (280) introduced head halter traction, followed in 1933 by Crutchfield's (69) introduction of tongs. Since then, several improvements have been made in this principle of skeletal traction. The most effective method for immobilization and, to some extent, for traction is the halo. This has been one of the landmark advances in the treatment of cervical spine trauma, deformity, and complex degenerative conditions.

Cervical Laminectomy

The Egyptians performed cervical laminectomies as part of the mummification process but never, it seems, for treatment. Paul of Aegina (3) removed laminae for spinal cord compression. Fabricus Hildanus (128) of Padua in about 1646 described his attempts to replace fracture dislocation of the neck by means of clamping the soft tissues and spinous processes with a special clamplike device and manipulating the cervical spine. He also did some open reductions but with limited success. Although a lot was written and spoken about laminectomy during the 1800s, few were attempted and none were successful. The first successful laminectomy after those of Paul of Aegina appears to have been done in 1829 by Alban Smith of Danville, Kentucky (263). It is interesting this should occur in what must have been a fairly unsophisticated area as regards medical development, whereas in the great centers of Europe, the surgeons shied away from it. Perhaps because he lived in what might be considered a frontier town, Dr. Smith didn't know that what he did was "impossible."

Posterior Fusion of the Cervical Spine

In 1891, Hadra (115) of Galveston, Texas, reported wiring the spinous processes of C6 and C7 for a dislocation in a baby. He did not fuse. The result was good, perhaps because healthy babies are indestructible.

Louis Pilcher (219) of Brooklyn, New York, in 1900 attempted to reduce a C1-C2 dislocation. Even though fusion was not intended, a great mass of callus developed. He later reported a 10-year follow-up on this patient, saying the patient was functioning well. Pilcher

published this case in 1910 in the *Annals of Surgery* as a companion article to one by Mixter and Osgood (193), who reported reducing a C1 on C2 dislocation by pulling on silk threads and tying the threads. No fusion was done in this case either.

William Rogers (238) of Boston established the modern principles of cervical fusion. He recommended operating under traction, reducing the fracture if necessary, fixing with wires around the spinous processes, and then fusing. This technique has remained the mainstay of posterior stabilization ever since. Robinson and Southwick (236) recommended fusing by wiring rods to the facets and Magerl (175) has developed a technique using screws through the lateral masses, attached to plates.

Atlanto-Axial Arthrodesis and Fixation of the Dens

In the late 1930s, W. Edward Gallie (100) of Toronto developed and popularized his landmark advance of C1-C2 fusion, using wire and a piece of ilium. Brooks and Jenkins (42) in 1978 reported a modification of Gallie's technique, which has made the operation easier. Bohler (28) in 1982 reported a method of reattaching the two fragments of the odontoid process through a transoral approach, using a screw.

Approaches to the Anterior Cervical Spine

Boudof (33) in 1864 reported using an approach to the cervical apophysis for drainage of abscesses and Dickson Wright (314) of Toronto in 1930 drained a tuberculous abscess through the pharynx. By the 1930s, otolaryngologists were approaching the front of the cervical vertebrae regularly to remove the huge osteophytes that sometimes grow on the front of the cervical vertebrae at about the C5 level and make swallowing difficult. Also, for years before orthopedists started approaching the area, cancer surgeons were stripping the lymphatics lying on the front of the vertebrae. But little interest was evidenced by orthopedists or neurosurgeons in this approach until 1955, when Robinson and Smith (235) reported anterior disc removal and fusion through this approach.

An important serendipitous result of the anterior cervical intervertebral fusion is the "melting" away of the osteophytes, which occurs if the fusion becomes solid.

In 1958, Ralph Cloward (53–55) of Honolulu presented his circular graft for anterior cervical interbody fusion. Two years later, Bailey and Badgley (16) of Ann Arbor reported their anterior cervical graft done for multiple level fusions.

While Robinson (235) and his group at Johns Hopkins were establishing anterior cervical discectomy combined with fusion as the procedure of choice, Hirsch (130) of Gothenburg, Sweden, in 1988 started doing discectomy alone without fusion for the same disease. In the case of "soft" disc disease where posterior bulging alone is causing the trouble, this does seem to be a good procedure. Tew and Mayfield (283,284) in a comparative study concluded that in select cases, the clinical results were about the same whether or not fusion was added following the discectomy.

Cervical Osteotomy

Osteotomy of the upper lumbar spine was first reported by Smith-Petersen and Larson in 1945 (264). However, the use of the procedure in the cervical spine was first reported by Mason et al. (179) in 1953. Herbert (125) also reported on the same procedure in 1954, as did Urist (289) in 1958. This is a seldom used procedure but, when indicated, can give great relief to the patient with the severe deformities of ankylosing spondylitis.

Cervical Spinal Stenosis

Spinal stenosis of the cervical spine has been recognized for about as long as stenosis of the lumbar spine. Like many other human diseases, spinal stenosis had been recognized in animals even before its description in humans. Wobbler's (129) disease in horses is due to spinal stenosis in the lower cervical spine.

The earliest mention of what was certainly spinal stenosis in the cervical spine was by Stookey (271) in 1928. He described compression of the cervical cord by what he surmised were multiple ventral extradural chondromas. In retrospect, these were undoubtedly enlarged, probably hard cervical discs bulging backward. In 1931, Elsberg (85) also came close to describing herniated cervical discs but, unfortunately, he classified them as tumors. Much later, in 1953, Mair and Druckman (177) gave the classic description of cervical spinal cord compression due to protruded discs in the neck, which they said caused clinical symptoms by compression of the anterior spinal artery.

First attempts at treatment of cervical spinal stenosis in humans was with massive bony posterior decompression, opening the dura, and often cutting the dentate ligaments. Later, anterior interbody fusion was popularized by Robinson and Smith (235). Simmons (261) channeled one or several bodies and then fused, using a keystone graft. Simmons's technique remains one of the popular alternatives in use today.

The laminoplasty was designed in 1971 by Hattori (123,124) and is being used in quite a few centers around the world. It was developed for the treatment of ossification of the posterior longitudinal ligament, a disease that was first recognized and reported on by Tsukimoto (288). Since then much has been written about the condition.

Acute Central Cervical Spinal Cord Injury

To Richard Schneider (253), a neurosurgeon at the University of Michigan, goes most of the credit for the description of the syndrome of acute central cervical spinal cord injury, which he reported in 1954. Schneider graciously gave credit to A.R. Taylor (281,282) for Taylor's description in 1948 of paraplegia due to hyperextension injury of the cervical spine without radiological change in the bony structures. Taylor also wrote a subsequent article in 1951 (280) on the mechanism of spinal cord injury "without damage to the bony vertebral columns."

The following is from Schneider's 1954 article (253):

> There is a syndrome of acute central cervical spinal cord injury characterized by disproportionately more weakness in the upper than in the lower extremities with some impairment of the bladder. Associated pain and temperature loss is found in early phases and in the more severe cases there may also be impairment of touch, motion, position, and vibration sensations.
>
> The prognosis for patients with such symptoms and lesions may be relatively good, with motor power returning in the lower extremities first, bladder function recovering next, and finally movement in the upper extremities. Motion of the fingers is the very last to return. Sensory recovery does not pursue an orderly pattern.
>
> The degree of recovery is directly proportional to the amount of edema as compared to hematomyelia, ranging from complete recovery to total destruction with ascending hematomyelia and death.
>
> The mechanism of production of such lesions is described with particular reference to hyperextension injuries of the spine. In a number of the cases cited, no bony injury to the spine could be demonstrated either by roentgenogram or at operation.

Whiplash Injury

This injury is believed to have been first described by Harold Crowe (68) of Los Angeles in 1928. It is a hyperextension injury. The term is a bit of a misnomer because it implies that it may be the forward snap that causes the damage, but the evidence is quite secure that it is the extension. Actual fractures are rare with this injury.

HISTORY OF DISORDERS OF THE LUMBAR SPINE

Human history is in essence a history of ideas.
—H. G. Wells (300)

Non-operative Treatment of the Lumbar Spine

In this section I will consider the treatment of low back pain due to degenerative disc disease, facet disease, spinal stenosis, and some less certain conditions such as internal disc disruption, musculoligamentous sprain and strain, etc. The history of idiopathic scoliosis, spinal cord injury, and cervical disorders have been dealt with previously in this chapter.

There is little doubt that low back pain and sciatica have been with us since antiquity. Skeletal remains contain an abundance of evidence of severe degeneration and other pathology that would surely have caused pain. Strangely, I found no mention of low back pain or sciatica in Nelson's concordance of the Bible. Perhaps in a day when terribly severe disease abounded, low back pain was not considered worthy of mention.

It has often been suggested (64) that the biblical passage from Genesis 32:25 refers to sciatica, but my ecclesiastical consultant (313) says it refers to a dislocated hip. The passage is as follows: "When the man saw that he did not prevail against Jacob, he touched the hollow of his thigh; and Jacob's thigh was put out of joint as he wrestled with him."

We find the following in Shakespeare's "Timon of Athens" (257), when Timon is raging against his false and fickle erstwhile friends in high places: "Thou cold sciatica, cripple our senators, that their limbs may halt as lamely as their manners." Thus, the term "sciatica" appears to have been commonly used for a long time.

Many of the great physicians of the past, even as far back as Hippocrates, have stressed the use of exercises for the treatment of back disease. Generally, these were prescribed more for the severe types of back diseases, such as scoliosis, kyphosis, or lordosis, rather than for low back pain. There was actually an institute founded in 1825 at Montpelier, France, that included a "back school."

Hot poultices, massage, various liniments, and some herbal sedative medications have been used for centuries. There is some evidence that even some manipulotherapy has been used since the days of Hippocrates or even before (4).

Osteopathy

To Andrew Still (270) (Fig. 17) (1828–1917), of Kirksville, Missouri, must go the credit for developing the theories of osteopathy. He was a practicing physician with about the usual amount of medical training for the frontier region where he lived. Seemingly, his concepts of manipulation as a mode of therapy didn't come to him suddenly, but he worked them out over a period of several years. By 1874, he was practicing and preaching his theories of osteopathy and was ready to present them at Baker University in Baldwin, Kansas.

To understand why osteopathy was developed, one must understand the condition of medicine in 1874. The tuberculosis bacillus would not be identified for another 8 years. Lister was still trying to introduce antiseptic sur-

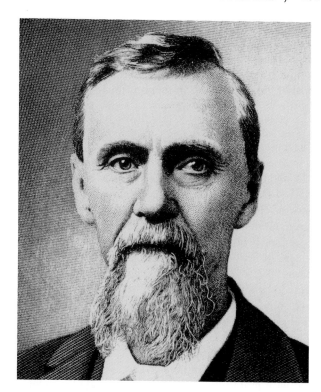

FIG. 17. Andrew Still (1828–1917), Kirksville, Missouri.

gery. X-rays would not be discovered for another 20 years. The sphygmomanometer for measuring blood pressure was 25 years away. Pasteur had promulgated the germ theory of disease only 10 years before, and few doctors subscribed to it. What drugs were available were crude and usually ineffective or, if effective, were usually used in far too large doses. Hertzler (126), author of *The Horse and Buggy Doctor,* who practiced during the latter fourth of the 1800s, made the comment that he often wondered if the country practitioners did more harm than good. He was, of course, being too hard on himself and his profession. But in fact the country physicians did massively overdose, deliver babies without washing their hands, lance boils on the upper lip, give violent purgatives to appendicitis patients, and many other things at which we would gasp today. The doctors who practiced manipulation did little harm at least.

This was also true of homeopathy (302), which became popular in the United States during the latter half of the nineteenth century. Homeopathy had been introduced by Samuel Hahnemann (116) in Meissen, Saxony, in 1796. The Hahnemann University Hospital was founded in Philadelphia in 1848. A school of homeopathy was instituted there the same year. Homeopathic therapeutics is based on two principles. The first and most important principle is; "Like is cured by like." The second principle is less important and is not subscribed to by all: "The more a drug is diluted, the more effective it becomes, even down to the millionths of dilutions." For example, if a patient is nauseated, he will be cured by an emetic. But the emetic may become more effective as the dose is reduced. This accounts for the infinitesimally small doses used by many homeopaths. These minute doses probably had as good a placebo effect as most of the drugs given in that day and certainly did no harm.

Chiropractic

Daniel David Palmer (D.D. Palmer, as he was known) (105) of Davenport, Iowa, is considered to be the originator of chiropractic. He held no medical degree or license but did do bone setting and something called "magnetic healing" (105). He was a rough-hewn frontier citizen. In September, 1985, in Davenport, Iowa, when he was 50 years old, he manipulated the spine of a patient named Harvey Lillard. The patient had a painful prominent spinous process in his cervicothoracic spine. The manipulation was performed by "using the spinous and transverse process as levers." He also gave the area a sharp thrust and he heard a snap. The patient was immediately better. With this clinical success, he continued to treat with manipulation and to promulgate his theories that subluxation of vertebrae caused nerve pressure. His methods of manipulation seem little different from those of the osteopath's. While the chiropractors have limited their work almost entirely to manipulation, the osteopaths have included allopathic medicine and their principles of treatment are based more on biologic disease.

Back Exercises

In 1937, Paul C. Williams (304,305) of Dallas published his famous exercises. This system of back flexion exercises to a large extent reigned supreme until Robin McKenzie (183–185) of New Zealand made his now classic observation that extension could reduce the pain of a herniated disc. Largely because of McKenzie's work, we have moved away from total concentration on flexion exercises and now include not only McKenzie extension type but also stabilization and even stretching exercises.

Epidural Blocks

The first use I came across of the epidural block for treatment of low back pain was by Evans in 1929 (88). In the years since, many articles have been written on this subject, which often conflict in their assessment of the efficacy of this treatment.

Two routes of injection are used: through the sacral hiatus and the direct lumbar epidural route. When cortisone became available, it was added to the anesthetic mixture, which is injected. Recently, the value of the added cortisone has come into question (20,142).

Trigger Point Injections

In 1938, Arthur Steindler and Vernon Luck (269) reported the use of procaine injection into trigger points in the lumbosacral area. This has continued to be an important adjunct to the treatment of low back pain and remains a landmark article in the non-operative treatment of the low back. Since their original description, lidocaine has replaced novocaine, and corticosteroid has been added to the injected material, but the basic premise remains unchanged.

Facet Syndrome

Goldthwait (109) in 1911 strongly implicated the facets as a cause of low back pain and sciatica, a viewpoint later emphasized by Putti in 1927. Ghormley and associates (104) in 1933 coined the phrase "facet syndrome" as a cause of low back pain with radiation into the leg. In the same year, Williams (304) recommended facetectomy for persistent back pain and Badgley (15) in 1941 wrote about the articular facets in relation to low back pain. Rees of Australia (231) in 1974 recommended percutaneous rhizolysis of the facets using a special knife and Shealy (258) in 1976 recommended percutaneous radiofrequency denervation of spinal facets. Mooney and Robertson (109) in 1976 recommended facet injection. Facet injection, much as Mooney recommended, has survived and is used often today. The techniques, especially those of Rees but also of Shealy, have largely been abandoned.

Back School

The person who deserves most credit for formulating the modern concept of the back school is Marianne Zacrisson, RPT (318,319). The first description of the modern-day back school was in 1979 (94). Several articles have been written on the subject since. Zacrisson's basic concept is that the back school "is for the purpose of understanding the relationship of pain to increased mechanical stress." The original training program consisted of four lessons in the form of individual or group education. The anatomy and physiology of the back are taught along with practical applications to the activities of daily living. This basic concept and curriculum remain largely unchanged. Still, the back school represents a major step forward in the non-operative treatment of low back pain.

One of the most unique and appealing institutions for training in back exercises was called a "back school" and was founded by J.M. Delpech (218) at Montpelier, France, in 1825. This is the first use of this term that I came across. However, his institution was largely for the treatment of spinal deformities. Treatment consisted of specific exercises for treatment of low back pain.

An interesting footnote is that on October 29, 1832, Delpech and his coachman were on their way home when they were shot by a deranged patient on whom Delpech had operated for a hydrocele. Both were killed instantly. The horses galloped off with the carriage and delivered their bodies to the institute.

All that remains of Delpech's institute is an atlas containing charming lithographs of cheerful young people engaged in therapeutic exercise.

Spine Pain Program

The Fellowship of those who bear the Mark of Pain. Who are the members of this Fellowship? Those who have learnt by experience what physical pain and bodily anguish mean, belong together all the world over; they are united by a secret bond.
—ALBERT SCHWEITZER

John Bonica (30) is considered the grandfather of modern pain control. His interest in pain control started in 1944 when he was chief of anesthesiology at Madigan Army Hospital. In addition to his regular duties, he was assigned the duty of seeing what he could do for the many injured soldiers who had severe, unremitting pain. In early 1945, he conceived the idea of the multidisciplinary approach to pain control. He gathered a group of specialists together and began using it. In 1946, he got out of the army and went into practice in Tacoma, Washington, where he immediately organized a multidisciplinary group. In civilian practice, the patients needing his new approach were largely ones who had had multiple back operations, but the same principles applied. At about this time, Bonica began working with Dr. Wilbert Fordyce (33), a clinical psychologist at the University of Washington in Seattle. Fordyce took B.F. Skinner's (262) ideas of behavior modification and applied them to humans (96–98).

B.F. Skinner (262), a professor at Harvard working with pigeons, enunciated the law of positive reinforcement in 1938. This law had stated "If a given behavior is followed by a pleasant consequence, that behavior will be repeated." Fordyce applied Skinner's principle in his spine pain program and termed it "operant conditioning." The basic premise when applied to a patient is that good (positive) behavior is rewarded, and bad (negative) behavior is ignored. Many pain programs continue to make use of this principle (8).

Biofeedback is yet another important modality and is part of most spine pain programs. Many workers have been involved in bringing biofeedback to clinical usefulness. Miller (190) did much of the animal research that forms the underlying rationale for biofeedback. Joseph Kamiya (145) instituted the use of the electroencephalogram as one method to monitor its effectiveness.

Of course, several other modalities of treatment are included in a good spine pain program, such as weaning the patient from narcotic and addictive drugs, training in back exercises to tolerance, instruction in body mechanics and back care, and counseling with the patient alone as well as with significant family members.

Intervertebral Disc Disease and Disc Surgery

In the hippocratic collection (4) there is a description of what would most certainly appear to be sciatica. The passage describes "hip ache at the end of the sacrum and the buttocks with radiation into the thigh." Andreas Vesalius (286) in 1543 gave a detailed account of the anatomy of the disc. It was an Italian physician, Domenico Cortugno (61), who in 1764 gave the classic description of sciatica. Cortugno was the first to implicate the sciatic nerve as the cause. This line is taken from his article describing sciatica: "For it seems to be an acrid and irritating matter, which lying on the nerve, preys on the stamina, and gives rise to pain." He did not incriminate the lumbar spine as the cause but believed that the pain arose from the nerve itself.

Charles Bell (22) in 1824 published a model description of post-traumatic disc herniation. Valleix (290) in 1841 described what he called a fractured disc. This was an autopsy finding in a patient who died after a severe injury. He also described the gross and microscopic details of the intervertebral disc. In 1858 Von Luschka (296) described a posteriorly protruded disc, but he attached no clinical significance to his finding. Babinski (14) pointed out the frequent absence of the Achilles reflex on the painful involved side. Brissaud (39) described the inclination of the spine associated with sciatica and coined the term "sciatic scoliosis." He recognized that at times the inclination was away from the side of the pain and at other times toward the painful side.

In 1880, the Lasegue test was described interestingly by J.J. Forst (95), a student of Charles Lasegue's. Forst made this test the subject of his doctoral thesis (Fig. 18) for admission to the faculty of medicine at the University of Paris. In this thesis, he graciously gave Lasegue, his professor, credit for "calling attention" to the possibilities of this maneuver; thus, the test will likely forever bear the name "Lasegue" rather than Forst (163). Some wag has promulgated the rumor that the idea of the test was really Forst's. Forst very much wanted and needed his doctorate, and Lasegue was an important professor at the university. At any rate, Forst got his coveted doctorate and Lasegue got credit for the sign. Perhaps justice was wrought.

In 1896 Kocher (157), a famous Swiss surgeon, reported a traumatic rupture of an intervertebral disc in a patient who had fallen 100 feet, landing in a standing position. The patient walked a few steps and then col-

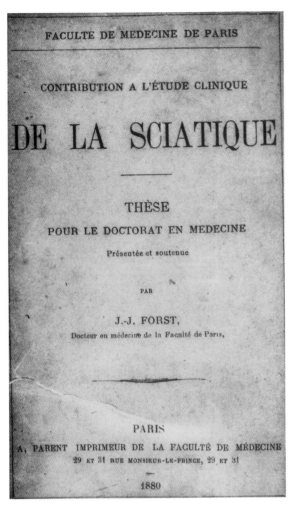

FACULTE DE MEDECINE DE PARIS

CONTRIBUTION A L'ÉTUDE CLINIQUE

DE LA SCIATIQUE

THÈSE

POUR LE DOCTORAT EN MEDECINE

Présentée et soutenue

PAR

J.-J. FORST,

Docteur en médecine de la Faculté de Paris,

PARIS

A, PARENT IMPRIMEUR DE LA FACULTÉ DE MÉDECINE
29 ET 31 RUE MONSIEUR-LE-PRINCE, 29 ET 31

1880

FIG. 18. Title page of Forst's thesis on the ''Lasegue'' test.

lapsed and died from visceral injuries. At autopsy Kocher found and described a posteriorly displaced disc between L1 and L2. He did not mention any possible connection between an extruded disc and sciatica.

Krause (212) in 1908 successfully removed what can be regarded with certainty as a ruptured disc. He made a low lumbar midline incision and reflected the paravertebral muscles from the laminae, which were then removed in one piece. The lesion was resected transdurally. It was thought to be an ''echondroma'' (Fig. 19).

In 1911 George Middleton, a practicing physician, and John Teacher, a pathologist at Glasgow University, described a case that was clearly a classical disc extrusion (188,189). A man had been lifting a heavy plate on the deck of a ship and felt a ''crack'' in the small of his back. He had intense pain and was unable to straighten up. Paraplegia developed, and the patient died 16 days later from bed sores and septic cystitis. At autopsy an extruded disc was found at about L1. Gross and microscopic studies confirmed that the extruded mass was nucleus pulposus that was pressing on the spinal cord. Middleton and Teacher described this extruded disc to perfection but, as did others, failed to connect the ruptured disc to backache and sciatica. It is easy to understand why these early physicians failed to make this connection even though sciatica had plagued mankind for centuries. We need only remember that these early observations were made from autopsy specimens mostly from patients dying after major trauma.

Joel Goldthwait (109) (Fig. 20), in an article published in 1911 on the lumbosacral articulation, showed how with loosening of the annulus fibrosus the pulpy nucleus

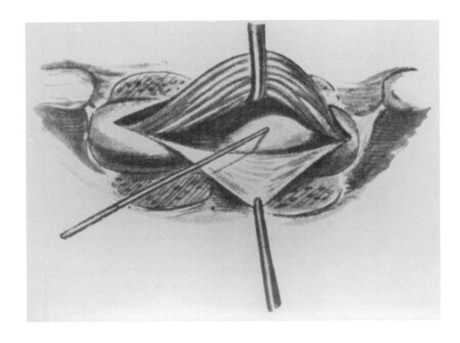

FIG. 19. Drawing of an ''extradurales echondroma'' by Krause in 1908. This was clearly a classical ruptured disc (231).

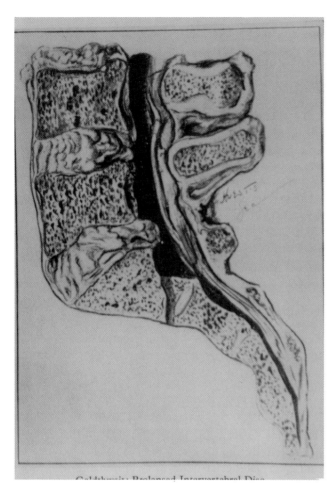

FIG. 20. Drawing of Goldthwait's conception of a herniated disc, published in 1911 (115).

could be projected backward to produce paralysis. He said that the time lapse for this displacement could be quite long or very short—sometimes weeks, sometimes days. He included in this article a lateral drawing of a sagittal section showing a classical disc rupture at L5. He, as had others before him, failed to clearly associate disc rupture with sciatica, but he came close because he did associate the ruptured disc with back pain.

In the 1920s, Murray Danforth and Phillip Wilson, Sr., in Boston did quite a number of spine dissections (73). They recognized bulging discs but, except for the hard bulging disc in the lateral canals, they did not connect them with sciatica. They also believed the spinal nerve, especially the L5 spinal nerve, could be compressed in its lateral tunnel to produce sciatica. They even recognized that it could be compressed by ligaments far laterally, even beyond the pedicles. They described the lumbosacral ligament and called it the "sickle ligament," which I think is a more appropriate name than the more commonly used "lumbosacral ligament." Danforth and Wilson were somewhat confused by the enlarged transverse processes noted in transitional verte-

brae, but tended to believe these structures could cause symptoms. This supposition is not surprising, since Bertolotti (23), an Italian, had written in 1917 about pressure on a spinal nerve due to enlarged transverse processes, which he believed could cause sciatica. This belief was popular for at least 20 years after Bertolotti published his paper.

Most of the surgeons of this era believed that a spinal nerve could be compressed in its lateral neurovascular canals by a build-up of osteophytes combined with narrowing of a foramen due to disc narrowing. In addition to Danforth and Wilson (73), Magnuson (176) in particular was a champion of this idea. Several surgeons even decompressed these nerves laterally by unroofing the lateral canals. A very modern concept, don't you think?

Walter Dandy (71) (Fig. 21), professor of neurosurgery at Johns Hopkins, discovered in 1929 that nodules of discal origin could produce sciatica by compression and that their removal would cure the pain. In 1929 he reported two such cases in the *Archives of Surgery* (72). His drawings in the article are beautiful examples of herniated discs. He described them to perfection, along with his technique for removal, and he described how these masses produced sciatica. He even thought that in many cases they might be produced by a series of small twisting injuries rather than by one major trauma. Unfortunately, he made the mistake of calling them "tumors" even though he was using the word in the generic sense, because, strictly speaking, any abnormal mass in the body can be called a tumor. Because of this small mistake in semantics, little attention was paid to his article and the profession had to await the report by Mixter and Barr (194) for "the shot heard 'round the world."

Demonstrating how knowledge seems to advance in a

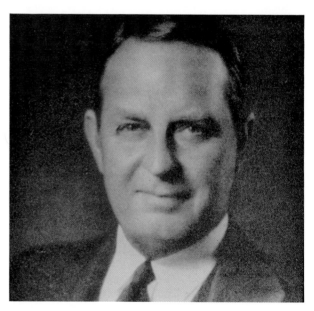

FIG. 21. Walter Dandy (1886–1946), Baltimore, Maryland.

parallel fashion in many countries, we read from an address given by Cauchoix (50) in 1978 that T.H. Alajouanine (5), a Parisian neurologist in 1929, had a female patient aged 20 years with pain and sciatica plus a certain amount of motor paralysis. A Lipiodol myelogram showed an "impression" at the level of the third lumbar disc on the left. Surgery was performed through a transdural approach by D. Petit Dutaillis (5), a general surgeon. A 7- to 8-mm projection was found, which was greater on the left side, and it was removed. Alajouanine and Dutaillis even said it came from the disc. They diagnosed the protrusion as a fibrocartilaginous lesion and called it a "disc tumor." The young woman recovered, but she continued to have weak ankle dorsiflexors. Again, the true nature of sciatica was not recognized, and again the relationship of ruptured discs to sciatica remained unclarified.

During the years before the publication of his classic work, George Schmorl (251,252) at the Dresden Institute of Pathology is said to have studied about 5,000 human spines grossly, radiographically, and microscopically. In 1932, the book by Schmorl and Herbert Junghanns, *The Human Spine in Health and Disease,* appeared. Dr. Joseph Barr (18), a young orthopedic surgeon just out of his residency at the Massachusetts General Hospital, was assigned the job of writing a critique on Schmorl and Junghann's new book.

During June of that year, Dr. Barr (Fig. 22) had a pa-

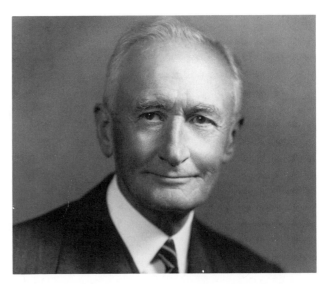

FIG. 23. William Jason Mixter (1880–1958), Boston.

tient with what would be recognized now as an extruded lumbar disc. He kept the patient in bed, trying various types of conservative treatment, for about 2 weeks. Since the patient was not getting well, he called in Dr. Jason Mixter (Fig. 23), who ordered a myelogram. Dr. Kubick did a Lipiodol myelogram and Dr. Mixter scheduled the patient for surgery. Dr. Barr reported (18) that he was not present during the operation (Dr. Mixter seemed to remember that he was); however, on the following Sunday, Barr stopped by to see his patient and found him to be doing well. Then Dr. Barr went to the laboratory and asked to see the microscopic slides of the "tumor" that Dr. Mixter had removed. Dr. Mallory (192) had made some excellent slides that he showed to Dr. Barr.

It is essential to this story to mention again that Dr. Barr was at that moment reviewing Schmorl's and Junghann's (251) new book. The book was in German and it took him a long time to "slog through it," as he later said. Incidentally, he memorized Schmorl's microscopic pictures of the disc. When Dr. Barr looked through the microscope that Sunday morning in June of 1932, he recognized immediately that the "tumor" was actually nucleus pulposus as Schmorl had so beautifully depicted in his photomicrographs. Dr. Barr and Dr. Mixter, along with Dr. Mallory, a pathologist at the Massachusetts General Hospital, studied the cases that had been done in the past few years that were called "chondromas," and related diagnoses. They decided that most of them were ruptured discs. On December 31, 1932, Dr. Barr and Dr. Phillip Wilson operated on the first patient for whom the preoperative diagnosis of "ruptured intervertebral disc" was made. A report of their observations relating to the disc was made on September 30, 1933, in an address by Drs. Mixter and Barr to the New England Surgical Society. Thus began the "dynasty of the disc," as Farfan (89) has so eloquently stated.

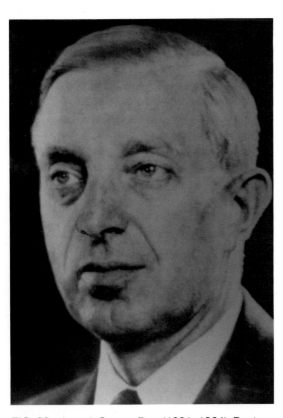

FIG. 22. Joseph Seaton Barr (1901–1964), Boston.

Surgeons throughout the world quickly rushed to adopt disc removal. Workers with a bent toward basic science studied the structural characteristics of the intervertebral disc. Keyes and Compere (150), and Coventry (64), in particular, of the Mayo Clinic conducted extensive studies of the microscopic characteristics of the disc. Arthur Naylor (205) of Britain and Carl Hirsch (130–132) of Sweden are also especially to be credited with contributing over the next 30 years to our basic knowledge of the intervertebral disc.

Love (170) of the Mayo Clinic, during the mid-1930s, developed a technique for extradural removal of the disc. He showed it was unnecessary to open the dura to perform successful disc surgery. Dr. Love (170) also presented a paper in 1939 that popularized the "key hole" laminotomy, which represents a precursor of the microdiscectomy. The use of the microscope had not yet been described for surgery in general.

While the relief of sciatica through lumbar disc excision was the central focus for some, others continued to search for alternative causes. For example, Shordania (259) in 1936 introduced the concept of the "piriformis syndrome." The idea was that spasm of the piriformis muscle could cause compression of the sciatic nerve and thus cause sciatica (19). Others presented favorable results after piriformis section. Although the diagnosis of piriformis syndrome continues to be made, treatment is now almost always by injection rather than by surgical section. In fact, the question of whether or not piriformis spasm has anything to do with sciatica is in serious doubt.

As the surgical treatment of disc disease evolved, alternative, less invasive options were pursued. Chemical dissolution of the disc was first introduced by Lyman Smith (312) in 1963. Dr. Smith got the idea for chymopapain dissolution of the disc from an article by Thomas (285). Thomas had injected papain into rabbits and noted that their ears drooped over. When he stopped giving the papain, their ears came upright again in a few days. Dr. Smith began his research in the late 1950s and published his first paper on chemonucleolysis in 1963. At present, chymopapain is being used fairly extensively throughout the world (208), but has limited popularity in the United States.

Another enzyme, collagenase, was advocated by Bernard Sussman in 1968 (275). Collagenase has not gained wide acceptance, but research on other potential chemonucleolytic agents is continuing.

The concept of using a microscope for microdiscectomy was introduced by Robert Williams (306) of Las Vegas, Nevada, in 1979. A small skin incision is used, and no bone is removed. His operation differs from Grafton Love's (170) in that an even smaller incision is made, the ligamentum flavum and the annulus are split rather than partially removed, and only the protruding portion of the disc is removed. McCulloch (182) and oth-

ers have modified the operation slightly. They still use a small incision, microdiscectomy instruments, and a microscope, but they decompress bone as necessary.

Basic Research in Lumbar Spinal Disease

In the past 50 years, and particularly during the past two decades, tremendous advances have been made in our understanding of the biology and biomechanics of the spine. Although a detailed history is beyond the scope of this chapter, there are some contributions that I feel merit special attention.

Vascular studies of the spinal cord have contributed a great deal to our ability to operate around the spine with safety. Important advances have been made by Adamkiewicz (2), Macnab (174), Dommisse (78,79), and Crock (66,67). The detailed and painstaking efforts that went into their studies are remarkable as models of elegant anatomic research.

It is my belief that the full import of the vascular supply to nerves in the spinal cord and the spinal nerves in their lateral canals has not been realized. Crock (66,67) has repeatedly stated that we are doing too much damage to the vessels that supply the spinal nerves when we do our decompressions. This damage may be producing a claudicant type of pain. How to avoid this damage to the vessels and still decompress remains to be learned.

The many years of painstaking research of Farfan (89) have been extremely important in explaining the biomechanics of the human spine. His concepts of rotary instability and the damage done by rotation were novel when first presented. They have proved to be correct and are of vital importance to our understanding of mechanical disorders of the spine. Similarly, Nachemson and his associates (202,203) have contributed greatly to our understanding of disc biomechanics.

There is little doubt that many others have contributed to the development of our surgical treatment of disc disease. Although most of the others did not describe actual surgical operations, their contributions have been vital. In particular, Roofe (239), Hult (138), Graham (111), Fraser (96), La Rocca (162), Andersson (9), Spengler (267), and Frymoyer (99) should be mentioned. These are only a few. The literature on the intervertebral disc is mountainous.

Lumbar Spinal Fusion

The history of spinal fusion really begins in New York with Fred Albee (6) (Fig. 24) and Russell Hibbs (127) (Fig. 25). Each published the results of his spinal fusions in 1911. However, Albee probably antedated Hibbs by a short time. The fusion methods that they devised had been preceded by the attempts of several other surgeons to stabilize portions of the spine (115,303).

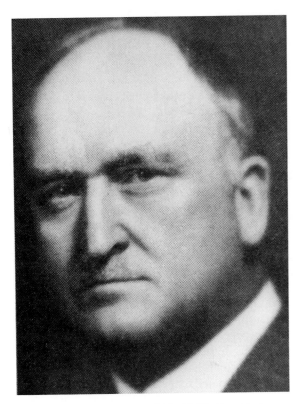

FIG. 24. Fred Albee (1876–1945), New York.

Albee's method of fusion consisted of obtaining a strip of autologous tibia, splitting the spinous processes sagittally, and laying the strip of tibia between the two halves of the spinous processes. He then sutured the soft tissues together securely. He even designed a sterilizable motor saw to aid in the removal of the strip of tibia. Hibb's concept was in some ways more advanced. He denuded the laminae and "feathered" the bone, overlapping the bony strips. He did not get bone grafts from other sources.

Willis Campbell (49) of Memphis described his method of trisacral fusion in the mid-1920s. In this operation he tamped bone out to the tips of the transverse processes of L5. He also used the principle of taking strips of iliac crest for graft. Later, it was natural to push bone out onto the transverse processes of L4 to S1 in performing lumbar spinal fusions. In a publication by Ghormley in 1933 (104), the use of iliac crest for graft was advocated and henceforth became the procedure of choice for most situations where autologous bone graft was needed. Strangely, it took 35 years after Campbell had described the placing of bone graft out to the tips of L5 in trisacral fusions before transverse process fusion became commonly used. Many older surgeons never stopped using simple posterior fusion as described by Hibbs, sometimes omitting iliac crest graft, even though other techniques, such as the transverse process fusion, improved the fusion rate remarkably.

In 1948, Cleveland and Bosworth (52) recommended repairing pseudarthrosis by going through the midline, exposing the transverse processes on only one side, and putting autologous iliac strips over this area. For some reason, in their early reports they did not describe placing graft on both sides. Obviously, using both sides was a simple progression of the technique (104).

Melvin Watkins (298) in 1953 became the first to recommend approaching the transverse processes from an approach just lateral to the sacrospinalis group of muscles. He recommended denuding the transverse process and the lateral masses and laying a large slab of iliac crest along this area, fixing this slab of bone with screws. However, as early as 1936, Mathieu and Demirleau (180), two French surgeons, had advocated far lateral grafting. They recommended driving a peg through a hole in the wing of the ilium and on over the transverse process. A small hole had to be made in the slab of graft to admit the transverse process. This procedure never gained popularity because it was technically difficult and fairly dangerous to the spinal nerves, which pass just anterior to the transverse process. The fact that such an operation could be done encouraged others to go out far laterally. Later, the sacrospinalis was split longitudinally in the cleft between the multifidus and the longissimus to reach the transverse processes and the lateral masses (310). As techniques have evolved, others have more carefully detailed the clinical outcomes.

Remarkable studies have been made in an effort to determine the effectiveness of spinal fusion in the relief of back pain. The work of DePalma and Rothman (76) and Rothman and Booth (240) in Philadelphia, Young (315,316) at the Mayo Clinic, and Frymoyer (98,99) at the University of Vermont should be mentioned.

Metallic Implants

Up until the mid-1930s, surgeons had struggled with various materials for internal fixation. Gold did not pro-

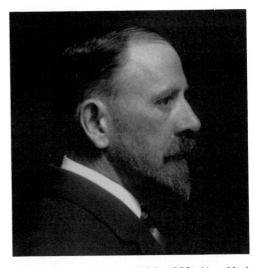

FIG. 25. Russell Hibbs (1869–1932), New York.

duce electrolysis, but it was too soft and too expensive. Nothing worked well, and most devices had to be removed before they had really done their work.

Charles Venable (291) of San Antonio, Texas, had been doing fracture work using these metals (and having the usual trouble). He was talking with his dentist and learned that the dentists were using an alloy called vitallium for dental braces. The dentist said it was inert. Electrolysis had previously caused the fillings to loosen and fall out, but with vitallium the fillings remained secure. This gave Venable an idea, and in 1939 he and Walter Stuck published their brilliant work (291) on the use of vitallium for external fixation. This was a remarkable step forward, because it made internal fixation feasible for the first time.

Stainless steel was developed in the late 1930s and, of course, other metals such as titanium and tantalum have come along since. Methylmethacrylate and other plastics as well as ceramics have been introduced in the last 30 years.

Internal Fixation of the Posterior Lumbar Spine

The first report of internal fixation of the spine that I could find was that of W.F. Wilkins (303) of Ottawa, Kansas, who described the following experience. In the summer of 1887, a severe tornado struck and destroyed the house of Mrs. G, who was in her eighth month of pregnancy. The corner of a table appeared to have hit her very hard in the abdomen. A day later she was delivered

of a male child with a peculiar "hunch on his back." Dr. Wilkins saw the child on the si-partum day. The "hunch" was the size of a goose egg. Dr. Wilkins operated, reduced the hunch, replaced the dural sac, brought the dislocated vertebrae, T12 and T1, into reduction, and fixed the spine with a carbolized silver suture that he passed around the pedicles of T12 and L1. The wound healed by primary intention and the child was practically well within 6 days (Fig. 26).

In 1891, Berthold Hadra (115) of Galveston successfully used wires wound around adjacent spinous processes in a case of fracture of the cervical spine. Fritz Lange (161) (Fig. 27) of Munich as early as 1909 tried to stabilize the spine by tying celluloid bars and later steel rods to the sides of the spinous processes, using silk and later steel wire. This was before the day of inert metals. When metal was used for internal fixation, it was a race between the bony healing and liquification of the bone around the internal fixation device. Interestingly, Fritz Lange's idea of using steel rods tied onto the spine with wire has a very modern ring, does it not? Thus, around the turn of the twentieth century, Wilkins (303), Hadra (115), and Lange (161) had used internal fixation in the spine. Albee's 1911 graft (6) was a form of internal fixation, but it was a slab of tibial bone.

In 1952, Phillip Wilson, Sr. (308), published his work describing the use of a plate that he bolted to the spinous processes, usually with a graft on one side and the plate on the other. However, this system was never successful. The next step in the use of internal fixation of the lumbar spine was made by Don King (151) of San Francisco,

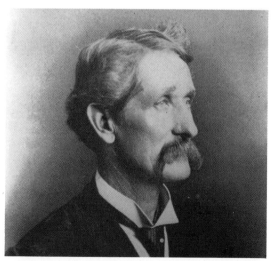

A

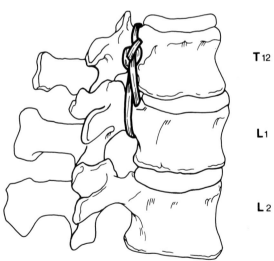

T12

L1

L2

B

FIG. 26. A: Captain W. F. Wilkins (1848–1935), soldier, lawyer, doctor, scholar, author, orator, civic leader, clinical researcher, master surgeon, and professor of medicine at the College of Physicians and Surgeons in Kansas City, Kansas. Truly a latter-day renaissance man, Dr. Wilkins is credited with performing the first operation on the spine where internal fixation was used. **B:** Drawing of Dr. Wilkins's operation performed on a newborn infant's spine. Carbolized silver wire was used to fix a fracture dislocation of T12 on L1. Note that the suture goes completely around the pedicles. The canal was dislocated and wide open so that Dr. Wilkins could safely pass a suture around the pedicles without injuring the spinal cord.

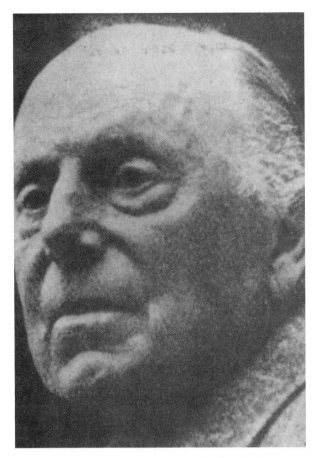

FIG. 27. Fritz Lange (1864–1952), Munich.

Arthur Steffee (268) of Cleveland, Ohio, has used a system of internal fixation by pedicle screws and plates since 1983. Working in Frymoyer's laboratory, Krag (156) has developed the Vermont system, which uses pedicle screws and connecting bars. The Edwards (83) system uses sacral screws fastened to Harrington-type rods. Zielke (320) has modified his screws slightly so they can be used in the pedicles and attached to his standard rods. Cotrel and Dubousset (62,63) have developed pedicle screws that can be attached to their posterior fixation rods. These are also valuable for reduction of scoliosis. Several other groups around the world are working on the development of pedicle screw fixation devices.

Saillant (247) Krag (159), Zindrick (321–323), and Misenhimer (191) have studied pedicle anatomy extensively, especially as to size, shape, and direction of the pedicles at various levels. They have measured pull-out strength of screw placements, including toggle strength and bone strengths, in human age groups.

Pedicle screws appear to have become safe enough for use by surgeons with special training in their insertion. Currently, there are many centers worldwide working on pedicle screws with either rods or plates. It is likely that the pedicle will be a most important area for attachment of screws to the vertebral body. Most of the knowledge necessary for successful internal fixation of the lumbar spine is now available. Recognizing that the population is getting older and that older spines collapse, it is imperative that we pursue a method of internal fixation that will produce stability, even in cases of wide decompression in which posterior bony stability has been sacrificed.

also during the early 1940s. He recommended using screws through the facets and first published his work in 1944. In 1959, Boucher (32) of Vancouver improved on the procedure by aiming the screws more medially so they went down into the pedicles; if driven further they would come out anterior to the base of the transverse processes. The plan, of course, was to keep them inside the bone. This was the first use of pedicle screws since King had put the screws through the facets only.

The next great advance in spinal internal fixation was made by Harrington (119–121). Although his rods are used much more extensively in scoliosis of the young, they may be used in the lumbar spine. Knodt (155) rods were developed in the 1950s and are used in the lumbar spine. The Luque (171,172) system, which consists of sublaminar wires and posterior rods, was developed during the 1970s. Roy-Camille (241,242) (Fig. 28) since 1963 and Rene Louis (169) of France since 1972 have pursued the use of pedicle screws but added plates between the screws. In the late 1970s, Magerl (175) developed a system in which he inserted Schanz screws into the pedicles either percutaneously or by open surgery. These are held in place by an external fixator resembling a Hofmann apparatus. This system has been modified by Dyck (82) and others so that the fixator is internalized.

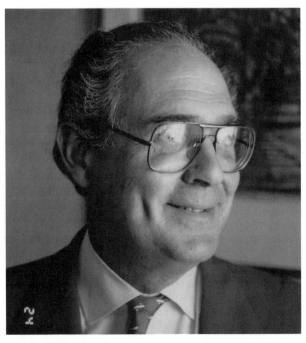

FIG. 28. Raymond Roy-Camille, Paris.

Anterior Interbody Fusion

In 1933, Burns (46) of Great Britain published a report in *Lancet* in which he described performing a successful interbody fusion on a case of spondylolisthesis in a 14-year-old boy. He drove an autogenous tibial peg from the abdominal aspect of the fifth lumbar vertebra into the sacrum. Although this appears to be the first report of interbody fusion, there is a report of a Russian surgeon performing a similar procedure almost concurrently; unfortunately, I have been unable to find the reference. In 1936, Jenkins (144) of New Zealand reported a similar case, but Jenkins attempted to reduce the spondylolisthesis by extension, traction, and then fusion. Walter Mercer (203) of Edinburgh also reported largely similar experiences in 1936.

In the years since, many modifications have been made. For instance, the retroperitoneal approach was described by Harmon (117) and has certain advantages. For the case of high-grade spondylolisthesis, Freebody (97) reported the use of a large iliac graft, nearly filling the bodies of L5 and S1, instead of the tibial peg. In most surgeons' experience, the Freebody operation has worked very well. However, because the graft is soft, the patient must be kept horizontal in plaster shells for 6 weeks. For cases of spondylolisthesis with virtually no slip, or for disc disease, the use of a hole saw and plugs has been reported. Paul Harmon (117) in particular has used this technique. More recently, Harry Crock (66,67) has developed an elegant system for interbody fusion using a hole saw and perfectly fitted grafts. His iliac grafts differ from others in that they are removed from the ilium from its crest downward.

Another surgeon who has been prominent in the development of the anterior interbody fusion is Hodgson (134) of Hong Kong. He started his work with tuberculosis but extended it to intervertebral disc disease.

Even as early as the 1880s, anterior approaches to the vertebral column for the draining of tuberculous abscesses were fairly common. It was Professor Ito (140) of Japan, however, who in 1934 refined the approach to the vertebral bodies to excise tuberculous tissue. His approach laid the groundwork for later surgeons' more complex procedures.

Horseshoe-shaped grafts from the iliac crest for use in the interbody area have been described by Goldner (106) and others. These grafts succeed well only if several grafts can be placed in the interbody space. They are best used in fusion for disc disease or for low-grade spondylolisthesis, since two opposing vertebral surfaces are needed. Obviously, these grafts are not suitable for cases of high-grade spondylolisthesis. Fibular pegs are very successful when inserted in the vertical position under heavy pressure. If they tilt onto their sides, however, the fusion will usually fail. Frank Raney (230) of San Francisco described his technique in the early 1960s. He placed a large rectangular-shaped iliac graft in the posterior portion of the interbody space and three to four fibular struts anteriorly. This technique succeeded well.

Humphries (139) of Cleveland was first to use a plate for anterior interbody fusion. During the 1950s, he designed a compression plate that was fastened onto the anterior surfaces of the vertebra by screws. These plates and screws were used especially at the lumbosacral joint. They have not been used to any great extent because of difficulty of application and possible danger to the great vessels.

Several plates have recently become available for use on the anterior or lateral aspects of the vertebral bodies. Those of Kaneda (147,148), Yuan (317), and Armstrong (11) are important contributions. The combined system of Kostuik (158) is also being used.

Posterior Lumbar Interbody Fusion

The first report on posterior lumbar interbody fusion (PLIF) was written by Briggs and Milligan (38) in 1944. In the early 1940s these surgeons began the practice of packing pieces of spinous process between the vertebral bodies after discectomy; but when fusion failed, they believed their procedure did not work. They found they were able to obtain solid fusion in most cases, however, when they combined this procedure with a posterior fusion. They did not extend their posterior fusion out onto the transverse processes but instead laid morcelled bone right onto the dura. This technique has not survived.

Cloward (53–55) reported that he had performed a posterior lumbar interbody fusion in 1940 but did not do another until 1943. Irwin Jaslow (143) published his experiences with posterior lumbar interbody fusion. These events began the PLIF. The Cloward operation is the classic example and the one that has survived. There were problems with Jaslow's method, as with other procedures where fragments of local bone were tamped in, because solid arthrodesis was usually not achieved. Because of the small amount of bone, this procedure probably fared no better for relief of pain than an ordinary discectomy. The technique also had the added disadvantage that pieces of graft could migrate posteriorly.

There have been several other modifications of the PLIF since Briggs and Milligan made their report. These include the use of large autologous iliac crest grafts, large homologous iliac crest or tibial grafts, and even small grapenut-like cancellous autologous or homologous grafts. Plug cutters were used posteriorly by Wiltberger (309) as early as 1957, and more recently, Ma and Paulson (173) have advocated box chisels to place grafts in the interbody area from the posterior route. Recently, Selby (255) has adapted the Crock system for use from a posterior approach. Steffee (268) has also developed a useful system.

Currently, the use of the PLIF is increasing in a number of centers throughout the world. It is another procedure that should be used only by those with a special interest in its technical details.

Fusion of the Sacroiliac Joint

In the 1920s, fusion of the sacroiliac joint was the surgical procedure of choice for low back pain and sciatica. Both Smith-Petersen (265) and Willis Campbell (49) described similar techniques of sacroiliac fusion. After surgery, the patient was kept in bed, usually in a cast for 6 weeks to 3 months, then allowed up in a corset. The results were fairly good and at least two reports indicate that good or excellent results were as high as 70%. It is highly likely that if we were to put our present-day disc patients to bed for 2 or 3 months, 70% would also declare themselves well.

With the description of the herniated disc by Mixter and Barr in 1934 (194,210), sacroiliac fusions for low back pain and sciatica stopped being done, but the procedure continued to be used for the fractured pelvis, tuberculosis of the sacroiliac joint, and a few other conditions.

For nearly 50 years, from 1932 to about 1980, the sacroiliac joint as a source of low back pain was largely ignored by orthopedic surgeons. However, in the past 10 years, it is being revisited. In particular, Kirkaldy-Willis (152) of Saskatoon, in conjunction with Cassidy of the same city, have revived the belief that the sacroiliac is a common source of pain. They believe this pain can frequently be relieved by manipulations, injections, or both. They have done considerable, very creditable research to validate their theories.

Reduction of Spondylolisthesis

The idea of reducing the slip in spondylolisthesis has held a fascination for orthopedic surgeons for many years (206). In 1936, Jenkins (144) tried to reduce slip by applying traction with the patient in extension, then fusing using interbody graft. Recently Ascani and Monticelli (13) and others have improved on Jenkins' methods but still advocate reduction by extension associated with spinal fusion. Paul Harrington (118–120) was the first in the United States to reduce spondylolisthesis with the use of rods. Matthiass (181) has used a plate with sacral hooks and pedicle screws to reduce the slip. David Bradford (35) and McPhee and O'Brien (186) have been using posterior decompression combined with fusion, then performing anterior fusion a few days later. Rene Louis plates, Steffee plates, and the Edwards device are being used to reduce the slip for single-level fusions.

Fusion of the Pars Fracture Only for Spondylolysis

Regarding fusion of the pars only for spondylolysis, Buck (45) was probably the first to attempt to fix the pars internally. He used a screw across the pars and grafted the defect. Scott (254) of Edinburgh advocates a technique of passing an 18-gauge wire around the base of the spinous process and the transverse process, bone grafting the pars, then twisting the wire tight. Morscher (200) has recently designed an apparatus with a hook that attaches to the lamina with a screw that goes into the lateral mass. He bone grafts the pars defect.

Spinal Stenosis

The condition we now recognize as spinal stenosis has, of course, been with us since antiquity. Several Egyptian mummies have been found to have the condition, even though the ancient Egyptians generally did not live to a ripe old age. Since spinal stenosis is usually a degenerative disease of the elderly, large numbers would not be expected to develop the condition.

Even some animals are afflicted with spinal stenosis (277). The dachshund and the Pekingese, in particular, frequently develop clinical symptoms due to spinal stenosis (277). German shepherds and Doberman pinschers develop the disease in the lumbar area. Wobbler's (277) disease in horses is due to stenosis in the cervicothoracic area. The veterinary literature abounds with reports of these conditions. However, for a surprisingly long time, it was not recognized in humans as an entity that caused symptoms and could be successfully treated by decompression.

Portal (222) of France seems to be the first to have studied spinal stenosis in 1803, when he analyzed the size of the vertebral canal as related to the cause of spinal compression. He noted that abnormal curvature of the spine might produce deformity of the canal to the extent that severe cord compression with paraplegia resulted.

In 1864, in a chapter on spinal cord compression due to spinal osseous processes, Jaccoud (141) discussed Portal's report: "Before terminating the subject I must recall that singular form of paraplegia which (described by Portal) results from compression of the spinal cord by a spinal canal which is too narrow."

During the latter part of the nineteenth century, a few authors wrote about a "strange condition" that seemed to respond only to opening the back and exposing the dura. One of the earliest examples of an operation to relieve spinal stenosis was reported by Arbuthnot Lane (160) in 1893. He had a patient with what was clearly degenerative spondylolisthesis producing cauda equina compression. He decompressed the lesion and relieved this patient. In 1893, Von Bechterew (295) proposed that there was a disease of the spine that produced pain, weakness in the legs, parasthesias, and the necessity of walking with the body bent forward, but he did not establish its pathological basis. Another early description of what was probably spinal stenosis was made in 1900 by Sachs and Frankel (246). Their patient had sacral and lumbar pain that caused him to walk bent forward. This patient was eventually relieved by a two-level laminectomy. The surgeon, A. Gerster (103), found neither tumor nor exudate but remarked on the unusual density of the laminae and the general thickness of the bone. After surgery, the patient could straighten up and walk well. Sottac (266) coined the term "intermittent claudication of the spinal cord" in 1896 to describe the symptoms and disease.

In 1910, Sumita (274) described narrowing of the vertebral canal due to achondroplasia. He showed a schematic drawing of a cross-section of the narrowed vertebral canal in one of his cases.

In 1911 Bailey and Casmajor described a patient with lower extremity pain and a weak left leg, who could walk only a short distance and who was obliged to walk with his body bent forward. He was cured after a laminectomy by Dr. Charles Elsberg (85), who again described the laminae as thicker than normal. No other explanation for the disorder could be found. Bailey and Casmajor stated that the spinal cord and the nerves of the cauda equina seemed susceptible to compression by arthritic abnormalities. They specifically emphasized the role of bony exostoses from articular processes and abnormalities of the ligamentum flavum that compressed the spinal roots from behind.

In 1913 Elsberg wrote of "a peculiar disease" (87) of the roots of the cauda equina with symptoms very much like those of tumor of the cauda equina, although no tumor was ever found at surgery. All the patients improved after operation, and the good result was ascribed to the wide laminectomy. A year later, in 1914, Kennedy (149) gave further information about 22 patients with the disease. The roentgenograms of many of them showed arthritic changes, and most were improved with laminectomy. In 1925, Parker and Adson (216) described spinal compression by hypertrophic arthritis, improved by laminectomy.

In 1931, Towne and Reichert (287) reported two cases of cauda equina compression improved by the removal of thickened, yellow ligaments at narrowed and hypertrophic interspaces.

In 1934, Cramer (65) described 26 patients, presumably those who had been operated on by Elsberg and who had been regarded as examples of the "peculiar disease" that later was called "cauda equina radiculitis." Cramer suggested that this tumor-like syndrome was secondary to arthritic changes in the spine, since arthritic changes were well advanced in two thirds of the cases. Most of these patients were improved after laminectomy. Many

others contributed to the increasing knowledge of the disease (252).

Sarpyener (270) of Istanbul must be credited with making a fundamental contribution to our understanding of spinal stenosis. His description of "the congenital structure of the spinal canal" published in 1945 came close to describing to perfection congenital spinal stenosis as we now understand it.

However, it was Henk Verbiest (292,293) (Fig. 29), a neurosurgeon in Utrecht, Holland, who finally brought spinal stenosis into focus. In 1949 he published his first article on the subject and has continued to study the condition extensively ever since. He probably has done more than anyone to delineate the condition and bring it to the attention of the medical profession.

Others who are prominent in the more recent development of our knowledge of spinal stenosis are Brodsky (40) and Ehni (84) of Houston. Kirkaldy-Willis (152–154) of Saskatoon is credited with creating a logical classification and with focusing our attention not only on the central canal, but on the lateral neurovascular canals as areas of compression. The lateral canals appear to be even more important than the central canal in the production of clinical symptoms.

In recent years, some surgeons have observed that a spinal nerve can be compressed even out beyond the lateral border of the pedicle (311). In a way, we are coming full circle. As mentioned earlier, Bertolotti in 1917 (23),

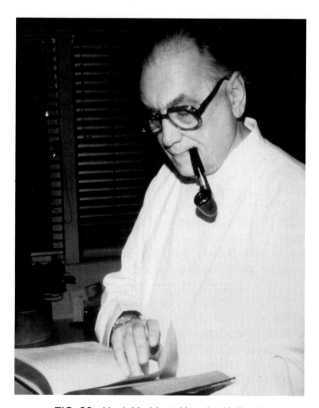

FIG. 29. Henk Verbiest, Utrecht, Holland.

Danforth and Wilson in 1925 (307), Ghormley in 1933, and Magnuson in 1944 (176) were suggesting that far lateral compression caused radiating pain into the leg.

Abdullah (1) in 1974 and, recently, Zindrick (323) in 1985 have reported on the finding of far lateral disc ruptures well out beyond the lateral border of the foramen. Because the spinal nerves are tightly bound in this far lateral area, an extruded disc lying underneath the nerve can cause identical symptoms to those of a ruptured disc in the central canal. These far lateral discs may well have been the "hidden discs" or the "phantom discs" referred to before the advent of the CT scan. The symptoms are often identical to those of a herniated disc in the lateral part of the central canal.

SUMMARY

The spine remains a most challenging subject. Every new advance in surgical technique or diagnostic capability opens up new possibilities for treatment. There is reason to believe that we are on the threshold of even greater moves forward.

Recently developed diagnostic techniques have been of immense value to spine surgeons. We have reached such a level of sophistication in our diagnostic capabilities that it is now unacceptable to "explore" the spine without knowing preoperatively what we are going to encounter. There should be few surprises during spine surgery. Our exact technique should be planned in detail ahead of time. Newer techniques of internal fixation of the spine have made it possible to do a more adequate decompression of entrapped neural tissue without jeopardizing stability.

Great advances have been made in the non-operative treatment of spinal disorders as well. Training in various types of exercises both for prevention and treatment of low back pain have improved back care. The back school is being used extensively throughout the world and is valuable in training people in the prevention of back disability.

As physicians charged with the medical and surgical treatment of the spine, we must continue to advance our specialty. Every spine surgeon's office can be a clinical research facility. Most spinal medicine and surgery today is done by groups of orthopedic surgeons and neurosurgeons, either in private practice or associated with university medical schools. These groups are ideally suited for clinical research. However, to do effective clinical research, it is mandatory that a computerized system of patient recall be available. Many of the large hospitals and virtually all the medical schools have research departments where more basic research can be done. If one has a bent for this type of investigation, one should take the opportunity to use these facilities. Setting aside a few hours or a day during the week for research is a welcome respite from our day-to-day practice and can be immensely rewarding.

As physicians, we should be alert to what is being done in other fields. We spend so much of our time reading the literature of our own specialty that we often neglect others and often find ourselves wasting time attempting to "reinvent the wheel."

Consideration should be given to new ideas, originating from even unlikely sources, if they seem to offer new hope. We must keep in mind that William Withering (51) in 1775 got the idea for digitalis from an old Shropshire woman who had a secret remedy for dropsy that consisted of a brew made of foxglove and some other herbs. Laennec (51), one day in 1816, got his idea for the stethoscope while watching children at play in a pile of wooden beams. One child would lay his ear against the end of a long beam and his friend would tap out a message on the other end. As Oliver Wendell Holmes (136) once reminded his fellow physicians:

> [Orthodox medicine] learned from a Jesuit how to cure agues, from a friar how to cut for the stone, from a soldier how to treat gout, from a sailor how to keep off scurvy, from a postmaster how to sound for the Eustachian tube, and from a dairymaid how to prevent smallpox.

Considered from the standpoint of the sheer number of patients affected by back pain, probably the most pressing need at the moment for spine surgeons is to find out why some discs in the early stages of degeneration hurt while others do not. Is there some chemical change in the painful disc that might be amenable to treatment?

And the crowning achievement: Perhaps we can learn to repair (or replace parts of) the spinal cord itself. Impossible? In a day when we can walk on the moon, send photographs back from distant stars, divide the atom into subatomic particles, and mathematically model the first 10^{-35} of a second after the birth of our universe, is it really impossible?

REFERENCES

1. Abdullah A, Ditto EW 3d, Byrd EB, et al. (1974): Extreme-lateral lumbar disc herniations. *J Neurosurg* 41:229–234.
2. Adamkiewicz AA (1881): Ueber die mikroskopischen Gefässe des menschlichen Rückenmarks. Transactions of the seventh session of the International Medical Congress L:155.
3. Adams F (1816): *Paulus Aeginata,* vol. 2. London; Syndenham Society, pp. 155–156, 193, 197.
4. Adams F (1939): *The genuine works of Hippocrates.* Baltimore; Williams & Wilkins, p. 231.
5. Alajouanine TH (1978): From the presidential address by Professor Jean Cauchoix before the annual meeting of the International Society for the Study of the Lumbar Spine, San Francisco, June, 1978.
6. Albee FH (1911): Transplantation of a portion of the tibia into the spine for Pott's disease. *JAMA* 57:885.
7. American Orthopaedic Association Research Committee (1941): End-result study of the treatment of idiopathic scoliosis. *J Bone Joint Surg* 23:963–977.
8. Anderson TP, Cole TM, Gullickman G, Hudgens A, Roberts AH (1977): Behavior modification of chronic pain. *Clin Orthop* 129: 96–100.

9. Andersson GB (1981): Epidemiological aspects on low back pain in industry. *Spine* 6:53–60.
10. Andry N (1743): *Orthopaedia or the art of preventing and correcting deformities in children.* Translated from the French. London.
11. Armstrong G (1989): Personal communication. Meeting of the American Orthopaedic Association, Colorado Springs, June 12–15, 1989.
12. Arnell S, Lidstrom F (1931): Myelography with skiodan (Abrodil). *Acta Radiol* 12:287–288.
13. Ascani C, Monticelli G (1975): Reduction of spondylolisthesis. Paper presented at Sicot Congress, 1975.
14. Babinski J (1896): Sur le reflexe cutané plantaire dans certaines affections organiques du système nerveux central. *Compt Rend Soc Biol* iii:207–208.
15. Badgely CE (1941): The articular facets in relation to low-back pain and sciatic radiation. *J Bone Joint Surg* 23:481–496.
16. Bailey RW, Badgley CE (1960): Stabilization of the cervical spine by anterior fusion. *J Bone Joint Surg [Am]* 42:565–594.
17. Ball JM (1910): *Andreas Vesalius.* St. Louis Medical Science Press.
18. Barr JS (1977): Lumbar disc lesions in retrospect and prospect. *Clin Orthop* 129:48.
19. Beaton LE, Anson BJ (1937): The relation of the sciatic nerve and of its subdivisions to the piriformis muscle. *Anat Rec* 70:1–5.
20. Beliveau P (1971): A comparison between epidural anaesthesia with and without corticosteroid in the treatment of sciatica. *Rheum Phys Med* 11:40–43.
21. Bell C (1839): *A system of operative surgery.* London, pp. 1807–1809.
22. Bell C (1824): *Observations on injuries of the spine and of the thigh bone.* London: Thomas Tegg.
23. Bertolotti (1917): *La Radiologia Medica.*
24. Bishop W (1968): *Familiar medical questions.* In: Strauss B, ed. Boston: Little Brown, p. 215A.
25. Bloch F (1946): Nuclear induction. *Physiol Rev* 70:460.
26. Blount WP (1958): Scoliosis and the Milwaukee brace. *Bull Hosp Joint Dis* 19(2):152–165.
27. Blount WP, Schmidt AC (1957): The Milwaukee brace in the treatment of scoliosis. *J Bone Joint Surg [Am]* 39:693.
28. Bohler J (1982): Anterior stabilization for acute fractures and non-unions of the dens. *J Bone Joint Surg [Am]* 64a:18–27.
29. Bohlman HH (1979): Acute fractures and dislocations of the cervical spine. *J Bone Joint Surg [Am]* 61:1119–1142.
30. Bonica JJ (1957): Management of myofascial pain syndromes in general practice. *JAMA* 164:732–738.
31. Bontecou RB (1887): *Transactions of the New York Medical Association,* vol. III:317.
32. Boucher HH (1959): A method of spinal fusion. *J Bone Joint Surg [Br]* 41b:248–259.
33. Boudof BG (1864): *Des resections des apopeses transverse des vertebraes.* Strausberg.
34. Bracewell R (1980): Quoted by Oldendorf WH, *The quest for an image of the brain.* New York: Raven Press.
35. Bradford DS (1979): Treatment of severe spondylolisthesis. *Spine* 4:423–429.
36. Bradford EH, Bracket EG (1904): Reduction of scoliosis. *Boston Med Surg J* March 17, 1904.
37. Breasted JH (1930): *The Edwin Smith surgical papyrus,* vol. 1. Chicago: University of Chicago, pp. 316–342.
38. Briggs H, Milligan PR (1944): Chip fusion of the low back following exploration of the spinal canal. *J Bone Joint Surg* 26:125–130.
39. Brissaud (1969): Quoted from Reynolds F, Katz S, Herniated lumbar intervertebral disc. *American Academy of Orthopaedic Surgeons symposium on the spine.* St. Louis: CV Mosby.
40. Brodsky AE (1969): Low back pain syndrome due to spinal stenosis and posterior cauda equina compression. Paper presented to the Hospital Joint Diseases Annual Scientific Alumni Meeting, Houston, October, 1969.
41. Brok AJ (1929): *Greek medicine.* London: J.M. Dent & Sons.
42. Brooks AL, Jenkins EB (1978): Atlantoaxial arthrodesis by the wedge compression method. *J Bone Joint Surg [Am]* 60a:279–284.
43. Brown RH, Nash CL Jr, Berilla JA, et al. (1984): Cortical evoked potential monitoring: a system for intraoperative monitoring of spinal cord function. *Spine* 9:256–261.
44. Buchanan F (1908): The electrical response of muscle to voluntary, reflex, and artificial stimulation. *Q J Exp Physiol* 1:211–242.
45. Buck JE (1970): Direct repair of the defect in spondylolisthesis. *J Bone Joint Surg [Br]* 52b:432–437.
46. Burns BH (1933): An operation for spondylolisthesis. *Lancet* 1:1233.
47. Calot JF: Des moyens de gueuir la bosse du mal de Pott. *France Med* 52.
48. Calot JF (1923): *L'ortopedie indispensible aux practiciens.* Paris: Meloine.
49. Campbell WC (1927): An operation for extra-articular fusion of sacroiliac joint. *Surg Gynecol Obstet* 45:218–219.
50. Cauchoix J (1978): Presidential address presented to the International Society for the Study of the Lumbar Spine, San Francisco, June, 1978.
51. Clendening L (1942): *Source book of medical history.* New York: Dover.
52. Cleveland M, et al. (1948): Pseudarthrosis in lumbosacral spine. *J Bone Joint Surg [Am]* 30a:302–312.
53. Cloward RB (1952): The treatment of ruptured intervertebral disc by vertebral body fusion. *Ann Surg* 136:987–992.
54. Cloward RB (1958): The anterior approach for removal of ruptured cervical disks. *J Neurosurg* 15:602–617.
55. Cloward RB (1982): *History of posterior lumbar interbody fusion.* Springfield: Charles C Thomas.
56. Cobb JR (1948): *Outline for the study of scoliosis,* vol. V. J.W. Edwards.
57. Compte A (1958): Positive philosophy. In: Strauss MB, ed. *Familiar medical quotations.* Boston: Little Brown, p. 213B.
58. Cooper A (1824): *A treatise on fractures and dislocations.* London, pp. 499–518.
59. Cooper A (1839): *Lecture on the principles and practice of surgery.* London: H. Renshaw, VIII:1824–1827.
60. Cormack (1980): Quoted by Oldendorf WH, *The quest for an image of the brain.* New York: Raven Press.
61. Cortugno D (1764): *De Ischiade Nervosa Canmentarius.* L. Naples, Simonocos Brothers.
62. Cotrel Y, Dubousset J (1984): Nouvelle technique d'osteosynthese rachidienne segmentioire par vole posterieure. *Rev Chir Orthop* 70:489–494.
63. Cotrel Y, Dubousset J (1985): The use of pedicle screws and universal instrumentation for spinal fixation. Paper presented to the AO Trauma Course, Davos, Switzerland, December, 1985.
64. Coventry MB (1968): Symposium: low back and sciatic pain. *J Bone Joint Surg [Am]* 50a:167–169.
65. Cramer F (1934): A note concerning the syndrome of cauda equina radiculitis. *Bull Neurol Inst NY* 3:501–505, 1934.
66. Crock HV (1976): Isolated lumbar disc resorption as a cause of nerve root canal stenosis. *Clin Orthop* 115:109–115.
67. Crock HV, Yashizawa H, Kame SK (1973): Observations on the venous drainage of the human vertebral body. *J Bone Joint Surg [Br]* 55:528–533.
68. Crowe HE (1928): Injuries to the cervical spine. Paper presented at the meeting of the Western Orthopaedic Association, San Francisco, 1928.
69. Crutchfield WG (1933): Skeletal traction for dislocation of cervical spine. *South Surgeon* 2:156–159.
70. Damadian R (1971): Tumor detection by nuclear magnetic resonance. *Science* 171:1151–1153.
71. Dandy WE (1918): Ventriculography following the injection of air into the cerebral ventricles. *Ann Surg* 68:5–11.
72. Dandy WE (1929): Loose cartilage from the intervertebral disc simulating tumor of the spinal cord. *Arch Surg* 19:660–672.
73. Danforth MS, Wilson PD (1925): The anatomy of the lumbosacral region in relation to sciatic pain. *J Bone Joint Surg* 7:109–160.
74. Davy SH (1799): *Researches, chemical and philosophical chiefly concerning nitrous oxide.* London: printed for J. Johnson, St. Paul's Churchyard, Briggs and Cottle, Bristol, XVI, 580 pp.
75. Denny-Brown D, Pennybacker JB (1938): Fibrillation and fasciculation in voluntary muscle. *Brain* 61:311–334.

76. DePalma AF, Rothman RH (1968): The nature of pseud-arthrosis. *Clin Orthop* 59:113–118.

77. Dewald RL, Ray RD (1970): Skeletal traction for the treatment of severe scoliosis. *J Bone Joint Surg [Am]* 52:233–238.

78. Dommisse GF (1975): *The arteries and veins of the human spinal cord from birth.* New York; Churchill Livingstone.

79. Dommisse GF (1972): The blood supply of the spinal cord at birth. Master's thesis, University of Cape Town, Cape Town, South Africa.

80. Drummond DS, Fowler JV, Ecoyer S, et al. (1976): Untreated scoliosis in the adult. *J Bone Joint Surg [Am]* 58a:136.

81. Dwyer AF, Newton NC, Sherwood AA (1969): An anterior approach to scoliosis. A preliminary report. *Clin Orthop* 62:192–202.

82. Dyck W (1985): Fixator interne. Paper presented to the AO Trauma Course, Davos, Switzerland, December, 1985.

83. Edwards WC (1985): The sacral fixation device: a new alternative for lumbosacral fixation. Paper presented at the meeting of the North American Spine Society, Laguna Niquel, California, July, 1985.

84. Ehni G (1969): Significance of the small lumbar spinal canal: cauda equina compression syndromes due to spondylosis. 1. Introduction. *J Neurosurg* 31:490–494.

85. Elsberg CA (1913): Experiences in spinal surgery. *Surg Gynecol Obstet* 16:117–132.

86. Elsberg CA (1928): Extradural spinal tumors. Primary, secondary, metastatic. *Surg Gynecol Obstet* 46:1–20.

87. Elsberg CA (1913): Tumors of the spinal cord and the systems of irritation and compression of the spinal cord and nerve roots. *Bull Neurol Inst NY* 1:350.

88. Evans W (1930): Intrasacral epidural injection in the treatment of sciatica. *Lancet* 2:1225–1229.

89. Farfan HF (1969): The effects of torsion on the intervertebral joints. *Can J Surg* 12:336–341.

90. Fleming A (1929): Experimental pathology.

91. Fordyce WE, Fowler RS, DeLateur B (1968): Application of behavior modification technique to a problem of chronic pain. *Behav Res Ther* 6:105–107.

92. Fordyce WE, Fowler RS, Jr, Lehmann JF, et al. (1968): Some implications of learning in problems of chronic pain. *J Chron Dis* 21:179–190.

93. Fordyce WE, Fowler RS Jr, Lehmann JF, et al. (1973): Operant conditioning in the treatment of chronic pain. *Arch Phys Med Rehab* 54:399–408.

94. Forssell MZ (1980): The Swedish Back School. *Physiotherapy* 66:112–114.

95. Forst JJ (1880): Contribution a l'étude clinique de la sciatique. Paris; doctoral thesis.

96. Fraser RD (1984): Chymopapain for the treatment of intervertebral disc herniation. The final report of a double-blind study. *Spine* 9:815–818.

97. Freebody D, Bendall R, Taylor RD (1971): Anterior transperitoneal lumbar fusion. *J Bone Joint Surg [Br]* 53b:617–627.

98. Frymoyer JW, Donagy RM (1985): The ruptured intervertebral disc. *J Bone Joint Surg [Am]* 67a:1113–1116.

99. Frymoyer JW, Hanley E, Howe J, Kuhlmann D, Matteri R (1978): Disc excision and spine fusion in the management of lumbar disc disease: a minimum ten year follow-up. *Spine* 3:1–6.

100. Gallie WE (1937): Skeletal traction in treatment of fractures and dislocations of the cervical spine. *Ann Surg* 106:770–776.

101. Garrett AL, Perry J, Nickel VL (1961): Stabilization of the collapsing spine. *J Bone Joint Surg [Am]* 43a:474–484.

102. Garrison F (1929): *Introduction to the history of medicine,* 4th ed. Philadelphia: W.B. Saunders.

103. Gerster (1900): Cited by Sachs B, Frankel J, Progressive ankylotic rigidity of the spine. *J Nerv Ment Dis* 27:1.

104. Ghormley RK (1933): Low back pain, with special reference to the articular facets with presentation of an operative procedure. *JAMA* 101:1773–1777.

105. Gibbons RW (1976): Chiropractic history. *ACAJ Chiropractic* (January).

106. Goldner JL, et al. (1969): Anterior disc excision and interbody spine fusion for chronic low back pain. American Academy of Orthopaedic Surgeons symposium on the spine. St. Louis: CV Mosby.

107. Goldstein LA (1966): Surgical management of scoliosis. *J Bone Joint Surg [Am]* 48a:167–196.

108. Goldstein LA (1969): Treatment of idiopathic scoliosis by Harrington instrumentation and fusion with fresh autogenous iliac bone grafts. *J Bone Joint Surg [Am]* 51a:209–222.

109. Goldthwait JE (1911): The lumbosacral articulation. *Boston Med Surg J* 164:365–372.

110. Gould GM (1903): Oliver Wendell Holmes. Medical discoveries by the non-medical. *JAMA* 40:1477–1487.

111. Graham CE (1975): Chemonucleolysis. A preliminary report on a double blind study comparing chemonucleolysis and intradiscal administration of hydrocortisone in the treatment of backache and sciatica. *Orthop Clin North Am* 6:259–263.

112. Gregory JC (1930): *The scientific achievements of Sir Humphrey Davy.*

113. Grundy BL, Nash CL Jr, Brown RH (1981): Arterial pressure manipulation alters spinal cord function during correction of scoliosis. *Anesthesiology* 54:249–253.

114. Guerin J (1839): Memoire sur les deviations simulees de l'epine et les moyens. *Gaz Med Paris* 7:241–247.

115. Hadra BE (1891): Wiring the spinous processes in Pott's disease. *Trans Am Orthop Assoc* 4:206–210.

116. Hahnemann University Medical School, Philadelphia, founded 1848.

117. Harmon PH (1960): Anterior etoneal lumbar disk excision and vertebral body fusion. *Clin Orthop* 18:169–184.

118. Harrington PR (1962): Treatment of scoliosis: correction and internal fixation by spine instrumentation. *J Bone Joint Surg [Am]* 44a:591–610.

119. Harrington PR (1972): Technical details in relation to the successful use of instrumentation in scoliosis. *Orthop Clin North Am* 3(1):49–67.

120. Harrington PR, Dickson JH (1976): Spinal instrumentation in the treatment of severe progressive spondylolisthesis. *Clin Orthop* 117:157–163.

121. Harrington PR, Tullos HS (1971): Spondylolisthesis in children. *Clin Orthop* 79:75–84.

122. Hart M (1978): *The 100 most influential persons of history.* New York: Hart Publishing Company, p. 95.

123. Hattori S (1973): A new method of cervical laminectomy. *Central Jap J Orthop Traum Surg* 16(3):792–794.

124. Hattori S (1980): Pathogenesis and surgical treatment of cervical spondylotic myelopathy. Special lecture presented at the meeting of the Japanese Orthopaedic Association, Tokyo, April, 1980.

125. Herbert JJ (1954): Reflexions sur la technique et les resultats de 42 osteotomies vertebrales. *Rev Chir Orthop* 73:357.

126. Hertzler AE (1938): *The horse and buggy doctor.* New York: Harper Brothers.

127. Hibbs RA (1911): An operation for progressive spinal deformities. *NY Med J* 93:1013.

128. Hildanus F (1672): Opera. In: Walker AE, ed. *A history of neurological surgery.* New York: Hatner Publishing Company, p. 366.

129. Hirabayashi K, Watanabe K, Wakano K, et al. (1983): Expansive open-door laminoplasty for cervical spinal stenotic myelopathy. *Spine* 8:693–699.

130. Hirsch C (1960): Cervical disk rupture, diagnosis and therapy. *Acta Orthop Scand* 30:172–186.

131. Hirsch C (1948–1949): An attempt to diagnose the level of disc lesion by disc puncture. *Acta Orthop Scand* 18:132.

132. Hirsch C, Schajowicz F (1953): Studies on structural changes in the lumbar annulus fibrosus. *Acta Orthop Scand* 22:184–231.

133. Hodes R, Larrabee MG, German WJ (1948): The human electromyogram in response to nerve stimulation and the conduction velocity of motor axons. *Arch Neurol Psychiatr* 60:340–365.

134. Hodgson AR, Stock FE (1960): Anterior spine fusion for treatment of tuberculosis of the spine. *J Bone Joint Surg [Am]* 42a:295–310.

135. Hoffa (1904): Reduction of scoliosis. *Boston Med Surg J* (March 17).

136. Holmes OW (1843): The contagiousness of puerperal fever. Reprinted in *Biol Med Libr Assn* 1943:31:319.

137. Houndsfield G (1980): Quoted by Oldendorf WH: *The quest for an image of the brain*. New York: Raven Press.

138. Hult L (1954): The Munkfors investigation. *Acta Orthop Scand* (suppl 16).

139. Humphries AW, Hawk WA, Berndt AL (1959): Anterior fusion of the lumbar spine using an internal fixation device. *J Bone Joint Surg [Am]* 41a:371.

140. Ito H, et al. (1934): A new radical operation for Pott's disease. *J Bone Joint Surg* 16:499–515.

141. Jaccoud S (1864): *Les paraplegics et l'atorie du mouvement*. Paris: Adriene Delahoye.

142. Jackson (1989): Comparison of clinical results of epidural injection with and without corticosteroid. Paper read at the meeting of North American Spine Society, Quebec, Canada, June, 1989.

143. Jaslow IA (1946): Intercorporal bone graft in spinal fusion after disc removal. *Surg Gynecol Obstet* 82:215–218.

144. Jenkins JA (1936): Spondylolisthesis. *Br J Surg* 24:80–85.

145. Kamiya J (1971): *Biofeedback and self control*. Chicago: Alume-Atherton.

146. Kane WJ, Moe JH, Lau CC (1967): Halo-femoral pin distraction in treatment of scoliosis. *J Bone Joint Surg [Am]* 49a:1018.

147. Kaneda K (1985): Personal communication (October).

148. Kaneda K, Abumi K, Fujiya M (1984): Burst fractures with neurologic deficits of the thoracolumbar-lumbar spine. *Spine* 9:788–795.

149. Kennedy F, Elsberg CA, Lambert CI (1914): A peculiar and undescribed disease of the nerves of the cauda equina. *Am J Med Sci* 147:645–667.

150. Keyes DC, Compere EL (1932): Normal and pathological physiology of the nucleus pulposus and intervertebral disc. *J Bone Joint Surg* 14:897–938.

151. King D (1948): Internal fixation for lumbosacral fusion. *J Bone Joint Surg [Am]* 30:560–565.

152. Kirkaldy-Willis WH (1983): Dysfunction: the sacroiliac syndrome. In: *Managing low back pain*, 2nd ed. New York: Churchill Livingstone.

153. Kirkaldy-Willis WH, McIvor GW (1976): Editorial: lumbar spinal stenosis. *Clin Orthop* 115:2–3.

154. Kirkaldy-Willis WH, Paine KW, Cauchoix J, et al. (1974): Lumbar spinal stenosis. *Clin Orthop* 99:30–50.

155. Knodt H, Larrick RB (1964): Distraction fusion of the lumbar spine. *Ohio State Med J* 12:1140–1142.

156. Koch R (1912): *Die actiologe Dr. Mitzbrand-Krankheit Klassker der Medizen*. Leipzig: J Barth.

157. Kocher T (1896): Die Verletzungen der Wirbelsaule zugleich als Beitrag zur Physiologie des menschlichen Rückenmarks. *Mitt Grenzgeb Med Chir* 1:415–480.

158. Kostuik JP, Errico TJ, Gleason TF (1986): Techniques of internal fixation for degenerative conditions of the lumbar spine. *Clin Orthop* 203:219–231.

159. Krag MH, Beynnon, BD, Pope MH (1986): An internal fixator for posterior application to short segments of the thoracic, lumbar or lumbosacral spine: design and testing. *Clin Orthop* 203:75–98.

160. Lane WA (1893): Case of spondylolisthesis associated with progressive paraplegia; laminectomy. *Lancet* 1:991.

161. Lange F (1910): Support for the spondylitic spine by means of buried steel bars, attached to the vertebrae. *Am J Orthop Surg* 8:344–361.

162. La Rocca H, Macnab I (1969): The value of pre-employment radiographic assessment of the lumbar spine. *Can Med Assoc J* 101(7):49–54.

163. Lasegue C (1864): Considerations sur la sciatique. *Arch Gen Med* 4(56):558–580.

164. Levacher AFT (1768): Nouveau moyen de prevenir et de guerir la courbure de l'epine. *Mem Acad R Chir* 4:596.

165. Lindblom K (1948): Diagnostic puncture of intervertebral discs in sciatica. *Acta Orthop Scand* 17(suppl 4):231–239.

166. Lindsley DB (1935): Myographic and electromyographic studies in myasthenia gravis. *Brain* 58:470–482.

167. Lister J (1867): On the antiseptic principle in the practice of surgery. *Br Med J* 2:246.

168. Long CW (1942): An account of the first use of sulphuric ether in inhalation as a anesthetic in surgical operations. In: Clendening

L, ed. *Source book of medical history*. New York: Dover, pp. 356–358.

169. Louis R (1986): Fusion of the lumbar and sacral spine by internal fixation with screw plates. *Clin Orthop* 203:18–33.

170. Love JG (1939): Removal of intervertebral discs without laminectomy. Proceedings of staff meeting. *Mayo Clin* 14:800.

171. Luque ER (1982): The anatomic basis and development of segmental spinal instrumentation. *Spine* 7:256–259.

172. Luque ER (1986): Interpeduncular segmental fixation. *Clin Orthop* 203:54–57.

173. Ma G, Paulson D (1982): Interbody fusion of the lumbar spine with the use of box chisels. Paper presented at the meeting of the Western Orthopaedic Association, October, 1982.

174. Macnab I, Dall D (1971): The blood supply of the lumbar spine and its application to the technique of intertransverse lumbar fusion. *J Bone Joint Surg [Br]* 53b:628–638.

175. Magerl F (1982): *External skeletal fixation of the lower thoracic and upper lumbar spine: current concepts of external fixation of fractures*. Berlin: Springer-Verlag.

176. Magnuson PB (1944): Differential diagnosis of causes of back pain accompanied by sciatica. *Ann Surg* 119:878–891.

177. Mair WGP, Druckman R (1953): The pathology of spinal cord lesions and their relation to the clinical features in protrusion of cervical intervertebral discs. *Brain* 76:70–91.

178. Malgaigne: *Traite des fractures et des luxations*, vol 1, pp. 410–426, vol. 2, pp. 318–391. Paris.

179. Mason C, Cozen L, Adelstein L (1953): Surgical correction of flexion deformity of the cervical spine. *Calif Med* 79:244–246.

180. Mathieu P, Demirleau J (1936): Surgical therapy of painful spondylolisthesis. *Rev Chir Orthop* 23:352–363.

181. Matthiass HH, Heine J (1986): The surgical reduction of spondylolisthesis. *Clin Orthop* 203:34–44.

182. McCulloch J (1985): Microdiscectomy. Paper presented at Surgery of the Spine Symposium, Melbourne, Australia, April, 1985.

183. McKenzie RA (1972): Manual correction of sciatic scoliosis. *NZ Med J* 76:194–199.

184. McKenzie RA (1979): Prophylaxis in recurrent low back pain. *NZ Med J* 89:22–23.

185. McKenzie RA (1981): *The lumbar spine: mechanical diagnosis and therapy*. Waikanae, New Zealand: Spinal Publications.

186. McPhee IB, O'Brien JP (1979): Reduction of severe spondylolisthesis. *Spine* 4(5):430–434.

187. Mercer W (1936): Spondylolisthesis. *Edinb Med J* 43:545–572.

188. Middleton GS, Teacher JH (1911): Extruded disc at the T12-L1 level: microscopic exam showed it to be nucleus pulposus. *Glasgow Med J* I(A):vlxxvi.

189. Middleton GS, Teacher JH (1911): Injury of the spinal cord due to rupture of an intervertebral disc during muscular effort. *Glasgow Med J* 76:1–6.

190. Miller NE, Banuazizi A (1968): Instrumental learning by cauterized rats of a specific visceral response, intestinal or cardiac. *J Comp Physiol Psychol* 65:1–7.

191. Misenhimer G, Peek R, Wiltse LL, et al. (1988): Anatomic analysis of pedicle cortical and cancellous diameter as related to screw size. Paper read at the meeting of the North American Spine Society, Colorado Springs, Colorado, July 27, 1988.

192. Mixter WJ (1949): Rupture of the intervertebral disk: a short history of its evolution as a syndrome of importance to the surgeon. *JAMA* 140:278–282.

193. Mixter SJ, Osgood RB (1910): Traumatic lesions of the atlas and axis. *Ann Surg* 51:193–207.

194. Mixter WJ, Barr JS (1934): Rupture of the intervertebral disc with involvement of the spinal canal. *N Engl J Med* 211:210–215.

195. Moe JH (1967): Methods and techniques of evaluating idiopathic scoliosis. American Academy of Orthopaedic Surgeons symposium on the spine November 1967. St Louis: CV Mosby, pp. 196–240.

196. Moe JH (1972): Methods of correction and surgical techniques in scoliosis. *Orthop Clin North Am* 3(1):17–48.

197. Moe JH, Winter RD, Bradford DS, et al. (1978): In: *Scoliosis and other deformities*. Philadelphia: W.B. Saunders, pp. 1–12.

198. Mooney V, Robertson J (1976): The facet syndrome. *Clin Orthop* 115:149–156.

199. Moore GE, Hinshaw WS (1980): Quoted by Oldendorf WH. In: *The quest for an image of the brain.* New York: Raven Press.
200. Morscher E, Gerber B, Fasel J (1984): Surgical treatment of spondylolisthesis by bone grafting and direct stabilization of spondylolysis by means of a hook screw. *Arch Orthop Trauma Surg* 103:175–178.
201. Morton WTG (1848): A memoir to the Academy of Sciences at Paris on a new use of sulphuric ether. *Littel's Living Age* 16(March 18):529–571.
202. Nachemson A (1960): Lumbar intradiscal pressure. *Acta Orthop Scand* 43(suppl):1–104.
203. Nachemson A (1965): The effect of forward leaning on lumbar intradiscal pressure. *Acta Orthop Scand* 35:314–328.
204. Nash CL Jr, Lorig RA, Schatzinger LA, Brown RH (1977): Spinal cord monitoring during operative treatment of the spine. *Clin Orthop* 126:100–105.
205. Naylor A (1962): The biophysical and biochemical aspects of intervertebral disc herniation and degeneration. *Ann R Coll Surg Engl* 31:91–114.
206. Newman PH (1965): A clinical syndrome associated with severe lumbosacral subluxation. *J Bone Joint Surg [Br]* 47b:472–481.
207. Nickel VL, Perry J, Garrett A, et al. (1968): The halo. A spinal skeletal traction fixation device. *J Bone Joint Surg [Am]* 50a:1400–1409.
208. Nordby EJ, Lucas GL (1973): A comparative analysis of lumbar disk disease treated by laminectomy or chemonucleolysis. *Clin Orthop* 90:119–129.
209. O'Brien JP (1975): The halo-pelvic apparatus. *Acta Orthop Scand* 163(suppl):1–188.
210. Ohry A, Ohry-Kossoy K (1989): Spinal cord injuries in the 19th century. *Paraplegia* 27(suppl 5):1–39.
211. Oldendorf WH (1961): Displaying the internal structural pattern of a complex object. *Trans Bio-Med Elect (BME)* 8:68.
212. Oppenheim H, Krause F (1909): Ueber Einklemmung bzw. Strangulation der cauda equina. *Dtsche Med Wchnschr* 35:697–700.
213. Oribasius (1862): *Oeuvres d'oribase,* vol. 4. Paris: Darenberg Edition, pp. 242–243, 394–395, 449–451.
214. Pare A (1958): *Oeuvres.* Paris, pp. 528, 551, 559.
215. Paris JA (1831): *The life of Sir Humphrey Davy.*
216. Parker, Adson (1969): Quoted in Reynolds F, Katz S, *Herniated lumbar intervertebral disc.* American Academy of Orthopaedic Surgeons symposium on the spine. St. Louis: CV Mosby.
217. Pasteur L (1863): Recherche sur la petrefaction comtes pednus domadaires. In: Vallery-Radot P, ed. *Oeuvres de Pasteur* (1922), 2 vols.
218. Peltier LF (1983): The "back school" of Delpech in Montpellier. *Clin Orthop* 179:4–9.
219. Pilcher LS (1910): Atlo-axoid fracture dislocation. *Ann Surg* 51:208–211.
220. Perkin WH (1885): Jean Baptiste Andre Dumas. *J Chem Soc (Lond).*
221. Piper H (1912): *Elektrophysiologie menschlicher Muskeln.* Berlin.
222. Portal A (1803): *Cours d'anatomie medicale ou elements de l'anatomie de l'homme,* vol. 1. Paris: Baudouin.
223. Pott P (1768): *Observations on the nature and consequences of those injuries to which the head is liable from external violence.* In: Hawes L, Carke W, Collins R, eds. London.
224. Pott P (1942): In: Clendening L, ed. *Source book of medical history,* New York: Dover, pp. 485–487.
225. Pott P (1779): *Remarks on that kind of palsy frequently found to accompany curvature of the spine.* London. Also in *Medical Classics* VI(4) December, 1936.
226. Proebster R (1928): Uber Muskulaskelationsstrome an gesunden und kranken Menschen. *Zeitschr Orthop Chir* 50:1.
227. Purcell EM, et al. (1946): Resonance absorption by nuclear magnetic moments in a solid. *Physiol Rev* 49:37–38.
228. Putti V (1927): New conceptions in pathogenesis of sciatic pain. *Lancet* 2:53–60.
229. Radon (1980): Quoted by Oldendorf WH, *The quest for an image of the brain.* New York: Raven Press.
230. Raney FL, Jr, Adams JE (1963): Anterior lumbar-disc excision and interbody fusion used as a salvage procedure. *J Bone Joint Surg [Am]* 45a:667–668.
231. Rees WS (1974): Multiple bilateral subcutaneous rhizolysis of segmental nerves in the treatment of intervertebral disc syndrome. *Ann Gen Pract* 26:126.
232. Reid A, Smith FW, Hutchison JM (1982): Nuclear magnetic resonance imaging and its safety implications: follow–up of 181 patients. *Br J Radiol* 55:784–786.
233. Richards DW (1968): Hippocrates of Ostia. *JAMA* 204:1049–1056.
234. Risser JC (1955): The application of body casts for the correction of scoliosis. American Academy of Orthopaedic Surgeons. Instructional Course Lectures 12:255–259.
235. Robinson RA, Smith GW (1955): Anterolateral cervical disc removal and interbody fusion for cervical disc syndrome. *Bull Johns Hopkins Hosp* 96:223.
236. Robinson RA, Southwick WO (1960): Indications and techiques for early stabilization of the neck in some fracture dislocations of the cervical spine. *South Med J* 53:565–579.
237. Roentgen C (1970): In: Talbott J, ed. *A biographical history of medicine.* Orlando: Grune & Stratton.
228. Rogers WA (1942): Treatment of fracture-dislocation of the cervical spine. *J Bone Joint Surg* 24:245–258.
239. Roofe PG (1960): Innervation of the annulus fibrosis and posterior longitudinal ligament. *Arch Neurol Psychol* 46(suppl):1.
240. Rothman RH, Booth R (1975): Failures of spinal fusion. *Orthop Clin North Am* 6:299–304.
241. Roy-Camille R, Roy-Camille M, Demeulenaere C (1970): Osteosynthesis of dorsal, lumbar, and lumbosacral spine with metallic plates screwed into vertebral pedicles and articular apophyses. *Presse Med* 78:1447–1448.
242. Roy-Camille R, Saillant G, Mazel C (1986): Internal fixation of the lumbar spine with pedicle screw plating. *Clin Orthop* 203:7–17.
243. Royle ND (1928): The operative removal of an accessory vertebra. *Med J Aust* 1:467.
244. Ruhrah J (1932): Nicholas Andry: 1658–1742. *Am J Dis Child* 44:1322–1326.
245. Rutherford (1980): Quoted by Oldendorf WH, *The quest for an image of the brain.* New York: Raven Press.
246. Sachs B, Frankel J (1900): Progressive ankylotic rigidity of the spine. *J Nerv Ment Dis* 27:1.
247. Saillant G (1976): Etude anatomique der pedicles vertebraux application chiruguale. *Rev Chir Orthop* 62:151–160.
248. Sarpyener MA (1945): Congenital stricture of the spinal canal. *J Bone Joint Surg* 27:70–79.
249. Sayre L (1876): *Lectures on orthopaedic surgery and diseases of the joints.* New York.
250. Schimmelbusch C (1894): *The aseptic treatment of wounds,* translated by T. Rake. London: H.K. Lewis.
251. Schmorl G (1926): Die Pathalogi der Wirbelsäule. *Dtsch Orthop Ges* 21:3.
252. Schmorl G, Junghanns H (1971): *Human spine in health and disease.* New York: Grune & Stratton, p. 22.
253. Schneider RC, Cherry GR, Pautek H (1954): The syndrome of acute central cervical spinal cord injury. *J Neurosurg* 11:546–577.
254. Scott J (1970): Fixation of spondylolysis with circumferential wire around the transverse processes and spinous processes. Paper presented to the combined meeting of the English speaking orthopaedists of the world, Edinburgh.
255. Selby D (1985): A modification of the Crock interbody fusion instruments for use in P.L.I.F. Personal communication.
256. Semmelweis, IP (1941): The etiology, the concept and the prophylaxis of childbed fever, translated by FP Murphy. In: *Medical Classics* 5:350.
257. Shakespeare W: *Timon of Athens,* Act 4, Scene 1, line 23.
258. Shealy CN (1976): Facet denervation in the management of back and sciatic pain. *Clin Orthop* 115:157–164.
259. Shordania JF (1936): Die chronische entzundung des musculus piriformis. *Med Welt* 10:999–1001.
260. Sicard JA, Forestier J (1921): Methode radiographique d'exploration de la cavité epidurale par le lipiodol. *Rev Neurol* 37:1264.

261. Simmons EH (1972): The surgical correction of flexion deformity of the cervical spine in ankylosing spondylitis. *Clin Orthop* 86: 132–143.

262. Skinner BF (1959): *Cumulative record.* New York: Appleton-Century Crofts, p. 430.

263. Smith AG (1829): Account of a case in which portions of three dorsal vertebrae were removed for the relief of paralysis from fracture, with partial success. *North Am Med Surg J.*

264. Smith FW (1983): NMR historical aspects. *Mod Neuroradiol* 2:7.

265. Smith-Petersen MN, Larson CB, Aufranc OE (1945): Osteotomy of the spine for correction of flexion deformity in rheumatoid arthritis. *J Bone Joint Surg* 27:1–11.

266. Sottac (1976): Intermittent claudication of the spinal cord. Reported by Verbiest H, *Neurogenic intermittent claudication.* Amsterdam: North Holland Publishing Co.

267. Spengler DM, Freeman CW (1979): Patient selection for lumbar discectomy. *Spine* 4:129–134.

268. Steffee AD, Biscup RS, Sitkowski DJ (1986): Segmental spine plates with pedicle screw fixation. *Clin Orthop* 203:45–53.

269. Steindler A, Luck V (1938): Differential diagnosis of pain in the low back. *JAMA* 110:106–113.

270. Still A, Northup GW (1966): *Osteopathic medicine: an American reformation.* Chicago: American Osteopathic Association, pp. 9–24.

271. Stookey B (1928): Compression of the spinal cord due to ventral extradural cervical chondromas. *Arch Neurol Psychiatr* 20:275–291.

272. Strain WH, Plati JT, Stafford LW (1942): Iodinated organic compounds as contrast media for radiographic diagnoses, iodinated aracyl esters. *J Am Chem Soc* 64:1436–1440.

273. Stryker H (1945): Personal communication, San Diego.

274. Sumita M (1910): Beitrage zur lehre von derchondrodystrophia foetalis (Kaufmann) und osteogenesis imperfecta (Vrolik) mit besonderer berucksichtingung der anatomischen und klinischen differential diagnose. *Dtsch Z Chir* 107:1–110.

275. Sussman BJ (1968): Intervertebral discalysis with collagenase. *J Nat Med Assoc* 60:184.

276. Tamaki T (1977): Clinical application of spinal cord action potentials. In Nash CL Jr, Brodkey JS, eds. *Proceedings of the workshop on clinical application of spinal cord monitoring for operative treatment of spinal diseases.* Cleveland: Case Western Reserve School of Medicine, pp 21–26.

277. Tarvin G, Prata RG (1980): Lumbosacral stenosis in dogs. *J Am Vet Med Assoc* 177(2):154–159.

278. Talbott VH (1970): *A biographical history of medicine.* New York: Grune & Stratton, pp. 67–69.

279. Tsuji H (1982): Laminoplasty for patients with compressive myelopathy due to so-called spinal canal stenosis in cervical and thoracic regions. *Spine* 7(1):28–34.

280. Taylor AR (1951): The mechanism of injury to the spinal cord in neck without damage to the vertebral column. *J Bone Joint Surg* [Br] 33b:543–547.

281. Taylor AR (1929): Fracture dislocation of the cervical spine. *Ann Surg* 90:321–340.

282. Taylor AR, Blackwood W (1948): Paraplegia in hyperextension cervical injuries with normal radiographic appearances. *J Bone Joint Surg* [Br] 30b:245–248.

283. Tew JM Jr, Mayfield FH (1972): The anterior interbody approach in the treatment of herniated cervical disc, spondylolysis, and fracture dislocation. Presented at the 22nd annual meeting of the Congress of Neurological Surgeons, Denver, Colorado, October 19, 1972.

284. Tew JM Jr, Mayfield FH (1975): Proceedings: anterior cervical discectomy a microsurgical approach. *J Neurol Neurosurg Psychiatry* 38(4):413.

285. Thomas L (1956): Reversible collapse of rabbit ears after intravenous papain, and prevention of recovery by cortisone. *J Exp Med* 104:245–252.

286. Thurwold J (1957): *The century of the surgeon.* New York: Pantheon Books, pp. 280–289, 418, 296–301.

287. Towne EB, Reichert FL (1931): Compression of the lumbosacral roots of the spinal cord by thickened ligamenta flava. *Ann Surg* 94:327–336.

288. Tsukimoto H (1960): An autopsied case of ossification within the spinal canal in the cervical region with myelopathy. *J Jap Orthop Assoc* 34:107.

289. Urist MR (1958): Osteotomy of the cervical spine. *J Bone Joint Surg* [Am] 40a:833–843.

290. Valleix (1969): Quoted in Reynolds F, Katz S, *Herniated lumbar intervertebral disc.* American Academy of Orthopaedic Surgeons symposium on the spine. St. Louis: CV Mosby.

291. Venable CS, Stuck WG (1939): Electrolysis controlling factor in the use of metals in treating fractures. *JAMA* 3(1):349.

292. Verbiest H (1949): *Sur certaines formes rares de compression de la queue de cheval: hommage a Clovis Vincent.* Paris: Malouie.

293. Verbiest H (1976): *Neurogenic intermittent claudication.* Amsterdam: North Holland Publishing Co.

294. Volkmann R (1889): Resektion von rippendtucker Scoliose. *Berl Klin Wehnschr* 50.

295. Von Bechterew W (1893): Steifigkeit der Wirbelsaule und ihre Verkrummung als besondere Erkrankungsform. *Neural Zentralb* 12:426–434.

296. Von Luschka H (1858): *Die Hagelenke des menschlichen Korpers.* IV. Berlin: G. Reimer.

297. Warren J (1957): *Century of the surgeon.* New York: Pantheon Books.

298. Watkins MB (1953): Posterolateral fusion of the lumbar and lumbosacral spine. *J Bone Joint Surg* [Am] 35a:1014–1018.

299. Wells CJ (1935): Horace Wells. *Anesthesia Analgesia* 14:176.

300. Wells HG (1920): *The outline of history,* chapter 40.

301. Wertheim-Salomonson JK (1895): Bijdrage tot de Diagnostick der kleinbersen Aandoeningen. *Neder Tidj Geneesk* 31:978.

302. Wheeler CE (1919): An introduction to the principles of homeopathy.

303. Wilkins WF (1888): Separation of the vertebrae with protrusion of hernia between the same-operation-cure. *St Louis Med Surg J* 54:340–341.

304. Williams PC (1937): Lesion of the lumbosacral spine, part II. *J Bone Joint Surg* 19:690–703.

305. Williams PC, Yglesias L (1933): Lumbosacral facetectomy for post-fusion persistent sciatica. *J Bone Joint Surg* 15:579–590.

306. Williams RW (1979): Microsurgical lumbar discectomy. Report to American Association of Neurology and Surgery, 1975. *Neurosurgery* 4(2):140.

307. Wilson PD, Danforth MS (1925): The anatomy of the lumbosacral region in relation to sciatic pain. *J Bone Joint Surg* 7:109–160.

308. Wilson PD, Straub LR (1952): The use of a metal plate fastened to the spinous processes. American Academy of Orthopaedic Surgeons Instructional Course Lecture, Ann Arbor, Michigan.

309. Wiltberger BR (1957): The dowel intervertebral-body fusion as used in lumbar disc surgery. *J Bone Joint Surg* [Am] 39a:284–292.

310. Wiltse LL, Bateman JG, Hutchinson RA (1968): The paraspinal sacrospinalis-splitting approach to the lumbar spine. *J Bone Joint Surg* [Am] 50a:919–926.

311. Wiltse LL, Guyer RD, Spencer CW, Glenn WV, Porter IS (1984): Alar transverse process impingement of the L5 spinal nerve: the far-out syndrome. *Spine* 9:31–41.

312. Wiltse LL, Rocchio PD (1975): Pre-operative psychological tests as predictors of success of chemonucleolysis in the treatment of the low-back syndrome. *J Bone Joint Surg* [Am] 57a:478–483.

313. Wiltsee, Lamont (1990): Personal communication, Pebble Beach, California.

314. Wright D (1985): Quoted in Fielding JW, Cervical spine surgery. *Clin Orthop* 200:287.

315. Young H, Love J (1959): End results of removal of protruded intervertebral discs with and without fusion. *The American Academy of Orthopaedic Surgeons Instructional Course Lectures,* Vol. 16. St. Louis: CV Mosby.

316. Young J (1906): *A manual and atlas of orthopaedic surgery.* Philadelphia: P. Blackston's Son & Co., pp. 596–597.

317. Yuan HA, Mann KA, Found EM, et al. (1988): Early clinical experience with the Syracuse I plate. *Spine* 13(3):278–285.

318. Zacrisson M (1979): The low back school, a sound-slide presentation. Danderyd Hospital, Sweden.

319. Zacrisson M (1980): see ref. 99, Frymoyer et al. (1978), *Spine* 3: 1–6.

320. Zielke K, Strempel AV (1986): Posterior lateral distraction spondylodesis using the twofold sacral bar. *Clin Orthop* 151–158.

321. Zindrick MR, Wiltse LL, Doornik A, Widdell EH (1987): Analysis of the morphometric characteristics of the thoracic and lumbar pedicles. *Spine* 12:160–166.

322. Zindrick M, Wiltse LL, Widell EH (1986): A biomechanical study of intrapeduncular screw fixation in the lumbosacral spine. *Clin Orthop* 203:99–112.

323. Zindrick MR, et al. (1985): Far lateral disc rupture beyond the pedicle zone. Paper presented to the meeting of the Los Angeles Chapter of the Western Orthopaedic Association, Arrowhead Springs, California, April, 1985.

The Adult Spine: Principles and Practice,
2nd edition, J.W. Frymoyer, Editor-in-Chief.
Lippincott-Raven Publishers, Philadelphia © 1997.

CHAPTER 3

The Future of Spinal Treatment

John W. Frymoyer, Thomas B. Ducker, Nortin M. Hadler, John P. Kostuik, James N. Weinstein, and Thomas S. Whitecloud III

Our focus should be to the patient who has a disease, and not to the disease which affects a patient.
—Sir William Osler

Five years ago, the editors of first edition of *The Adult Spine* concluded that future care for patients with spinal disorders would be shaped by advances in scientific and clinical knowledge as well as by powerful societal forces that are profoundly influencing how health care is financed and delivered. In the intervening five years, it has become evident that these societal and marketplace forces have influenced diagnosis and treatment more

than fundamental advances in scientific and clinical knowledge have. However, the advances occurring in science and technology will have a profound impact over the next decade. In particular, the rapidly exploding knowledge of the human genome and the molecular biologic basis of disease, as well as the rapid advances in computer technology, will have a great impact on how we diagnose and treat some spinal disorders.

In this chapter, we will examine the continuing societal forces, the possible proactive responses to these forces that can be made by health professionals, and the scientific and technological advances that will shape the care received by our patients. Finally, we will return to some basic values and principles directed at human beings, "the patient with a disease," who the editors feel should remain the focus for health professionals.

SOCIETAL FORCES

Health Care Delivery

In 1989 it was estimated that by the year 2000, the United States would utilize 15% of its gross national product for health care, compared with 5% four decades earlier. This figure was almost double that of other medically sophisticated industrialized nations, and it is rising rapidly (Fig. 1). On a *per capita* basis, the cost of health care in the United States was also almost double that of any other nation (Fig. 2). In a global economy, some predicted that as the United States moved towards a more government-based health financing system, other sys-

J. W. Frymoyer, M.D.: Dean, College of Medicine, Professor, Department of Orthopaedics and Rehabilitation, University of Vermont, Burlington, Vermont 05405.

T. B. Ducker, M.D.: Professor of Surgery, Department of Neurosurgery, Johns Hopkins Medical Institutions, Baltimore, Maryland 21205.

N. M. Hadler, M.D., F.A.C.P.: Professor of Medicine and Microbiology/Immunology, University of North Carolina at Chapel Hill; Attending Rheumatologist, University of North Carolina Hospitals, Chapel Hill, North Carolina 27599-7280.

J. P. Kostuik, M.D., F.R.C.S.(C): Professor, Department of Orthopaedic Surgery, Johns Hopkins Medical Institutions, Baltimore, Maryland 21287-0882.

J. N. Weinstein, D.O., M.S.: Division of Orthopedics and Neurosurgery, Senior Faculty Member, Center for Clinical Evaluative Sciences, Dartmouth Medical School, Dartmouth Hitchcock Medical Center, Hanover, NH 03755.

T. S. Whitecloud III, M.D.: Professor and Chairman, Department of Orthopaedic Surgery, Tulane University School of Medicine, New Orleans, Louisiana 70112.

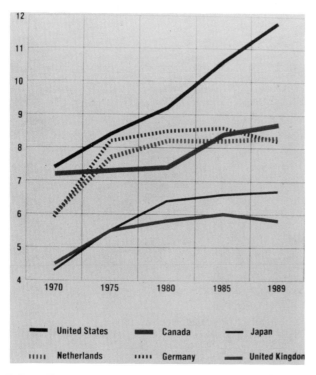

FIG. 1. Total health expenditures as a percentage of gross domestic product, selected countries, 1970–1989. In 1989, it was estimated that by the year 2000 the United States would utilize 15% of its gross national product for health care, compared with 5% four decades earlier. This figure was almost double that of other medically sophisticated industrialized nations and is rising rapidly. (From George Schieber and Jean-Pierre Poulier, Health Affairs 1991;10(1):109.)

tems would become more market based. The result would be a greater degree of similarity between nations (Fig. 3).

Many of these events predicted in 1989 have taken place to some degree (for example, the privatization of the socialized British system), although National Health

Reform, a cornerstone of the Clinton administration's agenda, substantially failed as a public policy. At the same time, new marketplace forces have become evident in the United States; health financing has progressively moved away from the traditional fee-for-service, toward capitated financing of care, often referred to as *managed care*. In this form of health-care financing, a fixed amount of dollars (expressed as dollars/member/month) is paid by an insurer intermediary, or directly by larger, self-insured industries, to providers (physicians, hospitals, physician–hospital organizations, or other organizations of providers) often referred to, usually inappropriately, as *integrated delivery systems*.

By changing the economic incentives, the health provider is forced into thinking about how to manage costs, rather than how to enhance revenues through the provision of additional services. Currently, more than 50 million Americans receive their medical care under such a financing system. In some states, this system of financing has been extended to federally funded systems such as Medicaid. In other states, capitated health-care financing is being developed for patients older than 65, who currently are funded by Medicare.

There are a number of very significant consequences of these changes in health-care financing. Capitated health-care financing has spawned a dramatic set of market-driven forces that are based principally on the ability of payers (insurers, industry) to achieve cost reduction by encouraging competition between health-care providers. These market forces and their impact on health-care delivery have been studied in some detail. Figure 4 shows the response that can be predicted to occur as a function of the proportion of a particular marketplace penetrated by capitated health-care financing systems.

There are significant regional variations in the rate of

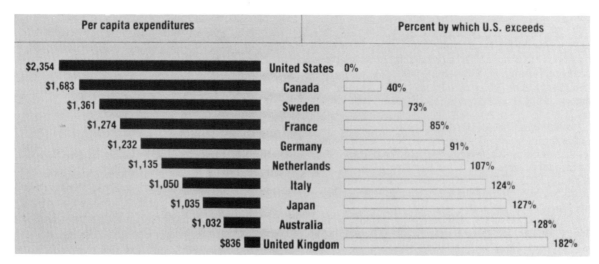

FIG. 2. Per capita health spending in U.S. dollars, selected countries, 1989. On a *per capita* basis, the cost of health care in the United States was also almost double that of any other nation. (From George Schieber and Jean-Pierre Poulier, Health Affairs 1991;10(1):113.)

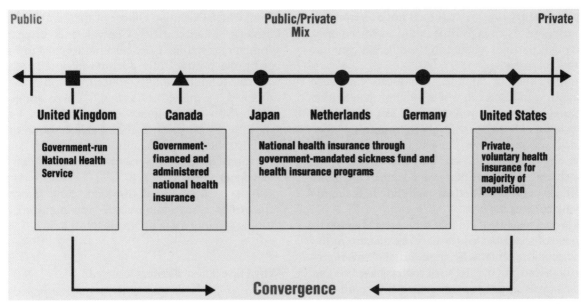

FIG. 3. The shrinking continuum. In a global economy, some predicted that as the United States moved towards a more government-based health financing system, other systems would become more market based, resulting in a greater degree of similarity between nations. (Courtesy of The Wyatt Company, 1991.)

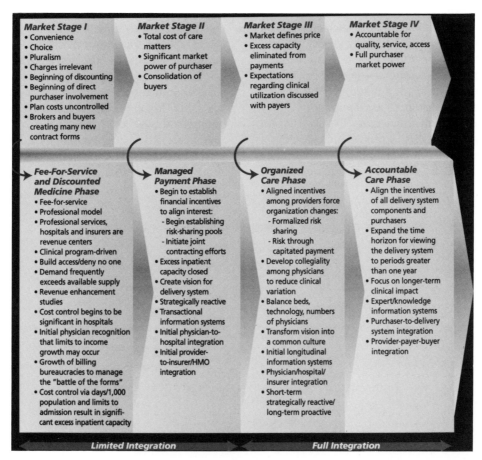

FIG. 4. A dynamic model for delivery system integration. The fairly predictable behavior that occurs as a function of the proportion of a particular marketplace penetrated by capitated health-care financing systems. (From "Integration: Market Forces and Critical Success Factors," Executive Summary, VHA Inc., Irving, TX, figure 4.)

marketplace change (Fig. 5). It should not be surprising that the response is strikingly different in advanced markets from that in states where capitated health care has made minimal inroads.

The implications of capitated health-care financing are profound with respect to where and how health care will be delivered and who will deliver it. For the past 50 years, the locus of health care has been hospitals. Under a capitated system of care, there are enormous shifts from the hospital setting to the outpatient setting and from the specialist to the primary care doctor. One result is the merging of hospitals and the reduction in the number of available hospital beds.

Since World War II, there has been a steady growth in the focus of sophisticated (tertiary) heath care in the academic medical centers. Because tertiary care represents the high-end cost of care, such centers have become particular targets in a capitated system of care. In fact, the lay press and publications from organizations such as the American Association of Medical Colleges point to the endangered state of the academic medical center. This is already leading to mergers of traditional rivals, with insurance groups buying out the health-care delivery arm of the academic medical centers, and there is considerable concern about the survival of local centers. The implications of these changes to the research and educational missions of these organizations are profound. [One of our editors (NH) suggests, however, that we should not mourn the academic medical centers, for we have lost sight of our mission to train people as compassionate physicians, instead of as technocrats.]

The number of specialists necessary to deliver health care is declining. Manpower estimates indicate that already there is an abundant oversupply, for example, in anesthesiology. An article in *Newsweek* quotes Samuel Thier, Chief Executive Officer of the combined Boston hospitals, Massachusetts General and Brigham and Women's, as stating, "The current ratio of 8 to 9 specialists to one primary care doctor will be altered to 1:1, while the total staff will be reduced." Another executive, unnamed, is quoted as saying, "We're going to get killed—Now the primary care physicians have the specialists by the short hairs!" Table 1 shows the possible distribution of specialists predicted by surveyors of managed-care delivery systems such as Kaiser Permanente.

In the area of spinal disorders, how many spinal surgeons does any nation need? How many specialized training programs will be required?

Why Have These Events Occurred?

There is little question that a driving force in the changes seen in health-care financing was that the cost of health care in the United States was unsustainable in a global economy. However, beneath the financing issue were two other critical issues. First, access to health care bears little relationship to the costs of health care. In nations with lower health care costs, all citizens have access to basic and essential health care, whereas in the United States, the number of individuals with inadequate or no access is estimated to be greater than 50 million. Second, the quality of health care, as measured by societal indicators such as immunization rate, infant mortality, life expectancy, incidence and prevalence of common disease, and reduction in work loss from injury, bears little relationship to the amount of money expended by different nations for health care. In fairness, some of these factors are largely beyond the control of

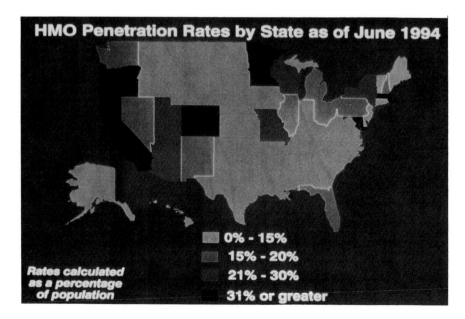

FIG. 5. There are significant regional variations in the rate of marketplace change. (Courtesy of Fletcher Allen Health Care.)

TABLE 1. *Six analysts' target numbers of full-time-equivalent physicians for 100,000 covered lives, listed by specialty[a]*

Specialty	Target number of MDs per 100,000 enrolled lives (low ratio)					
	California Pacific M.C.[b]	Kronick et al.	Penn	Kaiser Portland	Sentara	Sokolov
Primary care						
Adult	39.0			38.7		
Pediatric	9.0			14.9		
Subtotal	48.0	50.0	50.0	53.6	50.6	50.0
Obstetrics–gynecology	8.0	11.0		10.8		
Medicine						
Allergy	1.1			1.5		
Cardiology	2.0	3.0		2.8		
Dermatology	2.4			2.4		
Gastroenterology	1.2			1.5		
Neurology	1.6			1.2		
Oncology	1.6			2.2		
Pulmonary	1.0			1.3		
Other	1.4			3.0		
Subtotal	12.3			14.7		
Surgery						
CVS and thoracic	1.0	1.0		0.1		
General surgery	7.2	5.5		6.5		
Neurosurgery	0.6	0.5		1.3		
Ophthalmology	3.6			2.3		
Orthopedics	4.0	4.5		5.5		
Otolaryngology	2.0			3.2		
Plastic	0.4			0.3		
Urology	2.0	2.5		3.1		
Subtotal	20.8			22.2		
Other						
Anesthesiology	5.9	5.0		5.5		
Emergency med.	5.8	4.5		6.3		
Pathology	3.0			3.1		
Psychiatry	4.6	4.0		4.8		
Radiology	4.4	6.0		7.9		
All other	0.1	20.5[c]				
Subtotal	23.8					
Grand total	112.9	118.0		136.8	75.0	100.0

From: *Academic Medicine* 1995;70(7):574.

[a] The table's target ratios are estimates for integrated health care delivery systems. See the reference list items indicated by superscripts in the column headings above for sources of the six analysts' data. Covered lives, subscribers covered by the system.

[b] The data under "California Pacific M.C." reflect the contributions of nonphysician practitioners.

[c] Kronick listed "all other specialties" as ophthalmology, otolaryngology, dermatology, pathology, hematology and oncology, neurology, gastroenterology, allergy and immunology, pulmonary medicine, nephrology, endocrinology, infectious disease, and plastic and reconstructive surgery.

the health professional; for example, drug and other substance abuse is associated with teenage pregnancy, which in turn is associated with high-risk babies. However, much of health care *is* in the control of the health professionals. Nowhere is this more evident than in the management of spinal disorders.

One measure of quality is variation in the use of services. Keller and Atlas point out in chapter 6 that in tightly controlled, high-quality processes, the amount of variation generally has a predictable and fairly narrow range. In comparison, on an international basis, there are wide variations that are largely independent of the prevalence or incidence of spinal disorders or epidemio-

logic risk factors. In fact, the highest predictor is the number of spinal surgeons in the particular society. Similarly, there are wide variations in the rate of spinal surgery between regions of the United States and even within states (Fig. 6).

Value

In the normal competitive marketplace, consumers look for value, which is the relationship between the quality of the product, the quality of the service received, and the cost. Although these relationships are not strictly

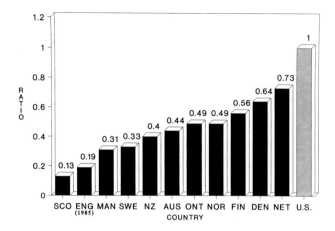

Ratio of back surgery rate in selected countries
to back surgery rate in the United States (1988-1989)

FIG. 6. There are wide variations in the rate of spinal surgery between countries.

quantitative or linear, conceptually they can be expressed by the equation shown in Figure 7A and the framework shown in Figure 7B.

The question then is, Is the care of spinal disorders achieving maximal value? Based on the available evidence, the answer must be no, although in fairness, elements of spine care and the cost of these elements are beyond the direct control of the physician or surgeon.

What is the evidence?

Cost

As outlined in chapter 8, the cost to society of spinal disorders in the United States is enormous and measurable in tens of billions of dollars. These costs are similarly enormous in other societies, and Nachemson has pointed out that in at least one, Sweden, the Socialist welfare state is driving itself towards bankruptcy because of ill-advised public policy that rewards continued disability.

Quality

As already pointed out, variance in the utilization of services suggests at the very least the absence of a systematic approach based on solid information and measurable outcomes.

WHAT IS THE OPPORTUNITY?

The opportunity for those genuinely interested in spinal disorders is to actively seek methods to maximize the value of care through explicit management of quality and cost. The economic arguments in defense of this objective are based on the concept of risk and care manage-

ment. As pointed out earlier, capitated systems of health care are based on a per-member-per-month financing charge, but it should be emphasized that this does not equal care management. In fact, most of so-called managed care is still based on some form of discounted fee-for-service and management of access through the use of the primary care "gatekeeper."

The concept of managing risk can be best explained by taking a real-life example. A fairly standard cost basis for capitation in the age group under 65 is $100/member/month. In not-for-profit environments, $10 of this is for insurance costs such as marketing and claims processing, and $90 is for health care delivery. Although a precise figure is unknown, let us presume that all spinal care capitation is $1.00/member/month. If a health-care system has responsibility for 1 million members, the amount available for spinal care is $1.00/member/month × 12 months × 1 million, or $12,000,000. If the providers responsible for spinal care are going to manage the risks and have an economic margin for future growth and development, there is a powerful incentive to reconceptualize the delivery of spinal care. This would require a truly integrated system of care management, very different from traditional health care. The steps involved in this reconceptualization are outlined by Plante, Rothwell, and Tufo in Chapter 5 and by Keller and Atlas in Chapter 6. The general attributes are:

1. Understanding each of the steps involved in the process of care for a patient with any given disorder.

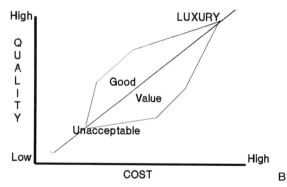

FIG. 7. In the normal competitive marketplace, consumers look for value, which is the relationship between the quality of the product, the quality of the service received, and the cost. These relationships are not strictly quantitative or linear and are expressed by the equation shown in **A** and the framework shown in **B**.

2. Establishing clear protocols for the management of these steps, with target performances.
3. Measuring the variance that occurs around the individual process steps, and adjusting the process based on the feedback of explicit information.
4. Explicit measures of value that take into account cost, quality of service, and quality of outcome, measured in functional terms.

There are examples of systems thinking already evident in the field of spinal disorders. Through the use of an explicit process and the measurement of the results, Boden et al. have demonstrated how the quality of spinal care can be improved in the notoriously difficult group of work-injured patients, while at the same time reducing the costs. Such systems of care are likely to be regionally based, and for the majority of spinal disorders, they are unlikely to be built around highly sophisticated one-stop shopping centers. This provocative conclusion is opposite to that contemplated in the first edition of *The Adult Spine* and is based on the premise that the majority of spinal disorders can be managed in a primary care setting, providing that the systems, the informational data bases, and the decision-making supports are in place. It is possible that specific and less common spinal disorders will be managed in such centers, providing they can demonstrate value.

Fundamental reengineering of the delivery of health care is just beginning, but its potential is an exciting offspring of new methods of financing health care.

TECHNOLOGICAL ADVANCES

There are three broad areas in which technological advances will influence spinal care: the development of information technology, the development of clinical techniques, and the application of discoveries in basic science.

Information Technology

Advances in information technology allow us to contemplate new care management systems, which require access to specific information regarding common medical records, decision analysis, variance analysis, and explicit outcome data with respect to value. The emergence of the capacity to transfer images and other visual data opens the pathway to obtaining information from geographically remote specialists and real-time consultation, making available to the clinician new information in a timely way.

Clinically Applicable Technology

Examples of new and exciting technology will be found throughout the second edition of *The Adult Spine.*

The majority of these technologies represent developments in imaging technology (for example, magnetic resonance imaging, and electrophysiologic techniques applicable to diagnosis and intraoperative management) or diagnostic tools or therapeutic approaches that are minimally invasive (for example, techniques for percutaneous discectomy and thoracoscopy, lasers, artificial disc devices, and percutaneous methods of achieving spinal fusion). Also, there are numerous examples of new techniques of spinal fixation applicable to the most complex deformities and other pathological conditions. The benefit of new imaging technology is to increase the sensitivity and specificity of diagnoses, and the benefits of new diagnostic and therapeutic techniques are to reduce morbidity, mortality, and presumably the costs of managing specific spinal disorders. However, there are two general cautions.

First, for many of the newer diagnostic techniques, there is only marginal evidence of measurably improved care for the vast majority of people who have benign, self-limited spinal disorders, or what Hadler terms *regional back pain.* In fact, there is disturbing evidence that many of these technologies may lead to misdiagnosis: an essentially normal aging change may be diagnosed as a pathological condition. However, there is no question but that these technologies are invaluable in the subset of people with major spinal pathology such as fractures, infections, and some tumors. The trick will be to better define the criteria on which to base the application of these diagnostic techniques.

Second, few of these new therapeutic techniques have been subjected to rigorous analysis with respect to outcome improvement. In fact, one of the more widely popular "least invasive" methods, percutaneous suction discectomy, has done poorly in comparison to chymopapain. Although the design of that experiment has been criticized, it emphasizes the crucial need for more explicit clinical research. It is also evident that federal funding agencies such as the National Institutes of Health are struggling with how to develop mechanisms to support better clinical research, including how to attract and retain clinical investigators.

It is also apparent there will be further coalescence of computer and surgical technology. The early developments in virtual reality technology suggest the future possibility of virtual reality surgery.

Basic Science

The most profound changes are occurring in molecular biology, and particularly around the Human Genome Project. Daily, new genes associated with well-known genetically determined conditions, as well as a variety of tumors and metabolic, neurological, and cardiovascular conditions, are discovered. Today there is unequivocal evidence to support a familial basis for relatively rarer conditions affecting the spine, as well as some of the more common ones, including possibly certain forms of degenerative disc disease. However, there are profound legal, ethical, and practical implications of discovering a well-defined and predictable predilection to degenerative disc disease. Should such individuals be precluded from physically demanding jobs? Should industry be made aware of the risk? If a person decides to pursue a particular job, should industry be relieved of liability?

The second part of these profound developments in molecular biology is their potential diagnostic and therapeutic implications. Two areas are of particular interest. First, rapid development in the understanding of neurological function opens enormous opportunities to understand the "pain experience" and potentially modify that experience through specifically targeted therapies. Second, the potential ability to treat metabolic conditions such as osteoporosis, tumors, and even degenerative diseases is enormous. Already, there is early evidence in peripheral degenerative joint disease of the ability to culture chrondrocytes *in vitro* and reimplant them into surface cartilage defects. It is well within the realm of possibility to contemplate specific treatments for symptomatic degenerative discs. The stimulation of spinal fusions through the application of genetic engineering techniques is already in clinical trials.

Ultimately, the litmus test for these newer developments will be how much they influence the value of the care we render to our patients with spinal disorders.

BIBLIOGRAPHY

Allis S, Dickerson JF, Reingold EM, Taylor E (1995): Teaching hospitals in crisis. *Time* 146(3):40–41.

American College of Physicians (1990): Position paper: access to heath care. *Ann Intern Med* 112(9):641–661.

Berwick DM (1989): Continuous improvement as an ideal in health care. *N Engl J Med* 320:53–56.

Bigos S, Bowyer O, Braen G, et al. (1994): *Acute low back problems in adults.* Clinical Practice Guideline #14. AHCPR Publication No.95-0642. Rockville, MD: Agency for Health Policy and Research, Public Health Service. U.S. Department of Health and Human Services.

Boden SD, Wiesel SW, Feffer JL (1993): A quality-based protocol for the management of low back pain and sciatica: a ten-year prospective outcome study. *Clin Orthop* 30:164–176.

Cherkin DC, Deyo RA, Loeser JD, Bush T, Waddell G (1994): An international comparison of back surgery rates. *Spine* 19(11):1201–1206.

Deyo RA (1993): Practice variations, treatment facts, rising disability. Do we need a new clinical research paradigm? *Spine* 18:2153–2161.

Ellwood PM (1988): Shattuck lecture. Outcomes management: a technology of patient experience. *N Engl J Med* 318:1549–1567.

Epstein A (1995): Sounding board performance reports on quality—prototypes, problems and prospects. *N Engl J Med* 333:57–61.

Frymoyer JW, Bordon SL (1989): *New perspectives on low back pain.* Chicago: American Academy of Orthopaedic Surgeons.

Frymoyer JW, Gordon SL (1989): Research perspectives in low back pain. Report of a 1988 workshop. *Spine* 14:1384–1390.

Frymoyer JW (1993): Quality: an international challenge to the diagnosis and treatment of disorders of the lumbar spine. *Spine* 18:2147–2152.

Greenberger NJ (1990): Universal access to health care in America: a moral and medical imperative. *Ann Intern Med* 112(9):637–638.

Graig LA (1991): *Health care of nations.* Chicago: The Wyatt Company.

Hadler NM (1994): Medicine's industrial revolution is here. Rally the Luddites. *J Occup Med* 36:1038–1040.

Henkel G (1995): Virtual hospital provides clinical decision support through the Internet [*Letter*]. *Spine* 2(5):1.

Integration: market forces and critical success factors. An executive report for VHA health care organizations. (1994) Irving, Texas: VHA Inc.

Keller RM, Soule DM, Wennberg JE, Hanley DF (1990): Dealing with geographic variations in hospital use: the experience of the Maine Medical Assessment Program's orthopaedic study group. *J Bone Joint Surg [Am]* 72A:1286–1293.

Lerner AN, McClendon J (1995): *Antitrust clouds work force solutions.* Bulletin of the American Academy of Orthopaedic Surgeons. 43:19–21.

MacDonald AS, Baloun ET, McKenna QL (1995): *Emerging models, integrated health systems.* GFP notes 8(1):1–5.

Nachemson A (1995): Will back pain doom the welfare State? The Swedish experience may be a warning for the U.S. *The Back Letter* 10:27.

Revel M, Papan C, Vallee C, et al. (1993): Automated percutaneous lumbar discectomy versus chemonucleolysis in the treatment of sciatica: a randomized multicenter trial. *Spine* 18:1–7.

Turner JA, Ersek M, Herron L, Haselkorn, Kent DL, Deyo R (1992): Patient outcomes after lumbar spinal fusion: a comprehensive literature synthesis. *JAMA* 268:907–911.

Volinn E, Mayer J, Diehr P, et al. (1992): Small area analysis of surgery for low back pain. *Spine* 17:575–581.

Wiesel SW, Feffer HL, Rothman RH (1984): Industrial low back pain: a prospective evaluation of a standardized diagnostic and treatment protocol. *Spine* 9:199–203.

PART I

EPIDEMIOLOGY, DISABILITY, AND SOCIETAL IMPACT

Editor: Nortin M. Hadler

The Adult Spine: Principles and Practice,
2nd edition, J.W. Frymoyer, Editor-in-Chief.
Lippincott-Raven Publishers, Philadelphia © 1997.

CHAPTER 4

Backache and Humanism

Nortin M. Hadler

The Adult Spine is designed to be a comprehensive and definitive treatise on axial neuromusculoskeletal disorders. The format, at first glance, seems constrained by a paradigm held sacrosanct by the Western physician since the dawn of modern medicine two centuries ago (12). In the early eighteenth century, Thomas Sydenham in London and later Hermann Boerhaave in Leyden perceived what we now consider the principle of differential diagnosis: any set of symptoms (the illness) can be ascribed to one of a finite number of possible anatomic or physiologic derangements (the disease). Without such a conceptual leap, catarrh (inflammation of mucous membranes) would still be considered a disease rather than an illness caused by a specific infection, and the modern physician would not have the satisfaction of curing a disease with the expectation that the illness would be alleviated. The quest for the disease, the pathophysiologic cause of the symptoms that are each patient's illness, is the diagnostician's banner. A person seeking medical care expects and is expected to enter into the exercise as the patient, *pari passu* the willing participant and the active collaborator. A satisfactory outcome of a patient–physician interaction is the diagnostic label; a satisfying outcome is a label that suggests meaningful intervention and prognostic insight; and a prideful outcome is a label that leads to a cure. Clinical treatises on a wide range of topics are either structured along these lines or are meant to be read for these insights. One can find recent volumes on infectious diseases, cancer, trauma, stroke, and many more—all embellished with pathophysiologic underpinning and epidemiologic context, but all expositions of diagnosis, prognosis, and cure.

The disease–illness paradigm has been so overwhelmingly successful that its shortcomings have been largely ignored for generations. This is no longer reasonable regardless of the category of disease (35) and it is not possible for *The Adult Spine.* Not every person with a spinal disorder seeks or needs to seek any care, let alone chooses to be a patient (18). Every labeling exercise is anxiety provoking at least and is justifiable only if the labeling leads to meaningful therapeutic or, arguably (35), prognostic inferences. Some justify the "laying on of diagnostic labels" as therapeutic in and of itself (31,32). However, physicians must be made aware of the considerable risks of the labeling exercise; it has the potential for iatrogenicity (6,11), particularly for provoking untoward physical and behavioral consequences in the setting of musculoskeletal complaints (16,20).

At this point in the history of Western medicine, the patient is seldom a free agent and the patient–physician relationship is seldom unfettered; layers of constraint and agendas from funding and regulatory agencies accompany the patient into the office. In order to fully understand the contemporary quandary that is backache, *The Adult Spine* does not focus just on the patient with spine disorders; intermixed is the person with axial symptoms and the claimant with axial symptoms whose requirements for medical care are coupled to the restraints imposed by others on fiscal redress.

N. M. Hadler, M.D., F.A.C.P.: Professor of Medicine and Microbiology/Immunology, School of Medicine, University of North Carolina at Chapel Hill, Chapel Hill, North Carolina, 27599-7280; Attending Rheumatologist, University of North Carolina Hospitals, Chapel Hill, North Carolina.

THE PERSON WITH A SPINAL DISORDER
(Fig. 1)

As is clear from the chapter that follows, axial discomfort is a ubiquitous, intermittent, and remittent predicament. Most people, most of the time, eschew the medical contact. Why they do so and how they choose among the alternatives is still poorly understood. But the fact of this behavior is undeniable. Usually they cope by relying solely on personal resources. Chapters throughout *The Adult Spine* attempt to offer insights into the rationale, methodology, and scanty validation of some of the myriad of alternative care modalities accessible to the sufferer. For example, spinal manipulation is reviewed by Haldeman et al. in Chapter 86, physical therapy in Chapter 83 by Witt, and back schools in Chapter 14 by Nordin and coauthors. Obviously these approaches may be initiated by medical prescription, orchestrated under medical supervision, or performed by physicians. However, they are available to people with a sore back or neck without medical intercession. Furthermore, every patient standing before a physician is aware of the alternatives, has considered them, and may have partaken in them. It is naive for a physician to think otherwise and unacceptable to be unaware.

THE PATIENT WITH A SPINAL DISORDER

Most of the text of this volume is committed to the diagnosis and treatment of disorders of the axial skeleton. Infections, fractures, tumors, and congenital anomalies should not long elude our elegant diagnostic machinations and should not escape without the benefit of our therapeutic algorithms. However, it is a rare patient indeed with a backache or neck pain who is well served by all this diagnostic activity. Most adults, most of the time, suffer a "regional backache" (17,22). These are individuals between 20 and 50 years of age who are otherwise well, who have suffered no traumatic precipitant involving external forces, and who are spared such neurologic catastrophes as cauda equina syndrome, myelopathy, or overt weakness of an extremity. The pain is typically abrupt in onset, relieved by recumbency, minimal on arising, and absent during sleep. As a corollary, the pain is exacerbated by usage of the spine, so that it increases during the course of the day.

Regional musculoskeletal illness (such as regional backache or regional neck pain) is the appropriate label for almost all people with these symptoms and almost all patients presenting for their first medical contact. All deserve kindness, empathy, insight (23), and advice; none deserves an anxiety-provoking diagnostic workup, because a meaningful yield is so likely to prove elusive. This should be reserved for the rare patient with a major neurologic catastrophe or systemic presenting features (22). Employing our growing wealth of diagnostic regalia indiscriminately is not cost effective. More troublesome and disturbing, the quest for a diagnosis establishes a patient–physician contract based on the assumption that an important disease underlies the pain and the implication that there is a need for intervention. The diagnostic

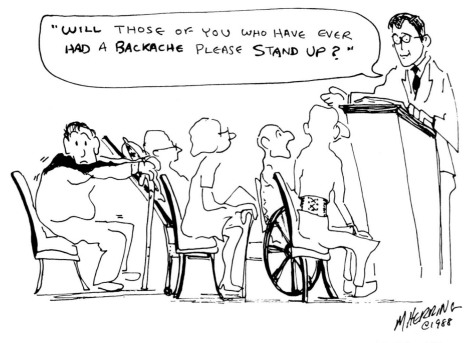

FIG. 1. With permission from the American College of Occupational Medicine (19).

contract and exercise can preempt patient autonomy and perturb clinical judgment, fomenting unproductive therapies. Chapters 20 by Andersson and Deyo, 25 by El-Khoury and Brandser, 82 by Deyo, and 89 by Frymoyer address the booming industry in unproductive, unproven, and unprovable interventions. Society must be re-educated about the implications of the regional backache. That is a major charge to the readership of *The Adult Spine;* the information is explicit and implicit throughout both volumes.

THE CLAIMANT WITH A SPINAL DISORDER (Figs. 2,3)

There is another patient–physician contract that is even more covert and has more malevolent potential than the diagnostic contract. Regional backache is always exacerbated by usage. Therefore, regional backache always carries a specter of some degree of incapacity. If the patient perceives himself as incapable of performing on the job, he has the illness of work incapacity. If his wage-earning capacity is sufficiently compromised, he then becomes eligible for benefits under one of several programs in every industrial nation. If he perceives his backache to have arisen out of and in the course of his employment, he is eligible for medical benefits under his Workers' Compensation insurance policy. Finally, if he is eligible for Workers' Compensation and has any degree of work incapacity, he is entitled to benefits that are almost always more liberal than other forms of disability insurance. The chapter that follows discusses the history and current status of these distinctions.

The moment a person chooses to seek care under Workers' Compensation, he or she is a claimant in an insurance scheme. At issue is whether he is injured, whether he is as well as he is likely to get, and whether there is residual illness or work incapacity. All three stipulations are inherently contentious for regional backache. The approach in the United States is discussed in Chapter 10. The American focus on the issue of causality is shared by most industrial nations but not all (25); Holland (19), for example, focuses on the last two issues and disregards causation entirely. If the physician treats a claimant under Workers' Compensation, the act certifies the accidental, putatively traumatic nature of the injury and the work relatedness of the onset of the illness. Seldom is this pathophysiologic assertion fully understood by the patient/claimant or the treating physician.

Workers' Compensation underwrites an impressive system of health care. For the worker who suffers a discrete traumatic event, a laceration or fracture or the like, the system is remarkably efficient from any perspective. However, for illnesses such as regional backache that conform poorly to the Workers' Compensation stipulation regarding causation, the system's track record is far less laudatory (21,24,29). The other major recourse for someone with the illness of work incapacity in the United States is the Social Security Administration, which operates the Social Security Disability Insurance (SSDI) and Supplemental Security Income (SSI) programs. These programs are modeled to some extent after

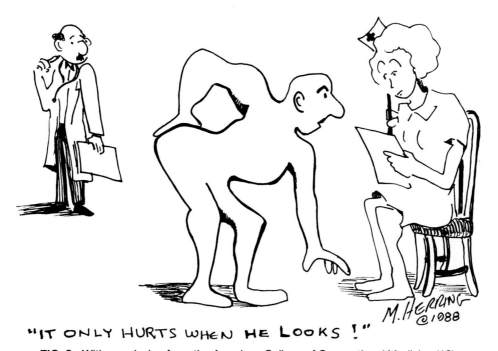

"IT ONLY HURTS WHEN HE LOOKS!"

FIG. 2. With permission from the American College of Occupational Medicine (19).

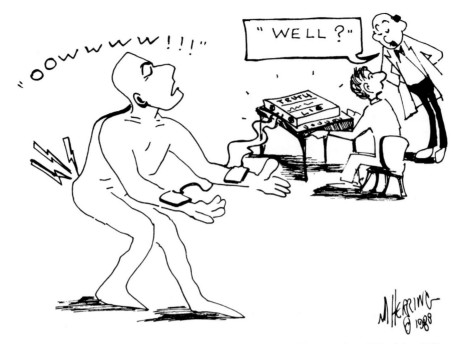

FIG. 3. With permission from the American College of Occupational Medicine (19).

the "invalid pensions" of Europe. For SSDI/SSI, causation is not an issue; consolidation is defined only in terms of duration rather than the "fixed and stable" consideration of Workers' Compensation insurance. But the critical distinction relates to the intent of the programs: Workers' Compensation is designed to insure against any loss of wage earning capacity, while SSDI/SSI kicks in if the illness of work incapacity is so severe that any "substantial gainful employment" is no longer feasible (25). SSDI/SSI provides a pension that is far less generous than Workers' Compensation programs and medical care under Medicare/Medicaid.

THE VORTEX OF DISABILITY DETERMINATION

Much of the health care dollar for backache relates to these two insurance schemes. Whenever one reads documents by econometricians, health policy administrators, epidemiologists, and others whose focus is the behavior of a population, rather than people behaving one at a time, it is crucial to question whether the data relate to people with backache, patients with backache, claimants with back injuries, or claimants with the illness of backache. Usually, such documents relate to claimants because those data are accessible from the insurance agencies. All too often, the writer is not aware or does not emphasize that the essay is describing the behavior of a population of claimants. Chapter 8 by Frymoyer and Durett discusses some of these issues.

Even more obfuscating, much of the surgical literature

on regional backache draws on the experience with claimants. It is only at the level of rehabilitation for the "failed back" or for "chronic back" that the distinction is drawn, as in Chapter 15 by Hazard and Chapter 17 by Turk and Stacey. The fact that the clinical sciences seem unaware of the special station in life occupied by the claimant until it is too late is unconscionable. The process of the claim is a gauntlet; the data suggest that too few negotiate it successfully (21).

The Workers' Compensation claimant with a regional backache who enters into the medical system under the guise of an injured patient is on the defensive from the outset. Since nothing special precipitated the backache, he must feel some degree of disquiet in asserting that he was injured and in responding to questions as to precipitants. Nonetheless, in nearly all jurisdictions, if he registers his complaint in the workplace, he is likely to be listed on the Occupational Safety and Health Administration (OSHA) 200 log as injured. (This log is a federally required recording of occupational illnesses and injuries, the reliability and validity of which is yet to be established.) The mandate for an identifiable, discrete precipitant has largely been abandoned in the United States. After all, regional backache is exacerbated by motion; it seems logical that usage is the precipitant as well. Such a liberalization of definitions is seductive because benefits, in terms of health care and salary compensation, are ready and adequate. Furthermore, most such claimants return to health and to the job in short order. However, the small minority of this enormous universe of claimants who do not heal rapidly find themselves in a special position. First, they carry some degree of resentment toward their workplace and employer as a natural outgrowth of the compensability of their backache. After all, they have been certified as injured on the job. In addition, as Bigos and Battié expound in Chapter 9, such claimants are not enamored with their work setting to begin with. Workers' Compensation is wedded to providing whatever medical care is necessary to return the claimant to work. As a result, the surgical community is long accustomed to making recommendations in this setting, with little resistance in terms of fee-for-service or in terms of patient dissent. The first reflects policy; the second, the defensive nature of the claimant's status. If the claimant refuses diagnostic or therapeutic interventions, his lack of cooperation may be construed to question the credibility of his persistent symptomatology. The contest of disability determination is joined.

The charge to the surgeon is to identify and repair the injury; the charge to the claimant is to prove he is still hurting in spite of passage of time and the interventions provided. In 1934, Mixter and Barr offered the world a remedial cause of the regional low back injury, the ruptured disc (28). Surgical zeal was unbridled in the face of a patient/claimant whose illness and expectations are perturbed by the contest. The results in this setting were disappointing to Barr himself by mid century (5) and have disappointed observers in every decade since (1,29,30). There is every reason to question the surgical algorithm (14,17) and *The Adult Spine* reinforces and expands on these arguments. However, the contest of disability determination has evolved to intertwine an enormous number of vested interests and to commandeer considerable resources. It still has a life of its own in spite of its track record and patent flaws.

When the claimant has submitted to all proffered interventions and still has the illness of work incapacity, the undercurrent of the entire gauntlet comes to the fore—disability determination. Is this worker really unable to return to his prior job (for Workers' Compensation) or to any job (for SSDI/SSI)? The decision is administrative, but the data sought are clinical. Workers' Compensation insurers are faced with considerable financial outlay if a worker is declared partially or totally disabled. That is why they traditionally grasp at any proffered cure and why they turn to various forms of rehabilitation programs before they will call a halt to the contest. Chapters 13 by Keefe and coauthors, 15 by Hazard, and 17 by Turk and Stacey discuss state-of-the-art programs of this nature. The reader should be aware that most of the "patients" in these programs are claimants, that they have spent months to years in a gauntlet that is the contest of disability determination. Hazard, Loeser, Keefe, and many others discover that such claimants are afflicted with considerable psychological disturbance. The very fact that they are covered by Workers' Compensation insurance bodes poorly for their recovery (9,13,24,33) regardless of the intervention. The work of

Bigos (Chapter 9) suggests that inherent psychological abnormalities do not predispose to becoming a claimant with a back injury. The work of Crown (8) suggests that psychological aberration is acquired as a consequence of negotiating the gauntlet of disability determination for Workers' Compensation. These studies leave a lot to be desired. However, the sadness that envelops the claimant with a back injury if he or she persists in the gauntlet is enough for me. This ostensibly ethical insurance paradigm is iatrogenic. It is hard, if not impossible, to get well if you have to prove you are sick. Even the rehabilitation and pain clinics, the functional restoration, and other programs serve this population unevenly if not poorly; they are funded to attempt to undo the psychological iatrogenicity of the gauntlet even before the claimant is out of the gauntlet (22). It is illogical.

DISABILITY DETERMINATION

In Chapter 11, Waddell and coauthors state the conundrum. Society is willing to go to great lengths to devise an objective measure of disability. The traditional approach is to invert the Sydenham paradigm: if the patient usually presents with an illness in quest of a valid diagnostic label, if the disease is present its subsequent course should be predictable and treatable. This is the banner of impairment rating; it is a tenet that dies slowly. If there is a sufficient quantity of physical damage, of demonstrable pathoanatomical abnormality, the inference of disability is alleged to be comfortable. Waddell and coauthors admit to the enormous difficulties inherent in this assertion, yet they remain convinced that it is basically valid and operational if one uses their descriptors to ferret out those who are less disabled than they claim (Chapter 11).

I, on the other hand, am equally convinced that the notion of impairment rating is fatally flawed and should be discarded! The illness of work incapacity is a necessary consequence only of global, catastrophic disease such as a massive stroke, terminal emphysema, end-stage Class IV heart disease, major spinal cord injuries, and the like. Short of such horrors, the illness of work incapacity is multivariate in precipitation and perpetuation. The work of Magora (27), Bigos et al. (2) (Chapter 9), and Deyo and Diehl (10) render this conclusion inescapable for low back pain; in fact, psychological and sociopolitical confounders overwhelm both disease and ergonomic measures in predicting the illness of work incapacity. A similar although less well understood phenomenon is apparent for disorders of the neck.

Nonetheless, impairment rating is the initial step in disability determination for SSDI/SSI. Furthermore, physicians performing contracted examinations on claimants seeking an award for disabling low back pain before the Social Security Administration conform to the principle of impairment rating in that they totally disregard symptoms in coming to a determination (7). In the United States, Workers' Compensation jurisdictions schedules for low back pain have largely been abandoned—but not reliance on impairment ratings in making a determination. This is quite remarkable and disturbing because some signs and most radiographic and electrodiagnostic findings are unreliable, insensitive, or nonspecific (22). No wonder surgeons seem to adopt their own idiosyncratic criteria for disability, which they offer to the insurer under the guise of impairment rating (4,15). In the United States, recourse is to the courtroom, usually before an administrative law judge within the system. Elsewhere, recourse is often before a panel of educated citizens, and more often impairment rating has been abandoned (25).

QUO VADIS

I suspect that every reader of *The Adult Spine* is already aware of the ramifications of the topic throughout our society. Being aware is insufficient if one wishes to care effectively for those afflicted with spinal morbidity; one must be keenly aware, truly cognizant, even expert. Because a goodly percentage of the readership are surgeons, I will close with a quote from Billroth, writing about German medical education in the mid nineteenth century (3):

> But the state, which trains competent physicians at such great sacrifice, has a right to demand that the physicians be not too completely unprepared for the questions it may put to them . . . The physician, as one of the most important members of the community, is expected not only to help in cases of individual sickness, but in community diseases as well. He is even expected to do his part in curing the stupidity and indifference of humanity. A beautiful task, but one that can be accomplished only by many generations of physicians and then only imperfectly! Before anyone can become interested in it, he must be filled with an almost sentimental enthusiasm for humanity in general.

Unfortunately, Billroth pales in the light of the social activism of his contemporary, Virchow. Billroth goes on to say,

> If the whole of Social Medicine must needs be part of the curriculum of the medical student, it must not take more than two hours per semester, let us say, during the last two semesters; otherwise it will surely be detrimental to his other studies.

If only Virchow were a spine surgeon instead of a pathologist!

REFERENCES

1. Beals RK, Hickman NW (1972): Industrial injuries of the back and extremities. *J Bone Joint Surg* [Am] 54:1593–1611.

2. Bigos SJ, Spengler DM, Martin NA, Zeh J, Fisher L, Nachemson A (1986): Back injuries in industry: A retrospective study. III. Employee-related factors. *Spine* 11:252–256.
3. Billroth T (1924): *The medical sciences in the German universities.* Translated by WW Welch. New York: Macmillan, pp. 89–90.
4. Brand RA, Lehmann TR (1983): Low-back impairment rating practices of orthopaedic surgeons. *Spine* 8:75–78.
5. Brown T, Nemiah JC, Barr JS, Barry H Jr (1954): Psychologic factors in low-back pain. *N Engl J Med* 251:123–128.
6. Burnum JF (1978): The worried sick [editorial]. *Ann Intern Med* 88:572.
7. Carey TS, Hadler NM, Gillings D, Stinnett S, Wallsten T (1988): Medical disability assessment of the back pain patient for the Social Security Administration: The weighting of presenting clinical features. *J Clin Epidemiol* 41:691–697.
8. Crown S (1978): Psychological aspects of low back pain. *Rheumatol Rehabil* 17:114–124.
9. Derebery VJ, Tullis WH (1983): Delayed recovery in the patient with a work compensable injury. *J Occup Med* 25:889–935.
10. Deyo RA, Diehl AK (1988): Psychosocial predictors of disability in patients with low back pain. *J Rheumatol* 15:1557–1564.
11. Eisenberg L (1980): What makes persons "patients" and patients "well"? *Am J Med* 69:277–286.
12. Foucault M (1975): *The birth of the clinic.* New York: Vintage Books.
13. Fredrickson BE, Trief PM, VanBeveren P, Yuan HA, Baum G (1988): Rehabilitation of the patient with chronic back pain: A search for outcome predictors. *Spine* 13:351–353.
14. Frymoyer JW (1988): Back pain and sciatica. *N Engl J Med* 318: 291–300.
15. Greenough CG (1993): Recovery from low back pain. *Acta Orthop Scand* 64(suppl 254):1–34.
16. Hadler NM (1985): A critical reappraisal of the fibrositis concept. *Am J Med* 81(suppl 3A):26–30.
17. Hadler NM (1986): Regional back pain [editorial]. *N Engl J Med* 315:1090–1092.
18. Hadler NM (1988): The predicament of backache [editorial]. *J Occup Med* 30:449–450.
19. Hadler NM (1989): Disabling backache in France, Switzerland, and the Netherlands: Contrasting sociopolitical constraints on clinical judgment. *J Occup Med* 31:823–831.
20. Hadler NM (1990): Cumulative trauma disorders—an iatrogenic concept. *J Occup Med* 32:38–41.
21. Hadler NM (1992): Back pain and the vortex of disability determination. *Semin Spine Surg* 4:35–41.
22. Hadler NM (1993): *Occupational musculoskeletal disorders.* New York: Raven Press, pp. 1–273.
23. Hadler NM (1994): The injured worker and the internist. *Ann Intern Med* 120:163–164.
24. Hadler NM (1994): Point of view. *Spine* 19:1116.
25. Hadler NM (1995): Disabling backache. An international perspective. *Spine* 20:640–649.
26. Haldeman S, Shouka M, Robboy S (1988): Computed tomography, electrodiagnostic and clinical findings in chronic workers' compensation patients with back and leg pain. *Spine* 13:345–350.
27. Magora A (1973): Investigation of the relation between low back pain and occupation. V. Psychological aspects. *Scand J Rehabil Med* 5:191–196.
28. Mixter WJ, Barr JS (1934): Rupture of the intervertebral disc with involvement of the spinal cord. *N Engl J Med* 211:210–215.
29. Rowe ML (1965): Disc surgery and chronic low-back pain. *J Occup Med* 7:196–203.
30. Taylor WP, Stern WR, Kubiszyn TW (1984): Predicting patients' perceptions of response to treatment for low-back pain. *Spine* 9: 313–316.
31. Trudge C (1980): In the end is the word. *New Scientist* 85:37–38.
32. Vaisrub S (1980): The magic of a name [editorial]. *JAMA* 243: 1931–1932.
33. Volinn E, Turczyn KM, Loesser JD (1994): Patterns in low back hospitalizations: Implications for the treatment of low back pain in an era of health care reform. *Clin J Pain* 10:64–70.
34. Webster BS, Snook SH (1994): The cost of 1989 Workers' Compensation low back claims. *Spine* 19:1111–1116.
35. Williams ME, Hadler NM (1983): The illness as the focus of geriatric medicine. *N Engl J Med* 308:1357–1360.

The Adult Spine: Principles and Practice,
2nd edition, J.W. Frymoyer, Editor-in-Chief.
Lippincott-Raven Publishers, Philadelphia © 1997.

CHAPTER 5

Managing the Quality of Care for Low Back Pain

Dennis A. Plante, Marilyn G. Rothwell, and Henry M. Tufo

One of the major issues affecting medicine today is the balance between cost and quality. Health care policy and control mechanisms are being established by government and insurance companies as a means to slow what is perceived as an unsustainable growth rate of health care costs. Industry and organized patient advocacy groups have also become major players in determining the type of medical care that will be delivered as well as the method of financing that care. The medical community finds itself less and less in control of policy and direction of patient care; yet the providers are ultimately held responsible for clinical outcomes.

In this context, patients with spinal disorders (particularly those with low back pain) are major contributors to health care costs (10). As pointed out in Chapter 8, spinal disorders affect a very large segment of the population and result in enormous socioeconomic consequences. It is not surprising that the prevention, diagnosis, and treatment methods of these conditions are coming under greater scrutiny. How does the physician maintain reasonable control of patient care while playing a positive

role in addressing the important socioeconomic issues (9)? We believe the answer lies in implementing explicit and measurable quality improvement systems. It is the purpose of this chapter to demonstrate how quality improvement systems can be applied to the care of patients presenting with spinal disorders. It is not our intent to present a comprehensive analysis of all spinal or low back problems. Rather, we have chosen the most common example, nonspecific acute low back pain (LBP) presenting in a primary care practice, as an example that can be applied to other aspects of back care (16).

QUALITY IMPROVEMENT

An Overview

Most providers and consumers of health care are familiar with the concept of quality assurance. In this model, outcomes are measured against a standard to eliminate or at least to recognize a suboptimal quality. This type of quality assurance, which relies on inspectors who have had limited experience in medical practice, is often seen by professionals as wasteful and counterproductive. In the progressive industrial sector, there has been a shift away from this narrow definition of quality because it has not been effective in motivating continuous improvement. These progressive industries have replaced it with a dynamic approach based on the concept of meeting customer needs without error. Moreover, en-

D. A. Plante, M.D.: Associate Professor of Medicine, University of Vermont; Given Health Care Center, Williston, Vermont, 05495.

M. G. Rothwell, R.N.C.: Given Health Care Center; Clinical Assistant Professor in Medicine, University of Vermont, Burlington, Vermont, 05401.

H. M. Tufo, M.D.: Given Care Center; Professor of Medicine, University of Vermont, Burlington, Vermont, 05401.

lightened managements in service and manufacturing industries seek to have a quality ethic permeate and improve all levels of the production process, a concept known as total quality management (TQM).

TQM is a "top down" commitment of an organization to define, measure, and implement a series of changes to ensure continuous quality improvement (CQI). The methods and tools required for TQM/CQI are based on quantitative statistics, which should easily become assimilated by physicians and other health care providers.

A central feature of TQM/CQI is termed the Shewhart P-D-C-A cycle (plan, do, check, act). In working on any area for improvement, an organization needs to develop a plan of action, do (or implement) the plan, check (that is, measure and analyze) the plan for the desired outcomes, and act to either revise the plan or to more broadly adopt it. Based on the feedback derived from monitoring quantitative and statistical information, the processes can be improved by removing variance, reducing errors, reducing unnecessary cost, and improving productivity.

An important principle of TQM/CQI is the empowering of all people involved in the process to contribute to change. In this context, LBP care is seen as a process built on a series of steps, which allows us to examine just how the steps should come together. Each step is designed to achieve error-free progress towards the desired outcomes. Many of the breakthroughs waiting to be discovered lie ultimately in the hands of the people who control a single step in the process of LBP care. Attaining outcomes of high quality depends not only on the overall process design, but also on the single inputs and outputs that occur between the individual steps.

The underlying working principle of the TQM/CQI process is understanding and controlling variance. All processes produce variance to a greater or lesser extent. Variance may be inherent in the process itself (*common variance*), caused by failure to follow the process steps (*special* or *attributable variance*), or it may result from uncontrolled influences (*random variance*). An example of random variance can be found when there is a genetic predisposition towards an illness or a particular type of response to therapy. When variations in pain control are accompanied by an unexpected, significant rate of serious side effects from a new anti-inflammatory medication, only monitoring will tell whether the variance inherent in the process (common variance) is acceptable or not. If the outcome, or rate of complication, is not always acceptable, the process must be modified to make it acceptable. Examples of special or attributable variance in medicine are the failure to transfer correct information about pain treatments or the failure to identify pertinent coexistent medical illnesses that influence the response to treatment. Such omissions often may lead to repetitive testing or a poor patient outcome.

One of the first tasks in any quality control system is to locate and eliminate special variance. The second is to continuously refine the process to reduce random variance. Continuous attention to the process and its outcomes should lead, over time, to quantum improvements in the process—breakthroughs that produce significant reductions in errors and marked reductions in costs.

Once such a system is in place, several attributes for success quickly become clear. Requirements must be clearly set forth. Every step in the process must be visible, explicit, and understood or there will be no way to track down and eliminate errors. In this context, the definition of quality is nothing more or less than conformance to requirements established by practitioners and their customers, patients, referring physicians, insurers, and, ultimately, society. In order to conform to these requirements, a specific, repeatable process must be in place. Only then is assessment of quality possible.

Translation to Patient Care

To demonstrate how we can transfer these techniques to patient care, we will discuss our experience with a quality improvement project for LBP within our multispecialty group practice. We studied the problem in our clinics and discovered substantial variance in the use of resources such as x-ray tests and medications as well as lack of clarity in documenting important elements of the clinical evaluation and outcomes. We assembled staff and provider teams to collaborate on a plan for managing the quality of LBP care. We have instituted an initial CQI plan and evaluated it, and we now propose a format that can be adopted for any location.

Planning for Change

We will use the FOCUS version of the Shewhart Cycle in planning for change (Fig. 1). In originating a plan, we begin with the following steps:

Find a process to improve. In this case, it is the evaluation and initial management of patients with acute LBP presenting to their primary care providers.

Organize a team of knowledgeable people. Pick people who can develop the relevant clinical hypotheses about how to diagnose, treat, and assess results in the care of patients with LBP. The team should include those with knowledge about implementing LBP care and others with knowledge about methods of measuring the results.

Clarify the process. Outline the interactions among the various providers who rely on one another in the evaluation and management of patients. This step includes developing both an inventory of information and services patients currently have available and an idealized array of opportunities one hopes to develop for them.

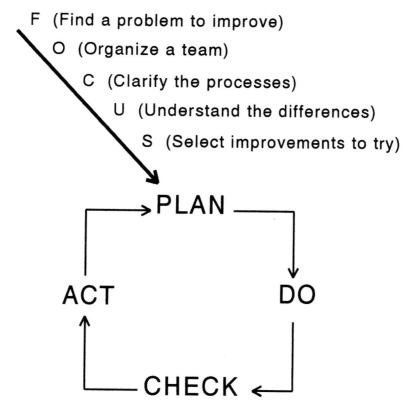

F (Find a problem to improve)
O (Organize a team)
C (Clarify the processes)
U (Understand the differences)
S (Select improvements to try)

FIG. 1. FOCUS variation of the Plan-Do-Check-Act cycle of Shewhart.

Understand the differences between the current care processes and the desired guidelines. To do so requires data to be gathered to understand the needs, expectations, and capabilities of the customers and suppliers in the process.

Establish quality outcome goals and select actions (known as key quality factors) that will meet the goals. In our own project, we started by defining quality outcome goals for a patient coming to the ambulatory practice with acute, nontraumatic back pain. Our goals included:

1. To limit bed-rest disability to 2 days (plus or minus 1).
2. To limit work disability to 7 days (plus or minus 1).
3. To not miss a serious life- or function-threatening disorder.
4. To prevent recurrences, within limits of what is known.
5. To control resource use; to achieve the first four goals as efficiently as possible.

Next, we established key quality factors that should lead us to achieve these goals.

1. Instructions to patient to have bed rest with movement, avoid sitting, and stop bed rest by day 3.
2. Instructions to patient and communications with company employer and supervisor about expected recovery.

3. Establishment of data base (history/physical examination/lab data) that will identify possible tumor, infection, fracture, future or present progressive neurologic defect, bladder/bowel dysfunction, or evidence of sciatica that will alter the recovery.
4. Establishment of educational program for patient (low back school) and work place–related education (see Chapter 16).

Select the improvements. The plan for achieving the quality goals needs to be developed. The concept of quality functional deployment defines the process of integrating customer needs and expectations with professional knowledge about what is achievable. We chose to accomplish this by designing a clinical algorithm. An algorithm is a clinical approach based on current knowledge of how diagnosis and treatment planning should proceed. It includes the decision options determined by the present condition of the patient and available resources to achieve these options (Figs. 2,3,4). An essential step is to document the algorithm to assure that the knowledge base is current and to provide the scientific clinical basis for the process steps (see Appendix A).

Algorithms are like any other medical device—they must be tested and redesigned on the basis of actual outcomes. This feature is an exciting aspect of quality improvement, because it provides the opportunity to turn practice into a learning laboratory while it improves the care of patients.

In other words, to manage quality, the clinical team must develop a uniform approach to the steps to take in diagnosing, treating, and following through on the diagnosis and treatment of patients with LBP. The approach must be agreed to by all users and then incorporated into the practice at each step of care. To help eliminate variation, tools such as standardized encounter or evaluation forms should be developed.

Do

With the algorithm completed, the team needs to create the system specifications and tools to facilitate each step of the process. Specifications are explicit, measurable statements of both the output goals and the (sub)-processes that will accomplish these goals. Specifications are the basis for managing quality because they are framed in terms of expectations of what is supposed to happen to meet the needs of the customer (the patient). When these specifications are achieved, quality is, by definition, present. Our team's next action, therefore, was to create the processes for providing care consistent with the algorithm.

The algorithm must be organized into actions that can be incorporated into the real-time work of the clinic. For example, to diagnose an infection masquerading as LBP requires that certain data base items be obtained: (a) a patient history of significant night pain; (b) risk factors such as steroid use, drug abuse, immunodeficiency, or recent urinary tract instrumentation; or (c) a history of systemic indicators of infection, such as chills, fever, weight loss, malaise.

To help achieve the specifications of the algorithm, we developed an acute care medical evaluation form that incorporates algorithm-based data and indications for diagnostic testing or specialty referral (Figs. 2–9). The designers of the tools (described in the section on Tools for Quality Care) need to work closely with the users (medical staff and providers) so that the tools reflect the users' own recommendations for an efficient, accurate clinical process.

Other specifications need to be incorporated into a process, such as appointment time, instructions for appointment secretaries, and educational material for patients. To help with documenting process problems in referring patients for specialty care, we developed a measurement/referral form. This tool has real value for primary care providers because it facilitates instructions to the secretaries about the type of referral to set up, with whom, and when, as well as what information must be transmitted to the specialist. The secretaries document on this form any process problems that may have occurred. A similar tool was created for the specialist, in which the specialty secretary documents the nature of the referral, whether the referral information was transmitted, and whether the provider evaluating the patient feels that the patient referral was appropriate or not.

Check

Remove *inappropriate variation.* Setting a goal of achieving 100% success in quality outcomes requires measuring progress toward that goal and documenting reasons that it has not been attained. TQM attempts to prevent mistakes by implementing those process steps that will prevent mistakes. However, we all know ideal outcomes may not occur even if we do everything right. Sometimes variation in outcome is unavoidable because we do not have the knowledge to prevent it. A major issue today in preventing recurrences of LBP is learning how to improve the process.

Checking uncovers quality output failures and inappropriate variations caused by failure to follow the process correctly. Getting rid of inappropriate variance may mean changing the process (for example, by designing new tools) so that the process steps can more easily be followed. Reviewing each case to see if the process is being used uncovers the sources of variation that need to be changed. Making the process more efficient increases adherence to the process specifications.

Once the process is clearly working and being followed, outcomes need to be measured to see if poor outcomes can be traced to specific components of the process. For example, patient education programs may not be clearly understood by patients or, indeed, it may be found the information was not handed out to patients at all. Once all inappropriate variation is removed, what remains is random or common variation. At this point, decreased variation in outcome (improved achievement of quality goals) or better productivity (goals achieved at lower cost) depends on experimenting with the process itself. Unfortunately, there will be times when it is not possible to control the application of key quality factors. For example, the patient may be ready to return to work but the employer may not be willing to make a workplace modification to enable the return.

The cost of checking is often mentioned as a real barrier for implementing TQM/CQI projects. However, as market changes to managed care occur, the cost of checking will become an important investment to ensure that health-care dollars are being spent wisely. We have been fortunate to have a college undergraduate statistician working with us to measure the initial outcomes following implementation of our low back pain CQI project.

Experience with Low Back Care Quality in Practice

We assume that the use of the acute care form (ACF) for LBP care is a key quality indicator, and as seen in

Table 1, we found the use of the ACF was poor early in the study (in June and July). The use of the ACF by providers ranged from 0% to 100%, a problem largely explained by inconsistent availability of the actual ACF at the different practice sites (attributable variance).

We then compared the outcomes of patients who were evaluated either by providers using the ACF or by providers not using the ACF (non-ACF). An important problem affecting the comparability of the two populations was that medical record documentation was incomplete in the non-ACF patients. Of the 197 variables contained in the ACF, 127 variables (64%) were more significantly commented on in the ACF patients than in the non-ACF patients. Most of these differences in responses resulted from negative responses in the ACF patients.

Only a small subset of the variables contained in the ACF were considered "essential" or "cannot afford to miss" items. Table 2 compares the frequency of responses of a subset of 38 essential variables. Again, the amount of information contained for the ACF patients was significantly greater than for the non-ACF patients. It is important to note in Table 2 that even with the ACF patients, the response rates (positive or negative) to important essential variables (such as strength, straight-leg raising, or deep tendon reflex variables) were far lower than the anticipated 100% rate.

Eleven percent of patients had lumbosacral (LS) spine x-rays performed after their initial primary care visit; the results of approximately half of the tests were missing in the medical records. Ultimately, 22% of patients had LS spine x-rays performed by the primary care provider. Only 2.4% of patients had computed tomography (CT)

scans ordered at their initial primary care visit, but eventually 11% of patients had CT scans. No patient had magnetic resonance imaging (MRI) scans performed after the initial visit; ultimately, 7.3% of patients had MRI scanning.

The patient population was also examined for underutilization and overutilization of radiological procedures. Ten percent of the patients had at least one indication for LS spine x-rays. Of these 10%, 60% had the x-rays performed, 40% did not (i.e., potential 40% underutilization of LS spine x-rays). Of the 90% of the patient population without an indication for LS spine x-rays, 8.7% had x-rays performed (representing a potential 8.7% overutilization of LS spine x-rays). Approximately 3% of patients had indications for CT/MRI scanning; however, none of these patients had the scans performed. Of the 97% of patients without CT/MRI scan indications, 3% actually had the scans performed. These data indicate possible underutilization and minimal overutilization of CT/MRI scanning. The overall frequency of obtaining a radiologic test is down from a preCQI project value of 41% (measured 2 years previously).

Availability of specialty referral was not documented as a process problem by the primary care staff. The specialty staff documented missing medical record information as the one process problem from primary care referring providers. Only one patient (5.6%) was felt by the specialists to have been inappropriately referred for evaluation.

A subgroup of 24 patients seen within the primary care practices were administered a telephone questionnaire approximately 4 to 6 weeks after their initial visit. Using a 10-point pain scale (0 = no pain, 10 = maximal possible pain), the average pain was 2.8 (range 0 to 9) during the week before the questionnaire, compared to 5.6 at the time of the initial visit ($p < 0.01$). Patients also rated the effectiveness of the care provided at their first visit on a 10-point scale (0 = ineffective, 10 = maximal effectiveness). The average rating was 6.4, with 29% of respondents indicating ratings of 10.

The majority of patients (83.3%) were primarily concerned with pain relief at their initial visit; 20% of patients reported dissatisfaction with the care they received for pain relief. Ninety percent of patients felt it was important to understand why their back pain had developed, and 92% of patients were satisfied with the explanations provided by the physicians.

Of those reporting, 22.2% were not able to work at the time of their initial visit, and all of these patients felt that the care they received had helped them return to work. No patients indicated that they were out of work because of back disability at the follow-up. Thirty-eight percent of patients expressed a desire for testing to be done at the initial visit but all were satisfied with the level of testing done over the course of their visits. This 38% contrasts

TABLE 1. *Non-use of the acute care form by provider and month*

Provider	% Non-use (total no. of patients)	Month	% Non-use per month
A	100 (2)	June	78.8
B	25 (8)	July	42.9
C	0 (9)	August	14.3
D	25 (4)	September	31.8
E	0 (1)	October	0
F	0 (2)	November	25
G	67 (6)	December	4.2
H	75 (4)	January	11.1
I	6 (16)	February	6.3
J	0 (9)	March	0
K	25 (12)		
L	55 (11)		
M	25 (4)		
N	0 (4)		
O	0 (5)		
P	6 (16)		
Q	10 (10)		

TABLE 2. *"Cannot afford to miss" parameters with and without the acute care form (ACF)*

Parameter	ACF (% evaluated)	Non-ACF (% evaluated)	Fisher's p value
Thigh pain radiation	78.8	36.0	<.0001
Calf pain radiation	67.4	16.0	<.0001
Pain affected by:			
Lying	84.7	12.0	<.0001
Sitting	88.8	12.0	<.0001
Standing	86.7	16.0	<.0001
Walking	82.7	12.0	<.0001
Bending	38.8	0	<.0001
Morning	74.5	0	<.0001
Night	66.3	4.0	<.0001
Bladder/bowel incontinence	86.7	12.0	<.0001
Workers' Compensation	38.3	8.0	.002
Disability/legal issues	30.6	0	.0003
Patient expectations:			
Pain relief	43.9	0	<.0001
Return of function	21.4	0	<.0001
Return to work	16.3	0	.0014
Testing	6.1	0	<.0001
Explanation of problem	19.4	0	.0012
Back examination:			
Extension	71.4	16.0	<.0001
Flexion	72.5	20.0	<.0001
Right/left bending	61.2	12.0	<.0001
Pain with axial loading	41.8	8.0	.0008
Strength testing:			
Knee bending	57.1	28.0	.0083
Heel walking	59.2	36.0	.032
Toe walking	55.1	36.0	.069
Deep tendon reflexes:			
Knee	68.4	32.0	.0011
Ankle	65.3	28.0	.0008
Straight leg raising:			
Seated	54.1	52.0	.514
Supine	69.4	48.0	.04
Return office visit:			
As needed	55.1	28.0	.013
1 week	21.4	16.0	.385
Therapy:			
Pain prescription	33.7	36.0	.697

with the 13.4% of patients who underwent x-ray testing after their initial visit.

The initial results of this QIP indicate a number of encouraging observations. First, the general use of the algorithm and the ACF for LBP care have increased over time. The case reviews clearly show that patient information is more thoroughly collected and that the indications for testing and referrals are more easily documented when the acute care form is used for patient care. Second, although direct comparative data are missing, the current care process has resulted in a relatively low rate of radiologic services, especially following the initial patient visit. Importantly, patient satisfaction ratings are high despite low rates of x-ray tests, implying that pro-

viders are educating their patients about the appropriate use of x-ray tests. Third, the changes have resulted in a low process problem rate of 4% (mostly missing record documentation), and a low inappropriate patient referral rate of 5.6%. Fourth, patients being seen in the primary care practices for acute LBP appear to have good return of function and are satisfied with the care they received.

Act

Redesign and implement changes that will promote "breakthroughs" in improving quality. The more stable the system becomes (by removal of inappropriate variation), the more it is available for experimentation by testing new approaches, which will produce either better outcomes or the same outcomes at lower cost (improved productivity). For example, when we reviewed our initial experience with an earlier version of the ACF, we found that providers wanted to have space on the form for at least one follow-up office visit. The redesigned form has improved its utilization—providers can efficiently document and compare two office evaluations on one ACF.

The results of the outcomes analysis and new ideas are incorporated into the process and then measured to see what gains have occurred. In this way, we have found a practice system can become a laboratory for improving care.

Discussion

Our experience suggests that the approach described above is effective in managing and improving quality in patient care (3). To date, the experience in quality improvement projects is limited in the treatment of spinal disorders. However, Choler (7) showed that an explicit process did positively affect the outcome of LBP. In her study, comparisons were made between subsets of the population of Gothenberg, Sweden. One group was managed under an algorithm similar to the one proposed here, while the other received traditional management without an explicit treatment process. The results of these differing interventions demonstrated a significant improvement in recovery from acute back pain as measured by an earlier return to work for those patients participating in protocol care. Resource use was inversely related, with non–protocol care patients consuming five times more resources than protocol care patients. Similarly, the program utilized for industry by Wiesel (30) had an explicit algorithm. The results of that intervention in comparison to historic controls were reduced work loss, reduced surgery, and significant cost savings.

However, there are important differences in quality as it is defined here and quality exemplified by the tightly controlled laboratory studies of Choler and Wiesel. In both studies there were historic controls; comparisons could, therefore, be made between two different treatment outcomes. In a quality improvement program, the outcome is the commitment to achieve stated goals; the intellectual stimulation is the achievement of these goals. If they are not achieved, the identification of the cause of variance and its correction become the laboratory for further understanding. The most important point in the process is under the physician's control. What we have proposed is a system applicable to a practice setting where process is agreed to by the providers and staff and there is an explicit commitment to reducing variance

and monitoring results. Such a system forms the basis for an internal quality improvement program. In comparison, the data suggest that Continuing Medical Education models have failed to improve the quality of back care (4,5).

CAN MANAGING QUALITY SAVE MONEY?

The questions are, of course, whose money can be saved and how can the savings be measured. In conventional research containing a cost analytic component, treatment A is compared to treatment B. However, such studies may not take into account all of the indirect costs found in actual patient care encounters. Determining who benefits involves measurement of the economic indicators elaborated in Chapter 8. For example, industry can benefit through diminished lost work time and compensation payments, and the payer can benefit through reduced payments for medical expenses, nonmedical expenses, and patient benefits.

Can these economic gains be quantified? Given today's base of knowledge, the answer is probably no, as measured by strict economic criteria. However, an estimation of the order of magnitude of overall savings is possible even though the beneficiary cannot be determined. For example, consider Choler's study and the difference in results between the protcol and traditional treatment groups.

Let us assume the following information based on the epidemiology and costs of LBP:

1. Four to five percent of the population have an acute low back episode each year. In the United States, this would comprise approximately 10 million adults.
2. The annual costs of LBP are approximately 50 billion dollars, as shown by Frymoyer and Durett in Chapter 8. It is reasonable to assume from the literature that 80% of these costs relate to those who have low back pain–related disability of greater than 3 months' duration.
3. Using the stated goals of our program, we are able to achieve the same improvement in outcome at a cost approximately 20% cheaper than that achieved by Choler, despite the differences between Sweden and the United States in industry, labor, and socioeconomic climates.
4. There are no confounding factors in the distribution of the various health care costs, such as expensive imaging studies, hospital treatment, and surgery, and the patients are a fairly homogeneous mix.

On the basis of these assumptions we can calculate the following costs and savings in acute LBP care:

1. Annual costs attributed to the acute LBP subset: $50,000,000,000 × 0.20 = $10,000,000,000
2. Annual costs per person with acute (i.e., less than 7 weeks' duration) LBP: $10,000,000,000/10,000,000 = $1,000
3. Savings per annum: $2,000,000,000

This is admittedly a superficial analysis but it gives an order of magnitude. A far more extensive analysis and mathematical modeling approach has suggested savings in the order of 6 billion dollars by a modest reduction in LBP disability extending beyond 3 months (see Chapter 8).

Does the doctor benefit? Studies of the quality improvement model in enlightened nonmedical industries consistently demonstrate two economic findings. Improvements in quality are clearly linked to both enhancement of market share and increased savings in the

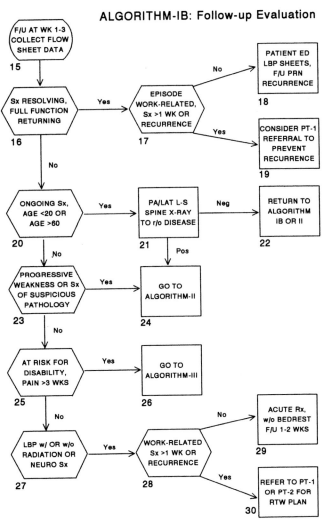

FIG. 3. Algorithm for follow-up evaluation of acute LBP. Reevaluate risk of progressive pain or neurologic symptoms versus return to full function.

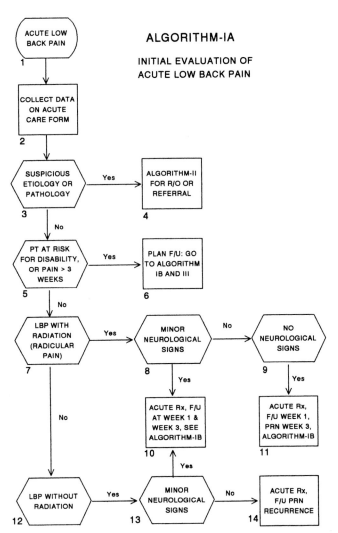

FIG. 2. Algorithm for the initial evaluation of acute LBP.

cost of producing a product or service. The greater the improvement in quality (fewer mistakes, less waste), the greater the efficiency. We contend that if the doctor gains financially from productivity gains (improved efficiency) rather than from resource utilization (more x-rays, more visits, etc.), then managing quality in this way will benefit the doctor, particularly in a managed care environment. More important, if a goal of medical care is to predictably improve outcomes for patients, then this approach is of critical importance to doctors. The quality improvement model described here is the basis for all outcome studies because fixing a process reveals the causal relationships of process to outcome. For example, failure to return to full activity within 30 days and failure to provide the necessary educational program to the patient may be linked.

SUMMARY

We have presented a translation of industrial quality improvement techniques to the care of LBP. The goals of this approach are improved outcomes for patients, high productivity (outcome goals achieved at lowest resource consumption), and efficiency for the practice. The key factors that make quality improvement work are identifying specifications of patient requirements, developing processes that achieve the requirements, committing to measurement of outcomes, removing inappropriate variance, and improving outcome attainment over time.

Quality theory is not magic. It is powerful mainly because it corresponds so well with the way most people function best: they want to do well, they need reliable feedback about the outcome of their efforts, and they need opportunities to do better. There are publications for those interested in understanding the many techniques used to design, monitor, and improve quality (1,8,15,21,27).

TOOLS FOR QUALITY CARE: ACUTE LBP PROTOCOL, ENCOUNTER FORM, REFERRAL FORM, AND PATIENT EDUCATION

Establishing Requirements and Specifications

As we have shown, quality care first defines a process that unites skillful individual performance with the best medical knowledge and then establishes a system to repeat the process consistently. The enduring value of the problem-oriented medical system, first described by Weed in 1969 (28), is reaffirmed as it provides the frame-

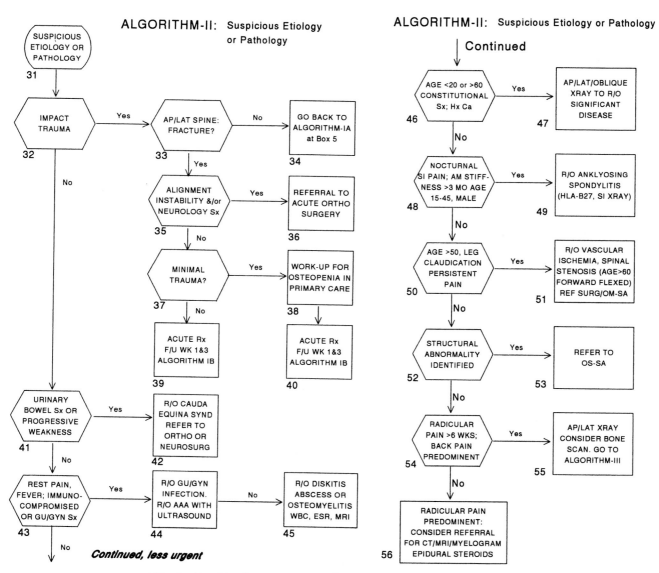

FIG. 4. Algorithm for assessment of suspicious etiology or pathology.

work for the information system in caring for acute LBP (20,24). A clinical data base of subjective (S) and objective (O) information leads to an assessment (A) about the nature of back pain which, in turn, is linked to plans (P) for follow-up and therapy. When outcomes are measured and the process is checked, we complete a cycle that matches Shewhart's Plan-Do-Check-Act.

The protocol, prepared by a small group and approved for practice-wide use by consensus of the entire group of clinicians responsible for low back care, serves as a reference to the critical knowledge about that condition. It consists of three algorithms, documented with annotations and a bibliography, that graphically illustrate each clinical step of the care process. Algorithm IA (Fig. 2) establishes the initial data base and triage decisions. Algorithm IB (Fig. 3) guides through a follow-up visit, while Algorithms II (Fig. 4) and III (Fig. 5) cover steps to identify suspicious pathology and risk for disability and recurrence, respectively. In quality improvement terms, each step (or box) is a key quality factor which, in turn, consists of specifications. To ensure that each specification will be part of the patient encounter, we have pre-

pared a comprehensive ACF (Fig. 6). It is the paper information tool that simultaneously directs the treatment and captures the data during the care process. It becomes a record of the encounter, a referral note, and the source for quality analysis. Patient education sheets (Figs. 7,8) provide uniform information on the nature of the problem, when to call for additional help, how to help recovery, and how to prevent recurrence. They assure the patient that he or she is part of the quality team.

There is also the referral form (Fig. 9) developed jointly by primary and specialty care providers and their scheduling teams. It specifies the indications for referral and identifies the appropriate specialty provider. Copies of the referral form and encounter form serve as the referral note, eliminating the need for dictation.

A word about the future. The information tool we are preparing for is a computerized record and knowledge base. Although the paper model establishes the principles of quality improvement, the computer with an information organizing system such as problem knowledge coupling (29) allows us to fully apply quality improvement to health care.

ALGORITHM-III: At Risk for Disability or Recurrence

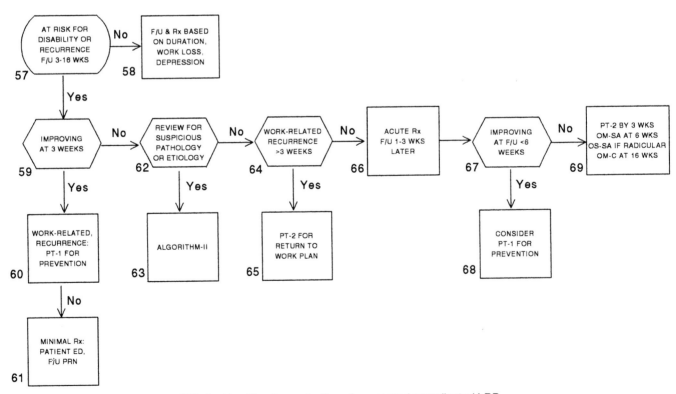

FIG. 5. Algorithm for evaluation of suspected complicated LBP.

SUBJECTIVE   Response Key: ⊞ Positive   ⊟ Negative   ☐ Not Evaluated

Initial Visit Date: _____

CC: _____
_____

HOW (trauma?[5]): _____
_____
_____
_____

DURATION: _____

PAIN: ☐ constant ☐ episodic
LOCATION: _____

RADIATES ☐ thigh ☐ calf/foot

	Worse	Better	No Effect
Lying			
Sitting			
Standing			
Walking			
Bending			
Morning			
Night			

THERAPY
Meds (names)
_____
_____
_____

Bed Rest			
Exercises			
Phys Ther			

COURSE: 0-10 today: _____
0-10 at worse (date): _____

ASSOCIATED Sx[5]:
☐ fever: _____
☐ weakness: _____
☐ numbness: _____
☐ incontinent bladder/bowel[4]
☐ abdominal pain: _____
☐ leg edema
☐ rash: _____
☐ other: _____

NAME: _____
BIRTH DATE: _____
TELEPHONE: _____

	Initial Visit	F/U Visit
Paramedic		
Provider		

Follow-up Date: _____

CURRENT Sx: _____
_____
_____
_____
_____
_____
_____

PAIN: ☐ constant ☐ episodic
LOCATION: _____

RADIATES ☐ thigh ☐ calf/foot

	Worse	Better	No Effect
Lying			
Sitting			
Standing			
Walking			
Bending			
Morning			
Night			

Meds (names)
_____
_____
_____

Bed Rest			
Exercises			
Phys Ther			

COURSE 0-10 today: _____

ASSOCIATED Sx[5]
☐ fever: _____
☐ weakness: _____
☐ numbness: _____
☐ incontinence bladder/bowel[4]
☐ abdominal pain: _____
☐ leg edema
☐ rash: _____
☐ other: _____

ASSOCIATED Hx:
☐ Arthritis/gout: _____
☐ H/O Cancer[5]: _____
☐ Weight loss[5]: _____
☐ Recent UTI or GU procedure
☐ Diabetes[1]
☐ Compromised host[1]: _____
☐ Stress[3]: _____
☐ Pt feels downhearted and blue[3]?
☐ other: _____

PAST Hx of Back Pain:
☐ Prior episode: _____
☐ Prior tests/results: _____
_____
☐ Prior treatment: _____
_____
☐ Spinal surgery: _____

WORK Data: (*Complete if Sx affect work*)
Occupation[2]: _____
☐ Unable to work since: _____
Job requirements: _____
_____
☐ Prolonged sitting (hrs): _____
☐ Prolonged standing (hrs): _____
☐ Repetitive bending/twisting
☐ Lifting (max. weight): _____
Satisfied with job: ☐ yes ☐ no:
_____
Employer willing to modify job
requirements? ☐ yes ☐ no:
_____
Pt feels who's at fault for back pain?:
☐ Self ☐ Emplr ☐ Other: _____
☐ Workers Compensation injury?
☐ Disability[3] or legal issues?
☐ Prior work loss: _____
  (occupation then: _____)

PATIENT Expectations:
Initial Visit   F/U Visit
☐ pain relief   ☐
☐ return of function   ☐
☐ return to work   ☐
☐ tests: _____   ☐
☐ explanation of problem   ☐
☐ other: _____   ☐

PATIENT Concerns: _____

FIG. 6. Acute care form for LBP, subjective data (Given Health Care Centers).

OBJECTIVE

T_____ BP_____ P_____ WT_____

	Initial Visit	F/U Visit
BACK INSPECTION		
trunk position (list R/L?)	☐	☐
forward bending	☐	☐
scoliosis/kyphosis/gibbus	☐	☐
iliac crest uneven	☐	☐
gluteal fold drop	☐	☐
spasm (location):	☐	☐
exaggerated response[3]	☐	☐

MOTION (standing) (N°)

	Initial	F/U
extension (30°):	___°	___°
flexion (90°):	___°	___°
Right lateral bend:	___°	___°
Left lateral bend:	___°	___°
axial load/trunk turn pain[3]	☐	☐

STRENGTH (1-5+)

	R	L	R	L
knee bend (L4)	__	__	__	__
heel walk (L5)	__	__	__	__
toe walk (S1)	__	__	__	__

DTRs (0-4+) (sitting)

	R	L	R	L
knee (L4):	__	__	__	__
ankle (S1):	__	__	__	__

SENSATION (touch)

	R	L	R	L
medial leg (L4)	__	__	__	__
lat leg (L5)	__	__	__	__
lat foot (S1)	__	__	__	__

Leg Pulses: __ __   __ __

SLR (L5/S1)

	R	L	R	L
seated[3] (causes leg pain)	___°	___°	___°	___°
supine (causes leg pain)	___°	___°	___°	___°
ankle dorsiflexion worse:	☐	☐	☐	☐
kneebend relief:	☐	☐	☐	☐
contralateral pain:	☐	☐	☐	☐

FABER (Hip/SI joint):   ☐ ☐   ☐ ☐

Femoral stretch (L3-4)   ☐ ☐   ☐ ☐

	Initial	F/U
abdomen (If age >50):	___	___
bruit[5] or pulsatile mass[5]	___	___
prostate (men age >60):	___	___
other: _____	___	___

AFFECT:

		Initial	F/U
	flat/sad[3]	☐	☐
	anxious[3]	☐	☐
	angry[3]	☐	☐
		☐	☐

ASSESSMENT

	Neuro signs absent	Neuro signs present
LBP only	☐[a]	☐[b]
LBP + leg pain	☐[c]	☐[d]

☐[e] Recurrent/persistent, legal, disability[3], occupational risks[2]

☐[f] Suspicious pathology[5] type:

_____
_____
_____
_____

F/U: ☐Better ☐Same ☐Worse

_____
_____
_____

PLANS

GOAL(S):

	Initial Visit	F/U Visit
☐ Pain relief		☐
☐ Problem definition		☐
☐ Improved function		☐
☐ Rehabilitation/Prevention		☐

DIAGNOSIS (O indications):

☐ AP/Lat X-RAYS: ☐
  O H/O impact/trauma/osteopor
  O Age < 20 or > 60
  O Fever or cancer concerns
  O Compromised host
  O Back pain > 6 weeks
  O Recurrent LBP
  O Other: _____

☐ CT OR MRI SCAN: ☐
  O Suspect cauda equina syndr
  O LBP w/radiculopathy >6 wks
  O Age >60, ? spinal stenosis
  O Other: _____

☐ BONE SCAN: ☐
  O Suspect cancer or O infection
  O Ongoing LBP w/out radiation
  O Other: _____

OTHER TESTS:
☐ WBC ☐ ESR ☐ urinalysis
☐ EMG: _____
☐ Other: _____
  O Indication: _____

RETURN OFFICE VISIT:

Initial Visit	F/U Visit
☐ 1-3 weeks: leg pain[c,d], neuro signs[b,d], work-related/disability, legal risk[e,] suspicious pathology[f]	☐
☐ Other: _____	☐

PHYSICAL THERAPY:

☐ Self-help program [PT-1] (non-suspicious recurrent LBP)		☐
☐ Multidiscipline program [PT-2]		☐

  O Work-related O Disability risk
  O LBP duration > 3 weeks
  O Recurrent, non-specific LBP

☐ SPECIALTY REFERRAL: ☐
  O Fracture/alignment problem[OS-A]
  O Suspect cauda equina syndr[OS-A]
  O Osteomyelitis/diskitis[OS-A]
  O Tumor, primary/metastatic[OS-A]
  O HNP on CT→ epidural Rx[OM-A]
  O LBP ± neuro sx >6 wks[OM-SA]
  O Work-related disability[OM-SA]
  O Workers Comp/Legal[OM-SA]
  O Other: _____

THERAPY: ☐ Pain:_____   ☐
☐ Inflammation: _____   ☐
☐ Spasm: _____   ☐
☐ Other: _____   ☐

OCCUPATION-Related:
☐ Restrictions: _____   ☐
☐ Return to work: _____   ☐

PT ED INFO: ☐ LBP ☐ exercises

NOTATIONS/EXPLANATIONS

1. Compromised Host: *diabetes, HIV immunosuppressants, ETOH abuse, splenectomy*
2. Occupational risks: *repetitive lifting in bent/twisted position, lifting beyond capacity, vibration, prolonged sitting or standing, job dissatisfaction*
3. Waddell's signs: *constant non-anatomic regional pain, emotional descriptors, whole leg pain, numbness/weakness, treatment intolerance, seated SLR better than supine, pain on axial loading or trunk turning*
4. Neurological Signs: *localized weakness, reflex asymmetry, sensory loss, loss of bladder or bowel function (Cauda Equina Synd)*
5. Suspicious Path: *pain (steady, writhing, worsening, persisting at night), Cauda Equina Synd, progressive weakness, severe trauma, fever, abdominal pain, compromised host, Hx CA or wt loss, known spine dx, rash, leg edema*

FIG. 6. (*Continued*.) Remaining sections of acute care form for LBP (Given Health Care Centers).

GIVEN
HEALTH CARE CENTERS

PATIENT INFORMATION SERIES

One South Prospect Street   Burlington, Vermont 05401   802/656-4531

87 Main Street   Essex Junction, Vermont 05452   802/878-8354

310 Pine Street   Burlington, Vermont 05401   802/864-0383

2 Blair Park   Williston, Vermont 05495   802/872-1470

LOW BACK PAIN

Four out of five Americans endure low back pain at one time or another. 15% of the sufferers have complications such as severe injury, herniated (ruptured) disk, tumors, arthritis or other diseases of the spine. Your back evaluation checks for these defects or diseases that require special treatment. In the other 85%, the specific cause of pain is not known but may be related to muscle or ligament strain from stressful positions and poor posture.

HOW DOES LOW BACK PAIN HAPPEN?

The spine, a column of thirty-three bones (vertebrae) protects the cable of nerves running through its center (spinal cord). Each vertebra, which fits into the groove (facet) in the back of the vertebra below, is cushioned in the front by a spongy disk. The entire spine is supported by side muscles and ligaments. Any of these components can cause an attack of low back pain but even today's technology cannot always identify the exact cause of back pain.

The stressful situations that cause the pain are: repetitive lifting in a bent, twisted position; lifting beyond capacity; vibration exposure of machinery or vehicles; and staying in one position for prolonged periods. We also recognize that feelings and unhappiness from job or personal problems keep us tense; that means tight muscles and more strain leading to pain, pain that takes longer to heal. When the muscles are weak and unexercised, they don't provide the support the spine needs--nor the protection from pain.

When slouching, bending or lifting in a rounded back position, you lose lordosis. Lordosis is the hollow in the low back, the curve that is key to preventing and curing most low back pain.

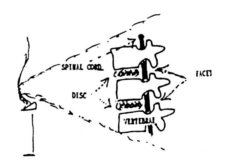

WHAT IS THE TREATMENT OF AN ATTACK OF LOW BACK PAIN?

Low back pain treatment reduces pain, spasm and inflammation, and allows you to resume normal activities as soon as possible. After recovery, the emphasis is on prevention of another attack with immediate home treatment if one does occur. Exercises, general body conditioning and proper lordosis position will increase back strength, flexibility and endurance. Working on stresses and adapting work positions or demands prevent continued strain.

Most people completely recover from low back pain within two weeks. Returning to work is good for the back as long as you can avoid the straining positions listed above. You may need to try light duty at first.

FIG. 7. Patient information sheet for LBP (Given Health Care Centers).

Immediate treatment is:

1) Up to 48 hours of lying flat on a firm surface may provide relief of pain. Surprisingly, pressure on the spine is higher when the head is propped to read or watch TV than when standing. More lying around isn't better; two days give as much benefit as seven days. Many experts feel absolute bed rest is not essential for healing. If rest doesn't relieve the pain or you can't take time to stay flat in bed, keep moving but do not lift, twist or stay in one position for more than a few minutes.

2) Try to keep the hollow in your back (lordosis) at all times by bending your knees and placing a small pillow or rolled towel around your waist when resting. Pain that worsens with lordosis may respond to lying on your side, knees to chest, and a rounded-out back.

3) Taking pain-killing, anti-inflammatory medication will relieve the discomfort and help you relax. Aspirin (2-3 tablets every 4-6 hours) or Ibuprofen (2 tablets every 6 hours) are usually effective. Be sure to take them with food or milk to avoid stomach irritation.

4) Local ice packs placed on top of your back for 15 minutes or so will often give pain relief. Heat that extends beyond your back such as a shower or bath is often more comforting than local heating pads. Use heat or ice to ease pain and start stretching.

5) When you can lie on the stomach with minimal pain, you should begin gentle stretching exercises as described on the exercise sheet. Of course you may have some pain as you begin to stretch and it's important to remember that moderate pain for short periods is a sign of stretching, not injury or permanent harm. Continuing exercises after the pain is over will help keep your back strong, flexible and free of pain. We can train you to get maximum benefit from the exercises.

WHEN TO CALL FOR AN APPOINTMENT

If you have been asked to return for an evaluation, please keep the appointment. If not, you should be rechecked when: you have pain, numbness or weakness that extends below your knees; the pain goes on longer than one week; you're having problems with the exercises; or you are not back to your previous level of activity by four weeks.

HOW TO AVOID ANOTHER ATTACK OF LOW BACK PAIN

In addition to a regular back and general exercise routine, you should follow some of these tips.

STANDING: Imagine being pulled up towards the ceiling by the top of your head. Keep shoulders relaxed and everything else should fall into line. During long periods of standing: shift your weight by leaning on one foot, then the other; put one foot up on a low stool or railing; do some twisting exercises from time to time; and avoid wearing high heels.

SITTING: Choose a chair with good height so that feet are flat on floor and hips and knees are at right angles. Support your back with a lumbar pillow or a rolled towel in the small of the back; support arms; change positions frequently; stand every half hour or so and do some standing back bends.

LIFTING: Use your legs and back; if you need to turn, pivot with your feet without twisting your back; keep feet wide apart and head up; and keep the load close to your body. If you've been sitting or riding for a long time, stretch before you lift.

SLEEPING: If you are comfortable when you sleep, don't change your position. If not, choose a firm mattress (water beds are not for everyone) and a pillow that supports your head and neck in a straight line. Placing a pillow under your knees may relieve the pressure on your back.

We recommend Robin McKenzie's TREAT YOUR OWN BACK published by Spine as a guide on back care.

FIG. 7. *Continued.*

GIVEN
HEALTH CARE CENTERS

PATIENT INFORMATION SERIES

One South Prospect Street	Burlington, Vermont 05401	802/656-4531
87 Main Street	Essex Junction, Vermont 05452	802/878-8354
310 Pine Street	Burlington, Vermont 05401	802/864-0383

EXERCISES FOR LOW BACK PAIN

Some of these stretching exercises may relieve your pain right away and all of them will help you recover from an attack of back pain. We now find that motion, not strict bed rest, is the treatment that will return you to full activity the fastest. Stretching is the safest way to start exercise; slow stretches with deep breathing to help relaxation are the best. You may have some discomfort when beginning a stretching program and improving your flexibility. Remember that short periods of aching are not a sign of harm; they're a sign that you're challenging and strengthening your muscles as you should be. If you are worried about the effect of the exercises, please call.
Choose a firm surface, exercise frequently (8-10 times a day) at first, then daily to keep flexible and prevent another attack.

EXTENSION

Lie on your stomach with your arms beside your body and your head turned to one side. Stay in this position for about 5 minutes, relaxing all muscles.

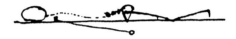

Raise your head up, support your upper body weight on your elbows for a count of 10 while your hips relax; then rest flat as above. Repeat, working up to 10 times. You may wish to hold this position longer at first.

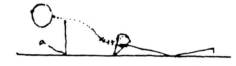

Still on your stomach, slowly raise your upper body until your arms are straight and your head as high as possible. This is a "press-up", not a push-up; all the lifting is above the hips. Work up to 10 press-ups per session, holding each for a count of 10.

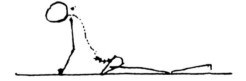

Stand upright with feet slightly apart, about shoulder width; place your hands in the small of your back; and bend backwards at your waist while keeping your legs as straight as possible. Hold for a count of 10, breathing in and out slowly, and then return to an upright position; repeat 10 times.

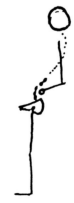

FIG. 8. Patient information sheet on exercises for LBP (Given Health Care Centers).

FLEXION

Lie on your back with knees bent up and feet flat on the floor or bed. Draw both knees up to your chest (it may be easier to do one at a time at first) and, with your hands, pull them slowly and firmly against your chest. Hold for a count of 10, then lower your legs without straightening your knees. Repeat 10 times.

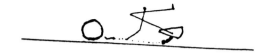

Sit on a firm chair, allow your back to slouch slightly for a count of 10, then sit up straight and hold a lordosis (hollow back) position for another count of 10. Repeat 15-20 times, remembering to breathe in and out slowly.

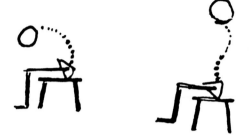

ROTATION

On your back with knees at chest and shoulders flat on floor with arms outstretched at shoulder level, roll your legs to rest on the floor at your left side. Hold for a count of 10, then bring your legs slowly, one at a time, to rest on the floor on the right side. Repeat 10 times.

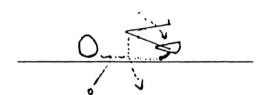

HOW TO AVOID ANOTHER ATTACK OF LOW BACK PAIN

In addition to a regular exercise routine, you should follow some of these tips.

STANDING: Imagine being pulled up toward to the ceiling by the top of your head. Keep shoulders relaxed and everything else should fall into line. During long periods of standing: shift your weight by leaning on one foot, then the other; put one foot up on a low stool or railing; do some twisting exercises from time to time; and avoid wearing high heels.

SITTING: Choose a chair with good height so that feet are flat on floor and hips and knees are at right angles. Support your back with a lumbar pillow or a rolled towel in the small of the back; support arms; change positions frequently; stand every half hour or so and do some standing back bends.

LIFTING: Use your legs and back; if you need to turn, pivot with your feet without twisting your back; keep feet wide apart and head up' and keep the load close to your body. If you've been sitting or riding for a long time, stretch before you lift.

SLEEPING: If you are comfortable when you sleep, don't change your position. If not, choose a firm mattress (water beds are not for everyone) and a pillow that supports your head and neck in a straight line. Placing a pillow under your knees may relieve the pressure on your back.

We recommend Robin McKenzie's **TREAT YOUR OWN BACK** published by Spine as a guide on back care.

FIG. 8. *Continued.*

LOW BACK PAIN REFERRAL MEASUREMENT FORM

Patient Name: _____ Patient DOB: _____ Today's Date: _____

PROVIDER SECTION: ## INDICATIONS FOR REFERRAL

OS-A   (Orthopedic Surgery (Krag, Grobler)—acute: requires prompt referral)
○ Impact trauma with fracture/alignment problem
○ Bladder/bowel dysfunction (?cauda equina) or progressive neuromotor sx
○ Other: _____

OS-SA (Orthopedic Surgery, sub-acute: referral needed within 1-2 weeks)
○ Structural abnormality identified on x-ray (e.g., spinal stenosis)
○ Other: _____

OS-C   (Orthopedic Surgery, chronic: referral without time constraints)
○ _____

OM-A   (Orthopedic Medicine (Hazzard, Talley, Gryzb), acute: prompt access)
○ Suspect facet syndrome (unremitting lordotic pain), evaluate for facet injection
○ Herniated disk with ongoing sx, no major neuromotor signs (consider epidural Rx)
○ Other: _____

OM-SA (Orthopedic Medicine, sub-acute: referral within 1-2 weeks)
○ Disability risk/legal case/work-related
○ Ongoing LBP signs/sx at 6 weeks
○ Other: _____

OM-C   (Orthopedic Medicine, chronic: time less critical for referral)
○ Ongoing LBP ≥16 weeks, for Rehab Program Evaluation
○ Other: _____

PT-1   (SpINE Self-Care Program): 1-3 visits over 4-6 weeks
○ Recurrent, non-specific LBP, signs/sx improving ≤3 weeks follow-up
○ Stress/depression-related, signs/sx still present ≥1 week F/U
○ Other: _____

PT-2   (SpINE Multidisciplinary Program): 12-15 visits over 4-6 weeks
○ Disability risk/legal case/work-related, signs/sx present ≥1 week F/U
○ Recurrent, non-specific LBP with signs/sx ≥3 weeks of follow-up
○ Other: _____

REFERRAL INSTRUCTIONS

Time for Referral: ○ ASAP   ○ 1-2 weeks   ○ 3-6 weeks   ○ >6 weeks

Copy/send to SpINE: ○ Acute care flow sheet   ○ Office notes from (date): _____
○ Problem List   ○ Other: _____

SECRETARY SECTION

Referral made (who, where, when): _____

Process Problems: _____

FIG. 9. Referral form from primary to specialty care (Given Health Care Centers).

APPENDIX A: DOCUMENTING THE PROCESS, ANNOTATIONS TO THE ALGORITHMS AND ACUTE CARE FORM

I. Algorithm IA: Initial evaluation of acute LBP (Fig. 2); using the acute care form (Fig. 6)

A. Box #1: Symptoms of acute LBP. Pain in the low back area (extending from the lower rib cage margin to the gluteal folds) arises from problems that may be classified on at least one of three levels. The levels are not mutually exclusive (12).

1. "Can't afford to miss" or "suspicious for medical pathology," including fracture, tumor, infection (spinal or visceral), intra-abdominal condition, progressive neurological deficit (limb or bladder/bowel), age over 60 or under 20.

2. "Recommend follow-up" or "suspicious for potential disability," including pain continuing longer than 3 to 6 weeks, recurrence of pain, sciatica with or without neurologic signs, positive Waddell's symptoms, occupational risks (25,26).

3. Self-limited and uncomplicated: nonspecific acute back pain with or without sciatica, but without major neurologic signs.

B. Box #2: Acute care form data.

1. Subjective information: Here are the key questions that characterize the pain and lead to assessment of possible cause. We expect 100% of items to be completed and provide the key of [+], [−], and [□] to allow quick recording of findings.

a. Chief complaint: How pain originated or manner of onset. This is an opportunity to present the patient's own description of the pain and how it began (12). Traumatic origin leads directly to "suspicious for pathology," Algorithm II. Emotional descriptors of pain may suggest an inappropriate response, one of Waddell's signs that leads to Algorithm III (25,26). Onset that is gradual is more suspicious than a sudden attack.

b. Duration: Classified as acute (<1 week), subacute (1 to 7 weeks), chronic (>7 weeks) (22). Although the initial evaluation of LBP of any duration begins with this review, 3 weeks of pain with little response to therapy automatically places the patient into the "suspicious" algorithms.

c. Constant/episodic: Intense, steady, writhing quality suggests back pain secondary to visceral infection or vascular cause (13). Constant, unrelieved pain without injury may also suggest a nonorganic cause (25).

d. Location: Location of pain varies with age: young, L5-S1; middle, L4-L5; older, L3-L4 (6). Nonorganic pain may extend over a wide area, whereas organic pain is usually in the specific and localized pattern of dermatomes (14).

e. Radiation to thighs or calves/feet: Sciatica is radicular pain along the nerve root. Neurologic claudication, often more generalized pain, is exacerbated by walking and relieved by spinal flexion. Both may be accompanied by numbness and weakness (12). Vascular claudication after walking is relieved by rest. Radiation to a regional area or entire limb suggests nonorganic origins (26).

f. Worse/better/no effect: Lying, sitting, standing, moving by walking, moving by bending, during inactivity, absent at night, and morning stiffness. Mechanical pain increases with motion, sitting, or standing, and lessens with rest (22). Pain with extension suggests facet origin while pain with flexion is usually from disc herniation, muscles, or ligaments. Pain persisting at rest suggests infection, tumor, or other bone disease (13). Ankylosing spondylitis pain worsens at rest, improves with exercise and is associated with morning stiffness (22). Nonorganic pain rarely responds to position changes (25).

g. Therapy: List measures (heat, rest, exercise, or medications) tried and their effects. Intolerance or failure of all therapies suggests nonorganic cause and inappropriate response (25).

h. Course: Ask patient to rate intensity of pain (1 = least, 10 = most) at this time and at its worst.

i. Associated symptoms: See notations under "suspicious for pathology" or "disability." Fever: Rule out (r/o) infectious cause. Sensory loss and/or weakness: Give location, asking patient to specify the nerve root or affected area on diagram. Incontinent bowel/bladder control: Known as cauda equina syndrome, increasing neuromotor deficit suggests epidural abscess or hemorrhage, intra- or extradural tumor, massive herniation (13). Abdominal pain: Visceral or vascular problem likely to be primary cause of pain (pyelonephritis, prostatitis, endometriosis, aortic aneurysm, pancreatitis) (13). Edema of legs: Consider venous thrombosis. Rash: Herpes zoster if along dermatome, or psoriasis rash accompanying psoriasis arthritis.

j. Associated history (19): Arthritis may involve the back, as in ankylosing spondylitis. Cancer/unexplained weight loss: r/o neoplasm/metastasis. Recent urinary tract infection (UTI) or genitourinary (GU) procedure: r/o UTI.

k. Compromised host (diabetes, immunosuppressants, HIV-positive, splenectomy, malnourishment, ethanol abuse): Increased risk of infection. Age under 20 or over 60: Back pain more likely a sign of systemic disease than regional backache (12). Stress: Disability risk. Downhearted/blue: The Medical Outcomes Study (MOS) (2,23) demonstrated that a five-item version of the Mental Health Inventory was effective in detecting most depression, affective, and anxiety disorders. The most powerful nonspecific detector for all of the five diagnostic clusters is this single question, which is included as a screen.

l. Past history of back problems: Prior episode/surgery/treatment/testing: 40% to 85% of LBP sufferers will have recurrence; prior disability predicts future disability and warrants early referral to physical therapy (PT). Plan follow-up to identify disability, reinforce preventive measures, or refer for multidisciplinary preventive measures (12).

m. Occupational history: Identify occupation. Note extent of interference with current activity, notably "unable to work," and duration. Estimate mechanical stress from occupation with approximate weight lifted regularly (or even occasionally), hours in sitting position, and tasks of repetitive motion, especially bending and twisting (12). Job satisfaction and possible job modification become critical if pain is prolonged.

  i. Workers' Compensation, disability, or legal issues: First, elicit patient's perception of fault for pain. If there are work or legal concerns, plan follow-up to promote return to full function and coordinate with em-

ployer as needed. Additional information required for employer, insurance agent, or attorney reviewing Workers' Compensation: Description of preinjury activities as baseline for future activity; preinjury status of prior injury or periods of disability; description of injury including location, time, and probable cause; postinjury treatment documentation; current status describing situation at the time of the primary evaluation or at later consultation. A back-to-work assessment should be completed. Detect pattern of prior work loss and occupation at that time.

  ii. Patient concerns and expectations: Record desire to return to work, alter job, or other concerns beyond pain relief. Successful planning depends upon agreement with goals of therapy.

2. Objective data: Each test or examination listed is required for a complete evaluation.

  a. Document vital signs.

  b. Back inspection: Area of inspection extends from costovertebral angle (CVA) along the spinous processes to the coccyx; it includes the interspinous ligaments, adjacent paravertebral muscles and iliac crests, sacroiliac junction and ligaments, and gluteal fold. Inspect while patient stands as erect as possible, noting trunk position (list or forward bend) if unable to stand erect. Extreme scoliosis (lateral curvature of the spine) and extreme lordosis (flattening or exaggeration of lumbar curve) contribute to mechanical LBP. Kyphosis (extreme thoracic convexity) is typical of osteoporosis, increased risk of fracture, and Scheuermann's disease. Gibbus (angular projection) is a sign of collapsed vertebrae. Iliac crests should be level, usually at the L4 point. Gluteal fold curvature should be symmetrical (12,22). Palpate and inspect for spasm: Note exaggerated response to exam as one of Waddell's signs.

  c. Motion/neurologic testing [nerve root tension, deep tendon reflex (DTR), and motor power]: Test to the point that pain commences (not to limit of endurance) to detect limitation of motion. Note degree of arc when pain appears; it is a protective mechanism that prevents further stretching of injured structures (12,22). Unlimited motion predicts a return to full function.

   i. Standing position testing: Extension (backward bend with legs straight and examiner supporting the lumbar spine) is usually possible to 30°, and flexion (forward bend with slight knee bend if necessary), to at least 90°. In unilateral radicular pain, the knee on the affected side will flex to relieve hamstring spasm and tilting of the pelvis. Lateral bending is limited by unilateral radiculopathy (12).

  ii. Two simulated tests (for Waddell's signs) that will not usually produce pain with organic cause, but may with nonorganic cause, are trunk turn (examiner slightly rotates hips and thorax as a unit; shoulders and pelvis kept in the same plane to avoid spine motion) and axial loading (examiner exerts slight pressure on top of the head) (25).

 iii. Testing for L-4: Impaired ability to perform single deep knee bend while hands are supported by examiner; eversion of each foot onto lateral edge (anterior tibialis). Testing for L-5: Heel walking with unequal foot lift; large toe lifts while standing (extensor hallucis longus). Testing for S-1: Toe walking on balls of feet with drooping heel suggests lesion; foot inversion by placing weight on medial edge of each foot (peroneus longus and brevis).

  iv. Seated testing: DTR unequal or missing at knee suggests L-4 lesion; at ankle, S-1.

   v. A distraction test (Waddell's) for suspected nonorganic cause is *straight-leg raising (SLR) in a seated position;* pain may be as severe as SLR pain in organic disease, whereas no pain is a positive Waddell's sign (25).

  vi. Sensation loss: Test for sensory reception (touch) of dermatome: L-4, along medial leg and foot; L-5, along lateral leg and dorsum of foot; and S-1, lateral foot. If regional responses cross dermatomes, suspect nonorganic cause (26). Check pedal pulses.

 vii. Supine testing (patient lying on back has less pressure on the disks than in sitting or standing position): SLR, passively raised: note angle when *radicular* pain appears. Hyperextension (dorsiflexion of the ankle at the point of pain) places tension on the sciatic nerve roots and hamstrings, causing increased radicular pain. Ligamentous strain and articular facet displacement cause minimal pain with ankle dorsiflexion. Knee bend at point of pain provides relief of radicular pain and confirms lumbosacral injury. Bent leg raising does not elicit pain. If SLR pain on affected side only, probable cause is LS root injury or disease with pain. If the opposite SLR also causes referred pain to the affected side (contralateral), there is an 89% chance of herniated disk. Herniated disk probability increases as the angle necessary to reproduce sciatica decreases.

viii. Faber test (flexion/abduction/external rotation) is passively bending the knee to a right angle, placing the foot on opposite patella, then pulling flexed knee laterally to rotate the hip joint. Passive flexion of the hips causes pain in sacroiliac (SI) or hip origins, nonorganic back pain, but not with LS injury or lesions.

  d. Abdominal exam: Inspect, palpate, and auscultate to r/o localized bruit, pain, aneurysm, mass. Perform on all with associated abdominal pain and all over 50 years old with back pain. Rectal exam on all men over 60 years to r/o prostate lesion.

  e. Prone testing (lying on stomach with pillow under pelvis): femoral stretch is passively raising straight leg, an extension that produces pain in the anterior thigh suggesting lumbar lesion above L-5.

  f. Mood/affect: Observation of mood as depressed, anxious, or angry.

3. Additional testing, imaging, and algorithm-based criteria.

  a. X-ray: Not shown to be helpful in uncomplicated LBP. Obtain anterior-posterior/lateral (AP/LAT) of LS spine if: serious or impact trauma; pain continuing more than 1 week and age under 20 or over 60; or unexplained pain without sciatica persists more than 7 weeks (12,13). Add oblique if known cancer, suspicion for spinal stenosis (19), or unexplained weight loss.

b. MRI: Differentiates soft tissue abnormalities (neoplasm, hematoma, infection). If osteomyelitis is suspected with positive erythrocyte sedimentation rate (ESR) and elevated white blood count (WBC), obtain MRI to r/o, and refer to orthopedic physician if positive. Other radiographic and imaging studies are not warranted at the initial primary care evaluation.

c. CT scan: Especially useful in evaluating persistent LBP (longer than 6 to 7 weeks) with sciatica, or if facet pain suspected.

d. Myelography: No longer considered a primary imaging modality for lumbar spine pathology, is reserved for multisegmental pathology or those with implanted metal fixation that interferes with imaging.

e. Invasive disc injection, CT discography, or injection studies of epidural, nerve root, or facet may r/o painful spine abnormalities, correlate symptoms with pathology, or predict surgical success, and these are reserved for orthopedic or neurologic evaluation (12).

4. Laboratory (15): Laboratory studies are reserved for suspected infection (WBC, urine analysis), inflammatory conditions (ESR), metabolic disease (Ca^{++}, PO_4, alkaline phosphatase, serum protein) or spondylitis (HLA-B27) and are noted in Algorithm II.

C. Box #3: Assessed as suspicious etiology or pathology. Positive key signs and symptoms suggest back pain arising from pathology (as distinguished from occupational or personal stresses) leading to prolonged recovery or disability. (See notations on acute care form: Suspected pathology and disability are not mutually exclusive in identifying causes of LBP; some patients may be in both tracks.) Signs and symptoms include pain (writhing, steady, worsening, persisting at night), severe trauma, fever, abdominal pain, compromised host, history of cancer or unexplained weight loss, known spinal disease, rash, edema, age over 60 or under 20, and cauda equina syndrome (bowel or bladder dysfunction). Generally, the more worrisome symptoms

for significant illness are pain at rest, nontraumatic origin, progressive intensity, or gradual onset. Less suspicious characteristics are pain with activity, moderately traumatic origin, stable intensity, or sudden onset.

D. Box #4: See algorithm II below and suspicious pathology on acute form for action on referral or further evaluation at the primary level.

E. Box #5: Assessed as suspicious for potential disability: Again, not mutually exclusive with possible pathologic causes, these symptoms and situations suggest a high potential for disability or prolonged recovery and warrant scheduled follow-up. Pain persisting longer than 3 weeks is sufficient reason for inclusion in this group.

1. Occupational body mechanics: Repetitive lifting in bent/twisted position; lifting beyond capacity; exposure to vibration of machinery/vehicles; sustaining a single position for prolonged periods; and job dissatisfaction (12).

2. Occupational or personal stress, anxiety, legal or disability concerns, depression: Characteristics of individuals at increased risk of prolonged work loss and disability (22,25).

3. Waddell's signs: Constant, nonanatomic, regional pain; emotional descriptors; whole leg pain, numbness, or weakness; intolerance of therapy; SLR improved with distraction; positive axial loading; positive trunk turn pain (25,26).

F. Box #6: See algorithms IB and III below for follow-up and referral. Other candidates for follow-up are: those with pain persisting longer than 3 weeks, of age under 20 or over 60, experiencing a recurrence, on Workers' Compensation, on narcotics, or with neurologic signs.

G. Boxes #7,8,9,11: Assessed as LBP with radiation, without neurological signs. True radicular pain extends down the posterior leg or anterior lower leg to the ankle or foot, or it affects the anterior thigh with pain to the knee. Posterior thigh or buttock pain without radiation to the foot or ankle is not radicular pain. Localization of pain to the nerve root and reproduction of pain with tension on the nerve root (positive SLR) confirms radicular pain.

H. Boxes #9,11: No neurologic signs: Treated with the standard acute phase therapy (see below) and reevaluated at 1 week to detect progressive power problems or worsening neurologic signs, and again at 3 weeks if not resolved or it recurs. See algorithm IB.

I. Box #8,10: Minor neurologic signs: Localized weakness, asymmetry of reflexes, or sensory loss also treated with standard therapy with checks at 1 and 3 weeks to r/o progressive neurologic or power problems. See algorithm IB.

J. Boxes #12,13,10: Assessed as LBP without radiation but minor neurologic signs present. If the pain has already persisted past the acute phase (1 week), begin standard therapy for a week and reassess. If there are neurologic signs, go to algorithm IB.

K. Boxes #12,13,14: Assessed as LBP without radiation or neurologic signs. Determined by the process of elimination, mechanical LBP is expected to resolve with basic acute therapy. Follow-up as needed (assessment box on acute form).

L. Box #14: Acute phase therapy (see patient education, Figs. 7 and 8). Basic regimen, acute phase, less than 7 days or reinforce for up to 4 weeks. Select goals.

1. Bed rest for 48 hours is as effective as for 7 days (11).

2. Ice or heat applications locally, whichever is more comfortable and effective in reducing pain. Nonsteroidal anti-inflammatories: ASA, 2 to 3 tablets (10 to 15 grains) QID, or ibuprofen, 400 to 800 mg TID, in decreasing amounts as discomfort eases. Narcotics and muscle relaxants may be beneficial during the first week. No narcotics beyond 4 weeks. Carisoprodol (Soma) 350 mg TID for 3 to 4 days may be warranted when there is considerable spasm.

3. Exercises using the McKenzie recommendations if they do not aggravate pain (17). General aerobic conditioning, especially walking, to improve endurance.

4. Patient education provides guidelines on re-evaluation and brief instruction on therapy, body mechanics, and exercises (see Figs. 7,8). If this is a recurrence and non–work related, self-care back school (see referral form for PT-1, Fig. 9) or purchase of McKenzie book recommended.

II. Algorithm IB reviews follow-up recommendations at 1 and 3 weeks as needed. The shaded column two provides space for easy comparison with the initial evaluation.

A. Box #15: Follow-up data: At each follow-up visit (usually 1 to 3 weeks after initial evaluation), review all subjective data and record in the shaded area of the encounter form. Retest any previously positive signs. Estimate status as better, worse, same.

B. Boxes 16,17,18,19: Resolving signs and symptoms. At least 50% will be able to answer *yes* af-

ter 1 week of acute therapy; by 4 weeks, 75% will be pain free. Only 10% will have persisting pain after 6 to 7 weeks, at which point the prognosis changes and the problem becomes chronic pain. It is this latter group that accounts for about 75% of expenditures for LBP care (22).

C. Box #18: If symptoms have resolved and no signs of inflammation remain, reassure patient that full recovery is expected and reinforce exercises and preventive measures (see patient education) to maintain recovery.

D. Box #19: If symptoms persisted longer than 1 week and the episode was a recurrence or work related, there is an increased risk for yet another recurrence. Consider referral to self-care (PT-1) for intensive prevention training (see referral form, Fig. 9). If symptoms or signs persist continue on through the algorithm.

E. Boxes #20,21: Patient age under 20 or over 60 with persistent symptoms or pain duration of 3 weeks or more. Candidates for nonmechanical origins of back pain warrant AP/LAT x-ray of spine after 1 week to r/o tumor, infection, or spine disease (see algorithm II).

F. Boxes #21,22: X-ray negative. Go to Box 23 or go to algorithm II.

G. Boxes #21,24: X-ray positive. Go to algorithm II.

H. Boxes #23,24: Progressive weakness or symptoms of suspicious pathology. Go to algorithm II.

I. Boxes #25,26: Pain longer than 3 weeks or suspicious for disability. Go to algorithm III.

J. Boxes #27,28,29,30: Continuing back pain, with or without radiation or minor neurologic signs. Since the above reviews for pathology and disability are negative, key factors for follow-up and planning are duration of pain, radiation, and work-related symptoms.

1. Pain for 1 week, stable with radiation: Reassure patient that radicular LBP is usually more persistent than nonradicular pain (12) but will resolve with therapy. Continue acute care therapy with gradually increasing activity and work plan. Follow-up at 3 weeks. If pain is work related or work loss continues beyond 1 week, consider referral to PT-2 to intensify therapy, and initiate a return to work (RTW) plan. Plan follow-up in primary care or have physical therapist report to primary care at 6 to 7 weeks.

2. Pain persisting 3 weeks or more: Go to algorithm III. Pain persisting 3 weeks or > is itself a criteria for suspected disability or prolonged recovery requiring intervention.

III. Algorithm II: Suspicious etiology or pathology.
   A. Box #31: Suspected pathology and risk for disability are not mutually exclusive causes of LBP; some patients may be in both tracks. The suspicious-for-pathology items are listed in Algorithm I, Box #3. Generally, the more worrisome symptoms for significant illness are pain at rest, nontraumatic origin, progressive intensity, or gradual onset, as listed under notations on the acute care form. Less suspicious characteristics are pain with activity, moderately traumatic origin, stable intensity, or sudden onset.
   B. Boxes #32,33,34: Impact trauma. Requires AP/LAT x-ray of the spine for significant impact trauma or suspected weakened bone strength with osteoporosis to r/o fracture. Oblique films are used only to r/o metastasis with known cancer or unexplained weight loss, or perhaps suspected spinal stenosis. If negative, return to Box #5.
   C. Boxes #32,33,35,36: Alignment/neurologic problems. Although simple radiographs are not sufficient to justify surgery, progressive neurologic injury (see below) or an alignment problem in addition to radiologically confirmed fracture warrants consideration of reduction and referral to OS-A (orthopedic surgery—acute care).
   D. Boxes #37,38,40: Fracture without alignment instability or neurologic signs. If trauma was minimal and resulted in fracture, treat in primary care with osteoporosis protocol.
   E. Boxes #37,39: None of the above; basic therapy and follow-up in 1 and 3 weeks Go to algorithm IB.
   F. Boxes #41,42: Symptoms of urinary, bowel, or sexual dysfunction, or increasing neuromotor deficit and/or progressive weakness. Suspicious for cauda equina syndrome; refer to OS-A for CT or MRI to confirm need for surgical intervention. If diagnosis is not confirmed by imaging, orthopedics will refer to neurosurgery.
   G. Boxes #43,44,45: Pain at rest, fever, compromised host, GU or gastrointestinal (GI) symptoms.
      1. Infection may be of GI or GU origin requiring WBC or urine culture or gynecologic examination. Treatment in primary care or by gyneologist as appropriate. Aortic aneurysm will cause similar pain without signs of infection: r/o with ultrasound.
      2. Suspicion of infection in bone or disc: r/o with ESR, WBC. If positive, obtain MRI to detect osteomyelitis (18). Consult with OM-A (orthopedic medicine-acute care) if positive (see referral form, Fig. 9).

   H. Boxes #46,47: Ages under 20 or over 60, history of cancer, constitutional symptoms. Use AP/LAT X-RAY to r/o neoplasm; refer or treat accordingly. This is seldom an orthopedic referral, usually primary care, oncology, or medicine.
   I. Boxes #48,49: Nocturnal, SI pain more than 3 months, morning stiffness, 15- to 49-year-old man. Suspicious for anklyosing spondylitis; r/o with SI x-ray and HLA-B27. Refer to rheumatology if positive.
   J. Boxes #50,51: Claudication, over age 50, persistent pain. Suspect spinal stenosis if forward-flexed spine along with claudication, x-ray, AP (supine) and LAT (standing). Refer to OM-SA (orthopedic medicine-subacute care) if positive (see referral form, Fig. 9). Suspect atherosclerotic ischemia if pain when walking, relieved with rest; initiate a vascular evaluation.
   K. Boxes #52,53: Structural abnormality identified. Refer to OS-A or SA (see referral form, Fig. 9).
   L. Boxes #54,55,56: Radicular pain more than 6 weeks. Distinguish between predominant back pain versus predominant radicular pain. Predominant back pain may represent systemic disease and should be evaluated with x-ray, bone scan, or dynamic films in consultation with OM. See algorithm III. The radicular pain group requires diagnostic tests for spinal cord pressure source. See Box #2, additional testing, above. When all testing is negative, consider chronic pain and algorithm III.

IV. Algorithm III: Suspicious for risk of disability. See Box #5 and notation 3 on acute care form. Again, not mutually exclusive with possible pathologic causes, these symptoms and situations, or simply pain prolonged past 3 weeks, suggest a high potential for disability or prolonged recovery that warrants scheduled follow-up.
   A. Boxes #57,58: At risk for disability or recurrence with follow-up over 3 to 16 weeks. Provide standard acute care treatment (see Box #15) and careful follow-up to detect disability and plan intervention early, including referral for PT-2 with psychological and return-to-work interventions. Key to planning: absence of signs of pathology, duration of pain, work loss, and positive Waddel signs or depression.
   B. Boxes #59,60,61: Improving at 3 weeks. Consider PT-1 if recurrence, work related, or more than 3 weeks of pain; otherwise, patient education for prevention. Follow-up as needed.
   C. Boxes #59,62,63: Continuing signs or symptoms. First, reevaluate for pathology and refer to algorithm II if positive.

D. Boxes #59,64,65,66: Continuing signs or symptoms plus recurrence, or work- or stress-related, at 3-week follow-up. Continuing symptoms and/or unimproved measurements in this high-risk group signal a need for follow-up and/or early intervention with a trained professional. The deciding factors for referral at the first follow-up are recurrence and work-related stress or injury. Refer to PT-2 (see referral form). PT intervention has been shown to decrease cost, lost work time, and recurrences. Schedule for 6- to 7-week follow-up to check on progress and effect of therapy or PT report. If pain is not work-related or a recurrence, continue acute care therapy without bed rest. Schedule for 1- to 3-week follow-up depending on severity of continuing symptoms. In either instance, a return-to-work plan should be initiated by 1 week; an adjusted early return is preferable to delay until full function is restored. Coordinate with employer as needed, a required step if Workers' Compensation is involved.

E. Boxes #66,67,68,69: Follow-up at 6 weeks. If symptoms are resolved and patient is back to full function, reinforce prevention and return to primary care as needed. Consider PT-1 referral for prevention, especially if this is a recurrence. If symptoms continue, refer to OM-S or PT-2 for psychological evaluation with return-to-work plan (see referral form). If radicular pain continues past 6 to 7 weeks, differentiate between LBP with sciatica predominant or LBP predominant. Go to algorithm II. Schedule for 12-week follow-up or PT report to review progress. At 12-week follow-up, PT referral. At 16 weeks, rehabilitation center referral (14).

REFERENCES

1. Berwick DM (1989): Continuous improvement as an ideal in health care. *N Engl J Med* 320:53–56.
2. Berwick DM, Murphy JM, Goldman PA, et al. (1991): Performance of a five-item mental health screening test. *Med Care* 29:169–176.
3. Bingham RL, Plante DA, Bronson DL, et al. (1990): Establishing a quality improvement process for identification of psychosocial problems in a primary care practice. *J Gen Intern Med* 5(4):342–346.
4. Cherkin DC, Deyo RA, Berg AO (1991): Evaluation of a physician education intervention to improve primary care for low-back pain. II: Impact on patients. *Spine* 16:1173–1178.
5. Cherkin DC, Deyo RA, Berg AO, Bergman JJ, Lishner DM (1991): Evaluation of a physician education intervention to improve primary care for low-back pain. I: Impact on physicians. *Spine* 16:1168–1172.
6. Cherkin DC, Deyo RA, Wheeler K, Ciol MA (1994): Physician variation in diagnostic testing for low back pain. Who you see is what you get. *Arthritis Rheum* 37:15–22.
7. Choler U, Larsson R, Nachemson A, Peterson L-E (1985): Ont i ryggen–niforsok med vardprogram for patienter med lumbala smarttillstand. *Spri Rapport* 188–198, ISSN 0586-1691.
8. Crosby PB (1980): *Quality is free: The art of making quality certain.* New York: New American Library.
9. Deyo RA (1983): Clinical strategies for controlling costs and improving quality in primary care of low back pain. *J Back Musculoskel Rehab* 3:1–13.
10. Deyo, Cherkin DC, Conrad D, Volinn E (1991): Cost, controversy, crisis: low back pain and the health of the public. *Annu Rev Public Health* 12:141–156.
11. Deyo RA, Diehl AK, Rosenthal M (1986): How many days of bedrest for acute low back pain? A randomized clinical trial. *N Engl J Med* 315:1064–1070.
12. Frymoyer JW (1988): Back pain and sciatica. *N Engl J Med* 318:291–300.
13. Hadler NM (1986): Regional back pain [editorial]. *N Engl J Med* 315:1090–1092.
14. Hazard RG et al. (1989): Functional restoration with behavioral support: a one-year prospective study of patients with chronic low-back pain. *Spine* 14:157–161.
15. Juran JM (1988): *Juran on planning for quality.* New York: Free Press.
16. Lawrence VA, Tugwell P, Gafni A, et al. (1989): *Acute low back pain and the community health perspective: the iterative loop approach.* Report from University of Texas at San Antonio, Department of Medicine, pp. 1–41.
17. McKenzie R (1980): *Treat your own back: How to safely, simply and scientifically relieve your own back pain.* Waikanae: New Zealand: Spinal Publications.
18. Meyers SP, Wiener SN (1991): Diagnosis of hematogenous pyogenic vertebral osteomyelitis by magnetic resonance imaging. *Arch Intern Med* 151:683–687.
19. Mooney V (1987): Where is the pain coming from? *Spine* 12:754–759.
20. Rothwell MG (1976): A patient-centered group practice. *Nursing Outlook* 24:745–748.
21. Ryan TP (1989): *Statistical methods for quality improvement.* New York: John Wiley & Sons.
22. Spitzer WO, LeBlanc FE, Dupuis M, et al. (1987): Scientific approach to the assessment and management of activity-related spinal disorders. A monograph for clinicians. Report of the Quebec Task Force on Spinal Disorders. *Spine* 12(7):S1–S59.
23. Stewart AL, Hays RD, Ware JE Jr. (1988): The MOS short-form general health survey: reliability and validity in patient population. *Med Care* 26:724–734.
24. Tufo H, Bouchard RE, Rubin AS, et al. (1977): Problem-oriented approach to practice. I. Economic impact. *JAMA* 238:414–417.
25. Waddell G (1986): A new clinical model for the treatment of low-back pain. *Spine* 12:632–641.
26. Waddell G, McCulloch JA, Kummel E, et al. (1980): Non-organic physical signs in low-back pain. *Spine* 5:111–119.
27. Walton M (1986): *The Deming management method.* New York: Dodd Mead.
28. Weed LL (1969): *Medical records, medical education and patient care.* Chicago: Year Book Medical Publishers.
29. Weed LL (1991): *Knowledge coupling: new premises and new tools for medical care and education.* New York: Springer-Verlag.
30. Wiesel SW, Feffer HL, Rothman RH, et al. (1984): Industrial low back pain: a prospective evaluation of a standardized diagnostic and treatment protocol. *Spine* 9:199–203.

The Adult Spine: Principles and Practice,
2nd edition, J.W. Frymoyer, Editor-in-Chief.
Lippincott-Raven Publishers, Philadelphia © 1997.

CHAPTER 6

Outcomes Research

Robert B. Keller and Steven J. Atlas

Over the last decade "outcomes research" has become a buzzword and much of the information produced has provided a significant stimulus to the health care reform debate. There seems little doubt that scientific publications, governmental analyses, and public testimony providing information from large data base analyses, small area analyses, and meta-analyses have raised issues that have added fuel to the fire of the health care reform agenda (26,42). The United States and other technologically advanced nations continue to be confronted with increasing health care costs. In 1993, 14% of the U.S. gross domestic product was expended on health care—the highest percentage in the world. This figure has been projected to rise to 18% or more by the year 2000. Outcomes research has defined and characterized the considerable clinical uncertainty and lack of solid evidence of therapeutic efficacy that characterizes much of current medical care. Policy makers have become increasingly aware that this variability and uncertainty contribute significantly to the cost of care.

While outcomes research has helped to define many of the current problems in medical care, it also offers the methods with which to seek their resolution. In this chapter we discuss the field of outcomes research and its

application to the wide range of spinal conditions and treatment methods that are covered in the text.

What Is Outcomes Research?

The field of outcomes research encompasses a number of techniques, all of which are based on methods of clinical and health services research. Some of these methods focus on epidemiologic analyses to study patterns of illness, utilization of medical and surgical care, and costs and outcomes resulting from the treatment of various conditions. The usual techniques include large data base analyses, small area variation studies, and meta-analyses of the literature.

A central feature of outcomes research characteristic of clinical research in general is the requirement of careful research design, proper statistical methodologies, and prospective patient evaluations. Clinical outcomes research is characterized by a focus on the outcomes of care from the perspective of patients, as opposed to evaluations by providers and measurements of "processes" of care.

Still other outcome methods include decision analysis and economic studies to determine cost effectiveness and cost benefit. Finally, there is hope that the information from high quality outcome studies will provide the information required to develop accurate and meaningful clinical practice guidelines.

A given outcomes research project could incorporate one or more of these concepts. The important factor is

R. B. Keller, M.D.: Maine Medical Assessment Foundation, Augusta, Maine; and Dartmouth Medical School, Hanover, Massachusetts.

S. J. Atlas, M.D., M.P.H.: Instructor in Medicine, Harvard Medical School; and Massachusetts General Hospital, Boston, Massachusetts 02114.

that each of these different techniques is characterized by well-defined and stringent methodologic processes. When studies are properly performed, it becomes possible for readers and analysts to evaluate the results accurately and compare the data across a number of studies.

Outcomes Research and Outcomes Assessment

In recent years, physicians in all types of practice settings have become increasingly interested in assessing the outcomes of the care they provide to patients. In part this has been stimulated by a scientific desire to learn more about the results of that care. Another important factor relates to the rapidly changing face of medical practice in this country. A new era of managed care, integrated health-care systems and competitive health plans has dramatically changed the practice landscape. As part of this evolution, practitioners correctly perceive that they will be required to provide to patients and payers definitive evidence of the outcomes of the care they provide.

Measurement of outcomes in this setting should not be characterized as research, but rather as assessment. Clinical outcomes *research* is characterized by the development of hypotheses, employment of strict statistical and research methods, and enrollment of a sufficient number of cases (power) to answer the question(s). Research of this kind requires expert multidisciplinary teams, organizational structures, and significant financial support.

Assessment of outcomes, using standardized evaluation instruments, will permit practitioners to collect patient outcome data (and other useful information) that can be analyzed and compared to data from other practices and/or large normative data bases. The information gathered in these settings may not reach statistical significance, but it will be of value to practitioners in better understanding their practices and in being able to provide credible evidence of the quality and appropriateness of care. This kind of information will also be a powerful ongoing educational tool.

It is important for physicians to understand the difference between research and assessment. Many of the same methods can be used for both purposes, but the end results may be different. One of the critical elements of both research and assessment relates to the way in which information is collected from patients. The development of high quality patient questionnaires, often referred to as instruments, which have been tested and validated, is an essential step in these processes.

Over the years, clinicians have developed many different tools and scoring systems for evaluating their clinical results. Unfortunately, few of these have ever been thoroughly tested and validated. For example, there are a number of measurement or scoring systems for hip arthroplasty. An analysis of them (3) indicates that when several scoring tools are applied to the same patients they produce very different measures of success or outcome of treatment. The same patient can appear to have either a good or bad result based on the scoring system used. Similarly, an evaluation of 34 different evaluation systems for knee arthroplasty revealed marked variability in design and utilization, and none of the systems had been tested for reliability and validity (14). Clearly, such systems are not helpful to those interested in determining the real outcome of hip and knee arthroplasty.

Similarly, there have been attempts to develop scores or questionnaires for spinal conditions. The Roland and Oswestry scores are well developed and tested examples (18,33). More recently, the North American Spine Society (NASS) has supported the development of a tested and validated low back pain outcomes assessment instrument. Some of the data elements of the Roland and Oswestry scores (as well as other questionnaires) have been incorporated in the NASS document. Under the auspices of the American Academy of Orthopaedic Surgeons (AAOS), this form will become the basis of a new instrument that will cover all spine conditions—lumbar, cervical, and deformity.

The availability of a high-quality, standardized, and broadly accepted assessment instrument will enable both researchers and physicians in practice to obtain reliable outcomes information and to do so in a manner that will produce standardized and comparable data. This will permit useful and valid comparisons of different treatment methods, practice outcomes, patient populations, and health systems.

Outcomes Research in Spine Treatment and Surgery

There is literally no field of medicine that does not need to involve itself in outcomes research. The requirement in spine care is especially urgent. The content of this textbook confirms the point. The editors of this text make this point in Chapter 3, The Future of Spinal Treatment: "From this perspective, the focus for research will be on outcome and efficacy. The health professional in or out of a larger system will have to demonstrate objectively his or her outcomes measured against standards of care." Hadler raises an important issue in Chapter 4, in which he defines the back pain "disease–illness paradigm" in which every symptom requires a diagnostic label and every label requires a treatment. As a result, there exist a myriad of treatments for these generally self-limited spinal disorders. Many of these treatments are part of the ever-growing field of "alternative" health care methods, and each of these methods has fervent advocates. Yet, as Deyo points out in Chapter 26, many current and accepted treatments have been proven ineffective when scientifically tested.

Within this text, significant differences in therapeutic

approaches are advocated by various authors. For example, the chapters on conservative treatment of low back disorders (Chapters 83 through 86) present discussions on a broad range of treatments including orthoses, manipulation, physical therapy, back school, and numerous other techniques. All of these methods have strong proponents, yet remarkably few have undergone rigorous clinical trials to prove or disprove their effectiveness.

Beyond the views noted above, there are two important lines of additional evidence to convince us of the need for an expanded and vigorous agenda of outcomes research in spine care, resulting from investigations using the specific techniques of outcomes research. With the development of computers and new methods of data analysis, epidemiologists and researchers have been able to undertake small area variation studies of the utilization patterns of lumbar and cervical disc procedures, lumbar fusion, hospitalization for low back conditions, and other treatments (as shown in the later section on small area analysis). The consistent finding has been that there are significant variations in population-based rates of all the kinds of spine care that have been studied.

For example, in northern New England in 1991 to 1992, there was a tenfold difference in the probability that residents would undergo a lumbar spine fusion when hospital service area utilization rates are compared across the three-state region (Fig. 1). Clinicians participating in the analysis of these data agree that the difference in rates is primarily attributable to the presence of surgeons with subspecialty training in spine surgery in high-rate communities. These surgeons appear to have different practice styles. Practice style can be defined as the process by which physicians evaluate clinical problems, process information, and make treatment recommendations to their patients. The variations in lumbar

fusion rates are clear evidence that the practice patterns of surgeons across northern New England are very different, and the result is a major difference in surgical rates.

Currently, we lack scientific information to indicate which of these different rates of lumbar fusion represents the "right" rate. High rates of surgery may result in healthier, happier, more functional citizens (29) or, conversely, lower rates may be more consistent with better outcomes. It should be clear that these remarkably different rates of fusion cannot all represent the best medical care. Either residents in the high-rate areas are being operated on too frequently, or citizens in the low-rate area not often enough, or something in between. At the present time, there is no solid information with which to answer this question.

As discussed in the section on data base analysis, variations in many methods of spine treatment have been elucidated in epidemiologic analyses of hospital service areas within states, and across states, large geographic regions, and countries. The problems they present and the issues that they raise cannot be disputed.

The second piece of evidence that has demonstrated the need for outcomes research in spine care results from meta-analyses of the scientific literature. Meta-analysis was originally developed as a technique to pool information from many randomized clinical trials in order to create a large base of information with greater validity and statistical significance. Two policy implications have resulted from the application of this technology.

First, true meta-analyses are difficult and occasionally impossible to conduct on the spine literature, not unlike most clinical literature in other disciplines. This is because scientific publications have used poor research methods, inadequate statistical measures and analyses,

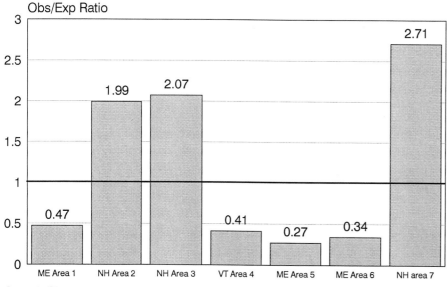

Obs/Exp Ratio

Source: UHDDS, All Significant @ p < 0.01

FIG. 1. The population-based rates of lumbar fusion for seven large hospital service areas in Northern New England vary tenfold—from 27% of the regional mean to 271% of the mean.

widely differing criteria to assess results, and measurement instruments that are not tested and validated. The result is that data from reports is often not accurate and/ or cannot be pooled to permit meta-analysis. While this represents a significant problem in applying the method, the more important consequence is that many of the conclusions (and subsequent treatment recommendations) derived from the current body of research may be faulty.

The second implication is that where it has been possible to conduct meta-analyses of various conditions or treatments, the results have raised significant questions about the value and appropriateness of many forms of medical care. The structured review of the lumbar spine fusion literature by Turner et al. (36) illustrates this problem. The authors do not conclude that lumbar fusion is an unproven procedure, but they do correctly state that the research that has been performed and published does not provide scientific support for most of the currently applied indications for surgery. They urge improvement in research methodologies and the conduct of appropriate clinical trials of this procedure. (The methods of meta-analysis are discussed in detail later in this chapter.)

Studies of large data base analyses and meta-analyses make it clear that there is a pressing need for outcomes research in the field of spine care. All parties involved— patients, physicians, payers, and regulators—have a legitimate interest in learning what works among the many treatment options for the wide range of spine conditions.

METHODS OF OUTCOMES RESEARCH

Large Data Base Analysis

Large health-care data bases maintained by various organizations are being increasingly utilized to examine clinical practice (Table 1). With the widespread availability of powerful microcomputers, the use of these data bases is growing rapidly. The appeal of using information derived from large data bases is readily apparent. One has access to information on large numbers of patients, frequently representing every hospitalized patient in a given geographic region or representing a given population (e.g., Medicare enrollees). There is less concern about bias in patient selection or whether or not findings are applicable only to a given institution or particular area. Many data bases are ongoing and will allow more refined comparisons over time. Results are often generalizable because the data may represent a well-defined population.

Large data bases are used in a variety of ways; the most common are (a) to assess rates and trends for various procedures and diagnoses, including variations across large and small regions (see section on small area analysis),

TABLE 1. *Examples of large data bases used for research purposes*

Government sponsored
  National
    National Center for Health Statistics
      National Hospital Discharge Survey
      National Ambulatory Medical Care Survey
      National Health Interview Study
      National Death Index
    Medicare Parts A and B
    Veterans Administration Hospitals
  Regional
    Washington State Commission Hospital Abstract
      Reporting System
    State Medicaid data bases
Registries (international, national, regional/local)
  International Bone Marrow Transplant Registry
  National Tumor Registry
  Mayo Clinic
Private insurance and HMO data bases
  Kaiser Permanente
  Blue Cross and Blue Shield
Other health-care data bases
  American Medical Association Physician Masterfile
  American Hospital Association Annual Survey

(b) to examine access to health care services for different populations, and (c) to assess complication rates and certain outcomes such as mortality, length of stay, and re-operations. Research in lumbar spine disorders has employed large data bases to examine several of these areas, as well as to provide preliminary data on which to base further studies. Specific criteria and computer algorithms have been devised to identify patients with low back pain, and hospitalization and procedure rates (5).

Using national or regional hospital discharge data bases from 11 countries and Canadian provinces in Europe and North America, Cherkin et al. recently compared international back surgery rates and demonstrated that rates in the United States were at least 40% higher than in any other country examined (4) (Fig. 2). Volinn et al. analyzed data from the U.S. National Hospital Discharge Survey over several years (40). Increasing rates of surgery, decreasing numbers of nonsurgical hospitalizations for low back pain, and regional differences in hospitalization and length of stay were identified. Data bases have also been used to compare complication rates according to age, diagnosis, and type of surgical procedure for a variety of lumbar spine conditions (11,12). Finally, the characteristics associated with re-operations after lumbar spine surgery in Medicare patients have been examined (6). Younger age, white race, previous spine surgery, recent hospitalization, and the diagnosis of a herniated disc (compared to other diagnoses) were associated with higher re-operation rates.

Large data bases also have significant limitations. The quality of the data may be variable, and often little is known about the accuracy or completeness of the medi-

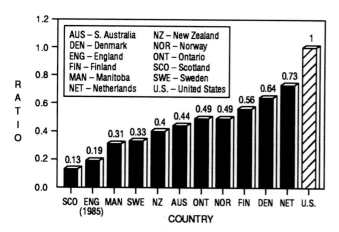

FIG 2. In comparison to a number of countries and Canadian provinces, more spinal surgery is performed in the United States—ranging from 40% to 670%. From ref. 4, with permission.

cal records on which they are based. It is difficult to assess the severity of illness from large data bases. This makes it hard to determine whether differences observed among groups are simply the result of one group having greater comorbidity or severity of illness. Despite these limitations, use of large data bases in spine disorders research offers many advantages including population-based rates of complications and resource utilization, as well as the characteristics associated with variation in rates. Those who conduct and publish these kinds of analyses must be scrupulous in their methods and must also be careful to acknowledge potential deficiencies and discrepancies.

Small Area Analysis

One of the first types of data base analysis that began to raise questions about the appropriateness and consistency of practice was based on the concept of small area variations. Wennberg and Gittelsohn refined older epidemiologic methods to assess the utilization of health care services of patients based on their place of residence (43). Using hospital discharge data bases and computer algorithms, they created "hospital service areas," defined as clusters of postal zip codes surrounding hospitals at which the majority (or plurality) of residents were hospitalized. Counting the number of admissions or procedures at the hospital or provider level is not helpful because patients may come from long distances to be treated by some institutions or physicians. Without knowing the denominator (i.e., the number of individuals at risk for treatment), one cannot calculate or compare the rates of services being utilized.

Small area analysis permitted the study of health care utilization among discrete populations. If these analyses had shown no significant differences across hospital service areas, the method would have been of only passing

interest. The findings, however, were a major step in changing the face of clinical research and medical practice itself. What Wennberg found was that for almost all of medical care there are striking differences in utilization rates among similar populations, but some medical conditions do not show these wide variations. In orthopedics, minimal variations are found for such conditions as hip fracture and polytrauma. However, for most medical and orthopedic conditions and procedures, significant variations across small and large areas have been observed.

Small area analysis has been used to examine rates of lumbar (23,39) and cervical spine surgery (16) in Washington State. Rates of lumbar spine surgery for low back pain varied a striking 15-fold among the state's 39 counties. For cervical spine surgery, rates varied 7-fold. Similar techniques have been used to show variation across many procedures and specialties (42). Again, while variation in clinical practice exists, this type of analysis cannot determine which population-based rate is correct. What is clear is that when rates vary greatly, some of them must be inappropriate. Variation is believed to result from physicians having different thresholds for recommending a particular treatment. The variations in lumbar discectomy, for example, are thought to reflect uncertainty about which of several therapeutic options represent optimal treatment. In general, financial incentives are not felt to be the major factor producing variations (21).

Meta-Analysis

Meta-analysis is a relatively new research tool that is used to combine data from a collection of individual studies in order to integrate the findings and improve the statistical power of the conclusions (19). Like traditional narrative literature review, meta-analysis attempts to summarize a given literature and arrive at conclusions about efficacy of a diagnostic test or therapeutic intervention. However, unlike narrative review, meta-analysis follows an explicit, structured approach. The major components of this methodology include (a) defining the study question and creating clear objectives, (b) performing a comprehensive literature search using specified criteria, (c) assessing the quality of the individual studies that meet inclusion criteria, and (d) determining whether the individual study results can be combined and, if appropriate, quantitatively pooling estimates and performing sensitivity analyses (Table 2).

While it is the pooled estimates of an outcome that are the goal of a meta-analysis, the methods used to review the literature and extract data are critical to evaluate the quality of this approach (25). The eligibility criteria for study inclusion may vary depending on the study's objective and the outcome to be assessed. Variables used

TABLE 2. *Meta-analysis methodology*

Formulate study question and specific objectives
Explicit research protocol
    Study inclusion and exclusion criteria
    Literature search strategy
    List papers included and excluded
    Use prospectively designed data extraction form
    Record study information
        Study characteristics (e.g., design, type of treatment/
           control, sample size)
        Patient characteristics (e.g., age, gender, insurance
           status)
        Outcomes (e.g., mortality, complications, re-operations)
Qualitative assessment
    Create prospective quality score
    Assess inter-reviewer reliability
    Perform analyses stratified by quality
Quantitative assessment
    Variation in study outcomes
        Test of homogeneity
        Graphic displays and stratified analyses
    Pooling of results of homogenous studies
    Sensitivity analysis

in the selection criteria can include study design (e.g., randomized, controlled, prospective, retrospective), sample size, outcome of interest, or the type of therapy. An explicit search strategy to identify relevant articles is required. Controversy exists about the use of unpublished data.

After identifying all relevant studies using predetermined criteria, the quality of each study should be assessed using a prospectively designed instrument. Ideally, study quality should be blindly assessed by at least two reviewers. The quality score can be correlated with the study outcome to assess the influence of study quality on results. Next, reviewers independently extract information on study characteristics and the outcome(s) of interest using a standardized protocol and data collection form. It is critical that measures of treatment effect be comparable. Consistency of the data extracted by reviewers should be assessed. Qualitative and quantitative tests to determine whether results of individual studies can be combined are then performed. The statistical methods to assess variation among studies, to create pooled estimates of outcome, and finally to perform sensitivity analyses are beyond the scope of this review (25).

Using meta-analysis, several attempts have been made to assess outcomes or predictors of outcomes for various lumbar spine disorders (20,24,36). In each, serious methodologic flaws have prevented the combining of individual results to achieve a pooled estimate of outcome or to determine predictors of outcome. Commonly, study design deficiencies included the absence of randomized studies, unblinded reporting of outcomes (often performed by the surgeon who did the procedure), and follow-up evaluations that were inconsistent and non-uniform. Most studies were retrospective and included

no comparison group. In one review, studies that prospectively followed patients had fewer satisfactory outcomes than studies in which patients were evaluated retrospectively (54.1% versus 72.6%) (36). Finally, the outcomes evaluated (e.g., pain relief, satisfaction, return to work) as well as the assessment methods (e.g., patient versus physician report) varied among studies.

For example, Turner et al. attempted a meta-analysis of outcomes for patients with lumbar spinal stenosis (37). A formal literature search was performed using explicit criteria. Each article was reviewed by two clinicians using a standardized data form. Because no single outcome measure was available, a range of outcomes were recorded. An outcome rating criterion was developed by the authors. Seventy-four of 625 articles met entry criteria. Of these studies, none was randomized and only three were prospectively assembled. While the authors concluded that surgery for lumbar spinal stenosis appears to be beneficial, satisfactory outcomes ranged from 26% to 100%. Wide variations in reported outcomes across the studies prevented the authors from pooling the results. The authors noted the widespread lack of rigorous study design, and they emphasized methods to better assess the relative benefits and risks of various treatments, both surgical and conservative, for well-defined patient groups.

Clinical Research Design

We have previously discussed the wide variations in rates of procedures for lumbar spine disorders identified using large data-base and small area analysis techniques. We have also examined the deficiencies in the lumbar spine literature uncovered by recent meta-analysis and structured literature reviews. In order to decrease variation in the treatment of common low back pain disorders, better information from high quality research studies is needed (10,22). To improve the quality of information available to clinicians, research studies must emphasize (a) adherence to rigorous research methods, (b) prospective data collection, (c) use of control populations, and (d) randomization of treatment allocation.

Research Methods

Significant effort must be made to identify clearly the research question, formulate hypotheses, and create study goals. The next crucial step is to focus on the patient characteristics needed to achieve these goals. Clear criteria for patient entry into the study must be specified. Ideally, all patients referred to a study but not enrolled should be recorded and the reason for exclusion given. Enrolled patients should have detailed baseline information collected, including demographic data such as age, gender, race, education, type of insurance, employment and compensation status, and comorbid conditions; past history such as number of prior episodes, length of current episode, and past treatments including surgery; symptoms such as location, frequency, and severity; physical examination and radiographic findings; and functional and disability status. The baseline information collected must be sufficient to appropriately classify patients into, for example, those with back pain alone, those with back pain and sciatica, and those with neurologic deficits.

Follow-up of patients must be complete and must be performed at uniform intervals. Enrolled patients later lost to follow-up must be identified, and the reason for not completing follow-up should be sought. To assess this potential bias better, baseline characteristics of patients completing and not completing follow-up must be compared. Every effort is needed to minimize the number of patients lost to follow-up, because outcomes of patients who do and those who do not complete follow-up may be quite different. For example, if patients who drop out do so because they have had a bad outcome, then outcomes in the remaining patients may be overstated.

The outcome measures employed in a study must be relevant to the patient. For example, if patients undergo lumbar spine surgery to decrease pain, then pain should be a major outcome variable. Because pain is a subjective outcome, it should be patient-reported. Other important outcomes to evaluate include changes in symptom frequency and severity in the back and/or leg, neurologic deficits, disability and functional status, satisfaction, complications of treatment, and employment or compensation status. Because patients may seek treatment for different reasons and thus have divergent goals, a variety of outcomes should be assessed. Finally, attempts to use standardized outcome measures should be encouraged to allow for comparisons among studies.

Prospective Design

The lumbar spine literature is dominated by retrospective studies. Retrospective implies that the event of interest, such as lumbar discectomy, occurred in the past. The patient is assessed for information, such as the outcome of surgery, at some point after the event. The advantage of such a study design is that one does not have to wait many years to measure outcomes. However, there are major problems, including limited or incomplete baseline information and loss of patients to follow-up. Because retrospective studies usually rely on review of clinical charts for baseline and follow-up information, important data are often missing. A review of spinal stenosis surgery found that even basic data such as age, sex, previous surgery, duration of symptoms, and neurologic deficits were frequently not reported (37).

In retrospective studies, it is often difficult to locate

and question all patients who had a specific treatment many years previously. As previously noted, biased follow-up and other factors may explain why retrospective studies often report more favorable outcomes than prospective studies (36). Prospective study design has the advantage of permitting the investigator to determine what data should be collected, as opposed to being limited to those that are available.

Control Groups

Most lumbar spine research studies retrospectively identify patients and can provide only descriptive analyses because they lack comparison groups. Such studies are referred to as case series and are used to examine individual patients with similar characteristics to generate hypotheses. Case series typically use historical controls, which can include patients from other published studies or patients treated by the same investigator or institution before the therapy of interest began to be used. Historical controls usually come from a different time period, one in which overall medical care, in addition to the treatment of interest, may have been different, or they may constitute a group with different characteristics. Consequently, the use of historical controls is subject to significant bias. For example, outcomes of a series of patients with lumbar disc herniation and sciatica treated by percutaneous discectomy initially seemed promising. However, subsequent controlled trials show that this technique is less effective than other treatment options (32).

While randomized studies are most commonly associated with the use of control groups, nonrandomized retrospective and prospective studies can also include control groups. A retrospective or case–control study identifies patients who, for example, underwent surgery at some time in the past. An appropriate control group would be patients who underwent an alternative treatment around the same time and for the same condition as the surgical patient. A prospective or observational cohort study identifies groups of patients with the same condition who are about to or have just undergone one of the alternative treatments being examined. They are then followed into the future for various outcomes.

Appropriate control groups to compare to patients undergoing a standard surgical treatment in either case–control or prospective cohort studies could include no treatment, nonsurgical treatment, or alternative surgical procedures. The choice of a control group depends in part on the study objectives and practical considerations. Regardless of the control group chosen, it should be evaluated concurrently with the index cases and should have similar baseline characteristics. Because a case–control or observational cohort study does not randomly assign treatment, differences between cases and controls are likely. For conditions whose treatment is clear (such as fractures), it would be impossible to select a comparable nontreatment cohort, although there are often instances in which competing treatment methods can be compared. However, for disorders with highly variable rates of surgery, such as lumbar disc herniation, it is known that physicians may choose surgical or nonsurgical treatment for similar types of patients. While surgical patients will generally be expected to have more severe disease than nonsurgical patients, sufficient overlap of patient characteristics can be expected to permit creation of comparison groups.

Randomization

While observational cohort studies have significant advantages over noncontrolled case series, cohort studies are likely to have different distributions of baseline clinical characteristics depending on treatment group. Without randomization of treatment assignment, one cannot definitely assert that any relative improvement or worsening does not result from differences among groups at baseline rather than from any effects of treatment. For this reason, randomized clinical trials (RCTs) remain the gold standard to assess efficacy of care. In RCTs, patients are randomly allocated into two or more treatment arms using strict protocols. If randomization is successful, baseline characteristics of treatment groups should be identical. It is the randomization process that differentiates RCTs from other prospective, controlled studies. The major advantage of an RCT is the assurance that bias is reduced in the comparison of treatment groups by equally distributing known and unknown patient characteristics that can influence outcome among groups.

Limitations of RCTs include the generalizability of findings to other patient populations. The entry criteria into randomized trials are often so rigid that it becomes very difficult to generalize the results to large populations. Additionally, both patients agreeing to randomization and physicians participating in RCTs may be different from the patients seen in community practice. Randomization alone does not eliminate potential biases. Blinding of patients only (single-blinded trials), or physicians and patients (double-blinded trials) to treatment assignments can minimize biased reporting of outcomes. However, when the treatments are surgery versus conservative care, it is impossible to blind without performing a sham procedure, which is usually unethical. Efforts to decrease this potential bias include using the patient and not the surgeon as the assessor of outcome, or using a blinded assessor. Other possibilities include randomly allocating patients to different physicians with different preferences for surgical procedures (34).

RCTs, while difficult and expensive to perform, should remain the cornerstone of efforts to assess effi-

cacy in lumbar spine disorders scientifically. The meta-analyses reviewed have documented the lack of RCTs in important conditions, such as spinal stenosis and use of lumbar fusion for various conditions. However, RCTs comparing standard discectomy to alternative treatments have been performed for herniated lumbar discs (3,17,30,35,38,41). Unfortunately, none are from the United States. Overcoming the difficulties inherent in performing RCTs remains of paramount importance in efforts to improve the information available to patients with, and physicians treating, lumbar spine disorders.

Cost-Effectiveness and Decision Analysis

Dramatic increases in national health-care expenditures, particularly in the U.S., have resulted in mounting pressure on medical professionals and others in the health care industry to control costs. The result has been increasing interest in cost-effectiveness studies to assess new and established diagnostic tests and therapeutic interventions. The terms *decision analysis* and *cost-effectiveness analysis* are often used interchangeably. Decision analysis refers to the process of critically appraising one of several alternative treatment strategies. Cost-effectiveness analysis is often used to refer to the decision analytic process as well as the unit of comparison, specifically the costs and benefits associated with alternative strategies. We will use cost-effectiveness analysis to mean the entire decision analytic process.

Cost-effectiveness analyses can be used to help set priorities for funding of health-care programs (9). They provide a means to compare the relative costs and benefits of different intervention strategies. Most importantly, cost effectiveness analyses allow different treatments, diagnostic tests, or programs to be compared to one another using a common unit of measure.

A cost-effective treatment strategy can have different meanings. It can mean that a strategy is cost saving with equal or better health outcomes compared to an alternative strategy. It can also refer to the more common situation in which a strategy has additional benefit and greater cost, but the benefit is worth the additional cost (13). What additional benefit of a given strategy justifies the additional dollar amount remains controversial. In cost-effectiveness analyses, costs are usually measured in dollars and benefits in years of life gained or quality-adjusted life years that take into account the relative health status of the person.

While the use of the term *cost-effective* is increasing, it is often used inappropriately or without sufficient documentation (13). In lumbar spine disorders, deficiencies in study methodology (see the section on meta-analysis) have resulted in a lack of uniform outcome measures. Not surprisingly, without uniform measures of benefit, few studies have assessed the relative benefits and costs of various treatment or diagnostic strategies for lumbar spine disorders (28). As an example of the inappropriate use of the term *cost effectiveness,* a study reported on the "cost effectiveness of chemonucleolysis versus laminectomy" in patients with herniated lumbar discs (31). Because there was no comparison of the relative benefits of each treatment, the authors should have referred to the treatment as being cost saving, not cost effective. This could be important if the less costly strategy were also associated with less benefit. If that were the case, one might not wish to endorse such a strategy.

Limitations of cost-effectiveness analysis include methodologic inconsistencies that question the validity and reliability of the calculated costs and benefits. Sensitivity analysis, the presenting of ranges of values for the costs and benefits used, is one attempt to address this uncertainty. Cost-effectiveness analysis is only important if resources are scarce, and choices have to be made among treatments or programs that cannot all be funded. Other considerations for allocating scarce resources other than cost-effectiveness may be appropriate. Programs with identifiable beneficiaries (e.g., transplant patients) are often favored over programs that may be more cost effective but where the beneficiary is never identified (e.g., disease prevention). Despite these limitations, cost-effectiveness analysis will continue to be used as a research and policy tool to help prioritize the allocation of health-care resources.

Practice Guidelines

Practice guidelines have been viewed by many as the solution to the myriad problems facing current medical practice. The belief is that guidelines could clarify and codify clinical practice so that variations in practice patterns would be eliminated, costs would be lower and more predictable, and quality of care would be improved. The U.S. Congress clearly had these objectives in mind when it created the Agency for Health Care Policy and Research (AHCPR). The development of clinical practical guidelines was mandated as a major task for the Agency (1).

In our view, the task of developing practice guidelines is far more difficult than originally anticipated, and the end result for many conditions will be less definitive than many would hope. There are several reasons for this opinion.

First, in order to develop guidelines for spine care, it is obvious that they must be based on accurate information about the outcomes of diagnosis and treatment of spinal conditions. As we have previously discussed, much of that information is not currently available. If many of the outcomes of spine care are not clearly known, how can guidelines be developed? The developers of the AHCPR guidelines for care of acute low back pain (2) used a method in which the quality of scientific evidence

was graded in developing their recommendations about numerous diagnostic measures and therapeutic treatments of this condition. Almost no randomized clinical trials were available for analysis, and the quality of evidence for most recommendations in the final guideline was marginal. As previously described, meta-analyses of conditions such as lumbar fusion have revealed an information base so deficient that it is clear that a scientifically based guideline for the procedure could not be written at this time. A low back guideline has recently been developed in the United Kingdom. Its authors incorporated some of the information from evidence tables created for the AHCPR guideline (2).

A second issue relates to the fact that there are many types of guidelines and many uses for them. For example, an insurance company can adopt a guideline on the preoperative testing or allowed length of hospital stay for a given condition. Such a guideline can be used for monitoring cost control but has little to do with the quality or outcome of care. One can develop guidelines for almost every aspect of medical care. Such guidelines can be inconsistent with each other, and this multiplicity of guidelines can lead to considerable confusion.

We believe that a useful way to categorize guidelines is to consider whether they have to do with *processes* or *judgements* about medical care. Process of care describes the operations or workings in medical treatments. For example, the use of an imaging study to determine if a patient has spinal stenosis can be defined as a process of care. Research can be (and has been) undertaken to determine if such procedures are useful for evaluating this condition (24). If they are, incorporation of this process of care (an imaging study) into a clinical guideline seems a useful and obvious strategy. There are many examples of widely accepted process guidelines in current use. Guidelines for anesthesia monitoring are an excellent example (15). Process guidelines can serve important purposes in considerations of the cost, quality, and appropriateness of care. Where available, their use should be encouraged, and where they are not yet developed, the necessary research to formulate them should be carried out.

Judgement guidelines can be defined as those in which there is patient choice among alternatives for health care. These are much more difficult to develop because the personal decision to undergo a given method of treatment involves a wide range of issues that cannot be easily covered in a guideline. Because most of medical care is elective and involves many alternatives, this becomes an important point. In the case of an emergent condition such as cauda equina syndrome, patient choice will likely not be an issue. The risk of a poor result without prompt surgery is well known, and, appropriately, the physician's recommendation will nearly always prevail. A guideline would be relatively easy to develop because patient choice is not a reasonable alternative.

More often we deal with conditions such as herniated lumbar disc with sciatica. In this situation there are choices. It is known that if a patient is willing to wait long enough, his or her symptoms usually resolve (41). On the other hand, discectomy is known to produce good results with few complications (20). In this situation the patient has a choice—surgery or watchful waiting. On the surface it would seem that a guideline to cover this situation could be written, and many have been (7). The problem is that the guideline cannot deal with the myriad variables that influence the choices that people make about their health care. There is nothing inherently wrong with available guidelines for lumbar discectomy, but neither are they very helpful in decision making by the ultimate user—the patient. Two patients presenting with sciatica could have identical symptoms, physical findings, and imaging studies. A surgeon seeing these two patients would probably make the same treatment recommendation to both. In this setting, the treatment decision is largely being guided by the preferences and beliefs of the surgeon (a concept referred to as delegated decision making), but the reality is that, given enough information, one patient might choose surgery and the other nonoperative treatment. A practice guideline cannot effectively deal with this issue.

The better strategy may be to focus on developing information systems by which patients are provided with an array of information that accurately describes the risks and benefits of alternative treatments and that permits them, in consultation with their physicians, to make informed choices that are based on their own appraisal of those risks and benefits. An interactive videodisk technology has been developed that in early experience appears to accomplish this goal (27).

Both practice guidelines and interactive patient decision-making systems must be underpinned with accurate information—information that will come about only as the result of outcomes research. We must also recognize that guidelines are an iterative and ongoing process. Regardless of the quality of an initial guideline, constant updating and revision will be required. The increasing knowledge base in basic science and pathophysiology along with the rapid development of new technologies will require ongoing outcomes research efforts and the incorporation of that new information into guidelines and decision-making systems.

Summary

In this chapter, we have defined and described the concept of outcomes research, particularly as it relates to the human spine. We have discussed the important differences between outcomes research and outcomes assessment and how they apply to physicians in their practices. Outcomes methodologies, such as small and large area

data analyses, and the state of clinical research have illuminated the problems confronting all physicians, including those involved in spine research and clinical care. This information has made clear the need to quickly expand and improve research in all aspects of this field.

There are many different methods that fall under the rubric of outcomes research. Large data base analysis, small area analysis, meta-analysis, clinical trials, and decision and cost-effective analyses all use specific techniques, but they are all characterized by well-established, validated, and statistically significant research methods. These concepts are described and illustrated. We discuss the role of practice guidelines as applied to spine care. For conditions for which patients have choices about the kind of care they can receive, it may be that methods that offer accurate, scientifically based information and data about the risks and benefits of alternative treatments will prove more useful than guidelines.

REFERENCES

1. Agency for Health Care Policy and Research (1990): *Purpose and programs.* Publication No. OM-0096. Rockville, MD: AHCPR.
2. Agency for Health Care Policy and Research (1994): *Acute low back pain problems in adults: assessment and treatment. Clinical practice guideline.* Publication No. 95-0643. Rockville, MD: AHCPR.
3. Andersson G (1972): Hip assessment: a comparison of nine different methods. *J Bone Joint Surg* 54B:621–625.
4. Cherkin DC, Deyo RA, Loeser JD, Bush T, Waddell G (1994): An international comparison of back surgery rates. *Spine* 19:1201–1206.
5. Cherkin DC, Deyo RA, Volinn E, Loeser JD (1992): Use of the international classification of diseases (ICD-9-CM) to identify hospitalizations for mechanical low back problems in administrative data bases. *Spine* 17:817–825.
6. Ciol MA, Deyo RA, Krueter W, Bigos SJ (1994): Characteristics in Medicare beneficiaries associated with reoperation after lumbar spine surgery. *Spine* 19:1329–1334.
7. American Academy of Orthopaedic Surgeons (1991): *Clinical policies.* Rosemont, IL: AAOS.
8. Crawshaw C, Frazer AM, Merriam WF, Mulholland RC, Webb JK (1984): A comparison of surgery and chemonucleolysis in the treatment of sciatica. A prospective randomized trial. *Spine* 9:195–198.
9. Detsky AS, Naglie IG (1990): A clinician's guide to cost-effectiveness analysis. *Ann Intern Med* 113:147–154.
10. Deyo RA (1993): Practice variations, treatment fads, rising disability. Do we need a new clinical research paradigm? *Spine* 18:2153–2162.
11. Deyo RA, Cherkin DC, Loeser JK, Bigos SJ, Ciol MA (1992): Morbidity and mortality in association with operations on the lumbar spine. *J Bone Joint Surg [Am]* 74:536–543.
12. Deyo RA, Ciol MA, Cherkin DC, Loeser JD, Bigos SJ (1993): Lumbar spinal fusion. A cohort study of complications, reoperations, and resource use in the Medicare population. *Spine* 18:1463–1470.
13. Doubilet P, Weinstein MC, McNeil BJ (1986): Use and misuse of the term "cost effective" in medicine. *N Engl J Med* 314:253–256.
14. Drake BG, Callahan CM, Dittus RS, Wright JG (1994): Global rating systems used in assessing knee arthroplasty outcomes. *J Arthroplasty* 9:409–417.
15. Eichorn JH, Cooper JB, Cullen DJ, et al. (1986): Standards for patient monitoring during anesthesia at Harvard Medical School. *JAMA* 256:1017–1020.
16. Einstadter D, Kent DL, Fihn SD, Deyo RA (1993): Variation in

the rate of cervical spine surgery in Washington State. *Med Care* 31:711–718.

17. Ejeskar A, Nachemson A, Herberts P, Lysell E, Andersson G, Irstam L, Peterson L-E (1983): Surgery versus chemonucleolysis for herniated lumbar discs. A prospective study with random assignment. *Clin Orthop* 174:236–242.

18. Fairbank JCT, Davies JB, Mbaot JC, O'Brien JP (1980): The Oswestry low back pain disability questionnaire. *Physiotherapy* 66: 271–273.

19. Glass GV (1976): Primary, secondary and meta-analysis. *Educ Res* 5:3–8.

20. Hoffman RM, Wheeler KJ, Deyo RA (1993): Surgery for herniated lumbar discs: a literature synthesis. *J Gen Intern Med* 8:487–496.

21. Keller RB, Chapin AM, Soule DN (1990): Informed inquiry into practice variations; the Maine Medical Assessment Foundation experience. *Qual Assur Health Care* 2:69–75.

22. Keller RB, Rudicel SA, Liang MH (1993): Outcomes research in orthopaedics. *J Bone Joint Surg [Am]* 75:1562–1574.

23. Keller RB, Soule DN, Wennberg JE, Hanley DF (1990): Dealing with geographic variations in the use of hospitals. *J Bone Joint Surg* 72(A):1286–1293.

24. Kent DL, Haynor DR, Larson EB, Keyo RA (1992): Diagnosis of lumbar spinal stenosis in adults: a meta-analysis of the accuracy of CT, MR, and myelography. *AJR* 158:1135–1144.

25. L'Abbe KA, Detsky AS, O'Rourke K (1987): Meta-analysis in clinical research. *Ann Intern Med* 107:224–233.

26. Letsch SW (1993): National health care spending in 1991. *Health Aff* 12:94–111.

27. Lyon HC, Henderson JB, Beck JR, et al. (1989): *A multipurpose interactive videodisc with ethical, legal, medical, educational, and research implications: the informed patient decision-making procedure.* Proceedings of the 13th Annual Symposium on Computer Applications in Medical Care, Washington, DC, November 5–8.

28. Malter AM, Larson DB, Deyo RA (1994): Surgical discectomy is cost-effective for the treatment of herniated lumbar discs unresponsive to initial medical therapy. *J Gen Intern Med* 9(S2):60.

29. Mark DB, Naylor CD, Hlatky MA, et al. (1994): Use of medical resources and quality of life after acute myocardial infarction in Canada and the United States. *N Engl J Med* 331:1130–1135.

30. Muralikuttan KP, Hamilton A, Kernohan WG, Mollan RAB, Adair IV (1992): A prospective randomized trial of chemonucleolysis and conventional disc surgery in single level lumbar disc herniation. *Spine* 17:381–387.

31. Ramirez LF, Javid MJ (1985): Cost effectiveness of chemonucleolysis versus chemonucleolysis in the treatment of herniated nucleus pulposus. *Spine* 10:363–367.

32. Revel M, Payan C, Vallee C, et al. (1993): Automated percutaneous lumbar discectomy versus chemonucleolysis in the treatment of sciatica. A randomized multicenter trial. *Spine* 18:1–7.

33. Roland M, Morris R (1983): Study of the natural history of back pain, part I: development of a reliable and sensitive measure of disability in low-back pain. *Spine* 8:141–144.

34. Rudicel S, Edsaile J (1985): The randomized clinical trial in orthopaedics: obligation or option? *J Bone Joint Surg [Am]* 67:1284–1293.

35. Tullberg T, Isacson J, Weidenheilm L (1993): Does microscopic removal of lumbar disc herniation lead to better results than the standard procedure? Results of a one-year randomized study. *Spine* 18:24–27.

36. Turner JA, Ersek M, Herron L, et al. (1992): Patient outcomes after lumbar spine fusions. *JAMA* 268:907–911.

37. Turner JA, Ersek M, Herron L, Deyo R (1992): Surgery for lumbar spinal stenosis. Attempted meta-analysis of the literature. *Spine* 17: 1–8.

38. Van Alphen HAM, Braakman R, Bezemer PD, Broere G, Berfelo MW (1989): Chemonucleolysis versus descectomy: a randomized multicenter trial. *J Neurosurg* 70:869–875.

39. Volinn E, Mayer J, Diehr P, Van Koevering D, Connell FA, Loeser JD (1992): Small area analysis of surgery for low-back pain. *Spine* 17:575–579.

40. Volinn E, Turczyn KM, Loeser JD (1994): Patterns in low back pain hospitalizations: implications for the treatment of low back pain in an era of health care reform. *Clin J Pain* 10;64–70.

41. Weber H (1983): Lumbar disc herniation. A controlled, prospective study with ten years of observation. *Spine* 8:131–140.

42. Wennberg JE, Freeman JL, Culp WJ (1987): Are hospital services rationed in New Haven or overutilised in Boston? *Lancet* 1:1185–1188.

43. Wennberg J, Gittelsohn A (1973): Small area variations in health care delivery. *Science* 182:1102–1108.

The Adult Spine: Principles and Practice,
2nd edition, J.W. Frymoyer, Editor-in-Chief.
Lippincott-Raven Publishers, Philadelphia © 1997.

CHAPTER **7**

The Epidemiology of Spinal Disorders

Gunnar B. J. Andersson

Epidemiology offers three insights critical to understanding back pain. It provides information on the magnitude of the problem and the resultant demand on medical and social resources (descriptive epidemiology), which is necessary to appropriate health resource allocations. Second, it provides information on the natural history,

which is important to patient counseling about prognosis and is a gold standard for determination of treatment effects. Third, it helps to determine associations between pain and individual and external factors, which allows risk factors to be identified and eliminated or modified.

G. B. J. Andersson, M.D., Ph.D.: Professor and Acting Chairman, Department of Orthopedic Surgery, Rush-Presbyterian-St. Luke's Medical Center, Chicago, Illinois, 60612.

HIGHLIGHTS

The author has faced a major challenge in writing this chapter. On the one hand, there is an enormous amount of epidemiologic information, particularly related to low back disorders, which is of particular importance to those with special interest in spinal epidemiology. On the other hand, the reader who wishes only a general sense of the issues may wish for only a brief overview. Therefore, I have created this "highlights" section to give an overview of the material as it relates to low back disorders. The serious student of spinal disorders will find it necessary to look within the chapter to truly understand the strengths and weaknesses of the data. There are remarkable similarities, but also differences, between various countries. The low back pain (LBP) portion of this chapter is organized such that the interested reader can analyze data from an international perspective.

Epidemiology of back pain (BP) is hampered by (a) lack of agreement on classification, (b) lack of objective evidence, (c) poor recall, (d) influence of legal, social, psychological, and work-related factors on morbidity and consequences, and (e) the intermittent nature of the problem. In short, there is a problem with validity and reliability, making the data, at best, approximate. Furthermore, most available data concern prevalence and are derived from case-control studies. While this permits calculation of odds ratios, causality cannot be determined directly. Also, most available data relate to the lumbar spine.

National statistics from the United States indicate a yearly prevalence in the 15% to 20% range. Back pain is the most frequent cause of activity limitation in people below age 45, the second most frequent reason for physician visits, the fifth most frequent for hospitalization, and the third ranking reason for surgical procedures. Nonsurgical hospitalizations decreased in the eighties, while surgical hospitalizations and procedures increased. About 1% of the U.S. population is chronically disabled because of BP and another percent is temporarily disabled. About 2% of the U.S. work force have compensable back injuries each year, for a total of over 500,000 injuries.

National statistics from European countries reveal that 10% to 15% of all sickness absence is due to back pain with rising absolute numbers of lost workdays per worker. The 1-year prevalence is 25% to 45%. Chronic BP is present in 3% to 7% of the adult population.

The lifetime prevalence of BP exceeds 70% in all industrial countries. Sciatica is present in about one-fourth of those with back problems. The average sickness absence for subjects with sciatica greatly exceeds that for subjects with BP. The lifetime prevalence of herniated lumbar discs is from 1% to 3%.

The annual rate of operations for herniated lumbar discs varies dramatically between countries. It is estimated that the rate per 100,000 is 10 in Great Britain, 20 in Sweden, 35 in Finland, and over 100 in the U.S. Over 95% of operations are at the L4 and L5 levels. The mean age at surgery is 40 to 45 years. Men are operated on twice as often as women.

The rate of all back surgeries is also higher in the U.S. than in other developed countries. In 1988–1989, the likelihood of having back surgery was 40% higher in the U.S. than in the Netherlands, which had the second highest frequency of back operations, and 5 times higher than in Scotland and England. The back surgery rates in two Canadian provinces were a third to a half of those in the U.S.

Over the 11-year period from 1979 to 1990, the number of adult low back operations in the U.S. increased by 55%, from 102 per 100,000 to 158 per 100,000. There are large regional variations in operative rates, however, from 113 per 100,000 in the West to 171 per 100,000 in the South. Over the same period (1979 to 1990), the nonsurgical hospitalizations decreased from 402 per 100,000 to 150 per 100,000.

As a subset, people with occupational LBP have received particular attention. Occupational risk factors are difficult to research because (a) exposure is usually uncertain, (b) the healthy worker effect can result in erroneous conclusions, (c) injury mechanisms are unclear, and (d) disability is influenced by work factors, individual factors, and legal and social factors. Despite these limitations, heavy physical work, lifting, static work postures, bending and twisting, and vibration are all physical work factors that have been associated with increased risk of BP. Additionally, psychological and psychosocial work factors, including work dissatisfaction, are important risk factors in low back disability.

In the nonoccupational setting, other risk factors are associated. The peak prevalence of LBP is between ages 35 and 55, indicating age-related risk. In women, there is some indication that the prevalence increases after menopause, but gender is of little importance with respect to low back symptoms.

Anthropometric data are contradictory. Generally speaking, there is no strong relationship between LBP and height, weight, or body build. Tallness appears to be a specific, but inconsistent, risk factor for sciatica and disc herniation. Posture is a risk factor only when extremely abnormal. Physical fitness is not a predictor of risk of acute LBP, but the physically fit have a lesser risk of chronic LBP and a more rapid recovery after a pain episode.

EPIDEMIOLOGIC RESEARCH ON BACK PAIN

Barriers

Epidemiologic research on back pain is difficult for several reasons. There is no general agreement on diagnostic classification. This makes comparison between studies difficult and precludes the development of general data bases. Moreover, it is well established that the response to the simple question of whether or not back pain is present at a certain time varies depending on the phrasing of the question. The situation further worsens when gathering data on previous back pain, because subject recall is imprecise. Also, there are often no objective signs in people complaining of back pain (377). For these reasons, some researchers have actually suggested that epidemiology of back conditions be restricted to studies of sciatica or disc herniations, where the definitions are easier and the classification is more uniform (187,406). This is also the reason why in this chapter I have divided the material into two sections; "all back pain" and sciatica. As will be apparent, the data on LBP are far more extensive than the data on cervical and thoracic pain.

Data Sources

Information on the prevalence and incidence of BP is available from numerous sources: national data, insurance and hospital data, interviews or questionnaires, and selective prospective and retrospective clinical studies. Unfortunately, the information is widely distributed in the scientific literature, and the quality of the data bases is rarely discussed. Wood and Badley (415) have reviewed the limitations of insurance and hospital data. Case definition is the main problem. Data on the consequences of BP also present problems, reflecting largely differences between societies and individuals. Mortality data are of no relevance. Sickness absence data are heavily influenced by work conditions (physical and psychological), and the diagnosis is of doubtful precision and accuracy. Data derived from workers' compensation claims are also affected by inherent biases (1): (a) all workers are not always covered by workers' compensation programs, (b) the claims data are mainly administrative, and therefore while accurate on absence and cost, they lack validity on diagnosis, and (c) all workers with BP do not file claims and many do not stay away from work. A further complication in using disability data is the poor correlation between tissue injury and disability, particularly long-term disability. In fact, it has been suggested that chronic disability in back pain is primarily related to a psychosocial dysfunction. This relationship might explain the observation that liberalization of compensation laws results in an increased rate of "injury" (418).

In questionnaire surveys, the occurrence of diseases and symptoms are usually underreported (147), which can be improved by better interview techniques. The validity and reliability of data on BP are uncertain and the data should be considered approximate (41,147, 238,354,355,402,403,405). Prospective studies are preferred, but the intermittent nature of back symptoms may result in omission of a significant number of cases (patients who have no back pain now, but had back pain a week ago), or in the same case being counted several times when performing a cross-sectional study. Further, prospective studies become very expensive. Retrospective studies, on the other hand, depend on recall and/or uncertain records but are the easiest and least expensive. Caution should be taken in overinterpreting available information. At best, these studies provide ideas about the frequency and impact of BP on the population. At worst they may actually reflect local practices in health care and local insurance and social systems.

DEFINITIONS

Incidence and prevalence are the two pivotal epidemiologic descriptions of any disease. Incidence is the rate at which people without a symptom or disease develop such over a specified time period. Incidence depends only on the rate at which a disease occurs. Prevalence, on the other hand, is a measure of the number of people in a given population who have a symptom or disease at a particular time. The 1-month prevalence of back pain, for example, is a measure of all those with BP identified over a 1-month period, irrespective of whether they had pain before the survey was started or not. Prevalence depends both on incidence and duration of disease. A change in prevalence therefore may result from a change in incidence or a change in duration of a disease (or symptoms), or both. Prevalence has the advantage that it can be determined by a single survey, while incidence requires following a population who were free of disease (or symptoms) at the onset of the study.

Prevalence is often determined in a cross-sectional study of a population sample. This sample should ideally be representative of all members of the population within defined limits. Prevalence can be related to other variables in the population gathered at the same time, to determine their effect on the disease. This information can generate etiologic hypotheses, but it is important to stress that these data do not prove causality (348). A frequently used cross-sectional study design is the case-control study; a group of cases (individuals with back pain) is compared to a control group. Factors of interest, such as occupational exposure, are recorded for cases and controls. Odds ratios (ORs) can then be calculated by comparing the number of subjects with a certain exposure who have BP to the number of subjects who also have BP but who have not been exposed. ORs can similarly be calculated for human factors. Some investigators use the term relative risk (RR) instead of OR to describe the relationship of disease rate in an exposed group to that in a nonexposed group. High ORs suggest, but do not prove, causality (348). Case-control studies have many advantages, including allowing the use of a smaller number of subjects and a shorter follow-up. Many exposures can be studied at once, and the cost is comparatively low. The main disadvantage is the possible bias from unblinded data gatherers, unverified exposures, inadequate recall, and imprecise diagnosis, to name a few of the methodologic issues posed in such epidemiologic research.

PREVALENCE OF "ALL" BACK PAIN/SCIATICA

National Statistics

United States

Cunningham and Kelsey (85) used the first Health and Nutrition Examination Survey (NHANES I) and found a prevalence of self-reported symptoms of 17%, whereas 15% had symptoms requiring a physician visit (Table 1). The peak prevalence was in middle age. They further estimated that 1% of all adults in the U.S. have or have had a disc disorder. Disc disorders were not associated with either education or income, while there was a tendency for "vertebrogenic pain syndrome" to be associated with higher education and income.

Deyo and Tsui-Wu (96,97) used the more recent NHANES II national survey (1976 to 1980), which included 27,801 subjects. The cumulative lifetime prevalence of LBP (lasting at least 2 weeks) was 13.8%, and 10.3% of respondents had BP within the previous year (Fig. 1). Sciatica was reported by 1.6% of the entire sample and by 12% of subjects with BP. At some time, 2% had been told that they had "a ruptured disc." Among subjects with previous or ongoing LBP, one-third had pain of 2 to 4 weeks duration, one-third for 1 to 5 months, and one-third for 6 months or longer. Severity of pain was mild in 21%, moderate in 43.5%, and severe in 34.5%. Age was an important factor as illustrated in Figure 1. There were also significant racial, regional, and educational influences, but women and men had equal lifetime prevalence (Table 2). The use of health professionals by subjects with BP is listed in Table 3. Overall, 84% of those with LBP had seen a health care profes-

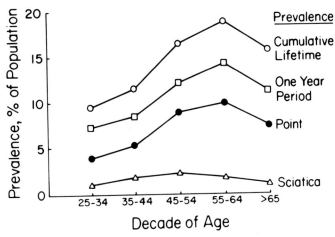

FIG. 1. Prevalence of low back pain. Only episodes lasting for at least 2 weeks are included. Sciatica is defined as pain radiating to the legs, increasing with cough, sneeze, or deep breathing. Redrawn from Deyo and Tsui-Wu (96).

sional, 30.9% had been admitted to a hospital because of LBP, and 11.6% had undergone surgery. The use of treatment modalities is listed in Table 4, of which the most common treatment was rest. Interestingly, 70% to 85% of subjects reported a benefit for any of the treatments listed, except for traction and cold application where the benefit was less certain.

Other data sources can be used to estimate the impact of LBP on the U.S. population. Among people below age 45, back problems are the most frequent cause of activity limitation, and among subjects 45 to 64, the fourth most frequent cause (274). The rate of physician visits is second only to heart problems among chronic conditions (270,273,274). Further, back problems are the fifth ranking reason for hospitalization, and the third ranking reason for surgical procedures (271,272,275). About 650,000 hospital discharges for BP were recorded annually in the U.S. between 1972 and 1978, accounting for 2.8% of all hospital discharges (Table 5) (127). In 1988, there were approximately 843,000 hospitalizations for back problems (310). Other data from the National Center for Health Statistics (NCHS) show that the annual "impairment of physical activity" resulting from a spinal condition rose from 0.8% to 1.6% in 1970–1971, to 1.4% to 2.5% in 1979–1980, i.e., almost doubled. Seven per-

TABLE 1. *Frequency distribution for NHANES I examinees (N = 6,913) and estimated prevalence among U.S. adults of self-reported musculoskeletal symptoms and physician-observed back abnormalities*

	Self-reported symptoms		Physician-observed abnormalities	
Part of body	HANES I examinees with symptoms Number (%)	Estimated prevalence among U.S. adults Number (%)	HANES I examinees with symptoms Number (%)	Estimated prevalence among U.S. adults Number (%)
Back	1,227 (17.7%)	18,388,000 (17.2%)	1,176 (17.1%)	16,121,000 (15.2%)

Source: ref. 85.

TABLE 2. *Lifetime prevalence of low back pain in selected NHANES II demographic groups (N = 10,404)*

	Unweighted (N)	Low back pain prevalence* (%)	Significance
Sex			
Male	4,904	14.2	NS
Female	5,500	13.4	
Race			
White	9,058	14.2	.005
Black	1,157	11.4	
Other	189	9.3	
Region			
Northeast	2,358	10.9	.0001
Midwest	2,707	14.5	
South	2,831	14.4	
West	2,508	15.0	
Education			
Elementary or none	2,422	17.3	<.0001
High school	5,076	14.4	
College	2,806	11.2	

Source: ref. 96.
* Weighted values, adjusting for probability of selection, non-response, and age, sex, and race composition of U.S. population.
NS = not significant, $p = 0.2$.

TABLE 3. *The use of health professionals by NHANES II subjects with LBP (N = 1,516)*

Health professional	Percentage
General practitioner	58.6
Orthopedist	36.9
Chiropractor	30.8
Osteopath	13.8
Internist	7.6
Rheumatologist	2.5
Any	84.6

Source: ref. 96.

LBP resulted in an average of 2.8 physician visits per affected person. Fifty percent of LBP sufferers had been hospitalized, and 22% had undergone surgery. Activity limitation in the previous year was also reported. Of subjects with LBP, 8.3% had been bedridden, and 8.0% had been off work.

Deyo and Tsui-Wu (97) used the NHANES II data to determine any functional disability due to BP. Activity limitations among subjects with LBP were common and strongly influenced by educational level. The higher the education level, the fewer the disability days. However, work absenteeism was most strongly correlated to income, and the rate increased as income decreased. Disability days were fewer among employed women than men, and in the women they correlated only weakly with education and income.

United Kingdom

Benn and Wood (28) found that the number of sickness absence episodes per 1,000 person-years was 11 for women and 22.6 for men. Wood (414) later attempted to calculate the impact of back problems on medical and social services (Table 6). Other surveys have shown that 25% of all British working men are affected by low back disorders each year (133). Annually, 1 out of 25 workers

cent of the adult population reported a disability due to the back alone or a combination of the back and other joint conditions. The mean number of days of restricted activity due to back problems was 23.5, and 8 days were lost from work. Chronic disability due to LBP was reported to affect 2.4 million Americans permanently, and an additional 2.4 million were temporarily disabled. Other NCHS data show that 14.3% of new patient visits to physicians are for LBP and each year there are close to 13 million physician visits for chronic LBP. Kramer et al. (201) used the 1976 National Health Interview Survey (NHIS) of 115,000 individuals to determine the social impact and medical care due to LBP. They found that

TABLE 4. *Use of specific treatments by NHANES II subjects with LBP (N = 1,516)*

Treatment	Percent who ever used this treatment	Of those using, percent who thought it helped	Of those who thought it helped, percent now using
Rest	80.8	85.5	48.5
Hot packs or heating pads	73.9	80.4	32.1
Aspirin	58.2	76.7	48.1
Stiff mattress	57.9	84.8	89.2
Exercises or physical therapy	40.5	78.1	43.0
Bedboard	36.1	84.8	63.6
Braces	27.0	70.8	28.1
Traction	20.7	62.9	9.6
Diathermy or paraffin	16.7	75.3	3.9
Cold packs or ice	7.2	55.9	15.5
Splints or casts	3.6	73.9	5.1

Source: ref. 96.

TABLE 5. *Estimated annual number of hospital discharges by first listed diagnosis in the United States, 1972–1978*

Annual discharges	Number
Total	650,000
Men	325,000
Women	325,000
Age < 15	5,000
15–44	292,000
45–64	263,000
65+	89,000
Hospital days (total)	6,694,000
Average duration (days/patient)	10.3

Source: ref. 127.

TABLE 6. *Back patients' need for medical and social services, expressed as rates per 1,000 persons at risk*

	Number of subjects
Handicapped/pension	2
General practitioner consultants	20 (58 visits)
Referrals	9
Admissions	1
Operations	0.1
Spinal symptoms	7

Source: ref. 28.

change jobs because of a back condition. In 1979, 79,000 persons were chronically disabled (140), and on any one day 0.05% of the work force has been chronically disabled for more than 6 months by a back problem (415). Wood and Badley (416,417) estimate that in 1978, one-third of all musculoskeletal complaints in Great Britain were due to BP, with 2.1% of the population reporting sick to work. The average absence period was 30 days. Patients with sciatica were on average off work for 40 days, while patients with LBP alone had a lower figure of 20 days. Frank (114) has recently reported that LBP was the largest single cause of sick leave in 1988–1989, accounting for 12.5% of the total number of sick days (which were 52.6 million). According to the National Back Pain Association (UK), there were 81 million certified back-related sick days in 1992–1993, and some 7 million visits to general practitioners for BP. During the same period, there were 33,000 work-related back "injuries".

Scandinavia

The fact that the Scandinavian countries have national health insurance systems makes it possible to obtain data on sickness absence from one source. Over a 10-year period from 1961 to 1971, 12.5% of all sickness absence in Sweden was related to a low back disorder, which accounted for 1% of all available work days (144). More recent data show that in 1983, 10.9% of all absence had a back diagnosis (Table 7) (317). The average sick-

ness absence period was 32 days and increased with advancing age (Table 8). Nachemson (263,264) calculated that in Sweden, a country of 8 million inhabitants and about 4.5 millions of working age, 14.8 million work days were lost in 1987 because of BP, representing 13.5% of all sickness absence days. Table 9 presents Swedish data on sickness absence for LBP and its resulting cost in terms of lost productivity.

A prospective Swedish review analyzed all patients who were sick-listed for LBP in a district of Gothenburg containing 49,000 subjects aged 20 to 65 years (74). A total of 7,526 sickness absence episodes for LBP were reported over an 18-month period; that is, about 10% of the population were off work for BP per year. Fifty-seven percent of patients recovered in 1 week, 90% in 6 weeks, and 95% after 12 weeks. At the end of 1 year, 1.2% remained work disabled. Those with sciatica were out of work for longer periods of time than patients who had BP only. Recurrent pain and disability were common and occurred in 12% over the 18-month period of observation.

Finnish National Health Interview Surveys show the prevalence of self-reported chronic BP to be 3.6% in 1964 and 7.1% in 1976 (193).

Canada

Lee et al. (222) analyzed data on musculoskeletal complaints identified by the 1978–1979 Canada Health Survey. The prevalence of "serious trouble with back and spine" was 4.4%. Table 10 shows the age distribution, again confirming an increase with advancing age. No difference was found between women and men. The to-

TABLE 7. *Sickness absence episodes with a back diagnosis per 100 insured: Swedish national data from 1983*

Sex	Age							
	16–19	20–29	30–39	40–49	50–59	60–64	65+	All
Men	4.1	11.4	12.0	14.0	15.3	10.4	3.2	12.2
Women	4.7	9.6	8.5	10.6	11.8	8.2	5.4	9.6
Both	4.3	10.6	10.3	12.4	13.4	9.3	13.2	10.9

Source: ref. 317.

TABLE 8. *Number of sickness absence days per sickness absence episode with a back diagnosis:*
Swedish national data from 1983

Sex	Age							
	16–19	20–29	30–39	40–49	50–59	60–64	65+	All
Men	4.9	22.3	22.3	25.9	74.2	110.4	176.3	62.3
Women	8.4	21.0	25.9	58.6	51.5	102.9	202.7	56.3
Both	7.9	22.2	24.5	47.7	62.9	108.4	186.6	58.7

Source: ref. 317.

tal number of disability days was estimated at 21.7 million, and the average duration of disability was 21.4 days per person per year.

Conclusions from National Prevalence Data

LBP is an enormously prevalent complaint with consistently high prevalence rates across countries. Affecting almost all people at some time in life, its annual prevalence rates range from 15% to 45% of the adult population. BP is a major cause of disability and is responsible for 10% to 15% of all sickness absence days in some countries. Chronic BP occurs in 2% to 7% of adults in industrialized countries. Little data is available on the occurrence of BP in developing countries.

Cross-Sectional Studies (Table 11)

United States

In 1973, Nagi, Riley, and Newby (266) determined the prevalence rates of persistent BP in a random sample of 1,135 residents of Columbus, Ohio, between 18 and 64 years old: 203 residents (18%) reported "often being bothered with pain in the back." Of those 203, 62% had had a spine radiograph, 26% had worn a back support, and 4% had had at least one back operation.

Frymoyer et al. (120,121) performed a retrospective cross-sectional analysis of 3,920 patients who had en-

rolled in a family practice facility in Vermont from 1975 to 1978, and the group later analyzed in more detail a subset of 1,221 men, 18 to 55 years of age (87). Almost 70% had had LBP. When the data from that study were extended to the 50 million working 18- to 50-year-old American males, it was calculated that 38.5 million workdays are lost annually. Patients with severe LBP had significantly more leg complaints, sought more medical care and treatment for LBP, and had lost more time from work when compared to subjects with no or moderate LBP. Sciatica-like symptoms had been present in 28.9% of the men with moderate LBP and 54.5% of the men with severe LBP. Of men with moderate LBP, 14% reported leg numbness and 17.5% weakness, compared to 37.4% and 44.0% among those with severe LBP. The utilization of health care services is given in Table 12.

Risk factors for severe LBP were heavy lifting, the use of jack hammers or machine tools, and the operation of motor vehicles. Those with moderate low back symptoms were more likely to be cigarette smokers, joggers, and cross-country skiers. Height, weight, body mass index, lumbar lordosis, and leg length inequalities were not found to be risk indicators, but those with BP had less trunk muscle strength (302).

The prevalence of LBP in persons 65 years and older was assessed in a survey of 3,097 persons living in rural parts of Iowa (212). In the year preceding the survey, 24% of the women and 18% of the men had suffered from LBP, with prevalence rates declining with age. Forty percent reported BP at the time of the interview. Of those reporting LBP, 75% had used health care services for

TABLE 9. *Estimated sick-listing for LBP and associated cost due to loss of production in Sweden*

Year	% of insured[1]	No. of days	Cost of loss of production[2] ($ million[3])
1970	1	20	51
1975	3	22	179
1980	4	25	285
1987	8	34	806

Source: ref. 263.
[1] 4.7 million
[2] Based on 1987 wages and social costs.
[3] Assuming $1 = 6 Sw. Cr.

TABLE 10. *Sex and age distribution of Canada Health Survey group with "serious trouble" with back or spine*

	Number (×1,000)	Percent of total population
Total (23,023)	1,015	4.4
Men (11,417)	497	4.4
Women (11,606)	518	4.5
Age (both sexes)		
15–24 (4,548)	116	2.6
25–34 (3,806)	167	4.4
35–54 (5,108)	388	7.6
55+ (4,030)	332	8.2

Source: ref. 222.

TABLE 11. *Prevalence and lifetime incidence of LBP in different cross-sectional studies*

Lifetime incidence (%)	Prevalence (%)		Study group			Comment	Reference
	Point	Period	N	Age	Sex		
62.6	12.0	—	449	30–60	M		Biering-Sørensen (34–40)
61.4	15.2	—	479	30–60	F		
48.8	—	—	692	15–72	F		Hirsch et al. (153)
60.0	—	—	1193	25–59	M	Industrial population	Hult (160)
69.9	—	—	1221	28–55	M		Frymoyer et al. (120, 121)
—	18.0	—	1135	18–64	M, F		Nagi et al. (266)
61	—	31	716	40–47	M	1 month period	Sevensson et al. (356–361)
67	—	35	1640	38–64	F	1 month period	
51.4	22.2	—	3091	20+	M		Valkenburg and Haanen (376)
57.8	30.2	—	3493	20+	F		
—	12.9	—	3316		M, F	8 work groups	Magora (239–244)
—	—	25		40–59	M	1 year period	Gyntelberg (132)

Source: ref. 303.

back symptoms, 25% had been hospitalized at least once for BP, and 5% had had low back surgery.

Scandinavia

The city of Göteborg (about 450,000 inhabitants) has been the source of much Swedish epidemiologic data. Hirsch, Jonsson, and Lewin (153) interviewed 692 women (15 to 72 years of age) from three census districts in this city, selected at random to represent the adult Swedish female population. The lifetime prevalence of LBP was 48.8% in the total sample; the percentage increased up to age 55 and then stabilized. This prevalence figure is almost identical to the 46.8% reported later for 276 nurses in Göteborg (93). Horal (157) and Westrin (403) compared a group of individuals previously (in 1964) sick-listed for LBP, to a matched control group of

people who had not been sick-listed for LBP. Sample data are given in Table 13. Interestingly, 49% of the control group had a history of BP and 27% of controls had BP at the time of the investigation. This illustrates that sickness absence data tend to underestimate the prevalence of a condition such as LBP that limits mainly physically heavy work.

Svensson and Andersson (356–358,360,361) performed cross-sectional studies of two groups of subjects, one consisting of 940 men 40 to 47 years old and the other of 1,760 women in the 38- to 64-year age range. Table 14 compares the prevalence of LBP in men and women as well as selected data on their use of medical services. The prevalence rates for all BP were quite similar between sexes: 40% of men and 47% of women with BP had sciatica. Neither the lifetime prevalence nor the one-month prevalence were influenced by age in the women. In men, the age range was too narrow to evaluate. The proportion of women with significant work disability was 2.6% among 38-to 49-year-old women, and it rose to 5.9% among those 50 and older. Insurance data were available for the men and permitted determination of work absenteeism and work recovery rates. Notably, one-fourth of the men who said they had never had BP had been off work with that diagnosis, albeit usually for 1 day only (355,357). This illustrates the difficulty of relying on memory in questionnaire data and interviews.

TABLE 12. *Type of health care services and treatment used by men with LBP in Vermont*

Health-care practitioner	Moderate LBP % (N = 565)	Severe LBP % (N = 288)
Family physician	30.5	66.7
Orthopedic surgeon	8.8	32.3
Neurosurgeon	2.7	9.5
Osteopath	7.0	23.8
Chiropractor	12.7	27.5
Physiotherapist	3.8	16.1
Other	5.0	12.1
Treatment		
Bed rest	35.1	72.8
Muscle relaxant	17.7	52.6
Prescription pain medication	21.1	58.0
Physiotherapy	9.5	23.9
Other conservative treatment	12.6	27.4
Operation	2.0	10.5

Source: ref. 120.

TABLE 13. *Low back pain in probands and controls*

	Probands (%)	Controls (%)
3–4 year period prevalence	95	49
Of which:		
Duration > 1 week	83	21
Pain medication	73	6
Physiotherapy	47	3
Brace or corset	18	1
Point-prevalence	53	27

Source: ref. 403.

TABLE 14. *Data on prevalence and use of medical services from two retrospective cross-sectional surveys in Göteborg, Sweden (%)*

	Men Age 40–47 (N = 940)	Women Age 38–64 (N = 1,760)
Lifetime prevalence	61	66
One-month prevalence	31	35
Chronic pain	3.5–4	—
Physician visit	40	38
Radiograph	23	30
Hospitalized	3.5	3.4
Operation	0.8	1.0

Sources: ref. 356 and 357.

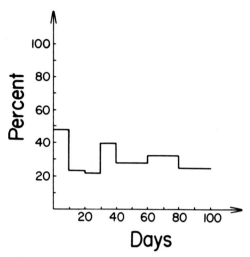

FIG. 3. Recovery from disability caused by sciatica. Percent of those absent at a given time who recover over the next 10 days. Redrawn from Andersson et al. (12).

The recovery rate was influenced by symptoms. In patients with LBP only (no radiation of pain), 60% recovered in 10 days (Fig. 2), whereas only 9% of patients with sciatica recovered in that time interval (Fig. 3) (12).

Bergenudd and Nilsson (30,31) studied a cross-sectional sample of 575 residents of Malmö, Sweden, 55 years of age. The point prevalence of BP was 29%. Of those with BP, 50% had had symptoms for more than 1 year. LBP exclusively was the most common complaint (12%), 5% had sciatica, and 2% had neck–shoulder pain. The remaining 10% had pain in several areas of the spine. In all, LBP was present in 25% of the sample. In another study from Malmö, Jacobsson et al. (166) reported an overall 1-year prevalence of 6% among 900 men and women who were 50 to 70 years old. Men were more often affected than women and the prevalence for both sexes decreased with increasing age.

Gyntelberg (132) reported the 1-year incidence of LBP among 4,753 residents of Copenhagen, Denmark, 40 to

59 years old: 25% developed LBP, 8% severe enough to warrant bed rest or require absence from work. Later, Biering-Sørensen (34–37) sampled 82% of all 30-, 40-, 50-, and 60-year-old inhabitants in Glostrup, Denmark. There were 449 men and 479 women who answered an extensive questionnaire and underwent objective measurements of spine function. Twelve months after the examination, 99% of the study population completed a follow-up questionnaire giving information about LBP in the intervening period. The lifetime prevalence of LBP is presented in Figure 19, along with the 1-year period and the point prevalence rates. The lifetime prevalence in men varied between 68% and 70%, and in women from 62% to 81%. In men, the prevalence was nearly constant within age groups, while in women the lifetime prevalence increased particularly for the 60-year age group. Table 15 shows sample data on symptoms and health care utilization among those with a lifetime history of BP. The 1-year incidence was 11% in the 30-year-olds and decreased in the older age groups (Table 16). The 1-year prevalence of LBP was 45% in both men and

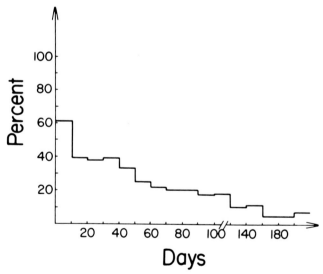

FIG. 2. Recovery from disability caused by low back pain. Percent of those absent at a given time who recover over the next 10 days. Redrawn from Andersson et al. (12).

TABLE 15. *Sample data on symptoms and health care utilization among individuals with a lifetime history of back pain in a Danish Community*

Symptoms and healthcare utilization	Patients using (%)
Daily symptoms	17
Work absence ever	22.5
Job accommodation ever	10
Physician consultation	60
Specialist consultation	25
Chiropractor consultation	15
Radiographs	30
Hospital admission	4.5
Surgery	1

Source: refs. 34–43.

TABLE 16. *One-year incidence of first time experience of LBP (%)*

Age (years)	Men	Women	Total
30	11	11	11
40	0	6	3
50	6	3	5
60	6	4	5
All	6	6	6

Source: ref. 34.

TABLE 18. *Sample data on symptoms and health care utilization among individuals with a lifetime history of low back pain in a Dutch community*

Symptoms and health-care utilization	Men (%)	Women (%)
Recurrences ever	85	85
3-month duration	30	30
Clinical disc prolapse	1.9	2.2
Work absence ever	50	33
Job change ever	8	4
Physician consult	28	42
Ever bedridden	30	30

Source: ref. 376.

women, and the 1-year incidence 17% in men and 16% in women. The prospective 1-year recurrence rate overall was 38% in men and 39% in women. A history of more recent and frequent LBP pain portended a greater risk of recurrences.

An analysis of risk factors was negative for occupation, while a history of previous BP, living alone, smoking, and motor vehicle transportation (public or private) were indicators of risk. Body height, obesity, leg length, and femoral epicondylar width were not found to be correlated to LBP (38). Poor isometric endurance of the trunk extensor muscles, and hyper-mobility of the spine were risk factors. A later analysis showed that gastric pain, daily smoking, and previous hospitalizations and operations were predictive of first time experience of LBP during the follow-up year (42).

Israel

Magora (239,241,244) and Magora and Taustein (246) performed investigations on 3,316 individuals taken at random from eight occupations. Present and previous LBP was determined: 429 (12.9%) were found to suffer from LBP at the time of the survey (point prevalence). Of those reporting current LBP (239), 92% (395 people) had suffered from pain on and off from 6 months to 11 years or more before the investigation, and they were analyzed further. Of the 42.2% who had been off work, 70.6% had absence periods exceeding 10 days. The highest prevalence of LBP was found in heavy industry workers, bus drivers, and nurses; the lowest in police-

men. Subjects who were unhappy about their occupation and who felt their work required a high degree of responsibility and mental concentration, had a higher prevalence of LBP than other subjects (241). Lifting and long-term sitting and standing also increased the risk, while leisure activities did not (240,242).

The Netherlands

Valkenburg and Haanen (376) reported on a study of 3,091 men and 3,493 women, 20 years of age and older, performed from 1975 through 1978 in Zoetermeer. A questionnaire, a physical examination, and radiographs were obtained. The lifetime prevalence of LBP was 51% in men and 58% in women, and the 1-year prevalence was about 30% in both sexes, increasing slightly with age up to 65 years and thereafter decreasing (Table 17). Table 18 reports selected data on symptoms and health care utilization among those with a lifetime history of BP.

Great Britain

A number of British studies report the annual frequency of consultations per 1,000 population to general practitioners for LBP and sciatica (Table 19) (19,98, 392,394). All studies report similar frequencies (20% to 25%), although the populations represent very different practices from rural to urban environments.

TABLE 17. *Low back complaints and work incapacity in the Zoetermeer study*

	Men (%)	Rel %	Women (%)	Rel %
Point-prevalence	22.2		30.2	
Lifetime incidence	51.4		57.8	
>3 months	14.3	28	19.6	34
Unfit for work	24.3	47	19.5	34
Work change	4.2	8	2.4	4

Source: ref. 376.

TABLE 19. *Annual frequency of consultations for LBP to general practitioners in Great Britain*

Reference	Sex	Consultations per 1,000
Walford (392)	M	21.4
Dillane et al. (98)	M	24.3
	F	20.3
Ward et al. (395)	M	22.8
	F	15.3
Barker (19)	Both	25.0

Belgium

A population-based survey of about 4,000 people was performed in Belgium to explore the influence of sociocultural and employment variables on self-reported LBP (343). The lifetime prevalence was 59%, while 33% had current LBP. Demographic and cultural factors influenced the risk of having the first episode of LBP, but were not associated with daily occurrence of LBP or severity of impairment. Age (OR > 2.0), female sex (OR = 1.42), living in a major city (OR = 1.18), and being French speaking (OR = 1.26) were associated with an increased risk of a LBP history.

A cross-sectional survey among the 4,256 employees (99.8% women) of the largest Flemish organization for family care was performed by Moens et al. (260), using a self-administered questionnaire. The 12-month prevalence was 18% [95% confidence interval (CI): 61.7 to 64.6] and the point prevalence was 18% (95% CI: 16.5 to 18.8). Among those with BP during the past year, 72% reported repeated episodes of pain. Of the those with pain, 29% stated that complaints interrupted their work during the past year. The mean sick leave for BP was 36 days and the median, 15 days.

Isolated Populations

The prevalence of lumbar and thoracic pain was determined among 1,381 migrants coming from the three Tokelau atolls, located south of the equator, who were resettled to New Zealand because of a severe hurricane (408). Almost 11% of men and 8.5% of women reported LBP, and an additional 1.5% of men and 3.1% of women reported pain in the thoracic area. BP prevalence was not influenced by age or sex but was positively associated with weight. BP among the migrants was compared with that of 811 Tokelauans who remained in the atolls (409). The only difference between the two samples was in the rate of thoracic BP in women, which was small and depended on small numbers. The rate of LBP was no more common in migrants, although compensation payments are available in New Zealand but not in the Islands.

Developing Countries

Waddell (391) has suggested that the introduction of Western-oriented cultures and medical practices may encourage, or legitimize, complaints related to BP that were almost unknown in the past, using Oman as an example. Unfortunately, there is insufficient information to reliably assess the magnitude of the problem in the developing countries. One study included 2,201 patients in a private clinic in Nairobi from 1982 through 1987 (261). All patients were carefully interviewed and received a standard x-ray examination. The point prevalence of LBP was 10%. The male to female ratio was 1: 1.7, and 38% were 31 to 40 years old.

The Industrial Problem

There are numerous reports on the prevalence of LBP in the workplace. Much of this information is difficult to evaluate because the work environment is highly selective (7,8,10,344). Only a small sample of the total number of published studies are reviewed here.

United States

Rowe (321–323) followed the employees at a plant in the state of New York over a 10-year period (1956 to 1965). LBP was second only to upper respiratory illness in terms of sickness absence; 35% of sedentary workers and 47% of workers with physically heavy work had made visits to the medical department because of LBP during the study period. Recurrences were frequent, occurring in about 85%. Data from the Liberty Mutual Insurance Company indicate annual rates of LBP ranging from less than 1% to over 15%, depending on occupation (344). Kelsey and White (187) estimate that about 2% of all employees in the U.S. have a compensable back injury each year. Back problems account for 19% of all Workers' Compensations claims in the U.S. (394), resulting in 400,000 such claims in 1978. Data from the Bureau of Labor Statistics supplementary data systems were used to calculate the incidence rate of "back sprains/strains" for 26 U.S. states in 1979. The average incidence rate was 0.75%, with large interstate differences ranging from 0.15% (New Mexico) to 2.08% (Washington). Men produced 76% of all claims, with the highest rates occurring in the 20- to 24-year age group (Fig. 4). The male to female risk ratio in that age group (20 to 24 years) was 3.0 and then decreased to 1.4 in the 55- to 64-year age group. Table 20 shows the events resulting in the injury. Manual handling activities dominate. The distribution according to industry employment is shown in Table 21, while Table 22 shows the distribution according to occupation. From both tables, the influence of work factors is obvious. Volinn et al. (389) have shown that large differences in incidence exist even between counties within a state; from 1.2% to 4.2% in the state of Washington in 1985.

Using the 1988 Occupational Health Supplement, which is part of the National Health Interview Survey, Behrens et al. (27) determined the prevalence of BP in the U.S. working population for specific occupational groups. The sample consisted of 30,074 individuals. Twelve-month prevalence rates were calculated for BP due to an injury and for BP due to repeated activities.

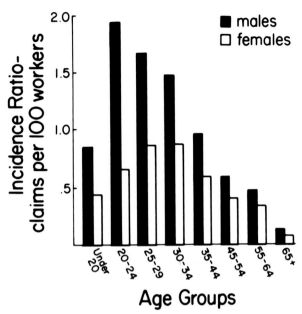

FIG. 4. Incidence ratio (claims per 100 workers) of compensation claims in 26 U.S. states due to strains/sprains of the back. Redrawn from Klein et al. (194).

Injury was defined as slipping, falling, twisting, lifting, or a car accident. The overall 12-month prevalence of BP due to an injury on the most recent job was 2.5%. For the population at large, this means that 2.62 million working people are injured annually. The highest prevalences were found among truck drivers (6.7%), operators of heavy machinery (5.6%), and people in the construction trades and other construction occupations (5.6%). The overall prevalence of BP due to repeated activity on the most recent job was 4.5%, representing 4.7 million U.S. workers. High prevalences were found among mechanics and repairers of engines and heavy equipment (10.5%), operators of heavy equipment (10.4%), and people in construction (10.1%)

The influence of insurance on the length of disability is obvious from a study by Sander and Meyers (332). When comparing time off work after injury on duty to that from injuries occurring off duty, statistically significant differences were found among comparable groups of railroad workers (Table 23). Compensation has also been found to influence the length of disability of patients receiving conservative care (128), as well as those receiving surgical treatment (113,137). Leavitt (221) found that work-related back symptoms resulted in a greater time loss than non-work-related even when controlling for the degree of physical work requirement.

Spengler et al. (347) conducted a retrospective analysis of injuries among 31,200 employees at the Boeing Company over a 15-month period in 1979 to 1980: 900 back injuries were reported (19% of all Workers' Compensation claims). The back injuries were responsible for 41% of cost, but 10% of more chronic back injuries were responsible for 79% of the cost. Material handling was the most common cause (46). Mechanics, maintenance and transportation employees, and clerks had the highest injury rates (3.8, 3.1, and 2.7 per 100 workers, respectively). Most injuries occurred in workers 25 years old and younger, but those injuries were typically more benign than injuries in the older population. In the prospective Boeing Study, which included 3,020 workers

TABLE 21. *Ratios (claims per 100 workers) of compensation claims for back strains/sprains in 26 states by industry*

Industry	Claims per 100 employees
Construction	1.6
Mining	1.5
Transportation	1.2
Manufacturing	1.0
Agriculture	0.9
Services	0.7
Wholesale/retail trade	0.6
Government (state and local)	0.2
Finance	0.2
Total	0.7

Source: ref. 194.

TABLE 20. *Workers' Compensation claims in 26 states for back strains/sprains by type of event or exposure*

Type	% of all back strains/sprains
Lifting objects	48.1
Overexertion, not elsewhere classified	9.0
Pulling or pushing objects	9.0
Voluntary bodily motions	6.6
Holding, wielding, throwing, or carrying objects	5.7
Involuntary bodily motions	4.7
Falls on working surfaces	4.3
Other exertions, not elsewhere classified	2.3
Others, individual less than 2%	10.4

Source: ref. 194.

TABLE 22. *Ratios of compensation claims in 26 states due to back strains/sprains by occupation*

Occupation	Claims per 100 workers
Miscellaneous laborers	12.3
Garbage collectors	11.1
Warehouse workers	9.3
Miscellaneous mechanics	5.6
Nursing aides	3.6
Nonspecific laborers	3.4
Material handlers	3.4
Lumber workers	3.3
Practical nurses	3.3
Construction laborers	2.8

Source: ref. 194.

TABLE 23. *Average number of months off work after injury until return to work*

	Injury on duty Months (No. of cases)	Injury off duty Months (No. of cases)
Lumbosacral sprain/strain		
All patients	14.9 (35)	3.6 (30)
Women	9.5 (3)	3.1 (7)
Men	4.5 (32)	38 (23)
Operated back		
All patients	9.3 (18)	4.4 (19)
Women	18.0 (1)	3.2 (3)
Men	8.8 (17)	4.6 (16)

Source: ref. 332.
All differences are statistically significant.

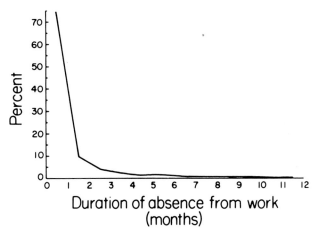

FIG. 5. Duration of work absence in workers with compensable back injury in Quebec, 1981. Redrawn from Spitzer et al. (349).

who were followed for about 4 years, 279 back injury reports were recorded (44). This means that just under 10% of the work force had a back injury over those years, or 2.4% per year assuming all injuries occurred in different workers. This number is similar to that of the retrospective study in which about 2.9% of the workers reported a back injury over a 15-month period.

In a prevalence study of back and joint problems among 5,903 employees in a chemical manufacturing company, 35.4% reported "any back or joint pain" in the previous year (60). BP lasting 30 days or more occurred in 5.3% of employees. There were no differences in prevalence between men and women or as a function of race. BP prevalence increased with increasing age.

Canada

Abenhaim and Suissa (1) studied the 1-year incidence of work-related LBP in the province of Quebec. In 1981,

the incidence of low back disability resulting in work absence was 1.4%. Of those disabled, 74% were off work for less than 1 month, whereas 7.4% were off work for 6 months or longer and were therefore responsible for 75% of all sickness absence days. Ten percent of the absentees accounted for 75% of the total direct cost (2,319). Prospective surveillance revealed a recurrence rate of 20% at 1 year, rising to 36.3% at 3 years. Men had a higher risk of recurrence than women, and subjects in the 25- to 44-year age group had the highest recurrence rate (Table 24). Occupation also influenced recurrence rate, the highest rates occurring in nurses and drivers and the lowest among white collar workers.

The recovery rate of the Quebec workers is illustrated in Figure 5. It is similar to that reported from other countries. At 1 year, 4.3% of workers remained absent from work (349). Incidence rates of compensated spinal disorders were computed by age and sex. For men, maximum rates (2.8%) were reached at 20 to 24 years of age; for women, 1.8% (Fig. 6). The difference between incidence rates in men and women was highly significant (1.9 for men versus 0.5 for women). The male to female RRs

TABLE 24. *Recurrence of back pain over a 3-year follow-up period: Risk of recurrence (risk ratio) calculated using a Poisson regression model*

	Recurrences (%)	Risk Ratio
Total	36.3	
Sex		
Male	38.0	1.85
Female	27.5	
Age		
15–24	35.0	
25–44	38.3	
45–64	31.8	
Occupation		
Driver	42.1	1.64
Nurse	39.6	2.62
Manual worker	36.6	1.26
Miner/lumber worker	36.4	1.14
White collar	28.6	1.00
Other	33.2	

Source: ref. 2.

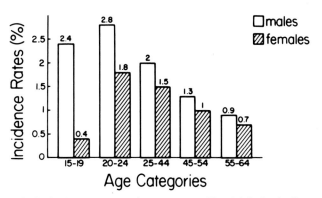

FIG. 6. Incidence rates of compensated back injuries in Quebec, 1981, by sex and age. Redrawn from Spitzer et al. (349).

Industrial Sector

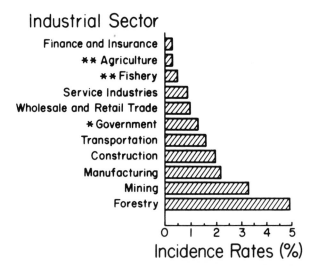

FIG. 7. Incidence rate of compensated back injury by industrial sector in Quebec, 1981. Redrawn from Spitzer et al. (349).

ranged from 5.6 at 20 to 24 years to 1.8 at 55 to 64 years, reflecting the reduced incidence rate in men with advancing age. One-year incidence rates per industrial sector are illustrated in Figure 7. Foresters and miners are at the top with 4.9% and 3.3%, respectively.

United Kingdom

In 1979, 50,000 British work injuries were classified as "overexertion etc." (369): 67% resulted from "lifting, carrying, wielding or throwing objects," and another 19% from pulling and pushing objects. Back injuries accounted for 61%, and 94% of these were labeled as sprains and strains. Back injuries accounted for 15% to 22% of all injuries for different industrial groups. David (91) studied the prevalence of "lumbar injuries and handling accidents" using the British Health and Safety Sta-

tistics for injuries resulting in work absence of at least 3 days. About 15% were back sprains and strains. The British Department of Health and Social Security (DHSS) reported 88,000 industrial back sprains and strains in 1977 to 1978. The median duration of the "spells" was 13 days (91,369). The highest rates for men were in mining and manufacturing industries, and for women in the timber and furniture industries (Table 25). The average annual incidence was 5.8 per 1,000 men employed, and 1.2 per 1,000 women employed. This resulted in an annual loss of 1.5 million working days in the U.K.

In a British survey of 2,685 male postal workers, Anderson (6) found that 23% had ongoing LBP, 7% had been referred to the hospital for their complaint, and 2% had been admitted. The annual absenteeism from work for LBP was 70 weeks per 100 men employed (7,8). Afacan (4) surveyed the medical records of 12 collieries of the National Coal Board. The study group comprised 12,125 men, 9,414 of whom were underground workers. During 1 year from 1976 to 1977, 14.8% of the total work force was absent from work because of back injuries. The number of new sickness absences was 19.1 for every 100 men employed.

Blow and Jackson (48) analyzed back injuries among dock workers in London resulting in sickness absence for at least 3 days. In 1967, the rate was 36 per 1,000 at risk with back injuries accounting for 28% of all reported injuries. Dock workers below age 25 had the highest annual incidence rate, 6%. Stubbs and Nicholson (351) performed a retrospective study of accidents occurring over 1 year in two large British construction companies. The annual back injury rate was 8.6 per 1,000 at risk. As in the studies by Blow and Jackson (48) and Afacan (4), the highest injury rates occurred in the younger age group.

Anderson (9) also analyzed cross-sectional data of 2,684 men from a range of occupations. The prevalence of current musculoskeletal complaints was 15%, while 25% had had musculoskeletal pain in the previous year.

TABLE 25. *Incidence of back injuries at work during 1977–1978*

Men		Women	
Industrial sector	Incidence of sprains and strains (per 1,000 employed)	Industrial sector	Incidence of sprains and strains (per 1,000 employed)
Mining and quarrying	28.3	Timber and furniture	3.3
Metal manufacture	9.7	Bricks, pottery, etc.	2.6
Bricks, pottery, etc.	9.4	Food, drink, and tobacco	2.3
Leather, etc.	8.9	Vehicles	2.3
Shipbuilding, etc.	8.3	Professional–scientific	1.8
Construction	7.7	Transport and communication	1.6
Transport and communication	7.5	Services	1.4
Gas and electricity	7.4	Chemical and allied industries	1.3
Distributive trades	6.1	Mechanical engineering	1.3
Public administration and defense	5.7	Other manufacturing	1.2
All industries	5.8		

Source: ref. 91.

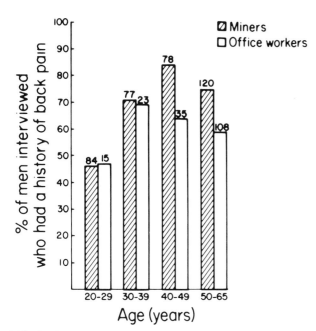

FIG. 8. Prevalence of back pain among miners and office workers, by age. Figures indicate absolute numbers. Redrawn from Lloyd et al. (229).

From this population, a cohort of 1,249 subjects with mixed jobs within a dockyard were followed for 2 years. The incidence rate of BP was 4.5%, and 8.9% of those affected at the start had at least one episode of sickness absence due to LBP over the 2 years. In another study, Lloyd et al. (249) surveyed 359 miners and 181 office workers at a Scottish colliery: 69% of the miners had had LBP at some time in life, 35% during the 3 months preceding the survey. The prevalence increased up to age 50 and then fell slightly (Fig. 8). The corresponding figures for the office workers were a lifetime prevalence of 58%, and a 3-month prevalence of 26%. Work loss in the 3-month period preceding the survey had occurred in 32% of miners with BP and 14% of office workers.

Nicholson (279) performed a detailed analysis of accident data from the telecommunications, electrical, and construction industries in Great Britain. Table 26 presents sample data on these accidents. Most injuries were due to material handling (50.5% to 70%), but falls were also a common cause. Subjects between 16 and 30 years of age had the highest rates among electrical workers and construction workers, while the 31- to 45-year age group had the highest rates in the telecommunications industry.

Scandinavia

In a classic early study, Hult (161) found that 60% of a sample of 1,193 Swedish men with different jobs had had BP at some time, 11% had been off work from 3 weeks to 6 months, and 4% had been off work for more than 6 months because of these symptoms. LBP was more frequent among heavy workers, occurring in 64.4% versus 54.7% for those with lighter work. Severe BP was reported by 6.8% of subjects with light physical work compared to 10.8% of subjects with heavy work. Disability because of LBP was almost twice as common among those with heavy physical jobs (43.5% versus 25.5%). The average yearly work absence was 2.93 days per 100 men, with an average sickness absence period of 24 days; 2.3% of subjects with light work and 4% of subjects with heavy work had been off work for more than 6 months.

Biering-Sørensen (40) reported the National Danish Statistics on work-related injuries. Overstraining was the main cause reported (57.6%). Particularly high accident rates were reported for workers in hospitals, home nursing, and patient treatment, who accounted for 42% of all injuries in 1979 to 1981. In a Danish Work Environment investigation of 10,000 workers representing 50 trade organizations, the prevalence of "low back pain when lifting" was 24%. The plumbers union (40%) and slaughterhouse workers union (38%) had the highest prevalences, and postal union (10%) and hospital laboratory technicians (8%) the lowest. Biering-Sørensen, in other studies (39,42), found high prevalence rates among truck drivers, hospital porters, and nursing aides.

A sample of 295 male Finnish concrete reinforcement workers were interviewed about musculoskeletal symptoms and radiologically examined (407,410). The lifetime prevalence of LBP was 80%. Radiographic evidence of disc degeneration was closely associated with the history of BP and sciatica, but was not associated with employment factors. In a later study based on a new sample, sciatica was significantly more common in concrete reinforcement workers than in a reference group of house painters, while "nonspecific" BP was equally common

TABLE 26. *All accident and back injury rates for three industries*

| Industry | No. at risk | Rates/1,000/year | | | |
		All accidents	Hand accidents	Back injuries	Back injuries from hand accidents
Telecommunications	100,931	22.4	7.3	5.6	3.6
Electrical	80,355	56.9	13.8	15.0	7.5
Construction	18,365	39.6	14.0	8.8	5.9

Source: ref. 279.

TABLE 27. *Cases of absenteeism per 1,000 man-years and percent of total absenteeism in occupational groups of the Dutch building industry in 1980*

Occupation	No. of injuries (per 1,000)	Absenteeism (% of all absences)
Carpenters	262	3.39
Bricklayers	410	5.78
Unskilled	438	6.67
Concrete workers	418	7.17
Roadmakers	481	5.92
Engine drivers	247	2.71
Supervisors	129	1.90
Total (average)	342	4.75

Sources: refs. 421 and 422.

in the two groups (314). In a Danish study from the construction industry, Damlund et al. (88,89) found a 1-year prevalence of 65% among construction workers, compared to 53% among warehouse workers.

A questionnaire survey of a random sample of 764 Finnish female nurses and 453 nursing aides revealed that symptomatic sciatica and disabling sciatica had affected nursing aides significantly more often than qualified nurses (383). Interestingly, there was no association between self-assessed workload and sciatica. Complaints of sciatica increased with the number of childbirths.

A postal survey of 12,000 Finnish farmers revealed that LBP was positively associated with a history of lifting and carrying heavy loads, whole body vibration, excess weight, and smoking (298).

The Netherlands

Zuidema (421,422) estimates, based on the Dutch Disablement Insurance System, that 12% of all cases with at least 1 year of disability in 1980 had a low back diagnosis. In the building industry, low back injuries were responsible for 23% of all absenteeism and 38% of all lost days in that year. Absenteeism was studied further in seven occupational groups. Bricklayers, road makers, concrete

workers, and unskilled workers had the highest injury rates, while supervisors had the lowest (Table 27). The percent of total absenteeism was highest among concrete workers.

Other Dutch statistics on occupational BP come from the Zoetermeer study (Table 28) (376). Unskilled workers had the highest prevalence rates among men, while among women the difference between occupations was less.

Belgium

Uyttendaele et al. (375) surveyed employees at a Belgian university and university hospital from 1971 through 1978. Sick-listing because of LBP increased from 0.4% of employees per year to 3.6% over the study period: 74% had LBP and 26% had sciatica. The mean duration of work absence for LBP was 11 days, and 39 days for sciatica. The incidence was significantly higher for women than for men, as was the average number of days off work. The highest incidence was among employees in the 25- to 35-year age range. Employees with a lower level of education and in heavy-lifting occupations had significantly higher incidence rates and also longer sick leaves.

Israel

Rotgoltz (320) determined the annual prevalence, severity, and duration of attacks of LBP in 208 workers in a pharmaceutical factory using a physician-administered questionnaire. Symptoms were cross-tabulated with job type, location, work requirements, sex, and years or work at the factory. LBP was reported by 66.3% of the workers. There was a significant and independent association between LBP and work in the packing or production department (OR = 2.03), with work requiring sitting or lifting (OR = 1.97), and with longer than 6 years employment (OR = 1.64).

TABLE 28. *Percentage of the Zoetermeer population with the clinical diagnosis of disc prolapse and lumbago, by sex and occupation*

Occupation	Men		Women	
	Disc prolapse	Lumbago	Disc prolapse	Lumbago
Unskilled	5.9	5.9	2.7	4.0
Skilled	2.1	3.3	2.3	4.0
Lower employees	1.5	4.0	1.0	5.5
Intermediate employees	0.3	3.2	0.9	4.7
Higher occupation	1.3	4.2	2.5	0.0
Self-employed	2.2	3.7	0.0	4.4
Unemployed	2.6	4.9	2.6	5.6

Source: ref. 376.

Summary

BP is a major industrial problem causing enormous costs to industry and society. Most studies are based on injury reports and medical claims, and, therefore, they reflect social, economical, legal, and individual factors. They also reflect only a small proportion of all BP. Most injuries are labeled as back sprains/strains or are of unspecified origin.

SCIATICA AND DISC HERNIATIONS

The definitions of sciatica used in epidemiologic surveys vary. Usually sciatica is defined as pain radiating along the sciatic nerve to one or both legs. A more specific definition is sometimes used in clinical reports. By this definition, pain radiates into the leg in a specific nerve root distribution and causes nerve root tension signs and neurologic findings. This form of sciatica is sometimes referred to as rhizopathy. Just as in LBP, sciatica is a symptom, not an etiologic entity. A herniated nucleus pulposus (HNP), on the other hand, is a specific pathologic entity defined as a situation wherein the disc protrudes from the normal annular border. HNP can be subdivided into complete prolapse (synonymous with ruptured disc, extruded disc, sequestered disc, and prolapsed disc) or an incomplete herniation. This type of herniation is also referred to as incomplete prolapse and contained disc herniation.

Incidence and Prevalence of Sciatic Symptoms

In early surveys undertaken by the Arthritis and Rheumatism Council in the United Kingdom in the 1950s, 40% of the men and 33% of the women 35 years and older gave a history of low back and leg pain (215,216). The pain was present at the time of the survey in 11% of men and 19% of women. Sciatica, suggesting a herniated lumbar disc, was found in 3.1% of all men and 1.3% of women (216). In the 55- to 64-year age group of men the prevalence was 9.6%, and in women the maximum prevalence of 5% occurred after the age of 64.

According to the combined results of several surveys conducted among 2,684 male British industrial employees, "disc disease" was recorded in 12.2% (6,9). The disc disease category was not clearly defined, however, and also included an unknown number of subjects with cervical disc syndromes. The prevalence of "disc disease" increased steeply with age, unlike the prevalence of "vague pains in back or neck." Of the patients with "disc disease," 43% had consulted a general practitioner because of pain in the back or neck during the past year, 12% had been hospitalized at some time, and 46% had

had at least one disabling episode lasting 3 weeks or more.

In an incidence study from a suburban general practice in southeastern London, Dillane et al. (98) recorded 605 attacks of LBP during 24,977 person-years. The incidence rates of HNP were 2.0 and 1.2 per 1,000 person-years for men and women, respectively.

In a representative sample of the 15- to 71-year-old female population of Gothenburg in Sweden, 13.8% of the women reported having had referred leg pains of the sciatic type (153). The lifetime history of sciatica was 3.6% in those younger than 25 but rose gradually to 22.4% among those aged 45 to 54.

Eleven percent of a sample of 4,753 men aged 40 to 59 years employed by large enterprises in Copenhagen reported the presence of sciatic pains during 1 year of observation (132).

In a sample of 295 male Finnish concrete reinforcement workers aged 15 to 64 years, 42% of all men and as many as 60% of those aged 45 or over reported a lifetime history of sciatica when first interviewed (407). Five years later, the lifetime prevalence had increased from 42% to 59% (315,316). In a reference group of house painters, the corresponding lifetime prevalence of sciatica at that time was 42%. The 5-year incidence of sciatica was 34% among the concrete workers and 23% among the house painters. Predictors of sciatica were occupation (RR = 1.5), back accidents (RR = 2.0), and previous LBP (RR = 3.9). Body height and stress were weakly associated with sciatic pain in the prospective survey, while abdominal and back muscle strength, body mass index, and smoking were not.

Random samples of 764 Finnish female nurses and 453 nursing aides were studied by postal questionnaire (383): 38% of the nurses and 43% of the nursing aides had experienced pain of sciatic distribution at least once previously. Reports of six or more previous episodes were given by 18% of the nurses and 23% of the nursing aides. Among 370 Finnish nursing school applicants (av-

TABLE 29. *Relative risk of herniated nucleus pulposus based on army hospital surgery at first admission*

Characteristic	Relative Risk
Craftsmen, foremen	1.47
Clerical	0.50
Married	1.33
Rural place of birth	1.53
Rural address	1.44
Good posture	1.00
Heavy frame	1.61
Ground combat specialty	1.53
2+ battle stars	0.67
Rank: staff-sergeant, sergeant	1.75
Rank: officer	0.80

Source: ref. 158.

TABLE 30. *Odds ratios for association between a prolapsed lumbar disc and lifting of 11.3 kg*

Variable	Frequency	Odds ratio
No lifting	—	1.0
Lifting	<5	0.8
	5–25	0.9
	>25	3.8
Lifting and twisting*	<5	3.0
	5–25	1.9
	>25	3.4

Sources: refs. 180–182.
* A twist occurs half or more of the time when lifting.

TABLE 31. *Prevalence (%) of lumbar disc syndrome and other low back syndrome by sex (age-adjusted)*

Diagnosis	Men	Women
Lumbar disc syndrome	5.3	3.8
Herniated nucleus pulposus (HNP)		
Definite	1.9	1.3
Probable	0.2	0.2
Sciatica		
Definite	1.9	1.3
Probable	1.3	1.0
Other low back pain (LBP)	12.5	13.2

Source: ref. 148.

erage age 22.1 years), 5% reported a previous history of sciatic pain (69).

Hrubec and Nashold (158) studied medical records of 1,095 army hospital admissions for HNP. The sample was matched for age and service period to other holders of Army National Service life insurance policies. Factors associated with admission for HNP were occupation of craftsman or foreman, married status, rural residence, excess height, excess weight, heavy frame, good posture, ground combat military occupation, and rank of sergeant or staff sergeant. A negative association was found with clerical occupation, earned battle stars, and officer rank. Essentially the same associations were found in the subgroup of subjects with surgically confirmed HNP (Table 29).

Kelsey (176-179,185) sampled women and men aged 20 to 64 years residing in the New Haven, Connecticut, area who had lumbar x-rays taken over a 2-year period for suspected HNP. She divided the sample into those with surgically confirmed herniated discs and those who had probable or possible herniated discs based on clinical signs and symptoms. A case-control design was used to determine risk factors for disc herniation. Two control groups were employed, and two controls selected for each case. One group was patients admitted to emergency rooms for reasons other than BP and matched for sex and age; the second was people who had radiographs of their spines, but who did not have symptoms and signs of a disc herniation. Associations were found between

disc herniations and sedentary occupations, driving of motor vehicles, chronic cough and chronic bronchitis, lack of physical exercise, participation in baseball, golf, and bowling, suburban residence, and pregnancy. Jobs involving lifting, pushing, and pulling were not found to be associated with increased risk of HNP (176-178,184,186).

Kelsey et al. (180,182,183) later performed another case-control study in Connecticut in 1979 to 1981 with minor methodological modifications. The study population was women and men aged 20 to 64 years who had had x-rays and myelograms at different health centers in New Haven and Hartford. As in the previous study, they were divided into those with surgically confirmed disc herniations, and those with probable or possible disc herniations. A control group of non-back patients admitted for in-hospital services was matched for sex and age. A number of possible risk factors were studied and odds ratios determined. Frequent lifting of heavy objects and twisting were both identified as significant risk factors (Table 30) (182). Lifting while twisting the body was found to increase the risk to particularly high levels (OR = 3.4). Even higher ORs (6.1) were calculated when lifting while twisting and keeping the legs almost straight. The number of hours spent in a motor vehicle and smoking were also associated with an increased risk, while pregnancy, height, weight, and participation in sports were not (180).

Other U.S. data on the prevalence of sciatica come

TABLE 32. *Age-standardized prevalences (%) of different handicaps in individuals with back syndromes*

Handicap	Lumbar disc syndrome (N = 326)	Other back syndrome (N = 927)	Attributable to lumbar disc syndrome (%)
Self-reported			
Abandon or reduce work duties	33.0	34.0	3.5
Cut down or reduce leisure activities	40.2	38.7	4.7
Clinical Exam			
Daily activities:			
Slightly reduced	55.6	53.4	3.7
Markedly reduced	21.1	23.7	2.5
Severely reduced	5.2	4.6	0.9

Source: ref. 148.

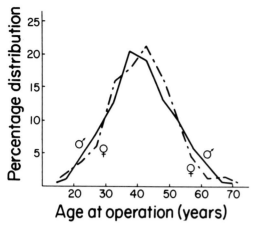

FIG. 9. Percent distribution of operations for herniated lumbar discs by age and sex.

TABLE 33. Multivariate relative risk (RR) of herniated intervertebral disc (HNP) or sciatica: Case-control studies

Factors	RR HNP	RR sciatica (including HNP)
Sex		
Women	1.0	1.0
Men	1.6	1.3
Occupation		
White collar	1.0	1.0
Men		
Motor vehicle drivers	2.9	4.6
Metal workers	3.0	4.2
Construction	2.4	3.1
Women		
Nurses	2.2	1.5
Housewives	0.4	0.8
Height		
Men (>180 cm)	2.3	
Women (>170 cm)	3.7	

Sources: refs. 145–148.

from the U.S. National Health Interview Surveys (1985 to 1988) (310) and show that annually 4.1 million persons report intervertebral disc disorders. Men are more likely to report disc disorders than women (2% compared to 1.5%). The highest prevalence rate was found in the 45- to 64-year age group (3.7 per 100 persons).

Heliövaara et al. (145-148) determined the prevalence rate of sciatica and its impact on society based on a sample of 8,000 persons representative of the Finnish population aged 30 or over. They carefully defined the diagnosis of lumbar disc syndrome based on medical history, symptom history, and a standardized physical examination, and they found it present in 5.3% of men and 3.7% of women. In both sexes, the prevalence rates were higher in the 45- to 64-year age group. The prevalences for definite herniated discs were 1.9% for men and 1.3% for women, while 0.2% of both sexes had a probable HNP. Low back syndrome other than sciatica was present in 12.5% of the sample of men and 13% of the women (Table 31). Disability due to lumbar disc syndrome (LDS) was estimated at 3.5% in men and 4.5% in women (Table 32). At clinical examination, 56% of the sample were slightly limited in their performance of daily activities, while 5% were severely limited. Approximately 6% of all work disability in the population was estimated to be attributable to LDS; 51% of patients with LDS needed long-term medical care, 2.1% of the total sample.

Hospitalizations and Operations

Sciatica usually resolves with conservative treatment, but it can lead to hospitalization and surgery. A number of studies are based on operative samples. Generalizations from these studies are difficult, because multiple factors other than disease severity influence the decision to perform surgery. Although diagnosis in these patients is more definite, a surgical sample is an incomplete representation of herniations.

In a review of 15,235 lumbar disc operations derived from multiple published reports, Spangfort (346) found that 46.9% involved the L5-S1 level, 49.8% the L4-L5

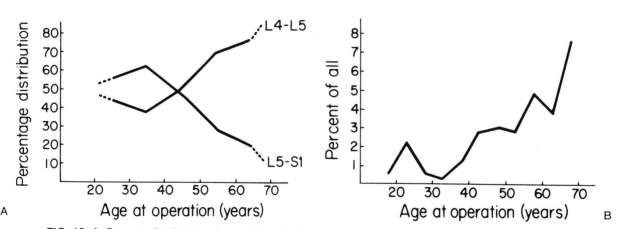

FIG. 10. A: Percent distribution of operations for herniated lumbar discs by age and level. **B:** Incidence of high lumbar herniations (above L4) by age at operation. Redrawn from Spangfort (346).

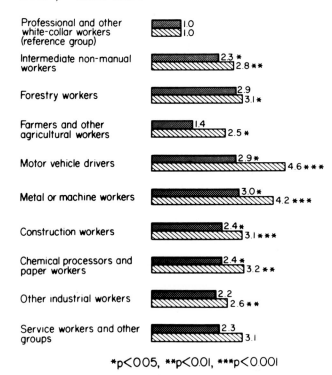

FIG. 11. Relative risk of herniated lumbar intervertebral disc (*dotted columns*) and of herniated disc or sciatica combined (*lined columns*) in men. Redrawn from Heliövaara (147).

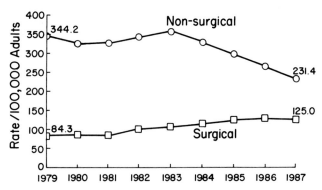

FIG. 12. Low back hospitalization in the U.S. per 100,000 adults. Based on Volinn et al. (390).

level, while 3.3% were performed at higher levels. In his own case material, which included 2,504 operations, the distribution was 50.5% L5-S1, 47.4% L4-L5, and 2.1% at higher lumbar levels. An increasing mean age at operation with the level of herniation in the cranial direction was noted (Figs. 9 and 10).

In 1974, about 5,000 persons (109.3 per 100,000 population) were discharged from Finnish hospitals with a diagnosis of either sciatica (3.1 per 100,000) or herniated intervertebral disc (78.3 per 100,000) (197). In 1977, the annual frequency of the diagnosis of herniated intervertebral disc in hospital discharge records for men aged 15 to 44 and 45 to 64 years were 126.1 and 262 per 100,000, respectively; the corresponding rates for women were 103 and 146. When comparing data from 1967 through 1977, no substantial changes were noted over the decade (280).

Heliövaara et al. (148) studied hospital admission records for HNP and sciatica in a group of 57,000 Finnish women and men who had participated in screening examinations over a period of 11 years (1966 to 1977). Using various social and health registers, they attempted to identify factors predicting back diseases. For each case accepted into the study, four control subjects matched for sex, age, and place of residence were selected. A total of 1,537 subjects were hospitalized because of back disease during the 558,074 person-years of follow-up. The discharge diagnosis was HNP in 30%, sciatica in 24%, and other back disease in 46%. Men had a 1.6-fold increased risk of HNP compared to women, and a 1.3-fold increased risk of sciatica (Table 33). Other back diseases were equally distributed between sexes. Among 592 cases with HNP or sciatica and their controls, ORs were calculated for different predictive factors (145–148). The risk of HNP was higher in tall people of both sexes, in obese men but not obese women, in industrial workers and motor vehicle drivers in men (Fig. 11), in women who did "strenuous work," were smokers, or had had multiple pregnancies, and in men and women with symptoms indicating physical distress. Marital status and leisure time physical activities were not risk factors. The relative risk of HNP and sciatica was lower in rural

TABLE 34. *Hospitalizations in the U.S. for back conditions in 1988, based on first-listed diagnosis by ICD.9.CM.Code (National Hospital Discharge Survey, 1988)*

Diagnosis	Hospitalizations (N)	ICD.9.Code
Intervertebral disc disorders	417,000	722
Other and unspecified back disorder	178,000	724
Fracture of the vertebral column	76,000	805
Spondylosis and allied disorders	75,000	721
Sprains and strains of other and unspecified parts of back	55,000	847
Sprains and strains of sacroiliac region	42,000	846

Source: ref. 310.

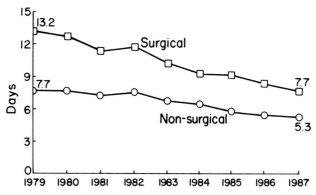

FIG. 13. Average length of stay for low back pain hospitalization in the U.S. per 100,000 adults. Based on Volinn et al. (390).

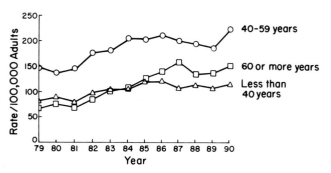

FIG. 14. Low back surgery rates per 100,000 adults, by age, 1979-1990. Based on Taylor et al. (364).

than in urban areas. Heliövaara concluded that the main influences on risk were sex, occupation, workload, and body height, while the other factors were of lesser predictive importance.

In the United States, 125 persons per 100,000 population were discharged from acute care hospitals in 1983, with a first-listed diagnosis of herniated lumbar intervertebral disc (190). Men were 1.5 times more often hospitalized than women. Younger people were less frequently hospitalized. The National Hospital Discharge data (310) show that intervertebral disc disorders are the most frequent musculoskeletal condition leading to hospitalization, with 417,000 episodes (Table 34). In the same year, there were 242,000 discectomies.

Volinn et al. (390) examined the National Hospital Discharge Survey for time trends (1979 to 1987), and for geographic variations (1987). The U.S. rate of lower back surgery increased 49% over the time period reviewed, while the rate of nonsurgical LBP hospitalization decreased by 33% (Fig. 12). The average length of stay decreased for both surgical and nonsurgical admissions (Fig. 13). Table 35 from Deyo et al. (95) further illustrates both the dramatic increase in back surgery in the U.S. and breaks it down into actual procedures. As can be seen, a comparatively larger increase occurred in fusions than in laminectomies or discectomies. Volinn et al. (390) also report large regional variation in hospitalization, surgical rates, and length of stay. They found that in 1987, the rate of surgery ranged from 77 per 100,000 adults in the northeast region to 146 per 100,000

in the southern region. This indicates that cultural differences and practice patterns have a major influence on hospitalizations and procedures. Taylor et al. (364) extended the review further by analyzing the National Hospital Survey Data from 1979 through 1990. The temporal trends up to 1987 presented in their report are the same as those reported by Volinn et al., but the data indicate a further increase in the number of surgical procedures from 1987 to 1990. Over the 11-year time period, adult low back operations increased by 55%, from 147,500 (1979) to 279,000 (1990). This corresponds to an increase from 102 to 158 per 100,000 adults. The rise was found to be particularly great for fusions, which increased by 100% from 13 to 26 per 100,000, but was large for the more common nonfusion operations as well (an increase of 47% from 89 to 131 per 100,000). In 1990, there were 46,500 lumbar fusions and 232,500 low back operations without fusion. The upward trends occurred among all age groups, but were particularly great for patients aged 60 and older (Fig. 14). Nonsurgical hospitalizations decreased from 402 per 100,000 in 1979 to 150 per 100,000 in 1990. The average back surgery rates for 1988 to 1990 were lowest in the West (113 per 100,000 adults) and highest in the South (171 per 100,000 adults) (Fig. 15). The same regional differences were found for nonsurgical hospitalizations as well.

Available data suggest marked intercountry variations in rates of back surgery (73,95). Nachemson (263) has reported that the number of operative procedures for HNP in Sweden has remained stable at 200 per million inhabitants per year from the mid 1950s through the 1980s. The corresponding numbers in Finland (1967 to

TABLE 35. *Rates of selected back operations in the U.S. per 100,000 general population*

Procedure	1979	1981	1983	1985	1987	% Increase from 1979 to 1987
Laminectomy	31	36	41	41	38	23
Discectomy	59	57	81	96	103	75
Lumbar fusion	5	9	10	18	15	200

Source: ref. 95.

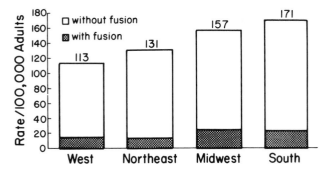

FIG. 15. Annual low back surgery rates per 100,000 adults divided by region (averages 1988–1990). Based on Taylor et al. (364).

1977) were 350 (148) and in Great Britain 100 (28,477). The number of people operated on for HNP per million per year in the U.S. has been variably assessed in the past as ranging between 450 to 900 (116,170,187). As discussed above, the rate in the U.S. for herniated discs in 1990 was 1,310 per million per year. A recent international comparison provides data on the rates of surgery in 13 countries. Figure 16 compares the back surgery rates and reveals that in the U.S. the rate is at least 40% higher than in any other country, and more than 5 times those of Scotland and England. Differences between countries were related to per capita availability of orthopedic surgeons and neurosurgeons (the higher the availability, the more procedures), but also to differences in hospital availability and health care systems. Differences in the underlying prevalence of BP was not felt to explain the differences in surgical rates.

OCCUPATIONAL RISK FACTORS

The relationship between occupational factors and LBP is not a simple research problem because exposure is usually difficult and sometimes impossible to quantify. It is also difficult to assess the effect of occupation or industry employment, because not everybody in the same occupation or industry performs the same job and is therefore not subject to the same exposure. Furthermore, the so-called healthy worker effect can result in erroneous conclusions. Healthy workers may well stay in the same occupation and job, while workers with LBP may leave a job and move to a less taxing one. The result is a shift in prevalence of BP from heavy to light jobs. Another problem is the definition of what is heavy and what is light. Traditionally, heavy physical jobs have been defined as jobs with high energy demand, and light as jobs with low energy demand. Many low energy jobs are static in nature, however, which as such can be a risk factor for LBP. Burdorf (61) reviewed 81 original epidemiologic articles to determine how well they assessed exposure to postural loading. In 58% there were no exposure data,

while in the remaining, exposure was based on questionnaire in 33%, observation in 9%, and direct measurement in 5% only. Throughout, it was felt that the quality of exposure data was poor.

The recall of exposure is even worse than the recall of previous pain and disability, and is often influenced by the insurance system. Subjects will tend to relate LBP to an injury or particular exposure if this results in compensation. Kelsey (177) found, for example, that 70.9% of men receiving compensation associated the onset of their problem with a specific event, compared to 35.5% of men not receiving compensation. Swedish and Canadian injury statistics would suggest the same. As stated by Frymoyer and Pope (119) "the Workers' Compensation System encourages workers to recall, if not perceive, an injury as causative of their backaches."

Further complicating the situation is the fact that exposure to several occupational risk factors often occurs in the same job. For example, a truck driver may have to load and unload his truck (lifting), sit for many hours in an unchanged posture (static loading), and be exposed to whole-body vibration. Despite these methodologic problems, meaningful information has been obtained about occupational risk factors.

Heavy Physical Work

Several investigations indicate an increase in sickness absence due to LBP, and also an increase in low back symptoms in individuals performing physically heavy work (10,344). A few will be discussed here.

Several of the studies discussed previously in this chapter compare prevalences among workers in physically heavy and light work. Sample data are listed in Table 36. Magora (239) found prevalence to vary greatly between occupations (Fig. 17). Uyttendaele et al. (375) found that

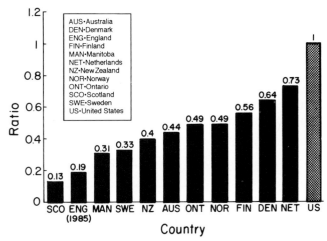

FIG. 16. Ratios of back surgery rates in 11 countries or Canadian states compared to the back surgery rate in the U.S. (1988–1989). Based on Cherkin et al. (73).

TABLE 36. *Prevalence of LBP in studies comparing physically heavy and light work*

Author (ref.)	Physically heavy (%)	Physically light (%)	N	Comment
Hult (160, 161)				
LBP	64.2	52.7		
Severe LBP	10.6	6.8		
Work absence	43.5	22.5		
Lawrence (223)	41.0	29.0	362	
Rowe (331, 333)	47.0	35.0		Medical visits
Ikata (164)	22.4	5.2		Sciatica
Magora (249)	21.6	10.4		
Lloyd et al. (239)	69.0	58.0		
	35.0	26.0		3 months

university and hospital employees with occupations demanding high physical strains were absent from work significantly more often due to LBP than those with light physical work (Fig. 18). Unskilled laborers had the highest prevalence rate for disc prolapse and lumbago in the Dutch study by Valkenburg and Haanen (376). Svensson and Andersson (358) found heavy physical work to be strongly associated with the occurrence of LBP; and the highest prevalence of LBP in their cross-sectional study was in men with physically heavy professions (Table 37). In a subsequent study in women, however, Svensson et al. (359) found only psychological variables, such as dissatisfaction with the work environment and the work tasks, and fatigue and worry at the end of the work day to be directly associated with LBP. More forward bending, more lifting, more standing, and more monotonous work correlated to LBP in the univariate analysis only.

Frymoyer and Pope (119) list incidence data of disabling back strains for workers in California. Industries with very high annual rates (defined as more than 1.5 per 100 workers) are listed in Table 38. In general, all these occupations must be considered physically heavy.

Klein et al. (194) found the highest rates of back sprain/strains among workers in physically heavy industries and with physically heavy occupations, as did Behrens et al. (27). Lloyd et al. (229) report a lifetime prevalence of 69% in miners and 58% in office workers; the 3-month prevalences were 35% and 26%, respectively. Leino et al. (224) followed a sample of Finnish employees in the metal industry over a 10-year period. LBP was more common among blue collar workers than among white collar workers. Among blue collar workers, however, only weak associations were found between morbidity and indices of physical work load.

Mitchell (258) surveyed LBP occurring in RAF (Royal Air Force) ground trades personnel. The male prevalence was 9.1% overall and increased with the severity of the job grade (Table 39). In all job grades, the prevalence was highest in the 40- to 49-year age group. The mean sickness absence period was 11.5 days, the median 5 days. Both sickness absence and frequency of employment restriction increased with the severity of the job grade.

Damlund et al. (88) reported on reasons for retirement among 157 construction workers in Denmark and 210 matched controls: 45% of the former construction workers and 25% of the controls said LBP was the reason.

Herrin et al. (151) analyzed musculoskeletal injury rates among 6,900 workers in 55 industrial jobs with almost 3,000 different manual tasks. The manual exertion requirements were determined using various job-stress indices, and 2-year retrospective as well as 1-year prospective medical reports were gathered. Musculoskeletal and overexertion medical problems were twice as common if predicted lumbosacral disc compression forces exceeded 6,800 N (newtons) (1,500 lb). Back problems were about 2.5 times higher in workers with performance requirements, which are met by only 10% of the U.S. work force.

Using the U.S. Quality of Employment Survey for 1972–1973, Leigh and Sheetz (223) found several variables likely to be associated with BP; they included physically heavy work, particularly farming (OR = 5.17). A cross-sectional survey at a U.S. oil company employing 10,350 full-time regular employees found the RR for a low back injury to be 1.57 in physically demanding jobs (374).

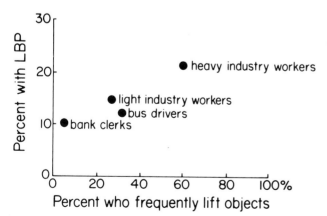

FIG. 17. Point prevalence of LBP in occupational groups in relation to frequency of lifting. Redrawn from Jensen (167).

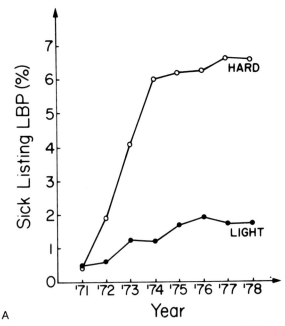
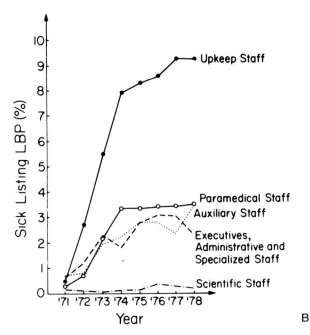

FIG. 18. Sicklisting because of LBP (**A**) in workers with heavy and light physical work and (**B**) according to employment. Redrawn from Uyttendaele (375).

Similar to LBP, sciatica has also an increased prevalence in physically heavy occupations. Wickström et al. (407) found a higher prevalence of sciatica in concrete reinforcement workers than in computer technicians, and higher rates of HNP have been reported in physically demanding occupations by Hrubec and Nashold (158), Kelsey et al. (180), and Videman et al. (383). Riihimäki (314) compared concrete reinforcement workers and house painters, reporting significantly higher prevalences of sciatica among the concrete workers. In a subsequent 5-year prospective study, the incidence was also found to be significantly higher among concrete workers. Hrubec and Nashold (158) found a negative association between HNP and clerical work, while craftsmen and foremen had a significantly higher than average risk.

Heliövaara (145) found that men had a significantly higher probability of being hospitalized for HNP if they were blue collar workers or motor vehicle drivers. A less dramatic difference between occupations was present in women, and in women the risk was also increased in those who felt their work was strenuous.

All these studies would seem to support heavy physical work as increasing the risk of LBP. Confounding factors may exist, however, and the level at which physical workload becomes a risk factor is not determined. Other studies are less clear. Lockshin et al. (230), Sairanen et al. (326), Porter (306), and Bigos et al. (45) did not find any differences in prevalence between heavy and light work. And occupational factors did not predict the incidence of LBP over a 1-year follow-up period in a Danish cross-sectional sample (42). It is not surprising in epidemiologic research of this type that some studies will be negative. The association between work load and LBP is relevant in time order, strong, dose-related (62,149,

TABLE 37. *Summary of work-related variables associated with LBP*

Variable	p value
Less overtime work	0.01
Diminished work satisfaction	0.01
Decreased potential to influence the work situation	0.01
Less demand on concentration	0.05
More monotonous/boring work	0.001
More physically demanding work	0.001
More lifting	0.001
Less sedentary work	0.05
More walking at work	0.05
More standing at work	0.05

Source: ref. 358.

TABLE 38. *Industries with high annual rates of disabling back strains per 100 workers in California, 1979*

Industry	Annual rate/100 workers
Lumber and wood	2.22
Stone, clay, glass	2.01
Food products	1.93
Metal products	1.73
Paper	1.67
Trucking and warehousing	2.29
Special trade contractors	1.53
Average all industries	0.78

Source: ref. 119.

TABLE 39. *Prevalence rate according to job grade among RAF ground trades personnel*

Trade group (job grades)	Population at risk	Prevalence rate (%)
Medium/heavy	3221	9.7
Medium/light	589	9.5
Light	369	7.6
Sedentary	316	7.6

Source: ref. 258.

206,311), consistent, and biologically coherent. Table 40 summarizes the annual rates per 100 workers reported by different investigators among different worker samples, using injury reports, registry statistics, questionnaires, and interviews. Although differences in research methods make data difficult to compare, the average prevalence rates range from a low of 0.75 to a high of 4.5; that is, large injury rates are reported everywhere. Prevalence rates are higher for workers in physically demanding jobs (Table 36). This reflects not only the risk, but also the difficulty of performing a heavy job with a painful lower back. It is obvious from the data, however, that BP is very frequent in physically light jobs as well. A change in the work environment, therefore, cannot be expected to solve the back injury problem completely.

Several studies concern nurses and nursing aides. The results do not allow definitive conclusions. Magora et al. (240) reported a higher prevalence of LBP in nurses than in farmers, bus drivers, and light industry workers. Cust et al. (86) compared the prevalence of LBP in nurses and teachers. While occupationally related LBP was more common in nurses, nonoccupational LBP was not, and therefore "all" LBP was similar in the two groups. Videman et al. (383) studied 862 qualified nurses and 318 nursing aides. Prevalence increased with age in both groups. Disability compensation was 3.4 times more common among the nursing aides who had a 4.5 times greater prevalence of sciatica. Chronic LBP was similar in both groups, however. Biering-Sørensen (40) reports that nurses have the highest injury rates of any occupations in Denmark, and Stubbs et al. (350) report a similar situation in England. Dehlin et al. (93), on the other hand, did not find a higher prevalence of BP among nursing aides in a geriatric hospital in Göteborg than in the female population at large.

Static Work Postures

It appears to be important to change one's work posture. Prolonged sitting, and bent-over work postures in particular, seem to carry an increased risk for BP. But there is considerable disagreement.

While many studies indicate an increased risk of LBP in subjects with predominantly sitting work postures (160,161,203,213,240,293), others do not (32,54,120,

145,146,316,358,359,403). Kelsey (176–178) and Kelsey and Hardy (184) found that men who spend more than half their workday in a car have a threefold increased risk of disc herniation. This could be due to the combined effect of sitting and vehicle vibration.

Magora (240) found that those who either sat or stood during most of the workday had an increased risk of LBP. Frequent changes in posture were also found to increase the risk of BP, however. Indeed, with respect to the predominant work posture (sitting or standing) the relationship appears U-shaped; frequent or infrequent, both increase the risk of BP.

Damkot et al. (87) studied the requirements of body postures at work in subjects with and without LBP: 40% of those with no pain, 36% of those with moderate pain, and 59% of those with severe LBP were required to stretch and reach. Standing and sitting per se were not associated with LBP.

Frequent Bending and Twisting

The association between low back symptoms and frequent bending and twisting is difficult to evaluate separately, as lifting is usually also involved. A large number of studies report an association between these movements in general and LBP (32,58,87,90,120,121,229, 235,368,407).

Troup, Roantree, and Archibald (372) found the combination mentioned above to be the most frequent cause of back injuries in England. Magora (242) established a connection between both excessive bending and occasional bending on the one hand and LBP on the other, and a similar finding was made by Chaffin and Park (72). Keyserling et al. (190) found LBP to be related to asymmetric postures in an automobile assembly plant, and Riihimäki et al. (316) report a relationship between sciatica and twisting and bending work postures, not only in physically heavy jobs, but in office workers as well. Further analysis of the data from the automobile assembly plant (311) revealed the following risks: mild trunk flexion (OR = 4.9, CI 1.4 to 17.4), severe trunk flexion (OR = 5.7, CI 1.6 to 20.4), and trunk twist or lateral bend

TABLE 40. *Annual prevalence of back sprains/strains (BS) and unspecified back injuries (BI) in selected studies*

Author (ref.)	Prevalence (%)	Comment
Hult (161)	2.9	BI. Worker samples
Blow/Jackson (48)	3.6	BI. Dockworkers
Stubbs/Nicholson (351)	0.9	BI. Construction workers
Klein et al. (194)	0.7	BS. General population
Anderson (9)	4.5	BI. Dockyard workers
Abenheim/Suiss (1)	1.4	BI. General population

(OR = 5.9, CI 1.6 to 21.4). The risk increased with exposure to multiple postures and with increasing duration of exposure. Thus, a combination of mild flexion and twist produced an OR of 7.4 (CI 1.8 to 29.4). The relationship of back disorders to nonneutral postures was not explained by nonoccupational factors such as sex, age, previous injury, or medical history in this carefully controlled study, where a biomechanical job analysis was performed.

Lifting, Pushing, and Pulling

It has been clearly established that BP can be triggered by lifting, but the frequency at which BP develops after lifting varies from 15% to 64% in these studies (32,46,161,164,176,177,194,229,239,240). Sudden unexpected maximal efforts were found by Magora (240) to be particularly harmful, and Glover (124), Tichauer (365), and Troup et al. (372) express the same opinion about lifting in combination with lateral bending and twisting.

Chaffin and Park (72) found that workers involved in heavy manual lifting had about 8 times the number of lower back injuries as those with a more sedentary work situation. Svensson and Andersson (358) found a direct association between occurrence of LBP and frequent lifting, as did Frymoyer et al. (121) and Hult (160,161). Snook (344) found that a worker was 3 times more susceptible to compensable low back injury if exposed to excessive manual handling tasks.

The National Institute of Occupational Safety and Health (NIOSH) estimated in 1981 (282) that one-third of the U.S. work force lifted in excess of what was considered acceptable, and that lifting was a major cause of LBP. They also concluded that the severity of injury rate while lifting was proportional to the weight of the object, the bulk of the object, the location of the object at the start of the lift, and the frequency of lifting.

Kelsey (177), on the other hand, in her first study found no indication that workers with herniated discs did more lifting on the job than workers without such symptoms. Further, there was no indication in that study that jobs requiring pushing, pulling, or carrying either increased or decreased the risk of herniated discs. In the second study (182), however, frequent lifting was identified as a risk factor for HNP, the risk increasing the heavier the weight lifted and the more frequent the lifts were performed (Table 30). Lifting while twisting increased the risk even further. The OR for HNP in subjects performing frequent lifting of heavy weights while twisting was 3.4.

Frymoyer et al. (120,121) found repetitive heavy lifting, pushing, and pulling to be associated with LBP in a retrospective study of a general practice population. Troup et al. (371) followed 802 workers over a 2-year

period. Half of the attacks of LBP were associated with a "back injury" and of those, 1 in 3 occurred from manual material handling. A cross-sectional survey in a small market town in the south of England correlated the lifetime occupational history of 545 adults with the prevalence of LBP (393). The strongest associations were for lifting and moving weights over 25 kg (RR = 2.0, CI 1.1 to 3.7). The same risk ratio was found for both men and women. Car driving also carried an increased risk for men (RR = 1.7, CI 1.0 to 2.9), but not for women. Overall, the prevalence of BP was 64% among the men, 61% among the women. When considering those individuals with severe, unremitting BP, the risk ratio for lifting increased to 5.3 among the men and 2.9 among the women.

Duration of employment may also be associated with BP, although the healthy-worker effect makes this difficult to evaluate. Magora (239) found an association with BP among workers doing heavy work, and Astrand (15) reports a direct relationship between BP and time of employment among 391 male employees in a Swedish pulp and paper industry.

Repetitive Work

Repetitive work increases, in general, the sickness absence rate. LBP seems to be no exception in this respect. This may explain, in part, why assembly line industries have a higher incidence of LBP among their manual workers than among their office employees (32).

Vibration Exposure

There are several studies suggesting an increasing risk of LBP in drivers of tractors (75–78,90,100–102, 159,318,339,340), of trucks (27,130,184,202,411), of buses (131,184), and of airplanes (112,338). These studies also suggest that LBP occurs at an earlier age in subjects exposed to vehicular vibration.

Kelsey and Hardy (184) found that truck driving increased the risk of disc herniation by a factor of 4, while tractor driving and car commuting (20 miles or more per day) increased the risk by a factor of 2. In a later study, the risk of HNP was related to the type of vehicle, indicating significant differences between different brands of cars (180).

Hulshof and van Zanten (159) have reviewed the epidemiologic data supporting a relationship between whole-body vibration and LBP. They concluded that vibration was a probable risk factor in helicopter pilots, tractor drivers, construction machine operators, and transportation workers. They were critical of the data, however, concluding that none of the many studies reviewed were adequate in terms of the quality of exposure data, effect data, study design, and methodology. Most

TABLE 41. *Radiographic changes of the spine in subjects exposed to whole-body vibration*

Author (ref.)	Vehicle exposure	No. of subjects	Prevalence (% exposed)	Prevalence (% controls)
Rosegger et al. (318)	Tractor	310	71	
Zimmermann (419)	Tractor	180	80	
Christ (77)	Tractor	211	50	
Dupuis et al. (100)	Tractor	137	69	
Dupuis et al. (101)	Tractor	106	80	
Schmidt (334)	Heavy truck	117	79	
Kristen et al. (202)	Light truck	94	83	
Kohne et al. (195)	Bus	352	81	
Fisher (110)	Helicopter	136	80	
Fisher (110)	Jet	143	47	
Hilfert et al. (152)	Earth mover	342	81	53

Source: ref. 138.

studies did not control for confounding variables, and only a few had control populations.

Dupuis and Zerlett (102), in a 10-year prospective study (1961 to 1971), describe an increased incidence of backache reports from 47% to 58% among tractor drivers. Hilfert et al. (152) found that 70% of 352 construction machine operators had periodic LBP compared to 54% in an unexposed control group. Gruber and Zipermann (131) compared 1,448 male interstate bus drivers to three control groups. Experienced drivers had a higher prevalence of spinal disorders than controls. A significant correlation was found between prevalence rates and exposure level. In a later study Gruber (130) compared 3,205 interstate truck drivers to 1,137 air traffic controllers. Prevalence among truck drivers was significantly higher than among traffic controllers. Behrens et al. (27) found the highest prevalence estimates for back injuries among U.S. occupational groups to occur among truck drivers. In a Danish study, 2,045 full-time male bus drivers in the three largest cities in Denmark were compared to 195 motormen (277). The prevalence of LBP was 57% versus 40%. Standardized morbidity ratio (SMR) was calculated for bus drivers discharged from hospitals from 1978 through 1984 with a diagnosis of a lumbar disc herniation as compared to the same discharge data for all Danish men. A significantly higher incidence was found among the bus drivers, the SMR being 137. Burdorf and Zondervan (63) found an OR of 3.6 for LBP among crane operators compared to controls.

Buckle et al. (59), Frymoyer et al. (121), Backman (17), Damkot et al. (87), Walsh et al. (393), and Biering-Sørensen and Thomsen (42) all report an association between automobile use and LBP. The risk of being hospitalized because of HNP was high among motor vehicle drivers in the Finnish Study by Heliövaara (146), and Pentinnen (298) and Riihimäki et al. (316) report an increased risk of sciatica with motor vehicle driving in other Finnish studies.

Studies of vibration-exposed populations have also indicated that radiographic changes occur in the spines of these subjects (Table 41). These studies are retrospective and usually limited to selected subject groups. It is therefore difficult to make cause–effect conclusions. Further, the radiographic findings are diverse and cannot all be explained by mechanical theory. Nonetheless the prevalence rates of radiographic changes are very high. Dupuis and Zerlett (102) followed a group of tractor drivers over a 10-year period. The prevalence rate and severity of radiographic changes increased over that time (Table 42). The absence of a control group unfortunately reduces the value of the study.

Psychological and Psychosocial Work Factors

Several psychological work factors have been implicated in LBP, including monotony at work, work dissatisfaction, and poor relationship to coworkers. These psychosocial factors have been found to increase the risk of complaining of LBP and reporting workers compensation claims (15,20,23,26,32,45,46,87,358–360). Monotony had a direct relationship to LBP in the study by Svensson and Andersson (358) while Bergquist-Ullman and Larsson (32) found that workers with monotonous jobs, requiring less concentration, had a longer sickness absence following LBP than the others. Diminished work satisfaction has also been found to be related to an

TABLE 42. *Radiographic changes over time in a group of tractor drivers*

	Year		
	0	5	10
Number studied	211	137	106
Age (mean; years)	18	23	29
Radiographic changes (%)			
Advanced	50.2	68.7	80.1
Moderate	22.3	10.2	8.5
Mild	14.7	13.1	5.7
None	12.8	8.0	5.7

Source: ref. 102.

increased risk of LBP by Westrin (402), Magora (241), and Svensson et al. (358). Bergenudd and Nilsson (30) found that middle-aged workers had an increased prevalence of BP if they had physically heavy jobs and that the association increased further when the workers were dissatisfied with their work. Individuals with BP had been less successful in a childhood intelligence test, and on average had a shorter education. Kelsey and Golden (183) point out that, since most of the studies are retrospective, it is difficult to determine whether psychological factors are antecedents or consequences of pain. Bigos et al. (46) and Battié et al. (23) in prospective studies concluded, however, that psychological work factors were more important than physical work factors as risk indicators of LBP. The reader is referred to their discussion in Chapter 11. Psychological factors are also further discussed below.

Summary

The seven most frequently discussed occupational risk factors are: heavy physical work; frequent bending and twisting; lifting, pulling, and pushing; repetitive work; static work postures; vibrations; and psychological and psychosocial factors. Among them, the first six physical work risk factors have been experimentally associated with the development of injuries in spinal tissues. Because they often occur together, the relative importance of each is difficult to determine. The seventh, "psychological and psychosocial work factors," is probably more related to disability claims than to occurrence of a specific organic pathology.

INDIVIDUAL FACTORS

Individual factors can, of course, influence the prevalence of LBP, and also its disabling effects. These differ from risk factors insofar as they are usually beyond the individual's or society's control, with a few exceptions such as obesity, physical fitness, and smoking.

Heredity

The relative roles of genetic and environmental factors in sciatica were studied in a nationwide Finnish cohort. Environmental factors explained more than 80% of the etiology of sciatica (142) and of LBP (382). Thus, the common low back syndromes seem to be mainly caused by environmental factors, although a familial predisposition to lumbar herniated discs has been reported (216,249,307,308,379). The wide variation in the occurrence of LBP by social class, degree of education, and occupational group (179,216,313,416) also suggests that environmental and behavioral factors play a primary role. Specific spinal disorders such as scoliosis, ankylos-

ing spondylitis, and spondylolisthesis may have genetic predispositions. Those disease entities are discussed elsewhere in this volume.

Age and Sex

LBP usually begins early in life (32,34,153,157, 160,161,326,358). The highest frequency of symptoms occurs in the age range of 35 to 55, while sickness absence and symptom duration increase with increasing age (10). Biering-Sørensen's data (36) indicate a difference in age pattern between women and men (Fig. 19). While men have a prevalence maximum at age 40, women have a large increase in prevalence and incidence from age 50 to 60 years. The most likely explanation for this is the earlier development of osteoporosis in women. However, other investigations have not confirmed Biering-Sørensen's observations. Svensson et al. (360) in their study of women in Göteborg, Sweden, did not find a significant age effect, although a trend was present. Hult (160) and Horal (157) report increasing prevalence up to age 50, but not thereafter. Age has a different influence on Worker's Compensation claims. In the prospective Boeing study (N = 3,200) Battié et al. (20,23) found a significantly higher risk of sickness absence due to LBP in younger workers. This confirms other reports on work-related injuries (194,347,349). Most patients admitted to hospital and operated on because of a disc herniation are between 35 and 50 years old (147,346).

Although sex seems to be of little importance with respect to low back symptoms (21,157,223,357,360,376), operations for disc herniations are performed about 1.5 to 3 times as often in men as in women (54,58,

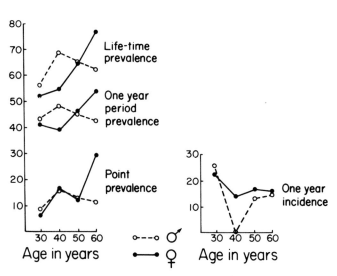

FIG. 19. *Top:* Prevalence rates of "low back trouble" by age and sex. Redrawn from Biering-Sørensen (34). *Bottom:* Incidence of "low back trouble" over one year in a general population. From Biering-Sørensen (38).

148,185,219,357,400), despite the observation that sciatica seems to be more equally distributed between sexes (147,185,362). However, U.S. men complain more frequently of disc disorder than women (310). Swedish insurance statistics indicate a much larger sickness absence in women with heavy physical work than in men doing the same job. A mismatch between the physical strength of the worker and the job requirements can be responsible for these differences. Brown (57) and Magora (239) report that women in heavy physical jobs have comparatively more back complaints than men in similar jobs. The period of sickness absence in Sweden at different ages was different between women and men. Women were absent more than twice as long as men in the 40- to 49-year age group, while men had a 30% longer absence period between ages 50 and 59 (317). Worker's Compensation claims in the U.S. are more common among men than women (194,347). Isthmic spondylolisthesis is about twice as common in men as in women (388), for reasons currently unexplained.

Posture

Postural deformities (scoliosis, kyphosis, hypolordosis, hyperlordosis, and leg length discrepancy) do not seem to predispose to LBP in general (22,35–37,139,156,157,161,244,302,323,345). Scoliosis has been particularly investigated, but there is no hard evidence of a true association with LBP, except in curves of 80° or more (23,24,53,80,198,199,262,281). Kostuik and Bentivoglio (198) reviewed 5,000 intravenous pyelograms in adults over the age of 20. An increase in prevalence of BP was found with increase in the magnitude of scoliotic curvatures. The prevalence was not related to age.

The degree of lordosis or kyphosis was unrelated to LBP in studies by Hult (161), Horal (157), and Rowe (323). Magora (239) found flattening of the spine (i.e., decreased lordosis) in patients with LBP. Because loss of the lumbar lordosis was frequently accompanied by muscle spasm, he concluded that the loss of lordosis was the cause of pain, rather than pain caused by lack of lordosis. Hansson et al. (139) determined the amount of lumbar lordosis from radiographs of 600 20- to 63-year old men. Three age-matched and occupationally matched groups of each 200 were compared: the first had no history of previous or present LBP, the second had experienced their first back injury ever, and third had chronic low back disability. There was no difference in the distribution of lordosis angles between the groups, nor was there an age-related difference. Leg length inequality is another area where considerable disagreement exists in the literature. Leg length discrepancy is quite common and appears to be related to an increase of LBP in studies by Rush et al. (324) and by Giles and Taylor (123). Other studies have shown no correlation (Table

43) (47). One of the major problems in determining the value of the leg length data is the accuracy of different measurement methods, which is poor.

Anthropometry

Anthropometric data indicate that there is no strong correlation between LBP and height, weight, or body build (35–37,72,157,160,161,264,301,302,322,323,358,360,395). Tallness, however, has been found to be associated with a higher-than-average risk of BP in some studies (23,132,176,177,213,223,363), sitting heights in other studies (106,213,256), and LBP (94) and sciatica (164) are more frequent in the very obese. Tables 44 and 45 summarize some of the studies on association between LBP and height, weight, and various body mass indices.

Westrin (403) studied several anthropometric factors in addition to height and weight, such as length of tibia and femur and width of femoral condyles and malleoli. None was related to risk of LBP. Biering-Sørensen (38) measured the femoral epicondylar width, the leg length, and the length of the upper body, and calculated the so-called Rohrers Index: weight in grams × 100 (height in meters)³. None of these measurements had prognostic value either for the first-time experience or for the recurrence of LBP. In a prospective study, Battié (20) found that in workers without previous back problems, no anthropometric measures were associated with LBP. In those with previous problems, however, taller men were at a slightly higher risk as were women of higher weight or greater obesity.

Hrubec and Nashold (158) found that body height predicted herniated lumbar discs among army recruits. Kelsey (176,177) and Kelsey et al. (181) did not observe differences in height between disc patients and controls, however. Heliövaara (145,147) found body height to be a significant predictor of HNP in both women and men. In tall men (above 179 cm) the RR was 2.3, and in tall women (above 169 cm) it was 3.7 in relation to subjects who were at least 10 cm shorter (RR = 1.0). Riihimäki et al. (316) found a weak correlation between tallness (<180 versus >169) and the lifetime prevalence of sciatica (RR = 1.7), but not with the 5-year incidence. A case-control study of 15-year-old children using magnetic res-

TABLE 43. *Studies of association of leg length inequality and low back pain (LBP)*

Leg length inequality:	LBP associated	LBP not associated
	Giles et al. (123)	Fisk et al. (111)
	Rish et al. (324)	Hult (160, 161)
		Fairbank et al. (106)
		Pope et al. (302)
		Battié et al. (23)

Source: ref. 20.

TABLE 44. *A sample of retrospective and prospective studies of association between height and back problems*

| | Reference | | | |
| | Back pain | | Herniated disc | |
Height	Associated	Not associated	Associated	Not associated
Standing	Lawrence et al. (213)	Hult (160,161)	Rowe (322)	Kelsey (176)
	Tauber (363)	Hirsch et al. (153)	Kelsey (176)	
	Merrian (256)	Pederson et al. (297)	Hrubec and Nashold (158)*	
	Mellin (255)	Fairbank et al. (106)	Heliövaara (145)*	
	Gyntelberg (132)*	Pope et al. (302)	Battié et al. (23)*	
		Mellin (255)		
		Biering-Sørensen (38)*		
Sitting	Merriam et al. (256)	Hult (160,161)		
	Lawrence et al. (213)			
	Burwell et al. (64)			
	Fairbank et al. (106)			

Source: ref. 20.
* Prospective study.
Some studies appear as Associated *and* Not associated because of difference between sexes.

onance (MR) identified more disc protrusions among taller children (327). In summary, tallness appears to be a risk factor for sciatica and herniated discs, while its relationship to LBP is uncertain.

Obesity was found to be associated with LBP in a U.S. industrial population (RR = 1.42) (374). Obesity was also a risk factor for non-low back musculoskeletal injuries, however (RR = 1.53). The significance of obesity to the occurrence of HNP appears complex. Heliövaara (145,147) found that a moderately increased body mass index predicted the development of HNP in men but not in women, whereas severe obesity appeared to carry less than moderate risk. Body mass index was not a predictor of risk of sciatica in the study by Riihimäki et al. (316). Hrubec and Nashold (158), on the other hand, report that high weight at enrollment into military service predicted higher risk of developing a lumbar disc herniation. Being overweight does add to the mechanical loading of the spine, and as such it may be more important as a factor contributing to the severity of existing pain than to its initial development.

The spinal canal diameter appears important in the development of symptomatic herniated discs. Thus, patients with sciatica or prolapsed discs have been found to have more narrow canals than control groups (150, 312,413). McDonald et al. (251) used ultrasound to determine the spinal canal diameter and attempted to predict future back injuries in 204 miners using this information. Although no definite conclusion could be made because of a high retirement rate due to work reduction, there was an indication that those who retired had smaller canals.

Muscle Strength

Poor strength in abdominal and back muscles has been found by some investigators in patients with BP

TABLE 45. *A sample of retrospective and prospective studies of association between weight and back problems*

| | Reference | | | |
| | Back pain | | Herniated disc | |
Weight	Associated	Not associated	Associated	Not associated
Pure	Pederson et al. (297)	Hult (160,161)	Hrubec and Nashold (158)	Rowe (322)
	Fairbank et al. (106)	Hirsch et al. (153)	Battié et al. (23)*	Kelsey (176)
	Mellin (255)	Pedersen et al. (297)		Kelsey et al. (181)
		Merriam et al. (256)		Battié et al. (23)*
		Pope et al. (302)		
		Mellin (255)		
		Biering-Sørensen (38)*		
Indexed		Hult (160,161)	Battié et al. (23)	Kelsey (176)
		Pope et al. (302)	Heliövaara (147)	Heliövaara (147)
				Battié et al. (23)

Source: ref. 20.
* Prospective study.
Some studies appear as Associated *and* Not associated because of difference between sexes.

(3,5,70,141,210,211,243,253,283,285,289,302,321). Others have found no differences from controls, or differences only in selected types of strength activities (33,35–37,265,297). A review of strength and endurance studies is given in Chapter 23.

The question of whether a weakness is primary or secondary to BP remains to be clarified. Chaffin and Park (72) evaluated isometric lifting strength in relation to job demands in 411 workers in 103 different jobs. During a 1-year follow-up, the incidence rate of LBP was 3 times higher in those individuals who did not have strength equal to or above that required by the job. However, the study population was small and the difference did not reach statistical significance. This study was later expanded by Chaffin et al. (71). They applied strength tests to 551 employees in six plants and followed them for 18 months. Again the 3:1 risk ratio was confirmed for jobs whose strength requirement approached or exceeded the worker's demonstrated strength.

Keyserling et al. (188) further evaluated the importance of isometric lifting strength in longitudinal studies. One study population in which the subjects were matched to the job based on the strength test tended to have fewer complaints during the follow-up year than a nonmatched group, and in another study population there was an increase in musculoskeletal accident reports in workers who were required to lift more than 75% of their maximum capacity. On the other hand, Battié et al. (22) did not find isometric strength to be a predictor of subsequent back injuries in their prospective study. The workers were not matched to their jobs, however, and the tests were not job specific. In a study of 902 Finnish employees in the metal industry, Leino et al. (224) did not observe any association between muscle function and either the 10-year incidence of chronic LBP, or the development of low back symptoms. For further discussion of this and other strength and endurance studies the reader is referred to Chapter 23.

Physical Fitness and Sports Activities

Subjects with a good state of physical fitness appear to have a lesser risk of chronic LBP and a more rapid recovery after a BP episode. Cady et al. (66,67) used several fitness factors to obtain an overall fitness score among 1,652 fire fighters in the Los Angeles area. The fittest fire fighters had fewer injuries than the less fit. Further, a significant decrease in worker compensation costs was reported following the introduction of the fitness program. Dehlin et al. (92) prospectively randomized nursing aides to fitness training and control treatment. Fitness improved but there was no difference in number of low back injuries. The fitness-trained nursing aides recovered more quickly after injury, however. Gyntelberg (132) and Troup et al. (370) did not find aerobic capacity to be predictive of future BP. Battié et al. (22) also concluded that cardiovascular fitness was not predictive of future

back injury reports. Long-term disabling BP appeared to be associated with a lower level of aerobic capacity, however. Nachemson et al. (263,264) found improved conditioning to have a significant effect on the recovery rate after acute LBP.

The role of physical exercises in the prevalence of LBP is difficult to determine. In Switzerland, a group of 739 recreational orienteers with a mean age of 33 years (range 10 to 65) had a cumulative occurrence of LBP of 47% (378). Kelsey (176,177) found "insufficient physical exercise," as well as baseball, golf, and bowling, to be associated with the occurrence of prolapsed lumbar discs. But Weber (398,399) reported an unexpectedly low percentage of physically active men in his study of patients with herniated discs. Svensson et al. (360) found LBP to be more common in men who were less physically active on their time off work, while Videman et al. (383) found the opposite in nurses. Frymoyer et al. (120) did not find sports activities in general to be a risk factor, although cross-country skiing did appear to be associated with an increased risk for mild LBP (122). Hurme et al. (163) found no difference in leisure-time activities between patients operated on for HNP and the general population. Granhed and Morelli (126) found no difference in the prevalence of BP between heavy weight lifters and referents. A Finnish–American study of the long-term effects of physical loading on back-related symptoms included 937 former athletes and 620 referents aged 36 to 64 years (385). The ORs for BP were lower among all former athlete groups than among controls (Table 46), and Leino (226) reported a negative correlation between physical activity and LBP in a longitudinal study. There were no statistically significant differences in the occurrence of sciatica (Table 47), back related pensions, or hospitalizations due to BP.

Spine Mobility

Spine motions are reduced in most subjects with BP (244,255,295,302,306,367). All movements are usually associated with some pain, particularly at the end of the range of motion. It appears quite unlikely that spine mobility is a factor in the causation of BP. Biering-Sørensen (35–37) found that reduced spine motion in subjects with previous LBP was associated with increased risk of recurrence. On the other hand, previously healthy subjects with less spine mobility had an increased risk for future LBP. Troup et al. (370) reported that flexibility was a poor predictor of future BP, while subjects with ongoing BP had poor sagittal flexibility. Battié et al. (24,25) found no association between either greater or poorer flexibility and subsequent BP. Bergquist-Ullman and Larsson (28) did not find spine flexibility to be associated with either the recovery from or the severity of acute LBP.

TABLE 46. *Back pain among former athletes and referents*

Sport	Occurrence (%)	OR adjusted for age and occupational loading	CI	Age-adjusted OR
Endurance	40.2	**0.62**	0.39–0.98	**0.57**
Sprint	39.0	**0.60**	0.37–0.96	**0.59**
Jumping	36.5	0.62	0.36–1.05	**0.54**
Throwing	43.7	0.73	0.43–1.22	0.73
Games	36.4	**0.60**	0.44–0.82	**0.54**
Contact	42.6	**0.67**	0.47–0.96	**0.69**
Weightlifting	44.0	0.62	0.33–1.18	0.72
Shooting	29.3	0.51	0.24–1.08	**0.38**
Referents	51.7	1.00	—	1.00

Source: ref. 384.
OR, occurrence rate; in bold type when statistically significant.
CI, 95% confidence interval.

Smoking

An association between smoking and HNP and LBP has been found by Kelsey (177), Kelsey et al. (180), Gyntelberg (132), Frymoyer et al. (120,121), Leigh and Scheetz (223), Svensson et al. (361), McFadden (252), Biering-Sørensen and Thomsen (42), Pentinnen (298), Deyo and Bass (94), Heliövaara (147), Tsai et al. (374), Boshuizen et al. (51), and O'Connor and Marlowe (286). Kelsey et al. (180) reported an increased risk of developing a herniated disc of 20% for each ten cigarettes smoked per day in the previous year (OR = 1.2). Battié et al. (22) reported an RR of back problems in smokers of 1.4 (95% CI 1.1 to 1.8), and Biering-Sørensen et al. (43), a relative risk of 2.6 for first-time incidence of LBP, and 2.0 for recurrence. All studies have not confirmed an association between smoking and BP, but the time order is relevant, the association consistent between countries, and there is evidence for a dose–response relationship (149,180,361).

Other risk factors that may confound the association between smoking and LBP have not been identified (104), yet smoking may be an indicator of other factors affecting the risk of LBP rather than a risk factor by itself.

Psychological Factors and Psychiatric Disorders

Psychological distress and psychiatric disorders appear to be risk factors for LBP (13,84,373,397). A number of cross-sectional studies indicate an association between psychological factors and the occurrence of LBP (30,49,50,87,117,149,169,241,315,359). These factors include anxiety, depression, somatization symptoms, stressful responsibility, job dissatisfaction, mental stress at work, negative body image, weakness in ego functioning, and poor drive satisfaction. The experience of stress, anxiety, and depression does not seem to be secondary to back problems, because in prospective studies various symptoms suggesting psychological distress predicted the development of back problems among people who did not have previous BP (16,42,45,132,148,225,299).

The possible etiologic importance of psychiatric disorders is particularly important in the case of chronic LBP.

TABLE 47. *Sciatica among former athletes and referents*

Sport	Occurrence (%)	OR adjusted for age and occupational loading	CI	Age-adjusted OR
Endurance	33.3	1.54	0.96–2.48	1.29
Sprint	21.2	1.01	0.59–1.73	0.81
Jumping	19.2	0.84	0.44–1.60	0.72
Throwing	30.6	1.20	0.67–2.15	1.34
Games	25.7	1.08	0.76–1.53	1.06
Contact	20.5	0.68	0.44–1.06	0.76
Weightlifting	33.3	1.46	0.76–2.80	1.43
Shooting	24.9	1.16	0.52–2.58	0.93
Referents	24.9	1.00	—	1.00

Source: ref. 384.
OR, occurrence rate.
CI, confidence interval.

Two hundred chronic LBP patients entering a functional restoration program were assessed for current and lifetime psychiatric syndromes using a structured psychiatric interview tailored to generate DSM-III-R diagnoses (300). Seventy-seven percent of patients met lifetime diagnostic criteria and 59% demonstrated current symptoms for at least one psychiatric diagnosis, most commonly depression, substance abuse, or anxiety disorders. In addition, 51% met criteria for at least one personality disorder. These prevalence rates were significantly greater than comparable rates in the general population. Fifty-four percent of patients with depression, 94% of those with substance abuse, and 95% of those with anxiety disorders had experienced these syndromes before the onset of their BP, indicating that substance abuse and anxiety disorders appear to precede chronic LBP, while depression may develop either before or after the onset of chronic LBP.

While the importance of psychiatric disorders for the occurrence of chronic LBP is more firmly established, the situation is less clear for acute LBP and sciatica.

A mental health survey was performed to determine the prevalence of psychiatric disorders among 15,538 individuals in five American communities, and at the same time data about 38 physical symptoms were collected (204). BP was the second most common reported symptom, with a lifetime prevalence of 32%. In 16% of the symptomatic cases, LBP was considered as sometimes due to psychiatric causes or to an unknown cause. Individuals with BP were more at risk of suffering from depression (OR = 2.0), dysthymia (OR = 2.1), panic disorder (OR = 1.9), somatoform disorder (OR = 3.9), and alcohol abuse (OR = 1.7). These data should be treated cautiously since this study was not primarily designed to assess physical symptoms and data on this subject topic were heavily dependent on self-reporting.

Other Somatic Diseases and Conditions

BP has been found to be associated with the presence of other somatic diseases and conditions, for example cardiovascular and respiratory diseases (42,132,149, 361). These associations, however, are quite weak and may be confounded by other risk determinants (149). There are more close associations between LBP and chronic neck pain (247) and osteoarthritis in the knee, hip, and hand (149). These associations are independent of work load and other known risk factors, suggesting a common etiology.

In contrast, decreased prevalence of chronic LBP has been observed among diabetics (149). This finding was unexpected, as diabetics are generally prone to a number of skeletal changes including osteoarthritis and hyperostotic spondylosis (341).

A number of studies have shown that pregnancy may increase the risk of LBP. Ostgaard et al. (292) have studied 855 pregnant women who were followed from the 12th week of pregnancy, every 2nd week until childbirth. They found a 9-month prevalence rate of 49% in this group, with a point prevalence rate of 22% to 28% from the 12th week until delivery. Back problems before pregnancy increased the risk of BP, as did young age at first pregnancy, multiparity, and several physical and psychological work factors including physically heavy work, lifting, twisting and bending, sitting, and poor work satisfaction (291,292). In other studies, similarly high rates of LBP during pregnancy have been reported (29,109, 136,248).

PREVALENCE OF BACK PAIN IN CHILDREN

LBP occurs much more frequently in children than often assumed. This is because disability does not occur, and generally fewer health care resources are employed for LBP in the child and adolescent. Severe LBP in children and teenagers must be addressed vigorously so as not to overlook a serious problem. Salminen (330) studied 310 Finnish children: 5% had a history of LBP interfering with physical activities and 27% had had LBP at some time. Similarly, Fairbank et al. (106) report that 26% of 446 pupils studied had had BP. The highest prevalence occurred at age 13 for boys and age 14 for girls; 14% of the sample had received some type of medical care (Table 48).

Balague et al. (18) followed a group of 1,715 Swiss school children, aged 7 to 17, prospectively using a questionnaire technique. The sample is small in the 7- to 8- and 16- to 17-year age groups. Overall, 33% had had LBP at some time, more than 50% in the 13-year and above age group. LBP had occurred more frequently in girls than in boys (38% versus 32%); 16% had had LBP in the week preceding the interview, and 14% had sought medical advice at least once because of BP. Among those with LBP, 27% had sought medical advice, 18% had had a radiograph, and 17% had been treated with physical therapy; 19% in the LBP group (10% of all children) said that pain had been disabling at some time. Factors associated with increased prevalence rates were (in addition to age and sex) time spent watching television and participation in sports. This later observation is in conflict with the study by Fairbank et al. (106) who reported that BP was more common in those who avoided sports. Salminen et al. (328) came to a similar conclusion and also found that children with BP had weaker trunk muscles. In an attempt to determine if leisure time physical activities and muscle strength were predictive of future LBP, Salminen et al. (329) followed a sample of 40 children with BP and 40 without from age 15 to age 18. There was no predictive value of either physical activity or strength. Anthropometric data also did not predict future LBP. Low frequency of leisure time physical activity, de-

TABLE 48. *Prevalence of LBP in children and adolescents*

	Reference		
	Salminen (330) N = 310	Fairbank et al. (106) N = 446	Balague et al. (18) N = 1715
Lifetime prevalence	27%	26%	33%
Point prevalence			16%
Lifetime disability	5%		10%
Medical consultation		14%	14%

creased spinal function (strength and mobility), and increased height in boys continued to characterize children reporting BP, however. The prevalence of LBP was also assessed in a cohort of 1,242 adolescents (aged 11 to 17) from an urban school district in Allegheny County, Pennsylvania (288). Overall, 30.4% reported LBP, with one-third of those with BP reporting activity limitations; 7.3% had sought medical treatment. Life table analysis demonstrated that by age 15, the prevalence of BP increased to 36%. Sex or race did not significantly influence the prevalence.

A few reports concern the subgroup of disc prolapse in children and adolescents (52,79,129,209,325). This is a rare event, where genetic factors as currently shown by family history may play a role. Prevalence rates cannot be determined from these studies. Girls are more often affected than boys, and congenital abnormalities of the spine occur more frequently than in the adult with an HNP.

LUMBAR DISC DEGENERATION

Disc degeneration has been studied using radiographs, autopsy material, discograms, and lately magnetic resonance imaging (MRI) techniques. The problem of defining disc degeneration when using radiographs is well known. Narrowing of the disc space is the usual indicator, but this is a sign of already quite advanced disc degeneration and difficult to detect until quite severe (11,228,304). Autopsies, on the other hand, have the problem of age and disease bias, and discograms are usually reserved for populations with back symptoms. MRI is a powerful technique, which potentially could be used for both case-control and prospective studies, but availability and cost so far have been prohibitive, although a few studies are now emerging.

Prevalence of Disc Degeneration

The degenerative process has been studied quite intensely over the past century. Early cadaver studies by Schmorl and Junghanns (335) revealed that significant disc degeneration was observed in most spines in the fourth decade and was present as early as the third.

Diffuse degeneration was found in 100% of autopsies in persons over 90 years of age. These observations were confirmed by Coventry et al. (81–83), Hirsch and Schajowicz (154), and others. Vernon-Roberts and Pirie (381) dissected about 100 spines and concluded that the degenerative process started early and progressed rapidly so that by age 50 it was present in all spines studied. Later on, Vernon-Roberts (380) reported on an enlarged sample and confirmed that disc degeneration always exists in the lumbar spine at age 50.

A clear association between increasing age and progressive degeneration of the spinal structures was established in all of the autopsy studies (Fig. 20). The influence of age on the prevalence of disc degeneration is obvious from radiographic studies as well (Fig. 21).

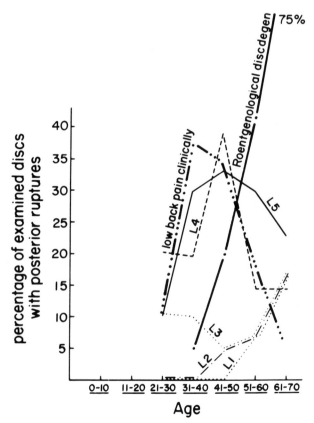

FIG. 20. Frequency of radiating posterior ruptures in the lumbar region compared with radiographic disc degeneration and prevalence of low back pain. From Hirsch (154).

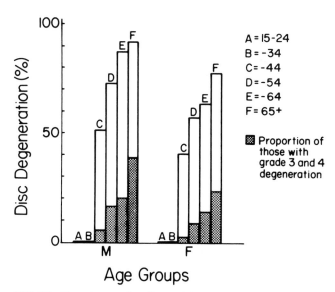

FIG. 21. Prevalence of radiographic disc degeneration. From Lawrence (215).

A = 15-24, B = -34, C = -44, D = -54, E = -64, F = 65+; Proportion of those with grade 3 and 4 degeneration

Disc Degeneration (%); Age Groups; M; F

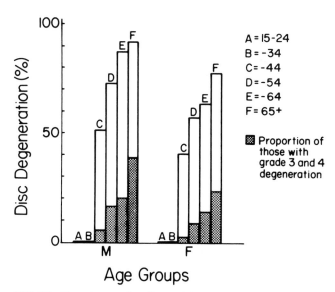

FIG. 21. Prevalence of radiographic disc degeneration. From Lawrence (215).

Kellgren and Lawrence (174) studied 204 men and 277 women aged 55 to 64 in the town of Leigh in northern England: 83% of men and 72% of women had radiographic changes of disc degeneration. In another study of a Jamaican rural population, Bremner et al. (55) surveyed 260 men and 268 women who were 35 to 64 years old. These subjects were compared to an age-matched group of 225 men and 240 women studied earlier in the United Kingdom. The prevalence of disc degeneration was similar in the two populations, with 65% of men and 56% of women having grade 2 to grade 4 degeneration on a scale from 0 (none) to 4 (severe). The Jamaicans more often had extensive disc changes involving more than three discs. A large number of studies confirm the age dependency of disc degeneration (160,161,214,217, 218,220,316,366,410).

While the influence of age is certain, the sex distribution varies between studies. In the two studies mentioned above (55,174), degenerative changes were more common in men than in women. Lawrence (213,215,216) and Hult (160,161) report similar data. Miller et al. (257) gathered data from published reports in which cadaver material had been used for mechanical testing to evaluate the presence of degenerative changes. They concluded that by age 50, 97% of all lumbar discs have degenerative changes. Further, they concluded that male lumbar discs start to degenerate already in the second decade of life, significantly earlier than the female discs, and that male discs were more degenerated than age-matched female discs at any age beyond age 10. Powell et al. (309) studied 302 women between 16 and 80 years of age using MR techniques. Disc degeneration was present in over one-third of the women aged 20 and increased linearly with increasing age (Fig. 22). Salminen et al. (327) report that disc degeneration as determined

more frequent among workers in physically heavy jobs than in light jobs. Wickström (405–407) reviewed the epidemiologic evidence for the effect of work on degenerative changes in the spine. He concluded that heavy physical work "may cause radiologically detectable spinal degeneration that develops up to 10 years prematurely." Injury and heavy lifting seemed to have the strongest degenerative effect. Hult (160,161) reported that both low back complaints and disc degeneration were more frequent in physically heavy jobs than in physically light jobs. In workers with heavy jobs in whom the healthy worker effect was unlikely because of a lack of job alternatives, the percentage of disc degeneration was 78, while 65% of heavy workers in communities where other types of jobs were available had disc degeneration. By comparison, 47% of light workers had radiographically detectable degeneration. Kellgren and Lawrence (174) studied male miners in the 41- to 50-year age group. Severe disc degeneration was found in 43% of the miners compared to 7% in a group of office workers. The difference was largest in workers who were between 21 and 40 years old but was consistent through all age groups. Lawrence et al. (220) compared disc degeneration in foundry workers and in controls, finding a 3-times-higher rate in the foundry workers. Other occupational studies include one by Mach et al. (233), in which lumbar disc degeneration was found in 55% of stevedores compared to 27% of an age-matched control group.

Wiikeri et al. (410) classified radiographs obtained from concrete reinforcement workers into four grades of disc degeneration from none (0) to severe (4). The degree of degeneration was strongly related to age but also to a history of BP and sciatica and to the length of work exposure. Caplan et al. (68) found disc degeneration in miners not to be related to age or duration of work experience but, on the other hand, it was related to a previously reported back injury. Osteophytic changes in contrast were related to age and work duration but not to a previous injury. Magora and Schwartz (245) compared 372 subjects with BP to 217 matched controls. They found no clear relationship between occupation and either the occurrence of degenerative changes of the disc or of the apophyseal joints. Biering-Sørensen et al. (39) related x-ray findings in 666 60-year-old men and women to BP history and physical measurements. Disc degeneration was significantly more common in those with BP than in those without. Heavy physical labor was significantly correlated to higher frequencies of disc degeneration and spondylosis. Evans et al. (105) used MRI techniques to compare 38 ambulating and 21 sedentary employees of a U.S. company. Disc degeneration was found to be significantly more frequent among sedentary women than among ambulating, while in the men there was no difference between the groups. This study is small, but it points to an interesting new possibility of studying the influence of work on disc degeneration.

Riihimäki et al. (314) studied the relationship of mechanical loading and lumbar disc degeneration in 216 concrete reinforcement workers and 201 house painters. Disc space narrowing occurred 10 years earlier, and spondylosis 5 years earlier, in the concrete workers. The RR for disc degeneration was 1.8, for spondylosis, 1.6. Earlier back accidents were found to increase significantly the risk of disc degeneration in a univariate analysis, but not in a multivariate.

Videman et al. (384) obtained careful occupational, recreational, and BP histories from the relatives of 86 individuals who came to autopsy, all deceased before age 65. A history of back injury was related to the occurrence of symmetric disc degeneration, annular ruptures, and vertebral osteophytosis. Symmetric disc degeneration was associated with sedentary work, and vertebral osteophytosis and annular ruptures with heavy work.

In summary, hard physical work in general and frequent lifting, stooping, and postural stress in particular, can be regarded as factors likely to result in degenerative changes of intervertebral discs.

Effect of Sports on Disc Degeneration

A variety of athletic activities place large mechanical demands on the spine. As discussed above, it does not appear that sports activities in general increase the risk of BP. Certain sports activities such as gymnastics, weight lifting, and soccer have been found to accelerate disc degeneration (168,173,352,353,385). Svard et al. (352) found a higher prevalence of degenerative changes in 19- to 29-year-old gymnasts (75%) compared to 23- to 36-year-old nonathletes (31%) using MRI. The gymnasts also had a higher prevalence of disc bulging, disc narrowing, Schmorl's nodes, and abnormal vertebral configuration. Videman et al. (385) performed MRI studies of former runners (N = 24), soccer players (N = 26), weight lifters (N = 19), and shooters (N = 25). Degenerative disc changes and disc bulging was more common among weight lifters throughout the lumbar spine, while soccer players had more degenerative changes than runners and shooters at L4-5 and L5-S1 (Fig. 23). Overall, however, the differences were relatively small considering the extreme difference in loading between weight lifters and shooters. The presence of disc narrowing and bulging was also higher among weight lifters. Salminen et al. (329) attempted to determine the influence of leisure time physical activity, trunk muscle strength, and anthropometry on the development of disc degeneration in 15-year-old school children. Forty children with LBP and forty controls were compared at baseline and followed for 3 years prospectively. MRI was used to determine if degeneration was present or not. At baseline (age 15), 31% of the sample had disc degeneration (327,328), which increased to 42% 3 years later. Disc protrusions and Scheuermann-like changes increased also. Degenerative changes were significantly more common in chil-

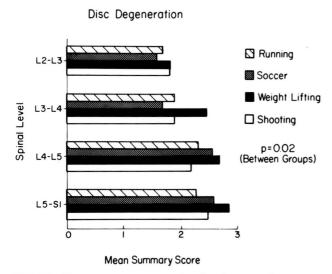

FIG. 23. Mean summary scores for disc degeneration among four groups of athletes. Weight-lifters had significantly greater degeneration scores. Based on Videman et al. (385).

dren with a LBP history and degeneration at age 15 predicted future LBP. Anthropometric data, leisure time physical activity, strength, and mobility were not predictive of degenerative changes.

Influence of Spinal Deformities on Disc Degeneration

In a 1971 paper (412), Wiltse reviewed the relationship between disc degeneration and different spinal deformities, concluding that spondylolisthesis, spinal tropism, and scoliosis contribute to an earlier and more severe development of degenerative disc changes. This has been confirmed by Farfan et al. (107,108) and by Noren et al. (284). Saraste (333) compared a group of 202 patients originally treated for spondylolysis and 170 age-matched controls without lumbar spine disorders. Disc space narrowing of the disc below the spondylolytic defect was significantly more common in the spondylolysis group.

SPONDYLOSIS AND FACET OSTEOARTHRITIS

The nomenclature regarding the term spondylosis is somewhat confused. It should be understood to refer to vertebral osteophytosis secondary to degenerative disc disease. Osteophytes occurring at the facet joints are different from osteophytes occurring on the vertebral margins adjacent to the discs because these joints are synovial joints.

Epidemiology of Lumbar Spondylosis

Since lumbar spondylosis is related to disc degeneration by definition, although the pathogenesis is not firmly established, the epidemiology of spondylosis

closely follows that of disc degeneration discussed above. Thus, the prevalence increases markedly with age. Lumbar spondylosis appears to occur somewhat later than disc degeneration, however, and is usually not seen until age 45 (227). Vernon-Roberts and Pirie (381) concluded, however, that some degree of osteophyte formation at the peripheral margins of the vertebral bodies was seen in all cases where degenerative changes occurred in the disc. Further, the more severe the degenerative changes in the disc, the more marked the osteophytes.

Prevalence of Facet Joint Osteoarthritis

The prevalence of facet joint osteoarthritis also increases with increasing age (65,160,161,165,175,227, 381). Several studies have sought to clarify the relationship between disc degeneration and facet joint osteoarthritis. Inglemark (165) found that marked changes in disc structure were always accompanied by significant facet joint osteoarthritis. Levin (227), on the other hand, concluded that apart from the L5-S1 motion segment, disc degeneration did not seem to be the sole or the dominant factor predisposing to the onset and development of osteoarthritis of the lumbar synovial joints. Vernon-Roberts and Pirie (381), when dissecting more than 100 lumbar spines, concluded that disc degeneration was the primary event leading to osteophyte formation and to apophyseal joint changes. They found that structural abnormalities in the discs were always accompanied by osteoarthritis in the associated facet joints, whereas osteoarthritis in the facet joints was absent or minimal when the discs were relatively normal or when only minor degenerative changes were present. The only exceptions in their studies were patients with structural abnormalities. They also determined that there was an inverse relationship between the severity of osteoarthritis and the preservation of the disc structure.

Butler et al. (65) used MRI to determine the degree of degeneration of discs and computed tomography (CT) scans of the same subjects to determine the occurrence of facet joint osteoarthritis. Disc degeneration without facet joint osteoarthritis was quite frequent, whereas all but one patient with facet joint degeneration also had disc degeneration. This one exception had advanced Paget's disease. Although it is not possible to determine the true sequence of events in a prevalence study, this would indicate that discs degenerate before facets.

Effect of Spinal Deformity on the Facet Joints

Osteoarthritis of the facet joints occurs more often in individuals with spondylolisthesis (412).

Relationship of Facet Joint Osteoarthritis to Work

There are no specific studies available in the literature allowing conclusions on this particular topic.

EPIDEMIOLOGY OF CERVICAL SPINE DISORDERS

Prevalence of Neck Pain

Much of the data presented previously in this chapter on "all" back pain includes pain in the cervical and thoracic spine as well as LBP. The proportion of symptoms attributable to the different regions of the spine is in many studies unknown. Some estimates can be made from those studies in which these symptoms have been separated by anatomic region. Svensson and Andersson (356) studied sick-listing among 917 men in Göteborg, Sweden. Among back diagnoses, 7% were due to neck problems, and only 0.2% to thoracic pain.

In studies more directly aimed at determining the prevalence of neck pain, neck symptoms are often poorly differentiated from pain in the shoulder region, and sometimes the two are combined. Although this makes it difficult to ascribe reported prevalence specifically to the neck, some useful information can be extracted. In a Swedish industrial survey, Hult (161) found prevalence rates of 35% to 71% in 15- to 49-year-old industrial and forest workers. Westerling and Jonsson (401) analyzed a random sample of 18- to 65-year-old men and women in Stockholm, Sweden. The sample size was 2,537, and the survey, which included an examination, was carried out from 1969 to 1971; 18% had suffered from neck–shoulder problems in the past 12 months, 16% of the men and 20% of the women. However, neck pain, tenderness, or stiffness without associated shoulder pain was present in 12% only. The frequency of problems increased with age. Physically demanding jobs were associated with a significantly higher prevalence, whereas lifting per se was not. Takala et al. (362) reported quite comparable data from a Finnish rural population of middle-aged women and men. The 1-year prevalence of pain, ache, or stiffness in the neck "occurring fairly often" was 18% in women, 16% in men. In another Finnish study of a general population sample (the Mini-Finland Study), four aspects of neck pathology were examined: the tension neck syndrome, cervical spondylosis, cervical disc herniation, and myelopathy. At least one of these conditions was present in 14% of the women and 9% of men 30 years and older (386). In a comparable large cross-sectional study of the Swedish work environment, 12.3% said they had symptoms from the upper spine–neck area almost daily (134). Bergenudd and Nilsson (30,31) reported a prevalence of shoulder–neck pain of 2% among 55-year-old residents of Malmö, Sweden.

Dvorak et al. (103) reviewed records from a Swiss accident insurance company that insures about two-thirds of the Swiss working population. Between 1978 and 1981, there were 11,423 patients with cervical spine injuries resulting in posttraumatic complaints, or 2,855 per year: 87.4% were soft tissue injuries, 53% resulted from motor vehicle injuries, and 45% from other types of injuries, mostly falls and sports accidents.

Cervical Herniated Discs

A few cross-sectional studies exist on the prevalence of cervical disc herniations. Kondo et al. (196) determined the incidence in Rochester, Minnesota, from 1950 through 1974, based on medical records from medical facilities. Residence in Rochester for at least 1 year was required. Both protrusions and herniations were accepted as long as they caused radicular symptoms. A total of 56 cases met the criteria. The annual incidence rates by sex were 6.5 per 100,000 for men and 4.6 for women, for a combined incidence of 5.5 per 100,000. The incidence for both sexes was highest between 45 and 54 years of age and slightly lower between 35 and 44. C5-C6 was the disc most frequently affected, followed by C4-C5 and C6-C7.

Kelsey et al. (180–182) surveyed people aged 20 to 64 years in New Haven and Hartford, Connecticut, who were identified as having a prolapsed cervical disc as determined by radiographs and myelograms performed between 1979 and 1981. Patients were divided into three groups: a surgical group, a probable group, and a possible group. The patients were compared to two control groups, one matched from the same medical services as the study patients and one obtained from a group of subjects who had cervical radiographs but no prolapse. People in the fourth decade of life were affected somewhat more often than individuals in other age groups. Men were more frequently affected than women; the ratio was 1.4. C5-C6 and C6-C7 were the affected discs in 75% of patients, and 23% were felt to be related to a car accident. ORs were calculated for a number of factors. Comparatively high ratios were found for frequent lifting, cigarette smoking, and frequent diving from a board (Table 49). Positive associations that were of borderline statistical significance or nonsignificant were operation of vibrating equipment and driving or time spent in motor vehicles. Factors not associated with increased risk were participation in sports other than diving, number of pregnancies and live births, frequent twisting of the neck at work, sitting work, wearing high heel shoes, and smoking of cigars and pipe.

Prevalence of Occupational Neck Pain

Classification and diagnostic criteria vary greatly between reports, and thus it is difficult to compare studies. Waris (396) divided occupational neck syndromes into cervical syndrome (CS) and tension neck syndrome (TNS). CS was defined as pain caused by degenerative changes in the cervical spine causing pain radiating from the neck into the shoulder(s) and arm(s). TNS was de-

TABLE 49. *Adjusted odds ratios for association between several factors and a prolapsed cervical disc*

Factor	Odds ratio
Lifting	
0 times	1.0
<5	1.6
5–25	2.7
>25	4.9
Smoking	1.7
Diving	
<10 times	1.0
10–25	2.3
>25	4.9
Golfing	2.0
Operating vibrating equipment	2.0

Source: ref. 181.

fined as pain, fatigue, and stiffness in the neck muscles. The thoracic outlet syndrome (TOS) was also considered a syndrome of cervicobrachial pain, characterized by weakness and sensory disturbances in the arms. Japanese investigators (234), on the other hand, created the special term "occupation cervicobrachial disorders" (OCD), which was specified as being of work-related pathogenesis (236,237,259,268). Other terms for these diffuse symptoms are repetitive strain injury, overuse syndrome (56), and fibromyalgia, which, however, has specific features discussed in Chapter 22. Kuorinka and Viikari-Juntura (208) discussed the classification and diagnosis problem, and concluded that agreement is impossible because etiology is uncertain, and because some symptom complaints never develop into clinical disease.

Using a modification of the classification by Waris (396), Hagberg and Wegman (135) reviewed the medical literature from 1966 to 1986 and calculated prevalence rates, ORs for occupational exposure, etiological frac-

tions, and their CIs based on over 200 reports. The etiological fraction is an estimate of the impact of exposure, that is, the proportion of exposed cases attributable to the exposure, estimated by: (OR − 1) divided by the OR. Table 50 presents prevalence rates and odds ratios of radiographically verified cervical spondylosis (degenerative changes of the cervical spine). ORs significantly exceeding 1 were found for meat carriers, dentists, miners, and heavy workers, while cotton workers were found to have fewer degenerative changes (both osteoarthritis and disc degeneration) than the general population. The point prevalence for cervical syndrome in these studies is listed in Table 51. Interestingly, civil servants were found to have a prevalence OR of 4.8 compared to iron foundry workers, with an etiological fraction of 0.79. The static nature of their work may account for this difference. Prevalence rates and ORs for TOS are given in Table 52. The rates vary considerably and none of the studies showed a significant OR. Pooling the groups together, an OR of 4.0 was found, with an etiological fraction of 0.75 for exposure to repetitive arm movements.

TNS was found to have the highest rates of all shoulder–neck disorders studied (Table 53) and was more frequent in women than in men. Thus, female industrial workers in the U.S. had an OR of 5.9 compared to male industrial workers. When pooling the keyboard operators together, the standardized OR was 3.0 with an etiological fraction of 0.67.

Although the review by Hagberg and Wegman (135) is exhaustive and helpful, they point out the difficulties in using published data. Confounding factors are poorly controlled, sample sizes can be inadequate, the healthy worker effect is unknown, exposure is often not quantified, and effect (disease) criteria are often not specified. In a subsequent analysis of the influence of work on cervical pain, Hagberg (134) concluded that although degenerative cervical spine changes were more common in some

TABLE 50. *Prevalence rates (number of cases per 100) and odds ratios of radiographically verified cervical spondylosis*

Occupational group	Sex	Prevalence study group	Prevalence reference group	Odds ratio	Reference
Meat carriers	M	84	33	8.4	Schroter & Rademacher (337)
Dentists	M	42	14	5.3	Schroter (336)
Miners	M	76	51	4.5	Newell (228)
Dentists	M	50	31	4.0	Katevuo et al. (171)
Miners	M	54	38	1.9	Kellgren & Lawrence (174)
Heavy workers	M	55	42	1.7	Hult (161)
Carriers	M	23	14	1.8	Schroter (336)
Manual workers	M	42	38	1.2	Kellgren & Lawrence (174)
Miners	M	13	14	0.91	Schroter (336)
Cotton workers					
Osteoarthritis	F	31	38	0.75	Lawrence (214)
Disc degeneration	F	56	70	0.69	Lawrence (214)
Osteoarthritis	M	41	53	0.61	Lawrence (214)
Disc degeneration	M	78	83	0.57	Lawrence (214)

Source: ref. 135.

TABLE 51. *Prevalence rates (number of cases per 100) and odds ratios of cervical syndrome (cervical disc disease)*

Occupational group	Sex	Prevalence study group	Prevalence reference group	Odds ratio	Reference
Slaughterhouse workers	M	5	1	8.5	Luopajarvi et al. (232) Viikari-Juntura (387)
Scissor makers	F	3	1	5.0	Kuorinka & Koskinen (207) Viikari-Juntura (387)
Civil servants	M	5	1	4.8	Partridge et al. (294) Viikari-Juntura (387)
Data entry operators	F	1	2	0.54	Kukkonen et al. (205)
Dockers	M	2	5	0.47	Partridge & Duthie (295)
Assembly line packers	F	1	2	0.27	Luopajarvi et al. (232)
Iron foundry workers	M	1	5	0.07	Partridge et al. (294) Partridge & Duthie (295)

Source: ref. 135.

occupations, the increased risk is small and the relationship of degenerative changes and symptoms uncertain. Further, he concluded that no studies showed a true relationship between occupational stress and neck disease, or between TOS and occupational stress. TNS, on the other hand, was felt to be more common in certain jobs.

In their review, Hagberg and Wegman (135) included only two of the many Japanese reports on OCD. This is understandable, because OCD was defined by the Japanese as "a functional and organic disorder occupationally produced on the basis of muscular and mental fatigue resulting from static and/or repetitive exertion of the arm and hand muscles," (172) and therefore does not fit well into the classification used. Indeed, it is questionable whether this is in fact a true neck disorder. Maeda (234), Aoyama et al. (14), Maeda et al. (235–237), Nagira et al. (267), O'Hara et al. (287), Miyaka et al. (259), Nakasiko et al. (268), and Kitayama (192) have reviewed this symptom complex and its prevalence and influence on the Japanese working population. The prevalence of complaints varies from 4.0% to 20.9%, with the highest rates in workers with repetitive or static work.

The Australian epidemic of RSI (repetitive strain injury) has been the subject of much controversy in recent years (155,191,231,250,276). At Telecom Australia, a telecommunications company with 90,000 staff members, the rate of RSI (neck and shoulder pain predominantly) began to rise late in 1983, peaked in late 1984 (at about 30 times higher levels than in 1982), and declined in 1985, reaching 1983 levels in 1987 (155). Hocking

(155) concluded that neither ergonomics, new technology, nor psychosocial theory fully explained the epidemic. Little evidence was found of a dose–response relationship of RSI to keystroke rate, age, and job duration. The condition was not related to new technology, and psychosocial factors could not explain the uneven distribution among similar groups of workers. Kiesler and Finholt (191) postulated that the RSI epidemic in Australia was more indicative of social problems than of workplace factors, and that dissatisfaction was a major contributor, as was social legitimization of the RSI complaints.

Whitaker et al. (404) compared the prevalence of neck symptoms among 248 urologists and 113 general practitioners in Great Britain. The prevalence was 47.6% and 43.4%, respectively. Significantly more urologists had severe symptoms and frequent attacks possibly caused by their head position during uroscopy. Dimberg et al. (99) analyzed 2,814 industrial workers in a mechanical industry in Sweden. Neck symptoms were present in 293 workers, or 18% of the women and 9% of men. Physical stress, vibrating hand tools, and mental stress were risk factors.

Prevalence of Degenerative Changes in the Cervical Spine

Degenerative changes of the cervical spine include spondylarthrosis, disc degeneration, and apophyseal

TABLE 52. *Prevalence rates (number of cases per 100) and odds ratio of thoracic outlet syndrome*

Occupational group	Prevalence study group	Prevalence reference group	Odds ratio	Reference
Assembly line packers	3	0	10	Luopajarvi et al. (232)
Assembly line workers	14	0	9.6	Sallstrom & Schmidt (331)
Assembly line workers	44	14	3.9	Sallstrom & Schmidt (331)
Slaughterhouse workers	1	0	2.5	Kuorinka & Koskinen (207) Viikari-Juntura (387)
Cash register operators	32	17	1.7	Sallstrom & Schmidt (331)

Source: ref. 135.

TABLE 53. *Prevalence rates (number of cases per 100) and odds ratios for tension neck syndrome*

Occupational group	Sex	Prevalence study group	Prevalence reference group	Odds ratio	Reference
Film-rolling workers	F	100	65	118	Onishi et al. (290)
Industrial workers	F	8	1	5.9	Silverstein (342)
Lamp assemblers	F	91	65	5.1	Onishi et al. (290)
Data entry operators	F	38	11	4.9	Hunting et al. (162)
Typists	F	35	11	4.2	Hunting et al. (162)
Scissor makers	F	61	28	4.1	Luopajarvi et al. (232) Kuorinka & Koskinen (207)
Terminal operators	F	28	11	3.2	Hunting et al. (162)
Data entry operators	F	47	28	2.3	Kukkonen et al. (205)
Office workers	F	80	65	2.1	Onishi et al. (290)
Assembly line packers	F	38	28	1.6	Luopajarvi et al. (232)
Slaughterhouse workers	M	5˙	28	0.15	Luopajarvi et al. (232) Viikara-Juntura (387)

Source: ref. 135.

joint osteoarthritis. Cervical degenerative changes have been found in 30-year-olds in autopsy studies and are present in almost all individuals at age 70 (143). Nathan (269) actually found degenerative changes in all 40-year-olds examined.

A number of radiographic studies have been performed. Hult (160,161) found degenerative changes in 61% to 100% of industrial workers and forest workers, the prevalence increasing with age (Table 54). Forest workers had significantly higher prevalence than industrial workers. The fifth cervical disc was the one most frequently degenerated, followed by the fourth and the sixth. This is in agreement with other investigations (115,218). Hult (160,161) found a strong correlation between cervicobrachial symptoms and increasing severity of degenerative changes, while Lawrence (218) found a significant relationship only when the degenerative changes were moderate and severe. Lawrence's results are in agreement with Kellgren and Lawrence (174) and Friedenberg and Miller (115). Gore et al. (125) determined the prevalence of degenerative changes in 200 asymptomatic men and women. By age 60 to 65, 95% of the men and 70% of women had at least one degenerative change. Although sex was a factor, age was the main factor increasing prevalence, and the C5-C6 and C6-C7 discs were the most often affected. The sex difference is a confirmation of previous data by Kellgren and Lawrence (174) and Lawrence (218,220). A discussion about the relationship of work and degenerative changes was given

above. Hagberg and Wegman (135) found ORs exceeding 1 for meat carriers, dentists, miners, and heavy workers.

Summary of Cervical Epidemiology

Neck disorders are common but often symptomatically related to shoulder disorders. In the literature of work-related neck disorders, exposure is rarely quantified. This makes it difficult to determine cause–effect relationships.

REFERENCES

1. Abenhaim L, Suissa S (1987): Importance and economic burden of occupational back pain: a study of 2500 cases representative of Quebec. *J Occup Med* 29:670–674.
2. Abenhaim L, Suissa S, Rossignol M (1988): Risk of recurrence of occupational back pain over three year follow-up. *Br J Ind Med* 45:829–833.
3. Addison R, Schultz A (1980): Trunk strengths in patients seeking hospitalization for chronic low back disorders. *Spine* 5:539–544.
4. Afacan AS (1982): Sickness absence due to back lesions in coal miners. *J Soc Occup Med* 32(1):26–31.
5. Alston W, Carlson KE, Feldman DJ, Grimm Z, Gerontinos E (1966): A quantitative study of muscle factors in the chronic low back syndrome. *J Am Geriatr Soc* 14(10):1041–1047.
6. Anderson JA (1971): Rheumatism in industry: a review. *Br J Ind Med* 28:103–121.
7. Anderson JA (1980): Back pain and occupation. In: Jayson MIV, ed. *The lumbar spine and back pain,* 2nd ed. Turnbridge Wells: Pitman Medical, pp. 57–82.
8. Anderson JA (1980): Occupational aspects of low back pain. *Clin Rheumat Dis* 6:17–35.
9. Anderson JA (1986): Epidemiological aspects of back pain. *J Soc Occup Med* 36:90–94.
10. Andersson GBJ (1981): Epidemiologic aspects on low back pain in industry. *Spine* 6:53–60.
11. Andersson GBJ, Schultz A, Nathan A, Irstam L (1981): Roentgenographic measurement of lumbar intervertebral disc height. *Spine* 6:154–158.
12. Andersson GBJ, Svensson HO, Oden A (1983): The intensity of work recovery in low back pain. *Spine* 8:880–884.
13. Andersson GBJ, Heliövaara M, de Girolami G (1994): *Epidemiology of low back pain.* WHO, Geneva, In press.
14. Aoyama H, Ohara H, Oze Y, Itani T (1979): Recent trends in

TABLE 54. *Prevalence of radiographic changes of disc degeneration in cervical discs*

Age	Industrial workers (%)	Forest workers (%)
35–39	61	70
40–44	68	82
45–49	80	100

Sources: refs. 160 and 161.

research on occupational cervicobrachial disorder. *J Human Er-gol* 8:39–45.

15. Astrand NE (1987): Medical, psychological, and social factors associated with back abnormalities and self reported back pain. *Br J Ind Med* 44:327–336.

16. Atkinson JH, Slater MA, Patterson TL, Grant I, Garfin SR (1991): Prevalence, onset, and risk of psychiatric disorders in men with chronic low back pain: a controlled study. *Pain* 45:111–121.

17. Backman AL (1983): Health survey of professional drivers. *Scand J Work Environ Health* 9:30–35.

18. Balague F, Dutoit G, Waldburger M (1988): Low back pain in school children. *Scand J Rehab Med* 20:175–179.

19. Barker ME (1977): Pain in the back and leg: a general practice survey. *Rheumatol Rehabil* 16:37–45.

20. Battié MC (1989): *The reliability of physical factors as predictors of the occurrence of back pain reports. A prospective study within industry* [Thesis]. Göteborg, Sweden: University of Göteborg.

21. Battié MC, Bigos SJ, Fisher LD, Hansson TH, Jones ME, Wortley MD (1989): Isometric lifting strength as a predictor of industrial back pain reports. *Spine* 14(8):851–856.

22. Battié MC, Bigos SJ, Fisher LD, Hansson TH, Nachemson AL, Spengler DM, Wortley MD, Zeh J (1989): A prospective study of the role of cardiovascular risk factors and fitness in industrial back pain complaints. *Spine* 14:141–147.

23. Battié MC, Bigos SJ, Fisher LD, Spengler DM, Hansson TH, Nachemson AL, Wortley D (1990): Anthropometric and clinical measurements as predictors of industrial back pain complaints: a prospective study. *J Spinal Disord* 3:195–204.

24. Battié MC, Bigos SJ, Fisher LD, Spengler DM, Hansson TH, Nachemson AL, Wortley D (1990): The role of spinal flexibility in back pain complaints within industry: a prospective study. *Spine* 15:768–773.

25. Battié MC, Bigos SJ, Sheehy A, Wortley MD (1987): Spinal flexibility and individual factors that influence it. *Phys Ther* 67:653–658.

26. Beals RK, Hickman NW (1972): Industrial injuries of the back and extremities. *J Bone Joint Surg* 54A(8):1593–1611.

27. Behrens V, Seligman P, Cameron L, Mathias CGT, Fine L (1994): The prevalence of back pain, hand discomfort and dermatitis in the U.S. working population. *Am J Public Health* 84:1780–1785.

28. Benn RT, Wood PH (1975): Pain in the back: an attempt to estimate the size of the problem. *Rheumatol Rehabil* 14:121–128.

29. Berg G, Hammar M, Moller-Nielsen J, Linden U, Thorblad J (1988): Low back pain during pregnancy. *Obstet Gynecol* 71:71–74.

30. Bergenudd H, Nilsson B (1988): Back pain in middle age; occupational workload and psychologic factors: an epidemiologic survey. *Spine* 13:58–60.

31. Bergenudd H, Nilsson B, Uden A, Willner S (1989): Bone mineral content, gender, body posture and build in relation to back pain in middle age. *Spine* 14:67:577–579.

32. Bergquist-Ullman M, Larsson U (1977): Acute low back pain in industry. A controlled prospective study with special reference to therapy and confounding factors. *Acta Orthop Scand* (Suppl) 170:1–117.

33. Berkson M, Schultz A, Nachemson A, Andersson GB (1977): Voluntary strengths of male adults with acute low back syndromes. *Clin Orthop* 129:84–95.

34. Biering-Sørensen F (1982): Low back trouble in a general population of 30-, 40-, 50-, and 60-year old men and women. Study design, representativeness and basic results. *Dan Med Bull* 29(6):289–299.

35. Biering-Sørensen F (1983): *The prognostic value of the low back history and physical measurements* [Dissertation]. Copenhagen, Denmark: University of Copenhagen.

36. Biering-Sørensen F (1983): A prospective study of low back pain in a general population. I. Occurrence, recurrence and aetiology. *Scand J Rehabil Med* 15:71–79.

37. Biering-Sørensen F (1983): A prospective study of low back pain in a general population. III. Medical service work consequence. *Scand J Rehabil Med* 15:89–96.

38. Biering-Sørensen F (1984): Physical measurements as risk indicators for low-back trouble over a one-year period. *Spine* 9:106–119.

39. Biering-Sørensen F (1985): The relation of spinal x-ray to low back pain and physical activity among 60-year-old men and women. *Spine* 10:451–455.

40. Biering-Sørensen F (1985): Risk of back trouble in individual occupations in Denmark. *Ergonomics* 28:51–60.

41. Biering-Sørensen F, Hilden J (1984): Reproducibility of the history of low-back trouble. *Spine* 9:280–286.

42. Biering-Sørensen F, Thomsen C (1986): Medical, social and occupational history as risk indicators for low-back trouble in a general population. *Spine* 11:720–725.

43. Biering-Sørensen F, Thomsen CE, Hilden J (1989): Risk indicators for low back trouble. *Scand J Rehabil Med* 21:151–157.

44. Bigos SJ, Battié MC (1992): Risk factors for industrial back problems. In: Wiesel SW, ed. *Seminars in Spine Surgery*, Vol. 4. Philadelphia: WB Saunders, pp. 2–11.

45. Bigos SJ, Battié MC, Fisher LD, Fordyce WE, Hansson TH, Nachemson AL, Spengler DM: A prospective study of work perceptions and psychosocial factors affecting the report of back injury. *Spine* 16:1–6.

46. Bigos SJ, Spengler DM, Martin NA, Zeh J, Fisher L, Nachemson A (1986): Back injuries in industry: a retrospective study. III. Employee–related factors. *Spine* 11:252–256.

47. Bjonness T (1975): Low back pain in persons with congenital club foot. *Scand J Rehabil Med* 7(4):163–165.

48. Blow RJ, Jackson JM (1971): Rehabilitation of registered dock workers. An analysis of back injuries in registered dock workers. *Proc R Soc Med* 64:753–757.

49. Bongers PM, de Winter CR, Kompier MAJ, Hildebrandt VH (1993): Psychosocial factors at work and musculoskeletal disease. *Scand J Work Environ Health* 19:297–312.

50. Boshuizen HC, Bongers PM, Hulshof CTJ (1992): Self-reported back pain in fork-lift truck and freight-container tractor drivers exposed to whole-body vibration. *Spine* 17:59–65.

51. Boshuizen HC, Verbeek JHAM, Broersen JPJ, Weel ANH (1993): Do smokers get more back pain? *Spine* 18:35–40.

52. Bradford DS, Garcia A (1969): Herniations of the lumbar intervertebral disk in children and adolescents. *JAMA* 210:2045–2051.

53. Bradford DS, Moe JH, Winter RB (1982): Scoliosis and kyphosis. Operative management of idiopathic scoliosis. In: *The spine*, 2nd ed., Rothman RH, Simeone FA, eds. Philadelphia: WB Saunders, pp. 346–348.

54. Braun W (1969): Ursachen des lumbalen Bandscheiberverfalls. *Die Wirbelsäule in Forschung und Praxis* 43. Hippocrates, Stuttgart.

55. Bremner JM, Lawrence JS, Miall WE (1968): Degenerative joint disease in a Jamaican rural population. *Ann Rheum Dis* 27:326–332.

56. Browne DW, Russell ML, Morgan JL, et al (1984): Reduced disability and health care costs in an industrial fitness program. *J Occup Med* 26:809–816.

57. Brown JR (1973): Lifting as an industrial hazard. *Am Industr Hyg Assoc J* 34(7):292–297.

58. Brown JR (1975): Factors contributing to the development of low back pain in industrial workers. *Am Industr Hyg Assoc J* 36:26–31.

59. Buckle PW, Kember PA, Wood AD, Wood SN (1980): Factors influencing occupational back pain in Bedfordshire. *Spine* 5:254–258.

60. Burchfiel CM, Boice JA, Stafford BA, Bond GG (1992): Prevalence of back pain and joint problems in a manufacturing company. *J Occup Med* 34:129–134.

61. Burdorf A (1992): Exposure assessment of risk factors for disorders of the back in occupational epidemiology. *Scand J Work Environ Health* 18:1–9.

62. Burdorf A, Govaert G, Elders L (1991): Postural load and back pain of workers in the manufacturing of prefabricated concrete elements. *Ergonomics* 34:909–918.

63. Burdorf A, Zondervan H (1990): An epidemiological study of low-back pain in crane operators. *Ergonomics* 33:981–987.

64. Burwell RG, Fraser MA (1981): *An anthropometric study of patients with low back pain syndromes.* Presented at the International Study of Lumbar Spine Meeting, Paris, France, May 1981.

65. Butler D, Trafimow JH, Andersson GBJ, McNeill TW, Huckman MS (1990): Discs degenerate before facets. *Spine* 15:111–113.

66. Cady LD, Bischoff DP, O'Connell ER, Thomas PC, Allan JH (1979): Strength and fitness and subsequent back injuries in fire fighters. *J Occup Med* 21(4):269–272.

67. Cady LD Jr, Thomas PC, Karwasky RJ (1985): Program for increasing health and physical fitness of firefighters. *J Occup Med* 27:110–114.

68. Caplan PS, Freedman LM, Connelly TP (1966): Degenerative joint disease of the lumbar spine in coal miners. A clinical and x-ray study. *Arthritis Rheum* 9(5):693–702.

69. Cedercreutz G, Videman T, Tola S, Asp S (1987): Individual risk factors of the back among applicants to a nursing school. *Ergonomics* 30:269–272.

70. Chaffin DB (1974): Human strength capability and low back pain. *J Occup Med* 16(4):248–254.

71. Chaffin DB, Herrin GD, Keyserling WM (1978): Preemployment strength testing. An updated position. *J Occup Med* 20(6):403–408.

72. Chaffin DB, Park KS (1973): A longitudinal study of low-back pain as associated with occupational weight lifting factors. *Am Ind Hyg Assoc J* 34:513–525.

73. Cherkin DC, Deyo RA, Loeser JD, Bush T, Waddell G (1994): An international comparison of back surgery rates. *Spine* 19:1201–1206.

74. Choler U, Larsson R, Nachemson A, Peterson LE (1985): Back pain. *Spri report* 188(in Swedish):1–100.

75. Christ W (1973): *Beanspruchung und Leistungsfahigkeit des Menschen bei underbrochener und Langzeit-Exposition mit stochastischen Schwingungen* [Dissertation]. Darmstadt: Technical University. VDI Ber 11:1–85.

76. Christ W (1974): Belastung durch mechanische Schwingungen und mögliche Gesundheitsschädigungen im Bereich der Wirbelsäule. *Fortschr Med* 92:705–708.

77. Christ W, Dupuis H (1966): Über die Beanspruchung der Wirbelsäule unter dem Einfluss sinusformiger und stochastischer Schwingungen. *Int Z Angew Physiol Einschl Arbeitsphysiol* 22:258–278.

78. Christ W, Dupuis H (1968): Untersuchung der Möglichkeit von gesundheitlichen Schädigungen im Bereich der Wirbelsäule. *Med Welt* 36:1919–1920; 37:1967–1972.

79. Clarke NM, Cleak DK (1983): Intervertebral disc prolapse in children and adolescents. *J Pediatr Orthop* 3:202–206.

80. Collis DK, and Ponseti IV (1969): Long term follow-up of patients with idiopathic scoliosis not treated surgically. *J Bone Joint Surg* 51A(3):425–445.

81. Coventry MB, Ghormley RK, Kernohan JW (1945): The intervertebral disc. Its microscopic anatomy and pathology. Part I. *J Bone Joint Surg* 27:105–112.

82. Coventry MB, Ghormley RK, Kernohan JW (1945): The intervertebral disc. Its microscopic anatomy and pathology. Part II. *J Bone Joint Surg* 27:233–247.

83. Coventry MB, Ghormley RK, Kernohan JW (1945): The intervertebral disc. Its microscopic anatomy and pathology. Part III. *J Bone Joint Surg* 27:460–474.

84. Crown S (1978): Psychological aspects of low back pain. *Rheumatol Rehabil* 17:114–124.

85. Cunningham LS, Kelsey JL (1984): Epidemiology of musculoskeletal impairments and associated disability. *Am J Public Health* 74:574–579.

86. Cust G, Pearson JC, Mair A (1972): The prevalence of low back pain in nurses. *Int Nurs Rev* 19:169–179.

87. Damkot DK, Pope MH, Lord J, Frymoyer JW (1984): The relationship between work history, work environment and low-back pain in men. *Spine* 9:395–399.

88. Damlund M, Goth S, Hasle P, Munk K (1982): Low-back pain and early retirement among Danish semi-skilled construction workers. *Scand J Work Environ Health* (Suppl) 8:100–104.

89. Damlund M, Goth S, Hasle P, Munk K (1986): Low back strain in Danish semi-skilled construction work. *Appl Ergonom* 17:31–39.

90. Daniel JW, Fairbank JC, Vale PT, O'Brien JP (1980): Low back pain in the steel industry: a clinical, economic and occupational analysis at a North Wales integrated steelworks of the British Steel Corporation. *J Soc Occup Med* 30:49–56.

91. David GC (1985): UK national statistics on handling accidents and lumbar injuries at work. *Ergonomics* 28:9–16.

92. Dehlin O, Berg S, Andersson GB, Grimby G (1981): Effect of physical training and ergonomic counseling on the psychological perception of work and on the subjective assessment of low-back insufficiency. *Scand J Rehabil Med* 13:1–9.

93. Dehlin O, Hedenrud B, Horal J (1976): Back symptoms in nursing aides in a geriatric hospital. *Scand J Rehabil Med* 8:47–53.

94. Deyo RA, Bass JE (1989): Lifestyle and low back pain. The influence of smoking and obesity. *Spine* 14:501–506.

95. Deyo RA, Cherwin D, Conrad D, Volinn E (1991): Cost, controversy, crisis: low back pain and the health of the public. *Ann Rev Publ Health* 12:141–156.

96. Deyo RA, Tsui-Wu Y-J (1987): Descriptive epidemiology of low-back pain and its related medical care in the United States. *Spine* 12:264–268.

97. Deyo RA, Tsui-Wu Y-J (1987): Functional disability due to back pain. *Arthritis Rheum* 30:1247–1253.

98. Dillane JB, Fry J, Kalton G (1966): Acute back syndrome. A study from general practice. *Br Med J* 2:82–84.

99. Dimberg L, Olafsson A, Stefansson E, Aagaard H, Oden A, Andersson GBJ, Hansson T, Hagert C-G (1989): The correlation between work environment and the occurrence of cervicobrachial symptoms. *J Occup Med* 31:447–453.

100. Dupuis H, Christ W (1966): *Untersuchung der Möglichkeit von Gesundheits-schädigungen im Bereich der Wirbelsäule bei Schlepperfahrern.* Research report. Bad Kreuznach: Max-Planck-Institute für Landarbeit und Landtechnik.

101. Dupuis H, Hartung E, Louda L (1972): Vergleich regelloser Schwingungen eines berenzten Frequenzbereiches mit sinusformigen Schwingungen hinsichtlich der Einwirkung auf den Menschen. *Ergonomics* 15:237–265.

102. Dupuis H, Zerlett G (1986): *The effects of whole-body vibration.* New York: Springer-Verlag.

103. Dvorak J, Valach L, Schmidt ST (1989): Cervical spine injuries in Switzerland. *J Manual Med* 4:7–16.

104. Ernst E (1993): Smoking, a cause of back trouble? *Br J Rheumatol* 32:239–242.

105. Evans W, Jobe W, Siebert C (1989): A cross-sectional prevalence study of lumbar disc degeneration in a working population. *Spine* 14:60–64.

106. Fairbank JC, Pynsent PB, Van Poortvliet JA, Phillips H (1984): Influence of anthropometric factors and joint laxity in the incidence of adolescent back pain. *Spine* 9(5):461–464.

107. Farfan HF, Cossette JW, Robertson GH, Wells RV, Kraus H (1970): The effects of torsion on the lumbar intervertebral joints: the role of torsion in the production of disc degeneration. *J Bone Joint Surg* 52A:468–497.

108. Farfan HF, Huberdeau RM, Dubow HI (1972): Lumbar intervertebral disc degeneration. *J Bone Joint Surg* 54A:492–510.

109. Fast A, Shapiro D, Ducommun J, et al. (1987): Low back pain in pregnancy. *Spine* 12:368–371.

110. Fisher V (1980): Vibrationsbedingte Wirbelsäulenschaden bei Hubschrankpiloten. *Arb Med Soz Med Prav Med* 7:161–163.

111. Fisk JW, Baigent ML (1975): Clinical and radiological assessment of leg length. *NZ Med J* 81:477–480.

112. Fitzgerald JG, Crotty J (1972): The incidence of backache among aircrew and groundcrew in the RAF, FPRC/1313.

113. Flynn JC, Joque MPA (1979): Anterior fusion of the lumbar spine. End result study with long-term follow-up. *J Bone Joint Surg* 61:1143–1161.

114. Frank A (1993): Low back pain. *Br Med J* 306:901–908.

115. Friedenberg ZB, Miller WT (1963): Degenerative disc disease of the cervical spine. A comparative study of asymptomatic and symptomatic patients. *J Bone Joint Surg* 45A:1171–1178.

116. Frymoyer JW (1988): Back pain and sciatica. *N Engl J Med* 318:291–300.

117. Frymoyer JW, Cats-Baril W (1987): Predictors of low back pain disability. *Clin Orthop* 221:89–98.

118. Frymoyer JW, Newberg A, Pope MH, Wilder DG, Clements J, MacPherson IB (1984): Spine radiographs in patients with low back pain. An epidemiological study in men. *J Bone Joint Surg* 66A:1048–1055.

119. Frymoyer JW, Pope MH (1987): Epidemiologic insights into the relationship between usage and back disorder. In: Hadler NM, ed. *Current concepts in regional musculoskeletal illness* Orlando: Grune and Stratton, pp. 263–279.

120. Frymoyer JW, Pope MH, Clements JH, Wilder DG, McPherson B, Ashikaga T (1983): Risk factors in low back pain. An epidemiological survey. *J Bone Joint Surg* 65A:213.

121. Frymoyer JW, Pope MH, Costanza MC, Rosen JC, Goggin JE, Wilder DG (1980): Epidemiologic studies of low-back pain. *Spine* 5:419–423.

122. Frymoyer JW, Pope MH, Kristiansen T (1982): Skiing and spinal trauma. *Clin Sports Med* 1:309–318.

123. Giles LGF, Taylor JR (1981): Low-back pain associated with leg length inequality. *Spine* 6(5):510–521.

124. Glover JR (1960): Back pain and hyperaesthesia. *Lancet* 1:1165–1169.

125. Gore DR, Sepic SB, Gardner GM (1986): Roentgenographic findings of the cervical spine in asymptomatic people. *Spine* 11:521–524.

126. Granhed H, Morelli B (1988): Low back pain among retired wrestlers and heavyweight lifters. *Am J Sports Med* 16:530–533.

127. Grazier KL, Holbrook TL, Kelsey JL, Stauffer RN (1984): *The frequency of occurrence, impact, and cost of musculoskeletal conditions in the United States.* Chicago: American Academy of Orthopaedic Surgeons. 1984.

128. Greenough CG, Fraser RD (1989): The effects of compensation on recovery from low back injury. *Spine* 14:947–955.

129. Grobler LJ, Simmons EH, Barrington TW (1979): Intervertebral disc herniation in the adolescent. *Spine* 4:267–278.

130. Gruber GJ (1976): *Relationships between whole-body vibration and morbidity patterns among interstate truck drivers.* U.S. Department of Health, Education and Welfare, DHEW (NIOSH) Publication No. 77-167.

131. Gruber GJ, Ziperman HH (1974): *Relationship between whole-body vibration and morbidity patterns among motor coach operators.* DHEW (NIOSH) Publication No. 75-104.

132. Gyntelberg F (1974): One year incidence of low back pain among male residents of Copenhagen aged 40-59. *Dan Med Bull* 21(1):30–36.

133. Haber LD (1971): Disabling effects of chronic disease and impairment. *J Chronic Dis* 24(7/8):469–487.

134. Hagberg M (1988): *The importance of the work environment to symptoms from neck and shoulder.* Stockholm: The Swedish Work Environment Fund, pp. 1–141.

135. Hagberg M, Wegman DH (1987): Prevalence rates and odds ratios of shoulder-neck diseases in different occupational groups. *Br J Ind Med* 44:602–610.

136. Hammar M, Berg G, Lilljeskold U, et al. (1986): Back pain during pregnancy (In Swedish). *Swedish Med J* 83:1960–1961.

137. Hanley EN, Shapiro DE (1989): The development of low-back pain after excision of a lumbar disc. *J Bone Joint Surg* 71A(5):719–721.

138. Hansson T (1989): *Low back pain and work.* Stockholm: The Swedish Work Environment Fund.

139. Hansson T, Bigos S, Beecher P, et al. (1985): The lumbar lordosis in acute and chronic low back pain. *Spine* 10:154–155.

140. Harris AI (1971): *Handicapped and impaired in Great Britain. Part I.* Social Survey Division. London: Office of Population Censuses and Surveys, Her Majesty's Stationery Office.

141. Hasue M, Fujiwara M, Kikuchi S (1980): A new method of quantitative measurement of abdominal and back muscle strength. *Spine* 5:143–148.

142. Heikkila JK, Koskenvuo M, Heliövaara M, Kurppa K, Riihimäki H, Heikkila K, Rita H, Videman T (1989): Genetic and environmental factors in sciatica. Evidence from a nationwide panel of 9,365 adult twin pairs. *Ann Med* 21:393–398.

143. Heine J (1926): Uber die Arthritis deformans. *Virchows Arch Pathol Anat* 260:521–663.

144. Helander E (1973): Back pain and work disability. *Socialmed Tidskr* 50:398–404 (in Swedish).

145. Heliövaara M (1987): Body height, obesity, and risk of herniated lumbar intervertebral disc. *Spine* 12:469–472.

146. Heliövaara M (1987): Occupation and risk of herniated lumbar intervertebral disc or sciatica leading to hospitalization. *J Chronic Dis* 40:259–264.

147. Heliövaara M (1988): *Epidemiology of sciatica and herniated lumbar intervertebral disc.* Helsinki: The Research Institute for Social Security, pp. 1–147.

148. Heliövaara M, Knekt P, Aromaa A (1987): Incidence and risk factors of herniated lumbar intervertebral disc or sciatica leading to hospitalization. *J Chronic Dis* 40:251–285.

149. Heliövaara M, Makela M, Knekt P, Impivaara O, Aromaa A (1991): Determinants of sciatica and low-back pain. *Spine* 16:608–614.

150. Heliövaara M, Vanharanta H, Korpi J, Troup JDG (1986): Herniated lumbar disc syndrome and vertebral canals. *Spine* 11:433–435.

151. Herrin GD, Jaraiedi M, Anderson CK (1986): Prediction of overexertion injuries using biomechanical and psychophysical models. *Am Ind Hyg Assoc J* 47:322–330.

152. Hilfert R, Kohne G, Toussaint R, Zerlett G (1981): Probleme der Ganzkörperschwingungs-belastung von Erdbaumaschinenführern. *Zentralblatt Arbeitsmedizin, Arbeitsschutz, Prophylaxe Ergonomie* 31:152–155.

153. Hirsch C, Jonsson B, Lewin T (1969): Low back symptoms in a Swedish female population. *Clin Orthop* 63:171–176.

154. Hirsch C, Schajowicz F (1953): Studies on structural changes in the lumbar annulus fibrosus. *Acta Orthop Scand* 22:184–231.

155. Hocking B (1987): Epidemiological aspects of repetition strain injury in Telecom, Australia. *Med J Aust* 147:218–222.

156. Hodgson S, Shannon HS, Troup JDG (1974): *The prevention of spinal disorders in dock workers.* Report to National Dock Labour Board, London.

157. Horal J (1969): The clinical appearance of low back disorders in the city of Gothenburg, Sweden. *Acta Orthop Scand* (Suppl) 118:1–109.

158. Hrubec Z, Nashold BS Jr (1975): Epidemiology of lumbar disc lesions in the military in World War II. *Am J Epidem* 102(5):367–376.

159. Hulshof C, van Zanten BV (1987): Whole body vibration and low back pain. A review of epidemiological studies. *Int Arch Occup Environ Health* 59:205–220.

160. Hult L (1954): The Munkfors investigation. *Acta Orthop Scand* (Suppl) 16:1.

161. Hult L (1954): Cervical, dorsal, and lumbar spinal syndromes. *Acta Orthop Scand* (Suppl) 17:1–102.

162. Hunting W, Laubi T, Grandjean E (1981): Postural and visual loads at VDP workplaces. *Ergonomics* 24:917–931.

163. Hurme M, Alaranta H, Torma T, Einola S (1983): Operated lumbar disc herniation: epidemiological aspects. *Ann Chir Gynaecol* 72:33–36.

164. Ikata T (1965): Statistical and dynamic studies of lesions due to overloading on the spine. *Shikoku Acta Med* 40:262.

165. Ingelmark BE (1959): Function of and pathological changes in the spinal joints. In: Spinal joint changes and dental infections. *Acta Anat* 38(Suppl 36):12–17.

166. Jacobsson L, Lindegarde F, Manthrupe R (1989): The commonest rheumatic complaints of over six weeks duration in a twelve-month period in a defined Swedish population. *Scand J Rheumatol* 18:353–360.

167. Jensen RC (1988): Epidemiology of work-related back pain. *Top Acute Care Trauma Rehabil* 2:1–15.

168. Jorgensen U (1984): Epidemiology of injuries in typical Scandinavian team sports. *Br J Sports Med* 18:66–78.

169. Joukamaa M (1986): *Low-back pain and psychological factors. A social-psychiatric study of the population of working age.* Turku, Publications of the Social Insurance Institution AL:28. (In Finnish with English summary).

170. Kane WJ (1980): Worldwide incidence rates of laminectomy for lumbar disc herniations. Presented at the annual meeting of ISSLS, New Orleans, LA.

171. Katevuo K, Aitasalo K, Lehtinen R, Pietila J (1985): Skeletal changes in dentists and farmers in Finland. *Community Dent Oral Epidemiol* 13:23–25.

172. Keikenwan SI (1973): Report of the Committee on Occupational Cervicobrachial Syndrome of the Japan Association of Industrial Health. *Jpn J Indust Health* 15:304–311 (in Japanese).

173. Keller CS, Noyes FR, Buncher CR (1987): The medical aspects of soccer injury epidemiology. *Am J Sports Med* 15:230–237.

174. Kellgren JH, Lawrence JS (1952): Rheumatism in miners: part II. X-ray study. *Br J Indust Med* 9:197–207.

175. Kellgren JH, Lawrence JS (1958): Osteoarthrosis and disk degeneration in an urban population. *Ann Rheum Dis* 17(4):388–397.

176. Kelsey JL (1975): An epidemiological study of acute herniated lumbar intervertebral discs. *Rheumatol Rehabil* 14(3):144–159.

177. Kelsey JL (1975): An epidemiological study of the relationship between occupations and acute herniated lumbar intervertebral discs. *Int J Epidemiol* 4(3):197–205.

178. Kelsey JL (1978): Epidemiology of radiculopathies. *Adv Neurol* 19:385–398.

179. Kelsey JL (1982): Idiopathic low back pain, magnitude of the problem. In: *Symposium on idiopathic low back pain.* White AA III, Gordon SL, eds. St. Louis: Mosby.

180. Kelsey JL, Githens PB, O'Connor T, et al (1984): Acute prolapsed lumbar intervertebral disc. An epidemiologic study with special reference to driving automobiles and cigarette smoking. *Spine* 9:608–613.

181. Kelsey JL, Githens PB, Walter SD, Southwick WO, Wert U, Holford TR, Ostfeld AM, Calogero JA, O'Conner T, White AA III (1984): An epidemiologic study of acute prolapsed cervical intervertebral disc. *J Bone Joint Surg* 66A:907–914.

182. Kelsey JL, Githens PB, White AA, et al (1984): An epidemiologic study of lifting and twisting on the job and risk for acute prolapsed lumbar intervertebral disc. *J Orthop Res* 2:61–66.

183. Kelsey JL, Golden AL (1988): Occupational and workplace factors associated with low-back pain. *Occup Med* 3:7–16.

184. Kelsey JL, Hardy RJ (1975): Driving of motor vehicles as a risk factor for acute herniated lumbar intervertebral disc. *Am J Epidemiol* 102(1):63–73.

185. Kelsey JL, Ostfeld AM (1975): Demographic characteristics of persons with acute herniated lumbar intervertebral disc. *J Chronic Dis* 28(1):37–50.

186. Kelsey JL, Pastides H, Bigbee GE Jr (1978): *Musculo-skeletal disorders: their frequency of occurrence and their impact on the population of the United States.* New York: Prodist.

187. Kelsey JL, White AA III (1980): Epidemiology and impact on low back pain. *Spine* 5(2):133–142.

188. Keyserling WM, Herrin GD, Chaffin DB (1980): Isometric strength testing as a means of controlling medical incidents on strenuous jobs. *J Occup Med* 22(5):332–336.

189. Keyserling WM, Punnett L, Fine LJ (1987): Postural stress of the trunk and shoulders: identification and control of occupational risk factors. In: *Ergonomic interventions to prevent musculoskeletal injuries in industry.* Chelsea, Michigan: Lewis Publishers, pp 11–26.

190. Keyserling WM, Punnett L, Fine LJ (1988): Trunk posture and back pain: identification and control of occupational risk factors. *Appl Ind Hyg* 3:87–92.

191. Kiesler S, Finholt T (1988): The mystery of RSI. *Am Psychol* 43:1004–1015.

192. Kitayama T (1982): Health care relating to the occupational cervicobrachial disorder. *J Human Ergol* 11:119–124.

193. Klaukka T, Sievers K, Takala J (1982): Epidemiology of rheumatic diseases in Finland in 1964-76. *Scand J Rheumatol* (Suppl) 47:5–13.

194. Klein BP, Jensen RC, Sanderson LM (1984): Assessment of workers' compensation claims for back strains/sprains. *J Occup Med* 26:443–448.

195. Kohne G, Zerlett G, Duntze H (1982): Ganzkörperswingungen auf Erdbaumaschinen. *Humanisierung des Arbeitslebens* 32:1–366.

196. Kondo K, Molgaard CA, Kurland LT, Onofric BM (1981): Protruded intervertebral cervical disc. *Minn Med* 64:751–753.

197. Koota K (1979): As quoted in ref. 147, Heliövaara M (1988): *Epidemiology of sciatica and herniated lumbar intervertebral disc.* Helsinki: The Research Institute for Social Security, pp. 1–147.

198. Kostuik JP, Bentivoglio J (1981): The incidence of low back pain in adult scoliosis. *Spine* 6:268–273.

199. Kostuik JP, Israel J, Hall JE (1973): Scoliosis surgery in adults. *Clin Orthop* 93:225–234.

200. Kozak LJ, Moien M (1985): Detailed diagnoses and surgical procedures for patients discharged from short-stay hospitals. United States, 1983. *Vital Health Stat* 13 (82).

201. Kramer JS, Yelin EH, Epstein WV (1983): Social and economic impacts of four musculoskeletal conditions. A study using national community-based data. *Arthritis Rheum* 26:901–907.

202. Kristen H, Lukeschitsch G, Ramach W (1981): Untersuchung der Lendenwirbelsäule bei Kleinlasttransportarbeitern. *Arb Med Soz Med Prav Med* 61:226–229.

203. Kroemer KH, Robinette JC (1969): Ergonomics in the design of office furniture. *Ind Med Surg* 38:115–125.

204. Kroenke K, Price RK (1993): Symptoms in the community. Prevalence, classification and psychiatric comorbidity. *Arch Intern Med* 153:2474–2480.

205. Kukkonen R, Luopajarvi T, Riihimäki V (1983): Prevention of fatigue amongst data entry operators. In: Kvalseth TO, ed. *Ergonomics of work station design.* London: Butterworths, pp. 28–34.

206. Kumar S (1990): Cumulative load as a risk factor for back pain. *Spine* 15:1311–1316.

207. Kuorinka I, Koskinen P (1979): Occupational rheumatic diseases and upper limb strain in manual jobs in a light mechanical industry. *Scand J Work Environ Health* 6(suppl 3):39–47.

208. Kuorinka I, Viikari-Juntura E (1982): Prevalence of neck and upper limb disorders (NLD) and work load in different occupational groups. Problems in classification and diagnosis. *J Hum Ergol* 11:65–72.

209. Kurihara A, Kataoka O (1980): Lumbar disc herniation in children and adolescents. *Spine* 5:443–451.

210. Langrana N, Lee CK (1984): Isokinetic evaluation of trunk muscles. *Spine* 9:171–175.

211. Langrana N, Lee CK, Alexander H, Mayott CW (1984): Quantitative assessment of back strength using isokinetic testing. *Spine* 9:287–290.

212. Lavsky-Shulan M, Wallace RB, Kohout FJ, et al (1985): Prevalence and functional correlates of low back pain in the elderly: the Iowa 65-Rural Health Study. *J Am Geriatr Soc* 33:23–28.

213. Lawrence JS (1955): Rheumatism in coal miners, Part III. Occupational factors. *Br J Ind Med* 12:249–261.

214. Lawrence JS (1961): Rheumatism in cotton operatives. *Br J Ind Med* 18:270–276.

215. Lawrence JS (1969): Disc degeneration: its frequency and relationship to symptoms. *Ann Rheum Dis* 28:121–138.

216. Lawrence JS (1977): *Rheumatism in populations.* London: Heinemann.

217. Lawrence JS, Aitken-Swan J (1952): Rheumatism in miners: part I. Rheumatic complaints. *Br J Ind Med* 9:1–18.

218. Lawrence JS, Bremner JM, Bier F (1966): Osteoarthrosis: prevalence in the population and relationship between symptoms and x-ray changes. *Ann Rheum Dis* 25:1–24.

219. Lawrence JS, Graft R, deLaine VAI (1983): Degenerative joint diseases in random samples and occupational groups. In: *The epidemiology of chronic rheumatism,* vol. I. Kellgren JH, Jeffrey MR, Bull J, eds. Oxford: Blackwell Scientific, pp. 98–119.

220. Lawrence JS, Molyneux MK, Dingwall-Fordyce I (1966): Rheumatism in foundry workers. *Br J Ind Med* 23:42–52.

221. Leavitt F (1992): The physical exertion factor in compensable work injuries. A hidden flaw in previous research. *Spine* 17(3):307–310.

222. Lee P, Helewa A, Smythe HA, Bombardier C, Goldsmith CH (1985): Epidemiology of musculoskeletal disorders (complaints) and related disability in Canada. *J Rheumatol* 12:1169–1173.

223. Leigh JP, Sheetz RM (1989): Prevalence of back pain among full-time United States workers. *Br J Ind Med* 4:651–657.

224. Leino P, Aro S, Hasan J (1987): Trunk muscle function and low back disorders: a ten-year follow-up study. *J Chronic Dis* 40:289–296.

225. Leino P (1989): Symptoms of stress predict musculoskeletal disorders. *J Epidemiol Community Health* 43:293–300.

226. Leino P (1993): Does leisure time physical activity prevent low back disorders? *Spine* 18:863–871.

227. Lewin T (1964): Osteoarthritis in lumbar synovial joints. *Acta Orthop Scand* (Suppl) 73:1–112.

228. Lindblom K (1951): Backache and its relation to ruptures of the intervertebral discs. *Radiology* 57:710–719.

229. Lloyd MH, Gauld S, Soutar CA (1986): Epidemiologic study of back pain in miners and office workers. *Spine* 11:136–140.

230. Lockshin MD, Higgins IT, Higgins MW, Dodge HJ, Canale N

(1969): Rheumatism in mining communities in Marion County, West Virginia. *Am J Epidemiol* 90:17–29.

231. Lucire Y (1986): Neurosis in the workplace. *Med J Austr* 145: 323–327.

232. Luopajarvi T, Kuorinka I, Virolainen M, Holmberg M (1979): Prevalence of tenosynovitis and other injuries of the upper extremities in repetitive work. *Scand J Work Environ Health* 6(suppl 3):48–55.

233. Mach J, Heitner H, Ziller R (1976): Die Bedeutung der beruflichen Belastung für die Entstehung degenerativer Wirbelsäulenveränderunger. *Z Hygiene Grenzgebiete* 22(5):352–354.

234. Maeda K (1977): Occupational cervicobrachial disorder and its causative factors. *J Hum Ergol* 6:183–202.

235. Maeda K, Harada N, Takamatsu M (1980): Factor analysis of complaints of occupational cervicobrachial disorder in assembly lines of a cigarette factory. *Kurume Med J* 27:253–261.

236. Maeda K, Hirayama H, Chang CP, Takamatsu M (1979): Studies on the progress of occupational cervicobrachial disorder by analyzing the subjective symptoms of work-women in assembly lines of a cigarette factory. *Jpn J Ind Health* 21:398–407.

237. Maeda K, Horiguchi S, Hosokawa M (1982): History of the studies on occupational cervicobrachial disorder in Japan and remaining problems. *J Hum Ergol* 11:17–29.

238. Magi M, Allander E, Bjelle A, Ragnarsson A (1984): Rheumatic disorders in a health survey: how valid and reliable are the reports? *Scand J Soc Med* 12:141–146.

239. Magora A (1970): Investigation of the relation between low back pain and occupation. 2. Work history. *Ind Med Surg* 39(12):504–510.

240. Magora A (1972): Investigation of the relation between low back pain and occupation. 3. Physical requirements: sitting, standing and weight lifting. *Ind Med Surg* 41:5–9.

241. Magora A (1973): Investigation of the relation between low back pain and occupation. 5. Psychological aspects. *Scand J Rehabil Med* 5:191–196.

242. Magora A (1973): Investigation of the relation between low back pain and occupation. 4. Physical requirements: bending, rotation, reaching and sudden maximal effort. *Scand J Rehabil Med* 6: 186–190.

243. Magora A (1974): Investigation of the relation between low back pain and occupation. 6. Medical history and symptoms. *Scand J Rehabil Med* 6:81–88.

244. Magora A (1975): Investigation of the relation between low back pain and occupation. 7. Neurologic and orthopedic condition. *Scand J Rehabil Med* 7:146–151.

245. Magora A, Schwartz A (1976): Relation between the low back pain syndrome and x-ray findings. 1. Degenerative osteoarthritis. *Scand J Rehabil Med* 8:115–125.

246. Magora A, Taustein I (1969): An investigation of the problem of sick-leave in the patient suffering from low back pain. *Ind Med Surg* 38:398–408.

247. Makela M, Heliövaara M, Sievers K, Impivaara O, Knekt P, Aromaa A (1991): Prevalence, determinants and consequences of chronic neck pain in Finland. *Am J Epidemiol* 134:1356–1367.

248. Mantle MJ, Greenwood RM, Curry HLF (1977): Backache in pregnancy. *Rheumatol Rehabil* 16:95–101.

249. Matsui H, Tsuji H, Terahata N (1990): Juvenile lumbar herniated nucleus pulposus in monozygotic twins. *Spine* 15(11):1228–1230.

250. McDermott FT (1986): Repetition strain injury: a review of current understanding. *Med J Aust* 144:196–200.

251. McDonald DB, Porter R, Hibbert C, et al. (1984): The relationship between spinal canal diameters and back pain in coal miners. Ultrasonic measurement as a screening test? *J Occup Med* 26:23–28.

252. McFadden JF (1985): Smoking cigarettes and lumbar disc pain. A preliminary report on 400 patients. *J Neurol Orthop Med Surg* 6:125–128.

253. McNeill T, Warwick D, Andersson G, Schultz A (1980): Trunk strengths in attempted flexion, extension, and lateral bending in healthy subjects and patients with low-back disorders. *Spine* 5: 529–538.

254. Mellin G (1986): Chronic low back pain in men 54–63 years of age. Correlations of physical measurements with the degree of trouble and progress after treatment. *Spine* 11:421–426.

255. Mellin G (1987): Correlation of spinal mobility with degree of chronic low back pain after correction for age and anthropometric factors. *Spine* 12:464–468.

256. Merriam WF, Burwell RG, Mulholland RC, Pearson JCG, Webb JK (1983): A study revealing a tall pelvis in subjects with low back pain. *J Bone Joint Surg* 65B:153–156.

257. Miller JA, Schmatz C, Schultz AB (1988): Lumbar disc degeneration: correlation with age, sex, and spine level in 600 autopsy specimens. *Spine* 13:173–178.

258. Mitchell JN (1985): Low back pain and the prospects for employment. *J Soc Occup Med* 35:91–94.

259. Miyake S, Himeno J, Hosokawa M (1982): Clinical features of occupational cervicobrachial disorder (OCD). *J Hum Ergol* 11: 109–117.

260. Moens GF, Dohogne T, Jacques P, VanHelshoecht P (1993): Back pain and its correlates among workers in family care. *Occup Med* 43:78–84.

261. Mulimba JO (1990): The problems of low back pain in Africa. *East African Med J* 67:250–253.

262. Nachemson AL (1968): Back problems in childhood and adolescence. *Lakartidningen* 65:2831 (in Swedish).

263. Nachemson AL (1989): Report to the Swedish Department of Economy (in Swedish). Manuscript, University of Goteborg, Goteborg, Sweden.

264. Nachemson A, Eck C, Lindstrom IL, et al. (1989): Chronic low back disability can largely be prevented: a prospective randomized trial in industry. AAOS 56th annual meeting, Las Vegas, p. 81.

265. Nachemson A, Lindh M (1969): Measurement of abdominal and back muscle strength with and without low back pain. *Scand J Rehabil Med* 1:60–63.

266. Nagi SZ, Riley LE, Newby LG (1973): Social epidemiology of back pain in a general population. *J Chronic Dis* 26:769–779.

267. Nagira T, Suzuki J, Oze Y, Ohara H, Aoyama H (1981): Cervicobrachial and low-back disorders among school lunch workers and nursery-school teachers in comparison with cash-register operators. *J Hum Ergol* 10:117–124.

268. Nakaseko M, Tokunaga R, Hosokawa M (1982): History of occupational cervicobrachial disorder in Japan. *J Hum Ergol* 11:7–16.

269. Nathan H (1962): Osteophytes of the vertebral column: an anatomical study of their development according to age, race and sex with considerations as to their etiology and significance. *J Bone Joint Surg* 44A:243–268.

270. National Center for Health Statistics (1975): *Physician visits, volume and interval since last visit, United States, 1971.* Series 10, Number 97.

271. National Center for Health Statistics (1976): *Inpatient utilization of short stay hospitals by diagnosis, United States, 1973.* Series 13, Number 25.

272. National Center for Health Statistics (1976): *Surgical operations in short stay hospitals, United States, 1973.* Series 13, Number 24.

273. National Center for Health Statistics (1977): *Limitation of activity due to chronic conditions, United States, 1974.* Series 10, No. 111.

274. National Center for Health Statistics (1981): *Prevalence of selected impairments, United States, 1977.* Series 10, No. 134.

275. National Center for Health Statistics (1982): *Surgical operations in short stay hospitals, United States 1978.* Series 13, No. 61.

276. National Occupational Health and Safety Commission (Worksafe Australia) (1986): *Repetition strain injuries (RSI): a report and model code of practice.* 1. Canberra: Australian Government Publishing Service.

277. Netterstrom B, Juel K (1989): Low back trouble among urban bus drivers in Denmark. *Scand J Soc Med* 17:203–206.

278. Newell DJ (1967): Prevalence, aetiology and treatment of pain in the neck and arm. *Trans Soc Occup Med* 17:104–106.

279. Nicholson AS (1985): Accident information from four British industries. *Ergonomics* 28:31–43.

280. Nikiforov O (1984): English summary: *General hospital care in Finland in the 1960s and 1970s.* Helsinki: Laakintohalliuksen tutkimuksia 32.

281. Nilsonne U, Lundgren KD (1968): Long-term prognosis in idiopathic scoliosis. *Acta Orthop Scand* 39(4):456–465.

282. NIOSH (1981): *Work practices guide for manual lifting.* DHHS (NIOSH) Publication No 81-122.

283. Nordgren B, Schel R, Linroth K (1980): Evaluation and prediction of back pain during military field service. *Scand J Rehabil Med* 12:1–8.

284. Noren R, Trafimow J, Andersson GBJ, Huckman MS (1991): The role of facet joint tropism and facet angle in disc degeneration. *Spine* 16:530–532.

285. Nummi J, Jarvinen T, Stambej U, Wickström G (1978): Diminished dynamic performance capacity of back and abdominal muscles in concrete reinforcement workers. *Scand J Work Environ Health* (Suppl 4) 1:39–46.

286. O'Connor FG, Marlowe SS (1993): Low back pain in military basic trainees. A pilot study. *Spine* 18:1351–1354.

287. Ohara H, Itani T, Aoyama H (1982): Prevalence of occupational cervicobrachial disorder among different occupational groups in Japan. *J Hum Ergol* 11:55–63.

288. Olsen TL, Anderson RL, Dearwater SR, et al (1992): The epidemiology of low back pain in an adolescent population. *Am J Public Health* 82:606–608.

289. Onishi N, Nomura H (1973): Low back pain in relation to physical work capacity and local tenderness. *J Hum Ergol* 2:119–132.

290. Onishi N, Nomura H, Sakai K, Yamamoto T, Hirayama K, Itani T (1976): Shoulder muscle tenderness and physical features of female industrial workers. *J Hum Ergol* 5:87–102.

291. Ostgaard HC, Andersson GBJ (1991): Previous back pain and risk of developing back pain in a future pregnancy. *Spine* 16:432–436.

292. Ostgaard HC, Andersson GBJ, Karlsson K (1991): Prevalence of back pain in pregnancy. *Spine* 16:549–552.

293. Partridge REH, Anderson JAD (1969): Back pain in industrial workers. *Proceedings of the International Rheumatology Congress.* Prague, Czechoslavakia, Abstract 284.

294. Partridge REH, Andersson JAD, McCarthy MA, Duthie JRR (1968): Rheumatic complaints among workers in iron foundries. *Ann Rheum Dis* 27:441–443.

295. Partridge REH, Duthie JJR (1968): Rheumatism in dockers and civil servants: a comparison of heavy manual and sedentary workers. *Ann Rheum Dis* 27:559–567.

296. Pearcy M, Portek I, Shepherd J (1985): The effect of low-back pain on lumbar spinal movements measured by three-dimensional X-ray analysis. *Spine* 10:150–153.

297. Pedersen O, Petersen R, Schack-Staffeldt E (1975): Back pain and isometric back muscle strength of workers in a Danish factory. *Scand J Rehabil Med* 7:125–128.

298. Pentinnen J (1987): *Back pain and sciatica in Finnish farmers.* Helsinki: Publications of the Social Insurance Institution, ML:71.

299. Pietri F, Leclerc A, Boitel L, Chastang J-F, Morcet J-F, Blondet M (1992): Low-back pain in commercial travelers. *Scand J Work Environ Health* 18:52–58.

300. Polatin PB, Kinney RK, Gatchel RJ, Lillo E, Mayer TG (1993): Psychiatric illness and chronic low-back pain. The mind and the spine—which goes first? *Spine* 18:66–71.

301. Pope MH (1989): Risk indicators in low back pain. *Ann Med* 21:387–392.

302. Pope MH, Bevins T, Wilder DG, Frymoyer JW (1985): The relationship between anthropometric, postural, muscular, and mobility characteristics of males, ages 18-55. *Spine* 10:644–648.

303. Pope MH, Frymoyer JW, Andersson GBJ (1984): *Occupational low back pain.* New York: Praeger.

304. Pope MH, Hanley EN, Matteri RE, Wilder DG, Frymoyer JW (1977): Measurement of intervertebral disc space height. *Spine* 2:282–286.

305. Pope MH, Rosen JD, Wilder DG, Frymoyer JW (1980): The relation between biomechanical and psychological factors in patients with low back pain. *Spine* 5:173–178.

306. Porter RW (1987): Does hard work prevent disc protrusion? *Clin Biomech* 2:196–198.

307. Porter RW (1986): Familial aspects of disc protrusion. Abstract from International Society for the Study of the Lumbar *Spine,* Dallas, May 28-June 2.

308. Postacchini F, Lami R, Pugliese O (1988): Familial predisposition to discogenic low-back pain. An epidemiologic and immunogenetic study. *Spine* 13:1403–1406.

309. Powell MC, Wilson M, Szypryt P, Symonds EM, Worthington BS (1986): Prevalence of lumbar disc degeneration observed by magnetic resonance in symptomless women. *Lancet* 2:1366–1367.

310. Praemer A, Furnes S, Rice DP (1992): *Musculoskeletal conditions in the United States.* Park Ridge, IL: Am Acad Orthop Surg, pp. 1–199.

311. Punnett L, Fine LJ, Keyserling WM, Herrin GO, Chaffin DB (1991): Back disorders and nonneutral trunk postures of automobile assembly workers. *Scand J Work Environ Health* 17:337–346.

312. Ramani PS (1976): Variations in the size of the bony lumbar canal in patients with prolapse of lumbar intervertebral discs. *Clin Radiol* 27:301–307.

313. Reisbord LS, Greenland S (1985): Factors associated with self-reported back-pain prevalence: a population-based study. *J Chronic Dis* 38:691–702.

314. Riihimäki H (1985): Back pain and heavy physical work: a comparative study of concrete reinforcement workers and maintenance house painters. *Br J Ind Med* 42:226–232.

315. Riihimäki H (1989): *Back disorders in relation to heavy physical work* [Thesis]. Institute of Occupational Health, Helsinki, Finland, pp. 1–72.

316. Riihimäki H, Wickström G, Hanninen K, Luopajarvi T (1989): Predictors of sciatic pain among concrete reinforcement workers and house painters. A five year follow-up. *Scand J Work Environ Health* 15:415–423.

317. Riksforsakringsverket (1987-1988): *Statistical information Is-1, 1987-8.* Stockholm, Sweden.

318. Rosegger R, Rosegger S (1960): Arbeitsmedizinische Erkenntnisse beim Schlepperfahren. *Arch Landtechn* 2:3–65.

319. Rossignol M, Suissa S, Abenhaim L (1988): Working disability due to occupational back pain: three-year follow-up of 2300 compensated workers in Quebec. *J Occup Med* 30:502–505.

320. Rotgoltz J, Derazne E, Froom P, Grushecky E, Ribk J (1992): Prevalence of low back pain in employees of a pharmaceutical company. *Israel J Med Sci* 28:615–618.

321. Rowe ML (1963): Preliminary statistical study of low back pain. *J Occup Med* 5(7):336–341.

322. Rowe ML (1965): Disc surgery and chronic low-back pain. *J Occup Med* 7(5):196–202.

323. Rowe ML (1969): Low back pain in industry. A position paper. *J Occup Med* 11(4):161–169.

324. Rush WA, Steiner HA (1946): A study of lower extremity length inequality. *Am J Roentgenol* 56:616–623.

325. Russwurm H, Bjerkreim I, Ronglan E (1978): Lumbar intervertebral disc herniation in the young. *Acta Orthop Scand* 49:158–163.

326. Sairanen E, Brushaber L, Kaskinen M (1981): Felling work, low back pain and osteoarthritis. *Scand J Work Environ Health* 7:18–30.

327. Salminen J, Erkintalo-Tertti MO, Paajanen HEK (1993): Magnetic resonance imaging findings of lumbar spine in the young: correlation with leisure-time physical activity, spinal mobility, and trunk muscle strength in 15-year-old pupils with or without back pain. *J Spinal Disord* 6:386–391.

328. Salminen JJ, Oksanen A, Maki P, Pentti J, Kujala UM (1993): Leisure time physical activity in the young: correlation with low-back pain, spinal mobility and trunk muscle strength in 15-year-old school children. *Int J Sports Med* 14:406–410.

329. Salminen JJ, Erkintalo MO, Laine M, Pentti J (1994): *Low back pain in the young: a prospective 3-year follow-up study of subjects with and without low back pain.* Manuscript. Finland, Univ of Turku.

330. Salminen JJ (1984): The adolescent back. A field survey of 310 Finnish schoolchildren. *Acta Paediatr Scand* (Suppl) 315:1–122.

331. Sallstrom J, Schmidt H (1984): Cervicobrachial disorders in certain occupations with special reference to compression in the thoracic outlet. *Am J Ind Med* 6:45–52.

332. Sander RA, Meyers JE (1986): The relationship of disability to compensation status in railroad workers. *Spine* 11:141–143.

333. Saraste H (1987): Long term clinical and radiological follow-up of spondylosis and spondylolisthesis. *J Pediatr Orthop* 7:631–638.

334. Schmidt U (1969): *Vergleichende Untersuchungen am Schwerlastwagenfahrern und Büroangestellte zur Frage der berufs-*

bedingte Verschleisschaden an der Wirbelsäule [Thesis]. Berlin, Germany, Humbolt University.

335. Schmorl G, Junghanns H (1971): *The human spine in health and disease.* New York: Grune and Stratton.

336. Schroter G (1959): Hat die berufliche Belastung Bedeutung für die Entstehung oder Verschlimmerung der Osteochondrose und Spondylose der Halswirbelsäule. *Deutsche Gesundheitswesen* 14: 174–177.

337. Schroter G, Rademacher W (1971): Die Bedeutung von Belastung und aussergewöhnlicher Haltung für das Entstehen von Verschleissschaden der HWSargestelt an einem Kollektive von Fleischabtragern. *Z Gesamte Hyg* 17:841–843.

338. Schulte-Wintrop HC, Knoche H (1978): *Backache in VH-ID helicopter crews.* AGARD-CP-255.

339. Seidel H, Bluethner R, Hinz B (1986): Effects of sinusoidal whole-body vibration on the lumbar spine: the stress-strain relationship. *Int Arch Occup Environ Health* 57:207–223.

340. Seidel H, Heide R (1986): Long-term effects of whole-body vibration: a critical survey of the literature. *Int Arch Occup Environ Health* 58:1–26.

341. Silberberg R, Adler HJ, Meier-Ruge W (1986): Effects of hyperinsulinism and of diabetes on proteoglycans of the intervertebral disc in weaning sand rats. *Exp Cell Biol* 54:121–127.

342. Silverstein BA (1985): *The prevalence of upper extremity cumulative trauma disorders in industry* (Thesis). Ann Arbor: University of Michigan, Occupation Health and Safety Engineering.

343. Skovron ML, Szpalski M, Nordin M, Melot C, Cukier D (1994): *Sociocultural factors and back pain: a population-based study in Belgian adults.* Spine 19:129–137.

344. Snook SH (1982): Low back pain in industry. In: *Symposium on idiopathic low back pain.* White AA, Gordon SL, eds. St Louis: Mosby, pp. 23–28.

345. Sorensen KH (1964): *Scheuermann's juvenile kyphosis* [Dissertation]. Copenhagen, Munksgaard.

346. Spangfort EV (1972): The lumbar disc herniation. *Acta Orthop Scand* (Suppl) 142:1–95.

347. Spengler DM, Bigos SJ, Martin NA, Zeh J, Fisher L, Nachemson A (1986): Back injuries in industry: a retrospective study. I. Overview and cost analysis. *Spine* 11:241–245.

348. Spitzer WO (1986): In: Troidl H, Spitzer WO, McPeek B, Mulder DS, McKneally MF, eds. *Principles and practice of research: Strategies for surgical investigators.* New York: Springer-Verlag.

349. Spitzer WO, LeBlanc FE, Dupuis M, et al (1987): Scientific approach to the assessment and management of activity-related spinal disorders: a monograph for clinicians. Report of the Quebec Task Force on Spinal Disorders. *Spine* 12:S1–S59.

350. Stubbs DA, Buckle PW, Hudson MP, Rivers PM, Worringham CJ (1983): Back pain in the nursing profession. I. Epidemiology and plot methodology. *Ergonomics* 26:755–765.

351. Stubbs DA, Nicholson AA (1979): Manual handling and back injuries in the construction industry: an investigation. *J Occup Accidents* 2:179–190.

352. Svard L, Hellstrom M, Jacobsson B, Nyman R, Peterson L (1991): Disc degeneration and associated abnormalities of the spine in elite gymnasts. A magnetic resonance imaging study. *Spine* 16:437–443.

353. Svard L, Hellstrom M, Jacobsson B, Peterson L (1990): Back pain and radiologic changes in the thoraco-lumbar spine of athletes. *Spine* 15:124–129.

354. Svensson HO (1981): *Low back pain in forty to forty-seven year old men: a retrospective cross-sectional study* [Thesis]. Goteborg, University of Goteborg.

355. Svensson HO (1982): Low-back pain in 40–47 year old men: socioeconomic factors and previous sickness absence. *Scand J Rehabil Med* 14:55–60.

356. Svensson HO, Andersson GBJ (1981): Sicklisting with diagnosis of injury or disease of the musculo-skeletal system. *Lakartidningen* 78:2761–2764 (in Swedish).

357. Svensson HO, Andersson GBJ (1982): Low back pain in forty to forty-seven year old men. I. Frequency of occurrence and impact on medical services. *Scand J Rehabil Med* 14:47–53.

358. Svensson HO, Andersson GBJ (1983): Low back pain in forty to forty-seven year old men: work history and work environment factors. *Spine* 8:272–276.

359. Svensson HO, Andersson GBJ (1989): The relationship of low-back pain, work history, work environment, and stress: a retrospective cross-sectional study of 38- to 64-year-old women. *Spine* 14:517–522.

360. Svensson HO, Andersson GBJ, Johansson S, Wilhelmsson C, Vedin A (1988): A retrospective study of low back pain in 38- to 64-year-old women. Frequency and occurrence and impact on medical services. *Spine* 13:548–552.

361. Svensson HO, Vedin A, Wilhelmsson C, Andersson GBJ (1983): Low back pain in relation to other diseases and cardiovascular risk factors. *Spine* 8:277–285.

362. Takala J, Sievers K, Klaukka T (1982): Rheumatic symptoms in the middle-aged population in southwestern Finland. *Scand J Rheumatol* (Suppl) 47:15–29.

363. Tauber J (1970): An unorthodox look at backaches. *J Occup Med* 12(4):128–130.

364. Taylor VM, Deyo RA, Cherkin DC, Kreuter W (1994): Low back pain hospitalization. Recent United States trends and regional variations. *Spine* 19:1207–1213.

365. Tichauer ER (1965): *The biomechanics of the arm-back aggregate under industrial working conditions.* ASME Rep No 65-WA/HUE-1.

366. Torgerson WR, Dotter WE (1976): Comparative roentgenographic study of the asymptomatic and symptomatic lumbar spine. *J Bone Joint Surg* 58A:850–853.

367. Triano JL, Schultz AB (1987): Correlation of objective measures of trunk motion and muscle function with low-back disability ratings. *Spine* 12:561–565.

368. Troup JD (1984): Causes, prediction and prevention of back pain at work. *Scand J Work Environ Health* 10:419–428.

369. Troup JDG, Edwards FC (1985): *Manual handling and lifting. An information and literature review with special reference to the back. Health and Safety Executive.* London: Her Majesty's Stationery Office.

370. Troup JDG, Foreman TK, Baxter CE, Brown D (1987): The perception of back pain and the role of psychophysical tests of lifting capacity. *Spine* 12:645–657.

371. Troup JD, Martin JW, Lloyd DC (1981): Back pain in industry: a prospective study. *Spine* 6:61–69.

372. Troup JDG, Roantree WB, Archibald RM (1970): Survey of cases of lumbar spinal disability. A methodological study. *New Scientist* 8:65–67.

373. Troup JDG, Slade PD (1985): Fear avoidance and chronic musculoskeletal pain. *Stress Med* 1:217–220.

374. Tsai SP, Gilstrap EL, Cowles SR, Waddell LC Jr, Ross CE (1992): Personal and job characteristics of musculoskeletal injuries in an industrial population. *J Occup Med* 34:606–612.

375. Uyttendaele D, Vandendriessche G, Vercauteren M, DeGroote W (1981): Sicklisting due to low back pain at the Ghent State University and University Hospital. *Acta Orthop Belgica* 47:523–546.

376. Valkenburg HA, Haanen HCM (1982): The epidemiology of low back pain. In: White AA, Gordon SL, eds. *Symposium on idiopathic low back pain.* St. Louis: Mosby, pp. 9–22.

377. Vallfors B (1985): Acute, subacute and chronic low back pain. Clinical symptoms, absenteeism and working environment. *Scand J Rehabil Med* (Suppl) 11:1–98.

378. Van der Linden SM, Fahrer H (1988): Occurrence of spinal pain syndromes in a group of apparently healthy and physically fit sportsmen (Orienteers). *Scand J Rheumatol* 17:475–481.

379. Varlotta GP, Brown MD, Kelsey JL, Golden AL (1991): Familial predisposition for herniation of a lumbar disc in patients who are less than twenty-one years old. *J Bone Joint Surg* (Am) 73A:124–128.

380. Vernon-Roberts B (1987): Pathology of intervertebral discs and apophyseal. In: Jayson MIV, ed. *The lumbar spine and back pain.* New York: Churchill-Livingstone, pp 37–55.

381. Vernon-Roberts B, Pirie CJ (1977): Degenerative changes in the intervertebral discs of the lumbar spine and their sequelae. *Rheumatol Rehabil* 16:13–21.

382. Videman T, Heikkila JK, Koskenvuo M, Heliövaara M, Kurppa K, Riihimäki H, Heikkila K, Rita H (1989): *The role of environmental factors in the development of back pain and sciatica. An epidemiological study with adult twin pairs.* International Society for the Study of the Lumbar Spine, Kyoto, May 15-19; Abstr. 19.

383. Videman T, Numminen T, Tola S, Kuorinka I, Vanharanta H,

Troup JDG (1984): Low back pain in nurses and some loading factors of work. *Spine* 9:400–404.

384. Videman T, Numminen M, Troup JDG (1990): Lumbar spinal pathology in cadaveric material in relation to history of back pain, occupation and physical loading. *Spine* 15:728–740.

385. Videman T, Sarna S, Battié MC, Koskinen S, et al. (1994): *The long term effects of physical loading and exercise lifestyles on back-related symptoms, disability and spinal pathology.* Volvo Award Presentation, International Society for the Study of the Lumbar Spine, Seattle, WA.

386. Viikara-Juntura E (1988): *Examination of the neck. Validity of some clinical, radiological and epidemiologic methods* [Thesis]. Helsinki, Finland: University of Helsinki, Institute of Occupational Health.

387. Viikari-Juntura E (1983): Neck and upper limb disorders among slaughterhouse workers. *Scand J Work Environ Health* 9:283–290.

388. Virta L, Ronnemaa T, Osterman K, Aalto T, Laakso M (1992): Prevalence of isthmic lumbar spondylolisthesis in middle-aged subjects from eastern and western Finland. *J Clin Epidemiol* 45:917–922.

389. Volinn E, Lai D, McKinney S, et al. (1988): When back pain becomes disabling: a regional analysis. *Pain* 33:33–39.

390. Volinn E, Turczyn KM, Loeser JD (1994): Patterns in low back pain hospitalizations: implications for the treatment of low back pain in an era of health care reform. *Clin J Pain* 10:64–70.

391. Waddell G (1987): A new clinical model for the treatment of low-back pain. *Spine* 12:632–644.

392. Walford PA (1962): Diseases of bones and organs of movement. In: *The General Register. Office studies on medical and population subjects, no 14.* Morbidity Statistics from General Practice III. London: Her Majesty's Stationery Office, pp. 77–87.

393. Walsh K, Varnes N, Osmond C, Styles R, Coggon D (1989): Occupational causes of low-back pain. *Scand J Environ Health* 15:54–59.

394. Ward T, Knowelden J, Sharrard WJ (1968): Low back pain. *J R Coll Gen Pract* 15:128–136.

395. Ward GM, Krzywicki HJ, Rahman DP, Quaas RL, Nelson RA, Consolazio CF (1975): Relationship of anthropometric measurements to body fat as determined by densitometry, potassium-40 and body water. *Am J Clin Nutr* 28:162–169.

396. Waris P (1979): Occupational cervicobrachial syndromes: a review. *Scand J Work Environ Health* (Suppl 5) 3:3–14.

397. Watson J (1979): Psychological and psychiatric aspects. In: Grahame R, ed: *Low back pain.* Volume 1. Annual Research Reviews. Westmount and St. Albans, Eden Press Inc, 50–56.

398. Weber H (1978): Lumbar disc herniation. A prospective study of prognostic factors including a control child, part I. *J Ospo City Hosp* 28:33–64.

399. Weber H (1978): Lumbar disc herniation. A prospective study of prognostic factors including a control child, part II. *J Ospo City Hosp* 28:89–120.

400. Weber H (1983): Lumbar disc herniation. A controlled, prospective study with ten years of observation. *Spine* 8:131–140.

401. Westerling D, Jonsson BG (1980): Pain from the neck-shoulder region and sick leave. *Scand J Soc Med* 8:131–136.

402. Westrin C-G (1970): Low back sick-listing. A nosological and medical insurance investigation. *Acta Soc Med Scand* 2:127–134.

403. Westrin C-G (1973): Low back sick-listing. A nosological and medical insurance investigation. *Scand J Soc Med* (Suppl) 7:1–116.

404. Whitaker RH, Green NA, Notley RG (1983): Is cervical spondylosis an occupational hazard for urologists? *Br J Urology* 55:585–587.

405. Wickström G (1982): Drawbacks of clinical diagnoses in epidemiologic research on work-related musculoskeletal morbidity. *Scand J Work Environ Health* (Suppl 1) 8:97–99.

406. Wickström G, Hanninen K (1987): Determination of sciatia in epidemiological research. *Spine* 12:692–698.

407. Wickström G, Hanninen K, Lehtinen M, Riihimäki H (1978): Previous back syndromes and present back symptoms in concrete reinforcement workers. *Scand J Work Environ Health* (Suppl 4) 1:20–29.

408. Wigley RD, Prim IAM, Salmond C, Stanley D, Pinfold B (1987): Rheumatic complaints in Tokelau. I. Migrants resident in New Zealand. The Tokelau Island Migrant Study. *Rheumatol Int* 7:53–59.

409. Wigley RD, Prior IA, Salmond C, Stanley D, Pinfold B (1987): Rheumatic complaints in Tokelau. II. A comparison in migrants in New Zealand and non-migrants. The Tokelau Migrant Study. *Rheumatol Int* 7:61–65.

410. Wiikeri M, Nummi J, Riihimäki H, Wickström G (1978): Radiologically detectable lumbar disc degeneration in concrete reinforcement workers. *Scand J Work Environ Health* (Suppl 1) 4:47–53.

411. Wilder DG, Woodworth BB, Frymoyer JW, Pope MH (1982): Vibration and the human spine. *Spine* 7:243–254.

412. Wiltse LL (1971): The effect of the common anomalies of the lumbar spine upon disc degeneration and low back pain. *Orthop Clin North Am* 2:569–582.

413. Winston K, Rumbaugh C, Colucci V (1984): The vertebral canals in lumbar disc disease. *Spine* 9:414–417.

414. Wood PHN (1976): Epidemiology of back pain. The lumbar spine and back pain. In: Jayson M, ed. *The lumbar spine and back pain.* London: Pitman, pp. 13–17.

415. Wood PHN, Badley EM (1980): Epidemiology of back pain. In: Jayson M, ed. *The lumbar pain.* London: Pitman, pp. 29–55.

416. Wood PH, Badley EM (1985): Musculoskeletal system. In: Holland WW, Detels R, Knox G, Greeze E, eds. *Oxford textbook of public health.* Vol 4. Specific applications. Oxford: Oxford University Press, pp. 279–297.

417. Wood PHN, Badley EM (1987): Epidemiology of back pain. In: Jayson M, ed. *The lumbar spine and back pain.* London: Churchill Livingstone, pp. 1–15.

418. Worrall JD, Appel D (1987): The Impact of workers compensation benefits on low back claims. In: Hadler NM, ed. *Current concepts in regional musculoskeletal illness.* Orlando: Grune and Stratton, pp. 281–298.

419. Zimmerman G (1966): *Gesundheitliche Schädigungen bei Tractorfahrern, unter besonder Berücksichtigung der Wirbelsäule.* Abstract 15. Int. Congress für Arbeitsmedicin, Vienna.

420. Zong LB, Ke JH, Andersson GBJ, et al.: In vivo measurement of water content in intervertebral discs in different age groups. *Spine*.

421. Zuidema H (1985): National statistics in the Netherlands. *Ergonomics* 28:3–7.

422. Zuidema H (1985): Risks of individual occupations in the Netherlands. *Ergonomics* 28:43–49.

The Adult Spine: Principles and Practice,
2nd edition, J.W. Frymoyer, Editor-in-Chief.
Lippincott-Raven Publishers, Philadelphia © 1997.

CHAPTER 8

The Economics of Spinal Disorders

John W. Frymoyer and Carol L. Durett

Back pain is a ubiquitous symptom affecting the majority of the adult population at one time or another. In the United States, as many as 60% of adults may have experienced back pain in the prior year, although for the majority, the symptoms are transient. Within industry, back pain is a serious cause of work loss, affecting 2% to 5% of the workforce in any given year and resulting in one million Workers' Compensation claims. At least 2.6 million people are disabled temporarily by back pain at any given time, and an additional 2.6 million are permanently disabled. Similar statistics are reported for most industrialized nations. Even though large numbers of people suffer from and are disabled by spinal disorders, accurate data regarding the cost of spinal disorders in the United States are rarely available, although the general consensus is that the cost is significant, measurable in tens of billions of dollars. There are many reasons for the lack of precision.

First, the data that are available have been recorded at different times, meaning a variety of technologies were used in the diagnosis and treatment of the spinal disorders. It has not been calculated precisely how these technologies have either increased or reduced costs. Second, there is a general impression, not yet proven by epidemiologic data, that indicates an increase in certain spinal disorders, particularly spinal stenosis, which can be attributed to changing demographics. Third, it may not be possible to extrapolate data obtained from one population base to another population base, because of variations in the utilization of surgical and nonsurgical treatments (Tables 1–3). Fourth, calculations that use assumptions about inflation are probably not accurate because of differential inflation and higher rates for medical services. Finally, managed care has grown substantially during the past 10 years, whereas traditional indemnity insurance has decreased; however, the impact of managed care on spinal disorders is not currently known.

J. W. Frymoyer, M.D.: Professor, Department of Orthopaedics and Rehabilitation; Director, McClure Musculoskeletal Research Center, University of Vermont, Burlington, Vermont, 05405.
C. L. Durett, M.B.A.: Department of Orthopaedics and Rehabilitation; McClure Musculoskeletal Research Center, University of Vermont, Burlington, Vermont, 05405.

ASSUMPTIONS USED IN THIS ANALYSIS OF COSTS

The most comprehensive data available for the cost of back disorders were presented by Grazier et al. (9) in 1984. Their data were calculated using NHANES I and

TABLE 1. *Estimated annual discharges from nonfederal, short-stay hospitals, United States, 1972–1978*

Diagnosis	Discharges			Total hospital days	Average length of stay (d)
	Women	Men	Total		
Back pain (all sites)	161,000	128,000	289,000	2,667,000	9.2
Prolapsed intervertebral disc	163,000	196,000	359,000	4,027,000	11.2
Fractures	45,000	42,000	87,000	1,064,000	12.2
Total	369,000	366,000	735,000	7,758,000	

Adapted with permission from ref. 9.

NHANES II (National Health and Nutrition Examination Surveys), which are based on a random sample of noninstitutionalized and nonmilitary sectors of the American population. Because of the difficulty in obtaining an accurate data base, we have used a number of assumptions that undoubtedly influence the precision of the calculated costs, although they probably do not influence the general magnitude calculated. To adjust historical data to 1995, we have assumed that the growth of services given for spinal disorders has occurred at the rate of population growth. Further, we have assumed no differential in age-specific growth for these services, because there is no accurate method to calculate these data, although it is likely that there are additional costs attributable to the older population. Inflationary increases have been adjusted, where appropriate, for the Medical Price Index (MPI), and physicians' services have been calculated based on the Physician Price Index (PPI). The Consumer Price Index (CPI) has been used for most of the indirect costs attributable to back disorders. The increases in these various indices are shown in Figure 1 and Table 4.

DIRECT COSTS: MEDICAL

Grazier et al. (9) used data shown in Table 1 to estimate the annual number of discharges for back pain at all sites, prolapsed intervertebral discs at all sites, and fractures of the vertebral column. According to their calculations, spinal disorders accounted for 2.8% of all hospital discharges. Certain spinal disorders had an increasing rate of hospitalization during the 1980s (Table 5).

Finally, Andrews et al. (1) reported in 1987 that the costs of spondylosis, intervertebral disc disorders, cervical disorders, and other back pain ranked as twelfth in the number of discharges from hospitals. From this information, it should be evident that there is no precise means to calculate the hospital costs for back disorders. Grazier et al. determined the figure as $4.5 billion in 1984. Because many variables may have influenced this figure, we have simply inflated it using the Hospital Price Index (HPI). Thus, without growth in the population, in 1994 the figure is $10.1 billion; when population growth is factored in, the figure is $11.3 billion.

Outpatient and Emergency Room Institutional Services

We can find no reliable information about the use of outpatient and emergency room services for spinal disorders. In 1984, the costs were estimated to be $260 million. Using the MPI, this figure is $522 million in 1994, and when adjusted for population growth it rises to $580 million.

Outpatient Diagnostic and Therapeutic Services

Since Grazier's report (9), there have continued to be major shifts in the availability of technology, including computerized tomography and magnetic resonance imaging, as well as new procedures now performed on an outpatient basis, such as percutaneous discectomy. Some of this technology may have increased costs, whereas some (myelography, for example) may have re-

TABLE 2. *Differences by race in utilization of laminectomy, excision intervertebral disc[a]*

Race	1980	1981	1982	1983	1984	1985	1986	1987	EAPC
Black	56.0	58.5	60.6	65.0	71.5	66.5	79.0	69.3	4.1
	(43.8, 68.3)	(47.2, 69.8)	(49.1, 72.1)	(52.9, 77.2)	(58.6, 84.4)	(52.8, 80.2)	(60.2, 97.7)	(52.1, 86.5)	(2.2, 6.0)
White	114.2	127.4	136.8	141.3	155.9	147.1	155.6	155.2	4.2
	(99.2, 129.3)	(111.9, 142.9)	(119.7, 153.9)	(125.5, 157.1)	(137.2, 174.7)	(130.1, 164.1)	(136.2, 174.9)	(136.6, 173.9)	(2.6, 5.8)

Source: Agency for Health Care Policy and Research, Center for General Health Services Intramural Research, Division of Provider Studies.
Adapted from ref. 8.
[a] Utilization rate per 100,000, estimated annual percent change (EAPC), and confidence interval in parentheses. Based on 20% of discharges from Hospital Cost & Utilization Project, 1980–87, weighted to obtain estimates, and age- and sex-adjusted to the 1970 resident US population.

TABLE 3. *Differences by region in utilization of laminectomy, excision intervertebral disc[a]*

Region	1980	1981	1982	1983	1984	1985	1986	1987	EAPC
United States	116.5 (103.4, 129.7)	129.6 (116.0, 143.1)	139.2 (124.3, 154.1)	144.5 (130.5, 158.6)	156.7 (140.3, 173.2)	147.1 (132.2, 162.1)	159.5 (141.8, 177.3)	160.1 (142.7, 177.5)	4.3 (2.8, 5.7)
Northeast	109.9 (88.3, 131.5)	121.3 (97.9, 144.6)	131.5 (108.2, 154.7)	132.9 (106.0, 159.8)	147.9 (116.3, 179.6)	145 (113.5, 176.5)	154.1 (118.7, 189.5)	153.5 (118.0, 189.0)	4.8 (3.6, 6.1)
North Central	124.6 (104.0, 145.2)	133.6 (111.2, 155.9)	139.2 (117.8, 160.7)	153.4 (127.1, 179.7)	159.7 (132.7, 186.7)	154.3 (125.0, 183.6)	142.1 (113.6, 170.6)	156.7 (126.8, 186.7)	2.7 (0.8, 4.7)
South	110.7 (81.3, 140.2)	123.4 (95.7, 151.1)	136.0 (103.1, 168.9)	146.3 (120.0, 172.6)	161.2 (125.9, 196.6)	145.7 (116.0, 175.4)	170.5 (132.7, 208.2)	166.9 (130.3, 203.5)	5.9 (3.9, 7.9)
West	124.6 (96.4, 152.9)	145.7 (112.9, 178.6)	155.0 (120.1, 189.9)	144.9 (111.9, 178.0)	155.7 (125.4, 186.0)	144.1 (119.9, 168.2)	170.2 (137.3, 203.0)	160.1 (130.8, 189.5)	2.9 (0.8, 5.0)

Source: Agency for Health Care Policy and Research, Center for General Health Services Intramural Research, Division of Provider Studies.

Adapted from ref. 9.

[a] Utilization rate per 100,000, estimated annual percent change (EAPC), and confidence interval in parentheses. Based on 20% of discharges from Hospital Cost & Utilization Project, 1980–87, weighted to obtain estimates, and age- and sex-adjusted to the 1970 resident US population.

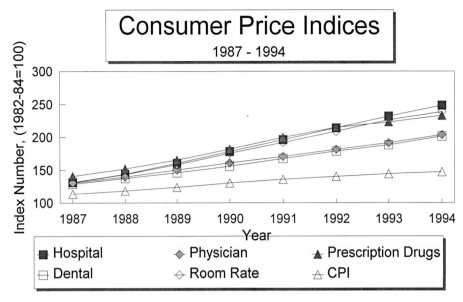

FIG 1. Consumer Price Indices from 1987 to 1994.

placed more costly technology. In other instances, it is uncertain whether there has been an increase or a decrease in costs. For example, Scavone et al. (19) estimated the costs of lumbar spinal radiography to be $600 million in 1981, but they did not include the costs of spinal radiographs obtained by chiropractors. [It is interesting to note that, despite being taken quite often, very few radiographs alter the course of treatment (12)]. In the first edition of *The Adult Spine,* we thought a reasonable estimate for spinal radiographs in 1990 was $1.79 billion. Grazier calculated outpatient diagnostic services to be $1 billion in 1984. Our recent calculations suggest that in 1994, costs are in the range of $2.03 billion and when adjusted for population growth are $2.26 billion.

Physician Inpatient Services

There is little reason to believe there has been any unusual increase in physician inpatient services other than for surgical procedures, and this varies highly according to the region of the country analyzed. However, there is a trend towards decreasing utilization of hospitals resulting, in part, from changes in technology and, more recently, from managed care financing. In Grazier's analysis (9), physician inpatient services were estimated to be $1.1 billion. Using the PPI and adjusting for population growth, the 1994 costs are estimated to be $2.28 billion.

Physician Outpatient Services

Grazier et al. (9) estimated that 11 million patient visits were made annually, including 9 million for "strains and sprains" and 2 million related to disc disorders. In 1987, Deyo and Tsui-Wu (7) calculated the number of visits to be 16 million per annum. They also noted a wide variations in the use of services for low back pain according to race, region, and education. Unfortunately, we have been unable to find reliable data about visits for cervical and thoracic disorders. For our 1990 calculation, we took Grazier's estimate (9) of $1.048 billion and adjusted it by a factor of 1.45 to account for the difference between his estimate of 11 million visits and Deyo's estimate of 16 million visits (7) to arrive at an adjusted cost of $1.5 billion. Using the PPI and adjusting for population growth brings this figure to $2.4 billion in 1990 and $3.2 billion in 1994.

Other Practitioner Services

In 1990, we concluded that the $234 million Grazier et al. calculated as the cost for other practitioners was a significant underestimate. The most significant omission was the impact of chiropractors, which for 1984 had been reported to account for 50 million visits per annum for back disorders (4). We assumed a nominal cost of $25

TABLE 4. *Changes in price indices: 1985–1984 (%)*

	1985	1986	1987	1988	1989	1990	1991	1992	1993	1994
Consumer Price Index change	3.6	1.9	3.6	4.1	4.8	5.4	4.2	3.0	3.0	1.9
Medical Price Index change	6.3	7.5	6.6	6.5	7.7	9.0	8.7	7.4	5.9	6.6
Hospital Price Index change	5.9	6.0	7.2	9.3	11.5	10.9	10.2	9.1	8.4	7.2
Physician Price Index change	5.9	7.2	7.3	7.2	7.4	7.1	6.0	6.3	5.6	6.4

Source: Statistical Abstract of the United States, 1994.

TABLE 5. *Procedure categories with significantly increasing rates for total US and regions:*
Hospital Cost and Utilization Project, 1980–1987[a]

Procedure category	United States	Northeast	North Central	South	West
Incision and excision of central nervous system	2.7	3.5	—	5.5	2.0
Extracranial ventricular shunt	5.9	3.9	—	10.9	4.7
Laminectomy, excision intervertebral disc	**4.3**	**4.8**	**2.7**	**5.9**	**2.9**
Corneal transplant	6.9	—	12.2	19.5	—
Procedures on the mouth and palate	2.4	3.4	—	3.3	—
Tracheostomy, temporary and permanent	3.1	3.1	—	4.9	—
Thoracentesis	5.5	7.9	—	8.8	—
Other procedures on respiratory system	2.1	3.9	—	4.0	—
Coronary artery bypass graft (CABG)	9.1	14.3	3.9	13.2	5.7
Percutaneous transluminal coronary angioplasty (PTCA)	69.5	70.2	51.9	92.4	84.5
Insertion of cardiac pacemaker	3.7	1.8	3.5	5.3	4.3
Peripheral vascular bypass	4.0	2.8	2.9	5.5	4.1
Hemodialysis	11.4	13.0	7.4	15.8	7.7
Injection or ligation of esophageal varices	46.9	44.3	37.5	98.1	43.7
Upper gastrointestinal endoscopy, biopsy	2.4	6.0	—	3.3	3.3
Gastrostomy, temporary and permanent	9.8	6.9	8.9	12.8	10.2

Adapted from ref. 9.
[a] Estimated percent of annual change.

per visit based on national data (5), and inflated Grazier's calculation by $1.25 billion to account for the use of chiropractic services. Using the PPI and adjusting for population growth, the figure is $1.6 billion in 1990 and $2.65 billion in 1994.

We also concluded that a variety of other caregivers have a significant impact on costs. Most notably, physical therapy for spinal disorders grew substantially during the 1970s and 1980s (Fig. 2). A total of 6,544,000 visits were made to physical therapists in 1981 (14). We took a cautious approach and inflated these 1981 figures by

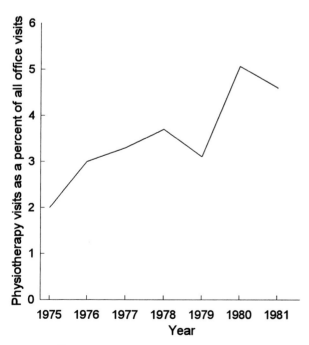

FIG. 2. Growth in the rate of utilization of physical therapy services, 1975–1981 (14).

population growth alone to arrive at a 1990 figure of 6,947,000 visits. To establish the costs of these services, we assumed a mean duration of 15 minutes for a visit at an average of $15.00 to arrive at a cost of $104 million in 1990. With adjustments, the figure in 1994 is estimated to be $137 million.

Another factor we believe may have been overlooked is the cost of neurologists and psychiatrists. Evidence exists that one third of all patients with a spinal disorder had on average one neurologic and one psychiatric consultation. We estimated that if 12.9 million back pain visits are the "floor," it is reasonable to assume that there were 4.3 million visits to psychiatrists and neurologists. Using the fee structures reported by the Paralysis Society of America (17) in 1988 ($110 for a neurologic consultation and $46.75 for a psychiatric consultation), we derived a cost basis of $673 million for 1984. Using the PPI and adjusting for population growth, the figure is $1.03 billion in 1994.

Finally, we took Grazier's 1984 figure of $324 million. Using the MPI and adjusting for population growth, we arrived at an estimated cost of $349 million in 1990 and $469 million in 1994. If the costs of chiropractic care ($2.65 billion), physical therapists ($137 million), and neurologists/psychiatrists ($1.03 billion) are added to the base cost of $469 million, the total estimated cost in 1994 is $4.29 billion.

Drugs

Grazier et al. (9) estimated the costs of drugs to be $121 million. In 1990, we were confident there had been no major breakthroughs in the pharmacologic management of back disorders, with the exception of antibiotics for spinal infections and chemotherapeutic agents for tumors, both relatively rare conditions. In 1994, there is little reason to believe there were further breakthroughs that would materially influence the costs. Thus, using the MPI and adjusting for population growth, we estimate the figure in 1994 to be $257 million.

Nursing Home Services

The calculated cost presented by Grazier et al. (9) was $3 billion, which some argued was too high. However, we could find no compelling evidence to change the figure and simply adjusted it using the MPI and growth in the general population as opposed to the differentially greater growth in the population over 65. The recalculated figure in 1994 is $6.56 billion.

Prepayment and Administration

The 1984 figure of $501.5 million has been adjusted by CPI and population growth to arrive at $791 million in 1994.

Non-Health-Sector Goods and Services

The 1984 figure of $1.28 billion has been adjusted by CPI and population growth to arrive at $2.0 billion in 1994.

Total Direct Medical Costs

Table 6 gives the total direct costs for spinal disorders as calculated by Grazier et al. (9) in 1984 and the calculations in 1994 derived from the preceding analysis.

TABLE 6. *Direct costs of back pain*

	Cost 1984 (×$1000)	Cost 1994 (×$1000)
Hospital services	4,462,770	11,289,109
Outpatient and emergency room	259,690	580,900
Outpatient diagnostic and therapeutic	1,010,590	2,260,588
Physician inpatient	1,075,750	2,277,666
Physician office, outpatient and ER	1,048,120	3,217,790
Other practitioner	233,630	4,368,155
Drugs	121,340	256,911
Nursing home	2,933,520	6,561,990
Prepayment	501,530	791,001
Non-health-sector goods and services	1,275,800	2,012,162
Total direct costs	12,922,740	33,616,273

DIRECT COSTS: NONMEDICAL

There are other direct costs that are not related to the delivery of health care and are difficult to derive, for example, legal services. In California, it was estimated that low back pain disability amounted to $600 million in 1989 (6). This figure represents 46% of all Workers' Compensation litigation in that state. California represents 11.5% of the United States population, and a straight calculation in 1990 suggested this figure was $5 billion. This extrapolation did not take into account any unusual propensity for Californians to sue more or less than other populations in the United States.

INDIRECT COSTS AND TRANSFER PAYMENTS

In 1990, we felt it was impossible to calculate the indirect costs (that is, productivity losses) of back disorders. From a societal point of view, transfer payments are not costs, although for insurers and employers they are. The estimates of total indirect and disability-related payments range from 2 times to 3 to 4 times the direct costs. For example, Levitt et al. (11) reported that medical costs account for only 33% of total Workers' Compensation disability payments. Webster and Snook (21) report similar figures of 31.5% for 1986 and 32.4% for 1989. By comparison, Grazier et al. (9) in 1984 calculated the total indirect cost of spinal disorders at $2.95 billion; $2.5 billion was for the lost earnings of wage earners and the remainder for lost earnings of homemakers. If this figure is adjusted for population growth and by the CPI, the calculation for 1994 is $4.6 billion.

Back pain represents 25% of all lost workdays in the United States, and back injuries represent 25% of all Workers' Compensation claims. This is more than twice the number of claims as the next most common cause of disability, finger injuries, which account for 11% (10).

One research group concluded that the disability-related cost of low back disorders was $43 billion in 1989. Another approach was used by Clark (6) who had access to accurate California data. He calculated the figure to be $4.3 billion, which, when extrapolated to the country as a whole, was estimated at $13.9 billion. Similarly, Webster and Snook (21) calculated the figure to be $11.4 billion for 1989. They also calculated that $3.6 million was for medical payments and the remaining $7.4 million for indirect costs.

The Impact and Growth of Disability Claims

Regardless of precise costs, considerable evidence demonstrates that a relatively small percentage of the back-injured patients account for the majority of the costs. For example, Spengler et al. (20) found that 10%

of the claims accounted for 79% of the costs. Webster and Snook (21) found almost identical figures, and the Quebec Task Force on Spinal Disorders (18) found that 7.4% of claims accounted for 76% of the costs.

The disproportionate cost of the chronically disabled includes both indirect and direct medical costs. The chronically disabled back pain patient uses significantly more medical services, including operations, although the probability of a successful outcome is significantly less (2,16).

Further, in many industrialized nations, the growth of disability claims for back pain has been explosive. In the United States, the average increase for all awards given by Social Security Disability increased 250% from 1957 to 1976, which was slightly greater than the rate of population growth. In comparison, disability awards for back pain went up 2800%, growth that was 14 times greater than that of the population (Fig. 3). In Sweden from 1952 to 1982, the growth in permanent disability was 2800% (15). This led Nachemson to conclude that low back disability in a socialized nation can lead to bankruptcy (13).

What Are the Indirect Costs of Spinal Disorders?

In 1990, we concluded it was impossible to calculate the indirect costs with any level of precision. Grazier's 1984 analysis extrapolated to 1994 using the Consumer Price Index (CPI) and adjusting for population growth is $4.6 billion. If the California data are extrapolated to the country as a whole, Clark (6) estimated that the cost to industry for low back disorders alone ranges from $32.1 to $55.7 million.

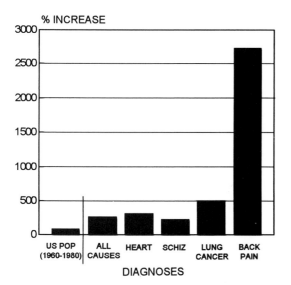

FIG. 3. Rate of increase for social security disability claims for spine compared to other chronic and often disabling disease processes as well as population growth, 1957–1976. Note the dramatic increase for spinal disorders.

WHAT ARE THE COSTS OF SPINAL DISORDERS?

In 1990, we were somewhat comfortable in our calculation of direct costs, estimated using a substantially greater national data base. At the same time, we recognized that there were a variety of assumptions about the growth (or shrinkage) of medical services.

Even less well known at this point is the impact of capitated care and more tightly controlled networks of health providers such as health maintenance organizations (HMOs). It is quite clear in markets such as California and Minnesota, which are heavily penetrated by managed care, that the costs have been driven down significantly as measured by the cost per member per month. However, there is little information to determine how great an impact this form of health financing has had on the costs of spinal disorders and on the high costs attached to disability in particular. There is also considerable evidence that more aggressive prevention methods and approaches such as tightly controlled case management can have a favorable impact on reducing the costs of Workers' Compensation. Finally, changes in public policy can be expected to affect some of the costs as well as the utilization of some forms of treatment rendered for spinal disorders. For example, the introduction of federal guidelines in the United States (3) will in all likelihood reduce the wide variations now identified in the use of spinal surgery for back pain.

There is even less certainty about the indirect costs of low back pain because of the absence of complete data bases.

Taking the available information, it would appear that approximate costs for back disorders could range from a low of $38 billion (representing the extrapolations of Grazier's data) to a high that is in excess of $50 billion. This latter figure is somewhat more conservative than the upper end figure we cited in 1990 of $100 billion.

CONCLUSION

Spinal symptoms are ubiquitous in all industrialized societies and have a very significant financial impact. The greatest source of costs, both direct medical costs and indirect costs, are associated with those disabled by their symptoms. Although it is impossible with existent data bases to give a precise estimate of these costs, a range of $38 billion to more than $50 billion seems reasonable. The costs of back pain are enormous, and therefore the prevention and treatment of these disorders deserves major attention.

REFERENCES

1. Andrews RM, Fox S, Elixhauser A, Coffey R, Raskin IE (1987): *The national bill for diseases treated in U.S. hospitals: 1987.* US

Department of Health and Human Services, Public Health Service, Agency for Health Care Policy and Research.

2. Berkowitz M, Greene C (1989): Disability expenditures. *Am Rehab* 15(1):7–15,29.

3. Bigos S, Bowyer O, Braen G, et al. (1994): *Acute low back problems in adults.* Clinical Practice Guideline No. 14, AHCPR Publication No. 95-6042. Rockville, MD: Agency for Health Care Policy and Research, Public Health Service, U.S. Department of Health and Human Services. December.

4. Brunarski DJ (1985): Clinical trials of spinal manipulation: a critical appraisal and review of the literature. *J Manipulative Physiol Ther* 7:243–249.

5. Bureau of National Affairs (1988): *Back injuries: costs, causes, cases, and prevention.* Washington, D.C.: Bureau of National Affairs.

6. Clark WC (1989): Personal communication.

7. Deyo RA, Tsui-Wu YJ (1987): Descriptive epidemiology of low-back pain and its related medical care in the United States. *Spine* 12:264–268.

8. Elixhouser A, Harris DR, Coffey RM (1994): *Trends in hospital procedures performed on black patients and white patients: 1980-87* (AHCPR Publication No. 94-0003) Provider Studies Research Note 20, Agency for Health Care Policy and Research, Rockville, MD. Public Health Service.

9. Grazier KL, Holbrook TL, Kelsey JL, Stauffer RN, eds. (1984): *The frequency of occurrence, impact, and cost of musculoskeletal conditions in the United States.* Chicago: American Academy of Orthopaedic Surgeons.

10. Klein BP, Jensen RC, Sanderson LM (1984): Assessment of workers' compensation claims for back strains/sprains. *J Occup Med* 326:443–448.

11. Leavitt SS, Johnston JL, Beyer RD (1971): The process of recovery: patterns in industrial injury. I: Costs and other quantitative measures of effort. *Ind Med Surg* 40:7–14.

12. Liang M, Komaroff AL (1982): Roentgenograms in primary care patients with acute low back pain: a cost-effective analysis. *Arch Intern Med* 142:1108–1112.

13. Nachemson A (1995): Will low back pain doom the welfare state? The Swedish experience may be a warning for the U.S. *The Back Letter* 10:27.

14. Nelson C (1986): Physiotherapy office visits: national ambulatory medical care survey: United States, 1980-1981. *NCHS Advance Data* 120.

15. Nettelbladt E (1985): Opuscula Medica. Sweden 30(2):54.

16. Norton WL (1986): Chemonucleolysis versus surgical discectomy. Comparison of costs and results in workers' compensation claimants. *Spine* 11:440–443.

17. Paralysis Society of America (1989): Research briefs, measuring the costs of medical care for SCI persons. Issue 3.

18. Quebec Task Force on Spinal Disorders (1987): Scientific approach to the assessment and management of activity-related spinal disorders. *Spine* 12(7):S1–S59.

19. Scavone JG, Latchaw RF, Rohrer GV (1981): Use of lumbar spine films. Statistical evaluation at a university teaching hospital. *JAMA* 246:1105–1108.

20. Spengler DM, Bigos SJ, Martin NA, et al. (1986): Back injuries in industry: a retrospective study. I. Overview and cost analysis. *Spine* 11:241–245.

21. Webster BS, Snook S (1994): The cost of 1989 workers' compensation low back pain claims. *Spine* 19(10):1111–1116.

The Adult Spine: Principles and Practice,
2nd edition, J.W. Frymoyer, Editor-in-Chief.
Lippincott-Raven Publishers, Philadelphia © 1997.

CHAPTER 9

The Impact of Spinal Disorders in Industry

Stanley J. Bigos and Michele Crites Battié

Spinal disorders exert a major impact throughout the industrialized countries of the world, that extends beyond the individual suffering and diminished quality of life experienced by affected workers and their families. Back pain has become the most expensive health-care problem of the 20- to 50-year age group, the most expensive musculoskeletal problem, and the most expensive industrial injury, primarily because it has become the most common cause of disability under age 45 (64,78,94). Thus, back problems are an increasing burden for society as industry incorporates higher insurance costs into the costs of goods and services, and more tax revenues are allocated to care for those declared disabled and their families (92,93).

Approximately 50% of people in the working age group admit to significant symptoms or to being limited by back symptoms for at least 1 day each year (15,98,100,103). However, only a small percentage, 2% to 5%, subsequently make the decision to seek medical care (104) or file a back injury claim (68,92,94). Furthermore, only about one-fifth of the patients with back problems can loosely associate the onset of their symptoms with an accident, injury, or unusual activity (40).

Back disorders are not limited to the industrialized countries of the world, yet their impact seems to be much less elsewhere. This expensive occupational and disability problem does not seem to occur in third world countries, where back pain is considered a part of life rather than an injury. While evidence is strong that people in these countries experience back symptoms, without experts to tell them that activity is dangerous or that back pain needs medical care, their problems show a better natural history for recovery than in the United States (1,110).

Treating work-related or compensation-related back symptoms tends to be more difficult than treating other back disorders (41,67). The likelihood of a good result following surgery in compensation cases has been reported to be one-fourth that in private cases (35). The compensation factor also seems to increase the chance of having residual back pain following disc surgery (46). There is also evidence that compensation delays recovery from back pain problems that are treated conservatively (41).

Most episodes of back pain do not seem to be caused by an injury in the typical sense of the word, but rather are a normal part of life and increase with advancing age. Back pain is extremely common; 85% of 50-year-olds recall having had back symptoms, and there is some indication that the remainder have forgotten such episodes (53; Holtman M., *personal communication,* 1989). The ability to set one's own work pace seems to impact the memory of those who have forgotten episodes, because in this circumstance pain less often threatens livelihood. Up to 25% of persons between ages 30 and 50 report the presence of back symptoms at the time of being surveyed (2,4,49,95,99). The usually transitory nature of back pain and its commonness has led some observers to question whether it should be called a disease (89). Questions also arise about the appropriateness of using an injury model when studying the onset of back problems. Onset is commonly gradual and does not relate to an accidental

S. J. Bigos, M.D.: Professor of Orthopedics and Environmental Health, University of Washington, Seattle, Washington, 98195.

M. C. Battié, Ph.D.: Professor and Chair, Department of Physical Therapy, University of Alberta, Edmonton, Canada T6G 2G4.

cause (40,86,89,105). A recent study of patients with acute, subacute, and chronic back symptoms showed that 77% of a patient population could not relate the onset of their symptoms to a time within 24 hours of an accident or unusual activity (40).

The failure of the injury model to explain industrial back problems has led to the cumulative trauma model, which is now proposed to explain musculoskeletal problems of gradual onset among workers. Unfortunately, the difficulties in monitoring off-work activities makes it virtually impossible to control all the factors needed to scientifically verify the cumulative model as an explanation of industrial back problems.

To add to our difficulties in explaining causation and rationally managing back problems, pathoanatomic diagnosis is determined in only 12% to 15% of patients (14,31). Thus, no objectively diagnosable condition is needed to explain back symptoms or to justify filing a back injury claim. Commonly used diagnostic terms such as back sprain or strain, myofasciitis, disc syndrome, facet syndrome, subluxation, and internal disarrangement are not objectively verifiable and for scientific purposes must be considered synonyms for idiopathic back pain. Thus, the basis for studying back problems is less objective than for studying more easily diagnosable problems such as fractures and lacerations.

Many unproved hypotheses have guided attempts at intervention and perhaps have been detrimental by distorting the perception of those experiencing the symptoms. For instance, recurrence is a widely expected aspect of the natural history of back symptoms; thus, a history of back symptoms tends to be a reasonably strong indicator of future risk and has nothing to do with re-injury. Other nonphysical factors having strong associations with future complaints include comorbidities, other types of symptom complaints, major psychological distress, and lower socioeconomic status (58). It is likely that lower socioeconomic status is a marker for a variety of potential risk factors such as lifestyle and occupational attributes that may increase the risk (13).

INDIVIDUAL RISK FACTORS

The majority of studies of suspected risk factors have been retrospective in nature, examining a variety of factors after back problems have been reported (2,92). Such studies do not allow the determination of cause or effect, and the potential for bias is great. In the case of individual physical function and psychological status, where findings can vary as a result of back problems, associations revealed in retrospective and cross-sectional studies can be particularly difficult to interpret. Thus, our discussion of the scientific literature related to suspected individual risk factors will center on the findings of prospective, longitudinal studies.

Unlike some well-defined disease processes, back problems are generally revealed only through symptom complaints, and the specific underlying pathology is unknown. Back problems generally have been defined and identified in one of three ways in the prospective, longitudinal studies conducted to date. Some have focused on back pain revealed on questionnaires (15–17,44,48,69–72,98,102), some have focused specifically on industrial incident reports or injury claims filed in the workplace (5,7,9–11,20–22,26,27,76,82,87), and others have investigated hospitalizations for the diagnosis of disc herniation (47,53). These different categories of back problems vary in incidence by approximately tenfold and will be examined separately.

Memorable Back Symptoms (Reported on Survey)

Gyntelberg, in 1974, reported one of the first prospective studies of risk factors for back problems. Nearly 4,700 Danish men between the ages of 40 and 59 years, were examined and then questioned 1 year later regarding back problems. Twenty-six percent of the subjects reported experiencing back problems during the 1-year period following their examination. Men reporting back problems were more likely to be slightly taller (greater than 181 cm), but they did not tend to be particularly obese or thin compared to men who did not report back problems. No association was found between fitness level, as judged through predicted maximal oxygen uptake, and back problems. However, an association was present between back pain complaints and reports of other symptomatic health problems (44).

Later, Biering-Sørensen reported on a study of more than 900 residents of Copenhagen who underwent a physical examination and were questioned about prior back trouble (15,16). One year later, the subjects were questioned about low back trouble experienced during the year since the examination. Anthropometric measurements were very poor predictors of low back trouble. The strongest indicators during this study were previous reports of similar problems. The few individual physical factors that were significantly associated with first-time low back troubles among men were diminished static back muscle endurance and greater lumbosacral flexion. Similar trends were not present among women. Maximum isometric strength in flexion and extension of the trunk were less in women reporting recurrent back problems than in those who reported only previous problems. Men did not exhibit similar differences.

In 1987, Troup and co-workers reported on a prospective study of the predictive value of a number of potential preemployment screening tests (98). Nearly 3,000 British men and women were questioned about their perception of physical exertion at work and about prior experiences of low back pain. They also underwent a battery of tests that included anthropometric measurements, back flexibility, maximal lifting strength, and psychophysical tests. None of the tests were of any value in predicting new cases of low back pain. A prior history of back trouble was the strongest predictor of subsequent back problems; once back pain history was known, the other variables slightly enhanced prediction.

Videman and colleagues (102) reported on risk indicators for back pain complaints among Finnish women who had completed their first year of nursing work. Of the factors considered, the incidence of sudden onset back pain was best explained by poorer patient handling skill, a poorer sit-up test, and heavier perceived workload. This was not the case, however, for back pain of gradual onset, which was the more common complaint. A high score on the hysteria scale from the Middlesex Hospital Questionnaire was associated with all types of back pain, including symptoms of gradual onset. Two other Scandinavian studies have investigated individual physical factors associated with back pain complaints among metal industry workers and military conscripts (48,69–72). Consistent with earlier reports, they found that muscle function tests were not highly associated with future experiences of notable back pain.

Judging from the prospective studies discussed above, basic anthropometric measures and individual physical capacities alone would appear to have little influence on risk of experiencing low back pain or troubles. Height and weight, strength as determined through isometric testing, psychophysical tests, flexibility in the sagittal plane, and estimated maximal aerobic capacity, among others, were deemed to be of little or no predictive value (16,44,98).

Hospitalizations for Herniated Discs

Two large prospective studies of hospitalizations for herniated lumbar discs have been reported. Hrubec and Nashold (53) examined anthropometric measurements obtained at the time of induction in 1,975 United States military recruits who later were hospitalized with a diagnosis of herniated disc. When compared to controls matched for age and period of military service, the hospital cases tended to be taller and heavier. A study by Heliövaara considered height, weight, and relative weight as potential risk factors for cases of hospitalizations for herniated discs; taller men and women were more likely to be hospitalized with a diagnosis of herniated disc during an 11-year follow-up period. An association between relative weight (wt/ht^2) and hospitalizations for disc problems was less clear (47). Both these studies found an association between hospitalizations for herniated discs and greater than average height. Heliövaara also found that certain blue collar occupations among men, symptoms suggesting psychological distress among women, and lower social class were risk indicators (47).

Industrial Back Injury Complaints

Several prospective longitudinal studies have attempted to identify risk factors specifically for back injury claims occurring at the work place (Table 1). In 1973, Chaffin reported on a longitudinal study of low back pain in association with isometric lifting strength and occupational lifting requirements (27). Isometric lifting strength in relation to job demands was evaluated among 411 persons employed in 103 different jobs. During the 1-year follow-up period, these subjects reported 25 low back incidents to the company medical department. The incidence rate was approximately 3 times greater in those who were unable to demonstrate strength equal to or greater than that required by the job, as compared to those demonstrating greater relative strength. However, this difference was not reported as statistically significant, perhaps because of the small number of subjects and back incident reports involved (27). Subsequently, additional prospective studies evaluated the effects of isometric lifting strength in relation to job requirements. Unfortunately, too few back problems were reported in these studies to allow for analysis of this subset of musculoskeletal complaints (65,66). There was no indication that strength exceeding job requirements provided any extra protection from musculoskeletal problems.

In 1979, Cady and caseworkers presented their finding from a prospective study of physical fitness in relation to subsequent back pain reports among 1,652 firefighters (26). An overall fitness score was derived from several isometric strength, flexibility, and cardiovascular endurance measures. They found an association between back pain reporting and fitness level, and they concluded that physical fitness and conditioning can prevent back injuries. Unfortunately, other potentially confounding factors that varied significantly between fitness groups, such as age, were not controlled during the analyses, making interpretation less clear.

Isokinetic lifting strength was investigated as a predictor of low back injury claims among nurses in a more recent study by Mostardi and colleagues (76). They found it to be a poor predictor of subsequent back symptom complaints and injury reports. Another study of back injury reports in nurses by Ready and colleagues (82) also found that isometric lifting strength failed to predict such reports, as did other general fitness parameters. The factors that discriminated most between the nurses who did and did not report subsequent back injuries were prior compensation pay, smoking status, and poorer job satisfaction. A history of compensation has been associated with work loss because of back problems in other studies as well (87).

One of the more comprehensive studies of back injury claims to date is the Boeing Study, a prospective, longitudinal investigation of industrial back pain complaints

TABLE 1. *Back symptom complaints in the workplace: Results of prospective, longitudinal studies*

	(3,6,18) U.S. aircraft mfrg. employees (3,020/4,027) 4	(22) Electronics mfrg. employees (411/?) 1	(21) Firefighters (1,652/1,900) 3	(44) Nurses (171/?) 2	(48) Nurses (131/574) 1.5	(53) Canadian aircraft mfrg. employees (269/395) 1
Reference: Study subjects: (Volunteers/# solicited): Follow-up duration (years):						
Factors considered						
Demographic						
Gender	0					
Age	↓	0				0
Education	0					
Anthropometric						
Standing height	↑ (men)	0			0	
Sitting height	0					
Arm span	0					
Weight	↑ (women)	0			↑	0
Obesity (relative wt.)	0				↑	
Lifestyle						
Smoking					↑↑	↑
Leisure time physical activity						0
Strength/endurance						
Isometric lifting	0	↓ (job-matched)			0	
Isokinetic lifting strength				0		
Estimated maximal aerobic capacity	0		↓		0	
Abdominal strength					0	
Flexion/ext. rotation					0	
Composite fitness score	0		↓			
Flexibility						
Lumbar flexion	0					
Lateral bending	0					
General flexion	0					
Other physical exam						
Decreased patellar reflex	↑					
Decreased achilles reflex	0					
Symptoms on SLR	↑↑					
Psychosocial						
Psychological distress	↑↑					
Health locus of control	0					
Family social support	0					
Stress level				0		
Work-related						
Social support/job satisfaction	↓↓			↓↓	↓↓	
Duration of employment					0	
# hours of overtime work					0	
Perceived physical demands	0					
Maximum weight loading	0					
Medical history						
Back pain history	↑↑	↑		↑		↑↑
Prior back-related compensation claim					↑↑	↑↑
Prior MVA					↑	
Health care utilization (for pain)	↑↑					

Modified from Battié and Videman (12), with permission.

↑, a positive association; ↑↑, a strong positive association; ↓, a negative association; ↓↓, a strong negative association; 0, not a predictor; SLR, straight-leg raising; MVA, motor vehicle accident.

in 3,020 aircraft manufacturing workers (5,7,9,10,20–22). The purpose of the study was to examine a wide variety of workplace and individual physical, demographic, and psychosocial variables suspected as risk factors for back pain reports. A detailed physical examination was conducted of all study volunteers at baseline, and medical history, demographic, and psychosocial information was requested. The study participants then were tracked for nearly 4 years during their employment with the Boeing Company, during which time 279 employees reported back problems. The incidence of back pain reporting was similar among men and women.

Younger employees were more likely to report back problems at the workplace than were older employees. Similar to several other studies of back problems, smoking was a risk indicator (17,29,38,39,47,64,96). The relative risk for a smoker was 1.4 times that of a nonsmoker for reporting an industrial back injury incident in the follow-up period (7).

Notably, none of the strength, flexibility, and aerobic capacity measures obtained were significantly associated with back pain reports (5,7,10). Furthermore, among employees without a history of prior back problems, no individual physical factors were associated with increased risk (9). Among subjects reporting a history of back problems, the only physical examination variable to be highly associated with future back pain reporting was back symptoms elicited on straight-leg raising (9,21).

A history of back problems has been recognized for some time as an important risk indicator for future problems. The Boeing study findings support this association: of all factors studied, the report of current or recent back problems was the variable most significantly related to future back injury reports. Additionally, a history of receiving medical care for back problems, chiropractic visits, doctor visits, and medical prescriptions for pain problems of any kind were associated with increased risk of industrial back injury reports (21).

One of the most interesting findings of the Boeing study was the influence of work perceptions and psychosocial factors on back pain complaints (20). Other than current or recent back problems, the strongest predictors of subsequent reports were perceptions of the workplace such as low job enjoyment and certain psychosocial responses identified on the Minnesota Multiphasic Personality Inventory (MMPI) (Fig. 1) (21). Responses on the Work APGAR questionnaire of hardly ever enjoying the job tasks and relatively high scale 3 scores on the MMPI, indicating tendencies toward somatic complaints and denial of emotional distress, were strongly associated with subsequent back injury reports. These findings demonstrate the multifaceted nature of factors affecting back pain reporting in industry.

Overall, the prospective studies of work-related back pain reports have been of limited scope, focusing on individual physical capacities among workers in occupations with high physical demands (Fig. 1). One study suggests an association between industrial back pain reports and insufficient isometric strength relative to job demands (27). A negative correlation between back incident reports and overall fitness, in terms of strength, flexibility, and cardiovascular fitness factors, may exist in firefighters (26) but has not been corroborated in other occupational groups with less extreme demand (5,7, 8,10,76,82). In the Boeing study, general lifting strength was not associated with reporting even when examined among employees working within the same job category (5). Perceptions of work and other psychosocial factors

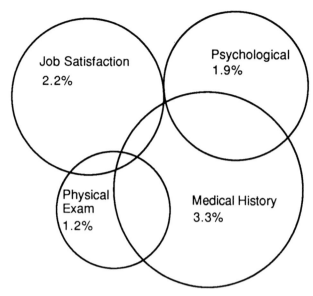

FIG. 1. Venn diagram of final multivariate model for predicting industrial back pain reports. Medical history explains 3.3% of the uncertainty in predicting a subject making or not making a report of industrial back pain, as compared with 1.2% explained by physical examination (straight-leg raising, SLR), 1.9% explained by psychological (MMPI and HLOC), and 2.2% explained by job satisfaction (modified Work APGAR) findings. The predictive value of medical history and physical examination together is 4.0%, of medical history and psychological findings together is 4.5%, and of medical history and job satisfaction together is 5.4%. The predictive value of psychological findings and physical exam considered together is 3.3%.

played a greater role in industrial back pain complaints than did the wide array of physical measures studied (21). These findings emphasize the importance of adopting a broader approach to understanding and dealing with the multifaceted problems of back pain complaints that interfere with work, and they offer an explanation as to why efforts focusing on purely physical or injury factors have met with little success.

THE WORK ENVIRONMENT

In the past, interest in the effects of the work environment on back problems centered on the physical attributes of the work site and job tasks. Today, there is increasing recognition that job satisfaction and sociocultural aspects of the work environment also may play a significant role in the filing of industrial injury claims. Thus, the work environment is now being examined in a broader sense to include both physical and nonphysical aspects.

Several studies have indicated that psychosocial factors associated with the work environment may influence spinal disorders. Gyntelberg reported a suggestion of a relationship in his 1974 study between stress at the work site and the development of back problems (44). In the Boeing study, a person's perceptions of support and acceptance from co-workers, and enjoyment of work tasks, affected risk for actively filing complaints of back pain, especially if the person had already reported distress according to the MMPI and had a previous history of back problems. Other studies have supported the importance of job enjoyment, as well as perceived psychological demands of work, and influence and control over work activities (42,45,57,59–62).

The role of physical loading in the production of back problems is controversial. Occupational exposures that have appeared frequently as suspected risk factors are vehicular vibration and physical loading involving heavy lifting, bending, twisting, and sustained nonneutral postures (3,32,37). Cross-sectional studies have reported associations between heavy physical work and low back pain and disability (55,56,75,84,96,99), but others have not (28,79,91). Prospective studies also have found mixed results (17,27,47,71). It is unclear whether variations in physical loading between individuals are important factors in the conditions underlying back symptoms, or whether they primarily serve to exacerbate symptoms from already existing conditions. Videman and colleagues controlled for the degree of degenerative changes and found that a history of back symptoms was correlated with physical loading (101). In the same Videman study, annular ruptures were more commonly found in subjects who engaged in occupations involving heavy physical loading, suggesting that heavy loading may lead to increased risk of some structural changes. However, Magnuson and colleagues (74) did not find back complaints at an assembly line related to peak loads, repetitive lifts, or large load doses while self reported exposures have been labeled as too crude to be a reasonable research tool (60,108). This finding supports the belief that loading exacerbates symptoms from existing conditions. Unfortunately, heavy work seems related to many lower socioeconomic factors that can impact the incidence of such age-related findings (13). A similar level of controversy surrounds the clinical importance of most degenerative changes identified on imaging studies because such findings are commonly found in symptom-free persons (22,23,50,88,107).

In the Boeing study, among the factors that were not associated with subsequent complaints were isometric lifting strength, maximal aerobic capacity, and range of motion in side bending and flexion. The strongest predictors of future back pain reports, other than having had current or recent back problems at the onset of the study, were negative perceptions of the workplace, including low job task enjoyment, low social support at the workplace, and emotional distress (Fig. 1) (21). The only factor from the baseline physical examination that was strongly associated with future reporting was back pain

elicited on straight-leg raise testing, which probably represents another aspect of recent or current back problems, which are known to influence future risk. These findings underline the multifaceted nature of back pain reporting in industry.

OCCUPATIONAL INJURY INSURANCE FACTORS

Some indicators show that medical insurance factors influence the response to spinal disorders in industry. Despite a lack of justification, there continues to be an emphasis on using an injury model to explain the onset of musculoskeletal problems that are more closely related to aging. For the most part, back pain is an unavoidable, normal part of life's experience. Yet, injury models continue to be used even though only approximately 20% of patients can even loosely associate their symptoms with an accident, injury, or unusual activity occurring within the last 24 hours before onset of pain (40). Furthermore, an injury model seems to ignore our inability to define the course of back complaints admitted annually by 50% of working persons, our inability to use objective physical factors to predict who will file a back injury claim (2% to 5% of the work force each year), and the evidence that factors other than the presence of symptoms incite the report of a back injury. For example, once a back problem is experienced, the chance of a recurrence and future interference with work probably depends upon numerous physical and situational factors (90). Nonphysical factors such as psychological distress and negative perceptions of the job are risk factors both for reporting back pain and for work interference (36,97).

Nonphysical factors are not fixed, stable states but dynamic situational factors that involve a person's self-perception in respect to his or her environment. As health-care providers we must accept that nonphysical stresses in life or work can influence the response to back symptoms. Symbolically, in relation to a back injury claim, back symptoms may be the last straw that breaks the back of the already burdened camel (Fig. 2). Concomitantly, not even the most ardent engineer would expect removal of that straw to bounce the camel right back to its feet (Fig. 3). Why should it be expected that concentrating on the back pain alone in an overburdened patient would be any more effective? In either case, concentrating only on the last straw does not seem to be the answer. Treating back pain alone may not spring the overburdened patient back to his or her feet, to work, or to the previous station in life. Back problems often seem many times to be only one aspect of the patient's total predicament.

An injury model may be suitable for insurance administration, but it is discordant with medical knowledge

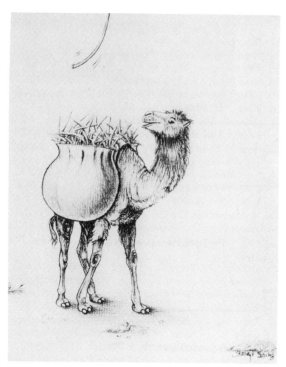

FIG. 2. Back pain (the proverbial last straw) relative to total problem of back injury claim.

about prevention and treatment. To date, the injury model has been unsuccessful as a basis for prevention or guiding treatment of patients with back problems.

Another shortcoming of the injury model is that it is based on implicit fault and thus provides the affected person with an expectation of entitlement as it relates to fault. If back pain is perceived to be caused by an external factor, the feelings of personal responsibility may diminish, thus altering treatment expectations and even recovery. Once symptoms have persisted for more than a few weeks, many patients have trouble accepting the fact that their backs will never feel or tolerate activity as if they were 18 years of age. Thus, embitterment, related to the belief that an external factor is responsible, can confound and emotionalize treatment and heighten the issues re-

lating to a demand for adequate fair compensation. The expectation of equitable redress and fairness, or insinuation of justice, seems commonly to lead to anger played out in the medical–legal system.

Overtreatment and prescribed inactivity are major problems in the care of spinal disorders. An expert's temporizing of surgical and nonsurgical recommendations has been found to be important to overcome a practitioner's exuberance to gain symptom control through inactivating the patient with rest or poorly warranted operations (106). Consultations between the treating physician and independent specialists seem to reduce excessive, questionable treatment. As Wiesel and co-workers found in the PEPCO study (107), the number of surgeries performed fell by 88% and the number of active cases open could be markedly reduced.

Another set of factors influencing spine disorders in industrial settings centers on hidden disincentives. The patient may have an incentive to negotiate an injury settlement as it relates to fault, but the employer's insurance provider tends to have few incentives to avoid such litigation. Poor incentives seem also to affect treatment providers as evidenced by the Kane study in Utah, where medical providers not covered by the state insurance program for injured workers did a much better job than those covered by the state program, at keeping the patients at work and returning them to work sooner (63). This study also found that the same type of treatment providers, when reimbursed by the state insurance fund rather than directly by the workers, became less effective at keeping their patients at work or returning them to work following back problems (42).

Figure 4 further denotes some of the complexities of patients' efforts to make decisions when symptoms first occur and the significance of decisions in various categories. They realize that eventually their decisions become passive if they have not taken an active role in recovery, but, as chronically disabled patients, they are waiting for society to provide recommendations to improve their condition. Not only does the injury insurance system have an impact on the type of decision-making process

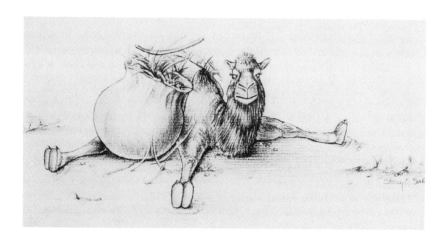

FIG. 3. Medical treatment models only attempt to lift "the last straw" (back pain). From Bigos and Battié (19), with permission.

**Levels of Back Problem
and
Related Decisions**

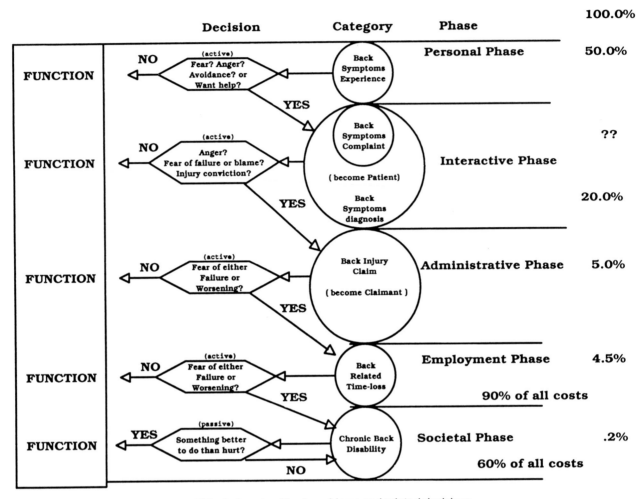

FIG. 4. Levels of back problems and related decisions.

the patient makes, but medicine also can make major contributions to the decisions made by patients once the experience of back pain becomes a back complaint, leading the person to become a patient and perhaps a claimant.

MEDICINE'S POTENTIAL CONTRIBUTIONS

Recent investigations have identified treatment approaches that significantly decrease the impact of spine disorders, especially back problems, on the industrial worker. The most recent Volvo study has disparaged the wisdom of acute care as commonly practiced, by reversing all debilitating prescriptions after 6 weeks of treatment, thereby activating the patient (73). Again from Sweden, a study by Gundewall et al. (43) has found that physically training the erector spinae muscles can have a

preventive impact on future back complaints in a cost-effective manner. These studies encourage us to do our part to caution workers, patients, and the general public about the debilitating aspects of excessively restricted activity, and to be realistic about medications and operations that are rarely warranted (30). Conversely, the importance of activities should be emphasized to avoid further debilitation and to provide protection in the future against further back problems (18,43). We also can overcome the emotions triggered by a fault-oriented injury model by reinforcing to patients that: (a) back pain is part of life, (b) the vast majority of patients get over their symptoms quickly, (c) no one at 50 years of age has a back that tolerates activity as was expected at age 18, (d) the extreme risk of being administratively labeled a low back loser is an avoidable consequence, and (e) many pitfalls are associated with trying to prove that a back problem is someone else's fault in the adversarial industrial insurance system that commonly has no money available for retraining after paying expensive professional consultants, evaluating medical professionals, and attorneys.

In the medical arena, we must gain the confidence and trust of workers to be able to help them with their problems. We can do so not only by providing them with the most effective and safest help with symptoms, but also by helping them to avoid debilitation resulting from inactivity by providing realistic conditioning to regain activity tolerance, while actively helping our patients realize their options regarding the reality of personal back symptoms and tolerance for work activity. Once patients have symptoms lasting more than a few weeks, they must understand that their back may never again tolerate life as was expected at 18 years of age. The dilemma focuses on helping workers understand reasonable activity tolerance relative to the physical demands of their job and to determine if it is realistic to expect to tolerate those demands until age 65. Workers commonly must also consider whether they will be wanted in a certain job situation until retirement. In any event, prolonged inactivity, work loss, and the unfortunate administrative label of low back loser are fates that we must help patients avoid.

In summary, medicine does not hold all the keys to returning a patient to work. The worker who is dissatisfied, not wanted, or incapable of holding a specific job until retirement has issues to address beyond the boundaries of back disorders. We can better avoid back pain disability by ministering to symptoms and helping patients identify their options. Back problems as confronted in the industrialized countries of the world seem to be linked to a balance between advancing age and the ability to tolerate strenuous activity. A variety of external factors explain why spinal disorders have become such an expensive, devastating problem. Trying to solve the back pain problem rather than dealing with the activity level and task tolerance rarely helps workers remain in unreasonably difficult job situations until age 65, nor does it make them desirable employees for certain tasks until retirement.

Adding nonphysical factors to industrial back problem complaints opens a door for a more educated approach to the needs of workers, employers, health-care providers, and society. It helps us to deal more realistically with many of the physical aspects. It also identifies situational factors that can be altered to the benefit of everyone by offering insight to this complex health problem reported as industrial back symptoms. To study such a complex entity with the many factors that have to be considered and to realize that in many instances workers are fighting to survive in their complex environments, may best explain why our simplistic linear models have failed to reverse the impact of spinal disorders and complaints in industry. Thus, it is difficult not to agree with

Dr. Bruce Hocking, who is now exploring the use of the chaos theory to create a more robust mathematical and statistical model for work-related illness (51).

REFERENCES

1. Anderson RT (1984): Orthopaedic ethnography in rural Nepal. *Med Anthropol* 8:46–59.
2. Andersson GBJ (1981): Epidemiological aspects of low back pain in industry. *Spine* 6:53–60.
3. Andersson GBJ (1991): The epidemiology of spinal disorders. In: Frymoyer JW, ed. *The adult spine: Principles and practice,* 1st ed. New York: Raven Press; pp 107–146.
4. Andersson G, Svensson HO (1979): Prevalence of low back pain. *S.P.R.I. Rapport* 22:11–23.
5. Battié MC (1989): *The reliability of physical factors as predictors of the occurrence of back pain reports: a prospective study within industry* (Thesis). Göteborg, Sweden: Gothenburg University.
6. Battié MC, Bigos SJ, Fisher LD, et al. (1987): Isometric lifting strength as a predictor of industrial back pain reports. *Spine* 14: 851–856.
7. Battié MC, Bigos SJ, Fisher LD, et al. (1989): A prospective study of the role of cardiovasular risk factors and fitness in industrial back pain complaints. *Spine* 14:141–147.
8. Battié MC, Bigos SJ, Fisher LD, Spengler DM, Hansson TH, Nachemson AL, Wortley D (1989): The role of spinal flexibility in back pain complaints within industry: a prospective study. *Spine* 15:768–773.
9. Battié MC, Bigos SJ, Fisher LD, Spengler DM, Hansson TH, Nachemson AL, Wortley MD (1990): Anthropometric and clinical measurements as predictors of industrial back pain complaints: a prospective study. *J Spinal Disord* 3(3):195–204.
10. Battié MC, Bigos SJ, Fisher LD, Spengler DM, Hansson TH, Nachemson AL, Wortley MD (1990): Anthropometric and clinical measurements as predictors of industrial back pain complaints: a prospective study. *Spine* 15(8):768–773.
11. Battié MC, Hansson T, Bigos SJ, Zeh J, Fisher LD, Spengler DM (1993): Scan ultrasonic measurement of the lumbar spine canal as a predictor of industrial back pain complaints and extended work loss. *J Occup Med* 35(12):1250–1255.
12. Battié MC, Videman T (1995): Back pain: epidemiology. In: Nordin M, Andersson G, Pope M, eds. *Work-related musculoskeletal disorders.* St. Louis: Mosby-Year Book.
13. Bergenudd H, Nilsson BO (1988): Back pain in middle age: occupational workload and psychologic factors: an epidemiologic survey. *Spine* 13(1):58–60.
14. Berkson MH, Nachemson A, Schultz AB (1979): Mechanical properties of human lumbar spine motion segments. Part II. Responses in compression and shear: influence of gross morphology. *J Biomech Eng* 101:53–57.
15. Biering-Sørensen F (1984): A one-year study of low back trouble in a general population: the prognostic value of low back history and physical measurements. *Dan Med Bull* 31:362–375.
16. Biering-Sørensen F (1984): Physical measurements as indicators for low back trouble over a one-year period. *Spine* 9:106–119.
17. Biering-Sørensen F, Thomsen C (1986): Medical social and occupational history as risk indicators for low-back trouble in a general population. *Spine* 11:720–725.
18. Bigos SJ, Battié MC (1987): Acute care to prevent back disability. Ten years of progress. *Clin Orthop* 221:121–130.
19. Bigos SJ, Battié M (1992): Risk factors for industrial back problems. *Semin Spine Surg* 4(1):2–11.
20. Bigos SJ, Battié MC, Fisher LD, Fordyce WE, Hansson TH, Nachemson AL, Spengler DM (1991): A prospective study of work perceptions and psychosocial factors affecting the report of back injury. *Spine* 16(1):1–6.
21. Bigos SJ, Battié MC, Fisher LD, Fordyce WE, Hansson TH, Nachemson AL, Spengler DM (1992): A longitudinal, prospective study of industrial back injury reporting. *Clin Orthop* 279:21–34.
22. Bigos SF, Battié MC, Fisher LD, Hansson TH, Spengler DM, Nachemson AL (1992): A prospective evaluation of commonly used pre-employment screening tools for acute industrial back pain. *Spine* 17(8):922–926.

23. Bigos SJ, Hansson TH, Castillo R, et al. (1992): The value of pre-employment radiographs for predicting acute back injury claims and chronic back pain disability. *Clin Orthop* 283:124–129.

24. Boden SD, Davis DO, Diana TS, et al (1990): Abnormal magnetic-resonance scans of the lumbar spine in asymptomatic subjects. *J Bone Joint Surg* 72:403.

25. Bond MB (1970): Low back injuries in industry. *Indstr Med Surg* 39:28–32.

26. Cady LD, Bischoff DP, O'Connell ER, et al (1979): Strength and fitness and subsequent back injuries in firefighters. *J Occup Med* 21:269–272.

27. Chaffin DB, Park KS (1973): A longitudinal study of low-back pain as associated with occupational weight lifting factors. *Am Ind Hyg Assoc J* 34:513–525.

28. Damkot DK, Pope MH, Lord J, Frymoyer JW (1984): The relationship between work history, work environment and low-back pain in men. *Spine* 9:395–399.

29. Deyo RA, Bass JE (1989): Lifestyle and low-back pain: the influence of smoking and obesity. *Spine* 14:501–506.

30. Deyo RA, Bigos SJ, Maravilla KR (1989): Diagnostic imaging procedures for the lumbar spine. *Ann Intern Med* 111(11):865–867.

31. Dillane JB, Fry J, Kalton G (1966): Acute back syndrome—a study from general practice *Br Med J* 2:82–84.

32. Editorial Reviews (1989): Risk factors for low back trouble. *Lancet* 1:1305–1306.

33. Fitzler SL, Berger RA (1982): Attitudinal change: the Chelsea back program. *Occup Health Saf* 51:24–26.

34. Fitzler SL, Berger RA (1983): Chelsea back program: one year later. *Occup Health Saf* 52:52–54.

35. Flynn JC, Hoque MA (1979): Anterior fusion of the lumbar spine. End-result study with long-term follow-up. *J Bone Joint Surg* [Am] 61:1143–1150.

36. Fordyce WE (1979): Use of the MMPI in the assessment of chronic pain. Clinical notes on the MMPI. In: Butcher M, Gynther B, Schofield W, eds. *Hoffman-Laroche monograph series* 3:1–13.

37. Frymoyer JW (1988): Back pain and sciatica. *N Engl J Med* 318:291–299.

38. Frymoyer JW, Pope MH, Clements JH, Wiler DG, MacPherson B, Ashikage T (1983): Risk factors in low-back pain. *J Bone Joint Surg* [Am] 65:213–218.

39. Frymoyer JW, Pope MH, Constanza MC, Rosen JC, Goggin JE, Wilder DG (1980): Epidemiologic studies of low-back pain. *Spine* 5:419–423.

40. Green M, Battié MC, Bigos SJ (1994): The role of acute back injuries in lower back pain. *J Spinal Disord* (submitted).

41. Greenough CG, Fraser RD (1989): The effects of compensation on recovery from low-back injury. *Spine* 14:947–955.

42. Greenwood JG (1985): Work related back and neck injury cases in West Virginia. *Orthop Rev* 14(2):53–61.

43. Gundewall B, Liljeqvist M, Hansson T (1993): Primary prevention of back symptoms and absence from work. A prospective randomized study among hospital employees. *Spine* 18(5):587–594.

44. Gyntelberg F (1974): One year incidence of low back pain among male residents of Copenhagen aged 40-59. *Dan Med Bull* 21:30–36.

45. Haber LD (1971): Disabling effects of chronic disease and impairment. *J Chronic Dis* 24:469–487.

46. Hanley EN Jr, Shapiro DE (1989): The development of low-back pain after excision of a lumbar disc. *J Bone Joint Surg* [Am] 71(5):719–21.

47. Heliövaara M (1987): Body height, obesity, and risk of herniated lumbar intervertebral disc. *Spine* 12:5:469–472.

48. Hellsing AL, Nordgren B, Shcéle R, Ahlborg B, Paulsson L (1986): Individual predictability of back trouble in 18-year-old men. *Manual Med* 2:72–76.

49. Hirsch C, Jonsson B, Lewin T (1969): Low back symptoms in a Swedish female population. *Clin Orthop* 63:171–176.

50. Hitselberger WE, Witten RM (1968): Abnormal myelograms in asymptomatic patients. *J Neurosurg* 28:204.

51. Hocking B, Thompson C: Chaos theory of occupational accidents. *J Occup Health Safety Aust NZ* 8:2:99–108, 1992.

52. Horal J (1969): The clinical appearance of low back pain disorders in the city of Gothenburg, Sweden. *Acta Orthop Scand* 118(Suppl):1–109.

53. Hrubec Z, Nashold BS Jr (1975): Epidemiology of lumbar disc lesions in the military in World War II. *Am J Epidemiol* 102:367–376.

54. Huddleson JH (1932): *Accidents, neuroses and compensation.* Baltimore: Williams and Wilkins.

55. Hult L (1954): Cervical, dorsal, and lumbar aspinal syndromes. *Acta Orthop Scand* 17(Suppl):1–102.

56. Hult L (1954): The Munksfors investigation. *Acta Orthop Scand* 16(Suppl):1–76.

57. Johansson JA (1994): The impact of decision latitude, psychological load and social support at work on musculoskeletal symptoms. *Eur J Public Health* (in press).

58. Johansson JA (1994): *Psychosocial factors at work and their relation to musculoskeletal symptoms* (Thesis). Göteborg, Sweden: Göteborg University.

59. Johansson JA (1994): Psychosocial work factors, physical work load and associated musculoskeletal symptoms among home care workers. *Scand J Psychol* 35:(in press).

60. Johansson JA (1994): Work-related and non-work-related musculoskeletal symptoms. *Appl Ergonom* 25:4:248–251.

61. Johansson JA, Nonas K (1994): Psychosocial and physical working conditions and associated musculoskeletal symptoms among operators in five plants using arc welding in robot stations. *Int J Hum Factors Manuf* 4:(in press).

62. Johansson JA, Rubenowitz S (1994): Risk indicators in the psychosocial and physical work environment for work-related neck, shoulder and low back symptoms: a study among blue- and white-collar workers in eight companies. *Scand J Rehab Med* 26.

63. Kane RL, Olsen D, Leymaster C, et al. (1974): Manipulating the patient. A comparison of the effectiveness of physician and chiropractor care. *Lancet* 1:1333.

64. Kelsey JL, White AA 3d (1980): Epidemiology and impact of low-back pain. *Spine* 5:133–142.

65. Keyserling WM, Herrin GD, Chaffin DB (1980): Establishing an industrial strength testing program. *Am Ind Hyg Assoc J* 41:730–736.

66. Keyserling WM, Herrin GD, Chaffin DB (1980): Isometric strength testing as a means of controlling medical incidents on strenuous jobs. *J Occup Med* 22:332–336.

67. Leavitt F (1992): The physical exertion factor in compensable work injuries. A hidden flaw in previous research. *Spine* 17:307–310.

68. Leavitt SS, Johnson TL, Beyer RD (1971): The process of recovery: patterns in industrial back injury. Part 1. Costs and the quantitative measures of effort. *Ind Med Surg* 40:7–14.

69. Leino P (1993): Does leisure time physical activity prevent low back disorders? A prospective study of metal industry employees. *Spine* 18(7):863–871.

70. Leino P (1989): Symptoms of stress predict musculoskeletal disorders. *J Epidemiol Community Health* 33:293–300.

71. Leino P, Aro S, Hasan J (1987): Trunk muscle function and low back disorders: a ten-year follow-up study. *J Chronic Dis* 40:289–296.

72. Leino P, Hasan J, Karppi S-L (1988): Occupational class, physical workload, and musculoskeletal morbidity in the engineering industry. *Br J Ind Med* 45:672–681.

73. Lindstrom I, Ohlund C, Eek C, Wallin L, Peterson L-E, Nachemson A (1989): *Work return and LBP disability: results of a prospective randomized study in an industrialized population.* Abstracts ISSLS Annual Meeting; Kyoto, Japan, May 15-19: p. 20.

74. Magnuson M, et al. (1990): The loads on the lumbar spine during work at an assembly line—the risks for fatigue injuries of the vertebral bodies. *Spine* 15(8):774–779.

75. Magora A (1970): Investigation of the relation between low back pain and occupation. II. Work history. *Ind Med Surg* 39:504–510.

76. Mostardi RA, Noe DA, Kovacik ME, Portfield JA (1992): Isokinetic lifting strength and occupational injury. A prospective study. *Spine* 17(2):189–193.

77. Nachemson AL (1982): The natural course of low back pain.

American Academy of Orthopaedic Surgeons symposium of idiopathic low back pain. St. Louis: Mosby, pp. 46–49.

78. Nachemson AL, Bigos SJ (1984): The low back. In: Cruess RL, Rennie WRJ, eds. *Adult orthopedics.* New York: Churchill Livingstone, pp. 843–937.

79. Partridge RE, Duthie JJR (1968): Rheumatism in dockers and civil servants. A comparison of heavy manual and sedentary workers. *Ann Rheum Dis* 27:559–568.

80. Porter R, Hibbert C, Wellman P (1980): Back-ache and the lumbar spine canal. *Spine* 5:99–105.

81. Porter R, Wicks M, Ottewell D (1978): Measurement of the spinal canal by diagnostic ultrasound. *J Bone Joint Surg* 60B:481–484.

82. Ready AE, Boreskie SL, Law SA, Russell R (1993): Fitness and lifestyle parameters fail to predict back injuries in nurses. *Can J Appl Phys* 18:1:80–90.

83. Riihimäki H, Mattson T, Zitting A, Wickstrom G, Hanninen K, Waris P (1990): Radiographic changes of the lumbar spine among concrete reinforcement workers and house painters. *Spine* 15(2):114–119.

84. Riihimäki H, Tola S, Videman T, et al. (1989): Low back pain and occupation. A cross-sectional questionnaire study of men in machine operating, dynamic physical work and sedentary work. *Spine* 14:204–209.

85. Riihimäki H, Videman T, Tola S (1989): Reliability of retrospective questionnaire data on the history of low back trouble. *ISSLS Abstracts,* Kyoto, Japan.

86. Roland M, Morris R (1983): A study of the natural history of low back pain. Part III. Development of guidelines for trials of treatment in primary care. *Spine* 8:145–150.

87. Rossignol M, Lortie M, Ledoux E (1993): Comparison of spinal health indicators in predicting spinal status in a 1-year longitudinal study. *Spine* 18:1:54–60.

88. Rothman RH (1984): A study of computer-assisted tomography: introduction. *Spine* 9:548.

89. Rowe ML (1969): Low back pain in industry. A position paper. *J Occup Med* 11:161–169.

90. Sachs BL, Sohail SA, LaCroix M, Olimpio D, Heath R, David J-A, Scala AD (1994): Objective assessment for exercise treatment on the B-200 isostation as part of work tolerance rehabilitation. A random prospective blind evaluation with comparison control population. *Spine* 19:49–51.

91. Sairanen E, Brüshaber L, Kaskinen M (1981): Felling work, low-back pain and osteoarthritis. *Scand J Work Environ Health* 7:18–30.

92. Snook SH, Campanelli RA, Hart JW (1982): Low back pain in industry. In: White AA, Gordon SL, eds. *Symposium on idiopathic low back pain.* St. Louis: Mosby, p. 23.

93. Social Security Statistical Supplement (1977–79) (1979): HE 3.3/3.979, Washington, DC. Government Printing Office.

94. Spengler DM, Bigos SJ, Martin NA, Zeh J, Fisher L, Nachemson A (1986): Back injuries in industry: a retrospective study. I. Overview and cost analysis. *Spine* 11:241–245.

95. Svensson HO, Andersson GBJ (1982): Low back pain in 40- to 47-year-old men. Frequency of occurrence and impact on medical services. *Scand J Rehabil Med* 14:47–53.

96. Svensson H-O, Andersson GBJ (1983): Low back pain in 40- to 47-year-old men: work history and work environment factors. *Spine* 8:272–276.

97. Taylor PJ (1968): Personal factors associated with sickness absence. A study of 194 men with contrasting sickness absence experience in a refinery population. *Br J Ind Med* 15:106–118.

98. Troup JD, Foreman TK, Baxter CE, Brown D (1987): Volvo award in clinical sciences: the perception of back pain and the role of psychophysical tests of lifting capacity. *Spine* 12:645–657.

99. Valkenburg HA, Haanen HCN (1982): The epidemiology of low back pain. In: White, AA, Gordon SL, eds. *Symposium on idiopathic low back pain.* St. Louis: CV Mosby, p. 9.

100. Vallfors B (1985): Acute, subacute and chronic low back pain: clinical symptoms, absenteeism and working environment. *Scand J Rehabil Med* 11:(Suppl)1–98.

101. Videman T, Nurminen M, Troup JDG (1990): Lumbar spinal pathology in cadaveric material in relation to history of back pain, occupation and physical loading. *Spine* 15:728–740.

102. Videman T, Rauhala H, Asp S (1989): Patient-handling skill, back injuries and back pain. An intervention study in nursing. *Spine* 14:148–156.

103. Vincente PJ (1988): The Nuprin report: a summary. Part I. *American Pain Society newsletter.*

104. Waddell G, McCulloch JA, Kummel E, et al. (1980): Nonorganic physical signs in low back pain. *Spine* 5:117–125.

105. Weber H (1983): Lumbar disc herniation: a controlled, prospective study with ten years of observation. *Spine* 8:131–140.

106. Wiesel SW, Feffer HL, Rothman RH (1984): Industrial low-back pain. A prospective evaluation of a standardized diagnostic and treatment protocol. *Spine* 9:199–203.

107. Wiesel SW, Tsourmas N, Feffer HL, Citrin CM, Patronas N (1984): A study of computer-assisted tomography: 1. The incidence of positive CAT scans in an asymptomatic group of patients. *Spine* 9:549–551.

108. Wiktorin C, et al. (1993): Validity of self-reported exposures to work postures and manual materials handling. *Scand J Work Environ Health* 19:208–214.

109. Wood DJ (1987): Design and evaluation of a back injury prevention program within a geriatric hospital. *Spine* 12:77–82.

110. World Health Organization (1986): *Epidemiology of work-related diseases and accidents.* Organization Technical Report Series 777. Copenhagen, Denmark.

The Adult Spine: Principles and Practice,
2nd edition, J.W. Frymoyer, Editor-in-Chief.
Lippincott-Raven Publishers, Philadelphia © 1997.

CHAPTER 10

Insuring Against Work Incapacity from Spinal Disorders

Nortin M. Hadler

Inability to support oneself or one's family is an age-old dread. Such individuals suffer the "illness of work incapacity."

THE HISTORY OF REDRESS FOR THE ILLNESS OF WORK INCAPACITY

The equally age-old remedies of charity, altruism, and philanthropy are as remarkable for their unevenness as for their magnanimity. In response to this dread, Poor Laws were first codified in Elizabethan England (12). These statutes required the nobility and landed gentry to identify the crippled and destitute on their lands and provide asylum care. Poor Laws represent the dawn of social legislation.

Just as they recognized a great human need, the Poor Laws also articulated a great Western scruple; only the deserving are to be helped—the unworthy are to be ferreted out. This stipulation is the first of the two great Western conundrums regarding redress for the illness of work incapacity. It survives today under the rubric of "disability determination."

Well into the eighteenth century, the exercise of distinguishing the worthy from the unworthy poor was pur-

sued with unconscionable zeal. Corporal punishment was specified for the malingerer or even "those whose defects make them an abomination." Under colonial American Poor Laws, a beggar, deemed by the gentry to be unworthy, could be "warned out of town" and punished upon returning with "36 lashes on the bare back if a man, 25 if a woman." The zeal tempered but the Poor Laws survived in Great Britain until they were finally superseded by the social insurance acts of 1911, shepherded through the Edwardian parliament by David Lloyd George. His condemnation of the Poor Laws, delivered in a speech at the Birmingham Town Hall on June 11, 1911, is memorable (7):

> You may say there is the poor law. Ah! Let me say this to the honour of the workers of this country, the last thing they pawn is their pride. There is no greater heroism in history as you find in the humble annals of those who fight through life against odds to maintain their self-respect and independence. They will suffer the last privation before they pin the badge of pauperism over their hearts, and certainly before they will put it on the breast of their children. . . .

So ended the English Poor Laws. They were a watershed in social consciousness, but the ethic they served was distorted by the often arbitrary nature of the determination of worthiness and the stigmatizing nature of their largesse. Besides, they were no match for the social ramifications of the industrial revolution. No longer was the worker's birthright and fate simply to work the land on which he was born; now he could or must seek em-

N. M. Hadler, M.D., F.A.C.P.: Professor of Medicine and Microbiology/Immunology, School of Medicine, University of North Carolina at Chapel Hill, Chapel Hill, North Carolina, 27599-7280; Attending Rheumatologist, University of North Carolina Hospitals, Chapel Hill, North Carolina.

ployment. Furthermore, it was held that the employer discharged all his responsibilities to the worker by payment of salary. Under common law, the employer was not liable even should the worker be injured or incapacitated on the job by virtue of three tenets (22):

1. Employment is voluntary. In accepting employment, the employee accepts the risks inherent in such employment.
2. If by his actions the employee contributes in any way to his accident, the employer is exonerated of all liability.
3. In 1837 Abinger articulated the "fellow servant" rule in the House of Lords, which was imported into Boston in 1842 by Judge Shaw: If a supervisor or other "fellow servant" intervenes between the intent of the employer and the injury of the worker, the supervisor and not the employer bears any liability. This rule effectively blocked nearly all redress for injured workers.

In 1862 a journalist, Henry Mayhew, published a collection of his essays as *London Labour and the London Poor,* which was recently republished by Dover Press (23). He had set out "to publish the history of a people, from the lips of the people themselves," the "people" being the street people of London. He argued that the numbers of such people were greatly underestimated, that civil law treated them in a prejudicial fashion, and that education was inaccessible to them. He urged compassion because it was the "effects of uncertain labour [that] drive the labourers to improvidence, recklessness, and pauperism." Mayhew, as did his contemporaries, categorized the street people into "those that will work, those that cannot work, and those that will not work." But Mayhew stood alone. Society was still wedded to a need to exclude the unworthy poor, "those that will not work," from compassion. And of those "that cannot work," the human cost of industrialization was weighing heavily on the community conscience. The injured worker, deprived of redress by the Abinger rule, was a voice not long to be denied (1).

The social reform legislated in Germany in 1884 under Bismarck and imported into England in 1897 under Russell Cecil, established two critical precedents: the continuing need to identify the unworthy by means of "disability determination," and the new need to single out those whose work incapacity is a consequence of accidental workplace injury for special treatment under Workers' Compensation programs. To this date in nearly all industrialized western countries, the latter category is maintained and the claimant so defined provided with considerably more redress and recompense. However, defining both "accident" and "injury" is the second great Western conundrum in providing redress for the illness of work incapacity.

THE SOCIOLOGY OF LOW BACK PAIN

The discussion that follows will explain the fashion in which industrialized countries provide redress for individuals who suffer the illness of work incapacity in the context of low back pain. It will become clear that the very act of seeking redress confounds the experience of backache. Prerequisite to this insight is an appreciation of the sociology and medical anthropology of the experience. The discussion will be restricted to individuals who are between the ages of 20 and 50, who suffer neither cauda equina syndrome nor severe leg weakness, whose backache was not precipitated by a discrete traumatic event involving external force, and who would be entirely well were it not for their backache. Such individuals suffer a regional backache; nearly every single one of us will join their ranks in the very near future according to several data sets.

For example, the Health in Detroit study was a pioneering survey of one adult from each of a probability sample of 589 white households in the Detroit metropolitan area conducted in 1978 and published by Verbrugge and Ascione in 1987 (26). After an initial interview, participants maintained a daily diary for 6 weeks up to the closing interview. During the 6-week period, the average adult had 16 symptomatic days; only 11% of men and 5% of women escaped symptom free. Musculoskeletal morbidity (Table 1) ranked second only to respiratory symptomatology. Nearly half the participants were experiencing musculoskeletal symptoms for 1 week out of 6! The quality of the experience and the response to this unfortunate happenstance are highlighted in Table 2.

Clearly, episodes of backache color our lives for more than a few days each year. Some of the episodes are of such impact, even import, that well over 10% of us can recall prolonged episodes occurring in the past year (5). Whenever we are faced with a backache, when we realize that the simplest of locomotor tasks can be confounded by increased pain, we have a *predicament* (11). There are three options available to us (Fig. 1). We have no choice but to consider these options, choose among them, and act accordingly. This sequence I have termed "processing the predicament."

The vast majority of the people sampled in the Health in Detroit survey chose to cope with their regional backache by relying on their personal resources (Table 2). This is advisable behavior (16), as the outcomes with the other alternatives are far more problematic. After all, the

TABLE 1. *The Health in Detroit survey: Incidence of musculoskeletal morbidity in 6 weeks (ref. 26)*

People experiencing musculoskeletal symptoms	51%
Days with musculoskeletal symptoms	11%
Average duration of symptoms	8 days

TABLE 2. *The Health in Detroit survey: Characteristics of people with musculoskeletal symptoms (26)*

The majority:
were suffering back or leg pain
were otherwise asymptomatic
thought they had "arthritis"
talked to their spouse
consumed OTC remedies
thought their symptoms were "not very serious"
Less than 10%:
experienced neck or hand pain
thought their symptoms were "very serious"
sought medical care (3%)
received medical care (0.3%)

majority of these predicaments remit spontaneously, albeit after challenging the sense of invincibility of more than one person so afflicted. Whether the average person can maintain sufficient self-confidence to cope within his personal sphere is itself problematic. Care, based usually on unproven remedies, is offered with conviction and a sense of urgency if not alarm by physicians and a myriad of alternative care givers. The sufferer is a market and the target of pervasive marketing in the United States.

One alternative is to cease to be a person with a predicament of backache and visit a physician. The moment one visits a physician, one is no longer a person with a predicament; one becomes a patient with the illness of backache. Although there are arguments questioning the approach (14,20), much of the interaction between the patient and physician relates to defining the cause of the backache in the hopes of effecting a cure. Backache is one of the most frequently encountered illnesses in office practice (6). The likelihood of a valid diagnosis of the underlying disease is exceedingly small; the likelihood of a diagnosis that leads to specific and reliably palliative intervention is vanishingly rare (11,25). Nonetheless,

contemporary medicine is wedded to this exercise for reasons that range from the self-serving to the service of the occasional patient who is benefited. Many of the chapters in this volume attempt to take the contemporary diagnostic and therapeutic posture to task. Furthermore, since the traditional approach to diagnosis and therapy is seldom definitive but often sacrificing of time, money, and healthfulness, the patient with the persistent incapacitating backache can well find himself afflicted with a confounding chronic illness, the illness of work incapacity. This fate, and the quest for a disability pension, will occupy our attention shortly.

There is a third option available to many with backache. If they perceive their backache to be a consequence of usage on the job, they can seek medical care as redress under Workers' Compensation statutes in all states and in most industrial countries. In so doing, they are no longer people with the predicament of regional backache; they transform into claimants with an injured back. Here the fate of a small percentage is also the chronic illness of work incapacity.

Between 1971 and 1975, the United States Health and Nutrition Examination Survey (HANES I) was carried out on a sample of noninstitutionalized adults (1). One segment of the survey involved a detailed history and physical examination of 6,913 adults aged 25 to 74 years. Table 3 presents the prevalence of backache lasting at least 1 month and occurring within 2 years of the survey. Table 3 also yields some insights into the magnitude of the risk of the illness of work incapacity 25 years ago. It is clear from the chapters that precede this one that the likelihood of choosing to be a claimant with a back injury and of suffering the illness of work incapacity has accelerated dramatically; it is equally clear that the likelihood of suffering the predicament or the illness of backache has not accelerated. After all, the predicament was already ubiquitous and the illness already overwhelmingly

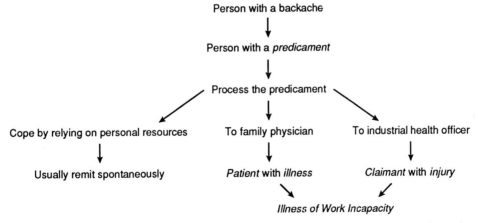

FIG. 1. Nearly all of us will be faced with low back pain in the near future and repeatedly throughout our lives. Those of us with regional backaches will be confronted with a predicament with every episode. We must choose among the options in this algorithm.

TABLE 3. *Prevalence of backache and consequent incapacity in the HANES I Survey (5)*

	Number
Total household sample	6,913
Recalled >1 month of backache in past 2 years	1,189
Recalled incapacity from axial pain	389
with moderate/severe restrictions	69
causing a job change	63
necessitating >5 days off work	55

common in medical practice. Something has perturbed the processing, and that something is the quest of the remainder of this chapter.

THE WORKERS' COMPENSATION PARADIGM

The turn of the century saw the rise of organized labor. Fueling the movement throughout the industrial world was the unconscionable lot of the average worker. Near the top of the list of grievances was the plight of workers who had been rendered "worthy poor" as a consequence of injuries suffered on the job. The Prussian statutes established the precedent for offering special treatment to such individuals. All 58 American Workers' Compensation jurisdictions offer an exclusive, no-fault remedy to those who suffer a personal injury that arises "out of and in the course of employment and occurred by accident." Such individuals are afforded medical care, suffer little financial compromise while mending, and are compensated, in theory, for any permanent loss of wage earning capacity. The vast majority of claimants have suffered discrete traumatic events such as lacerations, amputations, and the like. For these individuals, Workers' Compensation provides an efficient remedy, which has provoked little controversy and relatively little consternation regarding the cost/benefit ratio of the program up to the present. The controversies relate to coverage for "occupational diseases" and for disorders where the precipitant is less discrete or less overtly work related. The latter category includes such illnesses as "stress on the job," "cumulative trauma disorders" (11), and the like. The illness that has come to dominate in this regard is the regional backache. The compensable backache is a challenge for clinical medicine (8,10), econometrics (28), and labor relations (2). The challenge relates to two pivotal determinations, both of which masquerade as clinical constructs:

When is a regional backache an injury? Prior to World War II, regional backache was seldom conceptualized by the sufferer or by society as an "injury." Medicine provided an inventive differential diagnosis, but trauma was felt to be improbable. In 1934, two surgeons, Mixter and Barr (24), first described the syndrome of discal hernia-

tion in a series of patients, many of whom had cauda equina syndrome and several of whom improved following surgical intervention. They suggested that herniation was a common cause of regional backache, often amenable to surgical intervention. Their hypothesis took hold rapidly in the United States and began to pervade the remainder of the industrial world. At least as dramatic was the implication of their label for the disease, "rupture" of the disc. Everywhere, the judiciary held that if the clinical result was so violent as to be a "rupture," the details of the causal event should not be determinative of the accidental nature of the illness. In this fashion, regional backache became back injury, and backache occurring on the job and ascribed to discal herniation became compensable (15).

This line of reasoning dominates the administration of the American Workers' Compensation programs even today (27); a regional backache diagnosed as a ruptured disc almost always elicits an award from Workers' Compensation. That is not the case in other countries (13,17,19,21). Both New Zealand and Switzerland insure their entire adult populations separately for the clinical consequences of injury, regardless of work relatedness, with benefits that include medical care and compensation for lost wages. New Zealand provides ready, usually uncontested access to very short term benefits; Switzerland offers a severe gauntlet to access in terms of the assertion of accidental cause of the backache, but once access is gained, benefits are more liberal. France demands sudden onset at work corroborated by a witness before providing liberal benefits. These programmatic distinctions all reflect the need to come to grips with the issue of causality if one wishes to umbrella regional backache under a Workers' Compensation paradigm.

When is the worker's back injury as healed as it is likely to get? All schemes for redress for the illness of work incapacity encourage, support, even nurture the possibilities of healing and of sufficient recovery to return to gainful employment. Many schemes, particularly Workers' Compensation schemes, will expend considerable sums on medical care and income substitution as long as steady progress is being made or is likely to be made on the road to clinical recovery. The intent is noble. The pitfalls are obvious: therapeutic zeal is potentially unbridled and motivation toward rapid recovery is tested. The point of maximum healing is termed "fixed and stable" in the United States and often "consolidation" elsewhere. Its definition can be quite contentious, invoking the opinions of "independent medical examiners" (IMEs) in the United States, the "expert" in France, and sundry similar mechanisms in other jurisdictions (17). The IME is an expensive solution sharing all the shortcomings we shall discuss for contracted examinations in disability insurance schemes. Its supporters ar-

gue that it is more humane than the fixed cut-off employed by some countries.

DISABILITY INSURANCE SCHEMES

The distinction between a disabling backache and a disabling back injury is not trivial. In most countries, with notable exceptions such as Holland (17), disabling injuries that arise out of and in the course of employment are traditionally afforded more generous and more comprehensive benefits than similarly disabling illnesses whose pathogenesis is unrelated to employment. The distinction was drawn from the outset of the social legislation and is nowhere more dramatic than in the United States, where nearly half a century was to pass between writing Workers' Compensation statutes and national disability insurance.

"The American people," declared President Franklin D. Roosevelt in a message to Congress June 9, 1934,

want some safeguard against misfortunes which cannot be wholly eliminated in this man-made world of ours . . . I am looking for a sound means which I can recommend to provide at once security against several of the great disturbing factors in life—especially those which relate to unemployment and old age.

The issue of national disability insurance smoldered for nearly 20 years, awaiting the political opportunities of the early Eisenhower administration. In 1954, Social Security Disability Insurance (SSDI) was established. Wages were assessed, employers contributed, and the monies accumulated in a separate fund that was restricted, until recently, to the payment of disability benefits. Requirements as to how long or how much one must contribute to the Disability Insurance fund to be eligible for benefits in the event of disability have changed since 1954. Obviously, workers may become disabled after contributing for brief periods and some individuals with work incapacity may never have contributed. Rather than totally liberalize SSDI, the federal government assumed administration of the Supplemental Security Income (SSI) program in 1973. This program insures those who are ineligible for SSDI because of inadequate contributions and draws on general tax revenues.

The intent of SSDI/SSI is quite different from Workers' Compensation insurance (10,21); this program insures against poverty consequent to any illness, whereas Workers' Compensation insurance is designed with income substitution as a goal. To be eligible for SSDI/SSI one must be incapable of "any substantial gainful activity by reason of any medically determinable physical or mental impairment or impairments which can be expected to result in death or which have lasted, or can be expected to last, for a continuous period of not less than 12 months" (20 Code of Federal Regulations 404.1501).

Defining "substantial gainful activity" is administratively straightforward: the current operational definition is $300 per month. In other words, one must be so ill that he cannot earn even $300 per month in any job anywhere within reason. As we discussed above, these programs are attempting to ferret out the "unworthy," those who simply "will not work," and they therefore must establish some definition of the prerequisite illness. SSDI/SSI borrows from a tradition in Workers' Compensation that even Workers' Compensation administrations have largely abandoned—using impairment as the surrogate measure. Impairment "results from anatomical, physiological or psychological abnormalities which are demonstrable by medically acceptable clinical and laboratory diagnostic techniques. . . (Symptoms) are, alone, insufficient. . . ." (20 Code of Federal Regulations 404.1501). SSDI/SSI is attempting to establish quantifiable criteria for pathoanatomical abnormalities that are assumed to be highly sensitive and specific for the most severe illness of work incapacity rendering one incapable of earning even $300 per month (9). The criteria to be satisfied in order for a regional backache to qualify as disabling are given as Figure 2. If these criteria are met along with a determination that the claimant cannot maintain "substantial gainful employment," an award should follow. This is seldom the case (3); the vast majority of claimants are denied and share the fate of many disabled under Workers' Compensation. These individuals enter the contest of disability determination wherein they have to prove they are dreadfully ill.

THE CONTEST OF DISABILITY DETERMINATION

Every disability program, whether a Workers' Compensation program or an invalid pension program such as SSDI/SSI, defines disability as free from volition. If one has the choice to return to work, he is ineligible. How does one prove to the administrators that his quest for a pension relates to forces outside his control, that derive from his illness? In truth, impairment short of pathoanatomical catastrophe (such as coma) is seldom totally determinative of incapacity. In fact, as reviewed by Bigos

---

C. Other vertebrogenic disorders (e.g., herniated nucleus pulposus, spinal stenosis) with the following persisting for at least 3 months despite prescribed therapy and expected to last 12 months. With both 1 and 2:
  1. Pain, muscle spasm, and significant limitation of motion in the spine; AND
  2. Appropriate radicular distribution of significant motor loss with muscle weakness and sensory and reflex loss.

FIG. 2. Section 1.05C of the Social Security Administration's Handbook for Physicians. This is the "listing" for disabling regional backache.

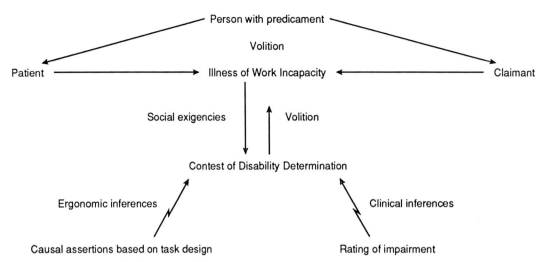

FIG. 3. The contest of disability determination. Whether patient or claimant, any individual faced with the illness of work incapacity may feel disaffected, bereft of any option other than to seek redress from a disability insurance scheme. Absent catastrophe, largesse is never readily forthcoming. The claimant has to prove illness beyond some preconceived notions of validity and veracity. The compensation claimant may also have to prove work-relatedness of the pathogenesis of the illness of work incapacity.

and Battié in Chapter 9, social exigencies in the workplace are major variables contributing to the processing of the predicament of backache as an injury claim (Fig. 1). Disability determination is not a bureaucratic fiat, it is a dynamic contest that places the claimant on the defensive. The claimant has to prove he is ill. Unsuspecting, under the mantle of social redress, with the encouragement of bureaucratic minions, physicians, and adjudicators, the claimant enters a contest that is itself iatrogenic. How can one possibly improve or heal if he has to prove he's ill (Fig. 3)? In SSDI/SSI to the extreme (4), but in all schemes to some extent (18), physicians will be testing the veracity of the claimant against invalid, unreliable standards, many of which are reviewed in Chapter 11 by Waddell, Allan, and Newton. The claimant under Workers' Compensation has the additional challenge of proving that his regional backache is an injury in the face of assertions and contentions based on marginal ergonomic data as reviewed by Bigos and Battié in Chapter 9. The entire unwieldy contest takes on a life of its own in which all parties seem to benefit except the claimant whose illness is so confounded that rehabilitation programs (Chapter 14) and pain clinics (Chapter 17) await him.

In SSDI/SSI, the claimant with a backache almost always loses the first round of the contest, played out before agency bureaucrats who review clinical records attempting to define impairment and apply the "substantial gainful employment" rule. Often the agency will purchase objective clinical data, the so-called "contracted examination," from a physician other than the claimant's physician. Over 250,000 contracted examinations are purchased each year. When analyzed as to their

intellectual content, it is clear that contracted examinations for backache are not clinical exercises in that they give little if any weight to the claimant's symptoms in assessing his disability; physical signs and radiographic findings hold sway (4). As reviewed in Chapter 9 and elsewhere (29), tying disability determination to impairment criteria is invalid. Without acknowledging this truth by programmatic change, SSDI/SSI has created a second level of the contest. Once denied by the agency (the fate of some 80% of claimants), there is ready recourse before an Administrative Law Judge in the Social Security Administration. Here the rules of the contest are expanded to permit the expression of symptoms, the corroboration of witnesses to the illness including the treating physicians, and the assistance of attorneys. Over 50% of contests are won before the Administrative Law Judge (9).

Disability insurance schemes are mandatory in an enlightened world. They must be made readily accessible and they must be salutary. We are now completing a century of experimentation and false starts. Let us hope the next generation of programs will show that the lessons have been learned.

REFERENCES

1. Bohlen FH (1912): A problem in the drafting of workmen's compensation acts. *Harvard Law Review* 25:328–348.
2. Burton JF (1985): Disability benefits for back disorders in workers' compensation. In: Hadler NM, Gillings DB, eds. *Arthritis and society.* London: Butterworths, pp. 89–103.
3. Carey TS, Hadler NM (1986): The role of the primary physician in disability determination for Social Security Insurance and Workers' Compensation. *Ann Intern Med* 104:706–710.

4. Carey TS, Hadler NM, Gillings D, Stinnett S, Wallston T (1988): Medical disability assessment of the back pain patient for the Social Security Administration: the weighting of presenting clinical features. *J Clin Epidemiol* 41:691–697.

5. Cunningham LS, Kelsey JL (1984): Epidemiology of musculoskeletal impairments and associated disability. *Am J Public Health* 74: 574–579.

6. Cypress BK (1983): Characteristics of physician visits for back symptoms: a national perspective. *Am J Public Health* 73:389–395.

7. Grigg J (1978): *Lloyd George: The people's champion, 1902-1911.* London: Eyre Methuen.

8. Hadler NM (1978): Legal ramifications of the medical definition of back disease. *Ann Intern Med* 89:992–999.

9. Hadler NM (1982): Medical ramifications of the federal regulation of the Social Security Disability Insurance program: Social Security and medicine. *Ann Intern Med* 96:665–669.

10. Hadler NM (1984): Occupational illness. The issue of causality. *J Occup Med* 26:587–593.

11. Hadler NM (1993): *Occupational musculoskeletal disorders.* New York: Raven Press, 1–273.

12. Hadler NM (1984): Who should determine disability? *Semin Arthritis Rheum* 14:45–51.

13. Hadler NM (1986): Industrial rheumatology. The Australian and New Zealand experiences with arm pain and backache in the workplace. *Med J Aust* 144:191–195.

14. Hadler NM (1986): Regional back pain [Editorial]. *N Engl J Med* 315:1090–1092.

15. Hadler NM (1987): Regional musculoskeletal diseases of the low back. Cumulative trauma versus single incident. *Clin Orthop Relat Res* (221):33–41.

16. Hadler NM (1988): The predicament of backache [Editorial]. *J Occup Med* 30:449–450.

17. Hadler NM (1989): Disabling backache in France, Switzerland, and the Netherlands: contrasting sociopolitical constraints on clinical judgment. *J Occup Med* 31:823–831.

18. Hadler NM (1992): Impairment rating in disability determination for low back pain: placing the AMA guides and the Quebec Institute Report into perspective. In: Burton J, ed. *Workers' Compensation desk book.* Horsham, PA: LRP Press.

19. Hadler NM (1994): Disabling backache in Japan. *J Occup Med* 36: 1110–1114.

20. Hadler NM (1994): The injured worker and the internist. *Ann Intern Med* 120:163–164.

21. Hadler NM (1995): Disabling backache—An international perspective. *Spine* 20:640–649.

22. Larson A (1972): *The law of workmen's compensation.* New York: Matthew Bender, section 4.30, pp. 25–32.

23. Mayhew H (1983): *London labour and the London poor,* vols. 1–4. London: Dover Press.

24. Mixter WJ, Barr JS (1934): Rupture of the intervertebral disc with involvement of the spinal canal. *N Engl J Med* 211:210–215.

25. Quebec Task Force on Spinal Disorders (1987): Scientific approach to the assessment and management of activity-related spinal disorders. A monograph for clinicians. Report of the Quebec Task Force on Spinal Disorders. *Spine* 12:S1–S59.

26. Verbrugge LM, Ascione FJ (1987): Exploring the iceberg. Common symptoms and how people care for them. *Med Care* 25:539–569.

27. Webster BS, Snook SH (1994): The cost of 1989 Workers' Compensation low back pain claims. *Spine* 19:1111–1116.

28. Worrall JD, Appel D (1987): The impact of Workers' Compensation benefits on low-back claims. In: Hadler NM, ed. *Clinical concepts in regional musculoskeletal illness.* Orlando: Grune & Stratton, pp. 281–298.

29. Yelin E, Meenan R, Nevitt M, Epstein W (1980): Work disability in rheumatoid arthritis: effects of disease, social, and work factors. *Ann Intern Med* 93:551–556.

The Adult Spine: Principles and Practice,
2nd edition, J.W. Frymoyer, Editor-in-Chief.
Lippincott-Raven Publishers, Philadelphia © 1997.

CHAPTER 11

Clinical Evaluation of Disability in Low Back Pain

Gordon Waddell, David B. Allan, and Mary Newton

Severity is one of the fundamental characteristics of any disease. Severity of symptoms and their interference with lifestyle are of fundamental importance both to the patient and to society, particularly in a chronic condition. Medical decisions about treatment, judgments of outcome, prognosis, and compensation awards all depend to some extent on assessment of severity.

Severity can be assessed clinically in terms of diagnosis, pain, disability, physical impairment, and ability to work. In most chronic disorders with a clearly understood and demonstrable pathologic basis—such as osteoarthritis of the hip—these can all be assessed reliably and different experts will agree. The patient's report of pain, disability, and ability to work is usually proportionate to the diagnosis and the objective physical findings. In a poorly understood condition such as chronic

G. Waddell, D.Sc., M.D., F.R.C.S.: Professor, Department of Orthopaedic Surgery, Western Infirmary, Glasgow G11 6NT, Scotland.
D. B. Allan, M.B., Ch.B., F.R.C.S.: Orthopaedic Department, Southern General Hospital, Glasgow G51 4TF, Scotland.
M. Newton, M.Ed., M.C.S.P.: Department of Physiotherapist, Clydebank Health Center, Clydebank G81, Scotland.

low back pain, however, where it is frequently impossible to make any pathologic diagnosis and may even be difficult to identify any physical basis for the patient's continuing symptoms, there is no generally agreed upon method of assessing low back disability or lumbar impairment. Yet, in view of the human, medical, and economic impact of low back pain, and despite the practical difficulties, medical assessment of severity is essential.

AN HISTORICAL PERSPECTIVE ON LOW BACK PAIN AND DISABILITY

Back pain is not new. Back pain has affected human beings throughout recorded history and probably long before. What is new is chronic disability due to simple low back pain. This historical background has been reviewed by Allan and Waddell (2).

The history of low back disability is closely linked to compensation legislation, and most modern definitions of disability imply a relationship to compensation. But it is wrong to imply that disability was caused by compensation. Indeed, the converse is true and compensation legislation was passed only after the need was recognized.

Our present forms of social insurance for sickness and

injury originated from the social, industrial, and medical revolutions of the nineteenth century. But compensation seems to be one of the earliest social and legal characteristics of civilization. Compensation predates written history, and examples such as the Code of Hammurabi (circa 1750 B.C.) and the Law of Moses (circa 800 B.C.) still survive. But these dealt purely with serious physical mutilation such as loss of a limb or an eye and there was certainly no compensation for back pain.

During the nineteenth century there was growing awareness of the social responsibility to care for the sick and disabled. The turning point was the building of the railroads which led to loss of life and limb, both by railway workers and to a lesser extent by passengers, on a scale previously unprecedented except in war. Public anxiety led to legislation making the railway companies responsible for accidents and this made it possible for the injured person to seek financial compensation through the courts. But fault still had to be proved and even by 1886 only 24% of accident victims made any claim and only 12% received any compensation.

The limitations of this system led to Workmen's Compensation legislation in most Western countries at the end of the nineteenth and the beginning of the twentieth century. This provided compensation regardless of fault and without redress to the courts. It was gradually extended to cover all workers and industrial diseases as well as accidents. Since that time, financial provision for disability has increasingly become a matter of social provision by the state, applying to all citizens. The right to civil litigation for additional compensation remains, but state benefits in one form or another now provide most of the support for the chronically sick and disabled.

These changes in the legal framework have been paralleled by and influenced by changed medical ideas about back pain. Two key concepts in the nineteenth century had a fundamental and lasting effect on our understanding of back pain: that back pain came from the spine and that it resulted from injury. Before that time back pain was regarded as one of life's "fleeting pains" or "rheumatics." In 1828, a paper on "spinal irritation" suggested for the first time that the vertebral column and the nervous system itself could be the source of back pain (11). It described a syndrome in young women which emphasized spinal tenderness and included a constellation of symptoms, many of which would now be regarded as psychosomatic. The concept of spinal irritation swept Europe and the U.S. and had a profound effect on medical thinking for nearly 30 years. The exact pathology was never shown and the diagnosis gradually disappeared. But the idea that the spine itself could be a source of pain was firmly established and the feeling that a painful spine must somehow be irritable remains to this day.

There can be few more distressing episodes in the history of back pain than the condition known as "railway spine" (17). This brought together the spate of railway accidents, the new compensation laws, and the concept of spinal irritation. By analogy with serious fracture dislocations of the spine, it was suggested that simple back pain might result from more minor injury or even cumulative trauma. It is difficult to appreciate today, but back pain was never previously regarded as a result of trauma. Since railway spine, back pain has been firmly linked to the idea of injury.

These medical ideas had profound social effects. By 1915, it was noted that "pain in the back as a result of injury is (now) the most frequent affection for which compensation is demanded from the casualty companies" (27). In the 1990s, low back pain is the largest single cause of chronic disability in the working years of life. We now have an epidemic of chronic disability resulting from low back pain in all Western societies.

Medical evidence is part of the basis for every legal or administrative decision about compensation for low back disability. But the limitations of that evidence have long been recognized; at least since 1916, "lawyers and judges appear to have a pretty generally formed opinion that a doctor's statement concerning disability of the lower back is largely a matter of guesswork" (72). Little has changed and there is clearly still a need to improve medical evidence in low back disorders.

DEFINITIONS

Pain and disability are not synonymous. Pain is a highly personal and subjective experience that can be communicated only poorly across the barriers of language. The best available definition is that adopted by the International Association for the Study of Pain: "An unpleasant sensory and emotional experience associated with actual or potential tissue damage, or described in terms of such damage" (43).

Unfortunately, every legislative and administrative body has felt the need to introduce its own terms and definitions for impairment, loss of faculty, disability, disablement, and handicap (16,73). The distinction between disability, disablement, and handicap is blurred and confused. But whatever the terminology of each system, the key concepts are physical impairment and disability. Impairment and disability are fundamentally different. The World Health Organization definition of impairment in general is "any loss or abnormality of psychological, physiological or anatomical structure or function" (73). In practical clinical terms, physical impairment is pathological, anatomical, or physiological abnormality of structure or function leading to loss of normal bodily ability (3,21,64). Disability is the resulting "diminished capacity for everyday activities and gainful employment" or the "limitation of a patient's performance compared to a fit person's of the same age and sex" (16,21,64). Impairment is assessed on objective structural limitation and is solely a medical responsibility. Disability is assessed largely on the patient's subjective report. The patient's subjective report of pain and disability must be clearly distinguished from the physician's objective assessment of physical impairment. Disability rating and compensation awards, however, are ultimately an administrative or legal, not a medical, responsibility, and are based on both the patient's report of disability and the physician's assessment of impairment. In practice, financial compensation is mainly but not exclusively for incapacity for work.

It is worth considering physical impairment in greater detail. The definition given above includes two fundamentally different aspects of impairment: pathological or anatomical loss or abnormality of structure and physiological loss or limitation of function. Many social security systems, like the U.S. Bureau of Disability Insurance (60), specify that impairment should be "demonstrable by medically acceptable clinical and laboratory diagnostic techniques," the main requirement being that it should be demonstrable or objective. In practice, and from this perspective, medical evaluation has emphasized anatomical or structural impairment, that is, tissue damage (62). In the context of pain, however, physiological loss and limitation of function may be equally important and still meet the definition of physical impairment, with the important proviso that any such functional limitation should again be objectively demonstrable on clinical evaluation.

THE MEDICAL EVIDENCE

It is a useful and instructive discipline to regard each piece of the medical data as evidence and to consider how well it would stand up to cross-examination in a court of law. Clinically, just as much as scientifically or legally, we should be able to substantiate our assessment.

Diagnosis

Diagnosis of pathology provides the clinical basis for medical treatment and prognosis. It also determines when rehabilitation is complete and what abnormality or loss may be considered permanent. Diagnosis gives a broad classification of the severity of the injury or disease, but different patients may be affected to widely varying degrees and it is illogical to rate equally all patients with a particular diagnosis. The more fundamental limitation is that in most patients with low back pain, it is impossible to reach any definite diagnosis. Diagnosis of injury to the bones or nerves of the spine is accurate and different doctors will reliably agree. Medical assessment of nerve root dysfunction is also accurate and reliable but this only applies in the minority of low back

disorders with nerve root pain. Clinical examination of the spine itself is much less satisfactory. Plain radiographs of the spine provide information about fractures but radiological changes of degeneration bear little relationship to low back pain. For these reasons, diagnosis and x-ray changes are of limited value in assessing the severity of most patients with uncomplicated low back pain.

Pain

Clinical practice emphasizes pain and most physicians and health professionals spend much of their working life treating pain. Some research workers have even suggested that the patient's report of back pain is the only possible measure of severity. But this is a naive oversimplification. When we see the complexity of pain and the difficulty of even defining pain, it is not surprising that we find pain difficult to measure in practice. Medical attempts to grade the severity of pain even as mild, moderate, or severe (1) have very limited usefulness and bear little relationship to any pathophysiologic change or to the patient's own assessment. They appear to be heavily influenced by objective pathology and impairment rather than pain. They are more the physician's estimate of what the pain should be and are prone to observer variation and bias. In principle, it must be accepted that only the sufferer can assess the severity of pain, accepting always the qualification that such a purely subjective assessment is open to psychological or conscious bias and must be compared with other more objective measures.

Disability

Disability can be defined and assessed much more readily than pain. It is agreed by a number of research groups around the world that in clinical practice, disability is best assessed on activities of daily living (6,18,44,53,64). These provide a basic and direct measure of function. The activities of daily living generally restricted by low back disorders include bending and lifting, sitting, standing, walking, travelling, social activities, sleep, sex life, and dressing, particularly putting on footwear. The level of disability in these basic activities can be applied to work, home, and leisure activities. Clinical questions about low back disability can be clear, precise, and easily understood and provide a very reliable and accurate assessment of disability as reported by the patient.

Physical Impairment

Assessment of impairment in an amputee is objective, standardized, and readily agreed upon between different medical experts. In low back pain, in contrast, clinical assessment of lumbar impairment is ill defined, observations are frequently subjective, and there may be wide disagreement between observers. Because of these practical problems, objective assessment of lumbar impairment is disparaged by some research workers. But some form of objective confirmation of the patient's report of pain and disability is logically, pragmatically, and legally indispensable.

These criticisms necessitate a fundamental reconsideration of how we assess lumbar impairment. First, physical impairment must by definition be based on objective physical characteristics of the low back disorder. Second, we must use reliable methods of clinical assessment (47,66). Third, these methods should also provide a real and valid measure of that particular physical characteristic. Objective physical characteristics should be clearly defined, specifically related to low back disorders, and should distinguish patients with low back pain from asymptomatic people. Some clinical signs such as standard neurological findings of nerve compression meet all these criteria. But many methods of clinical examination that are still routinely used are quite unreliable (39), and better techniques must be developed (48,70). Some, such as clinical tests of the sacroiliac joint (51) and many osteopathic palpations (8), are so unreliable that they should be discarded.

In addition, physical findings must be objective and psychological factors or conscious exaggeration must be excluded from the assessment of impairment. Much of physical examination consists of maneuvers that deliberately elicit pain, and the way that a patient reacts to examination is influenced by that individual's emotional response to pain and by any psychological disturbance. How patients respond to examination may also be modified by conscious or unconscious exaggeration related to a claim for compensation. Such psychological or conscious features must be clearly distinguished from the objective physical characteristics of impairment and a number of cross-checks must be built into the examination.

Work Loss

Work loss is the most important social and economic consequence of low back pain, although absence from work is influenced by many factors other than pain and disability. Accurate information about loss of time from work or modification of work is readily available and easily checked from the employer and sickness records. There is rarely any difficulty in assessing how much work time has been lost; the difficulty is in judging whether this is reasonable and what work capacity should be, now and in the future.

METHODS OF CLINICAL ASSESSMENT

Pain

A brief review of the assessment of pain has been prepared by Main and Waddell (32). The factors to be assessed are:

1. Time pattern: acute, recurring, or chronic. Acute and chronic pain are fundamentally different in kind (58,61). Acute pain bears a straightforward relationship to peripheral stimulus and tissue damage. There may be some anxiety about the meaning and consequences of the pain, but acute pain, acute disability, and acute illness behavior are usually proportionate to the physical findings. Chronic pain and chronic disability, in contrast, become increasingly dissociated from the physical problem and there may indeed be very little evidence of any remaining tissue damage. Instead, chronic pain and disability become associated with emotional distress, depression, disease conviction, and illness behavior. The chronic pain patient seems to adapt to chronic invalidity. Assessment of chronic pain must therefore include psychological and behavioral factors.

2. Anatomical pattern of pain. The pattern of pain is relevant to both diagnosis and assessment of severity. Patients may have back pain alone or associated with referred pain in the leg(s). True unilateral nerve root pain extending to the foot, approximating to a dermatomal pattern and often associated with sensory symptoms such as numbness or paresthesia, must be distinguished from the commoner, poorly localized, aching sclerotomal pain that may be referred to one or both buttocks or thighs. Neurogenic claudication is a specific description of radicular nerve root pain or neurological symptoms with a characteristic relationship to walking. Nonanatomical descriptions of whole leg pain, numbness, or giving way are more likely to be behavioral symptoms (63,65) and should be distinguished from the physical assessment (Table 1).

3. Pain scale. The simplest and most useful clinical method of measuring the severity of pain is some form of visual analogue pain scale (12,24,57) (Fig. 1). It is simple to administer and to score. The major difficulty is how to interpret what the pain scale measures. It is in no sense an absolute or objective measure of pain and it bears very little relationship to any physiological or pathological change. The patient's report of pain may include physical sensation, psychological distress, pain behavior, and communication. With these qualifications, it is obviously important not to overinterpret the pain scale but to accept it simply as a measure of how bad the patient tells the doctor the pain is. Words may be used to anchor the line at either end or numbers may be added below the line. A diagram of a thermometer may be used to clarify the concept of a scale (Fig. 1).

TABLE 1. *A comparison of the symptoms and signs of physical disease and abnormal illness behavior in chronic low back pain*

	Physical disease/ normal illness behaviour	Abnormal illness behaviour
Symptoms		
Pain	Anatomical distribution	Whole leg pain
		Tailbone pain
Numbness	Dermatomal	Whole leg numbness
Weakness	Myotomal	Whole leg giving way
Time pattern	Varies with time	Never free of pain
Response to treatment	Variable benefit	Intolerance of treatments
		Emergency admissions to hospital
Signs		
Tenderness	Anatomical distribution	Superficial
		Widespread, nonanatomic
Axial loading	No lumbar pain	Lumbar pain
Simulated rotation	No lumbar pain	Lumbar pain
Straight-leg raising	Limited on distraction	Improves with distraction
Sensory	Dermatomal	Regional
Motor	Myotomal	Regional, jerky, giving way

Adapted from ref. 63, with permission.

4. Pain ratings. Verbal rating scales are frequently used to describe the severity of pain (Table 2). It is, however, difficult to define the exact severity of each adjective used and the steps on the scale may not be equal. The fundamental limitation of both a visual analogue scale and the rating of pain severity is that no unidimensional scale can adequately reflect the complexity of the pain experience.

5. Pain descriptions. The quality of the pain can be assessed to some extent by the use of descriptive adjectives. The most widely used method is the McGill Pain Questionnaire (41). This was originally administered as an interview but is now usually given as a self-report questionnaire. The adjectives used to describe the pain

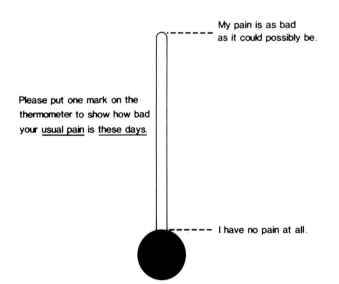

FIG. 1. The pain scale. The scale should be exactly 100 mm long, and the level marked by the patient is scored as a percentage. (From ref. 62, with permission.)

can be broadly separated into sensory and affective dimensions that provide some assessment of different qualities of the pain. A short-form McGill Pain Questionnaire has since been developed (42) that is more practical for routine use (Table 2).

Distress and Illness Behavior

Pain and suffering are not the same. The best measure of suffering may be psychological distress: (a) anxiety and increased somatic awareness, which can be measured by the Modified Somatic Perception Questionnaire (31), and (b) depressive symptoms, which can be measured by the Beck depressive inventory (5) or the Zung depressive inventory (74).

The physical symptoms and signs of disease must also be distinguished from behavioral symptoms and from signs of illness behavior. The concept of illness behavior is most simply illustrated by pain drawing (52): patients willingly draw the anatomical pattern of their pain on an outline of the body, but the way they draw their pain also reflects their psychological distress about the pain. Similarly, the physical and behavioral components of both clinical symptoms and responses to examination must be clearly distinguished (Table 1).

Illness behavior may be assessed clinically (69) by pain drawing (52), behavioral symptoms (65), nonorganic or behavioral signs (67), overt pain behavior (25,69), use of walking aids, and downtime (the average number of hours spent lying down between 7 A.M. and 11 P.M. (54).

Disability

Clinical assessment of disability must concentrate on loss of function rather than pain. The question is not, Is

TABLE 2. *The short-form McGill pain questionnaire*

Please tick which of these words describes your pain. Put the tick in the box which gives the intensity of that particular quality of your pain.

	None	Mild	Moderate	Severe
THROBBING	0) ___	1) ___	2) ___	3) ___
SHOOTING	0) ___	1) ___	2) ___	3) ___
STABBING	0) ___	1) ___	2) ___	3) ___
SHARP	0) ___	1) ___	2) ___	3) ___
CRAMPING	0) ___	1) ___	2) ___	3) ___
GNAWING	0) ___	1) ___	2) ___	3) ___
HOT-BURNING	0) ___	1) ___	2) ___	3) ___
ACHING	0) ___	1) ___	2) ___	3) ___
HEAVY	0) ___	1) ___	2) ___	3) ___
TENDER	0) ___	1) ___	2) ___	3) ___
SPLITTING	0) ___	1) ___	2) ___	3) ___
TIRING-EXHAUSTING	0) ___	1) ___	2) ___	3) ___
SICKENING	0) ___	1) ___	2) ___	3) ___
FEARFUL	0) ___	1) ___	2) ___	3) ___
PUNISHING-CRUEL	0) ___	1) ___	2) ___	3) ___

Please put a mark on the scale to show how bad your <u>usual pain</u> has been <u>these days</u>.

NO
PAIN _____

WORST
POSSIBLE
PAIN

How bad is your pain now?

0	NO PAIN	___
1	MILD	___
2	DISCOMFORTING	___
3	DISTRESSING	___
4	HORRIBLE	___
5	EXCRUCIATING	___

From ref. 42, with permission.
Note the scale is exactly 100 mm long.

that activity painful? but rather, Are you actually restricted in that activity? Does your back limit how much you do, or do you avoid that activity, or do you now require help with that activity? Restriction must have occurred only since the onset of back pain and because of back pain. The common or usual effect should be assessed, discounting occasional limitations or special efforts. Our studies (64) have shown the following limits to be most applicable in low back disorders:

Bending and lifting: Help required or avoid heavy lifting, such as 30 to 40 pounds, a heavy suitcase, or a 3- to 4-year-old child.

Sitting: Sitting in an ordinary chair generally limited to less than 30 minutes at a time before needing to get up and move around.

Standing: Standing in one position generally limited to less than 30 minutes at a time before needing to move around.

Walking: Walking generally limited to less than 30 minutes or 1 to 2 miles at a time before needing to rest.

Travelling: Travelling in a car or bus generally limited to less than 30 minutes at a time before needing to stop and have a break.

Social life: Social activities and normal social mobility regularly missed or curtailed (excluding sports, the missing of which implies a completely different level of disability).

Sleep: Sleep regularly disturbed by backache, two or three times per week.

Sex life: Reduced frequency of sexual activity because of pain.

Dressing: Help regularly required with footwear; tights, socks, or shoelaces.

Simple yes/no answers to these questions provide a simple, rapid and reliable disability score (number of yes answers out of nine) which is sufficient for clinical purposes. Although such scoring appears deceptively simple, the individual items add together to provide a statistically highly satisfactory total score (64). For formal disability evaluation, detailed questions can be asked about the exact level of restriction in each of the nine basic activities and how these interfere with each aspect of the patient's work, home and leisure activities. Although based on clinical interview and recorded by the physician, this must be clearly identified as the patient's subjective report of disability.

Similar questions about restricted activities of daily living can be presented as a self-report questionnaire. This may permit further distinction between activities that only increase pain and those that are actually limited or prevented by pain. A number of self-report questionnaires are now well established for measuring disability in activities of daily living due to low back pain (18,53).

Independent observation of disability may be carried out in an occupational therapy department or a rehabilitation unit. This can be more comprehensive and may examine specific work disabilities. It can attempt to introduce some measure of objectivity into the assessment of disability, but it remains limited by what the patient is prepared to do and by their cooperation and motivation.

PHYSICAL IMPAIRMENT

Although the principles of assessing lumbar impairment may be agreed upon, in practice it remains quite unsatisfactory. This is illustrated by the number of different systems that have been tried and the lack of agreement on any standard method. It is worth reviewing the problems of various well-known methods.

The first real attempt was by McBride (37), who developed a system of comprehensive evaluation of quickness, coordination, strength, severity, endurance, safety, and physique (38). Unfortunately, this was based entirely on subjective medical judgments of these ill-defined characteristics. Although many of McBride's concepts are worthy in principle, his system does not give reproducible results and has never gained wide acceptance.

More generally accepted methods of rating lumbar impairment were developed more than 30 years ago by the American Medical Association (AMA) (3) and the American Academy of Orthopaedic Surgeons (AAOS) (1). One survey found that 60%, 30%, and 5% of U.S. surgeons used the AMA, AAOS, and McBride system respectively (9). But both the AMA and the AAOS systems overemphasized diagnosis, and rating was best established and agreed upon in the few patients with a clear radiological abnormality, such as a fracture, a neurological abnormality, or previous surgery. The AMA method also included restriction of spinal movements, but it initially used an invalid method of measuring lumbar flexion. Neither method included much objective data applicable to the patient with uncomplicated low back pain. A recent revision of the AMA system now uses more valid methods of measuring range of movement using an inclinometer, but it still suffers the same fundamental limitations (4).

In an attempt to overcome these limitations, several clinical research groups have developed comprehensive evaluation systems (22,29,33). Unfortunately, these often fail to make a clear conceptual distinction between pain, disability, and physical impairment but instead try to combine them. Moreover, the method of scoring frequently has no statistical basis and the loadings applied are both arbitrary and subjective. More sophisticated recent attempts have identified many possible factors from a comprehensive literature review and then used a panel of experts to select the data that can most usefully be used to rate current impairment, as in the California disability rating schedule (14), or to predict future chronic disability (20). Such an approach can certainly give a consensus of current medical opinion. But complex mathematical scoring of the experts' votes is only an illusion of science. It is no substitute for hard clinical data or real understanding of the problem. Such a committee in the past would undoubtedly have proven statistically that boiling tar was the best possible treatment for amputation stumps!

Waddell and Main (64) tried to apply the above principles of impairment rating to an analysis of disability in 480 patients with chronic low back pain. They included only "objective physical characteristics," they used reliable methods of clinical examination, and they excluded nonorganic findings. They then used sophisticated statistical analysis to identify the following physical characteristics, which provided the best explanation of subjective disability:

anatomical pattern of pain
time pattern of pain
lumbar flexion
straight-leg raising (SLR)
nerve compression signs
previous lumbar surgery
spinal fractures.

The problem is that this is a very varied group of clinical characteristics, which reflect the patients in that study. Spinal fractures, nerve compression signs, and previous surgery are all structural impairments but are not relevant to the patient with uncomplicated low back pain who does not have neuropathology or previous back surgery. Moreover, in practice, this method is dominated by subjective reports of pain, which are clearly not physical impairments as originally defined.

The U.S. National Institute for Occupational Safety and Health (NIOSH) devoted a great deal of effort to developing reliable methods of clinical examination (48). An extensive literature review and an expert panel identified 105 clinical tests and measures. From these, reliability studies in different centers produced a final low back atlas of 19 carefully standardized tests to be used as the basis for future studies (49). Unfortunately, the only criterion was an almost unrealistically high level of reliability, so this produced a most unrepresentative group of tests. Six of the 19 tests were different measures of pelvic tilt and a further four were of lumbar lordosis! Yet there were no palpation findings and the only spinal movement measured was lateral flexion. Several measures of strength were included, but they were all of marginal reliability. However reliable this set of tests may be, they clearly provide a limited perspective on lumbar impairment and are of doubtful clinical validity or utility. Little further appears to have been done to turn the NIOSH atlas into a practical method of assessing impairment.

A METHOD OF ASSESSING LUMBAR IMPAIRMENT

We have attempted to develop a method of assessing lumbar impairment based on these principles and overcoming these problems (70). We confined our study to patients with chronic low back pain, excluding those with nerve root involvement, previous surgery, and structural radiological abnormalities such as fractures or spondylolisthesis. We included only objective findings from physical examination. We developed reliable methods of routine clinical examination. We identified and excluded nonorganic findings. Finally, we identified a group of physical signs that discriminated patients with low back pain from normal subjects and were associated with reported disability.

Examination Technique

The first step is to identify the anatomical landmarks (50,55,59) that can be palpated most easily with the patient lying prone with relaxed muscles. Horizontal marks are made on the skin in the midline at S2 and T12/L1. The inferior border of the posterior superior iliac spines lying at the bottom of the posterior part of the iliac crest just below and lateral to the dimples of Venus corresponds to S2. T12/L1 is identified by counting up the spinous processes, checking that the iliac crests approximate to the L4/5 level. Vertical marks are made in the midline over the spinous processes of T12 and T9.

The patient then performs warm-up exercises (26): flexion/extension twice, left/right rotation twice, left/right lateral flexion twice, and one more flexion/extension.

The examination positions must be carefully standardized (50,55,59). We found particular difficulty achieving a consistent erect position, but this is essential as reliable measurement of movement depends on a standard starting point. After personal discussion with Spangfort and Troup, we finally found the most satisfactory position to be: bare feet, heels together, knees straight with the weight borne evenly on the two legs, looking straight ahead, arms hanging at the sides, relaxed. If there is severe muscle spasm, the patient is asked

to get as close to that position as he or she can maintain comfortably for several minutes. The supine position is lying relaxed flat on the back, head lying on the couch without a pillow, arms at the sides with hips and knees as extended as possible without tension. The prone position is with no pillow, head and shoulders relaxed on the table, arms by the side.

The only equipment required is a ballpoint pen and an inclinometer. Although not essential, we find an electronic inclinometer more convenient (manufactured by Cybex Division of Lumex Inc, 100 Spence Street, New York, NY 11706).

The following tests can be carried out in any preferred order but it is most efficient to arrange them in sequence in the erect, prone, and supine positions.

Lumbar flexion is measured with the inclinometer (Fig. 2) (36). With the patient in the erect position, recordings are made at S2 and then at T12/L1. Holding the inclinometer on T12/L1, the patient is then asked to reach down with the finger tips of both hands as far as possible towards their toes, checking that they keep their knees straight. Keeping the patient fully flexed, the third recording is taken at T12/L1 and the fourth recording at S2. These four readings permit simple calculation of total flexion, pelvic flexion, and, by subtraction, lumbar flexion.

Lumbar extension is measured at T12/L1 (36). The first reading is obtained with the patient in the erect position. The patient is then asked to arch backwards as far as possible looking up to the ceiling. The examiner should support the patient with one hand on the shoulder to help maintain balance and give some feeling of security. The second reading is then obtained and subtraction gives the measure of total extension.

Lateral lumbar flexion is measured using a longer bar on the inclinometer. The first inclinometer reading is obtained in the erect position with the bar lined up tangentially with the spinous processes at T9 and T12. The patient is then asked to lean straight over to the side as far as possible with their fingertips reaching straight down the side of the thigh. The examiner should support the patient's shoulder with one hand and make sure that the patient does not flex forwards or twist around and that both feet stay flat on the ground.

Reliable examination of tenderness can only be achieved by particularly careful standardization of the technique (66). This is carried out with the patient prone and it is important to make sure that the muscles are relaxed. Palpation should be done slowly without sudden pressure and without hurting the patient unduly. Superficial tenderness to light skin pinch is behavioral in nature and invalidates palpation for deep tenderness (67). Local tenderness is then sought to firm pressure with the ball of the thumb over the spinous processes and interspinous ligaments within 1 cm of the midline from T12 to S2. It is important to use specific wording: Is that pain-

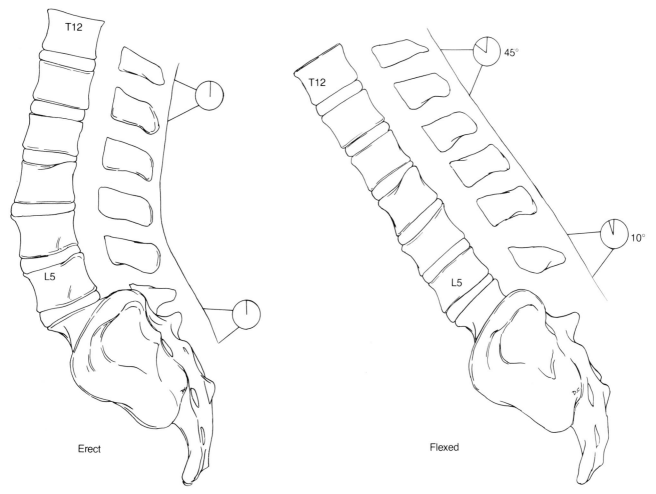

FIG. 2. The inclinometer technique of measuring flexion. The lower inclinometer measures pelvic flexion; the upper inclinometer measures total flexion; the difference between them is lumbar flexion. In this example, pelvic flexion = 10°, lumbar flexion = 35°, total flexion = 45°.

ful? *Any* response is taken as positive apart from a specific no. Any qualified response such as "only a little bit" is counted positive. If the patient is doubtful or does not answer, then the question is repeated: Is that painful when I do that? Widespread nonanatomical tenderness is again discounted as behavioral (67).

SLR is carried out with the patient supine, making sure that the head remains relaxed and that the patient does not look up to watch what is happening (modified from 10,36). The foot is held with one hand making sure that the hip is in neutral rotation. The inclinometer is positioned on the tibial crest just below the tibial tubercle with the other hand and set at zero. The leg is then raised passively by the examiner, whose other hand continues to hold the inclinometer in position and also holds the patient's knee fully extended. The leg is raised slowly to the maximum tolerated SLR (not just to the onset of pain) and the maximum reading is recorded. Limited SLR on formal examination should always be checked with distraction at a later stage of the examination and discounted if this is positive (67).

Bilateral active SLR is tested in the supine position (modified from 7). The patient is asked to lift both legs together with straight knees and hold the heels 6 inches off the couch for 5 seconds. Both heels and calves should be raised clear of the couch. The examiner should not count aloud or use verbal encouragement. The patient should not be allowed to use the hands to lift the legs. The patient may fail to lift the legs clear of the couch at all, lift clear but for less than 5 seconds, or manage to hold the legs clear for the full 5 seconds. Only the last is counted as successful.

Active sit-up is again tested in the supine position (modified from 7,30,49). The patient is asked to flex the knees to 90° and to place the soles of the feet flat on the couch. The examiner should hold down both feet with one hand. The patient is then instructed to reach up with the fingertips of both hands to touch (not hold) both knees and hold that position for 5 seconds. Again, the examiner should not count aloud or offer verbal encouragement. The patient may fail to reach the fingertips of both hands to the patellae, reach the patellae but for less than 5 seconds, or hold the position for the full 5 seconds. Only the last is counted as successful.

Interpretation of Physical Impairment

This is a comprehensive battery of objective clinical tests of spinal movements, SLR, spinal tenderness, and strength tests, which in our study discriminated patients with low back pain from normal subjects and explained low back disability (Table 3).

Interpretation of this scale requires fundamental reconsideration of our findings of physical impairment in terms of the original definition. In most patients with uncomplicated low back pain, it is not possible to identify any objective pathology or reach any definite diagnosis. The only permanent structural impairments demonstrated in previous studies have been structural deformities, fractures, surgical scarring, and permanent neurological deficits (64), but none of these apply to the patient with low back pain alone. The present method does provide an objective clinical evaluation, but it is not a measure of anatomical or structural impairment. Instead, the physical tests included in the final physical impairment scale are all measures of physical function, more specifically what Nagi (45,46) and Guccione (23) describe as "functional limitations" associated with pain and disuse. Movements and strength tests are clinical observations of what the patient does, or, more graphically, what Cassell (13) describes as the patient's "inability to do" because of pain. This may simply be the expression of the patient's "inability to do" in the context of clinical examination, whereas the measure of disability used in our study was the patient's self-report of "inability to do" in activities of daily living. These clinical observations will provide an objective cross-check on the patient's description of disability. It is however, a matter of perspective whether these findings are regarded as physiological im-

TABLE 3. *The final physical impairment scale*

Physical test	Cut-off
Total flexion	<87°
Total extension	<18°
Average lateral flexion	<24°
Average SLR	
Women	<71°
Men	<66°
Spinal tenderness	positive
Bilateral active SLR	<5 sec
Sit-up	<5 sec

From ref. 70, with permission.
Each test scored 0 or 1. Failing to achieve the cut-off results in a 1 score for impairment, to give a total score of 7.
SLR, straight-leg raising.

pairment as defined by the World Health Organization (73) or ultimately as clinical observation of the patient's behavior (19). In either event, these tests will depend on pain-inhibition, fear-avoidance (71), psychological distress (65), and illness behavior (68) just as much as on the physical or sensory disorder. Thus the patient's "inability to do" cannot necessarily be interpreted purely in terms of physical impairment (13).

In our study, all the tests included in the final scale were related to some degree to the behavioral signs (67). By the nature of the examination techniques, all these physical tests may also be open to conscious deception. It is never possible to separate clinical examination of pain entirely from such influences. Indeed, Spratt et al. (56) standardized physical examination to record pain behavior in response to such mechanical tests. In practice, the only safeguard is to assess the psychological and behavioral elements of disability separately and, if they are marked, to recognize that clinical evaluation of physical impairment is not possible in that patient at that point in time.

Finally, by the nature of these physical tests, they can only be measures of current impairment. Functional limitation may persist as long as pain lasts, and there is good clinical and epidemiologic evidence that after a period of time the chances of successful rehabilitation are low (40). But physically there remains at least the potential for improvement, and Cox et al. (15) have shown that these physical findings are reversible, even in people handicapped by chronic low back pain (35). For these reasons, this method should be regarded simply as providing an objective clinical evaluation of current functional limitation associated with chronic low back pain. In practice, assessment at one point in time is also limited by the absence of any pre-onset baseline of normal physical function for that individual, so that the individual patient can be compared only with the average of the normal population. Although this battery discriminates the groups reasonably well, discrimination between individual patients with chronic low back pain and normal subjects is limited. There is still a false-positive rate of 14% in normal subjects and a false-negative rate of 24% in patients, corresponding to a specificity of 86% and sensitivity of 76%.

If this interpretation is correct, it has profound implications both for health care and for compensation awards in chronic low back pain. The limitations of current knowledge must be recognized and due allowance made. Nevertheless, the lack of objective evidence of any permanent anatomical or structural impairment casts further doubt on traditional medical treatment for chronic low back pain based on the disease model and directed to tissue damage (61). It implies that most chronic low back pain still has the potential for rehabilitation. Recognition that the primary clinical findings are not of disease but of functional limitation, reinforces the need to direct medical management more to restoration of function based on a biopsychosocial model of disability (61). It illustrates the limitations of clinical evaluation and interpretation of the physical impairment associated with chronic low back pain. Finally, it questions the physical basis of permanent disability awards for chronic low back pain.

THE RELATIONSHIP BETWEEN PAIN, DISABILITY, AND PHYSICAL IMPAIRMENT

Disability must be assessed within a broad clinical framework. Assessment must start with diagnosis or at least the recognition of symptom clusters. It must allow for the coexistence of physical and psychological disturbances. Disability must then be balanced against personal requirements, such as work demands, coping abilities, and motivation (28). In addition to the practical problems, assessment at one point in time involves major conceptual difficulties (34). First, it assumes that disability is static rather than a dynamic process, yet all the above factors may vary with time. And it does not allow for prolonged inactivity and disuse producing a deconditioning syndrome that may itself cause disability. The potential for recovery and how much of current impairment is likely to be permanent is a separate issue that unfortunately remains a matter of clinical opinion and possible disagreement. Assessment in an adversarial system will also depend on the expert–claimant relationship and the possibility of observer bias must be recognized and discounted as far as possible.

Within this framework, pain and disability are logically and clinically related to physical impairment. There is considerable correlation between them, but it is certainly not a one-to-one relationship and there may be disproportion in the individual case (Fig. 3). It has to be repeated that the fundamental difference is that pain and disability are ultimately subjective and the patient's report may be influenced by psychological disturbances or conscious exaggeration, whereas physical impairment must be assessed on objective clinical findings. Even there, the clinical findings may depend to some extent on the patient's performance and behavior. Final judgment of severity in the individual case depends on the balance between the patient's report of pain, disability, and work loss and the physician's assessment of the nature of the injury, diagnosis, and objective physical impairment. Together, these provide a comprehensive evaluation, and, when all are proportionate, they can be combined to give unequivocal assessment of severity. The patient's report of his or her subjective symptoms and disability is then supported and substantiated by the objective medical evidence. If, however, there is a significant discrepancy between the patient's claimed pain, disability, and incapacity for work, and the physician's

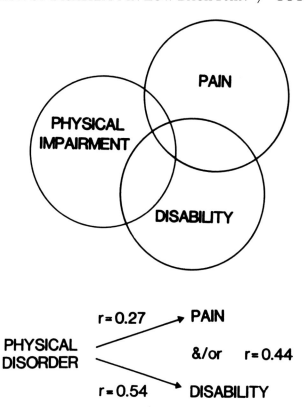

FIG. 3. The relation between pain, disability, and physical impairment, showing the correlation and overlap between them. r is the correlation coefficient, where 0 is no correlation and 1 is complete identity. (From ref. 62, with permission.)

assessment of injury, diagnosis, and physical impairment, then it is important to record this. Such a discrepancy may be explained either by psychological disturbances or by exaggeration related to a claim for compensation. A more comprehensive assessment is then required of the entire clinical picture and in particular of psychological and behavioral factors.

EXPERT MEDICAL OPINION

A medical report on lumbar impairment should meet specific legal and administrative needs for disability rating and compensation awards. It should draw clear, logical conclusions from the documented medical evidence and avoid unsubstantiated, subjective opinions that depend solely on the authority of the expert. The medical report should include separate and clearly identified descriptions of the patient's report of pain and disability, the physician's findings of physical impairment, and his or her expert opinion. The opinion should include:

1. A diagnosis with a rating of severity (e.g., a simple strain of the low back or a severe fracture of T12/L1), whether or not this is consistent with the reported injury, and the existence of any preexisting or predisposing condition.

2. The stage of recovery and whether or not a permanent state has been reached.

3. Duration of total and partial disability and work loss and whether or not this is consistent with the severity of the injury.

4. The present level of pain and disability and working capacity and whether or not this is consistent with and supported by the severity of the injury and the objective physical impairment.

5. Evidence of psychologic disturbance or conscious exaggeration or the absence of any such findings.

6. The likelihood of future improvement or deterioration including a time scale, the possibility of further treatment or rehabilitation, possible future complications, and probable future loss of time from work or employability.

ACKNOWLEDGEMENTS. We are grateful to the Chief Scientist Office of the Scottish Home and Health Department and to the Mactaggart Trust for their support of this work. Parts of this text were adapted with permission from Clinical Orthopaedics and Related Research 1987, 221:110–120, and from Spine 1992, 17:617–628.

REFERENCES

1. AAOS (1962): *Manual for orthopaedic surgeons in evaluating permanent physical impairment.* Chicago: American Academy of Orthopaedic Surgeons.
2. Allan DB, Waddell G (1989): An historical perspective on low back pain and disability. *Acta Orthop Scand* 60(suppl 234):1–23.
3. AMA (1958): A guide to the evaluation of permanent impairment of the extremities and back. American Medical Association. *JAMA* 166(suppl):1–122.
4. AMA (1988): *Guides to the evaluation of permanent impairment.* 3rd ed. Chicago: American Medical Association.
5. Beck AT, Ward CH, Mendelson MM, Mock J, Erbaugh J (1961): An inventory for measuring depression. *Arch Gen Psychiatry* 4: 561–571.
6. Bergquist-Ullman M, Larsson U (1977): Acute low back pain in industry. *Acta Orthop Scand* 170(suppl):1–117.
7. Biering-Sørensen F (1984): Physical measurements as risk indicators for low back trouble over a one year period. *Spine* 9:106–119.
8. Boline PD, Keating JC, Brist J, Denver G (1988): Interexaminer reliability of palpatory evaluations of the lumbar spine. *Am J Chir Med* 1:5–11.
9. Brand RA, Lehmann TR (1983): Low-back impairment rating practices of orthopaedic surgeons. *Spine* 8:75–78.
10. Breig A, Troup JDG (1979): Biomechanical considerations in the straight leg raising test. *Spine* 3:242–250.
11. Brown T (1828): On irritation of the spinal nerves. *Glasgow Med J* 1:131–160.
12. Carlsson AM (1983): Assessment of chronic pain. 1. Aspects of the reliability and validity of the visual analogue scale. *Pain* 16:87–101.
13. Cassell EJ (1995): The evaluation of disability due primarily to pain. In: Fordyce WE, ed. *International Association for the Study of Pain task force on pain in the workplace.* Seattle, IASP Press (*in press*).
14. Clark WL, Haldeman S, Johnson P, Morris J, Schulenberger C, Trauner D, White A (1988): Back impairment and disability determination. Another attempt at objective reliable rating. *Spine* 13: 332–341.
15. Cox R, Keeley J, Barnes D, Gatchel R, Mayer T (1988): *Effects of functional restoration treatment upon Waddell impairment/dis-ability ratings in chronic low back pain patients.* Presented to the International Society for the Study of the Lumbar Spine, Miami.
16. DHSS (1986): *Handbook for Industrial Injury Medical Boards.* London: HMSO.
17. Erichsen JE (1866): *On railway and other injuries of the nervous system.* London: Walton & Maberly.
18. Fairbank JCT, Mbaot JC, Davies JB, O'Brien JP (1980): The Oswestry Low Back Pain Disability Questionnaire. *Physiotherapy* 66: 271–273.
19. Fordyce WE (1976): *Behavioural methods for chronic pain and illness.* St Louis: CV Mosby.
20. Frymoyer JW, Cats-Baril W (1987): Predictors of low back disability. *Clin Orthop* 221:89–98.
21. Garrad J, Bennett AE (1971): A validated interview schedule for use in population surveys of chronic disease and disability. *Br J Prev Soc Med* 25:97–104.
22. Greenough CG, Fraser RD (1992): Assessment of outcome in patients with low back pain. *Spine* 17:36–41.
23. Guccione AA (1991): Physical therapy diagnosis and the relationship between impairments and function. *Phys Ther* 71:499–504.
24. Jensen MP, Karoly P, Braver S (1986): The measurement of clinical pain intensity: a comparison of six methods. *Pain* 27:117–126.
25. Keefe FJ, Block AR (1982): Development of an observation method for assessing pain behavior in chronic low back pain patients. *Behav Ther* 13:363–375.
26. Keeley J, Mayer TG, Cox R, Gatchel RJ, Smith J, Mooney V (1986): Quantification of lumbar function. Part 5: Reliability of range of motion measures in the sagittal plane and an in vivo torso rotation measurement technique. *Spine* 11:31–35.
27. King HD (1915): Injuries of the back from a medical legal standpoint. *Texas State J Med* 11:442–445.
28. Kuilman M (1989): Causes of work impairment and modern classification systems. Presented to the 16th International Congress of Life Assurance Medicine. *Ann Life Assur Med* (in press).
29. Lehmann T, Brand RA, O'Gorman TWO (1983): A low back rating scale. *Spine* 8:308–315.
30. Lloyd DCEF, Troup JDG (1983): Recurrent back pain and its prediction. *J Soc Occup Med* 33:66–74.
31. Main CJ (1983): The modified somatic perception questionnaire. *J Psychosomatic Res* 27:503–514.
32. Main CJ, Waddell G (1989): The assessment of pain. *Clin Rehab* 3:267–274.
33. Martinat EH (1966): Evaluation of permanent impairment of the spine. *J Bone Joint Surg* 48A:1204–1210.
34. Mayer TG (1987): Assessment of lumbar function. *Clin Orthop* 221:99–109.
35. Mayer TG, Gatchel RJ, Kishino N, et al. (1985): Objective assessment of spine function following industrial injury. A prospective study with comparison group and one-year follow-up. *Spine* 10: 482–493.
36. Mayer TG, Tencer AT, Kristoferson S, Mooney V (1984): Use of noninvasive techniques for quantification of spinal range of motion in normal subjects and chronic low back dysfunction patients. *Spine* 9:588–595.
37. McBride ED (1936): *Disability evaluation and principles of treatment of compensable injuries.* 1st ed. Philadelphia: JB Lippincott.
38. McBride ED (1963): *Disability evaluation and principles of treatment of compensable injuries.* 6th ed. Philadelphia: JB Lippincott.
39. McCombe PF, Fairbank JCT, Cockersole BC, Pynsent PB (1989): Reproducibility of physical signs in low back pain. *Spine* 14:908–918.
40. McGill CM (1968): Industrial back programmes: a control program. *J Occup Med* 10:174–178.
41. Melzack R (1975): The McGill pain questionnaire: major properties and scoring methods. *Pain* 1:277–299.
42. Melzack R (1987): The short-form McGill Pain Questionnaire. *Pain* 30:191–197.
43. Merskey R (1979): Pain terms: a list with definitions and notes on usage. *Pain* 6:249–252.
44. Million R, Haavik Nilsen K, Jayson MIV, Baker RD (1982): Evaluation of low back pain and assessment of lumbar corsets with and without back supports. *Ann Rheum Dis* 40:449–454.
45. Nagi SZ (1965): Some conceptual issues in disability and rehabilitation. In: Sussman MB, ed. *Sociology and rehabilitation.* Washington DC: American Sociological Association, pp. 100–113.

46. Nagi SZ (1969): *Disability and rehabilitation.* Columbus, Ohio: Ohio State University Press.
47. Nelson MA, Allen P, Clamp SE, de Dombal FT (1979): Reliability and reproducibility of clinical findings in low-back pain. *Spine* 4: 97–101.
48. Nelson RM, Nestor DE (1988): Standardized assessment of industrial low-back injuries: development of the NIOSH low-back atlas. *Top Acute Care Trauma Rehabil* 2:16–30.
49. NIOSH (1988): *National Institute for Occupational Safety and Health low back atlas.* Morgantown, West Virginia: U.S. Department of Health and Human Services.
50. Ohlen G (1989): *Spinal sagittal configuration and mobility. A kyphometer study* [Thesis]. Stockholm: Karolinska Institute.
51. Potter NA, Rothstein JM (1983): Intertester reliability for selected clinical tests of the sacroiliac joint. *Phys Ther* 65:1671–1675.
52. Ransford AO, Cairns D, Mooney V (1976): The pain drawing as an aid to the psychological evaluation of patients with low back pain. *Spine* 1:127–134.
53. Roland M, Morris R (1983): A study of the natural history of back pain. Part I: Development of a reliable and sensitive measure of disability in low back pain. *Spine* 8:141–144.
54. Rosensteil AK, Keefe FJ (1983): The use of coping strategies in chronic low back pain: relationships to patient characteristics and current adjustment. *Pain* 17:33–44.
55. Spangfort EV (1989): Personal communication.
56. Spratt KF, Lehmann TR, Weinstein JN, et al. (1990): A new approach to the low-back physical examination: behavioral assessment of mechanical signs. *Spine* 15:96–102.
57. Sternbach RA (1974): *Pain patients: traits and treatment.* New York: Academic Press.
58. Sternbach RA (1977): Psychological aspects of chronic pain. *Clin Orthop* 129:150–155.
59. Troup JDG (1989): Personal communication.
60. U.S. Bureau of Disability Insurance (1970): *Disability evaluation under Social Security. A handbook for physicians.* Washington, DC: U.S. Government Printing Office.
61. Waddell G (1987): A new clinical model for the treatment of low back pain. *Spine* 12:632–644.
62. Waddell G (1987): Clinical assessment of lumbar impairment. *Clin Orthop* 221:110–120.
63. Waddell G, Bircher M, Finlayson D, Main CJ (1984): Symptoms and signs: physical disease or illness behaviour? *Br Med J* 289:739–741.
64. Waddell G, Main CJ (1984): Assessment of severity in low back disorders. *Spine* 9:204–208.
65. Waddell G, Main CJ, Morris EW, Di Paola MP, Gray ICM (1984): Chronic low back pain, psychologic distress, and illness behaviour. *Spine* 9:209–213.
66. Waddell G, Main CJ, Morris EW, Venner RM, Rae PS, Sharmy SH, Galloway H (1982): Normality and reliability in the clinical assessment of backache. *Br Med J* 284:1519–1523.
67. Waddell G, McCulloch JA, Kummel E, Venner RM (1980): Nonorganic physical signs in low back pain. *Spine* 5:117–125.
68. Waddell G, Pilowsky I, Bond M (1989): Clinical assessment and interpretation of abnormal illness behaviour in low back pain. *Pain* 39:41–53.
69. Waddell G, Richardson J (1991): Clinical assessment of overt pain behaviour by physicians during routine clinical examination. *J Psychosomatic Res* 36:77–87.
70. Waddell G, Sommerville D, Henderson I, Newton M (1992): Objective clinical evaluation of physical impairment in chronic low back pain. *Spine* 17:617–628.
71. Waddell G, Sommerville D, Henderson I, Newton M, Main CJ (1993): A fear-avoidance beliefs questionnaire (FABQ): and the role of fear-avoidance beliefs in chronic low back pain and disability. *Pain* 52:157–168.
72. Wentworth ET (1916): Systematic diagnosis in backache. *J Bone Joint Surg* 8:137–170.
73. WHO (1980): *International classification of impairments, disabilities and handicaps.* Geneva: World Health Organization.
74. Zung WWK (1965): A self-rated depression scale. *Arch Gen Psychiatr* 32:63–70.

The Adult Spine: Principles and Practice,
2nd edition, J.W. Frymoyer, Editor-in-Chief.
Lippincott-Raven Publishers, Philadelphia © 1997.

CHAPTER 12

Practical Guide to Current United States Impairment Rating

A Critical Analysis

Timothy S. Carey

Back pain is a common problem, as other chapters in this volume have demonstrated. Death as a consequence of back pain is extremely rare, but disability is not. Multiple studies have assessed the functional status of individuals with symptomatic low back pain. These studies have indicated that during a symptomatic episode, the functional status of the sufferer is very poor (8). Indeed, it is equivalent to someone with severe congestive heart failure, metastatic cancer, or symptomatic acquired immune deficiency syndrome (17). Individuals with severe back pain have trouble bending, may not be able to put on their own shoes, have difficulty in ambulation, and cannot keep their own houses. What distinguishes individuals with low back pain from those afflicted with these other conditions is prognosis. Back pain essentially never shortens life. Acute back pain has a very benign prognosis, with over 90% of individuals returning to a functional status equivalent to their baseline status within 3 months of the onset of pain (9). Patients with chronic back pain have a significantly worse prognosis, but most cohort studies show that substantial numbers of chronic back pain patients improve over time with supportive therapy (19,20).

Society has elected to support disabled individuals.

T. S. Carey, M.D., M.P.H.: Associate Professor of Medicine, University of North Carolina at Chapel Hill; The Sheps Center for Health Services Research, Suite 210, Chapel Hill, North Carolina, 27599.

Back pain represents a special case in that the disability is nonlethal and there are no external stigmata of the functional impairment. No limb is severed, there is not obvious joint deformity as in rheumatoid arthritis. While the number of individual programs developed by society to financially support individuals temporarily or permanently disabled with back pain is very large, they can be divided into three broad categories.

1. State-based workers' compensation systems
2. Social Security Disability Insurance (SSDI)
3. Private disability insurance, including systems that insure income, mortgage payments, and time payments for appliances

Within each of these disability systems, a physician may function either to rate impairment or as a treating physician. Sometimes these roles are admixed. In all situations, the physician's and patient's interests are best served by clarity of communication between physician, patient, employer, and insurer.

WORKERS' COMPENSATION AND BACK PAIN

The history, structure, and overall rationale of the American Workers' Compensation system has been described previously in this volume. American Workers' Compensation is a no-fault system designed to pay the medical expenses of workers who undergo an injury or develop an illness arising out of gainful employment. This system also provides cash payments of a portion of the worker's income during the period of complete disability. Workers who are partially disabled may obtain long-term payments of the appropriate portion of their salary. Therefore, in American Workers' Compensation, three types of disability payments are possible: temporary total, permanent total, and permanent partial disabilities.

Temporary total disability indicates that the worker is unable to perform any gainful employment for a period of time. This is the most common circumstance in which payments are made under Workers' Compensation. The worker is ill or injured, receives treatment, recovers, and returns to work at full capacity. Permanent total disability indicates that the employee is so impaired that he or she is unable to pursue any gainful employment and that this condition is expected to persist indefinitely. A substantial period of time following an injury must pass before a worker can be assessed as permanently disabled. The greatest costs within state Workers' Compensation systems come from permanent partial disability (18). In permanent partial disability, the employee never recovers to baseline level of functioning, even after tests of time and treatment. Thus, while the employee can return to work, it may not be at the same employer or at the same job description. Great controversy exists as to the determination of the level of disability within partial disability.

The following comments regarding Workers' Compensation should be considered generic. Substantial variability exists among states regarding the exact apportionment of disability and the administrative process utilized. Each state has its own Workers' Compensation statutes, unlike the nationwide Social Security disability system.

An overriding paradigm of Workers' Compensation is the whole man concept. That is, if one is rendered completely unable to perform any gainful activity for pay, one is rendered 100% disabled. Using the whole man concept, partial disability awards can be apportioned (1).

The whole man concept has intuitive appeal, as well as some empiric validation, when applied to extremity injuries. If a digit or extremity is severed or rendered useless, that functional capacity is lost. The amount of functional capacity lost will be proportional to the number of digits lost or the weakness in the extremity. Industrial injuries of the early twentieth century were often associated with amputation or catastrophic injury. This probably led to the popularity of the whole man concept of disability (10). How can the whole man paradigm pertain to back problems? The type of impairment generated by back problems is qualitatively different from extremity injury. The impairment is global, persistent pain is a prominent characteristic, and quantification of the impairment is quite difficult. Despite these difficulties,

the American Medical Association (AMA) impairment rating guide does demonstrate detailed impairment rating for the back. Physicians who are performing impairment ratings for Workers' Compensation boards will need to be very familiar with this type of impairment rating. The focus of the AMA impairment rating guide is very much on the measurable. Range of motion is addressed in detail and in multiple axes (Fig. 1). Range of motion of the back is a difficult clinical measurement. Studies have shown that reliable range of motion measurements can occur only with practice and by using an inclinometer or goniometer (2,10,15,16).

This type of impairment rating for back trouble is clearly a square peg in a round hole: a system developed for extremity injury does not apply well to back pain. Unfortunately, there is no consensus as to what system would be an improvement. The state of California has been developing a substitute impairment rating system over many years. This system appears to have improved reliability (6,7). There is less emphasis on range of mo-

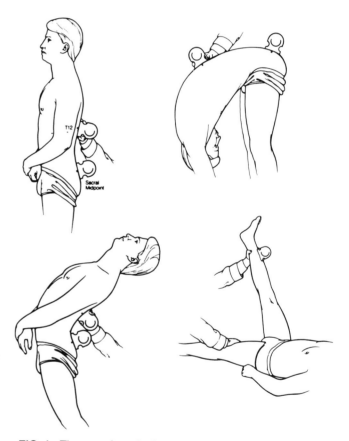

FIG. 1. The use of two inclinometers to measure back flexion and extension. The technique requires an initial marking of the skin for consistency of measurement. On flexion, the sacral (hip) inclination should be subtracted from the T12 inclination to obtain the true lumbar flexion angle. Inclinometers can be purchased from hardware stores. The instructions in the AMA Guide are explicit and should be consulted prior to performing measurements of back motion. From the AMA *Guide to the Evaluation of Permanent Impairment* (1).

gree to which patients attribute the pain to their own behavior. Patients scoring high on the Duration of Pain factor (i.e., who viewed their pain as permanent and constant) had lower self-esteem, higher levels of pain and somatic complaints, and poorer compliance with physical therapy and behavioral interventions than patients scoring low on this factor. Patients scoring high on the Pain as Mystery factor (i.e., who viewed their pain as an unexplainable mystery) had lower self-esteem, higher levels of personality disturbance, and poorer compliance with physical therapy than patients scoring low on this factor. Interestingly, patients scoring high on the Self-Blame factor of the PBAPI (i.e., who blamed themselves for their pain) rated their pain as lower than patients scoring low on this. The research by Williams and Thorn (121) suggests that the pain beliefs of chronic pain patients may have a significant relationship to psychological responses to pain and compliance with treatment.

Another important aspect of cognitive-behavioral assessment is examining the efforts patients make on their own to cope with, deal with, or minimize their pain (46,113). Rosenstiel and Keefe (93) developed the Coping Strategies Questionnaire (CSQ) to assess systematically the frequency with which patients use various strategies and the degree to which these strategies are perceived as effective. The CSQ has been found to be internally consistent and principal components analysis has revealed that three factors account for a large proportion of the variance in questionnaire responses (93). High scores on the first factor, Cognitive Coping and Suppression, indicate a conscious, cognitive effort to reinforce attempts to overcome pain as well as attempts to suppress pain by ignoring and reinterpreting pain sensations. High scores on this factor are related to lower levels of pain and depression and higher levels of functional impairment. High scores on the second factor, Helplessness, indicate a tendency to catastrophize when coping with pain and low ratings of coping strategy effectiveness. Patients scoring high on the Helplessness factor are significantly more depressed and anxious than patients scoring low on this factor. High scores on the third factor, Diverting Attention and Praying, indicate that patients are using attention diversion and praying or hoping strategies to cope with pain. High scores on this factor are related to higher levels of pain and higher levels of functional impairment. A study using the CSQ found that coping strategies were highly predictive of postsurgical outcome following lumbar laminectomy (39). It is noteworthy that in the above studies, the predictive validity of the CSQ was examined only after statistically controlling for demographic and medical status variables. The fact that coping strategies explain a significant proportion of variance in outcome measures after controlling for other important variables suggests that the CSQ provides valuable and unique information about low back pain patients.

Kerns, Turk, and Rudy (62) have developed a more general cognitive-behavioral questionnaire for use with chronic pain populations, the Multidimensional Pain Inventory (MPI). The MPI has nine clinical scales: Pain Severity, Interference, Life Control, Affective Distress, Support, Punishing Responses (by others), Distracting Responses (by others), Solicitous Responses (by others), and General Activity. Using cluster analysis, three profile types have been identified in several chronic pain populations (109). The first type, the Dysfunctional profile, is characterized by high pain severity, substantial interference of pain with daily lifestyle, high levels of affective distress, and low levels of activity and life control. The second type, the Interpersonally Distressed profile, is characterized by the perception of a pronounced lack of support from family members and significant others. The third profile type, the Minimizer/Adaptive Coper, is characterized by low levels of pain severity, interference, and affective distress and high levels of general activity and life control (109). Patients who exhibit either the Dysfunctional or Interpersonally Distressed profiles on the MPI have been found to have higher elevations on a number of MMPI scales as well as other measures of affective distress. Interestingly, traditional personality tests such as the MMPI had difficulty discriminating patients having Dysfunctional or Interpersonally Distressed MPI profiles, suggesting that the MPI provides information not available from these other instruments.

Comment

The application of cognitive principles to the assessment of chronic low back pain patients has considerable clinical value. Recent reviews of research in this area indicate that variables such as cognitive distortions, pain beliefs, self-efficacy, locus of control, and cognitive coping strategies are important predictors of both pain and disability in chronic low back pain patients (see Jensen, et al. [48] and Zautra and Manne [123]). Researchers are currently studying the development of cognitive distortions and pain beliefs in an attempt to find ways in which maladaptive cognitions can be easily identified and treated (58). Such research may lead to preventive interventions that reduce the psychological distress associated with persistent low back pain.

Psychophysiological Assessment

Abnormal psychophysiological responses are believed to be a major factor maintaining pain in many chronic low back pain patients (56). A number of assessment techniques have been developed to identify patterns of muscle tension and muscle spasm that may contribute to chronic back pain. Many investigators have examined paraspinal electromyographic (EMG) activity in chronic

low back pain patients (56). The diathesis-stress model proposed by Flor, Turk, and Birbaumer (24) postulates that low back pain may result from a predisposition to respond to personally relevant stressors with increased paraspinal muscle activity. These increases in muscle tension may lead to ischemia, reflex muscle spasm, oxygen depletion, and the release of pain-producing substances (e.g., histamine, substance P). It is proposed that this can create a vicious cycle in which movement-related anticipatory anxiety can produce muscular hyperactivity leading to increased pain and more anxiety.

To evaluate the role of paraspinal muscle activity in low back pain, a paraspinal surface EMG assessment is often performed (24). This typically involves bilateral placement of surface electrodes at the lumbar interspaces. Levels of muscle activity are then recorded while the patient is sitting, standing, involved in flexion, extension, or rotational maneuvers, and exposed to laboratory stressors (e.g., mental arithmetic). A number of methodological considerations need to be taken into account when evaluating such data (24). First, muscle activity may differ greatly depending on the age of the patient, duration of pain, or surgical history. Second, differences in procedures such as type of stressor and duration of activities, and differences in data analysis methods may produce varying results (24).

Despite these methodological considerations, studies of psychophysiological assessments of back pain patients show several consistent findings (24). First, low back pain patients do not display higher levels of baseline paraspinal muscle activity than controls. Second, there is little empirical support for the notion that low back pain patients have higher levels of paraspinal muscle activity during movement than controls. Finally, chronic low back pain patients may be hyperreactive to personally relevant emotional stressors and may show delayed return to baseline levels of muscle activity following termination of a stressor.

Comment

Psychophysiologic measures are useful in identifying excessive paraspinal muscle activity contributing to chronic back pain. Patients showing this pattern may respond to training in self-control interventions such as biofeedback and relaxation that are designed to teach them to reduce excessive muscle tension. It should be noted, however, that chronic low back pain populations are heterogeneous and abnormal psychophysiological responses are not apparent in all patients. Thus, this assessment may be best utilized to identify patients having neuromuscular abnormalities for whom psychophysiological treatment may be beneficial (57).

Psychiatric Diagnoses in Chronic Back Pain

The co-incidence of psychiatric disorder and chronic low back pain has long been recognized, and several investigators have reported an increased incidence of psychiatric disturbance in patients with low back pain (20,86). However, only recently have researchers employed rigorous methodology for diagnosing psychiatric disorder in low back pain patients. In one study of patients with nonspecific low back pain, 41% met criteria for a psychiatric diagnosis, with affective disorder being the most prevalent (11). Cluster analysis of these patients with psychiatric disorders revealed three subsets: (a) patients with high levels of nonorganic signs of low back pain but low mechanical features and physical findings; (b) those with high levels of mechanical features and physical findings, and few nonorganic signs; and (c) those with intermediate levels of both nonorganic and mechanical features. Thus, there are subgroups of back pain patients even among those with psychiatric disorders. Kinney et al. (63) compared rates of psychiatric disturbance in acute and chronic low back pain patients. When somatoform pain disorder was excluded (because 99% of patients met the criteria), chronic pain patients were found to have a much higher incidence (68%) of psychopathology than the acute pain group (23%). Similarly, Polatin et al. (85) reported that 77% of chronic low back pain patients in their sample met criteria for a psychiatric disorder in their lifetime and 59% met criteria at the time of evaluation. The most common diagnoses were affective disorders (e.g., depression), substance use disorders, and anxiety disorders. Interestingly, 57% of the patients met criteria for a psychiatric diagnosis prior to the onset of their back pain. Thus, while logic suggests that chronic pain may predispose individuals to psychiatric disorder, these data imply that the reverse may be the case. In this regard, a recent 10-year prospective study of industry workers found that self-reported depressive symptomatology was a significant predictor of subsequent musculoskeletal pain, but the reverse was not true (65). However, the proportion of variance in pain symptoms accounted for by depressive symptoms was quite small.

Comment

Recent studies using structured diagnostic interview indicate higher rates of psychiatric disturbance in chronic low back pain patients. Although temporal relationships between psychiatric diagnosis and pain have not been clearly established, it seems fair to conclude that psychiatric disturbance predates the development of pain in at least a portion of chronic back pain patients.

BEHAVIORAL AND PSYCHOLOGICAL TREATMENT OF LOW BACK PAIN

Initial interest in the behavioral treatment of back pain was sparked by a classic study by Fordyce and his colleagues (32) that demonstrated that increases in activ-

ity and decreases in pain medication intake could be achieved in chronic pain patients when they were treated in a specialized behavioral rehabilitation program. Since chronic low back pain is a complex problem, behavioral interventions are typically multimodal. Treatment packages typically combine a variety of operant–behavioral, cognitive–behavioral, and psychophysiological interventions. Recent controlled studies suggest that such multimodal treatments may be more beneficial than single modalities administered alone (61).

Operant–Behavioral Treatment

Operant conditioning, initially developed by B. F. Skinner (101), is based on the view that behavior is strongly influenced by its consequences. Behaviors that have positive consequences are likely to grow in strength and frequency. Conversely, behaviors that have aversive consequences are likely to weaken in strength and frequency. Fordyce (26) was one of the first to argue that pain behaviors may be acquired and maintained in some chronic pain patients by means of operant conditioning. In the case of an acute herniated lumbar disc, pain behaviors may simply reflect organic pathology. In some patients, though, pain behaviors persist long after the normal healing time. According to Fordyce (26), in this latter group of patients, pain behavior may be maintained by conditioning and learning. Patients may learn, for example, that the display of pain behavior is followed by positively reinforcing consequences such as delivery of a narcotic medication, avoidance of home or work demands, or solicitous attention from family members or health-care professionals.

Several studies of low back pain patients have examined the validity of the assumptions underlying the operant conditioning model of chronic low back pain (56). These studies suggest that: (a) pain behaviors in low back pain patients having an operant pain problem are not influenced by factors such as exercise, which one might expect would increase pain (66), (b) verbal and nonverbal pain behavior is significantly more likely to occur in patients having a solicitous spouse (5), and (c) pain behavior is higher in patients who report a high degree of satisfaction with social support (37) or in individuals who have been socially reinforced for pain complaints (68).

Daily activity patterns are a major target in the operant treatment of chronic low back pain. Chronic low back pain patients often live sedentary, restricted lifestyles, resulting in physical deconditioning, depression, and excessive anxiety regarding even simple everyday movements. Operant programs can be used to activate low back pain patients. As activity level increases, anxiety about physical performance decreases and improvements in mood occur.

Romano and her colleagues have recently conducted observational studies of patient–spouse interactions that provide support for the operant–behavioral model of pain (91,92). Patients and their spouses were videotaped as they engaged in a set of routine daily household activities (e.g., sweeping the floor and changing the bed). The tapes revealed that spouses of the chronic pain patients were much more likely to engage in solicitous responses than spouses of controls. Solicitous responses by spouses were also much more likely to precede and follow pain behavior displays in the pain patients than in control subjects (92).

Activity–rest cycling is one operant–behavioral method that can be used to increase activity in chronic low back pain patients (37). To establish a baseline level of activity, patients are asked to keep a daily activity diary of time spent sitting, standing or walking, and reclining. Patients are then asked to divide their daily uptime (time spent up and out of the reclining position) into cycles of activity and rest. A deactivated patient might be placed on an hourly activity–rest cycle consisting of 15 minutes up and out of bed, followed by 45 minutes of reclining in bed. The patient is encouraged to adhere to this schedule each hour if possible and, at a minimum, for 11 to 12 hours of the day. Each day, activity level is increased and time spent resting is decreased. Although controlled studies of activity–rest cycling are lacking, inpatient programs using such techniques have been able to achieve increases in uptime of 50% to 100% in low back pain patients having long histories of chronic pain (56).

Social reinforcement is a second operant–behavioral method that is widely used in the treatment of chronic low back pain patients (26). Social reinforcement in the form of therapist praise and attention is delivered to patients when they engage in well behaviors such as exercising, spending time out of bed, or becoming involved in vocationally relevant activities. At the same time that well behaviors are reinforced, there is an effort to minimize social reinforcement for excessive displays of pain behavior. Pain complaints are handled matter-of-factly, minimizing excessive attention. In many programs, spouses are systematically trained in social reinforcement methods for prompting and reinforcing well behavior (26).

A third operant–behavioral method used in the treatment of chronic low back pain is time-contingent pain medication (26). Many patients having chronic low back pain take their medication on a PRN or as needed basis. As a result, they have learned to associate high levels of pain and pain behavior with the delivery of potent narcotic medications. Switching the scheduling of narcotic medications from a PRN to a time-contingent basis breaks the association between severe pain and relief from pain. Time-contingent medications also produce more pain relief and lower levels of psychological distress (119). Time-contingent medication schedules have been found to be effective in withdrawing patients from narcotic medications (26,32).

Comment

Operant–behavioral interventions have successfully addressed two of the most important target behaviors of chronic low back pain patients: activity level and medication intake. Although there is little doubt that these methods can change such overt behavior patterns in chronic low back pain patients, their effects on pain ratings and other subjective responses are usually quite modest (56). Thus operant methods are frequently combined with cognitive–behavioral methods, which do appear to produce improvements in pain report and psychological distress.

Recently, operant–behavioral models of pain have been expanded to take into account the influence that individuals can play in controlling their own behavior. Theories such as Kanfer's self-regulation model (50) and Kanfer and Schefft's (51) general systems model have guided behavior therapists towards a greater use of techniques such as self-monitoring, self-reinforcement, and relaxation training. These techniques may be particularly useful in helping patients maintain and extend the gains obtained through operant behavioral treatment (51).

Cognitive–Behavioral Treatment

Cognitive–behavioral interventions for low back pain are designed to modify cognitive distortions, pain beliefs, and perceptions of coping strategy self-efficacy. The basic assumption underlying this approach is that changes in cognition will produce changes in behavior.

Cognitive restructuring is often used to modify cognitive distortions (107). In cognitive restructuring, patients are first taught to recognize the relationship among thoughts, feelings, behavior, and pain. They are then asked to monitor their thoughts and feelings in responses to pain. This assists the patient to identify negative or catastrophizing statements: "I am worthless. My life will never get any better. I can't stand this any longer." Patients are taught to modify these maladaptive thoughts by replacing them with more rational, calming self-statements.

Self-instructional training was originally developed to help individuals cope with acute pain (107). This training has recently been extended to the management of chronic low back pain. In self-instructional training, patients are taught to divide a severe pain experience into three phases: (a) preparing for intense stimulation before it becomes too strong, (b) confronting and handling intense stimulation, and (c) coping with the negative thoughts and feelings that arise. Patients are assisted to generate a list of calming self-statements to use during each of the three phases. Then patients practice using these statements during episodes of increased pain.

Practice in distraction and imagery techniques is another cognitive–behavioral intervention used in many pain management programs (72). Patients may be taught to distract themselves from pain by counting backward slowly, focusing on an aspect of their physical surroundings, or listening to music. Imagery is often presented in conjunction with relaxation training (111,112). Patients are asked to identify pleasant, relaxing images such as reclining on the beach or sitting in front of a fireplace, and then to practice diverting their attention from pain by imagining these scenes. One aspect of imagery that is particularly helpful to chronic pain patients is reinterpreting the pain stimulus as another sensation, e.g., as a dull or warm sensation (94).

Studies examining the efficacy of distraction and imagery suggest that these techniques are helpful, but that they work best for the control of low intensity pain stimuli (72). Reinterpretation appears to be more effective than distraction for severe pain, possibly because reinterpretation helps patients learn to cognitively reframe a perceptual experience that is difficult to ignore using distraction (72).

Psychophysiological Treatment

To address the muscular component of pain in low back patients, relaxation and biofeedback procedures are often included as part of a comprehensive behavioral program. Although a variety of forms of relaxation training are employed, progressive relaxation is most common. Most therapists use a form of Jacobson's approach which is similar to the procedures described by Bernstein and Borkovec (3). Relaxation is also thought to provide the patient with an effective competing response to fear, anxiety, and pain.

Biofeedback provides individuals with information about a physiological response in order to enable them to gain control over that response. In chronic low back pain patients, electrodes might be attached to the skin to record activity in the paraspinal muscles. Initial sessions usually focus on helping patients gain control over the target response under relatively easy conditions (e.g., reclining in a quiet room). In later sessions, emphasis is placed on helping patients gain control over the target responses while they are engaging in activities that tend to increase their pain (e.g., walking or stair climbing).

A recent study by Flor and Birbaumer (21) evaluated the long-term effects of biofeedback treatment for a mixed group of minimally disabled musculoskeletal pain patients, two-thirds of whom had back pain. Patients were randomly assigned to either EMG biofeedback, cognitive–behavioral therapy, or conservative medical treatment. Patients in the EMG biofeedback or cognitive–behavioral therapy group received eight, 60 minute sessions. At posttreatment, patients in all three groups

showed improvements, but those in the biofeedback group showed the best outcomes. By the 24-month follow-up, only patients in the biofeedback condition were able to maintain their improvements in pain, impairment, and stress-related reactivity of the affected muscles, and coping self-statements. These findings support the efficacy of biofeedback for patients with musculoskeletal back pain and agree with those reported in a review of EMG biofeedback (57), which concluded that controlled studies have demonstrated the efficacy of biofeedback for muscularly based low back pain.

Comment

Psychophysiological approaches to chronic low back pain, such as relaxation training, are central components of most behavioral treatment programs. Although these approaches are designed to alter maladaptive physiological responses, they also can produce changes in other target behaviors. Patients who are able to achieve significant reductions in lumbar paraspinal muscle activity through biofeedback training may also report changes in their beliefs about the controllability of their pain and expectations for the future. Patients who learn to use relaxation during daily activities may show a significant reduction in guarded movement, pain avoidance posturing, and other motor pain behaviors. Although psychophysiological approaches are helpful, it should be noted that the relationship between change in a psychophysiologic response such as muscle tension and improvement in pain is complex (24).

Comparative Treatment Outcome Studies

Recently, studies have begun to examine the relative efficacy of different behavioral treatment approaches to back pain. In one of the first studies, Turner (111) compared the relative efficacy of cognitive behavior therapy to relaxation training in mildly disabled low back pain patients. The cognitive behavior therapy intervention was superior on measures of pain, depression, disability, health care use, and absenteeism (111). More recently, Turner and Clancy (112) compared an operant–behavioral and a cognitive–behavioral intervention for low back pain. Although there were differential rates of improvement in physical and psychosocial disability over 12 months, there were no significant differences in outcomes at the 12-month follow-up (112).

In two studies, Turner and colleagues compared the separate and combined effects of cognitive therapy and relaxation to each alone, and a combination of behavioral therapy and exercise to each alone; again they found that each treatment resulted in significant improvement, but no differences in outcomes existed at follow-up (114,115). However, the combined approach of behavior therapy and exercise produced greater improvement from pre- to posttreatment than either treatment alone, on all patient self-report and observer-rated measures. Taken together, these studies suggest that a combined approach may achieve the greatest immediate improvements for mildly disabled low back pain patients, but further comparisons with larger samples are needed to confirm this hypothesis.

Nicholas, Wilson, and Goyen (78) recently compared the effectiveness of a combined cognitive–behavioral/physical therapy intervention to physical therapy alone in the treatment of a more disabled group of chronic back pain patients. The combined intervention was more effective than physical therapy alone in reducing functional impairment and medication use and in increasing self-efficacy and the use of active coping strategies. This study, like those by Turner cited earlier, underscores the utility of multimodal treatments in the management of chronic back pain.

Early and Brief Interventions

In behavioral treatment for low back pain, evidence has emerged that suggests that not only is the content of the treatment important, but also when and how treatment is delivered. Treatment can be administered before there is any sign of a pain problem (primary prevention), soon after the first occurrence of the pain problem (secondary prevention), or after the pain problem has become chronic (tertiary prevention). Data suggest that a person who misses work for 3 months because of low back pain has a very poor chance of recovery (49), underscoring the importance of primary or secondary prevention.

While it would be unwieldy to administer any preventive intervention to an entire population, primary prevention efforts may be beneficial for small-scale, high-risk populations. Hilyer and colleagues (44), for example, conducted a flexibility intervention with firefighters (whose leading on-duty injuries are musculoskeletal) and found that those who participated in the intervention demonstrated increased flexibility and lost significantly less time from the job when injured during the 2-year follow-up period. This intervention was conducted at the work site and involved a 30-minute exercise period each day led by bachelor-level fitness specialists. It was a relatively simple and inexpensive, yet helpful, intervention.

Gundewall, Liljeqvist, and Hansson (40) have demonstrated the benefits of primary prevention in the management of back pain in nurses. Nurses were randomly assigned to one of two groups. The experimental group participated in a supervised session involving endurance and strengthening exercise one to two times a week during work hours. The control group received no exposure

to the exercise program. After 13 months, subjects in the experimental group had fewer complaints of back pain and significantly less work absenteeism. The exercise intervention was also quite cost-effective.

Secondary prevention efforts with pain patients have also shown considerable promise in reducing pain levels and absenteeism from work (29). By intervening with patients before maladaptive behavioral patterns such as inactivity and overuse of analgesics are entrenched, treatment can be more effective and cost efficient.

In patients with no history of acute musculoskeletal pain (MSP), for example, delivery of an early outpatient behavioral treatment within a few days after the onset of pain resulted in less sick leave during a follow-up period than that for a control group and a group of patients with a history of MSP (69,70). The treatment consisted of maintenance of daily activities, practice of specified activities, and reinforcement of healthy behaviors by staff. In another study examining the effect of an intervention with nurses and nursing aides experiencing low back pain but still working, participants reported significantly less pain, fewer medications, and more activity at the 18-month follow-up (67). Both these studies represent substantial economic savings for the active intervention groups in terms of pain-related absenteeism.

Secondary prevention efforts can easily be carried out at the work site. For example, Donchin, Woolf, Kaplan, and Floman, (16) found that an exercise program (two times weekly for 45 minutes over 3 months) implemented for hospital employees resulted at 1 year in fewer "painful months" (4.5) than experienced by control subjects (7.4) or subjects in a back school intervention (7.3), as well as significant gains in abdominal muscle strength and trunk forward flexion. Sirles, Brown, and Hilyer (100) report that a back school intervention combined with exercise for back-injured municipal workers resulted in decreased anxiety, depression and pain perception at 3 months.

Given the current concern in the United States about cost containment in health care delivery, one important direction for chronic low back pain treatment research will be to evaluate ways of delivering behavioral treatments that are less expensive than repeated inpatient admissions or office-based, one-on-one, individual treatment. Modes of treatment for which there is initial support from other pain populations include home-based interventions, group interventions, and telephone contacts.

In home-based interventions, skills are introduced in the clinic, but the greater part of skill acquisition takes place at home, typically guided by treatment manuals and audio tapes. Home-based programs for headache, for example, generally require only three to four clinic therapy sessions, compared to 10 or more sessions in a routine clinic-based program. Group treatments employ as many treatment sessions as individual therapies, but maximize cost-efficiency through treating multiple patients simultaneously and reducing the cost for individual patients.

Use of these cost-contained interventions with other chronic pain populations is promising (81). A meta-analytic review of behavioral group treatment (six studies) and home-based treatment (ten studies) for headache revealed that intervention effects were equivalent to individualized intervention for tension headache (82) and for vascular headache (4). In osteoarthritis patients whose medical condition was stable, monthly telephone contact with trained nonmedical interviewers over 1 year was more effective than clinic visits in improving physical health and reducing pain (117,118) The telephone contacts consisted of reviewing medications, problems with joint pain, gastrointestinal symptoms, early warning signs for common chronic diseases, and scheduled outpatient visits, and patients were provided an evening/weekend clinic telephone number. The effects were maintained even in patients who had no change in drug treatment for their osteoarthritis and for whom physical therapy was not instituted over the year of the contacts (87).

Although some patients, such as those whose medical condition is unstable, those whose pain problem is particularly refractory to treatment, those who excessively use analgesic medications, and those who are clinically depressed, may continue to require more intensive treatments, home-based, group, or telephone interventions may be equally effective for other pain patients.

Relapse Prevention

There is growing recognition among cognitive–behavioral therapists that one needs to plan for maintenance of treatment effects rather than to hope that these effects will occur. A specialized area of study, termed relapse prevention, has been developed to examine issues in the maintenance of treatment effects (71). A major assumption of the relapse prevention model is that relapse is not an outcome (a treatment failure) from which patients cannot recover. Instead, lapses in coping efforts are assumed to be an integral component of long-term behavior change, and anticipating these lapses and adaptively responding to them will assist patients in maintaining treatment gains over time.

The relapse prevention model emphasizes the importance of a detailed analysis of relapse episodes. It is assumed that each patient will eventually face situations in which coping efforts become difficult, such as during a pain flare-up. Pain flare-ups can tax patients' coping efforts, decrease their confidence in continuing these coping efforts, and perhaps even lead them to stop their coping efforts. This sequence of events would be considered a relapse. As part of their training, patients learn

how to anticipate the series of events that can lead to relapse and how to restart their coping efforts.

Comment

There is a clear trend toward increased use of cognitive–behavioral interventions in the management of chronic low back pain. A major advantage of these interventions is their emphasis on self-control. Once patients master techniques such as cognitive restructuring or imagery, they can use these interventions on their own in a variety of situations. While controlled studies have demonstrated that cognitive–behavioral interventions help patients having chronic low back pain, the process by which these interventions work remains to be studied. Little is known, for example, about how changes in cognitions achieved during behavioral treatment relate to long-term improvements in pain and disability.

ISSUES IN ASSESSMENT AND TREATMENT

There are a number of clinical issues that one needs to be aware of in using psychological assessment and treatment methods with chronic low back pain patients (56). Two particularly important assessment issues are: (a) the relation of childhood trauma to back pain and (b) the relation of psychological factors to functional capacity measures. Three important treatment issues are: (a) preparing the patient for treatment, (b) matching treatment interventions to the needs of the patient, and (c) enhancing the generalization and maintenance of treatment effects.

Assessment Issues

The Relation of Childhood Psychosocial Trauma to Chronic Low Back Pain

Several researchers have noted that patients with chronic pain complaints report a history of abuse or trauma during childhood more frequently than do healthy subjects (15,122). This has recently been evaluated in patients with low back pain. Schofferman et al. (96) studied 86 patients who underwent spine surgery and determined whether they had had any of five types of childhood psychological trauma (sexual abuse, physical abuse, abandonment, a chemically dependent caregiver, or emotional neglect). Unsuccessful surgical outcome occurred in 85% of the patients who had three or more of the types of trauma, while only 5% of patients with no childhood trauma had unsuccessful outcomes. In a later study, these authors reported that chronic low back pain patients who had experienced three or more types of trauma were less likely to show structural pathology to account for their pain than patients experiencing two or less types of trauma (96,97).

These studies suggest that childhood psychological trauma may be a poor prognostic factor in patients with low back pain. However, the data must be interpreted cautiously, because base rates of childhood trauma in the general population are difficult to establish, and all research to date has relied on retrospective reporting of abuse in patients, which may be subject to considerable bias. Further research is needed to definitively establish the role of childhood psychological trauma in the development and maintenance of back pain.

Relation of Psychological Factors to Functional Capacity Measures

Recent advances in technology have increased the availability and utilization of biomechanical devices for assessing the functional capacities of the lumbar motion segment in low back pain patients (e.g., trunk strength, lumbar range of motion). Many clinicians consider the data generated by these testing procedures to be "objective" and hence more reliable and valid than patient-reported symptoms or "soft" clinical signs. Many of the testing protocols yield not only indices of strength and mobility but also measures of variability across repetitions; the increased variability is presumed to indicate submaximal effort. However, Robinson and colleagues have reported that submaximal efforts can be reliably produced, yielding relatively low coefficients of variability (88). These authors also found that pain-free subjects instructed to simulate a back injury produced consistent lumbar extension curves that were indistinguishable from their maximal efforts (89). These data call into question the ability of these testing procedures to identify submaximal effort using the coefficient of variation. Additionally, psychological variables may influence patients' performance in these types of testing procedures. Robinson et al. (90) reported, somewhat unexpectedly, that in low back pain patients, higher scores on measures of psychological distress were associated with lower torque variability in an isometric lumbar extension task. Also, Papciak and Feuerstein (80) found that in low back pain patients, psychological measures were associated with peak torque and torque variability in an isokinetic lumbar extension task. However, in this study, anxiety, catastrophizing, and somatization were negatively associated with peak torque, and catastrophizing was positively associated with the coefficient of variation.

Taken together, the above studies highlight the influence of psychological factors on the results of isokinetic and isometric trunk-strength testing. Thus, health-care professionals using biomechanical measures to assess function need to be aware that variables such as anxiety and somatization can have an impact on the outcome of their evaluations.

Treatment Issues

Patient Preparation

The psychological sophistication of patients having chronic back pain varies greatly. Many patients maintain an overly simplistic view of their pain, and find it difficult to admit that behavioral or psychological factors may affect the pain. These patients often view a referral for psychological evaluation or treatment as abandonment by the referring physician or an implication that their pain is entirely imaginary. Other patients are able to recognize the roles that environmental stressors or an overly solicitous spouse play in their adaptation to back pain and these patients are typically open to psychological intervention.

Given the variations in the degree to which chronic back pain patients are open to psychological intervention, careful preparation of the patient for referral to a psychologist is essential. Without such preparation, some patients will refuse referral or will be guarded and uncooperative. One important aspect of patient preparation is for the physician to assure the patient that the pain is a real and very complex problem. The patient then can be told that the focus of psychological evaluation is to help better understand and treat this problem. Behavioral treatment can be presented as a method of teaching patients how to alter their responses to pain in order to gain better control over pain. It is often helpful to mention that behavioral treatment methods have been found helpful for individuals having a clear-cut organic basis for pain such as children undergoing painful bone-marrow aspirations (56). This helps allay the suspicion held by many patients that if their pain is relieved by behavioral or psychological methods, then the pain must be psychological.

Matching Treatment to the Patient

As mentioned earlier, the current trend in psychological treatment of chronic back pain is to rely on treatment protocols that combine a variety of operant–behavioral, cognitive–behavioral, and psychophysiological interventions. Although some programs use a standard combination of interventions, most attempt to tailor treatment individually so as to address the unique problems experienced by a particular patient. Information gathered from psychological and behavioral assessment is quite useful in matching specific treatments to patient needs. For example, operant–behavioral methods are most likely to benefit patients who are deactivated, overly dependent on family members, or addicted to pain medications. Patients who are excessively anxious or depressed, in contrast, may require more intensive treatment with cognitive therapy techniques such as cognitive restructuring or self-instructional training.

One of the major advantages of individually tailored treatment is that it can reduce the time and costs of treatment. Patients who require instruction in cognitive therapy techniques, for example, may not need the intensive supervision and staff involvement needed by a patient placed on a strict operant program of activation and time-contingent medications. Streamlining the treatment process is important because many treatment methods require the involvement of a highly trained behavioral psychologist.

Maintenance and Generalization Issues

Cognitive–behavioral therapists are increasingly aware that planning for maintenance and generalization of treatment effects is necessary (107). Maintenance of treatment effects refers to the ability of treatment to produce lasting improvements in behavior. Generalization of treatment effects refers to the degree to which improvements in one target behavior (e.g., increases in activity) lead to improvements in other important target behaviors (e.g., improvements in mood and pain).

A variety of methods have been used in treatment programs for chronic back pain patients to enhance maintenance and generalization. First, most programs maintain contact with patients after they have completed their formal treatment, scheduling follow-up contacts at regular time intervals. This helps therapists avoid the tendency to respond to the patient only at times of crisis, thereby reinforcing high levels of pain behavior. It also provides opportunities to identify and reinforce changes in behavior that may not have been apparent during the initial stages of treatment. Second, follow-up visits may take the form of booster sessions in which the patient is provided with refresher training in a variety of treatment components (e.g., relaxation training, activation, cognitive coping skills). Third, social support for pain-coping efforts is an important part of follow-up, and to increase social support many programs use group therapy sessions as part of their follow-up contact with patients.

Spouse training is potentially one of the most effective methods for enhancing the maintenance and generalization of treatment effects. A major assumption of the behavioral approach is that patients do not change independent of their environment. Since the spouse often provides the most salient social contingencies in the patient's environment, spouses may function as a primary reinforcing agent and thus have significant effects on patient behavior (22,23,83,84).

Spouse training is accepted as pivotal in many pain treatment programs (77). Spouse training can instruct the spouse how to prompt and reinforce the patient's adaptive efforts to cope with pain during important functional activities such as walking and rising from a bed or a sitting position. The spouse can also help the patient overcome obstacles to practicing coping skills. Further,

spouse training can help prevent the spouse from unintentionally interfering with treatment goals by taking over tasks, enforcing inactivity or rest, and limiting social activities, all of which can result in excessive reinforcement of pain behavior and physical disability (26).

CONCLUSIONS

Psychological approaches to the assessment and treatment of chronic back pain are relatively recent. Most studies in this area have been carried out in the past 20 years. There is little doubt that the psychological and behavioral approaches to assessment discussed above have advanced our understanding of chronic back pain patients. The behavioral and psychological treatment methods we have reviewed have also reduced pain and suffering in many chronic back pain patients.

In the coming years we are likely to see a number of advances in the psychology of chronic back pain. The application of sophisticated multivariate statistical techniques such as cluster analysis may well lead to the identification of subgroups of chronic back pain patients who respond to particular treatment approaches. Psychological approaches to treatment are also likely to be used more widely. These approaches are currently restricted to patients having chronic pain and long-standing behavioral and psychological problems. Psychological approaches, however, could be applied earlier in the development of chronic pain so as to prevent maladaptive pain behaviors and psychological problems from becoming entrenched. In the future, treatment programs for acute back pain may combine behavioral approaches with medical and surgical interventions. Combined behavioral and medical treatment is one of the most promising methods for preventing the suffering and psychological distress that often accompany the chronic back pain experience.

ACKNOWLEDGMENTS. Preparation of this chapter was supported in part by grants AR35270 and AR42261 from the National Institute of Arthritis and Musculoskeletal Diseases.

REFERENCES

1. Armentrout D, Moore JE, Parker JC, Hewett JE, Feltz C (1982): Pain-patient MMPI subgroups: The psychological dimensions of pain. *J Behav Med* 5:201–211.
2. Beck AT (1972): *Depression: causes and treatment.* Philadelphia: University of Pennsylvania Press.
3. Bernstein DA, Borkovec TD (1973): *Progressive relaxation training.* Champaign, IL: Research Press.
4. Blanchard EB (1992): Psychological treatment of benign headache disorders. *J Consult Clin Psychol* 60:537–551.
5. Block AR, Kremer EF, Gaylor M (1980): Behavioral treatment of chronic pain: the spouse as a discriminative cue for pain behavior. *Pain* 9:243–252.
6. Blumetti AE, Modesti LM (1971): Psychological predictors of success or failure of surgical intervention for intractable back pain. In: Bonica J, Albe-Fissard D, eds. *Advances in pain research and therapy*, vol 1. New York: Raven Press.
7. Bradley LA, Prokop CK, Margolis R, Gentry WD (1978): Multivariate analysis of the MMPI profiles of low back pain patients. *J Behav Med* 1:253–272.
8. Bradley LA, Van der Heide LH (1984): Pain-related correlates of MMPI profile subgroups among back pain patients. *Health Psychol* 3:157–174.
9. Brennan AF, Barrett CL, Garretson HD (1987): The prediction of chronic pain outcome by psychological variables. *Int J Psychiatry Med* 16:373–387.
10. Calsyn DA, Louks J, Freeman CW (1976): The use of the MMPI with chronic low back pain patients with a mixed diagnosis. *J Clin Psychol* 32:532–536.
11. Coste J, Spira A, Ducimetiere P, Paolaggi JB (1991): Clinical and psychological diversity of non-specific low-back pain. A new approach towards the classification of clinical subgroups. *J Clin Epidemiol* 44:1233–1245.
12. Costello RM, Hulsey TL, Schoenfeld LS, Ramamurthy S (1987): P-A-I-N: a four cluster MMPI typology for chronic pain. *Pain* 30: 199–209.
13. Crisson J, Keefe FJ, Wilkins RH, Cook WA, Muhlbaier LH (1986): Self-report of depressive symptoms in low back pain patients. *J Clin Psychol* 42:425–430.
14. Crown S (1978): Psychological aspects of low back pain. *Rheum Rehab* 17:114–124.
15. Domino J, Haber J (1987): Prior physical and sexual abuse in women with chronic headache: clinical correlates. *Headache* 27: 310–314.
16. Donchin M, Woolf O, Kaplan L, Floman Y (1990): Secondary prevention of low-back pain: a clinical trial. *Spine* 15: 1317–1320.
17. Doxey NS, Dzioba RB, Mitson GL, Lacroix JM (1988): Predictors of outcome in back surgery candidates. *J Clin Psychol* 44: 611–622.
18. Dworkin RH, Hartstein G, Rosner G, Walther RR, Sweeney EW, Brand L (1992): A high-risk method for studying psychosocial antecedents of chronic pain: the prospective investigation of herpes zoster. *J Abnorm Psychol* 101:200–205.
19. Engel GL (1959): "Psychogenic" pain and the pain prone patient. *Am J Med* 26:899–918.
20. Fishbain DA, Goldberg M, Meagher BR, Steele R, Rosomoff H (1986): Male and female chronic pain patients categorized by DSM-III psychiatric diagnostic criteria. *Pain* 26:181–197.
21. Flor H, Birbaumer N (1993): Comparison of the efficacy of electromyographic biofeedback, cognitive–behavioral therapy, and conservative medical interventions in the treatment of chronic musculoskeletal pain. *J Consult Clin Psychol* 61:653–658.
22. Flor H, Kerns RD, Turk DC (1987): The role of spouse reinforcement, perceived pain, and activity levels of chronic pain patients. *J Psychosom Res* 31:251–259.
23. Flor H, Turk DC (1985): Chronic illness in an adult family member: pain as a prototype. In: Turk DC, Kerns RD, eds. *Health, illness, and families: A life-span perspective.* New York: Wiley.
24. Flor H, Turk DC, Birbaumer N (1985): Assessment of stress-related psychophysiological reactions in chronic back pain patients. *J Consult Clin Psychol* 53:354–364.
25. Follick MJ, Ahern DK, Laser-Wolston N (1984): Evaluation of a daily activity diary for chronic pain patients. *Pain* 19:373–382.
26. Fordyce WE (1976): *Behavioral methods for chronic pain and illness.* St. Louis: Mosby.
27. Fordyce WE (1985): On Rachlin's "pain and behavior": a lightening of the burden. *Behav Brain Sci* 81:58–59.
28. Fordyce WE, Brena SF, Holcomb RJ, DeLateur BJ, Loeser JD (1978): Relationship of patient semantic pain descriptions to physician diagnostic judgements, activity level measures, and MMPI. *Pain* 5:293–303.
29. Fordyce WE, Brockway JA, Bergman JA, Spengler D (1986): Acute back pain: a control-group comparison of behavioral versus traditional management methods. *J Behav Med* 9:127–140.
30. Fordyce W, Fowler R, DeLateur B (1968): An application of behavior modification technique to a problem of chronic pain. *Behav Res Ther* 6:105–107.
31. Fordyce WE, Fowler RS Jr, Lehmann JF, DeLateur BJ (1968):

Some implications of learning in problems of chronic pain. *J Chron Dis* 21:179–190.

32. Fordyce WE, Fowler RS Jr, Lehmann JF, DeLateur BJ, Sand PL, Trieschmann RB (1973): Operant conditioning in the treatment of chronic pain. *Arch Phys Med Rehab* 54:399–408.

33. Gatchel RJ, Mayer TG, Capra P, Barnett J, Diamond P (1986): Millon Behavioral Health Inventory: its utility in predicting physical function in patients with low back pain. *Arch Phys Med Rehab* 67:878–882.

34. Gentry WD (1982): Chronic back pain: does elective surgery benefit patients with evidence of psychologic disturbance? *South Med J* 75:1169–1170.

35. Gentry WD, Shows WD, Thomas M (1974): Chronic low back pain: a psychological profile. *Psychosomatics* 15:174–177.

36. Gil KM, Keefe FJ, Crisson JE, VanDalfsen PJ (1987): Social support and pain behavior. *Pain* 29:209–217.

37. Gil KM, Ross SL, Keefe FJ (1988): Behavioral treatment of chronic pain: four pain management protocols. In: France RD, Krishnan KRR, eds. *Chronic pain.* Washington, DC: American Psychiatric Press.

38. Graham JR (1987): *The MMPI: A practical guide,* 2nd ed. New York: Oxford University Press.

39. Gross AR (1986): The effect of coping strategies on the relief of pain following surgical intervention for lower back pain. *Psychosom Med* 48:229–241.

40. Gundewall B, Liljeqvist M, Hansson T (1993): Primary prevention of back symptoms and absence from work: a prospective randomized study among hospital employees. *Spine* 18:587–594.

41. Hamburgen ME, Jennings CA, Maruta T, Swanson DW (1985): Failure of a predictive scale in identifying patients who may benefit from a pain management program: Follow-up data. *Pain* 23:253–258.

42. Hanvik LJ (1951): MMPI profiles in patients with low-back pain. *J Consult Psychol* 15:350–353.

43. Hart RR (1984): Chronic pain: replicated multivariate clustering of personality profiles. *J Clin Psychol* 40:129–133.

44. Hilyer JC, Brown KC, Sirles AT, Peoples L (1990): A flexibility intervention to reduce the incidence and severity of joint injuries among municipal firefighters. *J Occup Med* 32:631–637.

45. Hoekstra DM, DeGood DE, Shutty MS (1987): *Beliefs about rehabilitative strategies and coping in chronic pain patients.* Paper presented at the Annual Meeting of the American Psychological Association, New York, NY.

46. Jensen MP, Karoly P (1991): Control beliefs, coping efforts, and adjustment to chronic pain. *J Consult Clin Psych* 59:431–438.

47. Jensen MP, Karoly P, Huger R (1987): The development and preliminary validation of an instrument to assess patients' attitudes toward pain. *J Psychosom Res* 31:393–400.

48. Jensen MP, Turner JA, Romano JM (1991): Coping with chronic pain: a critical review of the literature. *Pain* 47:249–284.

49. Johnson AD (1978): *The problem chain: an approach to early identification.* Department of Labor and Industries, State of Washington (USA), Internal report.

50. Kanfer FH (1971): The maintenance of behavior by self-generated stimuli and reinforcement. In: Jacobs A, Sachs LB, eds. *The psychology of private events.* New York: Academic Press.

51. Kanfer FH, Schefft BK (1988): *Guiding the process of therapeutic change.* Champaign, IL: Research Press.

52. Keefe FJ, Block AR (1982): Development of an observation method for assessing pain behavior in chronic low back pain patients. *Behav Ther* 13:363–375.

53. Keefe FJ, Brown C, Scott DS, Ziesat H (1982): Behavioral assessment of chronic pain. In: Keefe FJ, Blumenthal JA, eds. *Assessment strategies in behavioral medicine.* New York: Grune & Stratton.

54. Keefe FJ, Dunsmore J (1992): Pain behavior: concepts and controversies. *Am Pain Soc J* 1:92–100.

55. Keefe FJ, Dunsmore J (1992): The multifaceted nature of pain behavior. *Am Pain Soc J* 1:112–114.

56. Keefe FJ, Gil KT (1985): Recent advances in the behavioral assessment and treatment of chronic pain. *Ann Behav Med* 7:11–16.

57. Keefe FJ, Hoelscher T (1987): Biofeedback in the management of chronic pain syndromes: Biofeedback Society of America task force report. In: Hatch JP, Fisher JG, Rush JD, eds. *Biofeedback: studies in clinical efficacy.* New York: Plenum Press, 211–254.

58. Keefe FJ, Salley AN, Lefebvre JC (1992): Coping with pain: conceptual concerns and future directions. *Pain* 51:131–134.

59. Keefe FJ, Wilkins RH, Cook WA (1984): Direct observation of pain behavior in low back pain patients during physical examination. *Pain* 20:59–68.

60. Keefe FJ, Wilkins RH, Cook WA Jr, Crisson JE, Muhlbaier LH (1986): Depression, pain, and pain behavior. *J Consult Clin Psychol* 54:665–669.

61. Kerns RD, Turk DC, Holzman AD, Rudy TE (1986): Comparison of cognitive–behavioral and behavioral approaches to the outpatient treatment chronic pain. *Clin J Pain* 1:195–203.

62. Kerns RD, Turk DC, Rudy TE (1985): The West Haven-Yale Multidimensional Pain Inventory (WHYMPI). *Pain* 23:345–356.

63. Kinney RK, Gatchel RJ, Polatin, PB, Fogarty WT, Mayer TG (1993): Prevalence of psychopathology in acute and chronic low back pain patients. *J Occup Rehab* 3:95–103.

64. Lefebvre MF (1981): Cognitive distortion and cognitive errors in depressed psychiatric and low back pain patients. *J Consult Clin Psychol* 49:517–525.

65. Leino P, Magni G (1993): Depressive and distress symptoms as predictors of low back pain, neck-shoulder pain, and other muskuloskeletal morbidity: a 10-year follow-up of metal industry employees. *Pain* 53:89–94.

66. Linton SJ (1986): Behavioral remediation of chronic pain: a status report. *Pain* 24:125–141.

67. Linton SJ, Bradley LA (1992): An 18-month follow-up of a secondary prevention program for back pain: help and hindrance factors related to outcome maintenance. *Clin J Pain* 8:227–236.

68. Linton SJ, G'otestam KG (1985): Controlling pain reports through operant conditioning: a laboratory demonstration. *Percept Mot Skills* 60:427–437.

69. Linton SJ, Hellsing A, Andersson D (1993): A controlled study of the effects of an early intervention on acute musculoskeletal pain problems. *Pain* 54:353–359.

70. Linton SJ, Jensen I, Bradley LA, Hallman U (1987): Secondary prevention of chronic back pain: preliminary results of a controlled study [Abstr]. *Pain* 4(suppl):S121.

71. Marlatt GA, Gordon JR (1985): *Relapse prevention.* New York: Guilford Press.

72. McCaul KD, Malott JM (1984): Distraction and coping with pain. *Psychol Bull* 95:516–533.

73. McGill JC, Lawlis GF, Selby D, Mooney V, McCoy CE (1983): The relationship of Minnesota Multiphasic Personality Inventory (MMPI) profile clusters to pain behaviors. *J Behav Med* 6:77–92.

74. Melzack R, Wall PD (1965): Pain mechanisms: a new theory. *Science* 150:971–979.

75. Millon T, Green C, Meagher R (1982): *Millon Behavioral Health Inventory Manual,* 3rd ed. Minneapolis, MN: National Computer Systems.

76. Moore JE, Armentrout DP, Parker JC, Kivlahan DR (1986): Empirically derived pain-patient MMPI subgroups: prediction of treatment outcome. *J Behav Med* 9:51–63.

77. Moore JE, Chaney EF (1985): Outpatient group treatment of chronic pain: effects of spouse involvement. *J Consult Clin Psychol* 53:326–334.

78. Nicholas MK, Wilson PH, Goyen J (1992): Comparison of cognitive–behavioral group treatment and alternative non-psychological treatment for chronic low back pain. *Pain* 48:339–347.

79. Orme TJ, Brown CW, Richardson HD (1985): The use of the Millon Behavioral Health Inventory (MBHI) as a predictor of surgical suitability. *Proceedings of the International Society for the Study of the Lumbar Spine,* Sydney, Australia, April.

80. Papciak AS, Feuerstein M (1991): Psychological factors affecting isokinetic trunk strength testing in patients with work-related chronic low back pain. *J Occup Rehab* 1:95–104.

81. Penzien DB, Holroyd KA, Johnson CA (1991): Nonpharmacologic treatment of recurrent headache. *Pain Digest* 1:191–202.

82. Penzien DB, Rains JC, Holroyd KA (1992): A review of alternative behavioral treatments for headache. *The Mississippi Psychologist* 17:8–9.

83. Pinkston EM, Linsk NL (1984): Behavioral family intervention with the impaired elderly. *Gerontologist* 24(6):576–583.

84. Pinkston EM, Linsk NL, Young RN (1988): Home-based behavioral family treatment of the impaired elderly. *Behav Ther* 19: 331–344.

85. Polatin PB, Kinney RK, Gatchel, RJ, Lillo E, Mayer, TG (1993): Psychiatric illness and chronic low-back pain: the mind and the spine—which goes first? *Spine* 18:66–71.

86. Reich J, Tupin JP, Abramowitz SI (1983): Psychiatric diagnoses of chronic pain patients. *Am J Psychiatry* 140:1495–1498.

87. Rene J, Weinberger M, Mazzuca SA, Brandt KD, Katz BP (1992): Reduction of joint pain in patients with knee osteoarthritis who have received monthly telephone calls from lay personnel and whose medical treatmnt regimens have remained stable. *Arthritis Care Res* 35:511–515.

88. Robinson ME, MacMillan M, O'Connor PD, Fuller AK, Cassisi JE (1991): Reproducibility of maximal versus submaximal efforts in an isometric lumbar extension task. *J Spinal Dis* 4:444–448.

89. Robinson ME, MacMillan M, O'Connor PD, Fuller AK, Cassisi JE (1992): Effect of instructions to simulate a back injury on torque reproducibility in an isometric lumbar extension task. *J Occup Rehab* 2:191–199.

90. Robinson ME, O'Connor PD, MacMillan M, Shirley FR, Greene AF, Geisser ME, Fuller AK (1992): Physical and psychosocial correlates of test-retest isometric torque variability in patients with chronic low back pain. *J Occup Rehab* 2:11–18.

91. Romano JM, Turner JA, Friedman LS, Bulcroft RA, Jensen MP, Hops H (1991): Observational assessment of chronic pain patient-spouse behavioral interaction. *Behav Ther* 22:549–568.

92. Roman JM, Turner JA, Friedman LS, Bulcroft RA, Jensen MP, Hops H, Wright SF (1992): Sequential analysis of chronic pain behaviors and spouse response. *J Consult Clin Psychol* 60:777–782.

93. Rosenstiel AK, Keefe FJ (1983): The use of coping strategies in chronic low back pain patients: relationships to patient characteristics and current adjustment. *Pain* 17:33–44.

94. Rybstein-Blinchik E (1979): Effects of different cognitive strategies on chronic pain experience. *J Behav Med* 2:93–101.

95. Sanders SH (1980): Toward a practical instrument system for the automatic measurement of "uptime" in chronic pain patients. *Pain* 9:103–109.

96. Schofferman J, Anderson D, Hines R, Smith G, Keane G (1993): Childhood psychological trauma and chronic refractory low-back pain. *Clin J Pain* 9:260–265.

97. Schofferman J, Anderson D, Hines R, Smith G, White A (1992): Childhood psychological trauma correlates with unsuccessful lumbar spine surgery. *Spine* 17(suppl):S138–S144.

98. Schwartz DP, DeGood DE, Shutty MS (1985): Direct assessment of beliefs and attitudes of chronic pain patients. *Arch Phys Med Rehab* 66:806–809.

99. Shutty MS Jr, DeGood DE, Hoekstra D (1987): Assessment of chronic pain patients beliefs about rehabilitative strategies: relationship to coping styles and treatment outcome [abstr]. *Pain* 40: (Suppl) S326.

100. Sirles AT, Brown K, Hilyer JC (1991): Effects of back school education and exercise in back injured municipal workers. *AAOHN J* 39:7–12.

101. Skinner BF (1953): *Science and human behavior.* New York: Macmillan.

102. Smith TW, Aberger EW, Follick MJ, Ahern DK (1986): Cognitive distortion and psychological distress in chronic low back pain. *J Consult Clin Psychol* 54:573–575.

103. Smith TW, Follick MJ, Ahern DK, Adams A (1986): Cognitive distortion and disability in chronic low back pain. *Cog Ther Res* 10:201–210.

104. Sternbach RA, Wolff SR, Murphy RW, Akeson WH (1973): Aspects of chronic low back pain. *Psychosomatics* 14:52–56.

105. Sternbach RA, Wolff SR, Murphy RW, Akeson WH (1973): Traits of pain patients: the low-back "loser." *Psychosomatics* 14: 226–229.

106. Sweet JJ, Breuer SR, Hazelwood LA, Toye R, Pawl RP (1985): The Millon Behavioral Health Inventory: concurrent and predictive validity in a pain treatment center. *J Behav Med* 3:215–226.

107. Turk DC, Meichenbaum DH, Genest M (1983): *Pain and behavioral medicine: a cognitive–behavioral perspective.* New York: Guilford Press.

108. Turk DC, Flor H (1987): Pain behaviors: the utility and limitations of the pain behavior construct. *Pain* 31:277–296.

109. Turk DC, Rudy TE (1988): Toward an empirically derived taxonomy of chronic pain patients: integration of psychological assessment data. *J Consult Clin Psychol* 56:233–238.

110. Turk DC, Wack JT, Kerns RD (1985): An empirical examination of the "pain–behavior" construct. *J Behav Med* 8:119–130.

112. Turner JA (1982): Comparison of group progressive-relaxation training and cognitive–behavioral group therapy for chronic low back pain. *J Consult Clin Psychol* 50:757–765.

113. Turner JA, Clancy S (1986): Strategies for coping with chronic low back pain: relationship to pain and disability. *Pain* 24:355–364.

114. Turner JA, Clancy S, McQuade KJ, Cardenas DD (1990): Effectiveness of behavioral therapy for chronic low back pain: a component analysis. *J Consult Clin Psychol* 58:573–579.

115. Turner JA, Jensen MP (1993): Efficacy of cognitive therapy for chronic low back pain. *Pain* 52:169–177.

116. Turner JA, Romano JM (1984): Self-report screening measures for depression in chronic pain patients. *J Clin Psychol* 40:909–913.

117. Weinberger M, Tierney WM, Booker P, Katz BP (1991): The impact of increased contact on psychosocial outcomes in patients with osteoarthritis: a randomized, controlled trial. *J Rheumatol* 18:849–854.

118. Weinberger M, Tierney WM, Cowper PA, Katz BP, Booker PA (1993): Cost-effectiveness of increased telephone contact for patients with osteoarthritis: a randomized, controlled trial. *Arthritis Rheum* 36:243–246.

119. White B, Sanders SH (1985): Differential effects on pain and mood in chronic pain patients with timed versus pain-contingent medication delivery. *Behav Ther* 16:28–38.

120. Wilfling FJ, Klonoff H, Kokan P (1973): Psychological, demographic and orthopaedic factors associated with prediction of outcome of spinal fusion. *Clin Orthop* 90:153–160.

121. Williams DA, Thorn BE (1989): An empirical assessment of pain beliefs. *Pain* 36:351–358.

122. Wurtele K, Kaplan GM, Keairnes M (1990): Childhood sexual abuse among chronic pain patients. *Clin J Pain* 6:110–113.

123. Zautra A, Manne S (1993): Coping with rheumatoid arthritis: a review of a decade of research. *Ann Behav Med* 14:31–40.

124. Zung WWK (1965): A self-rating depression scale. *Arch Gen Psychiatry* 12:63–70.

The Adult Spine: Principles and Practice,
2nd edition, J.W. Frymoyer, Editor-in-Chief.
Lippincott-Raven Publishers, Philadelphia © 1997.

CHAPTER 14

Education: The Prevention and Treatment of Low Back Disorders

Margareta Nordin, Sherri R. Weiser, and Nachman Halpern

THE ROLE OF EDUCATION IN TREATING LOW BACK DISORDERS

Until recently, much of the responsibility for personal health has been assigned to medical professionals. Today, the rising cost of health care, the increasing number of chronically ill individuals, and advancements in our knowledge of health and illness make it necessary for individuals to take control and manage their health (59). Patient advocacy groups championing the patient's "right to know" have added to the demand for information about health and illness (15,99). Health education programs have proliferated in response to this demand.

Patient education programs have been successful in preventing and treating chronic illnesses (122). This model has been applied to low back disorders as well. During the first half of the twentieth century, attempts to prevent back injuries were limited to on-the-job training in lifting techniques. More recently, the concept of back education has broadened to include strength and fitness, ergonomics, physiology, personal lifestyle, and stress management (111).

The target of back education programs today includes the general population. The scope often goes beyond prevention to include treatment. Moreover, few education programs are limited to the presentation of information. Most are also concerned with changing attitudes, beliefs, and behavior in addition to imparting knowledge. The following is a description and review of low back education programs.

Who Needs To Be Educated?

Epidemiologic data from numerous studies show that lifetime prevalence of back pain in the general population of industrialized countries is between 45% and 85% (20). In workers, absence because of back pain fluctuates between 30% and 50% depending on the nature of the work task. In the working population, the annual incidence of compensable back injury is about 2% (1).

M. Nordin, R.P.T., Dr.Sci.: Adjunct Associate Professor, New York University School of Medicine, Director, Occupational and Industrial Orthopaedic Center, New York University Medical Center, Hospital for Joint Diseases, New York, NY 10014.

S. R. Weiser, Ph.D.: Occupational and Industrial Orthopaedic Center, New York University Center, Hospital for Joint Diseases, New York, NY 10014.

N. Halpern, M.A., C.P.E.: Occupational and Industrial Orthopaedic Center, New York University Medical Center, Hospital for Joint Diseases, New York, NY 10014.

Because most people afflicted with back pain are in the prime of their lives, back problems are more than a health concern. Industry suffers considerable economic strain in terms of increased insurance premiums and decreased productivity. This underscores the need for back education programs that address the population at risk for back disorders as well as those already injured.

Much effort has gone into identifying those at high risk for back injury (4,12,17,34). Personal risk factors based on prospective studies include previous history of low back pain, age, and cigarette smoking. In women, childbearing history is a risk factor. Height, various indices of obesity, poor muscle strength, and impact aerobic exercise have also been reported as risk factors, but the results of different studies are conflicting. Some risk variables for industrial back injury are recent job entry, amount of twisting and lifting, and job satisfaction (4,8,34,56,118). Studies that demonstrate associations between symptoms and job class characteristics may have difficulty demonstrating that a specific motion is actually causative because even a highly stereotyped task involves many complex motions.

While it is possible to target at-risk groups based on the findings described above, identifying a specific at-risk individual is more difficult. Consequently, some researchers called for directly measuring the relationship between individual symptoms and individual exposure (39). Even individuals who have every risk factor have only an increased probability rather than an absolute risk of injuring their backs. Therefore, in the workplace, pre-employment screening for potential back injury claimants presents legal and possibly ethical problems (42). A person may not be denied work because he or she is at risk. In order to exclude a candidate, the employer must demonstrate that the person cannot fulfill the physical requirements of the job at the time of employment.

THE PREVENTION OF LOW BACK DISORDERS THROUGH EDUCATION

In the case of low back disorders, it is widely recognized that prevention is the ideal treatment, but that it is often difficult to implement (73,90). Prevention programs are of three kinds: primary, secondary, and tertiary. Primary prevention aims at reducing the occurrence of low back pain before it occurs. Secondary prevention aims to reduce the severity or the recurrence of low back pain episodes. Tertiary prevention involves the reduction of disability and restoration of function in chronic low back pain patients. Each type of program will be discussed in turn.

Primary Prevention

Primary prevention programs for the population at large are uncommon for several reasons. As previously mentioned, accurate identification of at-risk individuals is difficult. Therefore, primary prevention programs have to address a substantial segment of the population. Given the magnitude of this task, funding for a public back injury prevention program is costly and difficult to justify. In addition, individuals who believe that the chance of becoming injured is remote may not be motivated to change their behaviors. Under these circumstances, intervention is fruitless. However, more focused primary prevention programs have begun to surface in the workplace, where back pain has taken a toll of about $6 billion each year in the United States (76,89,92,125, 126,131). Unlike traditional classes in proper lifting techniques, these programs include strength and fitness training, manual materials handling, personal lifestyle, stress management, and ergonomic principles. Each component will be discussed at length in the section entitled Review of Back Education Program Content. A recent critical review reveals that the literature on the success of training approaches is spotty at best (63). In two studies, there was a decrease in the number of reported back injuries and days lost following such a program (80,92). However, confounding factors made it difficult to credit the positive outcome to the back program alone.

In a 3-year prospective study by Versloot et al. (125) of 400 bus drivers in Holland, a significant decrease in absenteeism was achieved after a back injury prevention program was instituted. The average decrease in absenteeism was 6 days per employee per year. However, a similar study of 4,000 Swedish federal employees by Ljungberg and Sanne (76) did not support these findings. The conflicting results of these two studies may be attributed to system variables such as company support and the social security system, and program variables such as the use of model teachers and employee involvement. Further research is needed to clarify these questions.

Secondary Prevention

Secondary prevention programs are intended to reduce the severity and reoccurrence of an existing problem. They are usually aimed at the patient with acute (less than 1 month) or sub-acute (1 to 3 months) back pain. However, in the workplace, the target of these efforts may also be management and union members. Information may be imparted informally in the doctor's office or through more structured programs such as back schools. The following section describes secondary prevention programs for different target populations.

Back School

Back school is a structured education program aimed at changing the behavior and increasing the functional ability of patients who suffer from acute or intermittent

back problems. Delpech is generally believed to have initiated the Back School concept in the early part of the nineteenth century in Montpellier, France (96). Zachrisson-Forssell (32) is credited with developing the first formal back school in Stockholm in 1969. Since then, back schools have enjoyed great proliferation internationally (38,65,80).

Back schools are based on the premise that educating patients about proper back care can prevent and reduce the severity of future back pain episodes. The patient is expected to adopt health-promoting behaviors and take responsibility for recovery. As such, back schools represent a divergence from more conventional passive treatment modalities.

The group format provides an economical way to transmit information and fosters a supportive atmosphere in which students exchange ideas freely (Fig. 1). Classes generally consist of four to 12 patients who meet for five to seven sessions of approximately 1 hour in length. The term *school* is used to encourage learning and retention of information (111).

Back schools are most frequently taught by physical therapists but have also been taught by other health-care professionals. Topics covered include the causes of injury, physiology of the spine, fitness, posture, personal lifestyle, and the relationship between stress and pain (9,38,80). It is difficult to gauge the effectiveness of back schools because of the variation in teaching methods and topics covered in different programs. An additional obstacle has been the lack of controlled studies, often difficult to achieve in clinical settings (21,53,75). Nonetheless, Bergquist-Ullman and Larsson showed that back school is superior to passive treatment (physical therapy) or no treatment (9). Their prospective controlled studies

demonstrated that back schools effectively reduced the amount of lost work days in sub-acute low back pain (9) but had little effect on chronic back pain populations (65). Linton and Kamwendo, in a review of existing studies (75), also found conflicting results. These authors point out that the lack of positive results may have less to do with the content of back school than with the fact the students may not be retaining what they have learned. Efforts to assess knowledge and skills acquisition may be an important step in the evaluation of back schools. Others attribute positive results of back schools to the influence of authority figures and self-sufficiency rather than the content of the program (63). At most, back school by itself is marginally successful (13,58).

Health-Care Providers as Educators

Patient Interaction

Waddell (128) has emphasized the importance of the first contact between the patient and the health-care provider. It is here that trust between the two parties is established. It is here too that the patient's fear of a serious condition can be diminished and where simple instructions can be given that could prevent prolonged recovery.

Information that addresses the patient's greatest concerns increases the chances of an effective initial consultation. At the minimum, the patient with acute nonspecific low back pain should be given an explanation of the problem, a prognosis (the natural history of low back pain is very positive), recommendations for symptom control, and activity guidelines including both work and

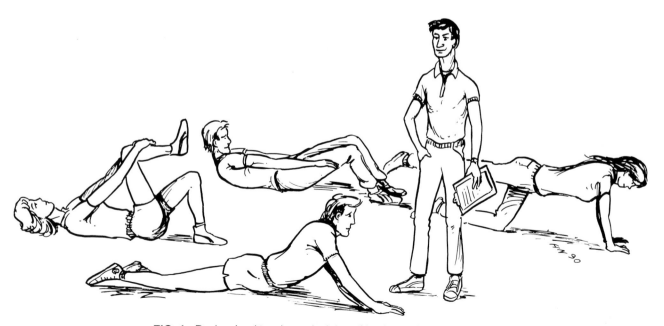

FIG. 1. Back school teaches principles of back care in a group setting.

leisure activities. This information should be given in conjunction with a thorough clinical evaluation (5).

The Team Approach and Early Care

Early care to prevent chronicity of nonspecific low back pain has been emphasized by several authors (20,71,72). Choler et al. (20) performed a controlled study of two urban populations. Individuals off from work 4 to 6 weeks because of nonspecific low back problems participated in a program emphasizing return to work. The program included careful evaluation, the Swedish back school, fitness training, a site visit at work by a physical therapist trained in ergonomics, and, when indicated, the judicious use of surgery. The treatment team included an orthopedic surgeon, a physical therapist, and a nurse. The reduction in long-term disability in this group was 90% greater than for back patients in another areas of the city where such a program was not provided. Lindstrom et al. (70–72) used a similar approach with Volvo company employees and found even better results. They concluded that the risk of delayed recovery (return to work) is decreased by an intensive approach including follow-up. These programs point out the importance of a multidisciplinary approach to nonspecific low back pain as early as 4 to 6 weeks after injury (31). They also emphasized the benefits of using activity and work as the primary objective. The relevance of these findings to other health-care systems is limited because these studies have yet to be replicated outside of Sweden.

Management/Union Education

In industry, most prevention efforts have focused on the worker. It has become evident that the cooperation of the management/union is a crucial component in the success of work-site health programs. Snook and White (111) point to the importance of training management in early detection and appropriate care of back disorders.

Management/union education includes the concept of creating a supportive environment where employees are encouraged to report new injuries, and then to manage them without work loss. Worker participation in on-site education programs also requires supervisor approval. Workers may participate more willingly if they are not penalized for lost work time. The management/union may also be educated in the benefits and pitfalls of temporarily reassigning an injured worker to a less physically demanding job (40a). In common practice, workers remain on disability leave until they are able to resume their normal responsibilities. However, statistics show that the likelihood of someone returning to work after 6 months of disability is slim (82,127).

Management can also learn ways of modifying the job to accommodate the worker (111). The benefits of such an approach may, in the long run, outweigh the costs (131).

Tertiary Prevention

It has been suggested that sub-acute pain becomes chronic as early as 6 to 7 weeks after onset (113). However, most pain centers classify pain as chronic after 3 months. At this point, the life of the patient may be seriously disrupted psychologically, socially, and financially. Education and training programs must take these factors into consideration in order to successfully rehabilitate the patient. Functional restoration programs and nonmedical pain management are two treatment modalities for chronic pain in which patient education is an important component.

Functional Restoration

Perhaps the greatest challenge in treating chronic pain (more than 4 months) is getting the patient to go back to work. Functional restoration and some work hardening programs are distinguished by their aggressive approach to rehabilitation and their emphasis on returning the chronic pain patient to gainful employment. These programs utilize a behavioral paradigm in which the physical functioning criteria are set by the instructor rather than the patient, and accomplishment of goals is rewarded. Additionally, many of these programs simulate actual physical work tasks in order to prepare the patient to return to work after rehabilitation.

In 1985, Mayer et al. popularized a comprehensive functional restoration program for chronic low back pain patients (81) (see Chapter 15). The program consisted of 54 hours of treatment per week for 3 weeks. It combined education, behavior training, physical fitness including endurance training, and work simulation. Objective functional capacity measurement techniques were used to guide the treatment program for pre- and postevaluation. Mayer et al. assessed the outcome of this program using a comparison group of patients who were unable to participate because they were denied insurance reimbursement (81). The study showed that 82% of the patients were reconditioned successfully and returned to work. In the no-treatment comparison group, only 40% of the patients returned to work. An identical functional restoration program was instituted at the New England Back Center with similar results (40) (see Chapter 15).

The return-to-work rates of these two programs are impressive. One must bear in mind, however, that the comparison groups in both studies were not randomly selected. Group differences may have resulted from factors unrelated to the program. Also, because of the multidisciplinary nature of these programs, it is difficult to isolate the factors that contributed to success. Clinically

controlled prospective studies, with and without the educational component, would be more informative in determining education's contribution to program success.

Nonmedical Pain Management

Pain of a chronic nature is rarely eliminated completely. Instead, chronic patients must learn how to reduce pain and come to terms with the pain that remains (112). Stress management techniques are used as a means of nonmedical pain management, with pain identified as the main stressor to learn to cope with.

Chronic pain patients are commonly characterized by disability disproportionate to their physical findings (116,127). Patients may remain sedentary because of fear of increased injury and pain, or because of secondary gains associated with pain behaviors (30,62).

Cognitive–behavioral techniques, where patients are rewarded for "well" behaviors, are taught to encourage return to pre-pain levels of functioning. These techniques also help to reassure the patient that normal activities will not exacerbate the injury (see Chapter 13).

REVIEW OF BACK EDUCATION PROGRAM CONTENT

All of the topics covered in back injury prevention programs are based on current knowledge about the etiology and risk factors associated with lumbar spinal disorders. Although there is not total agreement or scientific substantiation for all risk factors, the following are commonly included in designing curricula for education programs.

Manual Materials Handling

A number of handling techniques have been associated with back injury. The goal of manual materials handling (MMH) training is to teach techniques that put less strain on the back. Occupational groups such as healthcare workers, construction laborers, garbage collectors, truck drivers, and machinists have a high risk of injury (48). These groups are prime targets for MMH training.

Movements and postures associated with back injury compose the content of most training programs. They are frequent lifting (25 times per day), twisting while lifting, heavy lifting (11.3 kg or more), static postures, forward bending and twisting of the trunk, and muscle fatigue (19,34,41,43,55,64,94,100,106). Of all these motions, perhaps the most deleterious is simultaneous twisting and forward bending of the trunk. Kelsey et al. (56) showed a sixfold increase in reported back injuries as a result of this movement.

Several studies have attempted to train workers in proper handling techniques (18,23,91,110,126). MMH education has, so far, been unsuccessful in reducing injury rates. It is possible that broad generalizations concerning MMH cannot be made, considering the variety of the tasks involved. It is therefore questionable whether training recommendations used in many programs are applicable across industrial settings. Another reason for the arguable value of MMH training relates to instruction style. However, few of these studies attempted to assess the actual acquisition of new skills, or how the worker used the newly learned techniques on the job. For example, a 12- to 18-month follow-up after a 12-hour classroom training program revealed that orderlies in a geriatric hospital rarely used procedures from training in horizontal moves; these were used more frequently for vertical lifts (114).

The inconsistent record of training programs also may result from the fact that workers have only limited control of the way they handle materials. Some studies estimate that about 20% to 40% of all lifting motions can be attributed to individual worker technique (18,26,37). These studies suggest that avoiding twisting motions and maintaining the load close to the body (Figs. 2,3) (2) are the most important MMH concepts to promote in order to reduce back injuries. Other motions require ergonomic solutions, such as workplace redesign (Fig. 4).

Few studies have assessed MMH education in terms of motor skills acquisition. Such studies are important because they indicate which skills can be effectively taught. Motion analysis showed that trainees can learn to get a good grip on an object, move smoothly and avoid

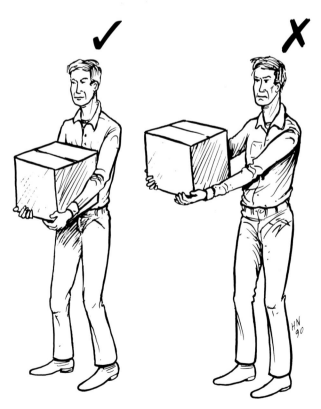

FIG. 2. The load should be kept close to the body.

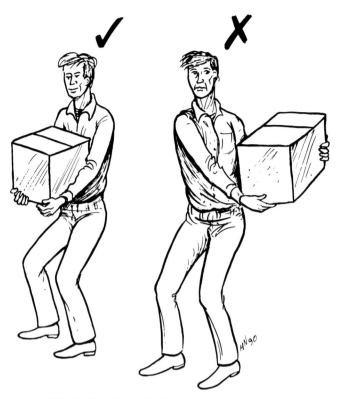

FIG. 3. Twisting while lifting should be avoided.

jerky motions, hold a load close to the body, and extend the knees and hips while keeping the trunk straight, particularly when handling heavy loads. The first two skills can be acquired in a 4-hour training program (18). The other skills require an intensive course of 35 hours (37). These findings limit the use of on-site training in industry. The long-term retention of new skills is also important. Hultman et al. (45) have shown that subjects remember to keep their trunks straight after 3 months. Long-term retention is probably most sensitive to feedback and on-site reinforcement (18,23,45,117,126).

More research is needed to examine the effectiveness of MMH training in reducing injury rates. Future studies should take into account the degree to which new motor skills have been acquired and retained, worker skill, and issues of compliance (60). In light of the estimate that 60% of reported back injuries could have been avoided by adopting safer moving techniques, MMH training remains justifiable (37). The training, however, should probably be job-specific rather than general.

The training in MMH should also address the issue of back support belts and corsets. These devices are not considered by OSHA as personal protective equipment but clothing equipment. It is not clear exactly how a belt could reduce back strain since the reactive forces and

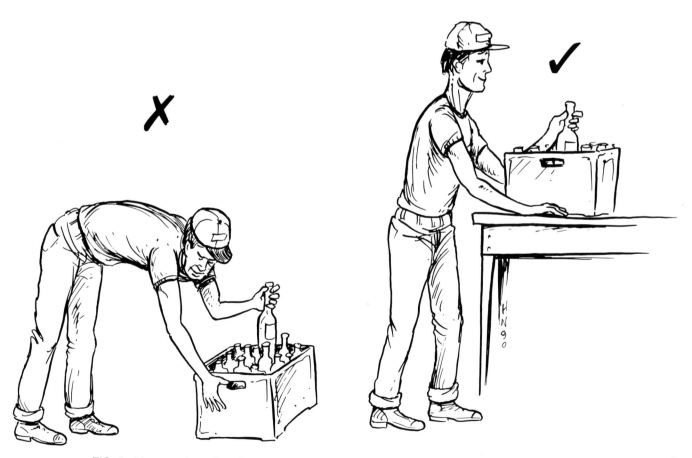

FIG. 4. Movements such as forward bending can be avoided by ergonomic workplace evaluations.

moments generated during lifting are imparted to the spine with or without a belt. The effects of the belt on intra-abdominal pressures are also not clear. In any event, the research on the role of intra-abdominal pressure in reducing back strain is contradictory. The experience gained so far with these devices indicates that training in proper use of the devices should be mandatory and include also instructions in lifting techniques, proper selection, and adjustment (47).

Strength and Fitness

Training in strength and fitness variably emphasizes musculoskeletal strength, cardiovascular fitness, aerobic capacity, endurance, and flexibility. While it is commonly believed that those in poor physical condition are prone to back injury, to date there is no scientific evidence to support this assertion (4,36,119). One study showed that firefighters who were fit were less likely to suffer back injuries over a 4-year period than their less fit coworkers (17). However, the failure of the investigators to control for such important baseline differences as age of subjects brings these findings into question.

In the largest prospective study to date, more than 3,000 employees underwent preemployment testing (4). After 3 years, it was shown that those with poor general isometric strength were as likely to report back pain as stronger workers. There was actually a trend for workers with greater strength to report increased back pain. These studies used generic isometric strength and endurance, and cardiovascular fitness testing unrelated to specific work tasks, as measures of strength. Strength testing more closely related to physical requirements of the job may be more predictive of initial back pain episodes. This idea was brought to light in one study where testing was biomechanically designed to reflect job demands (57). However, too few back problems were reported to allow for an accurate data analysis. Prospective studies of dynamic strength are needed to uncover the relationship between strength and low back pain.

Flexibility has also been found to be a poor predictor of onset and severity of low back pain (4,12,119). Nonetheless, fitness programs have been shown to reduce overall absenteeism and medical costs in industry (17). People may also benefit psychologically from feeling fit. Therefore, until it is known for certain that fitness has no relationship to back pain, it may be prudent to include some strength and conditioning concepts in a back pain prevention program.

Personal Lifestyle

A person's lifestyle may be defined as eating habits, activity level, sleeping patterns, tobacco and alcohol consumption, other substance use, and athletic pursuits. To the degree that these factors are under an individual's control, they are important to emphasize in education programs. Eating habits have an effect on low back pain, insofar as obesity is a risk factor for back pain and its chronicity. Deyo (24) has reported that individuals in the fifth quintile of weight are at greater risk. He also noted taller people were at risk, but height is beyond the control of the individual.

Some of the issues in activity level have been discussed in the preceding section, Strength and Fitness. Although the clinical data are inconclusive, there is a large body of basic information that demonstrates beneficial effects of aerobic activity on the metabolism and biomechanical integrity of muscles, ligaments, joints, and facets (33). This information lends credence to a clinical approach that stresses physical fitness not only in the prevention of back disease, but in overall health and well being.

As the antithesis of aerobic fitness, smoking appears to have a relationship to the incidence, severity, and resultant disability from low back disorders. In many cases, the clinical data are based on retrospective studies (34,118) and should therefore be viewed with some caution. Another study, also retrospective in design, showed a relationship of smoking to lumbar disc herniation (55). One prospective study found no relationship between smoking and onset of acute back pain (8), but in another study (4), smoking did have predictive value for future disability in a group of healthy subjects. The latter observation is consistent with cross-sectional epidemiologic surveys that show a significant interaction between smoking and disabling back complaints (103,104,124). In those same studies, alcohol consumption, drug use, poor eating habits, and sleep disturbances also were interrelated and predictors of disability. Thus, the question arises: is smoking a causal factor, or is it part of a broader set of psychosocial problems? Again the clinical data are unclear at this time, but basic disc research demonstrates a significant adverse effect of cigarette smoke and nicotine on intervertebral disc metabolism. Similarly, sleep disturbance has been related specifically to the clinical syndrome of fibromyositis. In fact, there is a school of thought suggesting that sleep disturbance is the primary event and back pain the outcome.

Last, some sports have been related to low back pain and even to sciatica. In particular, sports which involve twisting, such as golf, bowling, and tennis, have been associated with lumbar disc herniations (54). Other studies have suggested a relationship between mild, nondisabling back pain and jogging and cross country skiing. A special example is the relationship between isthmic spondylolisthesis and gymnastics, American football, and a number of other sports. The practical application of this knowledge in the prevention of back pain is limited. Certainly, no one would suggest a person give up sports to prevent back pain; conversely, a practical approach certainly would encourage both cessation of smoking and weight control.

Stress Management

There are a number of theories to explain the relationship between stress and pain. Muscle tension resulting from stress has been implicated as a causal factor in physiological theories (25,61,98,105). Psychological theories emphasize cognitive processes such as feelings of control and attitudes toward pain that moderate pain perception (11,35,52). Secondary gains that result from pain behaviors may also influence the subjective pain experience (30,62). Several authors have associated stress with back disorders (66,95,130). The Bureau of National Affairs (16) has also claimed a relationship between stress and accidents. Work dissatisfaction and work stress was related to reports of back problems in several studies (4,14,46). Leino and Lyyra (67) studied Finnish blue-collar workers and found that work stress and lack of social support predicted musculoskeletal complaints after 10 years in blue-collar workers, but not in white-collar workers. In one investigation, work satisfaction was the best predictor of outcome among demographic and health status variables in patients suffering from back pain (4).

Palliative stress reduction strategies modify the stress response but do not directly alter the stressor. In relaxation training, the person is taught deep breathing and directed concentration, which reduces muscle tension (7,10). Cognitive coping strategies are based on the premise that maladaptive or negative thoughts result in stress-related feelings and behaviors (6,27,85). Such techniques encourage a shift in perspective so that the individual may feel more in control or perceive the pain differently.

A robust literature attests to the effectiveness of relaxation and cognitive coping strategies in reducing chronic pain (11,28,50,93,112,120,121). Investigators are beginning to address the use of these techniques for the prevention and treatment of acute back disorders (73). Preliminary studies suggest that early education in stress management may forestall chronicity (31,51,88).

Active coping strategies focus on the effective management of the environment as a means of attenuating the degree and the nature of stressors. Strategies include time management, goal setting, problem solving, social skills training, and assertion training. There is insufficient literature linking these techniques to control of low back problems, but pain management programs that include active coping skills have found them to be a useful complement to palliative coping strategies (35,40).

Stress Management in the Workplace

Work-site stress management programs are increasing in popularity (29) and there is some evidence that they

are successful in decreasing accidents and preventing the development of low back pain (74,115). Often, the worker is chosen as the target for intervention. Identifying the workplace as the intervention site is an alternative approach and may result in innovations such as incentive programs, support groups, and modified workplace design. Since the worker and the work environment form an interactive system, it may be advisable to include elements of both approaches (84,95,107,123).

After reviewing a number of work-site stress reduction programs, Pelletier and Lutz (95) identified several ingredients for success: Participation should be limited to high-risk individuals who are motivated to learn. Classes should introduce a variety of stress management techniques, take place in a 4- to 8-week period, be of approximately 45 minutes in duration, and include 12 to 14 participants. Follow-up should include the reinforcement of skills as well as a method of program evaluation.

Ergonomic Principles

The ergonomic approach to injury control seeks to reduce the effect of biomechanical stress by eliminating the source of the hazard. The Proposed National Strategies for the Prevention of Leading Work-Related Diseases and Injuries (3) conclude that the ergonomic approach to workplace redesign may be the first choice for controlling musculoskeletal problems, with employee selection and training secondary (3). It has been estimated that almost half of all lifting motions are constrained by the design of the workstation. Therefore, it is not surprising that little improvement has been realized by training without the benefit of ergonomic changes in layout and object design (18,26,37).

Ergonomics education programs include the following topics: work physiology, anthropometrics/biomechanics, noise, job design, work organization, lifting, communication, and personnel issues. They are most effective in directing the trainees' attention away from management issues toward biomechanics and physiology as possible explanations for productivity problems (101). Evaluation of an in-plant lecture-based training in ergonomic principles revealed that the acquired factual knowledge was not readily translated into practical skills. Since trainees were sensitized to issues covered in the training, they tended to overrate work stress levels, in particular postural stress (69). This may be acceptable from a health and safety viewpoint, but it may not be economically acceptable. Consequently, the application of ergonomic principles becomes a matter of managing change in the workplace.

Management of ergonomic changes in the workplace is a critical issue that needs to be addressed in prevention programs. However, the line worker in a primary prevention training program, or the patient in a secondary and tertiary prevention program, has limited control over ergonomic changes. Therefore, these trainees may feel frustrated. This topic in particular requires context-specific examples (108). It is perhaps best to educate management in ergonomics (101). In fact, one long-term benefit of an ergonomic education program in primary prevention has been the growing number of ergonomic modifications initiated in the organization (49,68,101).

Similar to strength and fitness in secondary prevention, the application of ergonomic principles to MMH needs to be practiced. Luopajarvi describes an Early Rehabilitation Course for loggers in Finland. The 4-week course consisted of 29 hours of group education in body mechanics, planning, and logging techniques, and 26 hours of individual instruction practiced immediately. The course was effective in changing the logging trunk posture of the patients. The success was attributed to the participation of expert loggers in the training and the feedback on performance (78).

Few reports specify a reduction in musculoskeletal disorders as a result of ergonomic changes (15,97,109). Following an ergonomic education and workplace modifications program, Westgaard and Aaras (129) reported three results: a significant reduction of musculoskeletal-related sick leave, a reduction in labor turnover, and an increase in worker productivity. Other studies have supported these findings (68,97,109).

The voluntary training guidelines of OSHA provide a model for planning, executing, and implementing an ergonomics training program. The training should be provided at two levels. At minimum, a general awareness training should be provided for employees, including supervisors, management, engineers, purchasing agents, and safety and health personnel. Task- or risk-specific training should be developed for individuals and supervisors employed in high-risk jobs, as identified by worksite analysis and injury data (91).

It may be concluded that education and training in ergonomic principles is of value, particularly when used as part of an overall ergonomics management program (91). This may be particularly true for industries that require heavy and repetitive work. Little is known, however, about the efficacy of teaching ergonomic principles directly to employees. It is also not yet known whether these efforts directly affect back injuries.

ISSUES IN BACK EDUCATION AND TRAINING

Motivation and Learning

One of the most challenging aspects of health education is student motivation. Even the best program will fail if students are not interested in learning. A number of factors have been shown to facilitate learning and motivation in health education. One approach to ensuring a high level of motivation has been to offer programs on a voluntary basis, excluding those with no desire to learn. Indeed, in most cases this is intuitively logical. However, there are two problems with this approach. One problem is that a person may volunteer for reasons having little to do with learning, such as the opportunity to be a part of a group or to get additional free time from work.

An additional problem is that voluntary programs may not attract those individuals who are most likely to benefit from education. Programs that identify at-risk individuals usually have a higher success rate than broad-based approaches (95). In addition, the likelihood of injury in certain jobs is so great that a mandatory training program may be justified. The advantages and disadvantages of a voluntary program must be considered with regard to these issues. Regardless of the student's motivation level, certain principles of education and training have been shown to enhance learning. Students may learn best in group settings of three to 12 (99). Groups of this size permit the exchange of ideas and provide a supportive setting in which to learn. Patient education is also enhanced by the use of audio and visual aids (83,87) and the provision of relevant reading materials (83).

Programs that actively involve patients or students by emphasizing self-care and demonstrating treatments have been shown to be 1.5 to 3 times as successful as traditional education (99). Students are more likely to become involved in a topic that has relevance to them (132). The knowledge, beliefs, circumstances, and psychological status of the learner are important considerations in designing a program (86).

Studies have shown that patients' beliefs about their illness can differ substantially from those of health-care providers (C. Cedrashi, *personal communication,* 1989;77). For example, one study showed that 50% of participants believed that their problem would become chronic (76). In addition, another investigation found that patients, even after being educated, gave anatomically incorrect descriptions of their back problem (C. Cedrashi, *personal communication,* 1989;1). The educator must be sensitive to erroneous beliefs and attempt to correct them before introducing new information.

Two crucial tools for keeping students motivated are frequent feedback on performance (79) and positive reinforcement. Reinforcement not only enhances the learning process but is shown to improve fine and gross motor skills (102), which are often required for back injury prevention.

Finally, health behaviors are deeply rooted and resistant to change. A successful education program must acknowledge the need for frequent and ongoing reinforcement. Principles of proper back care must be incorporated into lifestyle practices. Most current programs are of brief duration. Clearly, short-term education will not provide long-term solutions.

Program Content and Instruction Method

Once the student is motivated to learn, another main issue in back education and training involves the transfer of information. Specifically, what information should be taught? In about 75% of all back injury cases, the cause of the problem is unknown. Therefore, most educators have used a trial and error approach to education, which reflects their basic beliefs about the etiology of back injury, as well as practical approaches to prevention.

Until more is known about how back pain develops, it is unlikely that one particular educational approach will be consistently effective. At this point, a multidisciplinary approach to back pain, particularly chronic pain, seems to be most reasonable, with one caveat. The importance of considering the individual characteristics and needs of the students cannot be underestimated. A successful educator will exercise sensitivity and flexibility in program content and emphasize the issues that are most appropriate to the students.

Furthermore, teaching methods are theoretically based and for the most part fail to emphasize the practical application of skills. The importance of practical information has been demonstrated in the success of functional restoration programs. Workplace intervention programs would be another example of this approach. More attention needs to be paid to translating information into the real life situation of the student.

Program Evaluation

Evaluations are a critical feature of any health education program and are done for several reasons. They allow the documentation of change and the justification of expense, and they provide feedback about how to improve the program (44). Considering evaluation at the start-up phase of training also helps the instructor define course objectives.

Programs should be evaluated on parameters determined by program objectives. Outcomes are easier to assess when put in operational terms. Traditionally, the goals of learning may be to increase understanding, change attitudes, change behavior, or reduce costs. Stated this way, it is unclear what quantifies a successful outcome. If, instead, the goal is to reduce absenteeism by, for example, 25%, the criteria for success can be clearly quantified.

Criteria for a successful program should be clearly decided on prior to the beginning of the course. Data can then be collected in such a way as to allow for before-and-after comparisons of these variables. It also helps to avoid post-hoc determinations of what defines a successful program.

Evaluation may be done using objective measures where certain behaviors or performances are quantified by observation. Subjective measures in a self-report format may also be used. Clearly, feelings and beliefs are more amenable to self-report, while knowledge and behavior are easier to observe. Since objective and subjective measures provide different information, it is best to use both (99).

Success criteria should, of course, be based on some meaningful quantity. The amount of change that makes the program worthwhile may be determined by a cost–benefit analysis. In general terms, costs may be quantified in terms of personnel, equipment, materials, and overhead. Benefits are the achievement of the course objectives. An education program may be considered successful when the benefits outweigh the costs.

A thorough discussion of program evaluation exceeds the scope of this chapter. A program evaluation done properly requires sophisticated knowledge and considerable skill. The reader is urged to consult reference material before undertaking an evaluation study (22).

SUMMARY AND CONCLUSIONS

Back education programs are an attempt to address the continuous rise in the prevalence and incidence of low back disorders. At present, the literature may be summarized as follows: There is no evidence that primary prevention programs are successful. There is research that suggests the effectiveness of secondary prevention approaches. Studies of patients 4 weeks post-injury engaged in active, multidisciplinary, goal-oriented programs are most encouraging. These programs may hold the most promise of reducing cost and suffering related to chronic low back pain syndrome. However, successful implementation of such a program in this country has yet to be demonstrated. Functional restoration programs as tertiary care may also be successful. Studies in this area require replication.

The following points highlight the issues of importance to consider when developing a back education program. Early education at the time of injury and follow-up at 4 to 6 weeks is probably the best way to avoid chronicity. Educators should take a goal-oriented approach and, in light of the findings mentioned here, adopt realistic expectations for outcome. While a multidisciplinary approach to education is advisable, it is equally important to be flexible in terms of program content depending on the target population.

In industry, it may be best to institute primary prevention programs to train the new employee. This way, the acquisition of poor working habits may be avoided. Ongoing prevention programs with frequent reinforcement must be implemented if a program is to succeed. Also, management must be educated about the importance of preventing and reducing the severity and recurrence of low back disorders.

Despite the paucity of conclusive findings in the area of back injury prevention education programs, it is too early to throw out the baby with the bathwater. As researchers and clinicians continue to elucidate the factors that result in a reduction in the severity and occurrence of back problems, better approaches to education and training will be developed. The educational approach reflects a belief in the individual's ability to participate in his or her own health care and may be the strongest weapon we have in the battle against low back disorders. It may be concluded that, conceptually, back education represents a sound approach to the prevention and treatment of low back disorders. Future work should build upon existing attempts to translate these concepts into successful practical approaches.

ACKNOWLEDGMENTS. We are most grateful to Dr. M. L. Skovron and Dr. P. Brisson for their critical review of the manuscript. We also thank Joan Kahn for her time devoted to this project. This project was supported by the HJD Research and Development Foundation.

REFERENCES

1. Andersson G (1979): Low back pain in industry: epidemiological aspects. *Scand J Rehab Med* 11:163–168.
2. Andersson G, Ortengren R, Nachemson A (1976): Quantitative studies of back load in lifting. *Spine* 1:178–185.
3. Association of Schools of Public Health (ASPH) (1986): *Proposed national strategies for the prevention of leading work-related diseases and injuries*, Part 1. Washington, D.C.: ASPH.
4. Battié M (1989): *The reliability of physical factors as predictors of the occurrence of back pain reporters: a prospective study within industry.* Doctoral dissertation. University of Gothenburg, Gothenburg, Sweden.
5. Battié M, Nordin M (1995): Backschool: state of the art. In: Wiesel S, ed. *The lumbar spine.* Philadelphia: W. B. Saunders.
6. Beck A (1984): Cognitive approaches to stress. In: Woolfolk R, Lehrer P, eds. *Principles and practice of stress management.* New York: Guilford, pp. 255–305.
7. Benson H (1975): *The relaxation response.* New York: Avon.
8. Bergenudd H (1989): *Talent occupation and locomotor discomfort.* Thesis, Lund University, Malmo, Sweden.
9. Bergquist-Ullman M, Larsson U (1977): Acute low back pain in industry. *Acta Orthop Scand* 170:1–117.
10. Bernstein D, Given B (1984): Progressive relaxation: abbreviated methods. In: Woolfolk R, Lehrer P, eds. *Principles and practice of stress management.* New York: Guilford, pp. 43–69.
11. Biedermann HJ, McGhie A, Monga TN, Shanks GL (1987): Perceived and actual control in EMG treatment of back pain. *Behav Res Ther* 25:137–147.
12. Biering-Sorenson F (1984): Physical measurements as risk indicators for low-back trouble over a one-year period. *Spine* 9:106–119.
13. Bigos S, Bowyer O, Braen G, et al. (1994): Acute low back pain problems in adults. Clinical practice guideline. No. 14. AHCPR Publication No. 95-0642. Rockville, MD: Agency for Health Care Policy and Research, Public Health Service, USDHHS.
14. Bigos SJ, Spengler DM, Martin NA, Fisher L, Zeh J, Nachemson A (1986): Back injuries in industry: a retrospective study: II. Injury factors. *Spine* 11:246–251.
15. Bille D (1981): Practical approaches to patient teaching. Boston: Little, Brown.
16. Bureau of National Affairs (1984): *Personal policies forum survey.* 132:3–11.
17. Cady LD, Bischoff DP, O'Connell ER, Thomas PC, Allen JH (1979): Letters to the editor: Authors' response. *J Occup Med* 21: 720–725.
18. Chaffin D, Gallay LS, Woolley CB, Kuciemba SR (1986): An evaluation of the effect of a training program in worker lifting postures. *Int J Ind Ergonom* 1:127–136.
19. Chaffin DB, Park KS (1973): A longitudinal study of low-back pain as associated with occupational weight lifting factors. *Am Ind Hyg Assoc J* 34:513–525.
20. Choler U, Larsson R, Nachemson A, Peterson LE (1985): *Back pain: a trial of case management for patients with unspecific low back pain.* Stockholm: SPRI Report 188 (in Swedish).
21. Cohen JE, Goel V, Frank JW, et al.: Group education interventions for people with low back pain: an overview of the literature. *Spine* 19:1214–1222.
22. Cook T, Campbell D (1979): *Quasi-experimentation design and analysis issues for field setting.* Chicago: Rand McNally.
23. Dehlin O, Hedenrud B, Horal J (1976): Back symptoms in nursing aides in a geriatric hospital. *Scand J Rehab Med* 8:47–53.
24. Deyo RA, Tsui-Wu YJ (1987): Descriptive epidemiology of low-back pain and its related medical care in the United States. *Spine* 12:264–268.
25. Dolce JJ, Raczynski JM (1985): Neuromuscular activity and electromyography in painful backs: psychological and biomechanical models in assessment and treatment. *Psychol Bull* 97:502–520.
26. Drury CG (1985): Influence of restricted space on manual materials handling. *Ergonomics* 28:167–175.
27. Ellis A, Harper R (1975): *A new guide to rational living.* Los Angeles: Wilshire.
28. Fernandez E, Turk DC (1989): The utility of cognitive coping strategies for altering pain perception: a meta-analysis. *Pain* 38: 123–135.
29. Fielding JE (1989). Work site stress management: national survey results. *J Occup Med* 31:990–995.
30. Fordyce WE (1988): Psychological factors in the failed back. *Int Disabil Stud* 10:29–31.
31. Fordyce WE, Brockway JA, Bergman JA, Spengler D (1986): Acute back pain: a control-group comparison of behavioral vs. traditional management methods. *J Behav Med* 9:127–140.
32. Forssell MZ (1981): The back school. *Spine* 6:104–106.
33. Frymoyer JW, Gordon S (1989): *New perspectives on low back pain.* Chicago: American Academy of Orthopaedic Surgeons.
34. Frymoyer JW, Pope MH, Clements JH, Wilder DG, MacPherson B, Askikaga T (1983). Risk factors in low back pain. *J Bone Joint Surg* [Am] 65:213–218.
35. Gottlieb H, Strite LC, Koller R, Madorsky A, Hockersmith V, Kleeman M, Wagner J (1977): Comprehensive rehabilitation of patients having chronic low back pain. *Arch Phys Med Rehab* 58: 101–108.
36. Gyntelberg F (1974): One year incidence of low back pain among male residents of Copenhagen aged 40–59. *Dan Med Bull* 21:30–36.
37. Hale A, Mason I (1986): L'Évaluation du role d'une formation kinetique dans la prevention des accidents de manutention. *Le Travail Humain* 49(3):195–208.
38. Hall H, Iceton JA (1983): Back school. An overview with specific reference to the Canadian Back Education Units. *Clin Orthop* 179:10–17.
39. Harber P, Bloswick D, Beck J, et al. (1993): Supermarket checker motions and cumulative trauma disorders. *J Occup Med* 35(8): 805–811.
40. Hazard RG, Fenwick JW, Kalisch SM, Redmond J, Reeves V, Reid S, Frymoyer J (1989): Functional restoration with behavioral support: a one-year prospective study of patients with chronic low-back pain. *Spine* 14:157–161.
41. Herrin GD, Jaraiedi M, Anderson CK (1986): Prediction of over-

exertion injuries using biomechanical and psychophysical models. *Am Ind Hyg Assoc J* 47:322–330.

42. Himmelstein JS, Andersson GB (1988): Low back pain: risk evaluation and preplacement screening. *State Art Rev Occup Med* 3: 255–269.

43. Holding D (1983): Fatigue. In: Hockey R, ed. *Stress and fatigue in human performance.* New York: John Wiley, pp. 145–165.

44. Holzemer W (1981): Evaluation of patient education programs. In: Bille D, ed. *Practical approaches to patient teaching.* Boston: Little, Brown, pp. 131–151.

45. Hultman G, Nordin M, Ortengren R (1984): The influence of a preventive educational program on trunk flexion in janitors. *Appl Ergonom* 15:127–133.

46. Hurri H (1989): The Swedish back school in chronic low back pain. II. *Scand J Rehab Med* 21:41–44.

47. Imker FW (1994): The back support myth. *Ergonom Design* (April issue):9–12.

48. Jensen R (1986): *Proceedings of the Human Factors Society, 30th Annual Meeting.* Santa Monica: The Human Factors Society.

49. Joseph BS (1986): *A participative ergonomic control program in a US automotive plant.* PhD Dissertation: University of Michigan.

50. Kabat-Zinn J, Lipworth L, Burney R (1985): The clinical use of mindfulness meditation for the self-regulation of chronic pain. *J Behav Med* 8:163–190.

51. Kamwendo K, Linton S (1986): Can pause-gymnastics prevent neck and shoulder pain? *Sjukgymnasten* 7:12–14.

52. Keefe FJ (1982): Behavioral assessment and treatment of chronic pain: current status and future directions. *J Consult Clin Psychol* 50:896–911.

53. Keijsers JFEM (1991): Validity and comparability of studies on the effects of back schools. *Physiother Theory Pract* 7:177–184.

54. Kelsey JL (1975): An epidemiological study of acute herniated lumbar intervertebral discs. *Rheumatol Rehab* 14:144–159.

55. Kelsey JL, Githens PB, O'Connor T, et al. (1984): Acute prolapsed lumbar intervertebral disc: an epidemiologic study with special reference to driving automobiles and cigarette smoking. *Spine* 9:608–613.

56. Kelsey JL, Githens PB, White AA 3rd (1984): An epidemiologic study of lifting and twisting on the job and risk for acute prolapsed lumbar intervertebral disc. *J Orthop Res* 2:61–66.

57. Keyserling WM, Herrin GD, Chaffin DB, Armstrong TJ, Foss ML (1980): Establishing an industrial strength testing program. *Am Ind Hyg Assoc J* 41:730–736.

58. Klingenstiena U (1991): Back schools/educational programs—a review. *Crit Rev Phys Rehab Med* 3(2):155–171.

59. Knowles J (1977): *Doing better and feeling worse: health care in the United States.* New York: Norton, pp. 1–8.

60. Komaki J, Heinzmann AT, Lawson L (1980): The effect of training and feedback: component analysis of a behavioral safety program. *J Appl Psychol* 65:261–270.

61. Kravitz E, Moore ME, Glaros A (1981): Paralumbar muscle activity in chronic low back pain. *Arch Phys Med Rehab* 62:172–176.

62. Kriegler JS, Ashenberg ZS (1987): Management of chronic low back pain: a comprehensive approach. *Semin Neurol* 7:303–312.

63. Kroemer K, Kroemer H, Kroemer-Elbert K (1994): *Ergonomics: how to design for ease and efficiency.* Englewood Cliffs, NJ: Prentice Hall, Chapter 10.

64. Lance BM, Chaffin DB (1971): The effect of prior muscle exertions on simple movements. *Hum Factors* 13:355–361.

65. Lankhorst GJ, Van de Stadt RJ, Vogelaar TW, Van der Korst JK, Prevo AJH (1983): The effect of the Swedish Back School in chronic idiopathic low back pain. A prospective controlled study. *Scand J Rehab Med* 15:141–145.

66. Leino P (1989): Symptoms of stress predict musculoskeletal disorders. *J Epidemiol Commun Health* 43:293–300.

67. Leino P, Lyyra A (1990): The effects of mental stress and social support on the development of musculoskeletal morbidity in the engineering industry. In: Sakurai H, Okajaki L, Omae I, eds. *Occupational epidemiology.* Amsterdam: Elsevier Science Publishers BV, 267–272.

68. Lifshitz YR, et al. (1989): The effectiveness of an ergonomics program in controlling work-related disorders in an automotive plant—a case study. In: *Proceedings of the International Conference on "Marketing Ergonomics."* The Netherlands: University of Twente.

69. Liker JK, Evans SM, Ulin SS (1990): The strengths and limitations of lecture-based training in acquisition of ergonomics knowledge and skills. *Int J Ind Erg* 5:147–159.

70. Lindstrom I, Ohlund C, Eek C, Wallin L, Peterson L-E, Nachemson A (1989): *Work return and low back pain disability: results of a prospective randomized study in an industrial population* [Abstract]. International Society for the Study of the Lumbar Spine (ISSLS), Kyoto, Japan.

71. Lindstrom I, Ohlund C, Eek C, et al. (1992): The effect of graded activity on patients with subacute low back pain: a randomized prospective clinical study with an operant-conditioning behavioral approach. *Phys Ther* 72(4):39–53.

72. Lindstrom I, Ohlund C, Eek C, et al. (1992): Mobility, strength, and fitness after a graded activity program for patients with subacute low back pain. *Spine* 17(6):641–652.

73. Linton SJ (1987): Chronic pain: The case for prevention. *Behav Res Ther* 25:313–317.

74. Linton SJ, Bradley LA, Jensen I, Spangfort E, Sundell L (1989): The secondary prevention of low back pain: a controlled study with follow-up. *Pain* 36:197–207.

75. Linton SJ, Kamwendo K (1987): Low back schools. A critical review. *Phys Ther* 67:1375–1383.

76. Ljungberg P, Sanne H (1986): *Ryggbesvar.* Göteborg, Sweden: Statshalsan.

77. Lorig KR, Cox T, Cuevas Y, Kraines RG, Britton MC (1984): Converging and diverging beliefs about arthritis: Caucasian patients, Spanish speaking patients and physicians. *J Rheumatol* 11: 76–79.

78. Luopajarvi T (1987): Workers' education. *Ergonomics* 30(2): 305–311.

79. Marteniuk R (1986): Information processes in movement learning: capacity and structural interference effects. *J Motor Behav* 18:55–75.

80. Mattmiller AW (1980): The California Back School. *Physiotherapy* 66:118–121.

81. Mayer TG, Gatchel RJ, Kishino N, et al (1985): Objective assessment of spine function following industrial injury. A prospective study with comparison group and one-year follow-up. *Spine* 10: 482–493.

82. McGill CM (1968): Industrial back problems: a control program. *J Occup Med* 10:174–178.

83. McKeachie W (1969): *Teaching tips: a guidebook for the beginning college teacher.* Lexington, KY: D.C. Heath.

84. McLeroy K, Green L, Mullen K, Foshee V (1989): Can we reduce stress in American workers? A review of programs. *Advances* 6(1): 16–19.

85. Meichenbaum D, Jarenko M (1983): *Stress reduction and prevention.* New York: Plenum.

86. Melvin J (1989): *Rheumatic diseases in adult and child: occupational therapy and rehabilitation.* Philadelphia: Davis.

87. Moll JM (1986): Doctor-patient communication in rheumatology: studies of visual and verbal perception using educational booklets and other graphic material. *Ann Rheumat Dis* 45:198–209.

88. Murphy L (1984): Stress management in highway maintainance workers. *J Occup Med* 26:436–442.

89. Myers J, Riordan R, Mattmiller AW, Pelcher A, Levenson BS, White A (1981): *Low back injury prevention at Southern Pacific Railroad: five years experience with a back school model.* International Society For The Study Of The Lumbar Spine (ISSLS), Paris, France.

90. Nachemson A (1983): Work for all: for those with low back pain as well. *Clin Orthop Rel Res* 179:77–85.

91. National Institute for Occupational Safety and Health (1993): Comments from the National Institute for Occupational Safety and Health on the Occupational Safety and Health Administration proposed rule on ergonomic safety and health management. 29 CFR Part 1910 Docket No. S-777. US DHS/CDC.

92. Nordin M, Frankel VH, Spengler DM (1981): *A preventive back-*

care program for industry [Abstract]. International Society for the Study of the Lumbar Spine (ISSLS), Paris, France.

93. Ost LG (1987): Applied relaxation: description of a coping technique and review of controlled studies. *Behav Res Ther* 25:397–409.

94. Parnianpour M, Nordin M, Kahanovitz N, Frankel V (1988): The triaxial coupling of torque generation of trunk muscles during isometric exertions and the effect of fatiguing isoinertial movements on the motor output and movement patterns. *Spine* 13:982–992.

95. Pelletier K, Lutz R (1989): Mindbody goes to work: a critical review of stress management programs in the workplace. *Advances* 6(1):28–34.

96. Peltier LF (1983): The "Back School" of Delpech in Montpellier. *Clin Orthop* 179:4–9.

97. Pope M (1987): Modification of work organization. *Ergonomics* 30(2):449–455.

98. Price JP, Clare MH, Ewerhardt FH (1948): Studies in low backache with persistent muscle spasm. *Arch Phys Med* 29:703–709.

99. Redmond BK (1988): *The process of patient education.* St. Louis: Mosby.

100. Riihimaki H (1985): Back pain and heavy physical work: a comparative study of concrete reinforcement workers and maintenance house painters. *Br J Ind Med* 42:226–232.

101. Rohmert W, Laurig K (1977): Increasing awareness of ergonomics by in-company courses. A case study. *Appl Ergonom* 8:19–21.

102. Rush D (1984): Peer behavior coaching soccer. *J Sport Psychol* 6:325–334.

103. Sandstrom J (1984): *Om kroniska landryggsbesvar.* Göteborg, Sweden: Göteborg Universitet.

104. Sandstrom J, Andersson GB, Wallerstedt S (1984): The role of alcohol abuse in working disability in patients with low back pain. *Scand J Rehab Med* 16:147–149.

105. Sargent M (1946): Psychosomatic backache. *N Engl J Med* 234:427–430.

106. Schultz A, Andersson GB, Ortengren R, Bjork R, Nordin M (1982): Analysis and quantitative myoelectric measurements of loads on the lumbar spine when holding weights in standing postures. *Spine* 7:390–397.

107. Seamonds B (1986): The concept and practice of stress management. In: Wolf S, ed. *Occupational stress.* Boston: PSG Publishing, pp. 153–163.

108. Silverstein BA, Richards SE, Alaseck K, et al. (1991): Evaluation of in-plant ergonomics training. *Int J Ind Erg* 8:179–193.

109. Simpson GC (1980): The economic justification for ergonomics. *Int J Ind Erg* 2:157–163.

110. Snook SH, Campanelli RA, Hart JW (1978): A study of three preventive approaches to low back injury. *J Occup Med* 20:478–481.

111. Snook SH, White AH (1984): Education and training. In: MH Pope, JW Frymoyer, G Andersson, eds. *Occupational low back pain.* New York: Praeger, pp. 233–244.

112. Spinhoven P, Linssen AC (1989): Education and self-hypnosis in the management of low back pain: a component analysis. *Br J Clin Psychol* 28(pt 2):145–153.

113. Spitzer WO, LeBlanc FE, DuPuis M (1987): Scientific approach to the assessment and management of activity-related spinal disorders. Report of the Quebec Task Force on Spinal Disorders. *Spine* 12:S1–S59.

114. St-Vincent M, Tellier C, Lortie M (1989): Training in handling: an evaluative study. *Ergonomics* 32:191–210.

115. Steffy B, Jones J, Murphy L, Kunz L (1986): A demonstration of the impact of stress abatement programs on reducing employee's accidents and their costs. *Am J Health Promot* Fall:25–32.

116. Sternbach P (1978): *The psychology of pain.* New York: Raven Press.

117. Stubbs DA, Buckle PW, Hudson MP, Rivers PM, Worringham CJ (1983): Back pain in the nursing profession: I. Epidemiology and pilot methodology. *Ergonomics* 26(8):755–765.

118. Svensson HO, Andersson GB (1983): Low-back pain in forty to forty seven year old men: work history and work environment factors. *Spine* 8:272–276.

119. Troup JDG, Foreman TK, Baster CE, Brown D (1987): The perception of back pain and the role of psychophysical tests of lifting capacity. *Spine* 12:645–657.

120. Turner JA (1982): Comparison of group progressive-relaxation training and cognitive–behavioral group therapy for chronic low back pain. *J Consult Clin Psychol* 50:757–765.

121. Turner JA, Clancy S (1988): Comparison of operant behavioral and cognitive–behavioral group treatment for chronic low back pain. *J Consult Clin Psychol* 56:261–266.

122. Upton A, Graber E (1993): *Staying healthy in a risky environment. The New York University Medical Center family guide: how to identify, prevent or minimize environmental risks to your health.* New York: Simon & Schuster.

123. Ursin H, Endresen IM, Svebak S, Tellnes G, Mykletun R (1993): Muscle pain and coping with working life in Norway: a review. *Work Stress* 7:247–258.

124. Vallfors B (1985): Acute, subacute and chronic low back pain: clinical symptoms, absenteeism and working environment. *Scand J Rehab Med* 11(Suppl):1–98.

125. Versloot JM, Schilstra AJ, Tolen FJ, van Akkervehen PF (1988): *Back school in industry, a prospective longitudinal controlled study (3 years).* [Abstract]. International Society for the Study of the Lumbar Spine (ISSLS), Miami, Florida.

126. Videman T, Rauhala H, Asp S, Lindstrom K, Cedercruetz G, Kampoc M, Tola S, Troup JD (1989): Patient-handling skills, back injuries, and back pain. An intervention study in nursing. *Spine* 14:148–156.

127. Waddell G (1987): A new clinical model for treatment of low back pain. *Spine* 12:632–644.

128. Waddell G (1992): Biopsychosocial analysis of low back pain. In: Nordin M, Vischer T, eds. *Common low back pain: prevention of chronicity. Bailliere's clinical rheumatology.* 6(3):523–555.

129. Westgaard RH, Aaras A (1987): The effect of improved workplace design on the development of work related musculoskeletal illnesses. In: Galer J, ed. *Applied ergonomics handbook,* 2nd ed. London: Butterworths, pp. 185–196.

130. Wolf S (1986): Common and grave disorders identified with occupational stress. In: Wolf S, ed. *Occupational stress.* Boston: PSG, pp. 47–53.

131. Wood DJ (1987): Design and evaluation of a back injury prevention program within a geriatric hospital. *Spine* 12:77–82.

132. Woodruff A (1961): *Basic concepts of teaching.* Scranton, PA: Chandler.

The Adult Spine: Principles and Practice,
2nd edition, J.W. Frymoyer, Editor-in-Chief.
Lippincott-Raven Publishers, Philadelphia © 1997.

CHAPTER 15

Functional Restoration of the Patient with Chronic Back Pain

Rowland G. Hazard

While the true incidence of back pain may not have changed significantly, disability from spinal disorders has increased explosively in Western countries since the turn of the century (14,41). As outlined in Chapter 8, "The Economics of Spinal Disorders," the financial impact of low back disability is astounding. Estimates of the annual cost of medical care, lost productivity, and wage compensation related to back disability in the United States range from $16 to $56 billion (2,37). National worker compensation costs alone have increased by 241% between 1980 and 1986 (42).

This epidemic of disabling back pain over the past several decades has defied the ministrations of a proliferation of medical technology. Diagnostic advances in electromyography, computerized axial tomography, and magnetic resonance imaging are widely available. Therapeutic developments such as discectomy, chemonucleolysis, and intervertebral fusion are commonplace. Despite these advances, however, a clear indisputable anatomic and pathophysiologic diagnosis is not evident in most cases of chronic back pain. A given patient's pain may be ascribed to segmental instability, disc space narrowing, muscular insufficiency, intervertebral subluxation, or simple lumbar strain, depending on the practitioner involved. The absence of a valid explanatory model for the patient's "disease" confounds the patient–

caregiver relationship. The patient may question the physician's credibility when clear diagnosis and subsequent cure are not forthcoming, or the patient may feel that his or her own credibility is questioned. Accusations of magnifying symptoms, if not malingering, may follow should the pain persist without a biological explanation. Without a diagnosis, the physician's ability to treat with confidence and advise regarding functional capacity and prognosis is severely limited. The physician may react to this uncertainty by warning the patient to avoid any painful activity until the injured tissue, whatever it may be, has healed. Prescriptions for bed rest may well last beyond the documented 2-day benefit (7). As pain and disability wear on, clinical decisions may be prompted more by the patient's behaviors than by the underlying pathophysiology. For instance, one patient with minor spondylolisthesis may plead for surgical fusion, while another with even greater displacement prefers to "live with the pain."

The skyrocketing costs and disability rates are all the more remarkable because fully 90% of all people suffering acute back pain recover comfort and function within 6 to 12 weeks (8,21,41). Patients with low back pain persisting beyond this acute phase develop complex biopsychosocial problems far beyond their initial anatomic nociceptive lesions. Patients whose pain disqualifies them from work and participation in key activities such as recreation and family life frequently suffer major deterioration of self-esteem. Depression is understandably a compounding feature of chronic back pain. Pain experience

R. G. Hazard: Associate Professor, Department of Orthopaedics and Rehabilitation, University of Vermont, Box 1043, Williston, VT 05495.

may be heightened by anxieties over occupational, financial, and family dynamic issues. Fear of re-injury, perhaps reinforced by warnings from physicians and family members, frequently results in avoidance of activities involving mechanical stress of the back. As the patient continues to avoid bending, trunk strain, and aerobic activity, trunk stiffness, weakness, and general deconditioning complicate the biological portion of the disability.

After several weeks of disability from low back pain, when the initial tissue injury might well be expected to have healed, the patient may have acquired such an array of psychosocial problems that eradication of the original lesion, even if possible, might not return him to normal function. At this stage, fewer than 5% of patients with persisting pain benefit from surgical intervention. Nonoperative therapies including medication, manipulation, massage, acupuncture, traction, etc., abound, but few have proven efficacy (6).

Medicine's failure to diagnose and cure while psychosocial problems accrue has staggering consequences. Snook (37) and Leavitt (24) have reported that the vast majority of costs devoted to patients with low back pain are consumed by relatively few complicated cases. More recently, Spengler (38) has reported that 10% of the cases

accounted for 79% of the total cost for occupational low back injuries. The majority of expenditures involve financial compensation for lost work and this indemnity increases significantly if the patient undergoes surgery (37). Clearly, the patient who is chronically disabled by low back pain poses the major medical and socioeconomic problems, and the magnitude of this cost bias is reflected in the recent focus of health, insurance, and industrial attention on the epidemic of chronic low back disability.

Two key features of the patient with chronic back pain confound our efforts to stem the tide of disability. First, we have no objective method for measuring pain. None of our imaging or electrodiagnostic techniques assesses pain severity, and assays of serum peptides and endorphins are disappointing in clinical use. We can observe and measure pain-related behaviors, but in the end we must rely on the patient's self-report of pain. Second, the correlation between the patient's report of pain and the observed physical capacity deteriorates with chronicity, as illustrated in Figure 1 (11,19). Since the primary concern in rehabilitation is with decreasing disability rather than with eradicating pain, this distinction is paramount. Once it is clear that a given patient's pain cannot be given an operational diagnosis and cured, quantification of function becomes essential to assessing rehabilitation needs and eventual fitness for work.

QUANTIFICATION OF SPINE FUNCTION

The deconditioning syndrome affecting practically all patients with chronic back pain includes trunk stiffness, weakness, intolerance for aerobic exercise, and loss of speed and coordination required for activities of daily living (28). Tests for these functional capacities and related psychosocial factors are outlined in Table 1.

Trunk flexibility has long been recognized as a major determinant of spinal impairment. Forward flexion may be measured by fingertip-to-floor, skin distraction, and radiographic techniques. The method currently recommended by the American Medical Association involves the use of two inclinometers (9). One inclinometer is placed over the sacrum and one over T1-T2. As the patient bends forward or backward, degrees of maximal movement are recorded. True lumbar movement is calculated by subtracting movement at the sacral level from movement at the thoracic level. Subject effort may be questioned if supine straight-leg raise exceeds hip flexion measured by the sacral inclinometer by over 10° (9,30).

Trunk strength may be measured in forward and side flexion, extension, and rotation. Resistance may be isokinetic (fixed speed), isometric (fixed position), isodynamic (controlled by preset torque minimum), and isoinertial (pulley-weight systems with fixed mass). Strength may be tested concentrically with muscles

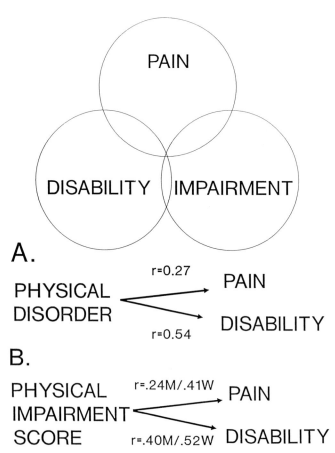

FIG. 1. Relationship between pain, impairment and disability in patients with chronic back injury. Correlation coefficients reported by Waddell (40) (**A**) and Hazard (19) (**B**).

TABLE 1. *Functional capacity evaluation: Typical measurements for assessing patients with chronic low back disability*

PHYSICAL FACTORS
    Trunk Flexibility: Inclinometry
        Effort factor: Hip motion—SLR > 30°
    Trunk Strength: Isokinetic flexion, extension, and rotation
        Effort factor: Curve variability
    Endurance: Cycle ergometry
        Effort factor: Heart rate response
SYMPTOM SELF-REPORTS
    Pain and Disability: Millon Visual Analogue Scale,
        Oswestry Pain Questionnaire, Pain Drawing
PSYCHOLOGIC FACTORS
    Personality Features: Minnesota Multiphasic Personality
        Inventory
    Disability Coping Style: Millon Behavioral Health Index
    Depression: Beck Depression Inventory
    Self-Perceptions, Family Dynamics, etc.: Clinical interview
OCCUPATIONAL FACTORS
    Employment History, Aptitudes, Goals: Interview
    Workers' Compensation, Litigation Status: Interview
    Interpersonal Work Behaviors: Interview

shortening as they contract, or eccentrically with muscles lengthening as they resist a given force. The variety of directions and modes in which trunk strength may be measured has led to a proliferation of testing devices, each touted for its safety, reliability, and biomechanical applicability, in testimony to considerable entrepreneurial effort. In reviewing the available devices, Mayer (27) has supported use of isokinetic extension/flexion and rotation devices until the various machines can be compared through unbiased research. To date there is no conclusive evidence proving the superiority of one testing mode over another, though there are great variations in cost and biomechanical applicability to daily tasks. An example of an isokinetic testing device, in which the subject exerts maximal force against resistance at a fixed speed, is illustrated in Figure 2. Torque/distance curves are recorded along with peak force, work, and power data.

The increased incidence of low back injuries among manual materials handlers has long suggested that lifting capacity is a key factor in assessing back impairment. Recent studies, reviewed by Bigos and Battié in Chapter 9, question this inference. They conclude that lifting capacity is not a major determinant of the likelihood of reporting a backache in an industrial setting. Deficient isolated trunk strength may constitute a weak link in the musculoskeletal lifting chain at work. However, lifting capacity once the back is hurting is directly applicable to the activities of daily living. Controversies in lifting evaluation include resistance modes, test safety, work capacity extrapolations, and indicators of subject effort (15,20,22). Again, comparative studies are lacking. Perhaps the simplest and most practical strategy is the Progressive Isoinertial Lifting Evaluation described by Mayer (26). In this

protocol, the subject lifts a crate with increasingly heavy loads from floor to waist until he or she reaches a safety maximum or reports inability to continue. Heart rate response may be a good indicator of the subject's effort level. While the ability of this test to predict future injury risk is unknown, it does have the advantage over isokinetic and isometric tests of being directly applicable to "real world" activities.

General endurance is most often tested in the rehabilitation setting with upper and lower extremity cycle ergometers and with treadmills. Cady (5) has demonstrated a lower incidence of back injury in physically fit firefighters, and Schmidt (36) has reported deficient aerobic capacity in chronic back patients.

Beyond the specific issues of flexibility, strength, and endurance, the more global assessment of tolerance for activities of daily living must be considered. Obstacle courses include pushing, pulling, crawling, climbing, bending, twisting, and balancing, and general speed and coordination may be estimated by timing a patient's performance. Tolerance for sustained trunk postures may be tested by timed sitting and crouching while the patient attends to simulated work tasks.

The patient's assessment of the problem on a psychosocial level may be recorded through a host of available self-rating tools. The Million Visual Analogue Scale contains 15 questions related primarily to the patient's pain (31). The Oswestry Pain Questionnaire has ten questions focusing on disability (10). Both of these tests are quickly and easily completed and scored. Comparison of these self-perceptions with the patient's measured physical capacity often elucidates the pain and function discrepan-

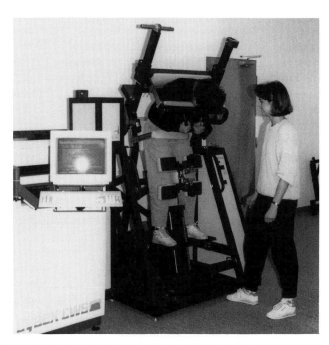

FIG. 2. Isokinetic trunk extension and flexion strength testing.

cies discussed above. The most common psychosocial barriers to recovery include depression, maladaptive coping styles, and a variety of personality problems. The Beck Depression Inventory is a 21-question screen for cognitive features of depression (3). Coping skills are addressed in the Millon Behavioral Health Index (32). The most commonly used test for personality features is the Minnesota Multiphasic Personality Inventory. Tests of intelligence and achievement are particularly helpful in recognizing underlying dysfunction, which may bear on future occupational planning and communication in the rehabilitation setting. Clearly the most important "test" of psychosocial function is the clinical interview. Family dynamics, substance use patterns, finances, compensation and other litigation status, work history, etc., must all be reviewed to identify barriers to recovery.

For the patient disabled by chronic back pain, this battery of physical, psychosocial, and self-assessment evaluations provides a foundation for rehabilitation. Pain, impairment, and disability outcomes commonly do not coincide following rehabilitation (19). If the patient's primary goal is pain relief, whatever functional gains may be made through exercise will not provide satisfaction. Medications that provide pain relief at the expense of mental clarity required by a patient's occupation will not satisfy, if the key goal is reemployment. Physical capacity goals may vary greatly between patients such as a 60-year-old seamstress and a 25-year-old package handler. Therefore, pretreatment setting of pain, physical capacity, and vocational goals is critical to successful rehabilitation. Active patient participation in setting these goals relieves the treatment staff from perceptions that they are forcing unwanted or otherwise inappropriate therapy upon the patient. Throughout the treatment program, repeated measurements of function can be used to gauge progress, alerting the therapist to unseen or uncorrected barriers to recovery when there is no progress toward the patient's stated goals. When rehabilitation is complete, these measurements give the best available justification for statements of work readiness.

DEVELOPMENT OF THE FUNCTIONAL RESTORATION APPROACH

With the recognition that large numbers of patients with chronic back pain and disability are not helped by the classical medical model of diagnosis and cure, a variety of alternative approaches have been developed over the past few decades. Most notably, over 1,000 pain centers have been established in the United States. These programs offer services ranging from behavioral modification to spinal injection therapy, and passive modalities such as manipulation, acupuncture, and ultrasound. While some pain centers use such modalities with a goal of reducing pain, the classic pain center approach in-

volves modifying behaviors stemming from the experience of pain. Various cognitive and behavioral techniques are designed to reduce pain behaviors through individual and family counseling, education, and stress management with or without biofeedback. Program content and pretreatment patient characteristics vary widely, making generalizations of outcome difficult. Improvements in activities of daily living, medication use, and other secondary behaviors have been reported, though the efficacy of the pain center approach in long-term pain reduction is controversial (1,12).

Over the past 15 years, work hardening programs have been developed for people with occupational disabilities. The cornerstone of this approach is graded, progressive rehabilitation through activities simulating the patient's anticipated work. Recognizing the biopsychosocial complexity of chronic disability, work hardening programs generally involve the disciplines of physical and occupational therapy along with psychology. Work hardening programs are designed to maximize the individual's ability to return to work. Reports of return-to-work rates following work hardening range from less than 50% to over 80%, perhaps resulting from variations in patient populations and program contents (33).

In the early 1980s, Dr. Thomas Mayer and his group of physical therapists, occupational therapists, and psychologists developed a program of "functional restoration" for patients with chronic low back disability. The key distinguishing feature of this approach was its reliance on repeated measurements of spine-related functional capacity. These measurements provided guidelines for a sports medicine approach to rehabilitating patients toward fitness for work. The physical training was integrated with work hardening, behavioral modification techniques, and education. This program at the Productive Rehabilitation Institute of Dallas for Ergonomics (PRIDE) reported an 86% return-to-work or training rate for the program treatment group compared to 45% for a nonrandom comparison group after a 1-year follow-up (28). Subsequently, a similar program was established at the New England Back Center (NEBC) (18). This program reported similar outcomes despite differences in socioeconomic settings. The remainder of this chapter describes the essential contents of these programs and outlines the results of their research and of subsequent related studies.

FUNCTIONAL RESTORATION WITH BEHAVIORAL SUPPORT: PROGRAM CONTENT

Functional restoration begins with an initial medical evaluation to ensure that the patient has been properly evaluated in order to rule out the presence of a surgically correctable cause for the pain and disability. Medical problems that might prove barriers to rehabilitation are screened for, and exercise tolerance testing is administered for patients who have significant cardiovascular risk factors or exceed 40 years of age. When consensus has been reached that surgery is not warranted, and there is no evidence for a severe psychiatric disorder precluding participation in group rehabilitation, the patient is introduced to the contents of the program. Once the patient expresses willingness to participate, insurance authorization is solicited for admission. Initial difficulties in procuring such authorization, apparently engendered by prior inadequate pain center accountability, have decreased with publication of functional restoration centers' outcomes.

Prior to entering the intensive phase of rehabilitation, patients may participate in an introductory phase of reconditioning. Kohles (23) has reported improved functional capacity outcomes for patients undergoing such initial reconditioning compared to those who enter the intensive program without it.

The formal program of functional restoration runs 8 to 10 hours per day, $5\frac{1}{2}$ days per week for 3 weeks. The program begins with approximately $1\frac{1}{2}$ days of functional, psychological, and occupational testing described above, and outlined in Table 1 above.

On the second day of the program, the medical, psychological, and physical and occupational therapy staffs each present test results. These presentations facilitate highly integrated multidisciplinary discussions of physical capacities and anticipated work demands, family dynamics and potential barriers to work return, personality features requiring special approaches in rehabilitation, and the like. Specific issues such as need for vocational training, uncooperative previous employers, overly supportive spouses, etc., are addressed and planned for. The cornerstone of these discussions is analysis of the patient's progress toward personal goals for recovery in the categories of pain and functional capacities. These staff meetings are repeated twice weekly for the remainder of the intensive program. The treatment program itself consists of three primary components: physical training, counseling and behavioral management, and work hardening with occupational counseling.

The physical training program begins with 1 hour of exercises designed to improve flexibility integrated with low impact aerobic exercise (Fig. 3). A second hour involves cardiovascular training with stationary arm and leg bikes, along with specific major muscle group strengthening through resistance training in a gym (Fig. 4). Patients are individually instructed in strengthening programs beginning below their performance levels on initial evaluation, and progressing toward their stated 3-week goals. The mutual understanding of these goals and the performance required to reach them by both therapist and patient is essential to the success of the physical rehabilitation. Deviations from this plan are viewed as reflections of either physical or psychosocial barriers to recovery. Medical, psychological, and socioeconomic re-evaluations may be necessary to uncover barriers such as fear of re-injury and compensation issues. In addition to flexibility exercises, strength training activities requiring speed and dexterity, such as volleyball and basketball, are included to encourage "unguarded" trunk stresses. These activities challenge the patient's fear of re-injury in addition to encouraging improvement in coordination and increasing appreciation for recreation.

Physical training is continued in the occupational therapy portions of the program. Progressing from spe-

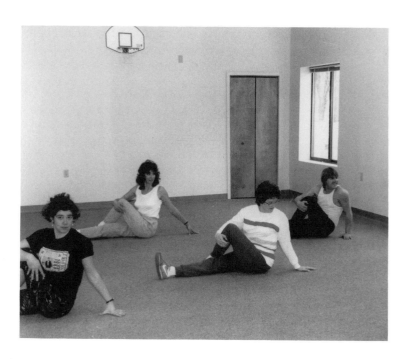

FIG. 3. General conditioning class in a functional restoration program.

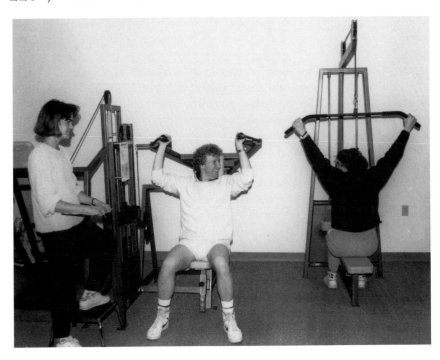

FIG. 4. Functional restoration patients are directed through individualized protocols of progressive resistance training in the gym.

cific flexibility, strength training, and cardiovascular endurance training, work hardening provides simulated work tasks: patients push and pull a sled loaded with concrete blocks. Awkward trunk postures are maintained while working on a mock automobile or "nuts-and-bolts" boards at varying heights (Fig. 5). Fixed ladders provide training in climbing. Prolonged sitting is required during computer terminal work. Repetitive bending with knees straight is accomplished through reaching over a saw-horse to pick up golf tees from the floor and placing them in pegboards on the wall. Crates are loaded with progressively greater weights to increase capacity for frequent lifting (Fig. 6). To some extent, these activities are geared toward the demands of the individual pa-

tient's anticipated work. However, a specific job is frequently not at hand, particularly early in the program, and more generic goals based on population norms are targeted. Floor exercises, gym participation, and work-related complex activities amount to approximately 5 hours per day in the program. Representatives of medical, psychological, occupational, and physical therapy disciplines teach classes in diagnostic technology, use and abuse of medications, compensation loss, spinal anatomy, and functional capacity measurement each day for 1 hour. Occupational therapists formulate return-to-work goals and plans with each patient. These plans may necessitate work aptitude and interest testing as well as considerable investigation of job availability,

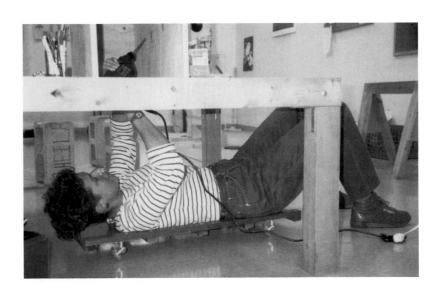

FIG. 5. Postural stresses required by a patient's anticipated work are simulated by tasks such as mock automobile repair.

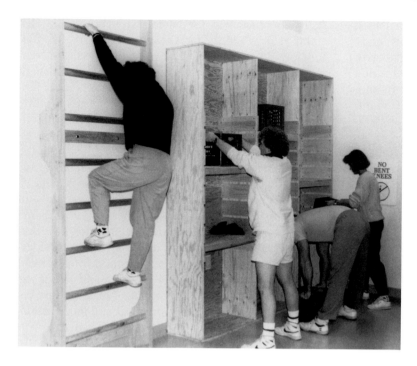

FIG. 6. Crates are loaded with progressively heavier loads to increase lifting capacity. Trunk extensor muscles may be targeted by training with straight-leg or "torso" lift.

often in coordination with a rehabilitation specialist who may follow the patient after discharge from rehabilitation. These plans must be realistically coordinated with the patient's observed functional capacities in the program.

The psychological portion of the program includes individual and group counseling sessions. Counseling is not directed at long-term "insight" techniques, but concentrates on immediate behavioral modification. Family dynamics are reviewed individually as needed, and with the family on a weekly basis. Observation of the patient's improved physical capacities by children and spouses often make cognitive impacts not possible through second-hand description. Depression may be treated with medication, though improvement in physical function frequently appears to create improvements in self-efficacy, mood, and affect. Stress management techniques are reinforced through biofeedback to combat the chronic anxieties often associated with persisting pain (Fig. 7). These techniques are also integrated with physical stretching exercises and breathing techniques in devising individual strategies for dealing with acute pain episodes. These instructions are particularly powerful when the patient suffers an episode of acute pain during rehabilitation, as they are direct proof of the patient's ability to recover through his or her own initiative. For 1 hour each day, didactic and participatory sessions address the advantages of assertiveness over passive-aggressive reactions to the disability syndrome, the theory and practice of stress management, and techniques for identifying unnecessary anxieties, particularly those associated with fear of re-injury.

The 3-week intensive portion of the program con-

cludes with a multidisciplinary staffing to discuss the patient's return-to-work plan and to assign responsibilities for patient follow-up, including rehabilitation specialist participation when appropriate.

On completion of the intensive portion of the pro-

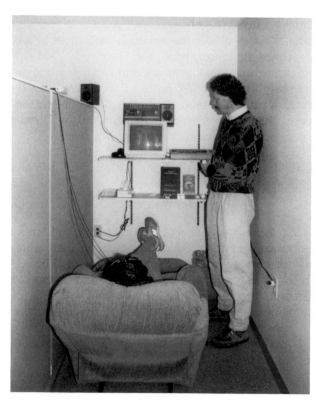

FIG. 7. Biofeedback using visual display of frontalis muscle tension to teach relaxation response techniques.

gram, the patient continues similar treatment for 1 to 2 days per week from 0 to 6 weeks, depending on functional capacity level, resolution of return-to-work barriers, and job availability. This follow-up program is designed to allow for integration of the improvements and behavioral changes generated during intensive treatment with the patient's return to the family, occupation, and other features of the "real world." Functional capacity testing and self-assessment questionnaires are administered at the time of discharge from the intensive program and thereafter at 6 weeks, 3 months, 6 months, and 1 year. Data from these re-evaluations are discussed with the patient and adjustments in work status and self-care programs are made as indicated.

CONTROVERSIES IN REHABILITATION OUTCOME

Difficulties in measuring rehabilitation outcomes for patients with chronic low back pain begin with the common discrepancies between self-reported symptom levels and measured functional capacities described above. The primary goal of rehabilitation is to improve the patient's functional capacity, so that quantification of physical capacity is clearly a key component of rehabilitation outcome assessment. However, subjective outcomes should be reported. Otherwise, positive physical capacity outcomes may be falsely encouraging for treatment approaches that, in fact, produce patients who are "doing better and feeling worse." A second consideration in assessing outcome reports is the natural history of recovery from acute back pain. Since 90% of patients with acute back pain recover comfort and function spontaneously within a few months of onset, therapies directed at patients in this time frame will have better outcomes than those directed at patients in the chronic phase of disability for whom prognosis is much worse.

To some extent, the relative importance of available treatment outcomes varies with the observer. While a given patient may be primarily concerned with pain relief, the employer and rehabilitation specialist are more concerned with the patient's physical capacity and ability to return to work. The patient's attorney may be more concerned with the physical measurements used in impairment evaluations in a Workers' Compensation setting, while asking for estimations of pain and suffering in the case of personal injury. Future health care utilization and compensation of costs may be paramount for the patient's insurance carrier. Documentation of such costs is difficult, particularly since the majority of expenditure is nonmedical, involving compensation payments, future wage loss, vocational rehabilitation, lost interest on savings, and so on.

Because of these difficulties in outcome measurement, return to work has been popularized as the best global statement of recovery for patients with chronic back disability (16). When the patient returns to work, it is presumably done in agreement with the physician, employer, attorney, and insurance carrier that sufficient comfort and physical capacity have returned for the performance of a particular job in the foreseeable future. This agreement is an appropriate basis for settling compensation and other legal issues in the patient's disability. However, return to work may be inappropriate as the sole measure of effectiveness for rehabilitation programs. After all, pretreatment patient characteristics such as age, pre-injury job satisfaction, education, and a host of motivational factors may vary considerably between one patient population and the next. Furthermore, measurements of return to work are not categorical; consideration of partial work return, participation in vocational training programs, and wage or work demand demotions must be taken into account. In spite of these caveats, return to work does provide a practical and facile assessment of rehabilitation outcomes for patients with chronic back pain and disability.

OUTCOMES OF FUNCTIONAL RESTORATION PROGRAMS

In 1985, Mayer et al. (28) evaluated 111 patients with chronic back disability referred to their practice, PRIDE. All these patients met the study requirements of greater than 4 months disability and lack of evidence for a surgically correctable cause of pain. Seventy-three of these patients were admitted to the functional restoration treatment program. Seven dropped out of the treatment program of their own volition, leaving 66 to graduate from the 3-week program. Of the original 111 patients, 38 were denied participation in the rehabilitation program by their insurance carriers, reportedly as a matter of policy rather than individual patient discrimination. This group formed a nonrandom comparison group. The initial treatment group characteristics outlined in Table 2 were comparable to those of the comparison group and drop-out group.

TABLE 2. *Initial mean patient characteristics of patients graduating from functional restoration programs at Productive Rehabilitation Institute of Dallas for Ergonomics (PRIDE) and New England Back Center (NEBC) (refs. 16,25)*

	PRIDE (n = 66)	NEBC (n = 59)
Age	36	37
Sex (% male)	64	64
Spinal surgeries	1.5	0.4
Months disabled	12	19
Workers' compensation (%)	90	91
Medications	1.2	1.1

All patients admitted to the program underwent the initial testing outlined in Table 1. Three months following the treatment program described above, program graduates underwent quantification of self-assessed pain, disability, and depression, and evaluation of functional capacity. One year following program completion, program graduates were interviewed by telephone regarding work status. At least partial data sets were available for 100% of the treatment group, 98% of the comparison group, and 86% of the drop-out group.

Eighty-six percent of the program graduates were either working or participating in a vocational training program 1 year after treatment. Only 45% of the comparison group and 20% of the drop-out group were similarly employed (Fig. 8). Only 7% of the program graduates underwent additional spinal surgery in the year following treatment, while 33% of the drop-out group and 6% of the comparison group were operated on. Of the graduates initially on worker compensation, 86% had settled their cases compared to 68% of the comparison patients and 67% of the drop-outs. Self-reports of pain intensity and disability improved significantly in the course of a 3-week treatment program. There were also significant improvements in self-reports of depression. Isokinetic trunk strength, frequent lifting, and trunk flexibility also improved significantly.

In a sequel to this study, Mayer (29) reported 2-year follow-up results of 116 program graduates and 72 comparison patients. Over 85% of the program graduates and comparison patients were included in the 2-year evaluation. While only 41% of the comparison group were employed at the end of 2 years, 87% of the program graduates were working. Additional surgery and health-care visits were more than twice as frequent for comparison patients. Furthermore, re-injury was only half as common in the program graduate group.

Hazard (18) subsequently reported similar outcomes in a different socioeconomic and geographic setting at the NEBC. Ninety patients meeting the PRIDE criteria of 4 months continuous disability and absence of a surgically correctable lesion were studied. In addition to the study design employed by Mayer, this study evaluated the correlation between year-end physical capacities and self-assessments with 1-year return-to-work status.

The original 90 patients included 59 program graduates, 5 drop-outs, and 17 comparison patients. Six patients were denied insurance authorization for the initial 6 months of the study, then authorized and treated and evaluated 6 months after treatment. Three patients refused participation in the treatment program. Initial program graduate patient characteristics are outlined in Table 2 above. The treatment group had a higher percentage of patients on Workers' Compensation, but the three patient groups were otherwise statistically similar in terms of age, sex, spinal surgeries, medications, smoking history, education, self-assessments of pain, disability, and depression, trunk flexibility, frequent lifting, isokinetic trunk strength, and cycling endurance.

Eighty-one percent of the program graduates, 40% of the program drop-outs, and 29% of the comparison group had returned to work 1 year following treatment (Fig. 8 above). The average time required for return to work following treatment was 1 to 2 weeks. All six of the cross-over patients were employed within 6 months following treatment. The program graduates who remained unemployed reported continuing pain, pregnancy, retirement, schooling, cardiac disability, and inability to find work.

In the course of the 3-week treatment program, self-assessments of pain, disability, and depression improved along with physical capacities (Table 3). These improvements persisted through 1 year of follow-up except for

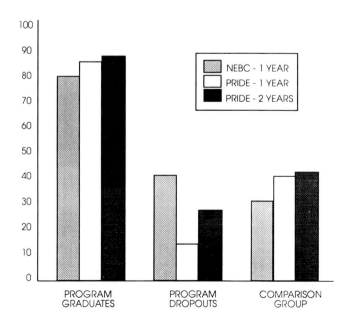

FIG. 8. Return to work outcomes at one- and two-year follow-ups by the New England Back Center (NEBC) and the Productive Rehabilitation Institute of Dallas for Ergonomics (PRIDE).

partial loss of gains in frequent lifting, cycling endurance, and isokinetic trunk extension strength. At year-end, program graduates who were working had lower Oswestry Pain Questionnaire scores, and greater trunk flexibility and cycling endurance compared to program graduates who remained unemployed. Other measurements of physical capacity and self-reported pain, disability, and depression were not significantly different between those who were working and those who were not. The most common criticism of these three studies has been the lack of a randomized and blinded study design (25). While there may be some bias introduced by the differences in insurance status between treatment and comparison groups, the similarity in initial patient characteristics in both studies strongly suggests that the treatment program was responsible for improved return-to-work outcomes for the graduates. In the weeks following program completion, NEBC graduates who returned to work were not significantly different from their unemployed peers by any self-assessment or physical capacity standards other than cycling endurance. While cardiovascular endurance may be important, it is far more likely that management of return-to-work issues was primarily responsible for helping the patients to return to work. In 1989, Tollison and colleagues reported results from a similar multidisciplinary, functional restoration program for patients with chronic low back pain and disability (39). Insurance company denial of treatment authorization was again used to separate the nontreatment comparison patients from those who participated in the treatment program. For the 72 program participants and the 41 comparison patients, the 18-month follow-up rates were 88% and 90%, respectively. Of the contacted program participants, 56% were working, whereas only 27% of the comparison patients were employed. The treated group had better than twice as good results in terms of medication use, additional spinal surgery, and hospitalization.

Oland and Tveiten (34) recently reported quite different results from their "modern active rehabilitation" program. This program involved less formal functional testing, less counselling, and more passive interventions than the programs previously described. Selection criteria also differed from the previous studies in that patients with fibromyalgia, olisthesis, prior spinal surgery, and somatoform disorder were excluded. The 66 patients in this study had no significant mean pain or disability score changes 6 and 18 months after treatment. Over half of the patients were receiving disability pensions at the time of the 18-month follow-up. The authors concluded that chronic back pain patients should be attended to by the Social Security system rather than through rehabilitation. However, it is more likely that integrated functional restoration programs such as those described above are more effective in reducing low back disability than the physically focused program of Oland and Tveiten. This conclusion is supported by the fact that their patients' pain and disability reports did not improve in the course of treatment.

Further refutation of the recommendation against rehabilitation for chronic back pain patients came from Bendix and colleagues in their report to the International Society for Study of the Lumbar Spine in 1993 (4). Their treatment program was a close facsimile of the functional restoration programs of Mayer and of Hazard, but their study design was superior. Their 118 chronically back-disabled patients were randomized to multidisciplinary functional restoration, physical training, or counselling with "warm up exercises." Patients in the multidisciplinary group had better self-assessed pain outcomes. Their 4-month employment (66%) and work feasibility (76%) rates were significantly better than those of the other two treatment groups.

Although the importance of individual physical, psychological, and occupational components of functional restoration programs is not clear, the integration of biological, social, and psychological approaches has been effective in helping people with long-standing disability from back pain return to work, in spite of the dismal prognosis for such patients. The cost of these intensive functional restoration programs, particularly if room and board are required, exceeds $5,000.00. Since most industrial back injuries resolve without intervention, this form of treatment is not appropriate for all back-injured workers. Fredrickson et al. (13) have found that patients over 50 years old are less likely than younger patients to return to work following intensive rehabilitation. Personality screens, pain drawings, trunk flexibility, strength, and endurance were generally poor predictors, although worker compensation and pending litigation predicted relatively poor outcome. Return-to-work prediction by a psychologist interviewing the patient before treatment and by the treatment staff on completion of treatment were relatively accurate. After considering 42 psychological, physical, and medical variables in patients undergoing functional restoration, Polatin (35) found that return to work was more common in patients with

TABLE 3. *Mean self-report scores and functional capacity measures at admission, discharge, and one-year follow-up from the New England Back Center program (ref. 16)*

	Admission	Discharge	One-year follow-up
Pain (Million):			
working	93	68	64
not working	92	72	88
Disability (Oswestry):			
working	39	24	20
not working	42	28	37
Depression (Beck):			
working	12.2	5.9	6.2
not working	10.9	5.6	11.2

comparatively low pretreatment self-assessments of pain, disability, and depression; low Millon Behavioral Health Inventory scores; a previous favorable surgical history; longer pre-injury work record; and job availability estimations. We hope intensive functional restoration programs can be more efficiently administered with better targeting of appropriate patients and perhaps through emphasis on specific physical and psychological program components to meet individual patients' needs. Patients who exaggerate their disability do not appear to have significantly different employment outcomes following rehabilitation (17). While patients who are unwilling to participate in rehabilitation undoubtedly get less out of such active care, people who appear less disabled than their self-reports might suggest should not necessarily be excluded from treatment.

REFERENCES

1. Aronoff GM, Evans WO, Erders PL (1983): A review of follow-up studies of multidisciplinary pain units. *Pain* 16:1–11.
2. Bauer WI (1985): Scope of industrial low back pain. In: Weisel SW, Feffer FW, Rothman RH, eds. *Industrial low back pain.* Charlottesville: Mitchie, pp 1–35.
3. Beck A (1967): *Depression: clinical, experimental and theoretical aspects.* New York: Harper and Row.
4. Bendix AF, Bendix T, Busch E, Ostenfeld S (1993): *Comparison of different active treatment programs for patients with chronic low back pain.* Abstract presentation. International Society for the Study of the Lumbar Spine. Marseilles, France.
5. Cady LD, Bischoff DP, O'Connell ER, Thomas PC, Allan JH (1979): Strength and fitness and subsequent back injuries in firefighters. *J Occup Med* 21:269–272.
6. Deyo RA (1983): Conservative therapy for low back pain: distinguishing useful from useless therapy. *JAMA* 250:1057–1062.
7. Deyo RA, Diehl AK, Rosenthal M (1986): How many days of bedrest for acute low back pain? *N Engl J Med* 315:1064–1070.
8. Dillane JB, Fry J, Kalton G (1966): Acute back syndrome: a study from general practice. *Br Med J* 2:82–84.
9. Engleberg AL, ed. (1988): *Guides to the evaluation of permanent impairment.* Chicago: American Medical Association.
10. Fairbank JC, Couper J, Davies JB, O'Brien JP (1980): The Oswestry low back pain disability questionnaire. *Physiotherapy* 66:271–273.
11. Fordyce W, McMahon R, Rainwater G, Jackins S, Questad K, Murphy T, DeLateur B (1981): Pain complaint–exercise performance relationship in chronic pain. *Pain* 10:311–321.
12. Fordyce WE, Roberts AH, Sternbach RA (1985): The behavioral management of chronic pain: a response to critics. *Pain* 22:113–125.
13. Fredrickson BE, Trief PM, VanBeveren P, Yuan HA, Baum G (1988): Rehabilitation of the patient with chronic back pain: a search for outcome predictors. *Spine* 13:351–353.
14. Hadler NM (1987): The language of diagnosis. In: Hadler NM, ed. *Clinical concepts in regional musculoskeletal illness.* Orlando: Grune & Stratton, pp. 3–24.
15. Hansson TH, Bigos SJ, Wortley MK, Spengler DM (1984): The load on the lumbar spine during isometric strength testing. *Spine* 9:720–724.
16. Hazard RG (1991): Functional restoration treatment outcomes. In: Mayer TG, Mooney V, Gatchel RJ, eds. *Contemporary care for spinal disorders.* Philadelphia: Lea & Febiger, pp 482–487.
17. Hazard RG, Bendix A, Fenwick JW (1991): Disability exaggeration as a predictor of functional restoration outcomes for patients with chronic low-back pain. *Spine* 16:1062–1067.
18. Hazard RG, Fenwick JW, Kalisch SM, Redmond J, Reeves V, Reid S, Frymoyer JW (1989): Functional restoration with behav-

19. Hazard RG, Haugh LD, Green PA, Jones PL (1994): Chronic low back pain: the relationship between patient satisfaction and pain, impairment and disability outcomes. *Spine* 19:881–887.
20. Hazard RG, Reid S, Fenwick J, Reeves V (1988): Isokinetic trunk and lifting strength measurements: variability as an indicator of effort. *Spine* 13:54–57.
21. Hult L (1954): The Munkfors investigation. *Acta Orthop Scand* 16(Suppl):1–76.
22. Kishino ND, Mayer TG, Gatchel RJ, et al. (1985): Quantification of lumbar function. Part 4: Isometric and isokinetic lifting simulation in normal subjects and low-back dysfunction patients. *Spine* 10:921–927.
23. Kohles S, Barnes D, Gatchel RJ, Mayer TG (1988): *Improved physical performance outcome following functional restoration treatment of chronic low back pain patients: early versus recent training results.* Colorado Springs: North American Spine Society.
24. Leavitt SS, Johnston TL, Beyer RD (1971): The process of recovery: patterns in industrial back injury. 1: Costs and other quantitative measures of effort. *Indus Med Surg* 40(8):7–14.
25. Lynn CK (1988): Restoration of function in industrial low back injury [letter]. *JAMA* 259:1181–1182.
26. Mayer TG, Barnes D, Kishino ND, Nichols G, Gatchel RJ, Mayer H, Mooney V (1988): Progressive isoinertial lifting evaluation. I. A standardized protocol and normative database. *Spine* 13:993–997.
27. Mayer TG, Gatchel RJ (1988): Objective trunk strength, endurance and aerobic capacity measurements. In: *Functional restoration for spinal disorders: the sports medicine approach.* Philadelphia: Lea & Febiger, pp 139–161.
28. Mayer TG, Gatchel RJ, Kishino N, Keeley J, Capra P, Mayer H, Barrett J, Mooney V (1985): Objective assessment of spine function following industrial injury: a prospective study with comparison group and a one-year follow-up. *Spine* 10:482–493.
29. Mayer TG, Gatchel RJ, Mayer H, Kishino ND, Keeley J, Mooney V (1987): A prospective two-year study of functional restoration in industrial low back injury. An objective assessment procedure. *JAMA* 258:1763–1767.
30. Mayer TG, Tencer AF, Kristoferson S, Mooney V (1984): Use of noninvasive techniques for quantification of spinal range-of-motion in normal subjects in chronic low-back dysfunction patients. *Spine* 9:588–595.
31. Million R, Hall W, Nilsen KH, Baker RD, Jayson MI (1982): Assessment of the progress of the back-pain patient. *Spine* 7:204–212.
32. Millon T, et al. (1982): *Millon behavioral health inventory manual,* 3rd ed. Minneapolis: National Computer Systems.
33. Neimeyer LO, Jacobs K (1989): *Work hardening: state of the art.* Thorofare, NJ: Slack.
34. Oland G, Tveiten G (1991): A trial of modern rehabilitation for chronic low-back pain and disability: vocational outcome and effect of pain modulation. *Spine* 16:457–59.
35. Polatin PB, Gatchel RJ, Barnes D, Mayer H, Arens C, Mayer TG (1989): A psychosociomedical prediction model of response to treatment by chronically disabled workers with low-back pain. *Spine* 14(9):956–961.
36. Schmidt AJ (1985): Cognitive factors in the performance level of chronic low back pain patients. *J Psychosom Res* 29:183–189.
37. Snook SH, Jensen RC (1984): Cost. In: Pope MH, Frymoyer JW, Andersson GBJ, eds. *Occupational low back pain.* New York: Praeger, pp. 115–121.
38. Spengler DM, Bigos SJ, Martin NA, Zeh J, Fisher L, Nachemson A (1986): Back injuries in industry: a retrospective study. I: Overview and cost analysis. *Spine* 11(3):241–245.
39. Tollison CD, Kriegel ML, Satterthwaite JR, Hinnant DW, Turner KP (1989): Comprehensive pain center treatment of low back workers' compensation injuries: an industrial medicine clinical outcome follow-up comparison. *Orthop Rev* 18:1115–1126.
40. Waddell G (1987): Clinical assessment of lumbar impairment. *Clin Orthop* 221:110–120.
41. Waddell G (1987): 1987 Volvo award in clinical sciences: a new clinical model for the treatment of low-back pain. *Spine* 12(7):632–644.
42. Webster BS, Snook SH (1989): *The cost of compensable low back pain.* Denver: Work Injury Management/CAIRE.

The Adult Spine: Principles and Practice,
2nd edition, J.W. Frymoyer, Editor-in-Chief.
Lippincott-Raven Publishers, Philadelphia © 1997.

CHAPTER 16

Work Hardening

Leonard N. Matheson

Work hardening is an occupational rehabilitation service that is provided as a secondary treatment intervention to people who are chronically disabled. Its primary purpose is to remediate occupational disability and return the chronically disabled person to work. In order to understand its value, a brief description of the societal and personal contexts of the problem of chronic disability resulting from occupational spinal injury is necessary.

SOCIETAL CONTEXT OF THE PROBLEM

In relation to the incidence of occupational spinal injuries, the prevalence of chronic disability among people who suffer an occupational spinal injury is low. Most people with occupational spinal injuries return to work within several days of the onset of the injury. The Quebec Task Force on Spinal Disorders (56) reported that 88% of all workers with industrial injuries resulting from activity-related spinal disorders returned to work within 3 months and an additional 5% returned to work within the next 3 months. Dixon (14) found that almost 50% of painful industrial injuries improve in a week and approximately 90% resolve within 1 month, regardless of treatment. Andersson, Svensson, and Oden (1) report that more than 70% of those who report back injury with back pain but without leg pain recover within 3 weeks and 90% recover within 6 weeks. However, the small

proportion of individuals who become chronically disabled due to spinal impairment are responsible for a disproportionate amount of the cost. In 1988, low back injuries accounted for 23% of the Workers' Compensation injuries in California and 34% of the cost of Workers' Compensation (6). Across the United States, back injuries account for an average of 21% of compensable work injuries and 33% of the Workers' Compensation expense (48). At Boeing Aircraft Corporation (55), back injuries have been reported to account for 41% of the Workers' Compensation expense.

Numerous studies have reported that approximately 10% to 15% of the people with low back injuries are accountable for 75% to 90% of the costs (26,28,42,54,60). These are the injured workers who are not able to successfully return after the primary treatment and require additional services, including surgery and rehabilitation. In turn, these cases cause occupational spinal injury to be the most costly major category of occupational injury.

The cost of medical care for occupational spinal injury is increasing at a rate that outstrips overall inflation. In 1986, the mean cost for low back pain claims against Liberty Mutual Insurance (60) was $6,807. This increased to $8,321 in 1989. This 22.2% increase exceeds the consumer price index increase over that period of 13.1% and the national weekly wage increase of 9.6% (12).

PERSONAL CONTEXT OF THE PROBLEM

The occupational spinal injury impairment is invisible to others. The pathology that results from an occupa-

L. N. Matheson, Ph.D.: Director, Employment and Rehabilitation Institute of California, Santa Ana, California, 92705.

tional spinal injury cannot be objectively quantified by current imaging techniques (35,39,40). The impairment itself fluctuates in response to involvement with activity, changes in the weather, and short-term effects of medication. Stress may also exacerbate the impairment. Its invisibility, combined with the intransigence of its symptoms in some people, causes it to be less than fully credible to many treaters, family members, and medical care underwriters.

For occupational spinal injury, the relationship between the impairment and the extent of functional limitations often is poor. Two people with similar levels of impairment may have vastly different functional limitations. The differences probably result from differences in pain tolerance and interpretation, fear of re-injury, and motivation, all of which are difficult to quantify given current technology. The inexact nature of the relationship between impairment and functional limitations in occupational spinal injury leads to frustration on the part of the caregiver and causes many to provide less than adequate guidance to the patient. Recommendations such as, "Don't do more than your back will let you" or "Avoid heavy lifting" are frequently provided to occupational spinal injury patients by primary caregivers. These appear to be innocuous and even helpful recommendations. However, the inadvisability of such recommendations is well known to secondary caregivers. When paired with the onerous experience of activity-related pain, such recommendations are adhered to assiduously by occupational spinal injury patients, resulting in conservative activity restrictions which, in and of themselves, are disabling. These restrictions quickly result in real changes in functional capacity, which have been termed the "deconditioning syndrome" (36). This problem is not a direct result of the pathology but an indirect result of the caregiver's attempt to resolve the inexact nature of the relationship between impairment and functional limitations in a manner that protects the patient from further harm. The iatrogenic nature of occupational spinal injury disability has yet to be adequately addressed in occupational spinal injury treatment. In fields such as cardiac rehabilitation, such recommendations are avoided in favor of specific activity recommendations and guidelines (31).

The fiscal costs of chronic spinal occupational disabilities are normally considered in terms of the medical treatment and indemnification for monetary damages (22). These costs are borne by the employer, insurance carrier, or governmental agency. Additional costs are also identified, related to welfare support which is provided by other governmental agencies (23).

In addition, however, substantial costs are borne by the many disabled persons and their families. In most jurisdictions in the United States, Workers' Compensation maintenance benefits are paid at a rate that is equal to two-thirds of the gross earnings of the injured worker up to a maximum that is roughly equivalent to the earnings of unskilled and semi-skilled workers but usually is substantially less than the earnings of skilled workers.

Unless these benefits are part of a wage-replacement program paid while the person is attempting to return to work on a light-duty basis, they are not taxed by the federal government and most other income tax agencies. The two-thirds tax-free ceiling creates a burden for some and a short-lived boon for others. It is unusual to find an individual who has been off of work for 6 months or longer who is not experiencing some important financial consequence. Rarely is the consequence neutral. Whether the income consequence produces an economic boon or an economic burden for the disabled person, it adds to the complexity of the rehabilitation problem and changes its character. The long-term costs are almost universally negative. In one study of occupational outcome after work hardening, only 14% of the returning workers experienced an increase in earnings, usually the result of improved skills (33). Of this sample, 52% experienced a loss of earnings rate that was measurable. Table 1 depicts the combined effects of degree of disability, gender, educational level, occupation, and race on lifetime earning capacity for those people who re-

TABLE 1. *Estimated lifetime loss of earning capacity as a consequence of partial disability due to occupational spinal impairment (All subjects returned to work in new occupations after rehabilitation)*

Factor	Subject A	Subject B	Subject C	Subject D
Age	26	34	38	29
Sex	Male	Female	Male	Female
Race	White	Black	Hispanic	White
Educational level	10 years	12 years	12 years	14 years
Disability rating	30%	50%	60%	30%
Occupation	Carpenter	School clerk	Electrician	Equip. technician
Pre-injury hourly earnings	$20.00	$14.00	$23.00	$16.50
Post-injury hourly earnings	$8.50	$10.00	$12.00	$10.50
Pre-injury annual earnings	$31,000	$29,120	$42,550	$34,320
Post-injury annual earnings	$17,680	$20,800	$24,960	$21,840
Pre-injury work life expectancy	31.34	18.97	23.33	25.11
Post-injury work life expectancy	24.58	12.99	14.86	21.30
Projected loss of lifetime earnings	$537,054	$282,318	$621,761	$396,564

turned to work at new occupations after becoming disabled resulting from occupational spinal injury. These cases from the author's recent practice depict a situation in which disability resulting from occupational spinal injury does not preclude return to work but restricts the level of work to which the person can return. In addition to a decrement in earning capacity, represented by an hourly wage, the disabled person experiences a truncation of expected worklife. These direct economic consequences are separate from and in addition to the ongoing medical care expense. Although figures such as these are very significant, they are rarely reported.

The societal and personal contexts of the problem of chronic disability resulting from occupational spinal injury are important to consider as intervention is attempted. However, the dynamics of the problem are of the greatest import to caregivers. In order to better understand the problem, let us turn now to its description.

DESCRIPTION OF THE PROBLEM

People who are treated in work hardening programs have been unsuccessful in primary treatment and have become chronically disabled. A preponderance of people in work hardening are disabled because of problems with the spine. Figure 1 depicts the make-up of the case load of the author's work hardening program. This represents more than 1,000 consecutive admissions during the late 1980s.

Work hardening is appropriate only for people who are chronically disabled. It is a secondary treatment program that should be used only when a primary treatment program has failed and the client presents certain characteristics that make it unlikely that return to work will be achieved by less comprehensive and expensive means.

There are seven intertwining problems that typically are encountered with people who are candidates for work hardening:

1. Functional deconditioning. If the work hardening client's physical capacity is adequate to the usual and customary job's demands, but the client has become substantially deconditioned as a consequence of avoiding pain-producing activity, a serious transient occupational disability will result (36). If this individual has been referred to work hardening, triage to a less intensive and expensive program is necessary. It is appropriate to attempt to remediate occupational disability for these individuals through the use of an exercise-oriented physical therapy, occupational therapy, or a work conditioning program. Involvement in a work hardening program is not only unnecessarily costly, it will expose the client whose only problem is physical deconditioning to other clients who have more serious impediments to rehabilitation. Although the effect of such exposure has not been studied, it is certainly a concern at the clinical level and, if it is not benign, it is certainly not helpful.

2. Erosion of self-efficacy (SE). The overriding goal of work hardening programs is the development of SE. Chronically disabled people suffer from problems with self-confidence, enthusiasm, and motivation. These problems develop gradually as a consequence of the gradual erosion of the individual's SE. SE is an important cornerstone of healthy adulthood. Bandura (4) points out that SE is based on the person's perception of competence and that these self-perceptions affect psychosocial function. Individuals' perceptions of their abilities affect how they behave, their level of motivation, thought processes, and emotional reactions to challenging circumstances. Christiansen (5) reports that "there is considerable agreement that the single characteristic of

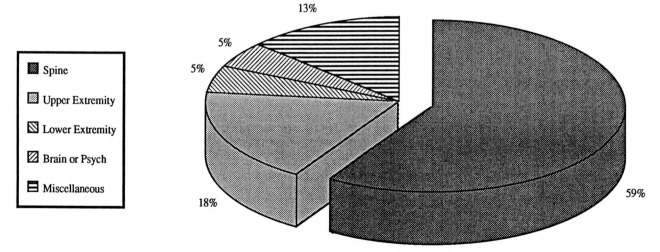

FIG. 1. Predominance of occupational spinal impairment in a work hardening case load at one California rehabilitation center.

the individual which has the greatest influence on performance is one's sense of competence." Whether problems with SE pre-dated the occupational spinal injury that resulted in the disability the client presents to the work hardening program, or whether the problems have arisen since than date, the program must be able to address this issue.

3. Abandonment of the occupational role. The work hardening patient's inadequacy for the demands of work extends beyond a mere mismatch of the individual's physical capacity and the job's physical demands to include the individual's inadequacies in terms of basic work habits and work behaviors. For example, individuals who are admitted to work hardening programs frequently demonstrate problems with attendance and timeliness in the early stages of the program (30). These problems pertain to jobs beyond the individual's pre-injury job or any new alternative job. These problems pertain to any job in any workplace for any employer and are fundamental to the individual's ability to return to the competitive labor market. The person who has been in the patient role for several months is often found to have given up the worker role and its attendant worker traits and behaviors. That is, the behaviors that this person displays are consistent with the patient role and inconsistent with the worker role. This is much more easily seen in a work hardening program when the client is provided with a work simulation task. Decrements in both the quantity and quality of productivity are often found. Problems with timeliness and adherence to a work schedule are also encountered frequently. Less frequent, but more troublesome problems are found with regard to willingness of the work hardening client to accept supervision as he or she would have in the usual and customary job. Objections to supervision are heard such as, "I shouldn't have to do this, I'm not getting paid for it." This is an example of a response to supervision that indicates that the work hardening client is well ensconced in the patient role. If this client is unable to identify the "pay-off" in performing an assigned therapeutic task, it may be that the patient role has become so well developed that return to the worker role is unlikely. For these people, work hardening is focused on returning the occupationally disabled individual to work by resolving problems with vocational feasibility and utilizing the individual's residual functional capacity.

4. Addiction to palliative measures. People who are disabled as a result of chronic spinal pain have been unsuccessful with a treatment program that usually has a substantial palliative component (30,35,36,40). Several strategies have been developed for primary treatment of spinal soft tissue injuries. Historically, treatment involved the use of bed rest, analgesics, muscle relaxants, and palliative physical therapy (65). However, more than 2 days of bed rest has been demonstrated to be counterproductive (13). Upon referral to the work hardening program, these people often report that "My pain won't let me go back to work." Upon inquiry, such beliefs are frequently stated by these patients. In the primary treatment program, pain is a convenient and dependable indicator of treatment effect. It provides direction to the treatment and encourages the patient's compliance with the regimen. If the patient's goal in the primary program is pain relief, exacerbation of pain through physically challenging activities may connote treatment failure. In this sense, the primary treatment program's paradigm may become a problem for a secondary treatment program such as work hardening.

5. Development of psychological disability. Among individuals who suffer from chronic pain, the incidence of major depression ranges from approximately one-third to more than one-half (17,25,27). Polatin, Kinney, Gatchel, Lillo, and Mayer (47) found that 97% of men and women who suffer from chronic low back pain also received a diagnosis of somatoform pain disorder. In addition, 64% fulfilled criteria for major depression, 36% for psychoactive substance use disorders, and 19% for anxiety disorders. All of the somatoform pain disorders were diagnosed after the injury; none were present prior to the injury. Twenty-nine percent of the patients developed depression after the injury with a modest preponderance of these being women. Feuerstein, Papciak, and Hoon (16) report that "many patients with chronic lumbar pain display a set of clinical features including affective pain experience, increased subjective distress, preoccupation with somatic concerns, low self-esteem, and disease conviction." Individuals who are appropriately admitted to work hardening programs after failure in primary treatment or less intensive secondary treatment programs often are psychologically disabled. In most cases, the psychological disability is depression, which has either occurred or is significantly exacerbated by the disabled role that the work hardening client has assumed. In fact, if the work hardening client does not have some problem with depression, a question should be raised concerning his or her adjustment to disability. Although it is certainly reasonable to adjust to a disability and to live life as a disabled person without depression, the individual who is actively involved in a work hardening program should be expected to be somewhat emotionally uncomfortable with his or her circumstance. This discomfort may become part of the motivation to participate, or it may lead to depression that will limit the motivation to participate. That the emotional discomfort also gives rise to depression makes the rehabilitation process more difficult and requires that it be addressed clinically. In the admission screening process, the person with chronic spinal impairment who is so comfortable with his or her circumstance that he or she is unwilling to put up with the discomfort and disruption of participation in the work hardening program, should be given a provisional admission. A 1-week trial in work

hardening for these people often allows the staff to identify the person who has made an adjustment to the disability role that is either permanent or will be so resistant to modification that the program's resources will not be adequate.

6. Development of behavioral disability. Problems with inappropriate behavior among disabled populations have been recognized for many years. Parsons (43) first defined the "sick role" as one that is conferred on the person who is ill and is actively involved in treatment. While the patient is in the sick role, he or she is allowed to temporarily escape from other role responsibilities. Mechanic (37) introduced the concept of "illness behavior" as an idiosyncratic response to symptoms given an individual's unique make-up and personality. This is a category of behaviors that are found by people in the sick role. Mechanic (38) reports that the purpose of illness behavior is "to make an unstable and challenging situation more manageable." Pilowsky (44–46) defines abnormal illness behavior as that which continues to dominate other social roles in spite of information provided to the patient concerning his or her disability indicating that active treatment has concluded and a return to modified or alternative social roles is now appropriate. The behaviors that make up the patient role appear to be learned within the context of a social support system (20). The familial context for such a role has been supported by research by Moss (41) and Rickarby, et al. (51). That such behavior is effective has been reported by Waddell and his colleagues (58,59). Matheson (34) de-

fines "symptom magnification syndrome" as a self-destructive pattern of behavior that is learned and maintained through social reinforcement. This pattern of behavior is composed of reports or displays of symptoms, the effect of which is to control the life circumstances of the sufferer. Behavior that is adaptive for the patient role often is inconsistent with the worker role. The work hardening program provides a transition between these roles to allow the person to abandon one role and resume the other.

7. Mismatch between residual capacity and job demands. Work hardening patients appear to be disproportionately represented in the heavier physical demand categories. Matheson (33) compared the proportion of jobs in the United States work force at each level of physical demand characteristics, with the usual and customary occupations of a sample of work hardening clients. Work hardening clients had jobs that typically were more physically demanding. Figure 2 depicts this relationship. This provides one important impediment to rehabilitation. The work hardening program must offer alternative vocational goals for these people in order to be successful. If the client is unable to participate in a conditioning program to the point that functional improvement occurs, success in the work hardening program is not likely unless an alternative vocational option is available. For some clients, the mismatch between the client's functional resources at entry to the work hardening program and the job's demands is so substantial that, even if the client has the capacity to eventually improve to a level

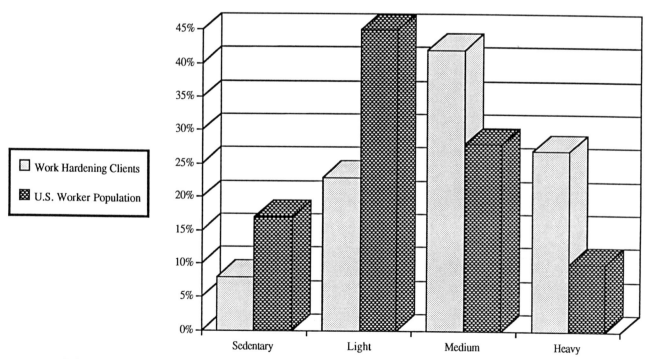

FIG. 2. Comparison of physical demand characteristics levels of jobs in the United States economy and the jobs of clients in one work hardening program.

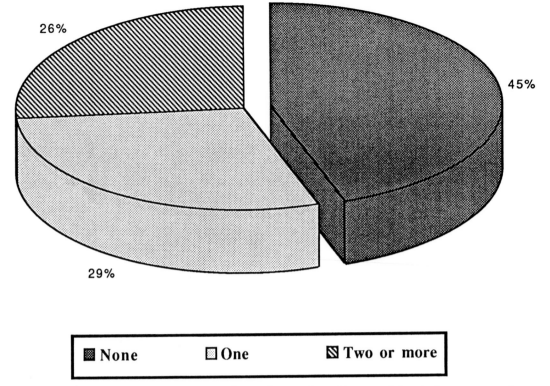

26%

45%

29%

■ **None**   ☐ **One**   ◩ **Two or more**

FIG. 3. Prevalence of prior injury among those clients referred to a work hardening program at one California rehabilitation center more than 1 year post injury.

that would allow return to the job, a more parsimonious approach is often to identify a less physically demanding vocational alternative. This is most often the case with clients whose impairments have recurred, especially if those impairments appear to have job demands as a contributing factor. Figure 3 describes the prevalence of prior injuries among those work hardening clients who have been off work for more than 1 year subsequent to the most recent injury.

The person who is occupationally disabled as a result of chronic spinal impairment presents unique challenges to the rehabilitation community. To the extent that this person is representative of an expensive and difficult-to-treat problem, this challenge offers unique opportunities as well.

HISTORICAL CONTEXT

The origins of work hardening are found in the United States in the early 1900s. Industrial rehabilitation began in response to the large number of World War I disabled veterans. Initially, rehabilitation services were provided within the context of Veterans Administration hospitals and large private medical rehabilitation centers. In 1920, the passage of the United States Vocational Rehabilitation Act provided funds to assist disabled workers to re-

turn to work by retraining the disabled worker "around the disability." Among the earliest efforts were programs in Industrial Therapy, which was defined as "the prescribed use of activities inherent to the hospital operation, planned for the mutual benefit of patient and institution" (53). Patients were assigned to work in keeping with aptitudes, interests, experience, and therapeutic goals (11,66). Treatment in these "curative workshops" was geared to restoration of the impairment. Graded activities, often planned along the lines of the physical demands of the patient's original job, were used to improve function. Therapeutic activities were adapted so that "the muscles he has always used and must use again in his job are brought into play and restored to the patient's functional and economic needs" (21).

In the 1940s, the first "work evaluation" program was established at the Rochester Rehabilitation Center in New York (57). This program was an evaluation center that supplied information for the identification of appropriate vocational goals. Individuals who had gained maximum physical restoration were admitted to the work evaluation program. In this program, clients were presented with a variety of industrial jobs in work conditions that simulated the industrial environment. Over the course of several weeks, clients would learn to work at maximum efficiency to meet industrial standards. Perhaps the best example of an early occupational rehabilitation program can be found in Wegg's (62) description of the work therapy program at the Morrison Center for Rehabilitation in San Francisco:

> This program consists of those activities which are simulations of actual on-the-job conditions which can be used both as an estimate of ability and as an exercise medium to develop work habits, confidence, increase physical and emotional tolerance, improve strength, range of motion, coordination, and dexterity. The familiar working situations promote good physiological effects. The clear treatment objectives provide motivation. The availability of the tools used in his trade allows the injured worker to begin developing the speed and skill he had attained during his employment. The occupational therapist is provided with an opportunity to grade activities as to length of time, resistances used, distances that weights are lifted and carried, positions of work, and so on.

In the late 1950s, there was movement toward using standardized vocational testing procedures, which led to the development of the profession of vocational evaluation. Vocational evaluation was seen as a comprehensive assessment process that used standardized work samples and psychometric tests to evaluate aptitudes, interests, temperaments, and skills. Prevocational programs, such as the Institute for the Crippled and Disabled in New York (52), helped develop a client's work habits, work tolerances, coordination, and productivity to levels acceptable for entry into vocational evaluation. The decision to undergo prevocational evaluation and training, begin vocational evaluation, or go directly into a job training program was made by the rehabilitation team. This team often used information gained from structured "work tests" (61) or from "physical capacity evaluations" (49) developed and administered by occupational therapists.

In 1976, work hardening was introduced as a new occupational rehabilitation program model (30). Developed at Rancho Los Amigos in California, this model utilized functional capacity evaluation to identify the appropriate level of physical challenge to be presented to the injured worker in graded work simulations and structured physical conditioning tasks. The purpose of work hardening was to assist the injured worker to develop the work tolerances, habits, and attitudes that were necessary to return to and remain in the competitive workplace.

In the late 1970s and the early 1980s, the Rancho model was adopted by other centers in California. The need became apparent for the development of standards of care. To this end, the California chapters of the American Occupational Therapy Association (AOTA) and the Vocational Evaluation and Work Adjustment Association convened an interdisciplinary committee to develop standards, which were subsequently published by each organization. Soon thereafter, these joint standards were circulated throughout the United States and Canada.

As the interest in work hardening increased during the 1980s, professional turf battles began to develop. The American Physical Therapy Association (APTA) (3) and the AOTA (10) each developed separate standards for work hardening programs. In addition, several large insurance carriers and state governmental underwriters of work hardening reported difficulties with lack of standardization. In response to this, the Commission on Accreditation of Rehabilitation Facilities (CARF) undertook development of standards. An interdisciplinary committee met in 1987 to draft standards that were subsequently circulated throughout the United States and Canada. Comments were received from more than 1,000 individuals and organizations. Recommendations that had a broad consensus were integrated into the proposed standards. The first CARF standards were implemented on July 1, 1988. These standards (8) included a definition with specific program standards that would need to be met by any program desiring CARF accreditation. Soon after the standards were published, organizations began to request accreditation. The growth in accreditation was more rapid than any experienced by CARF to that point, indicating a significant pent-up demand, as the chart in Figure 4 indicates. Figure 5 depicts variation in accreditation from region to region in the United States, independent of working-age population.

In 1991 and 1994, CARF undertook regular triennial revisions of the standards. In the most recent version, the term work hardening is replaced by Work Specific Industrial Rehabilitation. Nevertheless, the definition provided by CARF (9) is very similar to the two earlier CARF definitions. Work Specific Industrial Rehabilitation Programs are work-related, outcome-oriented, interdisciplinary, and individualized treatment programs that incorporate real or simulated work. These programs usually occur after an acute rehabilitation program, but they may occur without previous involvement in acute rehabilitation programs. The goals of the program include, but are not limited to, restoring physical, behavioral, functional, and vocational skills. These programs may be provided in hospital-based programs, freestanding programs, private or group practices, or in industry (jobsite).

In 1993, the APTA established guidelines for programs in industrial rehabilitation. Work hardening is defined as addressing the needs of patients with "vocational and behavioral dysfunction" and is contrasted with "work conditioning." Isernhagen (24) defines work conditioning as:

> a work-relevant, intensive, goal-oriented treatment program specifically designed to restore an individual's systemic, neuromusculoskeletal function (strength, endurance, movement, flexibility and motor control.) The objective of the work conditioning program is to restore the client's physical health and function so the client can return to work or for the client to become physically reconditioned so vocational rehabilitation services can commence.

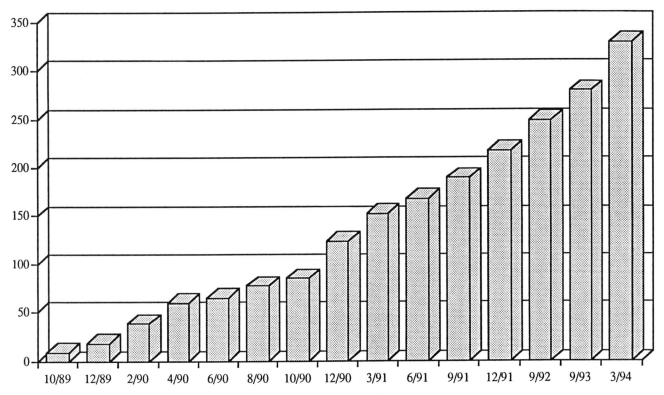

FIG. 4. CARF-accredited work hardening programs. Accreditation growth in terms of total number of programs, 1989 to 1994. Note: Accreditation must be renewed no less often than every 3 years.

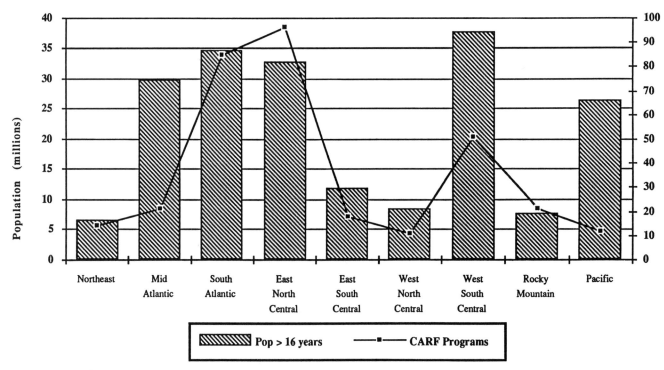

FIG. 5. Comparison of prevalence of CARF-accredited work hardening programs in terms of United States population over 16 years of age.

Work conditioning can be provided by a single discipline, while work hardening requires an interdisciplinary team. Work conditioning involves a combination of conditioning tasks and functional activities that are related to work, while work hardening uses real or simulated work activities to bring about therapeutic effect. Both programs are typically provided in multiple hour sessions beginning at 2 hours per day 5 days per week. Work conditioning sessions increase up to 4 hours per day, while work hardening sessions increase up to 8 hours per day.

The changes with time in the CARF standards as well as the development of other standards by the AOTA and the APTA have resulted in confusion. However, there are certain core attributes that are found in each work hardening program. These attributes are common to all of the standards and have survived from the first standards developed in California in the early 1980s. They include:

1. Work hardening is based on structured therapeutic activities which are available 5 days per week, several hours each day.

2. Work hardening uses work simulation on a graded basis to provide a therapeutic challenge.

3. Space and equipment for work simulation approximates a relevant work environment.

4. Work hardening services are provided by a coordinated interdisciplinary team. Depending on the needs of the client, the team is composed of an occupational therapist, physical therapist, psychologist, and vocational specialist. The interdisciplinary team is central to work hardening. Without the team, work hardening cannot be practiced.

WORK HARDENING STRATEGIES

Work hardening can be a very effective intervention for people who are chronically disabled as a result of occupational spinal injury. Work hardening programs use four strategies to assist the occupational spinal injury disabled person to return to work.

Occupational Role Development

Resumption of the lost occupational role is the primary goal of the work hardening program. The first step in this process is to develop an occupational goal. This strategy is implemented by two therapeutic activities; goal development and work simulation. Each of these is described below:

Goal Development

Goals help to define the individual's personal horizon. The healthy, growing individual sets goals that describe reasonable challenges and reflect his or her self-perceptions, values, and expectations for the future. A goal is a distinct, complete, and clear communication about one issue that makes life more satisfying. Occupational goals are integral to the healthy development of clients in work hardening programs. Unfortunately, work hardening clients either report no goals or describe goals that reflect an emphasis on palliative pain control. Resumption of the lost occupational role is not often a goal that is described by the work hardening client. If it is reported to be a goal, inquiry will reveal that often it is more of a pipe dream, described wistfully as something that cannot be attained but is wished for.

The goal development process is undertaken in a formal manner in some programs (32) and is less formal in other programs. All work hardening programs have a strong focus on occupational goals. Usually, the goal development process has these steps:

1. Listing of all occupationally-relevant goals. This is accomplished in a structured interview. The professional who is conducting the interview asks the client to respond to the questions, What are your goals? What do you want most out of a job? and records the client's responses. The listing process uses the client's words and separates each goal so that it is distinct, clearly stated, and positive.

2. Ranking of goals in terms of priority of importance. The client is assisted to rank each goal in terms of its importance within the context of the other goals. This is often performed from least important to most important.

3. Review of goals with significant others. The work hardening client is encouraged to review the ranked goals with at least one person who is trusted and who will provide honest feedback. Goals can be modified, deleted, or ranked differently during this step.

4. Formalization of the goal document. The ranked list of goals is typed and copied.

5. Distribution of the goal document. Copies of the list are circulated to those people who are important to the client, including the work hardening team members, physician, spouse, family members, and friends.

The goal development process takes place early in the therapeutic relationship. Through this process, the client reveals much of what is important about himself to the caregiver. The caregiver takes the client's goals seriously and respects the client's goals, thus modeling the behavior that the caregiver seeks from the client. The goal development process helps the client to establish a future orientation, develop a rational basis for planning, and receive positive feedback from the community. Perhaps the most significant value of this process to the client is that it assists the client to communicate clearly with the program staff those aspects of life that are important. Given this information, the client and program staff can work with greater coherence to move towards the client's goals.

Work Simulation

Occupational role development requires that the client be placed in a role that simulates the occupational role (30). While it is true that the client is no longer a patient, it is also true that he or she is not yet again a worker. The work hardening program provides the following to simulate work:

1. A relevant work environment. The physical space of the work hardening program is similar to a work environment. Most work hardening programs require large areas in order to provide environments that are relevant to the work environments of most of its clients. An industrial work environment will have concrete floors and will not be air-conditioned, while a clerical work environment will have carpeted floors and will be air-conditioned. The basic equipment relevant to the work environment will be found, including a time clock.

2. Work rules and hours. The hours of work and the rules regarding timeliness, safety, and interpersonal relations are identical to those found in a normal work environment and are integral to the work hardening program. Work hardening usually involves the patient 5 days per week, following a normal work schedule. The following work rules, which are consistent with the expectations of employers in the competitive labor market, must be adhered to:

Safety. Follow rules and instructions, do not exceed work restrictions, use proper body mechanics.

Interpersonal behavior. Accept supervisors' directions, get along with fellow workers.

Workplace tolerance. Start each morning on time. Take only scheduled breaks and return on time. Remain in the workplace for a full work day.

Productivity. Work at the maximum pace that will allow: (a) next day attendance, (b) completion of the scheduled workday, and (c) sustained activity without an unscheduled break from work.

3. Work procedures. In addition to simulating the physical and temporal structure of a work environment, the procedural structure of the program must simulate the work environment. The injured worker's day begins by selecting his time card from the time card rack, punching in on the time clock, and reviewing his clipboard on which his tasks for the work day are listed.

4. Work titles. Work hardening program staff are designated by occupational titles and industrial area designations: the evaluation technician is called the clerical supervisor and the occupational therapy assistant is called the woodshop superintendent. The client is called a client. This seems to be a title with which most people are somewhat uncomfortable, preferring either the safety of the patient designation or the status and independence of the actual work title, such as barber, secretary, or warehouseman.

5. Work tasks. The tasks that are performed by work hardening clients are similar to those performed in a competitive work environment. Task performance is quantified and graded in various manners relevant to the task itself. For example, a manual materials handling task is quantified in terms of the foot-pounds of work performed, while a typing task is quantified by the number of lines typed and the number of errors or corrections.

6. Equipment. Work hardening equipment includes work simulation tasks and the apparatus used for physical conditioning. The basic criteria are that all such equipment be safe, reliable, valid, practical, and useful. In terms of safety, occupational rehabilitation equipment must have a demand that can be measured and controlled by the professional in terms of duration, frequency, and load. The task must be able to be increased along these gradients as the patient demonstrates the ability to tolerate increased load. In terms of reliability, the equipment used in occupational rehabilitation must have a demand that can be replicated, performance that can be measured, and a reasonable expectation that the patient's performance can be replicated. In terms of validity, the equipment must sample critical content of the target job's demands or the demands of a job cluster. The better the sampling of such critical job demands, the higher the validity. In terms of practicality, this equipment must have a daily cost (capital plus staff) that is reasonable.

Wyrick et al. (67) described 192 work hardening and work adjustment programs throughout the United States. Work simulation tasks and other tasks with graded physical demands typically were utilized for therapy. Services were provided by occupational therapists or physical therapists, frequently in combination. To the degree that a work hardening program can simulate a relevant work environment, it will be better able to shape role-relevant behavior and encourage the client to resume behaviors that are appropriate to the worker role.

Self-Efficacy Development

A key aspect of being human is the need to feel competent. White (63) defines competence as "efficacy in meeting environmental demands." Competence is the ability to interact effectively with the environment while maintaining individuality and growth (64). White believed that there is an intrinsic drive in humans to influence the environment that provides motivation for exploring, manipulating, and acting on the environment. He used the term "urge towards competence" to emphasize the basic nature of this drive. Christiansen (5) notes that the development of competence is based on "the experience of occupation or doing . . . by learning skills and strategies necessary for coping with problems and adapting to limitations." The disabled person's perception of functional self-efficacy arises from experience. Christiansen reports that "the extent to which individuals are able to develop a positive sense of self and belief in their autonomy is largely based on their successes in dealing with environmental challenges. . . ." This strategy is implemented by two therapeutic activities: serial functional testing and progressive functional challenge. Each of these is described below.

Serial Functional Testing

Functional evaluation is an important part of the self-efficacy development process. Frequent functional evaluation helps the caregiver to properly pace the level of progressive challenge. In addition, evaluation provides feedback which allows the person's urge towards competence to generate correction. Correction can be suggested or shaped by the therapist who acts as a communicator and an interpreter of feedback and as a guide in the exploration of new alternative forms of responses. Most work hardening programs provide a structured functional capacity evaluation (FCE) of the client as the program gets underway. The initial FCE requires 2 to 6 hours to administer over 1 to 2 days. It begins with a musculoskeletal and/or cardiovascular screening. Subsequently, the client's perceived functional limits are assessed by interview or through the use of a standardized psychometric test. Subsequently, formal testing is undertaken of such factors as standing range of motion, lifting and carrying capacity, and sitting and standing tolerance. The client's symptomatic response to these activities is recorded along with his level of performance. During the course of the work hardening program, certain aspects of the FCE are repeated in order to measure progress.

Once the FCE has provided information concerning the baseline level of the client's function, particular emphasis is placed on those areas in which there is significantly greater functional limitation than should be expected given the diagnosis and impairment. Specific functional exercises are used to remediate difficulties in this specific area and to increase strength, endurance, and other area-specific factors.

Progressive Functional Challenge

Development of self-efficacy requires that the client be willing to face and overcome a meaningful challenge within a controlled clinical environment and have a means to measure his or her performance in response to

this challenge. Subsequently, the performance must be interpreted accurately by the evaluee.

A common method of work hardening involves a work simulation task that presents progressive demands to the client on a graded basis. The starting point and gradient of increase are controlled by the caregiver in order to develop a clear pattern of the relationship between activity and symptom. An excellent example of such a task is a progressive lifting test. The evaluee may begin at 10 pounds of load to perform a lift over a restricted vertical range and gradually increase the load and/or the vertical range and/or the frequency under the caregiver's direction. The purpose of this gradual increase is to not only identify the client's lifting capacity, but to develop a better understanding of the relationship between lifting tasks and the client's symptom response. Experience shows that the symptom response will not be idiosyncratic but will have a specific and dependable pattern. There are many other types of progressive demand tasks that can be used. The selection of the task depends on several factors. Early in the program, the task should relate to a symptom response that is relatively easily identified and controlled. This may not be the most important of the symptoms in a particular situation. However, success in developing negotiation strategies with a simple symptom–activity combination will generalize positively to more complex and difficult symptoms and activities.

Symptom Negotiation Development

Many work hardening clients do not effectively negotiate with their symptoms. Symptoms are perceived to be out of control or minimally controlled by the client. The disabled person's perception of function can be thought of in terms of "work function themes," the rules that guide participation in work activities. These rules are learned throughout life and are constantly modified, based on experience. Information that is gained in unique circumstances is generalized to other circumstances. As a new situation is approached, work function themes guide the client's participation.

The problem encountered by the person who has chronic activity-related pain can be interpreted in terms of the work function themes that have been developed by this person. Take the example of the warehouse person who has many years of experience in lifting and carrying heavy loads. If this person experiences a traumatic and painful low back strain, the experience itself will tend to modify the person's work function themes in a conservative direction. To the degree that the experience was painful, frightening, or generally aversive, the limitation of the work function theme will be irrational given the actual functional demands of the task. The ecological purpose of this limitation is to prevent a re-injury. Unfortunately, because the chronically pain-disabled person has only the aversive experience of the event as a guide, the self-limitation is often more pronounced than is appropriate. In order to develop rational work function themes, the chronically pain-disabled person must perform progressively demanding tasks successfully, experiencing pain that can be maintained within limits that he or she understands do not connote re-injury.

Symptom negotiating training is based on a simple idea: If symptoms can be predicted, they can be managed. In order to achieve this, the caregiver must set up situations in which the symptoms occur on a predictable basis and for which prediction and control of the symptoms can be accomplished by the client. One approach to this problem that has been especially effective in work hardening is to place the client into situations that exacerbate symptoms so that the specific causative factors can be identified. Once identified, strategies can be developed to be used by the client to provide behavioral control of the symptoms. Control will not be absolute but will be incremental. This is termed symptom negotiation and describes an ongoing process that many clients find useful and necessary beyond the work hardening environment. The responsibility for activity-related pain must be accepted by the patient and the pain must be interpreted as an indicator of a circumstance that may, but does not necessarily, limit activity. Behaviors that can be effective in negotiating with symptoms include both proper work pacing and the use of microbreaks and tool or job modification. These are described below.

Work Pacing and Microbreaks

A large majority of clients who are disabled by activity-related pain approach activity as an on-or-off experience. That is, the person works at one pace until he or she is no longer able to work and then stops. The caregiver can work with the client to slow the pace of work or, perhaps more effectively, interrupt the normal pace of work with microbreaks. Microbreaks last 30 to 90 seconds and can be scheduled every 5 to 15 minutes. They are intended to interrupt the flow of the activity in order to allow the person to stretch, change posture, lower the heart rate or cardiovascular work load, or in other ways decrease the immediate demand that the task is placing on the client. A kitchen timer with an alarm can be used to signal the microbreak. A token reinforcement behavior modification system may be useful to encourage the client to utilize the signal and take a microbreak.

Tool or Job Modification

Many clients who are disabled by activity-related pain have not learned the value of working smart rather than working hard. The client continues to perform the task in the same manner that he or she used prior to the injury or illness. While, is some cases, this may have been the most efficient means of performing the task, other means are available that may be nearly as effective or, in some cases, may be more effective. The focus of these means is to allow the client to return to a reasonable level of productivity through the completion of the task in a modified manner. Modification of hand tools, power work tools and stationary equipment, the work station, or the job tasks themselves, can be undertaken by the client with consultation from the caregiver. Modification of the job tasks so that they are within the injured worker's functional limitations is accomplished by both modification of the job tasks and modification of the injured worker's approach to the job tasks. Both job modification and worker training must be undertaken with reference to the injured worker's specific job. This usually begins in a simulated work environment and proceeds to the actual workplace. This often is quite inexpensive and easily accomplished. A survey in California (7) found that 81% of the job modifications that were utilized were either free or cost less than $500.

Additional Work Hardening Tasks

In addition to those tasks and activities designed to bring about the development of the disabled client in the areas described above, work hardening programs involve clients in other specific tasks and activities, the most important of which are described below.

1. Prior to admission to the program, a structured interview is conducted with the client which includes a review of his or her medical status, goals, and reported functional tolerances.

2. Early in the work hardening program, an FCE is performed that assesses the person's ability to participate safely in the program. The initial FCE establishes a benchmark in terms of the person's level of function in response to the expected demands of competitive employment. Subsequent FCE tasks that focus on one or two key functional tolerances are performed to measure progress.

3. As the work hardening program proceeds, it provides the client with education to teach safe job performance and to prevent re-injury. Work hardening clients also receive training in the issues of pathology and impairment concerning their diagnoses. In addition, spinal impaired patients often receive instruction in body mechanics, lifting techniques, and work pacing.

4. In order to prepare the client to return to a previous job, an assessment is made of the specific job requirements through worksite evaluation or job analysis. This information is used to structure the work simulation tasks to increase their validity and utility.

WORK HARDENING PROGRAM SURVEY

In April 1994, a total of 346 work hardening programs were asked to participate in a confidential mail survey, including all of the programs (n = 329) accredited by the CARF at that time. The purpose of the survey was to describe the current state of practice of work hardening in the United States. One of the important issues current in work hardening is the effect of the changes in program ownership on service delivery and program cost. In recent years, a few large multistate corporate health companies have purchased established work hardening programs from private practitioners.

Of the 83 programs that responded to the survey, 40 provided complete and detailed analyses of their operations. Eight of the programs were owned by physicians, twelve by physical therapists, eight by private for-profit health-care corporations, and the balance by community hospitals. Thirty-six of the programs were CARF accredited. In terms of the physical location of each program, eight were located in hospitals, six in medical office buildings, eighteen as stand-alone programs in industrial buildings, and the balance in professional office buildings. Most of the programs provide services 35 or more hours per week on a 5-days-per-week basis. A client's typical day begins at 8:00 A.M. to 8:30 A.M. and continues until 3:30 P.M. to 4:30 P.M. with a 30- to 60-minute break for lunch at midday. Fees range from $128 to $276 per day; the average program fee is $189 per day. The average cost for services ranges from $2,375 to $10,000 per case, with an average of $4,254 per case. Corporate health–owned programs were 40% more expensive than average, while physical therapy–owned programs were approximately 35% less expensive than average. The comparison of total cost to the length of stay is depicted in Figure 6. The corporate health programs have short lengths of stay, while the physician programs are the longest. Physical therapist total costs are the lowest, while physicians' total costs are the highest.

The mix of professionals in each of the work hardening programs seems to vary by the type of owner (hospital, physical therapist, corporate health, or physician). All of the programs use physical therapists, this being the predominant professional in hospital, corporate health, and physical therapist programs. Occupational therapists are involved to a similar degree in the physician programs, somewhat less in both the hospital and corporate health programs, and rarely in the physical therapist programs. Psychologists' involvement is highest in the physician programs, whereas corporate health and hospital programs have lower levels of involvement from psychologists. Vocational specialists' involvement varies significantly, with the hospital and physician programs having significant involvement from these professionals and the physical therapist and corporate health programs having very little. The mix of team members in terms of full-time equivalent workers (FTE) is depicted in Figure 7.

One of the most striking contrasts across categories of program ownership has to do with the employment of

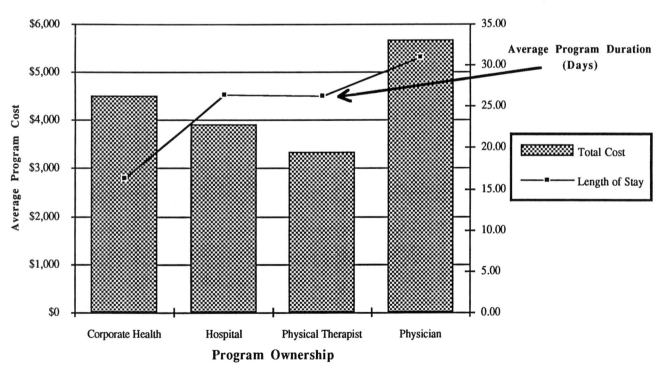

FIG. 6 Relationship between program duration and total program cost, compared across ownership groups.

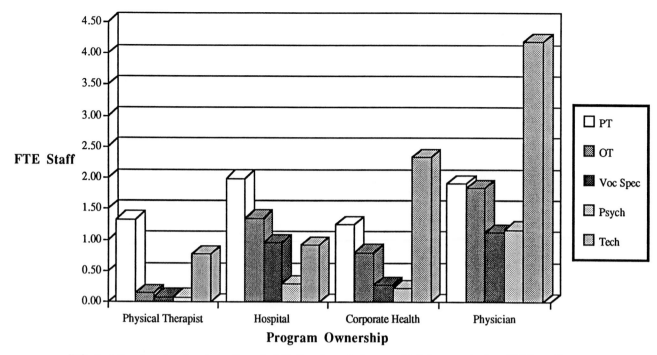

FIG. 7. Mix of professionals on the rehabilitation team in terms of full time equivalent (FTE) staff, compared across ownership groups.

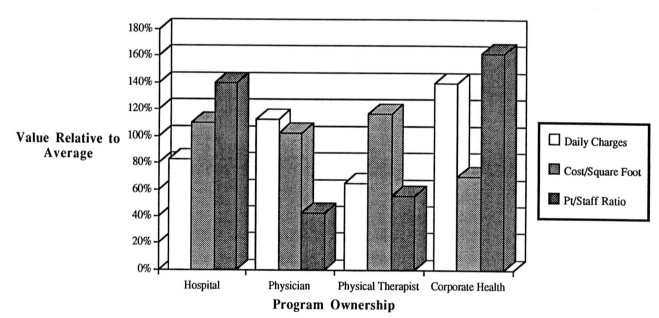

FIG. 8. Comparison of daily charges as a consequence of the two major expense areas, cost of space and the ratio of patients to staff. Each amount is presented in terms of the value relative to the average for that variable. That is, an 80% amount for daily charges is interpreted as 80% of the average daily charge for all programs sampled.

technicians. Physicians use four times as many technicians as either the hospital or physical therapist programs and twice as many as the corporate health programs. These workers do not supplant professionals, however, in that the physician-owned programs have high levels of involvement across all of the professional groups. In general, the physician-owned programs were the most balanced, while physical therapist–owned programs were the least well balanced.

The two most important costs involved with a work hardening program are the cost of space and the employees' salaries and benefits. The cost of space is fixed, whereas the cost of employees is variable above a minimum level, depending on the patient load. An analysis of the reported rent and the patient-to-staff ratio, each relative to the average for all programs, is presented in Figure 8. This describes substantial imbalance across program ownership. The daily charges in the corporate health–owned programs and the physical therapist–owned programs are closely related to the patient-to-staff ratio. Although programs owned by corporate health are the most expensive, they also have the highest patient-to-staff ratios. This is, of course, the opposite of what would be expected if quality of care were driving the daily charges. Both the physical therapist and physician programs offer the best patient-to-staff ratios, with the physical therapists appearing to provide the best value in terms of a comparison of staff availability to daily charges. Costs of space to house the various programs are similar for all but the corporate health program, which is approximately 20% less than each of the other programs.

WORK HARDENING PROGRAM OUTCOME

Although several established work hardening programs have assessed outcome, a uniform system for categorizing clients, services, or outcomes has never been followed. In addition, there are no studies on the efficacy of work hardening that utilize any random sampling or matching procedures. CARF-accredited programs are required to perform frequent program evaluation and should be able to provide the consumer with statistical descriptive information concerning program outcome, although this is, of course, not peer reviewed. Lechner (29) reviewed 12 published studies of work hardening and work conditioning and found that there were few randomized control studies or matched-case studies in which duration of treatment was also controlled and evaluations were conducted by blinded observers. She reports that there is tremendous variability in the research methods of the published studies. That greatly restricts comparison among models. She believes that, although each program reports successful outcome, work hardening program effectiveness has not yet been scientifically documented. This is in part because the difficulty of performing research in a clinical environment is significant. Figure 9 depicts one of the dilemmas that must be addressed if reasonable comparative data are to become available.

In Figure 9, the natural attrition of clients in the author's work hardening program is described. Depending on the point of reference one chooses, very different results will be reported. It is especially important to note

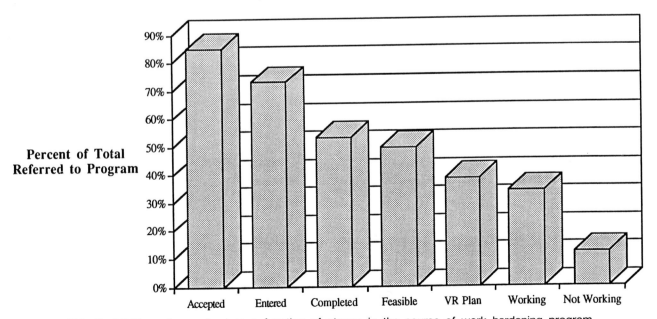

FIG. 9. Attrition of case load as a function of stages in the course of work hardening program involvement.

that slightly more than one-half of the clients who were referred to work hardening actually completed the program. Samples of published outcome reports from well-recognized programs are presented below:

1. The Work Assessment and Rehabilitation Program in Tuscaloosa, Alabama (19) reports that its work hardening program has an "85% rate of success for . . . either returning to the same job or to return to the same industry with restricted physical demands."

2. The Industrial Rehabilitation Program at Massachusetts General Hospital in Boston (18) presents the following outcome data:

Return to work same job, same employer 48%
Return to work different job, same employer 8%
Entry into a vocational training program 4%
Medical management 20%
Awaiting settlement 8%
No information 12%

3. The Work Hardening Program at the Irene Walter Johnson Institute at Washington University (50) reports that 70% of patients who have completed the work hardening program have returned to work.

4. The Work Employment Rehabilitation Center at Loma Linda University (2) reports that of those who have entered the work hardening program, 55% have returned to usual and customary work, modified work, or a new job immediately after discharge. An additional 15% have entered the vocational rehabilitation program to receive training. Twenty-six percent of the patients from the work hardening program returned for medical treatment.

5. The STEPS Rehabilitation Center program at Schwab Memorial Hospital in Chicago (15) reports an 88% return-to-work rate measured 30 days after discharge.

Although these data are not based on randomized control studies and provide no basis for matched comparisons, it is important to note that, in general, work hardening services are provided to people who had been found to be "rehabilitation failures."

SUMMARY

Injured workers who are chronically disabled as a result of occupational spinal injury require a disproportionate amount of health-care resources. Although these people are not working, they are often not so disabled that they cannot work if provided a work-oriented treatment program, such as work hardening.

This chapter has described an approach to treatment of chronically disabled people that can be effective in returning a significant number of them to work. Strategies of rehabilitation are presented that have been demon-

strated to be clinically efficacious. However, the efficacy of work hardening programs is much less evident. While attempts have been made to demonstrate efficacy using comparison group research methods (29,67), neither matched-control group studies nor randomly-selected group studies have been undertaken. Work hardening programs are at risk in this set of circumstances. The risk involves being caught up in wholesale cuts in health-care expenditures because the efficacy and cost-benefit of these programs has not been scientifically demonstrated.

If the anecdotal and descriptive statistical reports have any validity, it appears that work hardening can be useful in assisting one-third to one-half of the people who would otherwise continue to be disabled to return to work. This has important consequences for the successful individual, his or her family and employer, the service underwriter, and the welfare support agency. It is probably these consequences that have caused work hardening to have become a regular component of the strategy for treatment of occupational spinal injury for those people who are chronically disabled.

REFERENCES

1. Andersson GBJ, Svensson H-O, Oden A (1983): The intensity of work recovery in low back pain. *Spine* 8:880–884.
2. Anzai D, Wright M (1989): Freestanding work hardening programs affiliated with a hospital or rehabilitation facility. In: Ogden-Niemeyer L, Jacobs K, eds. *Work hardening: state of the art.* Thorofare, NJ: Slack.
3. APTA (1993): APTA guidelines for programs in industrial rehabiliation. *Phys Ther* 1(3):69–72.
4. Bandura A (1977): Self-efficacy: toward a unifying theory of behavioral change. *Psych Rev* 84:191–215.
5. Christiansen C (1991): Occupational therapy: intervention for life performance. In: Christiansen C, Baum C, eds. *Occupational therapy: overcoming human performance deficits*, chap I. Thorofare, NJ: Slack.
6. Clark WL, Haldeman S, Johnson P, Morris J, Schulenberger C, Trauner D, White A (1988): Back impairment and disability determination. *Spine* 13(3):332–341.
7. Collingnon F (1986): The role of reasonable accommodation in employing disabled persons in private industry. In: Berkowitz M, Hill MA, eds. *Disability and the labor market: economic problems, policies, and programs.* New York: ILR Press, 196–241.
8. Commission on Accreditation of Rehabilitation Facilities (1988): *Guidelines for work hardening programs.* Tucson, AZ: CARF.
9. Commission on Accreditation of Rehabilitation Facilities (1994): *Industrial rehabilitation standards.* Tucson, AZ: CARF.
10. American Occupational Therapy Association. Commission on Practice (1986): Work hardening guidelines. *Am J Occup Ther* 40: 841–843.
11. Cooke D (1937): Industrial therapy as applied in an occupational therapy department. *Occup Ther Rehabil* 6(1):39–42.
12. Department of Commerce Bureau of the Census (1993): *Statistical Abstract of the United States: 1993 (113th ed).* Washington, DC, Table 599, p. 379.
13. Deyo RA, Diehl AK, Rosenthal M (1986): How many days of bed rest for acute low back pain? A randomized clinical trial. *N Engl J Med* 315(17):1064–1070.
14. Dixon A (1973): Progress and problems in back pain research. *Rheum Rehab* 12:165–174.
15. Ellexson M (1989): S.T.E.P.S. Clinic, Schwab Rehabilitation Center. In: Ogden-Niemeyer L, Jacobs K, eds. *Work hardening: state of the art.* Thorofare, NJ: Slack.

16. Feuerstein M, Papciak AS, Hoon PE (1987): Biobehavioral mechanisms of chronic low back pain. *Clin Psych Rev* 7:243–273.

17. Fishbain D, Goldberg M, Meagher R, Steele R, Rosomoff H (1986): Male and female chronic pain patients categorized by DSM-III psychiatric diagnostic criteria. *Pain* 26:181–197.

18. Fortenbach M (1989): The industrial rehabilitation program at the Massachusetts General Hospital. In: Ogden-Niemeyer L, Jacobs K, eds. *Work hardening: state of the art.* Thorofare, NJ: Slack.

19. Fulper KE (1989): Work assessment and rehabilitation program. In: Ogden-Niemeyer L, Jacobs K, eds. *Work hardening: state of the art.* Thorofare, NJ: Slack.

20. Gil KM, Keefe FJ, Crisson JE, Van Dalfsen PJ (1987): Social support and pain behavior. *Pain* 29(2):209–217.

21. Gleave GM (1947): The Delaware curative workshop. *Am J Occup Ther* 1(5):306–307.

22. Hester EJ, Decelles PG, Keepper KL (1989): *A comprehensive analysis of private sector rehabilitation services and outcomes for workers' compensation claimants.* Topeka, KS: The Menninger Foundation.

23. Hester EJ, Decelles PG (1985): *The worker who becomes physically disabled: a handbook of incidence and outcomes.* Topeka, Kansas: The Menninger Foundation.

24. Isernhagen SJ (1991): Physical therapy and occupational rehabilitation. *J Occup Rehabil* 1(1):71–82.

25. Katon W, Egan K, Miller D (1985): Lifetime psychiatric diagnoses and family history. *Am J Psychiatry* 42:1156–1160.

26. Klein BP, Jensen RC, Sanderson LM (1984): Assessment of workers' compensation claims for back strains/sprains. *J Occup Med* 26:443–448.

27. Krishnan K, France R, Pelton S, et al. (1985): Chronic pain and depression. I: Classification of depression in chronic low back pain patients. *Pain* 22:279–287.

28. Leavitt SS, Johnston TL, Beyer RD (1971): The process of recovery: patterns in industrial back injury. Part I: Costs and other quantitative measures of effort. *Ind Med Surg* 40(8):7–14.

29. Lechner DE (1994): Work hardening and work conditioning interventions: Do they affect disability? *Phys Ther* 74(5):471–493.

30. Matheson LN, Ogden LD, Violette K, Schultz K (1985): Work hardening: occupational therapy in industrial rehabilitation. *Am J Occup Ther* 39(5):314–321.

31. Matheson LN, Selvester RH, Rice HE (1975): The interdisciplinary team in cardiac rehabilitation. *Rehabil Lit* 36(12):366–376.

32. Matheson LN (1994): Getting a handle on motivation: Self-efficacy in rehabilitation. In: Isernhagen SJ, ed. *Work injury management: the comprehensive spectrum.* Rockville, MD: Aspen.

33. Matheson LN (1991): *Job matching and vocational rehabilitation options after medical rehabilitation.* Occupational Spinal Disorders Conference: Prevention, Diagnosis & Treatment. Chicago, September.

34. Matheson LN (1991): Symptom magnification syndrome structured interview: rationale and procedure. *J Occ Rehab* 1(1):43–56.

35. Mayer TG, Gatchel RJ, Kishino N, Keeley J, Capra P, Mayer H, Barnett J, Mooney V (1985): Objective assessment of spine function following industrial injury: a prospective study with comparison group and one-year follow-up. *Spine* 10(6):482–493.

36. Mayer TG, Gatchel RJ, Mayer H, Kishino ND, Keeley J, Mooney V (1987): A prospective two-year study of functional restoration in industrial low back injury: an objective assessment procedure. *JAMA* 258(13):1763–1767.

37. Mechanic D (1975): Response factors in illness: the study of illness behavior. *Soc Psychiat* 1:11–20.

38. Mechanic D (1982): The concept of illness behaviour. *J Chron Dis* 15:189–194.

39. Mooney V (1987): Impairment, disability, and handicap. *Clin Orthop* 221:14–25.

40. Mooney V (1991): Surgical decision making: a system based on classification and symptom chronology. In: Mayer TG, Mooney JV, Gatchel R, eds. *Contemporary conservative care for painful spinal disorders.* Philadelphia: Lea & Febiger, 403–432.

41. Moss RA (1986): The role of learning history in current sick-role behavior and assertion. *Behav Res Ther* 24(6):681–683.

42. National Council on Compensation Insurance (1992): *Workers' compensation back claim study.* Boca Raton, FL.

43. Parsons T (1951): *The social system.* New York: Free Press of Glencoe.

44. Pilowsky I (1978): A general classification of abnormal illness behavior. *Br J Med Psych* 51:131–137.

45. Pilowsky I (1969): Abnormal illness behavior. *Br J Med Psych* 2:347–351.

46. Pilowsky I (1987): Abnormal illness behaviour. *Psychiatr Med* 5(2):85–91.

47. Polatin PB, Kinney RK, Gatchel RJ, Lillo E, Mayer TG (1993): Psychiatric illness and chronic low-back pain. The mind and the spine—Which goes first? *Spine* 18(1):66–71.

48. Pope MH, Andersson GBJ, Frymoyer JW, Chaffin DB, eds. (1984): *Occupational low back pain: assessment, treatment and prevention.* St. Louis: Mosby Year Book, 20–43.

49. Reuss EE, Raws DE, Sundquist AF (1958): Development of a physical capacities evaluation. *Am J Occup Ther* 12(1):1–14.

50. Rhomberg S (1989): Irene Walter Johnson Institute of Rehabilitation. In: Ogden-Niemeyer L, Jacobs K, eds. *Work hardening: state of the art.* Thorofare, NJ: Slack.

51. Rickarby G, Blyth D, Bennett DL (1987): Abnormal illness behavior as a required family role. *Psychiatr Med* 5(2):115–122.

52. Rosenberg R, Wellerson T (1960): A structured pre-vocational program. *Am J Occup Ther* 14(2):57–60, 106.

53. Shalik H (1959): *Introduction to industrial therapy.* Veterans Administration, Department of Physical Medicine and Rehabilitation, Washington, DC.

54. Snook SH, Webster BS (1987): The cost of disability. *Clin Orthop* 221:77–84.

55. Spengler DM, Bigos SJ, Martin NA, Zeh J, Fisher L, Nachemson A (1986): Back injuries in industry: a retrospective study. I. Overview and cost analysis. *Spine* 1(3):241–245.

56. Spitzer WO (1987): Quebec Task Force on Spinal Disorders. *Spine* (European ed suppl) 1:12(7S).

57. Stevens AL (1950): Work evaluation in rehabilitation. *Occup Ther Rehabil* 29(3):157–161.

58. Waddell G, Main CJ, Morris EW, Di Paola M, Gray ICM (1984): Chronic low-back pain, psychologic distress, and illness behavior. *Spine* 9(2):209–213.

59. Waddell G, Morris EW, Di Paola M, Bircher M, Finlayson D (1986): A concept of illness tested as an improved basis for surgical decisions in low-back disorders. *Spine* 11(7):712–719.

60. Webster BS, Snook SH (1994): The cost of 1989 Workers' Compensation low back pain claims. *Spine* 19(10):1111–1116.

61. Wegg L (1960): The essentials of work evaluation. *Am J Occup Ther* 14(2):65–69, 79.

62. Wegg L (1957): The role of the occupational therapist in vocational rehabilitation. *Am J Occup Ther* 11(4):252–254.

63. White RW (1959): Motivation reconsidered: the concept of competence. *Psych Rev* 66:197–333.

64. White RW (1971): The urge toward competence. *Am J Occup Ther* 25:271–274.

65. Wiesel SW, Feffer HL, Rothman RH (1984): Industrial low back pain: a prospective evaluation of a standardized diagnostic and treatment protocol. *Spine* 9(2):199–203.

66. Wilson SC (1951): Integration of occupational therapy and vocational rehabilitation. *Am J Occup Ther* 5(5):198–200, 216–217.

67. Wyrick JM, Niemeyer LO, Ellexson M, Jacobs K, Taylor S (1991): Occupational therapy work hardening programs: a demographic study. *Am J Occup Ther* 45:109–112.

The Adult Spine: Principles and Practice,
2nd edition, J.W. Frymoyer, Editor-in-Chief.
Lippincott-Raven Publishers, Philadelphia © 1997.

CHAPTER 17

Multidisciplinary Pain Centers in the Treatment of Chronic Back Pain

Dennis C. Turk and Brett R. Stacey

CHRONIC PAIN—A MULTIDIMENSIONAL PERSPECTIVE

Pain is an almost universal experience, yet there is little consensus how best to define it. Pain is a subjective experience, and there is currently no objective way to determine the extent of pain that an individual is experiencing or should experience. The clinician can only make inferences from the patient's voluntary (e.g., ambulation, facial expression) or involuntary (e.g., autonomic nervous system activity) behavior. A further difficulty is that pain is a symptom associated with many diseases and syndromes and may result from diverse pathology or even from no known pathology. Also, pain behavior is modulated by a range of psychosocial factors, each of which contributes to the interpretation of nociception as pain. Thus, pain is uniquely experienced by each individual. The complexity of pain is especially evident when pain persists over extended periods of time. Psychological, social, and economic factors interact with physical pathology to modulate the individual patient's report of pain and consequent disability.

In this chapter we will first consider those factors that contribute to pain and disability. We will then describe the development and evolution of clinics specifically de-

D. C. Turk, Ph.D.: Professor, Department of Psychiatry, Anesthesiology, and Behavioral Science, University of Pittsburgh School of Medicine, Pain Evaluation and Treatment Institute, Pittsburgh, PA 15213.
B. R. Stacey, M.D.: Assistant Professor, Department of Anesthesiology, University of Pittsburgh School of Medicine, Pittsburgh, PA 15213

signed to treat patients who suffer from chronic and often disabling pain. Next, we will examine the efficacy of these specialty pain treatment facilities, including the criticisms that have been leveled at them. Finally, we will identify unresolved issues and, in particular, what patient, with what set of characteristics is most likely to benefit from what types of treatment delivered in what way.

BIOMEDICAL CONTRIBUTIONS

The biologic model assumes that every pain originates from a specific physical cause. Physicians often spend inordinate time and effort (with the attendant cost) to establish a link between tissue damage and a pain complaint. The expectation is that once the physical cause has been identified, appropriate treatment will be able to eliminate the putative cause of the pain or the pain pathways will be successfully chemically or surgically disrupted.

There are several perplexing features of persistent pain complaints that do not fit neatly within such a biomedical model of an isomorphic association between tissue pathology and symptoms. A particular conundrum is the fact that pain may be reported even in the absence of identified physical pathology. This is particularly true in back pain, where in 80% to 85% of the patients, the cause cannot be given a definitive physical basis (34,174).

Contributing to the failure to identify the etiology of back pain may be the dubious reliability, sensitivity, specificity, and utility of many examinations and laboratory tests commonly used in the diagnosis of back pain (10). Furthermore, the clinical significance of identifiable structural abnormalities has been challenged. Many individuals with no history of back pain have radiographic evidence of degeneration, spondylolysis, lumbar lordosis, or congenital abnormalities; conversely, many people with low back pain show no abnormalities on radiographs and other imaging procedures. For example, many investigators have found on computed axial tomography (CAT) scans (175) and magnetic resonance imagining (MRI) (13) that abnormalities believed to be associated with pain can be identified in a significant number of asymptomatic patients. Moreover, substantial interobserver variability has been documented for various imaging and laboratory tests, including simple lumbar radiographs (35,84).

The sensitivity, specificity, and predictive value of myelography (71,72), plain radiographs (123,148), and MRIs (13,119) in the evaluation of back pain have all been challenged. A recent meta-analysis of studies on the accuracy of CAT, MRI, and myelography in the diagnosis of lumbar spinal canal stenosis concluded that the existing literature was poor in quality. Abnormal findings appeared in 4% to 28% of asymptomatic individuals (80).

In addition, to the questionable sensitivity, specificity, and utility of imaging and other diagnostic procedures, the inter-rater reliability between physicians has been shown to be problematic and may account for some of the inconsistencies in establishing the physical basis for pain reports. The reproducibility of clinical findings even among experienced physicians is low (107), and medical judgment as to organic versus nonorganic pain has only a moderate level of reliability between raters (1,53,107,169,179). This is true even for rating spine motion and muscle strength (1). Agreement between physicians has been shown to be better for items of patient history than for some items of the physical examination (179).

As is frequently the case in medicine, when physical examinations prove inadequate to explain symptoms, psychological etiologies are entertained as alternatives, particularly if the pain reported is disproportionate to objectively determined physical pathology or if the complaint is recalcitrant to "appropriate" treatment. The American Psychiatric Association (3) has created a psychiatric diagnosis, Pain Disorder Associated with Psychological Factors, based on the absence of sufficient (how to determine this is unspecified) physical pathology or other psychiatric disorders in the presence of reports of pain. The psychogenic view is posed as an alternative to a purely physiologic model. If the patient's report of pain occurs in the absence of, or is "disproportionate" to, objective physical pathology, then *ipso facto* the pain reports must have a psychological etiology.

ROLE OF ENVIRONMENTAL CONTINGENCIES

A conceptualization based on principles of learning, most notably operant conditioning, has been forwarded as an alternative to the more traditional somatogenic–psychogenic dichotomy (51). This model proposes that when an individual is exposed to a stimulus that causes tissue damage, the immediate response is reflexive, manifested by withdrawal and attempts to escape from that sensation. This may be accomplished by avoidance of activity believed to cause or exacerbate pain, or by help-seeking behavior to reduce symptoms. These pain behaviors displayed by overt expressions of pain, distress, and suffering such as limping, grimacing, and avoiding physical activities are observable. Such behavior elicits responses from significant others and serves to reinforce positively the pain behaviors and thereby increase the frequency with which they are displayed. Thus, pain behaviors serve a communicative function. From the operant conditioning perspective, it is these pain behaviors that should be the targets of intervention and not the pain per se.

According to the operant conditioning model, positive reinforcement such as attention, accompanied by avoidance of undesirable or feared activities, may serve to maintain the pain behaviors even in the absence of noxious sensory input. In this way, reflexive or respondent behaviors that occur following an acute injury may be maintained by reinforcement contingencies even after any tissue damage has resolved. Thus, pain behaviors are conditioned to occur in response to specific stimuli; pain behaviors and disability are maintained over time through reinforcement contingencies including the removal of aversive conditions such as stressful jobs or family circumstances.

A particularly important feature of conditioning models of pain is avoidance. Fordyce, Shelton, and Dundore (55) hypothesized that avoidance behavior does not necessarily require intermittent sensory stimulation from the site of bodily damage; environmental reinforcement or successful avoidance of aversive social activity can account for protective behaviors including the avoidance of movement. They suggested that protective behaviors can be maintained by *anticipation* of aversive consequences based on prior learning, since nonoccurrence of pain is a powerful reinforcer.

The learning principle of stimulus generalization is also important, as patients may come to avoid more and more activities that they believe are similar to those that previously produced pain. The consequent reduction of activity leads to greater physical deconditioning with the result that lesser activities elicit pain and even greater disability results. Moreover, it is quite probable that the deconditioning resulting from reinforced inactivity can result directly in increased noxious sensory input. Tissues that were involved in the original injury generally heal rapidly, but with underuse of the muscle they may become weakened and subject to noxious stimulation when called into action.

A variety of secondary biomedical features contribute to the pain experience, some of which are under the control of physicians. Several factors that may encourage maladaptive habit formation include advice to rest until recovered, loss of work or delegation of household duties to others, a solicitous and overprotective family that encourages dependence, and the desperate pursuit of further diagnosis and treatment. Consequently, the patient with chronic pain may become increasingly unfit, fearful of activity, and pessimistic about the prospects of pain relief. High fatigue and low stamina from physical deconditioning enhance sensitivity or decrease tolerance to pain, thus initiating a vicious circle of decreasing activity and increasing perception of pain, frustration, and a sense of helplessness and hopelessness.

The hallmark of treatment in the operant conditioning model is change of reinforcement contingencies such that activity and other well behaviors are positively reinforced, while pain behaviors are reduced or eliminated through lack of attention. Medication is prescribed on a round-the-clock basis rather than the customary "as needed," so that pain relief from medication does not serve to reinforce pain behaviors.

From this operant perspective, patients are encouraged to differentiate between hurt and harm. Once the likelihood of exacerbation of injury resulting from exercise is ruled out, patients are encouraged to continue despite pain. Patients are told that hurt does not mean that they are actually harming themselves but rather that the pain is associated with physical deconditioning and will diminish as they increase their muscles' tone, flexibility, and strength. Patients are encouraged to engage in activities according to a preset schedule regardless of pain rather than stopping when pain begins, as the cessation of activity at the onset of pain will only serve to provide positive reinforcement for termination of activity. Many pain clinics have adopted the operant conditioning perspective as an organizing basis for their treatment programs.

ROLE OF PSYCHOLOGICAL FACTORS

For the individual experiencing chronic back pain, there is a continuing quest for relief that often remains elusive and leads to feelings of demoralization and clinically significant depression, compromising all aspects of their lives. Health-care providers share these feelings of frustration as their patients' reports of pain continue despite their best efforts, often in the absence of physical pathology sufficient to account for the pain reported. Complaints of chronic back pain are equally sources of frustration for patients' families, employers, and third-party payers.

Patients with chronic back pain confront not only the stress of pain but also a cascade of ongoing stressors, such as financial and familial events, which compromise all aspects of their functioning. Moreover, the patient experiences "medical limbo," characterized as the presence of a painful condition eluding diagnosis that carries the implication of either psychiatric causation or malingering, or, on the other hand, the possibility exists of an undiagnosed, potentially progressive disabling condition that itself is the source of significant stress and psychological distress. Living with chronic pain tends to deplete one's emotional reserve and requires considerable emotional resilience.

Patients' inactivity leads to preoccupation with the body in pain. These cognitive-attentional changes increase the likelihood of amplifying and distorting pain symptoms. Patients perceive themselves as being disabled. At the same time, out of fear, the pain sufferer limits opportunities to identify activities that build flexibility, endurance, and strength without the risk of pain or injury. Moreover, distorted movements and postures used to avoid pain can cause further pain unrelated to any initial pathology. For example, when an individual limps, protection of muscles on one side of the back may stress the muscles on the other, producing a new painful condition. Thus, avoidance of activity, although it is a seemingly rational way to manage a pain problem, can actually play a significant role in increasing and exacerbating nociception, the chronic pain condition, and disability when maintained for extended periods of time.

Chronic pain sufferers often develop negative expectations about their own ability to exert any control over their pain. The negative expectations lead to feelings of frustration and demoralization when "uncontrollable" pain interferes with participation in recreational, occupational, and social activities. Pain sufferers frequently terminate efforts to develop new strategies to manage pain and instead turn to passive coping strategies such as inactivity, medication, or alcohol to reduce emotional distress and pain. They also absolve themselves of personal responsibility for managing their pain and instead rely on family and health-care providers.

The cognitive activity of back pain patients has been shown to contribute to the exacerbation, attenuation, or maintenance of pain, pain behaviors, affective distress, and dysfunctional adjustment to chronic pain (50,121,159). If psychological factors can influence pain in a maladaptive manner, they can also have a positive effect. Individuals who feel that they have a number of successful methods for coping with pain may suffer less than those who feel helpless and hopeless.

Some of the psychological interventions commonly used in pain clinics have been shown to be effective in helping people with persistent pain either to eliminate their pain, or, if pain cannot be eliminated, to reduce their pain, distress, and suffering. These studies have demonstrated that how patients think about their pain may mediate mechanisms associated with improvement (149). Moreover, it has been demonstrated that patients' interpretation of their ability to control pain may be more closely associated with improvement than either the extent of physical pathology or changes in actual behavior (78). Many pain clinics have incorporated efforts that do deal with patients' thoughts, attitudes, beliefs, and expectations as they may affect their reaction to ongoing pain and treatment failures.

The variability of patient responses to nociceptive stimuli and treatment is more understandable when consideration is given to the fact that pain is a personal experience influenced by attention, meaning of the situation, and prior learning history, as well as physical pathology. Biomedical factors, in the majority of cases, appear to instigate the initial report of pain. Over time, however, psychosocial and behavioral factors may serve to maintain and exacerbate the level of pain, influence adjustment, and prolong disability. It follows that back pain that persists over time should not be viewed as solely physical or solely psychological. Rather, the experience of pain is maintained by an interdependent set of biomedical, psychosocial, and behavioral factors.

In the case of chronic back pain, health-care providers need to consider both the physical basis of pain (the sensory or nociceptive component) and the patient's mood, fears, expectancies, coping resources, and coping efforts. In short, the health-care provider must consider the patient who is reporting pain and not just the physical cause of the symptom. Regardless of whether there is an identifiable physical basis for the reported pain, psychosocial and behavioral factors will interact to influence the nature, severity, and persistence of pain and disability. Given this overview, we can consider the development and evolution of specialty pain clinics.

PAIN CLINICS: HISTORICAL OVERVIEW

After World War II, a number of anesthesiologists developed pain clinics that predominantly involved nerve blocks as the primary model of diagnosis and therapy (126). These clinics rarely involved other medical specialties and did not include other health-care providers such as physical therapists or psychologists. In the 1950s only three multidisciplinary facilities existed (14). John Bonica, an anesthesiologist in Tacoma and later Seattle, Washington, pioneered the pain clinic movement and the scientific study of pain (15).

The poor results from all forms of treatment of chronic back pain patients, including peripheral and epidural nerve blocks, and often multiple neurosurgical and orthopedic surgical interventions, has been a further impetus for the development of pain clinics.

The American Society of Anesthesiologists (ASA) Committee on Pain Therapy conducted a survey and published a directory of pain clinics in 1977 in which 327 pain clinics were listed, with 73% of them located in the United States (90). The following year, the ASA committee identified an additional 100 pain clinics (90). By 1990, Bonica (14) estimated that there were 800 to 1,000 pain clinics in the United States, with another 1,000 pain facilities in some 36 countries world-wide. Also in 1990, the International Association for the Study of Pain (IASP) generated a report that provides criteria for the desirable characteristics of pain treatment facilities (89). Given this rapid proliferation of pain clinics, and the belief by some that these clinics are one of the most important advances in patients care during the past quarter century (104), the question remains, What is a pain clinic?

WHAT IS A PAIN CLINIC?

According to Bonica (14):

Complex pain problems could be more effectively treated by a multidisciplinary team, each member of which would contribute his/her specialized knowledge and skills to the common goal of making a correct diagnosis in developing the most effective therapeutic strategies.

There is no single model for a pain clinic; specific details may vary with the patient population, disciplines involved, general philosophy, and the combinations of therapeutic modalities and technology available. The IASP has detailed four levels of pain programs (Table 1) (89). The most comprehensive type of pain treatment facility is referred to as a Multidisciplinary Pain Center (MPC), which will serve as the focus of this chapter.

Several underlying concepts characterize MPCs. One fundamental concept is the understanding that patients with complex pain problems are best served by a team of specialists with different health-care backgrounds. Another concept is that the complaint of pain is not just the result of body damage but has cognitive, affective, and environmental origins as well. Equally important, MPCs treat not only the experience of pain but also associated patient distress, dysfunction, and disability (90). Implicit is a shift in responsibility from the health professional to the patient. Most MPCs aim to improve patients' physical performance and coping skills, and to transfer the control of pain and management of its related problems back to the individual.

The treatment plan is rehabilitative rather than investigative and curative. Treatments are designed to increase functional ability so that the patient can make further changes in life quality, environmental stressors, and the psychosocial factors such as self-esteem and mood,

TABLE 2. *General goals of multidisciplinary pain centers*

Identification and treatment of unresolved medical problems
Elimination of inappropriate medication
Symptomatic improvement
Restoration of physical functioning
Restoration of social and occupational functioning: social reintegration, return to productive employment
Reduction in use of health-care system
Improvement in coping and psychological functioning— fostering of independence

all of which will assist in pain control and management. Comprehensive care including drug detoxification, behavior modification, functional restoration, and rehabilitation serve as the basis for an integrated treatment plan.

The goals of MPCs are typically designed to be specific, definable, and realistic. As they have evolved, MPC treatments have become performance based, goal directed, and outcome driven. The general goals of MPCs are summarized in Table 2.

To accomplish these goals, the MPC assembles a team to assume responsibility for integrating the medical evidence related to the pain and physical impairment, with information concerning what the patient is doing or failing to do because of the pain, how these behaviors influence the patient's physical capacity, how others respond to the patient, the influence of psychosocial factors that contribute directly and indirectly to patient's physical and emotional status, and the potential for rehabilitation (i.e., degree of disability). The treatment team must build an alliance with the patient to instill motivation for self-management.

A multidisciplinary treatment team ideally consists of a core group of individuals. The general characteristics of these teams are summarized in Table 3. Bonica and Black (15) note that "to achieve maximum results, it is essential that the activities of the members of the clinic be finely coordinated so that the group functions as an efficient team, working on the common goal of making the correct diagnosis and formulating the most effective therapeutic strategy."

TABLE 1. *Classification of pain centers*

Multidisciplinary pain center: an organization of health-care professionals and basic scientists that includes research, teaching, and patient care related to acute and chronic pain. Includes a wide array of health-care professionals including physicians, psychologists, nurses, physical therapists, occupational therapists, and other specialty health-care providers. Multiple therapeutic modalities are available. These centers are usually affiliated with major health science institutions and provide evaluation and treatment.

Multidisciplinary pain clinic: a health-care delivery facility staffed by physicians of different specialties and other health-care providers who specialize in the diagnosis and management of patients with chronic pain. This differs from the multidisciplinary pain center in that it does not include research and teaching activities in its regular programs.

Pain clinic: a health-care facility focusing upon diagnosis and management of patients with chronic pain. A pain clinic may specialize in specific diagnoses or pain related to a specific region of the body such as headaches. This term is not used for a solo practitioner.

Modality-oriented clinic: a health-care facility that offers a specific type of treatment and does not provide comprehensive assessment or management. Examples include nerve block clinics and biofeedback clinics. There is no emphasis on integrated, comprehensive interdisciplinary approach.

Adapted from Loeser (89).

TABLE 3. *General features of multidisciplinary pain treatment teams*

They share a common conceptualization of chronic pain patients;
They synthesize the diverse sets of information based on their own evaluations, as well as those of outside consultants, into a differential diagnosis and treatment plan customized to meet the specific needs of each patient;
They work together to formulate and implement a comprehensive rehabilitation plan based on available data;
They share a common philosophy of disability management;
Perhaps most important, they act as a functional unit whose members are willing to learn from each other and modify, when appropriate, their own opinions based on the combined observations and expertise of the entire group.

Adapted from Turk and Stieg (161).

TABLE 4. *Commonalities of treatment at multidisciplinary pain clinics*

They reconceptualize the patients' pain and associated problems from uncontrollable to manageable.

Overt or covert efforts are made to foster optimism and combat demoralization.

Flexibility is the norm, with attempts to individualize some aspects of treatment to patient needs and unique physical and psychological characteristics.

They emphasize active patient participation and responsibility.

They provide training in the use of specific skills such as exercise, relaxation, and problem solving.

They encourage patient feelings of success, self-control, and self-efficacy.

They encourage patients to attribute success to their own efforts.

The integration of multiple modalities and disciplines for the treatment of pain has probably been the single most important advance in the modern care of the patient who suffers from chronic pain. MPCs were created because it had become evident that no one health-care provider is adequately trained to address the multitude of problems and needs of chronic pain patients. To achieve a successful outcome, the treatment team must be more than a group of individuals from different disciplines, each of whom is seeing the patient. There must be constant communication among team members and mutual reinforcement of the overall goals (161). Team members must reinforce each others' roles and efforts and communicate respect for each others' skills with the patients. They must maintain awareness of what other team members are doing, which will result in a consistent message to patients and their family. Often there is overlap among the professionals' activities. The apparent redundancy allows determination of consistency in patients' responses during evaluation and reinforces central rehabilitation components during treatment.

There is no standard way for treatment at an MPC to be delivered. Each program incorporates a broad range of modalities and is characterized by its idiosyncratic components (158). Some have criticized these programs for the diversity of techniques and strategies used (30); however, the general philosophy described above seems to characterize the majority of these programs (155). This is summarized in Table 4. Since there is wide diversity in treatment delivery, we will provide a general description of the roles of the treatment team but will base our description on the intensive rehabilitation program developed at the Pain Evaluation and Treatment Institute of the University of Pittsburgh Medical Center.

The Intensive Rehabilitation Program is a 3½ week, outpatient day program that is in operation 5 days per week, 9 hours per day. Table 5 contains a typical daily schedule.

Role of Physician

Medical issues including diagnosis and management of anatomic, pathologic, and physiologic processes relevant to the complaint of pain are the primary roles for physicians in MPCs. The physician who actually manages the patient must synthesize, interpret, and translate viewpoints of various medical consultants, monitor all medications and co-morbid medical conditions, and deal with any new symptoms that occur during the course of the treatment. Physical deactivation is almost always a part of the problem confronting the low back pain patient. The physician needs to sanction the physical activation program and endorse the emphasis on patient assumption of responsibility and self-management that will be promulgated by the other members of the treatment team.

Some MPCs also include physicians in the process of patient education. For example, at the Pain Evaluation and Treatment Institute at the University of Pittsburgh Medical Center, physicians lead educational sessions on topics related to basic physiology, the distinction between impairment and disability and cure and rehabilitation, doctor–patient relationships, and the rationale for the interdisciplinary self-management approach (see

TABLE 5. *Schedule for a typical day in the intensive pain rehabilitation program at the Pain Evaluation and Treatment Institute, University of Pittsburgh Medical Center*

8:00 A.M.–9:00 A.M.	Medical rounds and self-directed physical activities.
9:00 A.M.–10:00 A.M.	Physical therapy exercises.
10:00 A.M.–11:00 A.M.	Discussion lead by physician, nurse, PT, OT, or psychologist on topics such as medication, activity, and inactivity, gate control theory, life-style modification, or family involvement. On Monday, a review of weekend activities are conducted.
11:00 A.M.–12:00 noon	Individual treatment with PT or OT.
12:00 noon–12:30 P.M.	Lunch.
12:30 P.M.–1:00 P.M.	Self-directed physical exercises.
1:00 P.M.–2:00 P.M.	PT discussion regarding anatomy, body mechanics, posture, or use of heat and cold, or OT discussion of work-related activities, activities of daily living, or leisure time activities.
2:00 P.M.–3:00 P.M.	PT exercises.
3:00 P.M.–4:00 P.M.	Psychology session covering problem solving, coping, maladaptive attitudes, beliefs, behaviors, or relapse.
4:00 P.M.–5:00 P.M.	Monday through Thursday, pool therapy.

OT, occupational therapist; PT, physical therapist.

Table 3). These education sessions are designed to provide information and to be interactive so that patients become actively engaged in the processes rather than serving as passive recipients of information.

Role of the Nurse

Nurses play an important role in obtaining patients' histories and evaluating lifestyle issues affecting patients. They assist in monitoring and tapering medications. Nurses also provide instruction in medication side effects and interactions and in the use of over-the-counter drugs. They lead educational discussions on healthy lifestyle issues that are affected by chronic pain such as diet, weight, blood pressure, smoking, alcohol use, sexuality, and sleep.

When nerve blocks are used as a treatment modality (discussed below), nurses assist in patient preparation and during the procedure, and they monitor patients during the recovery phase. When patients return home, nurses maintain contact. Faucett (44) has recently described the results of a survey describing the many roles that nurses have assumed at different MPCs.

Role of Physical Therapist

The physical therapist (PT) assesses the patient's current capabilities and establishes treatment goals as well as the specific physical program. A comprehensive musculoskeletal evaluation is performed, including the examination of gait and postural abnormalities, joint range of motion, and neurological tests.

Treatment consists of a combination of instruction and exercises. Instructions focus on information regarding the anatomical and physiological basis of pain and of physical activity, proper body mechanics, the value of active exercise regimens and activity versus passive physical therapy modalities, the nature and role of poor posture and distorted gait on pain, and self-modalities for managing pain at home such as heat, ice massage, assistive devices, and physical distraction.

A carefully tailored program that addresses loss of flexibility, endurance, and strength is an essential part of treatment of patients with chronic pain. Patients are instructed in progressive daily exercises with a focus on stretching, flexibility, range of motion, strength and endurance, and general conditioning. Passive modalities tend to be de-emphasized while techniques that patients can use independently are emphasized. Self-control, self-responsibility, and self-management are emphasized throughout the program.

Role of Occupational Therapist

Occupational therapists (OT) often also play a central role in both assessment and treatment. Evaluations prior to and during treatment focus on body mechanics and energy conservation in activities of daily living, work, and leisure. OTs perform physical capacity evaluations and job assessments.

Like PTs, OTs provide information as well as design and supervise specific exercise programs. In contrast to the PTs, who focus on general conditioning, the OTs gear information and training toward energy conservation and functional activities related to common daily activities and work-related activities including movement patterns and vocational and leisure activities. OTs simulate the functional activities and supervise the progressive increase in the performance of these activities so that patients can return to as normal a level of functioning as possible. OTs often serve as the liaison between employers and injured workers and may develop job modifications that will permit injured workers to return to appropriate jobs.

Role of Psychologist

Psychologists assess psychosocial functioning, personality, social and relationship functioning, mental status, motivation, behavioral activities, past and current substance abuse (drugs and alcohol), response of significant others, patients' beliefs, attitudes, expectancies, and coping resources. The psychologist tries to determine if there are any contraindications to the patients' participating in a rehabilitation program, and to identify areas that need to be considered by the treatment team and possibly targeted in treatment. Structured interviews, self-report assessment instruments, and behavioral observations are all utilized in this assessment (156).

During treatment, psychologists attempt to facilitate a reconceptualization process emphasizing the patients' ability to exert control over their response to pain and even to the severity of the pain they perceive. Psychologists emphasize the role of stress and cognitive appraisals on pain perception and exacerbation. The role of significant others in the maintenance of pain (reinforcement), as well as the impact of the patient's pain on the significant others, is addressed.

Psychologists also deal with dysphoric mood, because 50% of pain clinic patients are depressed (124) or have interpersonal (family) problems. They teach coping skills, problem solving, stress management, and relaxation. They, along with the entire treatment team, focus on helping patients to reconceptualize their problems from hopeless to manageable.

A wide variety of techniques are used including problem solving, communication skills training, relaxation, and pleasant activity planning. Emphasis is usually placed on behavioral rehearsal and homework assignments rather than traditional psychotherapy and insight.

Patients are encouraged to learn new skills, to practice these skills, and to change their beliefs and expectations. Thus, both cognitive and behavioral strategies are used to bring about both cognitive and behavioral changes.

Psychologists frequently make use of cognitive coping skills training including distraction and imagery methods and identification and modification of maladaptive and self-defeating thoughts. Behavioral skills include controlling pain through the activity–rest cycle, setting realistic activity goals, and dealing effectively with spouse and family responses. Patients are encouraged to engage in creative problem solving and to practice new skills when appropriate. Any discussion by patients regarding their pain is discouraged. Self-control is consistently emphasized.

Vocational Specialist

Vocational issues usually loom large for patients with chronic back pain. Vocational counselors and rehabilitation nurses collect relevant data aimed at return to work and interact with third-party payers and claims managers.

TREATMENT APPROACHES

A broad range of treatment modalities are incorporated into MPCs. This makes it difficult to determine the necessary and sufficient components of treatment and to compare the outcomes of different treatment facilities. However, several general features appear to be relatively constant in treatment programs (see Table 4).

MPCs make extensive use of group activities (although not exclusively) to combat isolation and withdrawal and to give pain patients the sense that they are not alone in their difficulties. When modalities are employed, emphasis is usually placed on what patients can take with them when they leave the program, thus increasing independence and self-management skills.

Role of Nerve Blocks

The use of nerve blocks has been one of the mainstays of pain treatment since the earliest establishment of MPCs. Several MPCs have noted that they include nerve blocks as a central component of their treatment (21,23).

Many chronic pain patients respond to a nerve block with a brief diminution in pain intensity. However, pain intensity is only one aspect of the many effects of chronic pain; a more comprehensive outcome needs to be considered to establish the relative effectiveness of any treatment for this population (157). Unfortunately, many studies of nerve blocks and opioid medications (see below) in chronic pain patients report favorable outcome solely in terms of pain intensity, ignoring the other aspects of the patient's pain problem such as physical and psychological functioning. Given the subjective and complex nature of pain with alterations in all levels of patient functioning, treatment must consider functioning and not only symptomatic improvement.

Pain intensity has been shown to be only modestly correlated (r = .3 to .4) with functional measures (96,106,167). In addition to pain intensity, psychological distress, functional ability, activity level, employment status, use of medications, visits to health-care providers, pain behaviors, and cost-effectiveness should be considered, to establish the success of the outcome and the clinical utility of the treatment modality.

The evidence favoring nerve blocks over no treatment is somewhat divided, and the evidence favoring nerve block over other methods of treatment is even more scant. Numerous uncontrolled prospective studies exist, but for almost every "positive" study a "negative" study can be cited (136). Examples include the use of epidural steroids or local anesthesia for back pain (81), trigger point injection for back pain (57), sympathetic blocks for reflex sympathetic dystrophy (170), and facet injections (8) and blocks for herpes zoster and post-herpetic neuralgia (164).

Most of the conditions for which nerve blocks have been used are self-limited, mandating appropriate control groups to assess efficacy. Additionally, all of these chronic pain problems have been demonstrated to improve following a wide variety of alternative treatments including medications (131,172), conservative management (167), physical therapy (127), and chiropractic manipulations (100). Clearly the use of nerve blocks to treat these conditions represents, at best, one of the options for treatment that has not been adequately compared with alternative effective treatments.

Although adverse, immediate outcomes related to needles or the substances injected through them are well documented, and new complications are frequently reported (73), the psychological risk of nerve blocks is not often considered. Psychologists point out that every health-care provider–patient contact teaches the patient something (52). If the goals of rehabilitation include self-management and decreased use of the health-care system, can repeated nerve blocks (or any temporary pain relieving procedure) send a contradictory message (16)? Do some patients develop an unhealthy dependence on these procedures?

The appropriate use of nerve blocks in chronic pain may best be viewed as an adjunct to rehabilitation rather than as an alternative. Nerve blocks may provide some immediate, albeit short-lived, symptomatic relief that may permit the patient to engage in physical therapy exercises and increase ability to benefit from psychological interventions. A limited course of blocks may be helpful in this manner. However, it is important to inform the patients of the purpose of the blocks and to inform them that the relief experienced needs to be related to functional outcomes that will have a longer lasting result if they engage in an active rehabilitation program.

Role of Opioids: An Ongoing Controversy

A common goal of MPCs is elimination or significant reduction of opioid medications. Approximately 85% of patients treated at MPCs are taking medication for their pain; over 50% of patients take opioids at treatment onset (49). One study has reported that 85% of patients treated at the University of Virginia's MPC were taking opioid medication (19). Most studies report significant reductions in opioid use with either no change or significant reductions in pain (49).

Although significant proportions of patients taking opioids prior to treatment are able to terminate use of these drugs following treatment with no increase in pain, there are a minority of individuals who continue to report pain, and some increase their use of opioids after discharge. A critical concern for MPCs is improvement in functioning; symptomatic improvement is of limited value if the patient does not improve function. This issue has generated much controversy in the recent literature (153). A survey of physicians in the United States (154) reveals that the majority of the respondents maintained at least some chronic non-cancer pain patients on opioids for long periods of time.

There have been a number of papers examining the usefulness of opioids for over 750 chronic non-cancer pain patients (153). Although the results have generally been favorable, anywhere from 0% to 66% of patients have been reported to develop significant problems with addiction and side effects. No double-blind randomized control studies have been reported to date. Moreover, there are no data upon which to predict which patients are likely to develop problems when opioids are used (153).

Since pain clinics report the withdrawal of opioids for a large number of patients with few consequences, the potential benefit of symptomatic relief produced by opioids should be considered as an option. Careful monitoring is required. A number of authors have provided guidelines for long-term opioid therapy (153).

ARE MPCS EFFECTIVE?

Many questions have been raised as to the relative efficacy and cost effectiveness of specialty pain treatment facilities since their inception over a quarter of a century ago. A growing number of papers have appeared reviewing this approach in treating patients with persistent pain. A number of qualitative and quantitative reviews have summarized the literature (e.g., 11,48,49,88,163).

Although methodological concerns are always raised and each review calls for more and better research, the accumulated evidence does support the general efficacy of multidisciplinary pain clinics.

The success of MPCs depends on the criteria and on the nature of the patients treated. Some MPCs report success rates as high as 80% (94); others report little benefit for treated compared to untreated patients (140). What accounts for such discrepancies? Types of patients, the method of dealing with patients who do not complete treatment, inclusion-exclusion criteria and, importantly, the criteria for success all contribute to the interpretation of outcomes. Among the most common criteria used to evaluate treatment success are: (a) pain reduction, (b) reduction in addictive medication, (c) health-care utilization, (d) increased activity including return to work, (e) closure of disability claims, and (f) reduction in emotional distress. We will briefly review each of these below.

WHO IS REFERRED TO MPCS?

It is often assumed that patients referred to MPCs are representative of the population of patients with long-standing persistent pain. However, an examination of psychiatric diagnoses shows that up to 90% of patients treated at MPCs have at least one psychiatric diagnosis (86), over 60% have more than one diagnosis (47), and up to 59% have significant personality disorders (47). The differences between patients treated at specialized pain clinics and primary care facilities are especially dramatic. Typically, in MPC populations the prevalence of depression averages about 50% (124). In contrast, in a survey of pain patients treated in a health maintenance organization, Von Korff, Dworkin, LeResche, and Kruger (166) reported that the prevalence of major depression ranged from 6% to 10% depending on the type of pain.

Crook and her colleagues (27–29) studied chronic pain patients referred to MPCs and compared them to persistent pain sufferers in the community who were not referred to specialty pain treatment facilities. The persistent pain sufferers were more likely to:

suffer greater levels of emotional distress,
have work-related injuries,
report greater health-care utilization,
report more constant pain,
indicate more negative attitudes about the future,
be taking opioids,
have had surgery, and
report greater functional impairment.

Neither medical status factors such as duration of pain or pain location, nor socioeconomic and demographic factors significantly discriminated clinic from community pain samples. What most distinguished the patients referred to pain clinics was impairment in functioning and psychosocial difficulties.

When considering the success rates of specialty pain clinic programs, it is important to take into account the fact that the members of the population served have the most recalcitrant problems and are the least likely to benefit from intervention. As such, the population of pain patients referred to and treated at MPCs are at higher risk for failure for any treatment. It is against this backdrop that MPC outcome studies must be assessed.

CRITERIA OF SUCCESS

MPC treatment outcome studies have been criticized for the diversity in outcome measures (30). However, general conclusions can be extrapolated from the different criteria reported.

Pain Reduction

Published studies report reductions in pain from admission to discharge ranging from 14% (105) to over 60% (146) with an approximate average of 20% to 30% (49). Reductions in pain ratings appear to be reasonably well maintained at later re-evaluation or even to continue to decrease (49). It is important to acknowledge, however, that in at least two published studies there was no difference in reduction in pain between treated and untreated groups (33,140), and in a study by Newman et al. (109), 80 weeks following treatment termination, the majority reported that their pain was the same or slightly worse than it had been on admission (14.6% worse). Unfortunately, in this latter study, the authors did not report the actual changes in pain severity and there is no way to determine from patients' retrospective reports whether their pain had changed.

Some degree of relapse in pain severity following treatment has also been reported. For example, pain ratings were found to increase from discharge to follow-up for 14% (91,109) to 38% of patients (132).

Although in their meta-analysis Flor et al. (49) reported that pain reduction was statistically significant for patients treated at MPCs, it is unclear if these reductions are clinically significant. Some have suggested that at least a subset of patients treated at MPCs were dissatisfied with the level of pain reduction achieved (85). Patient satisfaction rather than exclusive reliance on statistical significance should be examined more fully, as dissatisfied patients are likely to seek additional treatments for their pain.

Elimination of Opioid Medication

Based on 65 studies containing over 3,000 patients, Flor et al. (49) determined that prior to treatment at MPCs over 50% of chronic pain patients were taking opioid medication for pain. Results indicate that up to 73% of patients decrease opioid use (91) and more than 65% remain medication free at 1 year (128,146).

Meilman, Skultety, Guck, and Sullivan (101) reported that patients evaluated from 18 months to 10 years following treatment reduced opioid medication significantly from 61% taking opioids at initial assessment to 22% at the long-term re-evaluation. Tollison (144) compared patients treated in a pain clinic with patients not treated because of denial by insurance companies. Sixty-nine percent of the treated patients were taking prescription analgesic medication before treatment compared with only 22% at 1-year follow-up. In contrast, untreated patients showed minimal change in the use of analgesics, reducing from 81% pretreatment to 75% at follow-up. In the Deardorff et al. (33) study, 64% of treated patients were medication free at follow-up compared to no change in medication reported by the untreated group. In general, the decreases in pain medication use have been found to be maintained at the 6- to 12-month follow-up (49).

On the negative side, Parris et al. (113) reported that although over half of patients decreased medication significantly, in 31% there was no change and 16% increased their medication intake. Some relapse was reported by Malec et al. (91), where the percentage of patients taking opioids at discharge was 0%, dropping from 73% pretreatment; however, by 6 months to 3 years, 23% reported using opioids for pain management. Sturgis et al. (140) reported no difference in the numbers of treated and untreated patients taking pain medication 2.5 years after treatment termination.

Interestingly, studies often report that reduction in opioid medication occurs with a concomitant reduction in pain and increased activity (113). These results suggest that the long-term use of opioids for many chronic pain patients treated at MPCs may be unwarranted and unnecessary. Recall, however, that patients referred to MPCs differ significantly from other pain patients. Thus, it is inappropriate to generalize from the results of MPCs to the larger population of patients with chronic pain.

Activity and Return to Work

An important criterion of success is increased activity following treatment, since most chronic pain patients have drastically reduced most physical activity. Peters et al. (116) examined activity levels of patients following treatment. They defined as inactive the patient who continued to receive compensation or was unable to manage at home. Prior to treatment, 78% of the patients were classified as inactive. At the re-evaluation 9 to 18 months following treatment, this number was reduced to 25%. In comparison, 33% of untreated patients were inactive prior to treatment and this number increased to 58% inactive by the time of the follow-up. Thus, not only should increased activity be considered but also the effectiveness of the pain clinic in preventing inactivity. Flor et al. (49) reported the results of a meta-analysis indicating dramatic increases in activity levels for treated versus untreated patients (65% versus 35% improvement for treated compared to untreated patients).

Some have suggested that the most important criterion of success is change in work-functioning. Unlike the other dependent measures, this variable is not susceptible to reporting bias as it can be confirmed by reports form other sources (e.g., insurance adjustors and rehabilitation counselors).

Return-to-work rates range from a low of 15% (17) to a high of 100% (117) with an approximate average of 50% of treated patients returning to employment or vocational rehabilitation (31,49) (Table 6). These outcomes can be compared with the 30% return to work for controls in the meta-analysis reported by Cutler et al. (31). Table 7 summarizes a set of studies that compared return-to-work rates for treated and untreated patients, with an average return to work of 24% for the untreated patients in comparison to 67% for the treated patients. These results are consistent with those reported in the Flor et al. (49) meta-analysis, which reported that patients treated in MPCs were twice as likely to return to work as conventionally treated patients, with 43% more patients working after treatment than before treatment.

The meta-analyses cited above (31,49) found that change in employment status at follow-up was highly significant ($p < .005$) for all groups examined. There was also a highly significant ($p < .001$) difference between those patients who were treated and those patients who were rejected from treatment because of lack of insurance coverage, and between treated patients and patients who dropped out of treatment. Moreover, it appears that the return-to-work rate may increase with longer follow-up (6,146). Fey et al. (45) showed the return-to-work rate to be 61% at the 1-year follow-up and 71% at the 2-year follow-up.

Fishbain et al. (48) have catalogued a range of methodological and logistical problems inherent in efforts to predict return to work. Definition problems such as difficulties in subcategorizing work outcome criteria to reflect full-time and part-time work, vocational training, change in functional job status, as well as movement in and out of the work force, complicate efforts to isolate variables predictive of return to work. Variation in follow-up time intervals and the percentage of respondents participating in follow-up times limits the ability to compare the effectiveness of various treatments.

Return to work is a problematic criterion of success, as a number of factors can influence employment status: local unemployment rates, disability compensation, job satisfaction, and the attitudes of employers towards persons with histories of pain. It becomes difficult to compare studies conducted in different localities and times. In addition, there has to be a job available and an employer who is willing to hire someone with a history of back pain (49). Finally, for managed-care companies, return to work may not be as important as reduction in the utilization of health services.

Utilization of the Health Care System

An important outcome, clearly, is the need to continue utilizing the health-care system for pain management following treatment in an MPC. Reports range from 62% (17) to 90% of the number of such patients who seek no additional treatment for their pain 3 to 12 months following discharge from an MPC (128,146).

Furthermore, low back pain patients in treatment MPCs require far fewer hospitalizations and less surgery. At a 2-year follow-up, Mayer et al. (97) found that pain-related visits for untreated back pain patients were more than twice as frequent (42 of 56 patients, 75%) than for the patients they treated (32 of 97, 33%). The mean total visits for the untreated group was 21 compared to a mean of 2.3 for the treated group, and at the 2-year follow-up, twice as many of the untreated patients (20%) as treated patients (9%) had had additional back surgery. Caudill et al. (22) treated 109 patients enrolled in HMOs in an MPC and reported a 36% reduction of clinic visits in the first year following treatment.

Cassisi et al. (20) reported that at follow-up, low back pain patients who were treated in the MPC underwent surgery far less frequently (3 of 39 patients versus 18 of 39) than untreated groups and had significantly fewer hospitalizations (5 of 39 patients hospitalized versus 25 of 76). Extrapolating from these numbers, 27 fewer surgeries per 100 back pain patients would be expected for patients treated at MPCs. In the experience of Tollison et al. (147), at 18 months following MPC treatment, 19% of the treated (n = 63) and 53% of the untreated (n = 37) patients required additional hospitalization. Additional surgeries were required in 13% of the treated compared to 32% of the untreated patients. In a subsequent study, Tollison (144) compared treated Workers' Compensation patients with low back pain with a group of patients who were denied insurance coverage. At the 1-year follow-up, only 18% of the treated patients required additional hospitalizations; whereas, 55% of the untreated patients were hospitalized. Similar results were reported for hospitalization; following treatment, 11% of patients required additional surgery, whereas 35% of the untreated patients had additional surgeries.

These reductions in health-care utilization for patients treated in MPCs are impressive. Untreated patients appear to be 3 to 6 times more likely to be hospitalized and to have surgery than treated patients.

TABLE 6. *Studies reporting on return to work*

Study (ref.)	Sample size	Follow-up	Patients working, pretreatment/ follow-up	Patients working at follow-up, % of those not working pretreatment
Swanson et al. (141)	21	6 mo	0/17[a]	81%
Anderson et al. (4)	31	6 mo–7 yr	0/23	74%
Gottlieb et al. (59)	72	6 mo	0/59[b]	82%
Ignelzi et al. (74)	142	2 yr	0/38	27%
Seres et al. (129)	71	4.5 yr	0/18	25%
Newman et al. (109)	36[d]	80 weeks	0/12	33%
Wang et al. (171)	407	1–3 yr	70 (17%)[c]/132	32%
Fey et al. (45)	188	2 yr	0/133	71%
Herman, Baptiste (70)	75	6 mo	15 (20%)[c]/36	60%
Malec et al. (91)	32	6 mo–3 yr	0/24[e]	75%
Vasusevan et al. (165)	149	1 yr	0/67	45%
Cairns et al. (17)	200[f]	1 yr	0/67	34%
Catchlove, Cohen (21)	30			
	15[g]	19.9 mo	0/4	27%
	15	9.6 mo	0/10	67%
Chapman et al. (23)	37	21 mo	0/9	24%
Podobnikar, Mackintosh (117)	19	6 mo	0/19	100%
Gottlieb et al. (60)	78	1 yr	0/35	45%
Moore et al. (105)	51	6 mo	12 (24%)[c]/23	59%
Meilman et al. (101)	35	6 mo	6 (17%)[c]/23	79%
Duckro et al. (38)	7	24–42 mo	4 (57%)[c]/5	33%
McArthur et al. (98)	78	1 yr	0/35	45%
Parris et al. (113)	95	3–21 mo	23 (24%)[c]/30	42%
Fredrickson et al. (56)	80	2.5 yr	0/50[h]	63%
Jamison et al. (75)	22	12 mo	0/9	41%
Snow et al. (133)	120	2 yr	0/47	39%
Cassisi et al. (20)	143	22 mo	19 (13%)[c]/92	74%
Cicala, Wright (24)	50	2 mo	0/24	48%
Talo et al. (143)	60	3–40 mo	0/20	33%
Wigley et al. (176)	102	4–5 yr	0/51	50%
Estlander et al. (43)	65	12 mo	35 (54%)[c]/30	86%
Tollison (144)	44	12 mo	0/26	59%
Dionne, Turcotte (37)	106	5 yr	0/75	71%
Altmaier et al. (2)	45	6 mo	0/26	57%
Peters et al. (116)	40	9–18 mo	9 (23%)[c]/23[j]	58%
Dieudonne et al. (36)	109	12 mo	28 (26%)[c]/23	28%
Jarvikoski et al. (77)	309	12 mo	157 (51%)[c]/86	57%
Tollison (145)	61	6 mo	0/31	60%
Total	3210	—	378 (12%)/1433	51%

[a] Five employed full time, 12 "had a gradual increase in work activity."

[b] Employed or in vocational training.

[c] Percentage of patients working at pretreatment.

[d] Return to work was not a goal for all patients, but the number is not specified.

[e] Employed or running a household.

[f] Inpatients (100) and outpatients (100).

[g] First 15 patients were given no explicit instructions regarding return to work; second set of 15 patients were given explicit instructions regarding expectations for return work.

[h] Working includes 54% employed and 9% involved in full-time schooling.

[i] This figure is based on a definition of employed as "fully employed at the same job." If a more liberal criterion is used (patient ". . . had returned to work part-time, was working full-time or part-time at the same job or at a lower level or was actively involved in training for a different job") then 81% (n = 36) of the treated patients would be identified as employed.

[j] Includes ability to manage at home.

Closure of Open Disability Claims

In addition to return to work, third-party payers often view success of treatment as enabling them to close disability cases. Several studies have reported on their success in allowing disability claims to be settled and cases to be closed following treatment. Painter, Seres, and Newman (112), at a follow-up of 2 years, on average, noted that 45% of treated patients were receiving compensation compared to 70% receiving compensation

TABLE 7. *Studies comparing employment following treatment for treated and untreated[a] groups*

Study (ref.)	Sample size (treated/untreated[a])	Follow-up period	Treated/untreated number working posttreatment (percent)
Roberts, Reinhardt (122)	26/20	1–8 yr	20 (77%)/1 (5%)
Sturgis et al. (140)	14/14	2.5 yr	4 (29%)/2 (14%)
Guck et al. (63)	20/20	1–5 yr	15 (75%)/5 (25%)
Finlayson et al. (46)	34/16	1 yr	22 (65%)/7 (44%)
Duckro et al. (38)	7/9	24–43 mo	5 (71%)/3 (33%)
Mayer et al. (97)	103/61	2 yr	90 (87%)/25 (41%)
Tollison et al. (147)	63/37	18 mo	35 (56%)/10 (27%)
Hazard et al. (69)	59/17	1 yr	48 (81%)/5 (29%)
Deardorff et al. (33)	25/7	10 mo	12[b] (48%)/0
Tollison (144)	44/20	12 mo	26 (57%)/4 (20%)
Peters et al. (116)	40/12	9–18 mo	15 (38%)/1[c] (8%)
Total number	435/259	—	292/63
Total percent	67%/24%		

[a] Untreated includes those denied treatment by third-party payer and those who dropped out of treatment prematurely.
[b] An additional 7 were involved in vocational rehabilitation.
[c] Does not include "home managers": 8 in the treated group, 4 in the untreated group.

prior to treatment. Fey et al. (45) reported that at the 24- to 36-month follow-up, 89% of Workers' Compensation cases were closed. Mayer et al. (94,95) reported that 86% of treated patients with Workers' Compensation had resolved litigation by the 1-year follow-up in contrast to 68% resolved litigations for the comparison group. Seres and Newman (128) noted that claims closure was recommended in 75% of chronic low back pain patients by 3 months postdischarge.

The results of reduction in disability compensation following MPC treatment can be contrasted with a study reported by White (173) of patients receiving compensation for their backs, where only 39% returned to work 4 years after surgery. The general experience has been that less than 50% of people who are disabled from work by their pain longer than 6 months ever return to work, and reemployment is almost nonexistent 2 years after work-related disability (99,167).

COST EFFECTIVENESS

An important criterion for success of MPCs is cost effectiveness. In our examination of cost effectiveness below, we have to make certain assumptions about the cost of disability, treatment costs, general inflation, and inflation in medical expenses. We will extrapolate treatment outcomes from the meta-analysis by Flor et al. (49).

The impressive reductions in health-care utilization reviewed above can be readily translated into monetary terms. For example, Simmons, Avant, Demski, and Parisher (130) reported a 58% reduction of medical costs as a result of treatment in an MPC. They noted that the costs for medical treatment of their patients in the year prior to treatment averaged $13,284 and in the year after

MPC treatment averaged $5,596, a total savings of $123,000 in medical costs for 16 patients.

If we extrapolate the savings reported by Simmons et al. (130) to the 2,318 patients successfully treated in MPCs reported in the meta-analysis (49), and correct for inflation of 3% per year, a savings of $20 million in medical expenses would accrue in the first year following treatment. If we assume the average cost for pain clinic treatment in 1988 was approximately $5,000 (the cost for treatment at the Pain Evaluation and Treatment Institute at the University of Pittsburgh), treating the entire MPC cohort of 3,089 (49), would cost approximately $15.6 million (again correcting for inflation), resulting in a net saving in medical expenses alone during the first year of $4.4 million. Although at first glance they appear rather modest, these savings are (a) only for the first year medical expenses and (b) in addition to savings in reduced disability payments, gains in productivity, and gains in revenue from taxes paid by the successfully treated patients.

The expense of long-term disability payments is estimated at $300,000 for Social Security and more than $600,000 for private disability insurance over a lifetime for an individual who becomes disabled at age 45. These costs, combined with loss of productivity and health-care costs, make treatment costs at MPCs seem reasonable (94,95). Flor et al. (49) reported that over 50% of patients treated in pain clinics were receiving some form of disability compensation. Extrapolating from data on return to work cited above, with approximately 50% of those treated returning to work following treatment, and assuming their disability cases are closed, then 744 patients will have their disability cases closed. This would result in savings in indemnity cost of over $223 million.

Steig and Williams' (139) analysis also argues for cost effectiveness. Although not all will agree with their assumptions, the cost for each compensation-covered man with a back injury on the job who was lost to permanent disability was an impressive $250,000. Moore et al. (105) reported that 25% of treated patients returned to full-time employment. A 46-year-old removed from the disability or compensation rolls on which he or she might otherwise be expected to remain for the next 19 years would save society in excess of $400,000 ($520,000 in 1994 dollars). Again, extrapolating from Flor et al. (49), an average saving of $520,000 × 774 (successfully treated patients) = $482,480,000. Subtract the cost of treatment [$6,200 (MPC charge corrected for inflation) × 3,089 (treated patients) = $19,151,800], and the total savings are well over $463 million.

It is important to underscore that in the past, patients who have been referred to MPCs consisted of those who did not respond to conservative treatment measures and surgical interventions. Thus, the easiest problems had already been solved. Those who are referred have the most refractory problems. In addition to the pain syndrome, these patients have concomitant medication dependency problems, emotional disturbance, and general life disruptions. Moreover, the mean duration of pain in pain clinics is over 7 years (49). McGill (99) found 25 years ago that a lengthy period of disability predicted a low chance of ever returning to work. Those out of work more than 6 months had a 50% probability of returning, those idled by disability for more than 1 year had only a 25% chance of returning, and those out of work for longer than 2 years were extremely unlikely to return.

The Flor et al. data suggest (49) that a significant number do return to work following treatment (43%). Long-term follow-up reveals that 56% of patients are doing better following treatment, and patients treated in pain clinics are functioning better than 75% of a sample that either is untreated or has been treated by conventional approaches (49). Flor et al. (49) concluded that "overall, . . . multidisciplinary pain clinics are efficacious. Even at long-term follow-up, patients who are treated in such a setting are functioning better than 75% of a sample that is either untreated or that has been treated by conventional, unimodal treatment approaches. In this light, the success rate is actually quite impressive."

Some have suggested that there is no reliable systematic research that convincingly demonstrates the effectiveness of MPCs (30); the data presented above belie this concern. The question is how to reconcile the positive results, which may be better than surgery in these disabled patients, with rather recent criticism of pain clinics by third-party payers and others (24,69,85,108). Historically, MPCs have been viewed as unresponsive to the needs of third-party payers. This is hard to justify, as even in the earliest studies reviewed above, return to work, health-care utilization, and settlement of disability claims were viewed as important outcomes.

The studies that have been published have been criticized because although there are a large number of MPCs in general, there have been few randomized controlled trials published from only a small number of MPCs, there has been a lack of standardization of treatments provided, patients are highly selected, and there is no agreement as to the most appropriate criteria of success. These criticisms deserve to be examined with care.

CRITICISMS OF RESEARCH

Attention has been drawn to a number of commonly occurring methodological problems in the MPC treatment outcome studies—the failure to use random assignment, high rates of attrition at follow-up, inadequate outcome measures, and outcomes evaluated by those providing the treatment—that may bias the results (48,110,158).

There are currently no validated criteria for evaluating pain clinics. The Commission of the Accreditation of Rehabilitation Facilities (CARF) and the American Pain Society have generated some guidelines largely related to the qualifications of the professional staff and record keeping, but at this point it is difficult to compare the treatments actually delivered.

The use of patients who are refused insurance coverage as an appropriate control for these programs has been criticized (160). None of the studies cited elaborate on the predicament of the patients, nor do they analyze the effects of being refused insurance assistance and the possible socioenvironmental consequences of such refusals. It seems reasonable to suppose that the patients might accumulate a wealth of anger and frustration as they find themselves locked into a disability role by financial constraints. Future studies need to compare different active treatments and to use random assignments of patients.

Cost is a major concern in health care, and the costs of MPCs have been challenged by many third-party payers. There is little information regarding the cost of MPC treatment compared to other commonly accepted treatments such as surgery. However, the savings in medical costs following treatment in MPCs cited above suggest that these programs are quite successful.

Another criticism raised about the efficacy of MPCs is relapse (158). Relapse (recidivism) rates over 1 to 2 years appear, however, to be surprisingly low, usually less than 10% (20,63,97,146), with the few longer follow-up studies supporting maintenance of gains from 2 to 8 years following treatment termination (46,56,98,133). However, at least one study reported relapse in 46.6% of successfully treated patients (92) and 33% of all patients who completed treatment at the 3-year follow-up. This raises another common concern, namely the number of patients available at follow-up. Turk and Rudy (158) note that it is not unusual for 50% or less of treated patients to be included in long-term follow-ups. In light of the relatively low percent of patients available at follow-up, the MPC treatment outcome results have to be interpreted with some caution.

Many treatments that have long been accepted as standard have never been proven efficacious. For example, the prescriptions for muscle relaxants or surgery for low back pain have never been subjected to well-designed random allocation, controlled studies, yet pain management programs are said not to have demonstrated their efficacy because of the lack of studies (90). To illustrate, Benzon (9) reviewed the use of epidural steroid injections for low back pain. He found five controlled studies of which three showed an advantage of epidural steroid over saline or local anesthetic. Outcome, however was reported purely in terms of subjective pain relief, with no attention to activity, medication use, or social/vocational rehabilitation.

The same concerns about MPC studies can be applied to more accepted treatments for back pain such as the host of surgical procedures currently performed. Millions of patients have undergone lumbar spine surgery, with over 200,000 procedures performed each year in the United States (178). Surgery is an alternative treatment for only a small subset of chronic low back pain patients, and even with liberal success criteria, only 30% to 40% of surgical interventions for chronic back pain are considered successful (42,168). Dvorak, Gauchat, and Valach (39) found in a 4- to 17-year surveillance of 575 patients operated on for lumbar disc herniation that 70% still complained of back pain. Carlson and Pellettieri (18) reported that at 8 to 24 months following spinal surgery, 31% of patients judged themselves to be worse than the ratings given by their surgeons. As many as 40%, however, fail to experience satisfactory long-term relief of symptoms after primary procedures (178). This figure rises to 66% after repeated procedures for failed back surgery syndrome (110). Steele-Rosomoff et al. (138) demonstrated that even failed back syndrome patients with three and more surgeries could be successfully treated in pain clinics.

In a retrospective study, North and colleagues (110) reported that at the 5-year follow-up, repeated surgery for low back pain was judged to be successful based on the criteria of at least 50% sustained pain relief and patient satisfaction in only about one-third of the cases. They noted that in the majority of cases, standard decompression and fusion procedures were not successful and "many patients experienced worsening in spite of or because of surgery." They reported that only 21% of those who were disabled or unemployed immediately prior to surgery returned to full-time work postoperatively, and of 38 patients working full-time before surgery, 14 retired prematurely (before age 60) or became disabled because of their low back condition during the 5-year mean follow-up period. Thus, the net gain in employment status was only 7% (7 patients of the 102 included in the study).

North et al. (110) reported that 23% of the back surgery patients underwent additional lumbosacral spine surgeries during the period of surveillance. In general, most patients studied reported no change in their abilities to work or engage in functional activities such as walking, going up stairs, sleeping, or driving, although there was some reduction in analgesic intake; neurological function, including strength, sensation, and bowel and bladder control, subjectively worsened more than it improved. The authors conclude that "most patients reported no change in their abilities to perform most activities. Overall, reported changes were as often favorable as they were unfavorable."

North, Ewend, Lawton, Kidd, and Piantadosi (111) reported a 5-year follow-up of patients who had spinal cord stimulators implanted. They noted that at follow-up, 47% of the patients were viewed as successes, determined by at least a 50% reduction in pain reported on a visual analog scale and patient satisfaction. In addition, the authors reported that the majority of patients reported significant gains in functional ability such as their ability to sit or walk up steps. Reduction or elimination of opioid medication was reported in over 75% of the patients. However, only 25% of patients returned to work following the implantation procedure. These results can be compared with MPC data where on all criteria of success they appear to be equal to or superior to surgery.

It is important to note that the patients in the North et al. (111) study had to have a demonstrated "objective" basis for their complaint of pain. Moreover, patients with behavior or drug habituation problems or with significant issues of secondary pain either were treated first in a behavioral program or were excluded. The authors do not indicate how many patients were excluded for each of these reasons.

Loeser (90) poses a challenge. Since there are virtually no data on other methods of treating chronic low back pain, one could suggest that proponents of any other form of treatment be asked to demonstrate its superiority to MPCs before it is utilized in uncontrolled clinical trials.

WHO IS TREATED AT MPCS: SELECTION AND SCREENING

Given the overall positive results, we should consider the characteristics of patients actually treated at MPCs, because as noted earlier, those patients who are referred to MPCs differ significantly from the general population of chronic pain sufferers, and of the referred, not all are accepted for treatment. From 15% (120) to 54% (4) of patients evaluated at pain clinics are denied treatment. Pain treatment programs use a wide variety of exclusion criteria to screen out patients who are unlikely to benefit from treatment. Exclusion criteria can be viewed as falling within seven domains: (a) medical status, (b) demographics, (c) psychopathology, (d) medicolegal, (e) motivation, (f) conceptual, and (g) financial (158).

The rationale for excluding patients is simple: screening out patients who appear unlikely to benefit from treatment is ethical, avoids frustrating the treatment staff, and is more cost efficient. However, the available research does not support the use of rigid selection criteria. For example, some programs exclude patients who show evidence of underlying tissue pathology that might be responsible for their pain (54), whereas other programs accept only patients who have documented tissue pathology (61). We will consider some of the common criteria used in deciding whether patients should be offered treatment at an MPC.

Duration of Pain

Several studies (45,79,141) have found that patients with relatively longer histories of pain respond poorly. For example, Maruta et al. (93) reported that unsuccessful patients had longer pain duration, more time off work, more prior surgical procedures related to pain, and higher levels of pain, and they were more dependent on medication. No differences were noted in regard to age, sex, or marital status. In contrast, Aronoff and Evans (5) found no significant differences between successful and unsuccessful patients at time of discharge when using the factors discussed by Maruta et al. (93). Other studies found that patients with long histories of pain had as good or even better outcomes (12,112). Thus, longer duration of pain does not appear to be an impediment to successful treatment.

Age

The effect of age on treatment outcome has been shown to make a difference in some studies (5,63, 79,125), with patients over age 50 less likely to return to work (56) and more likely to relapse (112). However, others studies have found age unrelated to outcome (32,64,105,120). As was the case for duration of pain, age does not appear to be an appropriate criterion for exclusion from treatment. Interestingly, however, it has been noted that older patients are underrepresented at MPCs (102,135).

Psychological Factors and Psychopathology

It has been suggested that optimal prediction of treatment response in chronic pain may be achieved by dividing patients into groups based on psychological characteristics. The support for the accuracy of psychological

factors to predict treatment success, however, is tenuous. In some studies depression is related to unsuccessful treatment outcome (41,118). Others have reported that the psychiatric diagnosis did not interfere with successful rehabilitation (58). Moreover, Painter et al. (112) found that those patients who were more depressed at pretreatment actually had higher success rates than those who were less depressed.

Dworkin et al. (41) studied treatment responses in groups of chronic pain patients who were and were not depressed. In the latter, beneficial response to treatment was related to number of treatment visits, not receiving Workers' Compensation, and fewer previous types of treatment. Patients with chronic pain and depression were more likely to benefit when they were employed at the beginning of the treatment and their pain was of shorter duration.

A number of studies have tried to use patients' responses on the Minnesota Multiphasic Personality Inventory (MMPI) to predict treatment success (93,122). Elevations on the MMPI indicating the presence of emotional problems, however, have not been shown to be consistently predictive of poor pain clinic treatment outcome (65,79,93,101,112,151). In fact, one study (83) reported that patients with elevations on MMPI Depression and Hysteria scales actually showed the greatest improvement with regard to pain and mood. King and Snow (82) similarly reported that patients with higher levels of psychological distress were the most likely to complete treatment, whereas those with lower degrees of psychological distress were the most likely to drop out of treatment prematurely. These results suggest that making treatment decisions based exclusively on psychological problems or psychiatric diagnosis may be unwarranted.

Disability Status

It has been suggested that because patients' income (e.g., Workers' Compensation benefits) may be contingent on reports of pain, compensation serves as a disincentive for successful pain treatment. Consequently, patients receiving compensation might be viewed as poorer risks for pain rehabilitation (62) and more likely to drop out of treatment (66,94). Therefore, it has been suggested that those patients receiving disability compensation are poor candidates for rehabilitation and should be excluded from treatment. In the Flor et al. (49) meta-analysis, 52% of patients treated at MPCs were receiving some form of disability compensation. Using disability status as an exclusion criterion would lead to rejection of an extremely large number of patients from treatment.

The effects of compensation on outcome, however, are not clear cut. Some studies have found little relationship between disability status and outcome (5,40,93,103,

112–114,143,150). Moreover, Barnes, Smith, Gatchel, and Mayer (7) reported that patients who were receiving the highest amount of compensation were the **most** likely to be successful in their rehabilitation programs.

Dworkin et al. (40) noted that in their examination of the relationships among compensation, litigation, employment, and short-term and long-term treatment response in 454 chronic pain patients, compensation benefits and unemployment status both predicted poor outcome. However, when employment and compensation were jointly used to predict outcome, only employment was a significant predictor of outcome. Those patients employed at the time of their initial evaluation had a better treatment response than those who were not. These studies suggest that there is only a weak association between treatment response and compensation and litigation. Thus, the suspicion with which litigating patients are often greeted may be unfounded.

Even those studies that report disability associated with poorer outcome report that a significant proportion of patients receiving compensation did respond to treatment at pain clinics. For example, Keefe et al. (79) found that proportionally more patients in a poor outcome group (45%) were receiving disability payments than were patients in the best outcome (23%). Although these results were statistically significant, it should be kept in mind that over 50% of the patients receiving disability had good outcomes and 25% of those without disability payments did poorly.

Litigation

Flor et al. (49) report that 21% of the over 3,000 patients included in their meta-analysis had litigation pending. Pending litigation has also been used as a criterion for exclusion, yet patients with pending litigation have shown improvements in physical functioning and subjective pain scores equal to patients not in litigation (5,112).

Solomon and Tunks (134) reported no significant differences in the amount of medication used, number of hours spent resting per day, or the number of individuals who returned to work, between litigant and nonlitigant patients. Trief and Stein (151) studied low back patients with litigation outcome and found that immediate beneficial effects of treatment in an MPC were significantly less for the group with pending litigation. Both groups improved from the treatment; however, the no-litigation group improved at a relatively faster rate and the improvement level remained stable up to the 3-month follow-up. Thus, they do not recommend withholding treatment until litigation is resolved.

There may be some interaction between type of compensation and litigation. Chapman et al. (181) and

Mayer et al. (94) reported that those receiving permanent disability compensation had much lower return-to-work rates as compared with those with pending litigation or time-limited compensation. Nonetheless, we feel excluding any patients solely on the basis of disability status or litigation may be inappropriate (5,23,150,151).

As has been noted, results regarding predictors of successful outcome are unclear. At the present time there are no criteria that consistently predict response to treatment at MPCs. A possible explanation for the current state of affairs is the tendency to treat all chronic pain patients as a homogeneous group. It has been suggested that there are subgroups of patients even with the same medical diagnoses and that treatment should be customized to unique subgroup characteristics (152). Additional research is needed to identify relevant patient characteristics and to address the question of what criteria should be used to select patients for this type of treatment.

UNRESOLVED ISSUES

Although the results reported tend to support the general efficacy of MPCs, there remain several issues that are unresolved.

Criteria of Success

One of the frequently voiced criticisms of MPC outcome studies is the lack of agreement on what criteria should be used to establish success (as discussed above). The failure to assess common domains in outcome interferes with the ability to compare across studies. The reliance on self-report measures has also been viewed as a serious limitation in assessing treatment efficacy. These criticisms are not specific to MPC treatment outcome studies. There is little consistency in the outcome measures used in studies of surgical outcomes for back pain, and often self-report of pain serves as the sole criterion of success.

Typical approaches to evaluating treatment outcome have relied on mean group comparisons. That is, pretreatment/posttreatment results are compared for a treated group and an untreated group. Comparing groups has a number of limitations (160). First, it obscures identification of the percentage of patients who improved. Average results can be greatly skewed by a few patients whose performance is at the extremes. This is especially a problem when small samples are used.

Group comparisons obscure determination of the clinical significance of the results by the statistical significance. One strategy that has been suggested is to establish *a priori* limits for clinical significance. Analyses can then be conducted that permit determination of the percentage of patients treated who achieve clinically significant changes.

Who Gets Better?

As reviewed above, a large number of studies have attempted to predict who will successfully respond to rehabilitation treatment at an MPC. At this point there are no predictors to identify which patients are likely to succeed. Research is needed to examine combinations of variables in an effort to be better able to prescribe treatment at an MPC.

Mode of Treatment Delivery

When MPCs were initially developed, the majority consisted of inpatient programs lasting 4 to 8 weeks. More recently, outpatient programs seem to have become the norm. The switch from inpatient to outpatient programs was driven by financial considerations (outpatient programs are cheaper) and by philosophical rationales (outpatient programs permit patients to function in more normal environments and thus may increase generalizability to the patient's natural environment).

Several studies compare the outcomes of inpatient to outpatient programs. Several studies that have randomized patients have been reported by a group in Finland. Jarvikoski et al. (76) reported initial advantages for the inpatient program, although differences between inpatient and outpatient programs were not discernible by the 1-year follow-up. Harkapaa et al. (67,68) reported superior 3-month and 6-month follow-up results for an inpatient treatment compared to an outpatient program. Williams et al. (177) reported that although both inpatient and outpatient treatments produced significant improvements in physical performance, psychological functioning, and reduction in medications, and these results were maintained at one-year follow-up, the inpatient programs achieved somewhat better results.

In contrast to the more favorable results reported for inpatient programs, Cicala and Wright (24), Peters and Large (115), and Peters et al. (116) reported essentially negligible differences between inpatient and outpatient programs. Thus, at this point the results favoring inpatient versus outpatient treatment are equivocal. The larger studies conducted in Finland (67,68) and England (177) do appear to support efficacy of inpatient program compared to outpatient programs. Future research needs to examine these differences in light of the significantly higher treatment costs for inpatient programs (24).

In addition to inpatient programs and intensive rehabilitation day-programs such as described earlier, alternative modes of delivery have been provided. For example, some MPCs offer less intense treatment such as several times a week for some specified time period, for example 2 months (87,142). Two studies conducted in Canada (25,26) demonstrated the merits of a program of long-term home-based treatment programs. the treatment described by Corey et al. (25) was of 6 months' duration, but since it made use of paraprofessionals supervised by specialists in pain management, it was significantly less expensive than many clinic-based pain treatment programs. However, because the treatments were of longer duration, insurance carriers had to continue paying disability for a period of time much longer than with traditional pain rehabilitation programs. Thus, these extended home-based programs trade off treatment expenses, indemnity payments, and the cost of keeping disability claims open. Variations that combine outpatient treatment with brief inpatient programs have also been reported (137).

To date, there has been no prospective attempt to customize treatment to patient characteristics (152). There have been some retrospective data suggesting that patients with more psychological distress do demonstrate better improvement in inpatient than outpatient programs (115). Research is needed to address this issue, as the current strategy of offering the same treatment package to all patients may underestimate the potential benefit of MPC treatment programs.

Results suggest a uniform efficacy of treatments despite different types of pain treated, dependent measures used, or patient characteristics. This evidence suggests that the effectiveness of these treatments may be attributable not to differences between treatments, but to the features that they share in common, such as the identification of psychological factors that exacerbate pain, contact with an empathic set of health professionals, combating demoralization, and the instillation of hope (155) (see Table 2). Further research is needed to isolate the shared components of different successful treatment programs (19,82,162).

Most MPCs include a broad range of components as a single package. When successful, there are currently no data demonstrating what the necessary and sufficient components of treatment are. Studies are needed to isolate the active components of pain treatment programs (158).

In sum, despite the criticisms and reservations raised, the body of literature available provides substantial evidence that MPCs improve overall functioning of chronic pain sufferers. These improvements are shown on meaningful objective measures such as employment status, medication use, utilization of the health-care system, cost, and closure of disability cases—not just on self-report measures. In contrast, patients who are left to rely on conventional medical support languish and even show deterioration (116). Surgical interventions have proven to have less than stellar results. Thus, from the standpoint of both patients and society, MPC treatments should be viewed more positively than seems to be the case by many third-party payers and claims adjusters (97,144). Seldom are other treatments for chronic back pain held to the same standards as MPCs.

MPCs are sometimes regarded as the treatment of last resort. The erroneous impression is beginning to change as more health-care providers recognize that early patient referrals may help eliminate needless or multiple operations, reduce health-care costs, and promote the patient's return to productivity. Earlier intervention would be expected to lead to even better outcomes.

REFERENCES

1. Agre JC, Magness JL, Hull KC, Baxter TL (1987): Strength testing with portable dynamometer reliability of upper and lower extremities. *Arch Phys Med Rehabil* 68:454–458.
2. Altmaier EM, Lehmann TR, Russell DW, Weinstein JN, Kao CF (1992): The effectiveness of psychological interventions for the rehabilitation of low back pain: a randomized controlled trial evaluation. *Pain* 49:329–335.
3. American Psychiatric Association (1994): *Diagnostic and statistical manual of mental disorders,* 4th ed. Washington, DC: American Psychiatric Association Press.
4. Anderson TP, Cole TM, Gullickson G, Hudgens A, Roberts AH (1977): Behavior modification of chronic pain: a treatment program by a multidisciplinary team. *Clin Orthop* 129:96–100.
5. Aronoff GM, Evans WO (1982): The prediction of treatment outcome at multidisciplinary pain center. *Pain* 14:67–73.
6. Aronoff GM, McAlary PW, Witkower A, Berdell MS (1987): Pain treatment programs: Do they return workers to the workplace? *Spine* 2:123–136.
7. Barnes D, Smith D, Gatchel RJ, Mayer TG (1989): Psychosocioeconmoic predictors of treatment success/failure in chronic low-back pain. *Spine* 14:427–430.
8. Barnsley L, Lord SM, Wallis BJ, Bogduk G (1994): Lack of effect of intraarticular corticosterioids for chronic pain in the cervical zygapophyseal joints. *N Engl J Med* 330:1047–1050.
9. Benzon HT (1986): Epidural steroid injection for low back pain and lumbosacral radiculopathy. *Pain* 240:277–295.
10. Bernard TN Jr, Kirkaldy-Willis WH (1987): Recognizing specific characteristics of nonspecific low back pain. *Clin Orthop* 217: 266–280.
11. Block AR (1982): Multidisciplinary treatment of chronic low back pain: a review. *Rehab Psychol* 27:51–63.
12. Block AR, Kremer EF, Gaylor M (1980): Behavioral treatment of chronic pain: variables affecting treatment efficacy. *Pain* 8: 367–375.
13. Boden SD, Davis DO, Dina TS, Patronas NJ, Wiesel SW (1990): Abnormal magnetic-resonance scans of the lumbar spine in asymptomatic subjects. *J Bone Joint Surg* 72A:403–408.
14. Bonica JJ (1990): Evolution and current status of pain programs. *J Pain Symp Management* 5:368–374.
15. Bonica JJ, Black RG (1974): The management of a pain clinic. In: Swerdlow M, ed. *Relief of intractable pain.* Amsterdam: Excerpta Medica, pp. 116–129.
16. Brena SF, Chapman SL, Sanders SH (1991): Needles and the brain. Psychophysiological factors involved in nerve blocks for chronic pain. *Clin J Pain* 7:245–247.
16a. Burke SA, Harms-Constas K, Aden PS (1994): Return to work/ work retention outcomes of a functional restoration program. A multi-center, prospective study with comparison group. *Spine* 19: 1880–1886.
17. Cairns D, Mooney V, Crane P. (1984): Spinal pain rehabilitation inpatient and outpatient treatment results and development of predictors for outcome. *Spine* 9:91–95.
18. Carlson H, Pellettieri L (1989): Doctors' versus patients' evaluation of results after neurosurgery. *J Neurol Neurosurg Psychiatry* 52:153–155.
19. Carron H, Rowlingson JC (1981): Coordinated outpatient management of chronic pain a the University of Virginia Pain Clinic. In: Ng LKY, ed. *New approaches to treatment of chronic pain: a review of multidisciplinary pain clinics and pain centers.* Rockville, Maryland: National Institute of Drug Abuse.
20. Cassisi JE, Sypert GW, Salamon A, Kapel L (1989): Independent evaluation of a multidisciplinary rehabilitation program for chronic low back pain. *Neurosurgery* 25:877–883.
21. Catchlove R, Cohen K (1982): Effects of directive return to work approach in the treatment of workman's compensation patients with chronic pain. *Pain* 14:181–191.
22. Caudill M, Schnabble R, Zuttermeister P, et al. (1991): Decreased clinic use by chronic pain patients: responsive to behavioral medical intervention. *Clin J Pain* 7:305–310.
23. Chapman SL, Brerna SF, Bradford LA (1981): The treatment outcome in a chronic pain rehabilitation program. *Pain* 11:255–268.
24. Cicala RS, Wright J (1989): Outpatient treatment of patients with chronic pain: an analysis of cost savings. *Clin J Pain* 5:223–226.
25. Corey DT, Etlin D, Miller PC (1987): A home-based pain management and rehabilitation program an evaluation. *Pain* 29:219–230.
26. Cott A, Anchel H, Goldberg WM, Fabich M, Parkinson W (1990): Non-institutional treatment of chronic pain by field management: an outcome study with comparison group. *Pain* 40: 183–194.
27. Crook, J, Tunks E (1985): Defining the "chronic pain syndrome": an epidemiological method. In: Fields HK, Dubner R, Cervero R, eds. *Advances in pain research and therapy,* vol 9. Raven Press: New York, pp. 156–168.
28. Crook J, Tunks E, Rideout E, Bowne G (1986): Epidemiologic consideration of persistent pain sufferers in specialty pain clinic and the community. *Arch Phys Med Rehabil* 67:451–455.
29. Crook J, Weir R, Tunks E (1989): An epidemiological follow-up survey of persistent pain sufferers in a group family practice and specialty pain clinic. *Pain* 36:49–61.
30. Csordas TJ, Clark JA (1992): Ends of the line: diversity among chronic pain centers. *Soc Sci Med* 34:383–393.
31. Cutler RB, Fishbain DA, Rosomoff HL, Abdel-Moty E, Khalil TM, Steele Rosomoff R (1993): Does non-surgical pain center treatment of chronic pain return patients to work? A review and meta-analysis of the literature [Abstract]. *Proceedings of the 7th World Congress of Pain.* Seattle, WA: IASP Press, p. 801–802.
32. Cutler RB. Fishbain DA, Steele-Rosomoff R, Rosomoff H (1994): Outcomes in treatment of pain in geriatric and younger age groups. *Arch Phys Med Rehabil* 75:457–464.
33. Deardorff WW, Rubin HS, Scott DW (1991): Comprehensive multidisciplinary treatment of chronic pain: A follow-up study of treated and non-treated groups. *Pain* 45:35–43.
34. Deyo RA (1986): The early diagnostic evaluation of patients with low back pain. *J Gen Intern Med* 1:328–338.
35. Deyo RA, McNiesh LM, Cone RO III (1985): Observer variability in interpretation of lumbar spine radiographs. *Arthritis Rheum* 28:1066–1070.
36. Dieudonne I, Richardson PH, Williams ACdeC, Featherstone J, Harding V (1993): Can pain management enable severely impaired chronic pain to return to work? [Abstract] *Proceedings of the 7th World Congress of Pain.* Seattle: IASP press, p. 138.
37. Dionne C, Turcotte F (1992): Coping with low-back pain: remaining disabilities 5 years after multidisciplinary rehabilitation. *J Occup Rehab* 2:73–88.
38. Duckro PN, Margolis RB, Tait RC, Korytnyk N (1985): Longterm follow-up of chronic pain patients: a preliminary study. *Int J Psychiatry Med* 15:283–292.
39. Dvorak J, Gauchat MH, Valach L (1988): The outcomes of surgery for lumbar disc herniation. I. 4-17 years follow-up with emphasis on somatic aspects. *Spine* 13:1418–1422.
40. Dworkin RH, Handlin DS, Richlin DM, Brand L, Vannucci C (1985). Unraveling the effects of compensation, litigation and employment on treatment response in chronic pain. *Pain* 23:49–59.
41. Dworkin RH, Richlin DM, Handlin DS, Brand L (1986): Predicting treatment response in depressed and non-depressed chronic pain patients. *Pain* 24:343–353.
42. Dzioba RB, Doxey NC (1984): A prospective investigation into

the orthopaedic and psychologic predictors of outcome of first lumbar surgery following industrial injury. *Spine* 9:614–623.

43. Estlander A-M, Mellin G, Vanharanta H, Hupli M (1991): Effects and follow-up of a multimodal treatment program including intensive physical training for low back pain patients. *Scand J Rehab Med* 23:97–102.

44. Faucett J (1994): What is the role of nursing in the multidisciplinary pain treatment center. *APS Bull* 4:6–8, 14.

45. Fey SG, Williamson-Kirkland TE, Fraugione R (1987): Vocational restoration in injured workers with chronic pain. *Pain* (Suppl 4):S379.

46. Finlayson RE, Maruta T, Morse RM, Martin MA (1986): Substance dependence and chronic pain: experience with treatment and follow-up results. *Pain* 26:175–180.

47. Fishbain DA, Goldberg M, Meagher BR, Steele-Rosomoff R, Rosomoff H (1986): Male and female chronic pain patients categorized by DSM III psychiatric diagnostic criteria. *Pain* 26:181–197.

48. Fishbain DA:, Rosomoff HL, Goldbert M, Cutler R, Abdel-Moty E, Khalil TM, Steele-Rosomoff R (1993): The prediction of return to the work to the workplace after multidisiciplinary pain center treatment. *Clin J Pain* 9:3–15.

49. Flor H, Fydrich T, Turk DC (1992): Efficacy of multidisciplinary pain treatment centers: a meta-analytic review. *Pain* 49:221–230.

50. Flor F, Turk DC (1988): Chronic back pain and rheumatoid arthritis: predicting pain and disability from cognitive variables. *J Behav Med* 11:251–265.

51. Fordyce WE (1976): *Behavioral methods for chronic pain and illness.* St. Louis: Mosby.

52. Fordyce WE (1988): Pain and suffering: a reappraisal. *Am Psychol* 43:276–283.

53. Fordyce WE, Brena SF, Holcomb R (1978): Relationship of semantic pain descriptions to physicians' diagnostic judgments, activity level measures, and MMPI. *Pain* 5:292–303.

54. Fordyce WE, Fowler, RS, Lehmann JR, DeLateur BJ, Sand PL, Trieshmann RB (1973): Operant conditioning in the treatment of chronic pain. *Arch Phys Med Rehabil* 54:399–408.

55. Fordyce WE, Shelton J, Dundore D (1982): The modification of avoidance learning pain behaviors. *J Behav Med* 4:405–414.

56. Fredrickson BE, Trief PM, VanBeveren P, Yuan HY, Baum G (1988): Rehabilitation of the patient with chronic back pain. *Spine* 13:351–353.

57. Garvey TA, Marks MR, Wiesel SW (1989): A prospective, randomized double-blind evaluation of trigger-point injection therapy for low-back pain. *Spine* 14:962–964.

58. Gatchel RJ, Polatin PB, Mayer TG, Garcy PD (1994): Psychopathology and the rehabilitation of patients with chronic low back pain disability. *Arch Phys Med Rehabil* 75:696–670.

59. Gottlieb H, Laban CS, Koller R, Madorsky A, Hockersmith V, Kleeman M, Wagner J (1977): Comprehensive rehabilitation of patients having chronic low back pain. *Arch Phys Med Rehabil* 58:101–108.

60. Gottlieb HJ, Koller R, Alperson BL (1982): Low back pain comprehensive rehabilitation program: a follow-up study. *Arch Phys Med Rehabil* 63:458–461.

61. Greenhoot JH, Sternbach RA (1974): Conjoint treatment of chronic pain. In: Bonica JJ, ed. *Advances in neurology,* volume 4. New York: Raven Press, pp. 595–603.

62. Guck TP, Meilman PW, Skultety FM, Dowd ET (1986): Prediction of long-term outcome of multidisciplinary pain treatment. *Arch Phys Med Rehabil* 67:293–296.

63. Guck TP, Skultety FM, Meilman PW, Dowd ET (1985): Multidisciplinary pain center follow-up study: Evaluation with a no-treatment control group. *Pain* 21:295–306.

64. Hallett EC, Pilowsky I (1982): The response to treatment in a multidisciplinary pain clinic. *Pain* 12:365–374.

65. Hamburgen ME, Jennings CA, Maruta T, Swanson DW (1985): Failure of a predictive scale in identifying patients who may benefit from a pain management program: Follow up data. *Pain* 23:253–258.

66. Hammonds W, Brena SF, Unikel I (1978): Compensation for work-related injuries and rehabilitation of patients with chronic pain. *South Med J* 71:664–666.

67. Harkapaa K, Mellin G, Jarvikoski A, Hurri H (1989): A controlled study on the outcome of inpatient and outpatient treatment of low back pain. Part I. Pain disability, compliance, and reported treatment benefits three months after treatment. *Scand J Rehab Med* 21:81–89.

68. Harkapaa K, Mellin G, Jarvikoski, A, Hurri H (1990): A controlled study on the outcome of inpatient and outpatient treatment of low back pain. Part III. Long-term follow-up of pain, disability, and compliance. *Scand J Rehab Med* 22:181–188.

69. Hazard RG, Fenwick JW, Kalisch SM, Redmond J, Reeves V, Reid S, Frymoyer JW (1989): Functional restoration with behavioral support. A one year prospective study of patients with chronic back pain. *Spine* 14:157–161.

70. Herman E, Baptiste S (1981): Pain control: mastery through group experience. *Pain* 10:79–86.

71. Hitzelberger WE, Witten RM (1968): Abnormal myelograms in asymptomatic patients. *J Neurosurg* 28:204–208.

72. Hudgens RW (1970): The predictive value of myelography in the diagnosis of ruptured lumbar disc. *J Neurosurg* 32:151–162.

73. Jackson KE, Rauck RL (1991): Suspected venous air embolism during epidural anesthesia. *Anesthesiology* 74:190–191.

74. Ignelzi R, Sternbach R, Timmermans G (1977): The pain-ward follow-up analyses. *Pain* 3:277–280.

75. Jamison RN, Matt DA, Parris WCV (1988): Effects of time-limited vs unlimited compensation on pain behavior and treatment outcome in low back pain patients. *J Psychosom Res* 32:277–282.

76. Jarvikoski A, Harkapaa K, Mellin G (1986): Symptoms of psychological distress and treatment effects with low-back pain patients. *Pain* 25:345–355.

77. Jarvikoski A, Mellin G, Estlander A-M, Harkapaa K, Vanharanta H, Hupli M, Heinonen R (1993): Outcome of two multimodal back treatment programs with and without intensive physical training. *J Spinal Dis* 6:93–98.

78. Jensen MP, Turner JA, Romano JM (1994): Correlates of improvement in multidisciplinary treatment of chronic pain. *J Consult Clin Psychol* 62:172–179.

79. Keefe FJ, Block AR, Williams RB, Surwit RS (1981): Behavioral treatment of chronic pain: clinical outcome and individual differences in pain relief. *Pain* 11:221–231.

80. Kent DL, Haynor DR, Larsen EB, Deyo RA (1992): Diagnosis of lumbar spinal stenosis in adults: A meta-analysis of the accuracy of CT, MR, and myelography. *Am J Radiol* 158:1135–1144.

81. Kepes ER, Duncan D (1985): Treatment of backache with spinal injections of local anesthetics, spinal, and systemic steroids. A review. *Pain* 22:33–47.

82. King SA, Snow BR (1989): Factors for predicting premature termination from a multidisciplinary inpatient chronic pain program. *Pain* 39:281–287.

83. Kleinke CL, Spangler AS (1988): Predicting treatment outcome of chronic back pain patients in a multidisciplinary pain clinic: methodological issues and treatment implications. *Pain* 33:41–48.

84. Koran LM (1975): Reliability of clinical methods, data, and judgements. *N Engl J Med* 293:642–645, 695–701.

85. Kotarba JA (1981): Chronic pain center: a study of voluntary compliance and entrepreneurship. *Am Behav Sci* 24:786–800.

86. Large RG (1980): The psychiatrist and the chronic pain patient: 172 anecdotes. *Pain* 9:253–263.

87. Linseen ACG, Zitman FG (1984): Patient evaluation of a cognitive-behavioral group program for patients with chronic low back pain. *Soc Sci Med* 19:1361–1365.

88. Linton SJ (1986): Behavioral remediation of chronic pain: a status report. *Pain* 24:125–141.

89. Loeser JD (1990): *Desirable characteristics for pain treatment facilities.* Seattle: International Association for the Study of Pain.

90. Loeser JD (1991): The role of pain clinics in managing chronic back pain. In: Frymoyer JW, editor-in-chief. *The adult spine: Principles and practice.* New York: Raven Press, pp. 211–219.

91. Malec J, Cayner JJ, Harvey RF, Timming RC (1981): Pain management: Long-term follow-up of an inpatient program. *Arch Phys Med Rehabil* 62:369–372.

92. Maruta T, Swanson DW, McHardy, MJ (1990): Three year follow-up of patients with chronic pain who were treated in a multidisciplinary pain management center. *Pain* 41:47–53.

93. Maruta T, Swanson DW, Swenson WM (1979): Chronic pain:

Which patients may a pain treatment program help? *Pain* 7:321–329.

94. Mayer TG, Gatchel RJ, Kishino N, Keeley J, Capra P, Mayer H, Barnett J, Mooney V (1985): Objective assessment of spine function following industrial injury. A prospective study with comparison group and one-year follow-up. *Spine* 10:484–493.

95. Mayer TG, Gatchel RJ, Kishino N, et al. (1985): Objective assessment of spine function following industrial low back injury. *JAMA* 258:1763–1767.

96. Mayer TG, Gatchel RJ, Kishino N, Keeley J, Mayer H, Capra P, Mooney V (1986): A prospective short-term study of chronic low back pain patients utilizing novel objective functional measurement. *Pain* 25:53–68.

97. Mayer TG, Gatchel RJ, Mayer H, Kishino ND, Keeley J, Mooney V (1987): A prospective two-year study of functional restoration in industrial low back injury. An objective assessment procedure. *JAMA* 258:1763–1767.

98. McArthur DL, Cohen MJ, Gottlieb HJ, Naliboff BD, Schandler SL (1987): Treating chronic low back pain. II. Long-term follow-up. *Pain* 29:23–38.

99. McGill CM (1968): Industrial back problems: a controlled program. *J Occup Med* 10:174–178.

100. Meade TW, Dyer S, Browne W, Townsend J, Frank AO (1990): Low back pain of mechanical origin: a randomized comparison of chiropractic and hospital outpatient treatment. *Br Med J* 300:1431–1437.

101. Meilman PW, Skultety FM, Guck TP, Sullivan K (1985): Benign chronic pain: 18-month to ten-year follow-up of a multidisciplinary program. *Clin J Pain* 1:131–137.

102. Melding PS (1991): Is there such a thing as geriatric pain? *Pain* 46:119–121.

103. Melzack R, Katz J, Jeans ME (1985): The role of compensation in chronic pain: an analysis using a new method of scoring the McGill Pain Questionnaire. *Pain* 23:101–112.

104. Melzack R, Wall PD (1982): *The challenge of pain.* New York: Basic Books.

105. Moore ME, Berk SN, Nypaver A. (1984): Chronic pain: inpatient treatment with small group effects. *Arch Phys Med Rehabil* 65:356–361.

106. Naliboff BD, Cohen MJ, Swanson GA, Bonebakker AD, McArthur DL (1985): Comprehensive assessment of chronic low back pain patients and controls: physical abilities, level of activity, psychological adjustment and pain perception. *Pain* 23:121–134.

107. Nelson M, Allen P, Clamp SE, deDombal FT (1979): Reliability and reproducibility of clinical findings in low-back pain. *Spine* 4:97–101.

108. Nepomuceno C, Richards JS, Urson JA (1989): Accountability of pain control programs in the United States. *South Med J* 88:1456–1466.

109. Newman RI, Seres JL, Yospe LP, Garlington B (1978): Multidisciplinary treatment of chronic pain: long-term follow-up of low back pain patients. *Pain* 4:283–292.

110. North RB, Campbell JN, James CS, Conover-Walker MK, Wang H, Piantadosi S, Rybock JD, Long, DM (1991): Failed back surgery syndrome: 5-year follow-up in 102 patients undergoing repeated operation. *Neurosurgery* 28:685–691.

111. North RB, Ewend MG, Lawton MT, Kidd BH, Piantadosi S (1991): Failed back surgery syndrome: 5-year follow-up after spinal cord stimulator implantation. *Neurosurgery* 28:692–699.

112. Painter JR, Seres JL, Newman RI (1980): Assessing benefits of the pain center: why some patients regress. *Pain* 8:101–113.

113. Parris, WCV, Jamison RN, Vasterling JJ (1987): Follow-up study of a multidisciplinary pain center. *J Pain Symp Management* 2:145–151.

114. Peck CJ, Fordyce WE, Black RG (1978): The effect of pendency of claims upon behavior indicative of pain. *Washington Law Rev* 53:251–278.

115. Peters JL, Large RG (1990): A randomized control trial evaluating in- and outpatient pain management programmes. *Pain* 41:283–293.

116. Peters J, Large RG, Elkind G (1992): Follow-up results from a randomized controlled trial evaluating in- and outpatient pain management programmes. *Pain* 50:41–50.

117. Podobnikar IG, Mackintosh S (1981): *Pain* center: A cost-effective approach to the treatment of chronic pain due to industrial injury [Abstract]. *Pain* (Suppl 1):S295.

118. Polatin P, Gatchel RJ, Barnes D, Mayer H, Arens C, Mayer TG (1989): A psychosociomedical prediction model of response to treatment by chronically disabled workers with low-back pain. *Spine* 14:956–961.

119. Powell MC, Wilson M, Szypryt P, Symonds EM, Worthington BS (1986): Prevalence of lumbar disc degeneration observed by magnetic resonance in symptomless women. *Lancet* 2:1366–1367.

120. Puder RS (1988): Age analysis of cognitive-behavioral group therapy for chronic pain outpatients. *Psychol Aging* 3:204–207.

121. Reesor KA, Craig KD (1988): Medically incongruent chronic back pain: physical limitations, suffering, and ineffectvie coping. *Pain* 32:35–45.

122. Roberts AH, Reinhardt L (1980): The behavioral management of chronic pain: Long-term follow-up with comparison groups. *Pain* 8:151–162.

123. Rockey JS, Tompkins RK, Wood RW, Wolcott BW (1978): The usefulness of X-ray examinations in the evaluation of patients with back pain. *J Fam Pract* 7:455–465.

124. Romano J, Turner JA (1985): Chronic pain and depression: Does the evidence support a relationship? *Psych Bull* 97:18–34.

125. Rossignol M, Suissa S, Abenhaim L (1988): Working disability due to occupational back pain: Three-year follow-up of 2300 compensated workers in Quebec. *J Occup Med* 30:502–505.

126. Rowlingson JC, Hamill RJ (1991): Organization of a multidisciplinary pain center. *Mt Sinai J Med* 58:267–272.

127. Schwartzman, RJ, McLellan TL (1987): Reflex sympathetic dystrophy: a review. *Arch Neurol* 44:555–561.

128. Seres JL, Newman RI (1976): Results of treatment of chronic low-back pain at the Portland Pain Center. *J Neurosurg* 45:32–36.

129. Seres JL, Newman RI, Painter RL (1977): Evaluation and management of chronic pain by nonsurgical means. In: Fletcher LJ, ed. Pain management symposium on the neurosurgical treatment of pain. Baltimore, MD: Williams and Wilkins.

130. Simmons JW, Avant WS, Demski J, Parisher D. (1988): Determining successful pain clinic treatment through validation of cost effectiveness. *Spine* 13:34–24.

131. Sklar SH, Blue WT, Alexander EJ, Bodien CA (1985): The treatment and prevention of neuralgia with adenosine monophosphate. *JAMA* 253:1427–1430.

132. Snow BR, Gusmorino P, Pinter I, Jimenez A, Rosenblum A (1988): Multidisciplinary treatment of physical and psychosocial disabilities in chronic pain patients: A follow-up report. *Bull Hosp Joint Dis Orthop Inst* 48:52–61.

133. Smith GT, Hughes LB, Duvall RD, Rothman S (1987): Treatment outcome of a multidisciplinary center for management of chronic pain: a long-term follow-up. *Pain* (Suppl. 4):S58.

134. Solomon P, Tunks E (1991): The role of litigation in predicting disability outcomes in chronic pain patients. *Clin J Pain* 7:300–304.

135. Sorkin BA, Rudy TE, Hanlon RB, Turk DC, Stieg RL (1990): Chronic pain in old and young patients: differences appear less important than similarities. *J Gerontol Psychol Sci* 45:64–68.

136. Stacey, BR (1991): Nerve blocks in chronic nonmalignant pain. *APS Bull* 1:4–6.

137. Stans L, Goosens L, Van Houdenhove B, Adriaesen H, Verstraeten D, Vervaeke M, Fannes V (1989): Evaluation of a brief chronic pain management program: effects and limitations. *Clin J Pain* 5:317–322.

138. Steele-Rosomoff S, Rosomoff HL, Fishbain DA, Cutler B, Abdel-Moty E (1993): Pain center treatment outcome for the "failed back syndrome" [Abstract]. *Proceedings of the 7th World Congress of Pain.* Seattle, WA: IASP Press, p. 604.

139. Stieg RK, Williams RC (1983): Chronic pain as a biosociocultural phenomenon: implications for treatment. *Semin Neurol* 3:370–376

140. Sturgis ET, Schaefer CA, Sikora TL (1984): Pain center follow-up study of treated and untreated patients. *Arch Phys Med Rehabil* 65:301–303.

141. Swanson DW, Floreen AC, Swenson WM (1976): Program for

managing chronic pain. II. Short-term results. *Mayo Clin Proc* 51:409–411.

142. Tait RC, Duckro PN, Margolis RB, Wiener R (1988): Quality of life following treatment: a preliminary study of in- and outpatients with chronic pain. *Int J Psychiat Med* 18:271–282.

143. Talo S, Hendler N, Brodie J (1989): Effects of active and completed litigation on treatment results: Workers' compensation patients compared with other litigation patients. *J Occup Med* 31:265–269.

144. Tollison CD (1991): Comprehensive treatment approach for lower back workers' compensation injuries. *J Occup Rehabil* 1:281–287.

145. Tollison CD (1993): Compensation status as a predictor of outcome in nonsurgically treated low back injury. *South Med J* 86:1206–1209.

146. Tollison CD, Kriegel ML, Downie GR (1985): Chronic low back pain: results of treatment at the pain therapy center. *South Med J* 78:1291–1295.

147. Tollison CD, Kriegel ML, Satterthwaite JR, Hinnant DW, Turner KP (1989): Comprehensive pain center treatment of low back workers' compensation injuries. *Orthop Rev* 18:1115–1126.

148. Torgerson WR, Dotter WE (1976): Comparative roentgenographic study of asymptomatic and symptomatic lumbar spine. *J Bone Joint Surg* 58A:850.

149. Tota-Faucette ME, Gil KM, Williams FJ, Goli V (1993): Predictors of response to pain management treatment. The role of family environment and changes in cognitive processes. *Clin J Pain* 9:115–123.

150. Trabin T, Rader C, Cummings S (1987): A comparison of pain management outcomes for disability compensation and noncompensation patients. *Psychol Health* 1:341–351.

151. Trief P, Stein N (1985). Pending litigation and rehabilitation outcome of chronic back pain. *Arch Phys Med Rehabil* 66:95–99.

152. Turk DC (1990): Customizing treatment for chronic pain patients: who, what, and why. *Clin J Pain* 6:255–270.

153. Turk DC: Clinician attitudes about prolonged use of opioids and the issue of patient heterogeneity. *J Pain Symp Management (in press).*

154. Turk DC, Brody MC, Okifuji A (1994): Physicians' attitudes and practices regarding the long-term prescribing of opioids for noncancer pain. *Pain* 59:201–208.

155. Turk DC, Holzman AD (1986): Commonalities among psychological approaches in the treatment of chronic pain: specifying the meta-constructs. In: Holzman AD, Turk DC, eds. *Pain management: a handbook of psychological approaches.* New York: Pergamon Press, pp. 269–275.

156. Turk DC, Melzack R, eds. (1992): *Handbook of pain assessment.* New York: Guilford.

157. Turk DC, Rudy TE (1987): Toward a comprehensive assessment of chronic pain patients. *Behav Res Ther* 25:237–249.

158. Turk DC, Rudy TE (1990): Neglected factors in chronic pain treatment outcome studies—Referral pattens, failure to enter treatment, and attrition. *Pain* 43:7–25.

159. Turk DC, Rudy TE (1992): Cognitive factors and persistent pain: a glimpse into Pandora's box. *Cogn Ther Res* 16:99–122.

160. Turk DC, Rudy TE, Sorkin BS (1992): Neglected factors in chronic pain treatment outcome studies: determination of success. *Pain* 53:3–16.

161. Turk DC, Stieg RL (1987): Chronic pain: the necessity of interdisciplinary communication. *Clin J Pain* 3:163–167.

162. Turner JA, Clancy S (1988): Comparison of operant behavioral and cognitive-behavioral group treatment for chronic low back pain. *J Consult Clin Psychol* 56:261–266.

163. Turner JA, Romano JM (1984): Evaluating psychologic interventions for chronic pain: issues and recent developments. *Advan Pain Res Ther* 7:257–296.

164. Vanagida H, Suwa K, Corssen G (1987): No prophylactic effect of early sympathetic blockage on postherpetic neuralgia. *Anesthesiology* 66:73–76.

165. Vasudevan SV, Lynch NT, Abram S (1981): Effectiveness of an ambulatory chronic pain management program [Abstract]. *Pain* (Suppl 1):S272.

166. Von Korff M, Dworkin S, LeResche L, Kruger A (1988): Epidemiology of temporomandibular disorders. II. TMD pain compared to other common pain sites. In: Dubner R, Gebhart GF, Bond MR, eds. *Proceedings of the 5th World Congress on Pain.* Amsterdam: Elsevier, pp. 506–511.

167. Waddell G (1987): A new clinical model for the treatment for low-back pain. *Spine* 12:632–644.

168. Waddell G, Kummer EG, Lotto, WN, Graham JD (1979): Failed lumbar disc surgery and repeat surgery following industrial injuries. *J Bone Joint Surg* 61A:201–207.

169. Waddell G, Main CJ, Morris EW, Venner RM, Rae PS, Sharmy SH, Galloway H (1982): Normality and reliability in the clinical assessment of backache. *Br Med J* 284:1519–1523.

170. Wang JK, Erickson RP, Ilstrup DM (1985): Repeated stellate ganglion blocks for upper extremity reflex sympathetic dystrophy. *Reg Anesth* 10:125–128.

171. Wang JK, Ilstrup DM, Nauss LA, Nelson DO, Wilson PR (1980): Outpatient pain clinic. A long-term follow-up study. *Minn Med* 63:663–666.

172. Watson PN, Evans RJ (1986): Postherpetic neuralgia: a review. *Arch Neurol* 43:836–840.

173. White AWM (1966): The compensation back. *Appl Therapeutics* 8:871–874.

174. White AWM, Gordon S (1982): Synopsis: workshop on idiopathic low back pain. *Spine* 7:141–149.

175. Wiesel SW, Tsourmas N, Feffer H, et al. (1984): A study of computer-assisted tomography. 1. The incidence of positive CAT scans in an asymptomatic group of patients. *Spine* 9:549–551.

176. Wigley RD, Carter M, Woods J, Ahuja M, Couchman KG (1990): Rehabilitation in chronic back pain: employment status after four years. *NZ Med J* 24:9–10.

177. Williams ACdeC, Nicholas MK, Richardson PH, Pither CE, Justins DM, Chamberlain JH, Harding VR, Ridout KL, Ralphs JA, Dieudonne I (1993): Inpatient vs outpatient pain management: results of a randomized controlled trial. *Proceedings of the 7th World Congress of Pain* [Abstract]. Seattle, WA: IASP publications, p. 138.

178. Wilkinson HA (1983): The role of improper surgery in the etiology of failed back syndrome. In: Wilkinson HA, ed. The failed back syndrome. Philadelphia: JB Lippincott, pp. 15–16.

179. Wood RW, Diehr P, Wolcott, BW, Slay L, Tompkins RK (1979): Reproducibility of clinical data an decisions in management of upper respiratory illnesses: comparisons of physicians and non physicians providers. *Med Care* 17:767–779.

The Adult Spine: Principles and Practice,
2nd edition, J.W. Frymoyer, Editor-in-Chief.
Lippincott-Raven Publishers, Philadelphia © 1997.

CHAPTER 18

The Pharmacologic Management of Chronic Back Pain

Marco Pappagallo and James N. Campbell

The natural history of the majority of cases of acute back pain is characterized by spontaneous resolution of the symptom within a few weeks of onset. Indeed, it has been reported that 90% of a large population of patients with acute low back pain returned to work within 2 months of the onset of their pain (21). A proportion of patients with acute low back pain do not improve. The patients in this subset, estimated to range from 5% to 10%, continue to have persistent symptoms. Some will ultimately respond to functional restoration methods of treatment as outlined in other chapters of this book. Others will require surgery for specific conditions, such as spinal stenosis. The remaining patients who do not respond to these techniques are usually referred to as having the "failed back syndrome." These patients represent a supreme therapeutic challenge. Some have undergone multiple operations, and others, exhaustive attempts at treatment. Some patients have specific diagnoses such as arachnoiditis, while in others the persistence of incapacitating pain has defied clear elucidation.

The management of chronic back pain with medications has traditionally centered on drugs other than opioids. This tenet was based on the belief that opioids are not safe or effective for long-term use. In recent years, however, the potential usefulness of opioids has been reconsidered. It has been recognized that the opioids represent the single most effective class of medications in the management of postoperative and cancer pain (8). It has also been noted that opioids may be used safely and effectively in the management of post-herpetic neuralgia, a chronic neuropathic pain syndrome (17).

Our clinical experience indicates that addiction (i.e., preoccupation with seeking and taking drugs for nontherapeutic purposes) and clinically significant tolerance to opioid analgesia occur rarely in patients who are given opioids for chronic pain. Notably, tolerance to most of the untoward side effects of opioids, such as nausea, vomiting, and drowsiness, usually develops quickly.

M. Pappagallo, M.D.: Assistant Professor, Department of Neurosurgery, Johns Hopkins Medical Institutions, Baltimore, Maryland 21287.

J. N. Campbell, M.D.: Professor of Neurosurgery, Johns Hopkins University School of Medicine, Baltimore, Maryland 21287.

Moreover, in terms of safety, opioids, unlike alternatives such as nonsteroidal anti-inflammatory drugs (NSAIDs), produce no organ damage, even after long-term treatment. Such observations are consistent with those gathered from the extensive experience with use of opioids in the management of patients suffering from cancer pain (19). Consequently, we have come to the belief that a large number of chronic back pain patients can be successfully managed with chronic opioid therapy.

To this end, we developed the Chronic Opioid Treatment Program for a selected group of patients with chronic nonmalignant pain syndromes. The majority of patients with failed back syndrome fall into this group, and we have considerable experience with successful management of these patients with opioid therapy. However, we must emphasize that selection of these patients requires extensive evaluation. Management of the patient on chronic opioid therapy by a single physician or by a group of associated physicians within the same medical center is recommended. The patients should be carefully monitored, and scrupulous logs of the prescribed drugs should be kept. It is extremely unusual for patients in pain to develop addictive behavior patterns after being enrolled in a chronic opioid treatment program with a well-structured protocol. Nevertheless, patients should be monitored for evidence of abnormal drug-seeking and -taking behavior, as discussed later in the chapter. Although this chapter is designed primarily to elucidate how opioids should be used, we also describe other potentially useful drugs such as NSAIDs, tricyclic antidepressants, and membrane-stabilizing agents.

OPIOIDS

Extensive clinical and experimental evidence has established that the sensation of pain in humans and "pain behavior" in animals can be modulated and counteracted by opioid analgesics. Opioids achieve a direct analgesic action by targeting the mu, kappa, and delta opiate receptors located at different levels along the central (16) and perhaps even peripheral pain pathways (23). At the spinal level, for example, opioids act at the incoming nociceptor nerve endings within the dorsal horn. In the brain, opioids are thought to act primarily in the periaqueductal and periventricular gray areas. Opioid analgesics may also have a synergistic effect when acting concurrently at multiple sites (i.e., supraspinal, spinal, and peripheral).

When it has been established that the patient is ready for a trial with opioids (see Appendix), the following factors become crucial for developing a successful long-term plan.

Choice of Opioid

Long-acting opioid preparations on around-the-clock dosing are used in order to (a) avoid daily mini-

withdrawals (see section on physical dependence), (b) achieve a steady level of satisfactory analgesia throughout the day, and (c) enhance the patient's compliance. The following schedules are appropriate: controlled release morphine, such as MS-Contin, every 8 or 12 hours; methadone and levorphanol every 8 hours; Duragesic, a transdermal fentanyl preparation, every 72 hours or, if necessary, every 48 hours; and slow-release oxycodone, hydromorphone, hydrocodone capsules (formulated and prepared by a compounding pharmacy) every 6 hours.

Short-acting opioid preparations such as Percocet, Tylox, Demerol, Darvocet, Talwin, etc. should not be the mainstay for long-term opioid treatment. In particular, short-acting analgesics such as Demerol (meperidine), Darvon/Darvocet (propoxyphene), and Talwin (pentazocine) have potentially toxic effects on the central nervous system (CNS) and are not recommended for chronic use. For example, normeperidine, an active metabolite of meperidine with a half-life of 12 to 16 hours, tends to accumulate and cause CNS toxicity, which is clinically characterized by irritability, tremors, multifocal myoclonus, and seizures. Norpropoxyphene, an active metabolite of propoxyphene with a half-life of 30 to 36 hours, tends to accumulate and cause CNS toxicity as well. Moreover, the half-life and toxicity of Demerol and Darvon increase in patients with mild hepatic and/or renal disease. Even at low doses, Talwin can cause acute CNS toxicity characterized by hallucinations and disorientation. Since it is a mixed agonist–antagonist agent, Talwin should not be used concurrently with pure opioid agonists because of the potential for inducing withdrawal symptoms.

In patients with renal insufficiency, morphine should also be used with caution because the morphine metabolite, 3-glucuronide, tends to accumulate and to interfere with the analgesic action of the active metabolite, morphine 6-glucuronide.

Dosing

Opioid analgesia is characterized by a dose–effect response with no predetermined ceiling dose. The doses are adjusted upward until satisfactory pain relief or unmanageable side effects occur. On the basis of our experience, the initial titration for each patient is arbitrarily aimed to reduce pain from severe to easily tolerated, with improvement in physical and social function. If minimal or no side effects are present, titration will be continued to achieve higher levels of relief and function. Dose adjustment may require several weeks. Close patient supervision is very important during the dose titration. Initially, it is useful to contact patients by telephone twice a week and to see them on a monthly basis for follow-ups. With elderly patients in particular, use of the long-acting opioids (e.g., Duragesic patch, methadone, levorphanol, and MS-Contin) and the compounded opioid preparations (e.g., oxycodone, hydromorphone, and hydrocodone compounded slow-release capsules) requires careful drug titration. In special situations, patients are hospitalized and placed on intravenous patient-controlled analgesia (PCA) to perform the initial opioid titration safely and effectively. When satisfactory analgesia has been achieved through the PCA, the parenteral opioid dose is converted to the equianalgesic oral or transdermal dose.

A large variability in maintenance doses exists. In our patient population, for example, the MS-Contin maintenance dose ranges from 30 to 600 mg/day.

Variability in Analgesic Effect and Side Effects

There is variability among different opioids in producing analgesia, side effects, and tolerance (i.e., incomplete cross-tolerance). Therefore if unmanageable side effects, poor analgesia, or clinically relevant tolerance occur during treatment, a different opioid preparation may be required. There is also considerable individual variability in terms of predisposition to opioid analgesia and side effects.

Toxicity

There is no evidence of organ damage from long-term opioid treatment (19). Opioid-related side effects are reversed when the medication is discontinued.

Cost

With respect to the cost of long-term opioid treatment, methadone is by far the least expensive among the recommended agents.

Side Effect Management

Most of the adverse side effects subside in time. Consequently, a patient may develop significant tolerance to the majority of the untoward effects, including nausea, vomiting, and drowsiness. In contrast, relevant tolerance to the analgesic effects of opioids is observed much less frequently. Because the management of opioid-related side effects is the most important single factor for a successful treatment outcome, this is considered in greater detail below.

PHYSICAL DEPENDENCE, ADDICTION, AND TOLERANCE

The reasons often given for not prescribing opioids for chronic pain syndromes of nonmalignant origin are fear of physical dependence, fear of addiction, and the common belief that analgesic tolerance will inevitably develop. These concerns are addressed below.

Physical dependence. Physical dependence exists if a withdrawal syndrome occurs when a drug is discontinued abruptly or a drug antagonist is given. In common with many other drugs, including steroids, benzodiazepines, and antiepileptic and antihypertensive drugs, opioids can cause physical dependence and withdrawal symptoms if they are stopped abruptly after chronic use.

The symptoms of withdrawal from opioids are often described by patients as similar to those of flu. The patient may develop diaphoresis, rhinorrhea, chills, myalgia, diarrhea, abdominal cramps, vomiting, insomnia, hyperthermia, and mydriasis. The opioid withdrawal syndrome is not life threatening; moreover it is self-limiting, usually lasting 3 to 7 days. If necessary, opioids can be safely and successfully tapered over a period of 2 weeks at any time during the long-term treatment, with minimal or no discomfort for the patient. During opioid tapering, the withdrawal symptoms can on occasion be managed with clonidine. We usually recommend a clonidine patch at the dose of 0.1 or 0.2 mg over 2 weeks. Of note, the withdrawal from methadone is characterized by less intense but more prolonged complaints, and in this case clonidine might be given orally or by transdermal patch for 3 weeks.

In management of chronic pain, physical dependence should not be of concern provided that the patient is informed and warned against sudden discontinuation of the medication. While the patient is receiving chronic opioid therapy, the concurrent use of a mixed agonist–antagonist opioid (e.g., Stadol, Talwin, etc.) should be avoided, as it could trigger withdrawal symptoms.

Addiction. Addiction is characterized by an abnormal drug-seeking or drug-taking behavior. For example, individuals with addictive behavior present with a manipulative attitude toward the physician and inconsistent behavior. These individuals show an overwhelming concern with procuring short-acting opioids, in particular injectable preparations. Typical behavior for addicts includes: forging prescriptions, injecting oral opioid preparations, selling or stealing drugs, use of illicit drugs, multiple episodes of prescription or drug loss, and multiple episodes of dose escalation without first consulting the treating physician. However, extensive clinical experience from the cancer pain population and several surveys from the chronic benign pain population have shown that addiction with opioids is very rare. In our experience, fewer than 2% of patients with chronic benign pain treated with opioids showed an abnormal behavior suggestive of addiction.

It should be stressed that patients with chronic pain who take opioids on a regular basis are not addicts; rather, opioids are necessary to maintain pain relief and to improve the patient's quality of life.

Tolerance. Tolerance is defined as the requirement for dose escalation to maintain the same effect. Tolerance to analgesia is therefore defined as the continued need for dose escalation in order to maintain the same level of pain relief. Contrary to the conventional belief, tolerance to opioid analgesia is not a common problem. Experience in the cancer pain population and in the management of chronic pain of noncancer origin supports this notion.

The mechanisms involved in the development of tolerance are not well understood and the following concepts are of interest: (a) Experimental evidence from animal studies indicates that chronic nociception may prevent development of tolerance to opioid analgesia (11); (b) Some experimental evidence suggests that development of tolerance to opioid analgesia may be prevented by N-methyl-D-aspartate (NMDA) receptor antagonists (16); and (c) Cross tolerance among several opioids is incomplete. The latter two observations provide clinical clues for management of tolerance in the unusual cases where it occurs. It is reasonable to use an alternative opioid if the patient shows clinically relevant tolerance to analgesia from a particular opioid preparation. Preliminary clinical experience suggests that the addition of an NMDA antagonist, such as the over-the-counter antitussive dextromethorphan, may be used to prevent or counteract analgesic tolerance.

The need for adjusting the opioid maintenance dose can arise for reasons other than tolerance. When an otherwise stable opioid dose ceases to be effective, the following factors need to be considered:

1. Progression or flare-up of the underlying disease.
2. Occurrence of a new pathology related or unrelated to the original disease.
3. Increased physical activity. Improvement of the patient's clinical status because of the opioid treatment may result in increased activity, which in turn provides an additional trigger for the underlying pain generator.
4. Compliance with oral medications. Missed doses may lead to mini-withdrawal problems as well as uneven analgesia. Dose escalation in the face of poor compliance is obviously to be avoided. Problems with compliance may also be related to factors such as high cost of medications, drug side effects, and the development of psychosocial problems during treatment. Thus, compliance should be carefully assessed and properly addressed.
5. Change of the medication brand name. In this instance, the actual opioid dose may be altered because of manufacturing differences, especially for controlled release morphine preparations (i.e., MS-Contin versus Oramorph SR).
6. Addition of new medications to the opioid regimen causing interference with intestinal absorption and/or the plasma clearance of opioids. For example, clearance of morphine and methadone can be doubled by concurrent use of estrogens or some antibiot-

ics such as rifampicin (24). In these situations, the decreased opioid serum level appears to be related to the drug-induced increased activity of the hepatic enzymes concerned with the opioid metabolism.

In any of the above conditions, the need for dose escalation is circumstantial and is not related to true tolerance to opioid analgesia. Therefore, clinical judgment must be used every time a patient reports less benefit from the treatment requiring a dose increase.

True tolerance to respiratory depression, drowsiness, nausea, and most of the other side effects of the opioids occurs much more commonly than tolerance to analgesia and constipation. For the side effects discussed below, unless otherwise stated, it may be assumed that tolerance develops quickly, usually within 2 to 3 weeks. If tolerance does not develop, trial with another opioid is warranted. Tolerance to the side effects constitutes a positive phenomenon that allows upward titration of the opioids to achieve satisfactory pain relief.

MANAGEMENT OF THE OPIOID SIDE EFFECTS

Nausea and vomiting. The opioids can cause nausea and vomiting via three mechanisms: (a) vestibular sensitivity, (b) stimulation of the medullary chemoreceptor trigger zone, and (c) gastroparesis. Tolerance may develop as quickly as 1 to 2 weeks. To counteract nausea, hydroxyzine, at a dose of 10 to 25 mg or more, can be given together with the opioid; transdermal scopolamine is also a useful anti-emetic agent. If nausea is primarily postprandial and associated with constipation, cisapride (Propulsid) or metoclopramide (Reglan) should be added before meals at the dose of 10 mg three times per day. Phenergan or Compazine suppositories can be used to relieve vomiting. Episodic epigastric pain secondary to opioid-induced biliary tract spasm may occur occasionally and can be relieved by sublingual nitroglycerin.

Respiratory depression. Respiratory depression is very rarely of clinical relevance, as it does not occur unless the opioids have induced profound sedation. For nonambulatory patients with significant pulmonary disease, careful titration is required.

Constipation. Prophylactic use of stimulants of intestinal motility (e.g., bisacodyl, senna) in combination with a surfactant agent (e.g., docusate sodium) is helpful. Alternatively, a trial with an osmotic laxative (e.g., lactulose) can be considered. Bulk-forming laxatives (e.g., psyllium, methyl cellulose), when taken as single laxative agents without sufficient liquid, can result in intestinal obstruction in opioid-treated patients and should be avoided. Indeed, fecal impaction may be a significant complication in the elderly, and major efforts should always be made to prevent it. Fecal impaction can be treated with enemas of commercially available solutions and/or with enemas of warm olive oil (20). If these measures fail, manual disimpaction may be necessary. If constipation is unmanageable, a trial with an alternative opioid is necessary.

Sedation. Proper titration and reassurance that drowsiness is likely to subside are recommended. Otherwise, use of stimulants, such as pemoline or methylphenidate, might be indicated.

Euphoria. This condition almost never occurs with the controlled release or long-acting opioid preparations, and if it does, tolerance develops quickly.

Confusion. Opioid-induced disorientation and confusion are common in patients with underlying encephalopathy or dementia. Organic hallucinosis has been reported. In patients suffering from dementia or encephalopathy, trials with short-acting opioid preparations, such as MSIR (morphine sulfate immediate release), oxycodone, hydrocodone, or hydromorphone are recommended.

Urinary retention. Urinary retention, although infrequent, may occur in elderly men. A temporary downward dose titration may be sufficient until tolerance develops. Otherwise a trial with a different opioid should be carried out.

Myoclonus. Multifocal myoclonus may occur and is best managed by reassurance until tolerance develops. For temporary use on an acute basis, a benzodiazepine, such as lorazepam, might be helpful.

Pruritus, flushing, diaphoresis, headaches, hypotension, pedal edema. Some or all of these side effects may be secondary to the release of histamine from mast cells and possibly from the release of neurogenic peptides. There is wide variability among the opioids in producing these side effects, and tolerance may not develop. Headaches more often occur in patients with a history of preexisting migraine disorder. Trials with nonsedating H_1 and H_2 histamine antagonists are recommended for the management of flushing and pruritus. More recently, we have successfully used oral cromolyn sodium (Gastrocrom) in the management of several of the above side effects (*unpublished observations*). Cromolyn sodium is an atypical anti-inflammatory agent that appears to have tachykinin antagonistic activity (6). Of note, pruritus may have a central origin when intraspinal opioids are used.

Allergy. It is very rare for a patient to develop an immune-mediated allergic reaction. If a typical anaphylactic response is seen, a trial with an alternative opioid is mandatory.

NONSTEROIDAL ANTI-INFLAMMATORY DRUGS AND ACETAMINOPHEN

The NSAIDs, which inhibit the enzyme cyclooxygenase, provide analgesia by decreasing the tissue levels of prostaglandins. There is evidence from animal studies that NSAIDs may also have a central analgesic effect, possibly by blocking the formation of cyclooxygenase products at the level of the dorsal horn (29). Moreover, some experimental evidence suggests that prostaglandins may stimulate bone resorption, which is an important pathogenetic factor in patients who have chronic back pain secondary to severe osteoporosis. By blocking the formation of prostaglandins, the NSAIDs might prevent further bone resorption. A study with diclofenac sodium, at a dose of 150 mg per day, has suggested a prophylactic role in decreasing postmenopausal bone loss (2).

Chronic use of NSAIDs, however, is limited by their gastrointestinal, renal, and platelet aggregation adverse effects. Because of the claimed reduction in gastrointestinal toxicity, nabumetone (Relafen), at a dose of 1000 to 2000 mg per day, or choline magnesium trisalicylate, at a dose of 1000 mg every 8 to 12 hours, may be useful. The NSAIDs are most valuable when administered for intermittent periods of 10 to 14 days. With longer use, gastrointestinal toxicity is common.

Acetaminophen is the active metabolite of phenacetin, the "coal tar" analgesic no longer available on the pharmaceutical market because of its presumed nephropathic effect (9). Acetaminophen is a mild analgesic with minimal anti-inflammatory action, and it has been traditionally included in the group of the NSAIDs. Acetaminophen is thought to have a predominantly central analgesic effect (18). Although acetaminophen has an excellent safety profile with regard to the gastroduodenal mucosa and platelet aggregation, it can cause hepatotoxicity in a dose-dependent manner at doses higher than 4 to 6 g per day. Acute intoxication with a dose higher than 15 g per day can cause fatal hepatic necrosis. Since most of the short-acting opioid agents are combined with acetaminophen, the total daily dose of acetaminophen must be carefully monitored to avoid hepatotoxicity.

Aside from the risk of organ toxicity, acetaminophen and NSAIDs are known to have a ceiling effect for analgesia, which means that beyond the recommended doses, no further pain relief occurs (5).

TRICYCLIC ANTIDEPRESSANTS AND SELECTIVE SEROTONIN RE-UPTAKE INHIBITORS

Over the past 20 years, TCAs have been used extensively in the management of depression, chronic pain states (in particular neuropathic pain), and secondary insomnia accompanying depression and chronic pain.

The analgesic mechanism of action of the TCAs remains unclear. The traditional hypothesis is that TCAs inhibit the re-uptake of norepinephrine and serotonin, which results in enhancement of the central endogenous analgesic system.

TCAs provide pain relief in nondepressed patients affected by neuropathic pain, such as painful diabetic neuropathy (14) and post-herpetic neuralgia (15). The beneficial effect of the tricyclics for chronic back pain was suggested in a 1986 study (26). In a recent clinical trial (28), however, the tricyclic nortriptyline appeared to improve pain and function only in chronic low back pain patients who were also depressed. Clinical depression has been identified in approximately 60% of chronic low back pain patients (N = 623) (25). It is possible that successful treatment of depression might very well improve the overall perception of pain in chronic back pain patients. In this regard, it is of interest that when Magni (12) and Max (13) reviewed the pertinent literature, they found that the data supporting the role of the TCAs as analgesics for chronic back pain were not convincing and minimal clinical benefit was reported (for review, see ref. 13).

In addition to questionable efficacy, the TCAs have never emerged as primary analgesics in the treatment of chronic low back pain because of their sometimes intolerable side effects such as: (a) anticholinergic effects such as dry mouth, confusion, memory loss, urinary retention, constipation, blurred vision, and atrioventricular (A-V) cardiac conduction abnormalities; (b) orthostatic hypotension, secondary to an alpha-adrenergic blocking effect; and (c) drowsiness, secondary to an antihistaminic effect. In the management of cancer pain, for example, the TCAs have been commonly relegated to the role of adjuvant analgesics.

Amitriptyline is the most commonly used tricyclic antidepressant. It should be started at the low oral dose of 10 to 25 mg at bedtime, which can be increased every 4 to 5 days as tolerated. A therapeutic blood level for depression should be achieved. Desipramine or nortriptyline may be an alternative if the patient is unable to tolerate the anticholinergic side effects of amitriptyline.

SSRIs are effective antidepressants and may be recommended for patients unable to tolerate TCAs. Occasionally an SSRI is added to enhance the antidepressant effect of the tricyclic drug. Of note, the SSRIs will increase tricyclic levels in serum, and hence close monitoring of the TCA level is needed. An example of an SSRI is fluoxetine, an agent that essentially lacks the anticholinergic, antihistaminic, and alpha-adrenergic blocking effects of the tricyclics. Fluoxetine can be started at a dose of 20 mg every other day and titrated to an everyday schedule, if needed. Sertraline and paroxetine, which are also effective antidepressants, are closely related to fluoxetine.

MEMBRANE-STABILIZING AGENTS

The oral local anesthetic mexiletine and the antiepileptic drug carbamazepine can be of some value in patients with back and lower extremity pain of neuropathic origin. The analgesic action of these drugs appears to be related to blockade of neuronal membrane sodium chan-

nels at the site of the nerve injury, where an "ectopic pain generator" has developed (4).

In patients who have ongoing burning or intermittent shooting pain in their lower extremities, a neuropathic mechanism can be suspected. For such patients, a trial with the oral antiarrhythmic mexiletine, structurally similar to lidocaine, is reasonable. A positive response to intravenous lidocaine has been suggested to predict a favorable response to oral mexiletine. In our center, we test this possibility by infusing lidocaine at a dose of 5 mg/kg over 1 hour. If the lidocaine infusion provides 50% or more pain relief without causing major side effects, a trial with oral mexiletine is recommended.

Mexiletine is contraindicated in the presence of second or third degree A-V block (if no pacemaker is present) and a baseline EKG is generally obtained prior to treatment. Mexiletine can be started at a dose of 150 mg per day and increased by 150-mg increments every 3 to 4 days to a total dose of 10 mg/kg/day, given three times per day. At therapeutic doses, the most common untoward side effects are nausea, vomiting, dizziness, tremor, and incoordination.

If no analgesic effect is reported, the mexiletine serum level can be determined. Further dose increments will be guided according to the serum level. An appropriate therapeutic range for the mexiletine serum level is 0.5 to 2.0 mcg/mL. When the serum level exceeds 2.0 mcg/mL, adverse central nervous system side effects, including short-term memory loss, hallucinations, and seizures, may occur.

The antiepileptic drugs may be useful for treatment of pain related to nerve root injury. Carbamazepine, for example, can be given at an initial dose of 100 mg twice a day and increased slowly over 2 weeks, for a total of 800 to 1200 mg per day, or until limiting side effects occur. The most frequent side effects, nausea, vomiting, dizziness, and drowsiness, usually subside in time. At doses of 800 to 1200 mg per day, the level of carbamazepine in serum should be measured. Further dose increments will be guided by the serum levels. Appropriate therapeutic levels are between 8 and 12 mcg/mL.

MUSCLE RELAXANTS, BARBITURATES, PHENOTHIAZINES, AND BENZODIAZEPINES

Muscle relaxants (e.g., Soma, Robaxin, Parafon Forte, Flexeril, Skelaxin, and Norflex), barbiturates (e.g., Fiorinal, Fioricet, Esgic), phenothiazines (e.g., Prolixin, Haldol, Mellaril), and benzodiazepines (e.g., Xanax, Valium, Librium, Ativan, Dalmane) generally play no role in the long-term management of chronic pain patients. As an exception, some clinicians use clonazepam (e.g., Klonopin), an oral benzodiazepine effective as an antiepileptic drug, for the treatment of neuropathic pain. However, despite their widespread use and indeed overuse, benzodiazepines may exacerbate the underlying depression commonly present in chronic back pain patients. Moreover, benzodiazepine may disrupt the patient's physiologic sleep and cause cognitive and psychomotor disturbances (7).

CONCLUSION

The medical treatment of chronic axial and radicular pain related to diseases of the spine has received little attention despite the magnitude and relevance of this problem. Traditionally, the most commonly used medications have been NSAIDs and acetaminophen. However, their use for the treatment of chronic back pain has been limited by low analgesic efficacy and organ toxicity. Other medications such as TCAs, SSRIs, and membrane-stabilizing agents appear to be effective only in a minority of patients.

This chapter focused on how long-acting opioids may be used in the treatment of chronic back pain. Over the past decade there has been an interesting shift toward an increasing acceptance of the use of opioids for chronic pain syndromes of noncancer origin. Concurrently, the issues of addiction liability, tolerance to opioid analgesia, and treatment safety have been addressed in depth and found to be of minimal clinical relevance. Moreover, tolerance to side effects allows the doses of opioids to be titrated to the point that effective pain relief can be achieved in the majority of patients.

In conclusion, we believe that chronic opioid therapy should be the mainstay of successful pharmacological management for a select group of patients with chronic back pain. These patients should be managed with a well-structured and controlled protocol and by physicians with experience in the treatment of chronic pain. The Appendix of this chapter describes in detail the Johns Hopkins Chronic Opioid Treatment Program and includes case histories, which provide data on the principles and efficacy of chronic opioid therapy.

APPENDIX A. THE JOHNS HOPKINS CHRONIC OPIOID TREATMENT PROGRAM

The majority of the chronic back pain patients referred to the Johns Hopkins Pain Treatment Center have failed multiple surgical, pharmacological, and rehabilitative interventions. We have established the Chronic Opioid Treatment Program for patients with chronic nonmalignant pain syndromes, including those with intractable chronic back pain. The protocol, which is followed strictly, is described below.

At the time of their first visit, patients undergo a physical and neurological examination and a routine blood work-up. As a mandatory first step, benzodiazepines, other sedatives, and muscle relaxants are tapered and discontinued. TCAs may be continued if their use is

deemed helpful. We do, however, determine the TCA serum level during the initial routine blood work-up and if necessary the TCA dose is adjusted to achieve a therapeutic range. Our patients are informed that they will undergo formal baseline assessments of:

1. pain by the Multidimensional Pain Inventory—Pain Intensity Subscale (10);
2. mood by the Beck Depression Inventory (1);
3. attention/psychomotor speed by the Digit Symbol Subscale from the Wechsler Adult Intelligence Scale—Revised (27); and
4. verbal learning by the Hopkins Verbal Learning Test (3).

If indicated, patients also receive a psychiatric interview by the Diagnostic Interview Schedule (22). Relative contraindications for the Chronic Opioid Treatment Program are a history of substance abuse and a severe personality disorder. Patients must agree to have their pain medications managed by a single physician. They will be withdrawn from the opioid program if they exhibit abnormal drug-seeking or drug-taking behavior. All patients must sign an informed consent form in which the issues of physical dependence, addiction, and tolerance to the opioids are addressed and discussed. The Johns Hopkins Pain Treatment Center Informed Consent for the use of opioids in the management of chronic benign pain syndromes is supplied at the end of this Appendix.

After giving informed consent, the patient is provided with a prescription for (a) a long-acting opioid, (b) hydroxyzine as needed for nausea, and (c) written guidelines for the management of constipation. For instance, a controlled-release oral preparation of morphine (i.e., MS-Contin) can be started at a dose of 15 mg orally twice a day; hydroxyzine can be given at a dose of 10 to 25 mg orally twice a day, as needed, to be taken each time together with MS-Contin. The patient is advised to take senna, 1 to 2 tablets per day, and Dulcolax, 2 to 3 tablets at bedtime as needed, for constipation.

Pain intensity is rated on a verbal scale of 0 to 10, where 0 is equal to no pain and 10 to the worst imaginable pain. Pain relief percentage (0% to 100%) and VAS score are obtained at subsequent visits. These two scales, the pain intensity 0 to 10 scale and the pain relief 0% to 100% scale, are not linearly related. Both outcome measures are important and useful to guide proper titration. Patients are asked about their overall level of functioning and occasionally about the level of specific activities (i.e., walking, shopping, reading, cleaning, etc.) before and during the opioid treatment. The levels of function can be measured on a scale of 0 to 10, where 0 means full disability and 10 means full function.

The patient is followed closely through phone conversations at least twice a week for the first 3 weeks of treatment and returns to the Outpatient Pain Treatment Center on a monthly basis for the first 3 months. The dose of the opioid is titrated upward, initially aiming at the arbitrary minimum level of 50% pain relief. At the end of the titration period and when the patient is thought to be in a stable condition, the follow-up assessment of pain, mood, attention, psychomotor speed, and verbal learning will be obtained. The formal baseline and follow-up assessments are conducted by an individual who is not involved in the patient's care.

APPENDIX B. CASE REPORTS

Principles in using opioids to control chronic back pain are exemplified by the following three cases.

CASE HISTORY #1. Ms. D. K., a 38-year-old woman, had a longstanding history of chronic back pain and severe osteoporosis (related to a total hysterectomy performed at age 24 to treat advanced endometriosis). In July 1992, x-rays and bone scan revealed compression fractures of the T-11 and L-1 vertebral bodies. In November 1992, the patient began treatment with calcitonin and transdermal estrogens. In April 1993, a diagnosis of costochondritis resulted in a series of steroid injections in her sternocostal junctions. Thereafter, her overall clinical picture worsened. She became unable to carry out her daily housekeeping activities and her part-time job as hairdresser. Trials with amitriptyline, acupuncture, and physical therapy were unsuccessful. She reported benefit from a back brace but, because of pain, was unable to follow a recommended comprehensive physical therapy program which included aquatic therapy and isometric strengthening exercises. Relafen, an NSAID, provided some pain relief, but, because of gastrointestinal intolerance, she was unable to take NSAIDs on a daily basis despite the use of H_2 antagonists. In the past, the patient reported 50% pain relief for about 2 hours after taking one tablet of Percocet (oxycodone plus acetaminophen).

At her initial visit at Johns Hopkins in December 1993, the patient had severe chronic mid and low back pain, neck pain, right shoulder pain, and diffuse joint pains as well as insomnia and chronic fatigue. In January 1994, she underwent baseline assessment of pain intensity, attention/psychomotor speed, and verbal learning (see Appendix C). On the same day, the patient entered the Chronic Opioid Treatment Program and was started on compounded slow-release oxycodone capsules at a dose of 15 mg orally, three times a day, and was given a prescription for hydroxyzine 25 mg orally, three times a day, to be taken with the oxycodone capsules as needed for nausea. She was started on the NSAID choline magnesium trisalicylate at a dose of 1,000 mg every 12 hours. The patient was followed by telephone conversations at least twice a week for the first 3 weeks. The dose of oxycodone was gradually titrated upwards to a maintenance dose of 30 mg every 6 hours. At that point, the patient reported 60% to 70% relief on the 0% to 100% pain relief

scale. She was able to tolerate the oxycodone capsules with no drowsiness or nausea. She complained of mild constipation, which was treated with senna, 1 tablet twice a day.

In April 1994, the patient returned for formal follow-up assessment, which showed her improvement not only in terms of pain intensity but also of psychometric scores (see Appendix C). She had resumed her part-time job and her daily housekeeping activities, and had become more involved in important projects, including both work and pleasure. In short, the overall quality of her life had improved.

CASE HISTORY #2. Mr. A. L., a 71-year-old patient, presented with a history of low back pain for more than 10 years. In 1983, he was diagnosed with spinal lumbar stenosis and underwent decompressive multilevel lumbar laminectomy, which did not relieve his symptoms. In 1984 and in 1992 the patient underwent, respectively, a lumbar laminectomy and a lumbar fusion. Neither procedure relieved his chronic low back and right hip pain, nor did multiple courses of physical therapy and rehabilitation and trials with NSAIDs and amitriptyline. He also failed the spinal cord stimulator trial. When first seen at the Johns Hopkins Pain Treatment Center in early July 1993, he was taking Tylenol with codeine, 2 to 3 tablets per day, with some pain relief, and he was wearing a back brace with some benefit. Physical activities, such as walking and standing, were very limited. Because of pain, the patient was unable to sleep at night and he was taking Dalmane, a benzodiazepine, 15 mg at bedtime.

The patient was allowed to continue the use of Tylenol with codeine, but the dose was increased to two tablets four times a day around the clock. Dalmane was tapered and discontinued. After baseline assessment of pain intensity, mood, attention/psychometric speed, and verbal learning (see Appendix C), he was enrolled in the Chronic Opioid Treatment Program and was started on the slow-release oxycodone compounded capsules at a dose of 3 mg every day. He was allowed to take two tablets of Tylenol with codeine every day as needed for breakthrough pain. The dose of oxycodone was gradually titrated upwards to 10 mg every 6 hours. The patient reported 40% pain improvement, but complained of persistent nausea and drowsiness. Hydroxyzine effectively controlled nausea, but intolerable drowsiness developed. One month later, oxycodone was changed to controlled release oral morphine (MS-Contin), at a dose of 15 mg every day, which the patient tolerated very well. Drowsiness and nausea subsided and the only side effect was constipation, which required daily use of laxatives (senna and docusate). Over the next 8 weeks, the dose of MS-Contin was gradually increased to 30 mg every morning, 15 mg every evening, and 15 mg at bedtime. At 6 months, the patient reported more than 50% pain relief (on the verbal scale of pain relief 0% to 100%) and

TABLE 1. *Psychological assessments for the Johns Hopkins chronic opioid treatment program*

Patient	38-yr-old women		71-yr-old men		44-yr-old men	
	Baseline	Follow-up (3 mo)	Baseline	Follow-up (10 mo)	Baseline	Follow-up (6 mo)
Pain intensity[a]	6	3.3	6	2	5.7	2.7
Depression[b]	NA	6	18	11	10.5	11
Attention and psychomotor speed[c]	61	71	45	50	44	53
Verbal learning[d]	27	28	29	28	20	21

[a] Multi-Dimensional Pain Inventory—Pain Intensity Subscale (scale 0 to 6, where score 6 corresponds to maximum level of pain intensity).

[b] Back Depression Inventory (a score of 18 indicates mild to moderate depression; scores of 11 or lower indicate no depression).

[c] Digit Symbol Subscale from the Wechsler Adult Intelligence Scale—Revised (higher scores indicate better performance).

[d] Hopkins Verbal Learning Test (scores 27 to 29 correspond to average verbal learning capacity).

NA, not available.

overall improvement in his daily physical and mental function. The dose of MS-Contin remained unchanged.

At 10 months, on formal follow-up evaluation, the patient reported improvement in the level of pain intensity and depression and achieved essentially the same or better psychometric scores (see Appendix C). He also reported a lower level of interference from his pain and an ability to fulfill his daily activities at a satisfactory level. Overall, Mr. A. L. benefited significantly from the chronic use of the long-acting opioid treatment.

CASE HISTORY #3. Mr. M. M., a 44-year-old patient, had a longstanding history of neck and upper back pain. In 1988, the patient sustained a work-related neck and upper back injury, after which he began to complain of left arm and neck pain. Magnetic resonance imaging (MRI) study revealed disc disease at the C6-7 level. In November 1988, the patient underwent a C6-7 anterior cervical fusion, which relieved the pain radiation to his left arm, but his neck pain persisted. A second unsuccessful anterior cervical fusion, this time at the C5-6 level was performed in August 1989. In 1991, he was diagnosed with cervical pseudoarthrosis, and in May 1992, he underwent revision of the fusions at C5-6 and C6-7 levels. Unfortunately, even his third surgery was unsuccessful. After failing multiple pharmacologic trials with NSAIDs and several courses of physical therapy, the patient was placed on permanent disability.

In March 1993, MRI of his cervical spine showed hypertrophic bone changes with bilateral foraminal stenosis at C5-6 and C6-7, as well as disc disease at the C2-3 level. At his first visit at Johns Hopkins, the patient was in moderate distress, complaining of depression, anger, anxiety, and insomnia. He was taking five to seven tablets of Vicodin (hydrocodone plus acetaminophen) per day with minimal pain relief, as well as Flexeril as needed.

In June 1993, the patient was started on nortriptyline titrated to a dose of 100 mg at bedtime. Three weeks later, he underwent the baseline assessment (see Appendix C) and was started on MS-Contin, 15 mg twice a day,

and Vicodin was discontinued. Over the following 6 weeks, MS-Contin was titrated upward to a maintenance dose of 60 mg three times a day. He did not require medications for nausea or constipation. He remained on the same dose of nortriptyline 100 mg at bedtime.

In January 1994, the patient returned to our Pain Treatment Center for the formal follow-up assessment (see Appendix C); pain intensity had declined and he had no cognitive impairment attributable to the long-acting opioid treatment. The patient stated that he had substantially increased the level of his daily activities.

APPENDIX C. PSYCHOLOGICAL ASSESSMENTS FOR THE JOHNS HOPKINS CHRONIC PAIN OPIOID TREATMENT PROGRAM

Table 1 describes these assessments.

APPENDIX D. INFORMED CONSENT FORM FOR CHRONIC OPIOID MANAGEMENT

The following issues pertain to the treatment of chronic pain with opioids (i.e., morphine-like drugs):

1. DRUG DEPENDENCE: There are two types of dependence.
   A. Physical Dependence is common to many drugs including steroids, blood pressure medications, anti-anxiety medications, anti-seizure medications, as well as opioids. Physical dependence poses no problem to the patient as long as the patient avoids abrupt discontinuation of the drug. The medication can be safely discontinued after a two- to three-week period of tapering off (see point #9).
   B. Psychological Dependence or Addiction is a rare occurrence in patients who have been diagnosed with an organic disease causing chronic pain. Addiction is seen in patients with a previous his-

tory of personality disorder (i.e., antisocial behavior) and in patients with a history of alcohol or drug abuse. Addiction is recognized when the patient abuses the drug to obtain mental numbness or euphoria, when the patient shows a drug-craving behavior or "doctor shopping," when the drug is quickly escalated without correlation to pain relief, and/or when the patient shows a manipulative attitude toward the physician in order to obtain the drug. If the patient exhibits such behavior, the drug will be tapered; such a patient is not a candidate for the opioid trial and he/she will be discharged.

2. TOLERANCE: Tolerance to pain relief is a much rarer phenomenon than was previously believed. It is defined as a need for a higher opioid dose to maintain the same effect. Usually, tolerance to sedation, euphoria, and nausea and vomiting will occur more commonly than tolerance to pain relief. There are several types of opioids. If the patient develops tolerance to one opioid medication, he/she can be switched to a different opioid. Tolerance can also be managed by adding a second, different, drug to the opioid management. If tolerance to opioids becomes unmanageable, the opioid will be discontinued.

3. SIDE EFFECTS: The most common side effects are nausea and vomiting (similar to motion sickness), drowsiness, and constipation. The less common side effects are mental slowing, flushing, sweating, itching, urinary difficulty, and jerkiness. These side effects occur at the beginning of the treatment and often spontaneously disappear within a few days. At the beginning of the opioid treatment, other medications may be given to counteract the above side effects. If, at the beginning of the treatment, the patient experiences severe sedation, it is imperative for the patient to hold the next medication dose and contact his/her physician.

4. DRIVING: If the patient develops drowsiness, sedation, or dizziness, he/she may not drive motor vehicles or operate machinery that can jeopardize his/her or other people's safety.

5. SINGLE PHYSICIAN: The opioids will be prescribed by a single physician. The patient must be aware that "doctor shopping" is an unacceptable behavior. The same physician will be managing the possible side effects during the first few weeks of the opioid treatment. The physician will be the only one to decide when and how the patient is to increase the opioid daily dose. If the physician decides to discontinue the use of opioids, he will follow the patient through the tapering-off period.

6. DOSE: The end point of the opioid trial will be significant degree of pain relief, unmanageable side effects, or lack of benefit because of tolerance. The opioid dose will be slowly titrated up over several days. Because of possible side effects, the opioid dose titration might be delayed. The physician will make use of either a slow release or a long-acting opioid medication, which will be given one to three times a day.

7. PERSONAL USE: The patient is informed that the opioid medication is strictly for personal pain relief. The opioid should never be distributed to others. Once the maintenance opioid dose has been achieved, the patient will be given a monthly supply and no exceptions will be made. The patient must call our office 5 to 7 days prior to running out of the medication. A new prescription will be mailed either to the patient or to his/her pharmacy.

8. COMMUNICATION: At the beginning of the opioid trial, the patient, however, is responsible for contacting the physician if at anytime excessive drowsiness or any other major side effect develops (see point #3). After office hours, the patient should contact the _____ resident on call at phone number _____ .

9. WITHDRAWAL SYNDROME: The patient is informed that he/she may not stop taking the opioid medication abruptly. If this happens, withdrawal symptoms usually occur 24 to 48 hours after the last dose. The patient may begin to experience yawning, sweating, watery eyes, runny nose, anxiety, tremors, aching muscles, hot and cold flashes, "goose flesh," or abdominal cramps and diarrhea. The withdrawal syndrome is self-limited and is not life threatening. It may last a few days. In order to avoid the withdrawal symptoms, the patient is informed that he/she is to contact the office 7 days prior to needing a new prescription.

10. DRUG INTERACTION: The patient is informed that he/she may not take other drugs such as tranquilizers, sedatives, or antihistamines without first consulting with his/her physician. The patient may not use alcohol. The combined use of the above drugs, alcohol, and opioids may produce profound sedation, respiratory depression, and blood pressure drop.

WARNING: During the opioid trial, the upward titration of the drug is conducted under the close supervision of the physician. It is imperative for the patient to follow the physician's directions and not to increase the opioid dose on his own. Drug overdose can cause severe sedation and respiratory depression.

I, _____ , have read the above information or it has been read to me and all my questions regarding the treatment of pain with opioids (i.e., morphine-like drugs) have been answered to my satisfaction. I hereby give my consent to participate in the opioid medication therapy.

Patient signature ——————————— Date ———————

Witness signature ————————————————————

Physician signature ————————————————————

Date/time of phone conference ————————————————

A phone conference has been arranged on the date and time noted above. If Dr. ——————————— is unable to contact you (i.e., patient's line busy, unforeseen emergency, patient not available, etc.), please call our office 30 minutes after scheduled time. Otherwise, a phone conference will be automatically scheduled for the next available date and time.

ACKNOWLEDGMENT. We would like to express our gratitude to Dr. Pamela Talalay, from the Departments of Neurology and Neurosurgery, Johns Hopkins University, for her assistance in editing this chapter; to Dr. Jennifer Haithorthwaite, from the Department of Psychiatry, Johns Hopkins University, for her help in the psychological assessment of patients; and to Dr. Donlin Long, Chairman of the Department of Neurosurgery, Johns Hopkins University, for his guidance in the development of the Chronic Opioid Treatment Program.

REFERENCES

1. Beck AT, Ward CH, Mendelson M, et al. (1969): An inventory for measuring depression. *Arch Gen Psychiatry* 4:561–571.
2. Bell NH, Hollis BW, Schary JR, et al. (1994): Diclofenac sodium inhibits bone resorption in postmenopausal women. *Am J Med* 96:349–353.
3. Brandt J (1991): The Hopkins Verbal Learning Test: development of a new memory test with six equivalent forms. *Clin Neuropsychol* 5:125–142.
4. Chabal C, Jacobson L, Mariano A, et al. (1992): The use of oral mexiletine for the treatment of pain after peripheral nerve injury. *Anesthesiology* 76:513–517.
5. Cherny NI, Portenoy RK (1994): Practical issues in the management of cancer pain. In: Melzack R, Wall PD, eds. *Textbook of pain* 3rd ed. London: Churchill Livingstone, pp. 1437–1467.
6. Crossman DC, Dashwood MR, Taylor GW, et al. (1993): Sodium cromoglycate: evidence of tachykinin antagonist activity in the human skin. *J Appl Physiol* 75(1):167–172.
7. Dellemijn PLI, Fields HL (1994): Do benzodiazepines have a role in chronic pain management? *Pain* 57:137–152.
8. Fields HL (1991): Group report: strategies for improving the pharmacological approaches to the maintenance of analgesia in chronic pain. In: Basbaum AI, Besson JM, eds. *Towards a new pharmacotherapy of pain.* New York: John Wiley & Sons, pp. 205–226.
9. Insel PA (1990): Analgesic-antipyretics and antiinflammatory agents: drugs employed in the treatment of rheumatoid arthritis and gout. In: Goodman Gilman A, eds. *The pharmacological basis of therapeutics,* 8th ed, New York: Pergamon Press, pp. 638–681.
10. Kerns RD, Turk DC, Rudy TE (1985): The West Haven–Yale Multidimensional Pain Inventory (WHYMPI). *Pain* 23:345–356.
11. Lyness WH, Smith FL, Heavner JE, et al. (1989): Morphine self-administration in the rat during adjuvant-induced arthritis. *Life Sci* 45:2217–2224.
12. Magni G (1991): The use of antidepressants in the treatment of chronic pain: a review of the current evidence. *Drugs* 42:730–748.
13. Max MB (1994): Antidepressants as analgesics. In: Fields HL, Liebeskind JC, eds. *Progress in pain research and management,* vol 1. Seattle: IASP Press, pp. 229–246.
14. Max MB, Lynch SA, Muir J, et al. (1992): Effects of the desipramine, amitriptyline, and fluoxetine on pain in diabetic neuropathy. *N Engl J Med* 326:1250–1256.
15. Max MB, Schafer SC, Culnane M, et al. (1988): Amitriptyline, but not lorazepam, relieves postherpetic neuralgia. *Neurology* 38:1427–1452.
16. Pasternak GW (1993): Progress in opiate pharmacology. In: Chapman CR, Foley KM, eds. *Current and emerging issues in cancer pain: research and practice.* New York: Raven Press, pp. 113–127.
17. Pappagallo M, Campbell JN (1994): Chronic opioid therapy as alternative treatment for postherpetic neuralgia. *Ann Neurol* 35:S54–56.
18. Piletta P, Porchet HC, Dayer P (1991): Central analgesic effect of acetaminophen but not aspirin. *Clin Pharmacol Ther* 49:350–354.
19. Portenoy RK (1990): Chronic opioid therapy in nonmalignant pain. *J Pain Symptom Manage* 5:S46–62.
20. *The Merck Manual* (1987): Berkow R et al., eds. General medicine, vol. 1, 15th ed., pp. 599–600.
21. Nachemsom A (1982): The natural course of low back pain. In: White AA, Gordon SL, eds. *Symposium on idiopathic low back pain.* St. Louis, MO: CV Mosby, pp. 46–51.
22. Robins LN, Helzer JE (1985): *The Diagnostic Interview Schedule (DIS): Version III-R.* St. Louis, MO: Mosby.
23. Stein C, Comisel K, Haimeri E, et al. (1991): Analgesic effect of intraarticular morphine after arthroscopic knee surgery. *N Engl J Med* 325:1123–1126.
24. Stockley IH (1994): *Drug interactions,* 3rd ed. Boston: Blackwell Scientific Publications.
25. Sullivan MJL, Reesor K, Mikail S, Fisher R (1992): The treatment of depression in chronic low back pain: review and recommendations. *Pain* 50:5–13.
26. Ward NG (1986): Tricyclic antidepressants for chronic low back pain. Mechanisms of action and predictors of response. *Spine* 11:661–665.
27. Wechsler D (1981): *Wechsler Adult Intelligence Scale-Revised (WAIS-R).* New York: The Psychological Corporation.
28. Williams RA, Atkinson JH, Slater MA, et al. (1993): *Efficacy of nortriptyline in the treatment of low back pain* [Abstract]. American Pain Society Twelfth Annual Meeting, Orlando, FL., Nov. 4–7.
29. Yaksh TL, Malmberg AB (1994): Interaction of spinal modulatory receptor systems. In: Fields HL, Liebeskind JC, eds. *Progress in pain research and management,* vol 1. Seattle: IASP Press, pp. 151–171.

The Adult Spine: Principles and Practice,
2nd edition, J.W. Frymoyer, Editor-in-Chief.
Lippincott-Raven Publishers, Philadelphia © 1997.

CHAPTER 19

Electrical Stimulation Techniques for Chronic Pain

Richard B. North

In one form or another, electrical stimulation has been used for its pain-relieving effects for thousands of years. In the first century B.C., Scribonius Largus described the application of a torpedo fish to an injured limb (127), and by the seventeenth century, artificially generated electrical currents were used in medical practice. However, the modern use of electrical stimulation devices has rapidly evolved over the last two decades. In part, the publication in 1965 of Melzack and Wall's gate theory (85) was the stimulus for renewed interest in electrical stimulation for pain management. In addition, solid-state electronics made portable devices such as transcutaneous electrical nerve stimulators (TENS) practical. Techniques for packaging implanted circuitry, originally developed for cardiac pacing, were applied to the development of spinal, peripheral nerve, and brain implants.

MECHANISMS OF ACTION

Although electrical stimulation devices are an important element in pain management, their mechanism of action remains controversial. According to the gate theory, pain sensation—the central transmission of neural activity signaling pain—is regulated by a spinal "gate." The gate opens in response to an excess of peripheral small fiber activity. Large fibers, which are more susceptible to depolarization by rectangular stimulation pulses, are then selectively recruited to cause the central gate to close. Such stimulation pulses may be directed along peripheral nerves (orthodromically) or via collateral processes from the dorsal columns of the spinal cord (antidromically).

Although the gate theory has been appraised critically (90), the clinical methods of electrical stimulation that it inspired are empirically successful and continue to grow in popularity. The gate theory has been countered by recent evidence that hyperalgesia is signalled by large fibers (19), allowing for the hypothesis that the analgesic effects of stimulation are mediated by a mechanism such as frequency-related conduction block acting on this fiber population (20). Although the peripheral nerve stimulation parameters employed clinically may (17,50) or may not (131) achieve this effect locally, branch points are particularly vulnerable. The effects of spinal cord stimulation may therefore occur at branch points of primary afferents into dorsal column and dorsal horn fibers. Such

R. B. North, M.D.: Associate Professor of Neurosurgery, Johns Hopkins University School of Medicine, Baltimore, Maryland, 21287-7713.

a mechanism, however, would not readily explain the prolonged latency and persistence of stimulation analgesia described by many patients with implanted spinal stimulators (92).

The precise mechanism(s) by which electrical stimulation produces analgesia is not clear; in fact, the mechanism of action may be different at differing parameters of stimulation. For instance, human studies show that the analgesic effects of TENS delivered at conventional low intensity (12 to 20 mA) and high frequency (50 to 100 Hz) are not reversible by the narcotic antagonist naloxone (1,40,140). Analgesia achieved with acupuncture-like low-frequency stimulation (2-Hz pulse repetition rate) (21) or burst repetition rate (125), however, is reportedly reversed by narcotic antagonist administration. Thus it would seem that these stimulation regimes have separate mechanisms.

TRANSCUTANEOUS ELECTRICAL NERVE STIMULATION

For over a century, commercially available, externally applied electrical stimulation devices have been used in pain management (127). It was not until 20 years ago, however, when their applicability as screening devices for spinal and peripheral nerve implants was being investigated (69), that they became important in the armamentarium for pain control. In fact, it was found that TENS alone proved to be adequate treatment for a substantial number of patients (68). In controlled trials using placebo stimulation, there is a rapid decline in the placebo effect shortly after institution of therapy. The profiles and incidence of overall patient response to TENS is similar to that found in pharmacologic studies (70,132). The importance of electrode placement, and the necessity for systematic testing for determination of optimal sites in individual patients, are well documented (75).

Like other forms of electrical stimulation for pain, TENS is a reversible, nondestructive, benign form of treatment, with few contraindications or significant adverse effects. Over the past two decades, the applications of TENS have expanded and now include postoperative pain (135) as well as acute and chronic pain caused by musculoskeletal, neurologic, and even visceral pathology (75). TENS can be a useful routine part of a conservative pain management program, despite the fact that only a minority of patients with chronic, intractable pain problems such as the failed back surgery syndrome (FBSS) achieve adequate analgesia with TENS alone (31,67). It is also an important tool in evaluation of patients who are being considered for implanted devices. However, it is important to remember that although failure to respond to TENS may be significant, it does not preclude a favorable response to an implant. In fact, it is only after TENS fails to provide satisfactory relief of pain that an implant should be considered.

Contraindications and Precautions

Despite its general safety, there are only a few patients for whom pain management with TENS is contraindicated. These include:

1. Patients with an implanted cardiac pacemaker in "demand" mode. In these patients, the pacemaker may be inhibited if an artifactual signal is not recognized as such by the R wave sensing circuitry. Any implanted cardiac pacemaker should be considered a contraindication to treatment with electrical stimulation, unless special arrangements can be made for cardiac monitoring or the pacemaker can be operated at "fixed rate."

2. Pregnant patients. Since there have been relatively few studies of the use of TENS in pregnancy (and in labor and delivery) (75), its use in these patients should be avoided until more data are available.

3. Patients who are unable to operate the device.

Additionally, the following precautions should be observed when using TENS:

1. Placement of TENS electrodes over the eyes, or in contact with mucous membranes, may cause injury.

2. Placement of TENS electrodes over or near the carotid sinus may provoke hypotension and/or bradycardia, particularly in patients with cardiac or cerebrovascular disease.

3. Although there are no reports of complications in patients with cardiac arrhythmias, TENS electrodes should not be placed over the anterior chest. Similarly, cephalic application should be avoided in epilepsy and stroke patients.

4. Skin irritation, resulting from chemical, mechanical, and sometimes allergic reactions to the TENS electrodes, is common. Careful routine hygiene is essential to avoid or minimize skin problems.

PATIENT SELECTION FOR IMPLANTABLE STIMULATORS

Intractable pain problems that do not respond to more conservative measures, including TENS, may in some cases be treated with implanted stimulation devices. Implantable devices for pain control are used most successfully in a multidisciplinary, comprehensive pain program. In addition to the technological advances in hardware and technique made over the past two decades, significant refinements have been made in the diagnosis and treatment of chronic pain syndromes. Also, specialized programs for pain management have been developed (13). A particularly important change has been the recognition of psychological factors in comprehensive pain management and in selection of appropriate candidates for implantation of stimulation devices (24,73).

The following, current criteria for treatment with an implanted stimulation device have evolved empirically:

1. The pain has an objective basis (e.g., myelographically demonstrated arachnoid fibrosis). When patients' original studies and records are available for the FBSS, it may be apparent that the indications for the original surgery were questionable (72). If objective pathology is demonstrable later in such patients, the outcome of treatment will be less favorable.

2. Alternative standard therapies, such as medically indicated decompression, stabilization, and ablative procedures, have been attempted and failed or are unacceptable.

3. Psychiatric evaluation has demonstrated a motivated patient capable of long-term commitment to functional rehabilitation and without major psychiatric or personality disorder, issues of secondary gain, serious drug habituation problems, or other abnormal illness behavior.

4. The topography of pain and its underlying pathophysiology are amenable to stimulation analgesia (e.g., spinal cord stimulation for radicular thoracic or lumbosacral pain, thalamic nucleus ventralis posterolateralis stimulation for radicular pain, and periaqueductal gray (PAG) stimulation for diffuse or axial topographies or nociceptive pain.) In addition, axial low back pain may be treated by spinal cord stimulation in a select groups of patients, with specialized methods (59).

Patient Screening and Temporary Trials

When the above criteria are met, candidates are routinely screened for responsiveness before receiving an implanted stimulator. TENS, electrophysiologic testing (137), and diagnostic peripheral nerve blocks (89) may be helpful. Demonstration of pain relief, sometimes required by third party payers for reimbursement, may be accomplished by a trial with a temporary percutaneous electrode. It is possible to meet the requirement of demonstrable pain relief, at least technically, by implantation of a permanent system in a procedure in which the patient reports pain relief intraoperatively (37). However, this method can only result in a higher rate of treatment failures and subsequent need for removal of the device. Temporary trials, consequently, are preferable except in deep brain stimulation, open peripheral nerve electrode implantation, and laminectomy placement of spinal electrodes, where the logistics and the morbidity of insertion of new electrodes preclude a less invasive trial. Temporary percutaneous extension wires are used for testing these systems; they are removed when the system is internalized (or the electrode is removed if the trial is unsuccessful) in a second stage procedure. In addition to its usefulness in patient selection, an extended stimulation trial with a temporary percutaneous electrode has the following advantages: (a) It provides an opportunity to thoroughly evaluate a greater number of promising stimulation sites, over a greater period of time. If the electrode is placed so as to allow incremental percutaneous withdrawal, even more sites can be tested; (b) This approach allows assessment of pain relief under a variety of conditions and body positions, away from the time constraints of the operating room; (c) The experience gained during a temporary trial not only enhances the technical results of implantation of the permanent device, it also expedites the surgical procedure, lowering the risk of infection; and (d) It affords greater flexibility in hardware choices. For example, if a fully implanted, primary cell device is under consideration, its longevity may be inferred from measurements of stimulation current requirements and duty cycle, using the temporary electrode.

During percutaneous testing and at follow-up after permanent implantation of a device, the clinical outcome should be assessed in the most objective fashion possible. Placebo effect can be assessed by crossover periods without stimulation, clarifying the cause and effect of the relationship between treatment and reported relief of pain. If this crossover is chosen, it must be recognized that technically adequate stimulation produces paresthesias; thus, blinding the patient to control periods is difficult. Criteria both for placement of a permanent implant and for long-term assessment of the results of treatment include direct estimates of pain relief using standard rating scales; comparison with effects of prior treatments; and indirect measures of effectiveness such as analgesic use, functional activity levels, ongoing health care needs, and employment status. When feasible, this information should be collected from the patient by an independent evaluator. In everyday clinical practice, nursing notes and medication records may be helpful ancillary sources of information. The author's practice is to proceed to permanent implantation in patients who report at least 50% relief of pain while demonstrating commensurate functional improvement and stable or reduced medication requirements, over a 2- to 3-day inpatient trial with a temporary electrode. The trial may be extended on an outpatient basis when appropriate—for example, in a patient with a percutaneous epidural electrode that is to be removed, who has no risk factors for infection, who is sufficiently reliable and compliant to be followed as an outpatient, and in whom the short-term response to trial stimulation is equivocal. The incremental benefit of extended trials remains to be studied.

PERIPHERAL NERVE STIMULATION

In 1967, Wall and Sweet (138), reported on the first clinical application of the gate theory in which patients received stimulation of large diameter afferents to manage pain. In this initial study, electrodes were placed directly on peripheral nerves. For chronic stimulation, open surgical technique allows direct visualization for peripheral nerve electrode placement. When possible, the procedure is performed under local anesthesia to permit isolation of appropriate sensory fiber populations. Electrode arrays backed by Silastic and/or Dacron are usually used. Multichannel programmable devices, as used for spinal cord and deep brain stimulation, allow isolation of the desired sensory effect by permitting noninvasive selection of electrodes from an array even after permanent implantation. Although this does ameliorate some of the problems associated with permanent implantation, the threshold for motor effects may be critically close to the threshold for sensory effects in a mixed peripheral nerve. This limits the usefulness of these devices.

Indications

Peripheral nerve stimulation (PNS) is most effective for pain in the distribution of a single nerve, attributable to a pathology distal to an accessible electrode implantation site. Peripheral nerve trauma or entrapment, treated with electrodes implanted proximal to the site of injury, has been the most consistently successful application of this technique. In contrast, treatment of disorders in which pain (e.g., sciatica) is caused by lesions proximal to the site of stimulation (e.g., lumbosacral radiculopathy), is not generally successful (18,86). Some cases of reflex sympathetic dystrophy may respond, but operating on the afflicted limb, even proximally, may be problematic.

Results

In 1968, Sweet and Wepsic (128) reported on selected patients from a larger series with chronically implanted devices. At extended follow-up in 1976, 19 of 31 patients (61%) reported sustained benefit (130). Other investigators (18,57,71,104,105,137) have reported comparable results (45% to 79%) at follow-ups of up to 10 years.

SPINAL CORD STIMULATION

Spinal cord stimulation (SCS), typically delivered via longitudinally oriented electrode arrays in the dorsal epidural space, is the most common application of implanted neural stimulation devices. Early electrodes (120) were fixed, flat arrays that required a laminectomy for implantation under direct vision (88,129). In the typical patient with FBSS or postlaminectomy syndrome, electrodes were implanted at upper thoracic levels to provide stimulation coverage of all segments below the array. Such broad coverage was often accompanied by uncomfortable thoracic radicular stimulation, and electrodes placed more caudally, which afford more selective

stimulation of the painful segments, have proven to be more effective. Optimum placement of electrodes is facilitated by intraoperative feedback from the awake patient. Implantation under local anesthesia is therefore advisable. This is cumbersome, however, when laminectomy is required, and when the appropriate level of electrode placement for an individual patient is not known preoperatively. Percutaneous electrode placement allows longitudinal mapping to address these issues.

Indications

In addition to the general criteria listed above for implantation of a stimulation device for pain management, the following spinal disorders have been identified as specific indications for spinal cord stimulation. These are presented in decreasing order of application and reported success rates.

1. Lumbar arachnoiditis or lumbosacral spinal fibrosis, presenting as a subset of patients with FBSS, and radiculopathic pain, which ideally predominates over axial and mechanical pain.
2. Spinal cord lesions, in particular, posttraumatic lesions with intractable, well-circumscribed segmental pain. Diffuse pain below a complete lesion is generally unresponsive.
3. Patients without spinal disease or those with spinal disease who have coexisting causalgia, phantom limb or stump pain, peripheral neuropathy, or peripheral vascular disease with ischemic pain all are candidates for SCS.

A preimplantation trial with a temporary percutaneous electrode [to determine the proper level of electrode placement and to demonstrate the analgesic effect prior to permanent implantation (35)] is commonly considered adequate when satisfactory relief is achieved for at least 2 to 3 days. Although a simple monopolar electrode is satisfactory in most patients, it may not adequately predict the results of bipolar stimulation, which has technical advantages as the routine method of chronic implantation (58). Patients commonly report that the topography of stimulation changes following electrode implantation, when they are no longer in an artificial, prone position. Use of multicontact electrodes, which are less vulnerable to these effects, is therefore advantageous even in the percutaneous trial phase.

Techniques

The techniques developed for placement of percutaneous temporary electrodes evolved into methods for implantation of permanent electrodes which often did not require laminectomy. A disadvantage of these techniques, however, was that multiple, individually inserted electrodes often migrated spontaneously, both with respect to one another and with respect to the spinal cord, requiring surgical revision (92). Multiple electrode arrays that can be inserted via Tuohy needle, and improvements in electrode anchoring techniques, have helped to minimize migration (61,95,99). In addition, programmable implanted pulse generators, which take full advantage of these arrays by noninvasively selecting combinations of stimulating anodes and cathodes, now permit optimization of the topography of stimulation coverage after surgery. Even hardware failures such as electrode migration may be amenable to noninvasive correction with these versatile devices.

There may be technical difficulties associated with the use of percutaneously inserted electrodes. In patients with prior laminectomy or with epidural scarring at the level of proposed electrode placement, and in those in whom the technical difficulty of percutaneous electrode insertion is confirmed at a trial procedure with a temporary electrode, implantation of fixed endodural and epidural electrode arrays (Fig. 1) via laminectomy should be considered. Although the risk of longitudinal migration with this technique is minimal, lateral migration or malpositioning is quite possible. For the typical FBSS patient, however, in whom postsurgical scarring is caudal to the usual T8-T11 electrode site, percutaneous placement is straightforward. As mentioned, currently available multiple electrode arrays, designed for insertion via Tuohy needle, are more resistant to migration (and immune, of course, to migration of one electrode with respect to another). Complemented by multichannel, programmable implants, which permit noninvasive

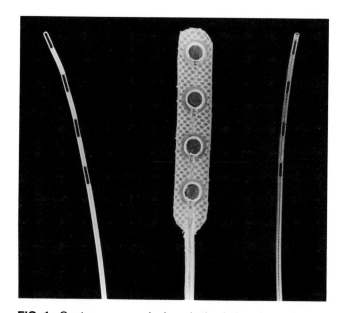

FIG. 1. Contemporary spinal cord stimulation electrodes are arrays with multiple contacts. Some require laminectomy; others may be placed percutaneously, through a Tuohy needle.

postoperative adjustments of stimulating electrode location, these rarely require surgical revision (93,99). By comparison with single-channel devices, these systems have a significantly lower electromechanical failure rate and significantly better long-term clinical results (99).

Results

The results of spinal cord stimulation for FBSS have been reported in a large number of series, summarized in Table 1. A variety of outcome measures have been used to evaluate the results; in general, at follow-up periods of up to twenty years (99), good or excellent results (i.e., at least 50% pain relief reported) have been obtained in most patients.

Outcomes have been reported not only in terms of pain relief and patient satisfaction, but also in terms of quality of life as reflected in activities of daily living, medication requirements, and neurologic function. Figure 2 presents our experience with a series of FBSS patients, followed for 5 years by disinterested third party interview.

Our retrospectively reviewed experience with SCS for FBSS (97) compares favorably with our experiences with repeated operation (96) and ablative surgery [dorsal root ganglionectomy (94) and radiofrequency (RF) facet denervation (100)]. Accordingly, we have undertaken a prospective, randomized study comparing SCS with reoperation. Patients who are candidates for the latter are randomly assigned to a trial of SCS first, proceeding to a permanent implant if the results are satisfactory, and crossing over to reoperation if the results prove unsatisfactory. Conversely, patients assigned to reoperation may cross over to SCS if postoperative pain warrants it. To date, results for this outcome measure (one among many to be compared) have been significantly better for SCS than for reoperation (101).

Complications

Major complications of SCS are rare; spinal cord injury and spinal infections have been reported in the literature in small numbers. The most common complications have been technical; most common of all has been electrode migration or malposition, so that stimulation paresthesias do not overlap the patient's distribution of pain. It can be difficult to distinguish electrode migration, unless radiographically obvious, from malposition. In either case, stimulation paresthesias do not satisfactorily overlap the patient's distribution of pain, and surgical revision of lead position is required. Figure 3 presents a Kaplan-Meier survival analysis, in which the statistical endpoint is a return to the operating room for surgical revision of electrode position; the two events are equivalent by this measure. Contemporary multicontact elec-

TABLE 1. *Comparison of studies*

Author (ref.)	Number implanted	Number screened	Number FBSS	Follow-up range
Bel, Bauer (9)	14	—	14	—
Blond et al. (10)	58	59	59	12–72 mo
Blume et al. (11)	20	—	20	up to 3 yr
Broseta et al. (14)	11	—	—	3–20 mo
Burton (15)	75	0	55	(Psych)
Burton (16)	198	—	186	—
Clark (22)	13	—	6	(Psych, TENS)
De la Porte, Siegfried (25)	36	94	36	3–96 mo
De la Porte, Van de Kleft (26)	64	78	78	1–7 yr
de Vera et al. (27)	110	124	18	(Psych, TENS × 1 mo)
Demirel et al. (28)	33	48	11	2–5 yr
Devulder et al. (29)	45	—	23	—
Devulder et al. (30)	69	—	43	up to 8 yr
Erickson, Long (36)	70	10	—	up to 10 yr
Hoppenstein (44)	27	—	12	(Obj dx, psych, TENS)
Hunt et al. (49)	13	—	5	9 mo–4 yr
Kälin, Winkelmüller (51)	—	—	77	—
Koeze et al. (52)	26	0	5	—
Krainick, Thoden (53)	91	126	5	up to 5 yr
Kumar et al. (55)	60	—	54	6–60 mo
Kumar et al. (56)	94	121	56	6 mo–10 yr
Law et al. (58)	81	—	—	—
Leclercq, Russo (60)	20	—	20	1– >24 mo
LeDoux, Langford (62)	26	32	32	up to 5 yr
LeRoy (64)	49	—	49	1–63 mo
Long, Erickson (68)	69	—	54	12–35 mo
Long et al. (71)	31	—	24	4–7 yr
McCarron, Racz (82)	22	—	—	3–24 mo
Meglio et al. (83)	64	109	19	(Psych)
Meilman et al. (84)	12	20	20	up to 3.5 yr
Mittal et al. (87)	26	31	21	—
Nielson et al. (91)	130	221	79	1– >35 mo
North et al. (97)	50	54	50	—
North et al. (100)	171	205	153	2–20 yr
Pineda (106)	76	—	56	—
Racz et al. (109)	26	0	18	12–42.7 mo
Ray et al. (111)	78	—	50	3–64 mo
Richardson et al. (114)	22	36	12	1–3 yr
Richardson, Shatin (113)	136	—	136	—
Robb, Robb (116)	79	65	22	6 mo–5 yr
Sanchez-Ledesma et al. (118)	33	49	0	—
Shatin et al. (119)	116	—	—	0.9–13.3 mo
Shealy (121)	80	0	—	7 mo–?
Shelden et al. (122)	27	—	3	—
Siegfried, Lazorthes (123)	89	191	75	1–8 yr
Simpson (124)	56	24	7	2 wk–9 yr
Spiegelmann, Friedman (126)	30	43	18	3–33 mo
Sweet, Wepsic (130)	98	100	33	(Psych)
Urban, Nashold (134)	7	20	9	—
Vogel et al. (137)	27	50	29	>3 yr
Waisbrod, Gerbershagen (138)	16	—	16	6–30 mo
Winkelmüller (140)	71	94	56	4 mo–7 yr
Young, Shende (142)	27	—	17	16–51 mo
Young (143)	51	14	25	12–67 mo

FBSS, failed back surgery syndrome; Psych, psychiatric testing done; Obj dx, objective diagnosis.
Modified and reproduced from North et al. (99), with permission.

of spinal cord stimulation for FBSS

Follow-up mean	Excellent/Good results (>= 50% relief)	Excellent/Good FBSS results	Third party follow-up
2 yr	60%	60%	
37 mo	89.5%	89.5%	
	70%	70%	
13 mo	64%		
1 yr	59%		y(mfr.)
	43%		
	54%	67%	
36 mo	60%		
4 yr	55%	55%	
	75%		
	18%		
	78%		
	55%		
	15–20%		y(60)
	58%	64%	
	15–31%	20–60%	
	88%	88%	
28 mo	46–62%		y
	18%		
	62%		
40 mo	66%		y
	36–80%		
	50%	50%	
	76% at 1 yr	76% at 1 yr	
30.7 mo	60%		n
	18%		y
	73% at 3 yr		y
	68%		
		23%	n
	60%	60%	
	46%		
	49%	46%	y
5 yr	47%	47%	y
7.1 yr	52%		y
	43%	43%	
	65%		n
19.4 mo	49%		
	56%		
45 mo	67%	67%	y (mfr.)
	72%	69%	
5.5 yr	57%		
	74% at 6 mo		y (mfr.)
	25%	15–45%	n
		67%	
~ 4 yr	37%		
29 mo	47%		
13 mo	60%		y
	21–42%	15–45%	y
	86%		
	18.6%		n
16 mo	75%		n
		69%	
	66% >= 50%		
38 mo	65% >= 50%		

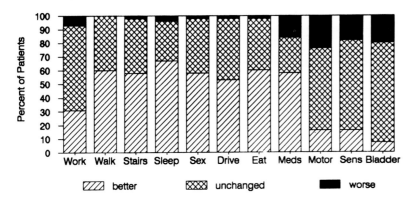

FIG. 2. A majority of patients with failed back surgery syndrome report improvement in many activities of daily living following spinal cord stimulation. Most have reported a decrease in daily medication usage. Neurologic symptoms progress infrequently and independently of treatment. Reproduced from North et al. (97), with permission.

trodes, supported by programmable, multicontact implanted pulse generators, require revision significantly less often than do nonprogrammable, single-channel devices. This translates into significantly better clinical results, as shown in Figure 4.

It has been proven empirically that patient perception of stimulation paresthesias, corresponding to the topography of pain, is a necessary condition for pain relief by somatosensory stimulators (peripheral nerve, spinal cord, and thalamic electrodes). In order to achieve specific stimulation coverage without uncomfortable sensory, reflex, or direct motor effects, careful attention must be paid to the position of surgically implanted electrodes (58). In any given patient, the final choice of stimulation parameters represents a compromise, and stimulation analgesia is often incomplete. At thoracic spinal cord levels, where electrodes are commonly placed to achieve coverage of multiple caudal segments, radicular thoracic effects may predominate. Anatomic factors contributing to these effects include (a) the proximity of entering dorsal root fibers to dorsal epidural stimulating electrodes; (b) the relatively superficial location of these

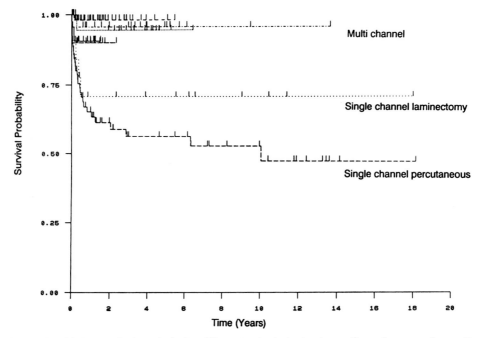

FIG. 3. Kaplan-Meier survival analysis for different spinal electrode configurations used over the past two decades. Technical failure requiring return to the operating room for surgical revision of electrode position is the statistical endpoint for this analysis. The uppermost curves represent contemporary multicontact percutaneous and laminectomy electrodes, which have been significantly more reliable than any bipolar single-channel configuration. The lowermost curve, which shows eventual technical failure in a majority of patients, represents dual, independently inserted percutaneous electrodes, which were vulnerable to longitudinal migration with respect to the spinal cord and with respect to one another. The middle curve represents bipolar electrodes implanted by laminectomy. Neither of these single-channel systems allowed noninvasive adjustment of anode and cathode positions. Reproduced form North et al. (99), with permission.

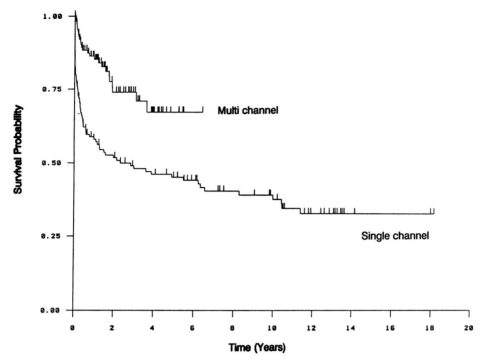

FIG. 4. Kaplan-Meier statistical analysis of the clinical reliability of single-channel and multichannel systems. The endpoint is a clinical failure, defined as patient no longer using device for pain control, for any reason. This includes electromechanical failure of the device without replacement, and failure of the device to relieve pain (which may occur without technical failure). Programmable, multichannel systems have been significantly more reliable ($p < 0.001$). Reproduced from North et al. (99), with permission.

fibers, within a few segments of their entry, in the dorsal columns (34); and (c) decreases in the mean diameter of fibers in fasciculus gracilis at cephalad levels (102).

Voltage and current profiles, which correspond well with *in vitro* measurements in primate and cadaver spinal cords for electrode configurations currently in clinical use (117), have been determined by finite element modeling of electrical fields applied to the spinal cord and surrounding structures (23,43). This model only addresses cathodal excitatory effects, however, and nerve stimulation does not necessarily result in excitation (110). In fact, with appropriate electrode geometries and stimulation waveforms, the result may be inhibition, blockade, or even unidirectional action potential propagation (134). In addition, specific subpopulations of fibers of varying diameters may be selectively stimulated (2).

DEEP BRAIN STIMULATION

The analgesic effects of stimulation via stereotaxic brain electrodes were first discovered about 30 years ago. Pool (108) and Heath and Mickle (41) reported on implants in human supraoptic nuclei and the septal area, and Mazars et al. (80) reported the successful treatment of deafferentation pain by stimulation of the spinotha-

lamic fasciculus. In the following years, similar successes were achieved by stimulation of specific sensory nuclei (45,81) and by stimulation of the internal capsule (3,39,45).

PAG stimulation was also found to have antinociceptive effects, first described by Reynolds in 1969 (112). In 1973, specific opiate receptors were discovered in the central nervous system (103) and were found in high concentration in PAG (54). These findings gave new impetus to studies of PAG stimulation. In animals, the phenomenon of stimulus-produced analgesia involves a descending inhibitory pathway, extending through the dorsolateral quadrant of the spinal cord. Reversal of the analgesic effects by the narcotic antagonist naloxone and the development of tolerance, with cross-tolerance to morphine, have both been described (7,66,76–79). The analgesic effect has been reported to be naloxone-reversible in humans as well (4,46). There are some reports of elevation of beta-endorphin levels in cerebrospinal fluid (5,47,146), thought at one time to be caused by an artifact produced by contrast ventriculography (32,38). Whether analgesia is mediated directly by endogenous opiate release or some other effect of stimulation, remains a matter of controversy. Nonetheless, the method has enjoyed continued clinical success in the management of chronic benign pain as well as cancer pain (33,48,113,143,144). Use of additional sites, for example the nuclei of Kölliker-Fuse, has been reported (42).

Indications

1. Deafferentation pain syndromes. These syndromes, treated by thalamic electrode placement, include chronic lumbosacral radiculopathy, pain of spinal cord injury, postcordotomy dysesthesia, and brachial or lumbosacral plexus lesions.

2. Nociceptive pain syndromes. These syndromes, treated by PAG electrode placement, include chronic axial low back pain (exclusive of radiculopathic/deafferentation pain) and cancer pain (exclusive of gross infiltration of the peripheral nervous system causing deafferentation pain). Pain responsive to narcotics, as determined by a morphine infusion test (48), may be an additional indication for deep brain stimulation (DBS), but this test may not be specific (145).

Techniques

Under local anesthesia, electrode implantation is performed stereotaxically, using standard ventriculographic or computed tomographic techniques (Fig. 5). In patients with unilateral, deafferentation pain, the electrode is placed in the contralateral sensory thalamus [in the ventral posterolateral (VPL) or ventral posteromedial (VPM) nucleus], depending on pain topography. Recording thalamic single unit activity is helpful in defining the target (63). Contralateral PAG or periventricular gray (PVG) is also accessible through the same burr hole. Once the electrodes have been placed, stimulation is delivered via percutaneous test leads to representative electrode combinations to assess patient response. If stimulation is ineffective, the electrode array is easily removed under local anesthesia. When stimulation is effective, analgesia may persist in some patients for 24 hours or more following stimulation. Since new electrode combinations may be assessed only when the patient's pain has returned, the number of combinations that may be tested acutely is limited for these patients. Once satisfactory stimulation analgesia is achieved, the system is adapted for chronic use by connection, under general anesthesia, of the existing electrodes to subcutaneously implanted electronics.

Results

A number of criteria have been used to analyze the results of treatment with DBS. Both direct estimates and indirect indicators of pain relief (such as analgesic use, patterns of stimulator use, functional capacity, and employment status) have been used. Young et al. (143) reviewed literature reports from 13 centers and found that

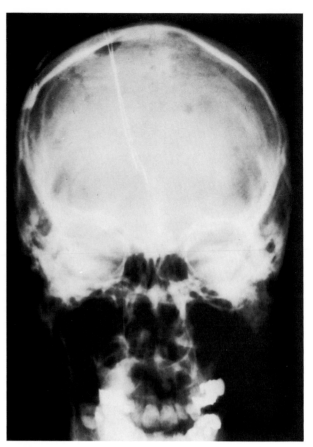

FIG. 5. Intracerebral electrodes are placed by standard stereotactic methods, via a frontal burr hole, where they are secured and connected to a pulse generator for use by the patient.

overall DBS was successful in 57% of 698 chronic pain patients treated with electrical stimulation of the brain. Thalamic stimulation was reported effective in from 50% (22) to 80% (123) of patients, and PAG/PVG stimulation was effective in from 0% (6) to 90% (12) of patients. In the most recent literature on the treatment of cancer pain with these techniques, success is reported in 70% to 76% of patients (48,144).

Complications

The complications of the procedure, and their frequency of occurrence in the largest published series (48,65,107,143), include:

1. Intracranial hemorrhage (2% to 4%), which is potentially fatal (0% to 2%). Accordingly, patients should be screened rigorously for clotting abnormalities, particularly if DBS is being considered for cancer pain.

2. Infection (3% to 6%), which may require removal of implanted hardware. The use of programmable, multichannel implants minimizes the duration of the

test phase with percutaneous leads, reducing the risk of infection.

3. Eye movement abnormalities (2% to 4%), which are not likely to occur when the tip of the electrode remains rostral to the iter of the aqueduct of Sylvius.

4. Hardware failures (2% to 12%), ranging from migration of implanted electrodes to electromechanical and electronic failures, which may require reoperation. Programmable, multichannel devices permit noninvasive adjustments to correct for certain faults, such as electrode migration or malposition, and to optimize therapeutic effects and minimize the side effects of stimulation. Histologic analysis of autopsy material has shown no deleterious effects, such as gliosis or parenchymal reaction along the trajectories or at the tips of the electrodes (8).

DBS represents a reversible, nonablative technique for central deafferentation pain states. Although associated with some serious complications, it represents a worthwhile alternative in patients refractory to PNS or SCS.

IMPLANTED STIMULATION DEVICES

The typical neural stimulation device, which has been implanted in a large population of patients over the past two decades, is shown in Figure 6. It is a passive RF re-

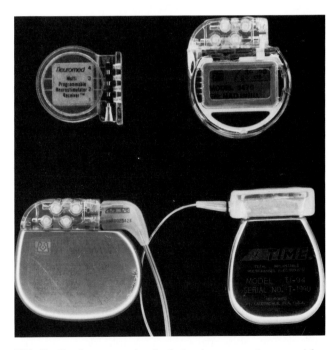

FIG. 6. Contemporary implanted pulse generators used for spinal cord stimulation allow noninvasive assignment of anode and cathode positions from an array of multiple electrodes. Some require or accept power from an externally worn device; others are powered by implanted primary cells (visible in this figure); one can use power from either source.

ceiver, with no battery or life-limiting components, and it functions only when powered by an external transmitter. The transmitter emits RF bursts of 455 kHz to 2 MHz. The stimulation waveform delivered to the electrodes by the implanted receiver (which functions as a simple AM demodulator) is determined by the amplitude, duration, and frequency (repetition rate) of these bursts. These stimulation parameters are adjusted by physician and patient to optimize analgesic effect.

As mentioned earlier, advances in cardiac pacemaker technology (primarily improvements in lithium batteries permitting lifespans of a decade for a pacemaker powered by a primary cell) fueled development of totally implanted neural stimulation devices. External hardware, required for control, commonly includes a permanent magnet for simple adjustments by the patient and a dedicated programming unit for a full range of adjustments by a physician. At present, primary cell devices are limited to fixed menus of stimulation parameters and do not have the flexibility (in accommodating novel stimulation regimes) of passive, RF-powered implants. In spinal applications, where energy requirements often exceed those of cardiac pacing by two orders of magnitude, currently available primary cell devices may not have acceptable longevity. In PAG stimulation, on the other hand, requirements are commonly restricted to a small charge per phase, at a low rate, with a duty cycle of minutes per day. These conditions are well within the design specifications of totally implanted neural stimulation devices for a lifespan of several years. Automatic cycling on and off (made possible because of the latency of analgesic effect after the stimulator is turned on and its persistence after the device is turned off) is one of the strategies for maximizing battery life.

In the past, with single-channel devices, variation of stimulation could be accomplished only by surgical revision. One of the greatest advantages of the latest, "multichannel" generation of devices is noninvasive selection of stimulating anode(s) and cathode(s) from an array of four to eight electrodes. This is a particularly important feature, since electrode position is a major determinant of the topography of stimulation paresthesias, and correspondence of topography with the patient's painful areas is important for maximum analgesic effect of all somatosensory stimulators (TENS, PNS, SCS, thalamic). In reported clinical applications to date, multichannel systems have been used not only to vary cathode position to optimize coverage (58), but also to achieve specific configurations of anodes and cathodes more complex than dipoles. A disproportionate number of SCS patients prefer "split anode" or "guarded cathode" configurations (95), presumably because of a favorable current distribution (23,43).

As a result of the greater flexibility and redundancy of current multichannel devices, implantation has been expedited, technical success and clinical results have been enhanced, and the number of failures requiring surgical revision has fallen dramatically. The cost of increases in the flexibility and number of stimulation channels, however, is greater complexity in the task of adjustment and electrode selection (e.g., testing the 50 working combinations of anodes and cathodes possible with four electrodes). General guidelines for determining the number of combinations are:

1. From an array of (n) electrodes, where n ≥ 2, the possible combinations of (m) active and (n − m) inactive electrodes is C(n,m) = n!/(n − m)!m!.

2. For each combination of m active electrodes, there are 2^m possible selections of anode(s) and cathode(s). This number includes two open circuit configurations (all anodes, all cathodes), and the number of useful configurations, therefore, is 2^{m-2}.

3. In aggregate, the number of unique electrode combinations totals:

$$\sum_{m=2}^{n} (2^m - 2)/(n - m)!m!$$

For example, four electrodes provide 50 combinations (12 + 24 + 14), and eight electrodes provide 6050 combinations (56 + 336 + 980 + 680 + 1736 + 1008 + 254).

If biphasic stimulation (alternating complementary electrode combinations) is considered, these figures increase by 50%.

As can be seen, increasing the number of available channels may make the task of thoroughly evaluating potentially useful electrode combinations impractical. Fortunately, in routine clinical practice, determination of appropriate commercial transmitter settings rarely requires exhaustive assessment of all possible combinations. In theory and in practice, electrode combinations that differ only in minor ways (addition or deletion of one among multiple anodes, for example) are often functionally equivalent and therefore redundant.

As with postoperative (and even intraoperative) adjustment of stimulation amplitude and pulse repetition rate, the patient (given appropriate means of control, constraints, supervision, and data collection) ultimately makes the decisions about electrode selection. To enhance this process, we have developed a personal computer interface to standard RF-coupled implants, with supporting user-friendly, expert system software for direct patient interaction (98) The system incorporates commercially available RF transmitters, and the pulse parameters available from the system are the same as those available from a transmitter in its usual, freestanding mode of operation. The computer and interface simply enhance selection of optimal settings by allowing automatic, rapid switching among standard pulse parameters. As illustrated in Figure 7, the patient uses simple controls designed for greater ease of operation than

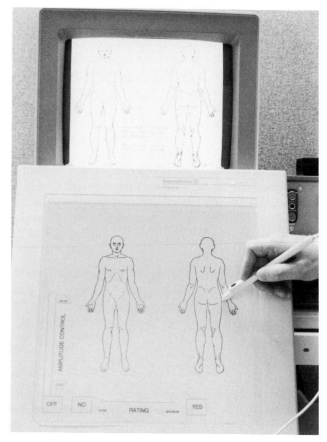

FIG. 7. Our patients use a graphics tablet and a contemporary personal computer to control standard radiofrequency-coupled spinal cord stimulation implants. This system's controls have been developed for easier operation than the available standard unit. "Pain drawings," corresponding drawings of the location of stimulation paresthesias, and associated 100 mm visual analog ratings are entered directly by the patient. Quantitative measures of stimulator performance are derived, to select settings for everyday clinical use. From North et al. (98).

those of the standard transmitter. Patient responses and impressions are entered through similar controls and through a simple graphics tablet which conveys topographic data. Comparisons of the perceived location of stimulation paresthesias with a patient's recorded pain topography may be made rapidly, automatically, and systematically, and psychophysical thresholds may be reproducibly determined. Protocols of varying complexity, which present stimulation parameters in random or pseudorandom order, may be implemented as required for each patient, and for each application.

With the computer interface, it is possible to change stimulation pulse parameters (amplitude, width, interpulse interval) and cathode or anode positions in as little as 1 millisecond. This is useful for research, and it permits, for example, interleaving pulses delivered from different electrode combinations with complementary effects. The system also allows modulation of pulse parameters in simple, deterministic patterns [as described in the literature on TENS (74)] as well as modulation by any scheme that may be coded in system software.

CONCLUSIONS

In appropriately selected patients, neural stimulation for chronic, intractable pain is used with increasing success. Although the precise mechanisms by which pain relief is achieved is only poorly understood, simple, monotonic sequences of pulses, of simple rectangular shape, delivered via simple electrode geometries, have been applied to complex neural systems with remarkable empirical success. Future advances in this form of treatment may come in the form of manipulation of the literally infinite number of possible stimulation regimens. The technology is now available to pursue both basic and clinical research to optimize this form of treatment.

REFERENCES

1. Abram S, Reynolds A, Cusick J (1981): Failure of naloxone to reverse analgesia from transcutaneous electrical stimulation in patients with chronic pain. *Anesth Analg* 60(2):81–84.
2. Accornero N, Bini G, Lenzi G, Manfredi M (1977): Selective activation of peripheral nerve fibre groups of different diameter by triangular shaped stimulus pulses. *J Physiol* 273:539–560.
3. Adams JE, Hosobuchi Y, Fields HL (1974): Stimulation of the internal capsule for relief of chronic pain. *J Neurosurg* 41:740–744.
4. Adams JE (1976): Naloxone reversal of analgesia produced by brain stimulation in the human. *Pain* 2:161–166.
5. Akil H, Richardson DE, Hughes J (1978): Enkephalin-like material elevated in ventricular cerebrospinal fluid of pain patients after analgetic local stimulation. *Science* 201:463–465.
6. Amano K, Kitamura K, Kawamura H (1980): Alterations of immunoreactive β-endorphin in the third ventricular fluid in response to electrical stimulation of the human periaqueductal gray matter. *Appl Neurophysiol* 43:150–158.
7. Basbaum AI, Fields HL (1978): Endogenous pain control mechanisms: review and hypothesis. *Ann Neurol* 4:451–462.
8. Baskin DS, Mehler WR, Hosobuchi Y, Richardson D, Adams J, Flitter M (1986): Autopsy analysis of the safety, efficacy and cartography of electrical stimulation of the central gray in humans. *Brain Res* 371:231–236.
9. Bel S, Bauer BL (1991): Dorsal column stimulation (DCS): cost to benefit analysis. *Acta Neurochir* 52(suppl):121–123.
10. Blond S, Armignies P, Parker F, Dupard T, Guieu JD, Duquesnoy B, Christiaens JL (1991): Sciatalges chroniques par désafférentation sensitive près chirurgie de la hernie discale lombaire: aspects cliniques et thérapeutiques. *Neurochirurgie* 37:86–95.
11. Blume H, Richardson R, Rojas C (1982): Epidural nerve stimulation of the lower spinal cord and cauda equina for the relief of intractable pain in failed back surgery. *Appl Neurophysiol* 45:456–460.
12. Boivie J, Meyerson BA (1982): A correlative anatomical and clinical study of pain suppression by deep brain stimulation. *Pain* 3:113–126.
13. Bonica JJ (1977): Basic principles in managing chronic pain. *Arch Surg* 112:783–788.
14. Broseta J, Roldan P, Gonzales-Darder J, Bordes V, Garcia-Salorio JL (1982): Chronic epidural dorsal column stimulation in the treatment of causalgic pain. *Appl Neurophysiol* 45:190–194.
15. Burton C (1975): Dorsal column stimulation: optimization of application. *Surg Neurol* 4:171–176.
16. Burton CV (1977): Session on spinal cord stimulation: safety and clinical efficacy. *Neurosurgery* 1:164–165.
17. Campbell J, Taub A (1973): Local analgesia from percutaneous electrical stimulation. *Arch Neurol* 28:347–350.
18. Campbell JN, Long DM (1976): Peripheral nerve stimulation in the treatment of intractable pain. *J Neurosurg* 45:692–699.
19. Campbell JN, Meyer RA (1986): Primary afferents and hyperalgesia. In: Yaksh TL, ed. *Spinal afferent processing.* New York: Plenum, pp 59–81.
20. Campbell JN, Davis KD, Meyer RA, North RB (1990): The mechanism by which dorsal column stimulation affects pain: evidence for a new hypothesis. *Pain* 5:S228.
21. Chapman C, Benedetti C (1977): Analgesia following transcutaneous electrical stimulation and its partial reversal by a narcotic antagonist. *Life Sci* 21:1645–1648.
22. Clark K (1975): Electrical stimulation of the nervous system for control of pain: University of Texas Southwestern Medical School experience. *Surg Neurol* 4:164–166.
23. Coburn B, Sin W (1985): A theoretical study of epidural electrical stimulation of the spinal cord. Part I: Finite element analysis of stimulus fields. *Biomed Engineer* 32(11):971–977.
24. Daniel M, Long C, Hutcherson M, Hunter S (1985): Psychological factors and outcome of electrode implantation for chronic pain. *Neurosurgery* 17(5):773–777.
25. De la Porte C, Siegfried J (1983): Lumbosacral spinal fibrosis (spinal arachnoiditis): its diagnosis and treatment by spinal cord stimulation. *Spine* 8(6):593–603.
26. De la Porte C, Van de Kelft E (1993): Spinal cord stimulation in failed back surgery syndrome. *Pain* 52:55–61.
27. de Vera JA, Rodriguez JL, Dominguez M, Robaina F (1990): Spinal cord stimulation for chronic pain mainly in PVD, vasospastic disorders of the upper limbs and failed back surgery. *Pain* 5(suppl.):S81.
28. Demirel T, Braun W, Reimers CD (1984): Results of spinal cord stimulation in patients suffering from chronic pain after a two year observation period. *Neurochirurgia* 27:47–50.
29. Devulder J, De Colvenaer L, Rolly G, Caemaert J, Calliauw L (1990): Spinal cord stimulation and the relief of chronic nonmalignant pain in 45 patients. *Pain* 5:S236.
30. Devulder J, DeColvenaer L, Rolly G, Caemaert J, Calliauw L, Martens F (1991): Spinal cord stimulation in chronic pain therapy. *Clin J Pain* 6:51–56.
31. Deyo R (1990): A controlled trial of transcutaneous electrical nerve stimulation (TENS) and exercise for chronic low back pain. *N Engl J Med* 322:1405–1411.
32. Dionne RA, Muller GP, Young RF, Greenberg P, Hargreaves KM, Gracely R, Dubner R (1980): Contrast medium causes the apparent increase in β-endorphin levels in human cerebrospinal fluid following brain stimulation. *Pain* 20:313–321.
33. Duncan GH, Bushnell MC, Marchand S (1991): Deep brain stimulation: a review of basic research and clinical articles. *Pain* 45:49–59.
34. Dyck PJ, Lais A, Karnes J, Sparks M, Dyck PJB (1985): Peripheral axotomy induces neurofilament decrease, atrophy, demyelination and degeneration of root and fasciculus gracilis fibers. *Brain Res* 340:19–36.
35. Erickson DL (1975): Percutaneous trial of stimulation for patient selection for implantable stimulating devices. *J Neurosurg* 43:440–444.
36. Erickson DL, Long DM (1983): Ten-year follow-up of dorsal column stimulation. In: Bonica JJ, ed. *Advances in pain research and therapy*, vol. 5. New York: Raven Press, pp. 583–589.
37. Feler C, Kaufman S (1992): Spinal cord stimulation: one stage? *Acta Neurochir* 117:91.
38. Fessler RG, Brown FD, Rachlin JR, Mullan S (1984): Elevated β-endorphin in cerebrospinal fluid after electrical brain stimulation: artifact of contrast infusion. *Science* 224:1017–1019.
39. Fields HL, Adams JE (1974): Pain after cortical injury relieved by electrical stimulation of the internal capsule. *Brain* 97:169–178.
40. Freeman TB, Campbell JN, Long DM (1983): Naloxone does not affect pain relief induced by electrical stimulation in man. *Pain* 17:189–195.
41. Heath R, Mickle WA (1960): Evaluation of seven years experience with depth electrode studies in human patients. In: Ramey

ER, ed. *Electrical studies on the unanesthetized brain*, pp. 214–247.

42. Hodge CJ, Apkarian AV, Stevens RT (1986): Inhibition of dorsal-horn cell responses by stimulation of the Kölliker-Fuse nucleus. *J Neurosurg* 65:825–833.

43. Holsheimer J, Strujik JJ, Rijkhoff NJM (1991): Contact combinations in epidural spinal cord stimulation: a comparison by computer modeling. *Stereotact Funct Neurosurg* 56:220–233.

44. Hoppenstein R (1975): Percutaneous implantation of chronic spinal cord electrodes for control of intractable pain: preliminary report. *Surg Neurol* 4:195–198.

45. Hosobuchi Y, Adams JE, Rutkin B (1975): Chronic thalamic and internal capsule stimulation for the control of central pain. *Surg Neurol* 4:91–92.

46. Hosobuchi Y, Adams JE, Linchitz R (1977): Pain relief by electrical stimulation of the central gray matter in humans and its reversal by naloxone. *Science* 197:183–186.

47. Hosobuchi Y, Rossier J, Bloom FE, Guilleman R (1979): Stimulation of human periaqueductal gray for pain relief increases immunoreactive β-endorphin in ventricular fluid. *Science* 203:279–281.

48. Hosobuchi Y (1986): Subcortical electrical stimulation for control of intractable pain in humans. Report of 122 cases (1970–1984). *J Neurosurg* 64:543–553.

49. Hunt WE, Goodman JH, Bingham WG (1975): Stimulation of the dorsal spinal cord for treatment of intractable pain: a preliminary report. *Surg Neurol* 4:153–156.

50. Ignelzi RJ, Nyquist JK (1976): Excitability changes in peripheral nerve fibers after repetitive electrical stimulation. *J Neurosurg* 45:59–165.

51. Kälin M-T, Winkelmüller W (1990): Chronic pain after multiple lumbar discectomies—Significance of intermittent spinal cord stimulation. *Pain* 5:S241.

52. Koeze TH, Williams AC, Reiman S (1987): Spinal cord stimulation and the relief of chronic pain. *J Neurol Neurosurg Psych* 50:1424–1429.

53. Krainick JU, Thoden U (1989): Dorsal column stimulation. In: Wall PD, Melzack R, eds. *Textbook of pain*. New York: Churchill Livingstone, pp. 701–705.

54. Kuhar M, Pert C, Snyder S (1973): Regional distribution of opiate receptor binding in monkey and human brain. *Brain* 245:447.

55. Kumar K, Wyant GM, Ekong CEU (1986): Epidural spinal cord stimulation for relief of chronic pain. *The Pain Clinic* 1(2):91–99.

56. Kumar K, Nath R, Wyant GM (1991): Treatment of chronic pain by epidural spinal cord stimulation: a 10-year experience. *J Neurosurg* 5:402–407.

57. Law JD, Swett J, Kirsch WM (1980): Retrospective analysis of 22 patients with chronic pain treated by peripheral nerve stimulation. *J Neurosurg* 45:692–699.

58. Law J (1983): Spinal stimulation: statistical superiority of monophasic stimulation of narrowly separated, longitudinal bipoles having rostral cathodes. *Appl Neurophys* 46:129–137.

59. Law JD, Kirkpatrick AF (1991): Pain management update: spinal cord stimulation. *Am J Pain Manage* 2:34–42.

60. Leclercq T, Russo E (1981): La stimulation epidurale dans le traitement el doleurs chroniques. *Neurochirurgie* 27:125–128.

61. Leclercq TA (1984): Electrode migration in epidural stimulation: comparison between single electrode and four electrode programmable leads. *Pain* 20(suppl. 2):78.

62. LeDoux MS, Langford KH (1993): Spinal cord stimulation for the failed back syndrome. *Spine* 18:191–194.

63. Lenz FA, Dostrovsky JO, Tasker RR, Yamashiro I, Kwan HC, Murphy JT (1988): Methods for microstimulation and recording of single neurons and evoked potentials in the human central nervous system. *J Neurosurg* 68:630–634.

64. LeRoy PL (1981): Stimulation of the spinal cord by biocompatible electrical current in the human. *Appl Neurophysiol* 44:187–193.

65. Levy RM, Lamb S, Adams JE (1987): Treatment of chronic pain by deep brain stimulation: Long-term follow-up and review of the literature. *Neurosurgery* 21:885–893.

66. Liebeskind JC, Guilbaud G, Besson JM, et al. (1973): Analgesia from electrical stimulation of the periaqueductal gray matter in the cat: behavioral observations and inhibitory effects on spinal cord interneurons. *Brain Res* 40:441–446.

67. Loeser JD, Black RG, Christman A (1975): Relief of pain by transcutaneous stimulation. *J Neurosurg* 42:308–314.

68. Long DM, Erickson DE (1975): Stimulation of the posterior columns of the spinal cord for relief of intractable pain. *Surg Neurol* 4:134–141.

69. Long DM (1976): Cutaneous afferent stimulation for relief of chronic pain. *Clin Neurosurg* 21:257–268.

70. Long D (1977): Electrical stimulation for the control of pain. *Arch Surg* 112:884–888.

71. Long DM, Erickson D, Campbell J, North R (1981): Electrical stimulation of the spinal cord and peripheral nerves for pain control. *Appl Neurophysiol* 44:207–217.

72. Long DM, Filtzer DL, BenDebba M, Hendler NH (1988): Clinical features of the failed-back syndrome. *J Neurosurg* 69:61–71.

73. Long DM (1991): A review of psychological considerations in the neurosurgical management of chronic pain: a neurosurgeon's perspective. *Neurosurg Quart* 1:185–195.

74. Mannheimer C, Carlsson CA (1979): The analgesic effect of transcutaneous electrical nerve stimulation (TNS) in patients with rheumatoid arthritis: a comparative study of different pulse patterns. *Pain* 6:329–334.

75. Mannheimer JS, Lampe GN (1984): *Clinical transcutaneous electrical nerve stimulation*. Philadelphia: F. A. Davis.

76. Mayer DJ, Wolfe TL, Akil H, et al. (1971): Analgesia from electrical stimulation in the brainstem of the rat. *Science* 174:1351–1354.

77. Mayer DJ, Liebeskind JC (1974): Pain reduction by focal electrical stimulation of the brain: an anatomical and behavioral analysis. *Brain Res* 68:73–93.

78. Mayer DJ, Hayes RL (1975): Stimulation-produced analgesia: development of tolerance and cross-tolerance to morphine. *Science* 188:941–943.

79. Mayer DJ, Price DD (1976): Central nervous system mechanisms of analgesia. *Pain* 2:379–404.

80. Mazars G, Roge R, Mazars Y (1960): Results of the stimulation of the spinothalamic fasciculus and their bearing on the physiopathology of pain. *Rev Neurol* 103:136–138.

81. Mazars GJ (1975): Intermittent stimulation of nucleus ventralis posterolateralis for intractable pain. *Surg Neurol* 4:93–95.

82. McCarron RF, Racz G (1982): *Percutaneous dorsal column stimulator implantation for chronic pain control*. Presented at North American Spine Society meeting, Banff, Alberta, Canada, June 25–28.

83. Meglio M, Cioni B, Rossi GF (1989): Spinal cord stimulation in management of chronic pain: a 9-year experience. *J Neurosurg* 70:519–524.

84. Meilman PW, Leibrock LG, Leong FTL (1989): Outcome of implanted spinal cord stimulation in the treatment of chronic pain: arachnoiditis versus single nerve root injury and mononeuropathy. *Clin J Pain* 5:189–193.

85. Melzack P, Wall PD (1965): Pain mechanisms: a new theory. *Science* 150(3699):971–978.

86. Meyer GA, Fields HL (1972): Causalgia treated by selective large fiber stimulation of peripheral nerve. *Brain* 95:163–168.

87. Mittal B, Thomas DGT, Walton P, Calder I (1987): Dorsal column stimulation (DCS) in chronic pain: report of 31 cases. *Ann R Coll Surg* 69(3):104–109.

88. Nashold BS Jr, Friedman H (1972): Dorsal column stimulation for control of pain, preliminary report on 30 patients. *J Neurosurg* 6:590–597.

89. Nashold BS, Goldner JL (1975): Electrical stimulation of peripheral nerves for relief of intractable chronic pain. *Med Instrum* 9(5):224–225.

90. Nathan PW (1976): The gate-control theory of pain: a critical review. *Brain* 99:123–158.

91. Nielson KD, Adams JE, Hosobuchi Y (1975): Experience with dorsal column stimulation for relief of chronic intractable pain. *Surg Neurol* 4:148–152.

92. North RB, Fischell TA, Long DM (1977): Chronic stimulation via percutaneously inserted epidural electrodes. *Neurosurgery* 1:215–218.

93. North RB, Fowler KF (1987): Computer-controlled, patient-interactive, multichannel, implanted neurological stimulators. *Appl Neurophys* 50:39–41.

94. North RB, Kidd DH, Campbell JN, Long DM (1991): Dorsal root ganglionectomy for failed back surgery syndrome: a five year followup study. *J Neurosurg* 74:236–242.

95. North RB, Ewend MG, Lawton MT, Piantadosi S (1991): Spinal cord stimulation for chronic, intractable pain: superiority of "multichannel" devices. *Pain* 44:119–130.

96. North RB, Campbell JN, James CS, Conover-Walker MK, Wang H, Piantadosi S, Rybock JD, Long DM (1991): Failed back surgery syndrome: five-year followup in 102 patients undergoing re-operation. *Neurosurgery* 28:685–691.

97. North RB, Ewend MG, Lawton MT, Kidd DH, Piantadosi S (1991): Failed back surgery syndrome: five-year follow-up after spinal cord stimulator implantation. *Neurosurgery* 28:692–699.

98. North RB, Fowler KR, Nigrin DA, Szymanski RE, Piantadosi S (1992): Automated 'pain drawing' analysis by computer-controlled, patient-interactive neurological stimulation system. *Pain* 50:51–58.

99. North RB, Kidd DH, Zahurak M, James CS, Long DM (1993): Spinal cord stimulation for chronic, intractable pain: two decades' experience. *Neurosurgery* 32:384–395.

100. North RB, Han M, Zahurak M, Kidd DH (1994): Radiofrequency lumbar facet denervation: analysis of prognostic factors. *Pain* 57:77–83.

101. North RB, Kidd DH, Lee MS, Piantadosi S (1994): Spinal cord stimulation versus reoperation for the failed back surgery syndrome: a prospective, randomized study design. *Stereotact Funct Neurosurg* 62:267–272.

102. Ohnishi A, O'Brien PC, Okazaki H, Dyck PJ (1976): Morphometry of myelinated fibers of fasciculus gracilis of man. *J Neurol Sci* 27:163–172.

103. Pert CB, Snyder SH (1973): Opiate receptor: demonstration in nervous tissue. *Science* 179:405–423.

104. Picaza JA, Cannon BW, Hunter SE, Boyd AS, Guma J, Maurer D (1975): Pain suppression by peripheral nerve stimulation. *Surg Neurol* 4:105–114.

105. Picaza JA, Hunter SE, Cannon BW (1978): Pain suppression by peripheral nerve stimulation. *Appl Neurophysiol* 40:223–234.

106. Pineda A (1975): Dorsal column stimulation and its prospects. *Surg Neurol* 4:157–163.

107. Plotkin R (1982): Results in 60 cases of deep brain stimulation for chronic intractable pain. *Appl Neurophysiol* 45:173–178.

108. Pool JL (1956): Psychosurgery in elderly people. *J Am Geriatr Soc* 2:456–465.

109. Racz GB, McCarron RF, Talboys P (1989): Percutaneous dorsal column stimulator for chronic pain control. *Spine* (141):1–4.

110. Ranck J (1975): Which elements are excited in electrical stimulation of mammalian central nervous system: a review. *Brain Res* 98:417–440.

111. Ray CD, Burton CV, Lifson A (1982): Neurostimulation as used in a large clinical practice. *Appl Neurophysiol* 45:160–206.

112. Reynolds DV (1969): Surgery in the rat during electrical analgesia induced by focal brain stimulation. *Science* 164:444–445.

113. Richardson DE, Akil H (1977): Pain reduction by electrical stimulation in man (Part I). *J Neurosurg* 47:178–183.

114. Richardson RR, Siqueira EB, Cerullo LJ (1979): Spinal epidural neurostimulation for treatment of acute and chronic intractable pain: initial and long term results. *Neurosurgery* 5(3):344–348.

115. Richardson DE, Shatin D (1991): *Results of spinal cord stimulation for pain control: long-term collaborative study.* Presented at American Pain Society, New Orleans, Louisiana, Poster #91240, program p. 56.

116. Robb LG, Robb MP (1990): Practical considerations in spinal cord stimulation. *Pain* 5:S234.

117. Sances A, Swiontek TJ, Larson SJ, Cusick JF, Meyer GA, Millar EA, Hemmy DC, Myklebust J (1975): Innovations in neurologic implant systems. *Med Instrum* 9(5):213–216.

118. Sánchez-Ledesma MJ, Garcia-March G, Diaz-Cascajo P, Gómez-Moreta J, Broseta J (1989): Spinal cord stimulation in deafferentation pain. *Stereotact Funct Neurosurg* 53:40–55.

119. Shatin D, Mullett K, Hults G (1986): Totally implantable spinal cord stimulation for chronic pain: design and efficacy. *PACE* 9: 577–583.

120. Shealy C, Mortimer J, Reswick J (1967): Electrical inhibition of pain by stimulation of the dorsal columns: a preliminary report. *Anesth Analg* 46:489–491.

121. Shealy CN (1975): Dorsal column stimulation: optimization of application. *Surg Neurol* 4:142–145.

122. Shelden CH, Paul F, Jacques DB, Pudenz RH (1975): Electrical stimulation of the nervous system. *Surg Neurol* 4:127–132.

123. Siegfried J, Lazorthes Y (1982): Long-term follow-up of dorsal column stimulation for chronic pain syndrome after multiple lumbar operations. *Appl Neurophys* 45:201–204.

124. Simpson BA (1991): Spinal cord stimulation in 60 cases of intractable pain. *J Neurol Neurosurg Psychiatry* 54:196–199.

125. Sjolund B, Eriksson M (1979): The influence of naloxone on analgesia produced by peripheral condition stimulation. *Brain Res* 173:95–301.

126. Spiegelmann R, Friedman WA (1991): Spinal cord stimulation: a contemporary series. *Neurosurgery* 28:65–71.

127. Stillings D (1975): A survey of the history of electrical stimulation for pain to 1900. *Med Instrum* 9:(6)255–259.

128. Sweet WH, Wepsic JG (1968): Treatment of chronic pain by stimulation of fibers of primary afferent neuron. *Trans Am Neurol Assoc* 93:103–107.

129. Sweet W, Wepsic J (1974): Stimulation of the posterior columns of the spinal cord for pain control. *Clin Neurosurg* 21:278–310.

130. Sweet WH (1976): Control of pain by direct electrical stimulation of peripheral nerves. *Clin Neurosurg* 23:103–111.

131. Swett J, Law J (1983): Analgesia with peripheral nerve stimulation: absence of a peripheral mechanism. *Pain* 15:55–70.

132. Thorsteinsson G, et al. (1978): The placebo effect of transcutaneous electrical stimulation. *Pain* 5:31–41.

133. Urban BJ, Nashold B (1978): Percutaneous epidural stimulation of the spinal cord for relief of pain: long term results. *J Neurosurg* 48:323–328.

134. Van den Honert C, Mortimer J (1979): Generation of unidirectionally propagated action potentials in a peripheral nerve by brief stimuli. *Science* 206:1311–1312.

135. Vanderark G, McGrath KA (1975): Transcutaneous electrical stimulation in treatment of postoperative pain. *Am J Surg* 130: 338–340.

136. Vogel HP, Heppner B, Hümbs N, Schramm J, Wagner C (1986): Long-term effects of spinal cord stimulation in chronic pain syndromes. *J Neurol* 233:16–18.

137. Waisbrod H, Gerbershagen HU (1985): Spinal cord stimulation in patients with a battered root syndrome. *Arch Orthop Trauma Surg* 104:62–64.

138. Wall PD, Sweet WH (1967): Temporary abolition of pain in man. *Science* 155:108–109.

139. Winkelmüller W (1981): Experience with the control of low back pain by the dorsal column stimulation (DCS) system and by the peridural electrode system (Pisces). In: Hosobuchi Y, Corbin T, eds. *Indications for spinal cord stimulation.* Amsterdam: Excerpta Medica, pp. 34–41.

140. Woolf CJ, Mitchell D, Myers RA, Barrett GD (1978): Failure of naloxone to reverse peripheral transcutaneous electro-analgesia in patients suffering from acute trauma. *S A Med J* 53:179–180.

141. Young RF, Shende M (1976): Dorsal column stimulation for relief of chronic intractable pain. *Surg Forum* 27:474–476.

142. Young RF (1978): Evaluation of dorsal column stimulation in the treatment of chronic pain. *Neurosurgery* 3:373–379.

143. Young RF, Kroening R, Fulton W, Feldman R, Chambi I (1985): Electrical stimulation of the brain in treatment of chronic pain: experience over 5 years. *J Neurosurg* 62:389–396.

144. Young RF, Brechner T (1986): Electrical stimulation of the brain for relief of intractable pain due to cancer. *Cancer* 57:1266–1272.

145. Young RF, Chambi VI (1987): Pain relief by stimulation of the periaqueductal and periventricular gray matter: evidence for a non-opioid mechanism. *J Neurosurg* 66:364–371.

146. Young RF, Bach FW, Van Norman AS, Yaksh TL (1993): Release of beta-endorphin and methionine-enkephalin into cerebrospinal fluid during deep brain stimulation for chronic pain. *J Neurosurg* 79:816–825.

PART II

GENERAL ISSUES OF SPINAL DISORDERS

Editor: James N. Weinstein

The Adult Spine: Principles and Practice,
2nd edition, J.W. Frymoyer, Editor-in-Chief.
Lippincott-Raven Publishers, Philadelphia © 1997.

CHAPTER 20

Sensitivity, Specificity, and Predictive Value: A General Issue in Screening for Disease and in the Interpretation of Diagnostic Studies in Spinal Disorders

Gunnar B. J. Andersson and Richard A. Deyo

The diagnosis of most spinal disorders depends on a detailed history and physical examination. Based on the results of this evaluation and the urgency of the patient's condition, additional hematologic, serologic, electrodiagnostic, and imaging studies may be obtained (see Chapters 25–32). Throughout this text, emphasis is placed on the importance of using these additional tests to confirm suspected diagnoses, rather than interpreting abnormalities independent of the patient's clinical condition. For example, it is well established that multiple congenital and acquired changes are frequently observed in spinal radiographs of asymptomatic volunteers, and post-mortem in subjects who have never had back pain. Similarly, myelograms, CT scans, and MR images of asymptomatic volunteers often show evidence of spinal stenosis and disc herniations.

This problem is even greater when populations are screened for future risk of spinal disease, as in school screening programs to identify scoliosis and other deformities. It has also been an issue in employment preplacement screening, in which some industries still use spinal radiographs to assess a potential employee's fitness for a job. To deal with these complexities, and to aid in the appropriate interpretation of tests, statistics have been developed, including sensitivity, specificity, and predictive value. The purpose of this chapter is to review the issues involved in these statistical methods from the perspectives of screening populations for diseases and of interpreting test results in a patient who is suspected of having a disease.

    G. B. J. Andersson, M.D., Ph.D.: Professor and Chairman, Department of Orthopedic Surgery, Rush-Presbyterian-St. Luke's Medical Center, Chicago, Illinois, 60612.
    R. A. Deyo, M.D., M.P.H.: Professor, Departments of Medicine and Health Service, Back Pain Outcome Assessment Team, University of Washington, Seattle, Washington, 98195.

SCREENING FOR DISEASE

Screening for disease is defined as the testing of asymptomatic individuals to detect either the presence of disease or factors that will place an individual at later risk for the disease (40) (Fig. 1). The term *screening* is also used to describe the testing of symptomatic individuals for diagnostic purposes (discussed later in this chapter). Screening for disease is worthwhile only if the disease being screened for is important in terms of death, impairment, or disability. It is particularly useful if it allows identification of risk factors that can be influenced by specific preventive measures. To justify screening, it should be established that early detection results in actual prevention or in a better long-term outcome than would treatment after the individual has overt disease. Thus, screening for hypertension and elevated serum cholesterol has been important in the prevention of cardiovascular disease, because such conditions can be favorably influenced by medication, exercise, and control of weight and diet. In spinal disorders, the best known example is screening for adolescent scoliosis, the value of which has been heavily debated in recent years (55).

To be successful, a screening program requires suitable screening tests. Ideally, such tests should be minimally invasive, cause minimal discomfort, and be inexpensive, easy to administer, safe, valid, reliable, and reproducible. Wilson and Jungner (56) identified ten requirements for a cost-effective screening program. As listed in Table 1, these fall into four main groups: knowledge of disease, feasibility, diagnosis and treatment, and cost. Although spinal disorders were not considered in their review,

TABLE 1. *Requirements for a screening program*

Knowledge of the disease
    The condition should be an important problem.
    There should be a recognizable latent or early symptomatic stage.
    The natural history should be adequately understood.
Feasibility of the screening procedure
    There should be a suitable test or examination.
    The test should be acceptable to the population.
    Case finding should be a continuing process, not a once-and-for-all project.
Diagnosis and treatment
    There should be accepted treatment for people with the disease.
    There should be facilities for diagnosis and treatment.
    There should be a clear policy on whom to treat.
Cost
    The cost of a case finding (including diagnosis and treatment) should be economically balanced in relation to the possible total expense of medical care.

From Wilson and Jungner (56).

these requirements need to be fulfilled to justify screening efforts in spinal diseases as well.

Validity

The validity of a screening test, that is, its ability to correctly identify people as diseased (risk-positive) or nondiseased (risk-negative), is measured by its sensitivity and specificity (Table 2). Sensitivity in screening for disease is defined as the proportion of those with disease (or risk of developing disease) who are correctly identified

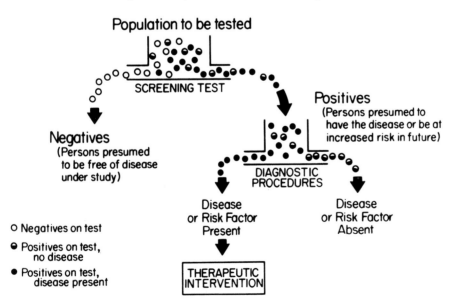

APPARENTLY WELL POPULATION
(Well persons plus those with undiagnosed disease)

Population to be tested

SCREENING TEST

Negatives
(Persons presumed to be free of disease under study)

Positives
(Persons presumed to have the disease or be at increased risk in future)

DIAGNOSTIC PROCEDURES

Disease or Risk Factor Present

Disease or Risk Factor Absent

THERAPEUTIC INTERVENTION

○ Negatives on test
◒ Positives on test, no disease
● Positives on test, disease present

FIG. 1. Flow diagram for screening examination. From Williams (55).

TABLE 2. *Results of a screening test*

Results of screening test (T)	Disease status (true diagnosis)		
	Positive	Negative	Total
Positive	a	b	a + b
Negative	c	d	c + d
Total	a + c	b + d	

$$\text{Sensitivity} = \text{Probability (T+Dx+)} = \frac{a}{a + c} =$$

$$\frac{\text{Persons with disease testing positive}}{\text{All those who have disease}}$$

$$\text{Specificity} = \text{Probability (T-Dx-)} = \frac{d}{b + d} =$$

$$\frac{\text{Persons without disease who tested negative}}{\text{All those who did not have disease}}$$

$$\text{PV+} = \text{Probability (Dx+T+)} = \frac{a}{a + b}$$

$$\text{PV-} = \text{Probability (Dx-T-)} = \frac{d}{c + d}$$

PV+, predictive value positive; PV−, predictive value negative.

by a test, that is, the probability of testing positive when disease (or pre-condition for disease) is truly present. As the sensitivity of a test increases, the number of subjects with disease who are missed, and are wrongly classified as test-negative (disease free), decreases. Conversely, specificity refers to the proportion of those without disease, or without risk of developing disease, who are correctly identified by a test, that is, the probability of screening negative if disease (risk) is truly absent. As the specificity of a test increases, the probability of being misclassified as having disease or risk of disease (a false positive) decreases.

Calculations of sensitivity and specificity are simple using the formulas in Table 2. Ideally, screening tests are both highly sensitive and specific. Usually, however, there is a trade-off between the sensitivity and specificity of a given test. This problem arises because there is almost always a gray zone between a clearly normal test (no risk) and clearly abnormal test (absolute risk). The cutoff for classifications of normal and abnormal for any given test is made arbitrarily. In order not to miss a true case, that is, to be 100% sensitive, it is common to place the cutoff such that a few persons without disease or risk will be misclassified as having disease. Lowering criteria for labeling a disease as present increases sensitivity but decreases specificity, whereas making the criteria more stringent has the opposite effect. Clearly, this means that decisions are made based on the consequences of having false negatives or false positives (Fig. 2). In general, sensitivity is increased at the expense of specificity when missing the diagnosis or the risk factor has disastrous

consequences. Specificity, on the other hand, should be increased when the costs and risks of evaluating false positives are unacceptably high.

In order to manage the trade-off better, several screening tests can be used together, either at the same time or sequentially. When more than one test is used at the same time, the procedure is called parallel. Parallel testing increases sensitivity but sometimes lowers specificity. An example in a back pain patient would be ordering an electromyogram (EMG) and a magnetic resonance imaging (MRI) test at the same time. When tests are administered sequentially, the appropriate term is serial testing, which in general leads to an increased specificity. An example would be ordering an MRI only in patients in whom an EMG is positive for radiculopathy.

Reproducibility

It is insufficient for a screening test to be valid; it must be reliable as well. In fact, validity depends on high reliability. This means that there should be consistency in results when examinations (tests) are repeated on the same person under the same conditions (reproducibility). Differences in test results can arise from (a) biological variation, (b) variation in test method (measurement), (c) intraobserver variability, which means differences over time when the same test is performed by the same observer, and (d) interobserver variability. Interobserver variability, or variation because of differences between different examiners in application and interpretation of a test, is reduced if end points are well

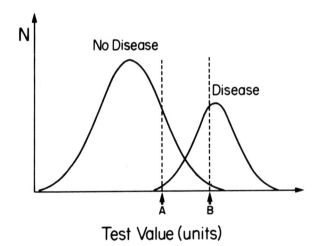

FIG. 2. In work screening tests there are patients who fall into a gray zone between clearly normal (no disease) and clearly abnormal (disease). To achieve high sensitivity, that is, not to miss true cases, the cutoff can be set at A. Setting the cutoff at B will lower the sensitivity but increase specificity, so that few healthy people will be test positive.

defined and quantifiable, and if the test results are few and simple (i.e., positive or negative).

Predictive Value

Sensitivity and specificity are theoretically independent of the characteristics of the population to which a test is applied. A critical factor in screening is the probability of the disease in the population being screened, or the disease prevalence. When a general population is surveyed, the prevalence is the same as the disease prevalence in the population as a whole. However, this is rarely the case, and variations in prevalence may result in major differences in predictive value. The predictive value of a positive or negative test takes prevalence into account as well as sensitivity and specificity. The predictive value provides the information we need for clinical decision making (given a test result, how likely is it to be correct?), whereas sensitivity and specificity alone do not.

The predictive value of a positive test (PV+) is the proportion of those with a positive test who have disease, or risk of disease, given the pretest probability of the disease in question. PV+ is calculated by the formula:

$$PV+ = \frac{\text{True positives}}{\text{True positives} + \text{False positives}}$$

It is important to remember the difference between sensitivity and positive predictive value. Sensitivity is a probability of a test result, predictive value the probability of disease.

The predictive value of a negative test (PV-), on the other hand, tells us the proportion of those with a negative test who are truly disease free, or have no risk of disease, given the pretest disease prevalence. PV- is calculated as follows:

$$PV- = \frac{\text{True negatives}}{\text{False negatives} + \text{True negatives}}$$

In general, a low disease prevalence means that there is an increased probability of many false positive tests. Assume, for example, that the prevalence is 1% (1/100 or 10/1,000), and that our screening test is 90% sensitive and specific. Of the 10 with disease, 9 will be identified correctly (1 will have erroneously positive tests), and of 990 without disease, 891 will be identified correctly (99 will be missed). This means that most positive tests (99 of 108) are false positives. Calculating the predictive values results in the following:

$$PV+ = \frac{9}{9 + 99} = 8.3\%$$

$$PV- = \frac{891}{1 + 891} = 99.9\%.$$

Since PV- is high, it means that the test was effective in ruling out disease (in identifying disease-free subjects) in this example. Only one subject with disease was not detected. The low PV+, however, indicates that definitive diagnosis cannot be made using this test. Only 9 subjects of 108 with a positive test actually had the disease. This means that for every subject who actually had the disease, 12 would be falsely suspected of having it, which could lead to unnecessary confirmatory procedures or unnecessary treatment. On the other hand, when the prevalence is high, the situation is different. For example, consider a condition whose prevalence (probability) is 80% (i.e., there are 80/100 or 800/1,000 with disease or risk of it) and the test is 90% sensitive and specific. The test will correctly identify 720 as test-positive, and 20 will test false positive. PV+ will be high,

$$PV+ = \frac{720}{720 + 20} = 95.9\%,$$

while PV- will be modest,

$$PV- = \frac{180}{80 + 180} = 69\%.$$

Table 3 illustrates the dependence of predictive value on the prevalence of disease. The chosen hypothetical test has high sensitivity (95%) and specificity (95%). When the prevalence is 50% or higher, the predictive value is very high. When the prevalence is below 10%, however, the ratio of true positives to false positives drops dramatically even with this excellent test, and the majority of those referred for diagnosis are normal. As in this example, most tests are most effective when the likelihood of disease is moderate: neither extremely high nor extremely low. The clinical evaluation is critical in selecting such a group.

Examples from Pre-Employment Screening for Low Back Pain

Pre-employment and pre-placement screening programs are being used by industry as preventive and cost-control measures. Screening tests are used to identify people with risk of future back problems. The difficulties

TABLE 3. *Predictive value of a positive test (95% sensitive and 95% specific) as a function of the disease prevalence*

Prevalence of disease (%)	Predictive value of positive test
1	16.1
2	21.2
5	50.0
10	67.9
15	77.0
20	82.6
25	86.4
50	95.0

TABLE 4. *Cumulative frequency of low back pain, by age (theoretical cohort of 1000 miners)*

Age (yr)	First attack	Cumulative frequency	Cumulative %
<30	25%	188	25%
30–40	24%	368	49%
40–50	38%	653	87%
>50	13%	750	100%

Based on MacDonald et al. (37).

of predicting risk for back pain have been discussed elsewhere in this book (see Chapter 11). A few examples of how sensitivity, specificity, and predictive value enter into this technology are presented here.

Himmelstein and Andersson (23) reanalyzed data from a study by MacDonald and co-workers (37) of 373 British coal miners to evaluate the implications of an accurate medical history as a predictive tool. MacDonald's group found that 75% of 50- to 60-year-old miners had suffered previous back pain. While this is not a true lifetime cumulative frequency, it should be a close estimate. On the basis of MacDonald's data, it was assumed that over a lifetime, 78% of those with back pain would ultimately lose some time from work (temporary disability). Of the 75% of miners suffering from back pain, the age distribution at the onset of the first attack and the cumulative incidence is shown in Table 4.

Table 4 assumes that one could take a cohort of 1,000 male miners of the same age and trace each miner through his lifetime, and that all workers with a previous history of low back pain would suffer recurrence. Based on those assumptions, Table 5 can be developed as follows. A questionnaire survey of 1,000 30-year-old miners would reveal that 188 (25% of 750) had already had an attack of low back pain. One hundred forty-seven (78% of 188) would be expected to lose time from work in the future. Therefore, screening at age 30 would identify only 147 out of 585 future cases of lower back disability (sensitivity is 147/585 = 0.25). Conversely, the screening test would fail to identify 438 of 585 future cases of lower back disability (the false negatives) and would identify 41 potential workers as at risk who would never experience disability (the false positives).

If the results of a screening program based on a history

TABLE 5. *Screening by previous history in subjects age 30*

Future LBD?	History of LBP?		
	Y	N	Total
Y	147	438	585
N	41	374	415
Total	188	812	1000

From Himmelstein and Andersson (23).
LBP, low pack pain; LBD, low back disability (assumed to occur in 78% of those with LBP).

of previous back pain were used as a way of "preventing" back disability by refusing employment to those at risk, we would need to deny employment to 188 applicants in the 30-year-old group in this example. The majority of future cases of lower back disability would not be identified, however.

Because the history of back pain is highly correlated with age in all cohorts studied, the majority of miners over the age of 50 would be identified as high risk; 750 out of 1,000 older workers would be denied employment. Therefore, the use of history of back pain as an independent screening tool would lead to systematic age discrimination, would be insensitive in the younger population that comprises the majority of new hires, and would have unknown effects on the ultimate morbidity of this population.

Another example cited by Himmelstein and Andersson (23) is an analysis of the use of x-rays for pre-employment screening performed by Rockey et al. (43). Rockey et al. assume that a random group of railroad workers will have 60% incidence of low back pain during their work lives, and that x-rays will be positive in 56% of those with low back pain (56% sensitive) and in 22% of those who will never have low back pain (76% specific). On the basis of these assumptions, Table 6 demonstrates that the value of a positive test for predicting future back pain would be 79% (336/424). In other words, with an underlying probability of a 60% cumulative incidence in the unselected population, the incidence of back pain among those with "positive" x-ray changes for degeneration would be 79%, compared to 46% (264/576) among those with "negative" x-rays.

Since the purpose of most programs is the prevention of disability, not pain, Rockey et al. (43) further analyzed this same hypothetical cohort in terms of the predictive value of x-rays for future lost time (disability) due to low back pain, assuming that 50% of those who experience pain will lose time from work. Table 7 demonstrates that the predictive value of a "positive" x-ray examination for estimating future time lost from work is 40% (168/424). Therefore, of the 424 who might be refused

TABLE 6. *Effects of an x-ray screening program on a hypothetical cohort of 1000 workers for the incidence of low back pain (LBP)*

	Will have LBP (N)	Will not have LBP (N)	Total
Positive low back x-ray	336 (true positives)	88 (false positives)	424
Negative low back x-ray	264 (false negatives)	312 (true negatives)	576
Total	600	400	1000

From Himmelstein and Andersson (23).
Assumptions: 60% cumulative incidence of LBP; 56% prevalence of positive x-rays in patients with LBP; 22% prevalence of positive x-rays in people with no LBP.

employment on the basis of abnormal x-rays, 256 (60%) would not have lost time from work because of low back pain. Conversely, of the 576 accepted, 132 (23%) would lose time from work for this reason. In this hypothetical cohort, then, there appears to be a clear differential susceptibility; workers with positive x-rays are nearly twice as likely (40%/23%) to experience subsequent lost time as those with negative x-rays. Furthermore, in perhaps as many as 56% (168/300) of workers who lost time, it might have been possible to prevent this loss by denial of employment to those with abnormal x-rays. On the other hand, of workers denied employment on the basis of low back x-rays, at least 20% will never have low back pain, and at least 60% will never lose time from work because of low back pain.

Rockey et al. (43) conclude that while strict financial accounting of this type of screening program may show it to be beneficial to the employer in terms of direct cost savings, there is likely to be negative social value resulting from false positive misclassifications.

Strength testing is another pre-employment screening tool intended to reduce the incidence and severity of back pain in industry. There is currently no study that permits calculations of absolute predictive values. Himmelstein and Andersson (23) used data from Chaffin et al. (12), which showed a relative risk of back injury of 3 for people whose strength did not equal or exceed that required by the job, and approximated the predictive value for a hypothetical cohort of workers required to do heavy material handling work. Table 8A summarizes the outcomes in a population of 1,000 workers with a yearly low back disability (LBD) incidence rate of 10 per 100 workers, a typical rate for the highest-risk jobs known, and a test positivity rate of 25%. Table 8B reproduces the same analysis except that the test positivity rate is only 20% (as would be true if the standard were lowered). Table 8C shows the effect of increasing the incidence rate to 20% per year, and Table 8D shows the effect of increasing

TABLE 7. Effects of an x-ray screening program on a hypothetical cohort of 1000 workers for the incidence of low back disability (LBD) (work absence)

	Will have LBP and lose time from work	Will never lose time from work because of LBP	Total
Positive low back x-ray	168 (true positives)	256 (false positives)	424
Negative low back x-ray	132 (false negatives)	444 (true negatives)	576
Total	300	700	1000

From Himmelstein and Andersson (23).
Assumptions: 60% cumulative incidence of LBP; 56% prevalence of positive x-rays in patients with LBP; 22% prevalence of positive x-rays in people with no LBP; 50% incidence of LBD among subjects with LBP.

TABLE 8. Predictive value of static strength-testing for a hypothetical cohort of workers with artificially varied rates and risks

A: Incidence rate = 0.1, test positivity rate = 0.25, relative risk = 3, predictive value = 0.20

	Future disability	No future disability	Total
Test positive	50	200	250
Test negative	50	700	750
Total	100	900	1000

B: Incidence rate = 0.1, test positivity rate = 0.2, relative risk = 3, predictive value = 0.25

	Future disability	No future disability	Total
Test positive	25	75	100
Test negative	75	825	900
Total	100	800	900

C: Incidence rate = 0.2, test positivity rate = 0.2, relative risk = 3, predictive value = 0.50

	Future disability	No future disability	Total
Test positive	50	50	100
Test negative	150	750	900
Total	200	800	1000

D: Incidence rate = 0.1; test positive rate = 0.1 relative risk = 10; predictive value = 0.53.

	Future disability	No future disability	Total
Test positive	53	47	100
Test negative	47	853	900
Total	100	900	1000

the differential susceptibility rate (relative risk) to 10. Even at this exceptionally high rate, the predictive value of a positive test would be only 53%, a dismally poor result given the significant disservice done to the employee denied a job on the basis of such testing.

DIAGNOSIS

Many of the principles discussed previously apply to diagnostic tests as well. Thus, a diagnostic test must be valid and reproducible, which unfortunately is by no means the case in many of the more commonly used tests employed for spinal disorders. When evaluating a test, it must be compared to a gold standard. For example, it has been common to compare results of myelograms, computed tomographic (CT) scans, and MRIs to operative findings.

The possible results of a diagnostic test compared to a gold standard are listed in Table 9. Sensitivity and specificity of the test are calculated from this table and vary from 0% to 100%. A test that is 100% sensitive and spe-

TABLE 9. *Determination of the diagnostic discrimination of a test*

Test	Gold standard positive	Gold standard negative
Positive	a = true positives	b = false positives
Negative	c = false negatives	d = true negatives

$$\text{Sensitivity} = \frac{a}{a+c}$$

$$\text{Specificity} = \frac{d}{b+d}$$

cific agrees completely with the gold standard. By definition, no test can be better than the gold standard. If a new test is actually better, this will be detected later based on outcome research, and then the new test becomes the gold standard.

Medical History

As with the diagnosis of any medical problem, the patient's history is, of course, extremely important. Certain elements of the history are particularly critical in order to exclude the occasional serious spine condition for which the prognosis is less favorable. Deyo et al. (16) analyzed the sensitivity and specificity of the patient's history for the diagnosis of tumors, spinal stenosis, spinal osteomyelitis, herniated discs, and compression fractures (Table 10). A previous history of malignancy was the most specific information for tumor (0.98) but had comparatively low sensitivity, whereas pain when resting in bed had high sensitivity (0.90) and low specificity. Sci-

atica was highly sensitive for a clinically important herniated disc, as was old age for spinal stenosis and compression fractures.

Physical Examination: Tests of Neurologic Dysfunction

The most common nerve disorder of the back in younger age groups is nerve root compression (or tension) by a herniated disc. In the older age groups, spinal stenosis becomes a more significant problem. Identification of neurologic impairment is important to the diagnosis and treatment of these disorders. Table 11 presents data on the importance of straight-leg raising (SLR) in the diagnosis of herniated lumbar discs. The gold standard here is the operative finding, which, although it is highly prone to subjective interpretation, is difficult to replace. Ipsilateral limitation in SLR is common but unspecific. In contrast, crossed SLR is less sensitive, but much more specific. Table 12 lists the validity of the neurologic examination as a test for lumbar disc herniation. Surgical findings are again the gold standard. While most neurologic tests have only moderate sensitivity and specificity, their accuracy is improved by considering combinations of the tests.

Lumbar Spine Radiographs

Plain radiographs are commonly obtained in patients complaining of low back pain. In 1979, it was estimated that 7 million such radiographs were performed in the United States (17), corresponding to about 11 million today. Yet it is generally agreed that the value of these

TABLE 10. *Performance characteristics of the medical history in the diagnosis of spine diseases causing low back pain*

Disease to be detected	Medical history	Sensitivity	Specificity	Sample
Cancer	Age ≥ 50 years	0.77	0.71	Unselected primary care
	Previous history of cancer	0.31	0.98	Unselected primary care
	Unexplained weight loss	0.15	0.94	Unselected primary care
	Failure to improve with a month of therapy	0.31	0.90	Unselected primary care
	No relief with bed rest	>0.90	0.46	Unselected primary care
	Duration of pain >1 mo	0.50	0.81	Unselected primary care
Spinal stenosis	Pseudoclaudication	.60–.90	?	Surgical case series
	Age ≥ 50 years	0.90?	0.70	Surgical case series
Spinal osteomyelitis	I.V. drug abuse, UTI, skin infection	0.40	?	Multiple case series
Herniated disc	Sciatica	0.98	0.88	Surgical case series (sens.); population survey of patients with back pain (spec.)
Compression Fracture[a]	Age ≥ 50 years	0.84	0.61	Primary care patients having x-ray
	Age ≥ 70 years	0.22	0.96	Primary care patients having x-ray
	Trauma	0.30	0.85	Unselected primary care
	Corticosteroid use	0.06	0.995	Unselected primary care

[a] From Deyo et al. (16), with permission. Previously unpublished data from 833 patients with back pain at a walk-in clinic, all of whom received plain lumbar roentgenograms.

UTI, urinary tract infection.

TABLE 11. *Straight-leg raising as a test for lumbar disc herniation*

Source (ref.)	Patients (N)	Criterion for positive test	Prevalence of disc herniation (%)	Sensitivity (%)	Specificity (%)
Ipsilateral SLR Charnley (13)	88	<40 degrees	84	72	66
Spangfort (47)	2504	leg pain	88	97	11
Hakelius (22)	1986	leg pain	75	96	14
Kosteljanetz et al. (34)	100	leg pain	58	76	45
		leg or back pain	58	91	21
Kosteljanetz et al. (33)	52	leg pain	86	89	17
		leg or back pain	86	95	14
Crossed SLR Spangfort (47)	2504	contra. leg pain	86	23	88
Hakelius (22)	1986	contra. leg pain	75	27	88
Hudgins (26)	274	contra. leg pain	83	24	96
Kosteljanetz et al. (33)	52	contra. leg pain	86	24	100
		contra. leg or back pain	86	42	85

All results are for surgical series; in every case the gold standard for disc herniation was the surgical finding.

TABLE 12. *Neurological examination as a test for lumbar disc herniation*

Neurological impairment	Population studied (ref.)	Patients (N)	Sensitivity (%)	Specificity (%)	Comments
Ankle dorsiflexor weakness	Surgery for HNP (47)	2504	49	54	70%–90% of patients with dorsiflexor weakness had HNP at L4/5 level.
	Surgery for HNP (22)	1986	20	82	
Great toe extensor weakness	Surgery for HNP (22)	1986	37	71	
	Surgery for HNP (32)	403	57		In 57% of cases with extensor weakness, HNP was at L5/S1, 32% at L4/5.
Ankle reflex	Surgery for HNP (47)	2504	50	62	HNP at L5/S1 level in 80%–90% for ages 20–45, and in 60% after age 50.
	Surgery for HNP (22)	1986	52	63	Absence of reflex has higher specificity than impaired reflex. Additional neurological deficit did not change predictive value.
	Upper lumbar HNP (3)	73	18		Impaired ankle reflex can occur with upper lumbar HNP.
Sensory loss	Surgery for HNP (33)	100	66	51	
	Surgery for HNP (32)	403	38	—	Most impairments in S1 dermatome. Area of sensory loss is poor predictor of level of HNP.
Patella reflex	Surgery for HNP (47)	2504	4	97	Sensitivity of 50% in L3/4 HNP. In 67% of cases of impairment, HNP is at L4/5 and L5/S1 levels.
	Surgery for HNP (22)	1986	7	93	If this is isolated finding, then sensitivity is worse.
	Surgery for HNP (32)	403	7	—	In 85% of cases of impairment, HNP is at L4/5 and L5/S1 levels.
	Upper lumbar HNP	73	50	—	
Quadriceps weakness	Surgery for HNP (22)	1986	<1	99	
Ankle plantarflexor weakness	Surgery for HNP (22)	1986	6	95	

HNP, herniated nucleus pulposus.

examinations is limited (30,36). The main reason to obtain plain films is to exclude systemic pathology. Waddell (51,52) calculated the negative predictive value to be 99%. Many other factors were equally predictive for negative pathology, however, including history, systemic symptoms, nonmechanical back pain, and elevated erythrocyte sedimentation rate (ESR) (>25 mm Hg). The positive predictive value in the same study was only 34%.

The most important consideration in spinal radiographs is perhaps the risk of missing spinal pathology in patients presenting with mechanical back pain. Tumors and infections are the two main conditions where a miss would be disastrous. Liang and Komaroff (36) estimate that there is a 0.2% probability that a person presenting with acute low back pain will have a specific treatable cause. Brolin (9) reviewed 68,000 spine radiographs obtained over a 10-year period, finding that only 1 in 2,500 patients had serious findings not suspected clinically. Deyo and Diehl (15), in a prospective study of 621 outpatients with low back pain, reported therapy-dependent findings in 3.8%, all of whom were either over 50 years old or had had a recent injury.

Other Imaging Techniques

Imaging studies do not reveal the source of pain but identify possible structural abnormalities thought to be consistent with the pain complaint (20). This simple concept is of importance in the clinical diagnosis and treatment of low back pain, as is a knowledge of the prevalence of structural abnormalities in the symptomatic and asymptomatic general population. The lumbar myelogram with water-soluble contrast used to represent the established standard for the diagnosis of lumbar disc herniation and spinal stenosis. CT scans began replacing myelography around 1980. CT scanning after the introduction of the contrast agent (the myelographically enhanced tomographic scan) provides enhanced visualization of the spinal canal, which is often useful additional information, particularly in planning for lumbar spinal surgery. This is most important in patients with suspected spinal stenosis. MRI became more widely used in the mid to late 1980s. It has appeal in that it is devoid of known biologic hazard. MRI is excellent for delineating soft-tissue structures, such as the intervertebral disc, but the technique is not quite as good in defining osseous structures. Still, with the proper choice of imaging parameters, this technique offers excellent diagnostic properties and has the advantages of noninvasiveness and absence of ionizing radiation. MRI also has the potential to give useful insight into the importance of degeneration within the involved disc, edema of the intrathecal and extrathecal nerves, degeneration of ligaments, and joint inflammation in the production of back pain (see Chap-

ter 28). For those reasons, this technique has largely replaced the others in the United States, while elsewhere its availability is less universal.

Myelography, CT, and MRI in Sciatica and Claudication

Imaging evidence of herniated disc and/or spinal stenosis is found in a large percentage of healthy individuals. Hitselberger and Witten (24) found that 24% of people with no history of back pain or sciatica showed significant abnormalities on myelography. Later, Wiesel et al. (54) reported that 35.4% of 52 CT scans obtained from asymptomatic individuals were abnormal. In individuals younger than 40 years, 19.5% had evidence of disc herniation, and in the over-40-year-old age group, 50% had spinal abnormalities (27% disc herniation, 35% stenosis, and 10% facet joint disease). More recently, Boden et al. (6) performed MRI studies of the lumbar spine in 67 individuals who had never experienced back pain or sciatica. In individuals younger than 60 years, 20% had herniated discs, and one had spinal stenosis. After age 60, the percentage of pathological findings increased to 36% with herniated discs and 21% with evidences of spinal stenosis. Bulging discs were even more common with increasing prevalence in the older population. The findings of Boden and collaborators (6) were confirmed by Jensen et al. (29). Their study involved 98 asymptomatic 20- to 80-year-old women and men. Fifty-two percent had bulging discs, 27% a protrusion, and one an extrusion. Thirty-eight percent had more than one level involved. In 14%, canal stenosis was present, while 8% had facet osteoarthritis. Only 36% of the 98 asymptomatic subjects had normal discs at all levels.

Similar findings have been made in the cervical spine. Teresi et al. (48) studied 100 symptom free individuals who had cervical MRI because of laryngeal disease. All were 45 years or older. Twenty percent of patients below age 64 had disc protrusions, compared to 57% in the older age group. Thirty-seven percent overall had spinal cord impairment, again with larger prevalence in the older age group. Boden et al. (7) studied 63 volunteers with no history of cervical disease. Abnormal MRI scans were found in 19%, 14% among those younger than 40, and 28% in those who were older. Of those younger than 40, 10% had a herniated disc and 4% had foraminal stenosis. Of those older than 40, 5% had a herniated disc, 3% a bulging disc, and 20% foraminal stenosis.

From an imaging point of view, these findings are true anatomic abnormalities, yet they are clinically irrelevant. From a clinical perspective, therefore, they are false positive. By this clinical definition, false positive imaging results can be expected in at least 25% of a healthy population, with larger percentages in older populations. This makes it critical to place an imaging finding in its proper clinical perspective. Combining the information from patient history, physical findings, and imaging studies is necessary to improve the accuracy of different imaging tests. Since most patients with a negative imaging test are never surgically explored (the gold standard), it is difficult to determine how prevalent false negative imaging is. Because CT and MRI examinations are static and typically performed with the patient supine, it is likely that false negative findings occur. This is particularly the case with spinal stenosis, where it has been demonstrated experimentally that extension can reduce the circumference of the thecal sack by as much as 20% (46).

Herniated Discs

The approximate sensitivity and specificity of imaging tests for herniated discs are given in Table 13. The table also includes common physical findings, allowing comparison. The selection of studies to be included in the table reflects quality, although other high-quality studies exist also (2,4,5,8,18,19,27,28,39,41,45,53,57). Predictive values are presented for two circumstances: one where the probability of a positive test is high (because the patients have clinical findings suggestive of a herniated disc), the other where it is low (the probability based on presenting symptoms and signs is low). The predictive values of imaging tests in the low probability patients are disappointing. As evidenced from the table, there is little difference between CT, MRI, and CT myelograms. The choice of test, therefore, depends on availability, cost, and complications. Thornbury and colleagues (49) recommend the following strategies for use of these tests: (a) In situations where the prior probability of a herniated disc is only moderate, a plain CT examination would be appropriate, based largely on cost; (b) In situations for which CT myelography would have been requested prior to the availability of MR (e.g., surgical planning), physicians should choose MR (based on sensitivity for rare neural tumors and noninvasiveness).

Masaryk et al. (38) established a set of criteria to diagnose sequestered discs by MRI, which is important to the choice of treatment. When prospectively applied to a group of 20 patients who were later operated on, an accuracy of 85% was reported. Janssen et al. (28) report that MRI is 93% accurate in identifying a sequestered fragment, compared to 71% for myelography and 31% for CT scans.

Spinal Stenosis

Table 14 shows representative estimates of sensitivity, specificity, and predictive value for imaging tests in spinal stenosis. Again, there are no major differences between CT and MRI. The use of CT myelography is attractive but has not been presented in sufficient detail in the literature to allow calculation of both sensitivity and specificity. Choice of test would again depend on availability, cost, and complications.

MRI in Metastatic Spine Lesions

Li and Poon (35) determined the accuracy of MRI in evaluation of the spinal cord and cauda equina in patients with known malignancies outside the CNS. The sensitivity for malignancy was 93%; specificity, 97%; and accuracy, 95%. The positive predictive value was 98%, and the negative predictive value was 91%.

In the same study, the ability of MRI to distinguish between benign and malignant vertebral collapse, using a signal intensity ratio, was outstanding. The sensitivity was 97.6%; specificity, 100%; and accuracy, 98.2%.

MRI and Radionuclide Bone Imaging in Vertebral Osteomyelitis

Because the clinical picture of vertebral osteomyelitis is so unspecific as to engender the label "the great mas-

TABLE 13. *Representative estimates of test accuracy for the diagnosis of herniated discs*

Test (ref.)	Sensitivity	Specificity	Positive predictive value, high prior probability[a]	Negative predictive value, high prior probability[a]	Positive predictive value, low prior probability[b]	Negative predictive value, low prior probability[b]
Ipsilateral SLR	0.80	0.40	0.67	0.57	0.04	0.99
Crossed SLR	0.25	0.90	0.79	0.44	0.07	0.98
Impaired ankle reflex	0.50	0.60	0.65	0.44	0.04	0.98
Plain CT (49, 54)	0.90	0.70	0.82	0.82	0.08	0.996
MRI (8, 49)	0.90	0.70	0.82	0.82	0.08	0.996
CT myelography (49)	0.90	0.70	0.82	0.82	0.08	0.996
Thermography (25)	0.90	0.60	0.77	0.80	0.07	0.995

From Deyo (14).

[a] High prior probability = 60% likelihood of herniated disc before test; typical of a patient with sciatica, positive straight-leg raising, and poor response to conservative therapy.

[b] Low prior probability = 3%; typical of a patient with no sciatica or neurologic signs/symptoms.

TABLE 14. *Representative estimates of test accuracy for the diagnosis of spinal stenosis*

Test	Sensitivity	Specificity	Positive predictive value, high prior probability[a]	Negative predictive value, high prior probability[a]	Positive predictive value, low prior probability[b]	Negative predictive value, low prior probability[b]
Plain CT	0.90	0.80–0.95	0.87	0.84	0.12	0.996
MRI	0.90	0.75–0.95	0.87	0.87	0.12	0.996
Myelography	0.77	0.70	0.79	0.67	0.07	0.990

From Deyo (14); tests as cited in Kent et al. (31).
[a] High prior probability = 60% likelihood of spinal stenosis before test; typical of a patient over age 50 with pseudoclaudication.
[b] Low prior probability = 3%; typical of a patient with no sciatica or neurologic signs/symptoms.

querader," diagnosis is often difficult. In one study, MR was found to have a sensitivity of 96% and a specificity of 92% (38). Bone scanning with 99m technetium had a sensitivity of 90% and a specificity of 78%. Plain radiographs had a sensitivity of 82% and a specificity of 57%. Thus, MR was at least as accurate as radionuclide bone scanning and substantially more accurate than plain radiographs in the detection of vertebral osteomyelitis. Three-phase bone scanning using 99m-TcMDP has been found in one study to be 89% to 100% sensitive and 94% specific, with an overall accuracy of 92%. Others have found substantially lower specificity and performance characteristics that are less favorable than MRI. Gallium and indium scans increase the specificity when used with a technetium scan, but are less sensitive when used alone (1).

Ankylosing Spondylitis

Different methods to diagnose ankylosing spondylitis (AS) have been tested for sensitivity and specificity. Calin

et al. (11) found a simple questionnaire to be 95% sensitive and 85% specific. Because of the very low prevalence of AS, the positive predictive value in industrial screening for disease was only 0.04, however. Table 15 summarizes data from three studies. In general, the sensitivity is low, but AS does not seem to debut after age 40. The screening questions of Calin et al. (10,11) had poor sensitivity and excellent specificity.

Measurements of Bone Mass

Measurements of bone mass are performed to determine the risk of vertebral fractures in osteoporosis. Ott et al. (42) used four different techniques and calculated sensitivity and specificity. At 90% specificity, the sensitivities of the tests were as follows: total body calcium (TBC) (neutron activation analysis), 34%; single photon absorptometry (SPA), 29%; dual photon absorptometry (DPA), 33%; and quantitative computed tomography (QCT), 36%. At 50% specificity, the sensitivity values were TBC 87%, SPA 84%, DPA 78%, and QCT 90%.

TABLE 15. *Accuracy of the history and physical examination in the diagnosis of ankylosing spondylitis*

Clinical finding	Sensitivity			Specificity		
	Study 1	Study 2	Study 3	Study 1	Study 2	Study 3
History						
4 out of 5 positive screening questions	—	0.38	0.23	—	1.00	0.82
Pain duration >3 mo, not relieved by rest	—	0.38	—	—	0.94	—
Pain duration >3 mo	—	—	0.71	—	—	0.54
Morning back stiffness	0.93	—	0.64	0.43	—	0.59
Age at onset <40 years	—	—	1.00	—	—	0.07
Pain or stiffness relieved by exercise	—	—	0.75	—	—	0.45
Hip pain or knee swelling	0.41	—	—	0.94	—	—
Pain not relieved lying down	—	—	0.80	—	—	0.49
Pain that made patient leave bed at night	—	—	0.65	—	—	0.79
Physical exam						
Flexion <3 cm, Schober test	0.49	—	—	0.37	—	—
Flexion <4 cm, Schober test	—	—	0.30	—	—	0.86
Flexion <5 cm, Schober test	—	0.52	—	—	0.89	—
Chest expansion <2.5 cm	—	0.10	0.09	—	1.00	0.99
Chest expansion <5 cm	0.34	0.60	—	1.00	0.67	—
Chest expansion <7 cm	—	—	0.63	—	—	0.53

From Gran (21), Sadowska-Wroblewska et al. (44), Van der Linden et al. (50).

SUMMARY

Statistical methods permit determination of the value of tests used for the screening of healthy populations and of diagnostic tests for patients with disease. Available data cast doubt on the use of screening tests for prevention. Parallel testing may offer better alternatives than are presently available. The controversy of who is at risk remains.

Available data also indicate the limited value of many tests used in current clinical practice. Only a few studies were mentioned in this chapter as examples, while others are mentioned throughout this text. Major decisions about treatment should not be made based on a single diagnostic test. The clinical picture combined with appropriate tests will permit diagnosis most of the time, but many current physical examination tests have poor reliability and validity. Structural examinations are grossly overused, with the associated costs to individuals and society. Public opinion, patient expectations, and legal issues perpetuate this unfortunate practice. Careful research on the true value of all diagnostic tests used in spinal disorders must continue.

REFERENCES

1. Adatepe MH, Powell DM, Isaacs GH, Nichols K, Cefola R (1986): Hematogenous pyogenic vertebral osteomyelitis: Diagnostic value of radionuclide bone imaging. *J Nucl Med* 27:1680–1685.
2. Anand AK, Lee BC (1982): Plain and metrizamide CT of lumbar disk disease, comparison with myelography. *AJNR* 3:541–567.
3. Aronson HA, Dunsmore RH (1963): Herniated upper lumbar discs. *J Bone Joint Surg* 45A:311–317.
4. Bell GR, Rothman RH, Booth RE, Cuckler JM, Garfin S, Herkowitz H, Simeone FA, Dolinskas C, Han SS (1984): Study of computer assisted tomography. *Spine* 9:552–556.
5. Bell GR, Rothman RH, Booth RE, et al. (1984): A study of computer-assisted tomography. II: Comparison of metrizamide myelography and computed tomography in the diagnosis of herniated lumbar disk and spinal stenosis. *Spine* 9:552–556.
6. Boden S, Davis DO, Dina TS, Patronas NJ, Wiesel SW (1990): The incidence of abnormal lumbar spine MRI scans in asymptomatic patients: a prospective investigation. *J Bone Joint Surg* 72A:403–408.
7. Boden SD, McCowin PR, Davis DO, et al. (1990): Abnormal Magnetic-resonance scans of the cervical spine in asymptomatic subjects. *J Bone Joint Surg* 72A:1178–1184.
8. Bosacco SJ, Berman AT, Garbarino JL, Teplick JG, Peysler R (1984): A comparison of CT scanning and myelography in the diagnosis of lumbar disk herniation. *Clin Orthop* 190:124–128.
9. Brolin I (1975): Product control of lumbar radiographs. *Lakartidningen* 72:1793–1795 (in Swedish).
10. Calin A, Kay B, Sternberg M, Antell B, Chan M (1980): The prevalence and nature of back pain in an industrial complex: questionnaire and radiographic and HLA analysis. *Spine* 5:201–205.
11. Calin A, Porta J, Fries JF, Schurman DJ (1977): Clinical history as a screening test for ankylosing spondylitis. *JAMA* 237:2613–2614.
12. Chaffin DB, Herrin CD, Keyserling WM (1978): Preemployment strength testing. An updated position. *J Occup Med* 20:403–408.
13. Charnley J (1951): Orthopedic signs in the diagnosis of disc protrusion with special reference to the straight leg raising test. *Lancet* 1:186–192.
14. Deyo RA (1995): Reliability of radiographic studies. In: Weinstein JN, Wiesel S, eds. *The lumbar spine*. Philadelphia: W. B. Saunders.
15. Deyo RA, Diehl AK (1986): Lumbar spine films in primary care: current use and effects of selective ordering criteria. *J Gen Intern Med* 1:20–25.
16. Deyo RA, Rainville J, Kent DL (1992): What can the history and physical examination tell us about low back pain? *JAMA* 268:760–765.
17. Eisenberg RL, Akin JR, Hedgecock MW (1979): Single well centered lateral view of lumbosacral spine: Is coned view necessary? *Am J Radiol* 133:711–713.
18. Firooznia H, Benjamin V, Kricheff II, Rafii M, Golimbu C (1984): CT of lumbar spine disk herniation: correlation with surgical findings. *AJR* 142:587–592.
19. Forristall RM, Marsh HO, Pay NT (1988): Magnetic resonance imaging and contrast CT of the lumbar spine, comparison of diagnostic methods and correlation with surgical findings. *Spine* 13:1049–1054.
20. Frymoyer JF, Gordon S (1988): *New perspectives in low back pain.* Park Ridge, IL.: Am Acad Orthop Surg, pp. 45–47.
21. Gran JT (1985): An epidemiological survey of the signs and symptoms of ankylosing spondylitis. *Clin Rheumatol* 4:161–169.
22. Hakelius A (1970): Prognosis in sciatica. *Acta Orthop Scand* (Suppl) 129:1–70.
23. Himmelstein JS, Andersson GBJ (1988): Low back pain: risk evaluation and preplacement screening. In: *Occupational medicine: state of the art reviews.* Philadelphia: Hanley and Belfus 3:255–269.
24. Hitselberger WE, Witten RM (1968): Abnormal myelograms in asymptomatic patients. *J Neurosurg* 28:204–206.
25. Hoffman RM, Kent DL, Deyo RA (1991): Diagnostic accuracy and clinical utility of thermography for lumbar radiculopathy: a meta-analysis. *Spine* 16:623–628.
26. Hudgins WR (1979): The crossed straight leg raising test: a diagnostic sign of herniated disc. *J Occup Med* 21:407–408.
27. Hudgins WR (1983): Computer-aided diagnosis of lumbar disc herniation. *Spine* 8:604–615.
28. Janssen ME, Bertrand SL, Joe C, Levine MI (1994): Lumbar herniated disc disease: comparison of MRI myelography and postmyelographic CT scan with surgical findings. *Orthopedics* 17:121–127.
29. Jensen MC, Brant-Zawdzki MN, Obuchowski N, et al. (1994): Magnetic Resonance Imaging of the lumbar spine in people without back pain. *N Engl J Med* 331:69–73.
30. Kelen GD, Noji EK, Dous PE (1986): Guidelines for use of lumbar spine radiographs. *Ann Emerg Med* 15:245–251.
31. Kent DL, Haynor DR, Larson EB, Deyo RA (1992): Diagnosis of lumbar spinal stenosis in adults: a meta-analysis of the accuracy of CT, MR, and myelography. *AJR* 158:1135–1144.
32. Kortelainen P, Puranen J, Koivisto E, Lahde S (1985): Symptoms and signs of sciatica and their relation to the localization of the lumbar disc herniation. *Spine* 10:88–92.
33. Kosteljanetz M, Bang F, Schmidt-Olsen S (1988): The clinical significance of straight-leg-raising (Lasegue's sign) in the diagnosis of prolapsed lumbar disc. *Spine* 13:393–395.
34. Kosteljanetz M, Esperen JO, Halaburt H, Miletic T (1984): Predictive value of clinical and surgical findings in patients with lumbago-sciatica: a prospective study (Part 1). *Acta Neurochir* 73:67–76.
35. Li KC, Poon PY (1988): Sensitivity and specificity of MRI in detecting malignant spinal cord compression and in distinguishing malignant from benign compression fractures of vertebrae. *Magn Reson Imag* 6:547–556.
36. Liang M, Komaroff AL (1982): Roentgenograms in primary care patients with acute low back pain. *Arch Intern Med* 142:1108–1112.
37. MacDonald EB, Porter R, Hibbert C, et al. (1984): The relationship between spinal canal diameter and back pain in coal miners. Ultrasonic measurement as a screening test? *J Occup Med* 26:23–28.
38. Masaryk TJ, Ross JS, Modic MT, Boumphrey F, Bohlman H, Wilber G (1988): High-resolution MR imaging of sequestered lumbar intervertebral disks. *AJR* 150:1155–1162.
39. Modic MT, Masaryk T, Boumphrey F, Goormastic M, Bell G (1986): Lumbar herniated disk disease and canal stenosis: prospective evaluation by surface coil MR, CT, and myelography. *AJR* 147:757–765.

40. Morrison AS (1986): *Screening in chronic disease.* New York: Oxford University Press.

41. Moufarrij NA, Hardy RW Jr, Weinstein MA (1983): Computed tomographic, myelographic, and opertaive findings in patients with suspected herniated lumbar disk. *Neurosurgery* 12:184–188.

42. Ott SM, Kilcoyne RF, Chesnut CH III (1987): Ability of four different techniques of measuring bone mass to diagnose vertebral fractures in post-menopausal women. *J Bone Miner Res* 2:201–210.

43. Rockey PH, Tompkins RK, Wood RW, Wolcott BW (1978): The usefulness of x-ray examinations in the evaluation of patients with back pain. *J Fam Pract* 7:455–465.

44. Sadowska-Wroblewska M, Filipowicz A, Garwolinska H, Michalski J, Rusiniak B, Wroblewska T (1983): Clinical symptoms and signs useful in the early diagnosis of ankylosing spondylitis. *Clin Rheum* 2:37–43.

45. Schipper J, Kardaun JW, Braakman R, Van Dongen KJ, Blaauw G (1987): Lumbar disk herniation: diagnosis with CT or myelography. *Radiology* 165:227–231

46. Schonstrom N, Lindahl S, Willén J, et al. (1989): Dynamic changes in the dimensions of the lumbar spinal canal. An experimental study in vivo. *J Orthop Res* 7:115–121.

47. Spangfort EV (1972): Lumbar disc herniation: a computer aided analysis of 2504 operations. *Acta Orthop Scand* (Suppl) 142:1–93.

48. Teresi LM, Lufkin, RB, Reicher MA, Moffit BJ, et al (1987): Asymptomatic degenerative disc disease and spondylosis of the cervical spine: MR imaging. *Radiology* 164:83–88.

49. Thornbury JR, Fryback DG, Turski PA, et al. (1993): Disk-caused nerve compression in patients with acute low-back pain: diagnosis with MR, CT myelography, and plain CT. *Radiology* 186:731–738.

50. Van der Linden S, Valkenburg HA, Cats A (1984): Evaluation of diagnostic criteria for ankylosing spondylitis: a proposal for modification of the New York criteria. *Arthritis Rheum* 27:361–368.

51. Waddell G (1982): An approach to backache. *Br J Hosp Med* (28)3:187–219.

52. Waddell G, Main CJ, Morris EW, et al. (1982): Normality and reliability in the clinical assessment of backache. *Br Med J* 284:1519–1523.

53. Weinreb JC, Wolbarsht LB, Cohen JM, Brown CE, Maravilla KR (1989): Prevalence of lumbosacral intervertebral disc abnormalities on MR images in pregnant and asymptomatic non-pregnant women. *Radiology* 170:125–128.

54. Wiesel SE, Tsourmas N, Feffer H, Ghui GM, Patronas N (1984): A study of computer-assisted tomography. I. The incidence of positive CAT scans in an asymptomatic group of patients. *Spine* 9:549–551.

55. Williams JI (1988): Criteria for screening: Are the effects predictable? *Spine* 13:1178–1186.

56. Wilson JMG, Jungner F (1968): *Principles and practice of screening for disease.* (Public Health Papers No. 34). Geneva, Switzerland: World Health Organization.

57. Zsernaviczky J, Juppe M (1989): A comparison of myelography and computer tomography in lumbar disc herniation. *Int Orthop* 13:51–55.

The Adult Spine: Principles and Practice,
2nd edition, J.W. Frymoyer, Editor-in-Chief.
Lippincott-Raven Publishers, Philadelphia © 1997.

CHAPTER 21

Clinical Evaluation of Patients with Suspected Spine Problems

Jeffrey D. Klein and Steven R. Garfin

The clinical evaluation of patients with suspected spine problems includes a local examination of both the cervical and the thoracolumbar regions, as well as a thorough neurologic assessment. In each case, the examination is modified by the specific environment in which care is provided. There are special considerations, for example, in the case of trauma and spinal cord injury. In all instances, the physical examination must be preceded by a thorough history.

HISTORY

A careful history is essential in the evaluation of patients with spinal disorders. Most diagnoses are made, or at least a differential diagnosis should be possible, at this stage. One must distinguish not only between the various primary disorders of the spine, but also differentiate them from systemic processes that can affect the spine, such as metastatic disease and the spondyloarthropathies.

J. D. Klein, M.D.: Hospital for Joint Disease, Orthopaedic Institute, New York, New York 10028.
S. R. Garfin, M.D.: Professor, Department of Orthopaedic Surgery, University of California at San Diego, San Diego, California, 92103-8894.

The location, quality, and chronicity of pain should be described. Coughing, sneezing, and straining cause an increase in intrathecal pressure. Radicular pain that occurs during these activities suggests the possibility of nerve root compression by a space-occupying lesion of the spinal canal, such as a herniated disc. In the cervical spine, axially located neck pain must be distinguished from arm pain. A radicular pattern should be sought. In the lumbar spine, back pain must be separated from leg pain (sciatica), while in the cervical spine one must distinguish neck pain from arm pain. This is important for diagnosis, though there are therapeutic and prognostic implications as well. This is particularly true in the degenerative processes, as leg or arm pain may have a time-dependent "window" to optimize the surgical results, whereas neck or back pain rarely does. Classically, the radiating sciatic type of pain extends below the knee. However, S1 and occasionally L5 irritation can localize to the buttock or posterior thigh. The patient may describe radiation of pain from the back, over the hip, and down the thigh and leg to the foot. Exact localization should be sought. For example, pain radiating to the dorsum of the foot and the great toe, particularly the first web space, suggest involvement of the L5 nerve root. Similarly, specific dermatomal patterns are identified in the cervical spine. Radicular pain should be distinguished from referred sclerotomal pain. Degenerative changes in the outer layers of the anuli fibrosi of the discs and degenerative changes in the lumbar facet joints are both potential sources of referred pain to the extremities. Such pain is typically less discrete than radicular pain in its distribution and tends to worsen throughout the day, partly as a function of increased physical loading. Figures 1 and 2 summarize the dermatomes of the upper and lower extremities.

Associated neurologic signs and symptoms should be sought. Dermatomal sensory loss, paresthesias, and localized motor weakness suggest radiculopathy. In contrast to isolated nerve root symptoms, generalized upper and lower extremity weakness, especially in conjunction with gait disturbance and bladder dysfunction, suggest myelopathy. The most common cause of myelopathy in those over 60 is cervical spondylosis (5). Early findings may include neck pain; numb, cold, or painful hands; decreased fine motor skills; and subtle gait disturbance (broad-based). Some patients may exhibit a mild scissoring gait or describe a perceived loss of control. Others describe a foot drop, or slapping, when they walk, or an inability to rotate internally or externally a lower extremity smoothly. Radiculopathy and myelopathy may also coexist.

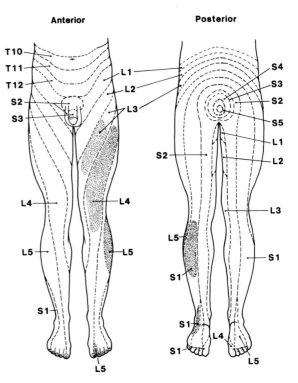

FIG. 2. Dermatomes of the lower extremity.

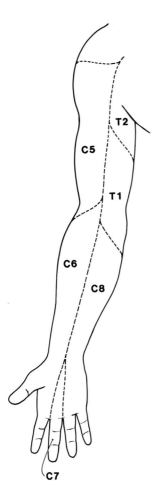

FIG. 1. Dermatomes of the upper extremity.

Disturbance of bowel or bladder function in the absence of upper motor neuron signs and symptoms demands immediate evaluation to exclude a diagnosis of a cauda equina syndrome. This is caused by compression of the nerve roots of the cauda equina by a space-occupying lesion, such as occurs with a large central disc herniation or a tumor. The presentation includes bowel or bladder dysfunction, saddle anesthesia, and variable loss of motor and sensory function in the lower extremities. In the older population the symptoms may be more subtle and sometimes confused with primary genitourinary disease. Urgent evaluation by appropriate neurodiagnostic imaging, followed by surgical intervention, is indicated.

In the lumbar spine, the pain of disc herniation tends to be worse when the patient is seated, presumably because of the increased intradiscal pressure which occurs in this position. In contrast, the neurogenic claudication of lumbar spinal stenosis is characterized by back pain and diffuse pain and numbness in the lower extremities. These symptoms are produced by standing, walking, and activities that require extension of the spine and are relieved by rest, including sitting down and leaning forward. This is explained by an increase in lumbar lordosis with standing and walking, associated with posterior disc compression and bulging into the canal, facet overriding, and increased buckling of the ligamentum flavum. These changes combine to encroach further upon the central canal and the neuroforamen, which are already narrowed by the hypertrophic facets and degenerative discs.

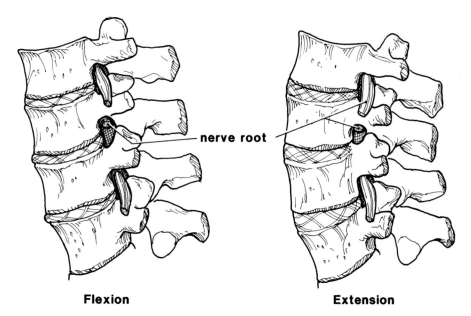

Flexion   **Extension**

FIG. 3. Lordosis and neural compression.

This is in contrast to the increased space available for the neural elements in both the lumbar canal and the neuroforamen when the spine is in flexion (Fig. 3).

The examining clinician must also differentiate neurogenic from vascular claudication. The leg pain of vascular claudication is slowly relieved by standing still, whereas in neurologic claudication postural changes (sitting, leaning forward) are required to produce relief. Walking uphill is poorly tolerated by those with vascular claudication, whereas walking downhill is painful in neurogenic claudication because of the increased lordosis associated with this activity. Bicycle riding is generally well tolerated by patients with neurogenic claudication, particularly with the spine in a flexed position, but it is not tolerated by those who suffer from vascular claudication (6). Walking distance is fairly constant with a fixed vascular lesion, and generally quite variable in individuals with spinal stenosis. Finally, the leg pain in vascular conditions tends to be crampy and involve the posterior calf, without foot radiation or numbness. These differences are summarized in Table 1.

In the evaluation of back pain, the type of work performed by the patient is important, as is any secondary gain associated with the condition. One must exercise caution in the treatment of work-related injuries, as the results of treatment, particularly surgical, are uniformly worse in the presence of Worker's Compensation claims (20). Age is also of importance when considering the diagnosis, as cervical and lumbar disc herniation are more common in adults under 55 years, and spinal stenosis is far more common in those over 60 years of age.

Constant, unremitting pain is suggestive of tumor or infection. Night pain is also classically associated with these medically significant diseases. Concurrent symptoms may include fever, malaise, and weight loss. Pyogenic vertebral osteomyelitis is seen more often in older, debilitated patients and intravenous drug users. A history of antecedent infection or immunologic compromise is common.

Inflammatory arthritides commonly involve the axial skeleton and may lead to pain complaints, as well as focal or generalized stiffness. The pain and stiffness of the spondyloarthropathies is typically most severe in the morning and improves throughout the day. Cervical spine involvement is common in patients with rheumatoid arthritis, especially those with longstanding polyarticular disease. Neck pain and occipital headaches are common complaints, and these patients must be followed carefully for the development of myeloradiculopathy. Low back pain is less commonly seen in rheumatoid arthritis, but it is a common presentation in the seronegative spondyloarthropathies.

Any previous or family history of spinal disorders should be noted. Concurrent medical and psychiatric illnesses are also important, as they may contribute to the symptoms and signs.

Visceral sources of referred pain to the lumbar spine

TABLE 1. *Characteristics of neurogenic versus vascular claudication*

	Neurogenic claudication	Vascular claudication
Palliative factors	Sitting, bending, leaning	Stop walking, standing
Walking uphill	Painless	Painful
Walking downhill	Painful	Painless
Bicycle test	Painless	Painful
Walking distance	Variable	Constant

and lower thoracic spine include peptic ulcers, cholecystitis, pancreatitis, retrocecal appendicitis, and dissecting abdominal aortic aneurysms in both genders, pelvic inflammatory disease and endometriosis in women, and prostate disorders in men. Angina, too, can be confused with cervical spine–related symptoms ("cervical angina"). However, the more difficult clinical problem is separating disorders of the shoulder and occasionally pulmonary disease such as Pancoast tumor from primary cervical disease.

THE CERVICAL SPINE

Examination of the cervical spine begins with inspection, including the patient's gait, posture, and head position. The patient should be seated and the neck viewed from the front, sides, and back for deformities. Head tilt may signify a muscular torticollis secondary to traumatic or inflammatory involvement of the sternocleidomastoid muscle. In this case, the head tilts towards the ipsilateral shoulder and rotates towards the contralateral side (Fig. 4). Head tilt may, however, reflect cerebellar dysfunction or an ophthalmological disorder. In the younger patient, congenital scoliosis or atlantoaxial rotatory subluxation are also considerations. The latter is a rotational and/or translational deformity involving the first and second cervical vertebrae, most often traumatic or inflammatory in nature.

It is extremely important, though frequently forgotten, to have the patient undress above the waist. This allows examination of the shoulder and back, anatomically related areas that can be sources of referred pain to the neck.

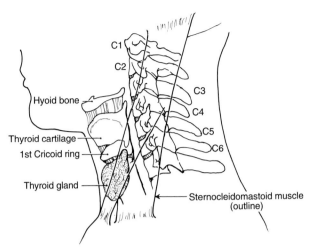

FIG. 5. The anterior bony and soft-tissue structures of the neck.

The examination proceeds with anterior and posterior palpation of the bony and soft tissue structures of the neck (Fig. 5). The hyoid bone lies anteriorly at the level of the C3 vertebral body. The thyroid cartilage marks the level of the C4 and C5 vertebral bodies. The first cricoid ring lies anterior to the C6 vertebral body. The thyroid gland lies over the thyroid cartilage at the C4-C5 vertebral level in the anterior midline. Tenderness or swelling of the sternocleidomastoid muscle may be traumatic or inflammatory in origin and can result in torticollis.

Occasionally, a cervical rib may be palpable in the supraclavicular fossa. This anomaly can be associated with thoracic outlet syndrome, which is characterized by intermittent vascular or neurologic compromise of the upper extremity resulting from compression of the subclavian vessels or the lower two nerve roots (C8, T1) of the brachial plexus. Additionally, compression of these neurovascular structures as they pass between the scalenus anticus and scalenus medius muscles can also cause this syndrome. One maneuver to assess this compression is Adson's test (Fig. 6). The patient's radial pulse is palpated and noted before and after the arm is passively abducted, extended, and externally rotated. Patients are then told to turn their heads towards the arm in question. Diminution or loss of the pulse suggests compression of the subclavian artery and a possible diagnosis of thoracic outlet syndrome.

Posteriorly, the spinous processes and interspinous ligaments should be assessed for tenderness. Such tenderness in the trauma patient suggests posterior ligamentous injury or a spinous process fracture. Generalized posterior cervical tenderness may also signify simple muscular strain. The spinous processes are aligned in the midline in the normal subject. A shift in alignment may signify a unilateral facet dislocation or a spinous process fracture.

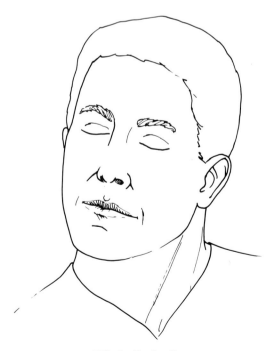

FIG. 4. Torticollis.

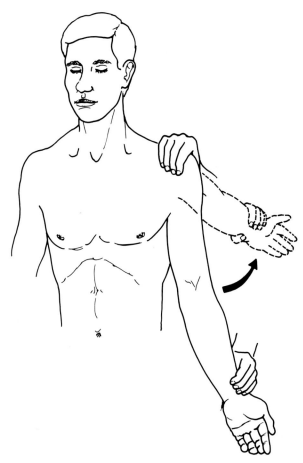

FIG. 6. Adson's test.

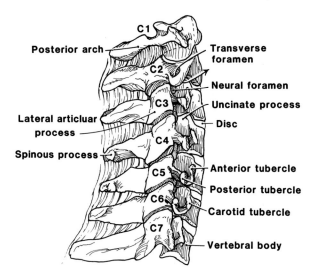

FIG. 7. The bony and ligamentous anatomy of the posterior cervical spine.

adult, for example, can touch chin to chest in flexion and bring the occiput to within three or four fingerbreadths of the dorsal spine in extension. Alternatively, a goniometer or inclinometer can be used for more precise angular measurements. Normal rotation is almost 90° (the chin should align with the shoulder) and lateral bending approaches 45° (Fig. 10). Approximately 50% of the flexion and extension in the cervical spine occurs at the occiput-C1 articulation and 50% of the rotation occurs across the C1-C2 motion segment.

Associated Tests

The cervical compression test is a provocative maneuver performed by applying axial pressure on the top of

However, these changes in alignment, or even the absolute levels of the structures, are often not easily discernible without radiographs. The C7 and T1 spinous processes are usually the most prominent and may serve as useful bony landmarks to the respective vertebral levels posteriorly. The bony and ligamentous anatomy of the posterior cervical spine is depicted in Figure 7.

The examiner may also encounter tenderness posterolaterally over the trapezius muscle. This may be due to direct injury or to spasm secondary to trauma, or it may be referred from an underlying cervical condition such as spondylosis, tumor, or infection. The greater occipital nerves represent the dorsal rami of C2 and may be tender at the base of the skull (Fig. 8).

Range of Motion

Active and passive range of motion should be noted. Qualitative descriptions of motion are probably more reproducible than specific numeric measurements. Measurement of the distance of the chin to the sternum in flexion and of the occiput to the dorsal spine in extension are helpful. This can be described in terms of fingerbreadths or measured with a ruler (Fig. 9). The normal

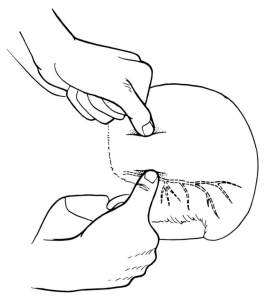

FIG. 8. The greater occipital nerve.

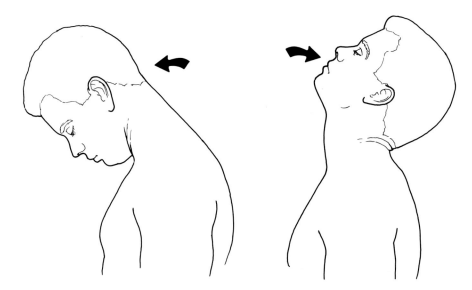

FIG. 9. Normal range of neck flexion and extension.

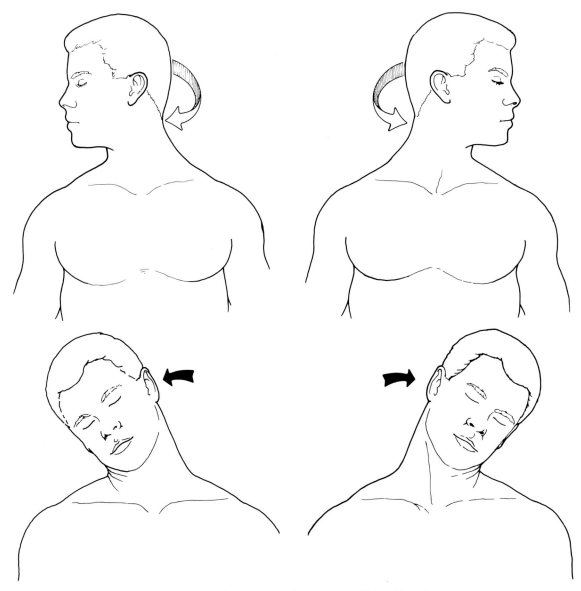

FIG. 10. Normal range of neck rotation and lateral bending.

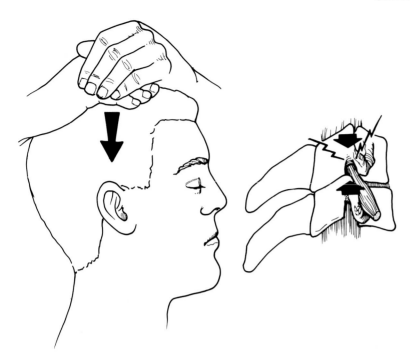

FIG. 11. The cervical compression test.

the patient's head (Fig. 11). A positive response includes neck pain, and more importantly, arm pain (note a radicular pattern if present). This is generally seen in patients with a disc herniation or neuroforaminal encroachment of the nerve root. Spurling's test includes compression of the head with the neck extended and rotated to the side of the radicular pain. A positive test includes complaints of reproduction of the radiating arm pain, and, again, it suggests spinal nerve root entrapment in the neuroforamen (18). The cervical distraction test is performed by gradually distracting the patient's head (Fig. 12). Patients with nerve root compression from herniated discs or neuroforaminal narrowing may note diminution of pain, as the distraction maneuver tends to en-

large the neuroforamen and decrease the load across the facet joints. The shoulder abduction test is performed by passively abducting the patient's involved arm. This reduces nerve root tension and relieves arm pain in 68% of patients with cervical radiculopathy due to extradural compression (4).

Neurologic Evaluation

Directly related to the physical examination of the cervical spine is the examination of the upper extremity by neurologic levels. Motor, sensory, and reflex activity, if appropriate, should be assessed at each root level. Muscle

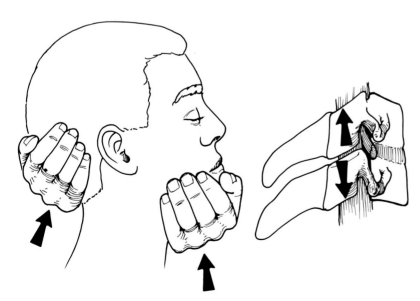

FIG. 12. The cervical distraction test.

TABLE 2. *Muscle grading*

Muscle gradations	Description
5—Normal	Complete range of motion against gravity with full resistance
4—Good	Complete range of motion against gravity with some resistance
3—Fair	Complete range of motion against gravity
2—Poor	Complete range of motion with gravity eliminated
1—Trace	Evidence of slight contractility; no joint motion
0—Zero	No evidence of contractility

strength is graded from 0 (no evidence of contractility) to 5 (complete range of motion against gravity with full resistance). A grade of 1 represents slight contractility, and 2, complete range of motion with gravity eliminated. A grade of 3 is complete range of motion against gravity, and 4, complete range of motion against gravity with some resistance. Table 2 summarizes the standard system for grading muscle strength. The critical importance of this examination warrants a review of these levels at this stage.

The C5 nerve root innervates the deltoid muscle and, along with C6, the biceps muscle. It supplies sensation to the lateral arm (over the shoulder) and is primarily responsible for the biceps reflex (Fig. 13). The C6 root innervates the wrist extensors and, along with C5, the biceps muscle. The C6 sensory distribution includes the lateral forearm, the thumb, the index finger, and occasionally part of the middle finger. The posterior rami of C6, C7, and C8 supply sensation to the region overlying the scapula. The associated reflex at this level is the brachioradialis (Fig. 14). The C7 motor distribution includes the triceps muscle, the wrist flexors, and the finger extensors. C7 provides sensation to the middle finger and is primarily responsible for the triceps reflex (Fig. 15). The C8 neurologic level includes motor innervation of the long finger flexors and the interossei. The sensory supply is to the ulnar side of the hand and the distal half of the ulnar aspect of the forearm. There is no reflex test for the C8 level (Fig. 16). The T1 level includes motor innervation of the interossei. Sensory supply is to the ulnar side of the proximal forearm and distal arm. There is no associated deep tendon reflex (Fig. 17). Figure 1 demonstrates the sensory supply of the upper extremity by root level, and Table 3 summarizes the neurologic levels of the upper extremity. It is important to note that the C4 sensory distribution includes the upper anterior chest wall. This is often confusing, because thoracic innervation occurs immediately below. The remainder of the cervical roots (C5 through C8) and the T1 root are, as noted above, represented along the arm and into the axilla. This distribution is related to the growth of the limb buds during embryonic development (14).

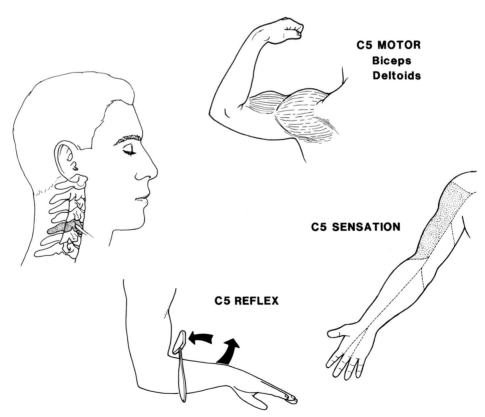

C5 MOTOR
Biceps
Deltoids

C5 SENSATION

C5 REFLEX

FIG. 13. The C5 neurologic level.

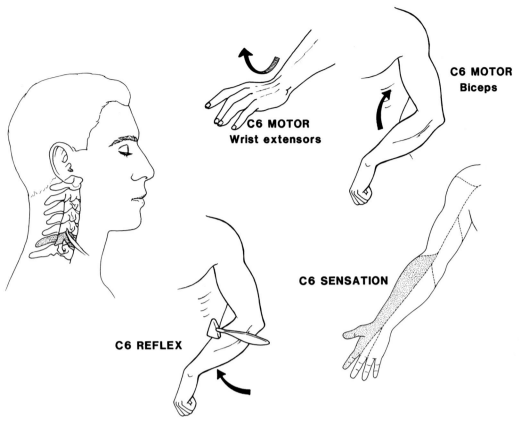

FIG. 14. The C6 neurologic level.

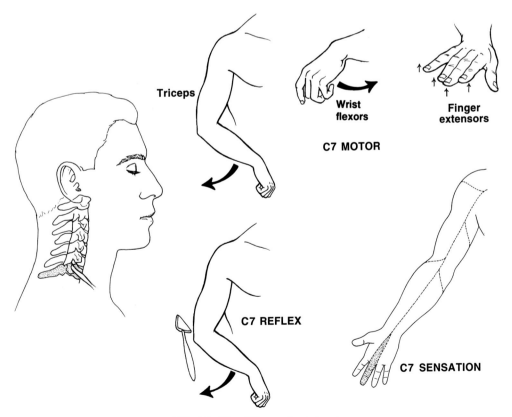

FIG. 15. The C7 neurologic level.

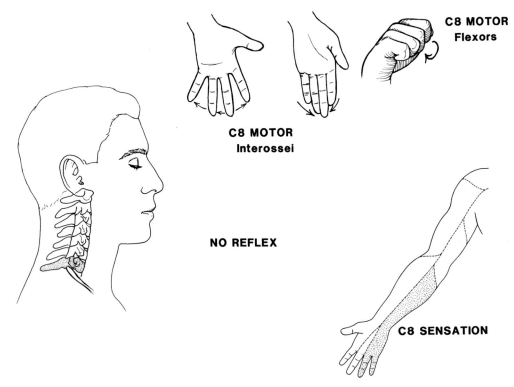

FIG. 16. The C8 neurologic level.

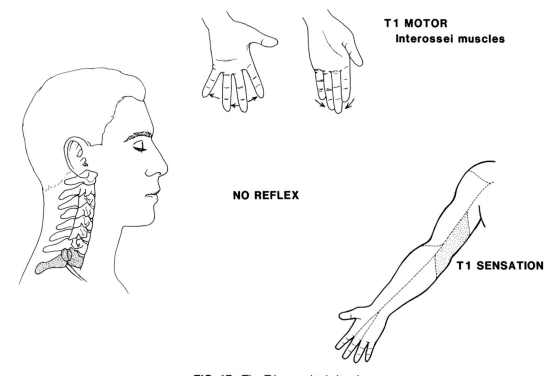

FIG. 17. The T1 neurologic level.

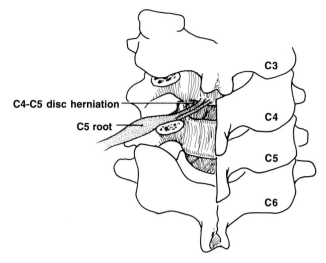

FIG. 18. Cervical disc herniation.

TABLE 3. *Neurologic levels of the upper extremity*

Root	Reflex	Muscles	Sensation
C5	Biceps reflex	Deltoid	Lateral arm
		Biceps	(Axillary nerve)
C6	Brachioradialis reflex	Wrist extensors	Lateral forearm
		Biceps	(Musculocutaneous nerve)
C7	Triceps reflex	Wrist flexors	Middle finger
		Finger extensors	
		Triceps	
C8	—	Finger flexors	Medial forearm
		Hand intrinsics	(Medial antebrachial cutaneous nerve)
T1	—	Hand intrinsics	Medial arm
			(Medial brachial cutaneous nerve)

The nerve roots in the cervical spine exit above the pedicle of the corresponding numbered vertebrae. There are eight cervical nerve roots and seven cervical vertebrae, thus changing this relationship at the cervicothoracic junction. Starting at T1 and throughout the remainder of the thoracolumbar spine, the numbered nerve root exits caudal to the pedicle of the corresponding vertebra. This has clinical implications in the evaluation of herniated discs. A typical posterolateral cervical disc herniation impinges on the nerve root exiting at the level of the disc. For example, a disc herniation at the C4-C5 level compresses the C5 nerve root and a C7-T1 herniated disc compromises the C8 root (Fig. 18). Occasionally, one may encounter an inconsistent or confusing level of neurologic involvement. In such a patient, consider the pos-

sibility of a prefixed (begins at C4), or postfixed (begins at C6), brachial plexus.

If the clinical setting warrants (trauma, rheumatoid arthritis, cervical spondylosis), it is important to test for pathologic upper motor neuron reflexes in both the upper and lower extremities, as well as other signs of myelopathy or spinal cord damage. Decreased vibratory sense and proprioception are subtle signs seen early in the course of myelopathy. Lhermitte's sign is characterized by shocklike pains radiating down the arms or legs with passive flexion and compression of the neck. Babinski's test involves firmly stroking the plantar surface of the foot with a sharp instrument, starting from the heel

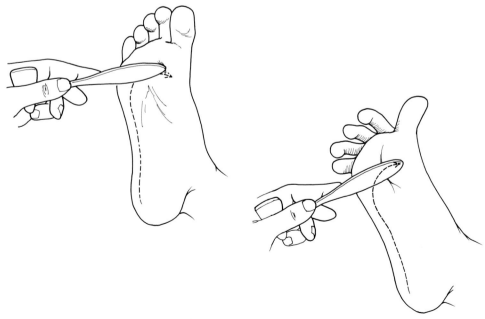

FIG. 19. The Babinski test.

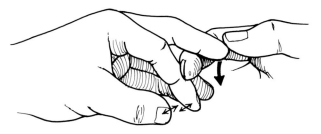

FIG. 20. Hoffman's sign.

and proceeding distally along the lateral aspect of the sole and then medially across the forefoot (Fig. 19). The normal, or negative, response consists of no movement or downward motion of the toes. A positive response consists of extension of the great toe and spreading (fanning) of the lesser toes. Oppenheim's sign is tested for by firmly running one's finger, or a hard object, distally along the crest of the tibia. A positive response is the same as for the Babinski test. This test is sometimes better tolerated than Babinski's test by those patients with very sensitive feet.

Generalized hyperreflexia is also associated with myelopathy (spinal cord compression), especially when in conjunction with a positive Babinski sign. Clonus is a rhythmic, repetitive oscillation of the foot at the ankle in response to sudden, maintained dorsiflexion of the foot and stretching of the tendo Achillis. The presence of clonus, too, is suggestive of myelopathy. Hoffman's sign is a pathologic reflex that is elicited in the upper extremity. The hand is held in a comfortable resting position and the nail of the middle finger is "flicked." A positive reaction consists of flexion of the terminal phalanx of the thumb and index finger (Fig. 20). If one elicits pathologic reflexes in the lower extremity, and Hoffman's sign is

negative, this may suggest that the problem lies below the level of the cervical spinal cord. This hypothesis can be further supported by hyperreflexia limited to the lower extremities.

Myelopathy hand refers to the loss of power of adduction and extension of the ulnar two or three fingers due to weak intrinsics (16). These fingers may spontaneously abduct giving rise to the "finger escape sign." These findings, together with hyperreflexia, are suggestive of cervical myelopathy, usually above the C6-C7 level (16).

THORACIC AND LUMBAR SPINE

Physical examination of the thoracic and lumbar spine includes observation of the gait and general movements of the patient. Any splinting, antalgia, circumduction, "drop foot gait," Trendelenburg gait, or awkward motions should be noted. Further inspection with the patient disrobed should seek evidence of abnormal skin markings or hairy patches that may be present at the base of the spine. These may signify a benign spina bifida, or they may be related to a more significant underlying anomaly, such as a diastematomyelia or tethered spinal cord.

The overall posture should be assessed and any deformities in the sagittal or coronal plane described. Scoliosis may be idiopathic or congenital in the child. Idiopathic scoliosis in the child is generally painless. Complaints of pain should prompt one to consider other concurrent diagnoses. An acute onset of scoliosis in an adult suggests either sciatica or tumor. A sciatic list to one side may indicate a contralateral lateral disc herniation or an ipsilateral axillary disc herniation (Fig. 21). In the child, serial clinical and radiographic examinations

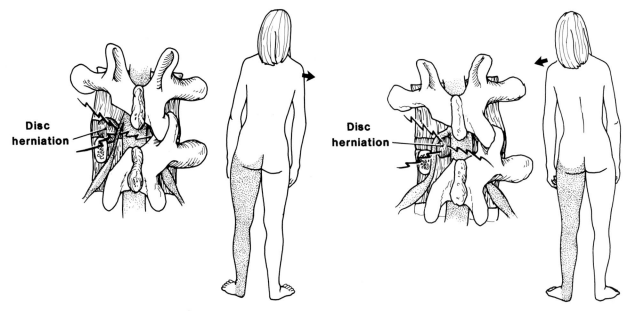

FIG. 21. Sciatic list and lateral bending in disc herniation.

are needed to document evidence of progression of any deformity. In the forward bend test, the examiner kneels in front and then behind the patient while the patient flexes forward at the waist, drops the hands, and flexes the neck. One inspects the spinal alignment and notes any rib or paravertebral muscle asymmetry, which reflects rotational deformity seen concurrently with scoliosis. By sighting down the spine, one can roughly measure the height of the rib prominence. A more accurate and reproducible assessment of the rotational deformity can be made with a scoliometer or inclinometer (Fig. 22).

The overall balance of the spine can be assessed by dropping a plumb line (a weighted string or tape measure) from the C7 vertebra or the occipital prominence. This straight line normally aligns with the gluteal cleft, indicating that the trunk is centered over the pelvis (is in balance). Distance in centimeters, lateral to the cleft, should be recorded (Fig. 23). Another method to assess alignment is to simply note the position of the trunk relative to the pelvis. It is important to exclude leg length inequality as a cause of pelvic obliquity and scoliosis. True leg lengths are generally measured from the ipsilateral anterior superior iliac spine to the medial malleolus, with the patient supine. The apparent, or functional, leg length is measured from the umbilicus to the medial malleolus (Fig. 24). Apparent leg length inequality may be secondary to fixed pelvic obliquity or from an adduction or flexion deformity of the hip.

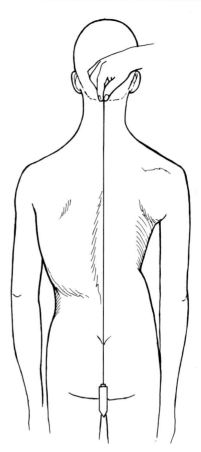

FIG. 23. The plumb line.

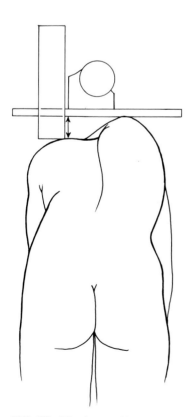

FIG. 22. The forward bend test.

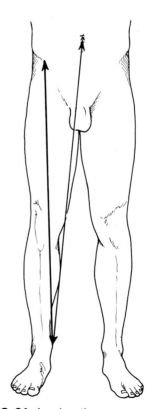

FIG. 24. Leg length measurement.

In contrast to childhood scoliosis, adult scoliosis is often more symptomatic, and back pain is a more common presenting complaint. Curves of large magnitude and lumbar curves are generally more painful. The etiology may be idiopathic, degenerative, posttraumatic, postsurgical, or neuromuscular, and it is sometimes associated with neuroforaminal and central stenosis. Thoracic curves greater than 65° may affect pulmonary function, especially if in combination with thoracic lordosis (15). In these individuals, baseline pulmonary function tests should be obtained as part of the examination.

The iliac crest and the posterior superior iliac spine are posterior bony landmarks that can aid in establishing approximate vertebral levels. The top of the iliac crest usually lies at approximately the level of the L4-L5 interspace, and the posterior superior iliac spine at the level of S2. The spinous processes and interspinous ligaments should be palpated and percussed for tenderness. In the trauma patient, tenderness or a palpable gap suggests ligamentous instability or fracture. A stepoff across the spinous processes suggests the possibility of spondylolisthesis. The paraspinal muscles should be palpated and any spasm or tenderness noted. Finally, the area over the sciatic nerve in the region of the sciatic notch should be palpated. Tenderness suggests irritation of contributing nerve roots, most commonly by a disc herniation, but occasionally by muscle spasm or direct trauma to the nerve.

Anteriorly, in a thin patient, one can, with deep pressure, palpate the sacral promontory and with difficulty the L4, L5, and S1 vertebral bodies. Palpation of the anterior abdominal muscles with the patient in a partial sit-up position can detect weakness or asymmetry in these segmentally innervated muscles. One should take this opportunity to examine the abdomen (routine evaluation including tenderness, masses, organomegaly, and aortic enlargement) in order to exclude sources of referred pain to the back. A rectal examination is important to perform in older patients in order to palpate the prostate gland, or in those complaining of coccygeal (tailbone) pain. A pelvic examination should be considered in women in order to exclude other sources of referred low back pain.

Range of Motion

Range of motion should be tested, and here, as in the cervical spine, qualitative descriptions are useful. Flexion can be measured by having the patient bend as far forward as possible, with the knees held straight, and noting the distance from the floor to the fingertips. The motion can be estimated in degrees or as a percent of total normal motion. It is important to note that much of the apparent flexion in the lower back occurs through the hips. The modified Schober's test attempts to identify those patients with true limitation of motion in the lumbar spine (12). With the patient standing, a 15 cm span is measured over the lumbar spine, beginning 10 cm above and extending 5 cm below the L5 spinous process. The test is considered positive if this span is not increased by at least 6 cm in full flexion.

Flexion and extension in the thoracic spine are limited because of the small size of the discs, the restraint imposed by the rib cage, and the coronal orientation of the facets. Rotation, however, is greater than across the lumbar spine. In the lumbar spine, the larger discs, the absence of ribs, and the sagittal alignment of the facets allow a large flexion and extension arc, though rotation is limited. Lateral bending should also be tested and has particular relevance in scoliosis wherein an attempt is made to distinguish between flexible and rigid curves. Lateral bending may also reproduce ipsilateral leg pain in the presence of a lateral disc herniation and contralateral leg pain with an axillary disc herniation (see Fig. 21).

Pain with, or limitation of, forward flexion is a rather nonspecific finding. Pain on extension or hyperextension also may be a nonspecific finding, but it can signify spondylolysis or spondylolisthesis in the younger, active patient. Spondylolysis most likely represents a stress fracture in the pars interarticularis resulting from repetitive hyperextension stresses in a genetically predisposed individual. It is the most common cause of low back pain in children and adolescents. Spondylolysis is rarely, however, symptomatic as an isolated, first-time presenting entity, in adults over 40 years of age.

In an older individual, pain (particularly reproduction of leg pain complaints) on extension may be seen with spinal stenosis. Such patients often find relief in the flexed, or seated, position. Peripheral pulses should be checked on these patients in order to rule out a vascular etiology for their claudication.

Neurologic Evaluation

The examination of the thoracic and lumbar spine by neurologic levels should be routinely performed, as it is for the cervical spine. As noted above, thoracic motor function is assessed with the patient performing a partial sit-up, in order to detect any asymmetry in the segmentally innervated rectus abdominus muscles. The upper portion of these muscles are supplied by the T5 to T10 roots, and the lower portion from T10 to L1. Weakness on one side only, causes the umbilicus to move in the opposite direction (positive Beevor's sign). The sensory dermatomes of the trunk are depicted in Figure 25. As a rough guide, the T4 dermatome lies at the level of the nipple line, T7 at the level of the xiphoid process, T10 at the umbilicus, and T12 at the inguinal crease. The superficial abdominal reflex is an upper motor neuron reflex based on the segmental innervation of the abdominal

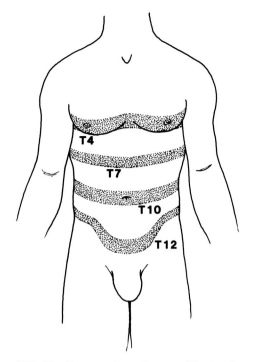

FIG. 25. Sensory dermatomes of the trunk.

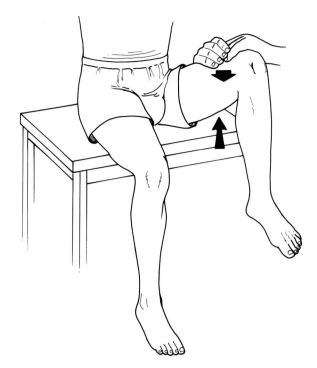

FIG. 26. Muscle test for the iliopsoas.

musculature. With the patient supine and relaxed, each quadrant of the abdomen is stroked. In the normal response, the umbilicus moves toward the stroked area. Lack of this superficial reflex suggests an upper motor neuron lesion. This is in contradistinction to the deep tendon reflexes, where increased reflexes would be expected in an upper motor neuron lesion.

Thoracic disc herniation is rare, and when present may cause cord, as well as root, symptoms. This process is more common in patients with underlying Scheuermann's kyphosis and tends to involve the mid to lower thoracic levels. If myelopathy is suspected from the clinical setting, pathologic upper motor neuron reflexes should be tested, as described for the cervical spine. In the adult patient with thoracic back and radicular pain, the differential diagnosis should include herpes zoster (shingles), noting that pain may precede the typical dermatomally distributed vesicular eruption.

The L1, L2, and L3 motor levels are tested by examining the iliopsoas muscle (primarily L1 and L2) (Fig. 26). This is performed manually by resisting hip flexion. The patient can also be observed stepping on and off a low platform. This may help detect a more subtle weakness. The corresponding sensory distribution includes the anterior thigh below the inguinal ligament. The superficial cremasteric reflex is another upper motor neuron reflex that tests the integrity of the T12 (efferent) and L1-L2 (afferent) neurologic levels. An intact reflex is characterized by unilateral elevation of the scrotal sac when the skin of the ipsilateral inner thigh is stroked (Fig. 27). The absence of this reflex suggests an upper motor neuron

lesion. The L2, L3, and L4 nerve roots innervate the quadriceps muscle (primarily L3 and L4) (Fig. 28). This is tested for by manually trying to flex the actively extended knee. A more subtle weakness may be detected by having the patient hold the knee in 5% to 10% of flexion, rather than full extension. The patient can also be ob-

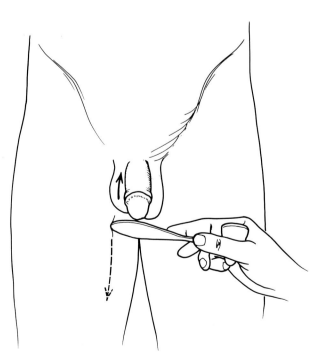

FIG. 27. The cremasteric reflex.

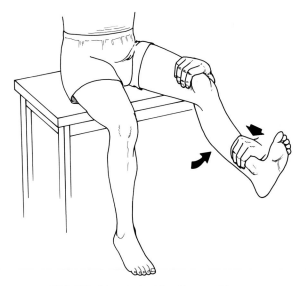

FIG. 28. Muscle test for the quadriceps.

served ascending and descending a series of steps. The sensory distribution courses along the anterior and anterolateral thigh.

The L4 nerve root innervates the tibialis anterior muscle in addition to the quadriceps. Heel walking is thus a test of the L4 motor level (additional contribution from the L5 innervated dorsiflexors of the great and lesser toes). The L4 root supplies sensation to the medial aspect of the leg and quite consistently to the skin overlying the medial malleolus. It is primarily responsible for the patellar reflex, though cross innervation occurs from L3, and to a lesser extent from L2 (Fig. 29).

The L5 root innervates the extensor hallucis longus. The patient is seated with both feet off the floor and is asked to actively dorsiflex both great toes against resistance (Fig. 30). Both toes are tested simultaneously to determine any asymmetry of strength. The L5 root is also the primary innervation of the hip abductors (with additional contribution from S1). In Trendelenburg's test, the patient is asked to alternately stand on one leg and then the other, while the examiner sits behind the patient with his or her hands on the patient's iliac crests. Normally, the pelvis remains level during this maneuver. Any drop of the pelvis on the side opposite the stance leg constitutes a positive sign (Fig. 31). A positive Trendelenburg sign implies weakness of the hip abductors on the weight-bearing side, resulting either from L5 root dysfunction or primary pathology of the hip joint. Any shift of the trunk over the stance leg during the performance of the test should be noted, as this maneuver generally indicates weakness of the abductor musculature.

The L5 root provides sensation to the lateral aspect of the leg and the dorsum of the foot, including the great toe. The first web space is uniformly attributable to L5 (Figs. 2,32). The associated reflex at this level is the tibialis posterior, if present. It is, however, difficult to elicit and the test is not routinely performed.

The S1 level includes motor innervation to the peronei and, along with S2, the gastrocsoleus muscle. Toe walking and repetitive toe raising are indications of the integrity of the S1 motor level. S1 provides sensation to the lateral aspect and sole of the foot, as well as the posterior leg. The associated reflex is that of the Achilles tendon (Fig. 33).

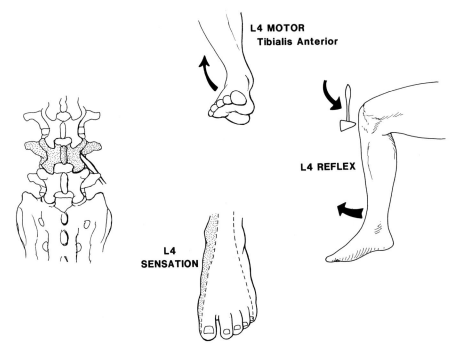

L4 MOTOR
Tibialis Anterior

L4 REFLEX

L4 SENSATION

FIG. 29. The L4 neurologic level.

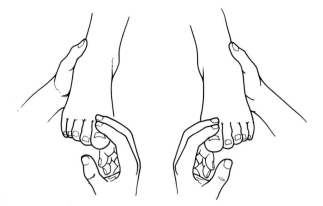

FIG. 30. Muscle test for the extensor hallucis longus.

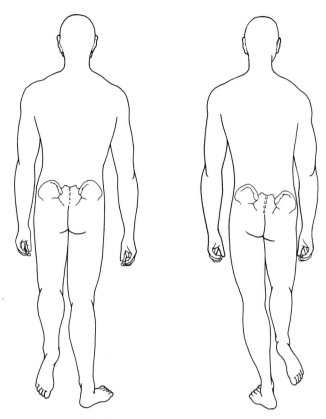

FIG. 31. The Trendelenburg test.

The S2, S3, and S4 levels supply the bladder, as well as the intrinsic muscles of the foot. The foot should be examined for cavus (high arch) as well as claw toe deformities. The innervation of the bladder can be assessed with urodynamic evaluation, if necessary. These levels also supply perianal sensation and provide innervation for the superficial anal reflex. Figure 2 depicts the sensory dermatomes of the lower extremity. Table 4 summarizes the neurologic levels of the lower extremity.

The nerve roots of the lumbar spine exit below the pedicle of the corresponding numbered vertebra and above the disc that is immediately caudal. A typical posterolateral disc herniation impinges on the nerve root that traverses over it, medial to the neuroforamen. For example, a disc herniation at the L4-L5 level most often affects the L5 nerve root (Fig. 34). However, a disc herniation lateral to, or at, the neuroforamen can affect the exiting nerve root above (for example, L4 for a far lateral

L4-L5 disc herniation), while a central herniation can affect one or more caudal nerve roots (Fig. 35). Lateral herniations are more common at L2-L3 and L3-L4, as opposed to typical posterolateral herniations, which are most common at L4-L5, followed by L5-S1. A large central herniation is a common cause of the cauda equina

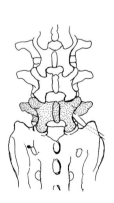

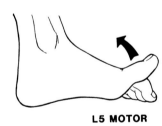

L5 MOTOR

Ext. Hal. Longus Lig.

NO REFLEX

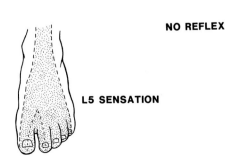

L5 SENSATION

FIG. 32. The L5 neurologic level.

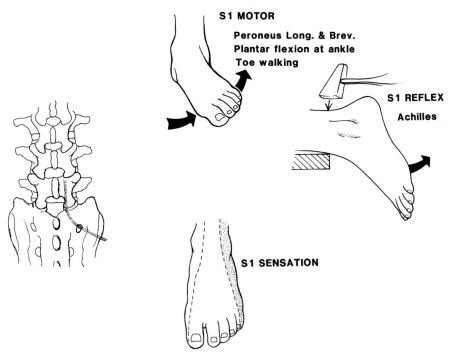

FIG. 33. The S1 neurologic level.

Nerve Root Tension Signs

Root tension signs are tests used to put the sciatic or femoral nerves on stretch. These are used primarily in the evaluation of the patient with suspected disc herniation and nerve root compression. The straight-leg raising test is performed with the patient supine, or sitting, on the examining table. The ankle is grasped and the leg lifted with the knee held in extension (Fig. 36). A positive test reproduces the patient's radicular pain. The degree of hip flexion at which hip or leg pain is experienced should be noted. Hamstring pain and tightness may cause posterior thigh pain. If there is any question, the knee can be flexed slightly from maximum extension and the foot dorsiflexed (the Lasègue maneuver) to again put the sciatic nerve on stretch and reproduce the patient's pain. Alternatively, with the knee slightly flexed, pressure can be applied to the tibial nerve in the region of the popliteal fossa (the bowstring test) (11). The con-

syndrome, and unlike most other disc herniations, represents a surgical urgency.

tralateral (well leg) straight-leg raising test is performed in the same fashion as the standard straight-leg raising maneuver, except that the uninvolved leg is elevated. A positive response reproduces pain in the opposite (involved) leg and suggests the possibility of an axillary disc herniation or a free fragment (17). The femoral stretch test is performed with the patient in either the prone or lateral decubitus position and involves extension of the thigh at the hip with the knee flexed (Fig. 37). Reproduction of the patient's pain (usually anterior or anterolateral thigh pain) is a tension sign suggesting involvement of the upper (L2, L3, and L4) nerve roots.

THE SACROILIAC JOINT

Sacroiliac joint pathology can be a cause of low back pain. One test for this is the Patrick or FABER (flexion, abduction, external rotation) test. With the patient supine, the knee is flexed and the foot placed on the opposite patella. The flexed knee is then pushed by the examiner as far laterally as possible. Any increased pain in the

TABLE 4. *Neurologic levels of the lower extremity*

Root	Reflex	Muscles	Sensation
L2	—	Iliopsoas	Anterior thigh, groin
L3	Patellar reflex	Quadriceps	Anterior and lateral thigh
L4	Patellar reflex	Anterior tibialis	Medial leg and medial foot; medial malleolus
L5	—	Extensor hallucis longus, hip abductors	Lateral leg and dorsum of foot; first web space
S1	Achilles reflex	Peroneus longus and brevis, gastroc. soleus	Lateral foot; little toe

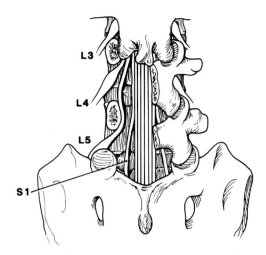

FIG. 34. Posterolateral lumbar disc herniation.

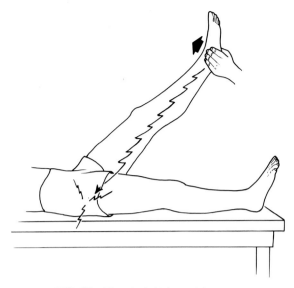

FIG. 36. The straight-leg raising test.

region of the sacroiliac joint is noted (Fig. 38). The pelvic rock test is also performed supine and involves compression of the iliac crests toward the midline of the body. This, too, may elicit pain with derangement of the sacroiliac joint.

THE HIP

The hip can also be a cause of referred pain to the back. This is further complicated by the fact that in older patients osteoarthritis of the hip frequently coexists with degenerative disease of the lumbar spine. Both can lead to hip and thigh pain. The former usually causes anterior groin and thigh pain proximal to the knee, while spinal stenosis is more often posterolateral, extending distal to the knee. Hip range of motion should be assessed, if hip joint pathology is in the differential. Even with neurodiagnostic studies, however, these clinical situations can be confusing. Occasionally, injection of local anesthetic into the hip, or conversely, an epidural steroid injection, can be helpful in distinguishing the source of the pain.

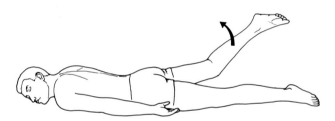

FIG. 37. The femoral stretch test.

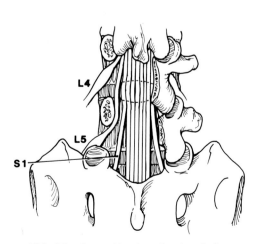

FIG. 35. Central lumbar disc herniation.

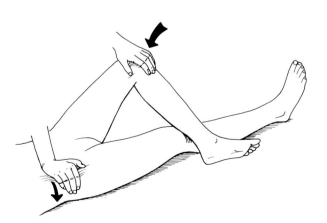

FIG. 38. The Patrick or FABER test.

NONORGANIC PHYSICAL SIGNS

When examining the patient with low back pain it is important to check for any nonorganic physical signs such as described by Waddell et al. (21). These five signs are an attempt to identify those patients who have a significant psychologic or socioeconomic basis for their pain. Nonorganic tenderness may include broad, superficial tenderness to light touch in the lumbar region, widespread deep tenderness in a nonanatomic distribution, or both. Simulation tests suggest to the patient that a specific examination is being performed, though in fact, it is not. For example, low back pain produced with either axial loading of the skull or shoulders, or passive rotation of the shoulders and pelvis in the plane through the hips, suggests involvement of nonorganic factors in the pain response. Distraction tests attempt to reproduce positive physical findings while the patient's attention is distracted. A positive supine straight-leg raising response may be suspect if the patient can flex the hip to 90° with the knee extended in the sitting position. This can be described to the patient as part of the routine knee examination. The supine straight-leg raising test as more commonly performed is described in all common texts and can be learned by the patient.

Regional disturbances are sensory and motor abnormalities that involve multiple regions and are unexplained on a neuroanatomic basis. "Give way" weakness, and sensory loss in a "stocking" rather than a dermatomal distribution, likely have a nonorganic component. Overreaction during examination may be the most frequently occurring, detectable, nonorganic physical sign. Disproportionate verbalization, inappropriate facial expression, tremor, collapsing, and sweating are all manifestations of this Waddell sign. The Waddell signs are summarized in Table 5.

Burns' test is another maneuver used to identify those patients who may be symptom magnifiers. In this test, the patient is asked to kneel on a chair and retrieve an object held below his reach. Patients with low back pain are generally able to perform this task by flexing at the hip, if necessary. Those who cannot perform this test may not be making a genuine effort to do so (7).

TABLE 5. *The Waddell signs*

Tenderness
  Superficial; nonanatomic
Simulation
  Axial loading; rotation
Distraction
  Straight-leg raising
Regional
  Weakness; sensory
Overreaction

THE MULTIPLY OPERATED LOW BACK

Patients who have had numerous low back operations are particularly difficult to evaluate and are sometimes referred to as failed-back patients. The objective is to identify those patients with a surgically correctable, mechanical lesion such as a recurrent herniated disc, spinal instability, or spinal stenosis. Patients with scar tissue (arachnoiditis or epidural fibrosis) and psychologic instability are best treated by nonsurgical means (1).

The length of the pain-free interval postoperatively is a useful historical point in the approach to these patients. Pain unchanged by surgery implies lack of adequate decompression, exploration of the wrong level, or possibly wrong choice of a patient. Pain that begins 6 to 12 months postoperatively suggests the possibility of a recurrent disc herniation at the same or different level. A pain-free interval between 1 and 6 months with gradual onset of pain is consistent with scar tissue formation (8). Scar and recurrent disc herniation are best differentiated with gadolinium-enhanced magnetic resonance imaging (MRI). Scar, which is vascular, enhances markedly, whereas disc, which is avascular, does not.

SPECIAL CONSIDERATIONS IN TRAUMA AND SPINAL CORD INJURY

In the case of spinal trauma, any subtle symptoms suggestive of neural injury, including transient numbness or paresthesiae, must be sought out. Conversely, in a patient with known spinal cord injury, any evidence of transient motor or sensory function after the injury is important and suggests an incomplete cord injury. The trauma evaluation must include inspection of the entire spine. It is safest to use a backboard or a log-rolling maneuver during lateral turning (13). Any tenderness, deformity, ecchymosis, or abrasions should be noted. Marks made by shoulder or seat belts should alert the examiner to the possibility of cervicothoracic or thoracolumbar spine injury, respectively. The lap seat belt may be associated with a characteristic thoracolumbar flexion–distraction type of injury. Unrestrained individuals ejected from a motor vehicle and motorcyclists are both at increased risk for thoracolumbar fracture–dislocation.

Suspect cervical spine trauma in any patient with significant craniofacial injury (9). It is essential to evaluate the entire spine, even with a known injury, as the incidence of noncontiguous spinal fractures is estimated at 5% to 10% (9,10). Missed spine injuries are most common in the presence of decreased level of consciousness, head injury, and in patients with multiple injuries. A careful neurologic examination is obviously critical in the setting of spinal cord injury. The exam should be re-

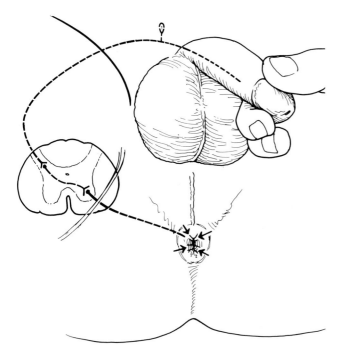

FIG. 39. The bulbocavernosus reflex.

peated serially in order to note any improvement or deterioration in the neurologic status.

After spinal cord injury, a period of variable length, termed spinal shock, is entered which is characterized by spinal cord dysfunction based on physiologic, rather than structural, disruption. Spinal shock is characterized by paralysis, hypotonia, and areflexia. The resolution of spinal shock is marked by the return of the reflex arcs below the level of injury. This is most commonly tested

by the bulbocavernosus reflex, which returns in 24 to 48 hours in 90% of patients (19). This reflex is mediated by the S3 and S4 nerve roots and involves squeezing, or pulling, the glans penis in male patients, or the clitoris in female patients, and noting contraction of the anal sphincter. This is sometimes easily performed by simply pulling on a Foley catheter (Fig. 39).

It is important to distinguish between complete and incomplete neurologic deficit as early as possible. Any evidence of motor function or sensory sparing below the level of spinal cord injury denotes an incomplete deficit and offers the hope of some functional recovery. This determination cannot be made until the period of spinal shock has ended (with return of the bulbocavernosus reflex, or lapse of more than 48 hours). Functional motor recovery is seen only rarely in patients presenting with complete neurologic deficits (3). Improvement of one nerve root level can be expected, however, in 80% of patients, and two root levels in 20% of patients with complete injuries (2).

Often the only indication that a spinal cord injury is incomplete is preservation of sacral function. Sacral sparing indicates at least some structural continuity of the long tracts and, thus, a chance for functional recovery. Findings may include perianal sensation, some rectal tone, and great toe flexion. Figure 40 depicts the cross-sectional anatomy of the cervical spinal cord. The sacral structures are the most peripherally placed in the lateral corticospinal tracts (motor), the spinothalamic tracts (sensory), and the posterior columns. This provides the anatomic basis for sacral sparing, as the peripheral sacral elements are commonly preserved, despite damage to the central fibers and cells of the spinal cord. Documen-

ANTERIOR

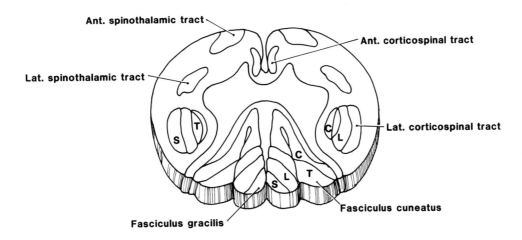

Ant. spinothalamic tract

Ant. corticospinal tract

Lat. spinothalamic tract

Lat. corticospinal tract

Fasciculus cuneatus

Fasciculus gracilis

POSTERIOR

FIG. 40. Cross section of the spinal cord in the cervical region.

TABLE 6. *Incomplete cord syndromes*

Syndrome	Frequency	Description	Functional recovery
Central	Most common	Usually quadriplegic with sacral sparing; upper extremities affected more than lower	75%
Anterior	Common	Complete motor deficit; trunk and lower extremity deep pressure and proprioception preserved	10%
Posterior	Rare	Loss of deep pressure, deep pain, and proprioception	—
Brown-Séquard	Uncommon	Ipsilateral motor deficit; contralateral pain and temperature deficit	>90%

tation of the presence, or absence, of sacral sparing is important prognostically in the evaluation of the patient with spinal cord injury.

The various specific types of incomplete neurologic syndromes are described in Table 6. The central cord syndrome is common (particularly in older patients) and is characterized by sacral sparing, and upper extremity greater than lower extremity involvement. Some functional recovery can be expected in approximately 75% of these patients. The anterior cord syndrome is relatively common and is characterized by a complete motor deficit below the level of injury and a very poor prognosis for functional recovery. In this instance, posterior column functions (deep pressure, vibration, and proprioception) are usually intact. The Brown-Séquard syndrome is characterized by ipsilateral motor deficit and contralateral pain and temperature loss, usually two levels below the insult. This is uncommon, is usually secondary to penetrating trauma to the cord through a lateral approach, and carries the best prognosis, with greater than 90% functional recovery.

The evaluation of the patient with spinal cord trauma proceeds with radiographic, and ultimately, neurodiagnostic studies. Nonetheless, the focus of the initial assessment of these patients remains an accurate history and thorough physical examination. These are essential in order to minimize the risk of further neurologic injury and maximize the potential for neurologic recovery.

REFERENCES

1. Armstrong JR (1951): The causes of unsatisfactory results from the operative treatment of lumbar disc lesions. *J Bone Joint Surg* 33B: 31–35.
2. Bohlman HH (1979): Acute fractures and dislocations of the cervical spine: an analysis of three hundred hospitalized patients and review of the literature. *J Bone Joint Surg* 61A:1119–1142.
3. Bracken MB, Shepard MJ, Hellenbrand KG, et al. (1985): Methylprednisolone and neurological function 1 year after spinal cord injury: results of the National Acute Spinal Cord Injury Study. *J Neurosurg* 63:704–713.
4. Davidson R, Dunn E, Metzmaker J (1981): The shoulder abduction test in the diagnosis of radicular pain in cervical extradural compressive monoradiculopathies. *Spine* 6:441–446.
5. Dillon WH, Watkins RG (1992): Clinical syndromes in cervical myelopathy. In: Rothman RH, Simeone FA, eds. *The Spine.* Philadelphia: WB Saunders, pp. 560–569.
6. Dyck P, Doyle JB (1977): "Bicycle test" of van Gelden in diagnosis of intermittent cauda equina syndrome. *J Neurosurg* 46:667–670.
7. Evanski PM, Carver D, Nehemkis A, Waugh TR (1979): The Burns' test in low back pain. *Clin Orthop Rel Res* 140:42–44.
8. Federowicz SG, Wiesel SW (1991): An algorithm for the multiply operated low back patient and treatment of operative complications. *Semin Spine Surg* 3:175–183.
9. Keenen TL, Benson DR (1992): Initial evaluation of the spine-injured patient. In: Browner BD, Jupiter JB, Levine AM, Trafton PG, eds. *Skeletal trauma.* Philadelphia: WB Saunders, pp. 585–604.
10. Kewalramani LS, Taylor RG (1976): Multiple non-contiguous injuries to the spine. *Acta Orthop Scand* 47:52–58.
11. Macnab I (1977): *Backache.* Baltimore: Williams and Wilkins.
12. MaCrae IF, Wright V (1969): Measurement of back movement. *Ann Rheum Dis* 28:584–589.
13. McGuire RA, Neville S, Green BA, et al. (1987): Spinal instability and the log-rolling maneuver. *J Trauma* 27:525–531.
14. Moore, KL (1977): *The developing human: clinically oriented embryology.* Philadelphia: WB Saunders.
15. Nachemson A (1979): Adult scoliosis and back pain. *Spine* 4:513–517.
16. Ono K, Ebara S, Fiji T, et al. (1987): Myelopathy hand. *J Bone Joint Surg* 69B:215–219.
17. Scham SM, Taylor TKF (1971): Tension signs in lumbar disc prolapse. *Clin Orthop Rel Res* 75:195–204.
18. Spurling RG (1956): *Lesions of the cervical intervertebral disc.* Springfield: Thomas.
19. Stauffer ES (1975): Diagnosis and prognosis of acute cervical spinal cord injury. *Clin Orthop Rel Res* 112:9–15.
20. Waddell G, Kummel EG, Lotto WN, et al. (1979): Failed lumbar disc surgery and repeat surgery following industrial injuries. *J Bone Joint Surg* 61A:201–207.
21. Waddell G, McCulloch JA, Kummel E, et al. (1980): Non-organic physical signs in low-back pain. *Spine* 5:117–125.

The Adult Spine: Principles and Practice,
2nd edition, J.W. Frymoyer, Editor-in-Chief.
Lippincott-Raven Publishers, Philadelphia © 1997.

CHAPTER 22

Evaluation of Muscle Function

Gunnar B. J. Andersson and Steven A. Lavender

The paravertebral supportive muscles are often considered to have etiologic significance in spinal disorders, and the extremity muscles also are affected by spinal disease. Examination of muscles, therefore, is part of a standard physical examination of the patient with spinal pain, dysfunction, or deformity. Routinely, the extremity muscles are investigated to determine loss of strength or atrophy, and trunk muscles are examined for tenderness, presence of "spasm," and asymmetry. However, the function of trunk muscles is inferred usually only as part of the range of motion examination. Historically, tests of strength and endurance were performed infrequently.

Today, the traditional approaches to the evaluation, diagnosis, and treatment of muscles are being reappraised as newer technologies become available. This chapter first describes the anatomy of the dorsal spinal muscles and their basic functional attributes, including strength, endurance, and coordination, and then critically assesses the newer technologies available to measure these attributes. Then the role of these muscles in spinal disorders is considered.

 G. B. J. Andersson, M.D., Ph.D.: Professor and Chairman, Department of Orthopedic Surgery, Rush-Presbyterian-St. Luke's Medical Center, Chicago, Illinois 60612.
 S. A. Lavender, Ph.D.: Assistant Professor, Department of Orthopedic Surgery, Rush-Presbyterian-St. Luke's Medical Center, Chicago, Illinois 60612.

THE ANATOMY OF SPINAL MUSCLES

The Anatomy of the Lumbar Back Muscles

A lumbar back muscle can be defined as any muscle lying in the posterior compartment of the spine that can exert a force on the lumbar vertebrae. This definition includes not only those muscles that attach to the lumbar vertebrae, but also those that cross the lumbar spinal column but lack any direct attachment to the vertebrae. The nomenclature of the posterior spinal muscles is confusing (216). The second edition of *Nomina Anatomica* defines the erector spinae muscles (ESM) as "all muscles of the back including the intertransversarii and interspinalis" (165). From the fourth edition onward, however, the ESM are considered to consist of the iliocostalis, longissimus, and spinalis only (166). This is the more common definition used today, although some authors still refer to the ESM as all muscles innervated by the dorsal rami of the spinal nerves, and consider the above three muscles a subgroup, the sacrospinal muscle group. It is not the purpose of this chapter to resolve this issue, only to explain why differences appear in the scientific literature that are based on definitions rather than physiology and function. Morphologically, the lumbar back muscles can be divided into short (intersegmental) muscles and long (polysegmental) muscles.

The intersegmental muscles are the interspinalis and intertransversarii. These muscles are small and can be found at every lumbar intervertebral joint.

There are only two polysegmental muscles of the lumbar spine, the multifidus and the erector spinae, as defined above. The lumbarmultifidus, which traditionally is described as a transversospinal muscle, is the most medial of the lumbar back muscles and consists of five segmental bands. Each segmental band stems from a spinous process and consists of several individual fascicles with various caudal insertions (215,217) (Figs. 1–3). The shortest fascicle in each band arises from the caudal edge of the spinous process and spans two intervertebral joints. Long fascicles arise from a common tendon from the tip of the spinous process and span three to five segments. The fascicles are inserted systematically into the mammilary processes of the lumbar vertebrae, the posterior superior iliac spine, and the dorsal surface of the sacrum and posterior sacroiliac ligament. Dissections have shown that all fascicles arising from a given spinous process are innervated by a single nerve, the medial branch of the dorsal ramus with the same segmental number as the spinous process (217). In other words, the fascicles arising from a given vertebra are innervated by the nerve that issues below that vertebra. The multifidus muscle is the largest muscle spanning the lumbosacral junction and is, because of its location and prominence, the lumbar muscle used for diagnostic electromyography and histochemical studies.

The erector spinae, in the lumbar region as discussed above, has traditionally been described as having three

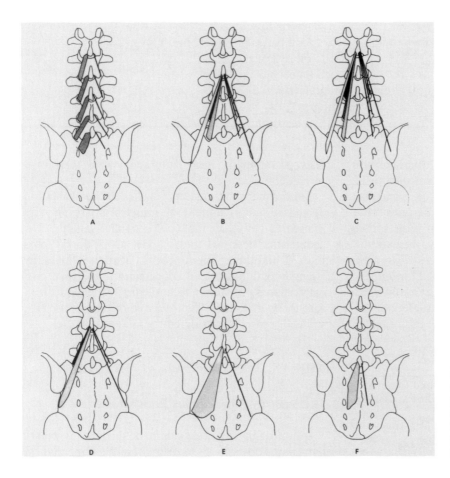

FIG. 1. Schematic illustrations of the fascicles of the lumbar multifidus as seen in a posteroanterior view. **A:** The laminar fibers at every level. **B–F:** The longer fascicles from the caudal edge and tubercles of the spinous processes at levels L1–L5. From Macintosh et al. (215), with permission.

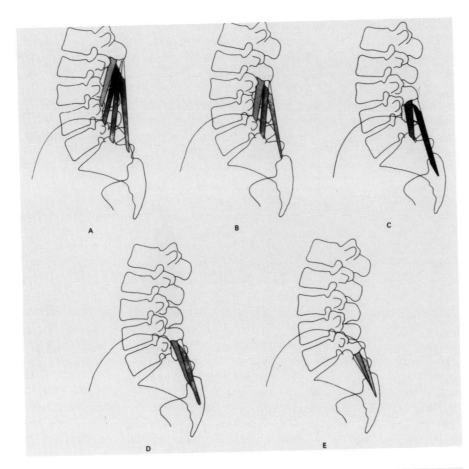

FIG. 2. Schematic illustrations of the fascicles of the lumbar multifidus as seen in lateral views. **A–E** show the fascicles present at levels L1–L5, respectively. From Macintosh et al. (215), with permission.

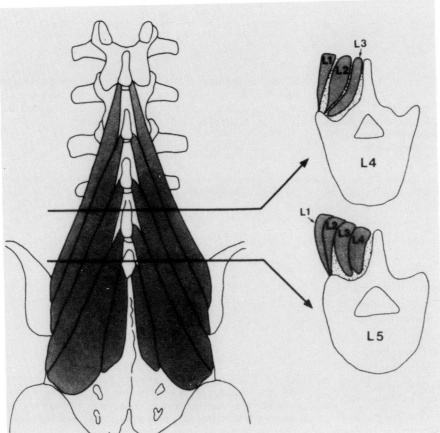

FIG. 3. A schematic illustration of the overlying structure of the lumbar multifidus. The dorsal surface of the intact muscle is formed by the dorsal-most fibers in each of the five bands that constitute the muscle. Each band is separated from its neighboring bands by distinct cleavage planes. In transverse sections, the overlapping arrangement of successive bands is evident. From Macintosh et al. (215), with permission.

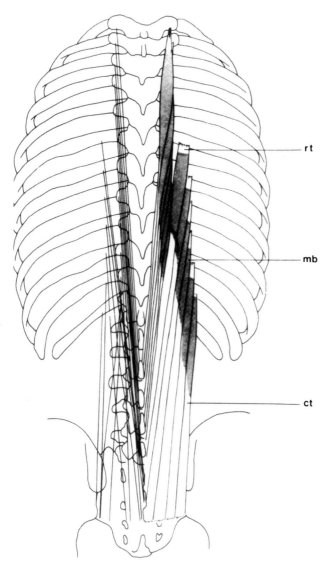

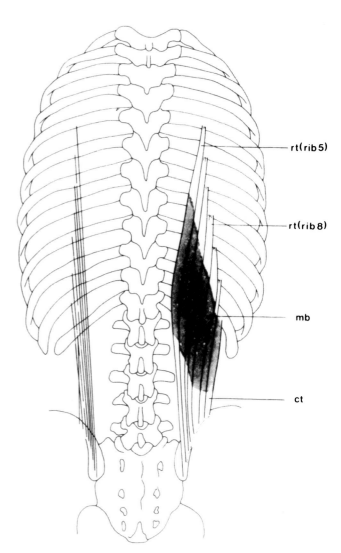

FIG. 4. A schematic illustration of the fascicles of the thoracic portion of longissimus thoracis. Each fascicle generally consists of a rostral tendon (*rt*), a muscle belly (*mb*), and a caudal tendon (*ct*) From Macintosh et al. (216), with permission.

FIG. 5. A schematic illustration of the thoracic fascicles of iliocostalis lumborum in a posteroanterior view, showing rostral tendon (*rt*), muscle belly (*mb*), and caudal tendon (*ct*). From Macintosh et al. (216), with permission.

parts: the longissimus thoracis, the iliocostalis lumborum, and the spinalis thoracis (or spinalis dorsi). The spinalis thoracis is relatively small and is principally a muscle of the thoracic region. Only its lowest fibers enter the lumbar region to insert onto the L1 to L3 spinous processes. Consequently, it has little functional role in lumbar spinal movements. The longissimus thoracis and iliocostalis lumborum, however, are massive muscles with substantial actions on the lumbar spine (Figs. 4–8). Topographically, the iliocostalis lumborum lies lateral to the longissimus thoracis and forms the lateral border of the erector spinae in the lumbar region. The longissimus thoracis lies adjacent to the multifidus, separated from it by a distinct, vessel-filled cleavage plane. In the lumbar region, the longissimus thoracis and iliocostalis lumborum muscles appear to form a single common muscle

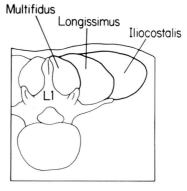

FIG. 6. Three columns of the lumbar back muscles in a transverse section through the spinous processes of L1, showing musculus multifidus, musculus longissimus, and musculus iliocostalis. Redrawn with permission from Gracovetsky (142); see also refs. 172 and 216.

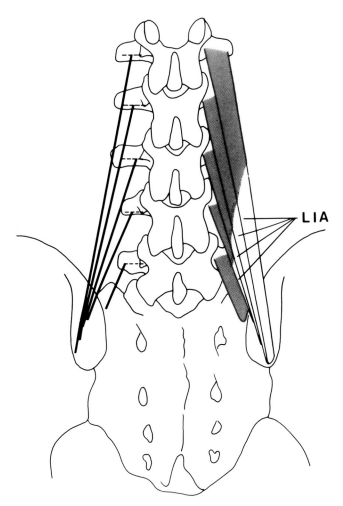

FIG. 7. A schematic illustration of the fascicles of the longissimus thoracis pars lumborum. Fascicles L1–L4 have long caudal tendons that form the lumbar intermuscular aponeurosis (*LIA*). The dotted lines mark the extent of the rostral attachments. From Macintosh et al. (216), with permission.

mass, but dissection reveals that the two are separated by a parasagittal aponeurosis, the lumbar intermuscular aponeurosis, with the longissimus lying medial to this aponeurosis and the iliocostalis lateral to it (216) (Fig. 6). In the thoracic region, the two muscles diverge and are separated distinctly by the iliocostalis thoracis.

Macintosh and Bogduk's (216) dissections have also shown that the longissimus thoracis and iliocostalis lumborum each consist of thoracic and lumbar fibers and may be described as having four parts: the longissimus thoracis pars thoracis, the iliocostalis lumborum pars thoracis, the longissimus thoracis pars lumborum, and the iliocostalis lumborum pars lumborum. The thoracic fibers arise from thoracic transverse processes or ribs, whereas the lumbar fibers arise directly from lumbar vertebrae.

The longissimus thoracis pars thoracis consists of multiple independent fascicles that arise from the transverse processes and ribs of the T1 to T12 segments

(Fig. 4). Each tendon fascicle consists of a short flat tendon, a short small muscle belly, and a long caudal tendon. These tendons insert serially into the lumbar and sacral spinous processes, the back of the sacrum, and the posterior superior iliac spine. The side-to-side aggregation of these caudal tendons forms the medial half or so of the lumbar part of the erector spinae aponeurosis.

The iliocostalis lumborum pars thoracis consists of eight fascicles that arise from the tubercles of the lower eight ribs. Each fascicle consists of a small muscle belly and a longer caudal tendon (Fig. 5). These tendons form the lateral part of the erector spinae aponeurosis and insert into the iliac crest.

The longissimus thoracis pars lumborum consists of five fascicles that arise from the accessory process of a lumbar vertebra and the adjacent medial four-fifths of the transverse process (Fig. 7). Caudally, the fascicles become aponeurotic and blend to form the lumbar intermuscular aponeurosis, which ultimately inserts into a small area on the medial aspect of the posterior superior iliac spine.

The iliocostalis lumborum pars lumborum consists of four fascicles that arise, one from each segmental level,

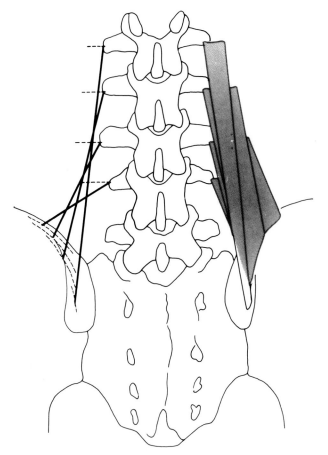

FIG. 8. A schematic illustration of the lumbar fascicles of iliocostalis lumborum. The dotted lines mark the extent of each attachment. From Macintosh et al. (216), with permission.

from the tips of the L1 to L4 transverse processes and the adjacent posterior surfaces of the middle layer of thoracolumbar fascia (Fig. 8). Caudally, each fascicle inserts directly into the iliac crest, lateral to the posterior superior iliac spine.

In summary, the lumbar erector spinae consists of four separate, recognizable parts. Only the thoracic fibers of the longissimus thoracis and iliocostalis lumborum contribute to the erector spinae aponeurosis. The lumbar fibers that form the bulk of the erector spinae in the lumbar region arise from individual lumbar vertebrae and insert into the iliac crest independent of the erector spinae aponeurosis. The fiber directions of the longissimus, iliocostalis, and multifidus muscles have been analyzed in some detail (86), as have some of the implications of the detailed anatomic information on the mechanical modeling of the spine (33,100).

The Weight of the Posterior Lumbar Back Muscles

The total weight of these muscles in the lumbar region is quite similar at each vertebral level (104), in spite of the fact that the lateral border is more medial at lower lumbar levels (171–173). This is because the anterior muscle mass increases from superior to inferior. Between muscles, the iliocostalis contributes the most. Both the longissimus and iliocostalis increase in weight caudally, whereas the multifidus decreases.

The Anatomy of the Abdominal Muscles

The space between the rib cage and the pelvis is covered by the four abdominal muscles: the rectus abdominis anteriorly and three flat muscles, the external and internal obliques, and the transverse abdominal muscle laterally (Fig. 9). The rectus abdominis runs from the fifth to seventh ribs and the xiphoid process to the pubic arch as a wide strong band. The muscle fibers of the rec-

tus do not extend all the way, however, but are interrupted by three to four transverse tendinous intersections. Further, the muscle is divided into two parts centrally by the linea alba, a small but strong tendinous band.

The internal and external oblique muscles are close together but with different fiber directions. The external oblique is the largest of the three lateral muscles and runs caudomedially from the ribs to the inguinal ligament, rectus sheath, and ilium. The internal oblique, on the other hand, is fan-shaped, running caudolaterally in the superior aspect and mediolaterally in the inferior. The attachments are the ribs and rectus sheath, and the origins the inguinal ligament and iliac crest.

The transversus abdominis muscle is deep to the obliques and runs mediolaterally (transversely) from the rectus sheath to the six lower ribs, the thoracolumbar fascia, and the ileum.

Additional Trunk Muscles

Several muscles are important functionally to the spine, yet do not fit directly into the classification systems typically used for trunk muscles. They include the quadratus lumborum, psoas, trapezius, and latissimus dorsi. The quadratus lumborum lies lateral to the spine, connecting the twelfth rib and transverse processes of the lumbar vertebrae to the pelvis. When contracting unilaterally, a lateral bending moment is exerted on the spine. The psoas muscle attaches to the dorsal part of the vertebral bodies of T12 to L5 as well as to the discs, and then combines with the iliacus muscle to form the iliopsoas, which attaches to the minor trochanter. The latissimus dorsi arises from the iliac crest and lower vertebral spinous processes (by way of tendinous fibers) and ribs to insert into the humerus (Fig. 10). Its effect on the lumbar spine is partly through the thoracolumbar fascia, the importance of which has recently been appreciated (105,142–144). The trapezius muscle, like the latissimus, is a superficial covering back muscle. Its superior, descending part runs from the back of the head and cervical spine to the clavicle; its middle, transverse part runs from the lower cervical and thoracic spine to the acromion; and its lower, ascending part runs from the thoracic spine to the spinal scapula.

The Anatomy of the Cervical Spine Muscles

The neck muscles are divided into anterior and posterior, and those two groups are in turn subdivided.

The posterior neck muscles are a continuation of the lumbar back muscles discussed previously. The iliocostalis muscle continues as the iliocostalis cervices inserting into the transverse processes of the four lower cervical vertebrae. The longissimus has two parts in the

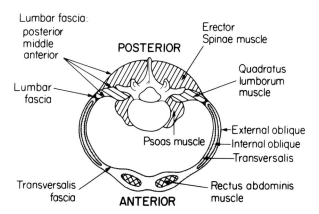

FIG. 9. Cross-section of the spine at the L3 level with posterior as well as abdominal muscles. From Andersson et al. (18), with permission.

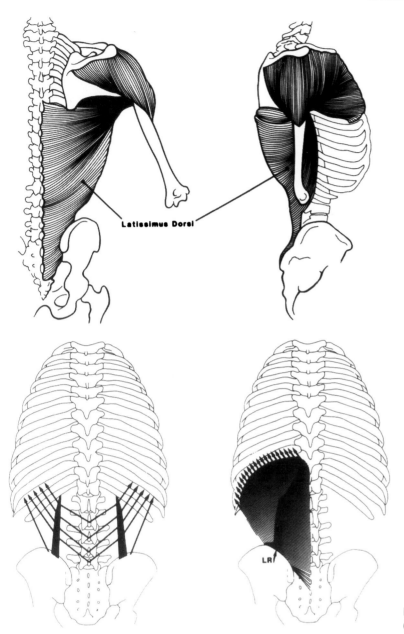

FIG. 10. Latissimus dorsi. From Gracovetsky (142), with permission.

cervical region: the longissimus cervices inserting into cervical transverse processes and the longissimus capitis inserting into the mastoid process. The spinalis muscle, which is absent in the lumbar region, is also divided into two parts: spinalis cervices connecting transverse processes, and spinalis capitis inserting into the occipital bone. The erector spinae part of the cervical muscles controls movements of both the neck and the head. It lies superficial to the semispinalis, multifidus, and rotator muscles covering them completely (Fig. 11). Those three muscles extend between transverse processes. The semispinalis capitis is the largest muscle mass of the back of the neck, extending from the midthoracic region and running all the way up to the occipital bone (Fig. 11). It is a powerful extensor of the head. The semispinalis

cervices insert into spinous processes in the neck, just medial to the semispinalis capitis. The multifidus muscle is small in the cervical region, overlying the rotators, which are the shortest of these three muscles.

In the upper part of the neck there are five muscle pairs, arising from the atlas and axis and inserting into the occipital bone. They lie deep to the semispinalis capitis and consist of: musculus rectus capitis major and minor, musculus rectus capitis lateralis, and musculus obliquus capitis inferior and superior. These muscles extend the head and rotate it and the atlas.

A fourth group of posterior neck muscles is sometimes referred to as the minor deep back muscles. They are the interspinales connecting adjacent spinous processes and the intertransversarii connecting adjacent transverse

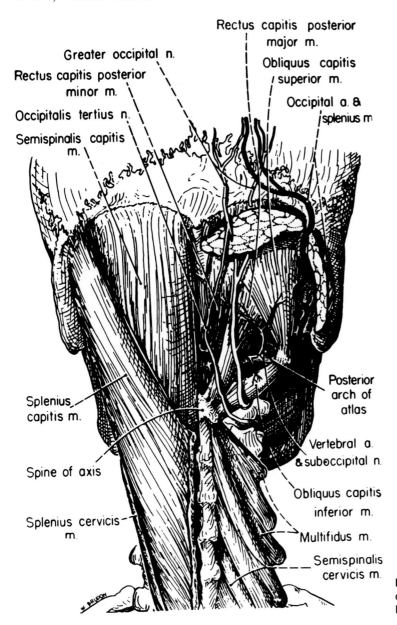

Rectus capitis posterior
major m.

Greater occipital n.

Obliquus capitis
superior m.

Rectus capitis posterior
minor m.

Occipital a. &
splenius m

Occipitalis tertius n.

Semispinalis capitis
m.

Posterior
arch of
atlas

Splenius
capitis m.

Vertebral a.
& suboccipital n.

Spine of axis

Obliquus capitis
inferior m.

Splenius cervicis
m.

Multifidus m.

Semispinalis
cervicis m

FIG. 11. The muscles of the back of the neck: the deeper suboccipital triangle is exposed on the right. From Woodburne (372), with permission.

processes. By contracting, they provide intrinsic stability to the spine.

The anterior neck is divided by the sternomastoid muscle into an anterior and a posterior triangle. The sternomastoid muscle is the most prominent of the anterior neck muscles arising from the sternum (medial head) and the clavicle (lateral head) and inserting into the mastoid process. This muscle is a strong rotator and lateral flexor of the head; in addition, when acting together, the sternomastoid muscles flex the neck.

The anterior triangle is divided by the hyoid bone into a supra- and an infrahyoid space. The suprahyoid muscles are small muscle pairs connecting the hyoid with the mandible or the skull. These muscles, the digastricus,

stylohyoid, mylohyoid, and geniohyoid, are important in controlling the mandible and oral space. Below the hyoid are the so-called strap muscles extending to the thyroid cartilage and sternum (Fig. 12A). The strap muscles are in two layers: superficially the sternohyoid and omohyoid, and deep the thyrohyoid and sternothyroid. These muscles control the location of the voice box.

Along the anterior surface of the neck vertebrae is a thin layer of muscles: the longus colli, rectus capitis anterior, and longus capitis (Fig. 12B). These muscles are weak because of their mass and location.

In the posterior triangle are a group of muscles called the scaleni. By location they are divided into anterior, middle, and posterior, extending from the first, second,

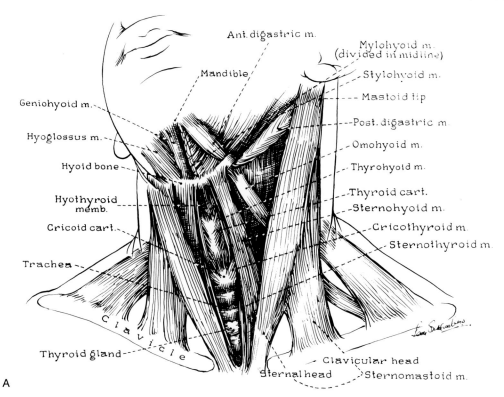

A

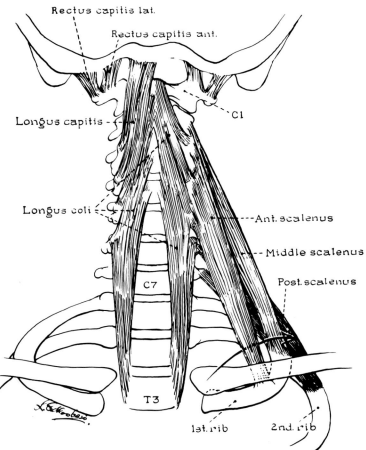

B

FIG. 12. A: Superficial muscles of the anterior neck. The sternomastoid divides the neck into the anterior and posterior triangles, and the hyoid presents a natural division between the muscles of the digastric triangle and the infrahyoid or strep muscles. From Rothman et al. (310), with permission. **B:** The deep muscles of the anterior neck, and the muscles of the posterior triangle. From Rothman et al. (310), with permission.

and sometimes third rib to the cervical transverse processes (Fig. 12B). Apart from their function on the cervical spine, they are also accessory inspiratory muscles.

THE FUNCTION OF THE TRUNK MUSCLES

The activities of the trunk muscles cannot be measured directly in mechanical terms but can be estimated indirectly, using electromyography. Because the relationship between electric output of muscles and force is monotonic, a calibration procedure will allow reasonably accurate transfer of EMG-activity measures into force quantities. Thus, quantitative measures of the myoelectric activities provide estimates of muscle forces provided the caveats of the techniques are known (43,49,77,222,251). Redfern (302) reviewed the general relationship between torque and myoelectric signal amplitude, and also discussed the length-tension and the velocity-tension effects on this relationship.

For the trunk muscles, the relationship between torque and myoelectric activity has been studied specifically by Stokes et al. (338). They found a linear relationship between the ESM electric activity and the extension moment, whereas a quadratic regression better described the relationship between abdominal muscle activity and flexion torque. Seroussi and Pope (320) found linear relationships for isometric extension efforts and for the difference between the left and right erector spinae myoelectric activity and the lateral bending moment. Vink et al. (364) placed 12 surface electrodes over the lumbar spine at L1, L3, and L5 levels to record myoelectric activity over the medial, intermediate, and lateral parts of the extensor muscles, corresponding topographically to the multifidus, longissimus, and iliocostalis muscles. When performing isometric extension efforts, a different relationship of force to myoelectric activity was found for the three muscle parts. Specifically, the multifidus muscles showed a linear relationship, and the longissimus and the iliocostalis muscles showed curvilinear relationships (Fig. 13). The authors speculated that this occurred because the medial part was mainly active in maintaining posture, whereas the lateral muscles are recruited mainly for movements.

Dolan et al. (98) regressed the paraspinal rectified and averaged electromyogram (EMG) on the extensor moment and found a strong linear relationship between these quantities when the spine was only slightly flexed ($r^2 = 0.94$) as well as when the spine was fully flexed ($r^2 = 0.81$). They noted that in both postures the intercepts of these functions were positive values, suggesting that passive tissues contributed to the extensor moment. This passive restorative moment was theorized to stem from disc, ligament, inactive muscle tissues, and possibly from intra-abdominal pressure. Although all

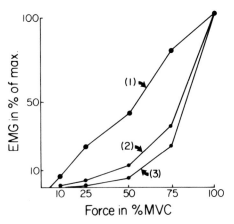

FIG. 13. The force/myoelectric activity curves computed for one of the test subjects. The force and myoelectric activity are both normalized in percentage of maximum. For the individual electrode pairs (i.e., the individual muscle) a different relationship is shown; 1) denotes the medial, 2) the intermediate, and 3) the lateral parts of the lumbar back muscles. From Vink et al. (364), with permission.

these studies support a monotonic relationship in flexion and extension efforts, it appears that the actual relationship varies between muscles and that passive tissue contributions can alter the precise relationship.

McGill (245) recorded muscle activities during static and dynamic twisting efforts. Peak muscle activity during maximal twisting efforts was low, compared to the maximum activity of all trunk muscles. Although generally a monotonic relationship occurred between torque and activity, the relationship was not consistently either linear or nonlinear. This is consistent with other studies by Pope et al. (288) and Thelen et al. (347). Thus, the relationship of torque and trunk muscle myoelectric activity while monotonic appears to vary from muscle to muscle, and to be influenced by the specific loading condition.

There is a temporal disparity between the initial myoelectric signal from a muscle and the initiation of a force output which is termed the *electromechanical delay*. Hinz and Seidel (158) calculated that the average delay for the erector spinae muscles was 65 msec, whereas Dolan and Adams (97) obtained delays of 60 to 80 msec during isometric contractions. Thelen et al. (347) quantified the delay by having subjects perform rapid attempted trunk flexion and extension cycles. However, these authors, because of the nature of the experimental protocol, could not separate the pure electromechanical delay from the dynamic phase shift due to the cyclic task. The average delays reported by these authors was longer, ranging from 111 to 218 msec depending upon the rate at which the cycles were performed and the effort level required. In general, the delays were greater for the trunk extensors than the trunk flexors and decreased as the task rate and the effort level increased.

Myoelectric Activity and Posture

The myoelectric activity of the trunk muscles in erect standing and in sitting postures has been studied extensively. Much of this work has been reviewed previously (11,12,15,161,276) and, therefore, we will review this topic as a broad overview.

Standing

Most studies of standing indicate slight myoelectric activity in the paraspinal muscles, usually more in the thoracic than in the lumbar and cervical regions (7,9,19,20,23,38,65,66,79,127,174,256,308,309,363). Asmussen and Klausen (31) found slight activity in erect standing posture in either the paraspinal muscles or the abdominal muscles, but not in both. This may result from the normal presence of postural sway. There is also slight activity in the vertebral portion of the psoas major muscle (17,38,255,258). Similarly, studies of the rectus abdominis and the external and internal oblique muscles reveal slight activity during relaxed standing, particularly of the internal oblique muscles (62,115,273,275,282).

Several authors have investigated the effects of applying external loads to the spine while subjects maintained an upright standing posture. These experiments have been useful in determining how muscles are recruited in response to variations in the magnitude of the applied load as well as the direction of the applied load (195,208,209,316,377). When the applied loads were symmetric about the body's midsagittal plane, the bilateral muscle recruitments were symmetric. When the orientation of these loads became asymmetric with regard to the midsagittal plane, the recruitment of the contralateral muscles increased whereas the ipsilateral muscles decreased. Thus, the loads were now being supported by fewer muscles thereby increasing the stress on the active contralateral tissues. Lavender et al. (209) quantified the cocontraction of eight trunk muscles in response to moments of 10, 20, 30, 40, and 50 nm applied from seven directions by computing the relative activation levels as a function of moment magnitude and direction. The relative activation level for a single muscle was defined as that muscle's percentage of the total normalized EMG activities from the eight muscles sampled. Although the totaled normalized EMG activity has no physiologic meaning, the relative activation level provided a means for determining the relative mix of the muscle contributions. The cocontraction pattern was fairly consistent as the moment magnitude increased, but a shift in moment direction resulted in substantial differences. This is shown schematically in Figure 14 where the pie slices represent each muscle's contribution to the total activity recorded. Thelen et al. (347) found that the cocontractions contributed an estimated 15% to 20% to the sum of all muscle forces when purely sagittal plane moments were generated. The cocontraction increased to between 35% and 45% of the total muscle forces as subjects attempted exertions in the frontal and transverse planes.

Ladin et al. (195,196) modeled lumbar muscle recruitment by defining active and inactive regions in a two-dimensional loading plane described by the magnitude of the sagittal and frontal plane moments. Any point in the plane was viewed as a loading point describing any combination of bending moments. The boundaries separating active or inactive states were called *switching curves* and derived on the basis of an optimization model. Validation studies indicated that the muscles' behavior was consistent with that predicted by the switching curves as the applied moments in the frontal and sagittal plane were manipulated. In a later refinement of their approach Ladin and Neff (197) created muscle activity maps, similar to contour maps, in which the lines drawn across the loading plane represent constant force output from a particular muscle. With this modification, the authors have developed a method for easily estimating not only whether a muscle will be on or off for a particular set of moment combinations but also for estimating its contraction level.

Sitting

The effects of sitting have received considerable attention, because of the common complaints of neck, shoulder, and low back pain in sedentary workers. Studies have been done to define optimal seating conditions. The activity of the lumbar paraspinal muscles is similar in standing and in unsupported sitting, whereas there is a somewhat higher level of activity in the thoracic region during sitting (17,19,20,23,65,115,175,214,308,309). Abdominal muscle activity in sitting has been studied much less frequently. Carlsöö (65) recorded slight activity in the anterior oblique muscles, but he did not investigate the rectus abdominis and transverse muscles. His results agreed with those of Schultz et al. (313) and Andersson et al. (24), who studied several supported sitting postures. They found slight activity in the rectus and oblique abdominal muscles, even though the posture was sagittally symmetric. The iliopsoas muscle is also slightly active when a sitting posture is assumed (23,117,255).

Andersson (13,14) summarized several studies of supported sitting and of work activities in sitting postures. These studies showed that the myoelectric activity of the trunk muscles was influenced by the posture of the seated subject, by supports incorporated into the chair, and by the specific work activities performed. The use of backrests was particularly important to reduce the muscle activity which is strongly influenced by the angle between the seat and the backrest (17,19,20,23). Levels of activity

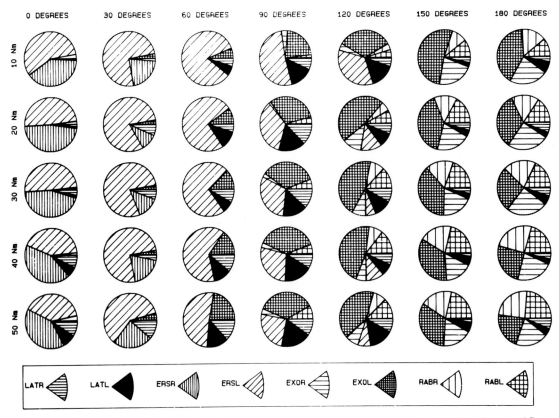

FIG. 14. The relative activations of eight trunk muscles in response to seven moment directions and five moment magnitudes. Relative activation level was defined as a particular muscle's normalized activity (under a specific moment magnitude and moment direction condition) divided by the totaled normalized EMG activity from the eight muscles sampled under that same condition. *LATR,* right latissimus dorsi; *LATL,* left latissimus dorsi; *ERSR,* right erector spinae; *ERSL,* left erector spinae; *EXOR,* right external oblique; *EXOL,* left external oblique; *RABR,* right rectus abdominis; *RABL,* left rectus abdominis. From Lavender et al. (208), with permission.

were quite low in all trunk muscles when the trunk was adequately supported by a reclining backrest (Fig. 15). A study by Hosea and associates (161) supported these findings and also confirmed that lumbar supports result in a lower level of activity in lumbar back muscles. However, a lumbar support that is too large tends to increase the activity (Fig. 16). Another study by Boudrifa and Davies (53) illustrates the importance of backrest angle and lumbar support which both influenced muscle activity when lifting in the seated posture.

The importance of the slope of the seat pan has also been studied to define optimal seating in the office setting. Yamaguchi et al. (374) found less muscle activity when the seat was inclined backward. Bendix et al. (44) studied the myoelectric activity of lumbar muscles when the subject sat in a chair with a posteriorly inclined seat, an anteriorly inclined seat, and a tiltable seat. There was no difference in activity, which throughout was low (Fig. 17). Soderberg et al. (336), on the other hand, recorded significantly lower levels of activity from the posterior back muscles with 10° and 20° of forward inclination of the seat pan compared to neutral. Their results apply to

both the lumbar and cervical regions of the back. Myoelectric activities directly measured during office work as well as model calculations of trunk forces suggest that, in general, the myoelectric signals are quite low and marginally influenced by table and chair adjustments

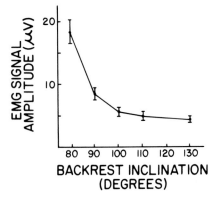

FIG. 15. The muscle activity of the lumbar erector spinae muscles decreases as the backrest inclination increases. From Andersson et al. (17).

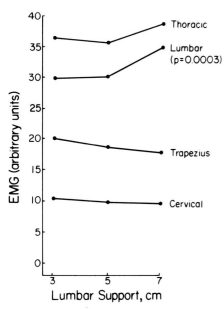

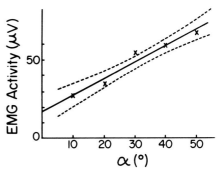

FIG. 16. Myoelectric activity (in arbitrary units) as a function of the horizontal size of the lumbar support. From Hosea et al. (161), with permission.

FIG. 18. The myoelectric activity of the lumbar back muscles increases linearly with the angle of flexion of the trunk. Mean values and 95% confidence limits. From Andersson et al. (21).

(13,14,26). It is not because of high muscle forces that back pain occurs in sitting postures. Most likely it is the long-term unchanged posture which is harmful.

Myoelectric Activity in Flexed Postures and During Forward Flexion

Studies of flexed postures have revealed an increase in the myoelectric activity of the back muscles, both when the angle of flexion is increased and when external load-

ing is increased at a fixed angle of flexion (Figs. 18 and 19) (21,206,257,272,313). In attempted flexion resisted by external forces, on the other hand, the abdominal muscles are strongly active while there are only low levels of activity in the lumbar part of the erector spinae muscle (135,136,314,316,377). When resisting extension moments in forward flexed postures, the abdominal muscle recruitment is greatly affected by the flexion moment created by the torso and upper body. Lavender et al. (206) showed that when the upper body balances an applied external extension moment the abdominal muscle activity comes close to baseline values.

Forward flexion of the trunk is a combined movement of the spine and pelvis (260,271). The first 50° to 60° are accomplished by motion of the lumbar spine and additional flexion primarily by rotation of the pelvis (64,105). The abdominal muscles are active only during the first few degrees of flexion, that is, when the movement is initiated (38,39,115,275). Thorstensson et al. (356) reported that when a rapid flexion motion was required, the action was initiated by a termination of the tonic activity in the back muscles and then a subsequent burst of abdominal muscle activity. However, when slow flexion

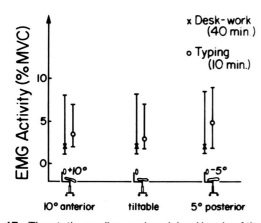

FIG. 17. The static, median, and peak load levels of the erector spinae muscle while sitting on each of the three chairs in the laboratory study. Each point is the mean of the values for nine subjects. No statistically significant differences between chairs were observed, but the static and median values were higher for typing than for desk-work. From Bendix et al. (44), with permission.

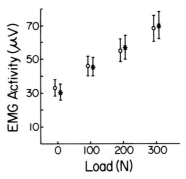

FIG. 19. The myoelectric activity of the lumbar back muscles increases as the load held by the hands increases. Measurements at 30° of trunk flexion. Mean and SEM for left and right sides. From Andersson et al. (21).

movements were required, the abdominal muscle activity was not observed, and there was only a decrease in the tonic activity in the back muscles.

The muscles of the trunk, pelvis, and thighs combine to control the movement pattern. During the first portion of a flexion movement, strong activity is found in the gluteus maximus, the gluteus medius, and the hamstring muscles (64,272); this muscle action locks the pelvis and prevents motion at the hip joints. As flexion progresses, the increasing trunk moment is balanced by a corresponding increase in back muscle activity. The gluteus maximus relaxes as full flexion is approached; the hamstring muscles are greatly active at first and remain active throughout the flexion movement. In the fully flexed position, however, lumbar myoelectric activity decreases and in some studies ceases almost completely (9,116,127,138,149,183,256,257,272,284,348,363). Floyd and Silver (116,117) called this the flexion-relaxation phenomenon of the back muscles and hypothesized that it results from stretch reflex inhibition. Other possible explanations are that in the fully flexed posture the trunk moment is resisted by structures other than muscles, such as the ligaments, thoracolumbar fascia, and facet joints.

Certainly the stretched extensor muscles also contribute. Valencia and Monroe (363), using wire electrodes, found a decrease in activity in full flexion only in subjects who reached their pre-experimental degree of trunk flexion. They thought many of the subjects were apprehensive about bending because of the wires and therefore did not bend fully. More recently, Dolan et al. (98) reported that 16% to 31% of the peak extensor moment is unrelated to the active tension of muscle tissue because it cannot be fully accounted for by recording of electromyographic signals. They further suggested that only a quarter of the passive extensor moment noted in their studies could be attributed to the discs and ligaments, and theorized that much of the passive restorative moment comes from the passive stretch of muscle tissue. Toussaint et al. (358) found significant activity in the thoracic component of the ESM during full flexion perhaps because the thoracic erector spinae provides extensor moment through its insertion into the dorsal fascia.

The main reason for the interest in the flexion-relaxation phenomenon is the potentially harmful effects of performing lifting and other work activities in flexed postures. It has been postulated that because the muscles are inactive in full flexion, the spine is unprotected. Further, the forces inside the spine increase because the moment arm acting on the ligaments is shorter. Farfan and Lamy (106), using a mechanical model, found stress on the ligaments in this position to be considerable and close to their calculated failure strength. Gracovetsky and associates (143,144) have suggested that the forces necessary to support the torso in an extremely flexed posture are

developed in the thoracolumbar fascia in addition to the ligaments. Adams and associates (2) examined the role of the lumbar intervertebral joints and thought they provided considerable stress shielding to ligaments. Schultz and associates (315) calculated the tissue tensions resulting from the flexion-relaxation phenomenon (Fig. 20). They also determined that the back muscles immediately become electrically active when exertions are performed in the fully flexed posture.

The mechanical loading of the spine itself becomes much more significant as the trunk is flexed. The increased bending moment from the torso mass requires much greater recruitment of the erector spinae for support. Many authors have shown that the compressive forces developed from the muscle recruitments can be of significant concern as individuals flex forward (75, 132,313). The degree to which shear forces are experienced by the spine in relation to muscle activities is not as clear. Potvin et al. (295) proposed that the lumbar erector spinae, when accurately modeled with regard to its line of action, is capable of developing a posterior shear force, thereby counteracting the anterior shear forces on the spine during trunk flexion.

Myoelectric Activity During Extension

When raising trunk from the flexed to the upright posture, the sequence of muscular activity is the reverse of

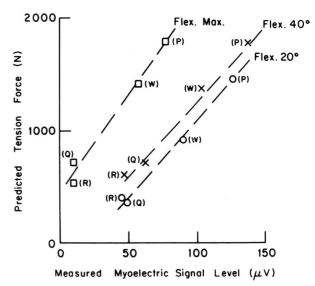

FIG. 20. Mean measured L3 level myoelectric activity versus mean predicted tissue tension force in the left side erector spinae muscles in various tasks. The tasks, performed at each of 20° and 40° and maximum degrees of flexion were quiet standing (Q), resist upward pull (R), hold weights anteriorly (W), and maximum voluntary upward pull (P). Results for the right side were similar. From Schultz et al. (315), with permission.

that when bending forward (9,21,99,115,117,127,256, 272). The gluteus maximus comes into action early together with hamstrings and initiates extension by a posterior rotation of the pelvis (272). The paraspinal muscles then become active and increase their activity until the movement is completed. It is noteworthy that extensor muscle activity is greater when the trunk is being raised than when it is being lowered, although in neither is it close to its maximum (127,174,272). The direction of the movement in relation to the weight forces of body segments is obviously important. Concentric contractions are known to require more muscle force than eccentric. Changes of the lumbar curvature itself also influence the activity. When adopting a forced lumbar lordosis, the myoelectric activity of the back muscles is increased (16,87,272). This is particularly interesting in light of work by Tveit et al. (361) showing that the moment arm of the erector spinae is significantly longer when a lordosis is maintained. With the increased mechanical advantage in the lordotic posture, the muscle would be expected to show reduced activity, however, as just described this was not the case. Thus, the maintenance of a lordotic posture during trunk extension requires substantial muscle force, especially during the early part of the extension motion (362).

When performing an extension movement, the erector spinae muscles have been found to be most active during the initial portion. The duration of their activity depends upon movement speed. In fast movements, the peak activity in the erector spinae has been found to be greater than during slower extensions, but the electromyographic activity ceased between 13° and 46° prior to an erect stance (356). Apparently the generated momentum accomplishes the rest of the movement. Conversely, with slow extension motions the same authors reported that the posterior muscle activity continued until the subject was between 4° of flexion and 5° of extension. Meanwhile, the anterior muscles also contract to slow the movement. In general, the faster the movement the earlier in the extension motion the anterior muscles will be recruited. For example, Thorstensson et al. (356) reported that the burst of anterior muscle activity could occur with the trunk between 17° and 58° of flexion during a rapid extension motion.

When the trunk is extended from the upright position, myoelectric back muscle activity is strong early on during the initial phase, but only after the gluteus maximus has become active. Both muscle groups are active in the position of full extension (9,79,117,256,284), whereas between these two extreme postures there is only slight activity. The abdominal muscles, particularly the rectus abdominis, show increasing activity throughout the extension movement (9,116). Extension of the trunk against resistance results in a marked increase in the activity of the muscles of the lumbar region of the back

(171,172,256,284,314,316,377). In fact, this is the activity in which the back muscles show their maximal activity.

Myoelectric Activity During Lateral Flexion and Twisting

When the trunk is flexed laterally, the myoelectric activity increases in the posterior back muscles on both sides of the spine. The main increase in activity in the lumbar region is on the side contralateral to the direction of lateral bend (64,117,127,294,308). This is also the case when the trunk is loaded in lateral flexion where comparatively higher levels of activity are found on the contralateral side of the lumbar region. In the thoracic region, on the other hand, the increase in muscle activity occurs mainly on the ipsilateral side (Fig. 21) (21). Muscle activity in the lumbar region is typically higher in the sacrospinal than in the transversospinal muscles (21). Jonsson (171–173) found the sacrospinal muscles to be active in lateral flexion, whereas the multifidi muscles, which are closer to the spine, were usually inactive. Intuitively, this observation makes sense. The response of the back muscles to a loading condition in which a weight is held in one hand during upright posture is equivalent to that in lateral flexion: the contralateral muscles contract strongly and in proportion to the lateral bending moment (21,24,53,117). Lavender et al. (202) found that the primary changes in muscle response to loads applied to

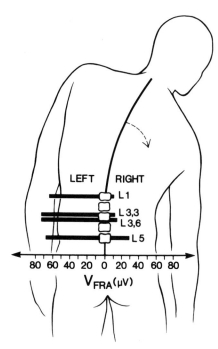

FIG. 21. When bending to the right, substantial muscle activity is recorded on the left side of the trunk. This activity is needed to maintain equilibrium. From Andersson et al. (21).

a torso which was laterally bent to the right occurred in the left and right external oblique and right erector spinae muscles. Figure 22 shows that the left external oblique muscle was active across a wide range of moment direction conditions, in part because it was that muscle which primarily supported the bending moment created by the upper body. It is interesting to note that the activity of the right erector spinae was elevated relative to neutral posture recordings when the applied load was laterally opposed to the direction of the lateral bend. This situation would be analogous to lifting a suitcase with the left hand and leaning to the right approximately 20°. Under these conditions the right posterior muscles have shortened and are at a less effective portion of the length-strength curve. Hence, an increased electromyographic response was observed.

The abdominal muscles are active in lateral flexion both ipsilaterally and contralaterally, with the level of activity higher on the contralateral side. Carlsöö (64) recorded strong activity in the gluteus medius and the tensor fasciae latae muscles on the ipsilateral side, which reflects the force necessary to rotate the pelvis.

McGill (246) modeled the spinal loads during static and dynamic lateral bending exertions with loads in the midfrontal plane. While he found recruitment patterns of the contralateral erector spinae and external oblique muscles similar to those described above, he also found significant coactivation of antagonistic muscles throughout the lateral extension motion. The significance of this contraction has been well described by McGill:

Even antagonistic activity as low as 8% MVC [maximum voluntary contraction] produces quite significant compressive load on the spine. Assuming similar muscle geometry, length, etc., between right-side antagonists and their left-side agonist counterparts, then an additional 8% MVC activation level is required. Thus, the resultant compressive penalty imposed on the spine is approximately twice the compressive load that is produced by the antagonistic muscle activity (page 412).

Part of the coactivation will be working to stabilize the spine in response to the varying moments created by the oblique architecture of the torso muscles. But during dynamic motions the coactivation serves to control movement, time, and speed (368,369).

Raftopoulos and associates (300) studied whether the flexion-silence phenomenon of back muscles observed in full flexion exists in lateral flexion as well. A relaxation phenomenon does seem to occur in the fully laterally bent trunk posture, but only in the trunk extensor muscles. The oblique abdominal muscles remain active.

Pope and associates (288,290) studied the myoelectric activity of trunk muscles when twisting was attempted, both with and without prerotation of the trunk. In general, a linear relationship was established between force output and myoelectric activity (Fig. 23). However, high levels of antagonistic activity were found in both abdominal and posterior back muscles. In some muscles, prerotation increased the antagonistic activity. In both of these experiments, the highest activity levels were found in the erector spinae and external oblique abdominal muscles.

Lavender and colleagues (207) investigated the changes in muscle recruitment as the torso was loaded in an axially rotated (twisted) posture. Bending moments were applied from 12 directions to a chest harness worn by the subjects. The myoelectric activities of the right erector spinae, right latissimus dorsi, and left external oblique responses were all greater in the right twisted posture than in the neutral nontwisted posture. Furthermore, the erector spinae response was shifted to be more active to directions opposite the twist, thereby making the muscles more responsive to left lateral bending moments. When the authors analyzed the coactivation, they found notable changes in the muscle recruitment pat-

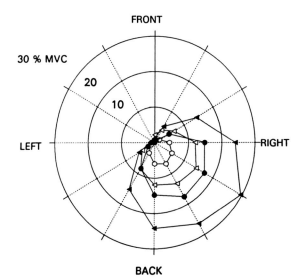

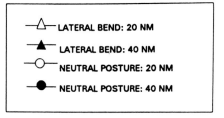

FIG. 22. The response of the left external oblique to moments of 20 and 40 nm applied to the torso in laterally bent and neutral postures. The location of each point corresponds to the applied moment direction and the magnitude of the normalized NOMG response (distance from the center) expressed as a percentage of the muscle's maximal response.

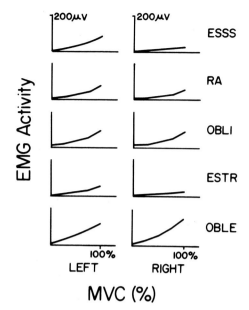

FIG. 23. Average myoelectric activity versus contraction level for the five muscle pairs: sacrospinal (*ESSS*), rectus abdominis (*RA*), oblique internus (*OBLI*), transversospinal (*ESTR*), and oblique externus (*OBLE*). From Pope et al. (288), with permission.

terns with applied moments of 20 and 40 nm, as well as with changes in moment direction, when the torso was twisted.

Myoelectric Activity During Lifting and Dynamic Exertions

Because of the common occurrence of low back strain with lifting, this topic has been of particular interest. The back muscles, the muscles of the buttocks, and the hamstring muscles are all myoelectrically active during a lift. The abdominal muscles are also active, but to a lesser degree. The levels of activity in these various muscles are directly related to the external moment and are, therefore, influenced by the weight lifted, the body posture, the location of the mass center of the weight, and the speed of the lift (9,22,24,32,37,42,52,67,99,106,117,142, 149,167,180,222,223,234,247,257,272,288,290,313,357).

At a practical level the question of whether the spine should be flexed or straight during the lift has been addressed using EMG measurement technique. Generally, in these studies, activity of the back muscles is similar in a leg lift (spine held straight) and a back lift (spine flexed) or, sometimes, is greater in the back lift (16,21,25, 57,88,149,257,272). Delitto et al. (87) analyzed two techniques of leg lifting and found higher ESM muscle activities during the first phase of the lift when lifting with lordosis than when lifting with lumbar kyphosis. Later in the lift the reverse was true. Overall, the highest activity levels occurred with lordotic lifts. The oblique abdominal muscles had comparable activity levels with both lift-

ing techniques. Similar results were reported by Vakos et al. (362). Potvin and associates (296), using an EMG-assisted model, reported that the restorative moment contributions of the lumbar erector spinae increased and the contributions from the thoracic erector spinae decreased as the lifting style was changed from a stooped to a squat type lift. Gallagher and Unger (130) reported that miners performing simulated mining material handling tasks showed greater erector spinae recruitment in kneeling versus stooped postures.

Several authors have shown, using biomechanical models, that the moments at L5/S1 increase with lifting speed (58,59,129). Marras and Reilly (231) documented the sequencing of the muscle recruitments through a range of trunk extension velocities that included 0 (isometric), 25, 50, 75, and 100% of each subject's maximum isokinetic velocity. They found that the recruitment sequences were dependent upon the trunk extension velocity, and that the anterior muscles showed the largest change in their onset and peak times as the velocity increased. Marras and Mirka (228) studied the myoelectric response of the trunk muscles to variation in trunk velocity, trunk position (both forward bending and asymmetric angle), and trunk exertion level. Their subjects produced constant torque about the lumbosacral junction while moving the trunk at constant angular velocities. Asymmetric conditions were varied between 0° and 30° by having subjects twist their torsos such that their shoulders were square to the dynamometer while their pelvises and lower extremities were rotated on a swivel base. Significant reactions to velocity, force level, and unique combinations of trunk angle and velocity were seen in all muscles of the trunk. Increasing trunk extension velocity increased the peak EMG amplitudes observed in both the posterior and the anterior muscles. These investigators also observed greater activity as the trunk, while maintaining constant torque, was extended through postures that were closer to upright. Thus, at least for the erector spinae muscles, their data suggest that the peak of length-strength relationship occurs when the trunk is flexed. Moreover, these investigators found that during the constant torque exertions there was greater activity in the concentric portion of the exertion than in the eccentric portion. De Looze et al. (88) found that the mean EMG across the seven muscles sampled during lowering was only 69% of the signal amplitude observed during the lifting trials. Therefore, they concluded that with the nearly equivalent joint moments occurring during lifting and lowering, the forces supported by the active muscle fibers must be substantially greater during the eccentric (lowering) component.

Freivalds et al. (122) showed that the rectified EMG signal increased during the acceleration phase of a lift. Marras and Mirka (227) found that all of the sampled muscles showed increased activity with greater acceleration. Asymmetric conditions enhanced this relationship for contralateral muscles. In a later study the acceleration levels were controlled (229). With the very low levels of acceleration tested there was little change in the EMG. The reader should be cautioned that these accelerations were much less than those observed in most industrial workplaces (224).

Boudrifa and Davies (53) studied back muscle activities when lifting while sitting. Generally, higher ESM activities occurred when the lift was performed to the side and further away from the body, thus confirming previous studies by Andersson et al. (24,26).

Bobet and Norman (51) measured EMG activity from the lumbar ESM when subjects carried a backpack placed either just below the midback or just above the shoulders. The high load placement resulted in significantly higher levels of muscle activity. Cook and Neumann (82) studied the effect of different load placement (anterior, posterior, and lateral) when subjects were walking. The lowest levels of activity occurred when carrying the load in a backpack. Carrying the load anteriorly resulted in significant increased erector spinae activity levels. Further, in this carrying mode, significantly higher levels of activity were found for women than for men. Side-carrying resulted in high contralateral muscle activities. The conclusion derived from these studies is that the lifting mode is less important than load placement and lifting speed.

Responses to Sudden Loading

The consequences of sudden unexpected loads or sudden changes in postural stability have been investigated as sudden loads were applied to the hands (63,230), as loads were applied to the torso directly (274), and during impending falls (307). All three types of events lead to increased loading of the spine and its supporting tissues. In sum, when the system is unexpectedly loaded a "startle response" is generated wherein the system overreacts (148). This response causes muscle recruitment and increases the mechanical loading of the spine.

Marras and associates (230) measured the activities of six back muscles when weights were dropped into a box that the subjects held in front of them. The weight drop was expected or unexpected, the latter produced by having the subjects blindfolded and wearing earplugs. The muscle activities generated under conditions of unexpected load were on average 70% higher than those when the subject anticipated the load. Thus, an individual's expectancies regarding the temporal occurrence of a loading event will significantly affect the magnitude of the startle response. Lavender et al. (205) reported that peak muscle response was inversely related to the amount of warning time which in their experiment varied from 0 to 400 msec. Similarly, expectancies as to the magnitude of the loading were theorized to develop. When subjects were led to expect a 25-pound lift, Khalil

et al. (182) found that the EMG response of the biceps to an actual 5-pound lift was equivalent to that of a 25-pound lift. Butler et al. (60) found a jerking motion and a significant increase in the peak L5–S1 moment, as detected via kinetic and kinematic analyses, when the magnitude of the lifted load was much less than anticipated. Patterson et al. (283) reported an oscillatory lifting pattern under such conditions while the body attempted to adjust its response based on the new information regarding the load's magnitude.

Carlson and associates (63) investigated the muscle activities necessary to maintain postural control in situations in which the body was subjected to sudden, unexpected loads in the sagittal and frontal planes. The latency of muscle activation was 61 to 91 msec. They concluded that the back muscles play a minor role in compensating for side perturbations since experiments with unblindfolded and blindfolded subjects revealed no differences. However, Lavender et al. (205) showed that when sudden loads were applied that would create forward bending and right lateral bending moments on the spine, collectively the peak responses of the contralateral (left) latissimus dorsi and erector spinae were observed to increase by 37%. In addition, the ipsilateral posterior muscles (right side) showed a 55% decrease in their peak combined response. These results indicate the extreme disparity between the left and the right sides of the body under such conditions. This type of loading would be expected to increase the lateral shear forces acting on intervertebral disks and the potential for injury.

The internal muscle responses before voluntary or anticipated involuntary motions have been observed using EMG. Several investigators have published data showing EMG activity in the gastrocnemius muscles prior to expected destabilizing perturbations (54,55,83). Similarly, subjects, when dropped from heights between 20 and 120 cm, showed an anticipatory activation of the soleus muscle before landing (148). The onset of the muscle activity in their study occurred at a consistent time before contact with the ground. Likewise, trunk muscle activity under sudden loading conditions has been shown to begin earlier when adequate warning time is available (205).

Lavender et al. (204) reported on the development of preparatory response strategies in four individuals exposed to multiple sessions of repeated sudden loadings. Subjects stood holding a lightweight container into which a 12-pound weight was dropped at regular 1-minute intervals. Over the experimental sessions all subjects developed preparatory response strategies which utilized increased trunk muscle coactivation. Furthermore, during the actual sudden loading the subjects reduced their trunk flexion and peak spine compression predicted with a biomechanical model (232). It was theorized that the temporal uncertainty increased coactivation during the preparatory period and resulted in the increased stiffness observed during the loading. The increased stiffness reduced the destabilizing effects of the loading, thereby reducing the internal forces acting on the spine. Lavender and Marras (203) also reported an experiment in which an analogue timing display was used to reduce the temporal uncertainty as to when the sudden loads would occur. The subjects increased their posterior muscle responses between 18% and 95% relative to a baseline session without the timing display. This resulted in a relative decrease in the coactivation response as the anterior muscles showed little change in their activity.

Trunk Myoelectric Activity During Physical Exercise and Walking

Studies performed to analyze different strengthening exercises commonly employed in rehabilitation have shown that for the deep back muscles the highest levels of activity occur when the back is arched with the subject in the prone posture (272,284). For the abdominal muscles, the highest activities were recorded in the "V-sit, basket hand, sidelying trunk raise, backward leaning, and curl-up" positions (113,282).

A few studies report on the myoelectric activity of the trunk muscles during walking (354). Battey and Joseph (40) recorded short periods of activity over the lateral part of the ESM; one at the start of stance phase, a second at the end. Using indwelling electrodes Waters and Morris (365), on the other hand, reported multifidus activity at heelstrike, and ESM activity at the time of contralateral heelstrike. Dofferhof and Vink (96), more recently, confirmed those findings recording short bursts of activity just before left and right heelstrike over both the multifidus and iliocostalis lumborum muscles. Perhaps the posterior back muscles are responding to a flexion moment occurring when the lower part of the body at heelstrike is decelerated. Load carrying altered the pattern of activity corresponding to the external moment resulting from load and its location.

Myoelectric Activity in Patients with Back Pain

As early as 1952, Golding reported myoelectric measurements in a series of patients with low back pain (138). Of 120 patients, 34 did not achieve the expected, and previously discussed, relaxation of the back muscles during complete flexion of the trunk. These findings were confirmed by Floyd and Silver (116) and Yashimoto and associates (375), who found that 84 of 104 patients had "abnormal" erector spinae activity, primarily an absence of the flexion-relaxation phenomenon. Triano and Schultz (359) studied the flexion-relaxation phenomenon in patients and control subjects and related those findings to disability rating scales. Almost 50% of

the patients did not exhibit flexion-relaxation, whereas all the control subjects did. A positive relationship was found between degree of disability and the loss of the flexion-relaxation phenomenon. These results are in agreement with studies by Ahern et al. (5) and Sihvonen et al. (325). Possible explanations include loss of reflex inhibition, abnormal muscle reaction to lengthening, and inability to flex fully because of pain. Ahern et al. (6) obtained videotape recordings of pain behaviors during flexion movements, and used those to determine the relationship of pain to flexion-relaxation. An absence of the flexion-relaxation response was found to be significantly associated with overt pain behavior. Paquet et al. (277) found that when flexion movements of patients were compared to movements of equivalent velocity made by a normal group, the expected relaxation at full flexion was not seen in the patients.

All these studies document the influence of back pain on the flexion-silence phenomenon. Other myoelectric studies include additional movements and functional tasks. Wolf and Basmajian (370) studied nine patients in various postures and during functional motions. Muscle activity was lower than, or the same as, that in a healthy control population. Wolf and associates (371) later collected data from 121 men and women without low back pain during dynamic and static conditions to provide a baseline for comparison with patients with back pain. Whereas the data is available, it is presently unclear that it has been used to that purpose. Soderberg and Barr (335) recorded myoelectric activities from the T10, L1, and L3 levels in healthy subjects and patients with chronic low back pain. When Valsalva maneuvers were performed, and when performing a sit-up, the healthy subjects increased their ESM activity, whereas the pain patients did not, or only very little. This would suggest that cocontraction of the trunk muscles does not occur as normally expected. When lifting weights of 4.5 and 16 kg, there were no measurable differences between patients and control subjects during the actual lift. The patient group maintained a higher level of myoelectric activity for a short period after the lift, however.

Nouwen and associates (270) studied 20 patients with low back pain and 20 pain-free control subjects during flexion, extension, lateral bending, and rotation. Patients with low back pain showed higher paraspinal and lower abdominal activity near full flexion than controls, as well as less paraspinal activity when returning to the upright standing position. No difference was noted between left-sided and right-sided paraspinal myoelectric patterns when patients and control subjects were compared, nor was there a significant difference during rotation and lateral bending activities.

Other studies have attempted to determine electromyographically whether or not patients with low back pain have a generally increased erector spinae muscle activity, since they often present with a clinical picture commonly termed *muscle spasm*. If increased muscle activity were a characteristic, biofeedback would be an alternative treatment method. Roland (306) pointed out a number of general problems associated with earlier studies. The patient populations were poorly described, and the degree of muscle spasm in the patients with low back pain was not quantified or often even specified. Also, technical difficulties existed, including positioning of the subjects and recording from selected muscles. This may explain the lack of agreement among studies. In some studies, patients with palpable abnormalities in their back muscles had increased myoelectric activity over those areas (29,92,102,103,110). On the other hand, Kraft and associates (189) found no increase in muscle activity over areas of muscle spasm. Holmes and Wolff (159) recorded myoelectric activities from 65 subjects with back pain and 10 healthy controls while they were undergoing a stressful interview. The back patients displayed continuous sustained muscle activity in contrast to healthy subjects. Similarly, Grabel (141) recorded higher levels of activity in back patients who were asked to "self-relax" than those found in healthy control subjects. Kravitz et al. (190), however, using modern signal analysis techniques to quantify the myoelectric activities, found no difference at rest between patients with low back pain and healthy controls. When asked to relax their back muscles while performing simple arm and leg muscle contractions, the patients were unable to reduce their ESM activity as much as the control subjects, however. This would indicate that the back muscles were used to control spinal posture even though the spine was not directly involved in the movement. Miller (250) found no difference in activity between a group of subjects with chronic low back pain and healthy control subjects. Their test positions were low-level activities, such as sitting, standing, and performing light unilateral upper extremity tasks while sitting. Similar results were obtained by Collins et al. (81). Hoyt et al. (162), on the other hand, found slightly higher activity levels in patients with chronic low back pain when standing, but not when sitting. Several studies of patients to determine activity levels and abnormality in activity pattern are summarized in Table 1. Clinical use of electromyography in diagnosis is reported in Chapter 33. Studies of back muscle fatigue in patients with low back pain will be discussed subsequently.

TABLE 1. *EMG studies of muscle activity in back pain patients*

Reference	Patients (no.)	Type of patient	Control	Activity changes
Denslow and Clough (92)	16	Osteopathic	Adjacent area	+
Denslow and Hassett (93)	17	Osteopathic	Adjacent area	+
Elliott (102)	8	Back pain	Adjacent area	+
Price et al. (298)	?	Acute/chronic	Normals	+/− abnormal
Holmes and Wolff (159)	65	Backache	Normals—10	+
Golding (138)	120	Back pain	—	No relaxation
Taverner (345)	?	?	—	No change
Floyd and Silver (115)	105	Back pain	Normals—45	No relaxation
Arroyo (29)	?	Fibrositis	Adjacent area	Continuous activity
DeVries (95)	8	Chronic back pain	Normals—4	+/−
Kraft et al. (189)	16	Fibrositis	—	−
Waylonis (366)	131	Cervical disc	—	+ (acute) No change (chronic)
England and Delbert (103)	10	Chronic back pain	Adjacent	+
Fowler and Kraft (121)	10	Chronic neck	Normals—35	+
Jayasinghe et al. (170)	7	Back pain	Normals—4	+
Wolf and Basmajian (370)	9	Chronic back pain	Normals—66	−
Kravitz et al. (190)	22	Back pain (>6 mo)	Normals—17	+ minimally
Hoyt et al. (162)	40	Back pain (>1 yr)	Normals—40	+
Collins et al. (81)	11	Back pain (>6 mo)	Normals—11	−
Soderberg and Barr (335)	25	Back pain (>3 mo)	Normals—20	+/− (no relaxation)
Flor et al. (114)	17	Back pain (>6 mo)	Normals—17	+
Fricton et al. (123)	16	Myofascial	Other area	+
Fischer and Chang (110)	9	Back pain (1–25 yr)	Normals—12	+
Yashimoto et al. (375)	104	?	—	No relaxation
Triano and Schultz (359)	?	Back pain	Normals	No relaxation
Ahern et al. (5)	?	Back pain	—	No relaxation
Nouwen et al. (270)	20	Back pain	Normals—20	Abnormal
Miller (250)	?	Chronic back pain	Normals	+/−

Adapted with permission from Roland (306).
+, increase; −, decrease.

Measurement of Intramuscular Pressure

Another measure of muscle function is intramuscular pressure. Intramuscular pressure provides a good estimate of muscle force under isometric (188,318) and dynamic conditions (278,339,340). Passive tension of a muscle increases the pressure at rest (184). Styf (339) used a microcapillary infusion technique to record intramuscular pressures in the erector spinae muscles. Pressure increased from 8 mm Hg at rest to as much as 265 mm Hg during contraction. Higher pressures were recorded during sitting as compared with standing, although there was considerable individual variation. Flexion of the trunk and lifting increased pressures. A further discussion of pressure measurements appears when compartment syndromes are discussed later in this chapter.

MUSCLE STRENGTH

Strength is the ability of a muscle or group of muscles to exert force, i.e., to develop tension actively. By definition, strength is not limited to one particular type of muscle contraction. However, the type of contraction will determine the force output and, therefore, must be described. Three types of contraction are distinguished: concentric contraction or shortening, isometric contraction where length is unchanged, and eccentric contraction or lengthening (Table 2). Strength in its broadest form is measured statically (isometrically) or dynamically. Measurements of dynamic strength are further subdivided into isotonic (concentric), eccentric, isokinetic, and isoinertial (Table 3).

Maximum strength is the greatest force that a muscle can exert on the skeletal system under a given set of loading conditions. The most frequently used clinical measure is maximum voluntary strength. Because strength varies as a function of muscle length, it is best defined as a curve displaying the force output as a function of the joint angle, often referred to as a *strength curve,* rather than by a single value (Fig. 24). Strength curves can be generated by repeated isometric measures at different joint angles or by dynamic measures in which strength is recorded continuously as a function of the joint angle. Strength and, therefore, strength curves are affected by a number of variables such as age, sex, subject motivation, pain, muscle and joint physiology, muscle geometry, and

exercise conditions. For purposes of reporting, therefore, all of these parameters need to be included. Conversely, failure to specify these conditions seriously limits the usefulness of the reported results.

In this chapter, trunk strength and lifting strength are purposely separated, because lifting strength refers to a physical whole-body activity, where the limiting muscle group may be other than trunk muscles. For example, in a squat lift (leg lift), the knee extensor muscles may be the limiting muscle group rather than the back muscles. The relationship of trunk strength to lifting strength is quite variable (253).

A short review of modes and techniques to measure muscle output will be given as background information to some of the data presented subsequently. No single testing mode is the best and most valid, and there is no proof that one testing mode has greater inferential capacity with respect to human function than others (312). Isometric techniques include manual muscle testing and the use of spring and strain gauges as well as dynamometers. A number of cable-attached spring and strain gauge systems have been developed for measurements of trunk strength over the years. Typically, the pelvis is strapped in and then the subject is fitted with a harness and asked to exert force against resistance. A recent system to measure isometric trunk strength more specifically was introduced by Medex (145–147). Other isometric equipment has been developed to measure static lift strength, as discussed subsequently. Generally, the advantages of the isometric systems are low cost and simple testing, but the cost increases with increasing sophistication of the measurement device. Data are also easy to interpret because they consist of one value or several discrete values which, combined, produce a strength curve. This means that accurate tests of strength can be performed through a full range of motion. Other advantages include a high degree of reliability (145). The disadvantages include the uncertain relationship of isometric strength to dynamic function. A number of studies, reviewed by Mital and Ayoub (253), indicate that dynamic strength is better correlated to task performance capabilities than static strength.

Isotonic strength measurement techniques include the use of free weights in a controlled movement system or the use of a constrained system that allows unequal effort. Most isotonic assessments are concentric. The lever arm and speed of movement are both important to an isotonic measurement. Because isotonic means the

TABLE 2. *Characteristics of muscle contraction*

Type	Action	Tension/unit area	Metabolic demand
Isometric	Tension but no motion	Medium	Related to intensity
Concentric	Moving a resistance while shortening (raising)	Low	High
Eccentric	Moving a resistance while lengthening (lowering)	High	Low

TABLE 3. *Definitions of muscle contractions*

Isometric	The external length of the muscle does not change. Same as *static*.
Isotonic	The internal force of the muscle does not change but the muscle shortens. Same as *concentric*.
Eccentric	The external force is greater than the internal force of the muscle, causing a lengthening of the muscle.
Isokinetic	A dynamic exercise where the speed of motion is constant.
Isoinertial	Contraction against a constant load. The torque generated by the muscle causes acceleration.

same force, a pure isotonic exercise would require a constant muscle tension throughout the exercise. To accomplish this, the resistance throughout the range of motion is changed in proportion to changes in moment arm, referred to as a *variable resistance exercise.* Although this can produce a constant external load, the internal forces are not constant, and thus not purely isotonic. There are currently several examples of constrained systems, including the Nautilus equipment. Isotonic data can be obtained inexpensively and easily. Assessment occurs throughout the range of motion, but reliability is a problem, and isotonic resistance is often an unfamiliar task to the patient. Also, in isotonic tests, maximum strength is determined by the weakest position in a range of motion.

Isokinetic assessment requires the subject to move the body (trunk or limb) at a constant controlled speed, preselected by the examiner. The systems are controlled through a dynamometer, which is either passive, allowing only concentric movement, or active, allowing both concentric and eccentric exercises. A large number of devices are currently available. Existing systems were evaluated by Malone in 1988 (219). All provide computer records of the tests, but some have incomplete normative data bases. The advantage of all of these isokinetic testing devices is that they test throughout the range of motion and at different speeds. Because the resistance is the func-

tion of the patient's efforts in the passive mode, these devices are considered safe. Disadvantages include cost, constraints in motion pattern, and the unfamiliar task of moving at a preselected speed. Because isokinetic tests include an acceleration phase in the early part of a range of motion, and a deceleration phase at the very end, information is lost during part of the movement. This is particularly important when testing at high speed.

Isoinertial (or isodynamic) testing is peculiar to the Isotechnology trunk assessment system (139). Essentially the test measures the maximum weight a person can move to an assigned point at a freely chosen speed. While resistance is controlled, acceleration is free and measured. Measurements can be obtained in a single plane (in three plane directions) or in a multiplane mode. Advantages include assessment throughout the range of motion in three planes, functional movements, and measures of acceleration and velocity. The disadvantages include cost and availability.

In addition to the dynamic test modes described, psychophysical strength testing is also used, where the maximum acceptable weight is determined as a measure of a person's dynamic strength (253).

Trunk Muscle Strength

Measurements of trunk muscle strength have been performed over many years both in healthy subjects and in patients. Strength has been measured isometrically (3,10,45,145–147,154,249,259,297,360), isotonically (112,192,193,249,291,360), isokinetically (43,85,154, 192,193,200,223,238,240,264,328,330,332,344,349, 353,355), and isoinertially (269,280) (Figs. 25–27). The

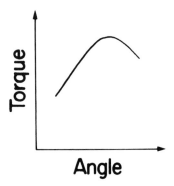

FIG. 24. Torque changes as a function of joint angle resulting in an angle-torque curve. The curve shape varies between joints. When performing isometric tests, the joint angle must be given.

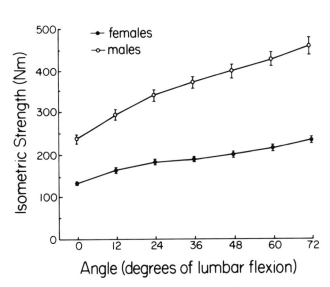

FIG. 25. Isometric trunk strength as a function of joint angle. Strength increases with increasing flexion. Men are significantly stronger than women at each angle. Adapted from Graves et al. (145).

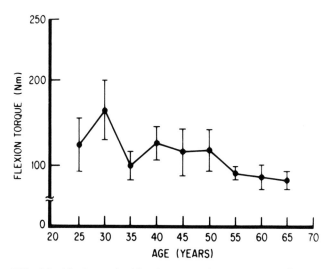

FIG. 26. Maximum isokinetic strength versus age: flexion (abdominal muscle) strength. From Langrana et al. (200), with permission.

equipment has varied from simple tensiometers to very sophisticated, computerized measurement devices. Because all measurements reflect voluntary efforts, it is important to remember that *voluntary* means that the effort is influenced by an individual's perception and tolerance of pain and discomfort. A patient who develops acute back pain will produce a lower force than he was capable of the day before his pain developed. This does not reflect a true loss of strength but rather a loss of functional strength.

Trunk Muscle Strength in Normals

Men as a group are stronger than women, but when strength is normalized to body weight, women may be as strong as men (177,259,330,331). The eccentric (lengthening) and isometric contractions produce higher levels of strength than concentric (shortening) contractions (269). Only a few studies comparing concentric and eccentric trunk exertions appear in the literature (323,327). Smidt et al. (327) found that eccentric strength exceeded concentric strength by 70 to 150 Nm. Reid and Costigan (303) report that subjects were able to exert 20% more eccentric force compared with concentric. The trunk extensors are normally stronger than the flexors. Indeed it appears that the trunk extensors in aggregate are the strongest muscle group in the body. In studies by Smidt and associates (329), the average moment of force generated for eccentric extensor muscle contractions was in excess of 400 Nm. Additional studies have revealed that trunk extensor strength in postmenopausal women is more than double the strength of the knee extensors (329). However, trunk strength seems to diminish significantly with age, beginning at 40 to 50 years (344).

Graves et al. (145,146) used a specially developed in-

strument to record isometric lumbar extension strength at different joint angles (Fig. 25). The pelvic fixation system restricted motion to the spine. Extension strength was found to be greatest in full flexion, and tests were highly repeatable. Men were stronger than women at each angle tested. The finding of greater strength in flexion confirms previous studies by Smidt et al. (330) and Marras et al. (223).

Kumar et al. (192) compared isometric trunk strength measured at different degrees of flexion to isokinetic flexion and extension. The posture had a significant influence on strength, leading to the conclusion that measurements made in one posture cannot be translated into capability or impairment in another posture. Isokinetic strength was 60–70% of the corresponding isometric values.

Langrana et al. (200) found the maximum muscle torques to be in the same order in isokinetic as in isometric tests. Motion was always found to be reduced in patients. Marras et al. (223) also examined the relationship between isometric and isokinetic torque. He found that the subjects were able to produce the greatest amount of torque under isometric conditions. As the speed of the movement increased, torque decreased. Trunk torque also varied as a function of the angle of the trunk; the greatest torques occurred at forward angled trunk positions. Later studies by Marras et al. (230) investigated trunk extensor torque in the sagittal plane under isokinetic velocity conditions ranging from 0 deg/sec to 90 deg/sec. They found that trunk torque was reduced by 0.55% of maximum for each deg/sec increase in trunk velocity.

Some of the test equipment available requires the person to be standing during the test, whereas others test the subject when sitting. Thus, it is important to know how

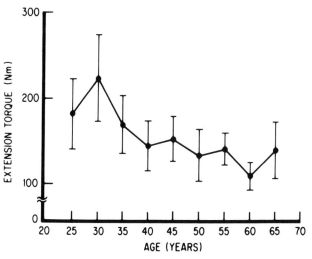

FIG. 27. Maximum isokinetic strength versus age: extension (paraspinal muscle) strength. From Langrana et al. (200), with permission.

body position alters the results. Langrana and Lee (199) compared sitting and standing measures (Fig. 28). They found that motion was reduced when sitting, and flexion strength was about two times greater in standing than in sitting. Extension strength was also greater, but only by about 20%. Cartas et al. (70) found the maximum isometric flexion strength to be significantly greater in standing than in semistanding or sitting. The maximum isometric extension strength, on the other hand, was not affected by the posture. The average power in standing, however, was twice that in the other two postures. There were no differences between semistanding and sitting in dynamic strength.

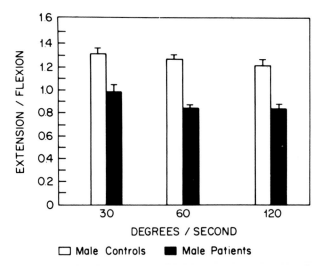

FIG. 29. Extensor/flexor ratios (expressed as a percent) for male normal control subjects versus male patients at multiple speeds. From Mayer et al. (240), with permission.

The symmetry of the test is also important to the measured strength. Marras and Mirka (225) reported that the reduction in strength with asymmetry was significantly affected by the trunk angular velocity. Kumar et al. (193) found progressively declining strength with increasing postural asymmetry. Asymptomatic volunteers and patients were significantly stronger in lateral flexion than in axial rotation (almost by a factor of 2). Isokinetic strength in these modes was 60–70% of isometric strength, and women were on average 30–40% weaker than men.

Trunk Muscle Strength in Patients

Using isometric techniques, it has been well established that patients have less trunk muscle strength than healthy control subjects. In healthy subjects, isometric trunk extension strength is greater than flexion strength (112,154,192,328,332,344,355). The ratio of the two has been used to determine abnormalities in patients (3,200,248,344,355,360). Mayer et al. (238,240,241) found a significant loss of both flexor and extensor muscle strength in chronic back patients compared to healthy controls, and also found that the main loss of strength was in the extensor muscles (Fig. 29). Hemborg (156) reported a drop in the ratio of extension to flexion from 1.54 to 1.29 when comparing healthy construction workers to those with chronic low back pain. These findings were later confirmed by Holmstrom et al. (160). Marras and Wongsam (233) found that back pain patients reduce the speed by which they move the trunk, and suggest that this is one of the first functional losses caused by pain. Shirado et al. (323) reported that while eccentric trunk strength was greater in normals than con-

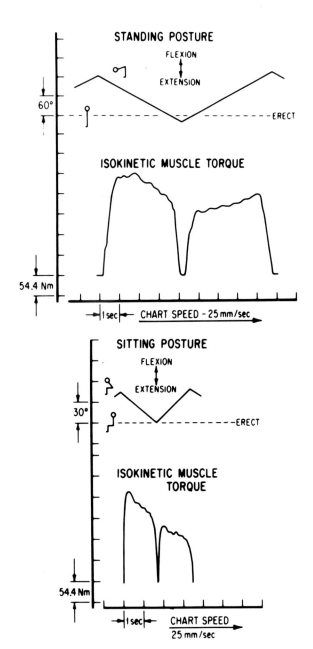

FIG. 28. An isokinetic recording in the standing and sitting postures. From Langrana et al. (200), with permission.

centric, this was not always the case in patients. Chronic low back patients always had weak extensors.

Isokinetic studies have been performed at various speeds, typically 30°, 60°, 90°, and 120° per second. Patients have consistently been found to have lower values in both flexion and extension, and the ratio between flexion and extension strength changes with back pain (Fig. 30).

Beimborn and Morrissey (43) summarized the literature up to 1987 on different methods to assess trunk muscle strength (Tables 4–6). They conclude that the strength hierarchy of the trunk muscles is from strongest to weakest; extension, flexion, side-bending, and rotation. The agonist to antagonist ratio for extension-flexion was on average 1.3 in the papers they reviewed. For rotation and side-bending, strength was equal between right and left side. Extension force was typically greater than flexion force irrespective of the mode of testing. All studies were not in agreement on this point, however. Pope et al. (289) found isometric trunk flexion to be greater than trunk extension, whereas Davies and Gould (85) found flexion strength to be greater than extension strength at 120° per second isokinetic speed, but not at other speeds tested.

Newton and Waddell (265) summarized the literature on isokinetic and isoinertial testing up until 1993, and concluded that there was insufficient scientific evidence to support the use of "iso-machines" in pre-employment screening, routine clinical assessment, and medicolegal evaluation. We agree with this position in general. Isometric trunk strength has also been used to predict risk of future low back pain. As with "iso-tests," the predictive value has been poor (48,305).

Surgery has a major negative effect on muscle strength. Kahanovitz et al. (178) found a decrease in strength of 30% or more for isometric and isokinetic extensor muscle strength 1 year after a surgical discectomy indicating the need for intense rehabilitation postoperatively.

Lifting Strength

Lifting strength has been used primarily in pre-employment testing to determine whether a person is capable of performing a job that involves lifting activities. It is different from trunk strength in the sense that the limiting muscle group in a lifting test may not be the trunk muscles but rather the leg or the arm muscles. Although this makes it a more realistic test for work capacity evaluation, it also means that these tests are of limited value in the guidance of physical rehabilitation of trunk muscles.

As a result of the extensive interest in pre-employment testing, many publications have developed on lifting strength over the past two decades (28,34,73–76,133, 150,179,181,191,220,268,299,304). In the early years, testing was primarily static (isometric). With the aim of standardizing tests, the American Industrial Hygiene Association published a guide providing advice on measurement techniques, subject information, description of exercise conditions, subject description, and data recording in static strength testing (61). The advantages of static strength testing are that it is easy to perform and the equipment cost is comparatively small. The method has been shown to be reproducible (181) and comparatively safe (72,376). Chaffin et al. (75) and Keyserling et al. (181) have shown that the test can be predictive of injury. However, the test must be job specific, otherwise its predictive value is low (41). Birch et al. (50) related isometric lift strength (ILS) to dynamic measures of muscular fitness, leg and back muscle strength, and muscle power. Significant correlations were found between ILS and back and leg strength, as well as standing, broad jump, and power output. This would indicate that ILS can be used to predict aspects of dynamic function.

The main disadvantage with isometric testing of lifting is that lifting in real life is a dynamic activity. Because static strength does not account for the effect of inertial forces, joint loading is underestimated compared to when a dynamic task is performed. With the aim of developing more realistic tests, therefore, isokinetic and isoinertial techniques have been introduced (84,179, 185,191,223,292,299).

Studies have shown that dynamic strength provides a better reflection of task performance capabilities than static (4,84,253). Dynamic strength testing is strongly influenced by factors such as posture, reach distance, arm orientation, speed of exertion, and duration of exertion. A review of current knowledge about the importance of

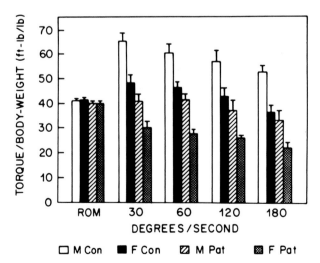

FIG. 30. Male patients (*M Pat*) and female patients (*F Pat*) versus normal male and female controls (*M Con* and *F Con*) on left rotation measures demonstrating range of motion in degrees and torque production normalized to body weight. From Mayer et al. (240), with permission.

TABLE 4. *Isometric tests*

Reference	Subjects	Equipment	E/F	E/F/SB	E/F/ROT	ROT
Addison and Schultz (3)	IM + F	Force-measuring load cells		X		
Alston et al. (10)	U	Harrison Clark cable tensiometer	X			
Asmussen and Heelboll-Nielsen (30)	UM	2 dynamometers	X			
Asmussen et al. (32)	UM + F	Dynamometer 1		X		
Backlund and Nordgren (35)	UM	Pressductor force transducer		X		
Davies and Gould (85)	UM + F	Cybex[a] II isokinetic dynamometer	X			
Hasue et al. (154)	UM + F IM + F	Cybex isokinetic dynamometer	X			
Heelboll-Nielsen (155)	UM + F	Dynamometer	X			
Langrana and Lee (199)	UM + F IM + F	Cybex II isokinetic dynamometer	X			
Langrana et al. (200)	UM + F IM + F	Cybex II isokinetic dynamometer	X			
Langrana and Stover (201)	UM + F IM + F	Cybex II isokinetic dynamometer	X			
Mayer et al. (238)	UM + F	Cybex F/E trunk strength tests	X			
Mayer et al. (238)	IM + F	Cybex F/E trunk dynamometer	X			
Mayer et al. (240)	UM + F IM + F	Cybex F/E trunk dynamometer	X			
Mayer et al. (241)	UM + F IM + F	Prototype isokinetic rotation unit			X	
McNeill et al. (248)	UM + F IM + F	Strain gauge load cells		X		
Nicolaisen and Jørgensen (266)	UM + F IM + F	Strain gauge dynamometer	X			
Pope et al. (291)	UM IM	Load cell	X			
Portillo et al. (293)	UF IF	Trunk strength measuring apparatus		X		
Smidt et al. (327)	UM	Iowa force table	X			
Smidt et al. (330)	UM + F	Iowa trunk dynamometer with Cybex II	X			
Smith et al. (332)	UM + F	Cybex II isokinetic dynamometer			X	
Suzuki and Endo (344)	UM	Cybex II isokinetic dynamometer	X			
Thorstensson and Arvidsson (353)	UM IM	Cybex II isokinetic dynamometer		X		
Thorstensson and Nilsson (355)	UM	Cybex II isokinetic dynamometer		X		
Troup and Chapman (360)	UM + F	Strain gauge	X			

After Beimborn and Morrissey (43).
I, injured; U, uninjured; M, male; F, female; F/E, flexion/extension; SB, side-bending; ROT, rotation.
[a] Cybex, Division of Lumex, Inc., Ronkonkoma, NY.

TABLE 5. *Isotonic tests*

Reference	Subjects	Equipment	E/F	E/F/SB
Flint (112)	UF IF	Dynamometer and 1 lift max	X	
Kluck (186)	UM + F	Elgin exercise unit	X	
Meyer and Greenberg (249)	UM + F	Swivel table with spring balance and precise gravity scale		X
Nachemson and Lindh (259)	UM + F	Spring balance Zadig dynamometer		

After Beimborn and Morrissey (43).
I, injured; U, uninjured; M, male; F, female; E/F, extension/flexion; SB, side-bending.

TABLE 6. *Isokinetic tests*

Reference	Subjects	Equipment	E/F	E/F/SB	E/F/ROT	ROT
Davies and Gould (85)	UM + F	Cybex II isokinetic dynamometer	X			
Hasue et al. (154)	UM + F	Cybex isokinetic dynamometer	X			
Langrana and Lee (199)	UM + F IM + F	Cybex II dynamometer	X			
Langrana et al. (200)	UM + F IM + F	Cybex II isokinetic dynamometer	X			
Langrana and Stover (201)	UM + F IM + F	Cybex II isokinetic dynamometer	X			
Mayer et al. (238)	IM + F	Cybex F/E trunk strength tests	X			
Mayer et al. (238)	IM + F	Cybex isokinetic dynamometer	X			
Mayer et al. (240)	UM + F IM + F	Cybex II isokinetic dynamometer	X			
Mayer et al. (241)	UM + F IM + F	Prototype isokinetic torso rotation table				X
Smidt et al. (327)	UM	Iowa force table	X			
Smidt et al. (330)	UM + F	Iowa trunk dynamometer with Cybex II	X			
Smith et al. (332)	UM + F	Cybex II isokinetic			X	
Suzuki and Endo (344)	UM IM	Cybex II isokinetic dynamometer	X			
Thompson et al. (350)	UM + F	Cybex II isokinetic dynamometer	X			
Thorstensson and Arvidsson (353)	UM	Cybex II isokinetic dynamometer		X		
Thorstensson and Nilsson (355)	UM	Cybex II isokinetic dynamometer		X		

After Beimborn and Morrissey (43).
I, injured; U, uninjured; M, male; F, female; E/F, extension/flexion; SB, side-bending; ROT, rotation.

these factors is provided in Mital et al. (253). Isokinetic pull strength is considerably higher in standing than in sitting postures. Reach distance influences the mechanical advantage of task performance and therefore influences strength. People are generally able to generate greater forces when lifting close to the body. Arm orientation also influences the mechanical advantage. As stated previously, the speed of motion is also important. Motion of body segments require muscle force simply to accelerate body mass and overcome inertia. During deceleration, on the other hand, the body's momentum reduces the need for muscle contribution to the force produced. The force-velocity property of muscle plays into this complex situation. Duration of lift is another influencing factor; the strength declines exponentially with the duration of a lift (253). Wheeler et al. (367) have developed a model to determine dynamic lifting capacity from a biomechanical analysis of a submaximal lift and a measure of maximum isometric trunk strength. This is an interesting approach which presently has only been tested in sagittally symmetric situations.

Psychophysical test methods have also been advocated to study lifting (333,334). The idea of using psychophysical techniques is that there is a relationship between perceived strength and actual strength, which can be described by a mathematical function. Psychophysical techniques have been used to determine acceptable weight lifting in industry (34,134,210,236,252,333). Psychophysical strength testing can be performed under realistic conditions and is quite reproducible. It is based on self-report of subjects, however, which obviously is influenced by factors other than the disease process. Moreover, Thompson and Chaffin (352) found that, in general, people were poor at perceiving the stress on the spine during lifting activities, thereby questioning the utility of the psychophysical approach.

There are also studies investigating external trunk strength as a function of asymmetric lifting. Garg and Badger (131) studied isometric lift strength at three asymmetric angles and found that strength decreased by 12% to 31% for asymmetric lift angles.

Whichever method is used, it has been clearly established that in pre-employment situations the test must be related to the job requirements to be predictive (40, 41,181).

TRUNK MUSCLE ENDURANCE

Another important attribute of muscles is their capacity to respond to repetitive loading, i.e., their endurance. Endurance is mechanically defined as the point at which fatigue of muscles is observable. This is when a contraction can no longer be maintained at a certain level (isometric fatigue), or when repetitive work can no longer be sustained at a certain output (dynamic fatigue). In both situations, the mechanical events are preceded by biochemical and physiologic changes within the muscle. However, these changes do not immediately influence the mechanical performance of the muscle. Moreover, the mechanical parameters of fatigue, such as failure to maintain a posture, an exertion, or pace of work, are highly subjective phenomena influenced by motivation. The biochemical and physiologic events, on the other hand, are not affected by motivation and, therefore, are of interest as objective measures. Whereas biochemical parameters must be sampled invasively, electromyography is a noninvasive method by which physiologic fatigue can be monitored using surface electrodes (Fig. 31) (89).

Mechanical tests of trunk muscle fatigue include maintaining a posture (47,48,160,266,269) or performing an activity repeatedly (154,281,330). Smidt et al. (330) studied dynamic endurance using a test in which the subjects moved a padded bar connected to an isokinetic dynamometer at a paced rate. Trunk flexor muscles were found to fatigue more rapidly than trunk extensor muscles; women were found to have a higher level of endurance than men. When comparing endurance levels for healthy subjects and chronic back patients, Smidt et al. found that the healthy subjects scored lower. Their findings would seem odd, but are explained by the fact that endurance was tested at a percentage of maximum torque levels and, therefore, the torque was much lower for the patients than for the healthy control subjects. Hasue et al. (154) developed an index relating the initial torque in an isometric and isokinetic device to the torque after a period of time. The trunk muscles were found to fatigue more easily when isometric contractions were performed, and the abdominal muscles were found to fatigue more easily than the back muscles. Biering-Sørensen (48), Nordin et al. (269), and Holmstrom et al. (160) used a postural endurance test in which the subjects maintained an unsupported trunk in a horizontal

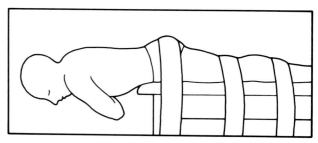

FIG. 32. Mechanical test of fatigue. The trunk is unsupported and the subject is trying to maintain the posture. Redrawn from Nordin et al. (269).

position for a defined period of time (Fig. 32). When using this postural test, Nicolaisen and Jørgensen (266) found that patients with ongoing low back pain had significantly shorter endurance time than healthy control subjects. Holmstrom et al. (160) obtained a similar result when testing construction workers with and without back pain. Significantly shorter endurance time was found both in workers with a definite low back disorder and in those with a probable back disorder. They found no correlation between maximum isometric trunk extensor strength and endurance. Nicolaisen and Jørgensen also used a test in which they measured the time during which a subject could maintain 60% of a maximum isometric voluntary contraction of the trunk muscles. Again, patients were found to fatigue earlier than controls. In a more recent study, Parnianpour et al. (281) used an isoinertial device to study the force output and movement pattern in three dimensions when subjects performed a flexion-extension movement. It was found that with fatigue, out-of-plane movements increased. In addition, torque, angular excursion, and angular velocity decreased. The neuromuscular adaptation to fatigue appears to include reduced accuracy, control, and speed of contraction.

Although electromyographic data analysis holds promise to be a more objective method of measuring muscle fatigue, it is still under development (46, 89,90,187,239,269,311,317,351). Early studies of back muscle fatigue using electromyography indicated a higher level of myoelectric back muscle activity in subjects with back pain during prolonged standing (95,170). These studies relied on the amplitude of the myoelectric signal as an indicator of muscle fatigue. Recent developments indicate, however, that the power density spectrum is a better indicator of fatigue, changing toward lower frequencies in sustained isometric contractions (89). Roy et al. (311) found significant differences in the speed by which the median frequency of the myoelectric signal changed in subjects with back pain compared to healthy control subjects (Fig. 33). These tests involved recordings of the myoelectric back muscle activity using six surface electrodes placed over the longissimus (at L1), iliocostalis (at L2), and multifidus (at L3) muscles. A

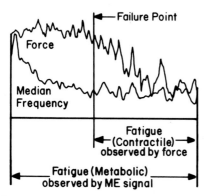

FIG. 31. Distinction between contractile fatigue and metabolic fatigue. In this case, the force was exerted during an isometric contraction of the first dorsal interosseous muscle. The task consisted of maintaining the force output at 50% of the maximal value for as long as possible, and when this was no longer possible, the subject attempted to produce as much force as possible. The failure point denotes the time when the force output was no longer maintained at the desired "average" value. The median frequency value was calculated from the power density spectrum of the myoelectric signal. The time duration of the contraction was 150 sec. From DeLuca (89), with permission.

lem in a rabbit model. Although an injured muscle retains enough strength to allow early rehabilitation, it is at risk for further damage should the exercise level be high. Rehabilitation, therefore, should be gradual with the purpose of maintaining muscle tone and range of motion. This study applies only to the immediate postinjury period. As healing progresses, rehabilitation can be more aggressive.

"Overuse" of Muscles

Throughout the history of spinal disorders, numerous attempts have been made to attribute common, activity-related, nonspecific neck and back pain to muscle injury or overuse. With few exceptions, the attempts to correlate these symptoms with a specific muscle lesion have been unrewarding, although MRI now offers a new and powerful research tool for noninvasive assessment (244,337). One obvious exception has been the post-traumatic cervical sprain, a topic that will be the focus of Chapter 59. The inability to define specific anatomic injuries has led to alternative proposed roles for muscles in the etiology of spinal pain. Based largely on studies of peripheral muscles, attention has been centered on the physiologic consequences of overuse and exercise. Included in these analyses have been the shifts that occur from aerobic to anaerobic metabolism after prolonged exercise. Detailed chemical analyses of peripheral muscles demonstrate increased concentrations of lactic acid, which occur in contracting muscles over time, accompanied by a decrease in local tissue pH, and the presence of enzymes that either facilitate anaerobic metabolism or have the capacity to promote local tissue inflammation. Hagberg et al. (152) studied serum creatinin kinase (SCK) in controlled exercises and work settings. They found significant elevations lasting 24 to 48 hours after "lifting work" but not after bicycle ergometry, despite the fact that the latter involved four times as much work. The mechanism of SCK release is theorized to result from sustained high load, especially static, which results in severe adenosine 5'-triphosphate (ATP) depletion, increased permeability, and release of SCK. After complete depletion, replacement of glycogen stores requires 24 to 48 hours (151).

In a review article, Edwards (101) proposed that occupational myalgia results from an imbalance between recruitment and relaxation of muscle motor units when muscles are used mainly for postural activity (holding or supporting fine movements) compared to phasic use in dynamic work. This would tend to move the emphasis away from the muscle itself to an alteration in central motor control, and would explain the apparent importance of mental stress to the occurrence of these disorders, and also why a more skilled worker seems to have less risk of symptoms than an unskilled worker.

Edwards's theory does not contradict the almost general agreement that muscle load is a major etiologic factor in spinal injuries (319). High loads on the muscles cause fatigue, followed by a number of changes in the muscles themselves. Muscle pain after exercise has been found to be associated with ultrastructural damage (125,261–263) and delayed inflammatory changes (173). There is also an increase in creatine kinase activity (152,254). Fatiguing contractions lead to depletion of local energy stores, with sometimes severe depletion of ATP in a small proportion of muscle fibers compared to a more modest average depletion (119). These local tissue events, rather than actual tissue disruption, are thought to cause pain, although the direct neurophysiologic pathways are not well established. Muscle injury is related to muscle fatigue. Lieber and Fridén (213) used a model of repetitive strain in the rabbit and demonstrated selective damage to fast glycolytic muscle fibers. They suggested that low oxidative capacity predisposed these muscle fibers to injury.

Another type of overuse, not to be confused with muscle strain, is the so-called delayed muscle soreness. This condition, which occurs 12 to 48 hours after an unusually vigorous (and typically eccentric) activity, is characterized by diffuse soreness in the muscle, tenderness to palpation, stiffness, and reduced range of motion. The symptoms disappear after 4 to 10 days, over which period there is a gradual decrease in symptom intensity. Increased levels of substance P have been measured in the muscle, and the urinary output of myoglobin and hydroxyproline has been observed (1). At electron microscopic levels, ruptures of Z-lines have been demonstrated and are perhaps responsible for the problem by releasing metabolites, causing edema and pain receptor stimulation (27,78,125,126,261). At a practical level, recovery from delayed muscle soreness is complete and treatment not indicated.

Laboratory research has demonstrated that eccentric muscle contractions damage skeletal muscle, particularly when they are not conditioned for the exercise. After only a few eccentric contractions, maximal isometric tetanic force may be reduced up to 50–60%, and recovery may take a week or longer. The magnitude of eccentric force, velocity of lengthening, and number of contractions seem to influence the loss of force. The magnitude of injury resulting from eccentric contractions depends on both the intensity and duration of the exercise (activity). From a prevention point of view, this information would suggest that eccentric contractions be controlled.

MRI studies of exhaustive biceps exercises, both concentric and eccentric, have shown evidence of muscle injury in muscles performing eccentric contractions, peaking on days 3 to 10 and lasting for as long as 75 days after the disappearance of symptoms (321,322). Symptoms and MR changes were initially closely related. Concentric contractions caused no MR changes.

In a review of their own and others' research, Fridén

and Lieber (124) suggest that the primary event of muscle damage involves the muscle fiber oxidative capacity and that fast glycolytic fibers fatigue within the first 10 minutes (or so) of an exercise. Being unable to regenerate ATP, these fibers enter a rigor or high-stiffness state. Subsequent stretch of the fiber causes mechanical disruption. The implication is that fatigue is important to eccentric muscle injuries, and that endurance training of muscles may have some preventive effect. These hypotheses are still untested.

Muscle Spasm

Another finding that is given etiologic significance is muscle spasm. Muscle spasm has long been associated with low back pain as a clinical phenomenon. It is usually defined as "contracted," "tight," or "hard" spinal muscles (91,94). Sometimes the contraction is asymmetrical, producing scoliosis. The occurrence and significance of muscle spasm have been poorly quantified because both definition and objective documentation are difficult (306). Magora (218) reported that 56 of 429 patients with low back pain (13%) had "tight or contracted" muscles. In other studies, significant interobserver errors have been reported, making the diagnosis unreliable (24,243).

Whether muscle spasm causes pain or is caused by pain is unclear. Mechanical stimulation of spinal structures in anesthetized cats causes electromyographically confirmed spasm in dorsal and hamstring muscles (287). Mooney and Robertson (254) injected hyperosmolar sodium chloride into the facet joints of human subjects and recorded reflex spasm in the hamstring muscles. Cobb and associates (80) also injected sodium chloride and produced spasm. These studies suggest that noxious stimulation of spinal structures can indeed cause reflex muscle spasm.

The idea that spasm is the cause of pain was suggested in 1920 by Lewis (211), who attributed this to the production of substance P in the muscle. Others have attributed pain to noxious substances that accumulate when there is decreased blood flow. Still others maintain that muscle spasm causes mechanical irritation of pain receptors within the walls of blood vessels in the contracted muscle (373).

The presence of spasm in muscles is the basis of several different treatment methods, including the use of muscle-relaxing drugs, biofeedback, physical therapy, and even analgesics. Mooney and Robertson (254) found that muscle spasm in the hamstring muscles decreased when local anesthetics were injected into facet joints. Clinical trials using muscle relaxants have arrived at conflicting results regarding therapeutic efficiency and mechanism of action (see Chapter 82). No study has as yet proven that the pain relief obtained with a muscle relaxant is the result of a direct effect on muscle spasm. Biofeedback, used to allow patients to relax their back muscles (120), was found in one study to reduce myoelectric activity levels in the back muscles of patients with low back pain while they were standing, and at the same time reduced their back pain (114). In another double-masked study, Nouwen et al. (270) confirmed the reduction in back muscle myoelectric activity, but did not find a reduction in pain. As evidenced by Table 1, conflicting data have been obtained by investigators over the years. Physical therapy, particularly stretching, has been reported to reduce the pain associated with muscle spasm (212), a claim that has yet to be supported scientifically.

In summary, it appears that back muscle spasm is a common clinical feature in low back pain. Pain can occur without spasm, however, and spasm can occur without pain. There appears to be support for the idea that a pain-spasm-pain cycle exists in some patients, and that therapy intended to reduce spasm is, therefore, of value. However, in the role of spasm, the causes of low back pain still remains poorly defined.

Deconditioning

A fourth mechanism of spinal pain related to muscles is the *deconditioning syndrome*. Physiologic measurements of motion, strength, cardiovascular fitness, and lifting capacity have all demonstrated a significant difference in performance between healthy control subjects and patients with chronic low back pain. This phenomenon has been referred to as the deconditioning syndrome (237), and forms the basis for a philosophy of functional restoration in those patients. Correction of the deconditioning has been found to lead to improved function, and is associated with reduced pain. The basic understanding that these changes are due to disuse has led to an increased awareness of the importance of activity in the treatment of back pain. Clearly, disuse has major negative consequences for muscle, including atrophy and loss of strength and endurance. Because atrophic muscles are more irritable and more easily overloaded, spasms and other adverse functional changes may develop. Significant recent scientific and clinical attention is directed not only to the understanding of the events that follow disuse, but how it can be measured and reversed (128,237) (see also Chapter 15).

Compartment Syndrome

A fifth, and probably rare, cause of muscle pain is the paraspinal compartment syndrome. The fact that the thoracolumbar fascia and its septa enclose the erector spinae muscles has raised the suspicion that a compartment syndrome can arise and cause acute or chronic low back pain (68,285,286,341,342). Carr et al. (68,69) found that the erector spinae muscles were encased by fascia, resulting in a clearly defined, well-developed compartment. Using a slit catheter, pressures were measured in eight healthy males performing some simple exercises. Spine extension was found to raise the pressure more than flexion, and a Valsalva maneuver induced a pressure increase, except in a 90° flexion. Isometric loading resulted in a sustained increase in compartment pressure. Styf and Lysell (341) used a different technique to measure pressure and concluded that chronic ESM compartment syndrome was uncommon based on a 4-year experience. They found only one patient with a unilateral compartment syndrome who was cured by a fasciotomy. Later, Styf (339) used pressure measurements to study the effect of isometric and concentric exercise on the erector spinae muscles. Significant pressure increase was recorded with exercise.

Fibromyalgia

Lastly, specific syndromes have been attached to muscles, such as the fibromyalgia and fibrositis syndromes. These topics will be considered in Chapter 41, where it will be apparent that these diagnoses and their treatment remain somewhat uncertain and controversial.

SUMMARY

To summarize, today's knowledge does not give a great deal of credence to muscles as the primary source of significant spinal disorders, yet there can be no doubt of their importance to the mechanical functioning of the spine, and only little doubt about the relevance of muscle deconditioning and reconditioning as an important aspect of spinal treatment.

REFERENCES

1. Abraham W (1979): Exercise induced muscle soreness. *Phys Sportsmed* 7:56–60.
2. Adams MA, Hutton WC, Stott JRR (1980): The resistance to flexion of the lumbar intervertebral joint. *Spine* 5:245–253.
3. Addison R, Schultz A (1980): Trunk strengths in patients seeking hospitalization for chronic low back disorders. *Spine* 5:539–544.
4. Aghazadeh F, Ayoub MM (1985): A comparison of dynamic and static strength models for prediction of lifting capacity. *Ergonomics* 28:1409–1417.
5. Ahern DK, Follick MJ, Council JR, Laser-Wolston N (1986): Reliability of lumbar paravertebral EMG assessment on chronic low back pain. *Arch Phys Med Rehabil* 67:762–765.
6. Ahern DK, Harmon DJ, Goreczny MA, Follick MJ (1990): *Correlation of chronic low back pain behaviour and muscle function: examination of the flexion-relaxation response.* Manuscript.
7. Akerblom B (1949): *Standing and sitting posture, with special reference to the construction of chairs* [Thesis]. University of Stockholm.
8. Alaranta H, Tallroth K, Soukka A, Heliövaara M (1993): Fat content of lumbar extensor muscles and low back disability: a

9. Allen CEL (1948): Muscle action potentials used in the study of dynamic anatomy. *Br J Phys Med* 11:66.
10. Alston W, Carlson KE, Feldman DJ, Grim Z, Gerontinos E (1966): A quantitative study of muscle factors in chronic low back syndrome. *J Am Geriatr Soc* 141:1041–1047.
11. Andersson GBJ (1974): *On myoelectric back muscle activity and lumbar disc pressure in sitting postures* [Thesis]. Göteborg, Sweden: University of Göteborg.
12. Andersson GBJ (1982): Measurements of loads on the lumbar spine. In: White AA III, Gordon SL, eds. *Symposium on idiopathic low back pain.* St. Louis: Mosby, pp. 220–251.
13. Andersson GBJ (1986): Loads on the spine during sitting. In: Corlett N, Wilson J, Manenica I, eds. *The ergonomics of working postures.* London: Taylor and Francis, pp. 309–318.
14. Andersson GBJ (1987): Biomechanical aspects of sitting: an application to VDT terminals. In: *Behaviour and information technology, vol. 6.* London: Taylor and Francis, pp. 257–269.
15. Andersson GBJ, Bogduk N, De Luca C, et al. (1989): Muscle: clinical perspective. In: Frymoyer JW, Gordon SL, eds. *New perspectives on low back pain.* Park Ridge, IL: American Academy of Orthopaedic Surgeons, pp. 293–334.
16. Andersson GBJ, Herberts P, Örtengren R (1976): Myoelectric back muscle activity in standardized lifting postures. In: Komi PV, ed. *Biomechanics 5-A.* Baltimore: University Park Press, pp. 520–529.
17. Andersson GBJ, Jonsson B, Örtengren R (1974): Myoelectric activity in individual erector spinae muscles in sitting. *Scand J Rehabil Med (Suppl)* 3:91–108.
18. Andersson GBJ, McNeill TW (1989): *Lumbar spinal syndromes.* Vienna: Springer-Verlag.
19. Andersson GBJ, Örtengren R (1974): Lumbar disc pressure and myoelectric back muscle activity during sitting. II. Studies on an office chair. *Scand J Rehabil Med* 6:115–121.
20. Andersson GBJ, Örtengren R (1974): Myoelectric back muscle activity during sitting. *Scand J Rehabil Med (Suppl)* 3:73.
21. Andersson GBJ, Örtengren R, Herberts P (1977): Quantitative electromyographic studies of back muscle activity related to posture and loading. *Orthop Clin North Am* 8:85–96.
22. Andersson GBJ, Örtengren R, Nachemson A (1976): Quantitative studies of back loads in lifting. *Spine* 1:178–185.
23. Andersson GBJ, Örtengren R, Nachemson A, et al. (1974): Lumbar disc pressure and myoelectric back muscle activity during sitting: I. Studies on an experimental chair. *Scand J Rehabil Med* 6:104–114.
24. Andersson GBJ, Örtengren R, Schultz A (1980): Analysis measurement of the loads on the lumbar spine during work at a table. *J Biomech* 13:513–520.
25. Andersson GBJ, Schultz AB (1979): Transmission of moments across the elbow joint and lumbar spine during work at a table. *J Biomech* 12:747–755.
26. Andersson GBJ, Schultz AB, Örtengren R (1986): Trunk muscle forces during desk work. *Ergonomics* 29:1113–1117.
27. Armstrong RB (1990): Initial events in exercise-induced muscular injury. *Med Sci Sports Exerc* 22:429–435.
28. Arnold JD, Ranschenberger JM, Soubel WG, et al. (1982): Validation and utility of a strength test for selecting steel workers. *Appl Psych* 67:588–604.
29. Arroyo P (1966): Electromyography in the evaluation of the reflex muscle spasm. *J Fla Med Assoc* 53:29–31.
30. Asmussen E, Heebøll-Nielsen K (1959): Posture, mobility and strength of the back in boys 7–16 years old. *Acta Orthop Scand* 28:174–189.
31. Asmussen E, Klausen K (1962): Form and function of the erect human spine. *Clin Orthop* 25:55.
32. Asmussen E, Poulsen E, Rasmussen B (1965): *Quantitative evaluation of the activity of the back muscles in lifting.* Copenhagen: Comm. National Association of Infantile Paralysis.
33. Aspden RM (1992): Review of the functional anatomy of the spinal ligaments and the lumbar erector spinae muscles. *Clin Anat* 5:372–387.
34. Ayoub MM, Mital A, Bakken GM, Asfour SS, Bethesda HJ (1980): Development of strength and capacity norms for manual

— radiographic and clinical comparison. *J Spinal Disord* 6:137–140.

materials handling activities. The state of the art. *Hum Factors* 22(3):271–283.

35. Backlund L, Nordgren L (1968): A new method of testing isometric muscle strength under standardized conditions. *Scand J Clin Lab Invest* 21:33–41.

36. Bagnall KM, Ford DM, McFadden KD, Greenhill BJ, Raso VJ (1984): The histochemical composition of human vertebral muscle. *Spine* 9:470–473.

37. Bartelink DL (1957): The role of abdominal pressure in relieving the pressure on the lumbar intervertebral discs. *J Bone Joint Surg [Br]* 39:718–725.

38. Basmajian JV (1958): Electromyography of iliopsoas. *Anat Rec* 132:127.

39. Basmajian JV, DeLuca CJ (1985): *Muscles alive.* Baltimore: Williams & Wilkins.

40. Battey CK, Joseph J (1966): An investigation by telemetering of the activity of some muscles in walking. *Med Biol Eng* 4:125–135.

41. Battié MC, Bigos SJ, Fisher LD, Hansson TH, Jones ME, Wortley MD (1989): Isometric lifting as a predictor of industrial back pain. *Spine* 14:851–856.

42. Bearns JG (1961): The significance of the activity of the abdominal muscles in weight lifting. *Acta Anat* 45:83.

43. Beimborn DS, Morrissey MC (1988): A review of the literature related to trunk muscle performance. *Spine* 13:655–660.

44. Bendix T, Winkel J, Jensen F (1985): Comparison of office chairs with fixed forwards and backwards inclining, or tiltable seats. *Eur J Appl Physiol* 54:378–385.

45. Berkson M, Schultz AB, Nachemson A (1977): Voluntary strengths of male adults with acute low back syndromes. *Clin Orthop* 129:84–95.

46. Biedermann HJ, Shanks GL, Forrest WJ, Inglis J (1991): Power spectrum analysis of electromyographic activity: discriminators in the differential assessment of patients with chronic low back pain. *Spine* 16:1179–1184.

47. Biering-Sørensen F (1982): Low back trouble in a general population of 30-, 40-, 50-, and 60-year old men and women. Study design, representativeness, and basic results. *Dan Med Bull* 29:289–299.

48. Biering-Sørensen F (1984): Physical measurements as risk indicators for low back trouble over a one-year period. *Spine* 9:106–119.

49. Bigland B, Lippold OCJ (1954): The relation between force, velocity and integrated activity in human muscles. *J Physiol (London)* 123:214–224.

50. Birch K, Sinnerton S, Reilly T, Lees A (1994): The relation between isometric lifting strength and muscular fitness measures. *Ergonomics* 37:87–93.

51. Bobet J, Norman RW (1984): Effects of load placement on back muscle activity in load carriage. *Eur J Appl Physiol* 53:71–75.

52. Boudrifa H, Davies BT (1985): The effect of backrest inclination, lumbar support and thoracic support on erector spinae muscles when lifting. *Eur J Appl Physiol* 54:538–545.

53. Boudrifa H, Davies BT (1987): The effect of bending and rotation of the trunk on the intra-abdominal pressure and the erector spinae muscle when lifting while sitting. *Ergonomics* 30:103–109.

54. Bouisset S, Zattara M (1981): A sequence of postural movements precedes voluntary movement. *Neurosci Lett* 22:263–270.

55. Branch TP, Patton D, Hutton WC (1991): Impulse dynamics: energy requirements, reflex response patterns and learning. 37th Annual Meeting, Orthopaedic Research Society, March 4–7, Anaheim, California.

56. Brodin H (1972): Die Viskoelastizität der Muskeln. *Man Med* 10:41–44 (in German).

57. Brown JR (1972): *Manual lifting and related fields: an annotated bibliography.* Toronto: Labour Safety Council of Ontario.

58. Buseck M, Schipplein OD, Andersson GBJ, Andriacchi TP (1988): Influence of dynamic factors and external loads on the moment at the lumbar spine in lifting. *Spine* 13:918–921.

59. Bush-Joseph C, Schipplein OD, Andersson GBJ, Andriacchi TP (1988): Influence of dynamic factors on the lumbar spine moment in lifting. *Ergonomics* 31:211–216.

60. Butler D, Andersson GBJ, Trafimow J, Schipplein OD, Andriacchi TP (1993): The influence of load knowledge on lifting technique. *Ergonomics* 36:1489–1493.

61. Caldwell LS, Chaffin DB, DuBobos FND, Kroemer KHE, Laubach LL, Snook SH, Wasserman DE (1974): A proposed standard procedure for static muscle strength testing. *Am Ind Hyg J* 35:201–206.

62. Campbell EJM, Green JH (1955): The behaviour of the muscles and the intra-abdominal pressure during quiet breathing and increased pulmonary ventilation: a study in man. *J Physiol (London)* 127:423–426.

63. Carlson H, Nilsson J, Thorstensson A, Zomlefer MR (1981): Motor response in the human trunk due to load perturbation. *Acta Phys Scand* 111:221–223.

64. Carlsöö S (1961): The static muscle load in different work positions: an electromyographic study. *Ergonomics* 4:193.

65. Carlsöö S (1963): *Table, chair and work posture.* Stockholm: Folksam and Facit AB. (In Swedish).

66. Carlsöö S (1964): Influence of frontal and dorsal loads on muscle activity and on the weight distribution in the feet. *Acta Orthop Scand* 34:299.

67. Carlsöö S (1975): *Lifting at work.* Stockholm: Folksam and Facit AB. (In Swedish).

68. Carr D, Frymoyer JW, Gilbertson L, Krag MH, Pope MH (1984): The lumbodorsal fascial compartment. *Trans Orthop Res Soc* 9:252.

69. Carr D, Gilbertson L, Frymoyer J, Krag M, Pope M (1985): Lumbar paraspinal compartment syndrome. A case report with physiologic and anatomic studies. *Spine* 10:816–820.

70. Cartas O, Nordin M, Frankel VH, et al. (1993): Quantification of trunk muscle performance in standing, semistanding and sitting postures in healthy males. *Spine* 18:603–609.

71. Chaffin DB (1969): A computerized biomechanical model: development and use in studying gross body actions. *J Biomech* 2:429–441.

72. Chaffin DB (1982): Functional assessment for heavy physical labor. In: Alderman MH, Hanley MJ, eds. *Clinical medicine for the occupational physician.* New York: Dekker, pp. 187–192.

73. Chaffin DB, Andersson GBJ (1984): *Occupational biomechanics.* New York: Wiley Interscience.

74. Chaffin DB, Andersson GBJ (1990): *Occupational biomechanics.* 2nd ed. New York: Wiley Interscience.

75. Chaffin DB, Herrin GD, Keyserling WM (1978): Preemployment strength testing. *J Occup Med* 20:403–408.

76. Chaffin DB, Park KS (1973): A longitudinal study of low back pain as associated with occupational weight lifting factors. *Am Ind Hyg Assoc J* 34:513–525.

77. Chapman AE, Troup JPG (1982): The effect of increased maximal strength on the integrated electrical activity of lumbar erectores spinae. *Electromyography* 9:263–280.

78. Clarkson PM, Tremblay I (1990): Exercise-induced muscle damage, repair and adaptation on humans. *J Appl Physiol* 65:1–6.

79. Clemmensen S (1951): Some studies on muscle tone. *Proc R Soc Med* 44:637–646.

80. Cobb CR, deVries HA, Urban RT, et al. (1975): Electrical activity in muscle pain. *Am J Phys Med* 54:80–87.

81. Collins GA, Cohen MJ, Naliboff BD, et al. (1982): Comparative analysis of paraspinal and frontalis EMG, heart rate and skin conductance in chronic low back pain patients and normals to various postures and stress. *Scand J Rehabil Med* 14:39–46.

82. Cook TM, Neumann DA (1987): The effects of load placement on the EMG activity of the low back muscles during load carrying by men and women. *Ergonomics* 30:1413–1423.

83. Cordo PJ, Nashner LM (1982): Properties of postural adjustments associated with rapid arm movements. *J Neurophysiol* 47:287–302.

84. Dales JL, MacDonald EB, Anderson JAD (1986): The "Liftest" strength test: an accurate method of dynamic strength assessment? *Clin Biomech* 1:11–13.

85. Davies GT, Gould JA (1982): Trunk testing using a prototype Cybex II isokinetic dynamometer stabilization system. *J Orthop Sports Phys Ther* 3:164–170.

86. DeFoa JL, Forrest WJ, Biedermann HJ (1989): Muscle fiber direction of longissimus, iliocostalis and multifidus: landmark derived reference lines. *J Anat* 163:243–247.

87. Delitto RS, Rose SJ, Apts DW (1987): Electromyographic analysis of two techniques for squat lifting. *Phys Ther* 67:1329–1334.

88. DeLooze MP, Toussaint HM, van Dieen JH, Kemper HCG (1993): Joint moments and muscle activity in the lower extremities and lower back in lifting and lowering tasks. *J Biomech* 26: 1067–1076.

89. DeLuca CJ (1985): Myoelectric manifestations of localized muscular fatigue. In: *CRC critical reviews in biomedical engineering*, West Palm Beach, FL. pp. 251–279.

90. DeLuca CJ (1993): Use of surface EMG signal for performance evaluation of back muscles. *Muscle Nerve* 16:210–216.

91. Denslow JS (1963): Palpation of the musculoskeletal system. *J Am Orthop Assoc* 63:1107–1115.

92. Denslow JS, Clough GH (1941): Reflex activity in the spinal extensors. *J Neurophysiol* 4:430–437.

93. Denslow JS, Hassett CC (1942): The central excitatory state associated with postural abnormalities. *J Neurophysiol* 5:393–402.

94. DeVries HA (1965): Muscle tonus in postural muscles. *Am J Phys Med* 44:275–291.

95. DeVries HA (1968): EMG fatigue curves in postural muscles. A possible etiology for idiopathic low back pain. *Am J Phys Med* 47: 175–181.

96. Dofferhof AS, Vink P (1985): The stabilising function of the mm. iliocostales and the mm. multifidi during walking. *J Anat* 140: 329–336.

97. Dolan P, Adams MA (1993): The relationship between EMG activity and extensor moment generation in the erector spinae muscles during bending and lifting activities. *J Biomech* 26:513–522.

98. Dolan P, Mannion AF, Adams MA (1994): Passive tissues help the back muscles to generate extensor moments during lifting. *J Biomech* 27:1077–1085.

99. Donish EW, Basmajian JV (1972): Electromyography of deep back muscles in man. *Am J Anat* 133:25.

100. Dumas GA, Poulin MJ, Gagnon M, Jovanovic M (1988): A three-dimensional digitization method to measure trunk muscle lines of action. *Spine* 13:532–541.

101. Edwards RHT (1988): Hypothesis of peripheral and central mechanisms underlying occupational muscle pain and injury. *Eur J Appl Physiol* 57:275–281.

102. Elliott FA (1944): Tender muscles in sciatica: electromyographic studies. *Lancet* 1:47–49.

103. England RW, Delbert PW (1972): Electromyographic studies: part I. consideration in the evaluation of osteopathic therapy. *J Am Osteopath Assoc* 72:221–223.

104. Etemadi AA (1974): Extensor power of different parts of the erector spinae muscles. *Z Anat Entwickl Gesch* 135:164–177.

105. Farfan HF (1975): Muscular mechanism of the lumbar spine and the position of power and efficiency. *Orthop Clin North Am* 6: 135–144.

106. Farfan HF, Lamy C (1975): *Human spine in the performance of dead lift*. Montreal: St. Mary's Hospital.

107. Fidler MW, Jowett RL, Troup JDG (1975): Myosin ATPase activity in multifidus muscle from cases of lumbar spinal derangement. *J Bone Joint Surg [Br]* 57:220–227.

108. Fischer AA (1987): Muscle tone in normal persons measured by tissue compliance. *J Neurol Orthop Med Surg* 8:227–233.

109. Fischer AA (1987): Tissue compliance meter for objective, quantitative documentation of soft tissue consistency and pathology. *Arch Phys Med Rehabil* 68:122–125.

110. Fischer AA, Chang CH (1985): Electromyographic evidence of paraspinal muscle spasm during sleep in patients with low back pain. *Clin J Pain* 1:147–154.

111. Flicker PL, Flechenstein JL, Ferry K, Payne J, Ward C, Mayer T, Parkay RW, Peshock RM (1993): Lumbar muscle usage in chronic low back pain. *Spine* 18:582–586.

112. Flint MM (1955): Effect of increasing back and abdominal strength in low back pain. *Res Q* 29:160–171.

113. Flint MM, Gudgell J (1965): Electromyographic study of abdominal muscular activity during exercise. *Res Q Am Assoc Health Phys Ther Educ* 36:29.

114. Flor H, Haag G, Turk DC, et al. (1983): Efficacy of EMG biofeedback, pseudo-therapy, and conventional medical treatment for chronic rheumatic back pain. *Pain* 17:21–31.

115. Floyd WF, Silver PHS (1950): Electromyographic study of patterns of activity of the anterior abdominal wall muscles in man. *J Anat* 84:132–145.

116. Floyd WF, Silver PHS (1951): Function of erectores spinae in flexion of the trunk. *Lancet* 1:133–134.

117. Floyd WF, Silver PHS (1955): The function of the erectores spinae muscles in certain movements and postures in man. *J Physiol (London)* 129:184–203.

118. Ford D, Bagnall KM, McFadden KD, Greenhill B, Raso J (1983): Analysis of vertebral muscle obtained during surgery for correction of a lumbar disc disorder. *Acta Anat* 116:152–157.

119. Foster CVL, et al. (1975): ATP distribution in single muscle fibers before and after maximal exercise in the thoroughbred horse. *J Physiol* 378:64P.

120. Fowler R (1974): *Techniques for healing selected pain problems using biofeedback*. Baimbridge Island, WA: J & J Enterprises.

121. Fowler RS, Kraft GH (1974): Tension perception in patients having pain associated with chronic muscle tension. *Arch Phys Med Rehabil* 55:28–30.

122. Freivalds A, Chaffin DB, Garg A, Lee KS (1984): A dynamic biomechanical evaluation of lifting maximum acceptable loads. *J Biomech* 17:251–262.

123. Fricton JR, Auviren MD, Dykstra D, Schiffman E (1985): Myofacial pain syndrome: electromyographic changes associated with local twitch response. *Arch Phys Med Rehabil* 66:314–317.

124. Fridén J, Lieber RL (1992): Structural and mechanical basis of exercise-induced muscle injury. *Med Sci Sports Exerc* 24:521–530.

125. Fridén J, Seger J, Ekblom B (1988): Sublethal muscle fiber injuries after high-tension anaerobic exercise. *Eur J Appl Physiol* 57: 360–368.

126. Fridén J, Sjöström M, Ekblom B (1983): Myofibrillar damage following intense eccentric exercise in man. *Int J Sports Med* 4:170–176.

127. Friedebold G (1958): Die Aktivität normaler Rückenstreckmuskulatur im Electromyogramm unter verschiendenen Haltungsbedingungen: eine Studie zur Skelettmuskelmechanik. *Z Orthop* 90:1.

128. Frymoyer JW, Gordon SL (1989): *New perspectives on low back pain*. Park Ridge, IL: American Academy of Orthopaedic Surgeons.

129. Gagnon D, Gagnon M (1992): The influence of dynamic factors on triaxial net muscular moments at the L5/S1 joint during asymmetrical lifting and lowering. *J Biomech* 25:891–901.

130. Gallagher S, Unger RL (1990): Lifting in four restricted lifting conditions. *Appl Ergonom* 21:237–245.

131. Garg A, Badger D (1986): Maximum acceptable weights and maximum voluntary isometric strengths for asymmetric lifting. *Ergonomics* 79:879–892.

132. Garg A, Chaffin DB (1975): A biomechanic computerized simulation of human strength. *AIIE Trans* (March 1–15).

133. Garg A, Mital A, Asfour SS (1980): A comparison of isometric strength and dynamic lifting capability. *Ergonomics* 23:13–27.

134. Garg A, Saxena U (1982): Maximum frequency acceptable to female workers for one-handed lifts in the horizontal plane. *Ergonomics* 25:839–853.

135. Garrett WE (1990): Muscle strain injuries: clinical and basic aspects. *Med Sci Sports Exerc* 22:436–444.

136. Garrett WE Jr, Duncan PW, Malone TR (1988): Muscle injury and rehabilitation. In: *Sport injury management* 1:3:1–76. Baltimore: Williams and Wilkins.

137. Garrett WE Jr, Nikolaou PK, Ribbeck BM, et al. (1988): The effect of muscle architecture on the biomechanical failure properties of skeletal muscle under passive extension. *Am J Sports Med* 16:7–12.

138. Golding JSR (1952): Electromyography of the erector spinae in low back pain. *Postgrad Med J* 28:401–406.

139. Gomez T, Beach G, Cooke C, Hrudey W, Goyert P (1991): Normative database for trunk range of motion, strength, velocity and endurance with the isostation B-200 lumbar dynamometer. *Spine* 16:15–21.

140. Gordon AH (1964): Method to measure muscle firmness or tone. *Res Q* 35:482–490.

141. Grabel JA (1973): Electromyographic study of low back muscle tension in subjects with and without chronic low back pain. *Dissertation Abstracts International* 34(B):2929-B.

142. Gracovetsky S (1988): *The spinal engine.* New York: Springer-Verlag.

143. Gracovetsky S, Farfan HF, Lamy C (1977): Mathematical model of the lumbar spine using an optimized system to control muscles and ligaments. *Orthop Clin North Am* 8:135–153.

144. Gracovetsky S, Farfan HF, Lamy C (1981): The mechanism of the lumbar spine. *Spine* 6:249–262.

145. Graves JE, Pollock ML, Carpenter DM, Leggett SH, Jones A, MacMillan M, Fulton M (1990): Quantitative assessment of isometric lumbar strength. *Spine* 15:289–294.

146. Graves JE, Pollock ML, Foster D, et al. (1990): Effect of training and specificity on isometric lumbar extension strength. *Spine* 15:504–509.

147. Graves JE, Pollock M, Leggett S, et al. (1992): Limited range-of-motion lumbar extension strength training. *Med Sci Sports Exerc* 24:128–133.

148. Greenwood R, Hopkins A (1976): Muscle responses during sudden falls in man. *J Physiol* 254:507–518.

149. Grieve DW (1974): Dynamic characteristics of man during crouch and stoop lifting. In: Nelson RC, Morehouse CA, eds. *Biomechanics,* 4th ed. Baltimore: University Park Press, pp. 19–29.

150. Griffin AB, Troup JD, Lloyd DC (1984): Test of lifting and handling capacity: their repeatability and relationship to back symptoms. *Ergonomics* 27:305–320.

151. Hagberg M (1984): Occupational musculo-skeletal stress and disorders of the neck and shoulder. *Int Arch Occup Environ Health* 53:269–278.

152. Hagberg M, Michaelson G, Ortelius A (1982): Serum creatine kinase as an indicator of local muscular strain in experiments and occupational work. *Int Arch Occup Environ Health* 50:377–386.

153. Hasselman CT, Best TM, Seabor AV, Garrett WE Jr (1995): A threshold and continuum of injury during active stretch of rabbit skeletal muscle. *Am J Sports Med* 23:65–73.

154. Hasue M, Masatoshi F, Kikuchi S (1980): A new method of quantitative measurement of abdominal and back muscle strength. *Spine* 5:143–148.

155. Heelboll-Nielsen K (1982): Muscle strength of boys and girls, 1981 compared to 1956. *Scand J Sports Science* 4:37–43.

156. Hemborg B (1983): *Intraabdominal pressure and trunk muscle activity during lifting* [Thesis]. Lund, Sweden: University of Lund, pp 1–79.

157. Hides JA, Stokes MJ, Saide M, Jull GA, Cooper DH (1994): Evidence of lumbar multifidus muscle wasting ipsilateral to symptoms in patients with acute/subacute low back pain. *Spine* 19:165–172.

158. Hinz B, Seidel H (1989): On time relation between erector spinae muscle activity and force development during initial isometric stage of back lifts. *Clin Biomech* 4:5–10.

159. Holmes TH, Wolff HG (1952): Life situations, emotions, and backache. *Psychosom Med* 14:18–33.

160. Holmstrom E, Moritz U, Andersson M (1992): Trunk muscle strength and back muscle endurance in construction workers with and without low back disorders. *Scand J Rehab Med* 24:3–10.

161. Hosea TM, Simon SR, Delatizky J, Wong MA, Hsieh C-G (1986): Myoelectric analysis of the paraspinal musculature in relation to automobile driving. *Spine* 11:928–936.

162. Hoyt WH, Hunt HH Jr, Depauw MA, et al. (1981): Electromyographic assessment of chronic low back pain syndrome. *J Am Osteopath Assoc* 80:728–730.

163. Hultman G, Nordin M, Saraste H, Ohlsen H (1993): Body composition, endurance, strength, cross-sectional area and density of mm erector spinae in men with and without low back pain. *J Spinal Disord* 6:114–123.

164. Hurme T, Kalimo H, Lehto M, Jarvinen M (1991): Healing of skeletal muscle injury: an ultrastructural and immunohistochemical study. *Med Sci Sports Exerc* 23:801–810.

165. International Anatomical Nomenclature Committee (1961): *Nomina anatomica.* 2nd ed. Amsterdam: Excerpta Medica.

166. International Anatomical Nomenclature Committee (1977): *Nomina anatomica.* 4th ed. Amsterdam: Excerpta Medica.

167. Iwasaki T, Ito H, Yamada M, et al. (1978): *Electromyogr Assoc* 4:52–61.

168. Jaarvinen M (1975): Healing of crush injury in rat striated muscle. *Acta Pathol Microbiol Scand* 83:269–282.

169. Jaarvinen M, Sorvari T (1975): Healing of a crush injury in rat striated muscle. *Acta Pathol Microbiol Scand* 83:259–265.

170. Jayasinghe WJ, Harding RH, Anderson JAD, Sweetman BJ (1978): An electromyographic investigation of postural fatigue in low back pain. A preliminary study. *Electroencephalogr Clin Neurophysiol* 18:191–198.

171. Jonsson B (1970): The functions of individual muscles in the lumbar part of the erector spinae muscle. *Electromyography* 10:5.

172. Jonsson B (1970): *The lumbar part of the erector spinae muscle: a technique for electromyographic studies of the function of its individual muscles* [Thesis]. Göteborg, Sweden: University of Göteborg.

173. Jonsson B (1970): Topography of the lumbar part of the erector spinae muscle. *Anat Entwicklungsgesch* 130:77.

174. Joseph J (1960): *Man's posture: electromyographic studies.* Springfield: Charles C Thomas.

175. Joseph J, McCall I (1961): Electromyography of muscles of posture: posterior vertebral muscles in males. *J Physiol (London)* 157:33–37.

176. Jowett R, Fidler MW, Troup JDG (1975): Histochemical changes in the multifidus in mechanical derangement of the spine. *Orthop Clin North Am* 6:145–161.

177. Kahanovitz N, Nordin M, Verderame R, Yabut S, Parnianpour M, Viola K, Mulvihill M (1987): Normal trunk muscle strength and endurance in women and the effect of exercises and electrical stimulation. Part 2. Comparative analysis of electrical stimulation and exercises to increase trunk muscle strength and endurance. *Spine* 12:112–118.

178. Kahanovitz N, Viola K, Gallagher M (1989): Long term strength assessment of postoperative patients. *Spine* 13:402–403.

179. Kamon E, Kiser D, Pytel JL (1982): Dynamic and static lifting capacity and muscular strength of workers. *Am Ind Hyg Assoc J* 43:853–857.

180. Karvonen MJ, Ronnholm N (1964): Electromyographic and energy expenditure studies of rhythmic and paced lifting work. *Ann Acad Sci Fenn* 106:3.

181. Keyserling WM, Herrin GD, Chaffin DB (1980): Isometric strength testing as a means of controlling medical incidents on strenuous jobs. *Occup Med* 22:332–336.

182. Khalil TM, Waly SM, Zaki AM (1990): The effect of load expectation on muscle recruitment. *Adv Ind Ergon Safety* 2:159–166.

183. Kippers V, Parker AW (1984): Posture related to myoelectric silence of erectores spinae during trunk flexion. *Spine* 9:740–745.

184. Kirkebo A, Wisnes A (1982): Regional tissue fluid pressure in rat calf muscle during sustained contraction of stretch. *Acta Physiol Scand* 114:551–556.

185. Kishino ND, Mayer TG, Gatchel RJ, McCrate-Parrish M, Anderson C, Gustin L, Mooney V (1985): Quantification of lumbar function. *Spine* 10:921–927.

186. Kluck DJ (1967): *A study of the strength ratio of the back extensors to the trunk flexors* [Master's thesis]. Iowa: University of Iowa.

187. Kondraske GV, Deivanayagam S, Carmichael T, Mayer TG, Mooney V (1987): Myoelectric spectral analysis and strategies for quantifying trunk muscular fatigue. *Arch Phys Med Rehabil* 68:103–110.

188. Körner L, Parker P, Almström C, et al. (1984): Relation of intramuscular pressure to the force output and myoelectric signal of the skeletal muscle. *Orthop Res* 2:289–296.

189. Kraft GH, Johnson EW, Laban MM (1968): The fibrositis syndrome. *Arch Phys Med Rehabil* 49:155–162.

190. Kravitz E, Moore ME, Glavros A (1981): Paralumbar muscle activity in chronic low back pain. *Arch Phys Med Rehabil* 62:172–176.

191. Kroemer KH (1983): An isoinertial technique to assess individual lifting capability. *Hum Factors* 25:493–506.

192. Kumar S, Dufresne RM, Shoor TV (1995): Human trunk strength profile in flexion and extension. *Spine* 20:160–168.

193. Kumar S, Dufresne RM, Shoor TV (1995): Human trunk strength profile in lateral flexion and axial rotation. *Spine* 20:169–177.

194. Laasonen E (1984): Atrophy of sacrospinal muscle groups in patients with chronic, diffusely radiating lumbar back pain. *Neuroradiology* 26:9–13.

195. Ladin Z, Murthy KR, DeLuca CJ (1989): Mechanical recruitment of low back muscles. *Spine* 14:927–938.

196. Ladin Z, Murthy KR, DeLuca CJ (1991): The effects of external bending moments on lumbar muscle force distribution. *J Biomech Eng* 113:284–294.

197. Ladin Z, Neff KM (1992): Testing of a biomechanical model of the lumbar muscle force distribution using quasi-static loading exercises. *J Biomech Eng* 114(4):442–449.

198. Lange M (1931): *Die Muskelharten.* München: Lehmann Verlag.

199. Langrana NA, Lee C (1984): Isokinetic evaluation of trunk muscles. *Spine* 9:171–175.

200. Langrana NA, Lee CK, Alexander H, Mayott CW (1984): Quantitative assessment of back strength using isokinetic testing. *Spine* 9:287–290.

201. Langrana NA, Stover CN (1979): Back strength assessment through isokinetic analysis. *Proceedings of the 7th Annual New England (North East) Bio. Eng. Conference,* Troy, New York, pp. 1345–1348.

202. Lavender SA, Chen I-H, Trafimow J, Andersson GBJ (1995): The effects of lateral trunk bending on muscle recruitments when resisting nonsagittally symmetric bending moments. *Spine* 20:184–190.

203. Lavender SA, Marras WS (1995): The effects of temporal warning signal on the biomechanical preparation for sudden loading. *J Electromyogr Kinesiol* (In press).

204. Lavender SA, Marras WS, Miller RA (1993): The development of response strategies in preparation for sudden loading to the torso. *Spine* 18:2097–2105.

205. Lavender SA, Mirka GA, Schoenmarklin RW, Sommerich CM, Sudhakar LR, Marras WS (1989). The effects of preview and task symmetry on trunk muscle response to sudden loading. *Hum Factors* 31(1):101–115.

206. Lavender S, Trafimow J, Andersson GBJ, Mayer RS, Chen I-H (1994): Trunk muscle activation: the effects of torso flexion, moment direction and moment magnitude. *Spine* 19:771–778.

207. Lavender SA, Tsuang Y-H, Andersson GBJ (1993): Trunk muscle activation and cocontraction while resisting applied moments in a twisted posture. *Ergonomics* 36:1145–1157.

208. Lavender SA, Tsuang YH, Andersson GBJ, Hafezi A, Shin CC (1992): Trunk muscle cocontraction: the effects of moment direction and moment magnitude. *J Orthop Res* 10:691–700.

209. Lavender SA, Tsuang Y-H, Hafezi A, Andersson GJ (1992): Co-activation of the trunk muscles during asymmetric loading of the torso. *Hum Factors* 34:239–247.

210. Legg SJ, Myles WS (1981): Maximum acceptable repetitive lifting workloads for an 8-hour work day using psychophysical and subjective rating methods. *Ergonomics* 24:907–916.

211. Lewis T (1920): *Pain.* New York: Macmillan.

212. Lewit S, Simons DG (1984): Myofascial pain: relief by postisometric relaxation. *Arch Phys Med Rehabil* 65:452–456.

213. Lieber RL, Fridén J (1988): Selective damage of foot glycolytic muscle fibers with eccentric contraction of the rabbit tibialis anterior. *Acta Physiol Scand* 133:587–588.

214. Lundervold AJS (1951): Electromyographic investigations of position and manner of working in typewriting. *Acta Physiol Scand (Suppl)* 84.

215. Macintosh JE, Bogduk N (1986): The biomechanics of the lumbar multifidus. *Clin Biomech* 1:205–213.

216. Macintosh JE, Bogduk N (1987): The morphology of the lumbar erector spinae. *Spine* 12:658–668.

217. Macintosh JE, Valencia F, Bogduk N, et al. (1986): The morphology of the human lumbar multifidus. *Clin Biomech* 1:196–204.

218. Magora A (1975): Investigation of the relation between low back pain and occupation. *Scand J Rehabil Med* 7:146–151.

219. Malone TR (1988): Evaluation of isokinetic equipment. In: *Sports injury management.* Baltimore: Williams and Wilkins, 1: 1:1–92.

220. Mandell PT, Weitz E, Bernstein JF, et al. (1993): Isokinetic trunk strength and lifting strength measures. *Spine* 18:2491–2501.

221. Mangold A (1922): Ein Verfahren zur physiologischen Hartenmessung besonders an Muskeln. *Dtsch Med Wochenschr* 48:1155.

222. Marras WS (1992): Overview of electromyography in ergonomics. *Selected topics in surface electromyography for use in the occupational setting: expert perspectives.* 2–4. Ed. G.L. Soderberg, US Department of Health, DHHS (NIOSH) 91-100, Washington, DC.

223. Marras WS, King AI, Joynt RL (1984): Measurement of loads on the lumbar spine under isometric and isokinetic conditions. *Spine* 9:176–187.

224. Marras WS, Lavender SA, Leurgans SE, Rajulu SL, Allread WG, Fathallah FA, Ferguson SA (1993): The role of dynamic three-dimensional trunk motion in occupationally-related low back disorders. The effects of workplace factors, trunk position, and trunk motion characteristics on risk of injury. *Spine* 18:617–628.

225. Marras WS, Mirka GA (1989): Trunk strength during asymmetric trunk motion. *Hum Factors* 31:667–679.

226. Marras WS, Mirka GA (1990): *A comprehensive evaluation of trunk response to asymmetric trunk motion.* Manuscript.

227. Marras WS, Mirka GA (1990): Muscle activities during asymmetric trunk angular accelerations. *Spine* 8:824–832.

228. Marras WS, Mirka GA (1992): A comprehensive evaluation of trunk response to asymmetric trunk motion. *Spine* 17:318–326.

229. Marras WS, Mirka GA (1993): Electromyographic studies of the lumbar trunk musculature during the generation of low-level trunk acceleration. *J Orthop Res* 11:811–817.

230. Marras WS, Rangarajulu SL, Lavender SA (1987): Trunk loading and expectation. *Ergonomics* 30:551–562.

231. Marras WS, Reilly CH (1988): Networks of internal trunk-loading activities under controlled trunk-motion conditions. *Spine* 13:661–667.

232. Marras WS, Sommerich CM (1993): A three-dimensional motion model of loads on the lumbar spine, II: model validation. *Hum Factors* 33:139–150.

233. Marras WS, Wongsam PE (1986): Flexibility and velocity of the normal and impaired lumbar spine. *Arch Phys Med Rehabil* 67: 213–217.

234. Marras WS, Wongsam PE, Rangarajulu SL (1986): Trunk motion during lifting: the relative cost. *Int J Indust Ergonom* 1:103–113.

235. Mattila M, Hurme M, Alaranta H, et al. (1986): The multifidus muscle in patients with lumbar disc herniation. *Spine* 11:733–738.

236. Mayer TG, Barnes D, Kishino ND, Nichols G, Gatchel RJ, Mayer H, Mooney V (1988): Progressive isoinertial lifting evaluation. *Spine* 13:993–997.

237. Mayer TG, Gatchel RJ (1988): *Functional restoration for spinal disorders: the sports medicine approach.* Philadelphia: Lea and Febiger.

238. Mayer TG, Gatchel RJ, Kishino N, Keely J, Capra P, Mayer H, Barnett J, Mooney V (1985): Objective assessment of spine function following industrial injury. *Spine* 10:482–493.

239. Mayer TG, Kondraske G, Mooney V, Carmichael TW, Butsch R (1989): Lumbar myoelectric spectral analysis for endurance assessment. *Spine* 14:986–992.

240. Mayer TG, Smith SS, Keely J, Mooncy V (1985): Quantification of lumbar function. Part 2. Sagittal plane trunk strength in chronic low back patients. *Spine* 10:765–772.

241. Mayer TG, Smith SS, Kondraske G, Gatchel RJ, Carmichael TW, Mooney V (1985): Quantification of lumbar function. Part 3. Preliminary data on isokinetic torso rotation testing. *Spine* 10: 912–920.

242. Mayer TG, Vanharanta H, Gatchel RJ, Mooney V, Barnes D, Judge L, Smith S, Terry A (1989): Comparison of CT scan muscle measurements and isokinetic trunk strength in postoperative patients. *Spine* 14:33–36.

243. McCombe PF, Fairbank JCT, Cockersole BC, Pynsent PB (1989): Reproducibility of physical signs in low-back pain. *Spine* 14:908–919.

244. McCully K, Schellock FG, Bank WJ, Posner JD (1992): The use of nuclear magnetic resonance to evaluate muscle injury. *Med Sci Sports Exerc* 24:537–542.

245. McGill SM (1990): *Electromyographic activity of the abdominal and low back musculature during the generation of isometric and dynamic axial trunk torque.* Manuscript, University of Waterloo.

246. McGill SM (1992): A myoelectrically based dynamic three-dimensional model to predict loads on lumbar spine tissues during lateral bending. *J Biomech* 25:395–414.

247. McGill SM, Norman RW (1986): Partitioning of the L4/L5 dynamic moment into disc, ligamentous and muscular components during lifting. *Spine* 11:666–678.

248. McNeill T, Warwick D, Andersson G, Schultz A (1980): Trunk strengths in attempted flexion, extension, and lateral bending in healthy subjects and patients with low-back disorders. *Spine* 5:529–538.

249. Meyer L, Greenberg BB (1942): Measurements of the strength of trunk muscles. *J Bone Joint Surg* 24:812–856.

250. Miller DJ (1985): Comparison of electromyographic activity in the lumbar paraspinal muscles of subjects with and without chronic low back pain. *Phys Ther* 65:1347–1354.

251. Mirka GA (1991): The quantification of EMG normalization error. *Ergonomics* 34:343–352.

252. Mital A, Garg A, Karwowski W, Kumar S, Smith JL, Ayoub MM (1993): Status in human strength testing and applications. *IIE Trans* 25:57–69.

253. Mital A, Ayoub MM (1980): Modeling of isometric strength and lifting capacity. *Hum Factors* 22(3):285–290.

254. Mooney V, Robertson J (1976): The facet syndrome. *Clin Orthop* 115:149–156.

255. Morinaga H (1973): Electromyographic study of the function of the psoas major muscle. *J Jpn Orthop Assoc* 47:351–365.

256. Morris JM, Benner G, Lucas DB (1962): An electromyographic study of the intrinsic muscles of the back in man. *J Anat* 96:509–520.

257. Morris JM, Lucas DB, Bresler B (1961): Role of the trunk in stability of the spine. *J Bone Joint Surg [Am]* 43:327–351.

258. Nachemson A (1966): Electromyographic studies on the vertebral portion of the psoas muscle. *Acta Orthop Scand* 37:177.

259. Nachemson A, Lindh M (1969): Measurement of abdominal and back extensor strength with and without low-back pain. *Scand J Rehabil Med* 1:60–65.

260. Nelson JM, Walmsley RP, Stevenson JM (1995): Relative lumbar and pelvic motion during loaded spinal flexion/extension. *Spine* 20:199–204.

261. Newham DJ (1988): The consequences of eccentric contractions and their relation to delayed onset muscle pain. *Eur J Appl Physiol* 57:353–359.

262. Newham DJ, Mills KR, Quigley BM, Edwards RH (1983): Pain and fatigue after concentric and eccentric muscle contractions. *Clin Sci* 64:55–62.

263. Newham DJ, Jones DA, Tolfree SE, Edwards RH (1986): Skeletal muscle damage: a study of isotope uptake, enzyme efflux and pain after stepping. *Eur J Appl Physiol* 55:106–112.

264. Newton M, Thow M, Somerville D, et al. (1993): Trunk strength testing with iso-machines. Part II: Experimental evaluation of the Cybex II Back Testing System in normal subjects and patients with chronic low back pain. *Spine* 18:812–824.

265. Newton M, Waddell G (1993): Trunk strength testing with iso-machines. Part 1: Review of a decade of scientific evidence. *Spine* 18:801–811.

266. Nicolaisen T, Jørgensen K (1985): Trunk strength, back muscle endurance and low back trouble. *Scand J Rehabil Med* 17:121–127.

267. Nikolaou PK, MacDonald BL, Glisson RR, et al. (1987): Biomechanical and histological evaluation of muscle after controlled strain injury. *Am J Sports Med* 15:9–14.

268. Nordgren B, Schele R, Lindroth K (1980): Evaluation and prediction of back pain during military field service. *Scand J Rehabil Med* 12:1–8.

269. Nordin M, Kahanovitz N, Verderame R, Parniapour M, Yabut S, Viola K, Greenidge N, Mulvihill M (1987): Normal trunk muscle strength and endurance in women and the effect of exercises and electrical stimulation. Part 1: Normal endurance and trunk muscle strength in 101 women. *Spine* 12:105–111.

270. Nouwen A, van Akkerveeken PF, Versloot JM (1987): Patterns of muscular activity during movement in patients with chronic low back pain. *Spine* 12:777–782.

271. Oddsson I, Thorstensson A (1990): Task specificity in the control of intrinsic trunk muscles in man. *Acta Physiol Scand* 139:123–131.

272. Okada M (1970): Electromyographic assessment of muscular load in forward bending postures. *J Faculty Sci (Tokyo)* 8:311.

273. Okada M (1972): An electromyographic estimation of the relative muscle load in different human postures. *J Human Ergol* 1:75–93.

274. Omino K, Hayashi Y (1992): Preparation of dynamic posture and occurrence of low back pain. *Ergonomics* 35:693–707.

275. Ono K (1958): Electromyographic studies of the abdominal wall muscles in visceroptosis. *Tohoku J Exp Med* 68:347.

276. Örtengren R, Andersson GBJ (1977): Electromyographic studies of trunk muscles with special reference to the functional anatomy of the lumbar spine. *Spine* 2:44–52.

277. Paquet N, Malouin F, Richards CL (1994): Hip–spine movement interaction and muscle activation patterns during sagittal trunk movements in low back pain patients. *Spine* 19:596–603.

278. Parker P, Körner L, Kadefors R (1984): Estimation of muscle force from intramuscular total pressure. *Med Biol Eng Comput* 22:453.

279. Parkkola G, Rytokoski R, Kormano M (1993): Magnetic resonance imaging of the disc and trunk muscles in patients with chronic low back pain and healthy control subjects. *Spine* 18:830–836.

280. Parnianpour M, Li F, Nordin M, Kahanovitz N (1989): A database of isoinertial trunk strength tests against three resistance levels in sagittal, frontal and transverse planes in normal male subjects. *Spine* 14:409–411.

281. Parnianpour M, Nordin M, Kahanovitz N, Frankel EV (1988): The triaxial coupling of torque generation of trunk muscles during isometric exertions and the effect of fatiguing isoinertial movements on the motor output and movement patterns. *Spine* 13:982–992.

282. Partridge MJ, Walters CE (1959): Participation of the abdominal muscles in various movements of the trunk in man: an electromyographic study. *Phys Ther* 39:791.

283. Patterson PE, Koppa R, Congleton J, Huchingson RD (1986): Low back stress, muscle usage, and the appearance of transient load movement during manual lifting. *Int J Indust Ergonom* 1:137–143.

284. Pauly JE (1966): An electromyographic analysis of certain movements and exercises: I. Some deep muscles of the back. *Anat Rec* 155:223.

285. Peck D (1981): Evidence for the existence compartment syndromes of the epaxial muscles. *Anat Rec* 119:198A.

286. Peck D, Nicholls PJ, Beard C, Allen JR (1986): Are there compartment syndromes in some patients with idiopathic back pain? *Spine* 11:468–475.

287. Pedersen HE, Blunck CHJ, Gardner E (1956): The anatomy of lumbosacral posterior rami and meningeal branches of spinal nerves (sinu-verterbral nerves). *J Bone Joint Surg [Am]* 38:377–391.

288. Pope MH, Andersson GBJ, Broman H, Svensson M, Zetterberg C (1986): Electromyographic studies of the lumbar trunk musculature during the development of axial torques. *J Orthop Res* 4:288–297.

289. Pope MH, Bevins TR, Wilder DG, Frymoyer JW (1985): The relationship between anthropometric, postural, muscular, and mobility characteristics of males ages 18–55. *Spine* 10:644–648.

290. Pope MH, Svensson M, Andersson GBJ, Broman H, Zetterberg C (1987): The role of prerotation of the trunk in axial twisting efforts. *Spine* 12:1041–1045.

291. Pope MH, Wilder DG, Stokes IA, Frymoyer JW (1979): Biomechanical testing as an aid to decision making in low back pain patients. *Spine* 4:135–140.

292. Porterfield JA, Mostardi RA, King S, Aroki P, Moats E, Noe D (1987): Simulated lift testing using computerized isokinetics. *Spine* 12:683–687.

293. Portillo D, Sinkora G, McNeill T, Spencer D, Schultz A (1982): Trunk strength in structurally normal girls with idiopathic scoliosis. *Spine* 7:551–554.

294. Portnoy H, Morin F (1956): Electromyographic study of postural muscles in various positions and movements. *Am J Physiol* 186:122.

295. Potvin JR, Norman RW, McGill SM (1991): Reduction in anterior shear forces on the L4/L5 disc by the lumbar musculature. *Clin Biomech* 6:88–96.

296. Potvin JR, McGill SM, Norman RW (1991): Trunk muscle and lumbar ligament contributions to dynamic lifts with varying degrees of trunk flexion. *Spine* 16:1099–1107.

297. Poulson E, Jørgensen K (1971): Back muscle strength, lifting and stooped working posture. *Appl Ergonom* 23:133–137.

298. Price JP, Clare MH, Ewerhardt RH (1948): Studies in backache with persistent muscle spasm. *Arch Phys Med Rehabil* 29:703–709.

299. Pytel JL, Kamon E (1982): Dynamic strength as a predictor for maximal acceptable lifting. *Ergonomics* 24:663–672.

300. Raftopoulos DD, Rafco MC, Green M, et al. (1989): Relaxation phenomena in lumbar trunk muscles during lateral bending. *Spine*.

301. Rantanen J, Hurme M, Falck B, et al. (1993): The lumbar multifidus muscle five years after surgery for a lumbar intervertebral disc herniation. Submitted to *Spine* 18:568–574.

302. Redfern MS: Functional muscle: effects of electromyographic output. In: *Selected topics in surface electromyography for use in the occupational setting: expert perspectives,* pp. 104–120. Ed. G.L. Soderberg, US Department of Health, DHHS (NIOSH) 91–100, Washington, DC.

303. Reid GJ, Costigan PA (1987): Trunk muscle balance and muscular force. *Spine* 12:783–786.

304. Reilly R, Zedeck S (1979): Validity and fairness of physical ability tests for predicting performance in craft jobs. *J Appl Psych* 64:262–274.

305. Riihimaki H, Wickstron G, Hanninen K, Loupajarvi T (1989): Predictors of sciatic pain among concrete reinforcement workers and house painters—a five-year follow-up. *Scand J Work Environ Health* 15:415–423.

306. Roland MO (1986): A critical review of the evidence for a pain-spasm-pain cycle in spinal disorders. *Clin Biomech* 1:102–109.

307. Romick-Allen R, Schultz AB (1988): Biomechanics of reactions to impending falls. *J Biomech* 21:591–600.

308. Rosemeyer B (1971): Electromyographische Untersuchungen der Rucken- und Schultermuskulatur im Stehen under sitzen under Berücksichtigung der Haltung des Autofahrers. *Arch Orthop Unfallchir* 71:59.

309. Rosemeyer B (1974): Die aufrechten Körperhaltungen des Menschen: eine vergleichende Untersuchung. *Z Orthop* 112:151.

310. Rothman RH, Simeone FA (1982): *The spine.* 2nd ed. Philadelphia: WB Saunders, pp. 75–78.

311. Roy SH, DeLuca CJ, Casavant DA (1989): Lumbar muscle fatigue and chronic lower back pain. *Spine* 14:992–1001.

312. Sapega AA (1990): Muscle performance evaluation in orthopaedic practice. *J Bone Joint Surg* 72A:1562–1574.

313. Schultz AB, Andersson GBJ, Örtengren R, et al. (1982): Analysis and quantitative myoelectric measurements of loads on the lumbar spine when holding weights in standing postures. *Spine* 7:390–397.

314. Schultz A, Cromwell R, Warwick D, Andersson G (1987): Lumbar trunk muscle use in standing isometric heavy exertions. *J Orthop Res* 5:320–329.

315. Schultz AB, Haderspeck-Grib K, Sinkora G, et al. (1985): Quantitative studies of the flexion-relaxation phenomenon in back muscles. *J Orthop Res* 3:189–197.

316. Schultz A, Haderspeck K, Warwick D, Portillo D (1983): Use of lumbar trunk muscles in isometric performance of mechanically complex standing tasks. *J Orthop Res* 1:77–91.

317. Seidel H, Beyer H, Brauer D (1987): Electromyographic evaluation of back muscle fatigue with repeated sustained contractions of different strengths. *Eur J Appl Physiol* 56:592–602.

318. Sejerstedt OM, Hargens AR, Kardel K-R, et al. (1984): Intramuscular fluid pressure during isometric contraction of human skeletal muscle. *J Appl Physiol* 56:287–293.

319. Sejerstedt OM, Westgaard RH (1988): Occupational muscle pain and injury. *Eur J Appl Physiol* 57:271–274.

320. Seroussi RE, Pope MH (1987): The relationship between trunk muscle electromyography and lifting moments in the sagittal and frontal planes. *J Biomech* 20:135–146.

321. Shellock FG, Fukunaga T, Mink JH, Edgerton VR (1991): Acute effects of exercise on MR imaging of skeletal muscle: concentric vs eccentric actions. *AJR* 156:765–768.

322. Shellock FG, Fukunaga T, Mink JH, Edgerton VR (1991): Exertional muscle injury: evaluation of concentric versus eccentric actions with serial MR imaging. *AJR* 179:659–664.

323. Shirado O, Kemeda K, Ito T (1992): Trunk-muscle strength during concentric and eccentric contraction: a comparison between healthy subjects and patients with chronic low back pain. *J Spinal Disord* 5:175–182.

324. Sihvonen T, Herno A, Paljarvi L, et al. (1993): Local denervation atrophy of paraspinal muscles in postoperative failed back syndrome. *Spine* 18:575–581.

325. Sihvonen T, Partanen J, Hanninen O, Soimakallio S (1991): Electric behavior of low back muscles during lumbar pelvic rhythm in low back pain patients and healthy controls. *Arch Phys Med Rehabil* 72:1080–1087.

326. Sirca A, Kostevc V (1985): The fibre type composition of thoracic and lumbar paravertebral muscles in man. *J Anat* 141:131–137.

327. Smidt GL, Amundsen LR, Dostal WF (1980): Muscle strength at the trunk. *J Orthop Sports Phys Ther* 1:165–170.

328. Smidt GL, Blanpied PR (1987): Analysis of strength tests and resistive exercises commonly used for low back disorders. *Spine* 12:1025–1034.

329. Smidt GL, Blanpied PR, White RW (1989): Exploration of mechanical and electromyographic response of trunk muscles to high intensity resistive exercise. *Spine* 14:815–830.

330. Smidt GL, Herring T, Amundsen L, Rogers M, Russel A, Lehmann T (1983): Assessment of abdominal and back extensor strength: a quantitative approach and results for chronic low-back patients. *Spine* 8:211–219.

331. Smidt GL, Rogers MW (1982): Factors contributing to the regulation and clinical assessment of muscle strength. *Phys Ther* 62:1283–1290.

332. Smith SS, Mayer TG, Gatchel RJ, Becker TJ (1985): Quantification of lumbar function. Part 1. *Spine* 10:757–764.

333. Snook SH (1978): The design of manual handling tasks. *Ergonomics* 21(12):963–985.

334. Snook SH, Irvine CH (1967): Maximal acceptable weight of lift. *Am Ind Hyg Assoc J* 28:322–329.

335. Soderberg GL, Barr O (1983): Muscular function in chronic low back dysfunction. *Spine* 8:79–85.

336. Soderberg GL, Blanco MK, Cosentino TL, Kurdelmeier CA (1986): An EMG analysis of posterior trunk musculature during flat and anteriorly inclined seating. *Hum Factors* 28:483–491.

337. Steinbach LS, Fleckenstein JL, Mink JH (1994): Magnetic resonance imaging of muscle injuries. *Orthopaedics* 17:991–999.

338. Stokes IAF, Rush S, Moffroid M, Johnson GB, Haugh LD (1987): Trunk extensor EMG-torque relationship. *Spine* 12:770–776.

339. Styf J (1987): Pressure in the erector spinae muscle during exercise. *Spine* 12:675–679.

340. Styf J, Körner L (1986): Microcapillary infusion technique for measurement of intramuscular pressure during exercise. *Clin Orthop* 297:253–262.

341. Styf J, Lysell E (1987): Chronic compartment syndrome in the erector spinae muscle. *Spine* 12:680–682.

342. Styf J, Suurkula M, Körner L (1987): Intramuscular pressure and muscle blood flow during exercise in chronic compartment syndrome. *J Bone Joint Surg [Br]* 69:301–305.

343. Sulemana CA, Suchenwirth R (1972): Topische Unterschiede in der enzymhistologischen Zusammensetzung der Skelettmuskulatur. *J Neurol Sci* 16:433–444.

344. Suzuki N, Endo S (1983): A quantitative study of trunk muscle strength and fatigability in the low-back pain syndrome. *Spine* 8:69–74.

345. Taverner D (1954): Muscle spasm as a cause of somatic pain. *Ann Rheum Dis* 13:331–335.

346. Taylor DC, Dalton JD, Seaber AV, Garrett JR (1993): Experimental muscle strain injury. Early functional and structural deficits and the increased risk for reinjury. *Am J Sports Med* 21:190–194.

347. Thelen DG, Schltz AB, Ashton-Miller JA (1994): Quantitative interpretation of lumbar muscle myoelectric signals during rapid cyclic attempted trunk flexions and extensions. *J Biomech* 27:157–167.

348. Thomas G, Rau E (1969): Über die Funktion der Rückenstreck-Muskulatur. *Z Orthop* 106:737.

349. Thomas LE (1984): Isokinetic torque levels for adult females: effects of age and body size. *J Orthop Sports Phys Ther* 6:21–24.

350. Thompson N, Gould JA, Davies GJ, Ross DE, Price SE (1985): Descriptive measures of isokinetic trunk testing. *J Orthop Sports Phys Ther* 7:43–49.

351. Thompson DA, Biedermann HJ, Stevenson JM (1993): Sensitiv-

ity of paraspinal EMG spectral analysis to training: two preliminary studies. *Spine* 18:2310–2313.

352. Thompson DD, Chaffin DB (1993): Can biomechanically determined stress be perceived? In *Proceeding of the Human Factors
and Ergonomics Society, 37th annual meeting,* 2:789–792.

353. Thorstensson A, Arvidsson A (1982): Trunk muscle strength and
low back pain. *Scand J Rehabil Med* 14:69–75.

354. Thorstensson A, Carlson H, Zomlefer MR, Nilsson J (1982):
Lumbar back muscle activity in relation to trunk movements during locomotion in man. *Acta Physiol Scand* 116:13–20.

355. Thorstensson A, Nilsson J (1982): Trunk muscle strength during
constant velocity movements. *Scand J Rehabil Med* 14:61–68.

356. Thorstensson A, Oddsson L, Carlson H (1985): Motor control of
voluntary trunk movements in standing. *Acta Physiol Scand* 125:
309–321.

357. Tichauer ER (1971): A pilot study of the biomechanics of lifting
in simulated industrial work situations. *J Safety Res* 3:98–115.

358. Toussaint HM, deWinter AF, deLooze YDHMP, Van Dieen JH,
Kingsma I (1995): Flexion relaxation during lifting: implications
for torque production by muscle activity and tissue stain at the
lumbo-sacral joint. *J Biomech* 28:199–210.

359. Triano JJ, Schultz AB (1987): Correlation of objective measure
of trunk motion and muscle function with low-back disability ratings. *Spine* 12:561–565.

360. Troup JDG, Chapman AF (1969): The strength of the flexor and
extensor muscles of the trunk. *J Biomech* 2:49–62.

361. Tveit P, Daggfeldt K, Hetland S, Thorstensson A (1994): Erector
spinae lever arm length variations with changes in spinal curvature. *Spine* 19:199–204.

362. Vakos JP, Nitz AJ, Threlkeld AJ, Shapiro R, Horn T (1994): Electromyographic activity of selected trunk and hip muscles during
a squat lift. Effect of varying the lumbar posture. *Spine* 19:687–
695.

363. Valencia FP, Monroe RR (1985): An electromyographic study of
the lumbar multifidus in man. *Electromyogr Clin Neurophysiol*
25:205–221.

364. Vink P, Van der Velde EA, Verbout AJ (1988): A functional sub-
division of the lumbar extensor musculature. *Electromyogr Clin
Neurophysiol* 28:517–525.

365. Waters RL, Morris JM (1972): Electrical activity of muscles of
the trunk during walking. *J Anat* 96:509–520.

366. Waylonis GW (1968): Electromyographic findings in chronic cervical radicular syndromes. *Arch Phys Med Rehabil* 49:407–412.

367. Wheeler DL, Graves JE, Miller GJ, et al. (1994): Functional assessment for prediction of lifting capacity. *Spine* 19:1021–1026.

368. Wierzbicka MM, Wiegner AW (1992): Effects of weak antagonist
on fast elbow movements in man. *Exp Brain Res* 91:509–519.

369. Wierzbicka MM, Wiegner AW, Shahani BT (1986): Role of agonist and antagonist muscles in fast arm movements in man. *Exp
Brain Res* 63:331–340.

370. Wolf SL, Basmajian JV (1977): Assessment of paraspinal electromyographic activity in normal subjects and in chronic back pain
patients using a muscle biofeedback device. In: Asmussen E, Jørgensen K, eds. *Biomechanics 6-B.* Baltimore: University Park
Press, pp. 319–324.

371. Wolf SL, Basmajian JV, Russe CTC, et al. (1979): Normative
data on low back mobility and activity levels. *Am J Phys Med* 58:
217–229.

372. Woodburne RT (1969): *Essentials of human anatomy.* London:
Oxford University Press, pp. 282–286.

373. Wyke B (1980): The neurology of low back pain. In: Jayson MIV,
ed. *The lumbar spine and low back pain.* London: Pitman, pp.
265–339.

374. Yamaguchi Y, Umezawa F, Ishinada Y (1972): Sitting posture:
an electromyographic study on healthy and notalgic people. *J Jpn
Orthop Assoc* 46:277.

375. Yashimoto K, Itami I, Yamamoto M (1978): Electromyographic
study of low back pain. *Jpn J Rehabil Med* 15:252.

376. Zeh J, Hansson T, Bigos S, Spengler D, Battié M, Wortley M
(1986): Isometric strength testing. Recommendations based on a
statistical analysis of the procedure. *Spine* 11:43–46.

377. Zetterberg C, Andersson GBJ, Schultz AB (1987): The activity of
individual trunk muscles during heavy physical loading. *Spine*
12:1035–1040.

378. Zhu XA, Parnianpour M, Nordin M, Kahanovitz N (1989): His-
tochemistry and morphology of erector spinae muscle in lumbar
disc herniation. *Spine* 14:391–397.

The Adult Spine: Principles and Practice,
2nd edition, J.W. Frymoyer, Editor-in-Chief.
Lippincott-Raven Publishers, Philadelphia © 1997.

CHAPTER **23**

Pain

James N. Weinstein

ANATOMY AND FUNCTION

Late nineteenth century anatomists and psychologists recognized that nerve fibers have anatomically distinct endings. Max Von Frey, a German physician, proposed that each anatomically distinct nerve ending responds to a different type of stimulus: touch, temperature, and pain. Pain was considered a specific sensation transmitted along a unique class of nerve fibers. Well before this, however, a seventeenth century French philosopher René Descartes wrote of the existence of specific pathways for transmitting pain information from an injured part of the body through the spinal cord to a pain center in the brain. This "telephone cable" view of how pain messages are transmitted has been accepted for many years. The fact that transecting this telephone cable that carries such pain messages will not consistently alleviate the pain reveals a very important concept about the generation of pain itself. Pain is, therefore, a complex perception and depends not only on the intensity of stimu-

lus but on the situation one has experienced, and more importantly upon the component parts of the individual who is experiencing the stimulus. Thus, it may be and often is a very subjective experience. In some cultures young men are asked to cross rivers with grappling hooks embedded in their stomachs to prove their manhood. In viewing pictures of these men, it is certainly not obvious that they are in pain. However, the expression of pain and the severity of pain differ from one individual to another.

It is the subjective experience of pain that makes the study of pain so difficult. Since the days of Descartes, a great deal of information has been accumulated in order to gain further understanding of how messages from injured tissue reach the brain. However, little information is available about the location in the brain where final decisions are made as to whether something is painful or not. In fact, little is known regarding the cortical mechanisms involved in one's perceptions of spinal pain. To date, investigators of such pain have been unable to communicate a clear understanding of the neuroanatomic mechanisms for their patients' back pain. Several investigators have even submitted to having their own nerves crushed, cut, or resutured in order to observe and describe their sensory experiences, but none of these investigators have ever agreed with each other.

J. N. Weinstein, D.O., M.S.: Division of Orthopedics and Neurosurgery, Senior Faculty Member, Center for Clinical Evaluative Sciences, Dartmouth Medical School, Dartmouth Hitchcock Medical Center, Hanover, NH 03755.

Definition

Before discussing the neuroanatomy of the functional spinal unit, it is important to have a definition of pain. The taxonomy committee of the International Association for the Study of Pain (1979) defined pain as "an unpleasant sensory and an emotional experience associated with actual or potential tissue damage, or described in terms of such damage" (80). The committee went on to say that pain is always subjective. Each individual learns, over time, the application of the word through experiences related to injury in early life. Pain often occurs in the absence of tissue damage and may in some instances be an emotional experience. If one regards his or her experience as painful and reports it in the same way as pain caused by direct tissue damage, then it should be accepted as painful. Thus, pain does not always have to be linked directly to a damaging stimulus.

To understand back pain, there must be a framework from which to work. The aim should be an understanding of the various neuroanatomical mechanisms, the nature of the spinal pain, and the rationale for its treatment. Only when one understands these mechanisms can one begin to institute rational treatments with predictable outcomes. The limitations of the verbalization of spinal pain are, as we know, restrictive. Unfortunately, spinal pain is what the patient feels and how he or she expresses those feelings.

The very nature of spinal pain and its impact upon industrialized countries has imposed a sense of urgency for a better understanding of the various pain pathways and neural mechanisms. At the present time, these issues are better understood for low back disorders than for other anatomic areas of the spine. This chapter focuses on the lumbar spine, but much of the neuroanatomy and physiology can be generalized. It is only through a better understanding of pain and its pathophysiology that responsible decisions can be made regarding treatment.

NEUROANATOMY OF THE FUNCTIONAL SPINAL UNIT

Dorsal primary rami provide nerve fibers which innervate each functional spinal unit of the spine. The distribution of medial branches from each dorsal ramus of the spinal nerve sends fibers to the vertebral periosteum, facet joint capsules, and ligamentous connections of the neural arches. The sinuvertebral nerve provides innervation to structures within the spinal canal. Most anatomic investigators (29,80,110,120,123,140) agree that the dorsal primary ramus is a branch off the spinal nerve just distal to the dorsal root ganglion and/or the dorsal section of the gray autonomic communicating ramus (Fig. 1). The largest component of the sinuvertebral nerve passes through the anterior superior part of each lumbar foramen cranial to the upper margin of the intervertebral disc and courses superomedially towards the posterior longitudinal ligament (Fig. 2). As it approaches the posterior longitudinal ligament, it divides into superiorly

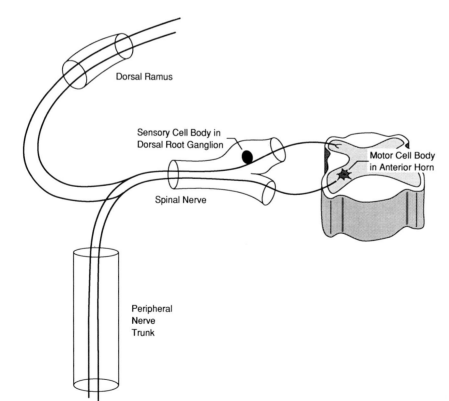

FIG. 1. Nerve roots, arising from anterior horn cells, and dorsal horn nerve roots, from sensory cell bodies in the dorsal root ganglion, form the spinal nerve. Beyond the dorsal root ganglion, the dorsal primary ramus and peripheral nerve trunk continue. From Rydevik et al. (106).

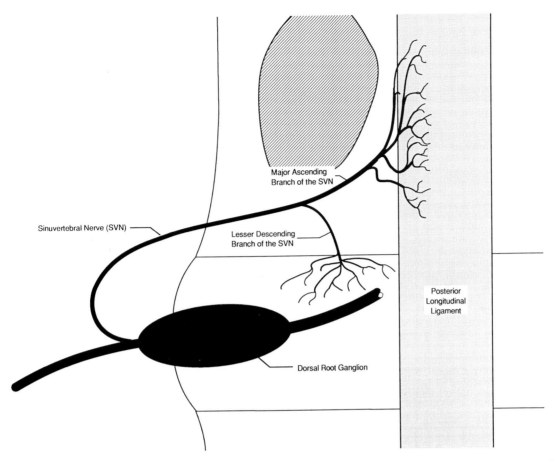

FIG. 2. The sinuvertebral nerve (SVN), which provides innervation to structures within the vertebral canal. The SVN has an ascending branch innervating the posterior longitudinal ligament and a lesser descending branch that also sends fibers to the posterior longitudinal ligament and annulus of the disc.

and inferiorly directed branches that in turn provide numerous finer branches to tissues in or around the posterior longitudinal ligament. Bogduk (8) and Parke (91) used dissections to show that each sinuvertebral nerve supplies at least two intervertebral discs. The inferiorly directed branch ramifies over the dorsum of the disc at the level of entry, while the longer superior branches course along the lateral margin of the posterior longitudinal ligament to reach the disc of the next superior level.

The posterior longitudinal ligament is the most highly innervated structure in the functional spinal unit with both complex encapsulated nerve endings and numerous poorly myelinated free nerve endings. Few investigators have emphasized the extent of the posterior longitudinal ligament with its lateral expansions from the midline laterally through the intervertebral foramen along most of the dorsal lateral aspect of the disc (92). Undoubtedly, the elevation of this highly innervated thin strap of connective tissue may provide a significant component in the production and perceptions of low back pain associated with lumbar disc herniations.

The sinuvertebral nerve pain fibers have been demonstrated by both clinical and laboratory experimentation.

Direct stimulation of the posterior longitudinal ligament is known to elicit back pain in humans. Pederson (97) showed that stimulation of these tissues in cats resulted in changes in blood pressure and respiration similar to those elicited by painful stimuli in other areas of the body.

The nerve endings associated with the sinuvertebral nerve and the posterior primary ramus of each functional spinal unit have been studied by various investigators (44,73,99). Three types of myelinated nerve endings have been identified: (a) free nerve endings terminating as single tapered tips, (b) complex unencapsulated endings usually terminating in multiple branches with expanded tips, and (c) encapsulated nerve endings of the Vater-Pacini type. Unmyelinated perivascular nerve networks have also been described. Malinsky identified two types of perivascular nerve endings in the immature annulus fibrosus: (a) simple, free termination of thin nerve fibers along capillary walls; and (b) more complex branching of thicker nerve fibers within blood vessel walls (73). In addition, plexiform and free unmyelinated nerve fiber terminals, not associated with blood vessels, are present. The structure of these various nerve endings significantly influences the type of sensation perceived as well as its intensity (123). Plexiform and freely ending unmyelinated nerve fibers respond to chemical or mechanical abnormalities and form the pain, or nociceptive, receptor system.

Encapsulated endings appear to be located primarily in the facet joint capsules and in the soft tissues along the anterolateral surfaces of the annulus fibrosus (44,99). The joint capsules also have free nerve endings and complex encapsulated endings. The anterior and posterior longitudinal ligaments, the supraspinous ligaments, and the interspinous ligaments have free nerve endings and complex unencapsulated endings (44,50). The posterior longitudinal ligament appears to have the greatest number of nerve endings (141). The cartilage end plates have perivascular nerves only (50). The vertebral periosteum is well supplied with free endings and complex unencapsulated nerve endings (49), and the vertebra has perivascular nerves as well as occasional solitary nerves (Table 1) (117). As stated previously, a number of investigators have reported that the peripheral layers of the annulus fibrosus have free fiber endings, but they did not find nerves in the inner regions of the annulus fibrosus or nucleus pulposus (44,50,73,103). However, Shinohara (118) reported free nerve fiber endings in the inner regions of the annulus and nucleus pulposus of degenerated discs. Another group (139) indicates that although unmyelinated nerves are present in fetal and neonatal discs, these nerves rapidly disappear with aging and growth. Thus, no nerves are present in the substances of normal mature human intervertebral disc material. Similarly, ultrastructural investigations have failed to identify nerves in the inner annulus of the normal disc.

The continuity between the peripheral nerves, the spinal nerve roots, and the spinal cord enables those patients perceiving pain to react through ascending and descending pathways. In the peripheral nervous system, three types of nerve fibers are found that transmit information from the body to the spinal cord and up to the brain (131). The largest peripheral nerves are called A-beta fibers, from 5 to 12 μm in diameter. These respond to non-noxious, noninjurious, and nonpainful stimuli. Because of their diameter, they transmit information very rapidly to the spinal cord from the peripheral tissues. A second type of fiber is the A-delta fiber, which ranges from 1 to 5 μm in diameter and transmits information much more slowly because of its smaller diameter. The smallest fibers, however, are the unmyelinated C-fibers. They are less than 1 μm in diameter and transmit information even more slowly than the A-delta fibers. The A-delta and the C-fibers are predominantly nociceptors; that is, they respond to injurious mechanical or thermal stimuli as well as endogenous neurogenic and non-neurogenically released chemicals from damaged tissue. When you bump your elbow, the first sharp pain experienced is due to the A-delta fibers, while the second diffuse throbbing pain, possibly burning pain, is transmitted by the C-fibers. One must remember that small C-fibers are exclusively activated by painful stimuli. However, large-diameter fibers must be present and play a significant role in appreciation of the quality of the stimuli to be preserved. In the absence of large fibers such as A-delta, a damaging stimulus might be perceived only as a burning sensation. It is possible, therefore, that in patients who have severe radicular symptoms, burning may be the most common complaint. A classic example is "causalgia," which literally means burning. If a damaging stimulus or injury has occurred, the "normal" C-fiber threshold for mechanical, thermal, and chemical stimulation may become altered, and these fibers, therefore, become sensitized, with a considerably lowered threshold for sending a pain signal to the spinal cord and brain. Therefore, patients with low back pain may complain of pain when they are up sitting or walking but find themselves very comfortable in an immobile supine position. On the other hand, in a patient who has no history of back pain and no history of injury to the back or surrounding structures, C-fiber thresholds may be normal,

TABLE 1. *Distribution of peripheral nerves to the three-joint complex and surrounding soft tissues*

Fiber type	Function	Location
Myelinated		
Free	Tissue or joint position	Facet joint capsules; anterior and lateral surfaces of annulus fibrosus; anterior/posterior longitudinal ligaments; supraspinous/intraspinous ligaments; periosteum
Complex unencapsulated	Tissue or joint position	Same as listed above
Complex encapsulated	Pressure	Facet joint capsules; anterior and lateral surfaces of annulus fibrosus; periosteum
Unmyelinated		
Perivascular	Vasomotor	Cartilage end plates; vertebrae; blood vessels
Simple	Vasosensory	
Complex	Nociceptor	
Free	Chemical Mechanical	Annulus fibrosus; facet joint capsules; ligaments
Plexiform	Nociceptor	

and, therefore, ambulating and sitting may never cause pain. Those who have had an injury and an altered thermostatic setting or threshold for pain often experience severe pain with even the slightest motions.

THE DORSAL ROOT GANGLION

As we move toward the spinal cord [central nervous system (CNS)] from peripheral nerves to the spinal nerve, we encounter the dorsal root ganglion, which I have termed the brain of the functional spinal unit (Fig. 3) (76,134). Lindblom and Rexed (66) were the first to implicate the dorsal root ganglion as the modulator of low back pain. Their cadaveric studies focused on compression of the dorsal root ganglion as a result of dorsolateral lumbar disc protrusions. In some specimens, enlarged facet joints were found to be an accessory factor in causing nerve injury. Such bony enlargement no doubt can cause similar damage to the dorsal root ganglion quite independent of a disc herniation. Today the importance of this compression is still uncertain.

The cells of the dorsal root ganglion were originally divided into two classes according to their diameters (65). The large diameter cells give rise to the large myelinated A-beta fibers while the small diameter cells give rise to the unmyelinated C-fibers and finely myelinated A-delta fibers. The central terminations of these primary afferent fibers, derived from the small ganglion cells, are primarily, but certainly not exclusively, in the substantia gelatinosa or lamina II of the spinal cord's dorsal horn.

The dorsal root ganglion manufactures several neurogenic peptides, including calcitonin gene-related peptide and substance P. Calcitonin gene-related peptide is the most abundant peptide discovered to date in the dorsal root ganglion (35). A great deal of information is available on the blood supply to the spinal cord, but little has been written about the blood supply to the dorsal root ganglion (4). Its vascular supply, venous and arterial, must play a significant role in its function. Bergman and Alexander (4) suggested that the aging and concomitant

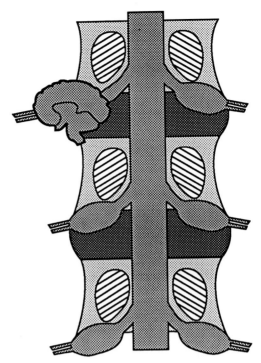

FIG. 3. The spine with the posterior elements removed demonstrates the critical location of the dorsal root ganglion at each functional spinal unit. Many of the peptides within the dorsal root ganglion co-locate; the functional significance of these co-stored peptides remains under investigation. This mechanically sensitive structure also may have a significant role in the modulation of activities in and around the functional spinal unit.

vascular changes of the dorsal root ganglion are associated with degeneration and changes in vibratory sensation. Because of the ganglion's vascular supply and tight capsule, Rydevik and associates (109) have suggested that mechanical compression of the ganglion may result in intraneural edema and a subsequent decrease in cell body blood supply, accounting for abnormal dorsal root ganglion activity and pain. In the spinal stenosis model developed by Delamarter, neurogenic claudication ap-

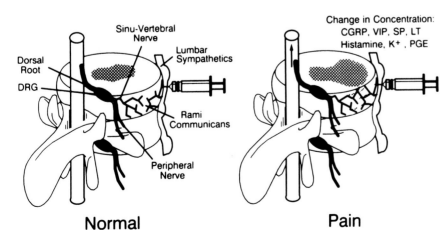

FIG. 4. Discography being performed in a normal (*left*) nonsensitized and an abnormal (*right*) sensitized disc. It is thought that sensitization of an abnormal disc allows chemical alterations to occur and thereby may be responsible for the perception of pain and/or furthering the degenerative process. From Weinstein et al. (133).

pears to begin with venous congestion of the nerve roots and the dorsal root ganglion distal to the induced constriction (23). Anatomically, the dorsal root ganglion serves as a vital link between the internal and external environment and the spinal cord. The primary sensory role of the spinal cord is to receive afferent stimuli in the form of action potentials and to relay the information transmitted to and from the brain.

This particular mechanism of pain transmission has attracted much attention. The classic hypothesis that the effects of nerves on target organs (bone, muscle, ligaments, cartilage) are mediated by chemicals released from those nerves was first studied in the peripheral nervous system and has now proven to be valid in the CNS as well (21,67). Thus, the dorsal root ganglion remains a vital link between the intrathecal spinal nerve and the extrathecal peripheral nerve (21,67). Nervi nervorum located on the dorsal root ganglion, as well as peripheral nerves, are mechanically sensitive nociceptors themselves. Therefore, the epineurium of the dorsal root ganglion may be directly activated by compression or mechanical stimulation of these nociceptors. These epineurally located nociceptors appear to respond in a similar way to cutaneous nociceptors in the peripheral nervous system (115).

In 1988, a study to assess the role of the dorsal ganglion in modulating the pain response associated with discography was reported (133). Lumbar discography is a commonly employed diagnostic tool, but important questions about it remain unresolved. Why is a morphologically abnormal discogram painful in one patient and not in another? This study was performed to investigate the changes in substance P (SP) and vasoactive intestinal peptide (VIP), found in the dorsal root ganglion, following discography in normal and abnormal canine lumbar intervertebral discs. The data from this study suggest that dorsal root ganglion SP and VIP are indirectly affected by manipulations of the intervertebral disc (Figs. 4 and 5). It may be that various neurochemical changes within the intervertebral disc are expressed by sensitized (injured) annular nociceptors and in part modulated by the dorsal root ganglion. Therefore, the concomitant pain sometimes associated with an abnormal discogram image may in part be related to the chemical environment within the intervertebral disc and the sensitized state of its annular nociceptors. In this study, immunohistochemical identification of SP, VIP, and calcitonin gene-related peptide was made in the outer annulus (Fig. 6).

LUMBAR NERVE ROOTS

Anatomy

As one moves from the dorsal root ganglion towards the spinal cord, the anatomy of the lumbar nerve roots themselves must be explained. Within the lumbar subarachnoid space, the dorsal and ventral lumbosacral nerve roots form the cauda equina. Nerve roots constitute the anatomic and physiologic connection between the central and peripheral nervous system. Anatomically, the nerve roots pass through confined spaces in the spine where pathological changes can cause mechanical deformation. Unlike the more homogeneous peripheral nerves, nerve roots are are composed of different anatomical and vascular structures (70,110). Therefore, nerve roots do not react to compression in the same fashion as peripheral nerves. A nerve root in the lumbar spine is not a single structure or entity but rather a complex arrangement consisting of the motor root, the sensory root, and the dorsal root ganglion, exiting through the neural foramen. The nerve roots in the spinal canal are enclosed by a thin, rich sheath. Outside the sheath is cerebral spinal fluid (CSF) and the spinal meninges. For each nerve root, the subarachnoid space ends at about the level of the dorsal root ganglion. It is at the dorsal root ganglion junction that the sensory nerve fibers mix with the motor fibers to form the spinal nerve. The dura is transformed at this point to be the epineurium of the peripheral nerve. The basement membranes that originate from the root sheath itself and the layer beneath the spinal dura and arachnoid form the perineurium of the spinal nerve, which eventually becomes a peripheral nerve.

It should be noted that nerve roots within the cauda equina lack perineurium and only have a very sparse epineurium (Fig. 7). Therefore, they may be more susceptible to compressive forces than peripheral nerves. On the other hand, nerve roots are surrounded by CSF and meninges, which have significant mechanical properties (105). The dorsal sensory roots are larger in diameter than the ventral motor roots. These roots vary in length from 6 to 17 cm, increasing from the L1 to S1 level (122). The axons making up the dorsal and ventral roots are extensions of the dorsal sensory root ganglion and ventral horn motor cells of the spinal cord, respectively. The

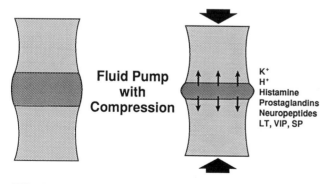

Fluid Pump with Compression

K⁺
H⁺
Histamine
Prostaglandins
Neuropeptides
LT, VIP, SP

FIG. 5. Axial loading of the disc and vertebrae affects intradiscal pressure and the transport of various neurogenic and non-neurogenic pain mediators. From Weinstein et al. (133).

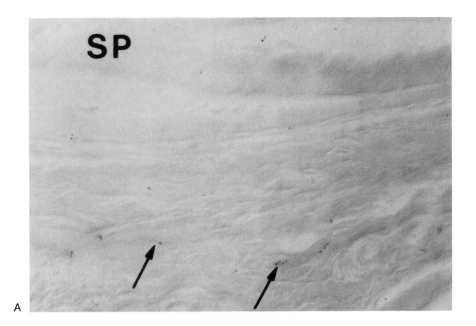

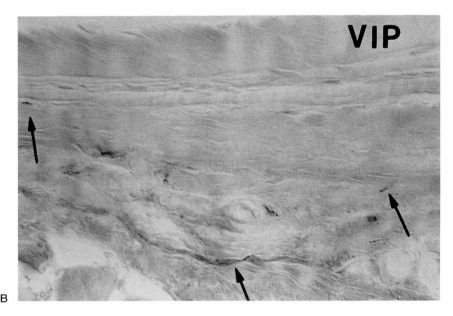

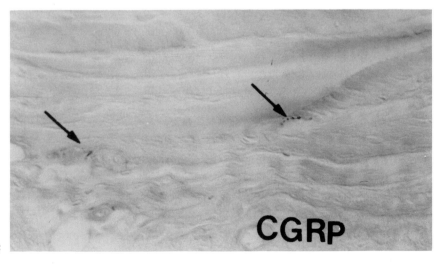

FIG. 6. Immunohistochemical demonstrations of the annulus fibrosus of rat disc. **A**: (*Top*) Substance P. **B**: (*Left*) Vasoactive intestinal peptide. **C**: (*Below*) Calcitonin gene-related peptide. From Sunderland (123).

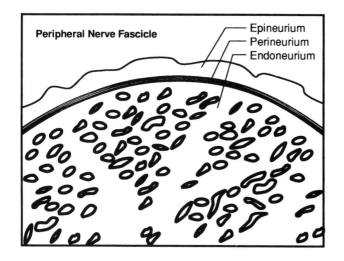

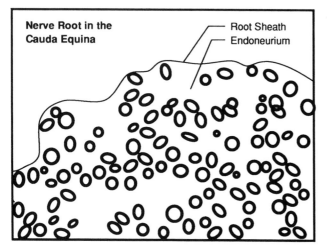

FIG. 7. Structural difference between nerves within the cauda equina and a peripheral nerve. Note that peripheral nerve fibers are located within the endoneurium, the fascicles are surrounded by the perineurium, and outside this sheath is the epineurium, which is a connective tissue stroma located around and in between the fascicles of the nerve trunk. Nerve roots of the cauda equina, however, have no epineurium and essentially no perineurium, just a very thin root sheath. From Rydevik et al. (106).

survival of these axons depends on the integrity of their parent cell bodies and the various axonal transport mechanisms.

Mechanics and Function

Most of our understanding regarding the pathophysiology of nerve roots is based on work done on peripheral nerves (20). That work has concentrated on mechanical compression resulting in ischemia and tension. Peripheral nerves respond to local compression by a total neural component reaction. At low pressure levels of 30 to 50 mm Hg, the first effect seen in a peripheral nerve is stagnation of venous blood flow (106). In the rabbit tibial nerve, this is seen in the 20 to 30 mm Hg pressure range.

Prolonged compression at such levels induces retrograde effects on the nutritive blood flow in the capillary circulation of nerve fascicles. As the amount of pressure and the duration of pressure increase, axonal transport becomes affected, and finally complete ischemia of the nerve is seen (106). Depending on the duration of compression, blood flow may be restored; however, postcompression edema within the endoneurium may have a negative effect on nerve function by either altering ionic balance or by increasing the pressure within the nerve fascicles (70).

Rydevik and his colleagues have speculated that longstanding edema can result in interneuronal fibrotic scar tissue where mast cells and fibroblasts may play a role (20). The neurophysiological events related to nerve root compression indicate that nerve roots might be more susceptible to compression than peripheral nerves (31,116). A model in the pig lumbosacral spine developed by Rydevik and associates (89,98) has allowed for an analysis of the effects of acute, graded compression on various physiologic and anatomic factors, such as intraneural blood flow, intraneural microvascular permeability, and impulse propagation in the nerve roots. Using vital microscopy of nerve roots, the researchers showed that compression of nerve roots within the cauda equina at very low pressures (5 to 10 mm Hg) induced acute changes in the intraneural microcirculation as measured by venous congestion (89). Total ischemia in the compressed nerve root was induced at 130 mm Hg pressure, which correlated well with the mean arterial pressure of these experimental animals. Analysis of neural transport using tritium-labeled methylglucose applied to the nerve root tissue during graded compression demonstrated that solute transport was reduced by nearly 45% when compressed at 10 mm Hg pressure (88). Intraneural edema was demonstrated when pressures 50 mm Hg for 10 minutes were applied. The edema formation was related not only to pressure but also to time of application. In essence, the more slowly the pressure was applied, the less edema was seen, whereas more rapid application at higher pressures compounded the problem. Compression at 100 mm Hg for 2 hours impaired nerve impulse conduction of sensory nerve roots by 75%. This was greater than the impairment seen in the motor nerve roots, which was 55%. Motor recovery was seen to be more rapid and more complete than sensory recovery after release of pressure.

Recently, the same authors assessed cauda equina function following intermittent and variably applied compression. Two different modes of compression were used. The pressure applied was proportional to the reduction of muscle action potentials for both compression modes. The reduction was most pronounced for the continuous/intermittent compression at 50 mm Hg. At 10 mm Hg there was no difference seen between the two compression modes. This low pressure level induced incomplete venous congestion, whereas at 50 mm Hg almost complete venous congestion was induced. Continuous compression at 50 mm Hg significantly reduced the ability of the cauda equina circulation to recover. Progressive functional impairment was associated with intermittent compression. It appeared from these studies that intermittent cauda equina compression may be more relevant clinically in regard to the pathophysiologic mechanisms of spinal stenosis (58).

Rydevik and his co-investigators have also pointed out that the endoneurial vessels of nerve roots and, in particular, the dorsal root ganglia are more permeable to plasma proteins than are the endoneurial vessels of peripheral nerves. There is then no effective blood–nerve barrier in nerve roots. In the peripheral nervous system, the perineurium can act as a diffusion barrier to macromolecules, while nerve roots lack this layer and are therefore relatively more exposed to substances and agents circulating within the blood and subarachnoid space (1,90) that might contribute to edema formation. The work of Schönström et al. (112) demonstrated that a decrease in the thecal sac diameter from 11.1 at L3 to 10.6 mm at L4 produced a critical point at which compression of nerve roots occurred. This compression was thought to be responsible for a number of neurophysiological changes that may be categorized by the following: (a) the biomechanics of nerve and nerve root injury; (b) intraneural blood flow alterations; (c) increased vascular permeability leading to intraneural edema; (d) effects on axonal transport; (e) inflammation accompanied by demyelination; and (f) atrophy with wallerian degeneration followed by regeneration. Sunderland (123) has discussed the mechanics of peripheral nerves quite well. He points out that peripheral nerves *in vivo* are under some tension, a fact reflected by the phenomenon that nerves retract about 10% to 20% of their original length if cut. Intraneural blood flow is gradually impaired as the peripheral nerve is stretched to about 8% beyond *in vivo* strain; in this range, circulatory changes start to occur. Intraneural blood flow ceases at about 15% beyond *in vivo* strain (71).

Conflicting opinions exist regarding which tissue component of the peripheral nerve is responsible for its tensile properties. Sunderland and Bradley (124) claim that the elasticity and tensile strength reside in the fascicular tissue, particularly in the perineurium, whereas Haftek (40) has concluded that the elasticity of the nerve trunk depends primarily on the epineurium, less on the perineurium, and only slightly on interfascicular tissue.

The nerve roots in the thecal sac generally lack epineurium and perineurium but under tensile loading exhibit both elasticity and tensile strength (125). The ultimate load of the ventral, motor, and spinal nerve roots from the thecal sac is between 2 and 22 newtons (N) and for dorsal and sensory nerve roots from the thecal sac is between 5 and 33 N (123,125). The mechanical properties of a human spinal nerve root are different depending on its location within the central spinal canal and/or the lateral intervertebral foramina. It has been estimated that ultimate loads are approximately five times higher for foraminal segments of spinal nerve roots than for the intrathecal portion of the same nerve roots under tensile loading (60).

Information on the direct effects of nerve root pressure and axonal function is derived from peripheral nerve compression models. There is deformation of the nerve fibers primarily at the edges of the compressed segment, and the nodes of Ranvier are displaced toward the noncompressed parts of the nerve (84). Nodal displacement is followed by demyelination and conduction block; this is reversible, although some axonal loss and wallerian degeneration may occur (84). Unmyelinated C-fibers are generally spared by this process, as compression primarily affects larger myelinated fibers. However, severe compression may produce degeneration across the spectrum of fiber diameter types.

Nerve roots are not static structures. They move with relative freedom within the CSF and at each functional spinal unit relative to the surrounding tissues. It is this micromotion that allows the nerve root to maintain its mechanical properties and receive nutrition. Chronic irritation and subsequent fibrosis around nerve roots secondary to a herniated disc or stenosis can impair this movement and effect repeated injury to the nerve roots even during their attempted normal movements. Tissue irritation may in some ways be responsible for the various symptom complexes encountered clinically.

Goddard and Reed (37) measured the normal range of movements of nerves in the human lumbar spine in cadaver experiments. They found nerve roots at the intervertebral foramina moved between 2 and 5 mm during a straight-leg maneuver. With this in mind, Spencer and colleagues developed a biomechanical model to explain the pathogenesis of symptoms induced by nerve root deformation (121). They demonstrated that the contact force between a simulated disc herniation in cadavers and a deformed nerve root is approximately 400 mm Hg pressure. When one looks at the work of Kwan (60), who demonstrated a normal root ultimate load to be around 70 N, the loads reported by Spencer are significant. Spencer went on to speculate that chymopapain relieves sciatica pain by decreasing disc height and therefore reducing nerve contact force and pressure.

Intraneural Blood Flow Alternations

Available evidence indicates that ischemia plays an important role in the clinical syndromes of nerve and nerve root compression. It is well known in those patients with spinal stenosis who undergo decompression and experience significant clinical relief. Similar immediate relief is seen after removal of a herniated nucleus pulposus (HNP) (24,25,107,138,139). Hypothetically, nerve roots lacking a well-developed endoneurial blood–nerve barrier are more susceptible to compression injury than peripheral nerves, with increased risk of endoneural edema formation.

Yoshizawa and colleagues have had a particular interest in blood nerve barrier functions. Specifically, their dog model was used to study the internal environment of the nerve root. Their model demonstrated changes in the blood–nerve barrier, which resulted in edema and increased endoneural fluid pressure within the nerve root. They also noted subsequent replacement of nerve root tissue by fibrous tissue (143).

Axoplasmic Transport

The transmission of axon potentials is a major function of nerve fibers. Transport of information from nerve cell bodies to the peripheral axon is also an important function. These mechanisms are energy-dependent processes that can be blocked by ischemia or compression (41,85). Chronic blockade of axoplasmic transport may lead to wallerian degeneration of a distal axon (41,85,108). This type of nerve injury may interfere with transport of neurotrophic factors from the periphery to the cell body and may produce chromatolysis or death of the cell body (38). Thus, interference with axoplasmic transport may produce degeneration both centrally and peripherally.

Inflammation Edema and Demyelination

Autoimmune mechanisms have been implicated in inflammatory tissue reactions seen around degenerating discs (6,32,75). It is these local inflammatory reactions in and around nerve roots in association with an intervertebral disc herniation that may be responsible for biochemical irritation from a mechanical stimulus.

Nerve Root Atrophy, Degeneration, and Regeneration

In spinal stenosis there is often a mixed lesion of the nerve roots. Atrophy, demyelination, and evidence of regeneration have all been documented (132). It has been demonstrated that compression of roots or ganglia is associated with increased amounts of connective tissue around the Schwann cells, signs of axonal and myelin degeneration, and proliferation of Schwann cells. Obviously if cell death predominates, the potential for recovery of nerve function is limited. It is well known that more proximal lesions are associated with more profound degeneration of the cell body, and lesions central to the dorsal root ganglion do not have a regenerative

potential equivalent to that of lesions peripheral to the ganglion (122,124). Therefore, an injury proximal to the dorsal root ganglion may produce serious and less reversible neurologic injury than an analogous injury in the periphery. To summarize, compression may produce a series of events resulting from ischemia, inflammation, demyelination, increased permeability, various blood-borne and CSF substances, and secondary endoneurial edema, followed by degeneration and regeneration of axons with chronic fibrosis. Thus, a degenerative spiral manifests itself as a syndrome that combines elements of functional loss and pain.

Neural Physiological Consequences of Nerve Injury

Nerve roots are not normally sensitive to mechanical stimulation. However, a nerve root at the site of chronic inflammation may produce radicular symptoms. This has been demonstrated in humans by placing ligatures or inflatable balloons around nerve roots at the time of surgery for a herniated disc and then mechanically stimulating the roots by traction or compression of the root postoperatively (72,119). Howe and associates (48) in an experimental model demonstrated that compression of normal roots induces only brief discharges. However, roots that are chronically inflamed and demyelinated produced long discharges similar to those observed in the normal dorsal root ganglion. Burchiel (10) and Wall and Devor (130) have shown that neurons of the dorsal root ganglion also become spontaneously active after lesion of their peripheral processes. In the rat, experimental compression of the dorsal root ganglion induced edema with increased tissue pressure in the ganglion (109). Such edema can lead to fibrosis, altered histologic characteristics, and abnormal function in the compressed ganglion. One can speculate that this abnormal function may result in the abnormal sensitivity of the dorsal root ganglion. It has been shown that lesions of the peripheral nerve, dorsal root ganglion, or nerve roots themselves can result in generation of ectopic impulses identical to those described in neuromas (83). Clinical data support the notion that spontaneous activity from such sites and within the spinal canal may be accompanied by pain and paresthesias.

The observation that activity in one nerve root fiber can induce activity in another fiber in cases of nerve injury has been previously reported (39). These artificial synapses, or ephapses, can be produced in areas of nerve root injury or demyelination (39,102). Cross-talk between demyelinated axons has been produced in the nerve roots of dystrophic mice (9,100). Cross-talk has also been demonstrated in experimental neurons (6,113). Studies have supported this mechanism as a coupling of action potential activity demonstrated in various combinations: A-fiber to A-fiber, A-fiber to C-fiber, C-fiber to C-fiber, and C-fiber to A-fiber (51,81). The significance of cross-talk as a mechanism of causalgia has been considered in some detail (12,13). Several observations, however, argue against this mechanism.

Another mechanism that might cause continuing pain after injury is mediated by the sympathetic nervous system. To date there are no well-documented cases of nerve root injury confined to the area within the spinal canal and in which the pain was shown to be sympathetically maintained. Nonetheless, we do know that the sympathetic nervous system may play an important role in nerve injury and therefore should be considered in the analysis. One hypothesis is that sympathetically maintained pain results from the development of the alpha nerve receptors and nociceptive afferent fibers (12).

In a series of experiments designed to develop and validate an animal model of lumbar radiculopathy, Kawakami and colleagues (54,55) developed a model of chronic neuropathic pain that represents a pioneering effort to develop a reproducible experimental model of lumbar radiculopathy. The model attempts to replicate clinical symptoms to help further understand the underlying neurochemical and neurophysiologic factors associated with radiculopathy. They have observed that rats treated with chromic gut ligature in large quantity demonstrated a different pattern of response consistent with lumbar radiculopathy. On the injured side, animals demonstrated significantly more thermal hyperalgesia. They also, for the first time, described an increase in the proto-oncogene c-fos. At 2 weeks postoperatively, there was a consistent trend towards baseline, and a return to baseline occurred by 12 weeks. Significantly greater levels of VIP concentration in the dorsal root ganglion were observed at 2 weeks postoperatively that did not resolve or tend toward baseline at 12 weeks follow-up. For the first time, a link was made between behavioral outcome and function with an underlying neurochemical process, specifically SP, VIP, and the proto-oncogene c-fos.

Neurochemical consequences of nerve root irritation provide a theoretical framework for hypothesizing about various types of mediating events that might explain how apparently similar pathologies (as in HNP) might reasonably lead to different behavioral consequences. To help unravel the pathomechanisms related to the clinical symptoms, especially pain, there was a need to develop such a model. The model holds promise in facilitating our understanding of both the injury and the repair process associated with neural injury, or radiculopathy (55).

Kawakami and associates also studied associated histologic changes following spinal nerve root irritation and concluded that mechanical constriction in and of itself causes a loss of myelinated fibers. However, this loss is not sufficient to produce the behavioral effects associated with the model of lumbar radiculopathy. Therefore, they hypothesize that chemical factors from the chromic gut itself (i.e., chromium salts) play a major role in the

pathophysiology and development of the behavioral changes. This appears to correlate nicely with clinical observations, whereas deformation and aberrancies seen on imaging, such as MRI of HNP, do not necessarily correlate with the clinical findings (54).

Chatani (18) also characterized thermal hyperalgesia using c-fos gene expression and alterations in neuropeptides following mechanical irritation of the dorsal root ganglion (DRG). In their model, they wanted to characterize the neurophysiological/neurochemical difference between the dorsal root ganglion and a nerve root, following mechanical irritation. They demonstrated thermal hyperalgesia occurring in rats with simple exposure of the DRG, as well as in rats with loose ligation of the DRG. This hyperalgesia was accompanied by an increase in c-fos expression and spontaneous pain-related behaviors. Observed alterations of neuropeptides within the DRG or spinal cord are likely related to the associated behaviors, but these changes were not correlated with the maintenance of thermal hyperalgesia. Microscopically, the associated nerve fibers revealed endoneurial edema and changes in nerve fiber composition.

Again, in this study the authors described an animal model wherein thermal hyperalgesia was accompanied by a change in c-fos gene expression and pain-related behavior. As expected, the DRG was more sensitive and its response was different from that of the nerve root (18).

Hayashi and colleagues (43) studied the effects of epidural steroid injections in their animal model of nerve root irritation as expressed by hyperalgesia. These authors attempted to experimentally explain the mechanism(s) whereby the clinical observations were associated with efficacious use of epidural steroids. Their work demonstrated a significant steroid effect on thermal hyperalgesia originating from nerve root irritation (see Fig. 1).

Pressure versus Chemical Agents

The response of lumbar dorsal nerve roots and dorsal root ganglion to locally applied pressure and various chemical agents continues to be studied *in vitro* (14–16). Studies by Cavanaugh et al. indicate that in an inflamed state, the nerve roots are much more mechanosensitive. Nerve excitation resulting from the application of HNP material suggest a probable role of chemical sensitization.

Cavanaugh and colleagues also looked at the facet joint response to loading. They found a relationship between tissue load and deformation and neural discharge in and around the lumbar facet joints. This relationship between facet joint deformation, loading, and neural response was observed with different loading directions. Loading associated with peak loads in the range of 4.8 to 6.3 N caused nerve discharge to increase from 30% to 73% over baseline rates. These data suggest that movement of the lumbar facet joints can cause large strains and increased neural discharge. One might suggest that excessive soft-tissue strain at this joint may in fact be a plausible cause for low back pain (14–16).

CHEMICAL MEDIATION OF NOCICEPTION

As previously stated, pain originating in the lumbar spine typically arises from mechanical or chemical irritation of primary sensory neurons. The site of activation may involve the peripheral terminal endings of these neurons and tissues such as muscles, joints, skin, periosteum, blood vessels, and meninges. Alternatively, it may involve a mechanical or chemical irritation to the dorsal root fiber or the soma within the dorsal root ganglion (141). Some of the endogenous chemical substances, particularly inflammatory mediators, can excite or increase the excitability of primary sensory neurons or otherwise alter their local environment.

Nociceptors are the peripheral terminal endings of sensory neurons that are selectively responsive to potentially or overtly injurious stimuli that cause pain in humans and cause affective painlike responses in animals.

Nociceptors have three important roles to play in the process of inflammation:

1. By evoking pain, they signal the presence of noxious physical or algesic chemicals, the latter when endogenous are inflammatory mediators originating from non-neural tissues such as mast cells and blood vessels and from peripheral endings of certain sensory afferent nerve fibers.

2. Some nociceptors become sensitized; that is, they develop a lowered response threshold and enhanced responses to suprathreshold stimuli after exposure to noxious physical stimuli or inflammatory mediators (5,11,42,73). There is evidence that nociceptor sensitization contributes to hyperalgesia, which is characterized by a lowered pain threshold or enhanced pain in response to normally painful stimuli (56).

3. It is probable that nociceptors responding directly to algesic stimuli serve as effectors and can release peptides and other neuromodulators that increase the excitability of neighboring nociceptors, modulate the inflammatory process, and promote tissue repair (96).

All three of these functions are protective; nociceptors therefore warn the CNS of danger, enhance local escape and avoidance reactions through the mechanisms of sensitization, and then contribute to the process of healing.

CHEMICAL MEDIATORS OF PAIN

Non-Neurogenic Pain Mediators

A variety of endogenous chemicals are released from non-neural tissues, all of which have pain-producing ca-

pabilities. These include bradykinin, serotonin, histamine, acetylcholine, prostaglandins E_1 and E_2, and leukotrienes (26,52,141). Serotonin and bradykinin excite heat-sensitive or mechanosensitive C- or A-fiber nociceptive afferents innervating the skin, joints, skeletal muscle, and visceral organs (3,17,42,45,52,56,77–79,126). There are various interactions among these chemicals and their physical stimuli as they affect nociceptor responses. Prostaglandins enhance the responses of C- or A-nociceptors in skin, joint, or muscle to heat, mechanical stimuli, or bradykinin (3,17,42,74,78,93, 94,101). Similarly, intradermal or subdermal injections of prostaglandin E_1 in humans produce mechanical tenderness and potentiate the pain from subdermal injections of bradykinin and the itch from histamine. Two other endogenous chemicals that have recently been shown to produce hyperalgesia are formed by the lipoxygenation of arachidonic acid: (a) dihydroxyeicosatetraenoic acid (diHETE), a 15-lipoxygenase product; and (b) leukotriene B_4, a 5-lipoxygenase product. Leukotriene B_4 is a chemotaxin for polymorphonuclear leukocytes that accumulate at locations of inflammation to destroy antigens (27). Leukotriene injected interdermally into the rat paw sensitizes C-nociceptors to mechanical stimuli and produces hyperalgesia. Further, this hyperalgesia is dependent upon the presence of polymorphonuclear leukocytes (59). The hyperalgesia resulting from these substances is not blocked by nonsteroidal anti-inflammatory drugs that block the cyclooxygenation of arachidonic acid (Fig. 8) (63). Levine and associates (64) provided evidence that diHETE injected interdermally into the rat paw produces a hyperalgesia equivalent in maximal effect to that produced by leukotriene B_4, bradykinin, or prostaglandin E_2. Saal et al. have suggested phospholipase A_2 activity may be extremely important in the presence of a clinical radiculopathy associated with an HNP (111).

Neurogenic Pain Mediators

For two decades, it has been known that a large number of primary afferent neurons produce neuropeptides such as SP (46). These neuropeptides are produced within the dorsal root ganglion in cell bodies of primary afferent neurons and delivered by axonal transport to both the central and peripheral processes of neurons. Although SP from primary afferent neurons has been demonstrated in response to intense electrical stimulation of peripheral nerves (142), as has the excitatory effect of SP on ascending projection neurons (137), it remains to be established whether SP (or any other neuropeptide within primary afferent neurons) is both necessary and sufficient as the chemical transmitter mediating nociception at the first synapse. This uncertainty stems from several sources. Capsaicin has been employed widely as a toxin for the reduction of peptides in primary afferent

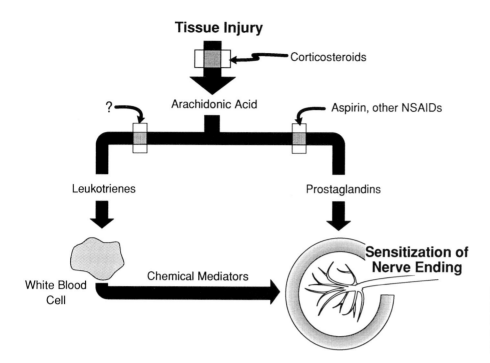

FIG. 8. The leukotrienes, non-neurogenic mediators, are not affected by nonsteroidal anti-inflammatory agents but do seem to be affected by steroids.

neurons. Studies using capsaicin have attempted to discern the role of neuropeptides in primary afferent neurons and nociception. Its limitation is that it may not destroy peptides in myelinated primary afferent nerve fibers (103,127–129). These residual myelinated peptineurgic fibers may play an important role in nociception and, therefore, confound the interpretation of experiments in which capsaicin is used.

The number of neuropeptides now known to occur in primary afferent neurons has been steadily increasing. In addition to SP, somatostatin, cholecystokininlike substance, VIP, calcitonin gene-related peptide, gastrin-releasing peptide, dynorphin, enkephalin, and galanin are neuropeptides predominantly produced by primary afferent neurons (22,28,30,33,34,36,57,61,62,69,86,91, 136).Each of these peptides is likely to be produced by a biosynthetic precursor that may, through posttranslational processing, give rise to additional biologically active peptides. Thus the potential number of biologically active peptides produced by primary afferent neurons is high; therefore, confounding this simple examination of their role or roles in nociception. Anatomic studies of neuropeptides in the DRG cells have found these neurons to contain enzymes that, by their presence, implicate their substrates as playing a role in neurotransmission or neuromodulation (for example, adenosine deaminase, which implicates purines, and fluoride-resistant acid phosphatase, whose substrate is unknown) (82). Neuropeptides are released from peripheral endings of nociceptive afferents as a result of noxious chemical or physical stimulation and can influence the inflammatory process (95). Antidromically induced release of neuropeptides by electrical stimulation of C-fibers can increase blood flow and vascular permeability. SP is believed to

act directly on the blood vessels to produce plasma extravasation and indirectly to produce vascular dilatation by releasing histamine. Antihistamines and SP antigens block the flare induced by histamine; however, it seems that SP antagonists do not block the flare produced by capsaicin, suggesting that the final vasodilator is not histamine. Another candidate mediator is calcitonin gene-related peptide which is a potent vasodilator and is co-localized with SP (62).

Neuropeptides are also known to stimulate the release from mast cells of leukotrienes and other factors that attract and stimulate polymorphonuclear leukocytes and monocytes (Fig. 9) (96). Certain pathologic conditions are accompanied by an increase in SP; for example, increased SP is seen in peripheral nerves supplying arthritic joints and in the CSF of patients with low back pain and chronic arachnoiditis (47). SP is released into joint tissues and stimulates proliferation of rheumatoid synovial sites and their release of prostaglandin E_2 and collagenase, thereby implicating this peptide in the pathogenesis of rheumatoid arthritis (68). In addition, it has been demonstrated that VIP can cause a dose-dependent increase of bone resorption by a cAMP-dependent mechanism. Neuropeptides such as calcitonin gene-related peptide and SP can also contribute to the repair of injured tissue by stimulating the proliferation of smooth muscle cells and fibroblasts (96).

In tissue culture, SP is known to stimulate endothelial cell proliferation and migration. Presence of NK-1 type SP receptors on blood vessels in the annulus fibrosis may indicate a role for SP in vasoregulation or in the neovascularization that often accompanies this degeneration. NK-1 is a tachykinin receptor subtype through which the vascular effects of SP are thought to be mediated (2).

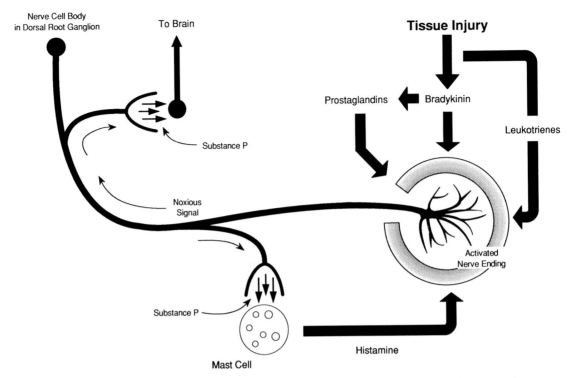

FIG. 9. The interaction between peripheral tissue injury and repair and the central neurogenic components. This scheme demonstrates how neurogenic mediators can affect non-neurogenic mediators through the stimulation of mast cells by substance P.

I have also demonstrated that degeneration of the lumbar spine secondary to vibration, a known epidemiologic cause of low back pain, may in part be related to neurogenic pain modulators (29,133,135). Work designed to establish and develop animal-based experimental paradigms and techniques for studying degeneration in the components of the functional spinal unit, has established that low frequency vibration causes changes in the amounts of SP and VIP in the DRG. The presence of these neuropeptides in the DRG as well as in the peripheral areas such as the disc annulus, facet joints, and blood plasma suggests exciting possibilities for explaining chronic degeneration of the spinal motion segment (133,135). Results from these studies have motivated the development of a working model explaining chronic functional spinal unit degeneration that hypothesizes causal links between environmental factors (e.g., vibration) and functional spinal unit degeneration mediated by biological events. The model is as follows: The release of neuropeptides from the DRG, induced by environmental and structural factors (i.e., vibrations), mediates a progressive degeneration of the functional spinal unit structures by stimulating the synthesis of inflammatory agents (e.g., prostaglandins E_2) and degradative enzymes (e.g., collagenase). The weakened functional spinal unit structures increase the susceptibility of the dorsal root ganglion to environmental factors, which, in turn, lowers the threshold necessary to stimulate neuropeptide activity, thereby creating a degenerative spiral (Fig. 10).

There is, however, no reason to believe that this degen-erative spiral could not be started by any of its component parts. As an example, Cornefjord and colleagues (19) demonstrated the effects of combining some nucleus pulposus with compression and made two important observations. First, a combination of nucleus pulposus and compression did not induce a more pronounced change than did application of either nucleus pulposus or compression alone. Second, the contralateral control route seemed to be affected in both series when nucleus pulposus was added, but not when only the constrictor (causing mechanical compression) was applied. The nerve root conduction velocities in their model averaged around 75 to 80 mm/sec. As judged from a second exposure 7 days later, it seemed likely that the nucleus pulposus was reaching the control route by diffusion. These results further emphasize the potential of nucleus pulposus in and of itself to induce changes in nerve roots after epidural application, and this material may by itself precipitate this degenerative spiral. The authors also noted an increase in SP levels in the dorsal root ganglion and nerve roots on the compressed nerve root side as compared to the noncompressed control side. A similar increase was not noted to be present for VIP. SP was mainly accumulated in the nerve root tissue, with less of an increase in the DRG after 1 week. This may indicate an initial increase in rate of synthesis of SP in dorsal root ganglion with a cranially directed axonal transport of the substance. However, after 4 weeks, SP begins to accumulate in the DRG itself, with lower levels in nerve root tissue.

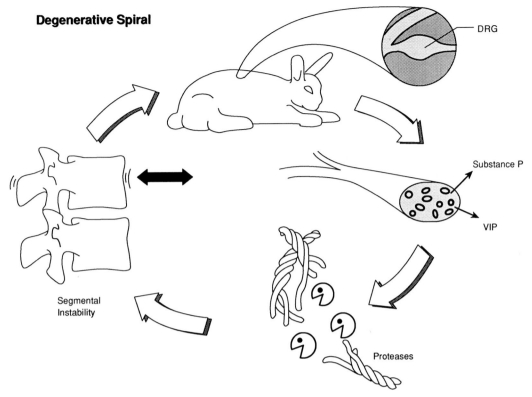

Degenerative Spiral

DRG

Substance P

VIP

Proteases

Segmental
Instability

FIG. 10. In a degenerative spiral, the functional spinal unit may undergo degeneration as a result of the interaction of mechanical and chemical stimuli seen in an injured or environmentally stimulated functional spinal unit.

In their model, compression occurred during the first 2 weeks. This was the result of using a constriction band that would swell over time. The change in axonal transport of SP in a cranial direction from the ganglion seemed to be blocked by 4 weeks. This would explain the lower nerve root levels and accumulation within the DRG. Since SP has been proposed to be related to pain perception, these results for the first time suggest an experimental basis for pain production in controlled nerve root compression (19).

Recently, metalloproteases, in particular gelatinase, which degrades gelatin, and caseinase (stromelysin), were shown to be produced by the intervertebral disc in culture. Gelatinase degrades gelatin and stromelysin degrades proteoglycans. One could hypothesize, therefore, that they have a role in the degradation of disc matrix and the degenerative process that is ongoing in the intervertebral disc. Additionally, various cytokines, for example IL-6 (interleukin-6) have been detected in very large amounts in the media of a herniated disc. In the literature, there is a suggestion that IL-6 is necessary in suppression of proteoglycan synthesis in normal articular cartilage. However, we do not currently know what its role is in the intervertebral disc, but it may be involved in the degenerative process. Nitric oxide production has also been seen in herniated disc cultures, and this has only recently been reported (53). Nitric oxide has been shown to play a role in immune regulation, inflamma-

tion, and in the pathophysiology of arthritis. We do not really know its role in intervertebral disc metabolism, but further investigation is being undertaken.

There has also been information regarding inflammatory cells associated with the nucleus pulposus versus control chambers without nucleus pulposus. These studies implicate the inflammagenic properties and chemotactic signals from the nucleus pulposus itself to the attraction of inflammatory cells (7). Results in these experimental studies indicate that the nucleus pulposus has inflammagenic properties unto itself. This observation might have direct implications on future research and therapeutic considerations, as it relates to intervertebral discs and disc herniations (87).

CONSCIOUS PERCEPTION OF PAIN

When a nerve root (as opposed to a peripheral nerve) is injured, DRG cells send an afferent barrage of signals to the CNS (130). Knowing how the CNS handles these messages is critical to our understanding of the relationship of nerve root injury and the realization of pain. Realizing that these nerve receptors can send false signals when they receive unusual messages from damaged peripheral tissues further compounds the problems. To this end, Melzack and Wall produced the gate control theory (Fig. 11) (76). Messages concerned with pain are transmitted by the nerve roots to the spinal cord by cen-

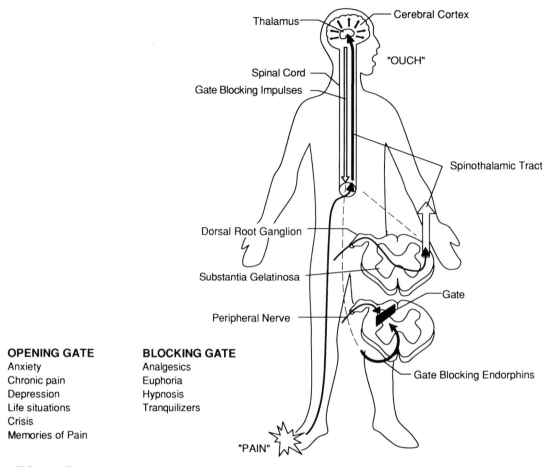

FIG. 11. The "gate control" theory of pain, as described by Melzack and Wall (76). Descartes first described such a pathway in 1664. As the figure depicts, first a toe is injured. This causes a release of various pain modulators, such as substance P and other chemicals. This starts the pain signal on its way as an electrical impulse. The message reaches the dorsal horn of the spinal cord (the substantia gelatinosa). It is relayed via the spinothalamic tract to the thalamus, the area of the brain where the painful stimulus first becomes conscious. The message then reaches the cerebral cortex where the location and intensity are perceived. Transmission of gate blocking impulses then descend from the brain stem via the spinal cord to provide pain relief. Chemicals like dynorphins and endorphins may be released to diminish the pain message from the injured toe.

tral cells in the dorsal horn of the spinal cord, specifically the substantia gelatinosa. This painful transmission within the spinal cord depends on three factors: (a) the arrival of nociceptive messages; (b) the convergent effect of peripheral afferent information, which may exaggerate or diminish the effects of nociceptive input message; and (c) the presence of controlled systems within the CNS which influence the central cells. Melzack and Wall emphasized the convergent controls that decide the fate of the arriving messages as they pass through every level of the CNS and eventually produce reaction, a sensation, and movement (76). From the dorsal horn of the spinal cord, the message is sent to its first level of consciousness, the thalamus. Then the message is sent to the postcentral gyrus of the brain wherein the nature and location of the pain is interpreted. The frontal lobe provides an affective component, whereas the temporal lobe provides stored memories from previous painful experiences. Some cells within the dorsal horn of the spinal cord, substantia gelatinosa, and lamina II learn to respond not only to a painful stimulus but also to an altering signal that says the noxious stimulus is about to happen. Thus, the signaling of injury by this central cell in the dorsal horn is dependent not only on the arrival of nociceptive afferent impulses but on other peripheral events occurring in and around the same zone, as well as on the current reaction of those cells within that zone and their state of excitability in relationship to their central and peripheral environment. These controls are contingent on one another and help to explain the variable responses to injury. The presence of such "gate" controls means that they themselves may become locked into a pathological position and can exaggerate or create pain. It is through these "gate" control systems that various therapeutic modalities have been used in the treatment of back pain (i.e., electrical stimulation, acupuncture, analgesics, and manipulation). The challenge is to have a better understanding of this complicated system and its peripheral influences (see Fig. 4).

CENTRAL MODULATION OF PAIN

Pain is not a one-way street. We are now beginning to formulate a better understanding of the descending influences on pain perception and modulation. At the site of the first synapses of the pain pathways in the dorsal horn of the spinal cord, neurotransmitters modulate nociceptive processing both pre- and postsynaptically. Both primary afferent neuron input and convergent peptineurgic input from local circuit neurons and descending bulbospinal neurons of the spinal cord and midbrain affect responses made at the first synaptic junction.

A great deal of attention has been given to opioidergic neurons in the spinal cord because of their ability to inhibit nociceptive transmission. However, neurotensin, a nonopioid neuropeptide found in the spinal cord, also has inhibitory capacities (104,114).

Neurons known to be peptidergic have been identified in the cerebral cortex and subthalamic, spinohypothalamic–telencephalic pathways. Surprisingly, however, the spinothalamic tract itself may not utilize neuropeptides for neurotransmission.

Families of endogenous, morphinelike opioids have been described. Most familiar, of course, are the β-endorphins. Other less well known, but not less important, endogenous chemicals are dynorphins. These act at several different types of receptors. Endorphins typically act at the mu-receptors, while the dynorphins have an affinity for the K-receptors. In the spinal cord, the principal sources of opioidlike peptides are the intrinsic dorsal horn neurons themselves. Most are local circuit interneurons.

SUMMARY

Pain is not a simple perception. Although millions of people suffer because of it, and billions of dollars are spent in trying to eradicate it, we are only in our infancy of understanding the very complex interactions necessary to perceive or distort our feelings of pain. In the future, we must not only continue to seek a better understanding of our patients' macroscopic impression of pain, but we must also look microscopically at each cell involved in the whole pain process. A time will come when our molecular understanding will provide us with the means to unlock the secrets of pain. Since the time of Descartes, we have come a long way in our understanding of the neurophysiology and anatomy of pain, but we have a great deal more work to do if we are going to provide our patients with better remedies in the future.

REFERENCES

1. Arvidson B (1979): Distribution of intravenously injected protein tracers in peripheral ganglia of adult mice. *Exp Neurol* 63:388–410.
2. Ashton IK, Walsh DA, Polak JM, Eisenstein SM (1994): *Substance P binding sites in the human intervertebral disc.* International Society for the Study of the Lumbar Spine Annual meeting, June 21–25, Seattle, Washington.
3. Beck PW, Handwerker HO (1974): Bradykinin and serotonin effects of various types of cutaneous nerve fibers. *Pflugers Arch* 347:209–222.
4. Bergmann L, Alexander L (1941): Vascular supply of the spinal ganglia. *Arch Neurol* 46:761–782.
5. Bessou P, Perl ER (1969): Response of cutaneous sensory units with unmyelinated fibers to noxious stimuli. *J Neurophysiol* 32:1025–1043.
6. Blumberg H, Janig W (1982): Activation of fibers via experimentally produced stump neuromas of skin nerves: ephaptic transmission or retrograde sprouting? *Exp Neurol* 76:468–482.
7. Bobechko WP, Hirsch C (1965): Auto-immune response to nucleus pulposus in the rabbit. *J Bone Joint Surg* [Br] 47:574–580.
8. Bogduk N, Twomey LT (1987): *Clinical anatomy of the lumbar spine.* Melbourne: Churchill Livingstone.
9. Bostock H, Sears TA (1978): The internodal axon membrane: electrical excitability and continuous conduction in segmental demyelination. *J Physiol* 280:273–301.
10. Burchiel KJ (1984): Effects of electrical and mechanical stimulation on two foci of spontaneous activity which develop in primary afferent neurons after peripheral axotomy. *Pain* 18:249–265.
11. Campbell JN, Meyer RA, LaMotte RH (1979): Sensitization of myelinated nociceptive afferents that innervate monkey hand. *J Neurophysiol* 42:1669–1679.
12. Campbell JN, Raja SN, Meyer RA: Painful sequelae of nerve injury. In: Dubner R, Gebhart GF, Bond MR, eds. Pain research and clinical management. Amsterdam: Elsevier (*in press*).
13. Campbell JN, Raja SN, Meyer RA, et al. (1988): Myelinated afferents signal the hyperalgesia associated with nerve injury. *Pain* 32:89–94.
14. Cavanaugh JM, Li QH, Ozaktay AC, King, AL (1994): *An initial investigation of the relationship between tissue load, deformation and neural discharge in and around the lumbar facet joint.* International Society for the Study of the Lumbar Spine Annual meeting, June 21–25, Seattle, Washington.
15. Cavanaugh JM, Vaidyanathan S, Ozaktay AC, Kallakuri S. (1994): *Response of lumbar dorsal roots and dorsal root ganglia to locally applied pressure and chemical agents: an in vitro neurophysiological study.* International Society for the Study of the Lumbar Spine Annual meeting, June 21–25, Seattle, Washington.
16. Cavanaugh JM, Weinstein JN (1994): Low back pain: epidemiology, anatomy and neurophysiology. In: Wall P, Melzack R, eds. *The third edition on pain.* New York: Churchill Livingstone.
17. Chahl LA, Iggo A (1977): The effects of bradykinin and prostaglandin E₁ on rat cutaneous afferent nerve activity. *Br J Pharmacol* 59:343–347.
18. Chatani K, Kawakami M, Weinstein JN, Meller ST, Gebhart GF (1995): Characterization of thermal hyperalgesia, c-fos expression, and alterations in neuropeptides after mechanical irritation of the dorsal root ganglion. *Spine* 20(3):277–290.
19. Cornefjord MD, Olmarker K, Farley DB, Weinstein JN, Rydevik B (1995): Neuropeptide changes in compressed spinal nerve roots. *Spine* 20(6):670–673.
20. Dahlin LB, Rydevik B, Lundborg G (1986): Pathophysiology of nerve entrapments and nerve compression injuries. In: Hargens AR, ed. *Tissue nutrition and viability.* New York: Springer-Verlag, pp. 135–160.
21. Dale H (1935): Pharmacology and nerve-endings. *Proc R Soc Med* 28:319–332.
22. Dalsgaard CJ, Vincent SR, Hokfelt T, et al. (1982): Coexistence of cholecystokinin- and substance P-like peptides in neurons of the dorsal root ganglia of the R2t. *Neurosci Lett* 33:159–163.
23. Delamarter RB, Bowman H, Dodge L, Biro C (1990): Experi-

mental lumbar spinal stenosis. *J Bone Joint Surg* [Am] 72:110–120.

24. Epstein BS, Epstein JA, Jones MD (1977): Lumbar spinal stenosis. *Radiol Clin North Am* 15:227–239.
25. Evans JG (1964): Neurogenic intermittent claudication. *Br Med J (Clin Res)* 2:985–987.
26. Ferreira SH (1972): Prostaglandins, aspirin-like drugs and analgesia. *Nature* 240:200–203.
27. Ford-Hutchinson AW, Bray MA, Doig MV, et al. (1980): Leukotriene B, a potent chemokinetic and aggregating substance released from polymorphonuclear leukocytes. *Nature* 286:264–265.
28. Franco-Cereceda A, Henke H, Lundberg JM, et al. (1987): Calcitonin gene-related peptide (CGRP) in capsaicin-sensitive substance P-immunoreactive sensory neurons in animals and man: distribution and release by capsaicin. *Peptides* 8:399–410.
29. Frymoyer J (1989): *New perspectives on low back pain.* Workshop, Airlie, VA: AAOS Publishers.
30. Fuxe K, Agnati LF, McDonald T, et al. (1983): Immunohistochemical indications of gastrin releasing peptide-bombesin-like immunoreactivity in the nervous system of the rat: codistribution with substance P-like immunoreactive nerve terminal systems and coexistence with substance P-like immunoreactivity in dorsal root ganglion cell bodies. *Neurosci Lett* 37:17–22.
31. Gelfan S, Tarlov IM (1956): Physiology of spinal cord, nerve root and peripheral nerve compression. *Am J Physiol* 185:217–229.
32. Gertzbein SD, Tile M, Gross A, et al. (1975): Autoimmunity in degenerative disc disease of the lumbar spine. *Orthop Clin North Am* 6:67–73.
33. Gibbins IL, Furness JB, Costa M (1987): Pathway-specific patterns of the co-existence of substance P, calcitonin gene-related peptide, cholecystokinin and dynorphin in neurons of the dorsal root ganglia of the guinea pig. *Cell Tissue Res* 248:417–437.
34. Gibbins IL, Furness JB, Costa M, et al. (1985): Co-localization of calcitonin gene-related peptide-like immunoreactivity with substance P in cutaneous, vascular and visceral sensory neurons of guinea pigs. *Neurosci Lett* 57:125–130.
35. Gibson SJ, Polak JM, Bloom SR, et al. (1981): The distribution of nine peptides in rat spinal cord with special emphasis on the substantia gelatinosa and on the area around the central canal (lamina X). *J Comp Neurol* 201:65–79.
36. Gibson SJ, Polak JM, Bloom SR, et al. (1984): Calcitonin gene-related peptide immunoreactivity in the spinal cord of man and of eight other species. *J Neurosci* 4:3101–3111.
37. Goddard MD, Reid JD (1965): Movements induced by straight leg raising in the lumbo-sacral roots, nerves and plexus, and in the intrapelvic section of the sciatic nerve. *J Neurol Neurosurg Psychiatry* 28:12–18.
38. Grafstein B (1975): The nerve cell body response to axotomy. *Exp Neurol* 48:32–51.
39. Granit R, Leksell L, Skoglund CR (1944): Fibre interaction in injured or compressed regions of nerve. *Brain* 67:125–140.
40. Haftek J (1970): Stretch injury of peripheral nerve: acute effects of stretching on rabbit nerve. *J Bone Joint Surg* [Br] 52:354–365.
41. Hahnenberger RW (1978): Effects of pressure on fast axoplasmic flow: an in vitro study in the vagus nerve of rabbits. *Acta Physiol Scand* 104:299–308.
42. Handwerker HO (1976): Influences of algogenic substances and prostaglandins on the discharges of unmyelinated cutaneous nerve fibers identified as nociceptors. In: Bonica JJ, Albe-Fessard D, eds. *Advances in pain research and therapy,* Vol. 1. New York: Raven Press, pp. 41–45.
43. Hayashi N, Weinstein JN, Kawakami M, Meller ST, Spratt KF, Lee HM, Gebhart GF (1994): *Morphometric changes of the DRG cells following nerve root irritation—an animal model.* International Society for the Study of the Lumbar Spine Annual Meeting, June 21–25, Seattle, Washington.
44. Hirsch C, Ingelmark BE, Miller M (1963): The anatomical basis for low back pain. *Acta Orthop Scand* 33:1–17.
45. Hiss E, Mense S (1976): Evidence for the existence of different receptor sites for analgesic agents at the endings of muscular group IV afferent units. *Pflugers Arch* 362:141–146.
46. Hokfelt T, Elde R, Johansson O, et al. (1976): Immunohistochemical evidence for separate populations of somatostatin-con-

taining and substance P-containing primary afferent neurons in the rat. *Neuroscience* 1:131–136.
47. Howe JF, Calvin WH, Loeser JD (1976): Impulses reflected from dorsal root ganglia and from focal nerve injuries. *Brain Res* 116:139–144.
48. Howe JF, Loeser JD, Calvin WH (1977): Mechanosensitivity of dorsal root ganglia and chronically injured axons: a physiological basis for the radicular pain of nerve root compression. *Pain* 3:25–41.
49. Ikari C (1954): A study of the mechanism of low-back pain. The neurohistological examination of the disease. *J Bone Joint Surg* [Am] 36:195.
50. Jackson HC, Winkelmann RK, Bickel WH (1966): Nerve endings in the human lumbar spinal column and related structures. *J Bone Joint Surg* [Am] 48:1272–1281.
51. Janig W: Pathophysiology of nerve following mechanical injury. In: Dubner R, Gebhart GF, Bond MR, eds. *Pain research and clinical management.* Amsterdam: Elsevier (*in press*).
52. Kanaka R, Schaible HG, Schmidt RF (1985): Activation of fine articular afferent units by bradykinin. *Brain Res* 327:81–90.
53. Kang JD, Georgescu HI, McIntyre L, Stefanovic-Racic M, Nita I, Donaldson WF, Evans CH (1994): *Herniated lumbar intervertebral discs make neutral metalloproteases, nitric oxide, and interleukin-6.* International Society for the Study of the Lumbar Spine Annual meeting, June 21–25, Seattle, Washington.
54. Kawakami M, Weinstein JN, Chatani K, Spratt KF, Meller ST, Gebhart GF (1994): Experimental lumbar radiculopathy: behavioral and histological changes in a model of radicular pain after spinal nerve root irritation with chromic gut ligatures in the rat. Part II. *Spine* 19(16):1795–1802.
55. Kawakami M, Weinstein JN, Spratt KF, Chatani K, Traub RJ, Meller ST, GF Gebhart (1994): Experimental lumbar radiculopathy: immunohistochemical and quantitative demonstrations of pain induced by lumbar nerve root irritation of the rat. Part I. *Spine* 19(16):1780–1794.
56. Keele CA, Armstrong D (1964): *Substances producing pain and itch.* London: Edward Arnold Ltd.
57. Khan AA, Raja SN, Campbell JN, et al. (1986): Bradykinin sensitizes nociceptors to heat stimuli. *Soc Neurosci Abst* 12:219.
58. Konno S, Olmarker K, Byrod G, Rydevik B, Kikuchi S (1994): *Intermittent cauda equina compression. An experimental study on the porcine cauda equina with analyses of nerve impulse conduction properties.* International Society for the Study of the Lumbar Spine Annual meeting, June 21–25, Seattle, Washington.
59. Kumazawa T, Mizumura K (1977): The polymodal receptors in the testis of dog. *Brain Res* 136:553–558.
60. Kwan MK, Rydevik BL, Brown R, et al. (1988): *Selected biomechanical assessment of lumbosacral spinal nerve roots.* Presented at the meeting of the International Society for the Study of the Lumbar Spine, April, Miami, Florida.
61. Leah JD, Cameron AA, Kelly WL, et al. (1985): Coexistence of peptide immunoreactivity in sensory neurons of the cat. *Neuroscience* 16:683–690.
62. Lee Y, Takami K, Kawai Y, et al. (1985): Distribution of calcitonin gene-related peptide in the rat peripheral nervous system with reference to its coexistence with substance P. *Neuroscience* 15:1227–1237.
63. Levine JD, Gooding J, Donatoni P, et al. (1985): The role of the polymorphonuclear leukocyte in hyperalgesia. *J Neurosci* 5:3025–3029.
64. Levine JD, Lam D, Taiwo YO, et al. (1986): Hyperalgesic properties of 15-lipoxygenase products of arachidonic acid. *Proc Natl Acad Sci USA* 83:5331–5334.
65. Lieberman AR (1976): Sensory ganglia. In: London DN, ed. *The peripheral nerve.* London: Chapman & Hall, pp. 188–278.
66. Lindblom K, Rexed B (1948): Spinal nerve injury in dorso-lateral protrusions of lumbar disks. *J Neurosurg* 5:413–432.
67. Loewi O (1921): Über humorale Übertragbarkeit der Herznervenwirkung. *Arch Gen Physiol* 193:201–213.
68. Lotz M, Carson DA, Vaughan JH (1987): Substance P activation of rheumatoid synoviocytes: neural pathway in pathogenesis of arthritis. *Science* 235:893–895.
69. Lundberg JM, Franco-Cereceda A, Hua X, et al. (1985): Coexistence of substance P and calcitonin gene-related peptide-like

immunoreactivities in sensory nerves in relation to cardiovascular and bronchoconstrictor effects of capsaicin. *Eur J Pharmacol* 108:315–319.

70. Lundborg G, Myers R, Powell H (1983): Nerve compression injury and increased endoneurial fluid pressure: a "miniature compartment syndrome." *J Neurol Neurosurg Psychiatry* 46:1119–1124.

71. Lundborg G, Rydevik B (1973): Effects of stretching the tibial nerve of the rabbit: a preliminary study of the intraneural circulation and the barrier function of the perineurium. *J Bone Joint Surg* [Br] 55:390–401.

72. Macnab I (1972): The mechanism of spondylogenic pain. In: Hirsch C, Zotterman Y, eds. *Cervical pain.* Oxford: Pergamon Press, pp. 88–95.

73. Malinsky J (1959): The ontogenetic development of nerve terminations in the intervertebral discs of man. *Acta Anat* (Basel) 38: 96–113.

74. Martin HA, Basbaum AI, Kwiat GC, et al. (1987): Leukotriene and prostaglandin sensitization of cutaneous high-threshold C- and A-delta mechanonociceptors in the hairy skin of rat hindlimbs. *Neuroscience* 22:651–659.

75. McCarron RF, Wimpee MW, Hudkins PG, et al. (1987): The inflammatory effect of nucleus pulposus: a possible element in the pathogenesis of low-back pain. *Spine* 12:760–764.

76. Melzack R, Wall PD (1965): Pain mechanisms: a new theory. *Science* 150:971–979.

77. Mense S (1977): Nervous outflow from skeletal muscle following chemical noxious stimulation. *J Physiol* 267:75–88.

78. Mense S (1981): Sensitization of group IV muscle receptors to bradykinin by 5-hydroxytryptamine and prostaglandin E_2. *Brain Res* 225:95–105.

79. Mense S, Schmidt RF (1974): Activation of group IV afferent units from muscle by analgesic agents. *Brain Res* 72:305–310.

80. Merskey, H (1979): Pain terms: a list with definitions and notes on usage. Recommended by the IASP subcommittee on taxonomy. *Pain* 6:249.

81. Meyer RA, Raja SN, Campbell JN, et al. (1985): Neural activity originating from a neuroma in the baboon. *Brain Res* 325:255–260.

82. Nagy JI, Daddona PE (1985): Anatomical and cytochemical relationships of adenosine deaminase-containing primary afferent neurons in the rat. *Neuroscience* 15:799–813.

83. Nordin M, Nystrom B, Wallin U, et al. (1984): Ectopic sensory discharges and paresthesia in patients with disorders of peripheral nerves, dorsal roots and dorsal columns. *Pain* 20:231–245.

84. Ochoa J, Fowler TJ, Gilliatt RW (1972): Anatomical changes in peripheral nerves compressed by a pneumatic tourniquet. *J Anat* 113:433–455.

85. Ochs S, Worth RM (1978): Axoplasmic transport in normal and pathological systems. In: Waxman SG, ed. *Physiology and pathobiology of axons.* New York: Raven Press, pp. 251–264.

86. O'Donohue TL, Massari VJ, Pazoles CJ, et al. (1984): A role for bombesin in sensory processing in the spinal cord. *J Neurosci* 4: 2956–2962.

87. Olmarker K, Blomquist J, Stromberg J, Nannmark U, Thomsen P, Rydevik B (1994): *Inflammatogenic properties of nucleus pulposus.* International Society for the Study of the Lumbar Spine Annual meeting, June 21–25, Seattle, Washington.

88. Olmarker K, Holm S, Hansson T, et al. (1986): Experimental graded compression of the pig cauda equina: effects of nerve root nutrition. Presented at the meeting of the International Society for the Study of the Lumbar Spine, May, Dallas, Texas.

89. Olmarker K, Rydevik B, Holm S, et al. (1989): Effects of experimental graded compression on blood-flow in spinal nerve roots. *J Orthop Res* 7:817–823.

90. Olsson Y (1972): The involvement of vasa nervorum in disease of peripheral nerves. In: Vinken PS, Bruyn GW, eds. *Handbook of clinical neurology: vol. 12, part 2, Vascular disease of the nervous system.* New York: American Elsevier, pp. 644–664.

91. Panula P, Hadjiconstantinou M, Yang HY, et al. (1983): Immunohistochemical localization of bombesin/gastrin-releasing peptide and substance P in primary sensory neurons. *J Neurosci* 3: 2021–2129.

92. Parke WW (1982): Applied anatomy of the spine. In: Rothman RH, Simeone F, eds. *The spine,* 2nd ed., vol. 1. Philadelphia: WB Saunders.

93. Pateromichelakis S, Rood JP (1981): Prostaglandin E_2 increases mechanically evoked potentials in the peripheral nerve. *Experientia* 37:282–284.

94. Pateromichelakis S, Rood JP (1982): Prostaglandin E_1-induced sensitization of A-δ moderate pressure mechanoreceptors. *Brain Res* 232:89–96.

95. Payan DG, McGillis JP, Goetzl EJ (1986): Neuroimmunology. *Adv Immunol* 39:299–323.

96. Payan DG, McGillis JP, Renold FK, et al. (1987): Neuropeptide modulation of leukocyte function. *Ann NY Acad Sci* 496:182–191.

97. Pedersen HE, Blunck CF, Gardner E: Anatomy of lumbosacral posterior rami and meningeal branches of spinal nerves (sinu-vertebral nerves) with experimental study of their functions. *J Bone Joint Surg* [Am] 38:377–391.

98. Pedowitz RA, Rydevik BL, Hargens AR, et al. (1988): Motor and sensory nerve root conduction deficit induced by acute graded compression of the pig cauda equina. *Trans Orthop Res Soc* 13: 134.

99. Ralston HJ III, Miller MR, Kasahara M (1960): Nerve endings in human fasciae, tendons, ligaments, periosteum, and joint synovial membrane. *Anat Rec* 136:137–147.

100. Rasminsky M (1978): Ectopic generation of impulses and cross-talk in spinal nerve roots of "dystrophic" mice. *Ann Neurol* 3: 351–357.

101. Reeh PW (1990): Sensory receptors in a mammalian skin-nerve in vitro preparation. *Prog Brain Res* (in press).

102. Renshaw B, Therman PO (1941): Excitation of intraspinal mammalian axons by nerve impulses in adjacent axons. *Am J Physiol* 133:96–105.

103. Roofe PG (1940): Innervation of the annulus fibrosus and posterior longitudinal ligament. *Arch Neurol Psych* 44:100–103.

104. Ruda MA, Coffield J, Dubner R (1984): Demonstration of postsynaptic opioid modulation of thalamic projection neurons by the combined techniques of retrograde horseradish peroxidase and enkephalin immunocytochemistry. *J Neurosci* 4:2117–2132.

105. Rydevik B, Brown MD, Lundborg G (1984): Pathoanatomy and pathophysiology of nerve root compression. *Spine* 9:7–15.

106. Rydevik B, Lundborg G, Bagge U (1981): Effects of graded compression on intraneural blood flow: an in vivo study on rabbit tibial nerve. *J Hand Surg* 6:3–12.

107. Rydevik B, Lundborg G, Nordborg C (1976): Intraneural tissue reactions induced by internal neurolysis: an experimental study on the blood-nerve barrier, connective tissues and nerve fibres of rabbit tibial nerve. *Scand J Plast Reconst Surg Hand Surg* 10:3–8.

108. Rydevik B, McLean WG, Sjostrand J, et al. (1980): Blockage of axonal transport induced by acute, graded compression of the rabbit vagus nerve. *J Neurol Neurosurg Psychiatry* 43:690–698.

109. Rydevik BL, Myers RR, Powell HC (1989): Pressure increase in the dorsal root ganglion following mechanical compression. *Spine* 14(6):574–576.

110. Rydevik B, Nordborg C (1980): Changes in nerve function and nerve fibre structure induced by acute, graded compression. *J Neurol Neurosurg Psychiatry* 43:1070–1082.

111. Saal JD, Dobrow R, White AH, Goldthwaite N, Franson R (1989): Biochemical evidence of inflammation in discogenic lumbar radiculopathy: analysis of phospholipase A_2 activity in human herniated disc. Presented at the International Society for the Study of the Lumbar Spine meeting, May, Kyoto, Japan.

112. Schonstrom N, Bolender NF, Spengler DM, et al. (1984): Pressure changes within the cauda equina following constriction of the dural sac: an in vitro experimental study. *Spine* 9:604–607.

113. Seltzer Z, Devor M (1979): Ephaptic transmission in chronically damaged peripheral nerves. *Neurology* 29:1061–1064.

114. Seybold VS, Elde RP (1982): Neurotensin immunoreactivity in the superficial laminae of the dorsal horn of the rat: I. Light microscopic studies of cell bodies and proximal dendrites. *J Comp Neurol* 105:89–100.

115. Shantha TR, Evans JA (1972): The relationship of epidural anesthesia to neural membranes and arachnoid villi. *Anesthesiology* 37(5):543–557.

116. Sharpless SK (1975): *Susceptibility of spinal roots to compression block: the research status of spinal manipulative therapy.* In: Goldstein M, ed. NINCDS monograph no. 15. Government Printing Office, 155–161.

117. Sherman MS (1963): The nerves of bone. *J Bone Joint Surg* [Am] 45:522–528.

118. Shinohara H (1970): Lumbar disc lesion with special reference to the histological significance of nerve endings of the lumbar discs. *J Jpn Orthop Assoc* 44:553–570.

119. Smyth MJ, Wright V (1958): Sciatica and the intervertebral disc: an experimental study. *J Bone Joint Surg* [Am] 40:1401–1418.

120. Spencer DL, Irvin GS, Miller JA (1983): Anatomy and significance of fixation of the lumbosacral nerve roots in sciatica. *Spine* 8:672–679.

121. Spencer DL, Mailler JA, Bertolini JE (1984): The effect of intervertebral disc space narrowing on the contact force between the nerve root and a simulated disc protrusion. *Spine* 9:422–426.

122. Sunderland S (1975): Avulsion of nerve roots. In: Vinken PJ, Bruyn GW, eds. *Handbook of clinical neurology: vol 25, part I, Injuries of the spine and spinal cord.* New York: American Elsevier, pp. 393–435.

123. Sunderland S (1978): Nerve and nerve injuries. In: *Peripheral sensory mechanism,* 2nd ed. New York: Churchill Livingstone.

124. Sunderland S, Bradley KC (1961): Stress-strain phenomena in human peripheral nerve trunks. *Brain* 84:102–119.

125. Sunderland S, Bradley KC (1961): Stress-strain phenomena in human spinal nerve roots. *Brain* 84:120–124.

126. Szolcsanyi J (1987): Selective responsiveness of polymodal nociceptors of the rabbit ear to capsaicin, bradykinin and ultra-violet irradiation. *J Physiol* 388:9–23.

127. Tuchscherer MM, Knox C, Seybold VS (1987): Substance P and cholecystokinin like immunoreactive varicosities in somatosensory and autonomic regions of the rat spinal cord: a quantitative study of coexistence. *J Neurosci* 7:3984–3995.

128. Tuchscherer MM, Seybold VS (1985): Immunohistochemical studies of substance P, cholecystokinin-octapeptide and somatostatin in dorsal root ganglia of the rat. *Neuroscience* 14:593–605.

129. Tuchscherer MM, Seybold VS (1989): A quantitative study of the coexistence of peptides in the varicosities within the superficial laminae of the dorsal horn of the rat spinal cord. *J Neurosci* 9: 195–205.

130. Wall PD, Devor M (1983): Sensory afferent impulses originate from dorsal root ganglia as well as from the periphery in normal and nerve injured rats. *Pain* 17:321–339.

131. Wall PD, Melzack R (1984): *Textbook of pain,* 1st ed. New York: Churchill Livingstone, 1–15.

132. Watanabe R, Parke WW (1986): Vascular and neural pathology of lumbosacral spinal stenosis. *J Neurosurg* 64:64–70.

133. Weinstein JN, Claverie W, Gibson S (1988): The pain of discography. *Spine* 13:1344–1348.

134. Weinstein JN, McLain RF (1994): Orthopaedic surgery. In: Wall P, Melzack, R, eds. *The third edition on pain.* New York: Churchill Livingstone.

135. Weinstein JN, Pope M, Schmidt R, Seroussi R (1988): Neuropharmacologic effects of vibration on the dorsal root ganglion. An animal model. *Spine* 13(5):521–525.

136. Wiesenfeld-Hallin Z, Hokfelt T, Lundberg JM, et al. (1984): Immunoreactive calcitonin gene-related peptide and substance P coexist in sensory neurons to the spinal cord and interact in spinal behavioral responses of the rat. *Neurosci Lett* 52:199–204.

137. Willcockson WS, Chung JM, Hori Y, et al. (1984): Effects of iontophoretically released peptides on primate spinothalamic tract cells. *J Neurosci* 4:741–750.

138. Wilson CB, Ehni G, Grollmus J (1971): Neurogenic intermittent claudication. *Clin Neurosurg* 18:62–85.

139. Wiltse LL, Kirkaldy-Willis WH, McIvor GW (1976): The treatment of spinal stenosis. *Clin Orthop* 115:83–91.

140. Wyke BD (1980): The neurology of low back pain. In: Jayson MIV, ed. *The lumbar spine and back pain,* 2nd ed. Kent: Pitman Medical, p. 265.

141. Wyke B (1982): Receptor systems in lumbosacral tissues in relation to the production of low back pain. In: White AA III, Gordon SL, eds. *American Academy of Orthopaedic Surgeons symposium on idiopathic low back pain.* St. Louis: CV Mosby, pp. 97–107.

142. Yaksh TL, Jessell TM, Gamse R, et al. (1980): Intrathecal morphine inhibits substance P release from mammalian spinal cord in vivo. *Nature* 286:155–157.

143. Yoshizawa H, Morita T, Kobayashi S, Nakai S (1994): *Chronic nerve root compression—pathophysiological mechanism of nerve root dysfunction.* International Society for the Study of the Lumbar Spine Annual Meeting, June 21–25, Seattle, Washington.

The Adult Spine: Principles and Practice,
2nd edition, J.W. Frymoyer, Editor-in-Chief.
Lippincott-Raven Publishers, Philadelphia © 1997.

CHAPTER **24**

Orthoses for Treatment of Cervical and Low Back Disorders

Malcolm H. Pope, Marianne Magnusson, Aaron J. Sandler, and Jiri Dvořák

HISTORICAL OVERVIEW

Mankind has been bracing backs for millennia, though the devices used have undergone many revisions. Lumbosacral corsets have probably been in use at least since the Minoan period, around the year 2000 B.C. (24). Women have used corsets for almost as long, to improve their figures. In the sixteenth century, Vesalius condemned the practice because of adverse effects on the abdominal viscera. During the latter part of the nineteenth century and the early twentieth century, corsets became widely advocated: "Wilson's magnetic appliances cure 90% of cases; Cure without medicine: No cure no pay" (44).

More rigid braces date back to Paul of Aegina in 500 A.D., who attempted to correct scoliosis by bandages and

M. H. Pope, D.M.Sc., Ph.D.: Iowa Spine Research Center, University of Iowa Hospitals and Clinics, Iowa City, Iowa, 52242.

M. L. Magnusson, Dr.Med.Sc.: Assistant Professor, Department of Orthopaedic Surgery, The University of Iowa Hospitals and Clinics, 200 Hawkins Drive, Iowa City, Iowa 52242-1088.

A. Sandler, B.S.: Spine Unit, Schulthess Clinic, Lengghalde 2, 8008 Zurich, Switzerland.

J. Dvořák, M.D., P.D.: Spine Unit, Schulthess Hospital, 8008 Zürich, Switzerland.

splints, and Ambroise Paré, who used a metal cuirass padded with rags. Sayre (67) popularized the use of plaster of Paris casts. The concept has undergone many revisions since then (45), and today there are more than 30 different types of back supports available for the care of spinal disorders (4,57). With the increase of back problems (7), so has there been an increase in use of these orthoses.

Back supports have enjoyed great acceptance by physicians. More than 99% of 3,410 orthopedic surgeons responding to a survey stated that they used supports for low back pain (LBP) sufferers (63). Usage of supports has increased to the point that 250,000 corsets were prescribed in Britain in a 1-year period (4). Deyo and Tsui-Wu (17) found that 27% of LBP patients use corsets or braces. Ahlgren and Hansen (1) showed that 75% of patients were still wearing corsets 4 years after they were prescribed. Indeed, some patients wear corsets for up to 20 years in the belief that they would not survive without them. Some patients are still provided with a spinal support as a placebo or because other measures have failed (34).

Recently, lifting belts, or, more properly, back supports, have been widely promoted as a prevention for both primary and secondary LBP (47).

Such widespread use of corsets and braces suggests the

need for a thorough understanding of their functions and applications in order to determine how and under what conditions to use them, what they can do and where they fall short, how they can help, and where, if misused or overused, they can cause problems.

CLASSIFICATION OF ORTHOSES

A convenient classification system would include:

1. Cervical orthoses
2. Trochanteric belts
3. Sacroiliac and lumbosacral belts
4. Corsets
5. Rigid braces
6. Hyperextension braces
7. Molded jackets
8. Lifting belts (back supports)

Cervical Orthoses

Cervical orthoses are used to provide neck stability for patients with various disorders in a number of circumstances including postsurgically, posttraumatically, and

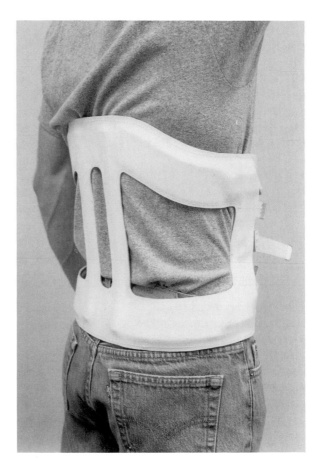

FIG. 2. The Knight or chair-back brace.

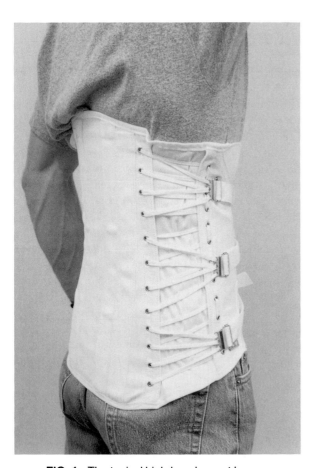

FIG. 1. The typical high-laced corset brace.

to stabilize an instability before, after, or instead of surgery.

A number of different models of orthoses are available, varying in cost, comfort, and design. Some of them appear to provide more stability than others, but most physicians rely on their own assessment of the orthoses; there are few studies that attempt to consider quantitatively the relative merits of different collars. Most often, the soft collar, the Philadelphia collar, the Philadelphia collar with extension, and the sterno-occipital mandibular immobilization (SOMI) device are utilized.

Trochanteric Belts

The trochanteric belt goes around the pelvis between the trochanter and iliac crests. The belt, which is usually between 5 and 8 cm wide, buckles at the front. The belt is usually prescribed for sacroiliac joint pain and pelvic fractures.

Sacroiliac and Lumbosacral Belts

The so-called sacroiliac (SI) belt and lumbosacral belt are usually made of heavy cotton reinforced by lightweight stays. They differ in width, the sacroiliac belt being 10 to 15 cm wide and the lumbosacral belt being 20 to 30 cm wide. Pressure is applied by means of the adjustable laces on the side or back. The sacroiliac belt is meant to prevent SI motion by squeezing the joints together. In practice, both belts are prescribed for LBP.

Corsets

Corsets (Fig. 1) usually extend over the buttocks and often have shoulder straps. Corsets have stays to provide rigidity, and laces at the back, side, or front. The shorter corsets are usually prescribed for LBP, whereas the longer corsets are used for problems in the mid thoracic and lower thoracic spine.

Rigid Braces

The rigid brace usually consists of posterior uprights contoured to the lumbar spine and often has pelvic and thoracic bands. Anterior pressure is applied by fabric and straps. Typical braces of this type are the Williams and Knight braces (Fig. 2). Both are usually prescribed for LBP or segmental instability. The Knight brace (chair-

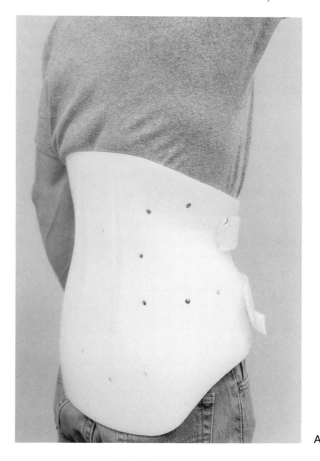

A

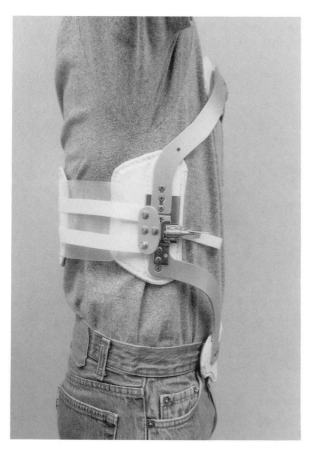

FIG. 3. The Jewett hyperextension brace.

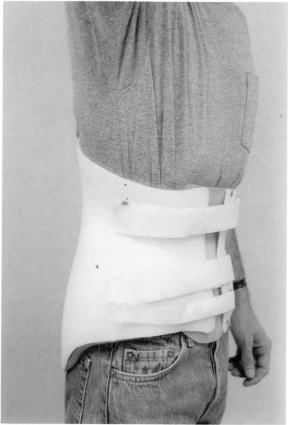

B

FIG. 4. Low, molded, anterior opening orthosis.

back type) functions to immobilize the lumbar spine in a neutral position. The Williams brace has no vertical uprights in the middle of the back and thus the low back can be pushed into flexion. The Raney flexion jacket, which reduces lumbar lordosis and holds the patient in pelvic tilt, is also commonly prescribed.

Hyperextension Braces

The anterior hyperextension brace (Taylor or Jewett) employs an anterior rectangular metal frame to apply pressure over the pubis and upper sternum, and counterpressure is applied at about the T-10 level (Fig. 3). It is designed to prevent excessive flexion and is often used for anterior compression fractures.

Molded Jackets

These devices were previously made from plaster of Paris, but molded plastic is now more commonly used (Fig. 4). Although the pressure is widely supported over the skin surfaces, local abrasion can be a problem. Some jackets are flexible and have anterior straps to provide

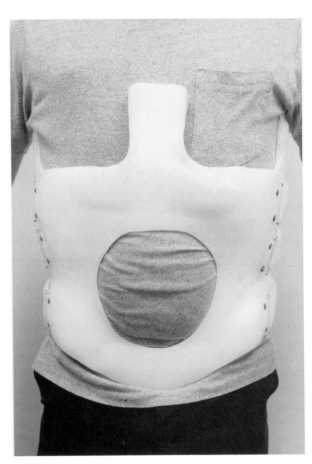

FIG. 6. Molded orthosis designed to increase hyperextension.

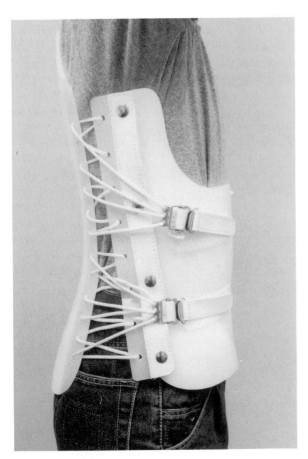

FIG. 5. Two-piece molded orthosis with adjustable side-lacing.

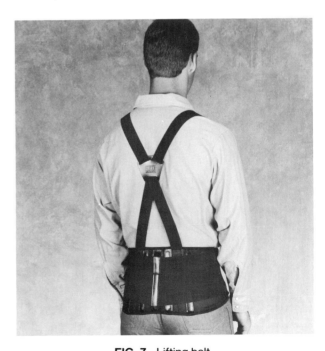

FIG. 7. Lifting belt.

access and support. These have been modified to provide greater flexibility in application (Fig. 5) or to provide hyperextension (Fig. 6).

Lifting Belts (Back Supports)

Like the SI belt, these differ in size. They are made of cloth and are without stays, but they sometimes have a lordosis pad (Fig. 7).

CLINICAL UTILIZATION

Rationale

Depending on the type chosen, braces and corsets may be designed to immobilize or support the spine in a neutral or upright, hyperextended, flexed, or sideways leaning position. Bracing of the lower back may be provided for LBP, trauma (e.g., fractures), infections, muscular weakness, and occasionally, metabolic bone disease such as osteoporosis. The majority of supports or braces, however, are prescribed for idiopathic LBP, prior to surgery or following the failure of surgery (51). Lucas (45) suggests that the objectives of spinal bracing are (a) control of pain, (b) protection from further injury, (c) assistance for muscle weakness, and (d) prevention and correction of deformity. Hipps (34) proposed that corsets and braces may promote a conditioned reflex and response reaction, which will develop tone and strength in weak abdominal muscles, improve patient posture, and decrease motion, thereby lessening pain. Million et al. (50) believed that the principal mechanism of symptom relief was the restriction of motion. Bugge and Biering-Sørensen (8) have suggested that proprioceptive stimuli, local temperature elevation, and an increased feeling of safety in braces may help LBP sufferers.

However, the most common rationale is that lumbar corsets and braces compress the abdomen, resulting in increased intra-abdominal pressure, which unloads the vertebral column itself (12,52–54). The topic of intra-abdominal pressure (IAP) is discussed further below.

TABLE 1. *Relation between subjective relief and type of corset*

| | Subjective relief | | | |
| | Excellent or good (%) | | Slight or negligible (%) | |
Type	Women	Men	Women	Men
Elastic (low)	7 (30)	7 (47)	16 (70)	8 (53)
Semirigid				
Low	5 (28)	5 (39)	13 (72)	8 (61)
High	16 (48)	2 (20)	17 (52)	8 (80)
Total	28 (38)	14 (37)	46 (62)	24 (63)

TABLE 2. *When did you last wear the corset?*

	Women (%)	Men (%)	All (%)
During the past week	32 (43)	13 (34)	45 (40)
2–4 weeks ago	13 (18)	9 (23)	22 (19)
1–2 months ago	10 (13)	4 (11)	14 (13)
3–4 months ago	8 (11)	6 (16)	14 (13)
6–9 months ago	3 (4)	2 (5)	5 (4)
9 months ago	8 (11)	4 (11)	12 (11)
Total	74 (100)	38 (100)	112 (100)

Clinical Trials

There is no unanimity of opinion among clinicians regarding the use of corsets and braces. Mooney and Cairns (51) state that they use lumbosacral supports in about 5% of outpatient care programs as an aid in controlling the acute problem. They do not advocate their use in chronic LBP. On the other hand, Alaranta and Hurri (2) suggest that a corset is in fact a reasonable therapy with patients with chronic LBP. A corset was found to be less expensive than other treatments. Likewise, Amundsen and Weber (5) found that the use of a three-point corset led to improved function in 53% of their patients with chronic LBP. However, the numbers were small and no control group was used. In an interesting study, Coxhead et al. (13) found greater improvement in patients who used four different simultaneous treatment modalities (including corsets) compared to those who received fewer treatment modalities, although this benefit was not sustained. Similarly, Larsson et al. (42) found that five simultaneous modalities worked better in the short run than either corset or bed rest alone. Noncomparative studies by Willner (75) support selected use of corsets.

Alaranta and Hurri (2) retrospectively studied 113 Finnish LBP patients. Thirty-seven percent of respondents claimed excellent or good relief from corsets. As shown in Table 1, men preferred the low, semirigid model. As shown in Table 2, the respondents had worn the corset quite recently.

Very few prospective trials have been reported. In a multicenter study, 456 British LBP patients were randomized into groups for treatment by manipulation, corset, physical therapy, or analgesics (20). There was no difference between groups at 3 and 6 weeks, 3 months, and 1 year. However, it was concluded that the corset alone was as effective as other treatments, less expensive than manipulation and physical therapy, and safer than drugs. Million et al. (50) found that spinal support (metal stays) in a lumbosacral corset was important in relieving symptoms. These investigators randomly allocated patients to a corset with or without support. Objective measures (straight-leg raising, lateral bend, flexion) did not differ between the groups, but subjective measures did.

Haugh et al. (33) conducted a 3-week randomized controlled clinical trial of transcutaneous muscle stimulation (TMS) compared to lumbosacral corset on patients with nonspecific, semiacute LBP. An interesting feature of this study was that a heat-sensitive compliance meter was sewn into the corset in an effort to measure compliance. Both treatment groups increased their muscle strength (assessed by maximum isometric extension contractions) by significant amounts and increased their fatigue times by insignificant amounts. Neither group changed in extension flexibility, and the difference in flexion flexibility between the groups was not statistically significant. The only group difference that was of statistical significance ($p < 0.05$) was the greater reduction in pain for the TMS group. Hansson et al. (32) reported that insulating corsets were prophylactic against LBP in construction workers.

Reddell et al. (64) completed a very comprehensive study of back belts in airline workers. There were no differences in injury rates between workers and controls. Some workers complained that the belts were too hot or caused soreness and shortness of breath, and they discontinued their use. However, these belts were narrow and did not fit over the pelvis. Also, those workers who lifted the heaviest weights subjectively reported a beneficial effect. Walsh and Schwartz (72) found that a back orthosis significantly decreased time lost from LBP at a follow-up of 6 months in warehouse workers.

It should be noted that the comprehensive Quebec Task Force report (43) concluded that there is no documented evidence to suggest that braces reduce the period of disability. In addition, Flor and Turk (26) concluded that corsets and braces, although widely used, have not been proven effective.

Perhaps the most important consideration is the correct indication. For example, Hipps (34) states that braces are more beneficial when (a) there is a localized area of spasm in an area of LBP, (b) there is a limited range of motion in a certain part of the back, usually in a painful area, and (c) pain occurs or is aggravated by the movements of the spine.

In summary, there are many hypotheses about the mechanism of action of braces and corsets. These include:

1. Increased abdominal pressure may have an analgesic effect.
2. The lower margin of a corset may provide circumferential support around the pelvic ring.
3. There is an unloading effect on the trunk by support through thoracic musculoskeletal structures.
4. They insulate the skin and the increased warmth decreases pain sensation.
5. Increased abdominal pressure results in hydraulic support for the painful back structures.
6. They physically limit the range of motion of the spine, thus decreasing stress to painful structures in the back.

7. Tactile stimulation from the device results in beneficial modification of muscle action, with decreased stress on the back.

Negative Aspects

In spite of the wide clinical use of back supports, their use is not without drawbacks. There is a possible loss of muscle function and psychological addiction to the device (69). These concerns are voiced by many clinicians, although neither of these effects has been proven. However, according to Kester (37), most patients should be able to eliminate the corset eventually.

MECHANICAL FUNCTION

The mechanical effects of braces and corsets have been measured by a variety of techniques.

Electromyography

Waters and Morris (73) found that while the subject was standing, both the chair-back brace and a corset slightly decreased or did not change erector spinae electromyographic activity (EMG). An inflatable corset reduced EMG, particularly during heavy load lifting. In slow or moderate walking, the EMG activity was increased if a rigid brace was worn. Similarly, Lumsden and Morris (46) found that a rigid brace actually increased intersegmental motion in rotation. Thus, the muscle activity might be an attempt to prevent the segmental rotation. Other investigations have produced equivocal results: Grew and Deane (29) and Morris and Lucas (53) noted decreased EMG activity with corsets, while Waters and Morris (73) and Nachemson et al. (56) found both increases and decreases depending on the task.

Magnusson and Pope (47), in a study of lifting set at the level of the new NIOSH guidelines, found that a back support reduced dorsal EMG, increased spine height, and was associated with subjective assessments of improved stability and enhanced lifting capacity.

Intradiscal Pressure

Nachemson and Morris (55) measured the intradiscal pressure (IDP) under a variety of circumstances. Subjects who experienced pain during different activities were found to have increased IDP. This supports the view that these patients have greater muscle contraction as a result of the muscles splinting the spine. Likewise, a Valsalva maneuver (a voluntary increase in intra-abdominal pressure with muscle contraction) actually increased IDP. Alternatively, an inflatable corset decreased the IDP by 25%.

Intra-abdominal Pressure

The abdominal cavity, as well as the thoracic cavity, is pressurized to a greater extent when the spine is placed under increased load (6,15,23,41). This cavity pressure has long been conjectured to decrease spinal loading by introducing an extension moment across the lumbar spine which reduces the tension required in the posterior spinal muscles. Based on controlled testing, however, Krag et al. (39) have shown that voluntary pressurization of the abdominal cavity causes the opposite effect, namely an increase of dorsal muscle activity.

Harman et al. (30) found that weight lifters who used a weight lifters' belt produced both a greater peak and a faster rise in IAP than without the belt. The authors concluded that a lifting belt increases IAP and reduces disc pressure.

Morris et al. (54) found that an inflatable corset increases the resting abdominal cavity pressure by about 10 to 15 mm Hg, but it does not raise the peak pressures during a controlled lift. Grew and Deane (29) concluded that over the period of treatment, a patient becomes accustomed to the brace or corset. It was suggested that when the spine is lightly stressed, the support reduces the activity of the abdominal muscles. Under stressful activity the brace strengthens the wall and enables the wearer to increase the IAP.

Krag et al. (38) compared lumbosacral corsets and Raney plastic jackets to no support in normal volunteers. They demonstrated that no significant effects were produced by either device, either for IAP or erector spinae EMG, during isometric extension efforts. Finally, Kumar and Godfrey (41) conducted a comparative evaluation of six commonly prescribed spinal supports. Volunteers were fitted with sacroiliac belt, lumbosacral corset, and Harris, Macnab, Knight, and Taylor braces in turn and were asked to perform sagittal, lateral, and oblique lifts, and same-level side-to-side weight transfers. The results show no significant difference in intra-abdominal pressure from different spinal supports in all activities studied. They concluded that there is no significant difference between the braces studied, as measured by IAP.

Motion

Most of these studies have been conducted for cervical orthoses. It is important that the prescribing physician understand the differences between the devices in order to make an informed judgment about which level of support is required and to provide the most cost-effective and comfortable solution for a given patient with a specific problem.

Many of the studies that do exist are primarily concerned with extrication collars and are therefore geared more toward emergency medical technicians than to specialists treating spinal disorders (48,65,71). It is generally accepted that soft collars provide little immobilization (10,31,36,58), but few studies have specifically compared them to hard collars, and many of these studies considered only flexion/extension motion (3,10,71) and lateral bending (48).

A recent study by Rosen et al. (65) used two different goniometric techniques and reported differences between the two techniques of up to 100% for flexion/extension measurements. Rosen et al. also emphasized emergency collars, not mentioning the soft collar or the SOMI brace, two widely used orthoses. Another study used a combination of roentgenograms and overhead photographs made at the extremes of active motion (36). Although over 15 years old, this study compared normal motion and several still widely used orthoses including the soft collar, the Philadelphia collar, and the SOMI brace. The results showed that the soft collar allowed 74% of normal flexion/extension, 83% of rotation, and 92% of lateral bending. The Philadelphia collar allowed 29%, 44%, and 66%, and the SOMI allowed 28%, 34%, and 66%, respectively. However, the study reports measurements taken only at the extremes of active motion, and it has the potential disadvantage of understating the amount of motion because the subject must hold his or her hand in an extreme position while the x-ray or photograph was taken. A newer technique allowing accurate measurements both passively and actively throughout the range of motion in real time is preferred, as it provides a better picture of the total range of motion (Table 3).

Sandler et al. (66) in a recent study compared the amount of motion allowed by four different orthoses with the amount of unrestricted neck motion in vivo (21,22) and found that there were no large differences between the collars, and that the collars did not restrict motion as much as previously reported.

They concluded that cervical orthoses do not provide a high level of mechanical restriction of motion but can be helpful for other reasons.

The efficacy of lumbar spinal braces in reducing lumbar intervertebral movements has been questioned by Norton and Brown (61). While gross movements are prevented, individual vertebral movements are sometimes increased. These investigators concluded that it was highly unlikely that any device applied to the exterior of the body can effectively splint the lumbosacral region. Lumsden and Morris (46) found a modified chair-back brace to be quite effective in restricting motion in standing, whereas a corset was quite ineffective. When the subject was walking, both the brace and the corset actually increased the axial rotation in the lumbar spine.

On the other hand, Fidler and Plasmans (25), on the basis of radiographic studies, state that corsets and braces do, in fact, decrease motion. Grew and Deane (29) concluded that in order to reduce spinal movements by an appreciable amount, a rigid form of bracing is required,

TABLE 3. *Amount of motion allowed by different cervical orthoses, in percent of unrestricted motion*

	No orthosis		Soft collar		Philadelphia collar		Philadelphia w/extension		SOMI device	
	%	(SD)	%	(SD)	%	(SD)	%	(SD)	%	(SD)
Flexion/extension										
Passive	100	(0)	93	(4)	63	(19)	53	(15)	42	(13)
Active	100	(0)	91	(7)	60	(21)	45	(22)	39	(21)
Axial rotation										
Passive	100	(0)	88	(8)	75	(9)	73	(12)	76	(19)
Active	100	(0)	88	(5)	72	(10)	73	(10)	70	(25)
Lateral bending										
Passive	100	(0)	89	(6)	90	(8)	79	(13)	77	(19)
Active	100	(0)	91	(6)	89	(18)	79	(18)	84	(26)

SD, standard deviation.

although a custom-fitted, less rigid brace is better than a non-custom-fitted, more rigid plastic shell. Corsets were said to provide little restriction of movement, although the location of the stays can enable specific painful movements to be influenced. The shorter corsets restricted movement better than the longer ones.

Temperature

Dixon et al. (18) found that chronic LBP responds as well to the wearing of an insulated belt as to an ordinary corset, and they suggested that the observed increase in lumbar and thoracic skin temperature was the cause of symptom relief.

Similar findings were reported by Grew and Deane (29). The workers found that thicker or padded material over the lumbar skin can be used to raise its temperature by almost 2°C. However, the material must be held in contact with the skin; apparently a rigid plastic jacket has a tendency to provide a cooling "funnel" that reduces its heating effectiveness. Hansson et al. (32) used an insulating corset to raise body temperature.

BIOFEEDBACK

Another proposed mechanism of action is that tactile stimulation from the brace or corset results in behavioral modification of muscle action, therefore improving active spinal support. EMG activity would presumably give evidence to this effect, but available reports are conflicting and show EMG activity to be increased (35), decreased (11), or unchanged (49) in persons with LBP. Two reviews, Dolce and Raczynski (19) and Nouwen (62), were equivocal.

It is accepted that LBP is often caused by mechanical stress (60). Clinical observations indicate that positions of decreased stress such as lying down sometimes improve pain temporarily. However, prolonged bed rest does not appear to help in the long run (16), perhaps because of simultaneous muscle deconditioning, bone loss, and increased degeneration.

Because decreasing stress appears to improve LBP, stress reduction by an orthosis would presumably be desirable. Tactile information from a corset, EMG signal, and inclinometer signal do not provide adequate information about flexion of the trunk, appropriate when standing but not when lying. Forward flexion either at the hips or in the trunk while standing proves a long lever arm for the force of gravity through the low back. With either movement, an inclinometer would be activated. When the trunk is partially flexed, EMG activity is increased, but with full flexion there is electrical silence (28). Holding an object while standing increases force and is countered by increased EMG activity (68,70) but would not activate an inclinometer. Force applied to the spine by the contraction of muscles in spasm (19) would be detected by EMG but not inclinometer.

Treatments involving EMG feedback have been reported as both effective (27,59) and not effective (9) in treating LBP. However, these reports focus on treatments applied for only 1 hour or less each day, in coordination with psychotherapy, rather than for longer treatment periods. Wolf et al. (76) and Nouwen (62) are the only two studies which involved longer periods of feedback; the latter showed no improvements, but the former, albeit dealing with only one patient, reported the treatment was superior. An inclinometer, a promising device for this application, has been used to monitor but not to treat persons with LBP (62). It has successfully improved head posture of children with cerebral palsy (77).

The feedback stimulus must be effective in changing behavior of the orthosis wearer. Feedback has been successfully used in ergonomics (14) applications. Wertsch (74), reviewing substitution of tactile for visual sensation, described auditory and visual feedback to patients with insensate feet but pointed out that stimuli are often ignored. It is apparent that there is some possibility of a specially designed biofeedback orthosis having some potential prevention of excessive forces or postural stresses.

FUTURE DIRECTIONS

Braces and corsets have been used for a very long time, but it is only recently that clinical trials have been run to test their efficacy and experiments proposed to assess their mode of action. The clinical trials that have been published were often not prospective or were poorly controlled and with small numbers of subjects.

It is not clear that present braces or corsets reduce spine load or immobilize the spine. However, the prophylactic use of industrial back supports is promising and deserves more study.

ACKNOWLEDGEMENT. We wish to acknowledge support from the Arbetsmiljöfonden.

REFERENCES

1. Ahlgren SA, Hansen T (1978): The use of lumbosacral corsets prescribed for low back pain. *Prosthet Orthot Int* 2:101–104.
2. Alaranta H, Hurri H (1988): Compliance and subjective relief by corset treatment in chronic low back pain. *Scand J Rehab Med* 20:133–136.
3. Althoff B, Goldie I (1980): Cervical collars in rheumatoid atlanto-axial subluxation: a radiographic comparison. *Ann Rheum Dis* 39:485–489.
4. American Academy of Orthopaedic Surgeons (1952): Braces, splints, show alterations. In: *Orthopaedic appliances atlas*, vol. 1. Ann Arbor: Edwards.
5. Amundsen T, Weber H (1982): Korsett-behandling av kronisk rygg. *Tidsskr Nor Laegeforen* 102:1649–1651
6. Bartelink DL (1957): Role of abdominal pressure in relieving pressure on lumbar intervertebral discs. *J Bone Joint Surg* [Bı] 39:718–725.
7. Benn RT, Wood PH (1975): Pain in the back: an attempt to estimate the size of the problem. *Rheumatol Rehabil* 14:121–128.
8. Bugge PM, Biering-Sørensen F (1987): Lumbar corset treatment. *Ugeskr Laeger* 149:577–579.
9. Bush C, Ditto B, Feuerstein M (1985): A controlled evaluation of paraspinal EMG biofeedback in the treatment of chronic low back pain. *Health Psychol* 4:307–321.
10. Colachis S, Strohm B, Ganter E (1973): Cervical spine motion in normal women: radiographic study of effect of cervical collars. *Arch Phys Med Rehabil* 54:161–169.
11. Collins GA, Cohen MJ, Naliboff BD, Schandler SL (1982): Comparative analysis of paraspinal and frontalis EMG, heart rate and skin conductance in chronic low back pain patients and normals to various postures and stress. *Scand J Rehabil Med* 14:39–46.
12. Coplans CW (1978): Conservative treatment of low back pain. In: Helfet AJ, Grubel LD, eds. *Disorders of the lumbar spine*. Philadelphia: JB Lippincott.
13. Coxhead CE, Inskip H, Meade TW, North WR, Troup JD (1981): Multicentre trial of physiotherapy in the management of sciatic symptoms. *Lancet* 1:1065–1068.
14. Cushman WH, Little RH, Lucas RL, Pugsley RE, Stevens JA (1983): Equipment design. In: Eastman-Kodak Company, Human Factors Section, *Ergonomic design for people at work*, vol. 1. Belmont: Lifetime Learning Publications.
15. Davis PR, Troup JDG (1964): Pressures in the trunk cavities when pulling, pushing and lifting. *Ergonomics* 7:465–474.
16. Deyo RA, Diehl AK, Rosenthal M (1986): How many days of bed rest for acute low back pain? A randomized clinical trial. *N Engl J Med* 315(17):1064–1070.
17. Deyo RA, Tsui-Wu YJ (1987): Descriptive epidemiology of low back pain and its related medical care in the United States. *Spine* 12(3):264–268.
18. Dixon ASJ, Owen-Smith BD, Harrison RA (1972): Cold sensitive, non specific, low back pain (a comparative trial of treatment). *Clin Trials J* 9:16–21.
19. Dolce JJ, Raczynski JM (1985): Neuromuscular activity and electromyography in painful backs. Psychological and biomechanical models in assessment and treatment. *Psychol Bull* 97(3):502–520.
20. Doran DM, Newell DJ (1975): Manipulation in treatment of low back pain: a multicentre study. *Br Med J* 2:161–164.
21. Dvorak J, Vadja E, Panjabi M, Grob D (1994): Normal motion of the lumbar spine as related to age and gender. ESJ (*in press*).
22. Dvorak L, Antinnes J, Panjahi M, Loustalot D, Bonomo M. (1992): Age and gender related normal motion of the cervical spine. *Spine* 17:393–398.
23. Eie N. Wehn P (1962): Measurements of the intra-abdominal pressure in relation to weight bearing of the lumbosacral spine. *J Oslo City Hosp* 12:205–217.
24. Evans A (1921): *The palace of Minos*, vol. 1. London: Macmillan, p. 503.
25. Fidler MW, Plasmans CM (1983): The effect of four types of support on the segmental mobility of the lumbosacral spine. *J Bone Joint Surg* [Am] 65(7):943–947.
26. Flor H, Turk DC (1984): Etiological theories and treatments for chronic back pain. I. Somatic models and interventions. *Pain* 19:105–121.
27. Flor H, Turk DC (1986): Long-term efficacy of EMG biofeedback for chronic rheumatic back pain. *Pain* 27:195–202.
28. Floyd WF, Silver PHS (1955): The function of the erector spinae muscles in certain movements and postures in man. *Physiologist* 129:184–203.
29. Grew ND, Deane G (1982): The physical effect of lumbar spinal supports. *Prosthet Orthot Int* 6:79–87.
30. Harman EA, Rosenstein RM, Frykman PN (1989): Effects of a belt on intra-abdominal pressure during weight lifting. *Med Sci Sports Exerc* 21:186–190.
31. Hartman J, Palumbo F, Hill B (1972): Cineradiology of the braced normal cervical spine. *Clin Orthop* :97–102.
32. Hansson T, Lindström I, Lindell V (1994): *An insulating corset to prevent low back pain*. Stoke, UK: Presented at Low Back Pain Society.
33. Haugh LD, Pope MH, MacDonald LP (1989): *Treatment of semi-acute low back pain by transcutaneous muscle stimulation or lumbosacral corset: a randomized clinical trial*. Presented at FCER meeting, Washington, DC, April.
34. Hipps HE (1967): Back braces: types, functions and how to order and use them. *Med Clin North Am* 51(5):1315–1343.
35. Janda U (1977): Muscle, central nervous motor regulation and a back problem. In: JM Korr, ed. *The neurobiological mechanisms in manipulative therapy*. New York: Plenum Press.
36. Johnson R, Hart D, Simmons E, Ramsby G, Southwick WO (1977): Cervical orthoses: a study comparing their effectiveness in restricting cervical motion in normal subjects. *J Bone Joint Surg* 59A:332–339.
37. Kester NC (1969): Evaluation and medical management of low back pain. *Med Clin North Am* 53(3):525–540.
38. Krag MH, Byrne KB, Miller L, Haugh L, Pope MH (1987): Failure of intra-abdominal pressure to reduce spinal loads without and with lumbar orthoses. *Proceedings of the Orthopedic Research Society, 33rd annual meeting*, San Francisco, CA.
39. Krag MH, Gilbertson L, Pope MH (1985): Intra-abdominal and intra-thoracic pressure effects upon load bearing of the spine (Proc Orthop Res Soc 31st annual meeting, Las Vegas, NV). *Orthop Trans* 9:358.
40. Kumar S, Davis PR (1973): Lumbar vertebral innervation and intra-abdominal pressure. *J Anat* 114:47–53.
41. Kumar S, Godfrey C (1986): Spinal braces and abdominal support. In: Karwowski M, ed. *Trends in ergonomics/human factors* III. New York: Elsevier.

42. Larsson U, Choler U, Lidström A, Lind G, Nachemson A (1980). Autotraction for treatment of lumbago-sciatica. *Acta Orthop Scand* 51:791–798.

43. Le Blanc F, Nachemson A, Norchin M, et al (1987): Scientific approach to the assessment and management of activity related spinal disorders. A monograph for clinicians. Report of the Quebec Task Force on Spinal Disorders. *Spine* 12(7):S1–S59.

44. Lewis L, Smith HJ (1982): *Oscar Wilde discovers America.* New York: Benjamin Blom, by arrangement with Harcourt, Brace and World.

45. Lucas DB (1969): Spinal bracing. In: Licht S, ed. *Orthotics.* Baltimore: Waverly Press, pp. 274–305.

46. Lumsden RM, Morris JM (1968): An in vivo study of axial rotation and immobilization at the lumbosacral joint. *J Bone Joint Surg* [Am] 50:1591–1602.

47. Magnusson M, Pope MH (1994): Does a back support have a positive biomechanical effect? *Appl Ergonom* (submitted).

48. McCabe JB, Nolan DJ. (1986): Comparison of the effectiveness of different cervical immobilization collars. *Ann Emerg Med* 15:50–53.

49. Miller DJ (1985): Comparison of electromyographic activity in the lumbar paraspinal muscles of subjects with and without chronic low back pain. *Phys Ther* 65:1347–1354.

50. Million R, Nilsen KH, Jayson MI, Baker RD (1981): Evaluation of low back pain and assessment of lumbar corsets with and without back supports. *Ann Rheum Dis* 40:449–454.

51. Mooney V, Cairns D (1978): Management in the patient with chronic low back pain. *Orthop Clin North Am* 9(2):543–557.

52. Morris JM (1974): Low back bracing. *Clin Orthop* 102:126–132.

53. Morris JM, Lucas DB (1963): Physiological considerations in bracing of the spine. *Orthop Prosth Appl* 37:44.

54. Morris JM, Lucas DB, Bresler B (1961): Role of the trunk in stability of the spine. *J Bone Joint Surg* [Am] 43:327–351.

55. Nachemson A, Morris JM (1964): In vivo measurements of intradiscal pressure. *J Bone Joint Surg* [Am] 46:1077–1092.

56. Nachemson A, Schultz A, Andersson G (1983): Mechanical effectiveness studies of lumbar spine orthoses. *Scand J Rehabil Med* (Suppl) 9:139–149.

57. Nattress LW, Litt BD (1962): *Report 2: survey to determine the state of services available to amputees and orthopedically disabled persons. Orthotic Services USA–1962.* Washington, DC: American Orthotics and Prosthetics Association.

58. Naylor J, Mulley G (1991): Surgical collars: a survey of their prescription and use. *Br J Rheumatol* 30:282–284.

59. Nigl AJ, Fischer-Williams M (1980): Treatment of low back strain with electromyographic biofeedback and relaxation training. *Psychosomatics* 21:495–499.

60. Nordin M (1982): *Methods for studying work load with special reference to the lumbar spine (thesis).* Goteborg, Sweden.

61. Norton PL, Brown T (1957): The immobilizing efficiency of back braces: their effect on the posture and motion of the lumbosacral spine. *J Bone Joint Surg* [Am] 39:111–139.

62. Nouwen A (1983): EMG biofeedback used to reduce standing levels of paraspinal muscle tension in chronic low back pain. *Pain* 17:353–360.

63. Perry J (1970): The use of external support in the treatment of low-back pain. *J Bone Joint Surg* [Am] 52(7):1440–1442.

64. Reddell CR, Congleton JJ, Huchingson RD, Montgomery JF (1993): An evaluation of a weightlifting belt and back injury prevention training class for airline baggage handlers. *Appl Ergonom* 23:319–329.

65. Rosen P, McSwain N, Arata M, Stahl S, Mercer D (1992): Comparison of two new immobilization collars. *Ann Emerg Med* 21:1189–1195.

66. Sandler A, Dvorak J, Thorsten H, Grob D, Daniels W (1995): The effectiveness of various cervical orthoses. *Spine* (submitted).

67. Sayre LA (1877): *Spinal disease and spinal curvature.* London.

68. Schultz AB, Andersson GB, Haderspeck K, Ortengren R (1982): Analysis and measurement of lumbar trunk loads in tasks involving bends and twists. *J Biomech* 15:669–675.

69. Selby DK (1982): Conservative care of nonspecific low back pain. *Orthop Clin North Am* 13(3):427–437.

70. Seroussi RE, Pope MH (1987): The relationship between trunk muscle electromyography and moments in the sagittal and frontal planes. *Proceedings of the Orthopedic Research Society 33rd annual meeting,* San Francisco, CA.

71. Solot J, Winzelberg G (1990): Clinical and radiological evaluation of vertebrace extrication collars. *J Emerg Med* 8:79–83.

72. Walsh NE, Schwartz RK (1990): The influence of prophylactic orthoses on abdominal strength and low back injury in the workplace. *Am J Phys Med Rehabil* 69:245–250.

73. Waters RL, Morris JM (1970): Effect of spinal supports on the electrical acitivty of muscles of the trunk. *J Bone Joint Surg* [Am] 52:51–60.

74. Wertsch J (1985): *Sensory substitution: state of the art and future technology.* Milwaukee, WI: Proc Clement Zablocky VA Medical Center.

75. Willner S (1985): Effect of a rigid brace on back pain. *Acta Orthop Scand* 56:40–42

76. Wolf SL, Nacht M, Kelly JL (1982): EMG feedback training during dynamic movement for low back pain patients. *Behav Ther* 13:395–406.

77. Woolridge CP, Russell G (1976): Head position training with the cerebral palsied child: application of biofeedback techniques. *Arch Phys Med Rehabil* 57:407–414.

Diagnostic Studies

The Adult Spine: Principles and Practice,
2nd edition, J.W. Frymoyer, Editor-in-Chief.
Lippincott-Raven Publishers, Philadelphia © 1997.

CHAPTER 25

Radiography of Spinal Disorders

Georges Y. El-Khoury and Eric A. Brandser

Despite the advances in imaging technology, plain radiography continues to be the mainstay of any diagnostic investigation for spinal problems. Shortly after Wilhelm Conrad Roentgen discovered x-rays in 1895, medical applications began to proliferate; radiography rapidly moved out of the physics laboratories to become an integral part of the medical profession. A good grasp of the physical principles of radiography is essential for health professionals utilizing this diagnostic modality in the evaluation of spinal disorders. Knowing these principles helps in obtaining high-quality radiographs and in protecting patients and medical staff from unnecessary radiation.

X-rays are a form of ionizing radiation belonging to the electromagnetic spectrum (92). In diagnostic imaging, the most useful components of the electromagnetic spectrum are x-rays and radio waves, both of which travel through the human body (36). Under proper predetermined conditions, x-rays and radio waves carry useful diagnostic information that can be captured by appropriate detectors; this information is then recorded on film or displayed on a television screen for evaluation by physicians. X-rays can be either generated in x-ray tubes or emitted spontaneously from the nuclei of radioactive

substances. Those generated in x-ray tubes are generally used in radiography, fluoroscopy, conventional tomography, and computed tomography (CT). X-rays emitted from radioactive isotopes are used in nuclear medicine and radiation therapy. Radio waves, which are less energetic than x-rays, are used primarily in magnetic resonance imaging (MRI) (36).

In diagnostic x-ray tubes, x-rays are produced when a fast stream of electrons is suddenly stopped by a target called the anode (the positive terminal). The electrons originate on the negative terminal of the tube, which is also called the cathode or filament (Fig. 1). The specific location on the target from which x-rays are emitted is called the focal spot. The size of the focal spot has an inverse relationship to image sharpness. Ideally, the focal spot should be a point source of x-rays in order to produce perfectly sharp images, but because this not physically possible, a reasonably small focal spot is selected for bone work (Fig. 2). Bone has a fine trabecular structure, and since early disease is often reflected as abnormalities of the trabeculae, image quality should be high. In practice, x-ray tubes purchased for bone work should have small focal spots, ranging in size from 0.3 mm to 1.0 mm. The ability of the x-ray tube to achieve high x-ray output is limited by the heat generated at the target or anode. To overcome this problem, the rotating anode was developed and is now universally used. The rotating anode allows the tube to withstand huge accumulations of heat generated during multiple exposures. Both the

G. Y. El-Khoury, M.D., Professor; E. A. Brandser, M.D., Assistant Professor: Department of Radiology, University of Iowa Hospitals and Clinics, Iowa City, Iowa, 52242.

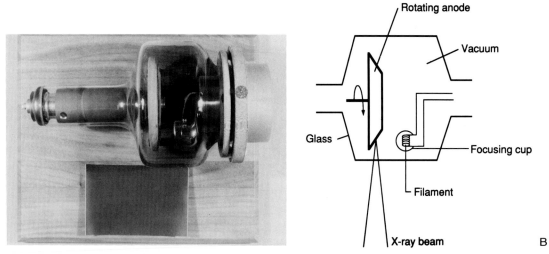

FIG. 1. X-ray tube. **A:** Photograph of an x-ray tube. **B:** Schematic diagram of an x-ray tube. Electrons are emitted from the filament and accelerated across the vacuum, striking the rotating anode. This generates the x-ray beam.

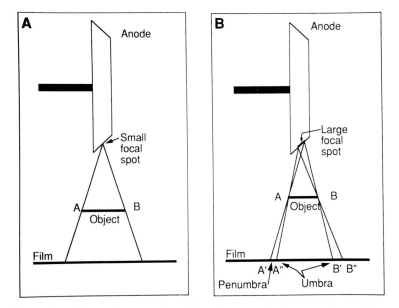

FIG. 2. Effect of focal spot size on image quality. **A:** With a small focal spot, edges of the object recorded on film are very sharp. **B:** With a large focal spot, the edges of an object recorded on film are unsharp. The amount of unsharpness is called the penumbra.

filament and the target are made of tungsten, which has a very high melting point.

After the x-ray beam is emitted from the focal spot, two essential processes manipulate the beam, both qualitatively and quantitatively. These are filtration and collimation. With every exposure, an x-ray beam is emitted that has of a wide spectrum of energies. Low-energy x-rays are not diagnostically useful and are actually harmful to the patient because the majority of these low-energy x-rays are absorbed by the tissues, resulting in cell damage and mutations; low-energy x-rays fail to reach the film or detector with any diagnostic information. Filtration changes the spectrum of energies present within the beam by eliminating low-energy radiation. Casings of x-ray tubes are designed with filters to remove low-energy radiation. Additional filtration is used to improve the quality of the beam, such that mainly high-energy radiation is allowed to reach the patient. Aluminum (1 to 3 mm thickness) is the most commonly used general purpose filter (19). There is a unique use of filters when radiographing the entire spine in patients with scoliosis: filters are used in this situation to equalize the radiographic density on the film when thin and thick body parts such as the chest and the abdomen are being exposed simultaneously.

To protect the public, it is now mandated by law that only the area or region of interest be irradiated during a radiographic examination. Thus, if a fracture is suspected in the cervical spine and the treating physician requests a radiographic examination of the cervical spine, only the cervical spine region would be included on the film. The collimator should be properly coned down limiting the beam to the region of interest. The fact that the collimator has been properly coned down is automatically marked and documented on the film at the time of the exposure. Equipment with malfunctioning collimators cannot be legally used on patients. Collimation also improves the quality of the image by reducing scatter which seriously degrades the image.

Physical principles governing the interaction of x-rays

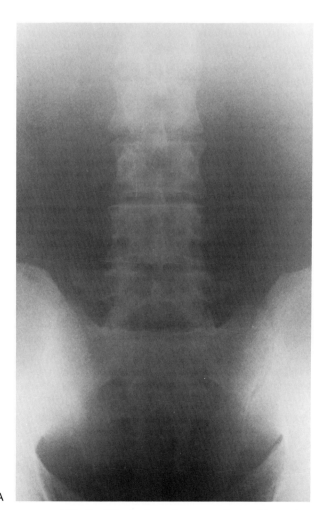
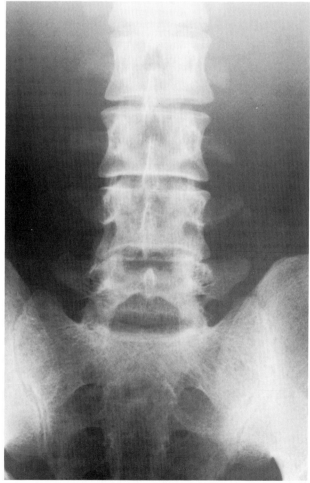

A

B

FIG. 3. Effect of scatter on radiographic quality. **A:** Radiograph of lumbar spine and pelvis phantom obtained without a grid. Note significant loss of bony architectural detail. **B:** Same pelvic phantom imaged with radiographic grid. Bony trabeculae are now visible and overall image quality is improved.

with tissues are complex and beyond the scope of this chapter. Generally, however, the interaction of x-rays with tissues is related to the energy of the x-rays used. High-energy diagnostic x-rays, produced by a high kilovolt setting on the x-ray machine, are generally favored because less radiation is absorbed by the patient; however, high-energy x-rays generate significant scatter, resulting in fuzzy images and diminished tissue contrast on radiographs (48). Without scatter control, especially when the x-rays have to traverse a thick body part such as the abdomen or pelvis, the information content of x-ray images is severely compromised (Fig. 3). Larger field size also results in more scatter and less tissue contrast on the images. Limiting the field size, that is, restricting the size of the beam to cover only the area of interest, achieves two important objectives: it reduces scatter and cuts the radiation dose to the patient.

Careful collimation has already been mentioned as a means to reduce scatter. However, the most effective way to control scatter is with the use of radiographic grids. The radiographic grid is an essential component of any radiographic equipment. Grids consist of lead strips separated by x-ray–transparent spacers (Fig. 4). Primary x-rays travel in a straight line from the tube to the image receptor. X-rays that interact with the tissues are deflected from a straight path and give rise to scattered radiation. The amount of scatter is proportional to the thickness of the part being radiographed and to the field size. Thicker body parts produce more scatter than thinner parts. The grid is positioned between the patient and the film. X-rays traveling in the main x-ray path (primary radiation) carry useful information and, for the

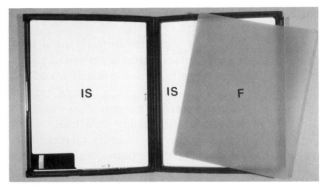

FIG. 5. Radiographic cassette. The radiographic film (F) is sandwiched between two image intensifying screens (IS).

most part, pass through the lucent strips of the grid, while scatter radiation, traveling obliquely in relation to the primary beam, is absorbed by the lead strips. About 85% to 95% of the scattered x-rays are absorbed by the grid (5). One disadvantage of grids is that they absorb some of the primary radiation emerging from the patient as well as most of the scattered radiation; therefore, it becomes necessary to increase the radiation to the patient in order to maintain adequate radiographic density on the film (5). Thin body parts, such as the cervical spine, produce little scattered radiation and can be radiographed without a grid. A caveat regarding the use of grids relates to the fact that grids are focused; therefore, proper alignment of the x-ray tube with the grid and using the proper distance from the x-ray tube to the grid should be always maintained; otherwise image quality quickly deteriorates (5,19). These standards are difficult to maintain when performing examinations in intensive care units, in the operating room, in the recovery room, or on the wards, where portable x-ray machines are used.

Radiographic films are loaded inside cassettes where they are sandwiched between two intensifying screens (Fig. 5). These screens function by changing x-rays into visible light which in turn exposes the radiographic film. Concepts controlling image formation are fundamental to the interpretation of radiographic images. The x-ray beam interacts with tissues as it passes through the patient. Variations in tissue composition give rise to differences in attenuation of the beam. X-rays passing through lungs inflated with air are only minimally attenuated, whereas most of the beam is absorbed as it passes through bone. Fat attenuates x-rays more than air, and water attenuates x-rays more than fat but less than bone. These alterations in the x-ray beam produce differences in the response, or visible light output, of the intensifying screen in the cassette. As more x-rays pass through the patient and reach the intensifying screen, more visible light is emitted from the screens, and the radiographic film becomes darker. Intensifying screens are essential because the sensitivity of radiographic film to x-rays is low compared with its sensitivity to visible light (5,55,91). The efficiency of the intensifying screen in

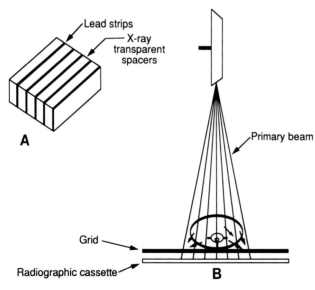

FIG. 4. Diagram of radiographic grid. **A:** A grid consists of very thin lead strips separated by x-ray transparent spacers. **B:** Primary beam radiation, which travels parallel to the lead strips, passes through the grid and reaches the radiographic cassette, whereas scattered radiation is absorbed by the grid.

converting x-rays to visible light is important in reducing the radiation dose to the patient. Highly efficient screens, which significantly reduce the radiation to the patient, tend to produce grainy images, whereas screens that produce images with fine detail tend to be less efficient. Selecting the proper screen–film combinations for different clinical situations is a technical skill requiring significant experience. The goal is to obtain the best images possible with the least amount of radiation to the patient. State-of-the-art radiography relies almost exclusively on the use of rare earth screen systems, which are much more efficient than the older calcium tungstate screens (5,55,91). In many institutions, digital radiography is slowly replacing film–screen radiography and in the foreseeable future all radiography will very likely become digital (digital radiography will be discussed in more detail).

FLUOROSCOPY

In fluoroscopy, the same physical principles apply as in radiography, except that the images are displayed on a TV screen instead of films. Judicial use of fluoroscopy is important both in the operating room and when performing needle procedures on the spine. Needle aspirations and biopsies for diagnosing spinal infections and tumors, as well as discography, facet injections, and epidural injections are all performed under fluoroscopy. Occasionally, biplane fluoroscopy is required for these procedures. In any fluoroscopic procedure, the length of time the patient is exposed to radiation should be limited to brief flashes, and the field of view should be restricted to the area of interest.

DIGITAL RADIOGRAPHY

An alternative to conventional film radiography is digital radiography. In this setting, images are primarily viewed on TV screens but can also be printed on film when necessary. This system has several advantages and in the near future it may replace the majority of conventional film radiography. Digital radiography is making headway at improving the way images are acquired, displayed, transmitted, recorded, and archived. Already, some authorities believe that digital radiography is the imaging technology of the future for studying patients with scoliosis, where the patient radiation is drastically reduced without compromising the quality of the images. In digital radiography, the conventional screen–film system is replaced with a storage phosphor plate, which is twice as efficient as the fastest rare earth screen–film combination. After the storage phosphor has been exposed in the same fashion as the regular cassette, a laser image reader extracts the latent image from the phosphor plate, and the data are handled by an image proces-

sor (a computer). Interactive workstations are connected to the image processor, replacing light boxes for viewing the images. Images can be manipulated to improve density and contrast, or they can be reduced or enlarged; images can also be transmitted from station to station. The radiation dose to patient is reduced because the storage phosphor is more sensitive to x-rays than the film–screen system. In addition, repeat exposures resulting from technical errors are nearly eliminated because image contrast and density can be electronically manipulated (63,73).

CONVENTIONAL TOMOGRAPHY

Conventional tomography continues to be an important imaging modality for evaluation of the spine. Radiographs are two-dimensional display of three-dimensional structures. Conventional tomography, also known as body section radiography, is a technique used to blur out superimposed structures and bring into focus structures of interest. The basic components of all tomographic units consist of an x-ray tube and a film cassette connected to a rigid arm. When the tube moves in one direction, the film moves in the opposite direction around a fulcrum or focal plane (Fig. 6) (17,19). The distance of tube travel is measured in degrees and is referred to as the tomographic angle. The plane of interest within the patient is positioned at the level of the fulcrum and is the only plane that stays in sharp focus. Structures within the patient above or below the fulcrum are blurred (17,19).

There are several types of tube motions available, but the one most commonly used in the evaluation of spinal problems is the circular motion, and to a lesser extent, the pluridirectional (or multidirectional) motion. Complex tube motions produce thorough blurring of structures outside the focal plane; however, complex motions expose the patient to more radiation, and the images produced with complex motion have diminished tissue contrast (17).

Other factors to consider in designing a protocol for a tomographic examination include section thickness and the interval between sections. The thickness of the tomographic section is inversely proportional to the distance of the tube travel measured in degrees. The more distance the tube travels, the thinner the section. The interval defines the distance between each tomographic section. The type of tube motion (linear, circular, or spiral), the distance of tube travel, and interval are predetermined for each examination depending on the size of the structure under evaluation. For example, an osteoid osteoma within a pedicle is best studied with thin sections, at intervals not exceeding 3 mm, whereas a large lytic or blastic lesion in the vertebral body can be studied with thicker sections at 5 to 8 mm intervals.

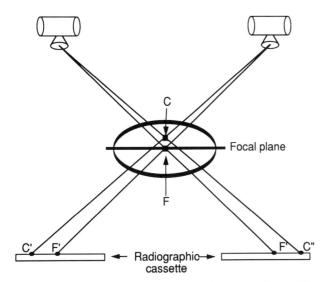

FIG. 6. Tomography. By moving both the x-ray tube and the radiographic cassette, only structures within the focal plane are well seen on the image. An object (F) within the focal plane is imaged on the same location of the cassette throughout the tomographic arc. However, an object out of the focal plane (C) is imaged in different places on the cassette and therefore blurred.

It is essential to be oriented when interpreting tomographic studies, so the films should be hung on the viewing box in the proper order. The numbers appearing on the films in a tomographic series indicate the distance between the focal plane and the film.

Many spine problems that were previously studied with conventional tomography are now evaluated with CT. However, segmentation anomalies, non-union related to failure of spinal fusion and nondisplaced dens fractures are still best studied with conventional tomography (Fig. 7).

BIOLOGIC EFFECTS OF RADIATION AND RADIATION PROTECTION

The use of x-ray examinations continues to increase in both the United States and other countries (43). In the evaluation of spine problems, radiographic examinations are often crucial in arriving at a specific diagnosis. Most physicians use ionizing radiation extensively in their diagnostic work; however, only a few are formally trained in handling ionizing radiation and in radiation

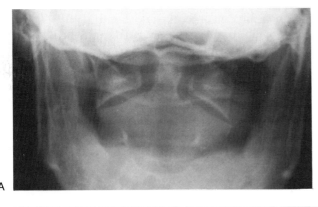
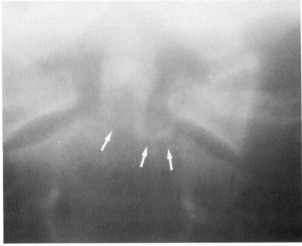
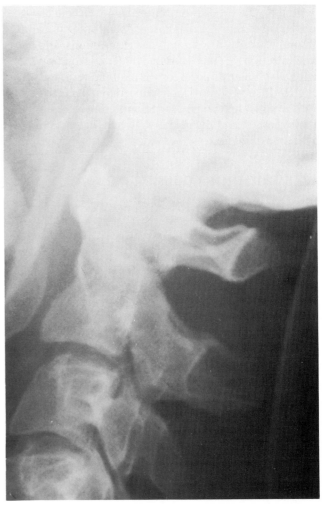

FIG. 7. Tomography of dens fracture. **A:** AP open-mouth view fails to demonstrate fracture. **B:** Lateral view demonstrates discontinuity of the posterior cortex of C2, but fracture is difficult to see. **C:** AP tomographic image shows nondisplaced type III dens fracture (*arrows*).

protection. Studies have shown that lack of technical training results in excessive population exposure to ionizing radiation (26). The exposure of patients to medical x-rays continues to command increased attention by society and public health officials (49). If basic principles of radiation protection are followed, the same level of diagnostic information can be achieved with reduced risk to patients and health workers.

X-rays absorbed by tissues exert their harmful effects on DNA by direct or indirect action. Direct action is DNA damage resulting from electrons being dislodged by the absorption of x-rays. In indirect action, the dislodged electrons interact with water molecules in the tissue to produce free radicals, which are highly reactive molecules that in turn damage the DNA. With diagnostic x-rays, the dominant harmful effects on DNA are produced by indirect action. Whether the action of x-rays on DNA is direct or indirect, there are three principal biologic effects of ionizing radiation on humans: (a) genetic effects, in which radiation causes mutations in germ cells that will be expressed in some future genera-

tion, (b) carcinogenesis, in which radiation affects somatic cells, causing malignant mutations, and (c) cell killing, which affects embryogenesis because the resulting cell depletion can adversely influence the developing embryo and fetus (43).

In terms of the genetic effects of radiation, exposure to radiation does not produce bizarre or unique mutations, but it does increase the frequency of mutations that occur naturally in the population (43,74). The radiation effects on a fetus depend on the stage of pregnancy. During preimplantation, or the first 10 days after conception, the main consequence is the death of the embryo. Radiation delivered during organogenesis, which occurs from 10 days to about 8 weeks after conception, leads to a broad spectrum of anomalies affecting organs and limbs. The natural prevalence of genetic disorders, however, is so high that small increments of fetal anomalies caused by radiation from diagnostic procedures are very difficult to measure directly (43,74). There is evidence to suggest that irradiation of the fetus later in pregnancy can result in the future development of leukemia. Present data in-

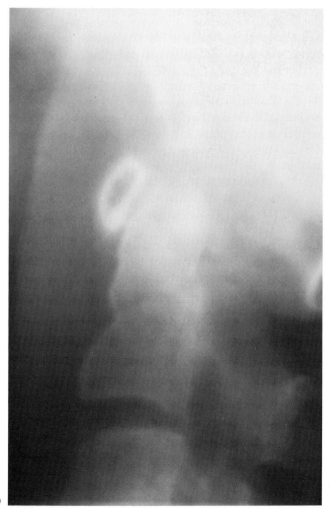

D

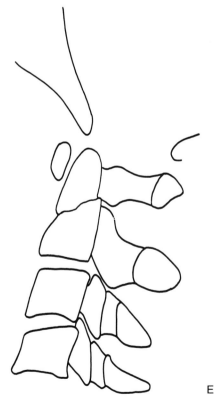

E

FIG. 7. (*Continued.*) **D:** Lateral tomogram demonstrates fracture line as well as discontinuity of the posterior cortex of C2. **E:** Diagram of lateral tomogram in D.

dicate that the risk of leukemia for a fetus exposed to more than 10 roentgens (R), or 10,000 milliroentgens (mR), increases from 1 in 3,000 to 1 in 2,000. To provide a basis for comparison, the average annual dose to the U.S. population from natural sources, or just from living in the United States, is 125 mR per year. The approximate fetal exposure from a chest x-ray to the mother is 1 mR, and an anteroposterior (AP) film of the lumbar spine is 50 mR (26,50). All estimates of the deleterious effects caused by radiologic procedures lead to the conclusion that the balance of risk versus benefit is heavily weighted in favor of benefits. If there is a valid medical indication to perform a diagnostic x-ray examination on a pregnant patient, the patient should not be denied the examination because of the pregnancy (74,98).

All health workers handling x-ray equipment, including physicians, should be familiar with the radiation protection guidelines at their institutions. The following are some general guidelines:

1. Appropriate personnel radiation-monitoring devices (PMDs) should be worn whenever there is a possibility of exposure to radiation.
2. PMDs should be worn only by the individual to whom they are assigned.
3. All exposure to the patient should be kept as low as reasonably possible by attempting to:
   a. Minimize the exposure time.
   b. Maximize the distance from the radiation source.
   c. Maximize filtration.
   d. Maximize film–screen speed (75).
   e. Use digital radiography when available or feasible.
   f. Use collimation.
   g. Use gonadal shielding.
   h. Eliminate unnecessary examinations and views (83,87).

TRAUMA

With the introduction of newer and more advanced imaging modalities, imaging of spinal trauma continues to undergo changes. Radiography, however, is still the first and best screening test for the initial evaluation of the patient suspected of a spine injury. There is now a strong body of evidence supporting the concept of screening the entire spine in patients with multiple trauma, especially if one fracture is detected (61,80,82). Often the second injury is not recognized early enough to prevent clinically significant extension of neurological deficit (14). Common sites for noncontiguous fractures are the upper cervical spine and thoracolumbar junction (14,42,85). Twenty-five percent of all craniovertebral junction fractures are reported to be associated with other fractures in the spine (61). Goldberg et al. (39) pointed out the utility of MRI in selected cases to survey long segments of the spine, therefore demonstrating noncontiguous multilevel fractures.

Cervical Spine

Radiography is an excellent screening examination in the emergency room where the prior probability of a fracture is high and the consequences of missing a fracture are severe. There are some drawbacks and limitations of radiography of the cervical spine related to difficulty in interpretation and relatively high rate of diagnostic error when interpretation is not performed by highly trained individuals. The consequences of missing a cervical spine fracture may be serious, resulting in deterioration of neurological function (80). In the series by Clark et al. (16), the most commonly missed injuries were undisplaced odontoid fractures (23%), facet fractures (14%), and hangman's fractures (10%). Some of the causes for the errors were poor quality radiographs, failure to do flexion and extension views even when these views are indicated, and misinterpretation of the radiographs. Under ideal conditions and using a three-film examination (lateral, AP, and open-mouth views) Streitwiesser et al. (94) reported a sensitivity of 93%, which is considered a high sensitivity for a screening test.

Some investigators argue that radiography for cervical spine trauma is overutilized and contributes to the high cost of medical care (58,72,82,103). In a comprehensive survey, Mirvis et al. (72) found that 96% of hospitals that handle trauma in North America follow the recommendations of the American College of Surgeons and obtain routine cervical spine radiographs on all major blunt trauma patients. Following such recommendations results in an unacceptably low yield of fractures (58). There are now specific clinical guidelines and indications being proposed to limit the use of radiography in the trauma patient (58,72,82,103). The goal is to improve the yield of the radiographic examination and reduce cost without compromising care. At our hospital, emergency physicians use the protocol developed by Ringenberg et al. (82) to select trauma patients who require evaluation with cervical spine radiography.

Other important issues that have received significant attention in the literature address how many radiographic views of the cervical spine are considered sufficient in the emergency setting, and when to perform flexion and extension views. The American College of Radiology has formed a task force to address issues related to appropriateness of radiographic examinations and recommendations should be available in 1996. Most centers perform either the three-view (lateral, AP, and open-mouth) or the five-view examination (lateral, AP, open-mouth, and both obliques). There is evidence in the literature that the three-view examination is basically sufficient and that there are no fractures or dislocations detected on the five-view series that are not seen or suspected on the three-view examination (34,67). Turetsky et al. (102), however, stress the importance of adding the two supine oblique views in order to demonstrate certain fractures that are not seen on the standard three-view series.

The question of when to perform flexion and extension views is not settled, but we believe that flexion and extension views should be performed in all patients with neck pain whose initial radiologic examination is normal (63). If the flexion and extension views are inadequate or do not provide any information in the acute phase because of pain and muscle spasm, the neck should be immobilized and the flexion and extension views should be repeated in 1 week. Flexion and extension views should not be performed on patients with obviously unstable cervical spine fractures such as a flexion tear-drop fracture or type II and III hangman's fracture.

In a multitrauma patient, the horizontal beam lateral

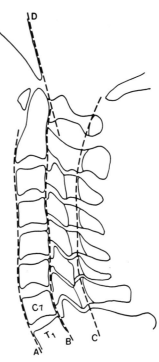

FIG. 9. Radiographic lines for cervical spine evaluation. See text for details.

view is the most important view of the cervical spine series. As soon as this film is developed, a physician should review it to make sure that it is technically adequate. The base of the skull, all seven cervical vertebrae, and the superior endplate of T1 should be included on the radiograph (Fig. 8). If the lower cervical segments are obscured by the shoulders, the examination should be repeated while pulling on the upper extremities. If this maneuver fails, a supine swimmer's view should be attempted. Unconscious or uncooperative patients and patients with fractures in the upper extremities may require CT to visualize the cervicothoracic junction.

To evaluate the lateral cervical spine, four lines (Fig. 9) are mentally drawn to ensure normal anatomic relationships of the bony structures:

1. A line drawn along the anterior surfaces of the vertebral bodies, starting at C2. This line has a gentle anterior curve and it should continue uninterrupted.
2. A line drawn along the posterior bodies should have an anterior gentle curve and should show no discontinuity. Special attention is paid to the region of the odontoid process (dens) and its junction to the body of C2. In fact, the lateral view is the best view for the evaluation of dens fractures. Contrary to common belief, it is better than the open-mouth view for assessment of these fractures. This line may show slight undulation at the junction of the dens with the body of C2. Interruption of this line at the base of the dens or sudden shifts in the position of the dens in relation to

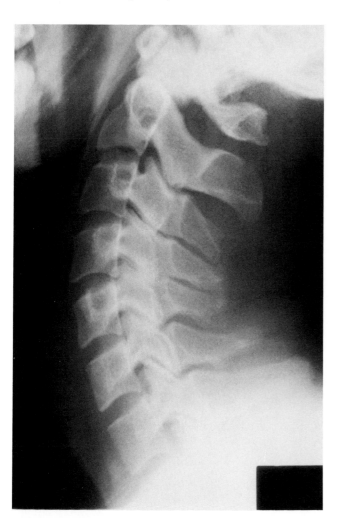

FIG. 8. Normal lateral radiograph of the cervical spine. Note that all seven cervical vertebrae, as well as the superior endplate of T1, are visible.

C2 suggests a dens fracture. As a caveat, the dens can normally be tilted posteriorly, which can be misinterpreted as a fracture; this is a normal variant (100).

3. The spinolaminar line is a line connecting the posterior aspect of the foramen magnum (inion) to the anterior cortex or base of all the cervical spinous processes as they connect with the laminae. As a normal variant, the smooth lordotic spinolaminar line may lie 2 to 3 mm anterior to the base of the C2 spinous process (53).

4. The basilar line of Wackenheim is important in defining the craniovertebral relationships. It is drawn along the posterior surface of the clivus, and its inferior extension should lie tangent or barely intersect the tip of the dens (105).

Close scrutiny of the vertebral body height is important to rule out compression or burst fractures. The vertebral height of C5 and C6 bodies is normally diminished compared to other vertebrae. Difference in the anteroposterior dimension between C7 and T1 may mimic subluxation (7). Below the age 10 years, vertebral bodies may look somewhat flattened, oval, or even wedged, but this is normal and should not be interpreted as compression fracture (100). Slight subluxation of C2 on C3 or C3 on C4 may be present in normal children and young adults up to 20 years of age (95,101).

The articular pillars are rhomboid in shape on the lateral view; the right and left articular pillars superimpose on a true lateral view. The articular surfaces of the facets are normally parallel; absence of this relationship should alert the observer to an articular pillar or pedicle fracture. When adjacent levels are evaluated and the articular pillars abruptly change from being superimposed to being separated (the bow tie appearance), a unilateral facet fracture with displacement or facet dislocation should be suspected. The normal indentation on the dorsal surface of C7 articular pillar, sometimes referred to as the dorsalization of C7, should not be mistaken for a fracture (52).

The distance between the adjacent spinous processes on the lateral view below C3 are almost equal. Increased distance between two spinous processes, especially when it persists on the extension view, usually indicates posterior ligamentous sprain.

The dens normally lies immediately below the tip of the clivus (opisthion), and the distance between the opisthion and the dens, on the lateral view, should not exceed 1.2 cm (46). Increased distance between these two structures can result from atlanto-occipital dislocation.

The retropharyngeal soft tissues, seen on the lateral view, should always be inspected in patients with cervical trauma. The thickness of the retropharyngeal soft tissues varies with body habitus and measurements are reliable only when performed between C2 and C4. Focal swelling is always abnormal, and patients with retropharyngeal

soft-tissue thickness exceeding 7 mm should be carefully studied for the possibility of a fracture.

The AP projection is viewed with special attention to the spinous processes that are aligned in the middle of the spine (Fig. 10). Widening of the interspinous distance at a particular level usually points to posterior ligamentous sprain or even bilateral facet joint disruption. Abrupt shift of a spinous process to one side usually indicates unilateral pillar fracture or facet joint dislocation at the level of the shift (Fig. 11). The articular pillars form the lateral border on each side of the cervical spine on the AP projection, and this border is normally wavy and uninterrupted. The orientation of the facet joints is about 45° from the vertical, and therefore facet joints should not be seen on the AP projection. If a facet joint is clearly identified on an AP projection, this should raise the suspicion of an articular pillar or pedicle fracture with rotation of the fractured fragment. Except for C7, where pedicles are often clearly identified, the pedicles in the cervical spine are oriented at 45° posterolaterally and thus are not well visualized on the AP projection. Finally, the air column in the pharynx and trachea should

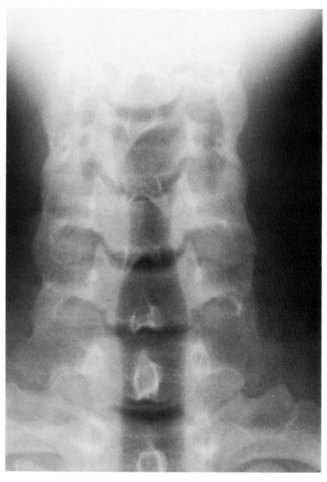

FIG. 10. Normal AP view of cervical spine. Note that the spinous processes are midline and that the distances between the spinous processes are similar.

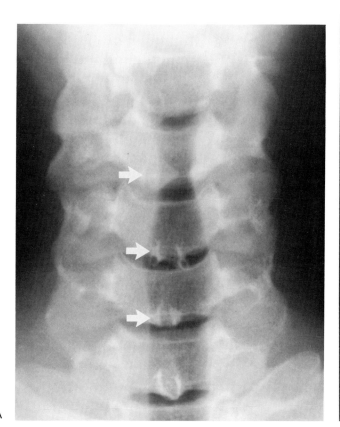

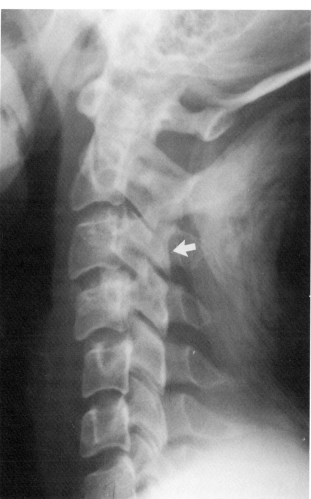

A

B

FIG. 11. Unilateral facet disc dislocation. **A:** AP view of the cervical spine demonstrates "jump" in the spinous process at the level of facet dislocation (*arrows*). **B:** Lateral view shows slight spondylolisthesis of C3 on C4. Facets inferior to dislocation are superimposed whereas above dislocation they are malaligned. "Bow tie appearance" at the level of the facet dislocation is noted (*arrow*).

project in the midline. A large pyriform sinus superimposed over the lateral masses may give the false impression of a lytic bone lesion.

The open-mouth view ideally demonstrates all of C1, the dens, and the superior facets of C2 (Fig. 12). This view is particularly helpful in diagnosing Jefferson fractures. Normally, the lateral borders of C1 and the lateral masses of C2 align. There are two instances when this rule fails: in children below the age of 4 years, when C1 may grow at a faster rate than C2, and in patients with congenital clefts in the anterior and posterior arches (37,97).

Supine oblique views are not as visually pleasing as views taken with the patient in the upright position, but in the emergency situation supine oblique views assist in verifying findings that are suspected on other projec-

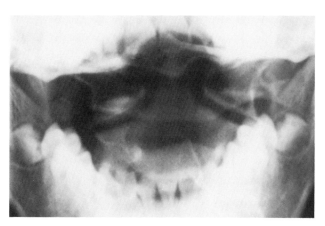

FIG. 12. Normal open-mouth view. Note that the lateral masses of C1 align with the superior facets of C2. The dens is well demonstrated.

tions. They are especially helpful in evaluating the articular pillars and facet joints.

Conventional tomography is useful in the evaluation of cervical spine trauma. Since there is a significant incidence of combined upper and lower cervical injuries, conventional tomography is especially helpful in patients in whom the entire cervical spine needs to be imaged to look for injuries suspected at separate levels. Conventional tomography is also the modality of choice for imaging dens and facet fractures.

Thoracic Spine

The thoracic spine is the largest segment of the spine, and it is a common site for trauma, especially in its lower

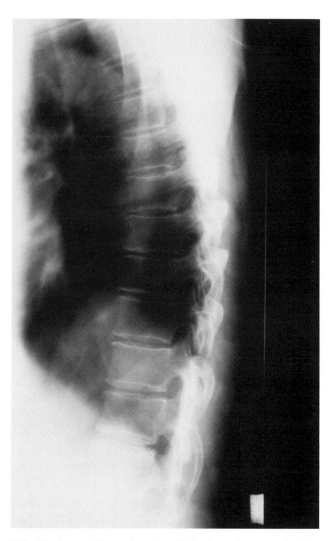

FIG. 14. Lateral thoracic spine. This view allows evaluation of vertebral body height and alignment as well as endplate irregularities or erosions. Note that the superimposed lungs and hemi-diaphragms are blurred by having the patient breathe during radiograph exposure.

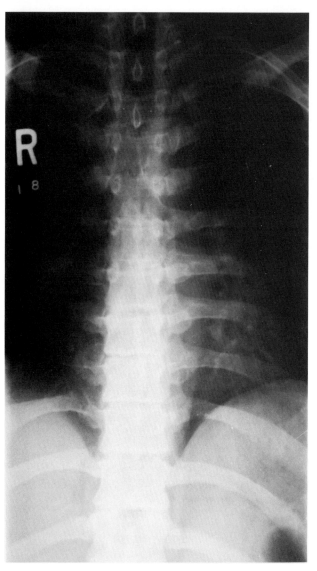

FIG. 13. AP view of normal thoracic spine. The AP projection is useful for evaluating vertebral body height, interpediculate distance, and alignment of spinous processes.

portion (T10-T12). AP and lateral radiographs are always required for evaluation of traumatized patients. AP radiographs can be easily obtained on supine patients; however, diagnostic lateral radiographs of the thoracic spine may be difficult to obtain in patients with multisystem trauma because the examination is performed in the supine position. A swimmer's view of the upper thoracic spine is often required when the upper thoracic vertebrae are not visualized.

AP radiographs (Fig. 13) are ideal for the evaluation of the vertebral bodies. The superior and inferior endplates of the vertebral bodies are seen as linear horizontal lines. The lateral margins are concave. Pedicles appear as oval structures projecting over the superior corners of the vertebral bodies. The articular facets and laminae are difficult to evaluate on the AP view. The transverse processes are visible as lateral extensions of the upper half of the vertebrae, whereas the costotransverse joints can be detected as two oblique lines close to the ends of the transverse processes. Rib heads are detected at the level of the intervertebral discs, articulating with the superior and inferior corners of adjacent vertebral bodies. The paraspinal soft tissues of the thoracic spine should be closely adherent to the vertebral bodies and only minimally visible. No focal swelling should be identified in the paraspinal soft tissues of the normal thoracic spine (29).

Lateral radiographs (Fig. 14) are helpful in assessing vertebral body height and alignment, disc height, end-plate irregularity, and erosions. On the lateral projection, vertebral bodies are seen as rectangular structures. The pedicles extend posteriorly from the superior half of the body. Located above and below the pedicles are the articular processes. The spinal canal and neural foramina are clearly delineated on the lateral radiographs. The inferior portions of the neural foramina are obscured by the heads of the ribs. The spinous processes are virtually impossible to visualize on the lateral view owing to the superimposition of the ribs (29). Anteriorly wedged vertebrae are usually considered abnormal in the clinical setting of trauma. However, normal wedging of the lower thoracic vertebral bodies, especially in men, is common (32,60). Fletcher (32) and Lauridsen et al. (60) proposed using a wedging ratio that compares heights of the anterior with the posterior vertebral bodies. Wedging ratios of 0.80 in men and 0.87 in women at the T8 to T12 levels are considered within normal limits.

AP and lateral views of the thoracic spine are helpful in assessing alignment. An abrupt change in alignment indicates spinal injury (Fig. 15). The presence of abnormal kyphosis, pleural fluid, paraspinal swelling, rib fractures, dislocations at the costovertebral joints, or widening of the interpediculate distance also suggests thoracic spine injury. The posterior aspects of the vertebral bodies are visible on lateral radiographs. Disruption, or bulging, of this line into the spinal canal is a reliable indicator of a burst fracture in the spine (Fig. 16). In a study of 114 patients with burst fractures, Daffner et al. (20) found

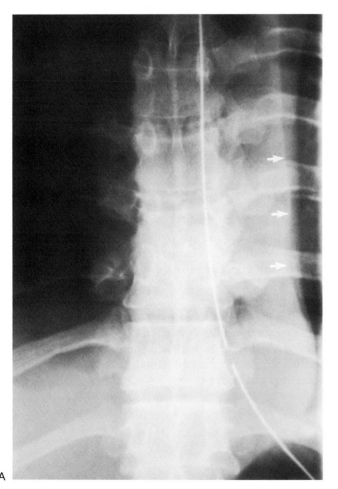

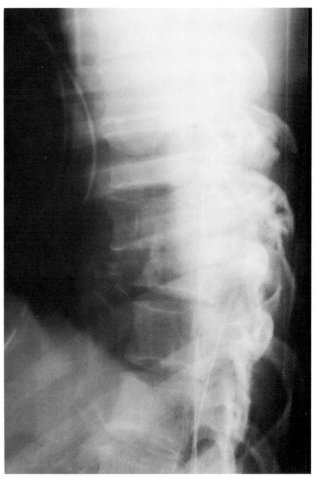

A

B

FIG. 15. Thoracic spine fracture. **A:** AP view of thoracic spine shows loss of intervertebral disc space at T8-9. Note also paraspinal fullness (*arrows*), representing hematoma. **B:** Lateral view demonstrates fracture dislocation of T8.

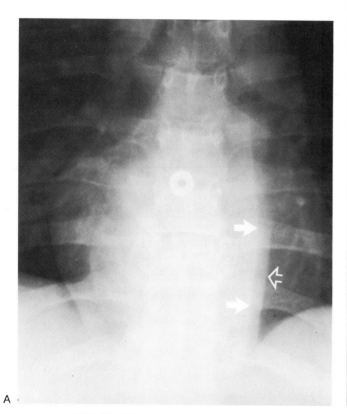

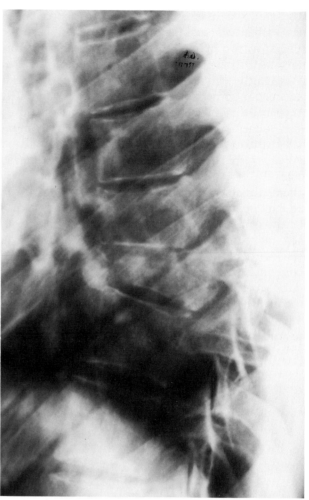

A

B

FIG. 16. Thoracic spine fracture. **A:** AP of lower thoracic spine shows widened interpediculate distance at T9. Note also paraspinal hematoma, (*closed arrows*), differentiated from descending aorta (*open arrow*). **B:** Lateral view demonstrates vertebral body fracture with loss of height. There is retropulsion of fracture fragments, with compromise of the spinal canal.

disruption of the posterior vertebral body line in all cases. This line should be carefully scrutinized in patients with trauma to the thoracic spine.

The spinous processes consistently project over the midline, and each tubercle (tip) of the spinous process extends slightly below the inferior endplate of its respective vertebral body. The double spinous process sign seen on the AP radiograph is a reliable indicator of a fracture of the spinous process (4,110).

Historically, fractures of the upper thoracic spine (T1–T10) have been considered analogous to fractures of the thoracolumbar junction and lumbar spine. However, these regions differ in both their neurologic and their osseous aspects (9). Bohlman drew attention to the unique features of trauma involving the upper thoracic spine and noted the following: (a) Because of its stiffness, considerable violence is necessary to produce fractures or fracture-dislocations in the upper thoracic spine; (b) The spinal canal in this region is narrow and injuries of the

upper thoracic spine are frequently associated with injuries of the spinal cord; and (c) Most of the osseous injuries occur in flexion and axial loading because very little rotatory motion occurs in the upper thoracic spine. Rogers et al. (85) recognized that fractures of the upper thoracic spine do not fit easily into the common fracture classifications and thus should be treated separately. In a review of 35 patients with acute injury to the upper thoracic spine and associated paraplegia, they found the basic pattern of injury, affecting 32 of 35 patients, consisted of an anterior fracture-dislocation involving two contiguous vertebrae.

Lumbar Spine

The thoracolumbar junction (T11–L2) is the commonest site for spinal fractures. Fractures in this region, the lower lumbar spine, and the sacrum are best evaluated with AP and lateral radiographs. In the trauma setting, these are obtained with the patient in the supine position. Alignment of vertebral bodies, pedicles, and spinous processes is demonstrated on the AP view. A sudden change in alignment raises the possibility of spinal injury. Wide interpediculate distance suggests the possibility of an unstable burst fracture with involvement of the posterior column. The lateral view is helpful in assessing the vertebral height and alignment, as well as retropulsion of bony fragments into the spinal canal. It is common practice to proceed with CT if a burst fracture is suspected on initial radiographs.

NEOPLASM

The vertebral column is the most common site of skeletal metastases; it is involved in approximately 40% of patients who die of cancer (1,11). Cord compression is among the most dreaded complications of cancer. The high prevalence of metastasis to the spine may be explained by the rich concentration of growth factors in the bone marrow stroma which have been shown to stimulate the proliferation of malignant cells *in vitro*. Another explanation is related to the vertebral venous plexus, which drains the thoracic, abdominal, and pelvic viscera when intra-abdominal pressure increases, such as during straining and coughing (1,11).

Primary bone tumors are far less common in the spine

than are metastatic lesions, particularly in adult patients. In older patients, primary spinal lesions are most frequently malignant, whereas in children and adolescents they are usually benign (106). Some lesions (osteoid osteoma, osteoblastoma) show a strong predilection for the posterior elements (Fig. 17); others (hemangioma, eosinophilic granuloma) are predominantly found in the vertebral body (Fig. 18). Radiographs are always indicated in patients with back pain and neurologic deficit of uncertain etiology. There is, however, some disagreement among authors as to the sensitivity of radiographs for detecting spinal tumors. Subtle lesions are especially difficult to visualize in the thoracic spine. Radiographs reveal vertebral metastases in approximately 85% of adult patients with metastatic epidural compression. The frequency of the bony abnormality depends on the type of tumor. Radiographs are abnormal in 94% of patients with breast cancer and 74% of those with lung cancer. Symptoms depend on the extent of epidural disease, and this correlates with the extent of vertebral metastasis. Grans et al. (41) found epidural lesions in 87% of vertebrae with more than 50% collapse and in 31% of those with pedicle erosion. Destruction of the vertebral pedicle is a valuable observation in the distinction of metastases from multiple myeloma (Fig. 19). CT is more sensitive in detecting and showing the extent of spinal metastases. CT findings of early metastatic spread to vertebral bodies rather than pedicles correlate well with pathologic findings. At autopsy, metastatic tumor may fill the marrow

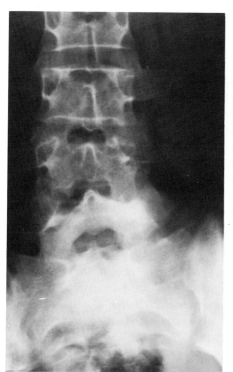
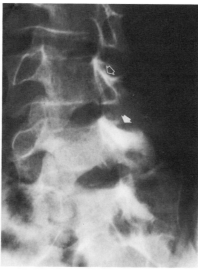
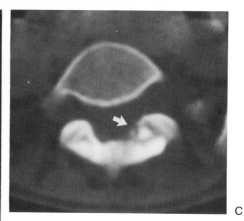

FIG. 17. Osteoid osteoma of L5. **A:** AP view demonstrates sclerosis of left pedicle at L5, with dextroscoliosis centered at same level. **B:** Oblique view better shows sclerotic pedicle (*arrow*), compared to normal pedicle at L4 (*open arrow*). **C:** CT scan at same level shows focal sclerosis with surrounding lucency (*arrow*), typical of osteoid osteoma.

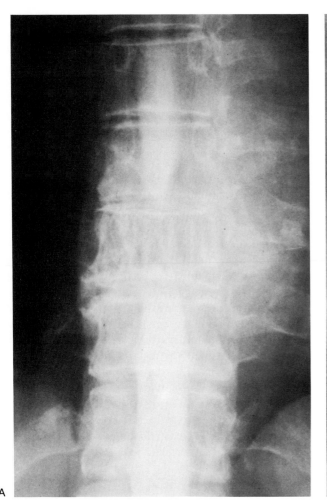
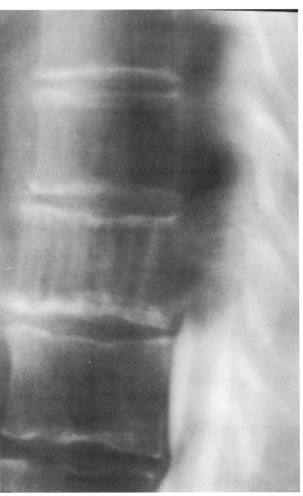

FIG. 18. Hemangioma of thoracic spine. **A:** AP view of thoracic spine during myelogram shows thick vertical trabeculations, typical of hemangioma. Note cord compression. **B:** Lateral view shows similar findings.

and leave cortical bone intact, a circumstance more easily detected by CT or MRI than conventional radiography.

LOW BACK PAIN

Low back pain is an extremely common disorder. It is second to upper respiratory tract symptoms as a reason for a visit to a physician (23). The prevalence of low back pain has been estimated at between 60% and 90% (35,44). The annual incidence is approximately 5% (35). Men and women are affected equally, but women tend to be affected later in life than men (35). It is the most expensive ailment in the 30- to 60-year-old population (44).

Most cases of low back pain are acute episodes without radicular symptoms and are related to muscle spasm (21). Only 1% to 1.5% of acute episodes have radicular symptoms (23,35). Acute back pain without radicular symptoms tends to improve on its own (35,44), with only 14% of cases of back pain lasting over 2 weeks (23). The vast majority of cases resolve by 6 weeks. Even patients with radicular symptoms tend to improve with time, and over 50% resolve within a month (35).

There is widespread agreement that routine radiographs of the spine are not indicated in the evaluation of patients with acute low back pain in the absence of radicular symptoms (21,23,35,44,64). Even in patients with sciatica, early radiographs are not needed, as many of these patients improve without treatment (18,35). In fact, in some states early radiographs are not reimbursed in the workup of patients with low back pain (30). Clinical examination is a better predictor of prognosis and outcome than a lumbar radiograph (30).

Subacute back pain refers to patients who still suffer after 6 weeks of conservative therapy. Approximately 10% of patients with low back pain will continue to have

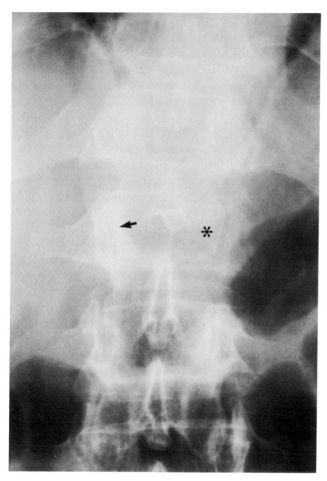

FIG. 19. Metastatic disease. AP view of the thoracolumbar junction in a patient with metastases. L1 vertebra is abnormal with absent left pedicle (*asterisk*). Note intact right pedicle (*arrow*).

symptoms beyond 6 weeks (35). This percentage is higher in patients with sciatica. Radiographs are recommended in these patients, searching for etiologies such as compression fracture, spondylolisthesis, spondylolysis, vertebral osteomyelitis, vertebral metastasis, degenerative changes, and spondyloarthropathy.

There are a number of factors that would indicate early radiographs. These include age over 50 or under 20, known history of neoplasm, history of serious trauma, significant weight loss, pain at rest, fever, alcohol or drug abuse, corticosteroid use, and clinical question of compression fracture (23,35). Imaging is also indicated when the clinical picture is atypical or unusual (35).

Patients with spinal stenosis usually have a different clinical course than patients with acute low back pain and disc-related disease. Duration of symptoms is longer, with the average duration being 4 years. The average patient age is 55 years old. Neurogenic claudication refers to radicular symptoms after walking, in patients with normal pulses, and is seen in patients with spinal stenosis (23).

The vast majority (98%) of neurologic symptoms are from the L4-L5 and L5-S1 levels (23). Clinical signs useful for radicular pain include a positive straight-leg raise test at 30° to 60°. A positive crossed straight-leg raise test (opposite leg raised produces symptoms) is a very specific test (23).

If lumbar spine radiographs are obtained, oblique views are not necessary. These views double the radiation dose to the patient, do not improve diagnosis, and increase the cost of the examination (35).

Choice of radiographic examination depends on the clinical suspicion. For example, MRI is probably better at diagnosis of disc disease, whereas some surgeons prefer the bone detail that CT gives when evaluating patients with spinal stenosis. In any case, AP and lateral radiographs of the lumbar spine are indicated. Disc space narrowing can be seen, and occasionally a herniated disc can be visible with rim calcification (Fig. 20).

Spondylolisthesis is best diagnosed by radiographs, and the degree of slippage is easily determined. The two commonest types of spondylolisthesis, degenerative and isthmic, are easily recognized on radiographs. Degenera-

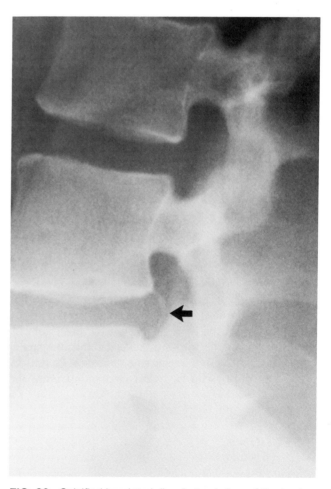

FIG. 20. Calcified herniated disc. Lateral view of the lumbar spine shows rim calcification of a disc protrusion at the L4-L5 interspace (*arrow*).

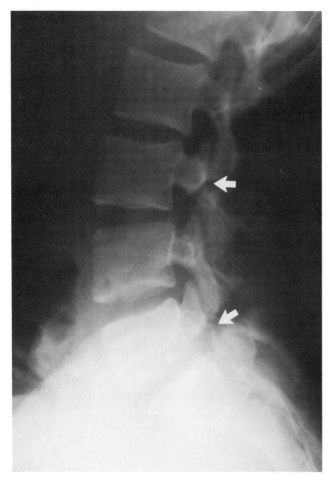

FIG. 21. Spondylolysis. Lateral radiograph of the lumbar spine demonstrates spondylolysis at both L3 and L5 (arrows). There is minimal spondylolisthesis at L5.

tive spondylolisthesis usually occurs at the L4-L5 level. As facet degeneration leads to instability, L4 slips forward on L5. This causes spinal stenosis as the posterior elements of L4 impinge on the posterior aspect of the L5 vertebral body. Isthmic spondylolisthesis results from a fracture of the pars interarticularis, called spondylolysis. This usually occurs at L5, but occasionally spondylolysis is seen at other levels (Fig. 21). The L5 vertebral body slips forward on the S1 segment, but the posterior elements of L5 remain in position. As a result, the spinal canal widens in AP diameter and stenosis does not occur. Tomography can be useful in demonstrating the spondylolysis.

INFECTION

Spinal osteomyelitis is fairly common, representing 1% to 2% of all cases of osteomyelitis. The incidence is also increasing (31,65). Many studies have shown that other modalities are more sensitive than radiography for

diagnosing vertebral osteomyelitis, including bone scintigraphy, CT, and MRI (31). However, radiography is often the initial modality with which this disease is diagnosed. Often, typical clinical signs such as elevated temperature, increased white count and sedimentation rate are absent, delaying the clinical suspicion of infection (13,31).

Most cases of vertebral osteomyelitis are pyogenic in origin, with *Staphylococcus aureas* found in 60% to 90% of cases (13,90,93). Nonpyogenic infections can be caused by tuberculous species, fungi, or syphilis (93). Most cases of vertebral osteomyelitis are from hematogenous seeding, affecting initially the endplate of a vertebral body. This is a result of the unique blood supply of the vertebral body (6,109). Arterial supply is from lumbar vessels, and these enter the body peripherally and course centrally. Venous drainage is from the periphery to the center in a treelike fashion to the central channel (6,109). These veins are interconnected via Batson's plexus, a network of valveless vessels running along the posterior aspect of the vertebral bodies along the spinal canal (6). The configuration of arterioles and veins creates a slow flow state, and this is why bacteria are thought to be deposited at the vertebral endplate.

Most cases of vertebral osteomyelitis are spontaneous. However, osteomyelitis may follow skin infection, urinary tract infection, respiratory tract infection, and instrumentation such as catheterization or cystoscopy (109). A history of intravenous drug abuse increases the risk of osteomyelitis (31). Direct implantation is usually iatrogenic and occurs after lumbar puncture, discography, myelography, discectomy, or spine surgery (65, 79,93). Infection of the posterior elements is uncommon (27).

Typical progression of disease is from the vertebral endplate into the intervertebral disc. Infection then spreads to the adjacent vertebral endplate and can also spread beneath the anterior spinal ligament (2). There may be anterior vertebral body erosion and paraspinal abscess formation. This is seen with tuberculous infections more than with pyogenic infection.

Radiographic findings follow the pathologic phases of vertebral osteomyelitis. Early in the disease, radiographs will be normal as radiographic findings lag behind disease onset by several weeks. Initially, the endplate of the infected vertebra becomes indistinct as bone destruction proceeds (2,31). Pyogenic infection, once it has spread to the intervertebral disc, will cause disc space narrowing (Fig. 22). Serial radiographs may show a rapid loss of height of the disc space. As the infection spreads to the adjacent vertebral body, that endplate will become indistinct as well. The bone attempts repair and a sclerotic area of the infected vertebral bodies may be seen. Rarely will paraspinal abscesses be visible on radiographs, but with tuberculous infection, one may see peripheral calcification surrounding the paraspinal collections (Fig. 23).

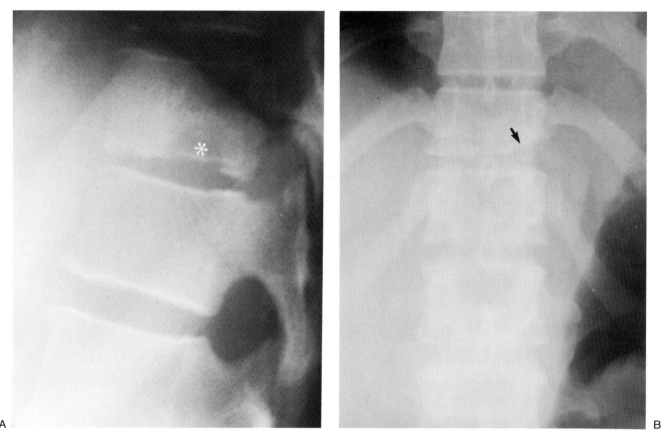

A   B

FIG. 22. Early pyogenic infection. **A:** Lateral view of the thoracic spine shows disruption of the inferior endplate of T11 (*asterisk*). Intervertebral disc at space T11-T12 is narrow compared to normal disc space at T12-L1. **B:** AP view also demonstrates disruption of cortical margin of left side of inferior endplate at T11 (*arrow*).

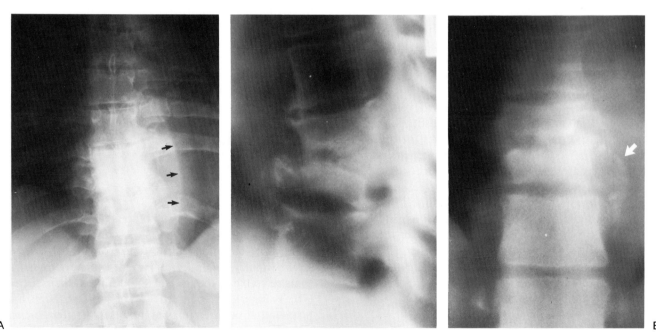

A   B,C

FIG. 23. Pott's disease. **A:** AP view of the thoracolumbar junction shows destruction at the T8-T9 level. Note paraspinal mass with displacement of paraspinal line (*arrows*). **B:** Lateral tomogram demonstrates adjacent vertebral destruction, reactive sclerosis, and wedge deformity. **C:** AP tomogram at same level shows calcification within the paraspinal abscess (*arrow*).

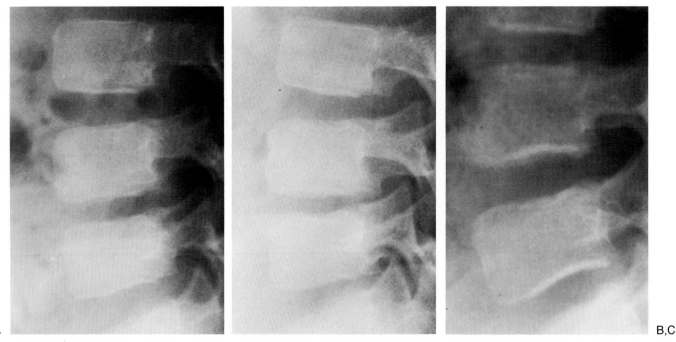

A   B,C

FIG. 24. Isolated discitis in a child. **A:** Lateral view of the lumbar spine in a 5-year-old child shows slight decrease in the L4-L5 intervertebral disc height. **B:** Similar radiograph obtained 6 weeks later shows interval loss of disc height. Patient was treated with antibiotics. **C:** Follow-up radiograph obtained 5 years later shows return of normal intervertebral disc height.

Gas within the disc space or vertebral body typically results from causes other than infection, but disc and vertebral body gas on radiographs has been reported on very rare occasions in patients with osteomyelitis due to gas-forming organisms (8). Another feature that distinguishes tuberculous from pyogenic infection is that the intervertebral joint space is often spared, and one can see two adjacent destroyed vertebrae with relatively preserved disc between them.

The long-term outcome of patients with vertebral osteomyelitis is variable. Complete reconstitution of the vertebra is possible, but usually residual deformity is present (93). Ankylosis of the adjacent vertebra is common. With untreated infection, complete bone lysis and collapse are possible, along with disc obliteration and resultant deformity of the vertebral column.

Discitis without adjacent vertebral osteomyelitis is encountered in children, in whom the disc has its own blood supply and isolated disc infection is possible (Fig. 24) (84,86,108). In most cases, no organism is isolated, even when cultures are obtained prior to antibiotic therapy (51,86,108).

INFLAMMATORY ARTHRITIS

Inflammatory arthritides that affect the spine include rheumatoid arthritis (RA) and a group of disorders called seronegative spondyloarthropathies; this group includes psoriatic arthritis, ankylosing spondylitis, Reiter's disease (reactive arthritis), and spondylitis associated with inflammatory bowel disease. Diagnosis of these diseases is not based purely on radiographic abnormalities but also includes history, physical findings, and laboratory studies. However, these diseases do have distinct patterns of radiographic abnormalities, and radiographs are therefore important for initial evaluation of patients where inflammatory arthritis is considered. In addition, radiographs are often used to follow patients, and they can help in diagnosing complications before clinical findings are present.

Rheumatoid Arthritis

RA commonly affects the spine, with cervical involvement more common than thoracic or lumbar disease. Approximately two-thirds of patients will develop symptoms referable to the neck at some time in their disease (76). Pannus leads to destruction of cartilage, bone, and ligaments at the occipitoaxial junction, the atlanto-axial articulation, the facet joints, and the uncovertebral joints. Radiographic findings in RA of the cervical spine can be divided into craniovertebral changes and subaxial disease. Craniovertebral changes include cranial settling and atlantoaxial (AA) subluxation.

Cranial settling occurs when pannus destroys the cartilage and bone at the occipitoaxial joint (89); ligamentous damage is less important here than in AA subluxation (99) (see below). The cranium articulates in an abnormally low position and as a result, the odontoid process protrudes through the foramen magnum. This can lead to impingement on the spinal cord or medulla oblongata and can cause occlusion of the vertebral artery. Sudden death has been reported (22). Cranial settling occurs in 5% to 8% of patients with severe rheumatoid arthritis and carries a graver prognosis than AA subluxation (28).

While MRI is important for evaluation of this condition, radiography is still the initial modality used to screen and follow patients with RA. Tomography provides excellent bone detail and is useful in evaluating patients with cranial settling. Radiographic features of cranial settling include protrusion of the dens through the

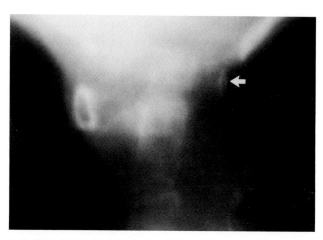

FIG. 26. Atlantoaxial subluxation in rheumatoid arthritis. Lateral tomogram shows striking decrease in the AP diameter of the spinal canal due to severe AA subluxation. Note position of posterior arch of C1 (*arrow*).

foramen magnum (Fig. 25). Important reference lines include Wackenheim's line, McGregor's line, and Chamberlain's line. Wackenheim's clival base line is drawn along the posterior margin of the clivus; the odontoid process should be tangent to or barely intersect this line (28,105). Chamberlain's line is a line from the posterior aspect of the hard palate to the posterior aspect of the foramen magnum. The tip of the dens should protrude no more than 3 mm above this line (15). McGregor's line is drawn from the posterior aspect of the hard palate to the inferior margin of the occiput. The tip of the dens should protrude above this line by less than 4.5 mm (68).

Atlantoaxial subluxation is present in between 15% and 36% of patients with RA and is therefore more common than cranial settling (15). There are synovial joints separating the dens from the anterior arch of C1 and from the cruciate ligament. A bursa is also present between the cruciate ligament and the posterior longitudinal ligament (68). Pannus leads to ligamentous destruction and bony erosion. During flexion, C1 slips anterior to the dens and the spinal canal diameter (from the posterior aspect of the dens to the posterior arch of C1) is reduced (Fig. 26). It is critical to do flexion and extension views to adequately demonstrate AA subluxation; standard lateral radiographs are insensitive (76). Some feel that all patients with RA should undergo flexion and extension examination prior to general anesthesia (15). With flexion, the AA space should not increase significantly; any space larger than 2.5 or 3 mm is considered abnormal (68,76).

Subaxial disease refers to changes from C2 through C7. Erosions occur at the facet joints, at the joints of Luschka (uncovertebral joints), and less commonly at the vertebral endplates. Intervertebral disc height can be reduced with overall loss of height of the cervical spine. Alignment abnormalities include spondylolisthesis,

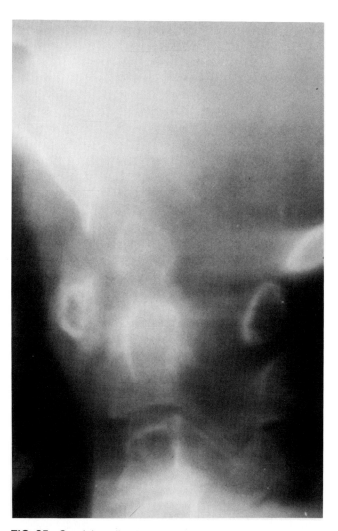

FIG. 25. Cranial settling in rheumatoid arthritis. Lateral tomogram of craniovertebral junction in a patient with rheumatoid arthritis. Dens projects above and posterior to Wackenheim's line. Also note atlantoaxial subluxation and erosions of the dens.

which, when extensive, gives the cervical spine a "step-ladder" appearance (Fig. 27) (76). Single-level involvement is usually at C3-C4 or C4-C5 (76). Vertebral endplate changes include sclerosis, erosions, and cystic areas. These can be mistaken for infection (76). While inconclusive, there is evidence that the discovertebral changes in RA may be related to chronic instability rather than inflammatory erosions (69).

Seronegative Spondyloarthropathies

The seronegative spondyloarthropathies are a group of rheumatic diseases that share a variety of clinical, radiologic, and genetic features. They include ankylosing spondylitis, psoriatic arthritis, Reiter's disease, and arthritis associated with inflammatory bowel disease. The common features in this group of diseases are a strong association with the genetically determined histocompatability antigen HLA-B27, inflammation at bony insertion of ligaments and tendons (enthesitis), spinal pre-

dilection resulting in sacroiliitis and spondylitis, onset at early age with male predilection in some of these diseases, and systemic manifestations.

The prototype of the seronegative spondyloarthropathies is ankylosing spondylitis (AS). Clinically, the disease begins insidiously (in 75% to 80%) and back pain is the most common complaint, seen in approximately 70% to 80% of patients. Peripheral joint involvement is seen in 10% to 20% of patients. Constitutional symptoms include anorexia, weight loss, and fever (81).

The arthritis associated with ulcerative colitis and Crohn's disease has radiographic features almost identical to those of AS (71,78). Although Reiter's and psoriatic arthritis each have unique radiographic characteristics, these two diseases resemble each other more than they resemble AS (71). The prevalence of AS is about 0.1% with the male-to-female ratio being between 4:1 and 10:1. The disease tends to follow a more benign course in women (77). Age of onset is 15 to 35 years, and the disease may be milder in women (10). Fewer than

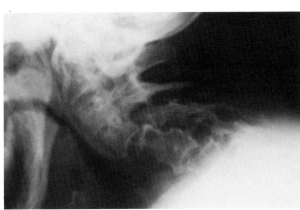

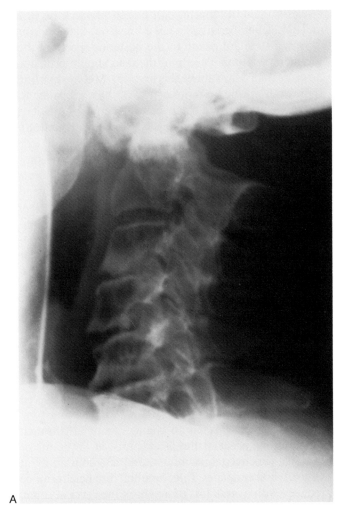

FIG. 27. Subaxial disease in rheumatoid arthritis. **A:** Lateral view of cervical spine shows uncovertebral erosions, disc space narrowing, and endplate irregularities. **B:** Different patient shows fusion at C5-C6, dramatic alignment abnormalities, and severe erosions of the facets and spinous processes.

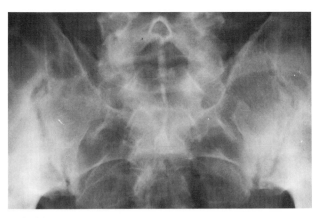

FIG. 28. Early sacroiliac erosions in ankylosing spondylitis.

20% of adult onset AS cases progress to significant disability (3).

AS is predominantly an axial disease affecting the sacroiliac (SI) joints and spine. Without involvement of the SI joints, it is not possible to make the diagnosis of AS. Spondylitis without sacroiliitis occurs in less than 1% of patients with AS (24). The disease in the SI joints starts with erosions on the iliac side of the joint associated with bony proliferation or sclerosis. Initially, the sacral side of the joint is protected from erosions because it is covered with thicker cartilage (Fig. 28). As a result of these erosions, early in the disease the joint may appear widened, but shortly after that, the joint starts to narrow and eventually it fuses (Fig. 29). The sacroiliitis may appear to be asymmetric early, but very quickly it becomes bilateral and almost always symmetric (88). These are important characteristics of sacroiliitis in AS. With time, fusion of

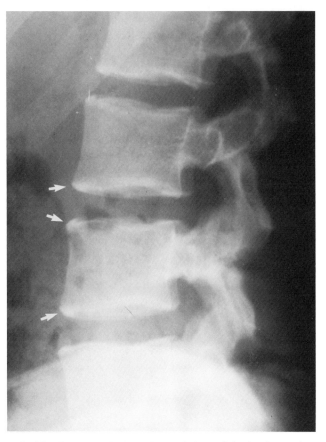

FIG. 30. Romanus lesions. Lateral view of the lumbar spine demonstrates sclerosis of the insertion of the annulus on the vertebral endplate (*arrows*). This has also been called shiny corners.

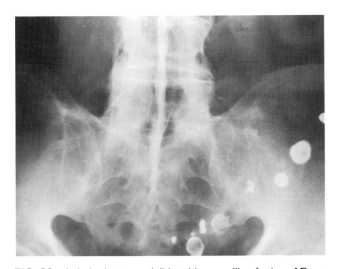

FIG. 29. Ankylosing spondylitis with sacroiliac fusion. AP radiograph shows complete fusion of the sacroiliac joints bilaterally. Bone density has returned to normal. Spinous processes have also fused, called the "dagger sign."

the SI joints is noted, and when completed the sclerosis disappears. Isolated sacroiliac abnormalities in long-standing AS are uncommon (81).

Spondylitis in AS is seen in about 50% of patients; early on it has a predilection for the thoracolumbar junction (88). Spine changes are almost never observed in the cervical or dorsal spine without lumbar involvement. Cases with "skip" involvement are more commonly seen in women (77). Enthesopathy in the spine manifests as small erosions at the insertion of the outer fibers of the annulus fibrosis. Vertebral corner erosions surrounded with bony sclerosis are evident in the early stages of the spondylitis; they are referred to as shiny corners or Romanus lesions (Fig. 30) (24). This is followed by ossification of the outer annular fibers and adjacent connective tissue fibers to form marginal syndesmophytes. This differs from osteophytes seen with degenerative disc disease and the paravertebral ossification (nonmarginal syndesmophytes) associated with Reiter's disease and psoriatic arthritis.

Marginal syndesmophytes extend from one corner of the vertebral body across the disc to the adjacent corner

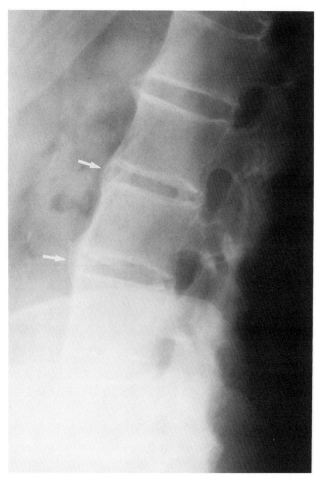

FIG. 31. Ankylosing spondylitis. Lateral view of the lumbar spine shows delicate, symmetric, marginal syndesmophytes (*arrows*).

(Fig. 31) (88). They are thin and delicate initially and are always symmetric in AS. Even when the disease starts early in life, syndesmophytes do not develop before the age of 20 years (24). The complete fusion of the vertebral bodies by these syndesmophytes results in what is called the bamboo spine (Fig. 32), which is characteristic of AS and colitic arthritis but not of Reiter's disease or psoriatic arthritis. Squaring of the vertebral bodies is also characteristic of AS and is at least partially caused by the corner erosions, but also by anterior apposition of periosteal new bone formation (88). Squaring is easier to appreciate in the lumbar spine where vertebrae are normally concave anteriorly; thoracic vertebrae normally have a straight anterior body.

When the spine fuses, osteoporosis sets in and even minor trauma puts the patient at risk for fracture (Fig. 33). Radiologists and clinicians should be alert when patients with longstanding AS and spinal fusion present with acute back pain; in this situation, fracture should be a primary consideration (33). These fractures are most common at the thoracolumbar junction and the thoracocervical junction and typically extend though all three columns. The fracture most commonly passes through an ossified intervertebral disc and also through the vertebral body adjacent to an endplate. Thirteen of 20 fractures occurred at the level of an intervertebral disc in one series, suggesting a selective vulnerability of an ossified disc (38). There is a high morbidity with these fractures; one series reported fractures in 12% of patients with AS and 8% with cord injury (107). AS increases the risk for cervical spine injuries above that present in the normal population (40). Acute fractures at the thoracocervical junction can result in paraplegia and even death (33).

Acute fracture can go undetected and proceed to nonunion and pseudoarthrosis. Pseudoarthrosis presents radiographically with discovertebral erosions and bone destruction, with an appearance resembling disc space infection. This is referred to as the Andersson lesion (Fig. 34) (24,25). This lesion is not only posttraumatic; it also

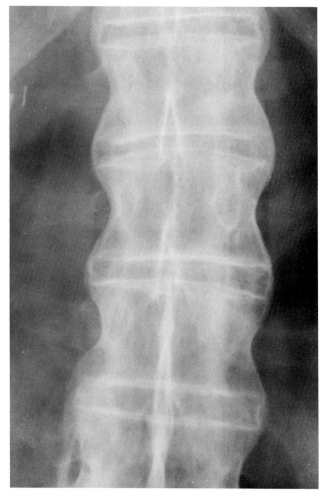

FIG. 32. Ankylosing spondylitis with "bamboo spine." When marginal syndesmophyte formation becomes pronounced, the lumbar spine resembles a bamboo stalk.

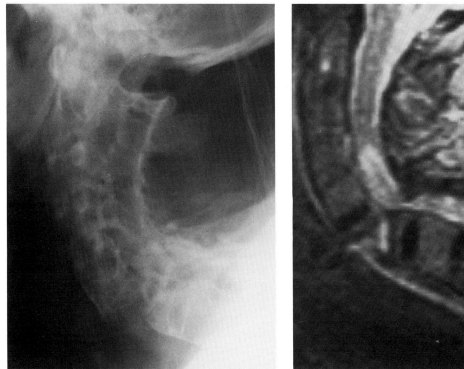
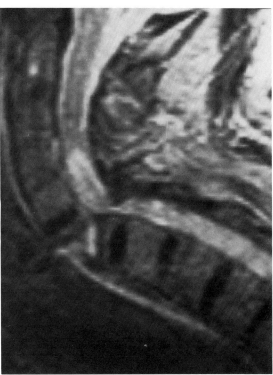

A B

FIG. 33. Fracture of cervical spine in ankylosing spondylitis. **A:** Lateral view of the cervical spine shows diffuse vertebral ankylosis and a fracture at C6. There is significant anterior displacement at the fracture. **B:** MRI (T2-weighted) shows fracture, compromise of spinal canal, and cord compression.

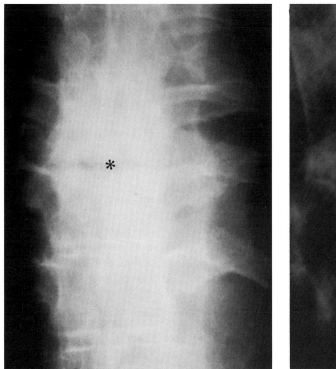
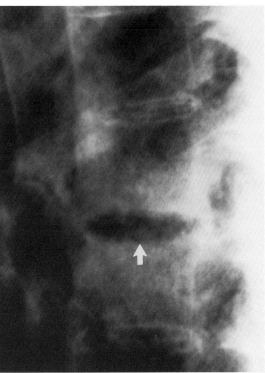

A B

FIG. 34. Andersson lesion. **A:** AP view of the thoracolumbar junction shows endplate sclerosis and loss of disc height (*asterisk*). **B:** Lateral view shows similar findings (*arrow*); this lesion should not be mistaken for vertebral osteomyelitis and discitis.

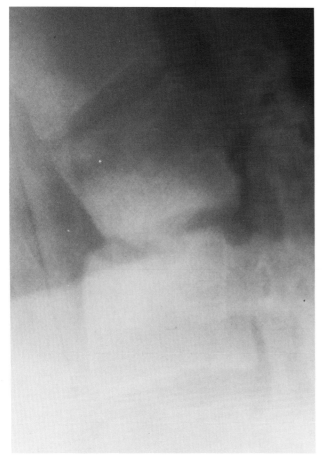

FIG. 35. Andersson lesion. Woman with 10-year history of ankylosing spondylitis. This level failed to fuse as the rest of the spine fused. Note acute angular deformity and sclerosis of adjacent endplates.

can develop at one or more levels during spinal fusion, with these levels failing to fuse as the remainder of the spine fuses (Fig. 35).

Apophyseal joint and costovertebral joint ankylosis is frequently seen in AS. Atlantoaxial subluxation is rarely seen (less than 2%) with AS (45), and it is not as common as in patients with rheumatoid arthritis. Subaxial subluxation is not seen in AS. In juvenile AS, radiological abnormalities are commonly present in the absence of specific symptoms referable to the SI joints. Initial evaluation of the SI joints is carried out when patients are examined for hip complaints or when spinal abnormalities are suspected (56).

Psoriatic arthritis (PA) is an asymmetric polyarticular disorder involving the upper and lower extremities with predilection for the interphalangeal joints of the hands and metatarsophalangeal and interphalangeal joints of the feet. PA is seen in approximately 5% of patients with cutaneous psoriasis. The male-to-female ratio is almost 1. Nail changes, especially pitting, are present in 80% of

patients with PA but occur in only 30% of patients with cutaneous psoriasis alone. Nail changes seem to correlate better with the arthritic changes than the skin disease. Skin changes usually antedate arthritis, but spondylitis can be seen as the presenting finding (66).

PA is included with the seronegative spondyloarthropathies because sacroiliitis or spondylitis develop in about 30% to 50% of patients with arthritis (47,96). Sacroiliac involvement is more commonly bilateral than unilateral (47). When bilateral, asymmetric involvement is typical, which differentiates this disease from the symmetric involvement of AS (Fig. 36) (71). Spondylitis is often associated with sacroiliitis (47) but spondylitis with normal sacroiliac joints is also a feature of PA (96). Ankylosis of the sacroiliac joints is uncommon in PA.

In the spine, PA presents with coarse, asymmetric, nonmarginal syndesmophytes, which have been termed paravertebral ossifications (PVO) (Fig. 37) (12,47, 54,66,96). The thoracolumbar junction is the most common site of spondylitis, with most cases involving the lower two thoracic and upper three lumbar vertebrae (96). The lower lumbar spine is usually spared (65). Unlike AS, PA often has discontinuous areas of involvement throughout the spine (96). The cervical spine is involved less commonly than the lumbar spine. Spinal fusion, vertebral body squaring, and apophyseal joint involvement are rare.

Reiter's arthritis is a subset of a collection of disorders termed reactive arthritides, occurring predominantly in HLA-B27– positive individuals. In classic Reiter's syndrome, nonspecific urethritis, arthritis, conjunctivitis, and mucocutaneous lesions appear within a month of sexual or enteric exposure (104). A number of organisms have been implicated, including *Chlamydia, Shigella, Salmonella* and *Yersinia.* HLA-B27 is the most readily identifiable marker in the predisposed host (10). It is present in approximately 90% of patients with urogenital infection and in 50% to 80% of those with enteric infection (104). Reiter's syndrome is being reported in patients with AIDS (104). Reiter's disease involves men more than women and most of the affected patients are young, ranging in age between 15 and 35 years.

Sacroiliitis is present in about 43% of patients with Reiter's disease (88) and it is more often asymmetric or unilateral. This is especially true early in the disease. Complete SI joint fusion is uncommon. Spondylitis of Reiter's disease is similar to psoriatic arthritis (70,71,88). The thoracolumbar junction is the most common location; changes are characterized by nonmarginal syndesmophytes (paravertebral ossifications) with asymmetric distribution. Reiter's spondylitis is a discontinuous, multifocal disease, differentiating it and psoriatic arthritis from ankylosing spondylitis (69,70). Cervical spondylitis is rare in Reiter's disease (88); however, cases of atlantoaxial subluxation have been reported (57,59).

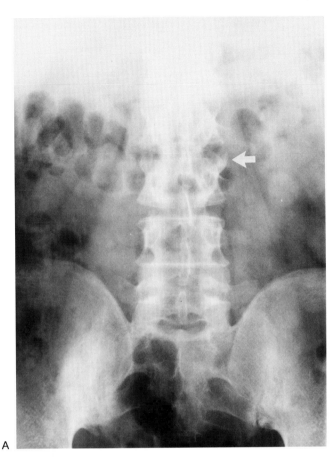

A

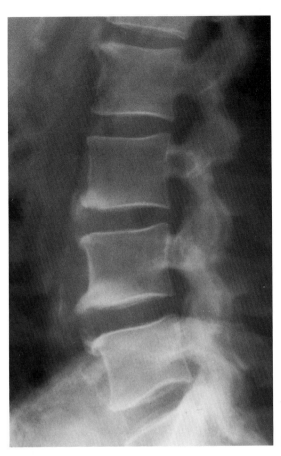

B

FIG. 36. Psoriatic sacrospondylitis. **A:** AP view of the lumbar spine and pelvis. Note asymmetric sacroiliac erosions. Paravertebral ossifications are present in the lumbar spine (*arrow*). **B:** Lateral view of lumbar spine demonstrating paravertebral ossifications, which are more horizontally oriented than syndesmophytes of ankylosing spondylitis.

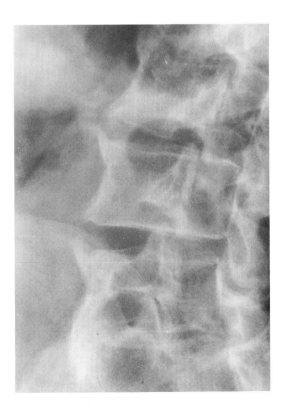

FIG. 37. Psoriatic arthritis with paravertebral ossification (PVO). Oblique view of the lumbar spine optimally shows that these ossifications originate away from the endplate margin.

CONCLUSION

Radiography remains a fundamental aspect of spine imaging, despite the development of many new imaging modalities. It is often the initial radiologic study performed, and radiographic findings dictate which other imaging studies should be utilized. This applies to many disease processes, including trauma, infection, neoplasm, inflammatory arthropathies, and evaluation of low back pain. A thorough understanding of how radiographs are generated, how to obtain high quality radiographs, and how to perform radiographic studies in a safe manner are all important features for anyone who plans to use radiography in clinical practice.

REFERENCES

1. Abrams HL, Spiro R, Goldstein N (1950): Metastases in carcinoma: analysis of 1,000 autopsied cases. *Cancer* 3:74–85.
2. Allen EH, Cosgrove D, Millard FJ (1978): The radiological changes in infections of the spine and their diagnostic value. *Clin Radiol* 29:31–40.
3. Arnett FC (1987): Seronegative spondylarthropathies. *Bull Rheum Dis* 37(1):1–12.
4. Baker BK, Sundaram M, Awwad EE (1991): Case report 88. *Skeletal Radiol* 20:463–464.
5. Barnes GT (1991): Contrast and scatter in x-ray imaging. *Radiographics* 11:307–323.
6. Batson OV (1957): The vertebral vein system. *AJR* 78(2):195–212.
7. Berquist TH (1988): Imaging of adult cervical spine trauma. *Radiographics* 8:667–694.
8. Bielecki DK, Sartoris D, Resnick D, Van Lom K, Fierer J, Haghighi P (1986): Intraosseous and intradiscal gas in association with spinal infection: report of three cases. *AJR* 147:83–86.
9. Bohlman HH (1985): Treatment of fractures and dislocations of the thoracic and lumbar spine. *J Bone Joint Surg* [Am] 67A:165–169.
10. Braunstein EM, Martel W, Moidel R (1982): Ankylosing spondylitis in men and women: a clinical and radiographic comparison. *Radiology* 144:91–94.
11. Byrne TN (1992): Spinal cord compression from epidural metastasis. *N Engl J Med* 327:614–619.
12. Bywaters EG, Dixon A (1965): Paravertebral ossification in psoriatic arthritis. *Ann Rheum Dis* 24:313–331.
13. Cahill DW, Love LC, Rechtine GR (1991): Pyogenic osteomyelitis of the spine in the elderly. *J Neurosurg* 74:878–886.
14. Calenoff L, Chessare JW, Rogers LF, Toerge J, Rosen JS (1987): Multiple level spinal injuries: importance of early recognition. *AJR* 130:665–669.
15. Clark CR, Goetz DD, Menezes AH (1989): Arthrodesis of the cervical spine in rheumatoid arthritis. *J Bone Joint Surg* (Am) 71(3):381–392.
16. Clark CR, Igram CM, El-Khoury GY, Ehara S (1988): Radiographic evaluation of cervical spine injuries. *Spine* 13:742–747.
17. Coulam CM, Erickson JJ (1981): Production of x-rays. In: Coulam CM, Erickson JJ, Rollo FD, James AE Jr, eds. *The physical basis of medical imaging*. New York: Appelton-Century-Crofts, p. 37.
18. Cowan NC, Bush K, Katz DE, Gishen P (1992): The natural history of sciatica: a prospective radiological study. *Clin Radiol* 46:7–12.
19. Curry TS III, Dowdey JE, Murry RC Jr (1990): *Christensen's physics of diagnostic radiology*, 4th ed. Philadelphia: Lea & Febiger, pp. 16–19, 222–225.
20. Daffner RH, Deeb ZL, Rothfus WE (1987): The posterior vertebral body line: importance in the detection of burst fractures. *AJR* 93–96.
21. Daffner RH, DeLuca SA (1983): What is radiology's role in low back pain? *Appl Radiol* Nov/Dec.
22. Davis, FW, Markley HE (1951): Rheumatoid arthritis with death from medullary compression. *Ann Int Med* 35:451–454.
23. Deyo RA, Rainville J, Kent DL (1992): What can the history and physical examination tell us about low back pain? *JAMA* 268(6):760–765.
24. Dihlmann W (1979): Current radiodiagnostic concept of ankylosing spondylitis. *Skeletal Radiol* 4:179–188.
25. Dihlmann W, Delling G (1978): Disco-vertebral destructive lesions (so-called Andersson lesions) associated with ankylosing spondylitis. *Skeletal Radiol* 3:10–16.
26. Doubilet PM, Judy PF (1981): Dosimetry of radiological procedures and dose reduction in diagnostic radiology. *Postgrad Radiol* 1:309–323.
27. Ehara S, Khurana JS, Kattapuram SV (1989): Pyogenic vertebral osteomyelitis of the posterior elements. *Skeletal Radiol* 18:175–178.
28. El-Khoury GY, Wener MH, Menezes AH, Dolan KD, Kathol ME (1980): Cranial settling in rheumatoid arthritis. *Radiology* 137:637–642.
29. El-Khoury GY, Whitten CG (1993): Trauma to the upper thoracic spine: anatomy, biomechanics and unique imaging features. *AJR* 160:95–102.
30. Enzmann DR (1994): On low back pain. *AJNR* 15:109–113.
31. Fernandez-Ulloa M, Vasavada PJ, Hanslits ML, Volarich DT, Elgazzar AH (1985): Diagnosis of vertebral osteomyelitis: clinical, radiological and scintigraphic features. *Orthopedics* 8(9):1144–1150.
32. Fletcher GH (1947): Anterior vertebral wedging: frequency and significance. *AJR* 57:232–238.
33. Fox MW, Onofrio BM, Kilgore JE (1993): Neurological complications of ankylosing spondylitis. *J Neurosurg* 78:871–878.
34. Freemyer B, Vnapp R, Piche J, Wales L, Williams J (1989): Comparison of fine view and three-view cervical spine series in the evaluation of patients with cervical trauma. *Ann Emerg Med* 18:818–882.
35. Frymoyer JW (1988): Back pain and sciatica. *N Engl J Med* 318(5):291–300.
36. Fullerton GD (1987): Magnetic resonance imaging signal concepts. *Radiographics* 7:579–596.
37. Gehweiler JA Jr, Daffner RH, Roberts L Jr (1983): Malformations of the atlas vertebra simulating Jefferson fracture. *AJR* 140:1083–1086.
38. Gelman MI, Umber JS (1978): Fractures of the thoracolumbar spine in ankylosing spondylitis. *AJR* 130:485–491.
39. Goldberg AL, Rothfus WE, Deeb ZL, Daffner RH, Lupetin AR, Wilberger JE, Prostko ER (1988): The impact of magnetic resonance on the diagnostic evaluation of acute cervicothoracic spinal trauma. *Skeletal Radiol* 17:89–95.
40. Goldberg AL, Keaton NL, Rothfus WE, Daffner RH (1993): Ankylosing spondylitis complicated by trauma: MR findings correlated with plain radiographs and CT. *Skeletal Radiol* 22:333–336.
41. Grans F, Krol G, Foley K (1985): Early diagnosis of spinal cord epidural metastasis (SEM): correlation with clinical and radiological findings [*abstract*]. *Proc Am Soc Clin Oncol* 4:269.
42. Gupta A, El Masri WS (1989): Incidence, distribution and neurological patterns. *J Bone Joint Surg* [Br] 71B:692–695.
43. Hall EJ (1991): Scientific view of low level radiation risks. *Radiographics* 11:509–518.
44. Hall FM (1980): Back pain and the radiologist. *Radiology* 137:861–863.
45. Hamilton MG, MacRae ME (1993): Atlantoaxial dislocation as the presenting symptom of ankylosing spondylitis. *Spine* 18(15):2344–2346.
46. Harris JH Jr, Carson GC, Wagner LK (1994): Radiologic diagnosis of traumatic occipitovertebral dislocation: 1. Normal occipitovertebral relationship on lateral radiographs of supine subjects. *AJR* 162(4):881–886.
47. Harvie JN, Lester RS, Little AH (1976): Sacroiliitis in severe psoriasis. *AJR* 127:579–584.
48. Hasegawa BH (1991): *The physics of medical x-ray imaging (or the photon and me: How I saw the light*, 2nd ed. Madison, WI: Medical Physics Publishing, pp. 36–37, 80–83.

49. Hendee WR (1991): Personal and public perceptions of radiation risks. *Radiographics* 11:1109–1119.
50. Hogan MJ, ed (1987): X-rays and the pregnant woman. *Mayo Clin Update* 3:1–2.
51. Jamison RC, Heimlich EM, Miethke JC, O'Loughlin BJ (1961): Nonspecific spondylitis of infants and children. *Radiology* 77(3):355–367.
52. Kattan KR (1976): The notched articular process of C_7 (dorsalization of C_7). *AJR* 126:612–616.
53. Kattan KR (1977): Backward "displacement" of the spinolaminal line at C_2: a normal variation. *AJR* 129:289–290.
54. Kellebrew K, Gold RH, Sholkoff SD (1973): Psoriatic spondylitis. *Radiology* 108:9–16, 1973
55. Kelsey CA (1985): *Essentials of radiology physics.* St. Louis: Warren H. Green, pp. 89–97.
56. Kleinman P, Rivelis M, Schneider R, Kaye JJ (1977): Juvenile ankylosing spondylitis. *Radiology* 125:775–780.
57. Kransdorf MJ, Wehrle PA, Moser RP (1988): Atlantoaxial subluxation in Reiter's syndrome: a report of three cases and review of the literature. *Spine* 13(1):12–14.
58. Kreipke DL, Gillespie KR, McCarthy MC, Mail JT, Lappas JC, Broadie TA (1989): Reliability of indications for cervical spine films in trauma patients. *J Trauma* 29:1438–1439.
59. Latchaw RE, Meyer GW (1978): Reiter disease with altanto-axial subluxation. *Radiology* 126:303–304.
60. Lauridsen KN, De Carvalho A, Andersen AH (1984): Degree of vertebral wedging of the dorso-lumbar spine. *Acta Radiol* 25:29–32.
61. Lee C, Rogers LF, Woodring JH, Goldstein SJ, Kim KS (1984): Fractures of the craniovertebral junction associated with other fractures of the spine: overlooked entity? *AJNR* 5:775–781.
62. Lee KR, Siegel EL, Templeton AW, Dwyer SJ III, Murphey MD, Wetzel LH (1991): State-of-the-art digital radiography. *Radiographics* 11:1013–1025.
63. Lewis LM, Docherty M, Ruoff BE, Fortney JP, Keltner RA Jr, Britton P (1991): Flexion-extension views in the evaluation of cervical spine injuries. *Ann Emerg Med* 20:117–121.
64. Liang M, Komaroff AL (1982): Roentgenograms in primary care patients with acute low back pain: a cost-effectiveness analysis. 142:1108–1112.
65. Lindholm TS, Pylkkanen P (1982): Discitis following removal of intervertebral disc. *Spine* 7(6):618–622.
66. Loebl DH, Kirby S, Ruffin Stephenson C, Cook E, Mealing HG, Bailey JP (1979): Psoriatic arthritis. *JAMA* 242(22):2447–2451.
67. MacDonald RL, Schwartz ML, Mirich D, Sharkey PW, Nelson WR (1990): Diagnosis of cervical spine injury in motor crash victims: how many x-rays are enough? *J Trauma* 30:392–397.
68. Martel W (1961): The occipito-atlanto-axial joints in rheumatoid arthritis and ankylosing spondylitis. *AJR* 86(2):223–239.
69. Martel W (1977): Pathogenesis of cervical discovertebral destruction in rheumatoid arthritis. *Arthritis Rheum* 20(6):1217–1225.
70. Martel M, Braunstein EM, Borlaza G, Good AE, Griffin PE (1979): Radiologic features of Reiter disease. *Radiology* 132:1–10.
71. McEwen C, DiTata D, Lingg C, Porini A, Good A, Rankin T (1971): Ankylosing spondylitis and spondylitis accompanying ulcerative colitis, regional enteritis, psoriasis and Reiter's disease: a comparative study. *Arthritis Rheum* 14(3):291–318.
72. Mirvis SE, Diaconis JN, Chirico PA, Reiner BI, Joslyn JN, Militello P (1989): Protocol-driven radiologic evaluation of suspected cervical spine injury: efficacy study. *Radiology* 170:831–834.
73. Murphey MD, Quale JL, Martin NL, Bramble JM, Cook LT, Dwyer SJ III (1992): Computed radiology in musculoskeletal imaging: state of the art. *AJR* 158:19–27.
74. Murphy PH (1991): AAPM tutorial. Acceptable risk as a basis for regulation. *Radiographics* 11:889–897.
75. Newlin N (1978): Reduction in radiation exposure: the rare earth screen. *AJR* 130:1195–1196.
76. Park WM, O'Neill M, McCall IW (1979): The radiology of rheumatoid involvement of the cervical spine. *Skeletal Radiol* 4:1–7.
77. Pastershank SP (1981): Ankylosing spondylitis in women. *J Can Assoc Radiol* 32:93–94.
78. Patton JT (1976): Differential diagnosis of inflammatory spondylitis. *Skeletal Radiol* 1:77–85.
79. Rawlings III CE, Wilkins RH, Gallis HA, Goldner JL, Francis R (1983): Postoperative intervertebral disc space infection. *Neurosurgery* 13(4):371–376.
80. Reid DC, Henderson R, Saboe L, Miller JDR (1987): Etiology and clinical course of missed spine fractures. *J Trauma* 27:980–986.
81. Resnick D, Dwosh IL, Goergen TG, Shapiro RF, Utsinger PD, Wiesner KB, Bryan BL (1976): Clinical and radiographic abnormalities in ankylosing spondylitis: a comparison of men and women. *Radiology* 119:293–297.
82. Ringenberg BJ, Fisher AK, Urdaneta LF, Midthum MA (1988): Rational ordering of cervical spine radiographs following trauma. *Ann Emerg Med* 17:792–796.
83. Roberts FF, Kishore PRS, Cunningham ME (1978): Routine oblique radiography of the pediatric lumbar spine: is it necessary? *AJR* 131:297–298.
84. Rocco HD, Eyring EJ (1972): Intervertebral disk infections in children. *Am J Dis Child* 123:448–451.
85. Rogers LF, Thayer C, Weinberg PE, Kim KS (1980): Acute injuries of the upper thoracic spine associated with paraplegia. *AJR* 134:67–73.
86. Sartoris DJ, Moskowitz PS, Kaufman RA, Ziprkowski MN, Berger PE (1983): Childhood diskitis: computed tomographic fingings. *Radiology* 149:701–707.
87. Scavone JG, Latshaw RF, Weidner WA (1981): Anteroposterior and lateral radiographs: an adequate lumbar spine examination. *AJR* 136:715–717.
88. Schumacher TM, Genant HK, Kellet MJ, Mall JC, Fye KH (1978): HLA-B27 associated arthropathies. *Radiology* 126:289–297.
89. Sherk HH (1978): Atlantoaxial instability and acquired basilar invagination in rheumatoid arthritis. *Orthop Clin North Am* 9(4):1053–1062.
90. Smith AS, Blaser SI (1991): Infectious and inflammatory processes of the spine. *Radiol Clin North Am* 29(4):809–827.
91. Sprawls P (1987): *Physical principles of medical imaging.* Rockville: Aspen, p. 25.
92. Sprawls P (1990): In: Gedgaudes-McClees RK, Torres WE, eds. The principles of computed tomography image formation and quality. Essentials of body computed tomography. Philadelphia: WB Saunders, pp. 1–9.
93. Stauffer RN (1975): Pyogenic vertebral osteomyelitis. *Orthop Clin North Am* 6(4):1015–1027.
94. Streitwieser DR, Knopp R, Wales LR, Williams JL, Tonnemacher K (1983): Accuracy of standard radiographic views in detecting cervical spine fractures. *Ann Emerg Med* 12:538–542.
95. Sullivan CR, Bruwer AJ, Harris LE (1958): Hypermobility of the cervical spine in children: a pitfall in the diagnosis of cervical dislocation. *Am J Surg* 95:636–640.
96. Sundaram M, Patton JT (1975): Paravertebral ossification of psoriasis and Reiter's disease. *Br J Radiol* 48:628–633.
97. Suss RA, Zimmerman RD, Leeds NE (1983): Pseudospread of the atlas: false sign of Jefferson fracture in young children. *AJR* 140:1079–1082.
98. Swartz HM, Reichling BA (1978): Hazards of radiation exposure for pregnant women. *JAMA* 239:1907–1908.
99. Swinson DR, Hamilton EB, Mathews JA, Yates DA (1972): Vertical subluxation of the axis in rheumatoid arthritis. *Ann Rheum Dis* 31:359–363.
100. Swischuk LE, Hayden CK Jr, Sarwar M (1979): The posteriorly tilted dens. A normal variation mimicking a fractured dens. *Pediatr Radiol* 8:27–28.
101. Townsend EH Jr, Rowe ML (1952): Mobility of the upper cervical spine in health and disease. *Pediatrics* 10:567–573.
102. Turetsky DB, Vines FS, Clayman DA, Northup HM (1993): Technique and use of supine oblique views in acute cervical spine trauma. *Ann Emerg Med* 22:685–689.
103. Vandemark RM (1990): Radiology of the cervical spine in trauma patients: practice pitfalls and recommendations for improving efficiency and communication. *AJR* 155:465–472.
104. Vaughan JH (1989): Infection and rheumatic diseases: a review. *Bull Rheum Dis* 39(1):1–7.

105. Wackenheim A (1974): *Roentgen diagnosis of the craniovertebral region,* 1st ed. New York: Springer-Verlag.
106. Weinstein JN, McLain RF (1987): Primary tumors of the spine. *Spine* 12:843–851.
107. Weinstein PR, Karpman RR, Gall EP, Pitt M (1982): Spinal cord injury, spinal fracture, and spinal stenosis in ankylosing spondylitis. *J Neurosurg* 57:609–616.
108. Wenger DR, Bobechko WP, Gilday DL (1978): The spectrum of intervertebral disc-space infection in children. *J Bone Joint Surg* [Am] 60(1):100–108.
109. Wiley AM, Trueta J (1959): The vascular anatomy of the spine and its relationship to pyogenic vertebral osteomyelitis. *J Bone Joint Surg* [Br] 41(4):796–809.
110. Zanca P, Lodmell EA (1951): Fracture of the spinous processes: A "new" sign for the recognition of fractures of cervical and upper dorsal spinous process. *Radiology* 56:427–428.

The Adult Spine: Principles and Practice,
2nd edition, J.W. Frymoyer, Editor-in-Chief.
Lippincott-Raven Publishers, Philadelphia © 1997.

CHAPTER **26**

Myelography

Charles Neuville Aprill III

HISTORY

The concept of altering the contrast of structures in the spinal canal to improve on radiographic images dates to the first quarter of the twentieth century. The introduction of gas (air) into the subarachnoid space as a contrast agent was originally introduced by Dandy (24). The application of this technique for localization of intraspinal pathology followed shortly (49). The era of positive contrast myelography was ushered in by accident: Sicard and Forrestier (89) inadvertently instilled iodized poppy seed oil (Lipiodol) into the subarachnoid space. The absence of an acute meningeal reaction or any other immediate untoward effects prompted the clinical use of this agent without experimental studies. It was not until later sequelae of severe meningeal irritation and crippling arachnoiditis became apparent that the need for safer contrast agents was realized (68).

Iophendylate (Myodil, Pantopaque) was developed in the 1940s (78). This oil-based agent was the preferred contrast material in Great Britain and the United States for over three decades. Pantopaque was tolerated and produced few severe acute reactions (74). This agent was employed to study the entire spinal subarachnoid space. It was used in evaluation of the cervical region in the United States until the late 1970s despite significant late meningeal pathology (16) (Fig. 1). The development of safe water-soluble agents led to the general cessation of its use.

Swedish investigators, unwilling to accept the risk associated with oil-based agents, employed absorbable contrast material (gas or water-soluble) like sodium methiodal (Abrodil), which was introduced in 1931 (2). For many years this agent was employed in Scandinavia for study of the lumbar subarachnoid space; however, it required a spinal anesthetic and the agent was quite toxic, inducing severe muscle spasms, sudden drops in blood pressure, and seizures.

The water-soluble ionic contrast material meglumine iothalamate (Conray) was studied as a potential myelographic agent in the 1960s (19). This agent was less toxic than Abrodil, but too toxic to be employed in the subarachnoid space above the level of the conus (30). Meglumine iocarmate (Dimer-X) proved superior to both Abrodil and Conray, becoming an acceptable myelographic agent in the early 1970s (33). Despite less neurotoxicity, these ionic contrast materials were associated with an unacceptably high incidence of meningeal irritation and central nervous system complications while complete evaluation of the spinal subarachnoid space was still not possible (35).

In contrast to the rapid and unstudied clinical use of Lipiodol, the development and deployment of water-soluble contrast agents was cautious. The first of the modern non-ionic water-soluble contrast agents, metrizamide (Amipaque) was introduced in the 1970s (1). This material proved to have acceptably low levels of toxicity (57). Clinical studies revealed much less meningeal reaction (46), and it could be safely brought into contact with the spinal cord (44).

The second generation of non-ionic water-soluble contrast agents includes iohexol (Omnipaque) and io-

C. N. Aprill III, M.D.: Diagnostic Conservative Management, Inc., New Orleans, Louisiana, 70115.

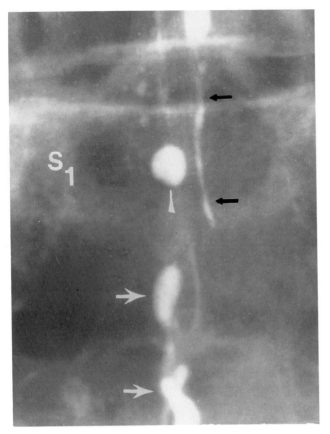

FIG. 1. Pantopaque myelogram showing arachnoiditis in a supine 36-year-old woman. Radiograph is centered at the level of the sacrum (right pedicle S1). Some residual Pantopaque globules are mobile (*arrowhead*), other collections are fixed (*white arrows*). Linear calcification (*black arrows*) is associated with thecal sac at the origin of left S2 nerve sheath.

pamidol (Isovue). These agents have been shown to be considerably less toxic than metrizamide (59). By the late 1980s, these agents became the contrast materials of choice and effectively eliminated the use of iophendylate and metrizamide.

A diagnostic advantage of a water-soluble, low-viscosity medium over oil contrast agents is better definition of the root sleeves and the intra-arachnoid structures (Fig. 2). Also, aqueous solutions may be introduced through smaller needles, and complete absorption from the spinal subarachnoid space eliminates the need to remove the agent, although partial removal has been advocated (45). These are now the contrast media of choice.

PATIENT CONSIDERATIONS

Myelography is usually an elective procedure and should in general be performed on patients who are healthy, based on a good screening history. It is important to question patients regarding any chronic or recurring infection, particularly related to dental, genitourinary, or skin problems. Systemic conditions such as diabetes (93), cardiovascular disease, and alcoholism may contraindicate myelography or alter the manner in which the study is performed. Either the condition or the medications employed to manage it may prompt a need for hospitalization or alteration in technique. Any past history of seizure is important. It is helpful to have a written list of the patient's medications and current doses. Allergies, particularly to radiographic contrast agents, should be noted and details of the reaction obtained. The

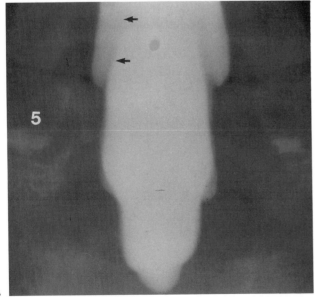

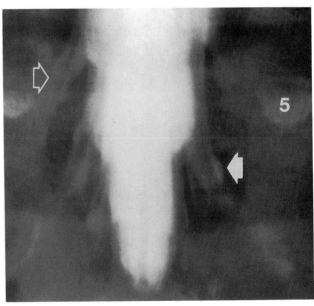

A   B

FIG. 2. Two prone erect myelograms. **A:** Pantopaque fills the caudal end of thecal sac, defining its margin. The viscous oil does not enter the dural root sleeves. Intra-arachnoid S1 rootlets are barely recognizable (*black arrows*). **B:** Metrizamide fills the thecal sac and dural root sleeves. Left L5 rootlets can be identified within the sleeve and left lateral recess (*open arrow*). Right S1 rootlets are identified in root sleeve just proximal to entry into radicular canal (*solid arrow*). Contrast material does not extend to the level of the dorsal ganglia.

possibility of pregnancy must be excluded in women of childbearing age. Screening examination by phone or in writing must be completed prior to the study. Many drugs lower seizure threshold. These include monoamine oxidase inhibitors, tricyclic antidepressants, and phenothiazines (5,94). When possible, they should be terminated several days prior to the study.

It is important not to restrict fluids prior to the examination (40). For early morning myelography, a clear-liquid breakfast is recommended. For late morning myelography, the patients may have a light breakfast and then clear liquids *ad lib.* If the study is performed in the afternoon, patients should be given a normal breakfast, a liquid lunch, and clear liquids.

Most patients undergoing myelography approach the exam with anxiety. Appropriate discussion of the procedure and postprocedure symptoms is essential. Ten to 15 minutes of discussion time employing models and drawings helps to allay patients' apprehension.

In most circumstances, the performance of lumbar myelography requires no premedication. However, in situations where seizure threshold may be reduced (age, alcoholism, past seizure history, neuroleptic drugs) or when large doses of contrast material are required, premedication is advisable. Diazepam has been effectively employed as a premedication in patients undergoing metrizamide cisternography (96). Diazepam in doses up to 5.0 mg or midazolam up to 2.5 mg administered intravenously immediately prior to the examination should be satisfactory premedication when the less toxic nonionic agents are employed.

In those patients whose clinical condition increases the risk of seizure, it is prudent not to perform myelography unless it is absolutely necessary, and then antiseizure precautions should be employed. Sodium phenobarbital has been shown effective in reducing neurotoxic reactions in animals exposed to metrizamide and neuroleptic drugs (31). It may be employed as a pre- and postmyelographic adjuvant. These patients require careful monitoring and should not be studied on an outpatient basis.

POSTPROCEDURE

After myelography, the patient should be placed on a stretcher, cart, or bed with the head elevated between 15° and 45° (based on patient comfort). The patient should remain at bed rest with the head elevated for the next 3 to 4 hours, especially if postmyelography computed tomography (CT) scanning is to be performed. This maintains the hyperbaric contrast material in the lumbar cistern for absorption via arachnoid villi and granulations of the lumbosacral root sleeves (51).

Postmyelographic CT scanning has proven to be an important adjunct to modern myelography. The scan should be delayed 3 to 5 hours after myelography. Scanning in the immediate postmyelogram period may in-

crease morbidity and result in an inferior examination. CT is performed with the patient supine, increasing the amount of contrast material entering the intracranial subarachnoid space. The delay of several hours allows time for some absorption and thus reduces the contrast material available for entry into the cranium. In addition, the decreased density of residual contrast material provides better CT visualization of intra-arachnoid structures.

If small needles are employed, patients should be allowed limited ambulation (55). If there is no nausea or vomiting, patients should resume usual diet with increased intake of fluids. Patients should be instructed to limit activities for 24 to 48 hours following the study.

Neurotoxic reactions have been reported to occur 4 to 6 hours after myelography (58). Although myelography is performed on an "outpatient" basis, patients should be observed for at least 6 hours. They must be accompanied by a responsible adult who can drive and report any problems or reactions. All patients should be provided with emergency phone numbers to contact the appropriate physician in the event of a postprocedure complication. Oral diazepam in low doses (5.0 mg t.i.d.) or phenobarbital (60.0 mg b.i.d.) for 1 to 2 days after the procedure may be helpful in limiting later complications. It is important to have outpatients "check in" the following day to report on their status. Inpatients may be discharged the day after myelography assuming there are no untoward effects.

It is obvious that postprocedure protocols must be individualized to the patient and condition. The elderly patient with diabetes, hypertension, spinal stenosis, severe spondylosis, or cord pathology may require much more pre- and/or postprocedure attention.

PROCEDURAL CONSIDERATIONS

Myelography is generally performed in routine radiographic/fluoroscopic suites. In many hospitals, these studies are carried out in the general radiology rooms, which are employed for all fluoroscopic procedures. Obviously a "clean" special-procedure room is preferable.

Lumbar puncture is easily performed with patients in the prone position (14). Direct posterior midline approach requires reduction of lordosis to separate the laminae and spinous processes; this is accomplished by placing a pillow or sponge (bolster) beneath the abdomen. Often the bolster produces an uncomfortable pressure sensation and occasional nausea. The procedure needle must traverse supraspinous and intraspinous ligaments. A relatively stiff needle (22-gauge) is required to maintain directional control.

If a slightly oblique paramedian approach is employed, lumbar puncture may be accomplished without the use of a bolster. By avoiding the ligaments, a smaller needle (25-gauge) may be easily directed into the subarachnoid space, through the ligamentum flavum. This reduces the incidence of post–lumbar puncture headache (36).

It is prudent to perform the puncture at the L2-L3 or L3-L4 segments and to approach from the side opposite the patient's dominant pain. The laminae and intralaminar notches of L2 through L4 vertebrae are identified by fluoroscopy. They are best seen with the patient in a slightly oblique position. The region selected for skin puncture should be thoroughly cleansed. Alcohol or antiseptic solutions should be employed and the area covered with sterile drapes (28).

Lumbar puncture can be accomplished with a 25-gauge needle in most patients. In larger individuals, it is necessary to employ 22-gauge needles to maintain control. A stylet must be in place (7). Local anesthetic infiltration into the skin and subcutaneous tissues is required only when 22-gauge needles are used. There is very little discomfort associated with skin penetration by a 25-gauge needle.

The skin puncture should be just off the midline and the needle directed slightly medially toward the inferior surface of the chosen lamina in an attempt to direct it into the intralaminar notch (Fig. 3). The ligamentum flavum is the first firm structure to be encountered. A

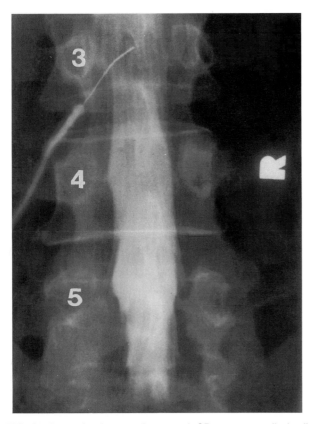

FIG. 3. Prone lumbar myelogram. A 25-gauge needle is directed beneath the left lamina of L3 via a paramedian oblique approach. Needle tip is in the center of the thecal sac.

change in resistance is recognizable when using 22-gauge needles, but a 25-gauge needle may penetrate the ligament with little noticeable change in resistance. Although the needle may be advanced fairly rapidly through the posterior subcutaneous and muscular tissues, it should be advanced slowly as the posterior arch is approached. Once the ligamentum flavum has been engaged and penetrated, the stylet should be removed and the head of the table elevated 10° to 15°. With experience, a single pass will result in satisfactory subarachnoid position, recognizable by the appearance of spinal fluid at the needle hub. Fluid appears quickly when 22-gauge needles are used. One to 2 minutes may elapse before fluid appears at the needle hub when 25-gauge needles are used. Collection of cerebrospinal fluid (CSF) for laboratory analysis is unnecessary except in specific clinical circumstances (82).

The posterior dura is not particularly sensitive and penetration is not usually associated with any complaint. Needle contact with intra-arachnoid rootlets will sometimes provoke pain, usually unilateral, extending into the lower extremity. The anterior dura is innervated and contact with it usually provokes complaint of back pain radiating into the hip or buttock region, often bilaterally. Complaints of pain are usually mild to moderate and, in response, the needle should be retracted slightly. In most instances, the discomfort stops with retraction of the needle.

The appearance of clear CSF at the needle hub indicates entry into the subarachnoid position. It is unnecessary to verify position with lateral filming. If the spinal fluid is slightly tinged with blood, injection of contrast material should be delayed until a few drops are collected to see if it clears. Examination with modern myelographic agents need not be postponed in the face of minimally blood-tinged CSF (40). In the event that the fluid is grossly bloody, needle position should be visualized in both the frontal and lateral planes. A needle placed immediately adjacent to the posterior aspect of a vertebral body may have penetrated an epidural vein. It should be retracted to the middle third of the spinal canal. Bloody fluid will usually clear and the examination may proceed. If the fluid does not clear and remains frankly bloody despite proper needle position, the approach should be abandoned, and puncture should be performed at another level, preferably two segments from the initial puncture site. The presence of frankly bloody fluid at a second puncture site implies hemorrhage into the subarachnoid space. This may be related to the nature of the primary pathology or may be the result of technical difficulties (9). The decision to continue or abort the myelogram must be based on the clinical situation, the experience and expertise of the myelographer, and the availability of other imaging modalities [CT, magnetic resonance imaging (MRI)].

Once a satisfactory lumbar puncture has been accomplished, contrast material should be instilled slowly into the subarachnoid space. The flow should be directly visualized by fluoroscopy early in the process to verify subarachnoid opacification. Elevating the head of the table promotes flow into the dependent lumbar cistern for easy verification. When small-gauge needles are used, instillation of fluid volumes necessary for myelography will require several minutes. Brief repeated fluoroscopic visualization is helpful to ensure the needle has remained in satisfactory position. By direct visualization, the examiner can determine the volume necessary to obtain a satisfactory exam. If the thecal sac is small, 8.0 to 10.0 cc may be sufficient. In a patient with a large thecal sac, 14.0 to 16.0 cc may be required. As a general rule, 10.0 to 14.0 cc is sufficient to opacify the lumbar thecal sac over three segments with the patient in the erect position (Fig. 4).

For lumbar studies, concentrations of 180 to 240 mg/cc are usually sufficient. When the dorsal spine is to be studied, the same concentrations may be employed, but the volume should be increased (up to 14.0 to 16.0 cc).

Cervical myelography may be performed following injection of contrast material into the lumbar subarachnoid space or by direct lateral cervical puncture. The lumbar approach is familiar to all myelographers and is relatively easy and safe and thus preferred by many. Ten cubic centimeters of contrast material at concentrations of 280 to 300 mg/cc is usually sufficient to provide adequate opacification of the cervical cistern when the myelographer is skilled and there are no unusual circumstances such as accentuated kyphosis or an uncooperative patient. Contrast material is directed into the cervical region by gravity.

Others have proposed direct lateral cervical puncture as the technique of choice for cervical myelography (84). The procedure is performed with the patient in the prone position and the neck extended. Direct lateral fluoroscopy is necessary for safe and efficient performance. The needle must be easily controlled: 22-gauge spinal needles are necessary because smaller needles are flexible and difficult to control with the precision required. The interspace between the C1 and C2 spinous processes is identified by lateral fluoroscopy, the skin entry point marked, and, after sterile skin preparation and draping, the skin and subcutaneous tissues are anesthetized. The needle is then directed horizontally to the posterior aspect of the central canal between the C1 and C2 processes. The needle should be advanced slowly and directed toward the junction of the middle and posterior third of the central canal. Repeated screening with lateral fluoroscopy is required to verify proper course (69). Advancement may be checked by vertical fluoroscopy. However, there is a definite tactile sensation associated with penetration of the dura. The stylet is removed and subarachnoid position verified by the appearance of CSF at the needle hub. Contrast material (8.0 to 10.0 cc at 280 to 300 mg/cc concentration) is slowly introduced.

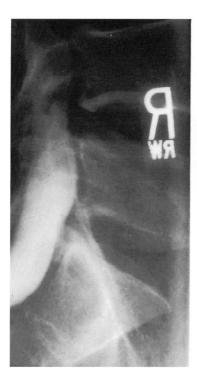
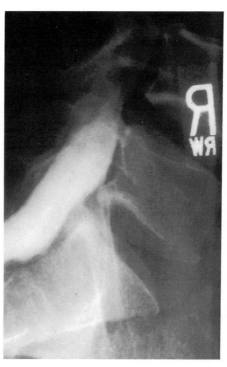
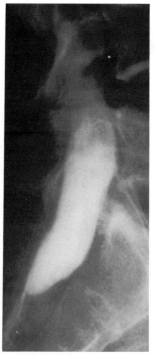

FIG. 4. Lateral myelograms, erect series. Although 8.0 cc of non-ionic contrast material results in good opacification, volume is inadequate for study of this normal but large lumbar cistern. Increasing the volume of contrast material to 14.0 to 16.0 cc at a concentration of 180 to 200 mg/cc should provide filling of the spine over the lower three lumbar motion segments for better functional assessment.

As with lumbar instillation, the volume of contrast material instilled into the cervical subarachnoid space should be individualized. This is accomplished by direct fluoroscopy during the instillation process. Malposition of the needle tip may be recognized early and position corrected for satisfactory subarachnoid delivery (Fig. 5). The cervical approach provides good filling of the cervical cistern and visualization is usually excellent. Precise control of contrast flow minimizes entry of concentrated contrast material into the cranial vault. C1-C2 puncture is a safe procedure in the hands of experienced practitioners. However, complications such as puncture of the cord have been reported (66). This technique is not recommended for practitioners with limited training and experience.

Dorsal and cervical myelography also can be performed by lumbar administration of contrast material. The procedure needle is removed once the material has been instilled into the lumbar subarachnoid space. Transfer of the contrast into the dorsal region is accomplished by placing the patient in a lateral decubitus position and tilting the head of the table down approximately 15°. It is important to move the table slowly and to elevate the patient's head by lateral bending of the neck. The head is supported on pillows. This maneuver prevents the rapid flow of contrast material into the cranial vault. Once the contrast has moved into the dorsal region, the patient is turned to the supine position and the table leveled for a dorsal spine examination. The contrast will pool in the dependent portion of the subarachnoid space.

Transfer of contrast material to the cervical region requires a different maneuver. Once the contrast material has moved into the dorsal region with the patient in the lateral decubitus position as described above, the patient is rolled into a prone position with the head of the table down 15°. The contrast material will flow into the now dependent cervical cistern. This maneuver requires careful and precise management of the patient's head and neck. The myelographer or a trained assistant must control the patient's head during the turn from the decubitus to the prone position. The head must be elevated and the neck maintained in extension.

An alternative method to transfer the contrast material from the lumbar to the cervical area is as follows: With the patient in the prone position and the neck fully extended and supported by sponges, the head of the table is turned down to 15°. A vertical fluoroscope is placed over the cervical region. The patient's hips are manually elevated approximately 6 inches above the table top. This will result in flow over the dorsal kyphosis. By observing the appearance of contrast material in the cervical region and changing the elevation of the patient's hips, the flow can be controlled. Maintaining a slow pace allows adequate opacification of the cervical cistern with little spill into the cranial vault. Lifting an average patient with this maneuver requires at least two adults of average strength and no back problems.

In patients with an exaggerated thoracic kyphosis or who have difficulty in obtaining a full extension of the neck, the lumbar approach may not be possible, and C1-C2 puncture may be the only appropriate route of administration.

Puncture of the subarachnoid space is not a totally innocuous procedure. Morbidity associated with lumbar puncture alone has been reported with occasional severe

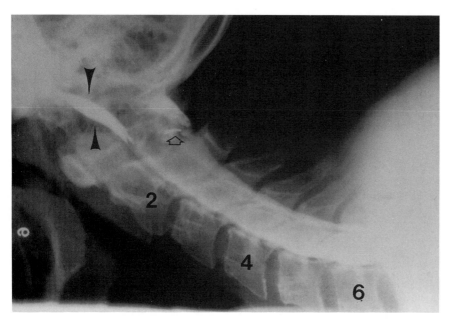

FIG. 5. Lateral cervical myelogram, C1-C2 puncture, patient prone. The needle is barely visible on horizontal lateral image. The tip is positioned in the subarachnoid space. The cervical cistern has been filled adequately (9.0 cc Iohexol, 300 mg/cc). Dense contrast material (*arrowheads*), posterior to the dens, is in the subdural/extra-arachnoid space. Recognition of unusual flow pattern at fluoroscopy during contrast instillation prompted slight manipulation to correct position of the needle tip.

consequences (38,62). The major problems associated with lumbar puncture are postprocedure headache and infection. The use of smaller gauge needles and pristine technique, and limiting the number of punctures will certainly reduce the incidence of significant spinal fluid leak and subsequent hydrostatic headaches. Obviously, infection of the subarachnoid space (meningitis) is a severe complication. It may occur in patients who have chronic, indolent infections. These should be detected on the pre-procedure screen. A break in sterile technique can result in inoculation of the subarachnoid space at the time of procedure. Strict adherence to the rules of aseptic technique must be observed.

Modern contrast agents are quite safe and outpatient myelography in appropriately selected patients is a reasonable procedure (73,101). Patients must be cautioned about potential adverse reactions to any contrast materials instilled into the subarachnoid space (58,91).

Another method to achieve CT myelography is low-dose intrathecal enhancement technique. The instillation of 3 to 5 cc of contrast material at low concentrations (180 to 200 mg/cc) is sufficient to provide excellent enhancement of the subarachnoid space if a later CT scan is performed. Scanning should begin immediately after instillation of the contrast material. Concentrations will remain sufficient for good visualization for 2 to 3 hours. When a low-dose approach with CT scanning is performed, handling of the patient depends on the primary area of interest. For lumbar scanning, the patient should be transported from the radiology suite to the CT scan area by stretcher and transferred to the CT couch in the supine position. Turning the patient through 360° disperses the contrast material. On the CT couch, the patient is turned to a lateral decubitus position, the prone position, the opposite decubitus, and finally the supine position immediately prior to scanning. If left in each of these positions for approximately 1 minute, there will be even dispersal of the contrast material in the regional subarachnoid space. This eliminates the problem of layering artifact. This artifact is particularly troublesome after myelography when the delay allows the hyperbaric contrast material to settle (Fig. 6). At times, the CSF can be isodense with the posterior disc, obscuring its margin. Occasionally, the artifact can simulate pathology.

For cervical or dorsal CT scanning, the contrast material should be delivered to the mid-dorsal region in the x-ray suite by the technique described above. The patient is transported to the CT area by stretcher in the supine position. If the dorsal spine is the area of interest, the patient handling is identical to that described for the lumbar study (the 360° maneuver).

For cervical scanning, the final step is to deliver contrast material to the cervical region. To accomplish this, the patient is transferred from the supine position on the stretcher to a prone position on the CT couch. However,

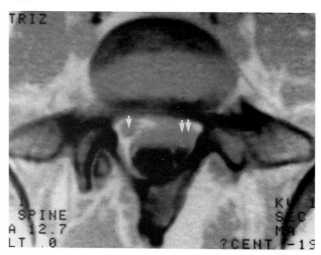

FIG. 6. Axial CT, L5-S1 interspace. Scan was acquired 4 hours after lumbar myelography (12.0 cc metrizamide, 180 mg/cc). The patient was transported from the hospital room by stretcher and transferred to the CT couch maintaining a supine position. Hyperbaric contrast material has settled, resulting in a "layering artifact" in the dependent portion of the lumbar cistern. Note asymmetry of the thecal sac. There is a composite left S1-S2 root sleeve (*double arrow*). Neither the composite root sleeve nor the right S1 root sleeve (*single arrow*) is opacified.

in the process of transfer, a folded pillow is placed under the abdomen. The patient maintains a modified knee-to-chest position for 1 to 2 minutes. This results in flow into the cervical region. Following this maneuver, the patient is returned to the supine position for cervical scanning. This technique has been employed for over 7 years in the performance of intrathecal enhanced cervical CT scans. There has been uniform success in obtaining satisfactory cervical intrathecal enhancement.

MYELOGRAPHY AND THE NEW TECHNOLOGIES

Increasing experience with high resolution CT scanning and the emergence of MRI as a primary imaging modality must prompt reassessment of the role of myelography in the evaluation of adults with spine disorders. This process begins with an understanding of what the myelogram demonstrates, particularly in comparison to CT and MRI.

Myelography is the positive contrast radiographic study of the spinal subarachnoid space. The inner margin of the thecal sac is usually defined over a length of three or more spinal segments. Structures contained within the subarachnoid space are recognizable. Each of the three major divisions of the spine may be evaluated.

Cervical Myelography

A standard cervical myelogram consists of frontal, oblique, and lateral views of the spinal subarachnoid space from the level of the foramen magnum to the cervicothoracic junction. The films are obtained with the patient in the prone position. Posteroanterior view demonstrates symmetrical filling of dural root sleeves and contained rootlets (Fig. 7). The width of the thecal sac is apparent, providing a general impression of canal volume. The size, shape, and position of the spinal cord are clearly defined. Slight enlargement of the cervical cord at the C5-C6 level is related to the afferent and efferent neural elements of the brachial plexus (53).

The size and configuration of the dural root sleeves are seen on the prone oblique views (Fig. 8). Adequate filling of the cervical cistern will result in visualization of the ipsilateral dural root sleeves and the posterolateral aspect of the thecal sac on the opposite side. Lesions involving the lateral recess and proximal foramen will deform the dural root sleeve. Large mass effects originating from the laminae or ligamentum flavum will deform the posterolateral aspect of the contrast column.

The horizontal beam lateral view best demonstrates the ventral surface of the contrast column (Fig. 9). With optimal filling of the cervical cistern, the posterior surface of the cord and the dorsal margin of the thecal sac are defined. Malalignment (retrolisthesis) and mass effects arising from disc or endplates are seen in profile. It is important to minimize the volume of contrast material entering the intracranial subarachnoid space (96). To prevent intracranial spill, the head and neck are maintained in extension for the duration of the examination. Unfortunately, this is an uncomfortable position for most patients with cervical spine pathology. Buckling of the ligamentum flavum and/or retrolisthesis of vertebral bodies may be accentuated in this position. These phenomena may increase discomfort, making it difficult for patients to maintain proper position. Patient motion or loss of contrast material into the cranial vault may result in a suboptimal study. Other patients may not be able to assume or maintain the extended position be-

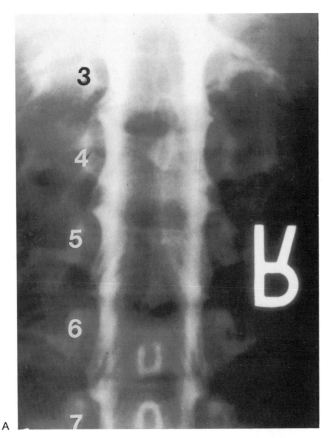
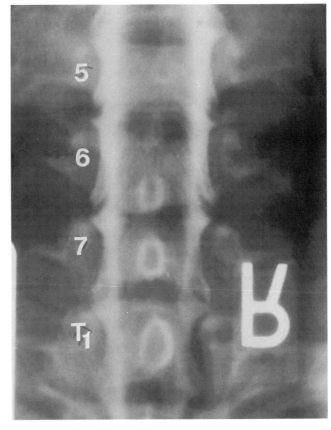

A

B

FIG. 7. Prone cervical myelogram, posteroanterior view. Iopamidol, 10.0 cc, 300 mg/cc, introduced via lumbar puncture. **A:** The downward course of the intrathecal rootlets becomes progressively more oblique at lower levels in the cervical region. **B:** At the cervicothoracic junction, the cervical cord is widest at C5-C6. Margins of the cord are clearly defined. The width of the subarachnoid space decreases.

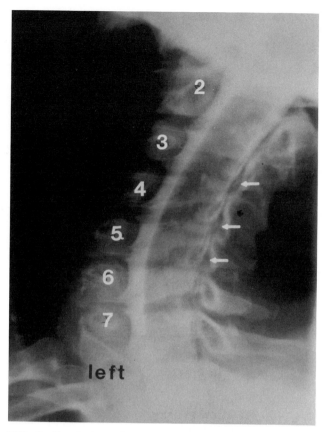

FIG. 8. Cervical myelogram, prone oblique view from left side. The left-sided dural root sleeves remain filled with this technique. The ligamentum flavum (*arrows*) on the right side of the canal interposed between the laminae defines the posterolateral aspect of the cervical central canal.

cause of anatomic circumstances such as severe cervical spondylosis or prior surgery (such as multilevel fusion). Finally, prolonged extension may be dangerous in the patient with a marginal-size canal and preexisting cord compromise.

Cervical myelography with water-soluble contrast material demonstrates extradural pathology to better advantage than myelography with oily contrast material (83,90). It is most accurate in monosegmental compression with radiculopathy (37,52) (Fig. 10). The radiographic finding may be definitive, but it is nonspecific (29,43). For this reason, CT has been recognized as an important adjunct to cervical myelography (21,54). Thin, contiguous sections are necessary for proper evaluation of the cervical motion segment (22). The axial or transverse images of the spine demonstrate the size and shape of the central canal. Intrathecal contrast enhancement provides direct visualization of the thecal sac, its dural root sleeves, and their relationship to bony elements (86). Extradural pathology is identifiable and may be characterized (4) (Fig. 11). The cord is directly visualized (60). CT myelography does accurately depict cord size (87) and shape (99). Delayed scanning can demonstrate cyst cavities in syringomyelia (3,50) and intramedullary enhancement in cervical spondylosis (48).

Intrathecal contrast enhancement is important for effective diagnosis of many cervical lesions, but full dose myelography is not necessary in most cases to obtain adequate subarachnoid opacification. Low-dose technique provides adequate information and may be employed as a primary study (6). This technique does not require the

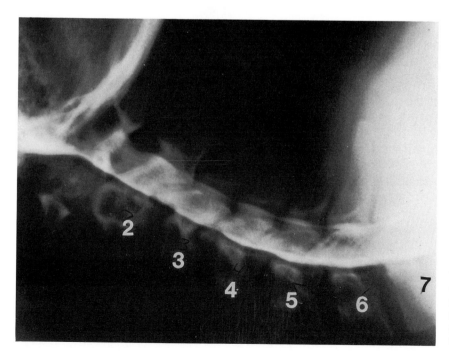

FIG. 9. Cervical myelogram, horizontal beam lateral view. The ventral margin of the thecal sac is defined. Small impressions at each disc space are normal. The shoulders obscure contrast column at the cervicothoracic junction. Additional film (Swimmer's view) is necessary for definition of this region (39).

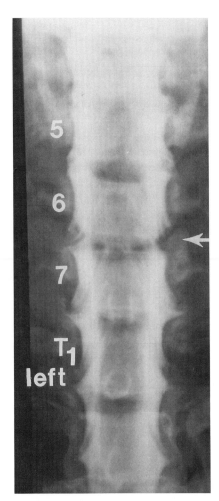

FIG. 10. Cervical myelogram, posteroanterior view, in a 36-year-old woman with chronic, severe right neck and upper extremity pain: a shooting pain down the right arm to the hand with altered sensation of the ulnar aspect of the forearm, paresthesias, and pain involving the long and ring fingers, with subjective weakness. Asymmetry is evident at C6-C7 with poor filling of the right-sided dural sleeve (*arrow*). The diagnosis is C7 radiculopathy secondary to foraminal compromise.

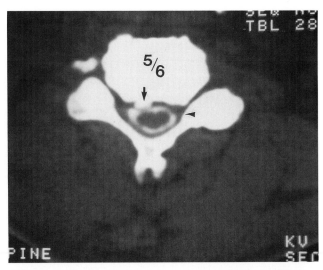

FIG. 11. Axial CT, low dose intrathecal contrast–enhanced, 2.0-mm-thick section through C5-C6 interspace, with soft tissue detail. Right parasagittal bony ridge impinges on the thecal sac abutting the right anterior cord (*arrow*). Poor filling (blunting) of the left C6 dural root sleeve (*arrowhead*) appears to be associated with soft tissue density in the lateral recess, effacing perineural fat. These findings suggest disc prolapse. The central canal is small by development. Representative mid-body, mid-sagittal measurements of 11.0 mm were recorded at C5 and C6.

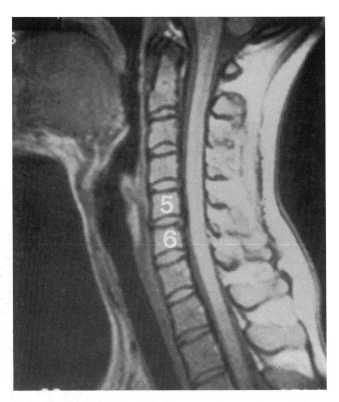

FIG. 12. Sagittal MRI, 0.6 Tesla, surface coil acquisition. Spin echo sequence, T1-weighted, EKG gated. Moderate-sized prolapse at C5-C6 abutting the cervical cord. Attenuation of posterior annulus at C4-C5.

neck extension of formal myelography, and the reduced dose of contrast material lessens the likelihood of neurotoxic complications.

Both myelography and enhanced CT scanning are of limited value at the cervicothoracic junction. The shoulders obscure the contrast column on lateral myelographic images. The increased density through the shoulders results in data starvation artifacts with loss of resolution on CT images. In stout subjects, or patients whose symptoms include neck and shoulder girdle muscle tension with upward retraction of the shoulders, this problem is significant. The result of these factors is that visualization of the lower cervical and cervicothoracic segments may not be adequate.

MRI is rapidly emerging as a primary diagnostic modality for evaluation of cervical spine disorders (64). Exquisite soft tissue detail, multiplanar capability, and its noninvasive character are major advantages of MRI. Limited availability and variation in the level of expertise (both technical and interpretive) are current disadvantages. A variety of artifacts can adversely affect image quality (34,42,56). Good-quality MRI is cost effective when compared to CT scanning and myelography.

MRI provides good visualization of the entire cervical spine. Extradural disease is nicely depicted (41) (Fig. 12). MRI is an ideal modality for evaluation of cord pathology. Intra-axial lesions are directly visualized (88,103) (Fig. 13). In addition to defining pathoanatomy, MRI provides important physiologic information. Alteration of signal from the cord may indicate early and potentially reversible changes secondary to compression (15,63,77). This information is not available by any other imaging technique.

However, obtaining consistently high-quality cervical MRIs is difficult. Image degradation may result from involuntary patient movement, common in patients suffering with pain related to cervical spine disorders. Physiologic motion, including vascular and CSF pulsations as well as simple swallowing, may severely distort images. Currently, MRI does not provide optimal visu-

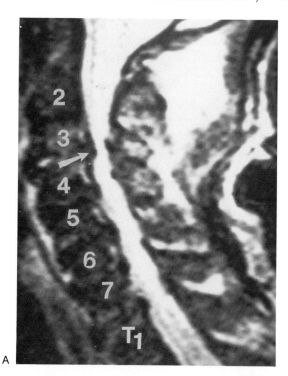

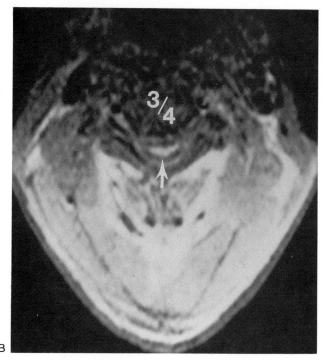

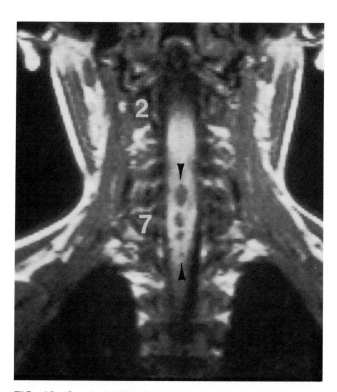

FIG. 13. Cervical MRI, 0.6 Tesla, surface coil acquisition. Spin echo, T1-weighted image, 4.0-mm-thick section, coronal plane. Multiple small syrinx cavities extend from C5 to C1 level (*arrowheads*). There is minimal alteration of cord size or contour.

FIG. 14. Cervical MRI, 0.6 Tesla, surface coil acquisition. **A:** Spin echo, T2-weighted image, mid-sagittal plane. Severe central canal stenosis at C3-C4 (*arrow*). Multilevel spondylitic pathology extending caudally to C7-T1 level. Irregular heart beat compromised EKG gating. Thick sections (6.0 mm) were required for rapid imaging, because of patient motion. Image quality less than optimal but sufficient for diagnosis. **B:** Spin echo, T1-weighted image, axial section at C3-C4 segment. Severe central spinal stenosis is verified in the axial plane. The cervical cord (*arrow*) is flattened at the level of maximum stenosis.

alization of subtle bony pathology, and techniques for adequately evaluating the lateral recesses and foramina are not widely available. However, even compromised studies often provide information adequate for diagnosis.

In difficult cases, myelography and MRI provide complementary data. Conventional myelography may demonstrate a complete block, whereas MRI may provide information regarding pathology above the level of the myelographic block. MRI demonstrates focal central stenosis and cord compromise (Fig. 14), whereas myelography demonstrates significance of pathology at lower levels and provides the managing physician with a global perspective of the disease process (Fig. 15).

Thoracic Myelography

Thoracic myelography is technically demanding. The contrast column is obscured by the complex of overlying

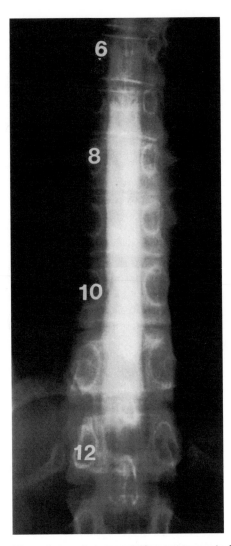

FIG. 16. Thoracic myelogram, supine anteroposterior view. Metrizamide (12.0 cc, 240 mg/cc) is pooled in the subarachnoid space of the dependent thoracic kyphosis. Extradural compression from the lateral aspect of the spinal canal at the lower half of the thoracic spine may be excluded.

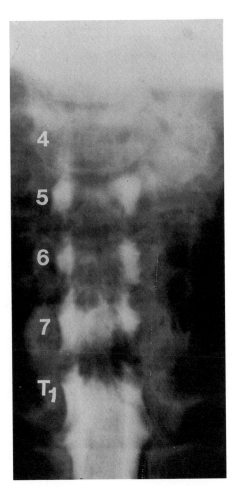

FIG. 15. Cervical myelogram of prone patient. Contrast introduced via lumbar puncture. Study reveals complete block of subarachnoid space at C4-C5. There is multilevel lateral stenosis with a particularly prominent lesion at C7-T1 on the left. Note the normal appearance of the upper thoracic region.

bony structures (ribs, scapulae). The natural kyphosis of the thoracic region prevents adequate prone myelography of the mid-thoracic region. The increased density through the region of the shoulder girdle severely compromises visualization of the contrast column in the upper third of the dorsal spine. In the supine position, subarachnoid contrast material pools in the dependent kyphosis. Supine (anteroposterior) view provides the best visualization of the thoracic subarachnoid space (Fig. 16). This view is insensitive to pathology affecting the ventral aspect of the thecal sac. Horizontal beam film with the patient in the lateral decubitus position provides fair visualization of the dependent side of the thecal sac. The use of conventional tomography aids visualization (84). However, despite these techniques, the results of thoracic myelography are often less than satisfactory.

The thoracic subarachnoid space may be compromised by lesions originating from both anterior and posterior arch structures (70). Myelography can demonstrate disc protrusions in the thoracic region (61), but extradural pathology affecting the thoracic region may not be detectable by myelography until the lesion is quite large.

In the lateral decubitus position, contrast material disperses longitudinally over a considerable length, and the full width of the thecal sac does not remain filled. There is dilution of the contrast material as it mixes with CSF. Together, these factors result in relatively poor opacification of the thoracic subarachnoid space. Myelography is relatively insensitive to small lesions in the thoracic region (Fig. 17). MRI, on the other hand, is effective in demonstrating these lesions (Fig. 18).

Thoracic disc herniation has been considered a rare lesion (20). Large lesions producing symptoms are not common (80). MRI demonstrates that thoracic disc protrusions are more common than previously realized. However, the clinical significance of many of these lesions is questionable (104).

Mass lesions in the thoracic spinal canal can result in devastating neurologic effects. Rapid progression of symptoms may prompt emergent evaluation. Quality MRI is not universally available. Plain CT does not visualize the cord directly (25), but intrathecal enhanced CT scanning provides excellent spatial resolution in the dorsal region. The cord, cerebrospinal space, and osseous and soft-tissue elements of the spine are well visualized (Fig. 19). The primary disadvantage of CT is the selec-

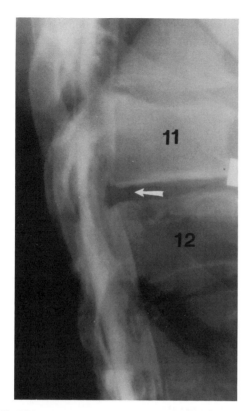

FIG. 17. This 45-year-old man, at 18 months after injury, had severe mechanical back pain in the low dorsal region, with no neurologic deficit. In this thoracic myelogram (left side down lateral decubitus position, lateral view), Iohexol (14.0 cc, 240 mg/cc) has been positioned for maximum opacification at T11-T12, where there is focal kyphotic angulation. Subtle attenuation of ventral contrast column (*arrow*) at level of the intervertebral disc suggests small protrusion.

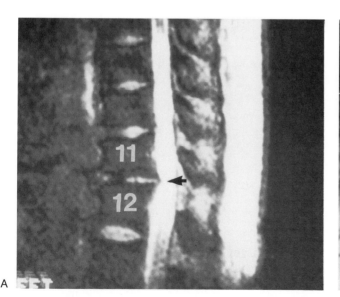

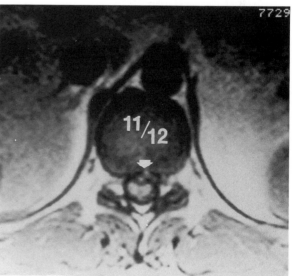

A   B

FIG. 18. Same patient as Fig. 17, MRI of the lower thoracic spine. **A:** Mid-sagittal section, spin echo, T2-weighted image. There is disc-space narrowing at T11-T12 and focal ventral impression on thecal sac with disc protrusion/prolapse (*arrow*). Note calcification in anterior third of nucleus (low signal zone). **B:** Axial section, spin echo, T1-weighted image of T11-T12 disc. Central/left paracentral disc prolapse (*arrow*) is clearly defined. Cord displacement and deformity are apparent.

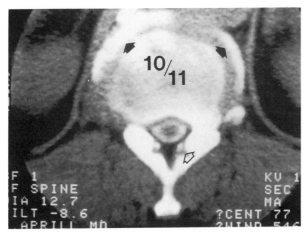

FIG. 19. Burst fracture, superior T11, in a 41-year-old man with a prior injury. Axial CT, T10-T11 interspace. Postmyelographic, intrathecal enhanced; 5.0-mm-thick section, soft tissue detail. Myelogram suggests marked narrowing of contrast column; CT demonstrates developmentally small central spinal canal. No cord displacement or deformity. Broad circumferential disc bulge is associated with superior T11 rim fracture (*closed arrows*). No posterior body or posterior arch fracture. Note calcification in ligamentum flavum (*open arrow*).

tion of the appropriate level for scanning. Conventional film myelography defines the level of the lesion and directs CT to the specific area of interest (12). Myelography alone is inadequate for determination of the exact size and extent of lesions (76) (Fig. 20).

Complete block of the subarachnoid space is not as commonly encountered with low-viscosity aqueous contrast agents as it was with oil-based agents. In most instances, sufficient contrast material can seep past the obstructing lesion to allow recognition by CT scanning. The superior margin of most lesions can be defined (27). When obstruction is complete, or there is reason to suspect multiple lesions, introduction of contrast by way of lateral C1-C2 puncture and descending myelography is required. The most common neoplastic lesions causing significant myelographic block in the thoracic region are meningiomas and primary benign neurogenic tumors. Myelography and Myelo-CT are effective in detecting these lesions (32) (Fig. 21). They are, however, conspicuous by MRI scanning (Fig. 22).

Intramedullary tumors of the thoracic cord are manifest on myelography by focal expansion of the cord (75). Tumors that have not yet resulted in enlargement of the cord are not evident (Fig. 23). MRI with gadolinium (Gd) enhancement allows recognition of the presence, location, and extent of the disease process (17,71). When available, high-resolution multiplanar MRI is the modality of choice in the investigation of patients with suspected thoracic spine pathology.

Lumbar Myelography

The lumbar cistern (Fig. 24) is the site of best visualization and greatest variation noted by myelography. The caudal limit of the subarachnoid space varies between S1 and S3 (84). The distal thecal sac may be broad and rounded at its termination, or long and thinly tapered. A wide ventral epidural space is common below

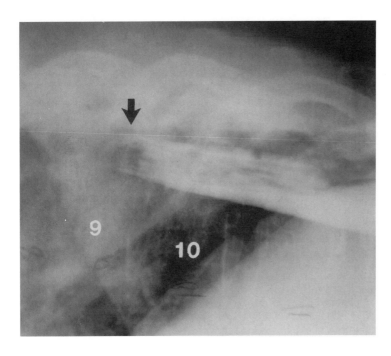

FIG. 20. Thoracic myelogram, horizontal lateral view, head down 20°. This 56-year-old woman with progressive paraparesis had severe lower dorsal pain. Myelogram (Iopamidol, 14.0 cc, 280 mg/cc) reveals complete block of contrast column at T9 body. Upper margin of lesion is not defined. Margin of the block (*arrow*) has "feathered edge," consistent with extradural mass. Diagnosis: epidural abscess secondary to vertebral osteomyelitis T8 and T9.

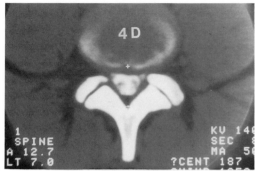

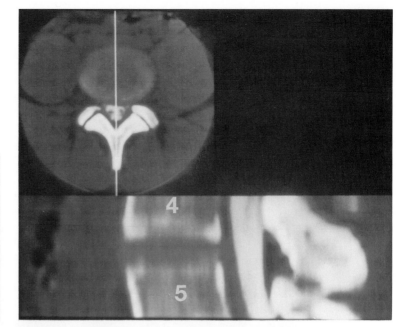

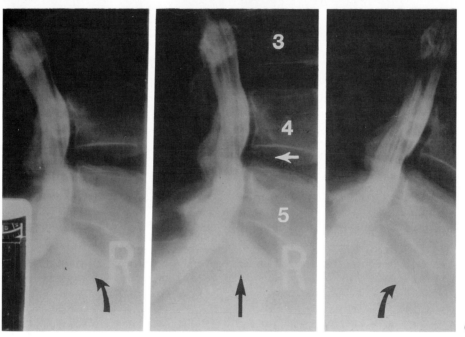

FIG. 28. A: Axial CT of L4-L5 motion segment, postmyelogram. Convex, slightly asymmetric posterior annular margin is prominent on left. Asymmetry of posterior joints: right wider than left. **B:** CT mid-sagittal re-formation of L4-L5 motion segment, postmyelogram. Normal appearance. No pathologic impression on ventral thecal sac at level of the disc. **C:** Lateral myelogram erect series: extension, neutral, and flexion. Definite ventral impression on thecal sac at L4-L5 disc (*white arrow*). Lesion is seen on all erect films but is most prominent on the extension view.

FIG. 26. Lumbar myelogram, prone 15° erect. This 46-year-old man, with a prior left L5 laminotomy, had recurrent back pain, right sciatica. Obvious broad extradural deformity (*open arrow*) of the left side of the thecal sac at the surgical site. Poor filling of left S1 root sleeve. Asymmetry of L5 dural root sleeves. Poor filling on right (*solid arrow*). Myelogram is indeterminate. Diagnosis: epidural scarring left L5-S1, extruded sequestered disc fragment right L5-S1 radicular canal (proven).

FIG. 27. Axial CT of L5-S1 interspace with low-dose intrathecal contrast enhancement. Right paracentral disc prolapse (*open arrow*) deforms the thecal sac. Note irregularity of posterior endplate, probably representing site of annular avulsion. Asymmetric width of posterior joints (left wider than right). Narrow joint on right (*closed arrow*).

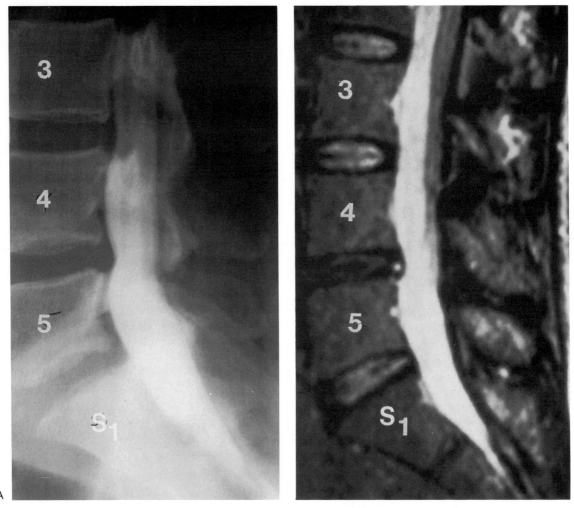

FIG. 29. A: Lumbar myelogram, lateral view, erect. Ventral impression on thecal sac at L4-L5 interspace is compatible with disc protrusion/prolapse. **B:** Lumbar MRI mid-sagittal section, spin echo T2-weighted image, 5.0-mm section. Ventral impression on thecal sac at L4-L5 interspace. Reduced nuclear signal. Bright signal in posterior annular substance indicative of annular pathology. Remaining discs are normal.

Currently, CT scanning is performed with patients supine, in as comfortable a position as possible, but the disadvantage is that there is no axial load on the spine and some lesions may not be demonstrated. In contrast, functional myelography has the capacity to demonstrate dynamic lesions (105,106). The ability to evaluate the effect of axial loading with erect flexion, extension, and lateral bending maneuvers is an advantage of lumbar myelography over both CT scanning and MRI (Fig. 28). For this reason, functional assessment should be routinely incorporated into the myelographic study of the lumbar region (72,85) and is particularly important in the assessment of spinal stenosis (100). Although CT scanning provides accurate assessment of central spinal canal sagittal diameter, the area of the thecal sac as determined by myelography may be even more sensitive in the evaluation of clinically significant stenosis (11).

The acceptance of MRI as an important modality for evaluating adult spinal disorders has increased seemingly in proportion to the deployment of the technology. According to Modic et al. (65), MRI is the primary imaging modality for study of the spine. This enthusiastic opinion is easily supported when a direct comparison of images is made (Fig. 29). Considering only the disc, MRI provides physiologic information relative to the health status of the nucleus. Degradation of the nuclear matrix decreases water-binding capacity, resulting in reduced signal intensity from the nuclear region of the involved disc. Direct visualization of the disc annulus makes MRI effective at the lumbosacral level, even in patients with a wide epidural space. Superior soft-tissue resolution makes intra-arachnoid structures conspicuous, effectively eliminating the need for invasive procedures in some patients (Fig. 30).

For these reasons, myelography can no longer be considered a primary imaging modality for the evaluation of lumbar spine pathology. Its use should be reserved for specific cases determined on an individual basis. As in the cervical region, the lumbar myelogram does provide a global perspective to multisegmental pathology. It should be employed in conjunction with CT scanning in presurgical staging of many patients with complex spine disorders.

Finally, there are some patients in whom MRI and CT scanning cannot be adequately performed (Fig. 31). The scatter artifacts associated with pedicle screws reduce the efficacy of CT scanning. Even small amounts of metal produce paramagnetic artifacts, frequently rendering MRI nondiagnostic. The growing use of metal instrumentation in the treatment of a variety of spine disorders ensures that the venerable technique of myelography will not be completely eliminated from the practice of spinal diagnostic medicine in the near future.

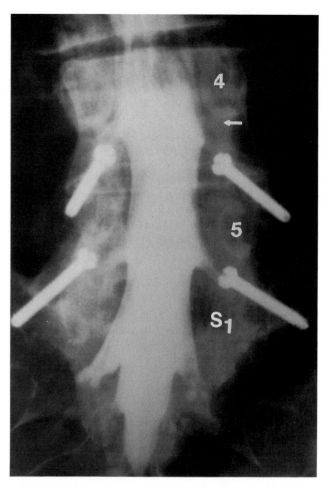

FIG. 31. Lumbar myelogram prone. This 52-year-old woman with prior two-level facet fusion with screws (12 years prior to myelogram) had back pain, and right leg pain and weakness. Poor filling of right L4 dural root pouch (*arrow*). Diagnosis: right L4 radiculopathy secondary to combined disc protrusion and foraminal stenosis.

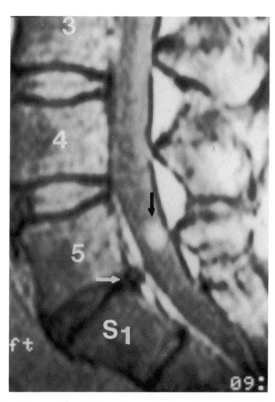

FIG. 30. Lumbar MRI mid-sagittal section, spin echo T1-weighted image, 5.0-mm section. This 32-year-old man had low back pain with radiation to his left leg. Reduced signal L5-S1 nucleus, and narrowing of the interspace and posterior annular protrusion (*white arrow*) indicate disc pathology. No impression on thecal sac, secondary to wide epidural space. Axial section demonstrated left posterolateral protrusion (surgically proven). Incidental finding is asymptomatic right S2 schwannoma (*black arrow*).

REFERENCES

1. Amundsen P (1979): The evolution of contrast media. In: Sackett J, Strother C, eds. *New techniques in myelography.* Hagerstown: Harper and Row, pp. 2–5.
2. Arnell S, Lidstrom F (1931): Myelography with Skiodan (Abrodil). *Acta Radiol [Stockh]* 12:287–288.
3. Auben MI, Vignaud J, Jordin C, et al. (1982): Computed tomography in 75 clinical cases of syringomyelia. *AJNR* 2:199–204.
4. Baleriaux D, Noterman J, Ticket L (1983): Recognition of cervical soft disc herniation by contrast enhanced CT. *AJNR* 4:606–608.
5. Banna M (1985): *Clinical radiology of the spine and spinal cord.* Rockville: Aspen, pp. 76,101.
6. Barrow DL, Wood JH, Hoffman JC (1983): Seizure after intrathecal administration of Iopamidol. *AJNR* 9:787–788.
7. Batnitzky S, Keucher TR, Mealey J, Campbell RL (1977): Iatrogenic intraspinal epidermoid tumors. *JAMA* 237(2):148–150.
8. Bauer D (1960): *Lumbar discography in low back pain.* Springfield: Charles C Thomas.
9. Bellamy EA, Perez DJ, Husband JE (1984): CT demonstration of spinal subarachnoid haematoma following lumbar puncture. *J Comput Assist Tomogr* 8:791–792.

10. Benner B, Ehni G (1978): Spinal arachnoiditis: the postoperative variety in particular. *Spine* 3:40–44.

11. Bolender NF, Schonstrom NSR, Spangler DM (1985): Role of computerized tomography and myelography in the diagnosis of central spinal stenosis. *J Bone Joint Surg [Am]* 67:240–246.

12. Bonatti G, Ortore P (1987): CT after myelography in complete spinal cord blocks. *Radiol Med [Torino]* 74(5):451–454.

13. Braun IF, Hoffman JC, Davis PC, et al. (1985): Contrast enhancement in CT differentiation between recurrent disc herniation and postoperative scar. *AJNR* 6:607–612.

14. Brinker RA (1973): Lumbar spinal puncture for neuroradiology procedures. *Am J Roentgenol* 118:674–676.

15. Brown E, Virapongse C, Gregorios JB (1989): MR imaging of the cervical spinal cord infarction. *J Comput Assist Tomogr* 13:920–922.

16. Burton CV (1978): Lumbosacral arachnoiditis. *Spine* 3:24–30.

17. Bydder GM, Brown J, Niendorf HP, Young IR (1985): Enhancement of cervical intraspinal tumors in MR imaging with intravenous gadolinium DTPA. *J Comput Assist Tomogr* 9:847–851.

18. Byrd SE, Cohn ML, Biggers SL, et al. (1985): The radiographic evaluation of symptomatic post operative lumbar spine patient. *Spine* 10:652–661.

19. Campbell RL, Campbell JA, Heimburger RF, Kalsbeck JE, Mealey J (1964): Ventriculography and myelography and absorbable radiopaque medium. *Radiology* 82:286–289.

20. Carson J, Gumpert J, Jefferson A (1971): Diagnosis and treatment of thoracic intervertebral disc protrusions. *J Neurol Neurosurg Psychiatry* 34:68–77.

21. Coin CG, Chan YS, Keranen V, Pennink M (1977): Computer assisted myelography in disk disease. *J Comput Assist Tomogr* 1:398–404.

22. Coin CG, Coin JT (1981): Computed tomography of cervical disc disease: technical considerations with representative case reports. *J Comput Assist Tomogr* 5:275–280.

23. Coughlin JR, Miller JD (1983): Metrizamide myelography in conjoined lumbosacral nerve roots. *J Can Assoc Radiol* 34:23–25.

24. Dandy WE (1919): Roentgenography of the brain after injection of air into the spinal canal. *Ann Surg* 70:397–403.

25. de Morpurgo P, Gozzi G, Pozzi-Mucelli F, Abbona M (1986): Findings in myelographic block: correlation with computerized tomography image. *Radiol Med [Torino]* 72(7,8):560–563.

26. Farfan HF (1973): *Mechanical disorders of the low back.* Philadelphia: Lea and Febiger.

27. Fink IJ, Garra BS, Zabell A, et al. (1984): Computed tomography with metrizamide myelography to define the extent of canal block due to tumor. *J Comput Assist Tomogr* 8:1072–1075.

28. Foens CS, Wenzel RP (1987): Questions and answers: skin preparation for lumbar puncture. *JAMA* 258(9):1241.

29. Fox AJ, Lin JP, Pinto RS, Kricheff II (1975): Myelographic cervical nerve root deformities. *Radiology* 116:355–361.

30. Gonsette R (1971): An experimental and clinical assessment of water-soluble contrast medium in neuroradiology: a new medium, Dimer-X. *Clin Radiol* 22:44–56.

31. Gonsette RE, Brucher JM (1977): Potentiation of Amipaque epileptogenic activity by neuroleptics. *Neuroradiology* 14:27–30.

32. Gozzi G, Pozzi M, deMorpurgo PL, et al. (1988): [Evaluation of expansive myelo-vertebral pathology using different radiologic modalities, magnetic resonance excluded]. *Radiol Med [Torino]* 75:577–583.

33. Grainger RG, Gumpert J, Sharpe DM, Carson J (1971): Watersoluble lumbar radiculography: a clinical trial of Dimer-X, a new contrast medium. *Clin Radiol* 22:57–62.

34. Haacke EM, Lenz GW (1987): Improving MR image quality in presence of motion by using rephasing gradients. *AJR* 148:1251–1258.

35. Hansen EB, Fahrenkrug A, Praestholm J (1978): Late meningeal effects of myelographic contrast media with special reference to metrizamide. *Br J Radiol* 51:321–327.

36. Harris LM, Harmel MH (1953): The comparative incidence of post-lumbar puncture headache following spinal anesthesia administered through #20 and #24 gauge needles. *Anesthesiology* 14:390–397.

37. Hartjes H, Roosen K, Grote W, et al. (1983): Cervical disc syn-

dromes: value of metrizamide myelography and discography. *AJNR* 4:644–645.

38. Hatfalvi BI (1977): The dynamics of post-spinal headache. *Headache* 17:64–66.

39. Hatten HP Jr (1982): Routine cervical myelography with overhead oblique projections and Pantopaque. *Spine* 7:512–514.

40. Haughton VM, Eldevik OP, Magnaes B, Amundsen P (1982): A prospective comparison of computed tomography and myelography in the diagnosis of herniated lumbar discs. *Radiology* 142:103–110.

41. Hedberg MC, Drayer BP, Flom RA, et al. (1988): Gradient echo (GRASS) MR imaging and cervical radiculopathy. *AJR* 150:683–689.

42. Heindel W, Friedmann G, Burke J, et al. (1986): Artifacts in MR imaging after surgical intervention. *J Comput Assist Tomogr* 10:596–599.

43. Herkowitz HN (1988): Cervical laminoplasty: its role in the treatment of cervical radiculopathy. *J Spine Disord* 1:179–188.

44. Hindmarsh T (1975): Myelography with the nonionic watersoluble contrast medium metrizamide. *Acta Radiol [Diag] [Stockh]* 16:417–435.

45. Hodges SD, Berasi CC (1987): Complications of myelography after partial metrizamide withdrawal. *Spine* 12:53–55.

46. Irstam L (1978): Lumbar myelography with Amipaque. *Spine* 3:70–82.

47. Irstam L (1984): Differential diagnosis of recurrent lumbar disc herniation and post operative deformation by myelography: an impossible task. *Spine* 9:759–763.

48. Iwasaki Y, Abe H, Isu T, Miyasaka K (1985): CT myelography with intramedullary enhancement in cervical spondylosis. *J Neurosurg* 63:363–366.

49. Jacobaeus HC (1921): On insufflation of air into the spinal canal for diagnostic purposes in cases of tumors in the spinal canal. *Acta Med Scand* 55:555–564.

50. Kan S, Fox AJ, Vinuela F, et al. (1983): Delayed CT metrizamide enhancement of syringomyelia secondary to tumor. *AJNR* 4:73–78.

51. Kido DK, Gomez DG, Pavese AM Jr, Potts DG (1976): Human spinal arachnoid villi and granulations. *Neuroradiology* 11:221–228.

52. Kikuchi S, Macnab I, Moreau P (1981): Localization of the level of cervical disc degeneration. *J Bone Joint Surg [Br]* 63:272–277.

53. Lamont AC, Zachary J, Sheldon PW (1981): Cervical cord size in metrizamide myelography. *Clin Radiol* 32:409–412.

54. Lee BC, Kazam E, Newman AD (1978): Computed tomography of the spine and spinal cord. *Radiology* 128:95–102.

55. Lestrange NR, Wolko HR, Tate CF, Astl AJ (1986): Advantages of ambulatory metrizamide myelography with contrast CT tomography. *Orthopaedics* 9:61–65.

56. Levy LM, DiChiro G, Brooks RA, et al. (1988): Spinal cord artifacts from truncation errors during MR imaging. *Radiology* 166:479–483.

57. Lindgren E (1977): Metrizamide-Amipaque: the nonionic watersoluble contrast medium. Further clinical experience in neuroradiology. *Acta Radiol [Suppl] [Stockh]* 355:1–432.

58. Lipman JC, Wang AM, Brooks ML, et al. (1988): Seizure after intrathecal administration of Iopamidol. *AJNR* 9:787–788.

59. MacPherson P, Teasdale E, Coutinho C, McGeorge A (1985): Iohexol versus Iopamidol for cervical myelography: a randomized double blind study. *Br J Radiol* 58:849–851.

60. Mawad ME, Hilal SK, Fetell MR, et al. (1983): Patterns of spinal cord atrophy by metrizamide CT. *AJNR* 6:611–613.

61. McAllister VL, Sage MR (1976): The radiology of thoracic disc protrusion. *Clin Radiol* 27:291–299.

62. McGruder JM, Cooke JE, Conroy JM, Baker JD 3d (1988): Headache after lumbar puncture: review of the epidural blood patch. *South Med J* 81:1249–1252.

63. Mirvis SE, Geisler FH, Jelinek JJ, et al. (1988): Acute cervical spine trauma: evaluation with 1.5 T. MR imaging. *Radiology* 166:807–816.

64. Modic MT, Masaryk TJ, Mulopulos GP, et al. (1986): Cervical radiculopathy: perspective evaluation with surface coil MR imaging, CT with metrizamide and metrizamide myelography. *Radiology* 161:753–759.

65. Modic MT, Masaryk TJ, Ross JS (1989): *Magnetic resonance imaging.* Chicago: Yearbook Medical.
66. Nakstad PH, Kjartansson O (1988): Accidental spinal cord injection of contrast material during cervical myelography with lateral C1-C2 puncture. *AJNR* 9:410.
67. Novetsky GJ, Berlin L, Epstein AJ, et al. (1982): The extraforaminal herniated disc detected by CT. *AJNR* 3:653–655.
68. Odin M, Runstrom G, Lindblom A (1929): Iodized oils as an aid to the diagnosis of lesions of the spinal cord and a contribution to the knowledge of adhesive circumscribed meningitis. *Acta Radiol [Suppl]* 7:1–86.
69. Orrison WW, Eldevik OP, Sackett JF (1983): Lateral C1-2 puncture for cervical myelography. III Historical, anatomic and technical considerations. *Radiology* 146:401–408.
70. Otani K, Yoshida M, Fujii E, et al. (1988): Thoracic disc herniation. Surgical treatment in 23 patients. *Spine* 13:1262–1267.
71. Parizel PM, Baleriaux D, Rodesch G, et al. (1985): Gadolinium DTPA: Enhanced MR imaging of spinal tumors. *AJR* 152:1087–1096.
72. Penning L, Wilmink JT (1987): Posture-dependent bilateral compression of L4 or L5 nerve roots in facet hypertrophy: a dynamic CT myelographic study. *Spine* 12:488–500.
73. Postacchini F, Massobrio M (1985): Outpatient lumbar myelography: analysis of complications after myelography comparing outpatients with inpatients. *Spine* 10:567–570.
74. Preacher WG, Robertson RC (1945): Pantopaque myelography: results, comparison of contrast media, and spinal fluid reaction. *J Neurosurg* 2:220–231.
75. Puljic S, Batnitzky S, Yang WC, Schechter MM (1975): Metastases to the medulla of the spinal cord: myelographic features. *Radiology* 117:89–91.
76. Raininko R (1983): The value of CT after total block on myelography. Experience with 25 patients. *Rofo Fortschr Geb Rontgenstr Neuen Bildgeb Verfahr* 138(1):61–65.
77. Ramanauskas WL, Wilner HI, Metes JJ, et al. (1989): MR imaging of compressive myelomalacia. *J Comput Assist Tomogr* 13:399–404.
78. Ramsey GH, French JD, Strain WH (1944): Iodinated organic compounds as contrast media for radiographic diagnoses: Pantopaque myelography. *Radiology* 43:236–240.
79. Raskin SP, Keating JW (1982): Recognition of lumbar disc disease: comparison of myelography and computed tomography. *AJR* 139(2):349–355.
80. Roosen N, Dietrich U, Nicola N, et al. (1987): MR imaging of calcified herniated thoracic disk. *J Comput Assist Tomogr* 11(4):733–735.
81. Ross JS, Masaryk TJ, Modic MT, et al. (1987): MR imaging of lumbar arachnoiditis. *AJNR* 149:1025–1032.
82. Rothfus WE, Latchaw RE (1983): Nonefficacy of routine removal of CSF during neurodiagnostic procedures. *AJNR* 5:797–800.
83. Sackett JF, Strother CM, Quaglieri CE, et al. (1977): metrizamide-CSF contrast medium. Analysis of clinical application in 215 patients. *Radiology* 123:779–782.
84. Sackett J (1979): Myelographic technique with water soluble contrast media. In: Sackett J, Strother C, eds. *New techniques in myelography.* Hagerstown: Harper and Row, p. 49.
85. Schumacher M (1986): [Stress myelography. A new functional study technique in diseases of the lumbar spinal canal.] *Rofo Fortschr Geb Rontgenstr Neuen Bildgeb Verfahr* 145(6):642–648.
86. Scotti G, Scialfa G, Pieralli S, et al. (1983): Myelopathy and radiculopathy due to cervical spondylosis: Myelographic-CT correlations. *AJNR* 4:601–603.
87. Seibert CE, Barnes JE, Dreisbach JN, et al. (1981): Accurate CT measurement of the spinal cord using metrizamide: physical factors. *AJNR* 2:75–78.
88. Sherman JL, Barkovich AJ, Citrin CM (1987): The MR appearance of syringomyelia: new observations. *AJR* 148:381–391.
89. Sicard JA, Forrestier JE (1922): Methode general d'exploration radiologique par l'huile iodee (Lipiodol). *Bull Mem Soc Med Hop Paris* 46:463–469.
90. Skalpe IO, Amundsen P (1975): Thoracic and cervical myelography with metrizamide. Clinical experiences with water-soluble, nonionic contrast medium. *Radiology* 116:101–106.
91. Sortland O, Nestvold K, Kloster R, Aandahl MH (1984): Comparison of iohexol with metrizamide in myelography. *Radiology* 151:121–122.
92. Sotiropoulos S, Chafetz NI, Lang P, et al. (1989): Differentiation between post operative scar and recurrent disk herniation: prospective comparison of MR, CT and contrast-enhanced CT. *AJNR* 10:639–643.
93. Steiner E, Simon JH, Ekholm SE, et al. (1986): Neurologic complications in diabetics after metrizamide lumbar myelography. *AJNR* 7:323–326.
94. Strother CM (1979): Cervical examination. In: Sackett J, Strother C, eds. *New techniques in myelography.* Hagerstown: Harper and Row, p. 121.
95. Strother CM (1979): Intracranial examination. In: Sackett J, Strother C, eds. *New techniques in myelography.* Hagerstown: Harper and Row, pp. 125–128.
96. Strother CM (1979): Adverse reactions. In: Sackett J, Strother C, eds. *New techniques in myelography.* Hagerstown: Harper and Row, pp. 186–201.
97. Tarlov IM (1938): Perineurial cysts of the spinal nerve roots. *Arch Neurol Psych* 40:1067–1074.
98. Teplick JG, Haskin ME (1984): Intravenous contrast enhancement of the post-operative lumbar spine: improved identification of recurrent disc herniation, scar, arachnoiditis and discitis. *AJNR* 5:373–383.
99. Thijssen HO, Keyser A, Horstink MW, et al. (1979): Morphology of the cervical spinal cord on a computed myelography. *Neuroradiology* 18:57–62.
100. Uden A, Johnsson KE, Jonsson K, Pettersson H (1985): Myelography in the elderly and the diagnosis of spinal stenosis. *Spine* 10:171–174.
101. Vezina JL, Fontaine S, LaPerriere J (1989): Outpatient myelography with fine-needle technique: an appraisal. *AJNR* 10:615–617.
102. Voelker JL, Mealey J, Eskridge JM, Gilmore RL (1987): Metrizamide enhanced computed tomography as an adjunct to metrizamide myelography in the evaluation of lumbar disc herniation and spondylosis. *Neurosurgery* 20:379–384.
103. Williams AL, Haughton VM, Pojunas KW, et al. (1987): Differentiation of intramedullary neoplasms and cysts by MR. *AJR* 149:159–164.
104. Williams MP, Cherryman GR, Husband JE (1989): Significance of thoracic disc herniation demonstrated by MR imaging. *J Comput Assist Tomogr* 13(2):211–214.
105. Wilmink JT, Penning L (1985): Influence of spinal posture on abnormalities demonstrated by lumbar myelography. *AJNR* 4(3):656–658.
106. Wilmink JT, Penning L, van den Burg W (1984): Role of stenosis of the spinal canal in L4-L5 nerve root compression assessed by flexion-extension myelography. *Neuroradiology* 26(3):173–181.
107. Wilmink JT (1989): CT morphology of intrathecal lumbosacral nerve-root compression. *AJNR* 10:233–248.

The Adult Spine: Principles and Practice,
2nd edition, J.W. Frymoyer, Editor-in-Chief.
Lippincott-Raven Publishers, Philadelphia © 1997.

CHAPTER 27

Computed Tomography of the Spine

S. James Zinreich, Kenneth B. Heithoff, and Richard J. Herzog

For the clinician who treats patients with spinal pathology, high-resolution computed tomography (CT) and magnetic resonance imaging (MRI) provide essential diagnostic information. To determine and institute appropriate early management of the patient with severe back pain and radiculopathy or myelopathy, such diagnostic information is of critical importance. Failure to establish a clear diagnosis can lead to delayed or improper therapy and increased overall patient management costs.

CT and MRI have become the primary modalities in diagnostic imaging of the spine. Myelography and, to a large extent, plain films have been relegated to a minor role. While the ability to visualize pathology with CT and MRI provides more precise information than myelography and plain films, it is not always possible to relate the visualized pathology to symptoms and to devise effective conservative treatment. The technological advances that CT and MRI provide, however, have been essential to new surgical techniques that demand precise anatomic definition and exact localization of a symptomatic lesion by preoperative imaging. In addition to confirming clinically a suspected disc herniation, the entire spine adjacent to the lesion(s) can be assessed, as well as the bony nerve root canals and spinal recesses. The visualization of the central canal and associated soft tissues, such as the ligamentum flavum, is also possible, and thus coexistent pathology can be excluded.

Neurosurgeons today rely on CT and MRI to provide answers to critical questions about the specific nature of spinal pathology. If there is a definite disc herniation, is it contained? If so, are outer annular fibers intact? If it is not contained, is it a free fragment? Is there definite nerve root compression? Are there other complicating lesions?

In this chapter, we will attempt to demonstrate the uses of the new CT techniques, including high-resolution CT, contrast-enhanced CT, and three-dimensional (3D) reconstruction methods. We will also show how these

S. J. Zinreich, M.D.: Associate Professor of Radiology, Department of Radiology/Neuroradiology, The Johns Hopkins University School of Medicine, Baltimore, Maryland 21205-0810.

K. B. Heithoff, M.D.: Center for Diagnostic Imaging, St. Louis Park, Minnesota, 55416.

R. J. Herzog, M.D.: Medical Director, San Francisco Neuro Skeletal Imaging, San Francisco Spine Institute, Daly City, California 94015.

techniques are used in clinical practice in conjunction with MRI, plain films, and myelography. CT continues to play a major role in the evaluation of patients with failed back surgery syndrome (FBSS). Its ability to define the bony architecture optimally affords a proper evaluation of the integrity of the central canal and lateral neural foramina. It also best displays mechanical obstruction as well as instability.

In this era of increasingly cost-conscious health care, it is crucial for the clinician to understand the appropriate selection and sequencing of tests. This will result not only in more cost-effective diagnosis, but also in better patient care and management.

SCANNING TECHNIQUES

High-resolution CT with multiplanar reformations (CT/MPR) transforms the standard axial CT examination of the spine into a more complete evaluative imaging study (38). The optimal delineation of spinal anatomy and pathology is obtained by studying the spine in complementary orthogonal planes. CT/MPR provides a standardized, integrated approach for evaluating the spine in the axial, sagittal, and coronal planes (37,65).

A high-resolution multiplanar CT exam requires thin contiguous axial sections of the cervical and thoracic spine and overlapping axial sections of the lumbar spine. The quality of the reconstructed images will be no better than the quality of the initial axial CT image data. The reconstructed CT images will have the same contrast resolution as the original axial images, but there will be at least some loss of spatial resolution resulting from the thickness of the initial axial sections (112). To prevent misregistration artifacts on the reconstructed images, the patient must remain motionless during the study. Because a complete CT/MPR study is performed in 25 minutes, it is usually not difficult for a patient to maintain a single position. With current rapid scanning techniques, patient x-ray exposure has been significantly reduced.

Anteroposterior (AP) and lateral CT scout images are obtained and serve as the plain films. They also are essential for orientation and correlation of the findings noted on axial images. Such scout images are adequate for detection of abnormalities of spinal alignment, loss of disc height, and gross degenerative changes and/or bony destruction, and these are reviewed as plain films are.

In the lumbar spine, the number of levels imaged is also an issue, and thus survey images are obtained at L1-L2 and L2-L3 if the lateral computed radiographs demonstrate abnormalities at those levels, or if the patient's pain drawing indicates groin or anterior thigh pain. This routine has been successful in detecting a number of lateral L2-L3 disc herniations, and a very occasional L1-L2 herniation (Fig. 1).

CT is dissimilar to plain films in that the beam is very tightly collimated and there is very little scatter radiation. The usual skin dose is 3–5 rads for a lumbar spine scan, with less exposure of internal structures.

By contrast, a full series of spine films with AP, lateral, and oblique views has equivalent direct radiation (3–5 rads), has considerable scatter radiation, and produces significantly more gonadal radiation than CT. Myelogra-

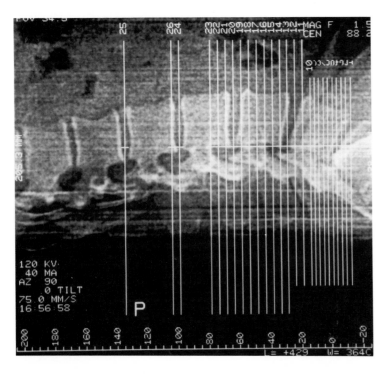

FIG. 1. Lateral computed radiograph of the lumbar spine showing our scanning technique. Note that the scans obtained at L5-S1 are 3-mm adjacent images and/or 5-mm images with 3 mm of table incrementation. Five-millimeter scans are obtained from the mid pedicle of L5 to the L3 pedicle, and survey images were obtained at L1-L2 and L2-L3. Survey images are obtained at L1-L2 and L2-L3 when there is evidence of degenerative disc disease on the lateral computed radiograph or when the patient has symptoms referable to the upper lumbar region, such as groin or anterior thigh pain. Axial adjacent images from L3 to S1 are obtained to provide continuous imaging of the lumbar anatomy and to allow sagittal reformatted images of the lower spine for quantification of lateral spinal stenosis.

phy has a considerably higher amount of primary and scatter radiation. The issues obviously are of far less concern in the cervical and thoracic levels.

When performing a CT/MPR study, there are only a few imaging parameters that must be determined at the time of image acquisition. On routine evaluation of the cervical spine, contiguous 1.5-mm thick sections are obtained from the pedicle of C3 or C4 to the pedicle of C7. Thin sections are necessary to delineate normal anatomy; in the thoracic spine, contiguous 3-mm thick sections are obtained in the area of interest. From 4 to 5 disc levels can be evaluated on a single thoracic CT/MPR study. In the lumbar spine, the routine examination includes overlapping 5-mm thick sections performed at 3-mm intervals from the pedicle of L2 or L3 through the L5-S1 disc level (Figs. 2,3).

After obtaining the initial axial images, computer-generated contiguous sagittal and coronal images are created with a spacing of 1.5 mm between images in the cervical examination and a spacing of 3 mm in the thoracic and lumbar examination. Approximately 20 sagittal and 20 coronal images are reconstructed from the axial data.

A multiplanar spinal exam must include contiguous sagittal and coronal reformations to evaluate the spine completely in complementary orthogonal planes. All images are photographed twice to optimally delineate soft tissue and osseous contrast. The strength of the CT/MPR exam is in its excellent spatial resolution and its superb delineation of calcified or osseous structures. The main limitations of CT/MPR are the radiation exposure, the slightly restricted field of view, and the poor delineation of intrathecal anatomy and pathology.

Initial axial CT data are reprocessed into additional tomographic projections when performing a CT/MPR examination. With recent advances in software technology, initial axial CT data can also be reconstructed into a 3D image. Most 3D CT images are produced using a surface contour method that permits evaluation of surface anatomy. The 3D CT image adds no new information compared to the multiplanar study, but with the new 3D perspective, pathological changes may be more

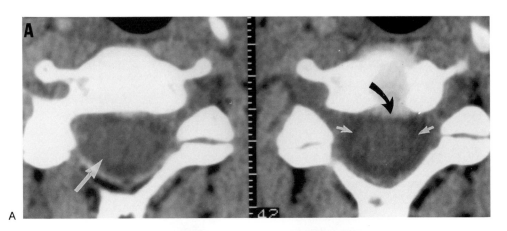

A

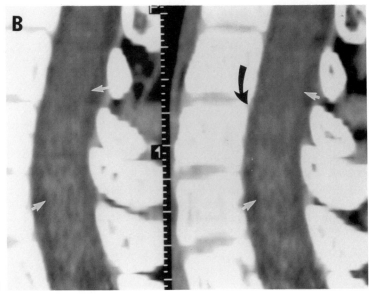

B

FIG. 2. A–E. Normal lumbar spine anatomy: CT/ MPR. On the axial (**A**) and sagittal (**B**) images, the spinal cord (*white arrows*) is delineated along with the posterior margin of the disc (*black arrow*). The images were photographed to optimize soft tissue resolution.

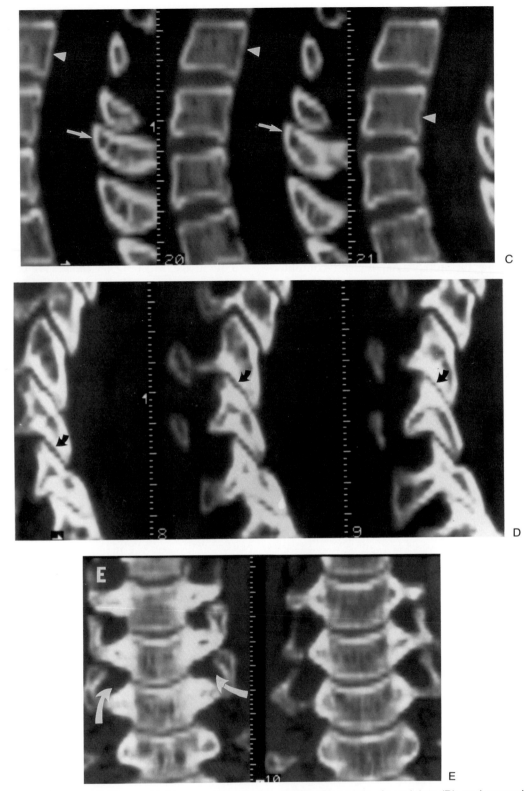

FIG. 2. (*Continued.*) The sagittal images through the midline (**C**) and the facet joints (**D**), and coronal images (**E**), were photographed to optimally evaluate the osseous structures. There is excellent delineation of the vertebral bodies (*white arrowheads*), the laminae (*straight white arrows*), the facet joints (*curved black arrows*) and the intervertebral canals (*curved white arrows*).

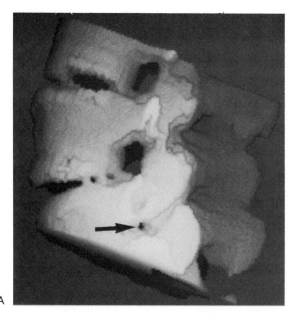
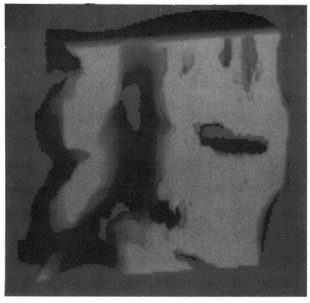

A

B

FIG. 3. Three-dimensional image of the lumbar spine. **A:** Lateral view of the 3D reconstruction of the lumbar spine from stacked axial images. Note the severe circumferential "pin-hole" lateral spinal stenosis at L5-S1 (*arrow*). **B:** Cut-away 3D image of the central spinal canal looking laterally toward the intervertebral nerve root canals. Note the extensive, irregular, osteophytic spurring extending into the left L5-S1 intervertebral nerve root canal, which produces severe bony lateral spinal stenosis. Three-dimensional reconstruction allows the surgeon a better appreciation of the position and extent of bony osteophytes that produce lateral spinal stenosis and can be helpful in planning surgery, as the osteophytic spur can be viewed with multiple cut-away views. More recent advancements allow 3D imaging of both bone and soft tissue.

easily appreciated. New 3D image displays employing noncontour data processing and semitransparent 3D displays offer potential new areas of application for 3D imaging (48).

LUMBAR CT SCANNING

Lumbar Anatomy and Anatomic Variants

A careful review of the normal lumbar spine anatomy and some of the common variations of soft tissue that may simulate disc herniation and nerve root edema is useful before pathological anatomy is discussed. Because of the inherent high contrast between the low-density fat and higher-density disc and nerve roots, high-resolution CT provides highly accurate and specific diagnoses of nerve root impingement by bony stenosis or soft-tissue entrapment by disc, fibrosis, inflammation, or neoplasm.

With the non-angled technique, and often with attempted angulation, visualization of a thin rim of L5-S1 disc posterior to the body of L5 is a normal finding, produced by angulation of the x-ray beam with respect to the plane of the disc. In normal patients, this visualized rim of disc is symmetrical, its prominence is directly proportional to the steepness of the lumbosacral angle, and it does not produce deviation or compression of the adjacent nerve roots or thecal sac.

Normal Variations

Several normal variations can lead to nerve root asymmetry, the most common being ectasia of the nerve root sheath. In these cases, nerve root asymmetry is the only finding of note, and no pathological impinging lesions such as a herniated disc or bony stenosis are identified. The attenuation values of this nerve root enlargement are low and near those of the cerebrospinal fluid (CSF). In cases of nerve root asymmetry and questionable nerve root impingement (such as a narrowed lateral recess), MRI or metrizamide-enhanced CT scanning is definitive.

Tarlov's sacral nerve root cysts also cause enlargement of the imaged nerve root/nerve root sheath complex. These cysts have the same density as CSF and are often associated with benign expansion of the sacral nerve root canals.

The conjoined nerve root is an anatomic variant of considerable interest and importance that most commonly occurs at the L5-S1 level. It is a common entity, present in 8% to 10% of patients. It arises from the thecal sac halfway between the nerve roots on the opposite side. The thecal sac is asymmetrical because the opposite, normal, more cephalad nerve root has exited the thecal sac and is surrounded by fat. The conjoined nerve root continues within the sac, producing a local anterolateral expansion of the thecal sac that contains a large, high-density nerve root mass. The attenuation values of the mass are increased (70 to 80 Hounsfield units). Because its density is near that of the disc, the conjoined nerve root may be mistakenly diagnosed as an asymmetrical disc protrusion herniation (85).

The conjoined nerve root mass arises more caudally than normal, courses directly laterally within the central spinal canal, and most often divides symmetrically with an equal amount of neural tissue exiting the intervertebral nerve root canal at that level and at the next level caudally. It can also be associated with a rounded enlargement of the lateral recess of the central canal.

At the L5-S1 level, the conjoined nerve root divides just medial to the pedicle, the S1 component of the L5-S1 conjoined nerve root mass is more lateral than normal, and no separate origin of the distal nerve root is identifiable. The conjoined nerve root is splayed over the pedicle and the lateral margin of the L5-S1 disc, lying directly dorsal to the disc in the caudal aspect of the L5-S1 nerve root canal (L5), and within the narrowest far lateral portion of the L5-S1 subarticular recess (S1). Thus the conjoined nerve root is fixed in the most restricted and narrowed portion of the L5-S1 nerve root canal and lateral recess, and very minimal disc bulges/herniations or bony hypertrophy of the superior articular process of S1 or hypertrophy of the S1 pedicle can cause it to be stretched or compressed (Fig. 4). Identifying an underlying disc protrusion may be difficult with CT because of the high density mass of the conjoined nerve root. Also, it is necessary to surgically free up the conjoined nerve root mass prior to removing the herniated fragment that underlies it to avoid nerve root damage, which otherwise occurs with disturbing frequency (115). Preoperative recognition of the conjoined nerve root is therefore of considerable importance to the surgeon and can directly contribute to the improvement of surgery in those patients with conjoined nerve root and concomitant disc herniation.

Epidural Hematoma

The characteristic CT features of an epidural hematoma consist of a rounded extradural mass lesion that is

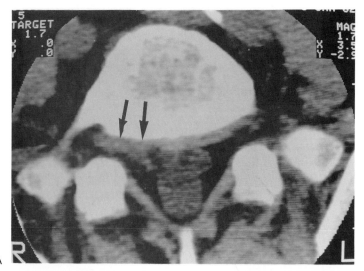

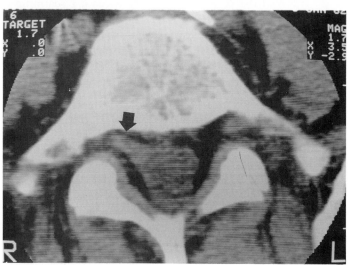

FIG. 4. L5-S1 conjoined nerve root. **A:** Note the asymmetry of the neural elements at L5-S1 with a prominence of the take-off of the right conjoined L5-S1 nerve root from the thecal sac (*arrow*). Note that the normal left L5 nerve root has already separated from the thecal sac. It is this more caudal take-off of the nerve root that is characteristic of the conjoined nerve root. **B:** More caudal axial CT of the same patient. Note that the conjoined nerve root now lies in the inferior aspect of the right side of the L5-S1 disc, and that it is the same density of, and on this single image could easily be mistaken for, a focal herniation. If in doubt, look at adjacent images for calcification. The abnormal caudal position of the L5 nerve root places it directly over the S1 pedicle, around which it is splayed, and directly dorsal to the L5-S1 disc in the more narrow caudal aspect of the nerve root canal. In this position, it is easily impinged upon. This is why conjoined nerve roots can become quite symptomatic with minimal degenerative overgrowth of the bony elements and mild lateral disc bulges. The abnormal position of an L5 conjoined nerve root directly dorsal to the L5-S1 disc is nicely illustrated on sagittal MR images.

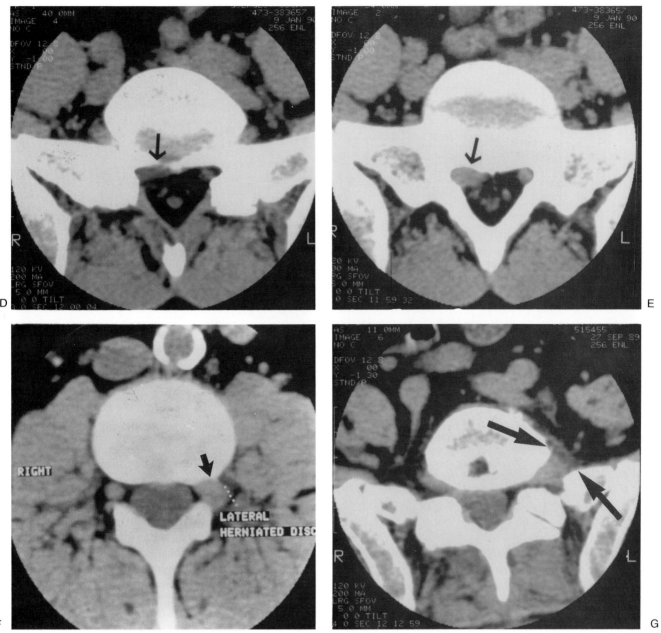

FIG. 8. *(Continued.)* **D,E:** Free fragment herniation at L5-S1 with severe compression of the right S1 nerve root. Note that the disc fragment enlarges as it extends caudally. This is the hallmark of a free fragment herniation as studied by CT. **F:** Axial CT showing a typical extruded lateral (foraminal) herniation at L4-L5 on the left with severe compression of the left L4 nerve root ganglia. **G:** Axial CT showing the typical appearance of a lateral disc herniation at L5-S1 on the left. Lateral disc herniations are most common at L4-L5, less common at L3-L4, and relatively rare at L5-S1. The typical triangular appearance of an extruded lateral disc herniation at L5-S1 results from the flattening of the lateral border of the herniation by the iliotransverse ligament, which extends from the lateral and inferior aspect of the L5 pedicle to the sacrum (*arrow*).

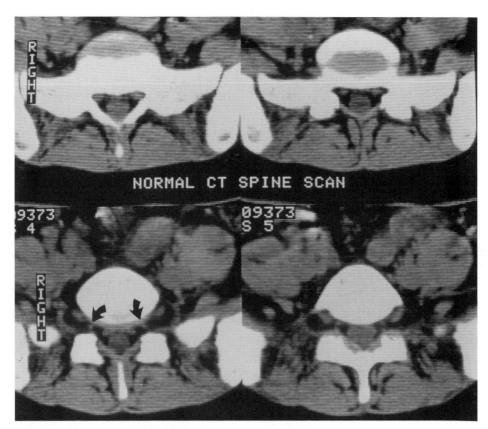

FIG. 9. Normal axial CT images of L5-S1. The visualization of a small circumferential rim of disc material dorsal to the L5 vertebra (*curved arrows*) is a normal finding resulting from the angulation of the disc with respect to the plane of this scan. This is a normal finding and should not be misconstrued as a degenerative disc bulge or central herniation. Note the normal appearance of the S1 nerve roots both adjacent to the disc and more caudally as they lie within the sacrum.

of the spine and a narrowed bony lateral recess (Figs. 11,12).

Since CT cannot differentiate annulus from nucleus as MRI can, it is difficult to differentiate accurately between a contained herniation (intact outer annulus and posterior longitudinal ligament) and a noncontained herniation. If the disc herniation is seen on CT scan as large, large and irregular, or extending significantly craniad or caudal to the disc, it can be assumed to be noncontained. However, when the disc is small or moderate in size and smoothly marginated, attempts to differentiate contained from noncontained by means of CT are guesswork. Therefore, it is necessary to perform MRI evaluation if percutaneous discectomy is contemplated.

MRI has enhanced our understanding of disc pathology and lends itself to a very specific and accurate nomenclature of degenerative disc disease. By this imaging technique, one can now clearly differentiate thickened, redundant annuli from diffuse, contained central disc herniations, and one can visualize complete and incomplete annular tears (both radial and circumferential) and inflammatory fluid within annular tears that may have significance in the prediction of symptomatic disc lesions.

MRI has shown that many of the nonspecific, symmetrical, central disc protrusions that, with the use of CT in the past, were conservatively called *annular bulges* are in fact contained central herniations with dorsal migration of nuclear material beyond the posterior margin of the vertebral body.

Lumbar Spondylosis and Stenosis

The pathogenesis of degenerative lumbar spondylosis and stenosis leads to a conglomerate of radiographic changes. Among them are (a) loss of disc height, (b) ligamentous laxity with rotational instability, (c) spondylolisthesis and retrolisthesis, (d) degenerative hypertrophy of the facets, (e) degenerative osteophyte formation, and (f) thickening of the ligamentum flavum. Therefore, a variety of configurations may be present that lead to nerve root entrapment (82).

Central spinal stenosis is usually seen at L4-L5 and above, while bony lateral spinal stenosis most often occurs at the lumbosacral level. Several entities occur commonly at this level that do not occur more proximally because of the configuration of the sacrum and the pres-

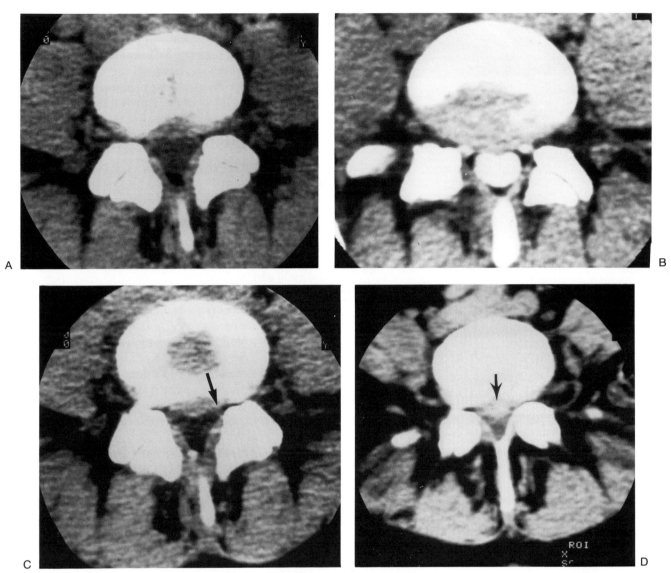

FIG. 10. CT of central protrusions. **A:** Mild broad-based symmetrical central disc protrusion with minimal flattening of the thecal sac. On the basis of CT examination, this would be called a simple annular bulge. On MRI, some of these discs show central annular tears and others may represent contained central disc herniation. Important to observe is the lack of any demonstrable nerve root impingement. **B:** Slightly larger symmetrical central disc protrusion with minimal flattening of the thecal sac and impingement on nerve roots. CT is unable to distinguish between thickening of the annulus and contained central disc herniation. **C:** More focal central disc herniation with irregular margination. On CT exam, this is a probable contained central disc herniation. **D:** Large triangular central disc herniation. This is a definite herniation, and it is suspect for an extruded herniation because of its large size; however, this is not definite on CT and would require MRI for differentiation.

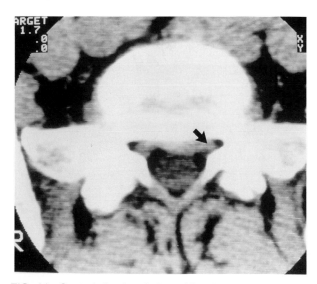

FIG. 11. Central disc herniation with subarticular nerve root impingement. Note the asymmetrical central and left-sided disc herniation with caudal extension into the subarticular recess. This surgically proven disc herniation is producing moderate subarticular compression of the left S1 nerve root (*arrow*) and mild impingement on the right S1 nerve root.

ence of unique anatomic degenerative (uncinate) spurs arising from L5.

The margins of the L5-S1 intervertebral nerve root canals are composed of the pedicles of L5 and S1 superiorly and inferiorly, the superior articular process of S1 dorsally, the L5 vertebral body and L5-S1 intervertebral disc ventrally, and the iliolumbar and corpotransverse ligaments laterally. Any one of these structures may interface with nerve roots and produce nerve root impingement. Morphologically, this may result in narrowing of the intervertebral nerve root canal in the cephalocaudad and anteroposterior dimensions, as well as in a circumferential narrowing, because of a combination of these lesions. The major classification of lateral spinal stenosis should be according to the anatomic narrowing (i.e., front-back stenosis and up-down stenosis) because these correspond to specific anatomic pathological entities.

Because of the plethora of diagnostic terms utilized, as well as differing understanding of the underlying pathology and appropriate surgical treatment, we recommend that the major classes of spinal stenosis be designated as central, subarticular (or spinal recess, as proposed by the 1988 Nomenclature Committee of the North American Spine Society), and lateral (Fig. 13). Burton suggests a "central zone, foraminal zone, and extraforaminal zone" classification. It is our belief that the term *extraforaminal* is a misnomer and actually refers to an up-down L5-S1 lateral stenosis occurring between the inferior margin of the pedicle of L5 and the sacrum or L5-S1 disc. This portion of the canal lies well lateral to the superior articular process of S1 because of the unique lateral flare of the L5 pedicle, but it is still part of the

canal, which terminates at the lateral margin of the L5 pedicle. This does not occur at more proximate levels. Very experienced surgeons have argued that they had encountered extraforaminal stenosis that lay beyond or lateral to the superior articular process of S1. The L5-S1 nerve root canal is a complex structure and is not truly a canal throughout its entire length. There is no posterior wall of the lateral one third of the canal lying between the lateral aspect of the superior articular process of S1 and the inferolateral margin of the L5 pedicle. The term *extraforaminal stenosis* arises out of a misunderstanding of the configuration and length of the canal. Surgeons who believe that they are extraforaminal after removing the L5-S1 facets fail to realize that the superior articular process of S1 is not the lateral border of the canal at L5-S1 as it is at other levels, because the pedicle of L5 flares laterally and lies considerably lateral to the superior articular process. Approximately one third of the L5-S1 intervertebral nerve root canal lies between the lateral superior articular process of S1 and the inferolateral border of the pedicle of L5, which is the true lateral border of the L5-S1 nerve root canal. By definition, if the nerve root is extraforaminal in location, it cannot be compressed, only displaced, since it is outside the nerve root canal. The importance of a spine surgeon understanding this concept cannot be overestimated, because the failure to remove up-down stenosis occurring lateral to the superior articular process of S1 but medial to or at the lateroinferior margin of the L5 pedicle is the most common error of omission.

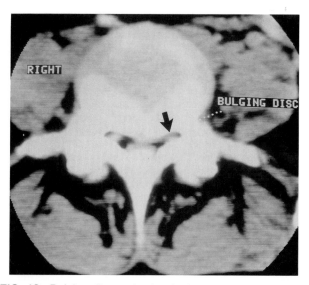

FIG. 12. Bulging disc and subarticular nerve root compression. The axial CT shows very narrowed lateral recesses in this patient with a congenital trefoil configuration of his central spinal canal. Broad-based bulging of the disc annulus, which is slightly more prominent to the left than to the right, is producing moderate subarticular compression of the left S1 nerve root. At surgery, there was merely bulging of the disc annulus without evidence of herniation, and a medial facetectomy was curative.

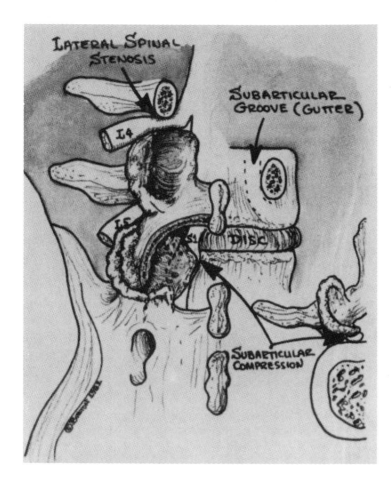

FIG. 13. Diagrammatic illustration of lateral and subarticular recess stenosis. Note the compression of the traversing S1 nerve root by the medial hypertrophy of the base of the superior articular process of S1 (*arrows*). In typical subarticular recess stenosis, pathological hypertrophy of the superior articular process projects into the central spinal canal to impinge on the traversing nerve root (S1 at L5-S1). In most cases, there is concomitant degenerative bulging of the disc annulus and associated thickening of the ligamentum flavum, which contribute to the subarticular impingement of the nerve root. Note also the depiction of the classical lateral spinal stenosis at L4-L5 with the margins of the canal being defined by the pedicle. The same definition of the canal by the pedicle by L5-S1 causes the L5-S1 canal to be elongated because the lateral flaring of the pedicle causes the canal to extend well beyond the lateral margin of the superior articular process. Stenosis in this more lateral aspect of the canal is responsible for the most common cause of FBSS due to residual lateral spinal stenosis (illustration copyright, Charles V. Burton, M.D.).

Another familiar term for this type of lateral stenosis is the *far-out stenosis* of Wiltse. Again, the L5 ganglia is compressed by the pedicle of L5, not the transverse process as reported, because the L5 nerve root emerges from the canal immediately adjacent to the vertebral body and courses anteriorly into the pelvis ventral and caudal to the more laterally situated transverse process.

Uncinate Spurs

Usually, lateral stenoses result from a multiplicity of degenerative and proliferative processes that cause the intervertebral nerve root canal to narrow in one or more of its several dimensions. It has become apparent that cephalocaudad stenosis at L5-S1 resulting from (uncinate) spurs arising from the dorsolateral aspect of L5 is the most common cause of lateral spinal stenosis at this level. In most cases, degenerative narrowing or collapse of the L5-S1 disc space is found in association with the development of these posterolateral osteophytes.

Uncinate spurs are anatomic correlates of the uncinate spurring found in the cervical spine. The etiology of uncinate spurs in the adult is believed to be the result of disruption or tearing of the annular and/or Sharpey's fibers from the vertebral endplates and the uncinate process. These osteophytes are visualized on standard CT

axial images as dense, rounded, bony structures that project dorsally and laterally into the intervertebral nerve root canal from the vertebral body of L5 (Fig. 14). The posterolateral location of these spurs correlates anatomically with the uncinate spurs found in the degenerated cervical spine. As they enlarge, they project into the intervertebral nerve root canal ventral and lateral to the superior articular process. Because they project into the ventral aspect of the nerve root canal and the L5 nerve root also lies ventrally, tightly opposed to the L5 vertebral body, the spur directly impinges on the caudal surface of the L5 nerve root or nerve root ganglion, causing compression of the ganglia against the caudal surface of the pedicle of L5. A surgeon will find these bony processes covered by tough, smooth tissue, ligaments, or portions of the annulus.

Up-Down Stenosis

As the spinal nerve root emerges from the thecal sac, anatomically proven small dural ligaments attach the nerve ventrally to the posterior longitudinal ligament, annulus, and fascia covering the posterior and lateral aspect of the vertebral body and intervertebral disc. The emerging neural structure (root, ganglia, and spinal nerve) remains relatively fixed in the ventral portion of

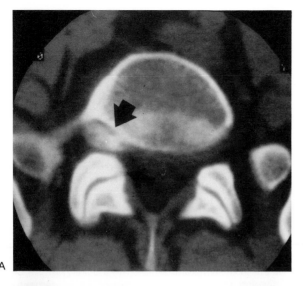

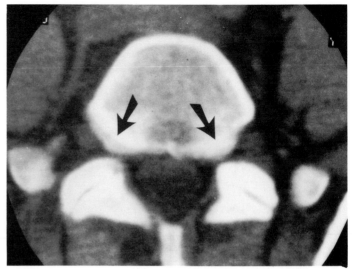

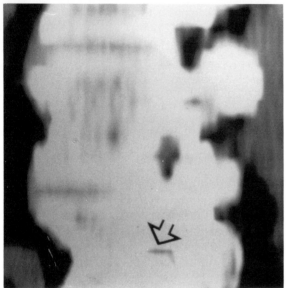

FIG. 14. Uncinate spur. **A:** The large right-sided uncinate spur occludes the right L5-S1 intervertebral nerve root canal and is producing severe compression of the exiting right L5 nerve root ganglia. The location and oval appearance of this osteophytic spur is typical both in appearance and location, being nearly identical from patient to patient. This reproducibility caused us to focus our attention on pathological spurring of an underlying process, which led to the discovery of the vestigial uncinate process at L5-S1. **B:** Bilateral typical dorsal lateral uncinate spurs at L5-S1 that produce moderate cephalocaudad bony lateral spinal stenosis. **C:** Sagittal reformatted image of the patient in A. Note the very severe cephalocaudad bony lateral spinal stenosis with only a residual slit-like foramen due to the presence of the large uncinate spur (*arrow*). Note for comparison the normal appearance of the L4-L5 foramen.

the canal because of (a) the close proximity of the root to the inferior aspect of the pedicle as it courses through the canal to exit beyond, (b) the filamentous fibrous extradural ligaments that anchor the nerve root sleeve as it traverses the canal, and (c) the normally slight outward traction of the spinal nerve.

The nerve lies against the vertebral body caudal to the pedicle, almost like a rope passing around a pulley. These natural structures may slide a bit in and out of their foramina, but they have little or no ventral–dorsal mobility. Posterolateral osteophytic (uncinate) spurs that arise from the vertebral body narrow that ventral portion of the canal where the nerve root structures are found, namely, the constricted space between the spur caudally and the pedicle cranially (Fig. 15). Conversely, the dorsal portion of the nerve root canal may be widely patent in these cases and may easily accept a surgical probe. There-

fore, surgical probing of a canal does not exclude significant lateral stenosis at L4-S1 because of uncinate spurring. Myelography is negative in these cases because compression of the nerve occurs at or beyond the ganglia distal to the termination of the nerve root sheath (Fig. 16). This makes preoperative CT diagnosis and evaluation essential.

The anteroposterior dimension of a CT scan of the craniad portion of the intervertebral nerve root canal that lies cephalad to this spur may be normal. A thin-section axial image obtained through this portion of the canal will not detect the osteophyte. The bony canal will appear normal, with epidural fat lying both anterior and posterior to the nerve root ganglia that lies within this cephalad aspect of the canal. In many cases, the only clue to cephalocaudad compression of the L5 nerve root ganglia is an asymmetrical enlargement on the affected side

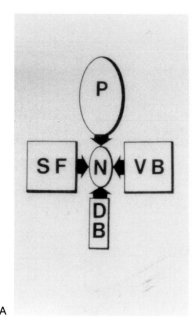

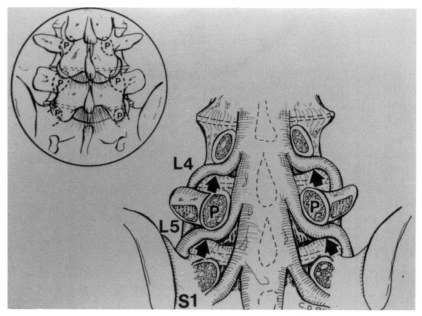

A

B

FIG. 15. A: Diagrammatic representation of the intervertebral nerve root canal demonstrating the structures responsible for up-down, front-back, and pin-hole stenosis: P, pedicle; V, vertebral body; DB, disc bar; SF, superior facet; N, neural canal. Loss of disc height or prominence of the disc and/or osteophytic spurring produces cephalocaudad stenosis, whereas overgrowth of the superior articular process or osteophytic spurring at the posterior margin of the vertebral body produces front-back stenosis. **B:** Diagrammatic illustration of uncinate spurring causing cephalocaudad lateral spinal stenosis. This occurs almost exclusively at L5-S1. As shown, the osteophytic spur arises from the posterior margin of the L5 vertebral body. The uncinate spur represents osteophytic overgrowth of a vestigial uncinate process of the L5 vertebral body resulting from traction on the process by the attachment of Sharpey's fibers. The uncinate spur projects in a craniad direction to produce a cephalocaudad compression of the exiting L5 nerve root ganglia against the undersurface of the pedicle as shown (*arrows*).

resulting from cephalocaudad compression of the ganglia. This compression produces an expansion of the ganglia in the axial plane. Sagittal reformatted images, however, clearly define the severity of the cephalocaudad narrowing and the position and degree of compression of the L5 nerve root ganglia. Similar cephalocaudad stenosis may be caused by osteophytes arising from the margin of the L5-S1 disc or by focal, irregular, and more laterally located osteophytes (Fig. 17).

Lytic Spondylolisthesis

Lytic spondylolisthesis is another entity commonly associated with up-down stenosis. Associated disc space narrowing on plain films is one accurate indicator of the presence of lateral stenosis or far-out stenosis in patients with lytic spondylolisthesis, because this condition is rarely detected in the absence of disc space narrowing. Conversely, lateral spinal stenosis commonly is present in patients with both lytic spondylolisthesis and degenerative disc space narrowing. In most patients, the forward slip of the vertebral body, pedicle, and pars of L5 is associated with a caudal settling of that vertebra as the disc

space narrows, resulting in entrapment and compression of the L5 nerve root between the pedicle and proximal pars cranially and the L5-S1 disc and body of S1 caudally (73,110).

Axial images of lytic spondylolisthesis show distortion of the intervertebral nerve root canal with elongation of the anteroposterior dimension of the canals because of the ventral slip of L5. Preimpingement swelling of the L5 nerve root often occurs. Sagittal reformatted images are the most useful in delineating nerve root compression both within the intervertebral nerve root canal and laterally between the transverse process of L5 and the sacrum (Fig. 18). Coronal and oblique reformatted images are occasionally useful.

Posterolateral bulging of the L5-S1 disc annulus and/or lateral disc herniations at L5-S1 may contribute to the L5 nerve root impingement. Marked narrowing of the cephalocaudad dimension of the intervertebral nerve root canal results in compression and flattening of the L5 nerve root ganglia, which can completely replace the epidural fat within the canal. Distinguishing between the density of the compressed nerve root ganglia and that of a degenerative bulging or laterally herniated L5-S1 disc is often difficult or impossible. Parasagittal reformatted

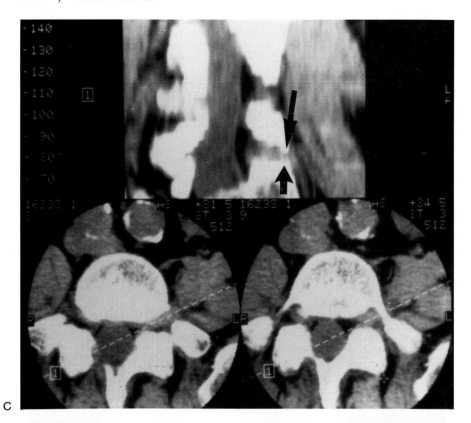

C

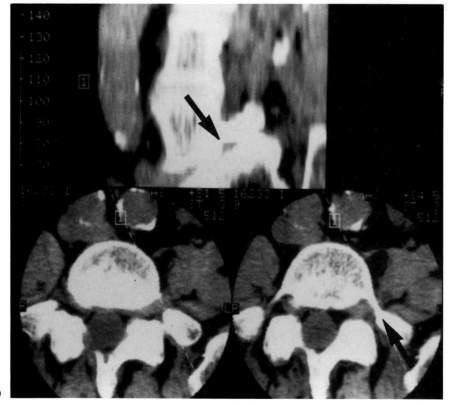

D

FIG. 15. (*Continued.*) **C:** Axial and oblique coronal reformatted images of far lateral, lateral spinal stenosis at L5-S1 on the left. Note the concave undersurface of the L5 pedicle (*large arrow*) with progressive narrowing of the intervertebral nerve root canal as one progresses laterally. The severe cephalocaudad bony lateral spinal stenosis in this patient occurred between the very lateral and inferior aspect of the pedicle of L5 and the superior margin of the endplate and laterally bulging L5-S1 disc (*arrows*). **D:** Oblique sagittal view paralleling the inferior margin of the L5 pedicle. Note the severe cephalocaudad far lateral, lateral stenosis caused by the descent of the lateral and inferior aspect of the pedicle of L5 onto the laterally bulging L5-S1 disc due to severe loss of disc height at this level (*arrows*).

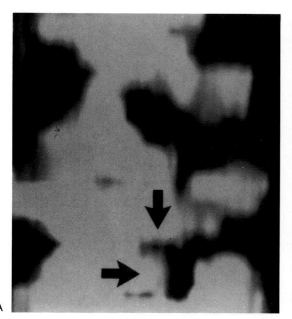
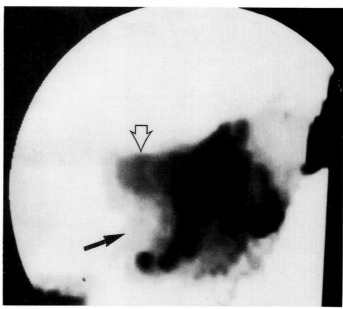

A

B

FIG. 16. A: Sagittal reformatted image of severe up-down lateral spinal stenosis. Note the large uncinate spur which produces severe up-down lateral spinal stenosis within the ventral half of the intervertebral nerve root canal (*horizontal arrow*). The exiting L5 nerve root ganglia are compressed between the undersurface of the pedicle and the superior aspect of the uncinate spur (*vertical arrow*). Note that both the ganglia and the uncinate spur lie within the ventral half of the intervertebral nerve root canal. The dorsal half of the canal is large and never contains neural elements. This case illustrates the potential pitfall faced by the surgeon who attempts to rule out lateral spinal stenosis by probing the intervertebral nerve root canal. The dorsal half of the canal is large enough to allow such probing with the false impression that there is no bony stenosis present. **B:** Three-dimensional reconstruction image of the L5-S1 intervertebral nerve root canal in a patient with a moderate-size uncinate spur (*large arrow*). Omnipaque within the nerve root sheath of the L5 nerve root identifies the ventral position of the exiting nerve root ganglia. Again, note the large size of the dorsal aspect of the canal and the abundant epidural fat within the canal which, if the significance of the uncinate spur is not realized, would lead the unwary radiologist to call the canal normal and the surgeon probing the canal to assume that no stenosis is present.

images may be helpful, and, when clinically indicated, MRI is definitive. MRI has shown that L5-S1 lateral herniation in these patients is not uncommon. Virtually all herniations occurring in these patients are more lateral in position than typical herniations, and, because of the more axial orientation of the L5-S1 disc in patients with lytic spondylolisthesis, a herniation at L5-S1 invariably extends in a cranial direction to compress the L5 nerve root and not S1.

With advancing age, the vertebral bodies frequently reduce in height but widen at the endplate margins. The pedicle, however, increases in diameter and may alter its normally oval configuration into a larger, more rounded shape. The changes are observed best on plain films of the lumbar spine. In effect, this represents an apparent relative descent of the pedicle in the vertebral body.

The pedicles approach each other downward, further restricting the cephalocaudad (up-down) diameter of the foramen. Disc margins, along which the annulus attaches, become more prominent and often calcified. These bars of the disc margin, especially the uncinate spur, further contribute to up-down narrowing.

Front-Back Stenosis

For some time, hypertrophy of the superior articular facet was considered the major cause of lumbar lateral spinal stenosis. As the disc space collapsed, it seemed plausible that the superior articular facet would rise up in the foramen and compress the nerve cephalad against the pedicle. Although facet hypertrophy is commonly associated with lateral stenosis, the hypertrophied superior articular process almost always lies dorsal to the nerve with resultant anteroposterior compression of the nerve ganglia against the dorsal aspect of the vertebral body by the enlarged facet. A combination of facet hypertrophy and osteophytic spurring may produce severe anteroposterior stenosis. This combination is the most common cause of front-back stenosis (Fig. 19).

In the most severe cases, all elements of bony hypertrophy (consisting of the dorsolateral osteophyte arising from the vertebral bodies, thickening of the pedicle, overgrowth of the superior articular process, and degenerative narrowing of the disc) are present and lead to severe multidimensional concentric bony stenosis. Sagittal

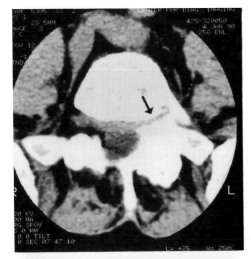

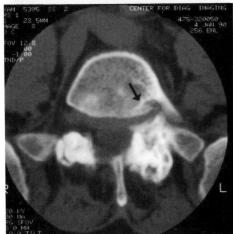

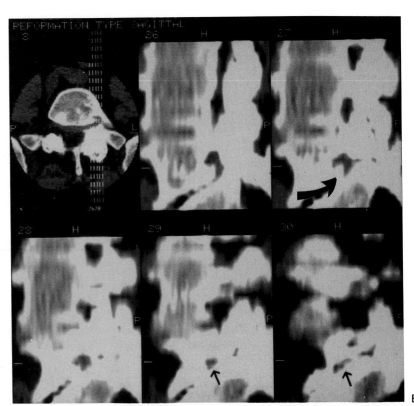

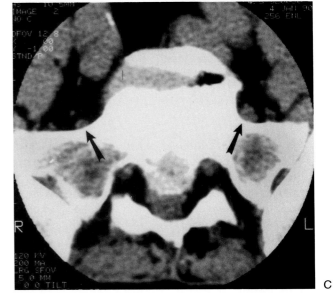

FIG. 17. Patient with severe left L5 radiculopathy. **A:** Axial CT showing severe lateral stenosis at L5-S1 on the left caused by a combination of uncinate spurring of L5 (*arrow*) as well as hypertrophic overgrowth of the superior articular facet of S1. **B:** Lateral computed radiograph of this patient shows an elongate lateral stenosis caused by the uncinate spur medially (*curved arrow*) and by severe loss of disc height and marginal osteophytes far laterally (*small arrows*). **C:** Axial CT in this patient showing postimpingement edema of the left L5 nerve root after it exits the severely stenotic left L5-S1 nerve root canal. The finding of nerve root swelling in conjunction with significant lateral stenosis is very highly correlative with radiculopathy.

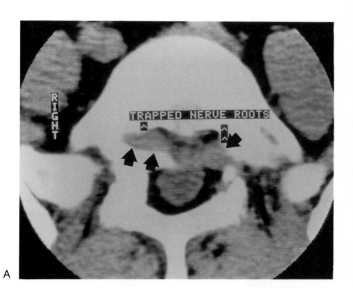

A

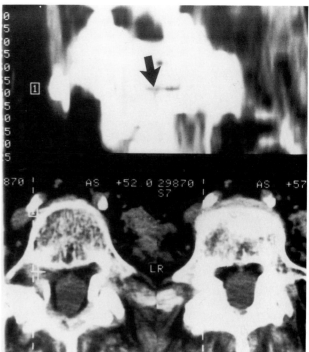

B

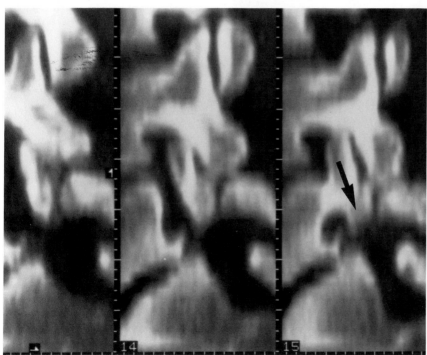

C

FIG. 18. Lytic spondylolisthesis with lateral stenosis at L5-S1. **A:** Axial CT shows typical preimpingement swelling of the L5 nerve roots in this patient with lytic spondylolisthesis, severe degenerative loss of disc height, and cephalocaudad compression of the L5 nerve root ganglia (*arrows*). **B:** Composite axial and sagittal reformatted images showing the elongate appearance of the L5-S1 nerve root canal on the axial image, and the very severe cephalocaudad (up-down) stenosis on the sagittal reformatted image (*arrow*). There is severe compression of the exiting L5 nerve root ganglia. **C:** Sagittal reformatted (CT/MPR) images demonstrating the pars fracture (*arrow*).

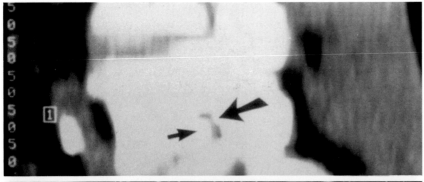

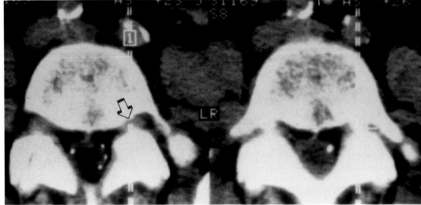

FIG. 19. Front-back stenosis. This is caused by a combination of hypertrophic overgrowth of the superior articular process (*large arrow*) and the presence of a moderate-size uncinate spur (*small arrow*). Note the anteroposterior flattening of the left L5 nerve root ganglia within the intervertebral nerve root canal (*open arrow*).

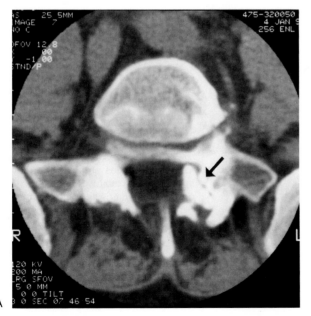

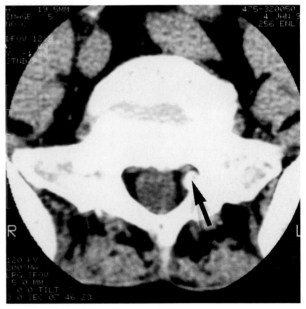

FIG. 20. Focal subarticular recess stenosis. **A:** Axial CT image showing focal bony subarticular recess stenosis caused by marked irregular hypertrophy of the left L5-S1 facet joint (*arrow*). **B:** Axial CT scan immediately caudal to the scan in A demonstrates flattening of the left S1 nerve root by the inferior aspect of the osteophyte (*arrow*).

reformatted images show a "pinhole" intervertebral nerve root canal in these instances.

Burned-Out Stenosis

CT with sagittal reformatted images accurately depicts the degenerative anatomic processes that lead to lateral spinal stenosis. With CT, degenerative processes that merely involve the facet joints without encroachment on the canal are clearly defined. In most cases, CT visualization of bony nerve root compression correlates closely with the clinical symptoms, particularly if swelling of the affected nerve root is observed. However, there are patients who have definite, and sometimes severe, bony stenosis without the associated clinical symptoms. Degenerative bony overgrowths and lateral stenosis result from chronic processes occurring over a span of years. Many of these patients, if questioned carefully, reveal a history of sciatica sometime in the past in the distribution of the affected nerve root. This may be followed by slow regression of symptoms, with or without conservative management. While the painful sciatica may disappear, some weakness or other loss of nerve function may remain. In

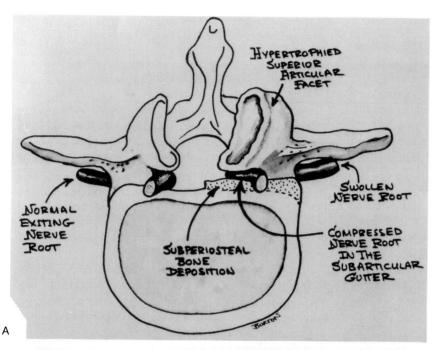

A

FIG. 21. Subarticular recess stenosis. A: Anatomic drawing depicting subarticular recess (gutter) stenosis resulting from hypertrophic overgrowth of the superior articular process and posterior osteophytic spurring. The subarticular recess stenosis occurs within the central spinal canal and medial to the pedicle and therefore is quite distinct from lateral spinal stenosis, which occurs within the intervertebral nerve root canal. Subarticular recess stenosis involves the traversing nerve root at that motion segment, whereas lateral spinal stenosis involves the exiting nerve root. There is often pre- or postimpingement swelling of the affected nerve root, as illustrated on this exam.

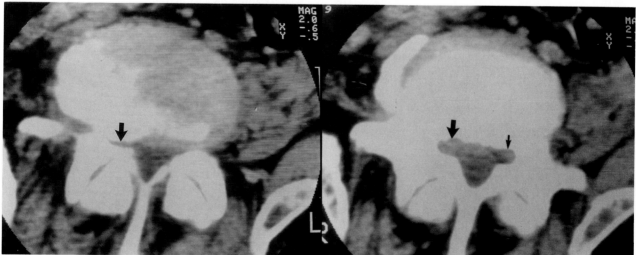

B   C

FIG. 21. (Continued.) B: Axial CT showing severe right-sided subarticular recess stenosis with marked compression of the traversing nerve root. The stenosis is predominantly a result of medial hypertrophic spurring of the base of the superior articular process (arrow). C: Axial CT image obtained just caudal to B showing moderate postimpingement edema of the right-sided nerve root (large arrow). For comparison, note the normal appearance of the left-sided nerve root.

some of these longstanding cases, the CT findings include a severe bony stenosis and a nerve root smaller than its companion on the opposite side. This suggests atrophy of the affected nerve root, and possibly it is the reason symptoms disappeared. This is one form of a burned-out sciatica syndrome.

Subarticular Stenosis

The subarticular recess is that space within the anterolateral portion of the central spinal canal lying ventral to the base of the superior articular process at its junction with the lamina and dorsal to the intervertebral disc. The subarticular recess is a lateral extension of the central canal and occurs when the canal has a trefoil configuration in conjunction with bulging of the disc or when there is medial hypertrophy of the base of the superior articular process or lamina. Not to be confused with the lateral recess of the intraosseous portion of a trefoil spine, the subarticular recess is a pathological entity not present in the normal spine.

Focal osteophyte overgrowth arising from the medial margin of the superior articular facet may produce subarticular recess impingement with entrapment of the nerve root as it traverses the intervertebral disc at that level (Fig. 20). In the more common form of subarticular recess stenosis or entrapment, the nerve is pressed dorsally by a disc bar against the superior ventral edge of the lamina or base of the superior articular process of the segment below (Fig. 21). With either form of subarticular recess, the nerve root exiting at that level is not affected, but the one exiting at the next lower level is.

As previously described, the extradural nerve root is tethered ventrally by ligamentous attachments to the posterior longitudinal ligament and disc margin. Although degenerative processes producing subarticular recess impingement are slowly progressive and chronic, the nerve root becomes entrapped within the subarticular recess because of its immobility.

When subarticular recess narrowing becomes severe, the affected nerve root often is not well visualized. Metrizamide-enhanced scans confirm the constant position of the affected nerve roots within the far anterolateral aspect of the central canal and clearly delineate their compression. Swelling of the affected nerve roots visualized within the nerve root sheath is strong evidence of the pathological significance of the subarticular narrowing and nerve root compression. Myelograms performed in the absence of CT show displacement and broadening of the affected nerve roots and often are misinterpreted as showing disc herniation.

Degenerative Spondylolisthesis

Degenerative spondylolisthesis occurs most commonly at the L4-L5 level. Hallmarks of this entity on axial images are (a) marked degenerative changes of the zygapophyseal joints, (b) severe hypertrophic overgrowth and fragmentation of the superior and inferior articular facets, and (c) erosion of the medial aspect of the superior articular processes with consequent anterior subluxation of the intact neural arch of the vertebral body above. This commonly produces severe central and subarticular recess stenosis (Fig. 22).

In addition to the bony constriction, thickening of the ligamentum flavum and degenerative bulging of the disc annulus occur (Fig. 23) (107). Also, the disc annulus becomes prominent because of the anterior subluxation of the vertebra above. Although the exiting nerve roots are usually indistinct as a result of compression by lateral

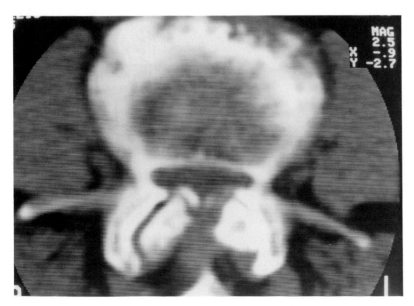

FIG. 22. Degenerative spondylolisthesis. Axial CT at L4-L5 showing the severe degenerative remodeling of the facets. There is ventral subluxation of the inferior facets due to the marked erosion and remodeling of superior articular facets. It is the forward subluxation of the intact neural arch of the craniad vertebra (usually L4) that causes central and subarticular recess stenosis as is seen in this patient. Conversely, lytic spondylolisthesis is rarely if ever associated with central stenosis but rather with lateral stenosis.

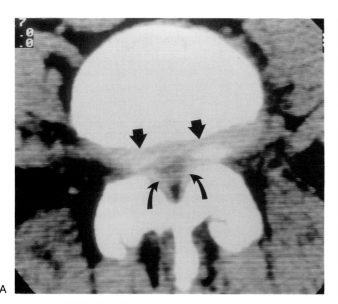

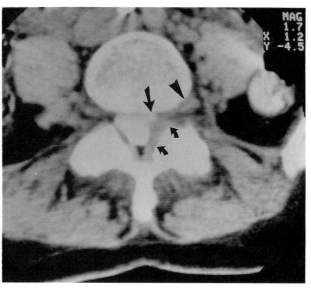

A

B

FIG. 23. Degenerative spondylolisthesis. **A:** Axial CT showing the contribution of the soft tissues to the central stenosis. Degenerative spondylolisthesis typically has marked thickening of the ligamentum flavum (*curved arrows*) and broad-based central disc protrusion which extends into the central canal and also laterally into the nerve root canals (*broad arrows*). **B:** Axial CT in a patient with focal thickening of the ligamentum flavum (*curved arrows*). This can progress to formation of a synovial cyst with subarticular compression of the traversing L5 nerve root (*large arrow*). Note the lateral extension of the L4-L5 disc into the caudal aspect of the intervertebral nerve root canal and displacement and indistinctness of the postganglionic portion of the left L4 nerve (*arrowhead*).

bulging or contained herniation of the severely degenerated disc into the intervertebral nerve root canals, bony lateral spinal stenosis is unlikely (Fig. 24).

It appears that lateral spinal stenosis is associated with degenerative spondylolisthesis only when there is an associated posterolateral osteophyte projecting into the intervertebral nerve root canal or rotational instability with more prominent anterior subluxation of the lamina and inferior facet on one side (Fig. 25).

Our classification of lateral stenosis is based on simple descriptions of the planes of narrowing of the lumbar neural foramina. By far, the most common is up-down stenosis, where the ganglion is pressed upward (cephalad) into the pedicle of that segment by a disc bar or spur immediately inferior (caudad). This was present in 95% of the 300 cases of lateral spinal stenoses at L5-S1 that we reviewed. This is an important concept, because at the L5-S1 level, the L5 nerve root is held within the ventral aspect of the L5-S1 intervertebral nerve root canal by surgically and anatomically definable ligamentous attachments. Thus, the L5 nerve root may be severely compressed in the cephalocaudad dimension within the ventral half of the intervertebral nerve root canal while the dorsal half of the canal remains devoid of neural tissue and filled with epidural fat. The operating surgeon unaware of this situation may conclude incorrectly that no stenosis is present after probing the patent uninvolved dorsal portion of the intervertebral nerve root canal.

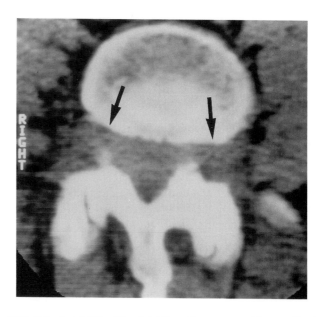

FIG. 24. Axial CT of the L4-L5 motion segment in a patient with the typical soft-tissue opacification of the intervertebral nerve root canals that occurs in degenerative spondylolisthesis. Prior to MRI, this was thought to represent fibrocartilaginous proliferation at the margin of the disc. However, MRI shows this to be a very redundant, thickened, and bulging annulus and/or contained disc herniation. The indistinctness results from the up-down compression of the L4 ganglia by the lateral extensions of these discs. Also, it is not infrequent to see degenerative spondylolisthesis complicated by lateral disc herniation.

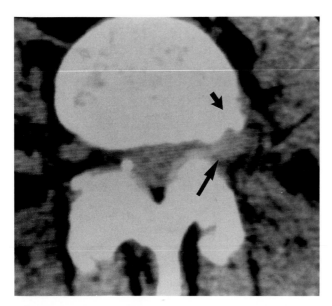

FIG. 25. Axial CT showing lateral stenosis complicating degenerative spondylolisthesis. Note the asymmetrical rotary subluxation of the left inferior articular facet to produce left L4-L5 subarticular and lateral stenosis. The lateral osteophyte arising from the inferolateral aspect of the L4 vertebral body (*small arrow*) also contributes to the lateral stenosis. Note the edema of the exiting left L4 nerve root (*large arrow*).

Therefore, lateral spinal stenosis cannot be excluded at surgery unless the nerve root is directly visualized and followed throughout the entire intervertebral nerve root canal. Since far lateral visualization requires extensive bony decompression, a preoperative CT/MPR scan of the lumbar spine is essential to exclude or clearly to define the etiology and location of the lateral spinal stenosis.

We believe that lateral stenosis is a commonly found entity and a natural concomitant of degenerative disc disease. Therefore, routine reformatting is essential. Intermittent or case-by-case image reformatting (in those cases in which the axial images suggest stenosis) should not be used, because axial images of pure cephalocaudal stenosis may appear normal.

THE SACROILIAC JOINTS

The sacroiliac joints are a bicompartmental articulation containing both a ventral synovial and a dorsal ligamentous compartment. Either component of the joint may be affected by a variety of arthropathies which affect osteotendinous and osteoligamentous junctions. Examination of the sacroiliac joints is most commonly performed to delineate radiographic changes of the seronegative spondyloarthropathies and degenerative joint disease. In the evaluation of the spondyloarthropathies, CT has been demonstrated to be more sensitive than plain film radiography in the depiction of early juxta-

articular osteopenia, joint space narrowing, subchondral sclerosis, and cystic changes. The involvement of the sacroiliac joints may initially be unilateral or asymmetrical, but typically bilateral symmetrical involvement of the joints will be delineated. Because of the relatively nonspecific nature of the response of the sacroiliac joints to an inflammatory process, radiologic discrimination of the variety of causes of sacroiliitis depends on the distribution of disease and additional clinical findings. The radiologic changes of degenerative diseases of the sacroiliac joints are quite different from the changes of the seronegative spondylopathies. The degenerative changes are frequently unilateral and present with osseous spurring and rarely cystic changes.

CERVICAL AND THORACIC CT OF DEGENERATIVE DISEASE

Unenhanced CT performed with 1.5-mm slice thickness imaging remains the procedure of choice for evaluating monoradiculopathy of the upper extremity when impingement of a cervical nerve root is suspected (15,16,28,44).

Images are routinely obtained from C7-T1 through C2. Slice thicknesses greater than 1.5 to 2.0 mm provide inadequate delineation of cervical discs and also inadequate delineation of the neural foramina. Despite the availability of an MR scanner, CT is the procedure of choice in cervical radiculopathy for two primary reasons: it is considerably less expensive than MRI, and the evaluation of narrowed foramina and differentiation of disc herniation from uncinate or posterior spurring is easier with CT at the present time (Fig. 26).

The utility of MRI in the evaluation of cervical radiculopathy is limited if the MR scanner employed cannot obtain thin-section images because of poor visualization of structures within pathologically narrowed foramina. Partial volume imaging present on wide (i.e., 5 mm) slice thickness scans, coupled with similarity of signal intensity of degenerated herniated disc material and uncinate spurring, makes these images all but uninterpretable, other than to state that they are abnormal. Quantitative data are difficult to extract from these images.

Axial images do provide excellent delineation and visualization of the central canal, cervical cord, and cord compression and displacement caused by cervical degenerative spurring and disc herniation.

Continued improvements in MRI, including recent software and hardware updates that allow 1.5-mm 3D stacked images of the cervical spine, have recently provided marked improvement in the imaging of the narrowed foramina by eliminating the problem of partial volume imaging. Certainly, MR images of normal foramina provide spectacular images of normal neural anatomy. However, when the nerve root canals become

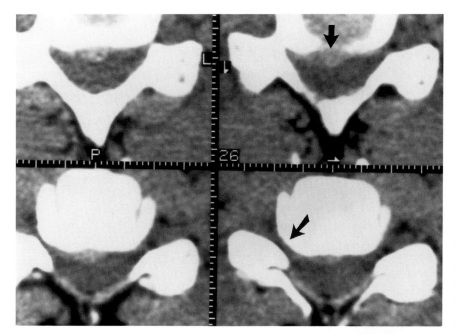

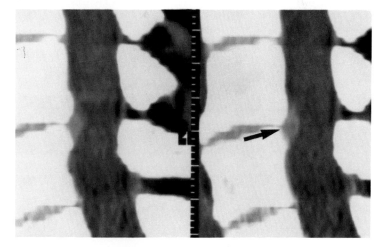

FIG. 26. A–F. CT of cervical degenerative disc disease and spondylosis. A: Axial CT of the cervical spine showing a focal central disc herniation with mild cord compression (*arrow*). There is associated right-sided uncinate spurring causing mild lateral stenosis (*angled arrow*).

FIG. 26. (*Continued.*) B: Sagittal reformatted CT (CT/MPR) showing the above disc herniation and cord compression (*arrow*).

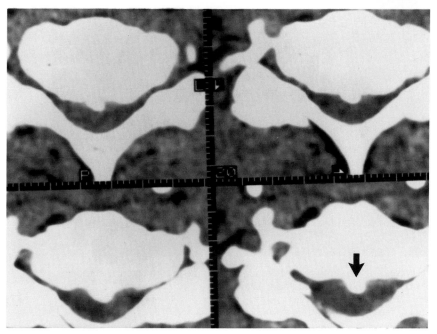

FIG. 26. (*Continued.*) C: Axial CT images of the cervical spine showing severe central and bilateral lateral stenosis due to severe posterior and bilateral uncinate spurring as well as calcification of the posterior longitudinal ligament in the midline (*arrow*). Note the marked cord compression.

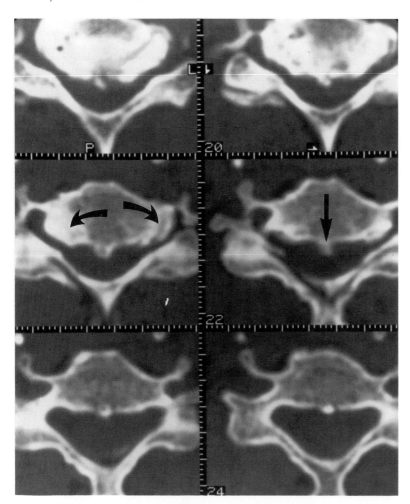

FIG. 26. (*Continued.*) **D:** Bone window axial CTs in this patient demonstrating the severe uncinate spurring (*curved arrows*) and the calcification of the posterior longitudinal ligament (*straight arrow*).

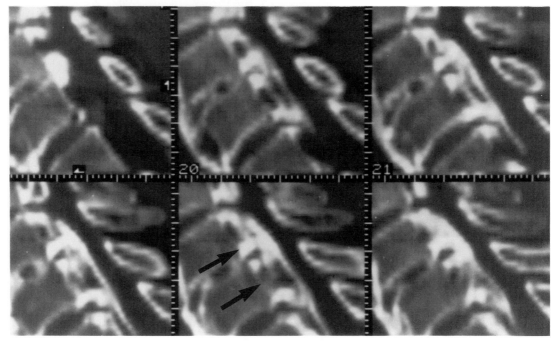

FIG. 26. (*Continued.*) **E:** CT/MPR images of the same patient demonstrating the marked central stenosis caused by the calcification of the posterior longitudinal ligament (*arrows*).

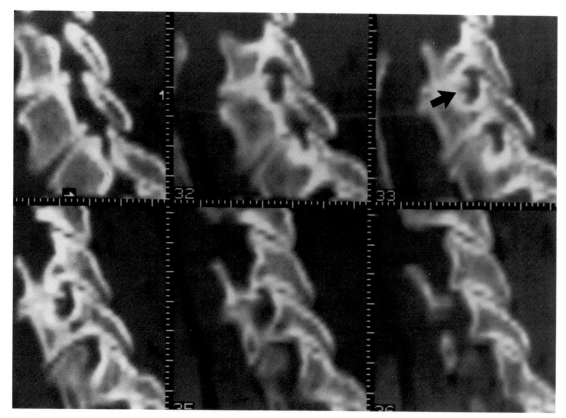

FIG. 26. (*Continued.*) **F:** CT/MPR images of the cervical spine demonstrating severe lateral stenosis secondary to uncinate spurring (*arrow*).

narrowed by either low-density disc herniation or osteophytes, and both are of similar low signal-intensity, MRI often cannot differentiate between them. This differentiation is more easily achieved at present with thin-section 1.5-mm CT imaging.

We have not found either intravenous (17) or intrathecal contrast enhancement of cervical 1.5-mm CT scans to be either necessary or useful when performed on a GE 9800 scanner (31,66,80,101,104,105). On the contrary, we have experienced cases in which the intrathecal contrast layered out and became isodense with a herniated disc and obscured the diagnosis. However, it must be understood that not all equipment is capable of providing 1.5-mm images or the resolution necessary for adequate definition of cervical disc pathology. When this is the situation, either intrathecal contrast should be used to supplement the CT, or MRI should be performed.

MRI has completely replaced CT in the study of degenerative disease of the thoracic spine. CT is used as an adjunct only to determine calcification of a disc herniation (1,2), to better define associated facet and bony abnormalities, and in cases of suspected antecedent trauma to define fractures.

MRI has also largely replaced CT in the study of spinal neoplasm, especially neoplasm associated with marrow involvement such as metastatic disease and myeloma

(45,52). MRI is also superior to CT in the study of epidural and intraspinal neoplasm (4,67,93) and paraspinous masses (20). CT retains utility in the study of primary bone neoplasms and calcified tumors (5,26,32, 33,51,61,76,114).

POSTOPERATIVE EVALUATION OF THE SPINE

It is estimated that as many as 25% to 40% of patients undergoing spinal surgery will have unsatisfactory results. Frequently these patients will require diagnostic imaging studies to determine the cause of persistent or recurrent spinal symptoms. With the yearly increase in the number of spinal surgical procedures performed in the United States, the number of diagnostic imaging studies evaluating the postoperative patient has also continued to rise.

Before the development of MRI, CT was the optimal imaging modality for the evaluation of the variety of causes of failed spinal surgery or new symptoms following a surgical procedure. These included persistent or recurrent disc herniations, epidural fibrosis, spinal stenosis, spinal malalignment, fusion complications, facet arthrosis or fracture, arachnoiditis, infection, epidural

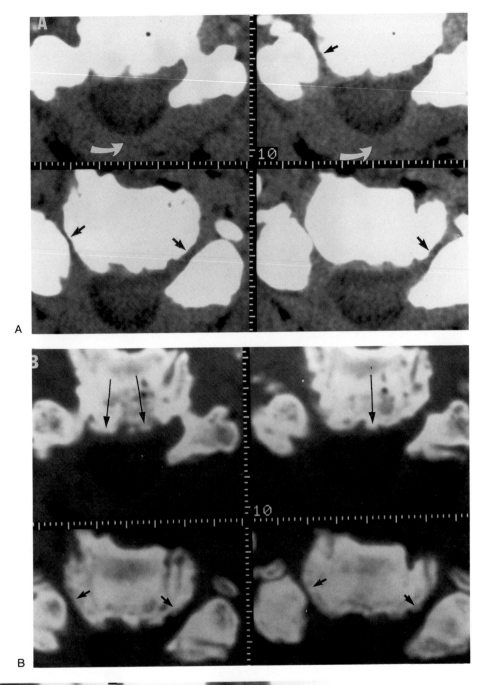

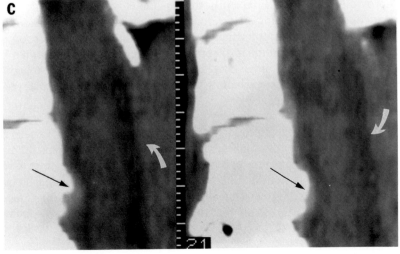

FIG. 27. Postoperative wide laminectomy from the C4-C5 disc level to the C6-C7 level for cervical myelopathy: CT/MPR. On the axial (**A,B**) and sagittal (**C**) images. postoperative changes from a wide laminectomy are identified (*curved white arrows*). At the C6-C7 disc level there is severe stenosis of the intervertebral canals bilaterally (*short black arrows*). Despite the wide laminectomy, there is persistent anterior impingement of the spinal cord by spondylotic ridges (*long black arrows*) at the C6-C7 disc level.

hematomas, and dural tears (109). MRI has replaced CT as the initial imaging modality in the evaluation of patients with suspected disc herniations (10,30,53), epidural fibrosis, stenosis secondary to fat grafts (72,89), epidural hematoma, pseudomeningocele (83), arachnoiditis (96), and infection (87). Currently, CT and CT/MPR are used for evaluation of the postoperative patient for stenosis, complications related to spinal fusion and instrumentation, instability, and facet arthrosis or fracture. Occasionally, CT and CT/MPR are also used for the evaluation of arachnoiditis and pseudomeningocele.

Cervical Spine

In one recent MRI study (95) of a group of symptomatic patients who had undergone anterior discectomy and cervical fusion, the most common findings that explained their persistent symptoms included bony stenosis at the fusion site and disc herniations at the first mobile segment above or below the fusion. MRI provided excellent delineation of disc herniations and encroachment of the central spinal canal, but the status of the interbody fusion was difficult to evaluate. In these patients, stenosis was secondary to hypertrophic bone from the fusion mass that encroached upon the central or inter-

vertebral canals. MRI is excellent in the delineation of the spinal cord, thecal sac, and soft tissues, but it lacks the osseous resolution of a thin-section CT study. In the preoperative evaluation of patients with cervical spondylosis, it is important to adequately evaluate the intervertebral canals because of the frequent association of central and intervertebral canal stenosis in patients with spondylitic symptoms (19) (Fig. 27). To achieve a successful surgical outcome in these patients, it may be necessary to decompress both the central and intervertebral canals to relieve neural impingement.

Postoperatively, CT/MPR is particularly helpful in the evaluation of osseous fusions (Fig. 28) and in the delineation of fractures (Fig. 29) or displacement of bone struts. CT/MPR also provides excellent delineation of disc herniations frequently identified at the first mobile segment adjacent to the levels fused (Fig. 30). In addition, CT/MPR provides excellent demonstration of spinal malalignment secondary to instability from multilevel laminectomies (56).

Lumbar Spine

In the evaluation of the causes of failed lumbar surgery, Burton et al. were among the first to stress the im-

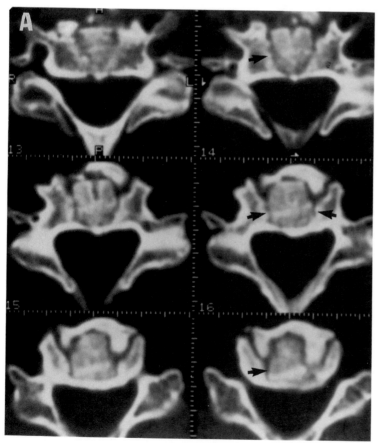

FIG. 28. A–C. Interbody at the C5-C6 and C6-C7 disc levels: CT/MPR. On the axial images (**A**), the bone plug from the Cloward procedure is identified (*black arrows*), but it is difficult to determine whether the fusion is solid.

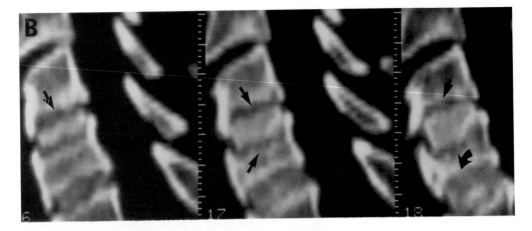

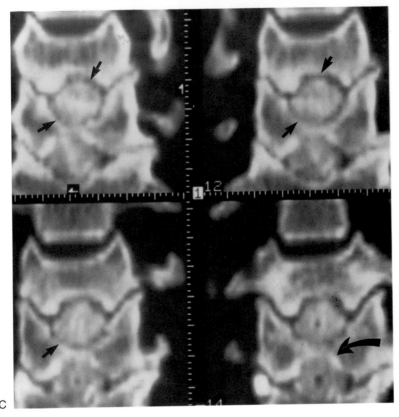

FIG. 28. (*Continued.*) On the sagittal (**B**) and coronal (**C**) reconstructed images, a pseudarthrosis is delineated at the C5-C6 disc level (*straight black arrows*). At the C6-C7 disc level, the bone plug is solidly fused to the C6 vertebral body (*curved black arrows*) but incompletely to the C7 vertebral body.

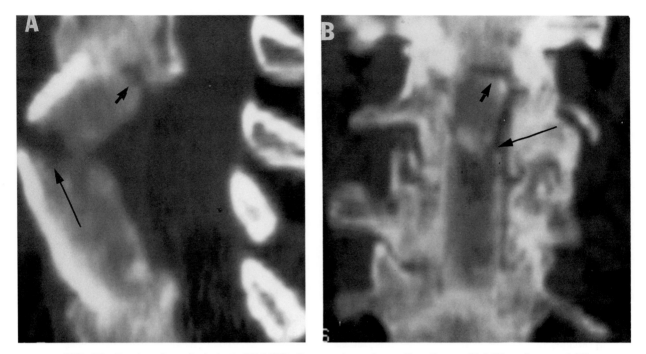

FIG. 29. Fractured cervical strut: CT/MPR. One week postoperative, the sagittal (**A**) and coronal (**B**) reconstructed images give excellent delineation of a fractured strut (*long black arrows*) in the cervical spine. There has been slight diastasis of the superior margin of the strut from the adjacent vertebral body (*short black arrows*).

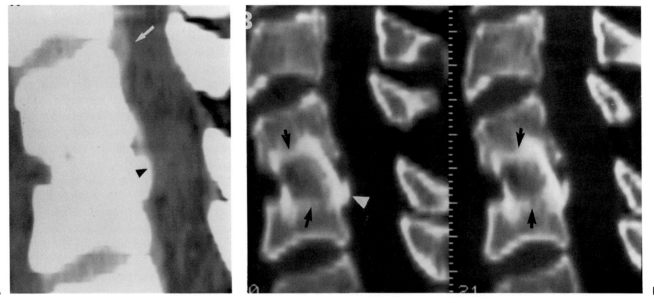

FIG. 30. Postoperative fusion at the C5-C6 disc level: CT/MPR. On the sagittal reconstructed images (**A,B**), a solid interbody fusion is identified at the C5-C6 disc level (*black arrows*). Posteriorly, at the fused segment, there still remain small degenerative spurs projecting into the central spinal canal (*arrowheads*). At the first mobile segment above the level of the fusion, a posterior midline disc herniation is identified (*white arrow*).

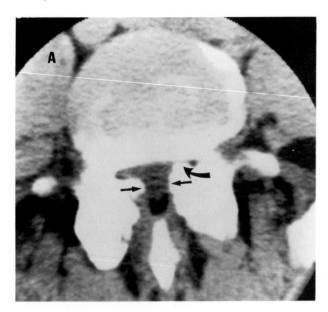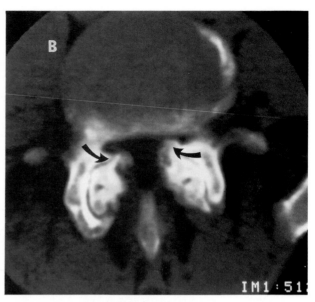

FIG. 31. Postoperative lumbar central and subarticular lateral recess stenosis. One year after laminotomy at the L4-L5 disc level, the patient was experiencing persistent left radicular pain. On the axial (**A,B**) images, severe facet degenerative changes are identified. In addition to facet hypertrophy, degenerative osseous spurring of the anteromedial margin of the facet joints is causing moderate central canal stenosis (*straight arrows*) and stenosis of the subarticular lateral recess (*curved arrows*).

portance of stenosis as the etiology for FBSS (12). At the Sister Kenny Institute, evaluation of patients with failed back surgery demonstrated lateral spinal stenosis in 58%, central spinal stenosis in 7%, arachnoiditis in 16%, recurrent or persistent disc herniation in 12%, and epidural fibrosis in 8%. An important point stressed in their clinical report was that in their 2-year review of high resolution lumbar CT scans in 500 patients with low back pain, lateral spinal stenosis was present in 53% of the cases. Stenosis was a common finding in patients at the time of their initial disc surgery, and the stenosis had to be adequately treated for a successful surgical outcome. In some patients, neural compression was caused only by the stenotic process.

Multiplanar CT still provides the greatest amount of information in the evaluation of spinal central and intervertebral canal stenosis (99). Postoperative central canal stenosis may be secondary to facet degenerative changes, including facet hypertrophy and hyperostotic spurring. The degenerative spurs projecting off the anteromedial margin of the facet joints may cause central stenosis with compression of the cauda equina or stenosis of the subarticular lateral recesses with resultant compression of the transiting nerve roots (Fig. 31). Postoperative instability and malalignment may cause further narrowing of the spinal, central, and intervertebral canals (54,68) (Fig. 32).

Stenosis of the intervertebral canals is typically secondary to osseous spurs projecting from the posterolateral margin of the vertebral body endplates (92). The degree of osseous stenosis is best delineated on sagittal reformatted CT images (Fig. 33). Narrowing of the intervertebral canal may also be secondary to facet degenerative changes (23) or to decreased cephalocaudal height of the intervertebral canal secondary to disc degeneration. At the L5-S1 disc level, it is not infrequent that degenerative spurs impinging the L5 nerve root at the exit zone of the intervertebral canal and in the paravertebral gutter are identified (Fig. 34). With the excellent delineation by CT/MPR of osseous structures, the exact etiology of the stenotic process can be defined, thereby indicating the appropriate surgical procedure if neural decompression is to be performed.

CT/MPR is also the initial examination of choice for patients who have been fused or instrumented and are presenting with persistent or recurrent back pain. In the evaluation of pseudarthrosis, sagittal and coronal reconstructed images are necessary to determine the status of the fusion mass (14,98) (Figs. 35,36). Because of the increased incidence of spinal degeneration at the first mobile segment adjacent to the area of fusion or instrumentation (8,69), this region must always be included when imaging these patients (Fig. 37). Potential complications of spinal instrumentation and fusion procedures, including strut displacement or fracture, fusion overgrowth or fragmentation (63), incorrect positioning (Fig. 38), or displacement of metallic devices (27) (Fig. 39), are optimally evaluated utilizing CT. CT/MPR also provides ex-

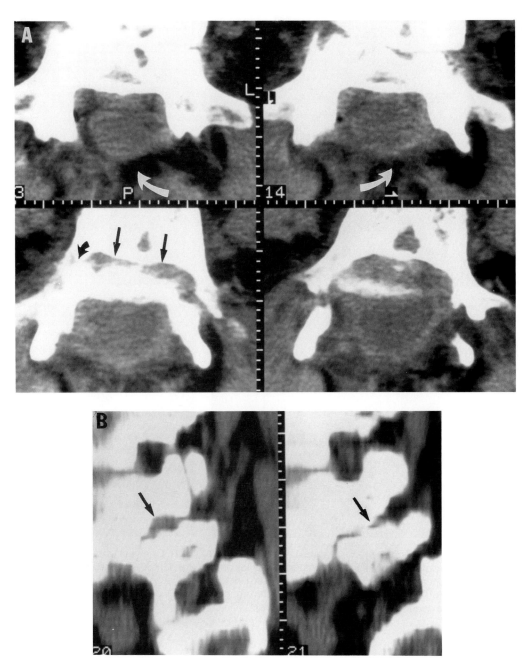

FIG. 32. Postoperative instability with an anterolisthesis at the L4-L5 disc level: CT/MPR. On the axial images (**A**), a wide posterior laminectomy (*curved white arrows*) is demonstrated. An anterolisthesis (*straight black arrows*) can be appreciated, but it is extremely difficult to determine the degree of stenosis of the right intervertebral canal (*curved black arrow*). On the sagittal reconstructed images (**B**), severe stenosis of the L4-L5 intervertebral canal (*arrows*) is delineated.

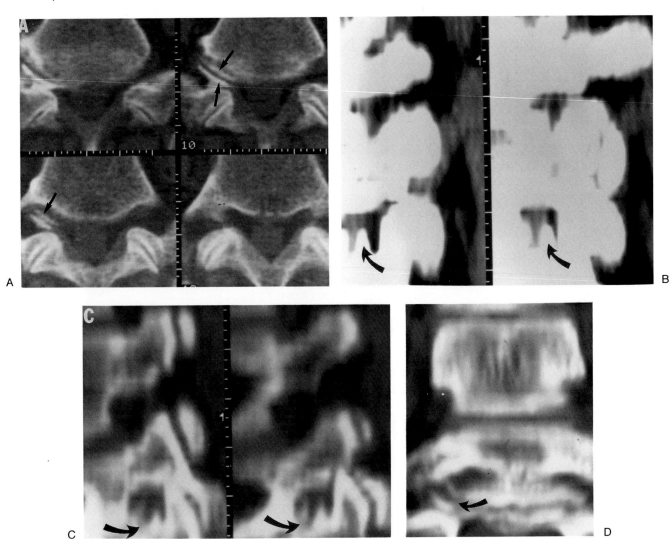

FIG. 33. Intervertebral canal stenosis at the L5-S1 disc level: CT/MPR. One year after discectomy at the L4-L5 level, the patient experienced persistent radicular pain in the right lower extremity. On the axial image (**A**), the spondylotic spurs (*straight arrows*) are identified projecting into the right intervertebral canal. The sagittal (**B,C**) and coronal (**D**) reconstructed images optimally delineate the degree of stenosis secondary to the degenerative spurs (*curved arrows*).

cellent delineation of postoperative spondylosis and facet fractures (100) (Fig. 40).

CT is occasionally needed in the evaluation of postoperative arachnoiditis and pseudomeningoceles (Fig. 41). MRI provides the initial screening evaluation for these complications, but CT-myelography is still occasionally obtained to delineate intrathecal nerve root anatomy in patients with suspected arachnoiditis and a normal MRI study, and to demonstrate the communication between a pseudomeningocele and the thecal sac.

Although MR is the procedure of choice for the evaluation of discitis and osteomyelitis, the diagnosis is often delayed or unsuspected and CT is obtained as the initial study.

Discitis and Osteomyelitis

MRI is more sensitive than CT in depicting changes within the vertebra resulting from infection and neoplasm, and it has become the procedure of choice in the study of discitis and osteomyelitis, as well as metastatic disease and myeloma of the spine.

Irregular erosion and destruction of the vertebral endplates are the hallmark of discitis and osteomyelitis on CT examination (Fig. 42). An associated, smoothly marginated, paraspinous mass paralleling the vertebral level is invariably present and present early (Fig. 42) (11,40,49,57,59,64,120). Psoas and retroperitoneal and epidural abscesses may complicate discitis and osteomy-

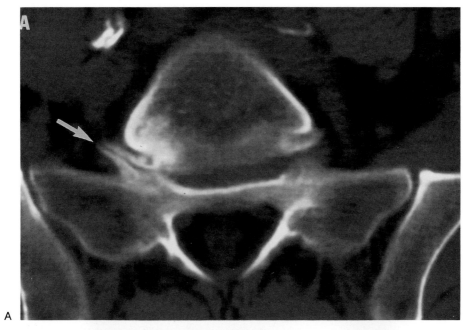

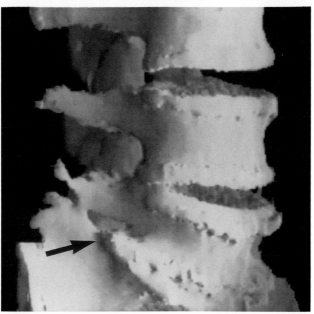

FIG. 34. Exit zone stenosis of the right intervertebral canal at the L5-S1 disc level: CT and 3D CT. On the axial CT image (**A**) of a patient with postoperative radiculopathy, spondylotic spurs (*arrow*) are present, projecting into the exit zone of the right intervertebral canal, lateral to the vertebral body endplates. The size and the position of the spondylotic spurs (*arrow*) are easier to appreciate on the 3D image (**B**) created from the CT data.

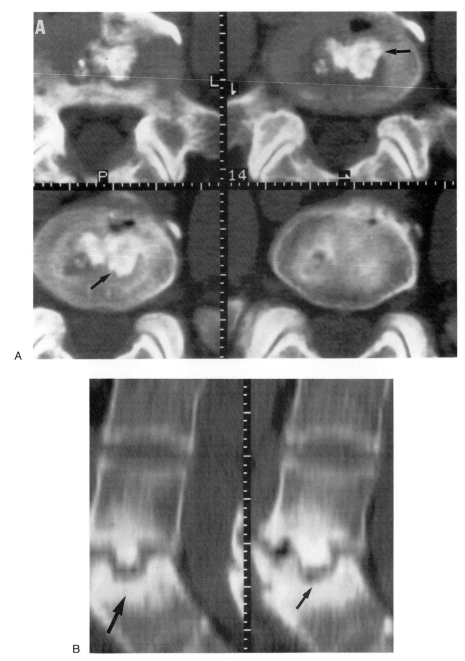

FIG. 35. A–F. Postoperative evaluation of anterior interbody fusions: CT/MPR. On the axial images (**A**) at the L5-S1 level, it is not possible to determine whether the interbody fusion (*arrows*) is solid. On the sagittal reconstructed images (**B**), a pseudarthrosis (*arrows*) is identified at the L5-S1 disc level.

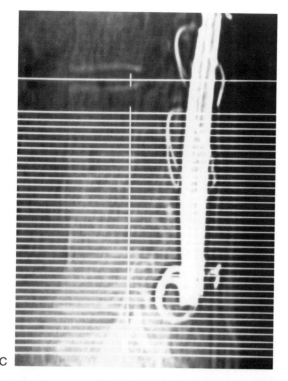

C

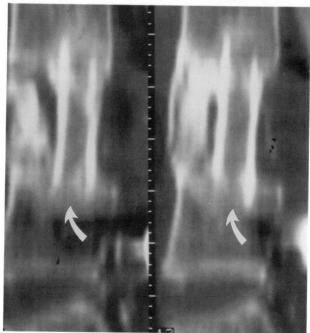

D

FIG. 35. (*Continued.*) On examination of another patient with posterior stabilization (**C**), the metallic instrumentation does not preclude the excellent delineation of the solid interbody fusion (*arrows*) demonstrated on the sagittal (**D**) reconstructed image.

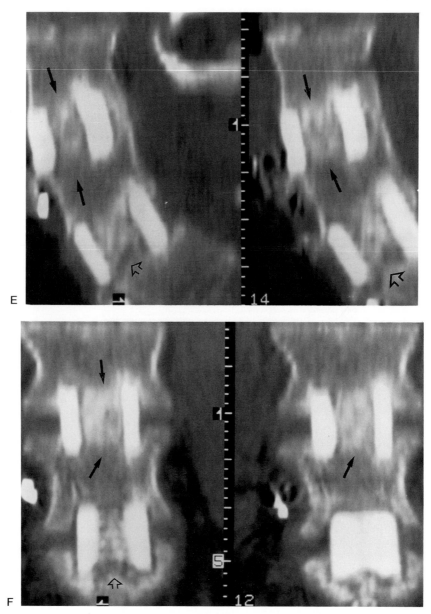

FIG. 35. (*Continued.*) The sagittal (**E**) and coronal (**F**) images from a third patient show a solid anterior interbody fusion at the L4-L5 disc level, with cancellous bone bridging from the bone strut to the adjacent vertebral bodies (*black arrows*). There is a pseudarthrosis at the L5-S1 disc level with incomplete bridging of the cancellous bone from the bone strut to the sacrum (*open black arrows*).

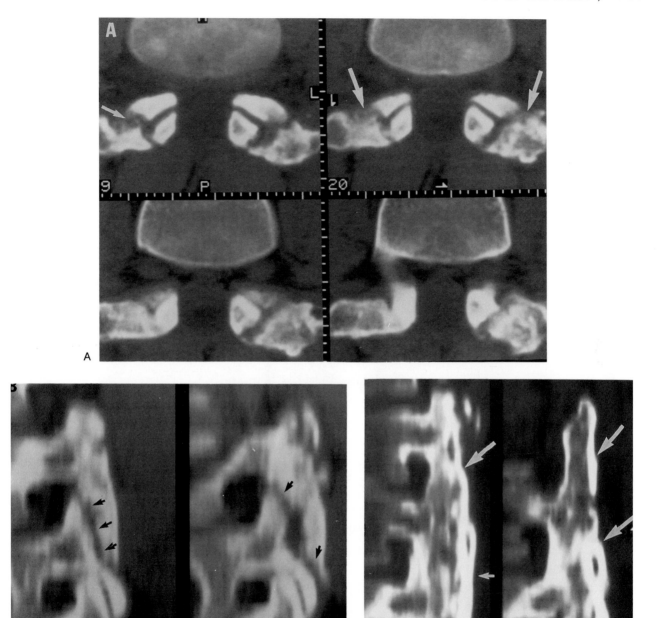

FIG. 36. Postoperative evaluation of a lumbar posterolateral fusion: CT/MPR. On the axial images (**A**), a posterolateral fusion is identified (*white arrows*), but it is difficult to delineate whether the fusion is solid. The sagittal reconstructed images (**B**) are needed to demonstrate the pseudarthrosis (*black arrows*) at the L4-L5 disc level. On examination of another patient, the sagittal images (**C**) give excellent delineation of a solid posterolateral fusion from L3 to L5 (*arrows*).

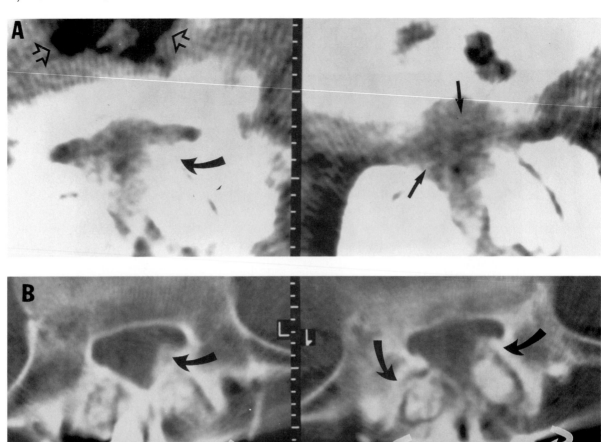

FIG. 37. Severe lumbar central canal stenosis at the first mobile segment above the level of instrumentation. On the axial images (**A,B**) at the L3-L4 disc level, there is severe central canal stenosis secondary to facet degenerative changes (*curved black arrows*) and prominence of the soft tissue (*straight black arrows*). There has been instrumentation from the L4-L5 level through the L5-S1 level, and the cephalad tips of the metallic rods are identified (*curved white arrows*). A prominent vacuum phenomenon (*open arrows*) is present, signifying chronic disc degeneration.

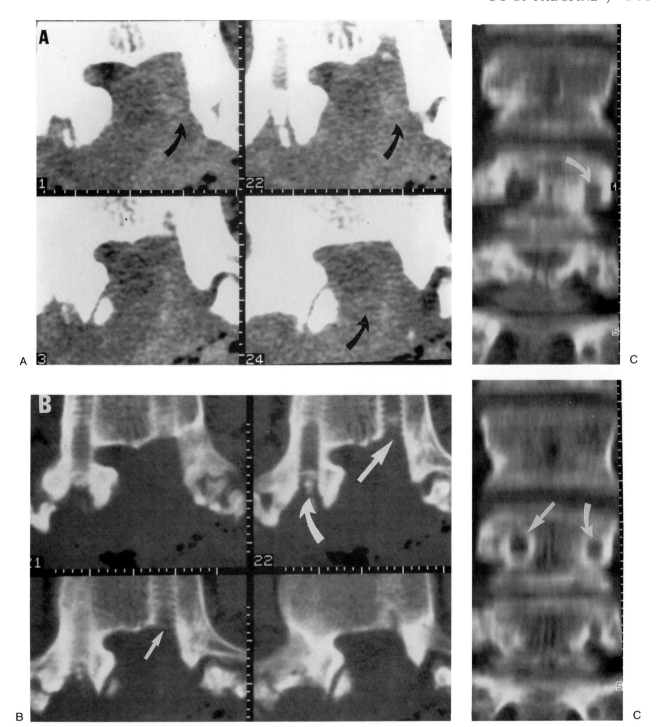

FIG. 38. Persistent left L4 radiculopathy after posterior stabilization procedure: CT/MPR. On the axial images (**A**), extensive perithecal fibrosis is identified at the surgical site (*curved arrows*). On the evaluation of the osseous structures on the axial (**B**) and coronal (**C**) images, an abnormal location of the previously positioned left pedicular screw is identified (*straight arrows*). The screw had been positioned medial to the left pedicle and was most likely impinging on the L4 nerve root. A normal location of the previously positioned right pedicular screw is identified (*curved arrows*).

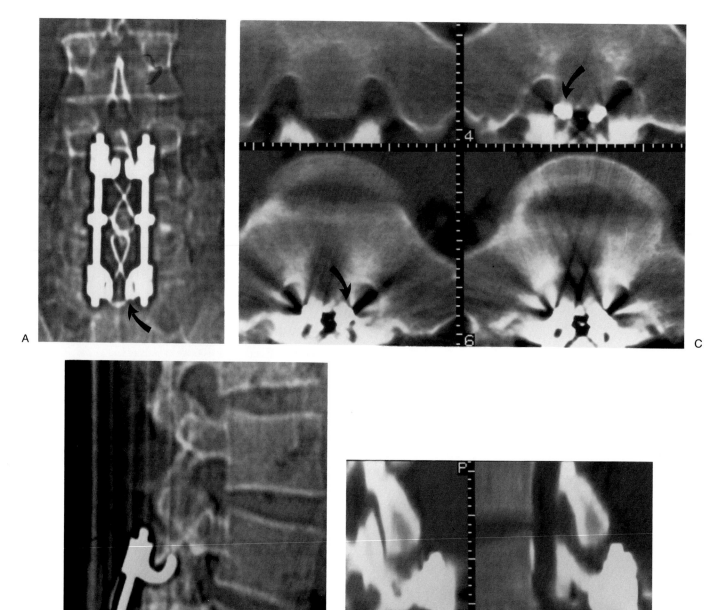

FIG. 39. Postoperative evaluation of a sacral radiculopathy in a patient with Knodt rods: CT/MPR. On the AP (**A**) and lateral (**B**) scout radiographs, the tip of the inferior hook of the Knodt rods (*curved arrows*) appears to be overlying the central spinal canal. The axial (**C**) and sagittal (**D**) reconstructed CT images demonstrate that a tip of the inferior hooks of the Knodt rods (*curved arrows*) is positioned in the central spinal canal in the region of the S2 nerve roots.

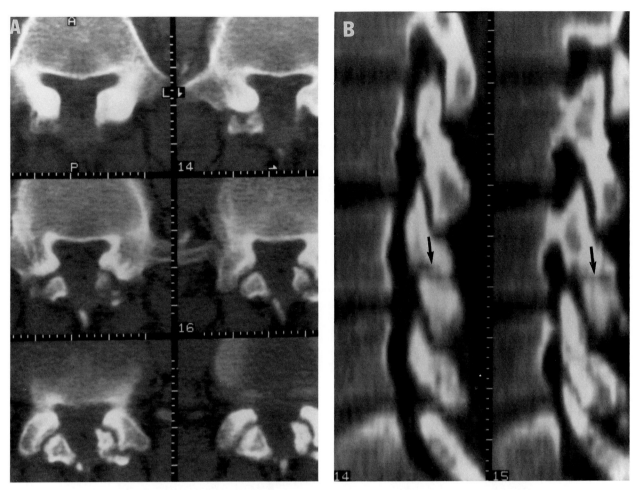

FIG. 40. Postoperative facet fracture at the L4-L5 disc level: CT/MPR. Two years after a surgical procedure, the patient reexperienced back pain. On the axial (**A**) images, it is extremely difficult to delineate the fracture of the left inferior articular process of L4 because of the horizontal orientation of the fracture. The sagittal (**B**) reconstructed image easily demonstrates the fractured inferior articular process (*straight arrows*).

elitis and are also detectable by CT. These inflammatory masses may extend into the nerve root canal and cause edema of the nerve roots within the lateral recess of the central canal. CT also is useful in diagnosing sacral and sacroiliar osteomyelitis (75,94).

The major role of CT and CT/MPR in the evaluation of the postoperative patient resides in their excellent delineation of osseous abnormalities. This is particularly important in evaluating spinal stenosis, the status of osseous fusions, and complications of spinal instrumentation.

SPINAL TRAUMA

In the evaluation of injury to the spinal column, advanced imaging techniques are frequently needed to optimally delineate spinal deformities. Before the

development and implementation of MRI, CT and CT-myelography were the primary imaging studies used to evaluate acute and subsequent traumatic changes in spinal pathology. With the improved soft-tissue imaging capabilities of MRI, particularly for the evaluation of the spinal cord, thecal sac, spinal ligaments, and paravertebral soft tissues (3,22,62,78,103,111), the role of CT has been greatly reduced.

Cervical Spine

In the cervical spine, the major application of CT and CT/MPR is in the evaluation of fractures of the posterior elements, displaced bone fragments into the central canal, and malalignment (78,111). Even with thin-section CT (1.5-mm thick sections), some fractures may be missed (84), but the excellent osseous detail of high-

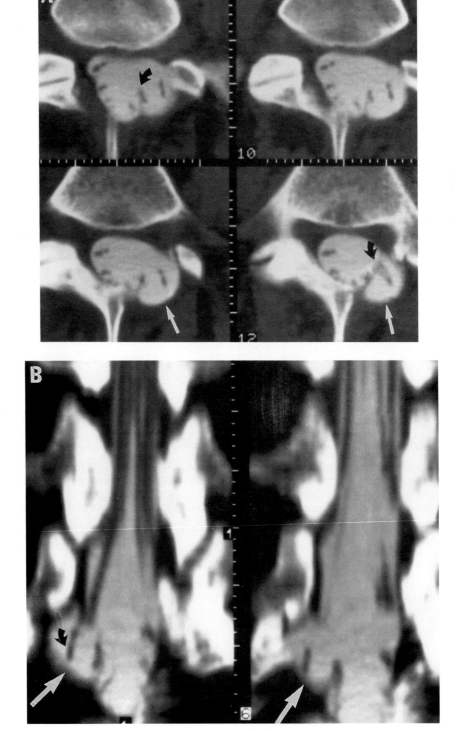

FIG. 41. Postoperative pseudomeningocele at the L5-S1 disc level: CT/MPR. On the CT/MPR myelogram, there is excellent delineation on the axial (**A**) and coronal (**B**) images of a small pseudomeningocele (*white arrows*) located at the L5-S1 disc level. The displacement of the nerve roots (*curved black arrows*) into the pseudomeningocele is demonstrated.

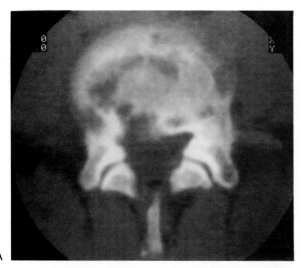

A

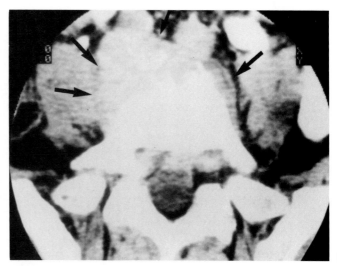

B

FIG. 42. Discitis and osteomyelitis. **A:** Axial CT image filmed with bone window shows the typical moth-eaten destruction of the endplates which is nearly pathognomonic of discitis and osteomyelitis. **B:** Axial CT image filmed with soft-tissue window showing the presence of a paravertebral soft-tissue mass (*arrows*). This is invariably present in patients with discitis and osteomyelitis. The paravertebral mass may be subtle and present as a thin indistinct rim around the vertebral body. One can be easily misled into thinking it is a simple bulging disc if one does not observe that it continues along the margin of the vertebral body on images taken away from the disc space. Interestingly, this paravertebral soft-tissue mass is often of low density on MR T2-weighted images, indicating that it is not abscess but presumably subperiosteal granulomatous reaction. This may explain the high incidence of negative attempted aspiration of these paravertebral masses.

resolution CT still offers a significant advantage over MRI in fracture delineation (Fig. 43). CT/MPR is particularly useful in evaluating posttraumatic malalignment (Fig. 44) and in demonstrating the exact position of displaced bone fragments. CT and CT/MPR also provide accurate measurements of the AP dimension of the central spinal canal (24,106) for the assessment of posttraumatic or developmental stenosis. Patients with a developmentally small spinal canal appear to be more prone to spinal cord injury due to the decreased functional AP diameter of their canal (21,71).

Recent studies have demonstrated MRI's superior capability (compared with CT-myelography) in delineating abnormalities of the spinal cord and intrathecal contents, thus obviating the need for intrathecal contrast in the majority of traumatized patients. CT-myelography still has a role in the evaluation of posttraumatic dural tears (79) and nerve root avulsions, and in the delineation of pseudomeningoceles (6) (Fig. 45). There are still situations in which a patient may not be able to undergo an MRI examination, and in these cases, CT-myelography offers an excellent alternative for evaluating spinal cord compression (6).

In the evaluation of the cervico-occipital junction and the C1-C2 motion segment, CT and CT/MPR are the optimal modalities to evaluate fractures and rotary subluxations. MRI has proved to be excellent in the delineation of atlantoaxial dislocations (9) and particularly useful in the demonstration of thecal sac encroachment and

spinal cord compression. MRI has also proven to be superior to CT-myelography in the evaluation of posttraumatic myelopathy (34,90).

Thoracolumbar Junction

The thoracolumbar junction is the second most common site of trauma to the spinal column after the cervical region. Burst fractures, compression fractures, and distraction injuries may potentially lead to instability and neural impingement (35,58). CT is optimal for defining the nature of the fracture deformity and for determining whether osseous encroachment of the central or the intervertebral canals is present (7,74,81). The decision for surgical decompression and stabilization is frequently based on these morphological changes along with the patient's presenting neural dysfunction (36,46).

CT/MPR is also excellent for reevaluating patients with a fracture deformity and for demonstrating evidence of instability or secondary degenerative changes. CT has the advantage that it permits an evaluation of osseous alignment in patients who have undergone instrumentation with metallic devices (41,116).

With the excellent delineation of the lower thoracic cord and conus medullaris by MRI, the only current indication for a CT-myelogram in the acutely traumatized patient is for the demonstration of dural tears that are associated with fractures of the posterior elements

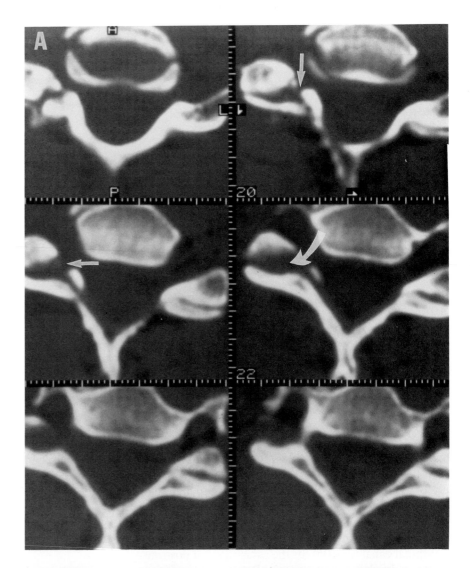

FIG. 43. Posterior element fracture and partial rotary subluxation at the C5-C6 disc level: CT/MPR. The axial images (**A**) identify a fracture involving the base of the right lateral mass of C6 (*straight arrows*) and diastasis of the right facet joint (*curved arrow*). It is extremely difficult to evaluate the degree of malalignment using only axial images. On the sagittal images (**B**), the anterior subluxation of the inferior articular process of C5 (*white arrows*) is delineated along with the impacted fracture of C6 lateral mass (*black arrows*). The diastasis of the C5-C6 facet joint (*curved white arrow*) is also well delineated. The coronal images (**C**) are optimal to delineate the orientation of the fracture (*arrows*) involving the base of the lateral mass of C6.

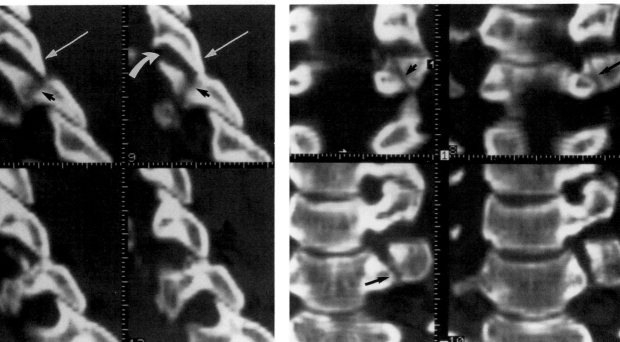

B

C

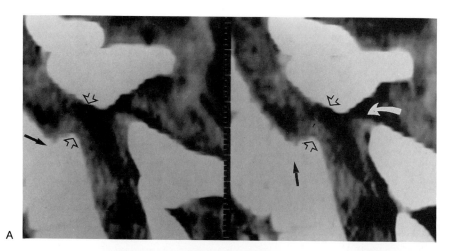

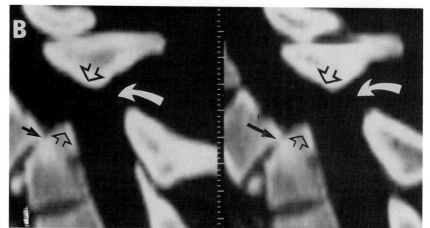

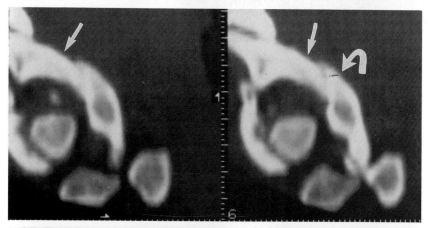

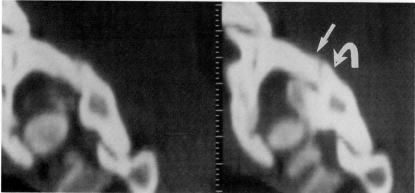

FIG. 44. Posttraumatic anterior subluxation of C7 on T1 associated with dislocation of the facet joints: CT/MPR. This 32-year-old patient presented 8 months after trauma with neck pain and leg weakness. Previous plain x-rays at the time of trauma had been interpreted as normal, but the C7-T1 relationship was not adequately evaluated on the lateral radiograph. On this CT/MPR study, on sagittal midline images (**A,B**) there is a grade II anterior subluxation of C7 on T1 (*solid black arrows*) associated with moderately severe central canal stenosis (*open black arrows*). Laminar diastasis (*curved white arrows*) is present. On the sagittal images through the facet joints (**C**), the anterior dislocation of the inferior articular facet of C7 (*straight white arrows*) is identified. The tip of the inferior articular process of C7 is locked anterior to the superior articular process of T1 (*curved white arrows*).

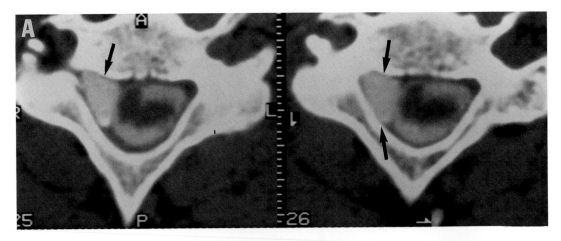

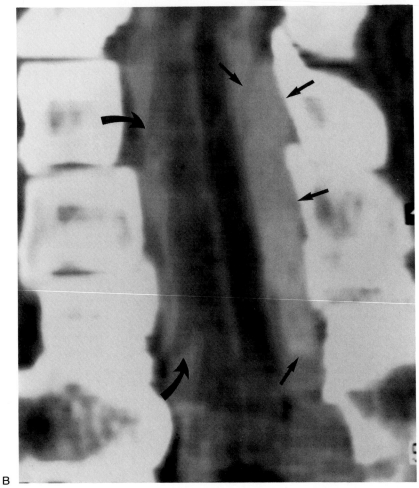

FIG. 45. Traumatic avulsion of the cervical nerve roots associated with a pseudomeningocele: CT/MPR. On axial (**A**) and coronal (**B**) images, the left cervical nerve roots are identified (*curved black arrows*). The right cervical nerve roots from the C5 through the C7 level have been avulsed, and a pseudomeningocele (*straight black arrows*) is present, causing mild cord compression.

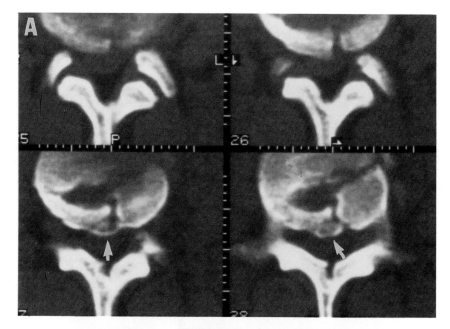

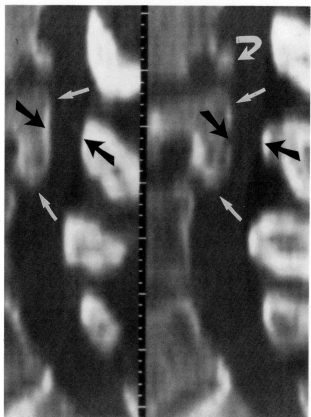

FIG. 46. Posttraumatic deformities of the lumbar spine: CT/MPR. On the axial (**A**) and sagittal (**B**) images, the fracture deformity of the L3 vertebral body is well delineated. As a result of the retropulsion of the L3 vertebral body (*straight white arrows*), there is moderately severe central canal stenosis (*black arrows*). Retropulsion of the posteroinferior rim of the L2 vertebral body (*curved white arrow*) is also present.

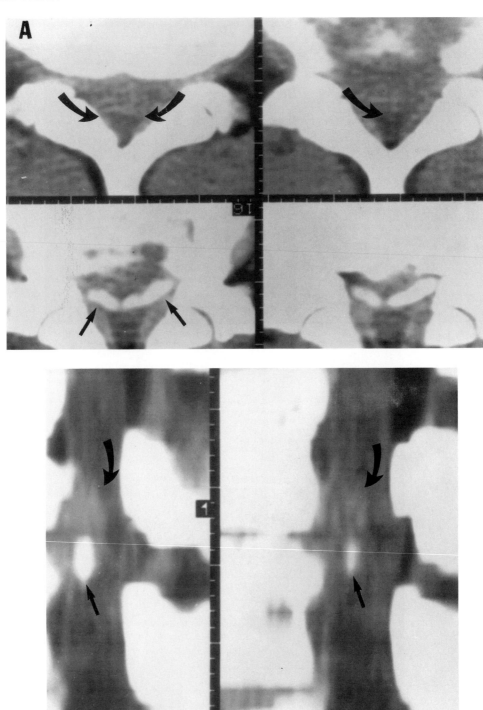

FIG. 47. Posttraumatic lumbar disc herniation: CT/MPR. After a fall, this 25-year-old patient developed acute bilateral leg pain. The axial (**A**) and sagittal (**B**) images demonstrate a large posterior disc herniation causing severe narrowing of the central spinal canal. In addition to the disc material (*curved black arrows*), the posterosuperior rim of the L5 vertebral body (*straight black arrows*) has been displaced posteriorly into the central spinal canal.

(13,86). Posttraumatic pseudomeningoceles have been reported at the thoracolumbar junction following a traumatic episode (102), and CT-myelography will help define the point of communication between the pseudomeningocele and the thecal sac.

The main advantage of CT/MPR in the evaluation of the thoracolumbar junction is in the delineation of vertebral morphology and alignment. Facet subluxations or dislocations are particularly difficult to assess in the axial plane, but with the benefit of sagittal and coronal reconstructed images, the nature of the deformity is clarified.

Lumbar Spine and Sacrum

In the lumbar spine, CT/MPR provides excellent delineation of posttraumatic vertebral deformities (Fig. 46). Posttraumatic spondylolysis and spondylolisthesis are optimally demonstrated on a CT/MPR study (97). After spinal instrumentation, CT is still the best modality in evaluating vertebral deformities or posttraumatic degenerative changes.

Traumatic disc herniations in the adolescent and young adult population may be associated with displacement of the posterior vertebral body rim into the spinal canal (18,108). The combination of disc material and bone in the spinal canal may cause marked compression of the thecal sac. With CT's excellent delineation of osseous material, it provides the optimal delineation of this traumatic deformity (Fig. 47).

The main strength of CT and CT/MPR in the evaluation of spinal trauma resides in its excellent delineation of osseous structures. Multiplanar imaging provides the optimal evaluation of spinal fractures and malalignment. MRI is now the examination of choice when evaluating the spinal cord, thecal sac, spinal ligaments, and paravertebral soft tissues.

Posttraumatic deformities of the sacrum may be extremely difficult to evaluate on routine radiographs. The undulating contour of the cortical surface, complex orientation of the sacroiliac joints, and the overlying pelvic contents frequently necessitate a CT evaluation in cases of spinal trauma to evaluate fractures and joint diastasis. The patient who has sustained major pelvic trauma may be in a body cast, which will seriously degrade routine radiographs, but which creates no problem with CT imaging. The CT evaluation of the sacrum uses 5-mm thick sections without angulation of the gantry. Each section is evaluated employing both soft tissue and bone windows. In elderly patients, stress fractures involving the sacral trabeculae are also optimally evaluated on a CT study.

MRI and CT/MPR are excellent in delineating disc herniations that occur with relative frequency in the cervical spine and occasionally in the lumbar spine in patients with acute spinal trauma.

FUTURE DEVELOPMENTS

Computers able to read CT and MRI information are currently in use in neurosurgical and ENT operating rooms. These computers, when coupled with a mechanical or light sensor system, can directly correlate the patient's anatomy with the radiographic data stored in the computer. Thus, the radiographic data obtained prior to the surgical procedure are used to guide the above-mentioned surgeries. In neurosurgery, it is proving to be very helpful because it provides a more accurate definition of the boundary between normal and pathological tissue. In ENT surgery, it is primarily used during endoscopic sinus surgeries where this instrumentation helps the surgeon identify the boundaries of the paranasal sinuses.

A small number of centers in the United States are currently using image guidance to orient the placement of spinal hardware. The orientation of pedicular screws can be guided with great accuracy. Image guidance also helps avoid many of the possible complications inherent to this procedure. With the development of improved registration methods, this technology may also be applicable in percutaneous discectomies. In this case, again, the instrumentation would help avoid complications.

SUMMARY

High-resolution CT of the lumbar spine led to a dramatic expansion of the understanding and knowledge of the normal and pathological anatomy of the lumbar spine. MRI adds considerably to this body of information and provides a clarity of soft-tissue resolution and certainty of diagnosis of disc disease and lateral stenosis. High-resolution CT is the diagnostic procedure of choice in the initial evaluation of patients with low back pain and sciatica. However, MRI is an invaluable diagnostic adjunct to CT in the study of the lumbar spine. It is used when high-resolution CT has not provided a clear diagnosis or there is a conflict between the CT findings and the clinical symptoms. MRI has proved most useful in the differentiation of soft-tissue abnormalities, such as spinal neoplasm, infection, and hematoma. MRI is the procedure of choice in differentiating recurrent herniation from fibrosis in the study of complicated disease in postoperative patients. It has proved very useful in the evaluation of the postoperative patient with recurrent sciatica and lateral nerve root entrapment, and in differentiating among recurrent disc herniation from conjoined nerve root, fibrosis, edematous ganglia, and inflammatory tissue.

The most common cause of FBSS has been the lack of adequate information before the first surgical procedure. High-resolution CT and MRI provide an accurate means of preoperatively assessing both the bony and soft-tissue disease of the spine. High-resolution CT and MRI allow the direct visualization of not only the pathological processes affecting the spine but also of the direct effect these lesions may have on the nerve roots and thecal sac. Together, they provide very clear images of the bony spinal canal and intervertebral nerve root canal as well as the soft tissues occupying those spaces. They can also identify herniated and sequestered discs; differentiate the various causes of FBSS (recurrent disc, fibrosis, stenosis, fusion overgrowth, and arachnoiditis); and define nerve root entrapment more accurately than previous imaging modalities used in the study of spine disease. Our experience has shown that 3D CT is the optimal choice not only for displaying spinal pathology but also for tracking a therapeutic course. We examined 100 consecutive patients with FBSS with and without fusion, evaluating them with direct CT, two-dimensional multiplanar imaging, and 3D imaging (122). The 3D images best displayed the surgical procedure and its extent, lateral neural foraminal narrowing, and fractures of the posterior elements.

The use of high-resolution CT and subsequently MRI with its improved soft-tissue imaging capabilities leads to increasingly accurate preoperative interpretation and diagnosis. MRI software improvements promise even more sophisticated and accurate evaluation of the spine in the near future.

There are many causes of spinal pathology, each with its unique radiographic appearance. An understanding of each of these processes will enable the radiologist to more clearly guide and focus the differential diagnosis and probable treatment of these patients. Three-dimensional CT of the spine offers the best choice for often complex pathology, and it is an integral component in the development of a comprehensive treatment plan aimed at restoring function and eliminating pain for the thousands of patients who suffer from spinal pathology.

REFERENCES

1. Alvarez O, Roque CT, Pampati M (1988): Multilevel thoracic disk herniations: CT and MR studies. *J Comput Assist Tomogr* 12:649–652.
2. Arce CA, Dohrmann GJ (1985): Thoracic disc herniation. Improved diagnosis with computed tomographic scanning and review of the literature. *Surg Neurol* 23:356–361.
3. Beers GJ, Raque GH, Wagner GG, Shields CB, Nichols GR II, Johnson JR, Meyer JE (1988): MR imaging in acute cervical spine trauma. *J Comput Assist Tomogr* 12:755–761.
4. Beres J, Pech P, Berns TF, Daniels DL, Williams AL, Haughton VM (1986): Spinal epidural lymphomas: CT features in seven patients. *AJNR* 7:327–328.
5. Bidwell JK, Young JW, Khalluff E (1987): Giant cell tumor of the spine: computed tomography appearance and review of the literature. *J Comput Assist Tomogr* 11:307–311.
6. Brant-Zawadzki M, Donovan-Post MJ (1983): Trauma. In: Newton TH, Potts DG, eds. *Computed tomography of the spine and spinal cord.* San Anselmo: Clavadel Press, pp. 149–186.
7. Brant-Zawadzki M, Jeffrey RB Jr, Minagi H, Pitts LH (1982): High resolution CT of thoracolumbar fractures. *AJR* 138:699–704.
8. Brodsky AE (1976): Post-laminectomy and post-fusion stenosis of the lumbar spine. *Clin Orthop* 115:130–139.
9. Bundschuh C, Modic MT, Kearney F, Morris R, Deal C (1988): Rheumatoid arthritis of the cervical spine: surface-coil MR imaging. *AJR* 151:181–187.
10. Bundschuh CV, Modic MT, Ross JS, Masaryk TJ, Bohiman H (1988): Epidural fibrosis and recurrent disk herniation in the lumbar spine: MR imaging assessment. *AJR* 150:923–932.
11. Burke DR, Brant-Zawadzki M (1985): CT of pyogenic spine infection. *Neuroradiology* 27:131–137.
12. Burton CV, Kirkaldy-Willis WH, Yong-Hing K, Heithoff KB (1981): Causes of failure of surgery on the lumbar spine. *Clin Orthop* 157:191–199.
13. Cammisa FP Jr, Eismont FJ, Green BA (1989): Dural laceration occurring with burst fractures and associated laminar fractures. *J Bone Joint Surg [Am]* 71:1044–1052.
14. Chafetz N, Cann CE, Morris JM, Steinbach LS, Goldberg HI, Ax L (1987): Pseudarthrosis following lumbar fusion: detection by direct coronal CT scanning. *Radiology* 162:803–805.
15. Coin CG (1984): Cervical disk degeneration and herniation: diagnosis by computerized tomography. *South Med J* 77:979–982.
16. Coin CG, Coin JT (1981): Computed tomography of cervical disk disease: technical considerations with representative case reports. *J Comput Assist Tomogr* 5:275–280.
17. DeSantis M, Crisi G, Folchi Vici F (1984): Late contrast enhancement in the CT diagnosis of herniated lumbar disk. *Neuroradiology* 26:303–307.
18. Dietemann JL, Runge M, Badoz A, Dosch JC, Beaujeux R, Bonneville JF, Wackenheim A (1988): Radiology of posterior lumbar apophyseal ring fractures: report of 13 cases. *Neuroradiology* 30:337–344.
19. Dillin WH, Watkins RG (1989): Cervical myelopathy and cervical radiculopathy. *Semin Spine Surg* 1:200–208.
20. Doubilet PM, Seltzer SE, Hessel SJ (1984): Computed tomography in the diagnosis and management of paravertebral masses. *Comput Radiol* 8:101–106.
21. Eismont FJ, Clifford S, Goldberg M, Green B (1984): Cervical sagittal spinal canal size in spine injury. *Spine* 9:663–666.
22. Emery SE, Pathria MN, Wilber RG, Masaryk T, Bohlman HN (1989): Magnetic resonance imaging of posttraumatic spinal ligament injury. *J Spinal Disord* 2:229–233.
23. Epstein JA, Epstein BS, Lavine LS, Carras R, Rosenthal AD, Sumner P (1973): Lumbar nerve root compression at the intervertebral foramina caused by arthritis of the posterior facets. *J Neurosurg* 39:362–369.
24. Eubanks BA, Cann CE, Brant-Zawadzki M (1985): CT measurement of the diameter of spinal and other bony canals: effects of section angle and thickness. *Radiology* 157:243–246.
25. Firooznia H, Benjamin V, Kricheff II, Rafi M, Golimbu C (1984): CT of lumbar spine disk herniation: correlation with surgical findings. *AJR* 142:587–592.
26. Firooznia H, Golimbu C, Rafi M, Reede DL, Kricheff II, Bjorkengren A (1986): Computed tomography of spinal chordomas. *J Comput Assist Tomogr* 10:45–50.
27. Foley MJ, Calenoff L, Hendrix RW, Schafer MF (1983): Thoracic and lumbar spine fusion: postoperative radiologic evaluation. *AJR* 141:373–380.
28. Fon GT, Sage MR (1984): Computed tomography in cervical disc disease when myelography is unsatisfactory. *Clin Radiol* 35:47–50.
29. Fries JW, Abodeely DA, Vijungco JG, Gaffey WR (1984): Lateral L3-4 herniated nucleus pulposus: clinical and imaging considerations. *Comput Radiol* 8:341–354.
30. Frocrain L, Duvauferrier R, deKorvin B, Ramee A, Pawlotsky Y (1988): Comparison of MRI and scanning coupled with myelography in the diagnosis of cervicobrachial neuralgia. *J Radiol* 69:99–102.
31. Frocrain L, Duvauferrier R, Husson JL, Noel J, Ramee A, Pawlotsky Y (1989): Recurrent postoperative sciatica: evaluation with MR imaging and enhanced CT. *Radiology* 170:531–533.
32. Gamba JL, Martinez S, Apple J, Harrelson JM, Nunley JA (1984): Computed tomography of axial skeletal osteoid osteomas. *AJR* 142:769–772.
33. Garfinkle W, Yudd AP (1982): Calcified intraspinal meningioma detected by computed tomography. *Comput Radiol* 6:305–307.

34. Gebarski SS, Maynard FW, Gabrielsen TO, Knake JE, Latack JT, Hoff JT (1985): Posttraumatic progressive myelopathy. *Radiology* 157:379–385.
35. Gellad FE, Levine AM, Joslyn JN, Edwards CC, Bosse M (1986): Pure thoracolumbar facet dislocation: clinical features and CT appearance. *Radiology* 161:505–508.
36. Gertzbein SD, Court-Brown CM (1989): Rationale for the management of flexion–distraction injuries of the thoracolumbar spine based on a new classification. *J Spinal Disord* 2:176–183.
37. Glenn WV Jr, Rhodes ML, Altschuler EM, Wiltse LL, Kostanek C, Kuo YM (1979): Multiplanar display computerized body tomography applications in the lumbar spine. *Spine* 4:282–352.
38. Glenn WV Jr, Rothman SLG, Rhodes ML, Kerber CW (1984): An overview of lumbar computed tomography/multiplanar reformations: What are its elements and how do they fit together? In: Donovan-Post MJ, ed. *Computed tomography of the spine.* Baltimore: Williams and Wilkins, pp. 135–154.
39. Godersky JC, Erickson DL, Sseljeskog EL (1984): Extreme lateral disc herniation: diagnosis by computed tomographic scanning. *Neurosurgery* 14:549–552.
40. Golimbu C, Firooznia H, Rafi M (1984): CT of osteomyelitis of the spine. *AJR* 142:159–163.
41. Golimbu C, Firooznia H, Rafi M, Engler G, Delman A (1984): Computed tomography of thoracic and lumbar spine fractures that have been treated with Harrington instrumentation. *Radiology* 151:731–733.
42. Greenough CG, Dimmock S, Edwards D, Ransford AO, Bentley G (1986): The role of computerized tomography in intervertebral disc prolapse. *J Bone Joint Surg [Br]* 68:729–733.
43. Guinto FC Jr, Hashim H, Stumer M (1984): CT demonstration of disk regression after conservative therapy. *AJNR* 5:632–633.
44. Halversen GL, Thoen DD, Satovick RM, Goldstein ML (1986): Value of high-resolution computed tomography in evaluating cervical herniated disks. *J Radiol* 67:423–429.
45. Harbin WP (1982): Metastatic disease and the nonspecific bone scan: value of spinal computed tomography. *Radiology* 145:105–107.
46. Hashimoto T, Kaneda K, Abumi K (1988): Relationship between traumatic spinal canal stenosis and neurologic deficits in thoracolumbar burst fractures. *Spine* 13:1268–1272.
47. Haykal HA, Wang AM, Zamani AA, Rumbaugh CL (1984): Computed tomography of spontaneous acute cervical epidural hematoma. *J Comput Assist Tomogr* 8:229–231.
48. Herman GT (1988): Three-dimensional imaging on a CT or MR scanner. *J Comput Assist Tomogr* 12:450–458.
49. Hermann G (1985): Role of x-ray computed tomography in infectious spondylodiscitis. A review article. *J Radiol* 66:13–20.
50. Hirofuji E, Tanaka S (1983): Computed tomography of lumbar disc herniation. *Spine* 8:300–304.
51. Hoeffken W, Traupe H, Heiss WD (1980): CT-visualization of an intraspinal osteoma-like mass in Paget's disease. *Neurosurg Rev* 3:179–182.
52. Holms CA, Genant HK (1982): Computed tomography in the early detection of skeletal involvement with multiple myeloma. *JAMA* 248:2886–2887.
53. Hueftle MG, Modic MT, Ross JS, Masaryk TJ, Carter JR, Wilber RG, Bohlman HH, Steinberg PM, Delamarter RB (1988): Lumbar spine: postoperative MR imaging with gadolinium-DTPA. *Radiology* 167:817–824.
54. Johnsson KE, Willner S, Johnsson K (1986): Post-operative instability after decompression for lumbar spinal stenosis. *Spine* 11:107–110.
55. Kaiser MC, Capesius P, Ohanna F, Roilgen A (1984): Computed tomography of acute spinal epidural hematoma associated with cervical root avulsion. *J Comput Assist Tomogr* 8:322–323.
56. Katsumi Y, Honma T, Nakamura T (1989): Analysis of cervical instability resulting from laminectomies for removal of spinal cord tumor. *Spine* 14:1171–1176.
57. Kattapuram SV, Phillips WC, Boyd R (1983): CT in pyogenic osteomyelitis of the spine. *AJR* 140:1199–1201.
58. Keene JS, Fischer SP, Vanderby R Jr, Drummond DS, Turski PA (1989): Significance of acute posttraumatic bony encroachment of the neural canal. *Spine* 14:799–802.
59. Kopecky KK, Gilmor RL, Scott JA, Edwards MK (1985): Pitfalls of computed tomography in diagnosis of discitis. *Neuroradiology* 27:57–66.
60. Kornberg M, Rechtine GR, Dupuy TE (1984): Computed tomography in the diagnosis of a herniated disk at the L5-S1 level. *Spine* 9:433–436.
61. Krol G, Sundaresan N, Deck M (1983): Computed tomography of axial chordomas. *J Comput Assist Tomogr* 7:286–289.
62. Kulkarni MV, McArdle CB, Kopanicky D, Minerr M, Cotler HB, Lee KF, Harris JH (1987): Acute spinal cord injury: MR imaging at 1.5 T. *Radiology* 164:837–843.
63. Laasonen EM, Soini J (1989): Low-back pain after lumbar fusion. *Spine* 14:210–213.
64. LaBerge JM, Brant-Zawadzki M (1984): Evaluation of Pott's disease with computed tomography. *Neuroradiology* 26:429–434.
65. Lancourt JE, Glenn WV Jr, Wiltse LL (1979): Multiplanar computerized tomography in the normal spine and in the diagnosis of spinal stenosis: a gross anatomic-computerized tomographic correlation. *Spine* 4:379–390.
66. Landman JA, Hoffman JC Jr, Braun IF, Barrow DL (1984): Value of computed tomographic myelography in the recognition of cervical herniated disk. *AJNR* 5:391–394.
67. Lapointe JS, Graeb DA, Nugent RA, Robertson WD (1986): Value of intravenous contrast enhancement in the CT evaluation of intraspinal tumors. *AJR* 146:103–107.
68. Lee CK (1983): Lumbar spinal instability (olisthesis) after extensive posterior spinal decompression. *Spine* 8:429–433.
69. Lee CK (1988): Accelerated degeneration of the segment adjacent to a lumbar fusion. *Spine* 13:375–377.
70. Levitan LH, Wiens CW (1983): Chronic lumbar extradural hematoma: CT findings. *Radiology* 148:707–708.
71. Matsuura P, Waters RL, Adkins RH, Rothman S, Gurbani N, Sie I (1989): Comparison of computerized tomography parameters of the cervical spine in normal control subjects and spinal cord-injured patients. *J Bone Joint Surg [Am]* 71:183–188.
72. Mayer PJ, Jacobsen FS (1989): Cauda equina syndrome after surgical treatment of lumbar spinal stenosis with application of free autogenous fat graft. *J Bone Joint Surg [Am]* 71:1090–1093.
73. McAfee PC, Yuan HA (1982): Computed tomography in spondylolisthesis. *Clin Orthop* 166:62–71.
74. McAfee PC, Yuan HA, Fredrickson BE, Lubicky JP (1983): The value of computed tomography in thoracolumbar fractures: an analysis of one hundred consecutive cases and a new classification. *J Bone Joint Surg [Am]* 65:461–473.
75. Merine D, Fishman EK, Magid D (1988): CT detection of sacral osteomyelitis associated with pelvic abscesses. *J Comput Assist Tomogr* 12:118–121.
76. Meyer JE, Lepke RA, Lindfors KK, Pagani JJ, Hirschy JC, Hayman LA, Momose KJ, McGinnis B (1984): Chordomas: their CT appearance in the cervical, thoracic, and lumbar spine. *Radiology* 153:693–696.
77. Mikhael MA (1983): High resolution computed tomography in the diagnosis of laterally herniated lumbar discs. *Comput Radiol* 7:161–166.
78. Mirvis SE, Geisler FH, Jelinek JJ, Joslyn JN, Gellad F (1988): Acute cervical spine trauma: evaluation with 1.5 T MR imaging. *Radiology* 166:807–816.
79. Morris RE, Hasso AN, Thompson JR, Hinshaw DB Jr, Vu LM (1984): Traumatic dural tears: CT diagnosis using metrizamide. *Radiology* 152:443–446.
80. Naksgawa H, Okumura T, Sugiyama T, Iwata K (1983): Discrepancy between metrizamide CT and myelography in diagnosis of cervical disk protrusions. *AJNR* 4:604–606.
81. O'Callaghan JP, Ullrich CG, Yuan HA, Kieffer SA (1980): CT of facet distraction in flexion injuries of the thoracolumbar spine: the "naked" facet. *AJR* 134:563–568.
82. Osborne DR, Heinz ER, Bullard D. Friedman A (1984): Role of computed tomography in the radiological evaluation of painful radiculopathy after negative myelography: foraminal neural entrapment. *Neurosurgery* 14:147–153.
83. Patronas NJ, Jafar J, Brown F (1981): Pseudomeningoceles diagnosed by metrizamide myelography and computerized tomography. *Surg Neurol* 16:188–191.
84. Pech P, Kilgore DP, Pojunas KW, Haughton VM (1985): Cervical spinal fractures: CT detection. *Radiology* 157:117–120.
85. Peyster RG, Teplick JG, Haskin ME (1985): Computed tomog-

raphy of lumbosacral conjoined nerve root anomalies. Potential cause of false-positive reading for herniated nucleus pulposus. *Spine* 10:331–337.

86. Pickett J, Blumenkopf B (1988): Dural lacerations and thoracolumbar fractures. *J Spinal Disord* 2:99–103.

87. Post MJ, Quencer RM, Montalvo BM, Katz BH, Eismont F, Green BA (1988): Spinal infection: evaluation with MR imaging and intraoperative US. *Radiology* 169:765–771.

88. Post MJ, Seminer DS, Quencer RM (1982): CT diagnosis of spinal epidural hematoma. *AJNR* 3:190–192.

89. Prusick VR, Lint DS, Bruder WJ (1988): Cauda equina syndrome as a complication of free epidural fat-grafting. *J Bone Joint Surg* [Am] 70:1256–1258.

90. Quencer RM, Sheldon JJ, Post MJ, Diaz RD, Montalvo BM, Green BA, Eismont FJ (1986): MRI of the chronically injured cervical spinal cord. *AJR* 147:125–132.

91. Quequet PM, Rosa A. Mizon JP (1987): Non-traumatic spinal epidural hematomas (2 cases): contribution of the CT scanner. *Rev Neurol* [Paris] 143:143–146.

92. Rauschning W (1987): Normal and pathologic anatomy of the lumbar root canals. *Spine* 12:1008–1019.

93. Roddy SC, Vijayamohan G, Rao GR (1984): Delayed CT myelography in spinal intramedullary metastasis. *J Comput Assist Tomogr* 8:1182–1185.

94. Rosenberg D, Baskies AM, Deckers PJ, Leiter BE, Ordia JI, Yablon IG (1984): Pyogenic sacroiliitis. An absolute indication for computerized tomographic scanning. *Clin Orthop* 184:128–132.

95. Ross JS, Masaryk TJ, Modic MT, Bohlman H, Delamarter R, Wilber G (1987): Postoperative cervical spine. MR assessment. *J Comput Assist Tomogr* 11:955–962.

96. Ross JS, Masaryk TJ, Modic MT, Delamarter R, Bohlman H, Wilbur G, Kaufman B (1987): MR imaging of lumbar arachnoiditis. *AJR* 149:1025–1032.

97. Rothman SL, Glenn WV Jr (1984): CT multiplanar reconstruction in 253 cases of lumbar spondylolysis. *AJNR* 5:81–90.

98. Rothman SL, Glenn WV Jr (1985): CT evaluation of interbody fusion. *Clin Orthop* 193:47–56.

99. Rothman SL, Glenn WV Jr (1985): The postoperative spine. In: Rothman SLG, Glenn WV Jr, eds. *Multiplanar CT of the spine.* Baltimore: University Park Press, pp. 255–292.

100. Rothman SL, Glenn WV Jr, Kerber CW (1985): Postoperative fractures of lumbar articular facets: occult cause of radiculopathy. *AJR* 145:779–784.

101. Russell EJ, D'Angelo CM, Zimmerman RD, Czervionke LF, Huckman MS (1984): Cervical disk herniation: CT demonstration after contrast enhancement. *Radiology* 152:703–712.

102. Sachdev VP, Huang YP, Shah CP Malis LI (1981): Posttraumatic pseudomeningomyelocele (enlarging fracture?) in a vertebral body: case report. *J Neurosurg* 54:545–549.

103. Schaefer DM, Flanders A, Northrup BE, Doan HT, Osterholm JL (1989): Magnetic resonance imaging of acute cervical spine trauma: correlation with severity of neurologic injury. *Spine* 14:1090–1095.

104. Scotti G, Scialfa G, Pieralli S, Boccardi E, Valsecchi F, Tonon C

(1983): Myelopathy and radiculopathy due to cervical spondylosis: myelographic-CT correlations. *AJNR* 4:601–603.

105. Sobel DF, Barkovich AJ, Munderloh SH (1984): Metrizamide myelography and postmyelographic computed tomography: comparative adequacy in the cervical spine. *AJNR* 5:385–390.

106. Stanley JH, Schabel SI, Frey GD, Hungerford GD (1986): Quantitative analysis of the cervical spinal canal by computed tomography. *Neuroradiology* 28:139–143.

107. Stollman A, Pinto R, Benjamin V, Kricheff I (1987): Radiologic imaging of symptomatic ligamentum flavum thickening with and without ossification. *AJNR* 8:991–994.

108. Takata K, Inoue S, Takahashi K, Ohtsuka Y (1988): Fracture of the posterior margin of a lumbar vertebral body. *J Bone Joint Surg* [Am] 70:589–594.

109. Teplick JG, Haskin ME (1983): Review. Computed tomography of the postoperative lumbar spine. *AJR* 141:865–884.

110. Teplick JG, Laffey PA, Berman A, Haskin ME (1986): Diagnosis and evaluation of spondylolisthesis and/or spondylolysis on axial CT. *AJNR* 7:479–491.

111. Tracy PT, Wright RM, Hanigan WC (1989): Magnetic resonance imaging of spinal injury. *Spine* 14:292–301.

112. Ullrich CG (1989): Three-dimensional CT of the cervical spine: introduction and clinical applications. In: TCSRSE Committee, eds. *The cervical spine.* Philadelphia: JB Lippincott, pp. 150–156.

113. Volle E, Kern A, Stoltenberg G, Claussen C (1988): CT reconstruction technique in lumbar intraneuroforaminal disc herniation. *Neuroradiology* 30:138–144.

114. Wang AM, Lipson SJ, Haykal HA, Weinberg DS, Zamani AA, Rumbaugh CL (1984): Computed tomography of aneurysmal bone cyst of the L1 vertebral body. *J Comput Assist Tomogr* 8:1186–1189.

115. White JG III, Strait TA, Binkley JR, Hunter SE (1982): Surgical treatment of 63 cases of conjoined nerve root. *J Neurosurg* 56:114–117.

116. White RR, Newberg A, Seligson D (1980): Computerized tomographic assessment of the traumatized dorsolumbar spine before and after Harrington instrumentation. *Clin Orthop* 146:150–156.

117. Wiesel SW, Tsourmas N, Feffer HL, Citrin CM, Patronas N (1984): A study of computer-assisted tomography. 1. The incidence of positive CAT scans in an asymptomatic group of patients. *Spine* 9:549–551.

118. Williams AL, Haughton VM, Daniels DL, Grogan JP (1983): Differential CT diagnosis of extruded nucleus pulposus. *Radiology* 148:141–148.

119. Williams AL, Haughton VM, Syvertsen A (1980): Computed tomography in the diagnosis of herniated nucleus pulposus. *Radiology* 135:95–99.

120. Wing VW, Jeffrey RB Jr, Federle MP, Helms CA, Trafton P (1985): Chronic osteomyelitis examined by CT. *Radiology* 154:171–174.

121. Zilkha A, Irwin GA, Fagelman D (1983): Computed tomography of spinal epidural hematoma. *AJNR* 4:1073–1076.

122. Zinreich SJ, Long DM, Davis R, Quinn CB, McAfee PC, Wang H. Three-dimensional CT imaging in postsurgical "failed back" syndrome. *J Comput Assist Tomogr* 14:574–580.

The Adult Spine: Principles and Practice,
2nd edition, J.W. Frymoyer, Editor-in-Chief.
Lippincott-Raven Publishers, Philadelphia © 1997.

CHAPTER 28

Diagnostic Disc Injection

I. Cervical Disc Injection

Charles Neuville Aprill III

Read not to contradict and confute, nor to believe and take for granted, nor to find talk and to discourse but to weigh and consider.
—FRANCIS BACON (2)

The use of direct puncture to study the intervertebral discs as a diagnostic procedure began over 40 years ago. In Scandinavia, Carl Hirsch (37) and Knut Lindblom (52) published studies describing techniques for lumbar disc puncture to localize symptomatic discs in patients with chronic low back pain. In the United States, techniques for study of the cervical discs were developed by George Smith (82) and Ralph Cloward (14). In the years following these initial reports, a dramatic polarization of opinion about discography developed. Diametrically opposed opinions as to the usefulness of these procedures are summed up in two papers published in 1968 (40,93).

The ensuing two decades witnessed major advances in imaging methods to evaluate the intervertebral discs. The development and deployment of minimally toxic contrast agents and improvements in techniques made myelography a much safer diagnostic procedure (89). Combining myelography, particularly when performed as a functional study, with postmyelographic computed tomographic (CT) scanning improves understanding of both modalities. Wilmink has shown that these proce-

dures provide supplementary information (95). Magnetic resonance imaging (MRI) and CT scanning have been recognized as primary modalities for investigating mass lesions (prolapse, extrusion, and sequestration) (42) as well as degenerative disease of the intervertebral disc (16). These modalities are the proper first tests to be employed in the study of cervical and lumbar discs. They provide accurate noninvasive assessment of anatomy and pathoanatomy. Disc injection has a role in the evaluation of patients with severe neck or back pain. Opinions and philosophies regarding discography reached the editorial stage by 1994 (59,62). Subspecialty societies joined the controversy, some taking positions of support (32). Others open the subject to scholarly debate (11).

HISTORY

In order to evaluate patients with chronic neck, shoulder girdle, and headache pain, Smith and Nichols developed a procedure for direct injection of the cervical discs in the early 1950s (82). Cloward reported a similar technique almost simultaneously (14). These investigators worked without knowledge of one another's researches (19). Both authors published additional papers (16,80) reporting indications. They pointed out that injection of an abnormal and symptomatic disc could reproduce the clinical symptoms. Both noted a high incidence of

C. N. Aprill III, M.D.: Spine Radiologist, Diagnostic Conservative Management, Inc., New Orleans, Louisiana 70115.

abnormal-appearing discs. The incidence of such degenerate discs seems related to patient age. Both considered the pain response on injection more important than the radiographic appearance of the disc. Cloward felt that the procedure was of specific value in differentiating discogenic from neurogenic pain (17). Both noted that normal discs accepted small volumes (0.1 to 0.3 cc), and the injection of such discs was not particularly painful.

Smith and Nichols, and Cloward developed surgical techniques for disc excision and fusion employing an anterior approach. Cervical disc injection (discography) was the diagnostic procedure employed in selecting the proper level for the surgical procedure (15,83).

In the following decade, a number of authors published reports questioning the value of cervical discography as a diagnostic technique (57,84,86).

The report of Earl Holt is often cited and warrants scrutiny (39). Holt studied asymptomatic volunteers. The subjects were 50 men selected from 200 who promptly volunteered when given an opportunity to participate in his experiment. All were inmates of the Missouri State Penitentiary. Cervical discography was performed by Holt in the radiology department of the penitentiary hospital. Fluoroscopy was not employed. In three instances, he reports two needles were introduced into the same disc space. In an additional two instances, he reports it was impossible to obtain a satisfactory puncture of a disc space. Injection of sodium diatrizoate (50%) produced great pain in every subject at every disc space. A tuberculin syringe (1.0 cc) was employed to inject through 22-gauge needles. One hundred ninety-eight routes of extravasation from the 148 discs were reported. The only figure in the paper demonstrates what appears to be filling of the cervical uncinate recesses. The patterns described suggest ten normal nucleograms, 126 with filling of the uncinate recesses (normal phenomenon), and ten with anterior leakage. No films demonstrating epidural leakage are presented in the published paper.

Holt concluded that cervical discography is "painful, expensive and without diagnostic value." However, in his final paragraph he states, "Whether or not cervical discography might be made relevant by a radical change in contrast media and techniques of performance is speculative." The purpose of this chapter is in part to address this speculation.

Klafta and Collis (48) evaluated cervical discography performed at the Cleveland Clinic. These authors found only 45 normal discs in 550 disc injections. Pain occurred in 490 of the 550 injections. Despite this incredibly high number of painful injections, these authors concluded that pain on injection was highly indicative of disc abnormality, but not diagnostic of protrusion. A small group of patients were evaluated at surgery by laminectomy and direct inspection of the posterior disc surface. In a subsequent paper, Klafta and Collis (47) specifically addressed the issue of pain response. He

concluded that induced pain, even if similar to presenting symptoms, was of no diagnostic significance. A conclusion that may be drawn from a review of both papers is that the authors considered symptoms to be related to cervical disc disease only when there was a mass effect, specifically a definable protrusion or prolapse.

A number of authors in North America and Europe support the use of cervical disc injection as a diagnostic study (1,5,30,35,46,55,65,74,85). Proponents have stressed the fact that the normal disc accepts a limited volume of solution and that distension does not provoke pain response. Excessive volume with decreased resistance and the presence of a pain response similar to the presenting complaints are indications of an abnormal and symptomatic disc. Recent studies raise questions as to the sensitivity and specificity of pain response in disc injections (13,77). The pattern of contrast dispersal has been recognized as the least important criterion in cervical discography. Gelehrter stressed the importance of the nucleogram (27). Posterior protrusion and free spill into the epidural space are significant radiographic findings.

In 1976, Roth reported on the use of local anesthetics injected into the cervical discs. Using relief of chronic pain as a criterion for selection of symptomatic levels, he reported a very high success rate for anterior disc excision and fusion (72). This analgesic technique was employed by Kofoed in differentiating upper extremity pain of discogenic origin from thoracic outlet syndrome (49). He concluded that analgesic cervical disc puncture was a valuable tool in the differential diagnosis of patients with suspected thoracic outlet syndrome.

NONINVASIVE IMAGING AND DISCOGRAPHY

Prompted by statements that modern myelography would eliminate the necessity for cervical discography, Hartjes et al. evaluated 100 patients by both myelography and cervical discography (34). The myelograms were performed with metrizamide introduced by lateral C1-C2 puncture. The authors concluded that discography was unnecessary in the evaluation of patients with clinical myelopathy. They state that there are two circumstances in which cervical discography is indicated: first, the patient with a specific radiculopathy and normal myelography; second, the patient with specific symptoms and multiple myelographic defects. In this latter instance, the authors felt that discography was important to determine which myelographic defect was related to the subjective symptoms. This comparison study suggested that discography is superfluous when symptoms of monosegmental radiculopathy correlate with a monosegmental myelographic abnormality. However, it has been reported that myelographic deformities correlate poorly with symptoms (26).

The development of postmyelographic CT scanning represents a natural evolution of the diagnostic process. Some clinical studies in the 1980s suggest that CT-myelography is effective and possibly superior to plain film myelography in the assessment of cervical pathology (3,23,60,75). In order to verify these reports, Penning et al. studied 80 patients with CT-myelography, and the significance of findings was assessed by correlation with patients' symptoms. They reported that a specific diagnosis could be made in about 40% of cases (67).

MRI is a technology in evolution. Techniques for reducing artifacts, especially those associated with physiologic motion, are improving spatial resolution. Development of new pulse sequences, particularly those with short acquisition times, improve signal-to-noise ratio. The ability to obtain thinner sections (less than 5.0 mm) cimproves conspicuousness of lesions on axial sections. MRI can be very sensitive to extradural pathology in the cervical region (88).

There is no doubt that the new technologies have provided the diagnostic physician with elegant methods of assessing the anatomic situation (45). But appearances may be deceiving. The images do not tell us whether or not the demonstrated pathoanatomy is symptomatic (Fig. 1). Correlation of symptoms with imaging data may

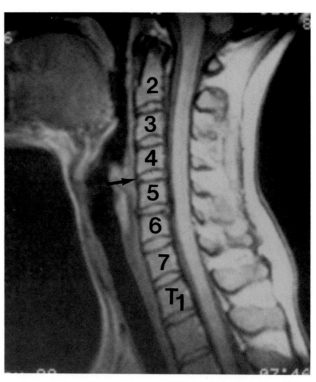

FIG. 2. MRI cervical spine. Mid-sagittal section, 0.6 Tesla, surface coil acquisition. Spin echo T1-weighted image with EKG gating. This is a 26-year-old woman with complaints of chronic neck and headache pain (cervical cephalalgia). There were no objective neurologic findings. The secondary complaint was shoulder girdle pain involving ascending and horizontal portions of trapezius muscles. This study demonstrates posterior prolapse at C5-C6. The appearance of the posterior annulus of the C4-C5 disc (level of *black arrow*) is different from that of the remaining cervical discs. Does this represent posterior annular attenuation? Is this a symptomatic lesion?

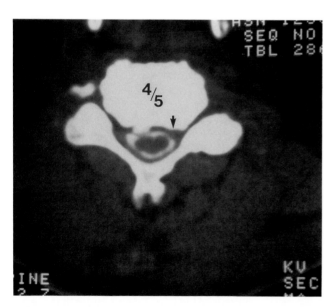

FIG. 1. Axial CT of C4-C5 motion segment. Low dose, intrathecal contrast enhanced, 2.0 mm thick section. Image photographed to provide optimal visualization of intrathecal contrast material. This is a 52-year-old man with obvious right paracentral endplate ridge deforming the thecal sac and abutting the right anterior cord. Clinically, left neck, shoulder girdle, and arm symptoms predominate. Pain and altered sensation suggest a C6 distribution (paresthesias involving thumb and index finger). Note the asymmetry of the thecal sac with blunting of the left dural root pouch *(arrow)*. The findings suggest a soft-tissue mass and possible disc prolapse. This lesion compromises the lateral recess near the origin of the left C6 segmental nerve.

not be sufficiently reliable to unequivocally determine the nature, location, and extent of symptomatic pathology (Fig. 2). A comparison study of cervical MRI and discography suggests a significant correlation between abnormality seen on MRI and pain response on discography. However, the false-positive and false-negative rates of MRI are high. The authors conclude discography is required to diagnose discogenic pain (64). This is particularly true in the patient whose dominant complaints are nonmyelopathic or nonradicular pain.

It is difficult to assess the accuracy of any given diagnostic modality. Surgical outcome studies are not conclusive, but they provide some indication of diagnostic accuracy. Diagnostic disc injection has been utilized to select levels for surgical disc excision and fusion for over two decades. Riley et al., employing cervical disc injection at the time of surgery, used discometry and the presence of epidural leakage as primary diagnostic factors. They report 72% good or excellent clinical results following disc excision and fusion in 93 patients (70). Simmons and Segil relied on pain response to saline distension and less on the discometric and radiographic appearance in the selection of symptomatic levels. These authors also report 72% good or excellent clinical results in 89 patients (79).

More recently, provocation/analgesic discography has been employed in evaluation of patients with chronic neck pain. Whitecloud and Seago carefully selected 40 patients with chronic discogenic symptoms using this technique (92). Patients with cervical spondylosis, radiculopathy, or myelopathy were excluded. Using the same criteria for evaluation of surgical results (63) as did Simmons, Whitecloud and Seago reported 70% good to excellent results with anterior disc excision and fusion. Siebenrock and Aebi reported 73% good or excellent results

in 27 similar patients selected for surgery on the basis of positive discography. Reported results in the literature in similar groups of patients without preoperative discography are less favorable with good or excellent results in the 35% to 46% range (78). Connor and Darden report only 46% good or excellent results in 22 patients following anterior cervical fusion (ACF) on the basis of "positive discography" (20). They also report an exceptionally high complication rate for discography in this series. Of the 31 patients, 13% having discography developed some complication of that procedure. Discography was used by Hubach in the preoperative staging of patients with discopathy and progressive neurologic findings. All levels with positive discography were fused. In this longterm study, good or excellent results approached 82%

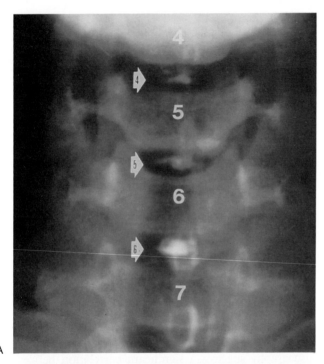

A

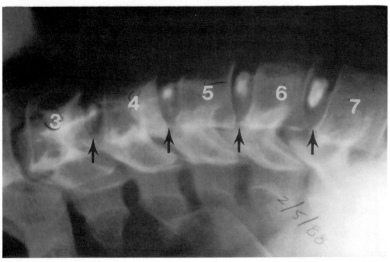

B

FIG. 3. A: Anterior/posterior spot film of the cervical spine following disc injection in a 30-year-old woman. Contrast material (arrows) is confined to the nuclear region of the discs. The nucleus of the C6-C7 disc is larger than the nucleus at other levels in this patient. This is a common phenomenon. The injected volume at each level was less than 0.5 cc. B: Lateral radiograph (horizontal beam) of the same patient. Contrast material is confined to the nuclear region of each disc (arrows). Contrast fills the entire nuclear space of the C5-C6 and C6-C7 discs. At C3-C4 and C4-C5, contrast is located in the anterior nuclear region with only a small volume in the posterior region. This dispersal pattern is not uncommon when saline is instilled into the nucleus for discometry prior to injection of contrast.

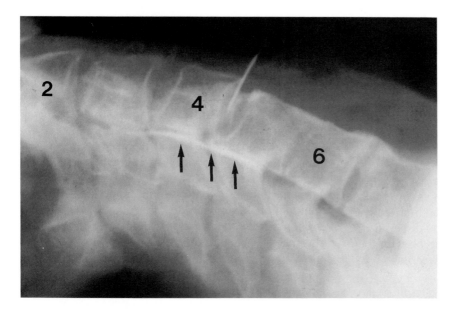

FIG. 4. Lateral radiograph of cervical spine during injection of C4-C5 disc. Contrast material escapes into the anterior epidural space *(arrows)*. This indicates a rent in the posterior annulus. This disc accepted in excess of 2.0 cc of solution (saline, contrast material, and lidocaine 1%) with little resistance. Note prior two-level fusion. There is complete arthrodesis at the C5-C6 interspace. At C6-C7, the appearance suggests that bony arthrodesis is not complete.

(41). These favorable surgical outcomes in a difficult patient population invite a closer look at the procedure of cervical discography.

THE DISCOGRAM

The volume of nucleus in the adult cervical disc has been reasonably well documented. In a cadaver study, Saternus and Bornscheuer found that the volume accepted by 75% of the discs at the C2-C3, C3-C4, and C7-T1 levels was less than 0.5 cc. Fifty percent of the discs at C4-C5, C5-C6, and C6-C7 levels accepted less than 0.5 cc. Those discs in which greater than 0.5 cc could be injected frequently demonstrated leakage from the posterolateral (uncovertebral) portions of the annulus (73).

Pressure/volume measurements have been made during discography at the time of cervical disc surgery (44).

Kambin et al. reported that 33 discs with a normal-appearing nucleus (Fig. 3) accepted 0.2 to 0.4 cc of solution while maintaining sustained high intradiscal pressures. Four discs demonstrated posterior escape of contrast material (Fig. 4). These discs accepted in excess of 1.5 cc of solution. Intradiscal pressures were relatively low and not sustained. The pressure/volume data and radiographic appearance confirmed significant leakage. Sixteen discs with radiographic and/or myelographic evidence of abnormality (degeneration, herniation) accepted 0.5 to 1.5 cc of solution at sustained pressures of an intermediate value. The nucleogram (Fig. 5) revealed some containment of the contrast material.

From these two studies, it may be concluded that the normal nucleus with an intact envelope will be filled by less than 0.5 cc of solution.

The uncovertebral articulations warrant special comment. The lateral and posterolateral portions of the cer-

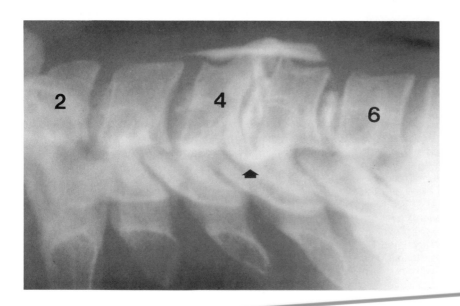

FIG. 5. Lateral radiograph of cervical spine post-disc injection at C4-C5 and C5-C6; normal nucleogram at C5-C6. Note contained posterior protrusion/prolapse at C4-C5 *(arrow)*. Anterior traction ridges are present in association with anterior superior annular fissure. The contrast material in the prevertebral space has escaped from the disc as a result of gross anterior annular degeneration and disruption.

vical disc annulus are relatively attenuated. This thinning of the annulus results in linear clefts that communicate with the nucleus (38,76). These have been called the joints of Luschka. Payne and Spillaine consider them to be "no more than uncovertebral fissures" of the annulus fibrosus (66). The uncovertebral recesses are not found in the human fetus, child, or adolescent. Filling of the uncinate recesses has not been observed in my limited experience with cervical discography in patients under the age of 20.

These clefts or recesses vary considerably in size and configuration and may fill asymmetrically in any given patient (Fig. 6). Opacification of one or both of the recesses is a common finding in adults. The dispersal of fluid into the uncovertebral recesses may account for the posterolateral leakage observed by Saternus and Bornscheuer (73).

This radiographic appearance is not the result of degeneration but reflects maturation of the cervical intervertebral disc. Misunderstanding of the nature and significance of this normal phenomenon will certainly lead to difficulty in interpreting the discographic image. Assuming that this is a pathologic phenomenon leads to the mistaken notion that these discs are degenerate.

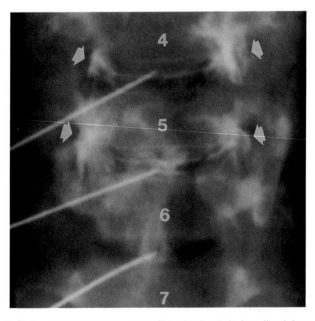

FIG. 6. Anteroposterior spot film obtained during disc injection at C4-C5 and C5-C6. Procedure needle is in place at C6-C7 but no contrast injection has been performed at that level. Lateral extension of contrast material to the right and left *(white arrows)* represents filling of the uncovertebral recesses (von Luschka joints). Note the asymmetry of filling and the irregularity on the left at C4-C5 and bilaterally at C5-C6. This is a normal phenomenon commonly seen in patients over the age of 20. In this instance, disc injection at C5-C6 provoked familiar neck and shoulder girdle pain. The disc accepted 1.2 cc of solution. The disc at C4-C5 accepted less than 1.0 cc of solution and injection was associated with no pain provocation.

PATIENT/PROCEDURE CONSIDERATIONS

The following recommendations are based on my personal performance of over 3,200 cervical disc punctures in over 3,000 patients in the 15-year period from 1979 to 1994.

Cervical disc puncture may be performed in any radiographic suite appropriate for the performance of myelographic studies. One special requirement is a C-arm fluoroscope (Fig. 7). The ability to directly visualize the cervical spine in both the frontal and lateral planes facilitates safe and efficient needle placement and speeds the examination, limiting needle time. Good visualization is essential. Disc puncture should not be performed at any interspace that cannot be adequately seen on a pre-procedural screening lateral fluoroscopic image.

The patient preparation, including pre-procedural screening and diet, is the same as for myelography (see Chapter 31). A detailed discussion of the patient's symptoms, focused physical examination, and an explanation of the procedure, including its risks, are essential.

Disc puncture is often performed at several levels. At best, this procedure is uncomfortable. At worst, it can be very painful. The expertise of the operator is a major factor in patient tolerance of this examination. In my opinion, patients should be sedated for diagnostic cervical disc puncture. Intravenous diazepam has been used as an effective sedative agent (36). Doses of 5.0 to 10.0 mg administered intravenously over 3 to 4 minutes are appropriate. It is important that all other sedative and pain medications be withheld for 4 hours prior to the procedure. Caution is important in that rapid (bolus) injection of diazepam in these doses may result in oversedation and respiratory depression (33). This effect is potentiated in the presence of narcotics or other sedative medications. Since 1985 (69), midazolam (Versed) has been used almost exclusively for over 2,000 invasive procedures. Intravenous doses of 3.5 to 5.0 mg are standard. This sedative is delivered slowly (over 3 minutes, by the clock) and the dose titrated by patient response. In older patients, the dose must be reduced. Often, 2.5 mg will suffice. Significant respiratory depression has not been observed in this series; however, capability for ventilatory support must be immediately available. Whatever pre-medication is chosen for sedation, it must allow the patient to be clearly conversant and responsive yet tolerant of the procedural discomfort (28). Midazolam is effective in this regard and frequently leaves the patient amnesic for events occurring immediately following administration of the drug. This is a beneficial side effect.

The sedative is usually administered with the patient in a supine position on a standard radiographic/fluoroscopic table. Neck extension is delayed until immediately prior to the procedure, as the position can be uncomfortable in patients with spine pathology. The neck is placed in full extension by elevating the upper trunk

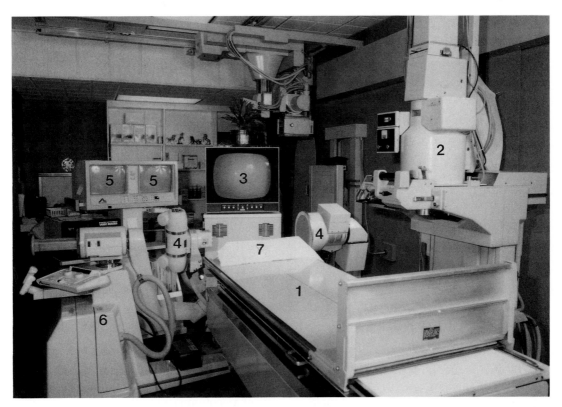

FIG. 7. Spine procedure suite (my outpatient clinic) set up for cervical disc injection. **1:** Standard movable fluoroscopic table. **2:** Image intensifier (vertical) mounted on standard spot film device. **3:** Fluoroscope monitor. **4:** C-arm fluoroscope (tube and image intensifier) set for direct lateral (horizontal) imaging. **5:** C-arm fluoroscope monitor. **6:** Mobile base of C-arm device. **7:** Triangular pillow for neck support during the procedure.

and placing a triangular sponge beneath the shoulders. The head is gently lowered to the table top or a small supporting sponge and the chin extended. A C-arm fluoroscope is positioned at the head of the table such that direct lateral horizontal fluoroscopy of the cervical spine can be performed. Some discographers employ only the C-arm for imaging, rotating it from the horizontal lateral to a frontal position. This technique allows for tilting of the C-arm so that the intervertebral disc spaces can be directly visualized at each level in the frontal plane and facilitates needle placement (51).

In my practice, disc puncture is usually accomplished using the fixed vertical imaging of the standard fluoroscopic system for frontal visualization. The C-arm may then be limited to horizontal imaging. This technique requires less movement of the equipment. The table top can be moved upward into the C-arm fluoroscope for direct lateral visualization (Fig. 8) and back downward for frontal visualization with the second fluoroscope (Fig. 9). All imaging systems must be operational and the patient's position checked to ensure adequate visualization of the spine before any needles are placed.

The skin of the anterior and anterolateral neck from the level of the mandible to the supraclavicular region is prepped in a fashion similar to that employed for mye-

lography. Sterile drapes, preferably with skin adhesive, are applied with their margins overlying the sternomastoid muscles. The drapes will cross in the midline just above the suprasternal notch and will extend alongside the neck. Covering the patient's shoulders is important so that the operator can participate in depressing the shoulders in order to improve visualization of the lower interspaces (C5-C6 through C7-T1) (Fig. 10).

The esophagus lies to the left of the spine at the level of C7 in most individuals, making a right-sided approach to the cervical discs natural. The level to be studied is identified at fluoroscopy. Digital pressure with the index and long finger of one hand is applied to the space between the trachea and medial border of the sternocleidomastoid muscle. Firm but gentle pressure will displace the laryngotracheal structures to the left. The right carotid artery is palpable directly beneath the fingers. The anterior surface of the spine can be palpated in most patients in this position. Pressure sufficient to displace the lateral margin of the larynx to the midline is sufficient.

The needle entry point should be adjacent to the medial border of the sternocleidomastoid but not through the muscle. Using the medial border of the muscle as a landmark, the skin puncture site will be more laterally placed at the C3-C4 level (an optimal position to avoid

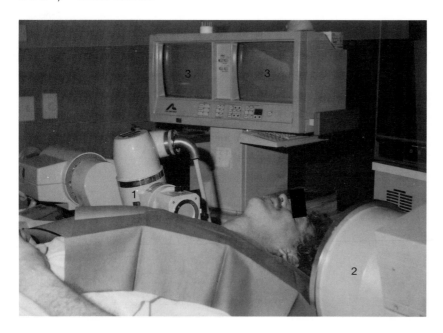

FIG. 8. Patient positioned for direct lateral visualization of the cervical spine with horizontal C-arm fluoroscope. **1:** Fluoroscopy tube. **2:** Image intensifier. **3:** C-arm fluoroscope monitors.

puncture of the hypopharynx) and more medially located at the C7-T1 level (better position to avoid puncture of the apex of the lung). Skin anesthesia is not necessary when 25-gauge needles are used (Fig. 11). Double-

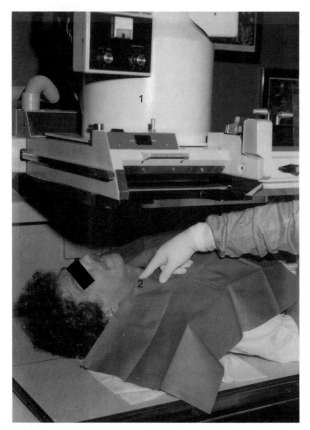

FIG. 9. Patient positioned for direct frontal visualization of cervical spine with standard vertical mounted fluoroscope. **1:** Image intensifier. **2:** Planned puncture site right anterior neck.

needle technique has been suggested (31), but I employ a single-needle technique. The procedure needle is directed obliquely toward the right anterior aspect of the vertebral column (Fig. 12).

It is advisable to direct the needle to the superior aspect of the vertebral body immediately below the disc to be studied. Contact with this bony structure determines the depth of the spine. Slight retraction and cephalad manipulation direct the needle onto the anterolateral surface of the disc annulus. Both maneuvers are uncomfortable as the periosteum of the vertebral body and the annulus itself are innervated. Local anesthetic should not be injected. The discomfort is transient and anesthetic injected in the periannular region may disperse along the course of the cervical sympathetic trunk, possibly altering pain response. The needle is advanced into the disc substance under direct lateral fluoroscopic visualization. All movements of the needle should be slow and deliberate. Documentary images of needle position prior to contrast injection are advisable (Fig. 13).

Standard 3½-inch spinal needles (22 or 25 gauge) are appropriate for cervical disc puncture. Shorter needles may not allow sufficient room for easy attachment and removal of syringes and may be dislodged by swallowing movements occurring during the examination. Larger-bore needles are unnecessarily painful; thinner needles are difficult to control with the precision required. Ideally, use 3.0-cc syringes with 22- and 25-gauge needles. The use of 5.0-cc (or larger) syringes is not recommended. The force required to instill solutions through small needles with large syringes is such that subtle pressure changes may not be appreciated. Use of 1.0-cc (tuberculin) syringes provides an overwhelming hydraulic advantage, making it difficult to detect normal disc resilience. Plastic syringes (Luer-Lok) are preferable to glass,

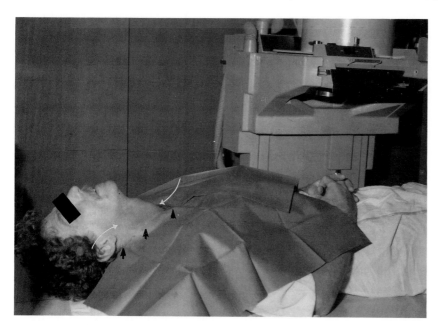

FIG. 10. Patient in position for cervical disc injection. Anterior edge of sterile drape *(black arrows)* is over sternocleidomastoid muscle. Shoulders are covered. Anterior and anterolateral neck has been cleansed and prepped with antiseptic solutions. Site of skin puncture for all disc injections from C2-C3 to C7-T1 will lie between the curved *white arrows*.

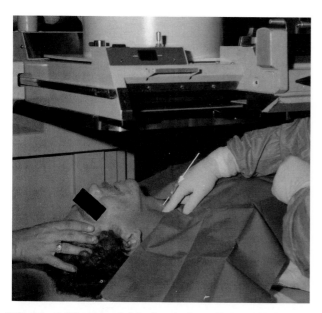

FIG. 11. A 25-gauge 3.5-inch spinal needle has been placed into the C5-C6 disc. The thin needle is highlighted *(white line)*. The needle hub *(white arrow)* is barely visible. The direction of the arrow defines the direction of needle insertion. Note that the needle course is parallel to the operator's right index finger. The assistant is adjusting the position of the patient's head to maintain true anteroposterior alignment.

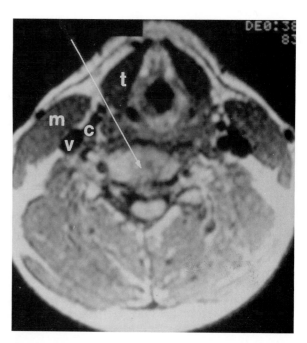

FIG. 12. Axial MRI of C5-C6 disc space. The thyroid (t) and laryngeal structures are displaced to the left. Skin puncture site is just medial to the sternocleidomastoid muscle (m). The carotid artery (c) and jugular vein (v) are displaced posterolaterally. The oblique needle course *(arrow)* traverses the platysma, longus colli muscles, and loose areolar tissues. This course will direct the needle to the center of the disc space. *Note:* This image was selected because of the natural eccentric position of the larynx simulating the displacement produced during performance of the procedure. There is a large central/left paracentral disc prolapse abutting the cervical cord. A lesion of this type does not require cervical disc injection for diagnosis. The image is to provide an example of the anatomic relationships.

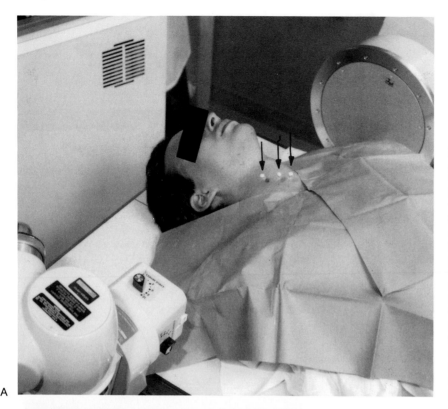

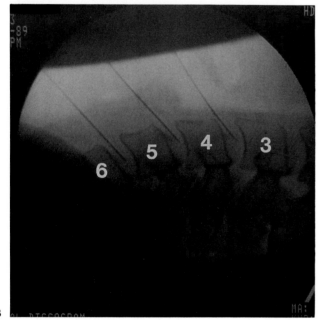

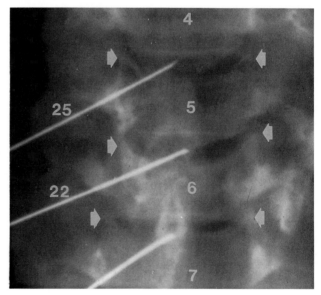

FIG. 13. A: Three 25-gauge needles *(black arrows)* have been placed into the C4-C5, C5-C6, and C6-C7 discs. Patient is in position for direct lateral fluoroscopic visualization of the spine. **B:** Lateral fluoroscopic image obtained at the time of needle placement: 25-gauge needles have been positioned in the center of the C3-C4, C4-C5, and C5-C6 interspaces. **C:** Anteroposterior spot film documents needle position prior to contrast injection. A 25-gauge needle has been used at C4-C5; 22-gauge needles were employed at C5-C6 and C6-C7. The needle tips are in the middle third of the interspaces almost equidistant from the uncinate processes *(arrows).*

as they do not freeze up with contrast material and the control of flow is more precise.

Four labeled 3.0-cc syringes are prepared prior to needle placement. They contain, in the usual order of use, normal saline, lidocaine 1% or 2% (without epinephrine), contrast material (preferably non-ionic aqueous agents), and a long-acting local anesthetic such as bupivacaine at 0.5% mixed with a steroid suspension (Depo-Medol, Celestone).

INJECTION TECHNIQUE

Injection should be performed under direct lateral fluoroscopic visualization (Fig. 14). Contrast material, preferably one of the non-ionic agents (iohexol or iopamidol) is the first agent instilled. Pressure on the syringe is increased slowly until the intrinsic disc pressure is exceeded. Volumes as small as 0.2 cc will cause visible separation of the vertebral bodies or realignment of the

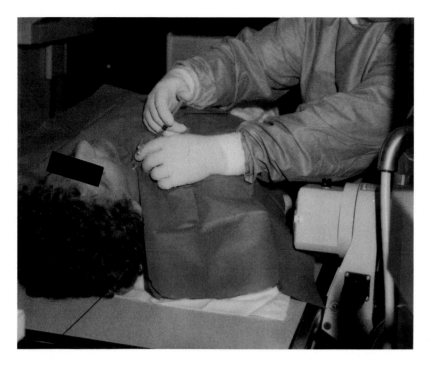

FIG. 14. Cervical disc injection at C6-C7. A 3-cc syringe is held in the right hand. The operator's left hand secures the procedure needle to prevent inadvertent movement of the tip. The operator's head is turned to observe the injection on the C-arm monitor at the initiation of the short injection phase.

slight retrolisthesis, which is common when patients are in the fully extended position. This vertebral movement is readily visible at fluoroscopy. Pain response should be recorded at the time of this distension. The discomfort may be verbalized or characterized by initiation of pain behaviors (e.g., grimaces, muscle contraction) (91). It is important to assess each disc injection response in comparison to injections at other levels in the same patient. All patients respond differently to painful stimuli. Accurate evaluation of the pain response is part of the art rather than the science of medical practice. This pain evaluation is akin to the evaluation of the abdomen in a child with suspected appendicitis. In that instance, the examiner must differentiate rebound tenderness from the simple discomfort of an abdominal exam in an irritable child. It is improved with experience and knowledge, as are most medical skills.

The volume that the disc accepts and the quality of resistance are noted. The normal disc offers firm resistance and accepts less than 0.5 cc of solution with little added discomfort at the time of distension. In the discometrically normal and painless disc, contrast material opacifies the nuclear space. Frontal and lateral radiographs are obtained and the needle removed.

If the injection provokes a pain response, the location, distribution of the pain, and an assessment of its relative intensity should be obtained by direct inquiry (91). It is helpful to enlist a trained assistant in the assessment of pain behaviors. Lidocaine 1% or 2% (0.5 cc) is instilled and usually reduces the induced pain in short order. The instillation of 0.5 cc of a long-acting local anesthetic and steroid suspension into any painful, anatomically abnormal disc is advocated (94).

POSTPROCEDURE CARE

Following uncomplicated cervical disc injection, patients are allowed to recover in an observation area under supervision of a trained nurse observer. An ice pack applied to the right anterior neck at the puncture sites makes patients more comfortable. Patients are offered liquids shortly after the procedure and encouraged to drink. As with any invasive procedure, vital signs are to be recorded both before and immediately after the examination and periodically in the recovery period.

Most patients can be studied on an outpatient basis and may be discharged approximately 2 hours after completion of the study, assuming they have recovered sufficiently from the sedative. Patients must be accompanied by a responsible adult who can drive and report any unusual occurrence. The patients are advised to rest for 24 to 48 hours and to expect the usual postprocedural symptoms such as discomfort with swallowing, local soreness of the right anterior neck, and increased stiffness of the neck. Procedural discomfort is often worst on the first postprocedure day. Discomfort subsides gradually over a 3- to 5-day period and usually resolves within a week. It is customary to provide narcotic pain medications (in limited amounts) at the time of discharge. An instruction form explicitly detailing the usual postprocedure symptoms and including emergency phone numbers is recommended.

The presenting symptoms are usually altered by the procedure. In some instances there is transient improvement (local anesthetic/steroid effect). An occasional patient will report complete relief of symptoms for periods of up to 2 weeks. In others cases there is a short-term exacerbation of chronic pain. Patients should be advised to record symptoms in a diary format on a daily basis for the first week following the procedure, and at 2 weeks postprocedure. Compliance with this request is facilitated if they are provided with a form and a self-addressed stamped enveloped at the time of discharge. Information obtained from the diary is useful both in understanding postprocedure symptoms and in the early detection of complications. A progressive increase or sudden change in the severity or character of pain should arouse suspicion, and further investigation may be warranted.

COMPLICATIONS

The major complications of diagnostic disc injection are neural injury and infection. On one occasion, the overly enthusiastic advancement of a needle by an inexperienced practitioner has been observed. The needle traversed the disc space and crossed the central canal with a single thrust. From the course of the needle, the spinal cord may have been impaled. The needle was quickly withdrawn. The patient survived this severely painful event with no apparent immediate neurologic deficit and remained neurologically intact at follow-up over 6 months after the procedure. Similar cord punctures without sequelae have been reported with lateral

C1-C2 cervical puncture for myelography (61). Careful deliberate advancement of the needle and good visualization prevent such technical problems and their potential catastrophic sequelae. The needle hub should be firmly grasped and its position fixed with one hand, while injection is performed with the other. This maneuver will prevent inadvertently advancing the needle into the spinal canal during the injection phase. This is particularly important when 25-gauge needles are used, as there is little resistance to their advancement.

Discitis is a rarely reported complication of disc injection. Roosen et al. reported their experience with 1,005 disc injections in 380 patients (71). There were two cases of disc space infection attributable to the procedure. Their report included a review of the literature, noting six cases of discitis in 4,237 disc injections for an overall incidence of 0.1% to 0.2% per disc. Recently, Guyer et al. reported two cases of cervical disc infection in 362 disc injections, for an incidence of 0.5% per disc (31). Some cases of cervical discitis appear to be self-limited and resolve spontaneously within a few months (31,90). I have observed two patients whose routine films revealed a dramatic change in the appearance of an interspace less than 4 months after a diagnostic disc injection (Fig. 15). In each instance, the patients reported severe neck pain beginning 3 to 5 days postinjection and continuing for 2 to 3 weeks. Neither case was diagnosed as discitis. Both patients indicated they were told that neck pain was to

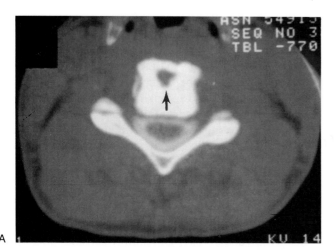
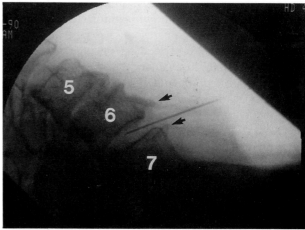

A   B

FIG. 15. A: Axial CT, 2.0-mm section through C4-C5 interspace (inferior C4 endplate). Low dose intrathecal contrast enhancement. The patient was referred with persisting severe neck pain. Diagnostic disc injection had been performed at another institution approximately 3 months prior to this scan. The discogram was reported to be negative. The irregular area of intermediate density *(arrow)* in the inferior C4 endplate was not present on a previous CT scan obtained prior to discography. This finding suggests endplate osteolysis and is presumed evidence of low-grade discitis. The segment underwent spontaneous fusion documented on later follow-up radiographs. **B:** Lateral fluoroscopic image of cervical spine. The patient was referred for diagnostic disc injection at C6-C7. A 25-gauge needle is in good position. Discography had been performed 4 months earlier at another institution. That study was reported negative at the C4-C5 and C5-C6 levels. The discographer was unsuccessful at obtaining satisfactory disc puncture at C6-C7, reportedly because of difficulty with anterior osteophytes *(arrows)*. Note the narrowed, sclerotic, irregular margins at the C5-C6 interspace. These changes were not present on the previous discographic films. They suggest probable discitis and developing arthrodesis at the interspace.

be expected following discography. No antibiotics were administered. In both instances, there was eventual relief of the acute episode, and within 4 months evidence of developing arthrodesis was noted at the involved segments. This relatively benign course suggests that discitis may be more common than is reported, as has been suggested by Crock (22) and Fraser (25). The true incidence of this form of self-limited discitis is not known.

Major infectious complications such as epidural abscess are rare and generally do not escape detection (4,68). Epidural and retropharyngeal abscesses may occur as sequelae of fulminant disc space infection. Lownie and Ferguson (53) reported a case of spinal subdural empyema following discography, and in that case, as well as the epidural/retropharyngeal abscess illustrated (Fig. 16), cultures revealed organisms indigenous to the oropharyngeal region. This supports the opinion of Cloward that such complications are the result of improper needle placement and penetration of the hypopharynx or esophagus (18).

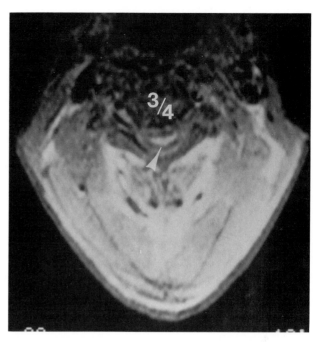

FIG. 17. MRI of cervical spine, axial image at C3-C4 interspace. This is a 70-year-old man with progressive myelopathy. MRI demonstrates flattening of the cervical cord (white arrow).

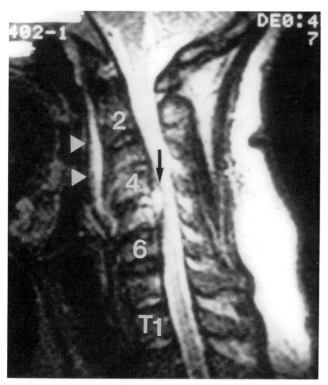

FIG. 16. MRI mid-sagittal section of cervical spine. Spin echo T2-weighted image. The patient underwent cervical discography at C3-C4, C4-C5, and C5-C6 at another institution 1 week prior to scan. The patient complained of severe neck pain within 48 hours of the study. MRI demonstrates retropharyngeal abscess (white arrowheads) extending anterior to the spine up to the level of the C2 body. The posterior mass (black arrow) is epidural abscess. Signal from the C3, C4, and C5 vertebral bodies is increased on T2 images consistent with vertebral hyperemia. Cultures at the time of surgical drainage revealed multiple organisms compatible with oropharyngeal flora.

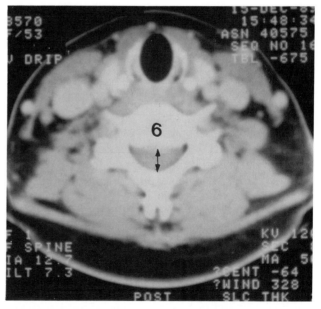

FIG. 18. Axial CT, mid-body C6. The sagittal diameter of the central canal in this patient is markedly reduced (developmental). Mid-sagittal mid-body measurements of 10.0 mm were recorded at each level from C3 through C7. The combination of a developmentally contracted central canal and superimposed spondylosis or disc prolapse are contraindications to performance of diagnostic cervical disc injection. Note: Accurate central canal measurements should be made on images photographed at wide window settings for optimal visualization of bony detail. This image, photographed at soft-tissue window settings, was selected for illustrative purposes (better demonstration).

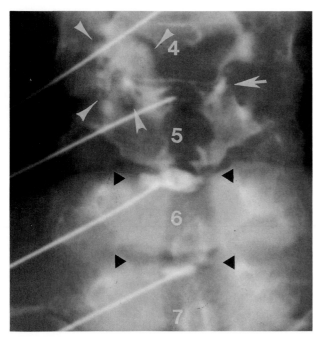

FIG. 19. Anteroposterior spot film of cervical spine. Procedure needles are in place in the C3-C4, C4-C5, C5-C6, and C6-C7 discs. Saline injection at C4-C5 and C5-C6 was painless. Nucleograms are normal *(black arrowheads)*. The injection of saline at the C4-C5 level provoked right-sided neck and shoulder girdle pain (reproducing symptoms). Contrast material is seen in the left uncinate recess of C4-C5 *(white arrow)*. Contrast material has leaked into the right-sided epidural space at C4 *(white arrowheads)* at the time of C4-C5 disc injection. Lateral view demonstrated contrast material in the epidural space and oblique view demonstrated flow into the right-sided C4-C5 intervertebral foramen. Preliminary CT and MRI scans demonstrated no disc protrusion.

Pneumothorax is a potential risk when discography is performed at the C7-T1 level. This possibility must be considered when study of the cervicothoracic region is required. Arterial and neural injury are theoretically possible; however, the use of fine needles and proper technique with good visualization will limit the occurrence of such complications.

Ill-advised performance of discography in patients with evidence of significant cord compression has resulted in catastrophic consequences (50). The diagnosis of cord compression does not require invasive testing (Fig. 17), and in fact, symptoms of myelopathy or cord compression on imaging studies are absolute contraindications.

High-resolution thin-section CT scanning and good quality MRI are primary imaging modalities. Cervical discography remains an adjunctive diagnostic procedure. The MRI and CT images must be reviewed by the discographer prior to disc injection. Discography may not be prudent in patients whose spinal canal is developmentally contracted (sagittal diameter of less than 11.0 mm) (Fig. 18), while the presence of segmental stenosis

(spondylitic ridges) reducing the canal diameter below 11.0 mm is a relative contraindication. Disc herniation resulting from discography is a rarely reported complication (81).

WHY DO CERVICAL DISC INJECTION?

Chronic cervical spine syndromes are difficult to evaluate. The clinician must be aware of the multiplicity of pain sources and the variety of clinical expressions (6) (Fig. 19). The cervical disc is innervated (12,56). Morphologically and functionally, the annulus resembles a ligament and, like ligaments, the annulus fibrosus is susceptible to injury. The common "whiplash" mechanism may, in fact, induce a variety of lesions, including injury to the disc resulting in mechanical dysfunction of the functional spinal unit (8,24,43,87).

Crock has proposed a biochemical mechanism for chronic pain (internal disc disruption syndrome) (22). Primary dural pain as a result of chemical irritation has been suggested as a possible cause of chronic cervical pain syndromes (7) (Fig. 20). There is no direct evidence that cervical discs suffer internal disc disruption as described in the lumbar spine.

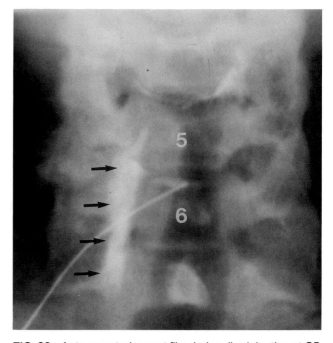

FIG. 20. Anteroposterior spot film during disc injection at C5-C6. This is a 48-year-old woman with chronic right-sided neck and right upper extremity pain. Working diagnosis: neck pain and right upper extremity sympathetic dystrophy. Disc injections at C4-C5 and C6-C7 were normal. Note contrast flow from C5-C6 disc to right paraspinous region adjacent to the neurovascular bundle of the right vertebral artery *(arrow)*. Saline injection provoked familiar neck and right upper extremity pain. Local anesthetic infiltration relieved the chronic pain in the immediate postprocedure period. The sympathetic dystrophy symptoms were improved following the procedure.

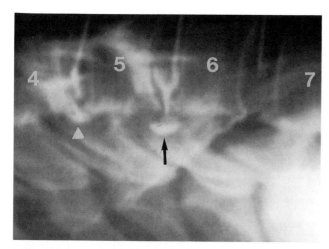

FIG. 21. Lateral radiograph of cervical spine. Disc injection demonstrates large contained posterior prolapse at C5-C6 *(black arrow)*. Injection provoked neck and shoulder girdle pain. There is a small posterior protrusion at C4-C5 *(white arrowhead)*. Saline injection provoked intense suboccipital pain; 0.5 cc bupivacaine 0.5% and 3.0 mg Celestone instilled into each disc. All symptoms were temporarily relieved following the procedure. Neck and shoulder girdle pain returned the following day. Headache was relieved for 10 days. The provocation/analgesic response implies two separate lesions acting in concert to produce the chronic cervical syndrome.

Intradural connections between adjacent cervical spinal nerves appear to be normal variants and can account for greater than expected overlap of dermatomal patterns of pain. Accordingly, symptoms may not always indicate the true level of pathology (54). The possibility of multiple lesions must always be considered (Fig. 21). The best quality imaging studies cannot be expected to demonstrate all pathology. Diagnostic cervical disc injection is a specialized procedure, and this examination may be indicated in patients with chronic pain of such severity that there is a clinical need to know the source of pain generation. Evaluation of discs adjacent to grossly abnormal segments as a presurgical staging procedure may be a limited second indication. Discography has been used to confirm herniation prior to cervical chemonucleolysis (29). When performed with impeccable technique and combined with clinical and imaging data, cervical discography is an aid in defining the level of symptomatic disc pathology in patients with chronic cervical syndromes (10).

REFERENCES

1. Altenstein G (1967): Erfahrungen mit der diskographie an hals und lendenwirbelsaule. *Z Orthop* 102:358–366.
2. Bacon F (1955): In: *The Oxford dictionary of quotations*, 2nd ed. London: Oxford University Press, p. 27.
3. Badami JP, Norman D, Barbaro N (1985): Metrizamide CT myelography in cervical myelopathy and radiculopathy: correlation with conventional myelography and surgical findings. *AJNR* 144: 675–680.
4. Baker AS, Ojemann RG, Schwartz MN, et al. (1975): Spinal epidural abscess. *N Engl J Med* 293:463–468.
5. Bettag W, Grote W (1969): Die bedeutung der diskographie fur die behandlung des "zervikalsyndroms." *Hippokrates* 40:138–141.
6. Bland J (1986): Searching for the cause of a pain in the neck-cervical spine syndromes. *J Musculoskeletal Med* Nov. 1986:23–41.
7. Bogduk N (1984): Neck pain. *Aust Fam Physician* 13:26–30.
8. Bogduk N (1986): The anatomy and pathophysiology of whiplash. *Clin Biomechanics* 1:92–101.
9. Bogduk N (1988): Neck pain: an update. *Aust Fam Physician* 17: 75–80.
10. Bogduk N (1988): The innervation of the intervertebral discs. In: Ghosh P, ed. *The biology of the intervertebral disc*, vol. I. Boca Ratan, Florida: CRC Press, pp. 145–147.
11. Bogduk N (1994): Discography. *APS Journal* III(3):149–154.
12. Bogduk N, Windsor M, Inglis A (1988): The innervation of the cervical intervertebral discs. *Spine* 13(1):2–8.
13. Bogduk N, Aprill C (1993): On the nature of neck pain, discography and cervical zygapophysial joint blocks. *Pain* 54:213–217.
14. Cloward RB (1958): Cervical diskography. Technique, indications and use in the diagnosis of ruptured cervical disks. *AJR* 79:563–574.
15. Cloward RB (1958): The anterior approach for removal of ruptured cervical disks. *J Neurosurg* 15:602–617.
16. Cloward RB (1959): Cervical diskography. A contribution to the etiology and mechanism of neck, shoulder and arm pain. *Ann Surg* 150:1052–1064.
17. Cloward RB (1963): Cervical discography. *Acta Radiol* [*Diag*] (*Stockh*) 1:675–688.
18. Cloward RB (1975): Cervical discography defended *(letter)*. *JAMA* 233:862.
19. Cloward R (1987): Presidential address. Annual meeting Cervical Spine Research Society, Washington, DC.
20. Connor P, Darden B (1993). Cervical discography complications and clinical efficacy. *Spine* 18(14):2035–2038.
21. Consensus Conference (1988): Magnetic resonance imaging. *JAMA* 259(14):2135.
22. Crock H (1983): *Practice of spinal surgery*. New York: Springer-Verlag.
23. Daniels DL, Grogan JP, Johansen JG, et al. (1984): Cervical radiculopathy: computed tomography and myelography compared. *Radiology* 151:109–113.
24. Davis S, Teresi L, Bradley W, et al. (1991): Cervical spine hyperextensive injuries. MRI findings. *Radiology* 180:245–251.
25. Fraser RD (1984): Chymopapain for the treatment of intervertebral disc herniation: the final report of a double blind study. *Spine* 9:815–818.
26. Fox AJ, Lin JP, Pinto RS, Kricheff II (1975): Myelographic cervical nerve root deformities. *Radiology* 116:355–361.
27. Gelehrter G (1975): The addition of nucleography to discography as an extended method of examination. *ROFO* 122(6):517–519.
28. Ginsberg G, Lewis J, Gallagher J, et al. (1992): Diazepam versus midazolam for colonoscopy: a prospective evaluation of predicted versus actual dosage requirements. *Gastrointest Endosc* 38:651–656.
29. Gomez-Castresana F, Vazquez-Herrero C, Baltex-Horche J (1995): Cervical chemonucleolysis. *Orthopedics* 18(3):237–242.
30. Grote W, Wappenschmidt J (1967): Uber technik und indikation zur-zervikalen diskographie. *ROFO* 106:721–727.
31. Guyer RD, Collier R, Stith WJ, et al. (1988): Discitis after discography. *Spine* 13:1352–1354.
32. Guyer R, Ohnmeiss B (1993): *Lumbar discography. Contemporary concepts in spine care*. North American Spine Society, July.
33. Hall SC, Ovassapian A (1977): Apnea after intravenous diazepam therapy. *JAMA* 238(10):1052.
34. Hartjes H, Roosen K, Grote W, et al. (1983): Cervical disc syndromes: value of metrizamide myelography and discography. *AJNR* 4:644–645.
35. Hatt MU (1969): Hohenlokalisation der cervicalen discushernie in klinik, elektromyographe (EMG) und myelographie. *Dtsch Zeitschr Nervenheilk* 197:56–65.
36. Hatton M, Williams D, Weis F (1987): A randomized double-blind pilot study to compare conscious sedation produced by Diazepam against sufentanil. *Anesthesiol Progress* 34:137–141.

37. Hirsch C (1948): An attempt to diagnose level of disc lesion clinically by disc puncture. *Acta Orthop Scand* 18:132–140.

38. Hirsch C, Schajowicz R, Galante J (1967): Structural changes in the cervical spine. A study on autopsy specimens in different age groups. *Acta Orthop Scand* (Suppl. 109) 7–77.

39. Holt EP Jr (1964): Fallacy of cervical discography. Report of 50 cases in normal subjects. *JAMA* 188:799–801.

40. Holt EP Jr (1968): The question of lumbar discography. *J Bone Joint Surg [Am]* 50:720–726.

41. Hubach P (1994): A prospective study of anterior cervical spondylodesis in intervertebral disc disorders. *Eur Spine J* 3(4):209–213.

42. Jensen M, Brant-Zawadzki M, Obuchowski N, Modic M, Malkasian D, Ross J (1994): Magnetic resonance imaging of the lumbar spine in people without back pain. *N Engl J Med* 33(2):69–73.

43. Jonsson H, Bring G, Rauschning W, et al. (1991): Hidden cervical spine injuries in traffic accident victims with skull fractures. *J Spinal Disorders* 4:251–263.

44. Kambin P, Abda S, Kurpicki F (1980): Intradiskal pressure and volume recording: evaluation of normal and abnormal cervical disks. *Clin Orthop* 146:144–147.

45. Karnaze MG, Gado MH, Sartor KJ, Hodges FJ 3d (1988): Comparison of MR and CT myelography in imaging the cervical and thoracic spine. *AJR* 150:397–403.

46. Kikuchi S, Macnab I, Moreau P (1981): Localisation of the level of symptomatic cervical disc degeneration. *J Bone Joint Surg [Br]* 63: 272–277.

47. Klafta LA Jr, Collis JS Jr (1969): The diagnostic inaccuracy of the pain response in cervical discography. *Cleveland Clin Q* 36:35–39.

48. Klafta LA Jr, Collis JS Jr (1969): An analysis of cervical discography with surgical verification. *J Neurosurg* 30:38–41.

49. Kofoed H (1981): Thoracic outlet syndrome. *Clin Orthop Rel Res* 156:145–148.

50. Laun A, Lorenz R, Agnoli AL (1981): Complications of cervical discography. *J Neurosurg Sci* 25:17–20.

51. Lazorthes Y, Richaud J, Verdie J, Bonafe A (1988): Chymopapain chemonucleolysis in cervical herniated discs. In: Bard M, Laredo J, eds. *Interventional radiology in bone and joint.* New York: Springer-Verlag, Wein, pp. 123–129.

52. Lindblom K (1948): Diagnostic puncture of intervertebral disks in sciatica. *Acta Orthop Scand* 17:231–239.

53. Lownie SP, Ferguson GG (1989): Spinal subdural empyema complicating cervical discography. *Spine* 14(12):1415–1417.

54. Marzo JM, Simmons EH, Kallen F (1987): Intradural connections between adjacent cervical spinal roots. *Spine* 12(10):964–968.

55. Massare C, Bard M, Tristant H (1974): Cervical discography. Speculation on technique and indications from our own experience. *J Radiol* 55:395–399.

56. Mendel T, Wink C, Zimny M (1992): Neural elements in the human cervical intervertebral discs. *Spine* 17:132–136.

57. Meyer RR (1963): Cervical diskography. A help or hindrance in evaluating neck, shoulder, arm pain? *AJR* 90:1208–1215.

58. Modic MT, Masaryk TJ, Mulopulos GP, Bundschuh C, Han JS, Bohlman H (1986): Cervical radiculopathy: prospective evaluation with surface coil MR imaging, CT with metrizamide and metrizamide myelography. *Radiology* 161:753–759.

59. Nachemson A (1989): Lumbar discography—where are we today? *Spine* 14(6):555–557.

60. Nakagawa H, Okurmura T, Sugiyama T, et al. (1983): Discrepancy between metrizamide CT and myelography in diagnosis of cervical disc protrusions. *AJNR* 4:604–606.

61. Nakstad PH, Kjartansson O (1988): Accidental spinal cord injection of contrast material during cervical myelography with C1-C2 puncture. *AJNR* 9:410.

62. North American Spine Society (1988): Position statement on discography. The Executive Committee of the North American Spine Society. *Spine* 13:1343.

63. Odom GL, Finney W, Woodhall B (1958): Cervical disk lesions. *JAMA* 166:23–28.

64. Parfenchuk T, Janssen M (1994): A correlation of cervical magnetic resonance imaging and discography/computed tomographic discogram. *Spine* 19(24):2819–2825.

65. Pascaud JL, Mailhes F, Pascaud E, et al. (1980): The cervical intervertebral disc: diagnostic value of cervical discography in degenerative and post-traumatic lesions. *Ann Radiol (Paris)* 23:455–460.

66. Payne EE, Spillane JD (1957): The cervical spine. *Brain* 80:571–596.

67. Penning L, Wilmink JT, van Voerden HH, Knol E (1986): CT myelographic findings in degenerative disorders of the cervical spine: clinical significance. *AJR* 146:793–801.

68. Ravicovitch MA, Spallone A (1982): Spinal epidural abscesses. *Eur Neurol* 21:347–357.

69. Reves J, Fragen R, Vinik H, et al. (1985): Midazolam pharmacology and uses. *Anesthesiology* 62:310–324.

70. Riley LH Jr, Robinson RA, Johnson KA, Walker AE (1969): The results of anterior interbody fusion of the cervical spine. Review of 93 consecutive cases. *J Neurosurg* 30:127–133.

71. Roosen K, Bettag W, Fiebach O (1975): Komplikationen der cervikalen diskographie. *ROFO* 122:520–527.

72. Roth DA (1976): Cervical analgesic discography. A new test for the definitive diagnosis of painful-disk syndrome. *JAMA* 235:1713–1714.

73. Saternus KS, Bornscheuer HH (1983): [Comparative radiologic and pathologic-anatomic studies on the value of discography in the diagnosis of acute intravertebral disc injuries in the cervical spine.] *ROFO* 139:651–657.

74. Schaerer JP (1968): Anterior cervical disc removal and fusion. *Schweiz Arch Neurol Neurochirurgie Psychiatry* 102:331–344.

75. Scotti G, Scialfa G, Pieralli S, et al. (1983): Myelopathy and radiculopathy due to cervical spondylosis: myelographic-CT correlations. *AJNRogy* 4:601–603.

76. Sherk H, Parke W (1983): Developmental anatomy. In: Bailey RW, ed. *The cervical spine.* Philadelphia: JP Lippincott, pp. 7–8.

77. Shinomiya K, Nakao K, Shindoh S, et al. (1993): Evaluation of cervical discography in pain origin and provocation. *J Spinal Disord* 6(5):422–426.

78. Siebenrock K, Aebi M (1994): Cervical discography and discogenic pain syndrome and its predictive value for cervical fusion. *Arch Orthop Trauma Surg* 113(4):199–203.

79. Simmons EH, Segil CM (1975): An evaluation of discography in the localization of symptomatic levels in discogenic disease of the spine. *Clin Orthop Rel Res* (108):57–69.

80. Smith GW (1959): The normal cervical diskogram with clinical observations. *Am J Roentg* 81:1006–1010.

81. Smith M, Kim S (1990): Herniated cervical disc restuling from discography: an unusual complication. *J Spinal Disord* 3(4):292–294.

82. Smith GW, Nichols P Jr (1957): Technic for cervical discography. *Radiology* 68:718–720.

83. Smith GW, Robinson RA (1958): The treatment of certain cervical-spine disorders by anterior removal of the intervertebral disc and interbody fusion. *J Bone Joint Surg [Am]* 40:607–623.

84. Sneider SE, Winslow OP Jr, Pryor TH (1963): Cervical diskography: Is it relevant? *JAMA* 185:163–165.

85. Stuck RM (1961): Cervical discography. *AJR* 86:975–982.

86. Taveras J (1967): Is discography a useful diagnostic procedure? *J Can Assoc Radiol* 18:294–295.

87. Taylor J, Twoomey L (1993): Acute injuries to the cervical joints: an autopsy study of neck sprain. *Spine* 18:1115–1122.

88. VanDyke C, Ross JS, Tkach J, Masaryk TJ, Modic MT (1989): Gradient-echo MR imaging of the cervical spine: evaluation of extradural disease. *AJR* 153:393–398.

89. Vezina JL, Fontaine S, LaPerriere J (1989): Outpatient myelography with fine needle technique: an appraisal. *AJNR* 10:615–617.

90. Volgelsang H (1973): Discitis intervertrablis cervicalis nach diskographie. *Neurochirurgia* 16:80–83.

91. Walsh T, Weinstein J, Spratt K, Lehmann T, Aprill C, Sayre H (1990): The question of lumbar discography revisited: a controlled prospective study of normal volunteers to determine the false-positive rate. *J Bone Joint Surg [Am]* [in press].

92. Whitecloud TS 3rd, Seago RA (1987): Cervical discogenic syndrome. Results of operative intervention in patients with positive discography. *Spine* 12:313–317.

93. Wiley J, Macnab I, Wortzman G (1968): Lumbar discography and its clinical applications. *Can J Surg* 11:280–289.

94. Wilkinson HA, Schuman N (1980): Intradiscal corticosteroids in the treatment of lumbar and cervical disc problems. *Spine* 5:385–389.

95. Wilmink JT (1989): CT morphology of intrathecal lumbosacral nerve-root compression. *AJNR* 10:233–248.

The Adult Spine: Principles and Practice,
2nd edition, J.W. Frymoyer, Editor-in-Chief.
Lippincott-Raven Publishers, Philadelphia © 1996.

Diagnostic Disc Injection

II. Diagnostic Lumbar Disc Injection

Charles Neuville Aprill III

HISTORY

In order to evaluate patients with clinical signs of neural compression but normal lumbar myelograms (Abrodil), Lindblom sought to develop a technique for directly evaluating the lumbar discs (99). The conceptual stimulus for this work was the original disc studies of Schmorl and Junghanns (165), and the presentation of a "discogram" by Lindgren in 1941. Lindblom performed anatomic studies, injecting red lead into the nucleus of cadaveric discs. He noted the presence of radial ruptures. However, clinical application of this technique was delayed by fear of damaging the disc by puncture. This fear was attributed primarily to a report of disc damage at lumbar puncture in children by Pease (152). These lumbar punctures were being performed on children with meningitis, and the discs were inadvertently punctured and presumably infected. Lindblom was encouraged by communications with Carl Hirsch, who noted no immediate prolapse or late effects in patients whose discs were punctured at the time of operation (74). Lindblom reported results on 15 disc injections in 13 patients in 1948 (100). Normal and abnormal patterns were described. The technique was employed on a number of patients and was the subject of three additional reports in the Scandinavian literature (101–103).

A body of pertinent literature was developing concomitantly. Arthur Steindler had noted in 1938 that sciatic pain could be relieved by injections of procaine into an intervertebral disc (175). Roofe had reported the innervation of the annulus fibrosus and posterior longitudinal ligament in 1940 (160). Hirsch reported pain provocation in 16 patients by injection of saline into the disc (74). Falconer stimulated discs at surgery under local anesthetic and noted induction of back pain (43). Experimental studies in animals (90) and in human cadavers (56,153) indicated that disc puncture was not harmful to the disc.

The work of Pierre Erlacher (41) is historically significant. Cadaveric studies documented the accuracy with which the contrast dispersal pattern defined the nuclear space. Using contrast material for radiographic visualization and the vital stains for anatomic correlation, his study revealed complete agreement between the radiograph and the actual dispersal pattern in 200 discs.

The first report of discography performed in the United States was that of Wise and Weiford (197). Shortly thereafter, Ralph Cloward reported on the technique and indications for lumbar discography (28) and developed a surgical procedure for the treatment of the abnormalities revealed (27).

The monograph of Ulf Fernstrom cites most of the pertinent reference material regarding discography, from Lindblom's original report in 1948, up to 1960 (48). This classic work is recommended reading for any student of low back pain. Fernstrom notes that back and leg pain can occur whether or not there is nerve compression. He suggests that there are both neurogenic (mechanical compressive) and discogenic (biochemical irritative) causes for the symptoms.

Collis and Gardner (31) enthusiastically claimed discography to be superior to myelography in evaluation of disc disease, reporting over 1,000 cases in which the procedure was employed. Feinberg (46) reported over 2,000 cases and defined patterns of abnormal discograms that remain valid today. He considered annular tear to be a significant lesion; back and leg pain could not be explained by nerve compression alone.

By 1965, Hirsch's enthusiasm for discography had waned (75). Earl Holt published his study on asymptomatic volunteers in 1968 (80). Because of its historical significance, Holt's report warrants and has received careful study (171).

Holt stated that the need for disc surgery in the absence of myelographically demonstrable posterior or posterolateral protrusion with nerve root impingement had not been established. He commented that the "abnormal" patterns described by other authors may be the normal changes of aging. He questioned whether internal derangement of the disc was an indication for surgery. A prospective study of asymptomatic volunteers was certainly in order. To this end, he enlisted volunteers from the inmate population of Menard Penitentiary in Chester, Illinois. The flaws in Holt's study include:

1. The selection of a suspect population. One must question the motivation of prisoners to join the study group. Is their history of no prior back problems accurate?

2. The high rate of technical failure (in part related to equipment available). Holt was unsuccessful in obtaining a discogram at 23% of the levels attempted, and some of his "successful" discograms may have been annular injections. Particular attention is called to Figure 4 of Holt's paper.

3. The use of irritant contrast material. Sodium diatrozoate (Hypaque 50) was the only contrast agent available, but it is extremely irritating (49,185). The Holt study was appropriate to its time, but its conclusions cannot be applied to modern discography.

In the same year—1968—Wiley et al. reported on 2,517 discograms (192). These authors believed that discography was most valuable in the assessment of patients with pain and no definite herniation. Gresham and Miller (67) noted in their cadaver study that 90% of the discs in subjects from 14 to 34 years of age were normal. By age 60, only 5% were normal.

Henry Farfan et al. (45) employed nucleography in studies of human cadaveric discs. Experimentally induced annular disruption is remarkably similar to the naturally occurring radial annular fissure. Recognition of the biomechanical effects of torsion overload on the lumbar motion segment is essential to understanding the torsion mechanism of injury.

The intervertebral disc is a complex structure and responds to injury in a variety of ways. The notion of "disc rupture" with pain secondary to nerve compression was immortalized by Mixter and Barr in 1934 (128). This popular belief was seemingly accepted by Lindblom, Collis, and Holt. However, the concept is not sufficient to explain the majority of back pain (76,82). Harry Crock suggested the probability of several different symptomatic disc lesions, including protrusion/prolapse, internal disruption, and isolated resorption (33). Each induced symptoms by a different mechanism. Discography was required to establish the diagnosis of internal disc disruption.

NEW TECHNOLOGY

The development of safe non-ionic contrast agents (163) and the emergence of computed tomography (CT) (125) and magnetic resonance imaging (MRI) (133) for primary noninvasive evaluation of disc pathology changed the role of discography in the evaluation of back pain.

CT scanning provides excellent visualization of disc contour in cross section (194). It is a satisfactory method for the diagnosis of disc herniation (Fig. 1) (193,202). There are lesions that can mimic intraforaminal disc herniation such as neurofibroma (12,95) and conjoined nerve root (78,154).

MRI is sensitive to the detection and characterization of a variety of disc lesions including prolapse and seques-

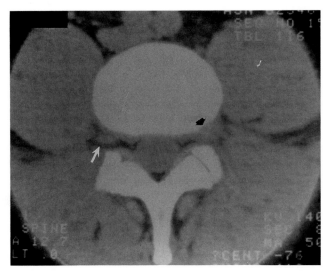

FIG. 1. Axial L4-L5 disc. Moderately large prolapse/extrusion of disc material into mid-radicular canal *(black arrow)*, normal dorsal ganglion on opposite side *(white arrow)*. The lesion does not disturb the thecal sac, epidural fat, or anterior internal vertebral veins.

tration (112). In the clinical setting of definitive neural compression correlating with a mass lesion, discography is superfluous (14,66).

In an ideal world, one would have the ability to perform clinical evaluation and predict the nature of structural lesions demonstrated on imaging studies. Haldeman, in an assessment of 100 patients with Workers' Compensation claims, found that this was not possible. Radiation of pain only to a point above the knee and negative straight-leg raising could be found in patients with marked CT abnormalities. Pain radiating below the knee and positive straight-leg raising occurred in some patients with normal CT scans (70). Asymptomatic herniations have been described in autopsy studies (122), by myelography (77), and by CT scanning (86).

Correlation studies of MRI and cryomicrotomed specimens improve understanding of the anatomy depicted and provide a basis for improving existing and developing new pulse sequences (159). Yu et al. (201) employed high-resolution thin section MRI to evaluate lumbar annulus fibrosus in 20 cadavers. They were able to identify three types of annular fissures: Type I, concentric outer annular tears; Type II, radial annular tears; and Type III, transverse fissures at the insertion of Sharpey's fibers. The Type I tears may represent a stage in the development of the myxomatous degeneration of the annulus described by Yasuma et al. (198).

A comparison study of discography and high-resolution, thin-section MRI in cadavers demonstrated MRI to be less sensitive than discography in the detection of annular fissures or tears. MRI (3.0-mm-thick sections) was able to detect 10 of 15 fissures demonstrated by discography (200). A second cadaver study revealed that not all peripheral annular lesions are detected by discography. Histologic studies indicate that rim lesions in the anterior annulus can be identified in 18% of the discs with normal discography (nucleogram). MRI was found to be less specific than discography in assessing this pathology (68). *In vivo* MRI has not yet evolved to the point where that degree of sensitivity is to be expected. Numerous studies comparing MRI to discography have documented an excellent correlation in terms of detecting disc degeneration (14,18,24,25,30,66,105,108,147,172).

Conventional MRI techniques do not distinguish the painful from the nonpainful disc in most instances. Ross et al. have reported the detection of annular tears on spin-echo (SE) T2-weighted images and with the use of gadolinium enhancement (161). Aprill and Bogduk described an MRI finding which is frequently seen in patients with back pain. It is highly specific and strongly predictive of a painful disc with outer annular disruption (7). An area of bright signal within the substance of the annulus on SE T2 images (Fig. 2) was detected in 28% of 500 patients referred for back pain. This high intensity zone (HIZ) appears to be a sign of severe annular fissure. Its sensitivity was modest, but specificity was high and

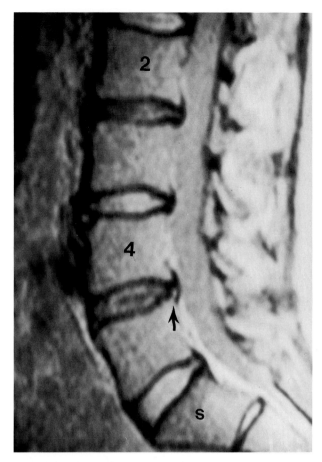

FIG. 2. Sagittal MRI spin-echo (SE) spin density. High intensity zone *(black arrow)* within posterior annular substance of L4-L5 presumably represents posterior annular fissure.

positive predictive value for disrupted painful disc was 86%. The sign has been noted in asymptomatic subjects (16), but the prevalence in the asymptomatic population has not yet been established. Complete radial fissures may occur in nondegenerated discs as a result of injury (2) or fatigue (3).

DISCOGENIC PAIN

The pathophysiology of discogenic pain is not known. Mechanical theories suggest instability and/or mass lesions compressing or deforming spinal nerves. Naylor (140) and Taylor and Akeson (179) described the internal biochemistry of the disc but only in the context of prolapse.

Fernstrom (48) noted back pain and sciatica in patients with annular fissures without neural compression. Crock (33) described a syndrome characterized by alteration of the internal structure of the disc as well as its metabolic activity. Goldner et al. (64) reported a similar syndrome. A number of authors have described lesions associated with severe and incapacitating back pain without neural compression. These include painful posterior annular fissure (150), acute traumatic interosseous herniation (115), isolated intervertebral disc resorption (84), and painful lumbar endplate disruption (81).

Nachemson (137) recorded low pH in the discs of several patients and found a significant correlation with the amount of perineural reaction. Leakage of catabolites or other breakdown products from the disrupted disc may incite inflammatory reaction in the adjacent epidural and perineural spaces (111,116). The possibility that disc proteins can reach the venous circulation by means of endplate capillaries and establish an autoimmune or hypersensitivity reaction has been postulated by Crock (35).

The intervertebral disc is innervated (17,199). Disc injury in some individuals may provoke activation of the sensory nociceptive system in the disc by chemical irritation. Degradation of the nucleus and annulus appears to be associated with an accumulation of extraordinary concentrations of inflammatory enzymes such as phospholipase A2 (51,91). This in turn may sensitize adjacent structures, including the dorsal ganglion (191). Such a mechanism may underlie the pain associated with disc injuries. Direct comparison studies with discography have shown MRI to be quite effective in detecting disc degeneration (60,167). Numerous authors have reported patients with severe back pain, normal MRI, and positive discography (18,93,147,172,203). Digital assessment of the MRI data appears to be superior to the subjective assessment of the brightness of disc signal by interpreters in terms of detecting degeneration, particularly in its early stages (187). Thus, diagnostic disc injection remains the only direct exam to differentiate symptomatic and asymptomatic discs (105).

DISC PUNCTURE/INJECTION

The following recommendations are based on my performance of over 6,700 disc punctures in over 2,750 patients in the 10-year period from 1979 to 1994.

The facilities required for lumbar disc puncture are no different from those utilized for cervical disc studies. A C-arm fluoroscope is not necessary for the techniques that will be described. Some feel that a C-arm facilitates approach to the disc space (96). Good visualization is essential. Catastrophic consequences have been reported as a result of subarachnoid injection of toxic substances resulting from inadequate visualization (39). The risk of such complications is nil in diagnostic disc injections with the use of non-ionic contrast materials. However, no solution should be instilled until the position of the needle tip is verified.

Patient preparation procedures including prescreening, interview, and exam; explanation of the procedure and potential risks; and pre-medication are identical to the cervical disc puncture technique, as already described.

To begin, the patient is placed in a prone position on the fluoroscopic table and a wide area prepped and draped as for any invasive procedure. The prep usually extends from the costal margin to the mid-buttock and includes the midline and flank on the side elected for puncture. As a general rule, the side selected is opposite the patient's dominant pain (120). In the case of dominant back, hip/buttock, or leg pain on the right, disc puncture should be performed from the left. This effectively eliminates any confusion regarding pain induction or annular leaking relative to the needle itself. There are exceptions to this general rule (129). If it is known that there is unilateral composite root sleeve (154), or cystic dilatation of a root sleeve (142) on the selected side, it is prudent to avoid puncture at that location. In such instances, disc puncture should be performed on the opposite side, the side of the patient's dominant pain. The presence of these normal variants is not a contraindication to diagnostic disc injection. If the anomaly is bilateral, then the procedure should be performed on the side opposite the dominant pain. Additional care in performance to avoid the neural elements in the case of composite root sleeves and the addition of lumbar puncture precautions to the postprocedure instructions in the case of cystic root sleeve dilatation are necessary.

In his description of discography technique, Lindblom (101) described a posterior transdural midline approach. This particular method of disc puncture was employed by many practitioners for diagnostic disc injection into the 1980s (126).

Erlacher (41) and Keck (89) described a "posterolateral technique" to theoretically avoid thecal puncture. In most instances, the thecal sac occupies the majority of space available in the central canal. Lindblom (103) recognized that this technique does not eliminate thecal puncture and places the segmental nerve sheath and the lateral recess in eminent danger. Initial reports (173) employing the posterolateral approach as described by Erlacher (41) noted a high incidence of postprocedure headache, presumably secondary to dural puncture.

In reality, there are two acceptable approaches to the lumbar disc: posterior (intrapedicular) and lateral (extrapedicular). The posterior approach is associated with all of the problems of lumbar puncture and will not be discussed here.

The lateral, extrapedicular approach is associated with its own particular risks. The lateral approach for puncture of the lumbar discs was described in the late 1960s (38,40). This approach was popularized by the development of chemonucleolysis as a treatment for lumbar disc disease (22,117,118,173).

McCulloch and Waddell (119) reported the use of an extrapedicular approach for diagnostic discography. They reported 20 dural punctures in 1,500 discograms. The primary advantage of the extrapedicular approach is

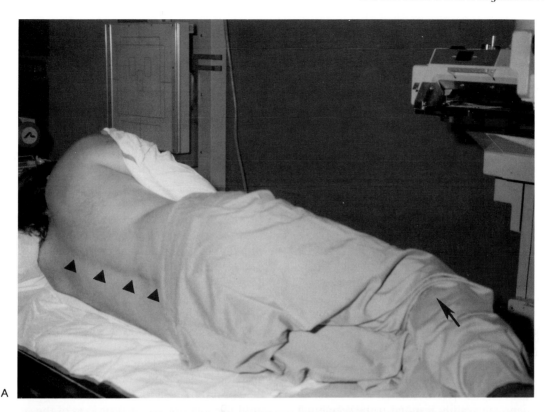

A

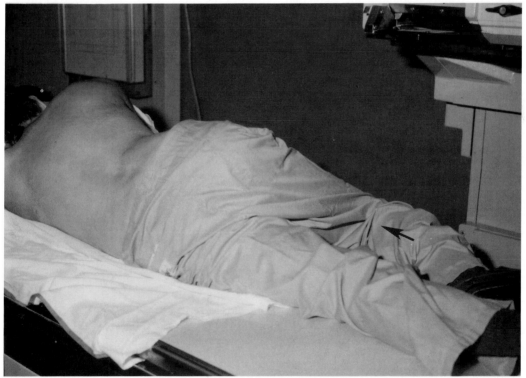

B

FIG. 3. Subject on fluoroscopy table prior to procedure. **A:** Left lateral decubitus position. Note the knees are one atop the other and slightly flexed *(arrow)*. The spine is relatively straight in this subject *(arrowheads)*. No bolus under the abdomen to level the spine is necessary in this case. **B:** Prone oblique position, right side up. Note the ipsilateral (right) knee is flexed and moved forward onto the table top, stabilizing the oblique position.

the avoidance of dural puncture (32). However, Dabezies and Murphy (37) noted that the frequency of dural puncture may be higher than expected even when the procedure is performed by an experienced practitioner. Benoist (9) pointed out the risk of bowel perforation with extreme lateral approaches. Review of axial images (CT and MRI) facilitates planning the approach to avoid such complications (141).

The extrapedicular approach directs the needle in close proximity to the segmental nerve. Knowledge of the course and position of the nerve is critical. The position of the dorsal ganglion is variable (71), but in general the segmental nerves occupy a cephalad position in the intervertebral foramen and course anterolaterally from the foramen. The anatomic relationships in the radicular canal of the lumbar spine have been described by Crock (34) and Rauschning (158).

Neural injury by direct needle trauma can occur (190). Konings and Veldhuizen have reviewed the anatomy in a cadaver study and point out that the discography needle should be kept relatively low in relation to the intervertebral foramen, entering the disc preferably below its midpoint (92). Significant neural injury is not likely to result from a procedure performed under local anesthesia, as the patient can readily respond if the segmental nerve is contacted.

Troisier has pointed out the advantages of the prone oblique position (183). A modification of this technique has been employed for diagnostic disc puncture in my practice at all lumbar levels above the lumbosacral junction for over 5 years with excellent success.

Once the decision is made as to the side of disc puncture, the patient is placed in the lateral decubitus position with the selected side up. A pillow is placed between the patient's head and the down-side arm, which is stretched out over the head so that the patient is lying directly on the chest wall along the axillary line (Fig. 3). While in this lateral decubitus position, a small sponge, folded towel, or other bolus material may be placed beneath the flank to reduce any side-bending of the lumbar spine. The patient is then gently rolled into a prone oblique position with the ipsilateral leg flexed. This is a stable position with the chest wall, hip, and knee acting to fix the patient. The sterile prep and draping are then completed. The drapes should be sufficiently large to allow the operator to move the patient and maintain sterility. From this basic position, the patient may be then rolled back to the lateral or forward to a more prone position during the procedure (Fig. 4).

By increasing or decreasing the degree of flexion of the ipsilateral leg, the hips and trunk can be rotated to find the optimum angle for approach. The patient is rotated until the superior articular process of the subjacent vertebra at the level selected is projected almost immediately between the anterior and posterior margins of the endplate of the vertebra above. A 3.5-inch 25-gauge nee-

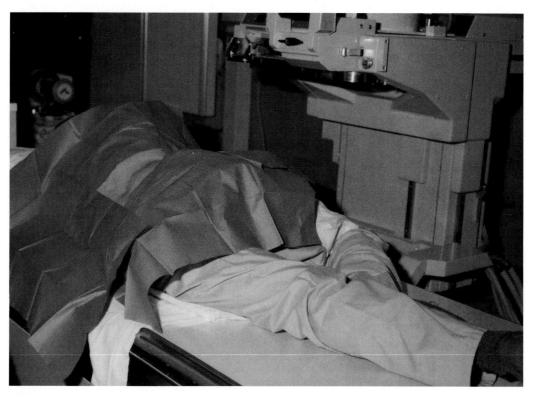

FIG. 4. Prone oblique position after completion of skin preparation and draping of the lumbar area prior to disc puncture via right extrapedicular approach.

dle is then directed vertically toward the anterior margin of the superior process (Fig. 5). In a thin subject, this needle may be long enough to reach the disc and complete the disc injection. More often, it is long enough to reach the superior process or peripheral margin of the disc. The needle is placed adjacent to the superior articular process and slowly withdrawn while injecting 3.0 to 5.0 cc of lidocaine 1%. A 6-inch spinal needle (25- or 22-gauge) can then be directed along the same course toward the disc (Fig. 6). If a bony obstruction is encountered, the patient is rolled to the lateral position to determine whether the needle has contacted the superior process or the vertebral endplate. Usually, a minor rotation of the needle is all that is required to proceed. Occasionally it is necessary to withdraw the needle 1 to 2 cm and slowly alter its path. By rotating the bevel, the direction of these thin needles can be altered slightly as they pass through tissues.

There is no mistaking the tactile sensation associated with penetration of the annulus. It is firm but resilient. The patient usually experiences a sharp, sudden aching or painful sensation in the back or hip as the annulus is contacted and penetrated. This is a momentary experience. After advancing the needle into the disc substance, its position must be checked in both the sagittal and frontal planes (Fig. 7).

This technique is satisfactory for examination of the lumbar discs above the lumbosacral level. It does not rely on measurements from the midline or determination of angles, but rather it is related to individual patient anatomy, which varies considerably. The maneuvers are simple and can be mastered quickly. With experience, disc puncture can be performed, the disc distended, and the needle removed in less than 2 minutes. Adherence to the principles of this technique avoids dural puncture and contact with the neural elements (Fig. 8).

Disc puncture at the lumbosacral level is challenging. The technique described below is similar to the method of Laredo et al. (96). To begin, the patient is in the lateral decubitus position. The lumbosacral angle is observed and a line projected back to the skin surface. This represents the transverse level at which the skin puncture will be made. The patient is then rolled to a prone or slightly prone oblique position. A point along the transverse level is selected that will allow the passage of a needle medial to the iliac crest and adjacent to the lateral margin of the superior articular process of the sacrum. A 25-gauge 3.5-inch spinal needle is then directed from the selected point caudally and medially toward the superior process. In most individuals, even those of robust body build, a 3.5-inch needle will suffice. Caution should be employed in subjects of average or slight build, as the 3.5-inch needle may be long enough to pass the process and contact the L5 segmental nerve at the level of the anterior ramus just distal to the foramen. In most pa-

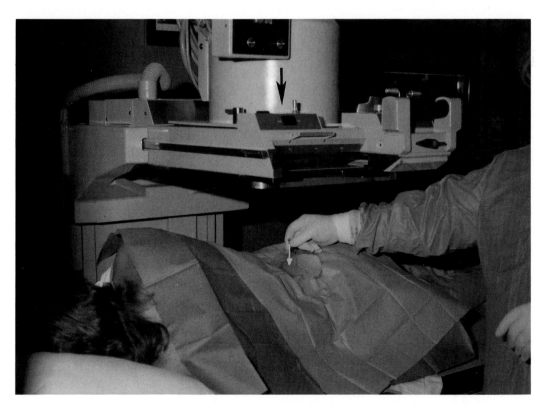

FIG. 5. Patient in prone oblique position. Image intensifier *(black arrow)* centered over target interspace (L4-L5). Needle is being directed toward the anterior aspect of the right superior articular process of L5. The thin needle (25-gauge) is barely visible on photograph and has been highlighted *(white arrow)*.

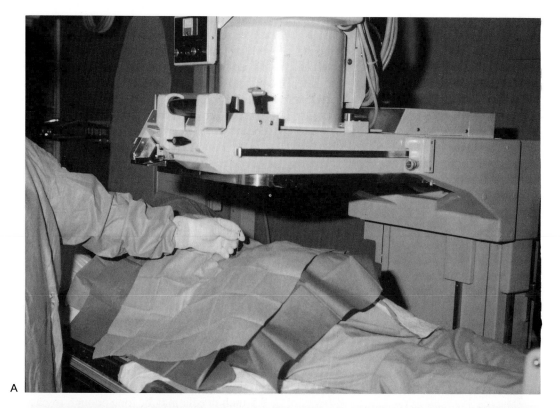

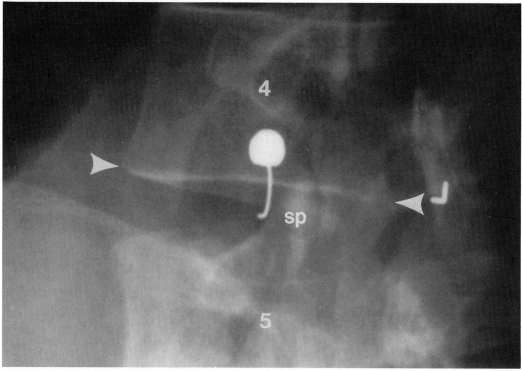

FIG. 6. A: Prone oblique position. Procedure needle (22-gauge) is directed toward the L4-L5 disc space. **B:** Prone oblique spot film of L4-L5 interspace. Patient is positioned so that the anterior aspect of the superior articular process (sp) is almost midway between the anterior and posterior margins of the inferior L4 endplate *(arrowheads)*. A 22-gauge needle has been directed vertically just anterior to the superior process into the disc space.

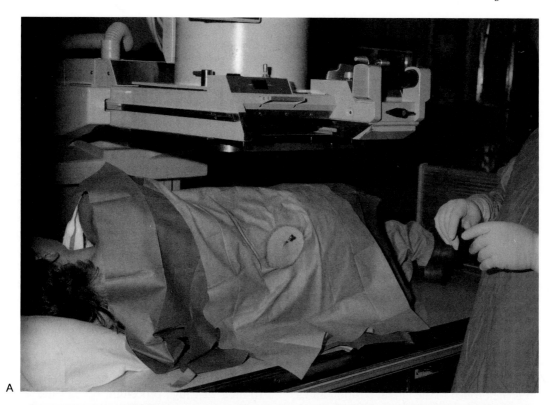

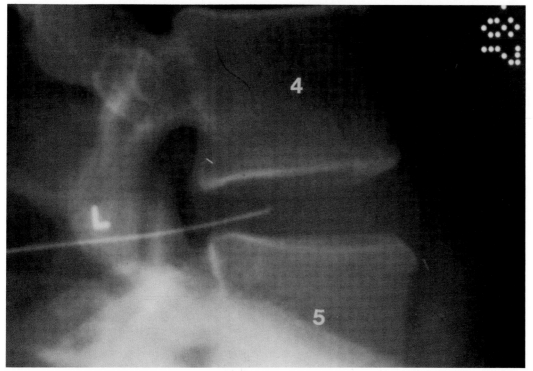

FIG. 7. A: Lateral decubitus position. Procedure needle is in place in L4-L5 disc. **B:** Lateral spot film of L4-L5 interspace. The needle is in good position at the junction of the posterior and the mid third of the interspace. Note that penetration is low in the annulus.

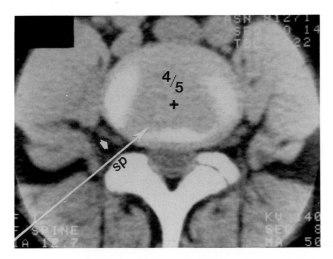

FIG. 8. Axial CT of L4-L5 disc. The extrapedicular approach allows the needle to traverse the center of the disc (+), avoiding contact with the adjacent L4 segmental nerve *(small arrow)*. The needle must pass immediately alongside the superior articular process (sp).

tients, the needle need only be advanced 2.5 to 3 inches to be adjacent to the superior process.

The patient is then rolled to the lateral position and a fluoroscopic check of the position is made. This determines whether the cephalocaudad angle is correct (in line with the disc space) and whether the needle depth is appropriate. Any changes in the angle or depth of the needle to place it immediately adjacent to the superior articular process should be made at this time. Once proper position has been established, this small needle is retracted while 5.0 cc of lidocaine 1% is instilled. The needle will traverse the lumbodorsal fascia, iliotransverse ligaments, and bands, which are sensitive; adequate local anesthesia is certainly helpful for patient cooperation. The maneuver with the 25-gauge needles serves several purposes: first, the depth to the superior articular process is established; second, the proper cephalocaudad angle can be selected; third, the regional tissues can be infiltrated with local anesthetic. If these goals are not accomplished with the first pass, the small needles may be reintroduced at a different angle with a minimum of trauma. This results in much less postprocedure discomfort than would occur if an 18- or 20-gauge guide needle were repeatedly introduced in order to establish proper position.

Disc puncture at L5-S1 by extrapedicular approach requires a double-needle technique. A guide needle is required because the procedure needle will be precurved to be directed into the nucleus of the disc. The use of an 18-gauge guide with 22-gauge procedure needle is advised until the technique is mastered. These heavier needles are fairly easy to control. A 20-gauge guide with 25-gauge procedure needles is less traumatic, but requires considerable finesse to control with precision (Fig. 9). The larger needles are required in obese or heavily muscled patients. On rare occasion, 6-inch 18-gauge guides and 10-inch 22-gauge procedure needles are necessary (for patients in excess of 300 pounds).

The optimum position of the guide needle is immediately adjacent to the anterolateral aspect of the superior articular process of the sacrum (Fig. 10A–C).

The procedure needle (6 inches) is precurved by hand. The tip should not be handled directly but should be wrapped in sterile gauze. The distal 2 to 3 cm of the needle is bent in a direction opposite the bevel. The amount of curve is based on operator preference and experience.

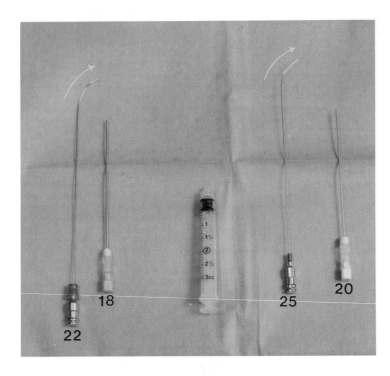

FIG. 9. Needles for disc puncture at L5-S1: 3.5-inch spinal needles (18- or 20-gauge) serve as guides; 6- or 5.5-inch procedure needles (22- or 25-gauge) are precurved at their tips *(white arrows)*.

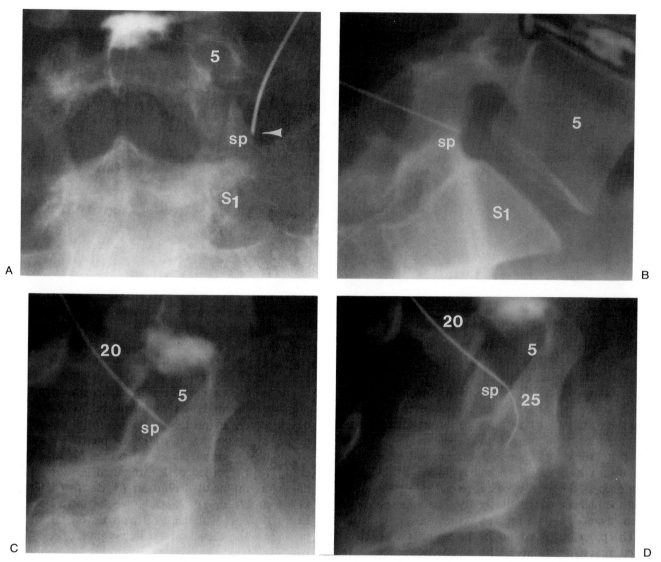

FIG. 10. A: Anteroposterior spot film of L5-S1 interspace. Tip of 20-gauge guide needle *(arrowhead)* lies immediately adjacent to the lateral margin of the superior articular process of S1 (sp). Note the bevel of the needle opens medially towards the interspace. **B:** Lateral spot film of L5-S1 interspace. Tip of the 20-gauge guide needle is adjacent to the anterior aspect of the superior process of S1 (sp). The angle of the needle is not perfect relative to the disc space but is satisfactory. **C:** Prone oblique spot film of L5-S1 interspace. Note the relationship of the guide needle to the superior process of S1 (sp). **D:** Prone oblique spot film of L5-S1 interspace. Tip of 25-gauge procedure needle is directed medially into the disc. The 20-gauge guide needle has been retracted slightly.

The procedure needle is then introduced into the guide needle and advanced. The inner needle may be difficult to advance because of the curve at its tip. It is necessary to secure the guide needle with one hand while advancing the inner needle with the other. This prevents the guide needle from being inadvertently advanced into the radicular canal.

The inner needle should be advanced slowly as it approaches the end of the guide needle. When the tip emerges, the bevels of the needles should be checked. The locking notch of the guide needle should be facing medially, opening the bevel toward the disc. The notch of the inner needle is 180° opposed.

With the patient in the oblique position, the inner needle is slightly advanced under direct fluoroscopic visualization. As it emerges, the guide needle is simultaneously retracted slightly. The result of this dual action is an unsheathing of the inner needle, which bows medially. The bevel and the curve of the needle direct it toward the disc space. Once the needle engages the annulus, it penetrates easily, moving toward the center of the disc (Fig. 10D). Position must be checked in both the frontal and lateral planes before injection (Fig. 11).

If the inner needle does not curve medially it will move forward, at best penetrating only the annulus, at worst contacting the L5 segmental nerve near the dorsal gan-

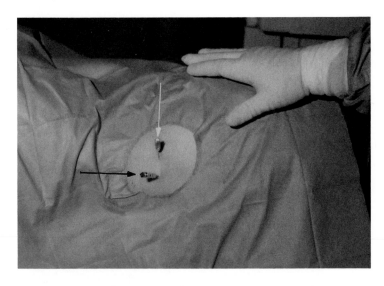

FIG. 11. Patient in left lateral decubitus position. Note the needle in the L4-L5 disc is directed vertically relative to the spine *(white arrow)*. The double needle system at L5-S1 (20/25-gauge) is angled caudally *(black arrow)*. In most instances, the skin puncture site for the L5-S1 approach is just medial to the puncture site for the L4-L5 approach.

glion or anterior ramus. This can be avoided by directly visualizing the emergence of the inner needle. If it does not curve medially, remove it and reform the curve. This problem is not common with 22-gauge needles, but is not rare with 25-gauge needles.

Should the procedure needle meet bony obstruction, the patient is turned to the lateral position to determine whether it has contacted the superior articular process or the vertebral endplate. If the needle has engaged the endplate, slight retraction and rotation will redirect the tip toward the disc. If the needle is blocked by the superior process, the inner needle is retracted into the guide and the pair are advanced slightly. The inner needle is then advanced and unsheathed as previously described.

This procedure is tedious for the beginner. Once mastered, it is quite effective, with a very high success rate even in large patients with deep-seated lumbosacral discs (Fig. 12) (162). Disc puncture employing CT for guidance as a primary procedure without use of fluoroscopy has been described (135). This technique is not yet in general use.

Syringes (3.0 cc) containing lidocaine 1%, bupivacaine 0.5% with Celestone or Depo-Medrol, and contrast material should be prepared prior to needle insertion. Although there is no contraindication to the use of the ionic contrast agent meglumine iothalamate (Conray) for discography, this agent is toxic if inadvertently instilled into the subarachnoid space (5). There are definite safety advantages in using non-ionic myelographic contrast agents (iohexol and iopamidol). It is prudent to use the safest available contrast material.

DISCOMETRY

Intrinsic disc pressure has been determined *in vitro* and *in vivo* (136,138). The intrinsic pressure within the disc varies, being lowest in the supine subject. Panjabi et al. (148) employed a standardized technique to evaluate the pressure/volume relationships (discometry) in 84 cadaveric discs. The intrinsic disc pressure is that pressure required to start flow of contrast material from the injection system into the nucleus (Fig. 13A). There is a direct relationship between intrinsic pressure and maximum pressure in normal discs. Quinnell and Stockdale (156) developed a standardized technique for *in vivo* evaluation of disc pressures. Intrinsic disc pressures in 40 discographically normal discs was less than 275 kPa. Walsh et al. (189) recorded peak intradiscal pressures in the discs of asymptomatic volunteers (30 discs) of 400 to 500 kPa using 22-gauge or 25-gauge needles and a 3-cc Luer-Lok syringe. It is difficult to maintain digital (thumb) pressure at these levels with a 3-cc syringe.

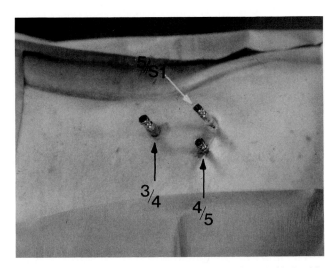

FIG. 12. Patient in prone position (viewed from left). In this large patient (5'9, 235 lb), 6-inch 22-gauge needles are advanced to their full length to reach the disc centers at L3-L4 and L4-L5 *(black arrows)*. Note the slightly medial position and relative caudal angulation of the 18/22-gauge double needle system employed to perform disc puncture at L5-S1.

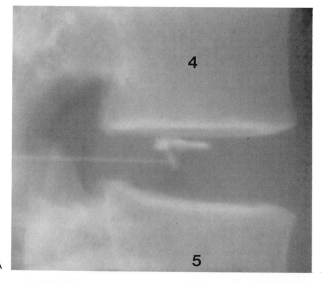

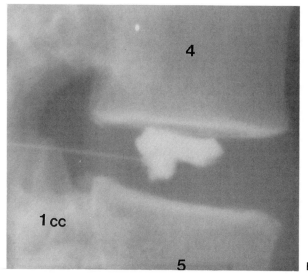

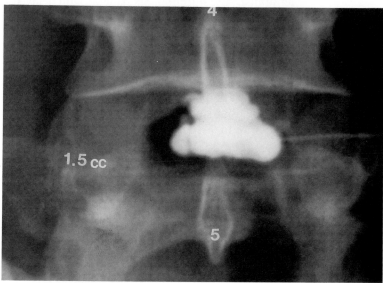

FIG. 13. **A:** Lateral spot film of L4-L5 disc: initial flow of contrast material into the nucleus. Direct fluoroscopic visualization verifies proper needle position in the nucleus. The pressure required to start flow into the nucleus is the intrinsic disc pressure. **B:** Lateral spot film of L4-L5 disc: 1.0 cc contrast material is easily instilled into the disc defining normal nuclear space, incompletely filled. **C:** Anteroposterior spot film of L4-L5 disc: rapid rise in resistance at volume of 1.5 cc. Additional volume of 0.5 cc to 1.0 cc can be instilled with increased pressure but refluxes back into the syringe when pressure is released. Resilience is a characteristic of the normal disc.

The normal disc accepts a limited volume of fluid varying from 1.5 to 2.5 cc (Fig. 13B,C) (1,41,157,186). The maximum pressure induced by a hand-held syringe is greater than intrinsic disc pressure but well below the maximum pressure of both normal and abnormal discs (85). When small-gauge needles and a 3.0-cc syringe are used, the procedure of disc injection is mechanically safe.

As fluid is instilled into the nuclear space, there is an outward bulge of the endplates and an overall increase in the width of the disc space. Endplate deflection (outward bulge) has been verified *in vitro* (72). This phenomenon is commonly observed in normal, asymptomatic discs. It is also observed in some symptomatic, minimally degenerate discs. This distraction of the vertebral bodies can be observed at fluoroscopy during disc injection in the lumbar area. Distraction results in a reduction of the disc circumference (20). The normal annulus does not bulge outward with injection.

Injection into the normal nucleus is accomplished by

gradually increasing thumb pressure on the syringe. The intrinsic disc pressure is easily overcome with a hand-held syringe, and contrast material flows into the nucleus. There is a rapid rise in pressure as the potential space of the nucleus is filled and the disc space height increased. Firm terminal resistance is encountered. Often there is resilience with recoil of the plunger of the syringe when pressure is released. It is important to fill the nucleus, but overfilling by applying excessive pressure is unnecessary. The tuberculin syringe does not hold sufficient contrast material to fill the lumbar intervertebral disc; 5.0-cc and 10.0-cc syringes require such digital pressure that there is a loss of the ability to note subtle changes in resistance and resilience. A 3.0-cc syringe is ideal for this procedure.

If firm resistance is encountered initially, the needle may be against the cartilage endplate or within the annulus itself. The position should be checked by fluoroscopy. Annular injection may or may not be painful. A pain response occurring with annular injection is not acceptable in the assessment of the disc. If any non-nuclear position is recognized, the needle should be manipulated into the nuclear region or removed and redirected to the nucleus (Fig. 14).

If there is little or no resistance to the injection of 1.0 cc of fluid, the injection should be observed under direct fluoroscopic visualization. Filling of venous structures or free spill into the epidural space is easily recognized (Fig. 15). Understanding the routes of communication between the injured disc and the surrounding spaces and neural structures is vital to proper interpretation of the studies (121,195). Pain response occurring during such injection may be evaluated but is not necessarily reliable.

PAIN RESPONSE

Accuracy in the interpretation of pain response at the time of injection is critical to the effective clinical use of discography. It is a great advantage to have a trained observer to aid in rating. Pain is an emotional response (123), and individuals respond to painful stimuli in different ways. It is not possible to completely standardize the interpretation of patient responses. Walsh et al.

(189) described a method of rating patient responses. The method includes:

1. Patient's self-reported pain intensity utilizing a visual analog scale.
2. Rater observation of pain behaviors (guarding/bracing/withdrawal, rubbing, grimacing, sighing, verbalizing).
3. Patient report of pain similarity to the chronic pain at the time of injection. The possible ratings are: (a) no pain; (b) similar, typical, or exact reproduction; and (c) different or atypical pain.

Pre- and postprocedure pain assessment is important in order to evaluate any analgesic effect resulting from instillation of local anesthetic into an abnormal disc. Analgesic response should be recorded prior to discharge.

Occasionally, patients develop severe pain shortly after lumbar disc injection. Six patients with delayed pain response to disc injection have been recently described (97). It is reasonable to delay the discharge of patients undergoing lumbar discography for several hours in order to observe this response. This is particularly important in patients with minimally painful disc injections and subtle annular abnormalities. The development of a pain response should prompt postinjection CT at that time, prior to discharge.

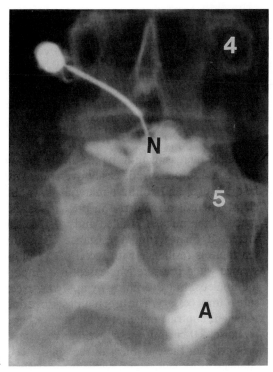
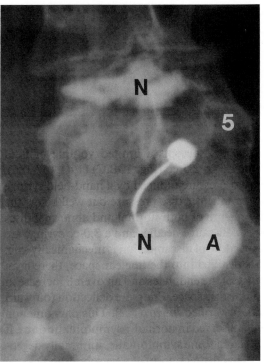

A

B

FIG. 14. A: Prone spot film lumbar discogram. Large patient (in excess of 300 lb). Initial attempt at L5-S1 disc puncture by right extrapedicular approach resulted in annular injection (A). The needles were removed. A posterior transdural approach to the L4-L5 disc was accomplished with 3.5-inch 18-gauge guide needle and a 7-inch 22-gauge procedure needle. This resulted in satisfactory filling of the nucleus (N). **B:** Posterior transdural approach with the same needle system was successful at L5-S1. The normal nucleus **(N)** and its relationship to the annular injection (A) is best visualized on the prone film.

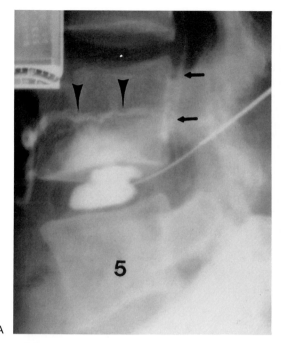
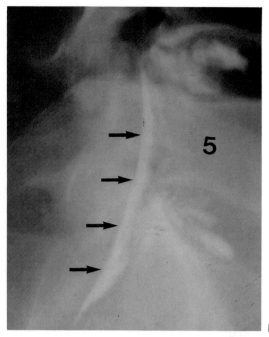

A

B

FIG. 15. A: Lateral spot film obtained during injection of L4-L5 disc. The nucleus is filled. Contrast material has flowed through the inferior L4 endplate into the vertebral marrow space. Anterior internal vertebral vein *(arrows)* and circumferential lumbar vein *(arrowheads)* are filled. There was little resistance to injection. **B:** Lateral spot film following disc injection. Epidural contrast material *(arrows)* flowed freely through the posterior annulus of the L5-S1 disc with no resistance.

NUCLEOGRAM

The appearance of the normal nucleus following contrast injection is unmistakable, with contrast confined to a central location within the interspace (Fig. 16). There are some normal variations in the size of the nuclear space (184). The shape of the normal nucleus is altered by extrinsic pressure. Lindblom (103) and Park (149) described shift in nuclear position with flexion and extension following discography. Schnebel et al. described a digitizing technique for study of the movement of contrast material within the disc with spinal motion (166). Discography accurately represents nuclear behavior of contrast material in the normal disc (Fig. 17).

The appearance of normal and abnormal discs has been classified by a number of authors (1,41,46,114). Not all abnormal patterns are associated with painful disc pathology. Common endplate lesions such as the limbus vertebra (59) can be identified but are rarely painful (63). Similarly, the Schmorl's node is frequently opacified with disc injection (102) but is rarely a symptomatic lesion (177). However, similar-appearing endplate abnormalities can be associated with painful disc pathology (81,115). Certain patterns are commonly associated with pain response. An example is contained radial fissures as described by Fraser et al. (52). Contrast material extends from the nucleus into the outermost annulus (Fig. 18). With disruption of the annular capsule, contrast material may spill freely into the epidural space (Fig. 19).

CT scanning after discography is discussed elsewhere in this text (Chapter 27). This is an integral part of the diagnostic disc infection. It is necessary if the study is to be complete and should be performed on any disc which is found to be painful on injection. The axial images verify that the injection has been performed into the nuclear

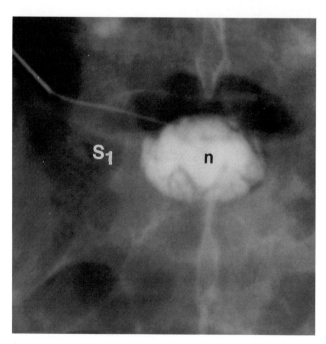

FIG. 16. Prone spot film L5-S1 discogram: 50-year-old woman, normal nucleogram, 1.5 cc, firm terminal resistance.

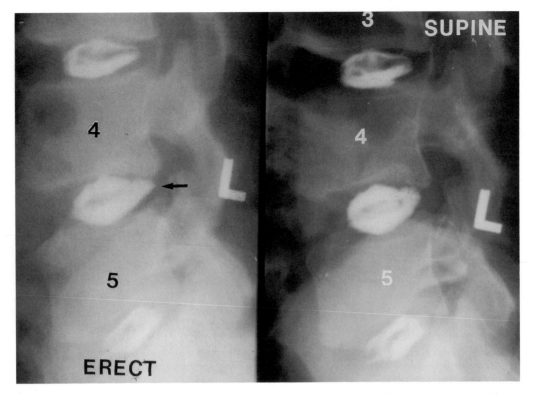

FIG. 17. Lateral spot film lumbar discography. Alteration of the nuclear configuration is most evident at the L4-L5 level. The change in configuration of the posterior nucleus *(arrow)* on the erect film is related to the increased axial load and is a normal phenomenon.

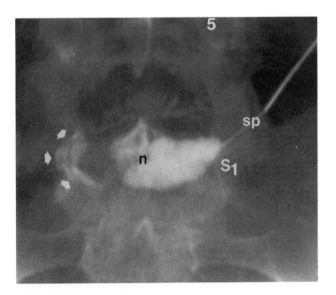

FIG. 18. Prone spot film of L5-S1 disc space. Nucleus (n) is filled. Note left outer annular fissure *(white arrows).*

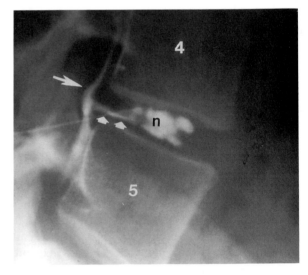

FIG. 19. Lateral spot film L4-L5 discogram. Nucleus (n) is filled. *Small arrows* denote radial annular fissure. *Large arrow* denotes protrusion and epidural contrast.

space (155). Numerous authors have reported on the value of postinjection CT in defining annular integrity (6,10,83,109,180), disc herniation (98,110,127,144), as a prelude to minimally invasive disc surgery (26,105, 130,131,174,182), and in repeat spinal surgery for recurrent herniation (11,79).

COMPLICATIONS

A variety of complications may occur. Many are iatrogenic and are likely related to the skill and experience of the operator (178). All patients should be screened for potential allergies. Neural injury is avoided by proper technique in a conscious but sedated patient.

The fear of disc space infection should be a major consideration of those who perform diagnostic disc puncture. The intervertebral disc is a large avascular structure with little ability to defend itself. Historically, discitis seems to have been rare or rarely reported. Collis and Gardner (31) report on 2,187 disc injections and mention only one intervertebral disc infection. Wiley et al. (192) reported a review of the literature revealing only 30 cases of discitis in approximately 5,000 disc injections. This is an incidence of 0.6% per disc.

Authors of major studies in the 1970s considered disc space infection a rare occurrence (21,117,170,196). Crock (35) suggested that the condition was more common than previously thought and postulated a chemical or aseptic etiology. A careful analysis of documented cases of discitis led Fraser et al. (54) to the conclusion that the diagnosis was underestimated for several reasons: (a) the long latent period between injections and onset of symptoms; (b) the lack of clinical contact between the patient and the radiologist; and (c) the lack of awareness on the part of clinicians.

The dominant characteristic of discitis is severe back pain, often accompanied by elevation of the sedimentation rate. Postoperative and postdiscographic clinical presentations are similar (13,54). Any postdiscogram patient with an increase in back pain or a change in the character of back pain should be evaluated clinically and a sedimentation rate obtained if there is any suspicion of postprocedure infection.

The development of new imaging technologies has changed the way the diagnosis is confirmed. Radionuclide scanning is more sensitive than routine radiographs (145). Though nonspecific in general, bone scans are very specific in a postdiscogram population (23) (Fig. 20). CT does play a role in the diagnosis of spine infection (73). Endplate destruction (osteolysis) is the earliest CT finding (65) (Fig. 21).

MRI is most effective in the detection of disc space infection (8,132). Szypryt et al. (176) evaluated MRI and radionuclide bone scanning in experimentally induced discitis in a rabbit model. MRI was superior with a 93% sensitivity, 97% specificity, and 95% accuracy overall.

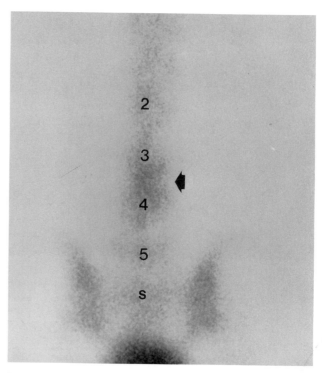

FIG. 20. Posterior camera view radionuclide bone scan (20 millicuries 99m Tc MDP). Lumbar/lumbosacral region of interest. Increased radionuclide localization at mid lumbar area *(arrow)*. Patient evaluated for increasing back pain following a three-level lumbar discogram 1 month earlier. The localizations suggest abnormality at the endplates of the L3-L4 motion segment. Sedimentation rate was elevated. No organism was cultured from blood or disc aspirate.

Twenty-two cases of discitis following disc puncture were evaluated by Agre et al. (4). In nine cases, the causative organism was isolated. *Staphylococcus aureus, S. epidermidis,* and *Escherichia coli* were the dominant organisms. In a series of nine patients with discitis after discography, Guyer et al. (69) reported positive culture in only two patients, both of whom were infected with *S. epidermidis.* The spectrum of organisms suggests inoculation with skin or surface organisms or technical misadventure (bowel perforation).

Fraser et al. (54) reviewed 432 cases and found an overall rate of infection of 2.3% per patient and 1.3% per disc. The study breaks down the incidence based on different techniques. The discitis incidence when 18-gauge needles without stylettes were employed was 2.7%. The incidence of infection fell to 0.7% when the same operator employed needles with stylettes and a double-needle technique. Fraser has recommended the use of a double-needle technique. The use of stylettes may be the most significant factor affecting the dramatic improvement in the rate of infection. The single-needle technique described earlier in this chapter has been employed for examination of approximately 2,000 patients between 1979 and 1989. We are aware of only one case

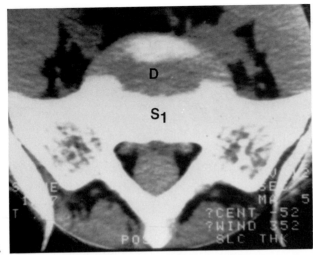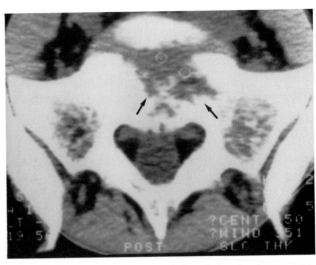

A   B

FIG. 21. A: Axial CT of L5-S1 junction: routine CT scan obtained during a work-up of chronic low back pain syndrome. Section demonstrates normal disc (D)/endplate (S1) interspace. **B:** Axial CT of L5-S1 junction: same patient, scan obtained 6 weeks following chemonucleolysis at L5-S1. Osteolysis of the superior S1 endplate is recognized by a geographic pattern of destruction *(arrows)*. Symptoms of increased back pain, elevated sedimentation rate, and an abnormal bone scan in conjunction with CT prompt the diagnosis of disc space infection. Blood culture and disc space aspiration revealed no organisms.

of acute postdiscographic discitis in that population (Fig. 22).

In the past 10 years, I have reviewed 17 cases of lumbar discitis. Two were spontaneous in onset with no disc intervention. Both were sterile on aspiration. The diagnosis was established by clinical findings and classic imaging findings, which were followed over time. Acute discitis occurring after discography and resulting from infection with virulent organisms (two cases of *E. coli,* one case of *S. aureus,* and one case of *Pseudomonas aeruginosa)* was associated with severe pain occurring within 48 hours of the procedure. These patients were septic. In each instance the diagnosis was established by culture (blood culture or disc aspiration).

In nine patients, including two from my practice, significant back pain did not develop until 2 weeks after the procedure. The diagnosis was established on clinical grounds, abnormalities of sedimentation rate, C-reactive protein, and imaging. Aspirations of the discs were negative. Three of these cases resolved spontaneously without antibiotics.

The studies of Fraser et al. on experimental discitis in a sheep model have provided convincing evidence that all discitis is initiated by infection (53). Once the endplates have been violated, the bacteria are rapidly removed by the patient's own defense systems.

The need to provide antibiotic coverage before or immediately after disc space infection has not yet been adequately evaluated. Fraser et al. feel that antibiotic infusion immediately prior to discography may have a

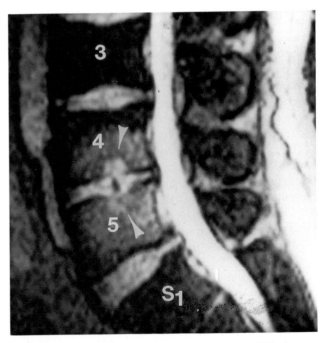

FIG. 22. Sagittal MRI of lower lumbar spine, 0.6 Tesla, gradient echo pulse sequence, 5.0-mm thick section. MRI was obtained 14 days after three-level diagnostic disc injection. A marked increase in back pain occurred 4 days following procedure. Sedimentation rate was elevated to 36 mm/hr at 6 days postprocedure. Blood culture 8 days following procedure revealed coagulase-positive *Staphylococcus aureus.* MRI demonstrates endplate destruction *(arrowheads)*, acute disc space narrowing, and altered signal in the adjacent marrow space of the involved vertebrae.

prophylactic effect (55). Strict adherence to aseptic techniques, including pre-procedure screening for potential chronic infection and utilization of pristine technique, will certainly keep the infection rate at a relatively low level. Following the recommendations of Osti et al. (146), I have added cefazolin to the contrast material employed for disc injection. The dose is low (less than 25 mg per cc of injectate). This technique has been used in over 250 patients, excluding those known to be allergic to the antibiotic. Over 620 discs in the cervical, dorsal, and lumbar regions have been injected in this manner. Careful follow-up in this group has detected no case of discitis.

For purposes of early diagnosis, it is a routine in my practice to provide patients with specific instructions as to what to expect in the immediate postprocedure period. Each is requested to maintain a pain journal over the 2-week interval following the procedure, and each is provided with a self-addressed stamped envelope. The patients are instructed to contact the clinic if their progress is different from that detailed in their postprocedure instructions. Any patient with increasing pain is evaluated clinically and blood work (CBC, sedimentation rate, and C-reactive protein) obtained. The sedimentation rate has been reported to be elevated in virtually all patients with discitis (47,104,181). However, there may be a form of infectious discitis that is less apparent clinically. Indolent infections caused by organisms of low virulence may account for less typical presentations of discitis, which might be overlooked (168). The actual incidence of such low-grade forms of discitis would be very difficult to determine.

DOES DISCOGRAPHY DAMAGE THE INTERVERTEBRAL DISC?

Discitis undoubtedly damages the intervertebral disc. In the absence of discitis, there does not appear to be significant evidence that discography is harmful.

The canine model has been employed to evaluate response to needle puncture and injection of various contrast agents. There is no convincing evidence that discography damages the canine disc (58,88,90,188).

There are a few histologic studies on human disc material removed surgically or at post mortem following diagnostic discography. None report significant inflammatory or pathologic changes to suggest disc damage (57,62,153).

It is unlikely that puncture of the disc annulus with a 22-gauge needle will result in herniation (56,74). Fernstrom, reporting some 1,500 disc injections, noted that six herniations occurred following discography that might be attributed to the procedure (48). Jayson et al. (85) studied bursting pressure. When the pressure is raised to the point of failure, failure occurs at the end-

plate and not through the disc annulus. Brinckmann (19) studied the effect of intradiscal injection on experimentally damaged discs. Intradiscal pressures such as those reached during diagnostic discography do not result in significant change in the disc bulge at the site of experimental annular injury. The disc annulus has limited healing potential. Trauma to the annulus should be kept at a minimum by using small-gauge needles and limiting the number of annular punctures (42).

Sporadic reports of patients undergoing repeat discography have appeared in the literature (67,113). Johnson (87) reported a retrospective analysis of 34 patients undergoing a second discogram at 80 lumbar levels. He concluded that there was no evidence that discography produced herniation of nuclear material or annular deterioration. The study did document the appearance of annular fissures in some previously normal-appearing discs. Johnson attributed these changes to factors other than discography, specifically the location of these discs adjacent to a solid fusion or compression fracture. Flanagan and Chung (50) surveyed a population of chemonucleolysis patients 10 to 20 years following their procedures. In this group, there were 36 patients in whom a normal discogram was obtained and no enzyme injected. The routine radiographs of these patients demonstrated no significant changes at these levels. The authors concluded that diagnostic discography of a normal disc does not initiate degenerative changes. On the basis of this combined evidence, it is reasonable to presume that diagnostic discography is a safe procedure in the absence of disc space infection.

DISC INJECTION: A STAGING PROCEDURE?

Several authors have employed discography in the selection of patients for surgical procedures (15,94,106, 107,143,164), reporting some success. The prospective study of Colhoun et al. (29) emphasizes the importance of pain response in selecting patients for surgery. Of the patients in whom discography revealed disc disease and provoked symptoms, 89% derived significant and sustained benefit from surgery; of patients who showed morphologic abnormality but no symptom provocation on discography, only 52% benefited.

Gill and Blumenthal reported 75% success rate for single-level anterior lumbar interbody fusion at the lumbosacral level in patients with positive discography as defined by pain provocation and abnormal disc morphology (fissure extending to the outer annulus) (61). The success rate for those patients whose discogram demonstrated a pattern defined as an inner annular fissure, not reaching the outer annulus, was only 50%. By contemporary standards, these should not be considered abnormal discograms. Disruption of the outer annulus is the major factor associated with primary discogenic pain

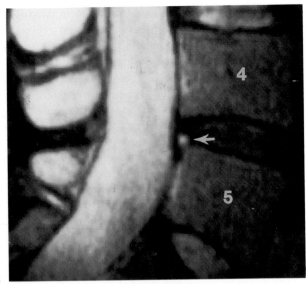 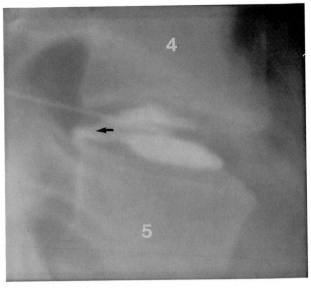

A

B

FIG. 23. A: Sagittal MRI of lower lumbar spine, SE T2-weighted image (TR 2000/TE 100). The L3-L4 and L5-S1 discs are normal. The L4-L5 disc is abnormal. Reduction of signal from the nuclear region reflects degradation of nuclear matrix. High signal intensity zone *(arrow)* within the posterior annular substance is consistent with an annular fissure or tear. There is no prolapse. B: Lateral spot film L4-L5 discogram. Nucleus is well organized. Posteroinferior radial annular fissure *(black arrow)* correlates with the lesion demonstrated on MRI scan. Injection provoked familiar pain.

(134). Primary discogenic pain is the cardinal feature of the internal disc disruption syndrome. The definitive diagnosis relies on two criteria: (a) provocation discography to reproduce the pain (36) and (b) CT/discography to reveal the internal disruption (10). These criteria have been for the Study of Pain in its taxonomy (124). The patients who did meet the criteria for the diagnosis of internal disc disruption fared better following the surgical procedure directed to that segment.

The primary purpose of diagnostic lumbar disc injection is the detection of painful abnormalities of the intervertebral disc. Modern imaging can detect annular pathology with great sensitivity (161,201). However, not all abnormalities are detected (200), and not all detected abnormalities are painful (189). Disc injection remains the sole procedure capable of correlating pathoanatomy and symptomatology (Fig. 23). It is the essential procedure to establish the diagnosis of primary discogenic pain (169).

REFERENCES

1. Adams MA, Dolan P, Hutton WC (1986): The stages of disc degeneration as revealed by discograms. *J Bone Joint Surg [Br]* 68: 36–41.
2. Adams MA, Hutton WC (1982): Prolapsed intervertebral disc. A hyperflexion injury. *Spine* 7:184–191.
3. Adams MA, Hutton WC (1985): Gradual disc prolapse. *Spine* 10: 524–531.
4. Agre K, Wilson RR, Brim M, et al. (1984): Chymodiactin postmarketing surveillance: demographic and adverse experience data in 29,075 patients. *Spine* 9:479–485.
5. Amundsen P (1979): The evolution of contrast media. In: Sackett J, Strother C, eds. *New techniques in myelography.* Hagerstown, Maryland: Harper & Row, pp. 2–5.
6. Antti-Toika I, Soini J, Tallroth K, et al. (1990): Clinical relevance of discography combined with CT scanning. A study of 100 patients. *J Bone Joint Surg [Br]* 72:480–485.
7. Aprill C, Bogduk N (1992): High intensity zones in the disc anulus: a sign of painful disc on magnetic resonance imaging. *Br J Radiol* 65:361–369.
8. Arrington JA, Murtagh FR, Silbiger ML, et al. (1986): Magnetic resonance imaging of post-discogram discitis and osteomyelitis in the lumbar spine: case report. *J Fla Med Assoc* 73:192–194.
9. Benoist M (1984): Positioning alternatives for chemonucleolysis: current concepts in chemonucleolysis. *J R Soc Med* 72:47–53.
10. Bernard T (1990): Lumbar discography followed by computed tomography. Refining the diagnosis of low back pain. *Spine* 15: 690–707.
11. Bernard T (1993): Repeat lumbar spine surgery. Factors influencing outcome. *Spine* 17:2196–2200.
12. Biondetti PR, Vigo M, Fiore D, et al. (1983): CT appearance of generalized von Recklinghausen neurofibromatosis. *J Comput Assist Tomogr* 7:866–869.
13. Bircher MD, Tasker T, Crashaw C, Mulholland RC (1988): Discitis following lumbar surgery. *Spine* 13:98–102.
14. Birney T, White J, Berens D, Kuhn G (1992): Comparison of MRI and discography in the diagnosis of lumbar degenerative disc disease. *J Spinal Disord* 5:417–423.
15. Blumenthal S, Baker J, Dossett A, Selby DK (1988): The role of anterior lumbar fusion for internal disc disruption. *Spine* 13:566–569.
16. Bogduk N (1991): The lumbar disc and low back pain. *Neurosurg Clin North Am* 2:791–806.
17. Bogduk N, Tynan W, Wilson AS (1981): The nerve supply to the human lumbar intervertebral disc. *J Anat* 132:39–56.
18. Brightbill T, Pile N, Eichelberger R, Whitman M (1994): Normal magnetic resonance imaging and abnormal discography in lumbar disc disruption. *Spine* 19:1075–1077.
19. Brinckmann P (1986): Injury of the annulus fibrosus and disc protrusions. *Spine* 11:149–153.
20. Brinckmann P, Horst M (1985): The influence of vertebral body fracture, intradiscal injection, and partial discectomy on the radial bulge and height of human lumbar discs. *Spine* 10:138–145.
21. Brodsky AE, Binder WF (1979): Lumbar discography. Its value in diagnosis and treatment of lumbar disc lesions. *Spine* 4:110–120.

22. Brown JE (1969): Clinical studies on chemonucleolysis. *Clin Orthop* 67:94–99.
23. Bruschwein DA, Brown ML, McLeod RA (1980): Gallium scintigraphy in the evaluation of disc-space infections: concise communications. *J Nucl Med* 21:925–927.
24. Buirski G (1992): Magnetic resonance signal patterns of lumbar discs in patients with low back pain. A prospective study with discographic correlation. *Spine* 17:1199–1204.
25. Buirski G, Silberstein M (1993): The symptomatic lumbar disc in patients with low back pain. Magnetic resonance imaging appearances in both a symptomatic and control population. *Spine* 18:1808–1811.
26. Castro W, Jerosch J, Happ R, Schulitz K (1992): Restriction of indication for automated percutaneous lumbar discectomy based on computed tomographic discography. *Spine* 17:1239–1243.
27. Cloward RB (1953): The treatment of ruptured lumbar intervertebral discs. *Am J Surg* 86:145–151.
28. Cloward RB, Busaid LL (1952): Discography. Technique, indications and evaluation of normal and abnormal intervertebral discs. *AJR* 68:552–564.
29. Colhoun E, McCall IW, Williams L, Cassar Pullicino VN (1988): Provocation discography as a guide to planning operations on the spine. *J Bone Joint Surg [Br]* 70:267–271.
30. Collins C, Stack J, O'Connell D, et al. (1990): The role of discography in lumbar disc disease: a comparative study of magnetic resonance imaging and discography. *Clin Radiol* 42:252–257.
31. Collis JS Jr, Gardner WJ (1962): Lumbar discography. An analysis of 1,000 cases. *J Neurosurg* 19:452–461.
32. Crawshaw C (1984): Needle insertion techniques for chemonucleolysis: current concepts in chemonucleolysis. *J R Soc Med* 72:55–59.
33. Crock HV (1970): A reappraisal of intervertebral disc lesions. *Med J Aust* 1:983–989.
34. Crock H (1981): Normal and pathological anatomy of the lumbar spinal nerve root canals. *J Bone Joint Surg [Br]* 63:47–49.
35. Crock H (1983): Practice of spinal surgery. New York: Springer-Verlag.
36. Crock H (1986): Internal disc disruption. A challenge to disc prolapse fifty years on. *Spine* 11:650–653.
37. Dabezies EJ, Murphy CP (1985): Dural puncture using the lateral approach for chemonucleolysis. *Spine* 10:93–96.
38. Day PL (1969): Lateral approach for lumbar diskogram and chemonucleolysis. *Clin Orthop* 67:90–93.
39. Dyck P (1985): Paraplegia following chemonucleolysis. A case report and discussion of neurotoxicity. *Spine* 10:359–362.
40. Edholm P, Fernstrom I, Lindblom K (1967): Extradural lumbar disc puncture. *Acta Radiol (Diagn) Scand* 6:322–328.
41. Erlacher PR (1952): Nucleography. *J Bone Joint Surg [Br]* 34:204–210.
42. Ethier D, Cain J, Yasemski M (1994): The influence of anulotomy selection on disc competence. A radiographic, biomechanical and histologic analysis. *Spine* 19:2071–2076.
43. Falconer MA, McGeorge M, Begg AC (1948): Observations on the cause and mechanism of symptom production in sciatica and low-back pain. *J Neurol Neurosurg Psychiatry* 11:13–26.
44. Farfan HF (1983): Mechanical disorders of the low back. Philadelphia: Lea and Febiger.
45. Farfan HF, Cossette JW, Robertson GH, Wells RV, Kraus H (1970): The effects of torsion on the lumbar intervertebral joints: the role of torsion in the production of disc degeneration. *J Bone Joint Surg [Am]* 52:468–497.
46. Feinberg SB (1964): The place of discography in radiology as based on 2320 cases. *AJR* 92:1275–1281.
47. Fernand R, Lee CK (1986): Postlaminectomy disc space infection. A review of the literature and a report of three cases. *Clin Orthop* 209:215–218.
48. Fernstrom U (1960): A discographical study of ruptured lumbar intervertebral discs. *Acta Chirurg Scand [Suppl]* 258:1–60.
49. Fischer HW, Redman HC (1971): Comparison of sodium methylglucamine diatrizoate contrast medium of minimal sodium content with a pure methylglucamine diatrizoate preparation. *Invest Radiol* 6:115–118.
50. Flanagan MN, Chung B (1986): Roentgenographic changes in 188 patients 10-20 years after discography and chemonucleolysis. *Spine* 11:444–448.
51. Franson R, Saal JS, Saal JF (1992): Human disc phospholipase A2 is inflammatory. *Spine* 17(Suppl):S190–S192.
52. Fraser J, McCall I, Park W, O'Brien J (1983): Discography in degenerating disc disease. *Orthop Trans* 7:466.
53. Fraser RD, Osti OL, Vernon-Roberts B (1986): Discitis following chemonucleolysis: an experimental study. *Spine* 11:679–687.
54. Fraser RD, Osti OL, Vernon-Roberts B (1987): Discitis after discography. *J Bone Joint Surg [Br]* 69:26–35.
55. Fraser RD, Osti OL, Vernon-Roberts B (1989): Iatrogenic discitis: the role of intravenous antibiotics in prevention and treatment. An experimental study. *Spine* 14(9):1025–1032.
56. Frieberg S (1941): Low back pain and sciatica by intervertebral disc herniation. Anatomical and clinical investigations. *Acta Chirurg Scand [Suppl]* 85:64.
57. Gardner WJ, Wise R, Hughes C, et al. (1952): X-ray visualization of the intervertebral disc with a consideration of the morbidity of disc puncture. *Arch Surg* 64:355–364.
58. Garrick JG, Sullivan CR (1970): Long-term effects of discography in dogs. *Minn Med* 53:849–850.
59. Ghelman B, Freiberger RH (1976): The limbus vertebra: an anterior disc herniation demonstrated by discography. *AJR* 127:854–855.
60. Gibson MJ, Buckley J, Mawhinney K, et al. (1986): Magnetic resonance imaging and discography in the diagnosis of disc degeneration. *J Bone Joint Surg [Br]* 68:369–373.
61. Gill K, Blumenthal S (1992): Functional results after anterior lumbar fusions at L5-S1 in patients with normal and abnormal MRI scans. *Spine* 17:940–942.
62. Goldie I (1957): Invertebral disc changes after discography. *Acta Chir Scand* 113:438–439.
63. Goldman A, Ghelman B, Doherty J (1990): Posterior limbus vertebrae: a cause of radiating back pain in adolescents and young adults. *Skeletal Radiol* 19:501–507.
64. Goldner JL, Urbaniak JR, McCullom DE (1971): Anterior disc excision and interbody fusion for chronic low back pain. *Orthop Clin North Am* 2:543–568.
65. Golimbu C, Firooznia H, Rafii I (1984): CT of osteomyelitis of the spine. *AJR* 142:159–163.
66. Greenspan A, Amparo E, Gorczyca D, Montesano P (1992): Is there a role for discography in the era of magnetic resonance imaging? Prospective correlation and quantitative analysis of computed tomography-discography, magnetic resonance imaging, and surgical findings. *J Spinal Disord* 5:26–31.
67. Gresham JL, Miller R (1969): Evaluation of the lumbar spine by discography and its use in selection of proper treatment of the herniated disc syndrome. *Clin Orthop* 67:29–41.
68. Gunzburg R, Parkinson R, Moore R, et al. (1992): A cadaveric study comparing discography, magnetic resonance imaging, histology, and mechanical behavior of the human lumbar disc. *Spine* 17:417–426.
69. Guyer RD, Collier R, Stith W, et al. (1988): Discitis after discography. *Spine* 13:1352–1354.
70. Haldeman S, Shouka M, Robboy S (1988): Computed tomography, electrodiagnostic and clinical findings in chronic worker's compensation patients with back and leg pain. *Spine* 13:345–350.
71. Hasue M, Kunogi J, Konno S, Kikuchi S (1989): Classification by position of dorsal root ganglia in the lumbosacral region. *Spine* 14(11):1261–1264.
72. Heggeness M, Doherty B (1993): Discography causes endplate deflection. *Spine* 18:1050–1053.
73. Hermann G, Mendelson DS, Cohen BA, Train JS (1983): Role of computed tomography in the diagnosis of infectious spondylitis. *J Comput Assist Tomogr* 7:961–968.
74. Hirsch C (1948): An attempt to diagnose level of disc lesion clinically by disc puncture. *Acta Orthop Scand* 18:131–140.
75. Hirsch C (1965): Efficiency of surgery in low back disorders. *J Bone Joint Surg [Am]* 47:991–1004.
76. Hirsch C, Inglemark BE, Miller M (1963): The anatomical basis for low back pain. *Acta Orthop Scand* 33:1–17.
77. Hitselberger WE, Whitten R (1968): Abnormal myelograms in asymptomatic patients. *J Neurosurg* 28:204–206.
78. Hoddick WK, Helms CA (1985): Bony spinal canal changes that differentiate conjoined nerve roots from herniated nucleus pulposus. *Radiology* 154:119–120.
79. Hodge J, Ghelman B, Schneider R, et al. (1994): Recurrent disc

versus scar in the postoperative patient: the role of computed tomography (CT)/discography and CT/myelography. *J Spinal Disord* 7:470–477.

80. Holt EP Jr (1968): The question of lumbar discography. *J Bone Joint Surg [Am]* 50:720–726.

81. Hsu KY, Zucherman JF, Derby R, et al. (1988): Painful lumbar end-plate disruptions: a significant discographic finding. *Spine* 13:76–78.

82. Inman VT, Saunders J (1947): Anatomicophysiological aspects of injuries to the intervertebral disc. *J Bone Joint Surg* 29:461–475.

83. Ito S, Yamada Y, Tsuboi S (1991): An observation of ruptured annulus fibrosis in lumbar discs. *J Spinal Disord* 4:462–466.

84. Jaffray D, O'Brien JP (1986): Isolated intervertebral disc resorption. A source of mechanical and inflammatory back pain? *Spine* 11(4):397–401.

85. Jayson MI, Herbert CM, Barks JS (1973): Intervertebral discs: nuclear morphology and bursting pressure. *Ann Rheum Dis* 32:308–315.

86. Johansen JG, Nestvold K, Sortland O (1988): Extraspinal pathology and incidental disc herniation in patients with sciatica. *Spine* 13(4):437–439.

87. Johnson RG (1989): Does discography injure normal discs? An analysis of repeat discograms. *Spine* 14(4):424–426.

88. Kahanovitz N, Arnoczky SP, Sissons HA, et al. (1986): The effect of discography on the canine intervertebral disc. *Spine* 11:26–27.

89. Keck C (1960): Discography. Technique and interpretation. *Arch Surg* 80:580–585.

90. Key JA, Ford LT (1948): Experimental intervertebral disc lesions. *J Bone Joint Surg [Am]* 30:621–630.

91. Kitano T, Zerwekh J, Usui Y, et al. Biochemical changes associated with the symptomatic human intervertebral disc. *Clin Orthop* 293:372–377.

92. Konings JG, Veldhuizen AG (1988): Topographic anatomical aspects of lumbar disc puncture. *Spine* 13(8):958–961.

93. Kornberg M (1989): Discography and magnetic resonance imaging in the diagnosis of lumbar disc disruption. *Spine* 14(12):1368–1372.

94. Kozak J, O'Brien J (1990): Simultaneous combined anterior and posterior fusion. An independent analysis of a treatment for the disabled low back pain patient. *Spine* 15:322–328.

95. Kumar AJ, Kuhajada FP, Martinez CR, et al. (1983): Computed tomography of extracranial nerve sheath tumors with pathological correlation. *J Comput Assist Tomogr* 7:857–865.

96. Laredo J, Busson J, Wybier M, Bard M (1988): Technique of lumbar chemonucleolysis. In: Bard M, Laredo J, eds. *Interventional radiology in bone and joint.* New York: Springer-Verlag, pp. 101–122.

97. Lehmer S, Dawson M, O'Brien J (1994): Delayed pain response after lumbar discography. *Eur Spine J* 3:28–31.

98. Lejeune J, Hladky J, Cotten A, et al. (1994): Foraminal lumbar disc herniation. Experience with 83 patients. *Spine* 19:1905–1908.

99. Lindblom K (1944): Protrusions of the discs and nerve compression in the lumbar region. *Acta Radiol Scand* 25:195–212.

100. Lindblom K (1948): Diagnostic puncture of the intervertebral discs in sciatica. *Acta Orthop Scand* 17:231–239.

101. Lindblom K (1950): Technique and results in myelography and disc puncture. *Acta Radiol Scand* 34:321–330.

102. Lindblom K (1951): Discography of dissecting transosseous ruptures of the intervertebral discs in the lumbar region. *Acta Radiol Scand* 36:12–16.

103. Lindblom K (1951): Technique and results of diagnostic disc puncture and injection (discography) in the lumbar region. *Acta Orthop Scand* 20:315–326.

104. Lindholm TS, Pylkkanen P (1982): Discitis following removal of intervertebral disc. *Spine* 7:618–622.

105. Linson MA, Crowe CH (1990): Comparison of magnetic resonance imaging and lumbar discography in the diagnosis of disc degeneration. *Clin Orthop* 250:160–163.

106. Linson M, Williams H (1991): Anterior and combined anteroposterior fusion for lumbar disc pain. A preliminary study. *Spine* 16:143–145.

107. Loguidice VA, Johnson RG, Guyer RD, et al. (1988): Anterior lumbar interbody fusion. *Spine* 13:366–369.

108. Loneragen R, Khangure M, McCormick C, Hardcastle P (1994): Comparison of magnetic resonance imaging and computed tomographic discography in the assessment of lumbar disc degeneration. *Aust Radiol* 38:6–8.

109. Maezawa S, Muro T (1992): Pain provocation at lumbar discography as analyzed by computed tomography/discography. *Spine* 17:1309–1315.

110. Marron J, Kopitnik T, Schulhof A (1990): Diagnosis and microsurgical approach to far lateral disc herniation in the lumbar spine. *J Neurosurg* 72:378–382.

111. Marshall LL, Trethewie ER, Curtain CC (1977): Chemical radiculitis. *Clin Orthop* 129:61–67.

112. Masaryk TJ, Ross JS, Modic MT, et al. (1988): High resolution MR imaging of sequestered lumbar intervertebral disc. *AJR* 150:1155–1162.

113. Massare C (1970): Reflexions sur la discographie après 500 cas. *J Radiol d'Electrol Med Nucleaire* (Paris) 51:571–574.

114. Massare C, Benoist M, Cauchoix J (1973): Le diagnostique des hernies discales lombaires et lombo-sacree interet de la discographie. *Revue de Chirurgie Orthopedique et Repatrice de L'Appareil Moteur (Paris)* 59:61–67.

115. McCall IW, Park WM, O'Brien JP, Seal V (1985): Acute traumatic intraosseous disc herniations. *Spine* 10:134–137.

116. McCarron RF, Wimpee MW, Hudkins PG, Laros GS (1987): The inflammatory effect of nucleus pulposus. *Spine* 12:760–764.

117. McCulloch JA (1977): Chemonucleolysis. *J Bone Joint Surg [Br]* 59:45–52.

118. McCulloch JA (1980): Chemonucleolysis: experience with 2,000 cases. *Clin Orthop* 136:128–135.

119. McCulloch JA, Waddell G (1978): Lateral lumbar discography. *Br J Radiol* 51:498–502.

120. McFadden JW (1988): The stress lumbar discogram. *Spine* 13:931–933.

121. McMillan J, Schaffer J, Kambin P (1991): Roots and incidence of communication of lumbar discs with surrounding neural structures. *Spine* 16:167–171.

122. McRae D (1955): Asymptomatic intervertebral disc protrusions. *Acta Radiol* 46:9–27.

123. Mersky H (1979): Pain terms: a list with definitions and notes on usage. Recommended by the I.A.S.P. Subcommittee on Taxonomy. *Pain* 6:249–252.

124. Mersky H, Bogduk N (1994): *Classification of chronic pain descriptions of chronic pain syndromes and definitions of pain terms.* Seattle: IASP Press, pp. 180–181.

125. Meyer GA, Haughton VM, Williams AL (1979): Diagnosis of lumbar herniated disc with computed tomography. *N Engl J Med* 301:1166–1167.

126. Milette PC, Melanson D (1982): A reappraisal of lumbar discography. *Journal de L'Association Canadienne des Radiologistes* 33:176–182.

127. Milette P, Raymond J, Fontane S (1990): Comparison of high resolution computed tomography with discography in the evaluation of lumbar disc herniations. *Spine* 15:525–533.

128. Mixter WJ, Barr JS (1934): Rupture of the intervertebral disc with involvement of the spinal canal. *N Engl J Med* 211:210–215.

129. Miyamoto M, Takemitsu Y, Harada Y, Iwahara T (1991): A case of recurrent extra-foraminal lateral lumbar disc herniation occurring at the same level and on the opposite site. *Spine* 16:996–998.

130. Mochida J, Alima T (1993): Percutaneous nucleotomy in lumbar disc herniation. A prospective study. *Spine* 18:2063–2068.

131. Mochida J, Toh E, Nishimura K (1993): Percutaneous nucleotomy in lumbar disc herniation. Patient selection and roles in various treatments. *Spine* 18:2212–2217.

132. Modic MT, Feiglin D, Pirano D, et al. (1985): Vertebral osteomyelitis: assessment using MR. *Radiology* 157:157–166.

133. Modic MT, Pavlicek W, Weinstein M (1984): Magnetic resonance imaging of intervertebral disc disease. *Radiology* 152:103–111.

134. Moneta G, Videman T, Kaivanto K, et al. (1994): Reported pain during lumbar discography as a function of anular ruptures and disc degeneration. A re-analysis of 833 discograms. *Spine* 19:1968–1974.

135. Murtagh F, Arrington J (1992): Computed tomographically guided discography as a determinant of normal disc level before fusion. *Spine* 17:826–830.

136. Nachemson A (1960): Lumbar intradiscal pressure. *Acta Orthop Scand Suppl* 43:1–104.

137. Nachemson A (1969): Intradiscal measurements of pH in patients with lumbar rhizopathies. *Acta Orthop Scand* 40:23–42.

138. Nachemson A, Elfstrom G (1970): Intravital dynamic pressure measurement in lumbar discs. *Scand J Rehabil Med Suppl* 1:1–40.

139. Nachemson A, Morris J (1964): In vivo measurements of intradiscal pressure. *J Bone Joint Surg [Am]* 46:1077–1092.

140. Naylor A (1962): The biophysical and biochemical aspects of intervertebral disc herniation and degeneration. *Ann R Coll Surg* 31:91–114.

141. Nazarian S (1985): Anatomical basis of intervertebral disc puncture with chemonucleolysis. *Anat Clin* 7:23–32.

142. Neave V, Wycoff R (1983): Computed tomography of cystic nerve root sleeve dilatation. *J Comput Assist Tomogr* 7:881–885.

143. Newman M, Grinstead G (1992): Anterior lumbar interbody fusion for internal disc disruption. *Spine* 17:831–833.

144. Ninomiya M, Muro T (1992): Patho-anatomy of lumbar disc herniation as demonstrated by computed tomography, discography. *Spine* 17:1316–1322.

145. Norris S, Ehrlich MG, Keim DE, et al. (1978): Early diagnosis of disc space infection using gallium-67. *J Nucl Med* 19:384–386.

146. Osti O, Fraser R, Vernon-Roberts B (1990): Discitis after discography. The role of prophylactic antibiotics. *J Bone Joint Surg [Br]* 72:271–274.

147. Osti O, Frasier D (1992): MRI and discography of annular tears and intervertebral disc degeneration. A prospective clinical comparison. *J Bone Joint Surg [Br]* 74:431–435.

148. Panjabi M, Brown M, Lindahl S, Istram L, Hermens M (1988): Intrinsic disc pressure as a measure of integrity of the lumbar spine. *Spine* 13(8):913–917.

149. Park W (1976): Radiologic investigation of the intervertebral disc. In: Jayson MIV, ed. *The lumbar spine and back pain*, 2nd ed. Bath, England: Pittman Medical Publishing, pp. 185–230.

150. Park WM, McCall IW, O'Brien JP, Webb JK (1979): Fissuring of the posterior annulus fibrosus in the lumbar spine. *Br J Radiol* 52:382–387.

151. Patrick BS (1975): Extreme lateral ruptures of the lumbar intervertebral discs. *Surg Neurol* 3:301–304.

152. Pease CN (1935): Injuries to the vertebrae and intervertebral discs following lumbar puncture. *Am J Dis Child* 49:849–860.

153. Perey O (1950): Contrast medium examination of intervertebral discs of the lumbar spine. *Acta Orthop Scand* 20(4):327–334.

154. Peyster R, Teplick G, Haskin M (1985): Computed tomography of lumbosacral conjoined nerve root anomalies. A potential cause of false-positive reading for herniated nucleus pulposus. *Spine* 10(4):331–337.

155. Quinnell R, Stockdale J (1980): An investigation of artifacts in lumbar discography. *Br J Radiol* 53:831–839.

156. Quinnell RC, Stockdale H (1980): Pressure standardized lumbar discography. *Br J Radiol* 53:1031–1036.

157. Quinnell RC, Stockdale HR, Willis DS (1983): Observations of pressures within normal discs in the lumbar spine. *Spine* 8(2):166–169.

158. Rauschning W (1987): Normal and pathologic anatomy of the lumbar root canals. *Spine* 12(10):1008–1019.

159. Reicher M, Gold R, Halbach V, Rauschning W, et al. (1986): MR imaging of the lumbar spine: anatomic correlations and the effect of technical variations. *AJR* 147:891–898.

160. Roofe PG (1940): Innervation of the annulus fibrosus and posterior longitudinal ligament. *Arch Neurol Psychiatry* 44:100–103.

161. Ross JS, Modic MT, Masaryk TJ (1989): Tears of the annulus fibrosus: assessment with Gd-DTPA-enhanced MR imaging. *AJNR* 10:1251–1254.

162. Sach B, Spivey M, Vanharanta H, et al. (1990): Techniques for lumbar discography and computed tomography/discography in clinical practice. *Orthop Rev* 19:775–778.

163. Sackett J, Strother C (1979): *New techniques in myelography*. Hagerstown, Maryland: Harper & Row.

164. Schechter N, France M, Lee C (1991): Painful internal disc de-

165. Schmorl G, Junghanns H (1959): *The human spine in health and disease*. New York, London: Grune and Stratton.

166. Schnebel BE, Simmons JW, Chowning J, Davidson R (1988): A digitizing technique for the study of movement of intradiscal dye in response to flexion and extension of the lumbar spine. *Spine* 13(3):309–312.

167. Schneiderman G, Flannigan B, Kingston S (1987): Magnetic resonance imaging in the diagnosis of disc degeneration: correlation with discography. *Spine* 12:276–281.

168. Schofferman L, Schofferman J, Zucherman J, Gunthorpe H (1989): Occult infections causing persistent low-back pain. *Spine* 14(4):417–419.

169. Schwarzer A, Aprill C, Derby R, et al. (1995): The prevalence and clinical features of internal disc disruption in patients with chronic low back pain. *Spine* 20 *(in press)*.

170. Simmons EH, Segil CM (1975): An evaluation of discography in the localization of symptomatic levels in discogenic disease of the spine. *Clin Orthop* 108:57–69.

171. Simmons J, Aprill C, Dwyer A, Brodsky A (1988): A reassessment of Holt's data on "The question of lumbar discography." *Clin Orthop* 237:120–124.

172. Simmons J, Emory S, McMillin J, et al. (1991): Awake discography. A comparison study with magnetic resonance imaging. *Spine* 16(Suppl 6):S216–S221.

173. Smith L, Brown JE (1967): Treatment of lumbar intervertebral disc lesions by direct injection of chymopapain. *J Bone Joint Surg [Br]* 49:502–519.

174. Solini A, Paschero B, Ruggieri N (1991): Automated percutaneous lumbar discectomy according to the Onic method: conclusive considerations. *Ital J Orthop Traumatol* 17:225–236.

175. Steindler A, Luck J (1938): Differential diagnosis of pain low in the back: allocation of the source of pain by procaine hydrochloride method. *JAMA* 110:106–113.

176. Szypryt E, Hardy J, Hinton C, Worthington B, Mulholland R (1988): A comparison between magnetic resonance imaging and scintigraphic bone imaging in the diagnosis of disc space infection in an animal model. *Spine* 13(9):1042–1048.

177. Takahashi K, Takata K (1994): A large painful Schmorl's node: a case report. *J Spinal Disord* 7:77–81.

178. Tallroth K, Soni J, Antti-Toika I, et al. (1991): Premedication and short term complications in iohexol discography. *Ann Chir Gynaecol* 80:49–53.

179. Taylor TK, Akeson WH (1971): Intervertebral disc prolapse: a review of morphologic and biochemic knowledge concerning the nature of prolapse. *Clin Orthop* 76:54–79.

180. Tervonin O, Lahde S, Rydberg J (1990): Lumbar disc degeneration. Correlation between CT and CT discography. *Acta Radiol* 31:551–554.

181. Thibodeau AA (1968): Closed space infection following removal of lumbar intervertebral disc. *J Bone Joint Surg [Am]* 50:400–410.

182. Tournade A, Patay Z, Tajahmady T, et al. (1991): Contribution of discography to the diagnosis and treatment of lumbar disc herniation. *J Neuroradiol* 18:1–11.

183. Troisier O (1982): Technique de la discographie extra-durale. *J Radiol* 63:571–578.

184. Tsuji H, Yoshioka T, Sainoh H (1985): Developmental balloon discs of the lumbar spine in healthy subjects. *Spine* 10:907–911.

185. Tuohimaa PJ, Melartin E (1970): Neurotoxicity of iothalamates and diatrizoates. II: Historadioautographic study of rat brains with 131-iodine-tagged contrast media. *Invest Radiol* 5:22–29.

186. Vanharanta H, Sach BL, Ohnmeiss DD, April C, et al. (1989): Pain provocation and disc deterioration by age. A CT/discographic study in a low back pain population. *Spine* 14(4):420–423.

187. Videman T, Nummi P, Battié M, Gill K (1994): Digital assessment of MRI for lumbar disc desiccation. A comparison of digital versus subjective assessments and digital intensity profiles versus discogram and macro-anatomic findings. *Spine* 19:192–198.

188. Wakano K, Kasman R, Chao EY, Bradford DS, Oegema TR

rangements of the lumbar spine: discographic diagnosis and treatment by posterior lumbar interbody fusion. *Orthopedics* 14:447–451.

(1983): Biomechanical analysis of canine intervertebral discs after chymopapain injection: a preliminary report. *Spine* 8:59–68.

189. Walsh T, Weinstein J, Spratt K, Lehmann T, Aprill C, Sayre H (1990): The question of lumbar discography revisited: a controlled perspective study of normal volunteers to determine the false-positive rate. *J Bone Joint Surg [Am]* 72:1081–1088.

190. Watt C (1977): Complications of chemonucleolysis for lumbar disc disease. *Neurosurgery* 1:2–5.

191. Weinstein J, Claverie W, Gibson S (1988): The pain of discography. *Spine* 13(12):1344–1348.

192. Wiley J, McNab I, Wortzman G (1968): Lumbar discography and its clinical applications. *Can J Surg* 11:280–289.

193. Williams AL, Haughton VM, Daniels DL, Grogen JP (1983): Differential CT diagnosis of extruded nucleus pulposus. *Radiology* 148:141–148.

194. Williams A, Haughton V, Meyer G, Ho K (1982): Computed tomographic appearance of the bulging annulus. *Radiology* 142:403–408.

195. Wiltse L, Fonseca A, Amster J, et al. (1993): Relationship of the dura, Hoffman's ligaments, Batson's plexus, and a fibrovascular membrane lying on the posterior surface of the vertebral bodies and attaching to the deep layer of the posterior longitudinal ligament. An anatomical, radiologic, and clinical study. *Spine* 18:1030–1043.

196. Wiltse LL, Widdell ER Jr, Yuan HA (1975): Chymopapain chemonucleolysis in lumbar disc disease. *JAMA* 231:474–479.

197. Wise RE, Weiford EC (1951): X-ray visualization of the intervertebral disc. Report of a case. *Cleve Clin Quart* 18:127–130.

198. Yasuma T, Makino E, Saito S, et al. (1986): Histological development of intervertebral disc herniation. *J Bone Joint Surg [Am]* 68:1066–1072.

199. Yoshizawa H, O'Brien JP, Smith WT, Trumper M (1980): The neuropathology of intervertebral discs removed for low back pain. *J Pathol* 132:95–104.

200. Yu SW, Haughton VM, Sether LA, Wagner M (1989): Comparison of MR and discography in detecting radial tears of the annulus: a post-mortem study. *AJNR* 10:1077–1081.

201. Yu SW, Sether LA, Ho PS, Wagner M, Haughton VM (1988): Tears of the annulus fibrosus: a correlation between MR and pathologic findings in cadavers. *AJNR* 9:367–370.

202. Yussen P, Swartz J (1993): The acute lumbar disc herniation: imaging diagnosis. *Semin Ultrasound CT MRI* 14(6):389–398.

203. Zucherman J, Derby R, Hsu K, et al. (1988): Normal magnetic resonance imaging with abnormal discography. *Spine* 13(12):1355–1359.

The Adult Spine: Principles and Practice,
2nd edition, J.W. Frymoyer, Editor-in-Chief.
Lippincott-Raven Publishers, Philadelphia © 1997.

CHAPTER 29

Magnetic Resonance Imaging of the Spine

Scott D. Boden, Roland R. Lee, and Richard J. Herzog

"What we observe is not nature in itself, but nature exposed to our method of questioning." Werner Heisenberg (209)

It frequently requires many years to evaluate the significance of a major scientific discovery. The phenomenon of magnetic resonance (MR) was first reported by Bloch (35) and Purcell (421) in 1946, but it was not until the early 1970s that Damadian (72) and Lauterbur (291) were able to construct images utilizing this technique. It quickly became apparent that the strength of magnetic resonance imaging (MRI) resided in its excellent soft tissue contrast resolution, direct multiplanar imaging, lack of ionizing radiation, and the potential capacity to directly characterize pathologic tissue (28,127,203,249,380). From 1970 to the present, there has been a continual stream of new technological advances (14,51,58,60,61,128, 132,157,163,215,260,272,282,293,434,469,498,502, 505,560,570,591) transforming the initial crude MR images into the current superb MRI examination.

The evolution of spinal imaging began with plain film radiography and was followed by axial tomography, myelography, discography, epidural venography, arteriography, radionuclide scanning, sonography, and computed tomography (216). The challenge in diagnostic imaging of the spine resides in the spine's complex osseous and soft tissue anatomy along with the myriad of disease processes that can affect it. The initial enthusiasm that MRI would be able to elucidate all facets of spinal pathomorphology thus obviating the need for other imaging studies has not yet been realized. In many imaging centers, MRI has quickly become the primary imaging modality in the evaluation of spinal dysfunction (30, 205,313,543) even though there have been few rigorous, prospective, controlled comparative studies to evaluate the true diagnostic efficacy of MRI examinations (93).

The purpose of this chapter is to define the current application of MRI in the evaluation of different pathologic processes involving the spine. Its perspective is based on imaging the spine with both high field strength (1.5 Tesla) and mid field strength (0.5 Tesla) MRI systems. In order to understand the current and potential applications of MRI, a fundamental knowledge of MRI physics is needed, but not until MRI is performed on a regular basis can the true nuances of MR imaging be un-

S. D. Boden, M.D.: Associate Professor of Orthopaedic Surgery, Director, The Emory Spine Center, Emory University School of Medicine, Decatur, Georgia 30033.

R. R. Lee, M.D.: Assistant Professor, Department of Radiology, Johns Hopkins Medical Institutions, Baltimore, Maryland 21287.

R. J. Herzog, M.D.: Medical Director, San Francisco Neuro Skeletal Imaging, San Francisco Spine Institute, Daly City, California 94105.

derstood. After a basic discussion of the physics and technical considerations relevant to MRI, the remainder of the chapter will concentrate on its clinical applications.

PHYSICS AND TECHNIQUE

An image of an object may be defined as a graphical representation of the spatial distribution of one or more of its properties (291). Whereas an image created using an x-ray source is the result of the electron density of the tissue being evaluated, MR images are a construct of totally different physical properties of tissue. If a nucleus of an atom contains either unpaired protons or neutrons, it will have a net spin and angular momentum (72). Each spinning nucleus will be surrounded by a magnetic field, and it can be thought of as a small bar magnet, or dipole, with a north and south pole. In the absence of an external magnetic field, all the magnetic dipoles in the body are randomly oriented, and thus there is no measurable net magnetization of the body. If a body is placed in a static external magnetic field, i.e., the MR magnet, the nuclear dipoles will align themselves along the vector of the externally applied magnetic field. By the laws of quantum mechanics, the magnetization vector of each nucleus (of spin $\frac{1}{2}$, such as hydrogen) will either be aligned antiparallel to the vector of the static field, this being the higher energy or excited state, or it will be aligned parallel to the static field, this being the lower energy or ground state. The parallel orientation, a lower energy level than the antiparallel, will be slightly favored after the body is placed in the external magnetic field, resulting in a slight excess of dipoles aligned parallel to the vector of the external magnetic field. The net magnetization vector of the tissue, which is the summation of all the dipoles, will thus be in the same direction as the applied static magnetic field, and this is considered the equilibrium state of the tissue.

When the spinning nuclei are aligned in the external magnetic field, they also precess (wobble) around the axis of the applied magnetic field. The frequency of this nuclear precession is called its resonant frequency and is proportional to the strength of the external magnetic field. At present, virtually all clinical MR imaging is performed by imaging hydrogen nuclei (proton imaging). Hydrogen is an ideal atom for imaging, comprising approximately two-thirds of all atoms in the body. It is the most abundant resonant nucleus in soft tissues and provides a strong MR signal. Other nuclei, such as sodium and phosphorus, may be imaged using high field strength systems but currently these images are of poor diagnostic quality. Magnetic field strength is measured in Tesla (T) units. MR field strength is broadly characterized as ultralow (less than 0.1 Tesla), low (0.1 to 0.3 Tesla), mid (0.3 to 0.6 Tesla), and high (0.6 Tesla or greater).

To create an MR image, radio waves of a specific radio frequency (RF) are pulsed into the body, which induces the transition of a fraction of the spinning protons from the lower into the higher energy state. With the termination of the RF pulse, the excited nuclei release energy and return to the lower energy state. This characteristic absorption and release of energy is called nuclear magnetic resonance. The transition between energy states is necessary for the construction of an MR image.

The process of returning from the excited to the equilibrium state is called relaxation and is characterized by two independent time constants, T1 and T2. T1 (longitudinal relaxation time) reflects the time required for excited protons aligned antiparallel to the main magnetic field to return to their parallel orientation. In time T1, 63% will return to their initial state; and in three T1, 95% will return to the equilibrium state. The T1 of most biologic tissue is in the range of 200–2,000 milliseconds (206).

When the hydrogen nucleus is excited by the application of an RF pulse, in addition to changing to a higher energy state, the initially random precession of the nuclei before excitation will become coherent, i.e., in phase, after excitation. This results in transverse magnetization which can be directly measured by a receiver coil. With the termination of the RF pulse, there is rapid loss of coherence of the precessing nuclei, and the T2 (transverse relaxation time) is the time reflecting the loss of the transverse magnetization. T2 relaxation is not affected by field strength and in most biologic tissue is in the range of 20–300 milliseconds (206).

T1 and T2 relaxation are intrinsic physical properties of tissue (60). The MR signal intensity is mainly dependent upon the T1, T2, and proton density, i.e., number of mobile hydrogen ions, of the tissue being evaluated. Flow also affects the signal intensity generated by body fluids (54,348,433). To obtain an anatomic image, spatial encoding of the energy released by the excited protons must be obtained in three anatomic planes. This is accomplished by creating small gradient magnetic fields within the larger static applied field. There are several excellent texts that describe this process in detail (57,72,353).

The imaging techniques for obtaining MR data are termed pulse sequences. Spin-echo (SE), inversion recovery (IR), saturation recovery (SR), and gradient-echo (GE) are currently the pulse sequences most often employed. Spin-echo pulse sequences are probably the most commonly used technique and are defined by TR and TE values. The repetition time (TR), the time between RF pulses, and the echo time (TE), the time between the application of the RF pulse and the time of recording the MR signal, are determined at the time of image acquisition. By varying the imaging parameters TR and TE, the relative contribution of T1, T2, and proton density of the tissue being evaluated will determine image contrast (55,210). A T1-weighted sequence, which emphasizes the T1 properties of the tissue, can be produced with a short TR (400–600 milliseconds) and short TE (5–30 milliseconds). A pulse sequence with a long TR (1,500–2,000 milliseconds) and short TE (5–30 milliseconds) is referred to as a proton-density or spin-density weighted sequence, and the signal intensity in the image reflects the absolute number of mobile hydrogen nuclei in the tissue being evaluated. A T2-weighted sequence, which emphasizes the T2 properties of the tissue, requires a long TR (1,500–3,000 milliseconds) and long TE (60–120 milliseconds). Multiecho sequences can be obtained using a long TR coupled with a short and long TE. This results in two sets of images: a proton-density weighted SE image from the long TR/short TE and a T2-weighted SE image resulting from the long TR/long TE.

Contrast resolution depends upon the difference in luminance between objects; therefore, differences in signal intensity are critical in contrast evaluation. The signal intensity and tissue characterization of both normal and abnormal tissue will depend upon the pulse sequences employed (Table 1).

T1-weighted images are ideal for evaluating structures containing fat, subacute or chronic hemorrhage, or proteinaceous fluid because these materials have a short T1 and yield a high signal on T1-weighted sequences. In some circumstances, calcification may appear T1-bright (213). T1-weighted images, frequently thought of as fat images, have the highest signal-to-noise ratio and are excellent in the delineation of anatomic structures and soft tissue interfaces.

The signal intensity on T2-weighted images is related to the state of hydration of the tissue being imaged. Free water or extracellular water has a long T1 and T2, and on T2-weighted sequences there is increase in signal intensity in any tissue which is rich in free or extracellular water, e.g., cerebrospinal fluid, cysts, necrotic tissue, fluid collections, intervertebral discs, and neoplasms. A great percentage of the water in soft tissues, e.g., muscle, is intracellular and has a shorter T1 and shorter T2 when compared to tissues primarily composed of extracellular water. As a result, signal intensity from soft tissue is usually intermediate between fat and cerebrospinal fluid. Hyaline cartilage is rich in extracellular water bound to a mucopolysaccharide matrix and has relaxation characteristics similar to cellular tissue with intermediate signal intensity on most MR sequences. Tissue with less water content and a higher concentration of collagen fibers, e.g., fibrocartilage, has a long T1 and very short T2 and, therefore, has a low signal intensity on both T1- and T2-weighted sequences similar to other tissue containing collagen, e.g., tendons and ligaments. Mineral rich tissue, e.g., bone, contains few mobile protons and consequently demonstrates very low signal intensity on all pulse sequences. Gas, having a density one-thousandth that of solids and liquids, will generate no MR signal. T2-weighted sequences are most helpful in evaluating tissue with increased fluid content, commonly seen in a variety of pathologic processes including ischemia, infarction, infection, neoplasm, and trauma.

Proton-density images are particularly useful in the evaluation of ligamentous structures and articular cartilage (187). Because of the wide variety of tissue types evaluated in spinal MR imaging, the typical examination will include T1-, proton-density, and T2-weighted sequences. With the wide choice of imaging parameters, there is also a wide spectrum in the appearance of normal and abnormal tissue. This is particularly evident with the development and application of fast scanning (gradient-echo) techniques (56,142,562).

It is not just signal intensity that differentiates normal from abnormal tissue, but also tissue and organ configuration. Spatial resolution, the ability to delineate fine detail, is determined by slice thickness, field of view (FOV), and the size of the acquisition and display matrices. Ideally, when imaging small structures, thin sections with a large matrix (256 × 256 or up to 512 × 512) should be utilized, but unfortunately MRI faces rather

TABLE 1. *Tissue and body fluid signal intensity on T1- and T2-weighted images*

Tissue or body fluid	T-1 weighted	T-2 weighted
Cortical bone	Low	Low
Tendons and ligaments	Low	Low
Fibrocartilage	Low	Low
Hyaline cartilage	Intermediate	Intermediate
Muscle	Intermediate	Intermediate
Non-neoplastic tumor	Low-intermediate	Low-intermediate (Occasionally high)
Neoplastic tumor	Low-intermediate	Intermediate-high (Occasionally low)
Free water (CSF)	Low	High
Proteinaceous fluid (abscess)	Intermediate	High
Adipose tissue	High	Intermediate-high
Hemorrhage	Variable	Variable

severe signal-to-noise constraints, and image degradation may result from low signal-to-noise ratios, S/N.

Improved spatial resolution can be achieved by using surface coils, with their higher signal-to-noise ratio, but at a cost of a smaller field of view, and a limited depth of visualization into the body (272,282). Fortunately, however, this presents no real limitation for spine imaging, because the structures of interest lie close to the posterior skin surface. Hence, essentially all present-day spine MRI protocols use posterior surface coils to receive the MR signals.

Furthermore, recent development of "phased-array" surface coils have solved the problem of small field of view in the rostrocaudal direction, by coupling many (4 to 6) such coils in a longitudinal array (444). This enables almost the entire spine (48 cm) to be imaged in a single acquisition, with good resolution (using a 512×512 matrix), rather than imaging the cervical, thoracic, and lumbar regions separately (Fig. 1).

To improve the signal-to-noise ratio (S/N), one may increase the signal by increasing the number of RF excitations, but this significantly lengthens the exam time and increases the risk of image degradation due to patient motion.

Another way to improve S/N is to reduce the noise. Surface coils, as described above, are one way to achieve this. Another method is to decrease the bandwidth over which the MR signals are received (571); most commercial MR manufacturers provide this variable-bandwidth option, especially useful for T2-weighted sequences.

Data acquisition in MRI is usually performed using a two-dimensional (2D) technique in which multiple adjacent images are simultaneously acquired. A small gap is usually present between successive images. Direct multiplanar images can be obtained without moving the patient, but a separate data acquisition set must be performed for each image plane. Three-dimensional (3D) acquisition techniques are also available, where any desirable imaging plane can be reconstructed from an initial volume of acquired data (498). This is currently the standard means of acquiring axial thin-section images of the cervical spine, where the relatively small size of the anatomic structures of interest mandates contiguous thin-section images (552,607).

As in all imaging procedures, artifacts can be a potential source of image degradation with significant loss of diagnostic information. The four general types of artifacts that can degrade MR images are: (a) static field artifacts, (b) RF magnetic field artifacts, (c) gradient artifacts, and (d) motion artifacts (14,25,30,541,543). The importance of specific artifacts will be covered in the clinical discussions where the artifact may obscure or mimic a disease process. Motion artifacts are probably the most common cause of image degradation for all types of MRI studies. Unlike CT, where patient motion results in degradation of a single image, movement causes degradation of all the MR images in a sequence; long scan times tend to promote the likelihood of movement artifacts. In order to decrease scan time, many fast-scanning methods have been developed, of which gradient-echo imaging was an early one. It currently has greatest utility in 3D-volumetric thin-section axial images of the cervical spine (552,607). The information obtained from gradient-echo sequences cannot be considered a simple replacement for the standard T1- and T2-weighted sequences, particularly in the evaluation of spinal cord pathology (562). Gradient-echo scans also tend to be more prone to artifacts from tissue and magnetic field inhomogeneity, and from motion (553).

A major development in fast-scanning, particularly useful in spine MRI, has been the RARE (Rapid Acquisition Relaxation Enhanced) sequence and variations thereupon, also known as fast spin-echo or turbospin-echo, first proposed by Hennig et al. (214,368). This sequence gives good T2-weighted contrast in a fraction of the time required for a true spin-echo acquisition, permitting better resolution and signal-to-noise than previously possible in reasonable imaging times (generally taking only a few minutes per sequence, rather than about 10 minutes for a true T2-weighted acquisition). RARE images exhibit less magnetic susceptibility sensitivity than true spin-echo images (247,368), which is an advantage in minimizing osteophytic bony artifacts (Fig. 2), and (to some extent) in reducing artifact from metal

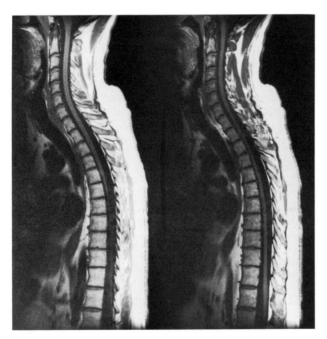

FIG. 1. Phased-array surface coil image of the entire spinal cord. Two contiguous 3-mm sagittal images using a 48 cm field of view and a 512×512 matrix (0.9 mm resolution) demonstrate superb resolution of the entire cord (C1 to L1) in a single 4-minute acquisition.

hardware (532). Possible disadvantages of RARE include bright signal from fat-containing structures, and decreased sensitivity to hemosiderin-containing blood products, as well as some blurring of images (172,214, 247,368).

Recent development of 3D RARE sequences promises thin-section, contiguous, high-resolution T2-weighted images which may be reconstructed in any plane, from a single relatively rapid acquisition.

The final step in the process of creating an MR image involves image display. Image display is rarely discussed in articles that describe MRI examinations, but it is frequently this last component of the MRI study that may cause the greatest loss of diagnostic information. Unlike CT where each gray scale value represents a single physical parameter, electron density, the digital gray scale values in an MR image are a construct of several physical parameters. Most MRI studies are photographed at one gray scale setting thus limiting the evaluation of the dynamic range of tissue contrast in the composite image. Because of the great range of contrast between normal and abnormal tissue, the selection of a single optimal gray scale representation is frequently difficult, particularly if the photographic process is controlled by a technologist who does not completely understand the pathomorphologic changes that are being evaluated.

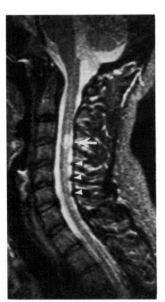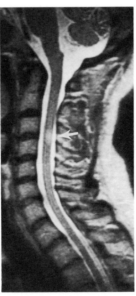

A,B

FIG. 2. The susceptibility artifact associated with small posterior degenerative osteophytes on the conventional T2-weighted image (**A**, small arrowheads), is significantly reduced on the fast-spin-echo (RARE) image (**B**). Note the improved signal-to-noise due to more acquisitions attainable with the RARE image (B), which was acquired in 3 minutes, as opposed to 7 minutes for (A). There is improved conspicuity between the cord and CSF due to magnetization transfer effect intrinsic in the RARE technique. However, the small patch of demyelination (large arrowhead) is more conspicuous on the conventional spin-echo image.

Various normalization algorithms are available to compensate for nonuniform signal intensities, such as the non-linear sensitivity inherent in surface coil receiver characteristics.

In order to appreciate the full dynamic range of the gray scale in the acquired image, an MR image optimally should be evaluated on a high resolution video display monitor which, with image manipulation, can easily display the full depth of gray scale values (18,125,228). Multiple monitors are needed to evaluate an entire MRI examination, and computer software is currently being developed which facilitates rapid evaluation of the MR images. Picture archival and communication systems (PACS) (45,158,178,231,304,311,336) allow for storage of all the digital MR data and for simultaneous viewing of the MRI study at multiple sites facilitating the consultative process. In the near future, this will improve the interpretation and communication of MRI evaluations.

SPINAL EXAMINATION PROTOCOLS

In order to maximize the information obtained from any imaging procedure, standard protocols must be developed for all diagnostic examinations. Only with a fixed, well-defined protocol is it possible to fine tune the quality of the examination and to be able to implement and assess the diagnostic efficacy of new technological advances. The optimal MRI examination of the spine is characterized by: (a) excellent contrast between neighboring structures, (b) maximum spatial resolution, (c) minimum noise and artifacts, (d) minimum acquisition time, and (e) adequate coverage. The primary imaging parameters that control the quality of the MRI examination include the pulse sequence employed (spin echo, gradient-echo, inversion recovery, etc.), the sequence parameters (TR, TE, flip angle, etc.), field of view (FOV), matrix size, slice thickness, and number of excitations (NEX) (55,400,433). The MRI exam must be tailored for the unique anatomy of the different parts of the spinal column. It is often tempting to shorten an imaging study when trying to answer a specific clinical question, but in the evaluation of spinal diseases, clinical symptoms and physical signs of neural dysfunction may not be easily localized to a specific motion segment (7,277,403) and can also be elicited by a variety of pathologic processes. For this reason, it is critical that in each spinal region evaluated, all spinal and paraspinal anatomy be completely examined and optimally displayed using sagittal, axial, and, when appropriate, additional nonorthogonal imaging sequences.

Before undergoing the MRI examination, each patient must be carefully questioned to determine if there are any contraindications to performing the study (254,495). Absolute contraindications include ferromagnetic cerebral aneurysmal clips (253,271), cardiac pacemakers, which may become dysfunctional in high magnetic fields (395), metallic foreign bodies in the orbit (261), and ferromagnetic cochlear or ocular implants. Pregnancy (252), recent cardiac or vascular surgery, transcutaneous electrical nerve stimulators, and severe claustrophobia are relative contraindications which must be managed on an individual basis to determine whether the benefit of the study outweighs the risk. There is no longer major concern of excessive heat production from ferromagnetic prostheses (495) as long as standard imaging times are maintained, and sequences with excessive gradient switching are avoided. Artifacts can be expected from a variety of metallic instrumentation devices (495) and from metallic particles in the body from previous trauma or surgery (207). It is difficult to predict the degree of image degradation from metallic devices, and frequently an MRI study will be helpful even in patients with spinal instrumentation. Titanium implants cause less artifact than steel (468).

Considering that the most frequent cause of image degradation is related to patient motion, the time of each imaging sequence and the total exam time should be kept to a minimum. Most patients can remain motionless for an imaging sequence of up to 12 to 14 minutes, and most current sequences should take significantly less time than this. The total exam time should be kept under one hour. Patient education concerning the nature of the study before the exam will frequently alleviate pretest anxiety and significantly reduce the number of exams that must be repeated or terminated (333). In one study, psychological preparation which included relaxation strategies was shown to be more effective in reducing anxiety during MR imaging than only providing patients with instructional information (425). Sedation is frequently given to pediatric patients (19,36,83,105,232) and occasionally will be needed with adults. Intravenous sedation should be used only if the patient can be closely monitored both during and after the examination is completed.

CERVICAL SPINE PROTOCOLS

One of the greatest challenges of MR spinal imaging is in the evaluation of the cervical spine. Due to its complex geometry and the small size of its anatomic components, imaging with high resolution surface coils is required (160). Thin sections (3–3.5 mm) with a small interslice gap in both axial and sagittal planes are necessary to delineate the normal neural structures in the spinal central and intervertebral canals (556). Considering that all intervertebral canals in the spinal column have a vertical and horizontal dimension as well as length (5 mm in the cervical to 12 mm in the lumbar) (31), the "canals" are a three-dimensional structure and should not be designated as "foramina."

The routine exam of the cervical spine must include both T1- and T2-weighted sequences to adequately evaluate all spinal and paraspinal anatomy (315,400,543). With high signal-to-noise and minimal cerebrospinal fluid (CSF) pulsation artifacts, T1-weighted images offer an excellent delineation of the cervical anatomy. A sagittal T1-weighted sequence covering from the cervicomedullary junction to the cervicothoracic junction provides an excellent survey of the vertebral bodies, intervertebral discs, spinal cord, thecal sac, and posterior elements (315). Axial T1-weighted sequences provide excellent evaluation of spinal cord morphology, intrathecal nerve root anatomy, vertebral bodies, posterior elements, intervertebral canals, and paraspinal soft tissues. However, conspicuity between CSF and degenerated disc or osteophytes is poor, so a T2-weighted gradient-echo sequence is necessary. To evaluate four disc levels on an axial sequence, it may be necessary to use a slightly longer TR to obtain adequate coverage. The slightly longer TR will yield a more proton-density weighted image, but will not compromise the quality of the anatomic delineation. On axial images, matrix size must always be optimized to achieve maximum anatomic detail (98).

The main limitation of the T1-weighted sequence is the lack of signal from the vertebral body cortex, the posterior annular-posterior longitudinal ligament complex, and the CSF in the adjacent thecal sac, resulting in poor differentiation between these structures (380). This makes the evaluation of small disc herniations, chondroosseous spurs, and hypertrophied or calcified ligaments extremely difficult. In order to achieve a contrast difference between the posterior margin of the discovertebral joint and the thecal sac, some form of T2-weighting (whereby the CSF is bright) is desired (357).

On standard T2-weighted sequences, CSF generates high signal intensity with a resultant CSF myelographic effect (144). The CSF–extradural interface is fairly well defined, as is the delineation of the spinal cord. The RARE (fast-spin-echo) sequence mentioned above gives a T2-weighted image with even better delineation of CSF from cord (at least partially due to an effect known as magnetization transfer [334]), and less susceptibility artifact from osseous/calcified structures than standard T2-weighted sequences. Furthermore, because of its more efficient use of imaging time, the RARE sequence can obtain both higher resolution and better signal-to-noise (more acquisitions) than conventional spin-echo imaging (247,460,532). (Fig. 2).

Unfortunately, due to the longer time required to generate conventional T2-weighted images, and due to the method in which the RARE sequence reconstructs images, the CSF pulsations in the cervical region and involuntary patient motion may cause significant artifacts which may degrade image quality (30,88,247,532). Cardiac gating, flow compensation, and special pulse sequences may decrease artifacts from pulsatile CSF

vertebral bodies and may occasionally detect cervical spine disease presenting as thoracic neural dysfunction (501). The initial sequence evaluating the thoracic spine consists of a sagittal T1-weighted localizer which includes an area from the cervicothoracic junction to the conus medullaris and may be obtained with the body coil or better, with a phased-array coil to achieve adequate coverage. This is followed by high resolution sagittal T1-weighted and flow compensated or cardiac-gated conventional or RARE T2-weighted sequences (Fig. 5). A surface coil is used to achieve high spatial resolution, and its field of view will usually be adequate to include an area from T1 or T2 to approximately T10 or T11. Using a phased-array surface coil, the entire cervicothoracic spine can be imaged in one acquisition, with excellent resolution. Sagittal sequences provide an excellent screening evaluation of thoracic anatomy and the pathologic processes affecting the vertebral bodies, intervertebral discs, and central spinal canal (307,457,586).

After the completion of the sagittal sequences, the examination should be reviewed by a radiologist to determine whether additional axial sequences are needed. These are obtained when a pathologic process is identified or if the patient's symptomatology suggests a specific location of a disease process, even though this area may appear normal on the initial sagittal images. This is particularly true in the evaluation of the intervertebral canals, paravertebral soft tissues, and posterior elements of the vertebrae which are not adequately evaluated utilizing only sagittal sequences (415). It is helpful to place lipid markers on the skin as localizers for the area of interest, but this should not preclude obtaining the initial sagittal sequence of the cervical spine which assures accurate numbering of the thoracic vertebral levels.

When performing axial sequences, thin sections should be obtained with a small interslice gap. T1-weighted images are used to evaluate thoracic cord anatomy, the central and intervertebral canals, vertebral body, and paravertebral soft tissues. Axial gradient-echo images or T2-weighted RARE images are helpful in the delineation of disc herniations and in evaluating degenerative changes which may encroach upon the central or intervertebral canals. Standard or RARE T2-weighted sequences are the primary imaging modality in the evaluation of spinal cord pathology.

In addition to the routine sequences, a coronal T1-weighted sequence is also frequently helpful in the evaluation of the spinal cord, extradural masses, scoliosis, and congenital anomalies. In some centers working predominantly with tumor patients, the initial screening study may also include an inversion recovery sequence which provides excellent delineation of abnormal vertebral marrow (124). Fast-spin-echo (RARE) inversion recovery gives good contrast in a fraction of the time. Fat-saturated RARE T2 and especially conventional T1-weighted images also depict abnormal marrow well (248). T2-weighted gradient-echo imaging has been particularly useful for myeloma (13). Chemical shift fat saturation T1 imaging has been useful to evaluate metastatic disease (554).

In summary, the standard screening MRI examination of the thoracic spine includes sagittal T1-weighted scout sequences of the cervical spine and thoracic spine down to the conus medullaris, followed by high resolution sagittal T1-weighted and flow compensated or cardiac gated conventional or RARE T2-weighted sequences. Selected axial T1-weighted or gradient-echo or T2-weighted sequences are obtained in areas of detected or clinically suspected abnormalities.

LUMBAR SPINE PROTOCOLS

Compared to the cervical and thoracic spine, the anatomic differences in the lumbar spine that directly affect the quality of MR images include: (a) the larger size of osseous, ligamentous, and cartilaginous components, (b) an increased volume of the thecal sac, and (c) increased epidural fat. To optimally evaluate the lumbar spine, sagittal T1 and sagittal and axial multi-echo T2-weighted sequences should be obtained. If fast-spin-echo (RARE) sequences are available, T1 and multi-echo RARE T2-weighted images should be obtained in the sagittal plane, followed by axial T1 and RARE T2 images (Figs. 6,7).

FIG. 4. Normal cervical spine anatomy. On the sagittal T1-weighted image (**A**), there is excellent anatomic delineation of the vertebral bodies, intervertebral discs (small black arrows), and spinal cord (white arrow). On the sagittal cardiac gated T2-weighted image (**B**), a myelographic effect is created by the increased signal intensity in the cerebrospinal fluid. There is an excellent interface between the posterior margin of the discovertebral joints (arrows) and the cerebrospinal fluid along with excellent delineation of the spinal cord. On the axial T1-weighted image (**C**), there is excellent delineation of the spinal cord (white arrow), ventral (short black arrow) and dorsal (long black arrow) nerve roots, and the intervertebral canals (curved black arrow). On the oblique T1-weighted image (**D**), the fat in the intervertebral canals outlines the neural (arrow) and vascular structures. On the axial gradient-echo image (**E**), a CSF myelographic effect is identified. The high signal intensity of the CSF produces excellent contrast for the delineation of the spinal cord (long arrow) and the posterior margin of the discovertebral joint (short arrow).

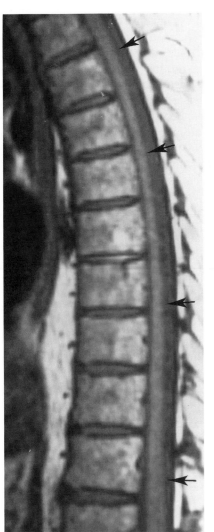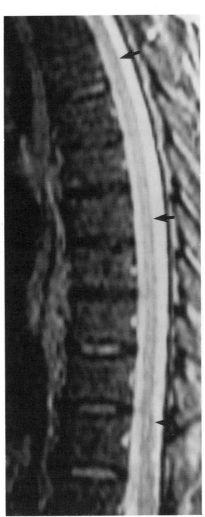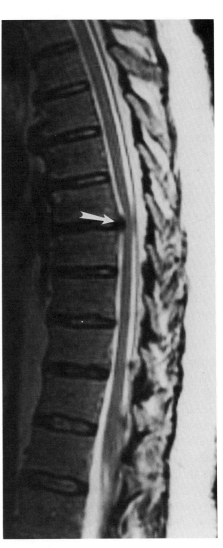

A,B   C

FIG. 5. Normal thoracic spine anatomy. On the sagittal T1-weighted image (**A**), there is excellent delineation of the vertebral bodies, intervertebral discs, and spinal cord (arrows). On the sagittal T2-weighted image (**B**), as a result of the myelographic effect, there is an excellent CSF-extradural interface and delineation of the thoracic spinal cord (arrows). On another patient (**C**), RARE (fast-spin-echo T2) sequence demonstrates increased conspicuity between cord and CSF compared to (B), and requires only about half the acquisition time. A disc protrusion resulting in cord deformity is well visualized (arrow).

As mentioned in the section on cervical spine imaging, gradient-echo images are inferior to T2-weighted images, especially given the availability of RARE sequences, which negate the only advantage of gradient-echo imaging (short imaging times). A further disadvantage of gradient-echo sequences in the lumbar spine is large chemical shifts (575). High resolution surface coils are standard for all lumbar exams (126), and the field of view on the sagittal sequences should include the area from the thoracolumbar junction, including the conus medullaris, to the sacrum (Fig. 8).

The high signal intensity of fat on T1-weighted images provides excellent contrast for the delineation of both normal spinal components and pathologic changes. Sagittal T1-weighted images are optimal in the evaluation of spinal anatomy, medullary bone, discovertebral joints, intervertebral canals, facet joints, thecal sac, conus medullaris, and the extradural space. Axial T1-weighted images provide excellent delineation of the thecal sac, extradural space, facet joints, ligamenta flava, nerve roots, intervertebral canals, and paraspinal soft tissue.

A major shortcoming of the T1-weighted axial image is poor conspicuity between the dark CSF and the dark desiccated disc annulus/herniation, which is the most common pathology presented on MR spine studies. For this reason, axial T2-weighted images are essential, with bright CSF clearly outlining the dark disc bulges/herniations, and dark nerve roots—the myelographic effect. A conventional multiecho axial sequence will give both the true T2-weighted myelographic image, as well as a

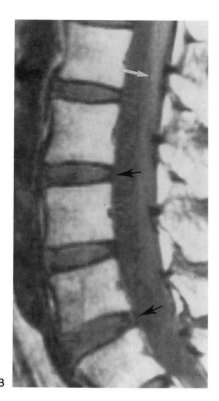
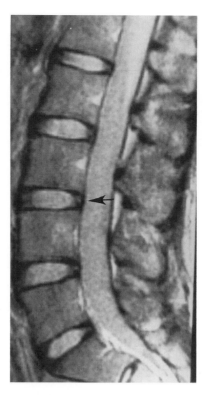
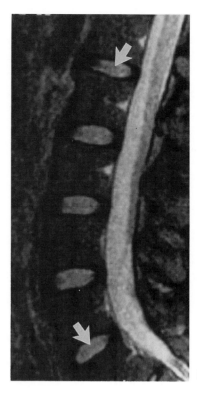

A,B

C

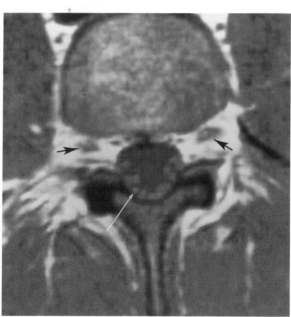

D

FIG. 6. Normal lumbar spine anatomy. On the sagittal T1-weighted image (**A**), there is excellent delineation of the vertebral bodies, intervertebral discs, thecal sac, lower thoracic cord, and conus medullaris (white arrow). The high signal intensity of the vertebral bodies is secondary to the fat in the cancellous marrow. The discs are slightly hyperintense with respect to the cerebrospinal fluid, but there is not a well-defined interface between the posterior outer annular fibers (black arrows) and the cerebrospinal fluid. On the sagittal proton-density weighted image (**B**), increased signal intensity in the disc is identified and increased signal intensity of the cerebrospinal fluid. This results in improved delineation of the posterior annular–posterior longitudinal ligament complex (arrow). On the sagittal T2-weighted image (**C**), increased signal intensity in the disc is identified along with a linear horizontal area of decreased signal intensity in the center of the disc representing the intranuclear cleft (arrows). There is increased signal intensity in the cerebrospinal fluid creating a myelographic effect and providing an excellent CSF-extradural interface. On the axial T1-weighted image (**D**), there is excellent delineation of individual nerve roots (long white arrow) in the thecal sac. The presence of fat in the extradural space and intervertebral canals provides an excellent soft tissue interface to evaluate nerve roots (short black arrows), ligaments, and osseous elements.

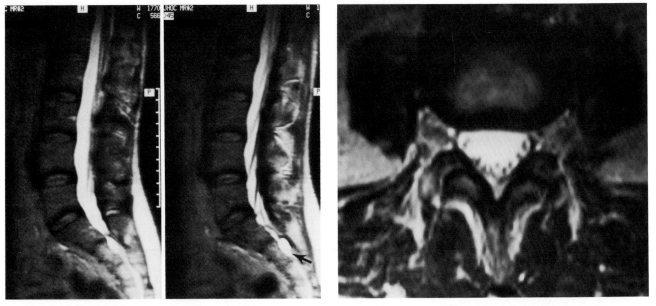

FIG. 7. Normal lumbar spine anatomy on RARE sequences. Consecutive 4-mm sagittal images (**A**) and axial image (**B**) show excellent delineation of nerve roots and normal anatomy, in a fraction of the time required for a conventional T2-weighted sequence such as Figure 6C. Incidental sacral Tarlov cyst (arrow) is noted in (A). Normally hydrated (T2-bright) discs are well demonstrated in both sagittal and axial planes.

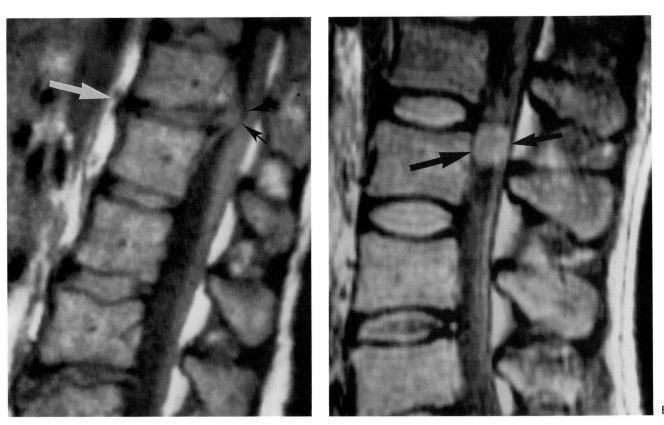

FIG. 8. On the sagittal T1-weighted image (**A**), on a patient presenting with a radicular syndrome, unsuspected cord compression by a posterior disc herniation (black arrows) is identified at the T12-L1 disc level (white arrow). On the evaluation of another patient with low back pain, the sagittal proton-density weighted image (**B**) demonstrated an unsuspected ependymoma (arrows) of the conus medullaris.

proton-density first echo which simulates a T1-weighted image, with bright fat outlining darker nerve roots in the neural canals. Thus this single multiecho sequence gives both T1-like and true T2-weighted information.

However, the invention of RARE sequences has dramatically improved lumbar spine imaging (460,532). Good T2-weighting can now be obtained in only a few (e.g. 3) minutes, as opposed to about 10 minutes for a true T2-weighted sequence. Higher resolution and more excitations (better S/N) may be achieved in a fraction of the time, allowing an additional sequence (axial T1-weighted) to be obtained, in less total time than a *single* T2-weighted sequence. So true T1- and T2-weighting may be obtained in *both* planes, with improved resolution and S/N, in very short imaging time (about 30 minutes total examination time, or less).

The importance of a sagittal T2-weighted sequence resides in the assessment of disc degeneration and herniation, marrow edema, abnormal fluid accumulations, and extradural masses. The T2-weighted sequence also creates a CSF myelographic effect for the evaluation of intra- and extradural disease. A sagittal proton-density sequence with a long TR (1,500–3,000 milliseconds)/short TE (30 milliseconds) is helpful in the evaluation of the posterior annular-ligamentous complex, ligamenta flava, the central and intervertebral canals, facet joints, and the posterior elements, and can be obtained as part of a multiecho sagittal sequence. Axial T1-weighted and conventional or preferably RARE T2-weighted sequences composed of sequential sections from the L2-3 or L3-L4 disc level through the L5-S1 disc level should be part of the routine examination (247,460,532). Slice thickness for the sagittal sequences is routinely 3–5 mm with an interslice gap of 1 mm, and on axial sequences slice thickness is routinely 4–5 mm with an interslice gap of 1–2 mm. A matrix size that optimizes spatial resolution should be used (272).

With the availability of multi-angle, variable interval scanning techniques (434), it is tempting to shorten the length of the examination time by imaging only the disc levels. This approach is fraught with potential problems. The goal of any imaging study is the ability to evaluate pathoanatomic abnormalities in two complementary orthogonal planes. With only selective angled sections, a large part of the central canal, vertebral body, posterior elements, intervertebral canals, and paravertebral soft tissues are not included on the axial sequence, resulting in limited diagnostic utility. True orthogonal axial images, perpendicular to the cephalocaudal axis of the central canal, are valuable in decreasing geometric distortion (154), but these axial images should only be obtained as an adjunct to the routine set of sequential axial images. When a patient is positioned in the scanner, it is helpful to have the knees and hips flexed as much as possible in order to reduce the lower lumbar lordosis. By straightening the lumbar curve, the amount of geometric distortion on the axial sequences is reduced. Coronal T1-weighted sequences are sometimes obtained to evaluate the conus medullaris, intra- and extradural masses, spinal alignment, sacroiliac joints, and paraspinal musculature and soft tissue (Fig. 9).

CSF motion artifacts are not as great a problem in the lumbar spine when compared to the cervical and thoracic MRI examinations. The amplitude of CSF pulsations is significantly less in the lumbar region, and flow artifacts can be easily prevented (467). Artifacts generated by abdominal motion can be significantly decreased with appropriate alignment of the phase encoded axis along with the use of surface coils (272) and by spatially saturating the protons of the abdominal contents. Patient motion is still the greatest cause of image degradation, and by keeping scan time to a minimum and patient comfort and education to a maximum, the potential for motion artifacts can be reduced.

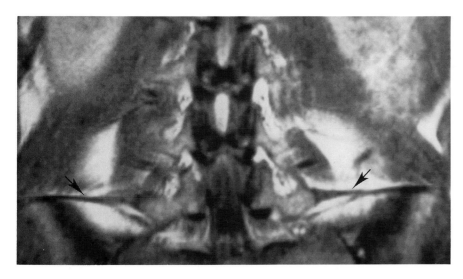

FIG. 9. On the coronal T1-weighted image, there is excellent delineation of the iliolumbar ligaments (arrows) traversing from the transverse processes of the L5 vertebra to the iliac crests.

In summary, the standard MRI examination of the lumbar spine should include sagittal T1- and multiecho T2-weighted sequences from the thoracolumbar junction, including the conus medullaris, to the sacrum, along with an axial multiecho T2-weighted sequence from the L2-L3 or L3-L4 disc level through the L5-S1 disc level. If RARE (fast-spin-echo) sequences are available, these should be employed in place of conventional T2-weighted images (460), and a T1-weighted axial sequence should be added. Gradient-echo imaging should not replace T2-weighted images (conventional or RARE) in the lumbar spine. Fat suppression techniques have increased the enhancement of epidural fibrosis, but have not increased the ability to distinguish recurrent herniated discs (345).

CLINICAL MRI APPLICATIONS

The purpose of an imaging study is to delineate and characterize normal and abnormal tissue. To maximize the information obtained from the MRI examination, it is first necessary to thoroughly understand normal spinal anatomy before intelligently evaluating the pathologic processes involving the spine (202,264,265,432,517). Considering that each MRI examination provides information about dynamic disease processes manifesting a spectrum of pathologic changes, optimal analysis of the radiologic data is possible only with a complete understanding of the natural history of the different spinal diseases (123). The transformation of data from an MRI exam into useful clinical information is directly related to the level of expertise of the clinician interpreting the study (138).

It is always important to try to answer the specific clinical question presented at the time of the exam, but this should not preclude a critical analysis of the entire area being examined. Clinical bias in the interpretation of an imaging study may have a positive or negative impact on diagnostic interpretation (27,136). For this reason, it may be useful for each MRI study to be interpreted twice, initially with no clinical history, followed by a second reading with the knowledge of the results of the prior studies and current clinical findings. The clinician ordering the MRI exam should also have a working diagnosis, including an idea of how likely it is that the patient truly has a specific disease. This "pretest" probability will frequently determine whether the MRI findings will be acted upon (86).

DEGENERATIVE SPINAL DISEASE

When describing the pathomorphologic changes in degenerative spinal disease, it is helpful to consider each disc level as a three joint complex or motion segment with the intervertebral disc and facet joints biomechani-

cally linked to form a functional spinal unit (1,198,266). This will promote a critical evaluation of the entire MR image when trying to understand spinal degenerative disease (436) and not simply a focus on one component, e.g., disc herniation when evaluating a patient presenting with pain or neural dysfunction.

Disc Degeneration

Both the nucleus pulposus and annulus fibrosus consist mainly of water, collagen, and proteoglycans, with the major difference between them being the relative concentration of the components and the particular type of collagen that predominates (47,174). In the young adult the normal nucleus pulposus is approximately 85% water and the annulus fibrosus approximately 70%. Even though the interface between the nucleus pulposus and inner annular fibers is well defined on pathologic specimens of young discs, it is not identified on MR imaging except in very young children. On T2-weighted images, the high signal intensity in the central portion of the disc originates from both the nucleus and inner annular fibers (223,608). The signal intensity in the disc is related to its state of hydration (217,392) and to the physicochemical state of the discal tissue (39,175). The fluid content of the disc is not an intrinsic property of the tissue, but responds to changes in external load (558). On T2-weighted images, the outer annular fibers demonstrate very low signal intensity as does the adjacent posterior longitudinal ligament (398).

With aging, there is a breakdown of the proteoglycans in the nucleus pulposus and gradual desiccation of the mucoid nuclear material (392). In the nucleus increased fibrocartilage is identified pathologically, and there is a loss of delineation between the nucleus and inner annular fibers (340). This change in discal structure appears to be part of the normal process of aging and probably should not be considered a sign of disc degeneration. Over age 30, an internuclear cleft is identified in normal discs on T2-weighted images. This cleft represents normal ingrowth of fibrous tissue (3).

On mid field strength systems, early disc desiccation may be identified on T1-weighted images as decreased signal intensity in the nucleus pulposus when compared to normal discs, but T2-weighted images are optimal on both high field and mid field strength systems for assessing the degree of disc desiccation (176,451,482). The decreased signal intensity of a degenerated disc, on T2-weighted images, appears somewhat exaggerated for the degree of water loss, and it is possible there are other physicochemical changes playing a role in the changes of signal intensity (39,152,354). Maturation of the annulus involves delamination of the concentric annular fibers with resultant infolding of the inner fibers along with cartilage metaplasia (301,419,477,604). This can lead to circumferential tears in the inner and outer annulus which are frequently identified in pathologic specimens (95,609). With aging, there is also an alteration in the distribution of Type I and Type II collagen in the annulus possibly secondary to altered mechanical loading (63). The signal intensity of the disc on the MRI evaluation is a construct of this dynamic physical state of discal tissue.

Disc degeneration and herniation may be considered to be an amplification of the normal maturation process (285). Both experimentally and clinically, it appears that the development of a radial annular tear may be the necessary step in the development of disc degeneration or herniation (302,609). Recent investigative work has demonstrated that posterior "bulging" of the annulus greater than 2.5 mm, even when maintaining its normal dorsal concavity, reflects pathologically an abnormal annulus containing radial tears (610). It is now possible with MRI to delineate small tears in the outer annulus on T2-weighted (Fig. 10) (608,612) and gadolinium-DTPA (Gd-DPTA) enhanced T1-weighted images (456). If these tears do not communicate with the nucleus pulposus, normal signal intensity of the disc may be maintained (608). There has been surgical documentation of radial tears extending through the outer annular fibers that did not communicate with the nucleus pulposus and were not demonstrated by discography (605). When the radial tear does communicate with the nucleus, the disc will begin to degenerate and demonstrate decreased signal intensity on T2-weighted images. With communicating radial tears, displacement of nuclear material is then

possible with resultant disc herniation (2). With the displacement of nuclear material into the region of the outer annular-posterior longitudinal ligament complex, there will be an alteration in the morphology of the periphery of the disc resulting in a focal protrusion of the disc beyond the margins of the vertebral end-plates (251). As long as the disc material is contained by outer annular fibers or the posterior longitudinal ligament, the herniation is designated a contained herniation. With the superb soft tissue resolution of MR imaging, it is frequently possible to determine whether the disc material is contained by the outer annular-ligamentous complex (Fig. 11) or has extruded through this complex becoming an extruded, noncontained, disc herniation (184) (Fig. 12). This information is extremely important with the implementation of percutaneous discectomy (135,343), performance of chemonucleolysis, and possibly as an indicator of surgical outcome for lumbar disc herniations (234). It is also possible to detect when the disc material has extended through the outer annular fibers, but not the posterior longitudinal ligament, particularly when disc material extends cephalad or caudad from the disc space in a subligamentous herniation. Rarely, disc material will penetrate the dura and present as an intradural mass (240,257,508).

The signal intensity of a disc herniation on T1-weighted images is frequently similar to the disc of origin and will usually be of an intermediate or low signal intensity. On T2-weighted images, the herniation may remain the same signal intensity as the disc of origin or demonstrate increased signal intensity. This is particularly common with sequestered disc fragments. The increased signal intensity probably reflects increased mobile hydrogen ions in the disc fragment, and current theories explaining this phenomenon include increased hydration secondary to granulation tissue (354), inflammatory reaction (285,329), or an autoimmune reaction (33). Epidural hematomas may have a similar appearance, and may be misdiagnosed as sequestered disc fragments (189). Considering that the herniated disc material is subjected to a decrease in axial compressive load compared to that of the disc of origin, it is possible that water imbibition into the disc fragment may explain the increased signal intensity identified. The differences in signal intensity in disc herniations may also depend upon the source of the herniated disc material, whether it is nuclear or annular in origin (197,301,604). Posterior disc herniations can be associated with fractures of the posterior rim of the vertebral body end-plates with resultant posterior displacement of a small amount of cortical bone (17,114,538) which also may affect the character of the signal intensity of the herniated disc. Acute traumatic disc herniations may extend into the adjacent vertebral body end-plates (328), and these are optimally delineated on the sagittal MRI sequences (275). With MRI's excellent soft tissue resolution, lateral herniations are

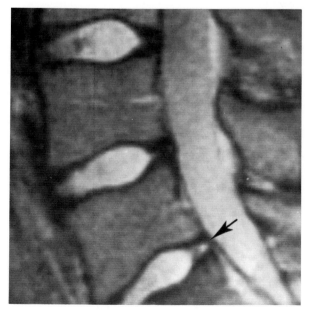

FIG. 10. On the sagittal T2-weighted image, at the L5-S1 disc level, there is a posterior annular fissure (arrow) demonstrating increased signal intensity.

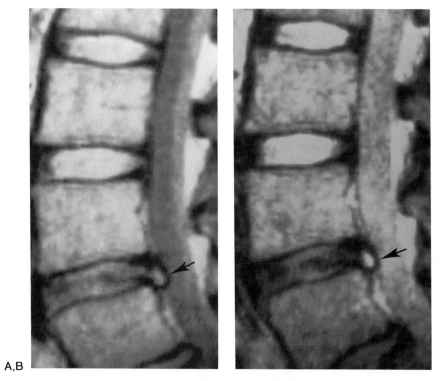

A,B

FIG. 11. On the sagittal T1-weighted image (**A**), at the L4-L5 disc level, there is a small posterior contained disc herniation (arrow) which is slightly hyperintense with respect to the adjacent disc of origin. On the sagittal T2-weighted image (**B**), there is now hyperintensity in the disc herniation compared to the disc of origin. The posterior annular–posterior longitudinal ligament complex is intact (arrow).

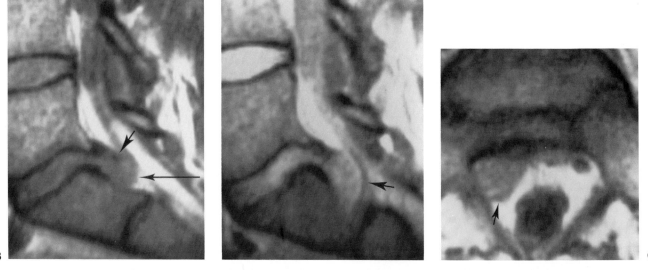

A,B

C

FIG. 12. L5-S1 disc extrusion. On the sagittal proton-density weighted image (**A**), at the L5-S1 disc level, there is a posterior disc extrusion (long arrow) which has penetrated through the posterior annular–posterior longitudinal ligament complex (short arrow). On the T2-weighted image (**B**), the right S1 nerve root (arrow) is identified being displaced posteriorly by the disc extrusion. On the axial T1-weighted image (**C**), it is difficult to separate the right S1 nerve root from the large disc extrusion (arrow).

easily defined on the axial T1-weighted images. Central or posterolateral herniations may be seen on T1-weighted images, but are better seen on axial T2-weighted images. Axial images are also optimal in the evaluation of neural displacement or impingement.

In the cervical spine, due to the lack of signal intensity in the posterior annular-ligamentous complex and the adjacent cerebrospinal fluid in the thecal sac, it may be difficult to delineate a small posterior disc herniation, particularly if it manifests low signal intensity. T2-weighted or gradient-echo images are necessary to delineate the exact position and size of these disc herniations. It is also difficult to evaluate the state of hydration of cervical discs given their small size. This information may be important in patients presenting with cervical discogenic syndrome without disc herniation (581). On the axial sequence, mass effect from the disc herniation, including displacement of the ventral roots or amputation of the root sleeve pouch can be identified (Fig. 13). Disc herniations into the intervertebral canals, lateral to the intervertebral canals, or sequestered fragments (310) are optimally evaluated on axial T1-weighted or especially 3D gradient-echo images. It is of interest how frequently central disc herniations are identified on MRI exams which is in contradistinction with the surgical literature where in one series central disc herniations constituted 1% of the herniations identified at surgery (491). At many centers, MRI has now completely replaced cervical myelography (404).

In the thoracic spine, it is also necessary to obtain sagittal T1-weighted and T2-weighted or gradient-echo sequences in the evaluation of disc herniations (7,30,581) (Fig. 14). Axial images are needed to determine the exact size and position of the herniation. Chemical shift artifacts have the potential of obscuring small disc herniations in the thoracic spine if there is posterior displacement of the fat signal from the vertebral body marrow (139).

In the lumbar spine, the increased amount of epidural fat creates a superb interface between the posterior annular-ligamentous complex, neural elements, and thecal sac. As a result, the standard sagittal T1- and T2-weighted sequences and an axial T1-weighted sequence are usually adequate to define the size and position of a disc herniation and to determine if neural impingement or compression is present. The recommended axial conventional or RARE T2-weighted images further increase sensitivity in detecting central or paracentral herniations (460). In studies comparing MRI to high resolution CT scans and myelograms, MRI was the most sensitive for identification of degenerative disc disease (126,356). In one study comparing MRI to contrast CT, in the evaluation of disc degeneration in 123 motion segments, MRI demonstrated degeneration in 60% whereas CT demonstrated degeneration in 22% (480). While some studies claim MRI to be as good as myelography, others still believe that the myelogram provides additional benefits (199,377).

After disc material has penetrated through the poste-

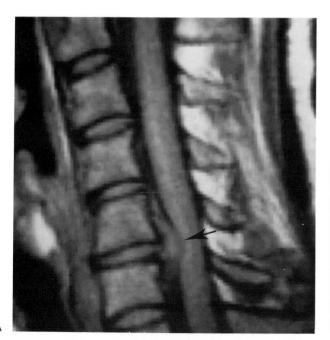

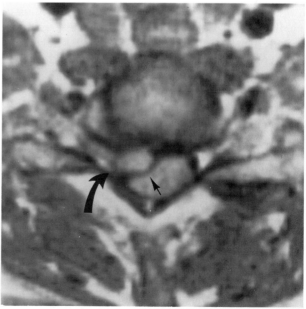

A

B

FIG. 13. C5-C6 disc herniation. On the sagittal T1-weighted image (**A**), there is a large posterior disc herniation (arrow) compressing the spinal cord. The axial T1-weighted image (**B**) is needed to assess the configuration of the herniation, degree of cord compression (short arrow), and obstruction of the entrance zone of the right intervertebral canal (long curved arrow).

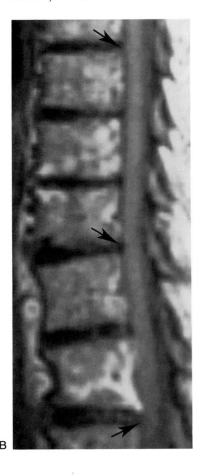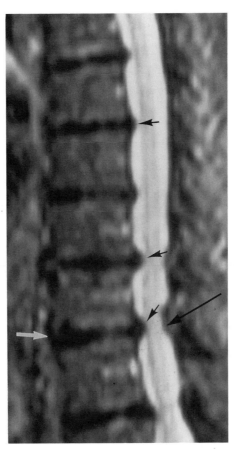

A,B

FIG. 14. Multilevel degenerative changes of the thoracic spine. On the sagittal T1-weighted image (A), multilevel degenerative changes are identified in the mid and lower thoracic spine. It is difficult to evaluate the anterior extradural space due to the isointensity of the posterior margin of the discovertebral joints (arrows) and the cerebrospinal fluid. On the sagittal T2-weighted image (B), with the increased signal intensity of the cerebrospinal fluid, multiple disc protrusions (short black arrows) are now identified. There is minimal impingement on the lower thoracic spinal cord. At the T9-T10 disc level (white arrow), thickening of the ligamentum flavum (long black arrow) is identified, with narrowing of the central spinal canal.

rior longitudinal ligament, it is possible for a portion of the disc material to separate from the disc of origin and become a sequestered fragment. These fragments may migrate either cephalad or caudad from the disc space and may present a variety of appearances on MR imaging. In one prospective study, 80% of sequestered disc fragments demonstrated hyperintensity on T2-weighted images compared to the degenerated disc of origin, whereas the remaining 20% were isointense (318). In the same study, the accuracy of MRI in differentiating sequestered disc fragments from other forms of lumbar disc herniation was 85% compared to a 65% accuracy for CT-myelography. If only proton-density and T2-weighted sagittal sequences are obtained in the screening exam, increased signal intensity in the cerebrospinal fluid may obscure a sequestered disc fragment manifesting high signal intensity (Fig. 15). In many cases the size of the herniated fragment will decrease over time with nonoperative management (53).

In an attempt to better determine which herniated discs visualized on MRI are likely to be symptomatic, observations have been made of the dorsal root ganglia (DRG) position as well as nerve root enhancement with gadolinium. When the DRG is more medial or proximal on the exiting root it is more likely to be symptomatic (194). Gadolinium enhancement of the compressed nerve root was observed in 92% of radiculopathy patients in one study and was noted frequently prior to discectomy in other studies (96,243,550). The false-positive rate and false-negative rate of this finding is not yet established. In addition, the time course of resolution of clinical symptoms and MRI root enhancement is also uncertain.

The differential diagnosis of a sequestered disc fragment includes epidural abscess, extradural tumor, conjoined nerve root, root sheath tumor or cyst (180), and epidural hematoma (189,210). Epidural abscesses are frequently associated with infections involving the disc space (415), and, therefore, the differentiation from a disc fragment is usually not difficult. Extradural tumors present more of a challenge, but their location, configuration, and possible enhancement after the intravenous administration of Gd-DTPA (531) may help differentiate a tumor from a sequestered fragment. Epidural abscess and extradural tumors are covered more completely in the following sections. Conjoined nerve roots (406) can be differentiated from a sequestered disc fragment on axial T1-weighted images. Root sheath cysts demonstrate characteristic morphology and are isointense with CSF on T1- and T2-weighted sequences. Gd-DTPA may result in pseudoenhancement of a herniated disc due to large veins or granulation tissue (9). Dilated foraminal veins can mimic far lateral disc herniations (184).

Chronic epidural hematomas also must be considered

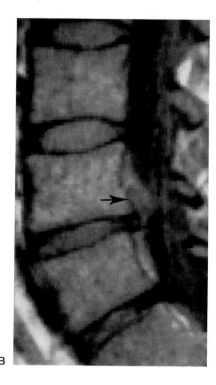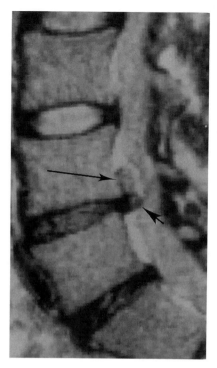

A,B

FIG. 15. Sequestered disc fragment. On the sagittal T1-weighted image (**A**), there is an oblong anterior extradural disc fragment (arrow) positioned immediately cephalad to the L4-L5 disc level. The disc fragment is slightly hyperintense compared to the L4-L5 disc. Decreased height of the L4-L5 disc is present along with slight decreased signal intensity in the disc compared to the normal L3-L4 disc. On the sagittal T2-weighted image (**B**), the sequestered disc fragment (long arrow) is hyperintense with respect to the L4-L5 disc and isointense with respect to the cerebrospinal fluid making delineation of the fragment difficult. A posterior disc herniation (short arrow) is now identified at the L4-L5 disc level along with further decreased signal intensity in the L4-L5 disc compared to the T1-weighted image.

in the differential diagnosis of sequestered disc fragments (52,189,294). A patient with a chronic lumbar epidural hematoma may present with symptoms of disc herniation or spinal stenosis (375) and not with the acute catastrophic symptoms which acute, spontaneous epidural hematomas frequently manifest in their more typical thoracic or cervical location (397,462). An epidural hematoma is usually delineated as a soft tissue hyperintense mass on T1- and T2-weighted sequences, but the appearance of the hematoma may vary depending upon its age (Fig. 16). In the lumbar spine, an epidural hematoma may have tapered margins, extend beyond one disc

level, and be adjacent to a normal disc space which helps in its differentiation from a sequestered disc fragment. Both sequestered disc fragments (473) and epidural hematomas may regress in size on follow-up examinations; therefore, decrease in size is not a distinguishing feature. Secondary epidural hematomas are associated with trauma (577), coagulopathies, tumors, arteriovenous malformations, infections, anticoagulant therapy (397), and Paget's disease (195).

Following herniation, the disc will continue to degenerate and lose signal intensity. Disc herniations associated with normal signal intensity (106) in the disc have

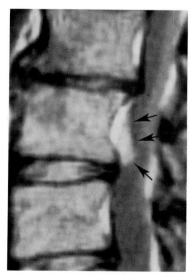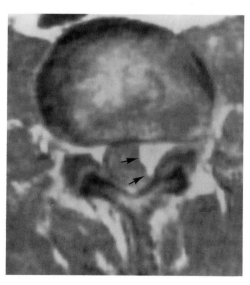

B

FIG. 16. Epidural hematoma. On the sagittal proton-density weighted image (**A**) and the axial proton-density weighted image (**B**), there is an epidural hematoma (arrows) effacing the left anterior margin of the thecal sac. The epidural hematoma is isointense with respect to the extradural fat and hyperintense with respect to the cerebrospinal fluid. The epidural hematoma is delineated by its mass effect on the thecal sac.

been reported, and one study demonstrated normal signal intensity in discs that were shown to be abnormal morphologically on discography (615). To date, there has been no prospective study to determine the length of time necessary for a normally hydrated disc to become desiccated after it herniates. In one MR study evaluating 246 patients suffering from persistent back and leg pain, degenerative disc changes were seen to increase with age until approximately the fifth decade. Very few discs with a normal signal intensity were herniated, and disc dehydration was associated with an increase in the occurrence of herniation (106).

In the natural history of disc degeneration, there is loss of the normal architecture of the nucleus and annulus along with ingrowth of granulation tissue (95). With progressive disc degeneration, there is concomitant loss of signal intensity in the disc on T2-weighted sequences. Occasionally there may be fluid-containing fissures in the degenerated disc which, along with ingrowth of granulation tissue (94), can result in increased signal intensity in the disc on T2-weighted images, and the granulation tissue may enhance with contrast. This increased signal intensity and enhancement should not be confused with an inflammatory process (354). In addition to gross changes of desiccation, fissuring, and osteophyte formation, pathologic specimens in severely degenerated discs have demonstrated osteophytic-like cartilage near the end-plates (339). These changes may also influence the characteristics of the signal intensity on the T2-weighted images. Degenerated discs may calcify or occasionally form gas-containing clefts. These findings may be difficult to detect on T2-weighted sagittal images because of the decreased signal intensity in the severely degenerated disc along with lack of signal from the calcium or gas

(126,185). T1-weighted or gradient-echo images are frequently more useful in delineating a vacuum phenomenon or disc calcification (354). In one pathologic study, intervertebral disc changes with aging in the cervical spine appeared similar to those described in the lumbar spine (382).

In addition to delineating the degenerative changes in the disc, MRI is extremely sensitive to alterations in the vertebral body end-plates at a degenerating discovertebral joint (109). Due to the thinness of the hyaline cartilage (441) it is difficult to delineate isolated degenerative changes of cartilage. In addition, there may be chemical shift artifacts at the discovertebral junction which distort the appearance of the cartilage end-plate (185,398). In an excellent pathoanatomic study, Modic (358) has demonstrated altered vertebral body marrow adjacent to the end-plate of discs undergoing degeneration. He refers to type I end-plate changes when there is prominent fibrovascular tissue in the marrow spaces which has replaced the normal marrow fat of the subchondral bone. As a result, on the T1-weighted image, there is decreased signal intensity in the cancellous bone and on the T2-weighted image increased signal intensity, probably secondary to the fluid content of the fibrovascular tissue. Type II end-plate degenerative changes are depicted by increased fat in the subchondral bone which, on T1-weighted images, demonstrate hyperintensity and, on T2-weighted images, slight hyperintensity or isointensity when compared to the normal marrow (Fig. 17). On RARE T2-weighted sequences, because fat is relatively bright (247,248,460), type II end-plate changes appear relatively hyperintense. Type I end-plate changes may progress to type II, but the reverse has not been reported. Type III end-plate changes represent coarsening and

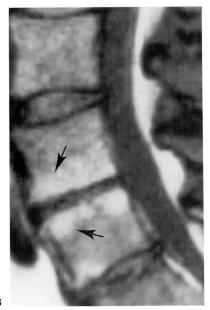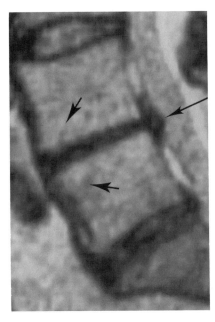

A,B

FIG. 17. On the sagittal T1-weighted image (**A**), at the L4-L5 disc level, type II end-plate degenerative changes are identified (arrows) with increased signal intensity in the marrow adjacent to the inferior end-plate of L4 and superior end-plate of L5. Changes of disc degeneration are present with moderately severe decreased disc height. On the sagittal T2-weighted image (**B**), the signal intensity in the marrow (short arrows), adjacent to the L4-L5 disc, has become isointense with the normal marrow. With the improved conspicuity of the extradural space, a posterior disc herniation (long arrow) is now identified.

thickening of the subchondral trabeculae with formation of woven bone, which is depicted on T1- and T2-weighted images as decreased signal intensity (Table 2).

Vertebral body end-plate changes have also been reported (316) in discogenic vertebral sclerosis (512) and hemispherical spondylosclerosis (242). On the MRI evaluation of these two processes, the altered marrow signal intensity was similar to type I end-plate degenerative changes with hyperintensity in the region of the sclerotic bone on the T2-weighted sequence. It is of interest that the biopsy in the case of hemispherical spondylosclerosis showed only mild marrow hypercellularity without evidence of fibrovascular changes. Type I end-plate changes frequently develop after the injection of chymopapain and may progress to type II changes (316,533). Gradient-echo sequences are not as sensitive as standard spin-echo T1- and T2-weighted sequences to the signal intensity changes within the disc or in the adjacent vertebral body marrow associated with disc degeneration (354), and hence should be avoided.

In addition to the evaluation of end-plate abnormalities associated with degenerative disc disease, MRI may also be of benefit in the evaluation of the natural history of end-plate changes and disc degeneration in Scheuermann's disease (521) and of traumatic spondylodystrophy at the thoracolumbar junction. There have been several reports describing young patients presenting with mechanical type back pain, vertebral body end-plate irregularities, and disc degeneration at the thoracolumbar junction (183). The incidence of end-plate changes appears to be particularly high in young elite athletes who repetitively axial load their spines (229,526). It is of interest that both these patients (183) and patients with Scheuermann's disease (383) have an increased incidence of spondylolysis.

With the excellent MRI characterization of the nor-

mal and the abnormal disc, it should now be possible to noninvasively study the natural history of disc degeneration and herniation. The sensitivity of MRI to early changes of disc degeneration should help in the evaluation of patients with intervertebral disc resorption (238) or internal disc disruption (38) possibly obviating the need for discography. Multiple studies have been reported describing the excellent sensitivity, specificity, and accuracy of MRI in the diagnosis of discal disease (126,162,535). A few studies have reported discs with normal appearance on MRI that had annular tears evident on discogram (387,456,615). Even though a disc herniation is identified, it is always important to realize the relatively common occurrence of asymptomatic disc herniations in the cervical (Table 3) (43,332,542), thoracic (586), and lumbar spine (Table 4) (40,221,332, 418,576,582). A recent article again documents the common frequency of asymptomatic bulges and protrusions, but suggests that asymptomatic extrusions are much more rare (241). With the increased utilization of MRI, it has also become clear that disc degeneration and herniation afflict the adolescent age population (17,75, 148,153,177,389) and young adults as well as patients over the age of 30. There are also congenital anomalies of the spine that may predispose to disc herniation (81). The greatest challenge in the evaluation of degenerative disc disease is to understand when normal maturation is transformed into abnormal degeneration and to determine which pathomorphologic changes may explain the clinical symptomatology.

TABLE 2. *MRI and the differential diagnosis of discitis and degenerative disc disease*

	Marrow			Disc		
	T1	T2	T1-Gd	T1	T2	T1-Gd
Degenerative disc disease						
Type I	−	+	+	I	−	I
Type II	+	I/+	I	I	−	I
Type III	−	−	I	I	−	I
Discitis	−	+	+	−	+	+

a MR signal characteristics in the intervertebral disc space and adjacent vertebral bone marrow in degenerative disc disease on unenhanced T1-weighted (T1), more T2-weighted (T2), and contrast-enhanced T1-weighted (T1 + Gd) images (354, 358, 506).

b Intensity of signal is reported relative to the same structure at an adjacent normal level. I = isointense; − = hypointense; + = hyperintense.

TABLE 3. *Percentage of asymptomatics with cervical spine MR abnormalities (n = 63)*

	Occurrence by age		
Finding	<40 yr old (%)	>40 yr old (%)	Total (%)
Herniated disc	10	5	8
Disc bulge	0	3	2
Foraminal stenosis	4	20	9
Total	14	28	19

From Boden et al., ref. 43.

TABLE 4. *Percentage of asymptomatics with lumbar spine MR abnormalities (n = 67)*

	Occurrence by age		
Finding	20–39 yr (%)	40–59 yr (%)	60–80 yr (%)
Herniated disc	21	22	36
Spinal stenosis	1	0	21
Disc bulge	56	50	79
Disc degeneration	34	59	93

From Boden et al., ref. 40.

Facet Arthrosis

As part of the three joint complex, the facet joints are biomechanically linked to the discovertebral joint (99,121,198). The size and orientation of the facet joints differ at different levels of the spine, and being diarthrodial joints are subject to painful degeneration (46,80, 198,364,540). Degenerative changes of the facet joints which can be resolved by MRI include facet hypertrophy, osteophytic spurring, cartilage narrowing, joint effusions, synovial cysts (237,303,500), and capsular hypertrophy. In the cervical spine, the facet joints are oriented obliquely to the axial and coronal planes and, therefore, optimally delineated with sagittal images (611). Cervical facet joints, including their menisci, are best evaluated with a long TR/short TE (proton-density) sequence utilizing 3 mm thick sections with a 256 × 256 matrix (611). In the thoracic spine, there appears to be a pathoanatomic association between facet joint orientation and degenerative changes, particularly at the thoracolumbar junction (308). In the lumbar spine, the orientation of the facet joints changes from a more sagittal orientation in the upper and mid lumbar segments to a more coronal orientation at the lumbosacral junction (561). For this reason, there is no single plane to optimally evaluate the facet joints on an MRI study, and the axial and sagittal images offer complementary information (187). In one recent study, the best delineation of the morphology of hyaline cartilage and the cancellous-cortical bone complex of the facet joint was obtained using a long TR/short TE sequence. A short TR/short TE sequence was optimal to evaluate the fat–soft tissue interface of the facet capsule and characterization of the medullary bone (187). The anterior facet capsule, which represents a lateral extension of the ligamentum flavum, appears as an intermediate signal intensity structure on both T1 and proton-density images. The capsule is slightly hypointense when compared to the more medial portion of the ligamentum flavum (222).

The most common degenerative changes identified involving the facet joints are osteophytic spurring and facet hypertrophy (Fig. 18). Cartilage thickness is difficult to measure accurately because of partial volume averaging and chemical shift artifacts (187). Gradient-echo sequences may prove useful in the evaluation of facet degenerative changes, particularly in the evaluation of articular cartilage (Fig. 19). MRI can image the facet joint capsule and synovium well (597). Degenerative synovial cysts may appear slightly hyperintense or isointense on T1-weighted sequences and may be hyper- or hypointense on T2-weighted sequences (303). MRI has also been reported to detect an early defect in the pars interarticularis before visualization by CT or plain radiography (601).

Spinal Stenosis

In the natural history of spinal degeneration, the degenerative processes affecting the various components of the spinal column may eventually lead to spinal stenosis. Spinal stenosis is defined as local, segmental, or generalized narrowing of the central or intervertebral canals by bony or soft tissue elements that may lead to encroach-

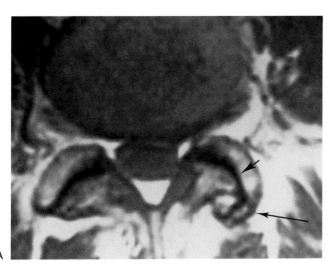
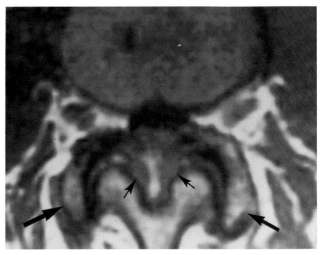

A

B

FIG. 18. Lumbar facet joint degeneration. On the axial proton-density weighted image (**A**), degenerative changes of the left facet joint are identified with narrowing of the articular cartilage (small arrow) and osteophytic spurring of the dorsal surface (long arrow) of the left superior articular process. On the axial T1-weighted image (**B**), degeneration of the facet joints is identified with facet joint hypertrophy (large arrows) and prominence of the ligamenta flava (small arrows). This is causing mild to moderate narrowing of the central spinal canal.

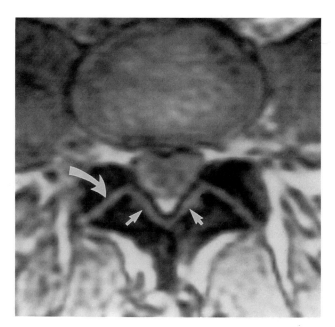

FIG. 19. On the axial gradient-echo image, the ligamenta flava (short arrows) is well defined due to its intermediate signal intensity compared to the adjacent hypointensity of the osseous structures and increased signal intensity of the posterior epidural fat. The articular cartilage (long curved arrow) of the facet joint is identified due to its intermediate signal intensity.

ment of the neural structures. The narrowing may involve the bony canal alone or the dural sac, or both (10). The degenerative changes most often associated with stenosis include hyperostotic spurring of the vertebral body end-plates, uncinate processes, and facet joints, along with hypertrophy of the ligamenta flava and anterior facet capsule (6,222,227,306,396,432,584,606). The initial size of the central and intervertebral canals is an important factor in determining whether degenerative changes will lead to neural impingement or compression. The goal of MRI in the evaluation of the patient presenting with radiculopathy, myeloradiculopathy, or myelopathy is not just to demonstrate that stenosis is present, but to define the relative contributions of each component of the stenotic process.

Before the development of MRI, myelography and CT-myelography were the standard examinations in the evaluation of cervical myelopathy and myeloradiculopathy (104,490,511). Thin-section high resolution CT has been an excellent screening exam of the cervical spine (349), but does not directly demonstrate neural impingement or compression, and thus is frequently followed by a contrast study in the preoperative evaluation. In several series, excellent results with MRI compared to CT-myelography and myelography have been demonstrated in the evaluation of patients with radiculopathy (205,352) and myelopathy (65,235) thus obviating the need for an invasive myelographic exam (312,445).

In the evaluation of the cervical spine, in addition to the routine sagittal MRI sequences, axial 3D thin-section gradient-echo sequences are beneficial in defining the exact etiology of stenosis (552,607). Initially, there was great enthusiasm that MRI would delineate the difference between osseous spurs and disc protrusions, but this has been somewhat tempered by the difficulty in making that distinction. The difficulty is predominantly related to the range of signal intensity present in abnormal disc material and degenerative spondylotic ridges (553,607). On standard T1-weighted images, the signal intensity of a degenerative ridge may be hyperintense compared to the adjacent vertebral body and disc if the degenerative spur contains abundant fatty marrow, or it may be isointense or hypointense depending upon the structure and amount of cortical bone in the degenerative ridge (352). In one prospective study comparing the accuracy of MRI, myelography, and CT-myelography in evaluating patients with cervical radiculopathy, MRI was as sensitive as CT-myelography in the identification of the degenerative level, but not as specific for type of disease. The major advantage of CT-myelography was its ability to distinguish bone from soft tissue degenerative changes and the presence of contrast in the thecal sac was not necessary to acquire this additional information. Myelography was the least specific for disease type, and the authors concluded that MRI complemented by plain computed tomography provides a thorough examination of the cervical region (352). Though the differentiation between disc herniations and spondylotic spurs as the cause of neural impingement may make no difference in surgical outcome (115), the differentiation may be important in determining what type of conservative therapy is useful with a patient presenting with stenotic symptoms, and in the determination of which patient may eventually require a surgical procedure.

In the cervical spine, there is a strong association pathologically between degenerative changes of the discovertebral joint and uncinate spurs at the same motion segment (227) (Fig. 20). Many patients presenting with myelopathy secondary to spondylotic changes will also have an associated radiculopathy. In evaluating patients with radiculopathy, if axial and sagittal images do not demonstrate the cause of the radicular symptoms, additional anatomic delineation of the intervertebral canals can be obtained with oblique T1-weighted (Fig. 21) or gradient-echo images (355). In one study, oblique images of the intervertebral canal added important information not available on the sagittal images or clarified changes seen on the axial images (355,458,459). In a recent report with patients presenting with radicular symptoms, an MRI study using gradient-echo imaging gave equal or more detailed information compared to CT-myelography in all cases in which both were performed. Surgical correlation with the gradient-echo images was excellent (205). Intravenous infusion of Gd-DTPA may also help

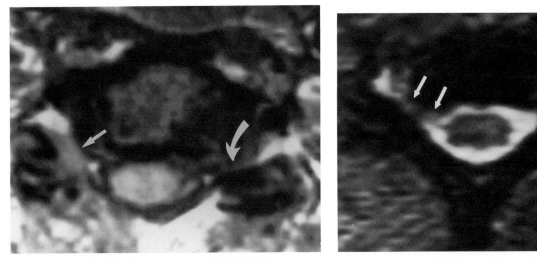

FIG. 20. **A:** Cervical intervertebral canal stenosis. On the axial T1-weighted image, at the C5-C6 disc level, there is impingement on the right dorsal root ganglion by an uncinate spur (short arrow), and severe osseous stenosis of the left intervertebral canal (long curved arrow). **B:** On the axial gradient-echo image of another patient, at C6-7, a bony uncovertebral osteophyte (arrows) narrows the right intervertebral canal and impinges on the exiting right C7 nerve root, in agreement with this patient's symptoms.

define intervertebral canal pathology by enhancing the extradural and intracanalicular venous channels, nerve root sheath, and dorsal root ganglia (101,450,458,459). This parallels the information formally obtained with intravenous contrast infusion followed by thin-section high resolution CT (208,470,471).

In the evaluation of patients with myelopathy or mye-loradiculopathy, it is important to determine the size of the central spinal canal. There have been a plethora of roentgenographic studies (70,179,218,219,443,594) depicting the normal sagittal diameter of the cervical spine, but only CT scanning with axial imaging orthogonal to the long axis of the cervical canal or multiplanar CT imaging with sagittal reformations can accurately delineate

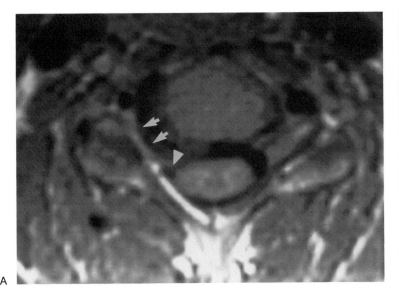
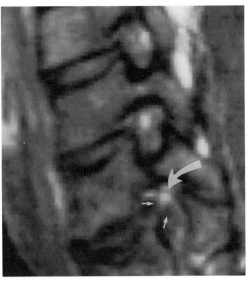

FIG. 21. Cervical intervertebral canal stenosis. On the axial T1-weighted image (**A**), at the C6-C7 disc level, prominent degenerative changes are identified involving the right uncovertebral joint causing moderately severe narrowing of the right intervertebral canal (short arrows) along with effacement of the right C7 nerve root sleeve (arrowhead). On the oblique T1-weighted image (**B**), uncinate spurs (small arrows) at the C6-C7 disc level are causing moderate to moderately severe stenosis of the intervertebral canal (curved arrow).

the true osseous mid sagittal diameter. The developmental mid sagittal diameter, which is not affected by degenerative changes, is measured from the middle of the posterior surface of the vertebral body to the closest point of the adjacent spino-laminar line. The degenerative sagittal diameter, also referred to as the spondylotic AP diameter (130,131), is measured from the posterior margin of end-plate degenerative spurs to the closest point of the adjacent spino-laminar line and this usually represents the smallest AP diameter of the central canal in a patient with cervical spondylosis.

In one CT study, the measurements of the normal sagittal developmental diameter from C3 to C6 measured 14–14.5 mm with one standard deviation of 1.3–2.1 mm (519). If relative stenosis is defined as one standard deviation below average and absolute stenosis as two standard deviations below average, then an AP diameter of less than 12.5 mm would be considered relative stenosis and less than 10.5 mm absolute stenosis, and would closely parallel the terminology describing lumbar stenosis. MR measurements of the cervical cord and spinal canal have been made (226,497).

It is well known that osseous stenosis does not necessarily cause cervical myelopathy, and the great advantage of MRI over CT in the evaluation of stenosis is to determine what effect the degenerative processes and/or a developmentally narrowed central canal has on the neural structures. Patients presenting with myelopathic symptoms will frequently have degenerative spondylotic changes superimposed on a developmentally narrowed central canal (130,131,370,563) (Fig. 22) but, in addition, a developmentally small central canal with decreased reserve capacity may be a cause of myelopathy, even without superimposed degenerative changes (146,218,220,361). In recent studies, it appears that the best predictor of the clinical course in myelopathic patients, impact of surgical intervention, and pathologic changes of the spinal cord is the degree of cord compression and measurement of cord volume (166,167,384, 537,613). MRI is ideally suited to give this information, but to date there have been no MRI studies determining which sequence is the most accurate in evaluating cord measurements although the RARE T2-weighted sequence, with its superb CSF/tissue delineation and good spatial resolution, would be a good candidate (226). In one study comparing MRI to myelography and CT-myelography in 57 patients with suspected cervical myelopathy, MRI was more informative than myelographic studies in 23%, equally informative in 73%, and less diagnostic in 4% of patients studied (317). This study was performed early in the development and application of surface coils, and it would be expected that the advantages of MRI would be significantly improved with current imaging techniques. A recent MRI study evaluated 668 patients with chronic cervical cord compression and demonstrated high signal intensity within the spinal cord

on T2-weighted or proton-density images in 14.8% of the patients. This finding was directly related to increased spinal cord compression and to the severity of clinical myelopathy. Patients with high signal intensity areas responded less favorably to surgical or medical treatment (537). Other studies have confirmed the poor prognosis with increased cord signal (320). MRI has also been useful in defining the stage of compressive myelomalacia and has demonstrated the potential reversibility of the early stages (430).

Dynamic changes in the shape of the spinal cord, alignment of vertebral elements, and alteration of spinal canal volume have been demonstrated in experimental (401,574) and clinical (204,443) studies evaluating normal and myelopathic patients (204). A potential exciting application of MRI is in the dynamic evaluation of the cervical spine in flexion and extension (92,151). Dynamic studies of the cervical spine may also be of benefit in the post-traumatic evaluation of patients with neural dysfunction and normal plain x-rays, as well as with patients with developmental stenosis, who appear to have a predisposition to cord injury secondary to cervical trauma (287,549). MRI is also excellent in the delineation of additional pathologic processes that may cause central canal stenosis including ossification of the posterior longitudinal ligament (325,341,369,386,388,602), diffuse idiopathic skeletal hyperostosis (DISH) (5,437), pseudotumors (528), Paget's disease (580), vertebral hemangiomas (455), rheumatoid arthritis, and in the exclusion of disease processes that may mimic spondylotic cervical myelopathy including spinal cord tumors, metastatic disease (510), and demyelinating processes.

CSF flow can be qualitatively and quantitatively measured by MRI, because the phase of the precessing nuclei in the magnetic field gradients is very sensitive to motion. In particular, the oscillatory motion of CSF in the brain and spinal canal (especially in the cervical region) which is driven by brain expansion and contraction during the cardiac cycle, may be visualized by phase-contrast cine imaging (141,172,295,378,422). This technique may be useful to assess the degree of blockage of CSF within the thecal sac, for example, from congenital stenosis as from achondroplasia (Fig. 23). Other possible uses include making the distinction between intradural subarachnoid cyst vs. normally widened spinal canal, although the interpretation of such studies has yet to be perfected (172).

In the thoracic spine, the most common etiology of compressive myelopathy and radiculopathy includes metastatic disease, spinal cord tumors, post-traumatic deformities, disc herniations, and chronic inflammatory processes. With decreased mobility of the thoracic motion segments, degenerative stenosis of the central or intervertebral canals is unusual (131). In one report MRI underestimated the size of calcified thoracic herniated discs (573). Ossification of the posterior longitudinal lig-

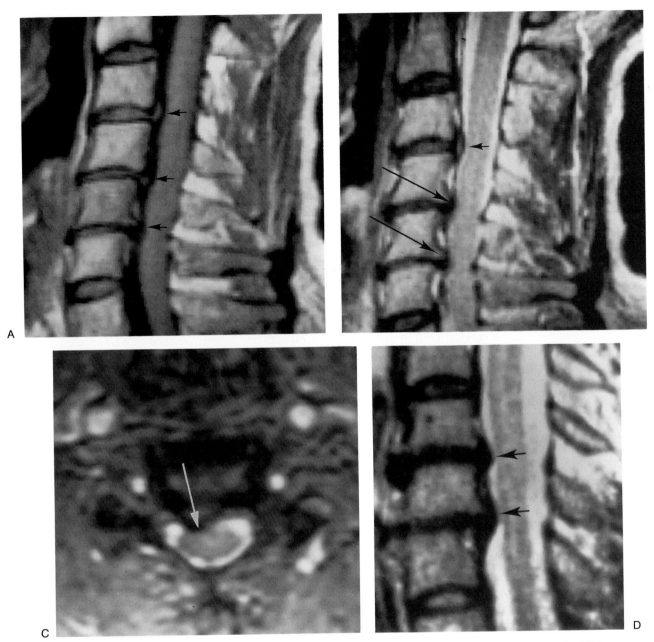

FIG. 22. Multilevel cervical spondylosis superimposed on developmental stenosis. On the sagittal T1-weighted image (**A**), degenerative changes are identified at the C3-C4, C4-C5, and C5-C6 disc levels (arrows). The extradural space is poorly defined due to the isointensity of the cerebrospinal fluid, posterior annular–posterior longitudinal ligament complex, and vertebral body cortex. On the sagittal cardiac gated T2-weighted image (**B**), with the increased signal intensity in the cerebrospinal fluid, a posterior disc herniation causing minimal cord impingement is now identified at the C3-C4 disc level (short arrow). Changes of cervical spondylosis are present at the C4-C5 and C5-C6 disc levels with spondylotic ridges (long arrows) causing mild cord impingement. There is decreased AP diameter of the central spinal canal from the C3-C4 level through the C6-C7 level on a developmental basis with resultant decreased functional spinal canal volume predisposing to cord impingement. On the axial gradient-echo image (**C**), a spondylotic ridge (arrow) causing minimal cord impingement is delineated. On another patient, the sagittal cardiac gated T2-weighted image (**D**) demonstrates spondylotic ridges (arrows) at the C5-C6 and C6-C7 disc levels. The spinal canal volume is normal and there is no spinal cord impingement by the degenerative ridges.

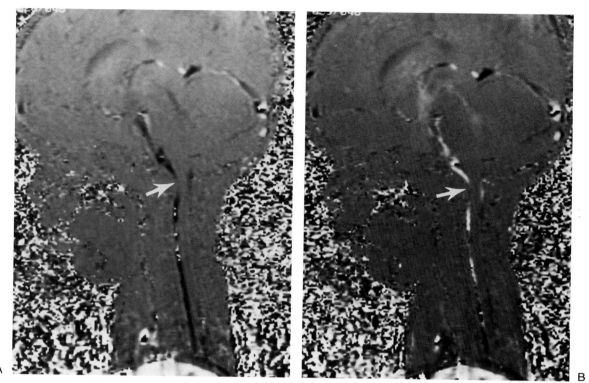

FIG. 23. CSF flow study in 14-month-old achondroplast. Phase-contrast images obtained during different phases of brain and CSF pulsation demonstrate CSF flow anterior to the cord as black (rostral flow, **A**) or white (caudal flow, **B**). There is mild obstruction to CSF flow at the foramen magnum at the level of the dens (arrows).

ament (369), ligamenta flava (525), and thickening of the laminar arch and facet joints (600) have been reported causing narrowing of the thoracic central canal. There have also been several case reports of epidural lipomatosis involving the thoracic spine in patients presenting with myelopathic symptoms (73,118,424,515). Cord compression secondary to disc herniation and thoracic kyphos have been reported in patients with Scheuermann's disease (599). Osteopenic compression fractures which are extremely common in the thoracic spine rarely result in cord compression, but there have been scattered reports of this occurrence (474).

In the lumbar spine, the importance of spinal stenosis as the cause of nerve root and cauda equina compression has been demonstrated by Verbiest's excellent clinical and investigative work (564–569). Patients of any age presenting with disc herniations may have superimposed stenosis (201), and isolated stenosis may also be the only finding in patients presenting with leg and back pain (391). Without a firm understanding of the normal anatomy of the central and intervertebral canals (31,50,87, 97,202,338,432,481,488) it is extremely difficult to reach a cogent diagnosis when imaging a patient with a plethora of degenerative changes (87,133,267,268).

The classification of spinal stenosis as congenital, developmental, and acquired is extremely helpful when

evaluating a small spinal canal. Whatever its etiology, the diagnosis of stenosis can only be made by means of accurate measurement (569) and not by a general impression when interpreting an imaging study. Congenital stenosis is due to disturbed fetal development and may occur as one element of a congenital malformation of the lumbar spine (485). Developmental stenosis (89,413, 439,567) is a growth disturbance of the posterior elements, involving the pedicles, lamina, and articular processes resulting in decreased volume of the spinal canal. A true midline osseous sagittal diameter measuring less than 12 mm is considered relative stenosis and measurements of less than 10 mm are considered absolute stenosis (567). The diameter is measured from the middle of the posterior surface of the vertebral body to the point of junction of the base of the spinous process and laminae. With relative stenosis, the reserve capacity of the spinal canal is reduced and a small disc herniation (Fig. 24) or early degenerative changes may result in symptomatic stenosis in both the young (150,201,268) and the older population (145,147,212,276,411,412,592). Developmental lumbar stenosis has been reported in several siblings in one family (417), and there is a reported increased incidence of developmental stenosis of the lumbar spine associated with developmental stenosis of the cervical spine (131). Acquired stenosis represents

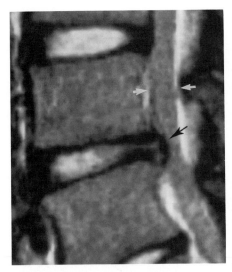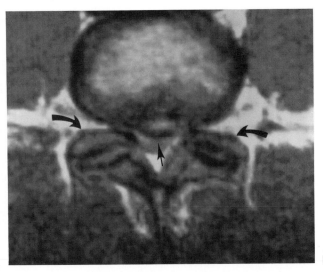

B

FIG. 24. On the sagittal (**A**) and axial (**B**) T1-weighted images, a posterior contained disc herniation (black arrow) is identified at the L4-L5 disc level causing moderate thecal sac effacement. The degree of thecal sac effacement is amplified due to a developmentally small central spinal canal. The developmental sagittal diameter (white arrows) measures 12 mm. On the axial image (**B**), the facet joints (curved arrows) are prominent, but there are no facet degenerative changes.

narrowing of the central or intervertebral canals by degenerative changes of the discovertebral joint, facet joints, and ligamenta flava (222,566).

When evaluating the stenotic spinal canal by MRI, it is important to determine the exact etiology of the stenotic process in order to try to explain clinical symptomatology and to direct surgery if indicated. Before the development of MRI, the diagnosis of structural spinal stenosis was determined by myelography (22,555), functional myelography (516), CT (557), CT-myelography (351,480), and ultrasonography (11,544). In a prospective study, 60 patients with suspected lumbar disc herniations and/or central stenosis were studied with surface coil MRI, CT, and/or myelography, and the results were compared to the findings at surgery. Surgical findings of stenosis agreed with the MRI findings in 77%, CT findings in 79%, and myelographic findings in 54%. This study did not differentiate between central and intervertebral canal stenosis (351). In a retrospective study comparing MRI and contrast CT, there was 96.6% agreement between MRI and contrast CT in the diagnosis of spinal stenosis (480). In recent reports, it appears that the cross-sectional area of the thecal sac correlates best to stenotic symptoms (49,472,483). With direct multiplanar imaging, MRI is ideally suited to evaluate the true sagittal dimension of the thecal sac along with thecal sac cross-sectional area (226,497), thus obviating the need for an invasive myelographic procedure (225,435). In addition, all the components of the stenotic process can be adequately assessed with the standard MRI sequences. Sagittal T1- and multiecho sequences and axial T1-weighted and RARE (fast-spin-echo) T2-weighted sequences are

optimal in the evaluation of spinal morphometry, degenerative changes of the vertebral bodies and facet joints, thickening of the ligamenta flava, and evaluation of the posterior epidural fat pad (187). T2-weighted sequences are of value to assess the effects of the stenotic process on the thecal sac (Fig. 25). A potential application of MRI would be in the dynamic evaluation of neural impingement in the central and intervertebral canals, particularly in extension (393,402,484,536).

The importance of intervertebral canal stenosis as a cause of radicular symptoms (410) has been well documented, as well as its significance in failed back surgery (71). Any component of the intervertebral canal may impinge on or compress the nerve root (Fig. 26). With the abundance of fat in the intervertebral canal, sagittal T1- and proton-density weighted images are optimal for defining normal and pathologic changes (187). The intervertebral canal at the L5-S1 disc level is unique in its morphometry (202) and due to its length may be stenotic at its entrance, mid, or exit zone. The most common cause of stenosis at this level is osteophytic spurs projecting off the inferior end-plate of L5 and less commonly the superior end-plate of S1 (48,432) (Fig. 27). These probably represent enthetic spurs secondary to abnormal biomechanics of a degenerative disc leading to increased traction by Sharpey's fibers (499). With disc degeneration, there is decreased attenuation of compressive forces associated with increased anisotropic distribution of radial tension which may explain the development of enthetic spurs in the intervertebral canals. In one study, narrowing of the intervertebral canals by osseous spurs and disc protrusions was associated with venous conges-

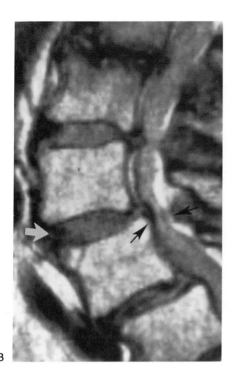 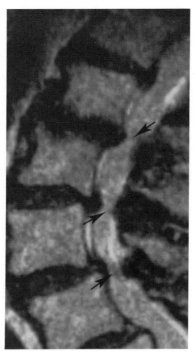

A,B

FIG. 25. Multilevel degenerative changes associated with an anterior degenerative spondylolisthesis at the L3-L4 and L4-L5 disc levels. On the sagittal proton-density weighted image (**A**), multilevel degenerative changes are identified. A degenerative spondylolisthesis is present at the L3-L4 disc level (white arrow) causing moderately severe central canal stenosis (black arrows). On the sagittal T2-weighted image (**B**), disc degeneration and loss of signal intensity is identified at all disc levels. Increased signal intensity in the thecal sac facilitates the evaluation of the degree of multilevel central canal stenosis (arrows).

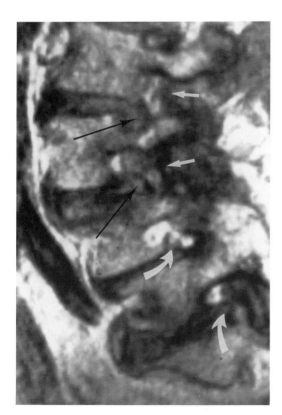

FIG. 26. Multilevel intervertebral canal stenosis. On the sagittal proton-density weighted image, stenosis of the intervertebral canals is identified secondary to end-plate spurs (curved white arrows), disc herniations (long black arrows), and hypertrophied facet joints (straight white arrows).

tion in the intervertebral canal along with neural and perineural fibrosis. The intervertebral canals may also be small on a developmental basis (89,567) which predisposes to neural impingement by a degenerative process. Extracanalicular ("far-out") (588,589) stenosis may also occur at the L5-S1 level in patients with spondylolisthesis or elderly patients with scoliosis (188) and disc degeneration. This stenosis is secondary to apposition of the base of the transverse process of L5 to the adjacent sacral ala. In addition, osseous spurs may project off the lateral margin of the vertebral body end-plates of L5 and S1 which can impinge on the L5 nerve root in the paravertebral gutter.

Degenerative spondylolisthesis is an important cause of central canal stenosis (236,305,360) and most frequently involves the L4-L5 disc level (305). Disc degeneration associated with degenerative changes of sagittally oriented facet joints (476) may result in a degenerative spondylolisthesis. Patients with both (left and right) facet joints oriented at an angle greater than 45° (relative to the coronal plane) may have a 24 times increased risk of degenerative spondylolisthesis (44). The spondylolisthesis rarely progresses beyond a grade I slip due to the intact neural arch. Hyperostotic spurs projecting off the anteromedial margin of the facet joints, hypertrophy of the ligamenta flava, annular redundancy, synovial cysts (237,303,500), and the spondylolisthesis can result in severe central canal and subarticular lateral recess stenosis. There is usually at least mild narrowing of the interver-

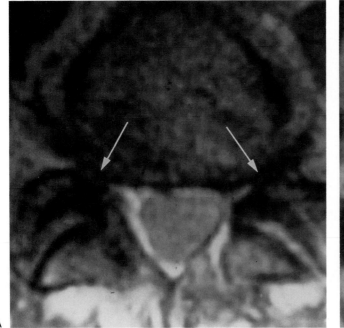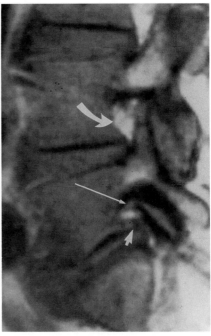

A   B

FIG. 27. Intervertebral canal stenosis. On the axial proton-density weighted image (**A**), at the L5-S1 disc level, degenerative ridges are projecting into the intervertebral canals bilaterally (arrows). It is difficult to determine the degree of stenosis on the axial image. On the sagittal T1-weighted image (**B**), at the L5-S1 disc level, the osseous spurs (short arrow) are identified projecting into the intervertebral canal causing moderate stenosis. There is also prominence of the superior articular process of S1 which is impinging on the L5 nerve root (long arrow). The intervertebral canal (curved arrow) at the L4-L5 disc level is normal for comparison.

tebral canals in the cephalocaudal direction secondary to the decreased disc height and the spondylolisthesis, but osteophytic spurring causing neural impingement of the nerve root in the intervertebral canal is an unusual finding. At the L5-S1 disc level, congenital spondylolisthesis associated with dysplastic or sagittally oriented articular processes can be associated with severe central canal narrowing (578). Spondylolisthesis at the L5-S1 disc level has also been described in association with childhood discitis (596).

Isthmic spondylolysis represents a fracture of the pars interarticularis, but since the presenting symptoms of adult patients with spondylolysis are usually related to secondary degenerative changes it has been included in this section on degenerative disease. In patients with isthmic spondylolysis and spondylolisthesis, there are several potential etiologies for neural impingement (590). Fragmentation and hypertrophy of the pars interarticularis can lead to a narrowed central spinal canal (578). Stenosis of the intervertebral canals (129) is frequently identified and may be secondary to the spondylolisthesis, the hypertrophied pars interarticularis, degenerative spurs projecting off the vertebral body end-plates, and disc or soft tissue encroachment. Spondylolysis and spondylolisthesis at the L5-S1 disc level will frequently lead to stenosis of the intervertebral canals in a cephalo-

caudal direction which can compress the L5 nerve root between the pedicle of L5 and the posterosuperior rim of S1 (210) (Fig. 28). The detection of spondylolytic defects with MRI is optimal on a sagittal T1-weighted image (186,246), but MRI has limitations in identifying the degree of pars fragmentation and in delineating small spondylolytic defects (186). MRI is excellent in the evaluation of associated disc degeneration which appears more prevalent in patients with spondylolysis at both the level of the spondylolytic defects (534) and at the superjacent disc level (186,463).

In addition to osseous degenerative changes which may lead to stenosis of the spinal canal, other osseous abnormalities which may narrow the central spinal canal include post-traumatic deformity (Fig. 29), overgrowth of a spinal fusion (268), Paget's disease (580), fluorosis, vertebral hemangiomas (455), and diffuse idiopathic skeletal hyperostosis (256). Soft tissue elements in the central spinal canal can also compress the cauda equina. Hypertrophy and ossification of the posterior longitudinal ligament and ligamenta flava (283) have been associated with stenotic symptoms. Compression of the thecal sac secondary to epidural fat has been documented in both morbidly obese patients (15,518) (Fig. 30), patients with elevated cortisol levels, and in postoperative patients with autogenous fat grafts (324,420). The noncom-

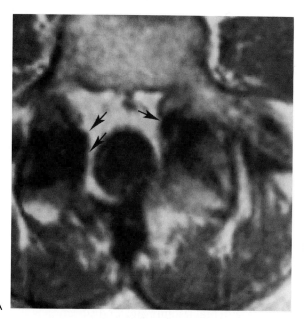
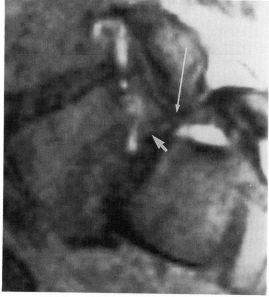

A

B

FIG. 28. Isthmic spondylolysis. On the axial T1-weighted image (**A**), there is a deformity of the L5 pars interarticularis bilaterally (arrows) suggesting a bilateral spondylolysis. On the sagittal T1-weighted image (**B**), the spondylolysis (long arrow) is better defined along with the severe cephalocaudal narrowing of the intervertebral canal. The L5 nerve root (short arrow) is compressed between the pedicle of L5 and the posterosuperior rim of the S1 vertebral body.

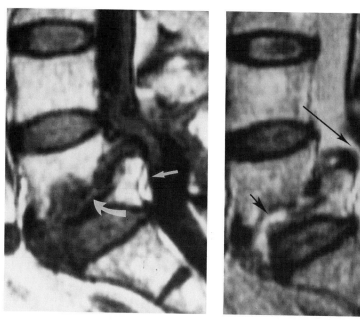

A

B

FIG. 29. On the sagittal T1-weighted image (**A**), there is marked deformity of the L4-L5 discovertebral joint (curved arrow) and marked deformation of the adjacent vertebral body end-plates. A severe compression deformity of the L5 vertebral body (straight arrow) is identified along with a grade I spondylolisthesis. On the sagittal T2-weighted image (**B**), increased signal intensity is identified in the disc space (short arrow) but not in the adjacent vertebral bodies. These changes were secondary to chronic compression fractures associated with severe degenerative changes of the intervertebral disc and not to infection. The T2-weighted image optimally delineates the severity of the central canal stenosis (long arrow).

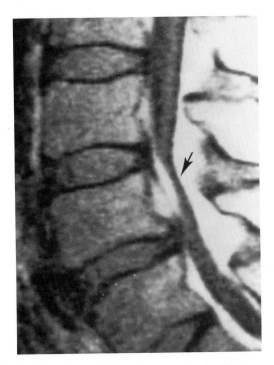

FIG. 30. Central canal stenosis associated with exogenous obesity. On the sagittal T1-weighted image, posterior to the midbody of L4, there is severe circumferential narrowing of the thecal sac (arrow) secondary to prominent epidural fat.

pliance of the normal posterior epidural fat and its potential role in compressing the thecal sac has been demonstrated on dynamic CT evaluation of the spine (402). Facet joint degenerative changes along with facet joint hypertrophy may be associated with anterior displacement of the posterior epidural fat resulting in posterior compression of the thecal sac (Fig. 31). MRI is also excellent in excluding disease processes that may present with neurogenic claudication, or radicular symptoms, including intracanalicular (322) and intraspinal synovial cysts (20,237,284,303), intra- and extradural tumors (170,330,603), multiple myeloma (Fig. 32), and metastatic disease (13).

SPINAL TRAUMA

The optimal treatment of cervical cord injury secondary to vertebral fracture and/or dislocation is still in evolution (108,239). MRI provides the first noninvasive imaging procedure to directly assess the degree of dural and spinal cord compression along with pathologic spinal cord changes. Traumatic injury to spinal ligaments, soft tissues, and osseous structures can also be evaluated on the standard MRI exam (270). The coexistence of cervi-

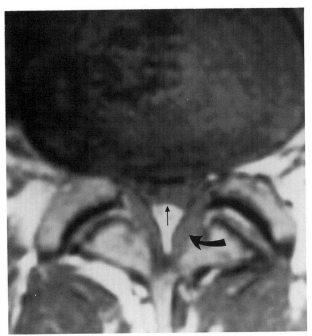
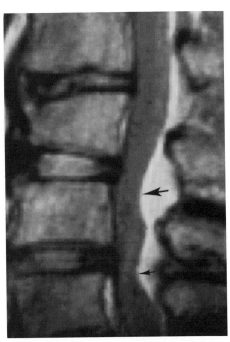

FIG. 31. On the axial T1-weighted image (**A**), there is prominence of the facet joints and thickened ligamenta flava (curved arrow). The posterior epidural fat (small straight arrow) is effacing the posterior margin of the thecal sac. This is better demonstrated on the sagittal proton-density weighted image (**B**), where the posterior compression of the thecal sac by the posterior epidural fat (arrows) is identified at the L3-L4 and L4-L5 disc levels.

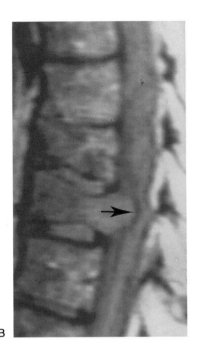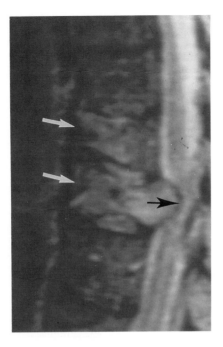

A,B

FIG. 32. Multiple myeloma. On the sagittal T1-weighted image (**A**), a compressed and deformed T12 vertebral body is identified which is causing severe stenosis (arrow) of the central spinal canal. On the sagittal T2-weighted image (**B**), increased signal intensity is identified in the T11 and T12 vertebral bodies (white arrows) compatible with metastatic disease or myeloma. With increased signal intensity of the CSF, there is improved delineation of the thoracic spinal cord and the degree of cord compression is now delineated (black arrow).

cal fracture/dislocations and disc herniations is higher than once thought and is easily seen on MRI (120,438).

It is now possible to closely monitor the acutely injured patient during an MRI examination (327,346,461). The value of MRI in diagnosing spinal cord hemorrhage and edema along with neural compression has been well documented (21,281,326,347,551). In two studies, patient outcome was directly related to the presence of spinal cord hemorrhage, contusion, or edema at the time of the initial injury. Neurologic recovery was insignificant in patients with intramedullary spinal cord hemorrhage; however, patients with spinal cord edema or contusion recovered significant neurologic function (281,479). While a sagittal T1-weighted image may demonstrate altered spinal cord morphology, a sagittal T2-weighted image is the most important in delineating abnormal signal intensity in the spinal cord. Gradient-echo sequences are the most sensitive in detecting hemosiderin, due to their increased sensitivity to magnetic susceptibility effects.

The appearance of hemorrhage in the spinal cord can vary depending upon the state of hemoglobin breakdown (191,347). Decreased signal intensity on T2-weighted images in an acutely injured spinal cord most likely represents deoxyhemoglobin in acute hemorrhage, whereas increased signal intensity represents changes of contusion and edema (191). Another recent study evaluating acute cervical spine trauma demonstrated that MRI findings of an intramedullary hematoma or spinal cord contusion involving more than one spinal segment were associated with severe neurologic deficit (159,478, 479). One study comparing MRI to CT-myelography demonstrated MRI to be superior except in the evaluation of cervical spine fractures. Employing T1- and T2-weighted sequences, MRI was sensitive in the evaluation

of vertebral body fractures and malalignment but was limited in the evaluation of fractures of the posterior elements (347). The benefit of the CT study was only in fracture delineation, obviating the need for intrathecal contrast. The same study demonstrated a high incidence of chronic disc disease in the acutely injured patient, and the disc herniations and spondylotic changes were better delineated on the MRI exam. In one study comparing MRI to high resolution CT in the evaluation of subluxation and spinal canal measurements, MRI provided similar measurements of subluxation compared to CT and also provided additional information in the evaluation of disc, spinal cord, and ligamentous injury (551). Four of the patients in that series sustained acute penetrating spinal injuries and in two patients the location of metallic foreign bodies was demonstrated with MRI. Neither patient with metallic foreign bodies deteriorated during or after the MRI examination. In a recent study evaluating acute post-traumatic ascending myelopathy, magnetic resonance imaging demonstrated intrathecal hemorrhage within the first 2 weeks following injury followed by cord atrophy within 4 weeks of the initial trauma (598).

Patients with cervical developmental spinal stenosis (134,287,321) or spondylosis (149) appear to be more prone to spinal cord injury because of the decreased functional AP diameter of their central canals. The decreased sagittal diameter appears to be more important than the cross-sectional area in predicting the potential of cord injury (321). The evaluation of the cervico-occipital junction and C1-C2 relationship in patients with an atlantoaxial dislocation (273) can also be easily assessed with MRI evaluation.

In the evaluation of the chronically injured spinal

cord, MRI has been more accurate than CT-myelography in the characterization of intramedullary abnormalities (262). The difference between myelomalacia and post-traumatic cysts is frequently difficult to determine with delayed CT-myelography, but can be delineated by MRI (169,423).

The MRI evaluation of patients with either acute spinal cord trauma or post-traumatic myelopathy requires, at a minimum, axial and sagittal T1-weighted sequences to optimally evaluate the vertebrae, disc, ligamentous anatomy, and cord morphology. Sagittal and occasionally axial T2-weighted sequences are needed for the optimal evaluation of intramedullary cord pathology, compressive deformation of the thecal sac, and posterior ligamentous disruption. If a limited number of MRI sequences are obtained, it may be difficult to delineate the exact origins of the epidural abnormalities (21). MRI is also the optimal modality to evaluate patients with persistent cranial or neural symptoms after a cervical injury. In one study, patients presenting with cranial symptoms of the Barré-Lieou syndrome having also sustained previous whiplash neck injuries had lateral disc herniations demonstrated at the C3-C4 level (539).

The second most common region for spinal trauma is at the thoracolumbar junction with burst fractures, wedge compression fractures, and flexion distraction injuries potentially leading to neural impingement (12,173). The correlation between the acute traumatic deformation and the eventual neurologic outcome is still under investigation (173,200,259), particularly since remodeling of the traumatic deformity has been documented (155). By its excellent delineation of the thecal sac and conus medullaris, MRI has been helpful in delineating the degree of encroachment of the spinal canal (Fig. 33). In one study, neurologic morbidity was related to the level of the conus medullaris and patency of the ventral subarachnoid space demonstrated on the MRI examination (37). Patients with a conus located above the level of the fracture and a patent ventral subarachnoid space experienced the least neurologic injury. In one recent study, MRI had a sensitivity of 90% and a specificity of 100% for predicting disruption of the posterior ligaments (137). With MRI, it is also possible to demonstrate extradural collections of fluid secondary to dural lacerations. Dural lacerations have been associated with laminar fractures at the thoracolumbar junction (76,407). The same imaging sequences used in the cervical spine are employed in the evaluation of the thoracolumbar junction. In addition, axial conventional or RARE T2-weighted or gradient-echo sequences are needed to define the position and configuration of extradural fluid accumulations. In the lumbar spine, post-traumatic vertebral deformity and stenosis may also occur and the approach to MR imaging would be similar to the evaluation of the thoracolumbar junction. In addition to post-traumatic stenosis, there have been iso-

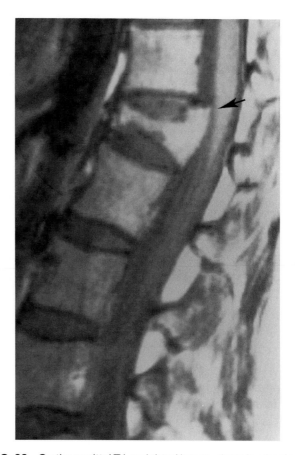

FIG. 33. On the sagittal T1-weighted image, there is a benign compression fracture of the L1 vertebral body with retropulsion of the vertebral body causing minimal impingement of the conus medullaris (arrow). Diffuse decreased signal intensity in the cancellous bone of the L3, L4, and L5 vertebrae is present and represents metastatic disease.

lated reports of post-traumatic arachnoid cysts in the lumbar spine which MRI accurately defined (344).

SPINAL TUMORS

Patients with tumors involving the central spinal canal or vertebrae may present with a rapidly progressive myeloradiculopathy, but most frequently their symptomatology is subacute or chronic in nature. In the evaluation of spinal tumors, it is helpful to classify tumor location as: (a) intramedullary, (b) intradural-extramedullary, (c) extradural, and (d) osseous. Some tumors will be located in two sites, particularly metastatic disease involving the vertebral body and extending into the extradural space.

MRI has rapidly become the imaging study of choice in the assessment of intramedullary lesions of the spinal cord (116,161,250,414,514,530). In addition to delineating morphologic alterations of the spinal cord, MRI is able to characterize the nature of the intramedullary pathology due to the differences in signal intensity of blood, tumor, and cyst compared to the normal spinal cord. Intramedullary cord tumors may be isointense or hypointense on T1-weighted sequences and isointense or hyperintense on T2-weighted sequences when compared to the normal spinal cord (Fig. 34). A true T2-weighted sequence with flow compensation or cardiac gating is needed to optimally evaluate the spinal cord for intramedullary pathology. An additional gradient-echo sequence may also help characterize spinal cord pathology, particularly if there is a hemorrhagic component to the pathologic process (Fig. 35).

It may be difficult to differentiate between a malignant versus a benign spinal cord syrinx on a standard MRI exam. On standard T2-weighted sequences, a benign syrinx may be associated with increased signal intensity in the spinal cord immediately adjacent to the syrinx, which pathologically represents areas of gliosis. The administration of Gd-DTPA, which penetrates the regions of blood-brain barrier breakdown, improves characterization and delineation of malignant processes (74,394, 529,530,559) and is particularly helpful in the delineation of tumor margins and in the differentiation between a malignant versus a benign syrinx (504,530,585) (Fig.

36). The limits of the tumor may not be precisely defined by Gd-DTPA due to intra-axial infiltration of the tumor beyond the region of breakdown of the blood-brain barrier (116). Gd-DTPA has also proved useful in the evaluation of patients who have undergone an operative procedure or radiation therapy and are being reevaluated for the possibility of tumor recurrence. Enhancement with Gd-DTPA has been helpful in distinguishing between cord edema, demyelination, and gliosis versus recurrent tumor (530). In addition to primary and metastatic malignant tumors in the spinal cord, enhancement with Gd-DTPA has also been reported with spinal cord infarcts, myelomalacia, myelitis, multiple sclerosis (314), sarcoidosis (376), arteriovenous malformations (116), and intramedullary metastases (164).

In the evaluation of intradural-extramedullary tumors, the intravenous injection of Gd-DTPA transforms a relatively insensitive standard MRI examination (280) into an extremely effective exam in depicting leptomeningeal spread of tumors (29,486,520,527). In addition to the detection of small tumor nodules, thickening and clumping of the nerve roots has also been detected in cases of leptomeningeal disease (527). Compared to myelographic studies, standard MRI examinations have

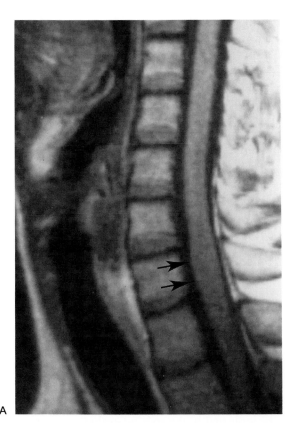 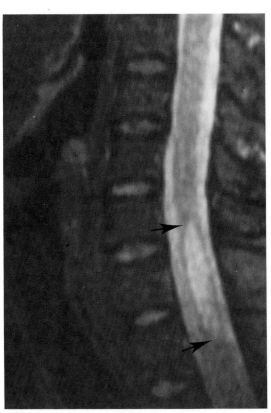

A   B

FIG. 34. Cervical glioma. On the sagittal T1-weighted image (**A**), there is widening of the cervical spinal cord (arrows) at the cervicothoracic junction and slight decreased signal intensity in the central portion of the spinal cord. The sagittal cardiac gated T2-weighted image (**B**) is needed to optimally evaluate the abnormal signal intensity in the spinal cord and to delineate the extent of the tumor (arrows).

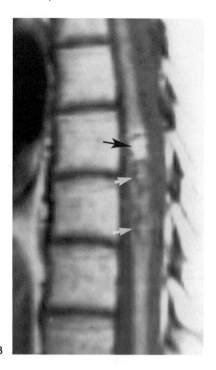 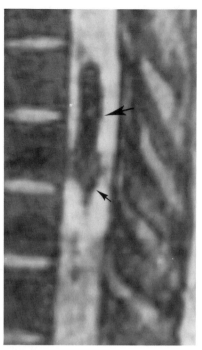

A,B

FIG. 35. Intramedullary mass of the mid-thoracic spinal cord, probably cavernous hemangioma. On the sagittal T1-weighted image (**A**), an intramedullary mass in the thoracic spinal cord is identified which is causing mild cord widening. There is increased signal intensity in the cephalad portion (black arrow) of the mass probably related to hemoglobin breakdown products. The remainder of the mass is isointense or hypointense (white arrows) with respect to the normal spinal cord. On the sagittal gradient-echo image (**B**), there is diffuse decreased signal intensity in the mass (arrows) compatible with blood breakdown products causing signal loss from tissue susceptibility effects.

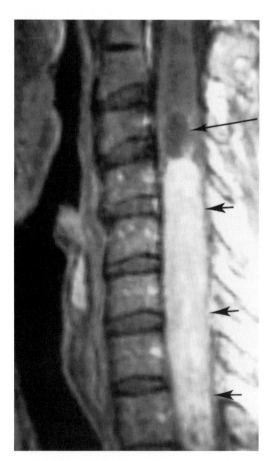

FIG. 36. Cervical glioma. The sagittal T1-weighted sequence, after an intravenous injection of Gd-DTPA, helps differentiate the intramedullary tumor with high signal intensity (short arrows) from the adjacent benign cystic changes (long arrow).

also provided a more complete evaluation of meningiomas, neurofibromas (69,323,489) (Fig. 37), and fatty tumors (362,546). On T1-weighted sequences, Pantopaque in the subarachnoid space demonstrates high signal intensity and should not be mistaken for an intradural fatty tumor or hemorrhage (309,524). A study comparing MRI to myelography in the evaluation of patients with extradural masses causing cord compression demonstrated a sensitivity of 92% and specificity of 90% with MRI, compared to 95% specificity and 88% accuracy with myelography. For extradural masses without cord compression, the sensitivity of MRI was 73% and the specificity 90% versus a sensitivity of 49% and a specificity of 88% for myelography. The authors recommended that MR imaging should be the initial study in the evaluation of spinal cord compression due to metastatic disease (78). MRI has also been very helpful in delineating noncontiguous extradural masses which can easily be missed by myelography in patients with high grade blocks of the subarachnoid space. In patients with extradural masses, it is frequently helpful to obtain additional sagittal T1-weighted sequences of the remaining spinal column to exclude unsuspected metastatic deposits. Use of the phased-array surface coil with a large (48 cm) field of view and a 512 × 512 matrix permits a high resolution scan of essentially the entire spine in a single acquisition of less than 5 minutes.

The administration of Gd-DTPA does not appear to be indicated in the routine evaluation of extradural spinal tumors. One recent study demonstrated no improved detection rate of neoplastic involvement of the vertebrae or epidural space (531), and in some cases, the

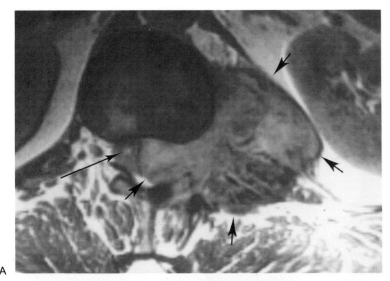

A

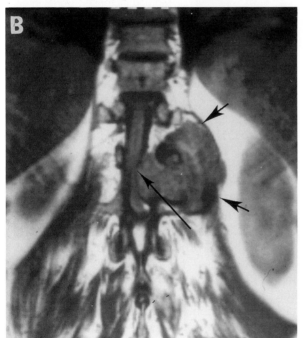

B

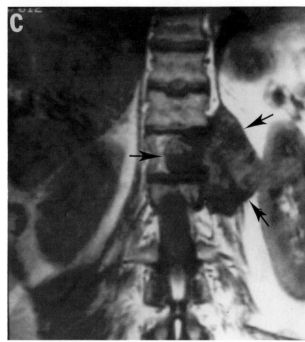

C

FIG. 37. Neurofibroma. On the axial T1-weighted image (**A**), a large extradural neurofibroma (short arrows) is identified displacing the conus medullaris (long arrow) to the right. The neurofibroma extends through the left intervertebral canal and into the left paraspinal space. On the coronal T1-weighted images (**B**) and (**C**), the degree of cord displacement (long arrow) along with the tumor margins (short arrows) are well-delineated.

Gd-DTPA-enhanced images obscured metastatic osseous deposits by transforming lesions that were hypointense to the adjacent bone marrow on precontrast images to isointense lesions on postcontrast images, rendering them no longer detectable (520,531) (Fig. 38). Gd-DTPA may be of benefit in selecting the biopsy site of extradural tumors and in differentiating tumor versus disc herniation (62). Chemical shift imaging (fat saturation) utilizing paramagnetic contrast material (171,502,548) and inversion recovery sequences (124,520) has demonstrated these sequences to be more effective in the evaluation of extradural tumors and bone metastases when compared to standard T1 and T2 sequences. These additional sequences may become an important adjunct in

the evaluation of patients presenting with myelopathy or suspected of having metastatic disease. MRI can detect bone lesions even when the bone scan is negative (90).

Neurologic dysfunction secondary to arteriovenous malformations (AVM) of the spinal cord most frequently presents in the adult population and rarely in the pediatric age group (390). MRI has been successful in distinguishing between extradural, dural, and intradural arteriovenous malformations (112,119,319,342,545). In addition, MRI is able to evaluate the status of the spinal cord adjacent to the malformation (342). In one study, Gd-DTPA infusion helped delineate the margins of the AVM and demonstrated enhancement in the adjacent spinal cord (545).

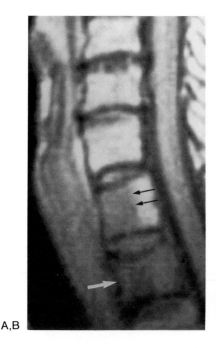 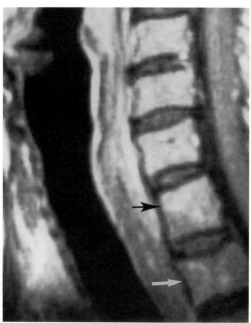

A,B

FIG. 38. Metastatic prostate carcinoma. On the sagittal T1-weighted image (**A**), the anterior two-thirds of the C7 vertebral body (black arrows), and the entire T1 vertebral body (white arrow) are hypointense compared to the normal C6 vertebra. After the intravenous injection of Gd-DTPA, on the sagittal T1-weighted image (**B**), the anterior two-thirds of the C7 vertebral body (black arrow) is now isointense compared to normal marrow, making the diagnosis of metastatic disease extremely difficult if there was no precontrast T1-weighted image for comparison. Mottled increased signal intensity is identified in the T1 vertebral body (white arrow) compared to the T1-weighted image.

MRI (especially using a gradient-echo sequence sensitive to susceptibility of hemosiderin) is excellent at screening intramedullary AVMs. However, with extramedullary vascular malformations, a small draining vein of a spinal-dural arteriovenous fistula may be missed on MRI, due to its small size, as well as pulsation artifact within T2-bright CSF, and lack of conspicuity with T1-dark CSF. In such cases, meticulously performed plain myelography (with the patient supine) may be needed to detect the dilated draining vein on the dorsum of the cord.

Benign cystic lesions involving the spinal cord, subarachnoid (503), and extradural spaces (371) are optimally evaluated with MRI (82,180,274,292,409,496, 583,585) (Fig. 39). In the evaluation of syringomyelia and hydromyelia, it is possible to quickly determine the extent of the cystic cavity and to evaluate the adjacent spinal structures determining whether spinal malformations are present (107). Thin-section sagittal and axial T1-weighted images clearly delineate the dark-appearing syrinx from the relatively bright cord parenchyma. The sequencing parameters of an MRI examination are important to prevent syrinx-like artifacts (truncation errors) (64,100,296) and may also be helpful in investigating fluid dynamics in cystic lesions (140). Extradural cysts most often occur in the lower thoracic spine and may compress the adjacent spinal cord or nerve roots (182). MRI has been successful in delineating the extent of each of these cystic processes (182,408,503) and in determining the degree of neural compression.

In the evaluation of spinal dysraphism, MRI has quickly become the initial screening examination for evaluating the spinal cord, position of the conus medul-laris, morphology of the filum terminale, and for identifying associated lipomatous traction lesions (19,105, 372,427,587) (Fig. 40). Coronal and sagittal T1-weighted images are frequently obtained for a rapid screening exam, but additional multiplanar sequences are necessary for a more complete evaluation of a dysraphic myelopathy (19). Axial T1- and T2-weighted images are needed to diagnose focal syringohydromyelia and myelomalacic abnormalities located near the conus. These abnormalities have been identified in some patients with a tethered cord (427). Axial T2-weighted images are also frequently needed to distinguish between diastematomyelia and small hydromyelic cavities (105). Imaging of pulsatile cord motion may also be clinically useful when evaluating diseases restricting cord motion or changing the status of parenchymal compliance (297).

VERTEBRAL BODY MARROW DISORDERS

The basic microstructure of bone marrow consists of a trabecular bone framework surrounding fat cells, hematopoietic cells, reticulum cells, nerves, and vascular sinusoids. MR imaging of marrow depends upon the chemical components of the two types of marrow: red marrow which contains approximately 40% water, 40% fat, and 20% protein, and yellow marrow which contains approximately 15% water, 80% fat, and 5% protein (572). T1-weighted sequences optimize the signal from fat (117,431) and provide excellent anatomic detail. Any pathologic process which replaces fat in the marrow can be delineated by decreased signal intensity of the marrow on a T1-weighted image, but T2-weighted sequences are

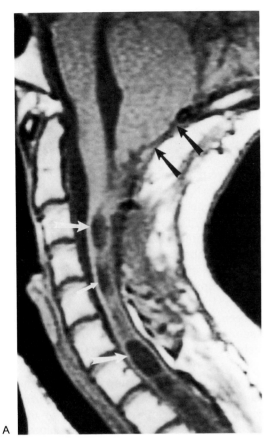
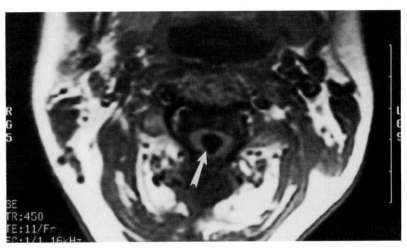

A

B

FIG. 39. Arnold-Chiari malformation with holocord syrinx. Sagittal T1-weighted image (**A**) shows pronounced cerebellar tonsillar herniation below the foramen magnum (black arrows), and postoperative changes from decompressive laminectomy. Syrinx containing septations is well demonstrated on T1-weighted sagittal (**A**) and axial (**B**) images (white arrows).

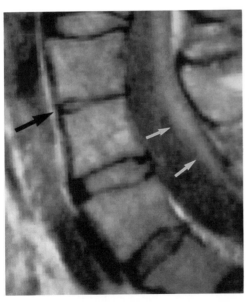
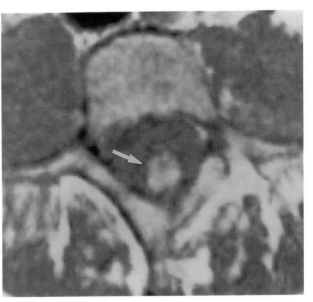

A

B

FIG. 40. Tethered spinal cord in a middle-aged male presenting with a short history of radicular symptoms. On the sagittal (**A**) and axial (**B**) T1-weighted images, a tethered spinal cord is identified (white arrows). A segmentation anomaly at the L3-L4 disc level is present (black arrow) along with increased AP diameter of the lower central spinal canal. There is a spina bifida of L5 and S1 with absence of the spinous processes.

needed to characterize the abnormal tissue. A pathologic process with increased free water or unbound intracellular water will demonstrate hyperintensity on T2-weighted images compared to the normal fatty marrow. In addition to the standard T1- and T2-weighted sequences recommended for the evaluation of vertebral marrow (510), inversion recovery, gradient-echo (492), chemical shift imaging (446,593), and various fast-spin-echo sequences (248) are being utilized in the evaluation of marrow disorders. Fat-saturated post-gadolinium T1-weighted sequences may improve lesion conspicuity (171,548).

Any disease process that infiltrates or replaces red or yellow marrow can accurately be delineated on standard T1- and T2-weighted images. This includes benign and malignant tumors (91,455,510), leukemia (365), lymphoma (299), myeloma (102), infection, thickened trabecular bone (440), focal fat deposition (193), marrow abnormalities associated with degenerative disc disease (109), and avascular necrosis (373). T1-weighted gradient-echo images and fat-suppressed sequences such as short T1 inversion recovery (STIR) are also useful to image multiple myeloma (13,298,367,428,429). MRI is extremely sensitive to alterations in the vertebral body marrow, but lacks specificity as to the etiology of the various pathologic processes (523). Any disorder or therapeutic procedure resulting in loss of myeloid elements,

such as aplastic anemia (509) or radiation therapy (431), may demonstrate increased T1 signal intensity in the marrow secondary to fatty replacement of hematopoietic tissue. MRI is also excellent in delineating the vertebral and paravertebral extent of tumor (78,192,289,359, 487,510) which is important information when planning radiation therapy or surgical decompression (579). Thin-section (3 mm) T1-weighted sagittal images using the phased-array coil with large field of view (48 cm) and large matrix (512 × 512) permit screening of essentially the entire spine for vertebral metastases in a single acquisition. Fast-spin-echo (RARE) sagittal T2-weighted images (for myelogram effect), and axial T1 or RARE-T2 images through regions of tumor complete the screening MRI in a total exam time of 30 minutes (Fig. 41). In addition, Gd-DTPA enhanced MRI may be helpful in defining the response of leukemic and myelomatous bone marrow to therapy and for evaluating the possibility of recurrence (331,385,429).

There have been conflicting reports on the value of MRI in distinguishing between benign and malignant causes of vertebral compression fractures (16,614) (Fig. 42), and a large prospective study is needed to determine the accuracy of MRI to predict the causes of compression deformities. One study reported chronic benign fractures had a homogeneous isointense marrow signal on T1 and T2-weighted images (16). Pathologic vertebral fractures

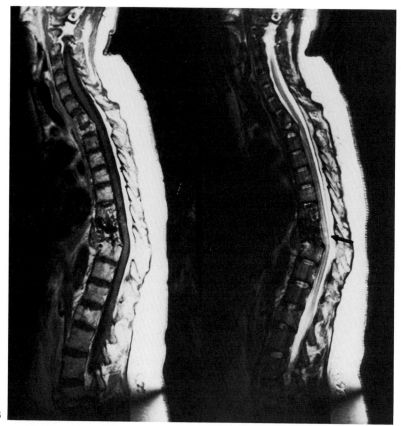

A,B

FIG. 41. Screening study for cord compression in a patient with metastatic lung cancer. Large field-of-view images using the phased-array surface coil cover essentially the entire spine in a single rapid acquisition. Sagittal T1 (**A**) and RARE-T2 (**B**) images show a compression fracture at T2, with kyphotic angulation and slight posterior displacement of the cord, and prior fusion of tumor-infiltrated bone from T7-T9, with kyphotic angulation at T9-10. Note a tiny focus of post-traumatic myelomalacia at the level of T9 (arrow). For purposes of counting vertebrae, note that the occipito-atlantal (C1) junction is well demonstrated at the top of Figure 41A.

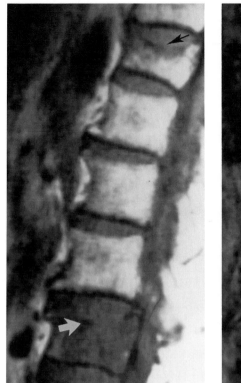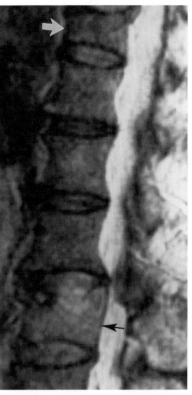

A   B

FIG. 42. Benign and malignant vertebral compression fractures. On the sagittal T1-weighted image (**A**), there is a benign compression fracture of the T12 vertebral body. Except for a small hemispheric region of decreased signal intensity in the superior segment of T12 (black arrow), the signal intensity in the superior segment of the T12 (black arrow), the signal intensity in the cancellous bone of T12 is isointense with respect to the normal L1 vertebral body marrow. There is a malignant compression fracture of the L4 vertebral body (white arrow), and in contrast to the T12 vertebra the marrow signal intensity of L4 is diffusely hypointense with respect to the normal marrow. On the sagittal T2-weighted image (**B**), the normal vertebral marrow fat has become less intense compared to its appearance on the T1-weighted image. The metastatic process involving the L4 vertebra (black arrow) has become slightly hyperintense compared to the normal vertebral bodies making it difficult to delineate the abnormal cancellous bone on the T2-weighted image compared to the T1-weighted image. The signal intensity of the T12 vertebra (white arrow) remains isointense with the normal vertebrae.

were characterized by decreased signal intensity on T1- and increased signal intensity on T2-weighted images, and had posterior-convex deformity of the vertebral body. Acute benign compression fractures also had increased signal intensity on T2-weighted images, but were inhomogeneous.

SPINAL INFECTION

In the adult, infection of the spinal column usually involves the vertebral bodies and intervening disc. Staphylococcus is the most common organism causing spinal infection, but in diabetics, intravenous drug users, and immunosuppressed patients, a variety of organisms, both aerobic and anaerobic, may be the source of infection. The diagnosis of vertebral osteomyelitis based on MRI includes: (a) confluent decreased signal intensity in the vertebral bodies and intervertebral disc with inability

to discern a margin between the disc and the adjacent vertebral bodies on T1-weighted images, (b) increased signal intensity in the vertebral bodies adjacent to the intervertebral disc on T2-weighted images (TR 2,000–3,000 milliseconds, TE 120 milliseconds), and (c) abnormal configuration and increased signal intensity of the intervertebral disc, along with the absence of the intranuclear cleft (3) on a T2-weighted image (TR 2,000–3,000 milliseconds, TE 120 milliseconds) (Fig. 43). The altered signal intensity in the disc and adjacent vertebral bodies is probably secondary to the inflammatory infiltrate and vascular ischemia in the infected vertebrae (350).

In the diagnostic evaluation of osteomyelitis, MRI has a reported sensitivity of 96%, a specificity of 93%, and an accuracy of 94%, equaling the results of a combined bone scan and gallium study (350). The main advantages of MRI over radionuclide studies included significant anatomic information concerning the spinal cord, thecal

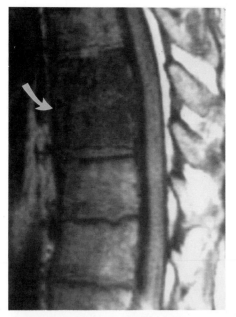

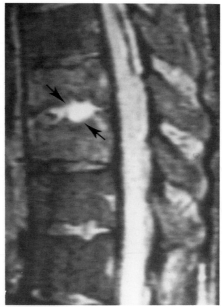

A

B

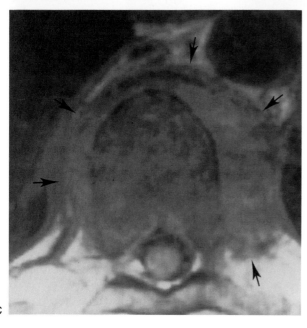

C

FIG. 43. Pyogenic vertebral osteomyelitis. On the sagittal T1-weighted image (**A**), there is a confluent area of decreased signal intensity involving the T7 and T8 vertebral bodies and the intervening disc (arrow). On the sagittal T2-weighted image (**B**), increased signal intensity is identified in the disc space (arrows) along with diffuse increased signal intensity in the adjacent vertebral body marrow. The axial T1-weighted image (**C**) is needed to demonstrate the degree of extension of the inflammatory process into the paravertebral soft tissue (arrows).

sac, and paravertebral soft tissues. MRI was also useful in following the resolution and possible recurrence of the inflammatory process. The hyperintensity of the infected disc on T2-weighted images may not be as prominent in patients receiving antibiotics. In follow-up studies, the abnormal signal intensity in the disc appeared to resolve more quickly than the abnormal signal intensity changes in the adjacent vertebral bodies (350). In the adult, isolated discitis is usually the result of iatrogenic intrusion of the disc space and has been reported following surgery (32,103,300), discography (190), and percutaneous nucleotomy (34). Theoretically, in a child isolated discitis can occur due to the presence of direct vascular communications into the disc. With MRI evaluation of

childhood discitis (168), it is possible to determine whether discitis is truly limited to the disc space.

The MRI findings of nonpyogenic osteomyelitis may be different from the findings of pyogenic infections (24). In one small series, the presentation of tuberculous spondylitis suggested neoplasm rather than infection because of the involvement of the posterior margin of the vertebral body and posterior elements and the lack of involvement of the disc and vertebral body end-plates (507). Brucellar spondylitis may also present with MRI abnormalities confined only to the vertebral body. In one series comparing the presentation of brucellar versus tuberculous spondylitis, tuberculosis had a propensity to involve the thoracic spine and brucellosis to involve the lumbar spine, but when tuberculosis involved the lumbar spine, the two disease processes appeared quite similar (493). Tuberculosis did have a tendency for greater extension into the spinal canal and paravertebral space (Fig. 44). A coronal sequence will frequently help delineate the degree of paraspinal involvement (24,110,494).

MRI has quickly become the screening exam for the evaluation of epidural abscesses (8,415,475) (Fig. 45). In several studies, MRI findings were diagnostic for osteomyelitis with disc space infection associated with epidural abscesses, and obviated the need for CT-myelography when there was no concomitant meningitis (381,547). Axial T2-weighted images were needed to delineate the margins and extent of the epidural abscess, but it was not possible to determine whether an abscess was acute or chronic. An epidural abscess is usually iso- or hypointense on T1, hyperintense on T2, hyper- or isointense on T2* GRE images, and enhances with gadolinium, often containing nonenhancing foci of pus, surrounded by enhancing inflammatory tissue (278, 416,475). Fat-saturated post-gadolinium images may enhance conspicuity of the abscess (171,548). Fifteen percent of the epidural abscesses were not associated with vertebral osteomyelitis. The location of the epidural abscesses was ventral or ventral-lateral to the thecal sac which is in contrast to the typical dorsal location reported in other studies (415). In the same series (collected in 1987), if a patient had an epidural abscess and meningitis, the abscess was poorly defined by MRI, requiring CT-myelography to make the definitive diagnosis. With current MR technology, both signal-to-noise and resolution are significantly improved since this study was performed in 1987, so the need for confirmatory CT-myelography is lessened or obviated. Epidural abscesses have also been reported in association with pyogenic osteomyelitis of a facet joint (442).

Transverse myelitis may present as an isolated inflammatory process involving the spinal cord (335) or associated with epidural abscesses (415), demyelinating processes, collagen-vascular disease, and paraneoplastic syndromes (335). The findings on MRI have included widening of the spinal cord on T1-weighted images, and on T2-weighted images, isointensity (335) or hyperintensity (415) of the abnormal spinal cord segment compared to the normal spinal cord. In the cervical spine, multiple sclerosis plaques may demonstrate similar findings (Fig. 46), and an MRI examination of the brain is needed to help differentiate the two disease entities (314), although multiple sclerosis may present with spinal plaques in the absence of brain plaques. MRI is also excellent in the delineation of spinal cord atrophy which is a potential sequela of acute myelitis.

A,B
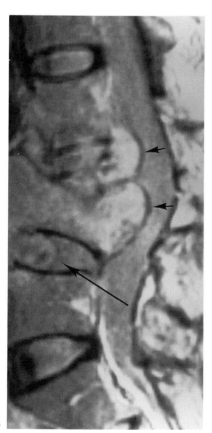
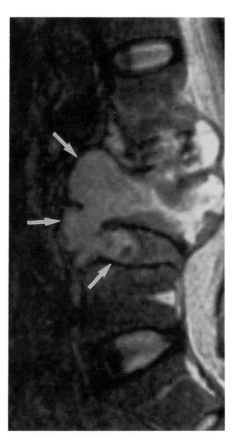

FIG. 44. Tuberculous spondylitis. On the sagittal proton-density weighted image (A), a large inflammatory mass is identified involving the L3 and L4 vertebrae and the intervening disc. The mass extends posteriorly, where it is causing moderately severe thecal sac effacement (short arrows). Inferior extension of the inflammatory mass under the anterior longitudinal ligament is present along with extension of the inflammatory process into the anterior compartment of the L4-L5 disc space (long arrow). On the sagittal T2-weighted image (B), there is increased signal intensity in the large abscess (arrows) involving the L3 and L4 vertebral bodies and the intervening disc. The extension of the abscess into the anterior compartment of the L4-L5 disc space is well delineated.

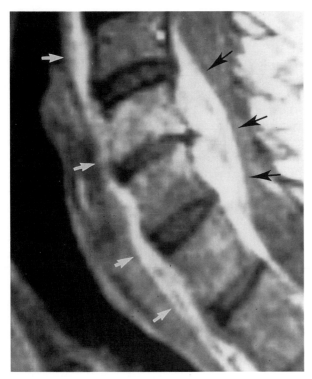

FIG. 45. Epidural abscess of the cervical spine. On the Gd-DTPA enhanced sagittal T1-weighted image, at the C5-C6 disc level, there is a hyperintense fusiform anterior epidural abscess (black arrows) which is causing severe compression of the spinal cord. There is slight increased signal intensity in the C5 vertebral body, but no evidence of an infection involving the C5-C6 disc space. Increased signal intensity is identified anterior to the cervical vertebral bodies (white arrows) secondary to extension of the inflammatory process.

POSTOPERATIVE EVALUATION OF THE SPINE

As many as 15% of patients who have undergone spinal surgery may experience persistent or recurrent symptoms. In one series, the most frequent findings accounting for failed spine surgery included central or lateral canal stenosis, recurrent or residual disc herniation, arachnoiditis, instability, and discitis (71). In the evaluation of recurrent symptoms following surgery, the challenge is to distinguish mechanical and nonmechanical causes of pain. Mechanical lesions such as spinal stenosis, disc herniation, and discitis can all produce symptoms by pressure on neural elements and are generally amenable to surgical intervention. Nonmechanical entities such as epidural fibrosis, psychosocial instability, or medical disease are not amenable to surgery.

The most important and difficult challenge of postoperative spinal imaging is to distinguish epidural scar from recurrent or residual disc material. When unenhanced CT is used in this assessment, scar can be separated from disc in 43–60% of cases (59,156). CT with intravenous contrast increases the likelihood of overall correct diagnosis to 70–83% (59,67,156,513). Unenhanced MR is reported to have an accuracy comparable to that of contrast-enhanced CT, 76–89% (67,68,224,233,513). The diagnostic accuracy of contrast-enhanced MR has been reported as high as 100% (233,448).

It is important to distinguish normal postoperative changes from findings that can result in persistent or recurrent symptoms. For example, studies in the lumbar spine have shown that 44% of asymptomatic postoperative patients show persistent herniated disc and other CT findings which are indistinguishable from those of symptomatic postoperative patients (84,363). Studies with unenhanced MR have revealed that 69% of early (<10 days) postoperative discectomy patients had intermediate intensity epidural signal with mass effect mimicking the preoperative herniated disc (454). The timing of the MRI study is important as the appearance improved in 90% of these cases on the late postoperative study. In this small series, there was no correlation between postoperative appearance and patient symptomatology, and it was concluded that the MRI examination in the immediate postoperative period is not useful to explain the causes of persistent pain.

A variety of postoperative findings are delineated when evaluating patients with recurrent back pain or failed back surgery syndrome. Epidural fibrosis is frequently present at the operative site and typically demonstrates intermediate signal intensity on T1-weighted images and increased signal intensity on T2-weighted images. Most fibrosis is poorly marginated and demonstrates no mass effect. Recurrent disc herniations typically are contiguous with the disc space, are well-marginated, and, compared to the disc of origin, demonstrate isointensity or hypointensity on T1-weighted images and isointensity or hyperintensity on T2-weighted images (67,224). Depending upon the size of the recurrent herniation, mass effect may be demonstrated with impingement on the neural elements or thecal sac. Sequestered disc fragments may be difficult to differentiate from epidural fibrosis. On T1-weighted images, sequestered fragments are frequently hyperintense to the disc of origin and may be slightly hyperintense to epidural fibrosis, and on T2-weighted images sequestered fragments may be isointense with epidural fibrosis and the thecal sac. In two studies utilizing the criteria of epidural location, morphologic configuration, signal intensity, and mass effect, MRI was extremely accurate in differentiating between disc herniation and fibrosis (67,165). In one prospective study of 14 patients evaluating the efficacy of MRI imaging in the differentiation of epidural scar versus herniated disc material, 86% of the MRI findings fully agreed with the findings at surgery (67). A complete MRI exam included a sagittal T1- and T2-weighted sequence along with axial T1-, proton-density, and T2-weighted sequences.

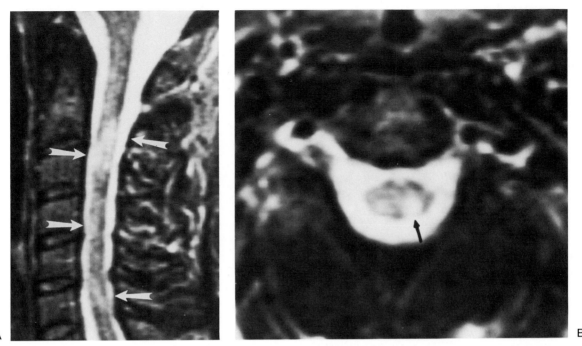

FIG. 46. Multiple sclerosis. On the sagittal (**A**) and axial (**B**) T2-weighted images, there are multiple focal regions of increased signal intensity (arrows) in a morphologically normal spinal cord.

The intravenous administration of Gd-DTPA has also been helpful in the differentiation between a disc herniation and epidural fibrosis (448). T1-weighted images obtained immediately after the intravenous administration of Gd-DTPA will demonstrate increased signal intensity in perithecal fibrosis (Fig. 47) but not in disc material (Fig. 48). Fat-saturation technique used in conjunction with gadolinium has been reported to improve conspicuity of enhancement (171,548). In one series evaluating 30 patients with failed back surgery syndrome, MRI with

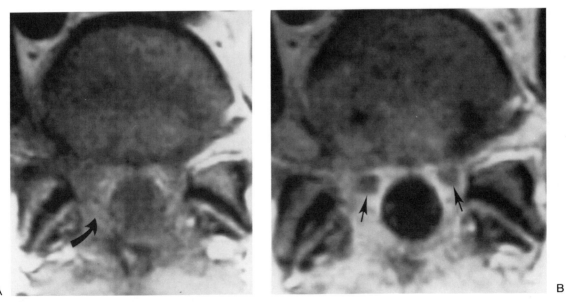

FIG. 47. Postoperative perithecal and perineural fibrosis. On the axial T1-weighted image (**A**), at the L5-S1 disc level, there is loss of signal intensity in the epidural fat secondary to postoperative fibrosis (arrow). This results in obscuration of the margins of the thecal sac and S1 nerve roots. After the intravenous injection of Gd-DTPA, the repeat axial T1-weighted image (**B**), there is homogeneous increased signal intensity in the fibrosis resulting in excellent delineation of the thecal sac and S1 nerve roots (arrows).

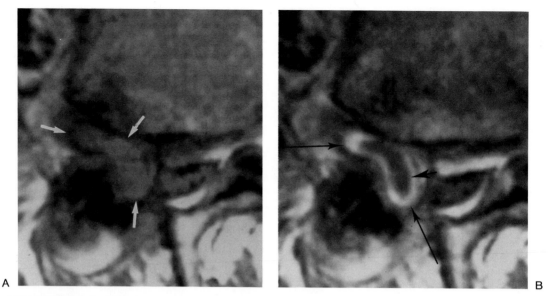

FIG. 48. Postoperative sequestered disc fragment. On the axial T1-weighted image (**A**), there is a large soft-tissue extradural mass (arrows) interposed between the right lateral margin of the thecal sac and the right facet joint. The mass extends through the right intervertebral canal. After the intravenous administration of Gd-DTPA, on the repeat axial T1-weighted image (**B**), a large sequestered disc fragment (short arrow) with low signal intensity is now identified surrounded by epidural fibrosis (long arrows) with high signal intensity.

Gd-DTPA was used to differentiate between disc herniation and fibrosis. In the 17 patients who eventually came to surgery, the precontrast MRI study had a sensitivity of 100%, specificity of 71%, and accuracy of 89%, which was improved to a 100% specificity and accuracy after the administration of Gd-DTPA (233). In one large series evaluating postoperative patients, imaging with sagittal and axial spin-echo sequences was more accurate than Gd-DTPA enhanced studies in defining the presence of disc versus fibrosis (211). Considering the additional cost of Gd-DTPA, a well-controlled large prospective study is still needed to adequately evaluate its efficacy compared to routine MRI studies.

In a recent prospective investigation, Boden et al. de-

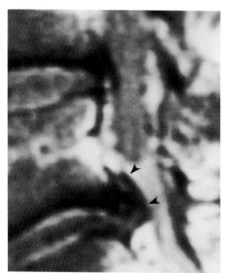
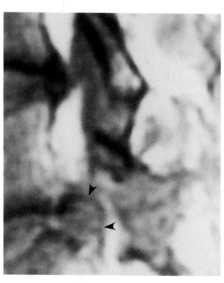
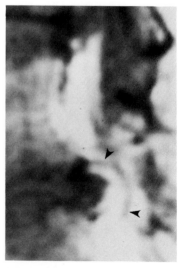

FIG. 49. Sagittal views of magnetic resonance scans from a patient who underwent uncomplicated lumbar discectomy and experienced immediate and complete relief of symptoms. **A:** Preoperative T1-weighted image shows a herniated L5-S1 disc (arrowheads). **B:** Unenhanced T1-weighted image 3 weeks after disc surgery demonstrates a large mass contiguous with the operated disc space which is at least as large as the original disc herniation. **C:** Gadolinium-enhanced image at 3 weeks shows a peripheral enhancement pattern (arrowheads) strongly suggestive of residual disc material rather than scar. From Boden et al. (41).

TABLE 5. *Postoperative epidural mass effect (n = 16)*

Neural compression[a]	No. of levels (%)		
	3 weeks	3 months	6 months
No smaller	4 (25%)	2 (13%)	2 (13%)
Little smaller	5 (31%)	3 (19%)	3 (19%)
Much smaller	6 (38%)	10 (63%)	10 (63%)
Bigger	1 (6%)	1 (6%)	1 (6%)

From Boden et al., ref. 41.

[a] Size of postoperative epidural mass effect relative to the preoperative herniated disc in patients following successful (complete resolution of symptoms) lumbar discectomy.

scribed the normal sequence and timing of gadolinium-enhanced MR changes following successful lumbar disc surgery (asymptomatic postoperative patients) (41). A reproducible sequence of enhancement of facet joints, paraspinal muscles, and nerve roots at the involved level was observed. The most clinically relevant postoperative MR finding was that of anterior epidural intermediate-intensity signal tissue contiguous with the disc space which mimicked the mass effect of the preoperative disc herniation (Fig. 49). Although such mass effect had been previously reported in a postoperative series with unenhanced MR, 75% of the patients in that series had persistent symptoms (454). In this prospective series, anterior epidural mass effect was noted postoperatively in all pa-

tients despite complete relief of leg pain. The tendency was for this mass effect to shrink in size over the initial 6-month postoperative period. Based on the timing of the appearance and shrinking of this finding, we surmise that it represents normal postoperative hematoma which then changes to immature (avascular) and then mature (vascular) epidural scar tissue (Table 5).

In the early postoperative period, the finding of anterior epidural mass can easily be misinterpreted as recurrent or residual disc material (Fig.50). Gadolinium does not solve this problem either, because 38% of the asymptomatic postoperative patients had a peripheral enhancement pattern consistent with disc rather than scar (67,68,224,233,449,513). It was even more disappointing to note that there was no correlation of the size of the postoperative mass effect with the presence of mild transient radicular symptoms in the few patients who experienced them.

Another aspect of postoperative imaging that is receiving increased attention is nerve root enhancement. In a prospective study of patients who were asymptomatic after disc surgery, Boden et al. described extradural nerve root enhancement as a high signal intensity of a nerve root outside the dural sac (41). This finding was different from dorsal root ganglion enhancement, which can be seen normally. Unilateral extradural root enhancement was seen at the operated level in 81% of patients early (3 weeks postoperatively) and was still present in nearly

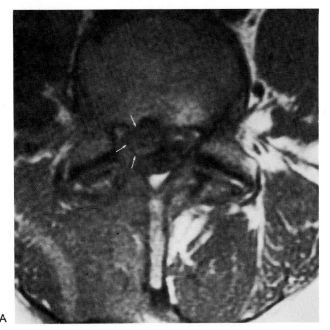
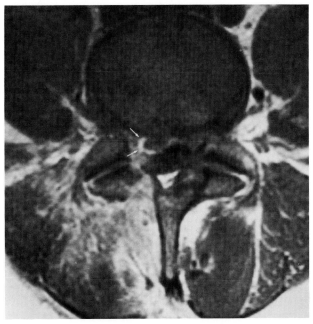

A   B

FIG. 50. Axial magnetic resonance images 3 weeks after routine discectomy from a patient with immediate complete relief of symptoms. **A:** Unenhanced T1-weighted image shows a large intermediate-intensity anterior epidural mass at the site of the original L4-5 disc herniation with compression of the thecal sac. **B:** Gadolinium-enhanced study at the same time demonstrates a peripheral rim enhancement pattern (arrows) consistent with disc material rather than scar. This patient remained asymptomatic following surgery. From Boden et al. (41).

one-third of patients at 6 months. In contrast, intradural nerve root enhancement was seen on the operated side tracking proximally from the operated level in 62% at 3 weeks but was not seen in any of the asymptomatic patients at 6 months. Other studies have observed that nerve root enhancement may signify root dysfunction and may be correlated with symptoms in the chronic (>6 months) postoperative phase (244).

Despite the use of gadolinium enhancement, MR studies in the initial postoperative period (6 months) are difficult to interpret because of the normal sequence of changes. Even in successfully decompressed (asymptomatic) patients, residual mass effect on the neural elements with an enhancement pattern suggestive of disc may be seen in about 45% of cases during the first 3–6 months after surgery. Decision about further surgery made on the basis of MR examinations during this period must be carefully contemplated.

To shorten examination time when evaluating postoperative patients, some centers are currently only performing pre- and postcontrast (Gd-DTPA) T1-weighted sequences. By utilizing only T1-weighted sequences, other potential causes of back pain in these patients may be overlooked. An axial T2-weighted sequence is important to exclude epidural abscess, pseudomeningocele (Fig. 51), and arachnoiditis (245,452). With arach-noiditis, MRI may demonstrate abnormal morphology and position of the nerve roots with either central clumping, peripheral adhesions (empty sac), or marked distortion of the thecal sac (452,454) (Fig. 52). In a study comparing MRI, myelography, and CT-myelography, MRI had a 92% sensitivity, 100% specificity, and 99% accuracy in the diagnosis of arachnoiditis compared to the myelographic procedures. Neoplastic seeding of the CSF can produce findings identical to arachnoiditis; however, the nerve roots in arachnoiditis were generally smooth and tapered in contrast to the nodular nerve root contours identified with CSF seeding (452). Nerve root enhancement with gadolinium is often seen in arachnoiditis, but gadolinium is generally not needed to make the diagnosis (245).

In the MRI evaluation of the postoperative patient, the routine MRI study includes sagittal T1- and T2-weighted sequences followed by an axial (conventional or RARE) T2-weighted sequence. The T2-weighted axial images are especially helpful if infection, arachnoiditis, or pseudomeningocele is clinically suspected. Gd-DTPA is administered if there is difficulty in interpreting the pathologic changes, especially to distinguish between residual/recurrent disc and epidural scar tissue.

In patients undergoing lumbar percutaneous nucleotomies, it appears that the outcome of the procedure

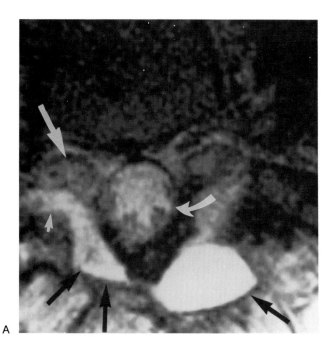
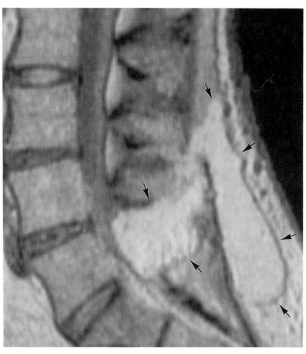

FIG. 51. Postoperative pseudomeningocele. On the axial T2-weighted image (**A**), there is a collection of fluid (black arrows) posterior to the thecal sac (curved white arrow). The fluid extends into the right intervertebral canal (short white arrow) where it is positioned posterior to an enlarged dorsal root ganglion (large white arrow). The nerve roots in the thecal sac have a normal appearance. On a different patient, on the sagittal proton-density weighted image (**B**), there is a large pseudomeningocele extending posteriorly from the L5 vertebral level into the subcutaneous tissue (arrows).

cannot be predicted from the appearance of the follow-up MRI evaluation. In one study, 9 of 11 successful outcomes and 6 of 7 demonstrated no change in size or configuration of the disc herniation (111).

Considering the high reported incidence of stenosis in patients with failed back surgery, an axial T1- or RARE T2-weighted sequence and sagittal T1- and RARE T2-weighted sequences are needed to optimally evaluate the central and intervertebral canals. In patients with low back pain after lumbar fusion, a multiplanar CT study should probably be the initial examination of choice to evaluate for possible fragmentation of the fusion mass, pseudarthrosis, or spinal stenosis. These findings were the most frequent indications for re-operation in one series of patients with spinal fusion (286). The delineation of postoperative fractures of the lumbar articular facets may also be difficult to demonstrate with MRI and probably requires multiplanar CT to be detected (464).

One study has suggested that MRI may be useful to assess the status of lumbar spine fusion (288). This investigation observed subchondral vertebral bands on either side of the disc space that was attempted to be fused. In most patients with a solid fusion, the subchondral bands were hyperintense on T1-weighted sequences whereas most of the pseudarthroses had hypointense bands.

In the evaluation of the postoperative cervical spine, the most common findings in a group of patients who had undergone anterior discectomy and fusion and presented with recurrent symptoms included bony stenosis at the fusion site and disc herniations at the first mobile segment above or below the fusion site (Fig. 53). A wide spectrum of graft and vertebral body signal changes were identified, but by 2 years it was possible to identify solid bony fusions as areas of continuous marrow signal, without evidence of the original intervertebral disc space or deformable bone graft. Stenosis was secondary to hypertrophic bone from the fusion mass which encroached upon the central or intervertebral canals. The hypertrophic bone demonstrated varied signal intensity when compared to the vertebral body marrow (453).

Postoperative MRI changes after various cervical spine procedures have also been retrospectively described (453). A spectrum of bone graft and vertebral body changes were seen up to 2 years after surgery. The

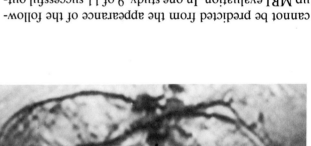

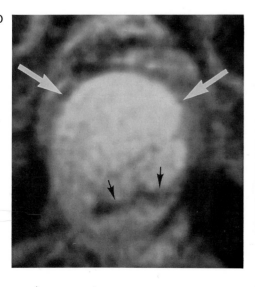

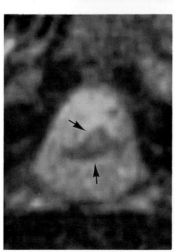

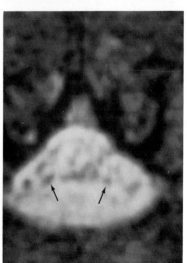

FIG. 52. Arachnoiditis. On the axial T2-weighted image (A), above the level of the surgical procedure, the nerve roots (arrows) have a normal appearance. Further caudally (B), the nerve roots (arrows) are clumped in the central portion of the thecal sac. At the level of disc surgery (C), the nerve roots (arrows) are clumped and positioned anteriorly in the thecal sac. There is ectasia of the thecal sac (white arrows) at the laminectomy site. In another patient with six prior spine surgeries, RARE-T2 axial images (D) show an empty-appearing thecal sac, with thickened nerve roots adherent to the posterior and lateral walls of the thecal sac (arrows). There is excellent signal-to-noise, acquired in half the time of conventional T2-weighted sequences. Note the distortion of anterior soft tissues due to hardware-associated metallic susceptibility artifact.

retrospective nature and variety of surgical techniques precluded a precise definition of the normal time sequence of cervical MR changes.

Postoperative metal artifact is a relatively common problem either from metal debris left at the initial surgery or from metallic internal fixation devices. Use of plastic rather than metal suction tips can decrease the debris from a burr used to decorticate the end-plates or remove spurs (405). In addition titanium implants result in less artifact (468). These artifacts can mimic neurologic compression and appear as a "black-out" area on T1- and T2-weighted images. Although posterior wires for cervical fusion cause distortion in the posterior soft tissues, the anterior portion of the spinal canal is usually not affected.

Another major advantage of MRI lies in the diagnosis of postoperative disc space infection. The most common error regarding postoperative discitis is not to think of the diagnosis because the entity is so rare. Furthermore, the usual clinical signs of fever, leukocytosis, and wound infection are seen in only the minority of cases. The second most common error is to assume that T2-bright MR signal changes seen in the disc space of a postoperative patient are normal postsurgical changes. In reality, there are very few "normal" MR changes within the disc space following uncomplicated discectomy, especially several months after surgery.

The most predictive MR finding of postoperative discitis may be gadolinium enhancement of the adjacent vertebral bone marrow on each side of the affected disc, with very T2-bright signal within the disc (42). End-plate enhancement after disc surgery may be normal (181). Marrow enhancement is a more reliable finding than decreased signal on T1, and increased signal on T2, unenhanced sequences. Gadolinium enhancement of the disc space and/or posterior annulus fibrosus may also be suggestive of early discitis (Fig. 54).

It is also important to examine all paradiscal marrow changes in light of the differential diagnosis of degenerative disc disease and neoplasia (Table 2). Whereas tumors tend to spare the cartilaginous disc space and involve most of the vertebral body, marrow changes from degenerative disc disease can mimic the findings of early discitis and tend to involve only the half of the vertebral body on either side of the involved disc (354,358,506). In questionable cases, look for the preoperative MR scans to determine if marrow changes associated with degenerative disc disease were present, since degenerative disc changes are more common than postoperative discitis.

A knowledge of the time course of the MR changes of discitis is important to avoid unnecessary surgical intervention. The MR findings of postoperative discitis frequently appear to worsen before improving, even when appropriate treatment is administered and clinical symptoms improve. The bone marrow changes usually resolve

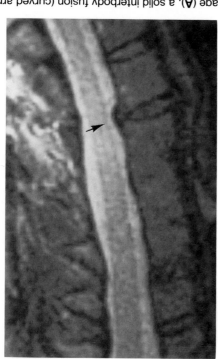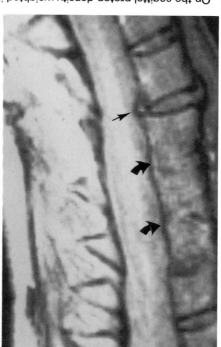

FIG. 53. On the sagittal proton-density weighted image (A), a solid interbody fusion (curved arrows) is identified from C3 through C6. At the first mobile segment caudad to the fusion, a posterior disc herniation (small straight arrow) is delineated. The sagittal cardiac gated T2-weighted image (B) is needed to demonstrate the relationship of the disc herniation to the spinal cord (arrow).

as evaluating C1-C2 and subaxial subluxations (99). MRI has also provided an objective assessment of joint changes in rheumatoid patients while on therapy (26).

In patients with ankylosing spondylitis presenting with spinal pseudarthrosis or fracture dislocations, MRI may be of benefit in delineating vertebral malalignment and determining whether neural compression by soft tissue or osseous structures (85,196). In patients with longstanding ankylosing spondylitis who develop the cauda equina syndrome, the classic findings of a dilated thecal sac with erosion of the posterior elements are well demonstrated on MR, obviating the need for myelography (263) (Fig. 56).

Patients on long-term hemodialysis may occasionally present with spinal arthropathy which may mimic osteomyelitis. MRI has been shown to be helpful in these cases to exclude an inflammatory process (426). In patients with neuropathic spinal arthropathy who present with progressive joint degeneration, bone fragmentation, and ligamentous instability, MRI may also be of benefit to exclude a superimposed infection and to assess the degree of stenosis (255).

MRI: A CLINICIAN'S PERSPECTIVE

The past two decades have brought a technological explosion in the field of neuroradiologic imaging. We have seen the development of new noninvasive imaging mo-

after 2–4 months with the disc space enhancement persisting longer in many cases.

SPONDYLOARTHROPATHIES

The spine, a composite of amphiarthroses, diarthroses, and entheses, may be affected by a variety of arthritic processes. MRI is particularly useful in evaluating patients with rheumatoid arthritis (258,595) affecting the cervical spine, who present with symptoms of myelopathy or myeloradiculopathy secondary to vertical subluxation of the odontoid, atlantoaxial subluxation, or subaxial subluxation (66) (Fig. 55). MRI has been shown to be useful in the evaluation of spinal cord impingement in these cases and particularly helpful in demonstrating the degree of pannus formation which may contribute to the central canal stenosis (122). In one study, with patients having severe chronic rheumatoid arthritis who underwent stabilization for atlantoaxial subluxation, MRI demonstrated a reduction in the periodontal pannus after stabilization (290). A sagittal T1-weighted sequence in flexion and extension has been of benefit to determine the degree of instability and spinal cord compression at the malaligned segments (23,122,279). In clinical studies evaluating patients with rheumatoid arthritis, MRI was comparable to pluridirectional tomography in evaluating the atlantodental interval, dens erosions, and osteophytes of the upper cervical spine as well

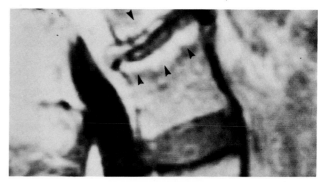

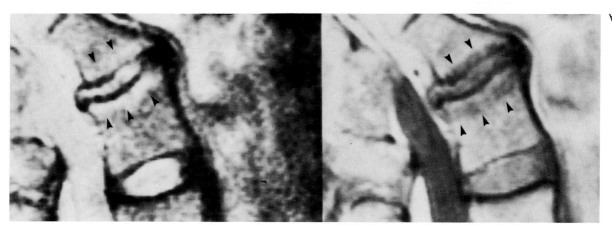

FIG. 54. A: Magnetic resonance scans from a patient with back pain and spasm 4 weeks after lumbar discectomy. The classic findings of postoperative discitis are well demonstrated. T1-weighted sequence (left) demonstrates decreased signal of the bone marrow adjacent to the affected disc. More T2-weighted sequence demonstrates increased marrow signal as well as increased signal within the disc space itself. B: Gadolinium enhancement of the adjacent marrow and the posterior disc space is consistent with discitis. From Boden et al. (42).

dalities as well as refinements in older modalities. This ability to obtain better noninvasive anatomic resolution of the spine is a double-edged sword and imaging studies can be the spine surgeon's best friend or worst enemy.

The most efficient treatment for complications of spine surgery is to avoid them. Often unnecessary complications are created due to errors in decision-making prompted by imaging studies. Such errors may occur in three general areas: (a) the indications used to obtain the study; (b) the timing of the study acquisition during the clinical course; and, (c) the actual interpretation of the imaging study.

What is the appropriate role of diagnostic imaging studies in spine patients? Diagnostic tests should be used to confirm the core of information gathered from a thorough history and physical examination (138). While there are many imaging modalities available, each with its own place in the temporal sequence of the evaluation of spine disorders, none of them should be used for general screening. Most imaging modalities are overly sensi-

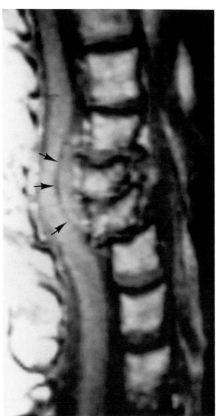

FIG. 55. Rheumatoid arthritis with subaxial subluxation and cord compression. On the sagittal T1-weighted image, there is subluxation at the C4-C5, C5-C6, and C6-C7 disc levels. In addition to the vertebral body malalignment, a soft tissue mass (arrows) identified in the anterior extradural space causes moderately severe compression of the adjacent spinal cord. The soft tissue mass most likely represents a reactive process secondary to chronic instability of the motion segments.

tive and relatively unselective. ''Let's get an MRI to see if there is anything wrong with the spine'' is a dangerous thought process. Many of the iatrogenic catastrophes in the management of patients with back and neck pain can be attributed directly to excessive reliance on diagnostic studies without precise clinical correlation. The potential exists for this problem to become even more common because the resolution of magnetic resonance scans is so good that any pathoanatomy looks obvious to even the novice reader. A recurring theme of this chapter emphasizes that pathology visualized on any imaging study is not necessarily painful, and may not be the cause of a particular patient's pain.

To evaluate the true clinical value of any diagnostic study, one must know its sensitivity which is a reflection of the false negatives, or the ability of the test to detect disease when it is present. One example of this problem is the use of the Cobb angle to follow patients with scoliosis and define surgical criterion. Recent studies have suggested that the measurement of the Cobb angle from a single plain radiograph may not have the sensitivity or precision to detect the magnitude of changes it has been assumed to measure (77,366).

More relevant to the avoidance of complications is the specificity, which is a reflection of the false positives, or the ability of the test to remain negative in the absence of clinical disease. Most frequently the specificity and false-positive rate are measured in a population of symptomatic patients who have undergone surgery to confirm the imaging predictions; however, often there is a much higher rate of false positives when an asymptomatic group is studied. Since technically the pathoanatomy of an asymptomatic MRI-evident herniated disc does exist, it is not really a false-positive finding, but since there is no clinical disease it is not a true positive either. Thus, we use the term *clinical false positives* to refer to imaging abnormalities that are present in asymptomatic subjects. It is essential to understand the spectrum and frequency of imaging abnormalities that can exist without causing symptoms in order to better interpret such findings in symptomatic patients.

The physician's challenge is to select diagnostic tests on the basis of their performance characteristics so that the correct diagnosis is obtained with minimal cost and morbidity. More important is the use of restraint in ordering these expensive tests routinely or too early in the treatment of conditions such as acute low back pain which have a natural history of improvement in the vast majority of cases. Finally, any imaging finding must correlate precisely with clinical signs and symptoms if reliable results from surgery are to be expected.

The most recent data suggest that MRI is more accurate in the detection of degenerative disc disease than discography or myelography and that it is unsurpassed for the imaging of infection, tumor, and trauma which all rely on its superior ability to image soft tissues.

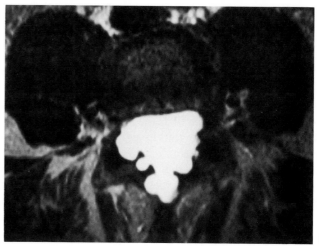

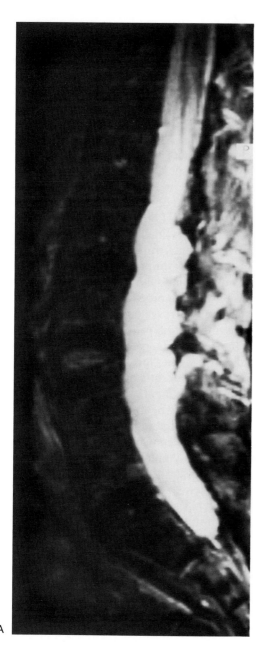

FIG. 56. Cauda equina syndrome in ankylosing spondylitis. Sagittal (**A**) and axial (**B**) RARE-T2 images show a dilated lumbar thecal sac, with eroded, scalloped posterior elements. Inflamed, scarred nerve roots adhere to the walls of the thecal sac.

The problem with many imaging/surgical correlation studies used to determine accuracy is the lack of long-term clinical follow-up documenting resolution of symptoms. Mere visualization of MR-evident pathology at the time of surgery does not guarantee that the visualized pathoanatomy was the cause of the patient's pain. This point cannot be better illustrated than in a recent series of patients with extra-spinal causes of lumbar radiculopathy. Several of the patients had imaging studies consistent with spinal stenosis or disc herniation and despite lumbar decompression they died from intrapelvic or retroperitoneal tumors which were the true cause of their symptoms (269).

As with the other diagnostic imaging modalities discussed, MR has also been shown to have a significant clinical false-positive rate in asymptomatic individuals (241). In one study, in the lumbar spine 22% of the asymptomatic subjects under age 60 and 57% of those over age 60 had significantly abnormal scans (herniated disc or spinal stenosis) (40). In addition, the prevalence of "disc degeneration" on T2-weighted images was found to approach 93% in subjects over the age of 60 (Table 4). Therefore, we must seriously reconsider any alteration of surgical procedures solely on the basis of an MR finding such as decreased disc signal on T2-weighted sequences, when it is a ubiquitous finding in asymptomatic individuals. Significant abnormalities were also seen on cervical spine MR examinations in 19% of asymptomatic individuals (43). Increasing age was associated with a higher prevalence of MRI abnormalities in both studies (Table 3). In one recent study analyzing lumbar MRIs of asymptomatic individuals, the prevalence of bulges increased with age, but not the prevalence of protrusions. Asymptomatic extrusions were, however, rare (241). The lower prevalence of asymptomatic MR abnormalities in the cervical spine when compared with the lumbar spine may be due to the smaller amount of excess space in the cervical canal as well as the increased sensitivity of spinal cord (central nervous tissue) versus spinal nerves (peripheral nerve tissue).

It should be obvious by now that the most dangerous errors in decision-making using these neurodiagnostic imaging studies do not come from faulty interpretation of the images, but rather from the lack of effort or precision in documenting specific anatomic correlation with a patient's clinical symptoms and physical signs. These tests should never be used to "screen" patients for spinal disease. A patient with a negative history and physical examination for a spinal lesion has a 1-in-3 chance of having a surgically treatable CT or MR finding. If the decision for surgery is based only on the scan results, there is a 30% chance that the patient will undergo an unnecessary and unsuccessful operation. Even worse, such a patient assumes all of the risks of surgery with no chance for any of its benefits. Alternatively, if the patient's clinical picture correlates well with the imaging pictures, the neuroradiologic studies can be appropriately used as a confirmatory diagnostic tool.

CONCLUSION

With the rapid development of new technology, it is always tempting to ask, "What will it offer tomorrow?" A more cogent question is "How can current technology be optimally utilized?" At this time, the complexity of MR technology and application has outpaced the level of understanding of most physicians ordering and interpreting MRI exams. It is necessary for more radiologists to become subspecialists in the evaluation of organ systems, such as the spine, if we hope to maximize the information we can obtain from this complex diagnostic modality. With subspecialization, the radiologist can become an integral part of the team of physicians caring for patients with spinal dysfunction. Our goal should be a greater understanding of the natural history of spinal disorders, which will only be achieved with a multidisciplinary approach.

To muse a moment about the future: Advances in computer software and hardware will result in the improvement of spatial and contrast resolution. There will be continued development and application of 3D acquisition techniques giving further flexibility to imaging protocols, and continued improvement in fast-imaging sequences. It is possible that MR spectroscopy will ad-

vance to the level of accurately defining abnormal metabolic pathways in a discrete anatomic location (4,51,337,374,447). By optimizing our imaging sequences which are exquisitely sensitive to alterations in tissue hydration, we may be able to delineate areas of neural or muscular ischemia, hyperemia, or edema more precisely (79,230,399,471,522). Perhaps by integrating the pathophysiology and pathoanatomy, we may finally help answer the most challenging question, "Where is the pain coming from?"

From the clinician's standpoint, neurodiagnostic imaging studies should be used to confirm the anatomic location and extent of clinically suspected pathology in the spine. Many errors in decision-making with imaging studies do not come from misinterpretation of what is seen on the images, but instead are related to how the imaging information is used and integrated into the clinical decision-making process. Because all neurodiagnostic imaging studies reveal abnormalities in at least one-third of asymptomatic people, the use of these tests for general screening is dangerous. Furthermore, obtaining these expensive studies too early in the treatment of self-limited disorders is costly and often misleading to both the physician and patient.

When interpreting neurodiagnostic imaging studies of the spine it is essential to have an understanding of the spectrum and frequency of abnormalities that can exist without causing symptoms. On preoperative imaging studies it is necessary to distinguish imaging abnormalities that are likely to be clinically significant from those which are part of the normal aging process. Similarly, on postoperative images it is important to distinguish imaging abnormalities that are symptomatic from those which are part of the normal sequence of postoperative imaging changes. The guiding light in making all these distinctions must be the meticulous correlation of the anatomic location of imaging abnormalities with clinical signs and symptoms in each patient as well as the exercise of restraint in obtaining these tests until appropriate conservative management has failed. This philosophy should help avoid many of the common problems in decision-making following MRI investigations of the spine.

ACKNOWLEDGMENTS. We especially want to thank Sandra Pinkerton, Ph.D., and Janet Schuster for their contribution to this chapter in the first edition, and Thelma Snider for reading and editing the current version of the manuscript at different stages and for coordinating the preparation of the references.

REFERENCES

1. Adams MA, Hutton WC (1981): The relevance of torsion to the mechanical derangement of the lumbar spine. *Spine* 6:241–248.

2. Adams MA, Hutton WC (1985): Gradual disc prolapse. *Spine* 10: 524–531.

3. Aguila LA, Piraino DW, Modic MT, Dudley AW, Duchesneau PM, Weinstein MA (1985): The intranuclear cleft of the intervertebral disk: Magnetic resonance imaging. *Radiology* 155:155–158.

4. Aisen AM, Chenevert TL (1989): MR spectroscopy: clinical perspective. *Radiology* 173:593–599.

5. Alenghat JP, Hallett M, Kido DK (1982): Spinal cord compression in diffuse idiopathic skeletal hyperostosis. *Radiology* 142: 119–120.

6. Allen KL (1952): Neuropathies caused by bony spurs in the cervical spine with special reference to surgical treatment. *J Neurol Neurosurg Psychiatry* 15:20–36.

7. Alvarez O, Roque CT, Pampati M (1988): Multilevel thoracic disk herniations: CT and MR studies. *J Comput Assist Tomogr* 12:649–652.

8. Angtuaco EJ, McConnell JR, Chadduck WM, Flanigan S (1987): MR imaging of spinal epidural sepsis. *AJR* 149:1249–1253.

9. Araki Y, Ootani M, Furukawa T, Yamamoto T, Tsukaguchi I, Mitomo M (1992): Pseudoenhancement of intervertebral disc herniation. *Neuroradiology* 34:271–272.

10. Arnoldi CC, Brodsky AE, Cauchoix J, Crock HV, Dommisse GF, Edgar MA, Gargano FP, Jacobson RE, Kirkaldy-Willis WH, Kurihara A, Langenskiold A, Macnab I, McIvor GW, Newman PH, Paine KW, Russin LA, Sheldon J, Tile M, Urist MR, Wilson WE, Wiltse LL (1976): Lumbar spinal stenosis and nerve root entrapment syndromes: Definition and classification. *Clin Orthop* 115: 4–5.

11. Asztely M, Kadziolka R, Nachemson A (1983): A comparison of sonography and myelography in clinically suspected spinal stenosis. *Spine* 8:885–890.

12. Atlas SW, Regenbogen V, Rogers LF, Kim KS (1986): The radiographic characterization of burst fractures of the spine. *AJR* 147: 575–582.

13. Avrahami E, Tadmor R, Kaplinsky N (1993): The role of T2-weighted gradient echo in MRI demonstration of spinal multiple myeloma. *Spine* 18:1812–1815.

14. Babcock EE, Brateman L, Weinreb JC, Horner SD, Nunnally RL (1985): Edge artifacts in MR images: Chemical shift effect. *J Comput Assist Tomogr* 9:252–257.

15. Badami JP, Hinck VC (1982): Symptomatic deposition of epidural fat in a morbidly obese woman. *AJNR* 3:664–665.

16. Baker LL, Goodman SB, Perkash I, Lane B, Enzmann DR (1990): Benign versus pathologic compression fractures of vertebral bodies: Assessment with conventional spin-echo, chemical-shift, and STIR MR imaging. *Radiology* 174:495–502.

17. Banerian KG, Wang A-M, Samberg C, Kerr HH, Wesolowski DP (1990): Association of vertebral end plate fracture with pediatric lumbar intervertebral disk herniation: Value of CT and MR imaging. *Radiology* 177:763–765.

18. Barnes GT, Lauro K (1989): Image processing in digital radiography: Basic concepts and applications. *J Digit Imaging* 2:132–146.

19. Barnes PD, Lester PD, Yamanashi WS, Prince JR (1986): MRI in infants and children with spinal dysraphism. *AJR* 147:339–346.

20. Baum JA, Hanley EN Jr (1986): Intraspinal synovial cyst simulating spinal stenosis. *Spine* 11:487–489.

21. Beers GJ, Raque GH, Wagner GG, Shields CB, Nichols GR II, Johnson JR, Meyer JE (1988): MR imaging in acute cervical spine trauma. *J Comput Assist Tomogr* 12:755–761.

22. Bell GR, Rothman RH, Booth RE, Cuckler JM, Garfin S, Herkowitz H, Simeone FA, Dolinskas C, Han SS (1984): A study of computer-assisted tomography II. Comparison of metrizamide myelography and computed tomography in the diagnosis of herniated lumbar disc and spinal stenosis. *Spine* 9:552–556.

23. Bell GR, Stearns KL (1991): Flexion-extension MRI of the upper rheumatoid cervical spine. *Orthopedics* 14:969–973.

24. Bell GR, Stearns KL, Bonutti PM, Boumphrey FR (1990): MRI diagnosis of tuberculous vertebral osteomyelitis. *Spine* 15:462–465.

25. Bellon EM, Haacke EM, Coleman PE, Sacco DC, Steiger DA, Gangarosa RE (1986): MR artifacts: A review. *AJR* 147:1271–1281.

26. Beltran J, Caudill JL, Herman LA, Kantor SM, Hudson PN, Noto AM, Baran AS (1987): Rheumatoid arthritis: MR imaging manifestations. *Radiology* 165:153–157.

27. Berbaum KS, El-Khoury GY, Franken EA Jr, Kathol M, Montgomery WJ, Hesson W (1988): Impact of clinical history on fracture detection with radiography. *Radiology* 168:507–511.

28. Berger PE, Atkinson D, Wilson WJ, Wiltse L (1986): High resolution surface coil magnetic resonance imaging of the spine: Normal and pathologic anatomy. *Radiographics* 6:573–602.

29. Berns DH, Blaser S, Ross JS, Masaryk TJ, Modic MT (1988): MR imaging with Gadolinium-DTPA in leptomeningeal spread of lymphoma. *J Comput Assist Tomogr* 12:499–500.

30. Berns DH, Blaser SI, Modic MT (1989): Magnetic resonance imaging of the spine. *Clin Orthop* 244:78–100.

31. Berry JL, Moran JM, Berg WS, Steffee AD (1987): A morphometric study of human lumbar and selected thoracic vertebrae. *Spine* 12:362–367.

32. Bircher MD, Tasker T, Crawshaw C, Mulholland RC (1988): Discitis following lumbar surgery. *Spine* 13:98–102.

33. Bisla RS, Marchisello PJ, Lockshin MD, Hart DM, Marcus RE, Granda J (1976): Auto-immunological basis of disk degeneration. *Clin Orthop* 121:205–211.

34. Blankstein A, Rubinstein E, Ezra E, Lokiec F, Caspi I, Horoszowski H (1987): Disc space infection and vertebral osteomyelitis as a complication of percutaneous lateral discectomy. *Clin Orthop* 225:234–237.

35. Bloch F (1946): Nuclear induction. *Phys Rev* 70:460–474.

36. Bloomfield EL, Masaryk TJ, Caplin A, et al (1993): Intravenous sedation for MR imaging of the brain and spine in children: Pentobarbital versus propofol. *Radiology* 186:93–97.

37. Blumenkopf B, Juneau PA III (1988): Magnetic resonance imaging (MRI) of thoracolumbar fractures. *J Spinal Disorders* 1: 144–150.

38. Blumenthal SL, Baker J, Dossett A, Selby DK (1988): The role of anterior lumbar fusion for internal disc disruption. *Spine* 13:566–569.

39. Bobest M, Furo I, Tompa K, Pocsik I, Kuncz A (1986): ^{1}H Nuclear magnetic resonance study of intervertebral discs. *Spine* 11:709–711.

40. Boden SD, Davis DO, Dina TS, et al (1990): Abnormal magnetic resonance scans of the lumbar spine in asymptomatic subjects: A prospective investigation. *J Bone Joint Surg* 72-A:403–408.

41. Boden SD, Davis DO, Dina TS, et al (1992): Contrast-enhanced MR imaging performed after successful lumbar disk surgery: Prospective study. *Radiology* 182:59–64.

42. Boden SD, Davis DO, Dina TS, et al (1992): Postoperative discitis: Distinguishing early MR findings from normal postoperative changes. *Radiology* 184:765–771.

43. Boden SD, McCowin PR, Davis DO, et al (1990): Abnormal magnetic resonance scans of the cervical spine in asymptomatic subjects: A prospective investigation. *J Bone Joint Surg* 72A:1178–1184.

44. Boden SD, Riew KD, Yamaguchi K, et al (1995): Lumbar facet joint orientation: Defining "normal" and the relationship to spinal disease. *J Bone Joint Surg* (In press).

45. Boehme JM II, Choplin RH (1992): PACS mini refresher course: Systems integration: Requirements for a fully functioning electronic radiology department. *Radiographics* 12:789–794.

46. Bogduk N, Marsland A (1988): The cervical zygapophysial joints as a source of neck pain. *Spine* 13:610–617.

47. Bogduk N, Twomey LT (1987): *Clinical anatomy of the lumbar spine.* Melbourne: Churchill Livingstone.

48. Bohatirchuk F (1955): The aging vertebral column (macro- and historadiographical study). *Br J Radiol* 28:389–404.

49. Bolender NF, Schonstrom NS, Spengler DM (1985): Role of computed tomography and myelography in the diagnosis of central spinal stenosis. *J Bone Joint Surg [Am]* 67:240–245.

50. Bose K, Balasubramaniam P (1984): Nerve root canals of the lumbar spine. *Spine* 9:16–18.

51. Bottomley PA (1989): Human in vivo NMR spectroscopy in diagnostic medicine: Clinical tool or research probe? *Radiology* 170:1–15.

52. Boyd HR, Pear BL (1972): Chronic spontaneous spinal epidural hematoma: Report of two cases. *J Neurosurg* 36:239–242.

53. Bozzao A, Gallucci M, Masciocchi C, Aprile I, Barile A, Passariello R (1992): Lumbar disk herniation: MR imaging assessment of natural history in patients treated without surgery. *Radiology* 185:135–141.

54. Bradley WG Jr (1989): Magnetization: Physical basis for T1 and T2, Part 2. *MRI Decisions* (January/February):17–25.

55. Bradley WG Jr, Tsuruda JS (1987): MR sequence parameter optimization: An algorithmic approach. *AJR* 149:815–823.

56. Bradley WG (1988): When should GRASS be used? *Radiology* 169:574–575.

57. Brant-Zawadzki M, Norman D, eds (1987): *Magnetic resonance imaging of the central nervous system.* New York: Raven Press.

58. Brasch RC, Weinmann H-J, Wesbey GE (1984): Contrast-enhanced NMR imaging: Animal studies using gadolinium-DTPA complex. *AJR* 142:625–630.

59. Braun IF, Hoffman JC, Davis PC, Landman JA, Tindall GT (1985): Contrast enhancement in CT differentiation between recurrent disk herniation and postoperative scar: Prospective study. *Am J Neuroradiol* 6:607–612.

60. Breger RK, Rimm AA, Fischer ME, Papke RA, Haughton VM (1989): T1 and T2 measurements on a 1.5-T commercial MR imager. *Radiology* 171:273–276.

61. Breger RK, Williams AL, Daniels DL, Czervionke LF, Mark LP, Haughton VM, Papke RA, Coffer M (1989): Contrast enhancement in spinal MR imaging. *AJR* 153:387–391.

62. Briceno CE, Fazl M, Willinsky RA, Gertzbein S (1989): Sequestrated lumbar intervertebral disc associated with vertebral erosion. *Spine* 14:898–899.

63. Brickley-Parsons D, Glimcher MJ (1984): Is the chemistry of collagen in intervertebral discs an expression of Wolff's law? A study of the human lumbar spine. *Spine* 9:148–163.

64. Bronskill MJ, McVeigh ER, Kucharczyk W, Henkelman RM (1988): Syrinx-like artifacts on MR images of the spinal cord. *Radiology* 166:485–488.

65. Brown BM, Schwartz RH, Frank E, Blank NK (1988): Preoperative evaluation of cervical radiculopathy and myelopathy by surface-coil MR imaging. *AJR* 151:1205–1212.

66. Bundschuh C, Modic MT, Kearney F, Morris R, Deal C (1988): Rheumatoid arthritis of the cervical spine: Surface-coil MR imaging. *AJR* 151:181–187.

67. Bundschuh CV, Modic MT, Ross JS, Masaryk TJ, Bohlman H (1988): Epidural fibrosis and recurrent disk herniation in the lumbar spine: MR imaging assessment. *AJR* 150:923–932.

68. Bundschuh CV, Stein L, Slusser JH, et al (1990): Distinguishing between scar and recurrent herniated disk in postoperative patients: Value of contrast-enhanced CT and MR imaging. *AJNR* 11:949–958.

69. Burk DL Jr, Brunberg JA, Kanal E, Latchaw RE, Wolf GL (1987): Spinal and paraspinal neurofibromatosis: Surface coil MR imaging at 1.5 T. *Radiology* 162:797–801.

70. Burrows EH (1963): The sagittal diameter of the spinal canal in cervical spondylosis. *Clin Radiol* 14:77–86.

71. Burton CV, Kirkaldy-Willis WH, Yong-Hing K, Heithoff KB (1981): Causes of failure of surgery on the lumbar spine. *Clin Orthop* 157:191–199.

72. Bushong SC (1988): *Magnetic resonance imaging: Physical and biological principles.* St. Louis: Mosby.

73. Buthiau D, Piette JC, Ducerveau MN, Robert G, Godeau P, Heitz F (1988): Steroid-induced spinal epidural lipomatosis: CT survey. *J Comput Assist Tomogr* 12:501–503.

74. Bydder GM, Brown J, Niendorf HP, Young IR (1985): Enhancement of cervical intraspinal tumors in MR imaging with intravenous gadolinium-DTPA. *J Comput Assist Tomogr* 9:847–851.

75. Callahan DJ, Pack LL, Bream RC, Hensinger RN (1986): Intervertebral disc impingement syndrome in a child: Report of a case and suggested pathology. *Spine* 11:402–404.

76. Cammisa FP Jr, Eismont FJ, Green BA (1989): Dural laceration occurring with burst fractures and associated laminar fractures. *J Bone Joint Surg [Am]* 71:1044–1052.

77. Carman DL, Browne RH, Birch JG (1990): Measurement of scoliosis and kyphosis radiographs: Intraobserver and interobserver variation. *J Bone Joint Surg* 72-A:328–333.

78. Carmody RF, Yang PJ, Seeley GW, Seeger JF, Unger EC, Johnson JE (1989): Spinal cord compression due to metastatic disease: Diagnosis with MR imaging versus myelography. *Radiology* 173:225–229.

79. Carr D, Gilbertson L, Frymoyer J, Krag M, Pope M (1985): Lumbar paraspinal compartment syndrome: A case report with physiologic and anatomic studies. *Spine* 10:816–820.

80. Carrera GF, Haughton VM, Syvertsen A, Williams AL (1980): Computed tomography of the lumbar facet joints. *Radiology* 134:145–148.

81. Castellvi AE, Goldstein LA, Chan DPK (1984): Lumbosacral transitional vertebrae and their relationship with lumbar extradural defects. *Spine* 9:493–495.

82. Castillo M, Quencer RM, Green BA, Montalvo BM (1988): Syringomyelia as a consequence of compressive extramedullary lesions: Postoperative clinical and radiological manifestations. *AJR* 150:391–396.

83. Cauldwell CB, Fisher DM (1993): Sedating pediatric patients: Is propofol a panacea? *Radiology* 186:9–10.

84. Cervellini P, Curri D, Volpin L, Bernardi L, Pinna V, Benedetti A (1988): Computed tomography of epidural fibrosis after discectomy: A comparison between symptomatic and asymptomatic patients. *Neurosurgery* 23:710–713.

85. Chan F-L, Ho EK, Chau EM (1988): Spinal pseudarthrosis complicating ankylosing spondylitis: Comparison of CT and conventional tomography. *AJR* 150:611–614.

86. Chang PJ (1989): Bayesian analysis revisited: A radiologist's survival guide. *AJR* 152:721–727.

87. Ciric I, Mikhael MA, Tarkington JA, Vick NA (1980): The lateral recess syndrome: A variant of spinal stenosis. *J Neurosurg* 53:433–443.

88. Citrin CM, Sherman JL, Gangarosa RE, Scanlon D (1987): Physiology of the CSF flow-void sign: Modification by cardiac gating. *AJR* 148:205–208.

89. Clark GA, Panjabi MM, Wetzel FT (1985): Can infant malnutrition cause adult vertebral stenosis? *Spine* 10:165–170.

90. Colletti PM, Dang HT, Deseran MW, Kerr RM, Boswell WD, Ralls PW (1991): Spinal MR imaging in suspected metastases: Correlation with skeletal scintigraphy. *Magn Reson Imaging* 9:349–355.

91. Colman LK, Porter BA, Redmond J III, Olson DO, Stimac GK, Dunning DM, Friedl KE (1988): Early diagnosis of spinal metastases by CT and MR studies. *J Comput Assist Tomogr* 12:423–426.

92. Condon BR, Hadley DM (1988): Quantification of cord deformation and dynamics during flexion and extension of the cervical spine using MR imaging. *J Comput Assist Tomogr* 12:947–955.

93. Cooper LS, Chalmers TC, McCally M, Berrier J, Sacks HS (1988): The poor quality of early evaluations of magnetic resonance imaging. *JAMA* 259:3277–3280.

94. Coventry MB, Ghormley RK, Kernohan JW (1945): The intervertebral disc: Its microscopic anatomy and pathology Part II. Changes in the intervertebral disc concomitant with age. *J Bone Joint Surg* 27:233–247.

95. Coventry MB, Ghormley RK, Kernohan JW (1945): The intervertebral disc: Its microscopic anatomy and pathology Part III: Pathological changes in the intervertebral disc. *J Bone Joint Surg* 27:460–474.

96. Crisi G, Carpeggiani P, Trevisan C (1993): Gadolinium-enhanced nerve roots in lumbar disk herniation. *AJNR* 14:1379–1392.

97. Crock HV (1981): Normal and pathological anatomy of the lumbar spinal nerve root canals. *J Bone Joint Surg [Br]* 63:487–490.

98. Curtin AJ, Chakeres DW, Bulas R, Boesel CP, Finneran M, Flint E (1989): MR imaging artifacts of the axial internal anatomy of the cervical spinal cord. *AJR* 152:835–842.

99. Cyron BM, Hutton WC (1980): Articular tropism and stability of the lumbar spine. *Spine* 5:168–172.

100. Czervionke LF, Czervionke JM, Daniels DL, Haughton VM (1988): Characteristic features of MR truncation artifacts. *AJR* 151:1219–1228.

101. Czervionke LF, Daniels DL, Ho PS, Yu S, Pech P, Strandt J, Williams AL, Haughton VM (1988): Cervical neural foramina: Correlative anatomic and MR imaging study. *Radiology* 169:753–759.

102. Daffner RH, Lupetin AR, Dash N, Deeb ZL, Sefczek RJ, Scha-

piro RL (1986): MRI in the detection of malignant infiltration of bone marrow. *AJR* 146:353–358.

103. Dall BE, Rowe DE, Odette WG, Batts DH (1987): Postoperative discitis. *Clin Orthop* 224:138–146.

104. Daniels DL, Grogan JP, Johansen JG, Meyer GA, Williams AL, Haughton VM (1984): Cervical radiculopathy: Computed tomography and myelography compared. *Radiology* 151:109–113.

105. Davis PC, Hoffman JC Jr, Ball TI, Wyly JB, Braun IF, Fry SM, Drvaric DM (1988): Spinal abnormalities in pediatric patients: MR imaging findings compared with clinical, myelographic, and surgical findings. *Radiology* 166:679–685.

106. DeCandido P, Reinig JW, Dwyer AJ, Thompson KJ, Ducker TB (1988): Magnetic resonance assessment of the distribution of lumbar spine disc degenerative changes. *J Spinal Disorders* 1:9–15.

107. DeLaPaz RL, Brady TJ, Buonanno FS, New PF, Kistler JP, McGinnis BD, Pykett IL, Taveras JM (1983): Nuclear magnetic resonance (NMR) imaging of Arnold-Chiari type I malformation with hydromyelia. *J Comput Assist Tomogr* 7:126–129.

108. De La Torre JC (1981): Spinal cord injury. *Spine* 6:315–335.

109. de Roos A, Kressel H, Spritzer C, Dalinka M (1987): MR imaging of marrow changes adjacent to end plates in degenerative lumbar disk disease. *AJR* 149:531–534.

110. de Roos A, van Persijn van Meerten EL, Bloem JL, Bluemm RG (1986): MRI of tuberculous spondylitis. *AJR* 147:79–82.

111. Deutsch AL, Mink JH, Goldstein T, Delamarter R (1989): MR imaging in percutaneous lumbar diskectomy. *Radiology: 75th Anniversary Scientific Assembly and Annual Meeting Radiological Society of North America.* Chicago. 173(P) Supplement:43.

112. Di Chiro G, Doppman JL, Dwyer AJ, Patronas NJ, Knop RH, Bairamian D, Vermess M, Oldfield EH (1985): Tumors and arteriovenous malformations of the spinal cord: Assessment using MR. *Radiology* 156:689–697.

113. Di Chiro G, Fisher RL (1964): Contrast radiography of the spinal cord. *Arch Neurol* 11:125–143.

114. Dietemann JL, Runge M, Badoz A, Dosch JC, Beaujeux R, Bonneville JF, Wackenheim A (1988): Radiology of posterior lumbar apophyseal ring fractures: Report of 13 cases. *Neuroradiology* 30:337–344.

115. Dillin W, Booth R, Cuckler J, Balderston R, Simeone F, Rothman R (1986): Cervical radiculopathy. *Spine* 11:988–991.

116. Dillon WP, Norman D, Newton TH, Bolla K, Mark A (1989): Intradural spinal cord lesions: Gadolinium-DTPA-enhanced MR imaging. *Radiology* 170:229–237.

117. Dooms GC, Fisher MR, Hricak H, Richardson M, Crooks LE, Genant HK (1985): Bone marrow imaging: Magnetic resonance studies related to age and sex. *Radiology* 155:429–432.

118. Doppman JL (1989): Epidural lipomatosis. *Radiology* 171:581–582.

119. Doppman JL, Di Chiro G, Dwyer AJ, Frank JL, Oldfield EH (1987): Magnetic resonance imaging of spinal arteriovenous malformations. *J Neurosurg* 66:830–834.

120. Doran SE, Papadopoulos SM, Ducker TB, Lillehei KO (1993): Magnetic resonance imaging documentation of coexistent traumatic locked facets of the cervical spine and disc herniation. *J Neurosurg* 79:341–345.

121. Dunlop RB, Adams MA, Hutton WC (1984): Disc space narrowing and the lumbar facet joints. *J Bone Joint Surg [Br]* 66:706–710.

122. Dvorak J, Grob D, Baumgartner H, Gschwend N, Grauer W, Larsson S (1989): Functional evaluation of the spinal cord by magnetic resonance imaging in patients with rheumatoid arthritis and instability of upper cervical spine. *Spine* 14:1057–1064.

123. Dwyer AJ (1989): Time and disease: The fourth dimension of radiology. *Radiology* 173:17–21.

124. Dwyer AJ, Frank JA, Sank VJ, Reinig JW, Hickey AM, Doppman JL (1988): Short T1 inversion-recovery sequence: Analysis and initial experience in cancer imaging. *Radiology* 168:837–841.

125. Dwyer SJ III, Stewart BK, Sayre JW, et al (1992): PACS mini refresher course: Performance characteristics and image fidelity of gray-scale monitors. *Radiographics* 12:765–772.

126. Edelman RR, Shoukimas GM, Stark DD, Davis KR, New PF, Rosenthal DI, Wismer GL, Brady TJ (1985): High-resolution surface-coil imaging of lumbar disk disease. *AJR* 144:1123–1129.

127. Edelman RR, Stark DD, Saini S, Ferrucci JT Jr, Dinsmore RE, Ladd W, Brady TJ (1986): Oblique planes of section in MR imaging. *Radiology* 159:807–810.

128. Edelman RR, Wedeen VJ, Davis KR, Widder D, Hahn P, Shoukimas G, Brady TJ (1986): Multiphasic MR imaging: A new method for direct imaging of pulsatile CSF flow. *Radiology* 161:779–783.

129. Edelson JG, Nathan H (1986): Nerve root compression in spondylolysis and spondylolisthesis. *J Bone Joint Surg [Br]* 68:596–599.

130. Edwards WC, LaRocca H (1983): The developmental segmental sagittal diameter of the cervical spinal canal in patients with cervical spondylosis. *Spine* 8:20–27.

131. Edwards WC, LaRocca SH (1985): The developmental segmental sagittal diameter in combined cervical and lumbar spondylosis. *Spine* 10:42–49.

132. Ehman RL, McNamara MT, Brasch RC, Felmlee JP, Gray JE, Higgins CB (1986): Influence of physiologic motion on the appearance of tissue in MR images. *Radiology* 159:777–782.

133. Eisenstein S (1977): The morphometry and pathological anatomy of the lumbar spine in South African negroes and caucasoids with specific reference to spinal stenosis. *J Bone Joint Surg [Br]* 59:173–180.

134. Eismont FJ, Clifford S, Goldberg M, Green B (1984): Cervical sagittal spinal canal size in spine injury. *Spine* 9:663–666.

135. Eismont FJ, Currier B (1989): Surgical management of lumbar intervertebral disc disease. *J Bone Joint Surg [Am]* 71:1266–1271.

136. Eldevik OP, Dugstad G, Orrison WW, Haughton VM (1982): The effect of clinical bias on the interpretation of myelography and spinal computed tomography. *Radiology* 145:85–89.

137. Emery SE, Pathria MN, Wilber RG, Masaryk T, Bohlman HN (1989): Magnetic resonance imaging of posttraumatic spinal ligament injury. *J Spinal Dis* 2:229–233.

138. Enzmann DR (1994): On low back pain. *AJNR* 15:109–113.

139. Enzmann DR, Griffin C, Rubin JB (1987): Potential false-negative MR images of the thoracic spine in disk disease with switching of phase- and frequency-encoding gradients. *Radiology* 165:635–637.

140. Enzmann DR, O'Donohue J, Rubin JB, Shuer L, Cogen P, Silverberg G (1987): CSF pulsations within nonneoplastic spinal cord cysts. *AJR* 149:149–157.

141. Enzmann DR, Pelc NJ (1991): Normal flow patterns of intracranial and spinal cerebrospinal fluid defined with phase-contrast cine MR imaging. *Radiology* 178:467–474.

142. Enzmann DR, Rubin JB (1988): Cervical spine: MR imaging with a partial flip angle, gradient-refocused pulse sequence: Part I. General considerations and disk disease. *Radiology* 166:467–472.

143. Enzmann DR, Rubin JB (1988): Cervical spine: MR imaging with a partial flip angle, gradient-refocused pulse sequence: Part II. Spinal cord disease. *Radiology* 166:473–478.

144. Enzmann DR, Rubin JB, Wright A (1987): Cervical spine MR imaging: Generating high-signal CSF in sagittal and axial images. *Radiology* 163:233–238.

145. Epstein BS, Epstein JA, Lavine L (1964): The effect of anatomic variations in the lumbar vertebrae and spinal canal on cauda equina and nerve root syndromes. *AJR* 91:1055–1063.

146. Epstein JA, Carras R, Hyman RA, Costa S (1979): Cervical myelopathy caused by developmental stenosis of the spinal canal. *J Neurosurg* 51:362–367.

147. Epstein JA, Epstein BS, Lavine L (1962): Nerve root compression associated with narrowing of the lumbar spinal canal. *J Neurol Neurosurg Psychiatry* 25:165–176.

148. Epstein JA, Epstein NE, Marc J, Rosenthal AD, Lavine LS (1984): Lumbar intervertebral disk herniation in teenage children: Recognition and management of associated anomalies. *Spine* 9:427–432.

149. Epstein N, Epstein JA, Benjamin V, Ransohoff J (1980): Traumatic myelopathy in patients with cervical spinal stenosis without fracture or dislocation: Methods of diagnosis, management, and prognosis. *Spine* 5:489–496.

150. Epstein NE, Epstein JA, Carras R (1988): Spinal stenosis and disc herniation in a 14-year-old male. *Spine* 13:938–941.

151. Epstein NE, Hyman RA, Epstein JA, Rosenthal AD (1988):

Technical note: "Dynamic" MRI scanning of the cervical spine. *Spine* 13:937–938.

152. Erkintalo M, Laato M, Aho H, Paajanen H, Komu M, Kormano M (1989): Correlation of MR imaging, radiographic, biochemical, and histologic changes in healthy and degenerated human intervertebral lumbar disks. *Radiology: 75th Anniversary Scientific Assembly and Annual Meeting of the Radiological Society of North America.* Chicago. 173(P) Supplement:314.

153. Erkintalo M, Salminen JJ, Paajanen H, Terho P, Kormano M (1989): Disk degeneration in 14-year-old children: MR imaging study on low back pain and asymptomatic groups. *Radiology: 75th Anniversary Scientific Assembly and Annual Meeting of the Radiological Society of North America.* Chicago. 173(P) Supplement:313.

154. Eubanks BA, Cann CE, Brant-Zawadzki M (1985): CT measurement of the diameter of spinal and other bony canals: Effects of section angle and thickness. *Radiology* 157:243–246.

155. Fidler MW (1988): Remodelling of the spinal canal after burst fracture. *J Bone Joint Surg [Br]* 70:730–732.

156. Firooznia H, Kricheff II, Rafii M, et al (1987): Lumbar spine after surgery: Examination with intravenous contrast-enhanced CT. *Radiology* 163:221–226.

157. Fisher MR, Barker B, Amparo EG, Brandt G, Brant-Zawadzki M, Hricak H, Higgins CB (1985): MR imaging using specialized coils. *Radiology* 157:443–447.

158. Fisher P, Grover B, Brauer G, Ritchie G (1989): Digital image display station performance requirements based on physician experience with a prototype system. *J Digit Imaging* 2:150–155.

159. Flanders AE, Schaefer DM, Doan HT, Mishkin MM, Gonzalez CF, Northrup BE (1990): Acute cervical spine trauma: Correlation of MR imaging findings with degree of neurologic deficit *Radiology* 177:25–33 [see comments *Radiology* 177:18–20].

160. Flannigan BD, Lufkin RB, McGlade C, Winter J, Batzdorf U, Wilson G, Rauschning W, Bradley WG Jr (1987): MR imaging of the cervical spine: Neurovascular anatomy. *AJR* 148:785–790.

161. Fontaine S, Melanson D, Cosgrove R, Bertrand G (1988): Cavernous hemangiomas of the spinal cord: MR imaging. *Radiology* 166:839–841.

162. Forristall RM, Marsh HO, Pay NT (1988): Magnetic resonance imaging and contrast CT of the lumbar spine: Comparison of diagnostic methods and correlation with surgical findings. *Spine* 13:1049–1054.

163. Frahm J, Haase A, Matthaei D (1986): Rapid three-dimensional MR imaging using FLASH technique. *J Comput Assist Tomogr* 10:363–368.

164. Fredericks RK, Elster A, Walker FO (1989): Gadolinium-enhanced MRI: A superior technique for the diagnosis of intraspinal metastases. *Neurology* 39:734–736.

165. Frocrain L, Duvauferrier R, Husson JL, Noel J, Ramee A, Pawlotsky Y (1989): Recurrent postoperative sciatica: Evaluation with MR imaging and enhanced CT. *Radiology* 170:531–533.

166. Fujiwara K, Yonenobu K, Ebara S, Yamashita K, Ono K (1989): The prognosis of surgery for cervical compression myelopathy: An analysis of the factors involved. *J Bone Joint Surg [Br]* 71:393–398.

167. Fujiwara K, Yonenobu K, Hiroshima K, Ebara S, Yamashita K, Ono K (1988): Morphometry of the cervical spinal cord and its relation to pathology in cases with compression myelopathy. *Spine* 13:1212–1216.

168. Gabriel KR, Crawford AH (1988): Magnetic resonance imaging in a child who had clinical signs of discitis. *J Bone Joint Surg [Am]* 70:938–941.

169. Gebarski SS, Maynard FW, Gabrielsen TO, Knake JE, Latack JT, Hoff JT (1985): Posttraumatic progressive myelopathy. *Radiology* 157:379–385.

170. Gennuso R, Zappulla RA, Strenger SW (1989): A localized lumbar spinal root arteriovenous malformation presenting with radicular signs and symptoms. *Spine* 14:543–546.

171. Georgy BA, Hesselink JR (1994): Evaluation of fat suppression in contrast-enhanced MR of neoplastic and inflammatory spine disease. *AJNR* 15:409–417.

172. Georgy BA, Hesselink JR (1994): MR imaging of the spine: Recent advances in pulse sequences and special techniques. *AJR* 162:923–934.

173. Gertzbein SD, Court-Brown CM (1989): Rationale for the management of flexion-distraction injuries of the thoracolumbar spine based on a new classification. *J Spinal Disorders* 2:176–183.

174. Ghosh P, ed. (1988): *The biology of the intervertebral disc, vol. I.* Boca Raton: CRC Press.

175. Ghosh P, ed. (1988): *The biology of the intervertebral disc, vol. II.* Boca Raton: CRC Press.

176. Gibson MJ, Buckley J, Mawhinney R, Mulholland RC, Worthington BS (1986): Magnetic resonance imaging and discography in the diagnosis of disc degeneration. *J Bone Joint Surg [Br]* 68:369–373.

177. Gibson MJ, Szypryt EP, Buckley JH, Worthington BS, Mulholland RC (1987): Magnetic resonance imaging of adolescent disc herniation. *J Bone Joint Surg [Br]* 69:699–703.

178. Goldberg MA, Rosenthal DI, Chew FS, Blickman JG, Miller SW, Mueller PR (1993): New high-resolution teleradiology system: Prospective study of diagnostic accuracy in 685 transmitted cases. *Radiology* 186:429–434.

179. Gore DR, Sepic SB, Gardner GM (1986): Roentgenographic findings of the cervical spine in asymptomatic people. *Spine* 11:521–524.

180. Goyal RN, Russell NA, Benoit BG, Belanger JM (1987): Intraspinal cysts: A classification and literature review. *Spine* 12:209–213.

181. Grand CM, Bank WO, Baleriaux D, Matos C, Levivier M, Brotchi J (1993): Gadolinium enhancement of vertebral endplates following lumbar disc surgery. *Neuroradiology* 35:503–505.

182. Gray L, Djang WT, Friedman AH (1988): MR imaging of thoracic extradural arachnoid cysts. *J Comput Assist Tomogr* 12:646–648.

183. Greene TL, Hensinger RN, Hunter LY (1985): Back pain and vertebral changes simulating Scheuermann's disease. *J Pediatr Orthop* 5:1–7.

184. Grenier N, Greselle JF, Vital JM, Kien P, Baulny D, Broussin J, Senegas J, Caille M (1989): Normal and disrupted lumbar longitudinal ligaments: Correlative MR and anatomic study. *Radiology* 171:197–205.

185. Grenier N, Grossman RI, Schiebler ML, Yeager BA, Goldberg HI, Kressel HY (1987): Degenerative lumbar disk disease: Pitfalls and usefulness of MR imaging in detection of vacuum phenomenon. *Radiology* 164:861–865.

186. Grenier N, Kressel HY, Schiebler ML, Grossman RI (1989): Isthmic spondylolysis of the lumbar spine: MR imaging at 1.5 T. *Radiology* 170:489–493.

187. Grenier N, Kressel HY, Schiebler ML, Grossman RI, Dalinka MK (1987): Normal and degenerative posterior spinal structures: MR imaging. *Radiology* 165:517–525.

188. Grubb SA, Lipscomb HJ, Coonrad RW (1988): Degenerative adult onset scoliosis. *Spine* 13:241–245.

189. Gundry CR, Heithoff KB (1993): Epidural hematoma of the lumbar spine: 18 surgically confirmed cases. *Radiology* 187:427–431.

190. Guyer RD, Collier R, Stith WJ, Ohnmeiss DD, Hochschuler SH, Rashbaum RF, Regan JJ (1988): Discitis after discography. *Spine* 13:1352–1354.

191. Hackney DB, Asato R, Joseph PM, Carvlin MJ, McGrath JT, Grossman RI, Kassab EA, DeSimone D (1986): Hemorrhage and edema in acute spinal cord compression: Demonstration by MR imaging. *Radiology* 161:387–390.

192. Haggstrom JA, Brown JC, Marsh PW (1988): Eosinophilic granuloma of the spine: MR demonstration. *J Comput Assist Tomogr* 12:344–345.

193. Hajek PC, Baker LL, Goobar JE, Sartoris DJ, Hesselink JR, Haghighi P, Resnick D (1987): Focal fat deposition in axial bone marrow: MR characteristics. *Radiology* 162:245–249.

194. Hamanishi C, Tanaka S (1993): Dorsal root ganglia in the lumbosacral region observed from the axial views of MRI. *Spine* 18:1753–1756.

195. Hanna JW, Ball MR, Lee KS, McWhorter JM (1989): Spontaneous spinal epidural hematoma complicating Paget's disease of the spine. *Spine* 14:900–901.

196. Hansen ST Jr, Taylor TK, Honet JC, Lewis FR (1967): Fracture-dislocations of the ankylosed thoracic spine in rheumatoid spondylitis: Ankylosing spondylitis, Marie-Strumpell disease. *J Trauma* 7:827–837.

197. Harada Y, Nakahara S (1989): A pathologic study of lumbar disc herniation in the elderly. *Spine* 14:1020–1024.
198. Harris RI, MacNab I (1954): Structural changes in the lumbar intervertebral discs: Their relationship to low back pain and sciatica. *J Bone Joint Surg [Br]* 36:304–322.
199. Hashimoto K, Akahori O, Kitano K, Nakajima K, Higashihara T, Kumasaka Y (1990): Magnetic resonance imaging of lumbar disc herniation: Comparison with myelography. *Spine* 15:1166–1169.
200. Hashimoto T, Kaneda K, Abumi K (1988): Relationship between traumatic spinal canal stenosis and neurologic deficits in thoracolumbar burst fractures. *Spine* 13:1268–1272.
201. Hasso AN, McKinney JM, Killeen J, Hinshaw DB Jr, Thompson JR (1987): Computed tomography of children and adolescents with suspected spinal stenosis. *J Comput Assist Tomogr* 11:609–611.
202. Hasue M, Kikuchi S, Sakuyama Y, Ito T (1983): Anatomic study of the interrelation between lumbosacral nerve roots and their surrounding tissues. *Spine* 8:50–58.
203. Haughton VM (1988): MR imaging of the spine. *Radiology* 166:297–301.
204. Hayashi H, Okada K, Hamada M, Tada K, Ueno R (1987): Etiologic factors of myelopathy: A radiographic evaluation of the aging changes in the cervical spine. *Clin Orthop* 214:200–209.
205. Hedberg MC, Drayer BP, Flom RA, Hodak JA, Bird CR (1988): Gradient echo (GRASS) MR imaging in cervical radiculopathy. *AJR* 150:683–689.
206. Heiken JP, Glazer HS, Lee JKT, Murphy WA, Gado M (1986): *Manual of clinical magnetic resonance imaging*. New York: Raven Press.
207. Heindel W, Friedmann G, Bunke J, Thomas B, Firsching R, Ernestus RI (1986): Artifacts in MR imaging after surgical intervention. *J Comput Assist Tomogr* 10:596–599.
208. Heinz ER, Yeates A, Burger P, Drayer BP, Osborne D, Hill R (1984): Opacification of epidural venous plexus and dura in evaluation of cervical nerve roots: CT technique. *AJNR* 5:621–624.
209. Heisenberg W (1958): *Physics and philosophy*. New York: Harper & Row.
210. Heithoff KB (1988): Magnetic resonance imaging of the lumbar spine. In: WH Kirkaldy-Willis, ed. *Managing low back pain*. New York: Churchill Livingstone, pp. 183–208.
211. Heithoff KB, Burton CV, Fritts HF, Schellhas KP (1989): MRI in the evaluation of postoperative recurrent disc herniation versus fibrosis. *International Society for the Study of the Lumbar Spine*. Kyoto, Japan, pp. 43–44.
212. Heliovaara M, Vanharanta H, Korpi J, Troup JD (1986): Herniated lumbar disc syndrome and vertebral canals. *Spine* 11:433–435.
213. Henkelman RM, Watts J, Kucharczyk W (1991): High signal intensity in MR images of calcified brain tissue. *Radiology* 179:199–206.
214. Hennig J, Nauerth A, Friedburg H (1986): RARE imaging: A fast imaging method for clinical MR. *Magn Reson Med* 3:823–833.
215. Herman GT (1988): Three-dimensional imaging on a CT or MR scanner. *J Comput Assist Tomogr* 12:450–458.
216. Hesselink JR (1988): Spine imaging: History, achievements, remaining frontiers. *AJR* 150:1223–1229.
217. Hickey DS, Aspden RM, Hukins DWL, Jenkins JPR, Isherwood I (1986): Analysis of magnetic resonance images from normal and degenerate lumbar intervertebral discs. *Spine* 11:702–708.
218. Hinck VC, Gordy PD, Storino HE (1964): Developmental stenosis of the cervical spinal canal: Radiological considerations. *Neurology* 14:864–868.
219. Hinck VC, Hopkins CE, Savara BS (1962): Sagittal diameter of the cervical spinal canal in children. *Radiology* 79:97–108.
220. Hinck VC, Sachdev NS (1966): Developmental stenosis of the cervical spinal canal. *Brain* 89:27–36.
221. Hitselberger WE, Witten RM (1968): Abnormal myelograms in asymptomatic patients. *J Neurosurg* 28:204–206.
222. Ho PS, Yu S, Sether LA, Wagner M, Ho KC, Haughton VM (1988): Ligamentum flavum: Appearance on sagittal and coronal MR images. *Radiology* 168:469–472.
223. Ho PSP, Yu S, Sether LA, Wagner M, Ho KC, Haughton VM (1988): Progressive and regressive changes in the nucleus pulposus, Part I. The neonate. *Radiology* 169:87–91.
224. Hochhauser L, Kieffer SA, Cacayorin ED, Petro GR, Teller WF (1988): Recurrent postdiskectomy low back pain: MR-surgical correlation. *AJR* 151:755–760.
225. Hollis PH, Malis LI, Zappulla RA (1986): Neurological deterioration after lumbar puncture below complete spinal subarachnoid block. *J Neurosurg* 64:253–256.
226. Holsheimer J, den Boer JA, Struijk JJ, Rozeboom AR (1994): MR assessment of the normal position of the spinal cord in the spinal canal. *AJNR* 15:951–959.
227. Holt S, Yates PO (1966): Cervical spondylosis and nerve root lesions: Incidence at routine necropsy. *J Bone Joint Surg [Br]* 48:407–423.
228. Horii SC (1992): PACS mini refresher course: Electronic imaging workstations: Ergonomic issues and the user interface. *Radiographics* 12:773–787.
229. Horne J, Cockshott WP, Shannon HS (1987): Spinal column damage from water ski jumping. *Skeletal Radiol* 16:612–616.
230. Hoyland JA, Freemont AJ, Jayson MI (1989): Intervertebral foramen venous obstruction: A cause of periradicular fibrosis? *Spine* 14:558–568.
231. Huang HK, Taira RK, Lou SL, et al (1993): Implementation of a large-scale picture archival and communication system. *Comput Med Imaging Graph* 17:1–11.
232. Hubbard AM, Markowitz RI, Kimmel B, Kroger M, Bartko MB (1992): Sedation for pediatric patients undergoing CT and MRI. *J Comput Assist Tomogr* 16:3–6.
233. Hueftle MG, Modic MT, Ross JS, Masaryk TJ, Carter JR, Wilber RG, Bohlman HH, Steinberg PM, Delamarter RB (1988): Lumbar spine: Postoperative MR imaging with gadolinium-DTPA. *Radiology* 167:817–824.
234. Hurme M, Alaranta H (1987): Factors predicting the result of surgery for lumbar intervertebral disc herniation. *Spine* 12:933–938.
235. Hyman RA, Edwards JH, Vacirca SJ, Stein HL (1985): 0.6 T MR imaging of the cervical spine: Multislice and multiecho techniques. *AJNR* 6:229–236.
236. Inoue SI, Watanabe T, Goto S, Takahashi K, Takata K, Sho E (1988): Degenerative spondylolisthesis. *Clin Orthop* 227:90–98.
237. Jackson DE Jr, Atlas SW, Mani JR, Norman D (1989): Intraspinal synovial cysts: MR imaging. *Radiology* 170:527–530.
238. Jaffray D, O'Brien JP (1986): Isolated intervertebral disc resorption: A source of mechanical and inflammatory back pain? *Spine* 11:397–401.
239. Janssen L, Hansebout RR (1989): Pathogenesis of spinal cord injury and newer treatments: A review. *Spine* 14:23–32.
240. Jenkins LE, Bowman M, Cotler HB, Gildenberg PL (1989): A case report: Intradural herniation of a lumbar intervertebral disc. *J Spinal Disorders* 2:196–200.
241. Jensen MC, Brant-Zawadzki MN, Obuchowski N, Modic MT, Malkasian D, Ross JS (1994): MRI of the lumbar spine in people without back pain. *NEJM* 331:69–73.
242. Jensen ME, Hayes CW, DeBlois GG, Laine FJ (1989): Hemispherical spondylosclerosis: MR appearance. *J Comput Assist Tomogr* 13:540–542.
243. Jinkins JR (1993): MR of enhancing nerve roots in the unoperated lumbosacral spine. *AJNR* 14:193–202.
244. Jinkins JR, Osborn AG, Garrett D Jr, Hunt S, Story JL (1993): Spinal nerve enhancement with Gd-DTPA: MR correlation with the postoperative lumbosacral spine. *AJNR* 14:383–394.
245. Johnson CE, Sze G (1990): Benign lumbar arachnoiditis: MR imaging with gadopentetate dimeglumine. *AJNR* 11:763–770.
246. Johnson DW, Farnum GN, Latchaw RE, Erba SM (1989): MR imaging of the pars interarticularis. *AJR* 152:327–332.
247. Jones KM, Mulkern RV, Schwartz RB, Oshio K, Barnes PD, Jolesz FA (1992): Fast spin-echo MR imaging of the brain and spine: Current concepts. *AJR* 158:1313–1320.
248. Jones KM, Schwartz RB, Mantello MT, Ahn SS, Khorasani R, Mukherji S, Oshio K, Mulkern RV (1994): Fast spin-echo MR in the detection of vertebral metastases: Comparison of three sequences. *AJNR* 15:401–407.
249. Just M, Thelen M (1988): Tissue characterization with T1, T2

and proton density values: Results in 160 patients with brain tumors. *Radiology* 169:779–785.

250. Kaffenberger DA, Shah CP, Murtagh FR, Wilson C, Silbiger ML (1988): MR imaging of spinal cord hemangioblastoma associated with syringomyelia. *J Comput Assist Tomogr* 12:495–498.

251. Kambin P, Nixon JE, Chait A, Schaffer JL (1988): Annular protrusion: Pathophysiology and roentgenographic appearance. *Spine* 13:671–675.

252. Kanal E, Gillen J, Evans JA, Savitz DA, Shellock FG (1993): Survey of reproductive health among female MR workers. *Radiology* 187:395–399.

253. Kanal E, Shellock FG (1993): MR imaging of patients with intracranial aneurysm clips. *Radiology* 187:612–614.

254. Kanal E, Shellock FG, Talagala L (1990): Safety considerations in MR imaging. *Radiology* 176:593–606.

255. Kapila A, Lines M (1987): Neuropathic spinal arthropathy: CT and MR findings. *J Comput Assist Tomogr* 11:736–739.

256. Karpman RR, Weinstein PR, Gall EP, Johnson PC (1982): Lumbar spinal stenosis in a patient with diffuse idiopathic skeletal hypertrophy syndrome. *Spine* 7:598–603.

257. Kataoka O, Nishibayashi Y, Sho T (1989): Intradural lumbar disc herniation: Report of three cases with a review of the literature. *Spine* 14:529–533.

258. Kawaida H, Sakou T, Morizono Y, Yoshikuni N (1989): Magnetic resonance imaging of upper cervical disorders in rheumatoid arthritis. *Spine* 14:1144–1148.

259. Keene JS, Fischer SP, Vanderby R Jr, Drummond DS, Turski PA (1989): Significance of acute posttraumatic bony encroachment of the neural canal. *Spine* 14:799–802.

260. Kelly WM, Clark JA (1988): MRI fast scan in neurodiagnosis: Practical clinical applications, Part 2. *MRI Decisions* (September/October): 17–26.

261. Kelly WM, Paglan PG, Pearson JA, San Diego AG, Solomon MA (1986): Ferromagnetism of intraocular foreign body causes unilateral blindness after MR study. *AJNR* 7:243–245.

262. Kerslake RW, Jaspan T, Worthington BS (1991): Magnetic resonance imaging of spinal trauma. *Br J Radiol* 64:386–402.

263. Kerslake RW, Mitchell LA, Worthington BS (1992): Case report: CT and MRI of the cauda equina syndrome in ankylosing spondylitis. *Clin Radiol* 45:134–136.

264. Kikuchi S, Hasue M, Nishiyama K, Ito T (1984): Anatomic and clinical studies of radicular symptoms. *Spine* 9:23–30.

265. Kirkaldy-Willis WH (1984): The relationship of structural pathology to the nerve root. *Spine* 9:49–52.

266. Kirkaldy-Willis WH (1988): The pathology and pathogenesis of low back pain. In: WH Kirkaldy-Willis, ed. *Managing low back pain.* New York: Churchill Livingstone, pp. 49–75.

267. Kirkaldy-Willis WH, Paine KW, Cauchoix J, McIvor G (1974): Lumbar spinal stenosis. *Clin Orthop* 99:30–50.

268. Kirkaldy-Willis WH, Wedge JH, Yong-Hing K, Reilly J (1978): Pathology and pathogenesis of lumbar spondylosis and stenosis. *Spine* 3:319–328.

269. Kleiner JB, Donaldson WI, Curd JG, et al (1991): Extraspinal causes of lumbosacral radiculopathy. *J Bone Joint Surg [AM]* 73:817–821.

270. Kliewer MA, Gray L, Paver J, Richardson WD, Vogler JB, McElhaney JH, Myers BS (1993): Acute spinal ligament disruption: MR imaging with anatomic correlation. *JMRI* 3:855–861.

271. Klucznik RP, Carrier DA, Pyka R, Haid RW (1993): Placement of a ferromagnetic intracerebral aneurysm clip in a magnetic field with a fatal outcome. *Radiology* 187:855–856.

272. Kneeland JB, Hyde JS (1989): High-resolution MR imaging with local coils. *Radiology* 171:1–7.

273. Kobori M, Takahashi H, Mikawa Y (1986): Atlanto-axial dislocation in Down's syndrome: Report of two cases requiring surgical correction. *Spine* 11:195–200.

274. Kokmen E, Marsh WR, Baker HL Jr (1985): Magnetic resonance imaging in syringomyelia. *Neurosurgery* 17:267–270.

275. Kornberg M (1988): MRI diagnosis of traumatic Schmorl's node. *Spine* 13:934–935.

276. Kornberg M, Rechtine GR (1985): Quantitative assessment of the fifth lumbar spinal canal by computed tomography in symptomatic L4-L5 disease. *Spine* 10:328–330.

277. Kortelainen P, Puranen J, Koivisto E, Lahde S (1985): Symptoms and signs of sciatica and their relation to the localization of the lumbar disc herniation. *Spine* 10:88–92.

278. Kricun R, Shoemaker EI, Chovanes GI, Stephens HW (1992): Epidural abscess of the cervical spine: MR findings in five cases. *AJR* 158:1145–1149.

279. Krodel A, Refior HJ, Westermann S (1990): The importance of functional magnetic resonance imaging (MRI) in the planning of stabilizing operations on the cervical spine in rheumatoid patients. *Arch Orthop Trauma Surg* 109:30–33.

280. Krol G, Sze G, Malkin M, Walker R (1988): MR of cranial and spinal meningeal carcinomatosis: Comparison with CT and myelography. *AJR* 151:583–588.

281. Kulkarni MV, McArdle CB, Kopanicky D, Miner M, Cotler HB, Lee KF, Harris JH (1987): Acute spinal cord injury: MR imaging at 1.5 T. *Radiology* 164:837–843.

282. Kulkarni MV, Patton JA, Price RR (1986): Technical considerations for the use of surface coils in MRI. *AJR* 147:373–378.

283. Kurihara A, Tanaka Y, Tsumura N, Iwasaki Y (1988): Hyperostotic lumbar spinal stenosis: a review of 12 surgically treated cases with roentgenographic survey of ossification of the yellow ligament at the lumbar spine. *Spine* 13:1308–1316.

284. Kurz LT, Garfin SR, Unger AS, Thorne RP, Rothman RH (1985): Intraspinal synovial cyst causing sciatica. *J Bone Joint Surg [Am]* 67:865–871.

285. Kurz LT, Herkowitz HN (1989): The pathogenesis and natural history of lumbar disc disease: disc degeneration and herniation. *Sem Spine Surg* 1:2–7.

286. Laasonen EM, Soini J (1989): Low-back pain after lumbar fusion. *Spine* 14:210–213.

287. Ladd AL, Scranton PE (1986): Congenital cervical stenosis presenting as transient quadriplegia in athletes. *J Bone Joint Surg [Am]* 68:1371–1374.

288. Lang P, Chafetz N, Genant HK, Morris JM (1990): Lumbar spinal fusion: Assessment of functional stability with magnetic resonance imaging. *Spine* 15:581–588.

289. Laredo JD, Reizine D, Bard M, Merland JJ (1986): Vertebral hemangiomas: Radiologic evaluation. *Radiology* 161:183–189.

290. Larsson E-M, Holtas S, Zygmunt S (1989): Pre- and postoperative MR imaging of the craniocervical junction in rheumatoid arthritis. *AJR* 152:561–566.

291. Lauterbur PC (1973): Image formation by induced local interactions: Examples employing nuclear magnetic resonance. *Nature* 242:190–191.

292. Lee BC, Zimmerman RD, Manning JJ, Deck MD (1985): MR imaging of syringomyelia and hydromyelia. *AJR* 144:1149–1156.

293. Lenz GW, Haacke EM, Masaryk TJ, Laub G (1988): In-plane vascular imaging: Pulse sequence design and strategy. *Radiology* 166:875–882.

294. Levitan LH, Wiens CW (1983): Chronic lumbar extradural hematoma: CT findings. *Radiology* 148:707–708.

295. Levy LM, Di Chiro G (1990): MR phase imaging and CSF flow in the head and spine. *Neuroradiology* 32:399–406.

296. Levy LM, Di Chiro G, Brooks RA, Dwyer AJ, Wener L, Frank J (1988): Spinal cord artifacts from truncation errors during MR imaging. *Radiology* 166:479–483.

297. Levy LM, Di Chiro G, McCullough DC, Dwyer AJ, Johnson DL, Yang SS (1988): Fixed spinal cord: Diagnosis with MR imaging. *Radiology* 169:773–778.

298. Libshitz HI, Malthouse SR, Cunningham D, MacVicar AD, Husband JE (1992): Multiple myeloma: Appearance at MR imaging. *Radiology* 182:833–837.

299. Linden A, Zankovich R, Theissen P, Diehl V, Schicha H (1989): Malignant lymphoma: Bone marrow imaging versus biopsy. *Radiology* 173:335–339.

300. Lindholm TS, Pylkkanen P (1982): Discitis following removal of intervertebral disc. *Spine* 7:618–622.

301. Lipson SJ (1988): Metaplastic proliferative fibrocartilage as an alternative concept to herniated intervertebral disc. *Spine* 13:1055–1060.

302. Lipson SJ, Muir H (1981): Proteoglycans in experimental intervertebral disc degeneration. *Spine* 6:194–210.

303. Liu SS, Williams KD, Drayer BP, Spetzler RF, Sonntag VK

(1990): Synovial cysts of the lumbosacral spine: Diagnosis by MR imaging. *AJR* 154:163–166.

304. Lou SL, Huang HK (1992): Assessment of a neuroradiology PACS in clinical practice. *AJR* 159:1321–1327.

305. MacNab I (1950): Spondylolisthesis with an intact neural arch, the so-called pseudo-spondylolisthesis. *J Bone Joint Surg [Br]* 32: 325–333.

306. MacNab I (1975): Cervical spondylosis. *Clin Orthop* 109:69–77.

307. Maiman DJ, Daniels D, Larson SJ (1988): Magnetic resonance imaging in the diagnosis of lower thoracic disc herniation. *J Spinal Disorders* 1:134–138.

308. Malmivaara A, Videman T, Juosma E, Troup JDG (1987): Facet joint orientation, facet and costovertebral joint osteoarthrosis, disc degeneration, vertebral body osteophytosis, and Schmorl's nodes in the thoracolumbar junctional region of cadaveric spines. *Spine* 12:458–461.

309. Mamourian AC, Briggs RW (1986): Appearance of pantopaque on MR images. *Radiology* 158:457–460.

310. Manabe S, Tateishi A (1986): Epidural migration of extruded cervical disc and its surgical treatment. *Spine* 11:873–878.

311. Mankovich NJ, Taira RK, Cho PS, Huang HK (1988): Operational radiologic image archive on digital optical disks. *Radiology* 167:139–142.

312. Mapstone TB, Rekate HL, Shurin SB (1983): Quadriplegia secondary to hematoma after lateral C-1, C-2 puncture in a leukemic child. *Neurosurgery* 12:230–231.

313. Maravilla KR, Hartling RP (1988): Imaging decisions in degenerative spinal disease: A practical approach. *MRI Decisions* 2:2–13.

314. Maravilla KR, Weinreb JC, Suss R, Nunnally RL (1985): Magnetic resonance demonstration of multiple sclerosis plaques in the cervical cord. *AJR* 144:381–385.

315. Mark AS, Atlas SW (1988): MRI of the cervical spine and cord. *MRI Decisions* 2:23–32.

316. Masaryk TJ, Boumphrey F, Modic MT, Tamborrello C, Ross JS, Brown MD (1986): Effects of chemonucleolysis demonstrated by MR imaging. *J Comput Assist Tomogr* 10:917–923.

317. Masaryk TJ, Modic MT, Geisinger MA, Standefer J, Hardy RW, Boumphrey F, Duchesneau PM (1986): Cervical myelopathy: A comparison of magnetic resonance and myelography. *J Comput Assist Tomogr* 10:184–194.

318. Masaryk TJ, Ross JS, Modic MT, Boumphrey F, Bohlman H, Wilber G (1988): High-resolution MR imaging of sequestered lumbar intervertebral disks. *AJR* 150:1155–1162.

319. Masaryk TJ, Ross JS, Modic MT, Ruff RL, Selman WR, Ratcheson RA (1987): Radiculomeningeal vascular malformations of the spine: MR imaging. *Radiology* 164:845–849.

320. Matsuda Y, Miyazaki K, Tada K, Yasuda A, Nakayama T, Murakami H, Matsuo M (1991): Increased MR signal intensity due to cervical myelopathy. Analysis of 29 surgical cases. *J Neurosurg* 74:887–892.

321. Matsuura P, Waters RL, Adkins RH, Rothman S, Gurbani N, Sie I (1989): Comparison of computerized tomography parameters of the cervical spine in normal control subjects and spinal cord–injured patients. *J Bone Joint Surg [Am]* 71:183–188.

322. Maupin WB, Naul LG, Kanter SL, Chang CS (1989): Synovial cyst presenting as a neural foraminal lesion: MR and CT appearance. *AJR* 153:1231–1232.

323. Mayer JS, Kulkarni MV, Yeakley JW (1987): Craniocervical manifestations of neurofibromatosis: MR versus CT studies. *J Comput Assist Tomogr* 11:839–844.

324. Mayer PJ, Jacobsen FS (1989): Cauda equina syndrome after surgical treatment of lumbar spinal stenosis with application of free autogenous fat graft. *J Bone Joint Surg [Am]* 71:1090–1093.

325. McAfee PC, Regan JJ, Bohlman HH (1987): Cervical cord compression from ossification of the posterior longitudinal ligament in non-orientals. *J Bone Joint Surg [Br]* 69:569–575.

326. McArdle CB, Crofford MJ, Mirfakhraee M, Amparo EG, Calhoun JS (1986): Surface coil MR of spinal trauma: Preliminary experience. *AJNR* 7:885–893.

327. McArdle CB, Wright JW, Prevost WJ, Dornfest DJ, Amparo EG (1986): MR imaging of the acutely injured patient with cervical traction. *Radiology* 159:273–274.

328. McCall IW, Park WM, O'Brien JP (1985): Acute traumatic intraosseous disc herniation. *Spine* 10:134–137.

329. McCarron RF, Wimpee MW, Hudkins PG, Laros GS (1987): The inflammatory effect of nucleus pulposus: A possible element in the pathogenesis of low-back pain. *Spine* 12:760–764.

330. McGuire RA, Brown MD, Green BA (1987): Intradural spinal tumors and spinal stenosis. *Spine* 12:1062–1066.

331. McKinstry CS, Steiner RE, Young AT, Jones L, Swirsky D, Aber V (1987): Bone marrow in leukemia and aplastic anemia: MR imaging before, during, and after treatment. *Radiology* 162:701–707.

332. McRae DL (1956): Asymptomatic intervertebral disc protrusions. *Acta Radiol* 46:9–27.

333. Melendez JC, McCrank E (1993): Anxiety-related reactions associated with MRI examinations. *JAMA* 270:745–747.

334. Melki PS, Mulkern RV (1992): Magnetization transfer effects in multislice RARE sequences. *Magn Reson Med* 24:189–195.

335. Merine D, Wang H, Kumar AJ, Zinreich SJ, Rosenbaum AE (1987): CT myelography and MR imaging of acute transverse myelitis. *J Comput Assist Tomogr* 11:606–608.

336. Meyer-Ebrecht D (1993): Digital image communication. *Eur J Radiol* 17:47–55.

337. Michaelis T, Merboldt K-D, Bruhn H, Hanicke W, Frahm J (1993): Absolute concentrations of metabolites in the adult human brain in vivo: Quantification of localized proton MR spectra. *Radiology* 187:219–227. [Erratum: *Radiology* 188:288].

338. Mikhael MA, Ciric I, Tarkington JA, Vick NA (1981): Neuroradiological evaluation of lateral recess syndrome. *Neuroradiology* 140:97–107.

339. Milgram JW (1982): Osteoarthritic changes at the severely degenerative disc in humans. *Spine* 7:498–505.

340. Miller JAA, Schmatz C, Schultz AB (1988): Lumbar disc degeneration: Correlation with age, sex, and spine level in 600 autopsy specimens. *Spine* 13:173–178.

341. Minagi H, Gronner AT (1969): Calcification of the posterior longitudinal ligament: A cause of cervical myelopathy. *AJR* 105:365–369.

342. Minami S, Sagoh T, Nishimura K, Yamashita K, Fujisawa I, Noma S, Itoh K, Togashi K, Oda Y, Matsumoto M, Yamagata S, Kikuchi H, Nakano Y, Konishi J (1988): Spinal arteriovenous malformation: MR imaging. *Radiology* 169:109–115.

343. Mink JH (1989): Imaging evaluation of the candidate for percutaneous lumbar discectomy. *Clin Orthop* 238:83–103.

344. Mirich DR, Hall JT, Carrasco CH (1988): MR imaging of traumatic spinal arachnoid cyst. *J Comput Assist Tomogr* 12:862–865.

345. Mirowitz SA, Shady KL (1992): Gadopentetate dimeglumine-enhanced MR imaging of the postoperative lumbar spine: Comparison of fat-suppressed and conventional T1-weighted images. *AJR* 159:385–389.

346. Mirvis SE, Borg U, Belzberg H (1987): MR imaging of ventilator-dependent patients: Preliminary experience. *AJR* 149:845–846.

347. Mirvis SE, Geisler FH, Jelinek JJ, Joslyn JN, Gellad F (1988): Acute cervical spine trauma: evaluation with 1.5 T MR imaging. *Radiology* 166:807–816.

348. Mitchell DG, Burk DL Jr, Vinitski S, Rifkin MD (1987): The biophysical basis of tissue contrast in extracranial MR imaging. *AJR* 149:831–837.

349. Miyasaka K, Isu T, Iwasaki Y, Abe S, Takei H, Tsuru M (1983): High resolution computed tomography in the diagnosis of cervical disc disease. *Neuroradiology* 24:253–257.

350. Modic MT, Feiglin DH, Piraino DW, Boumphrey F, Weinstein MA, Duchesneau PM, Rehm S (1985): Vertebral osteomyelitis: Assessment using MR. *Radiology* 157:157–166.

351. Modic MT, Masaryk T, Boumphrey F, Goormastic M, Bell G (1986): Lumbar herniated disk disease and canal stenosis: Prospective evaluation by surface coil MR, CT and myelography. *AJR* 147:757–765.

352. Modic MT, Masaryk TJ, Mulopulos GP, Bundschuh C, Han JS, Bohlman H (1986): Cervical radiculopathy: Prospective evaluation with surface coil MR imaging, CT with metrizamide, and metrizamide myelography. *Radiology* 161:753–759.

353. Modic MT, Masaryk TJ, Ross JS (1994): *Magnetic resonance imaging of the spine.* 2nd ed. St. Louis: Mosby-Year Book.

354. Modic MT, Masaryk TJ, Ross JS, Carter JR (1988): Imaging of degenerative disk disease. *Radiology* 168:177–186.

355. Modic MT, Masaryk TJ, Ross JS, Mulopulos GP, Bundschuh CV, Bohlman H (1987): Cervical radiculopathy: Value of oblique MR imaging. *Radiology* 163:227–231.

356. Modic MT, Pavlicek W, Weinstein MA, Boumphrey F, Ngo F, Hardy R, Duchesneau PM (1984): Magnetic resonance imaging of intervertebral disk disease. *Radiology* 152:103–111.

357. Modic MT, Ross JS, Masaryk TJ (1989): Imaging of degenerative disease of the cervical spine. *Clin Orthop* 239:109–120.

358. Modic MT, Steinberg PM, Ross JS, Masaryk TJ, Carter JR (1988): Degenerative disk disease: Assessment of changes in vertebral body marrow with MR imaging. *Radiology* 166:193–199.

359. Mohan V, Gupta SK, Tuli SM, Sanyal B (1980): Symptomatic vertebral haemangiomas. *Clin Radiol* 31:575–579.

360. Moiel R, Ehni G (1968): Cauda equina compression due to spondylolisthesis with intact neural arch. *J Neurosurg* 28:262–265.

361. Moiel RH, Raso E, Waltz TA (1970): Central cord syndrome resulting from congenital narrowness of the cervical spinal canal. *J Trauma* 10:502–510.

362. Monajati A, Spitzer RM, LaRue WJ, Heggeness L (1986): MR imaging of a spinal teratoma. *J Comput Assist Tomogr* 10:307–310.

363. Montaldi S, Fankhauser H, Schnyder P, et al (1988): Computed tomography of the postoperative intervertebral disc and lumbar spinal canal: Investigation of twenty-five patients after successful operation for lumbar disc herniation. *Neurosurgery* 22:1014–1022.

364. Mooney V, Robertson J (1976): The facet syndrome. *Clin Orthop* 115:149–156.

365. Moore SG, Gooding CA, Brasch RC, Ehman RL, Ringertz HG, Ablin AR, Matthay KK, Zoger S (1986): Bone marrow in children with acute lymphocytic leukemia: MR relaxation times. *Radiology* 160:237–240.

366. Morrissy RT, Goldsmith GS, Hall EC, et al (1990): Measurement of the Cobb angle on radiographs of patients who have scoliosis: Evaluation of intrinsic error. *J Bone Joint Surg [Am]* 72:320–327.

367. Moulopoulos LA, Varma DG, Dimopoulos MA, Leeds NE, Kim EE, Johnston DA, Alexanian R, Libshitz HI (1992): Multiple myeloma: spinal MR imaging in patients with untreated newly diagnosed disease. *Radiology* 185:833–840.

368. Mulkern RV, Wong STS, Winalski C, Jolesz FA (1990): Contrast manipulation and artifact assessment of 2D and 3D RARE sequences. *Magn Reson Imaging* 8:557–566.

369. Murakami J, Russell WJ, Hayabuchi N, Kimura S (1982): Computed tomography of posterior longitudinal ligament ossification: Its appearance and diagnostic value with special reference to thoracic lesions. *J Comput Assist Tomogr* 6:41–50.

370. Murone I (1974): The importance of the sagittal diameters of the cervical spinal canal in relation to spondylosis and myelopathy. *J Bone Joint Surg [Br]* 56:30–36.

371. Nabors MW, Pait GT, Byrd EB, Karim NO, Davis DO, Kobrine AI, Rizzoli HV (1988): Updated assessment and current classification of spinal meningeal cysts. *J Neurosurg* 68:366–377.

372. Naidich TP, McLone DG, Mutluer S (1983): A new understanding of dorsal dysraphism with lipoma (lipomyeloschisis): Radiologic evaluation and surgical correction. *AJR* 140:1065–1078.

373. Naul LG, Peet GJ, Maupin WB (1989): Avascular necrosis of the vertebral body: MR imaging. *Radiology* 172:219–222.

374. Negendank WG, Crowley MG, Ryan JR, Keller NA, Evelhoch JL (1989): Bone and soft-tissue lesions: Diagnosis with combined H-1 MR imaging and P-31 MR spectroscopy. *Radiology* 173:181–188.

375. Nehls DG, Shetter AG, Hodak JA, Waggener JD (1984): Chronic spinal epidural hematoma presenting as lumbar stenosis: Clinical, myelographic, and computed tomographic features; A case report. *Neurosurgery* 14:230–233.

376. Nesbit GM, Miller GM, Baker HL Jr, Ebersold MJ, Scheithauer BW (1989): Spinal cord sarcoidosis: A new finding at MR imaging with Gadolinium-DTPA enhancement. *Radiology* 173:839–843.

377. Neuhold A, Stiskal M, Platzer C, Pernecky G, Brainin M (1991): Combined use of spin-echo and gradient echo MR-imaging in cervical disk disease. Comparison with myelography and intraoperative findings. *Neuroradiology* 33:422–426.

378. Nitz WR, Bradley WG, Watanabe AS, Lee RR, Burgoyne B, O'Sullivan RM, Herbst MD (1992): Flow dynamics of cerebrospinal fluid: Assessment with phase-contrast velocity MR imaging performed with retrospective cardiac gating. *Radiology* 183:395–405.

379. Nordqvist L (1964): The sagittal diameter of the spinal cord and sub-arachnoid space in different age groups: A roentgenographic post-mortem study. *Acta Radiol Diagn Suppl* 227:1–96.

380. Norman D, Mills CM, Brant-Zawadzki M, Yeates A, Crooks LE, Kaufman L (1983): Magnetic resonance imaging of the spinal cord and canal: Potentials and limitations. *AJR* 141:1147–1152.

381. Numaguchi Y, Rigamonti D, Rothman MI, Sato S, Mihara F, Sadato N (1993): Spinal epidural abscess: evaluation with gadolinium-enhanced MR imaging. *Radiographics* 13:545–559. Discussion follows.

382. Oda J, Tanaka H, Tsuzuki N (1988): Intervertebral disc changes with aging of human cervical vertebra, from the neonate to the eighties. *Spine* 13:1205–1211.

383. Ogilvie JW, Sherman J (1987): Spondylolysis in Scheuermann's disease. *Spine* 12:251–253.

384. Ogino H, Tada K, Okada K, Yonenobu K, Yamamoto T, Ono K, Namiki H (1983): Canal diameter, anteroposterior compression ratio, and spondylotic myelopathy of the cervical spine. *Spine* 8:1–15.

385. Olson DO, Shields AF, Scheurich CJ, Porter BA, Moss AA (1986): Magnetic resonance imaging of the bone marrow in patients with leukemia, aplastic anemia, and lymphoma. *Invest Radiol* 21:540–546.

386. Ono K, Ota H, Tada K, Hamada H, Takaoka K (1977): Ossified posterior longitudinal ligament, a clinicopathologic study. *Spine* 2:126–138.

387. Osti OL, Fraser RD (1992): MRI and discography of annular tears and intervertebral disc degeneration. A prospective clinical comparison [published erratum appears in *J Bone Joint Surg [Br]* 1992 Sep 74(5):793]. *J Bone Joint Surg [Br]* 74:431–435.

388. Otake S, Matsuo M, Nishizawa S, Sano A, Kuroda Y (1992): Ossification of the posterior longitudinal ligament: MR evaluation. *AJNR* 13:1059–1067.

389. Paajanen H, Erkintalo M, Kuusela T, Dahlstrom S, Kormano M (1989): Magnetic resonance study of disc degeneration in young low-back pain patients. *Spine* 14:982–985.

390. Padovani R, Tognetti F, Laudadio S, Bernardi B (1986): Arteriovenous malformations of the spinal cord in the pediatric age group. *Spine* 11:23–25.

391. Paine KW, Haung PW (1972): Lumbar disc syndrome. *J Neurosurg* 37:75–82.

392. Panagiotacopulos ND, Pope MH, Krag MH, Block R (1987): Water content in human intervertebral discs, Part I. Measurement by magnetic resonance imaging. *Spine* 12:912–917.

393. Panjabi MM, Takata K, Goel VK (1983): Kinematics of lumbar intervertebral foramen. *Spine* 8:348–357.

394. Parizel PM, Balériaux D, Rodesch G, Segebarth C, Lalmand B, Christophe C, Lemort M, Haesendonck P, Niendorf HP, Flament-Durand J, Brotchi J (1989): Gadolinium-DTPA-enhanced MR imaging of spinal tumors. *AJR* 152:1087–1096.

395. Pavlicek W, Geisinger M, Castle L, Borkowski GP, Meaney TF, Bream BL, Gallagher JH (1983): The effects of nuclear magnetic resonance on patients with cardiac pacemakers. *Radiology* 147:149–153.

396. Payne EE, Spillane JD (1957): The cervical spine: An anatomico-pathological study of 70 specimens (using a special technique) with particular reference to the problem of cervical spondylosis. *Brain* 80:571–596.

397. Pear BL (1972): Spinal epidural hematoma. *AJR* 115:155–164.

398. Pech P, Haughton VM (1985): Lumbar intervertebral disk: Correlative MR and anatomic study. *Radiology* 156:699–701.

399. Peck D, Nicholls PJ, Beard C, Allen JR (1986): Are there compartment syndromes in some patients with idiopathic back pain? *Spine* 11:468–475.

400. Peck WW (1989): Current status of MRI of the cervical spine. *Appl Radiology* 18:17–30.

401. Penning L, van der Zwaag P (1966): Biomechanical aspects of spondylotic myelopathy. *Acta Radiol Diag* 5:1090–1103.

402. Penning L, Wilmink JT (1987): Posture-dependent bilateral com-

pression of L4 or L5 nerve roots in facet hypertrophy: A dynamic CT-myelographic study. *Spine* 12:488–500.

403. Penning L, Wilmink JT, van Woerden HH, Knol E (1986): CT myelographic findings in degenerative disorders of the cervical spine: Clinical significance. *AJNR* 7:119–127.

404. Perneczky G, Bock FW, Neuhold A, Stiskal M (1992): Diagnosis of cervical disc disease. MRI versus cervical myelography. *Acta Neurochir* 116:44–48.

405. Peterman SB, Hoffman JC Jr, Malko JA (1991): Magnetic resonance artifact in the postoperative cervical spine: A potential pitfall. *Spine* 16:721–725.

406. Peyster RG, Teplick JG, Haskin M (1985): Computed tomography of lumbosacral conjoined nerve root anomalies: Potential cause of false-positive reading for herniated nucleus-pulposus. *Spine* 10:331–337.

407. Pickett J, Blumenkopf B (1989): Dural lacerations and thoracolumbar fractures. *J Spinal Disorders* 2:99–103.

408. Pierot L, Dormont D, Oueslati S, Cornu P, Rivierez M, Bories J (1988): Gadolinium-DTPA enhanced MR imaging of intradural neurenteric cysts. *J Comput Assist Tomogr* 12:762–764.

409. Pojunas K, Williams AL, Daniels DL, Haughton VM (1984): Syringomyelia and hydromyelia: Magnetic resonance evaluation. *Radiology* 153:679–683.

410. Porter RW, Hibbert C, Evans C (1984): The natural history of root entrapment syndrome. *Spine* 9:418–421.

411. Porter RW, Hibbert C, Wellman P (1980): Backache and the lumbar spinal canal. *Spine* 5:99–105.

412. Porter RW, Hibbert CS, Wicks M (1978): The spinal canal in symptomatic lumbar disc lesions. *J Bone Joint Surg [Br]* 60:485–487.

413. Porter RW, Pavitt D (1987): The vertebral canal I. Nutrition and development: An archaeological study. *Spine* 12:901–906.

414. Post MJD, Quencer RM, Green BA, Montalvo BM, Tobias JA, Sowers JJ, Levin IH (1987): Intramedullary spinal cord metastases, mainly of nonneurogenic origin. *AJR* 148:1015–1022.

415. Post MJ, Quencer RM, Montalvo BM, Katz BH, Eismont FJ, Green BA (1988): Spinal infection: Evaluation with MR imaging and intraoperative US. *Radiology* 169:765–771.

416. Post MJ, Sze G, Quencer RM, Eismont FJ, Green BA, and Gahbauer H (1990): Gadolinium-enhanced MR in spinal infection. *J Comput Assist Tomogr* 14:721–729.

417. Postacchini F, Massobrio M, Ferro L (1985): Familial lumbar stenosis. *J Bone Joint Surg [Am]* 67:321–323.

418. Powell MC, Szypryt P, Wilson M, Symonds EM (1986): Prevalence of lumbar disc degeneration observed by magnetic resonance in symptomless women. *Lancet* 2:1366–1367.

419. Pritzker KP (1977): Aging and degeneration in the lumbar intervertebral disc. *Orthop Clin North Am* 8:66–77.

420. Prusick VR, Lint DS, Bruder WJ (1988): Cauda equina syndrome as a complication of free epidural fat-grafting. *J Bone Joint Surg [Am]* 70:1256–1258.

421. Purcell EM, Torrey HC, Pound RV (1946): Resonance absorption by nuclear magnetic moments in solids. *Phys Rev* 69:37–38.

422. Quencer RM, Donovan Post MJ, Hinks RS (1990): Cine MR in the evaluation of normal and abnormal CSF flow: Intracranial and intraspinal studies. *Neuroradiology* 32:371–391.

423. Quencer RM, Sheldon JJ, Post MJD, Diaz RD, Montalvo BM, Green BA, Eismont FJ (1986): MRI of the chronically injured cervical spinal cord. *AJR* 147:125–132.

424. Quint DJ, Boulos RS, Sanders WP, Mehta BA, Patel SC, Tiel RL (1988): Epidural lipomatosis. *Radiology* 169:485–490.

425. Quirk ME, Letendre AJ, Ciottone RA, Lingley JF (1989): Evaluation of three psychologic interventions to reduce anxiety during MR imaging. *Radiology* 173:759–762.

426. Rafto SE, Dalinka MK, Schiebler ML, Burk DL, Kricun ME (1988): Spondyloarthropathy of the cervical spine in long-term hemodialysis. *Radiology* 166:201–204.

427. Raghavan N, Barkovich AJ, Edwards M, Norman D (1989): MR imaging in the tethered spinal cord syndrome. *AJR* 152:843–852.

428. Rahmouni A, Divine M, Mathieu D, Golli M, Dao TH, Jazaerli N, Anglade MC, Reyes F, Vasile N (1993): Detection of multiple myeloma involving the spine: Efficacy of fat-suppression and contrast-enhanced MR imaging. *AJR*, 160:1049–1052.

429. Rahmouni A, Divine M, Mathieu D, Golli M, Haioun C, Dao T,

430. Anglade MC, Reyes F, Vasile N (1993): MR appearance of multiple myeloma of the spine before and after treatment. *AJR* 160:1053–1057.

430. Ramanauskas WL, Wilner HI, Metes JJ, Lazo A, Kelly JK (1989): MR imaging of compressive myelomalacia. *J Comput Assist Tomogr* 13:399–404.

431. Ramsey RG, Zacharias CE (1985): MR imaging of the spine after radiation therapy: Easily recognizable effects. *AJR* 144:1131–1135.

432. Rauschning W (1987): Normal and pathologic anatomy of the lumbar root canals. *Spine* 12:1008–1019.

433. Reicher MA, Gold RH, Halbach VV, Rauschning W, Wilson GH, Lufkin RB (1986): MR imaging of the lumbar spine: Anatomic correlations and the effects of technical variations (ARRS Executive Council Award Paper). *AJR* 147:891–898.

434. Reicher MA, Lufkin RB, Smith S, Flannigan B, Olsen R, Wolf R, Hertz D, Winter J, Hanafee W (1986): Multiple-angle, variable-interval, nonorthogonal MRI. *AJR* 147:363–366.

435. Rengachary SS, Murphy D (1974): Subarachnoid hematoma following lumbar puncture causing compression of the cauda equina. *J Neurosurg* 41:252–254.

436. Resnick D (1985): Degenerative diseases of the vertebral column. *Radiology* 156:3–14.

437. Resnick D, Guerra J Jr, Robinson CA, Vint VC (1978): Association of diffuse idiopathic skeletal hyperostosis (DISH) and calcification and ossification of the posterior longitudinal ligament. *AJR* 131:1049–1053.

438. Rizzolo SJ, Piazza MR, Cotler JM, Balderston RA, Schaefer D, Flanders A (1991): Intervertebral disc injury complicating cervical spine trauma. *Spine* 16:S187–S189.

439. Roberson GH, Llewellyn HJ, Taveras JM (1973): The narrow lumbar spinal canal syndrome. *Radiology* 107:89–97.

440. Roberts MC, Kressel HY, Fallon MD, Zlatkin MB, Dalinka MK (1989): Paget disease: MR imaging findings. *Radiology* 173:341–345.

441. Roberts S, Menage J, Urban JPG (1989): Biochemical and structural properties of the cartilage end-plate and its relation to the intervertebral disc. *Spine* 14:166–174.

442. Roberts WA (1988): Pyogenic vertebral osteomyelitis of a lumbar facet joint with associated epidural abscess: A case report with review of the literature. *Spine* 13:948–952.

443. Robinson RA, Afeiche N, Dunn EJ, Northrup BE (1977): Cervical spondylotic myelopathy: Etiology and treatment concepts. *Spine* 2:89–99.

444. Roemer PB, Edelstein WA, Hayes CE, Souza SP, Mueller OM (1990): The NMR phased array. *Magn Reson Med* 16:192–223.

445. Rogers LA (1983): Acute subdural hematoma and death following lateral cervical spinal puncture: Case report. *J Neurosurg* 58:284–286.

446. Rosen BR, Fleming DM, Kushner DC, Zaner KS, Buxton RB, Bennet WP, Wismer GL, Brady TJ (1988): Hematologic bone marrow disorders: Quantitative chemical shift MR imaging. *Radiology* 169:799–804.

447. Ross BD, Kreis R, Ernst T (1992): Clinical tools for the 90s: Magnetic resonance spectroscopy and metabolite imaging. *Eur J Radiol* 14:128–140.

448. Ross JS, Delamarter R, Hueftle MG, Masaryk TJ, Aikawa M, Carter J, VanDyke C, Modic MT (1989): Gd-DTPA-enhanced MRI of the postoperative lumbar spine: Time course and mechanism of enhancement. *AJR* 152:825–834.

449. Ross JS, Modic MT, Masaryk TJ, et al (1989): Assessment of extradural degenerative disease with Gd-DTPA-enhanced MR imaging: Correlation with surgical and pathological findings. *AJNR* 10:1243–1249.

450. Ross JS, Modic MT, Masaryk TJ, Carter J, Marcus RE, Bohlman H (1990): Assessment of extradural degenerative disease with Gd-DTPA-enhanced MR imaging: Correlation with surgical and pathological findings. *AJR* 154:151–157.

451. Ross JS, Tkach J, Van Dyke C, Modic MT (1991) Clinical MR imaging of degenerative spinal diseases: pulse sequences, gradient-echo techniques, and contrast agents. *J Magn Reson Imaging* 1:29–37.

452. Ross JS, Masaryk TJ, Modic MT, Delamater R, Bohlman H, Wil-

bur G, Kaufman B (1987): MR imaging of lumbar arachnoiditis. *AJR* 149:1025–1032.

453. Ross JS, Masaryk TJ, Modic MT (1987): Postoperative cervical spine: MR assessment. *J Comput Assist Tomogr* 11:955–962.

454. Ross JS, Masaryk TJ, Modic MT, Bohlman H, Delamater R, Wilber G (1987): Lumbar spine: Postoperative assessment with surface-coil MR imaging. *Radiology* 164:851–860.

455. Ross JS, Masaryk TJ, Modic MT, Carter JR, Mapstone T, Dengel FH (1987): Vertebral hemangiomas: MR imaging. *Radiology* 164:165–169.

456. Ross JS, Modic MT, Masaryk TJ (1990): Tears of the anulus fibrosus: Assessment with Gd-DTPA-enhanced MR imaging. *AJR* 154:159–162.

457. Ross JS, Perez-Reyes N, Masaryk TJ, Bohlman H, Modic MT (1987): Thoracic disk herniation: MR imaging. *Radiology* 165:511–515.

458. Ross JS, Ruggieri PM, Glicklich M, Obuchowski N, Dillinger J, Masaryk TJ, Qu Y, Modic MT (1993): 3D MRI of the cervical spine: Low flip angle FISP vs. Gd-DTPA TurboFLASH in degenerative disk disease. *J Comput Assist Tomogr* 17:26–33.

459. Ross JS, Ruggieri PM, Tkach JA, Masaryk TJ, Paranandi L, Dillinger JJ, Modic MT (1992): Gd-DTPA-enhanced 3D MR imaging of cervical degenerative disk disease: Initial experience. *AJNR* 13:127–136.

460. Ross JS, Ruggieri P, Tkach J, Obuchowski N, Dillinger J, Masaryk TJ, Modic MT (1993): Lumbar degenerative disk disease: Prospective comparison of conventional T2-weighted spin-echo imaging and T2-weighted rapid acquisition relaxation-enhanced imaging. *AJNR* 14:1215–1223.

461. Roth JL, Nugent M, Gray JE, Julsrud PR, Berquist TH, Sill JC, Kispert DB (1985): Patient monitoring during magnetic resonance imaging. *Anesthesiology* 62:80–83.

462. Rothfus WE, Chedid MK, Deeb ZL, Abla AA, Maroon JC, Sherman RL (1987): MR imaging in the diagnosis of spontaneous spinal epidural hematomas. *J Comput Assist Tomogr* 11:851–854.

463. Rothman SL, Glenn WV Jr (1984): CT multiplanar reconstruction in 253 cases of lumbar spondylolysis. *AJNR* 5:81–90.

464. Rothman SL, Glenn WV Jr, Kerber CW (1985): Postoperative fractures of lumbar articular facets: Occult cause of radiculopathy. *AJR* 145:779–784.

465. Rubin JB, Enzmann DR (1987): Optimizing conventional MR imaging of the spine. *Radiology* 163:777–783.

466. Rubin JB, Enzmann DR, Wright A (1987): CSF-gated MR imaging of the spine: Theory and clinical implementation. *Radiology* 163:784–792.

467. Rubin JB, Wright A, Enzmann DR (1988): Lumbar spine: Motion compensation for cerebrospinal fluid on MR imaging. *Radiology* 167:225–231.

468. Rupp R, Ebraheim NA, Savolaine ER, Jackson WT (1993): Magnetic resonance imaging evaluation of the spine with metal implants: General safety and superior imaging with titanium. *Spine* 18:379–385.

469. Rusinek H, Mourino MR, Firoozina H, Weinreb JC, Chase NE (1989): Volumetric rendering of MR images. *Radiology* 171:269–272.

470. Russell EJ, D'Angelo CM, Zimmerman RD, Czervionke LF, Huckman MS (1984): Cervical disk herniation: CT demonstration after contrast enhancement. *Radiology* 152:703–712.

471. Rydevik B, Brown MD, Lundborg G (1984): Pathoanatomy and pathophysiology of nerve root compression. *Spine* 9:7–15.

472. Rydevik BL, Hansson TH, Garfin SR (1989): Pathophysiology of cauda equina compression. *Sem Spine Surg* 1:139–141.

473. Saal JA, Saal JS, Herzog RJ (1990): The natural history of lumbar intervertebral disc extrusions treated nonoperatively. *Spine* 15:683–686.

474. Salomon C, Chopin D, Benoist M (1988): Spinal cord compression: An exceptional complication of spinal osteoporosis. *Spine* 13:222–224.

475. Sandhu FS, Dillon WP (1991): Spinal epidural abscess: evaluation with contrast- enhanced MR imaging. *AJNR* 12:1087–1093.

476. Sato K, Wakamatsu E, Yoshizumi A, Watanabe N, Irei O (1989): The configuration of the laminas and facet joints in degenerative spondylolisthesis: A clinicoradiologic study. *Spine* 14:1265–1271.

477. Scapinelli R, Little K (1970): Observations on the mechanically induced differentiation of cartilage from fibrous connective tissue. *J Pathol* 101:85–91.

478. Schaefer DM, Flanders A, Northrup BE, Doan HT, Osterholm JL (1989): Magnetic resonance imaging of acute cervical spine trauma: Correlation with severity of neurologic injury. *Spine* 14:1090–1095.

479. Schaefer DM, Flanders AE, Osterhold JL, Northrup BE (1992): Prognostic significance of magnetic resonance imaging in the acute phase of cervical spine injury. *J Neurosurg* 76:218–223.

480. Schnebel B, Kingston S, Watkins R, Dillin W (1989): Comparison of MRI to contrast CT in the diagnosis of spinal stenosis. *Spine* 14:332–337.

481. Schneck CD (1985): The anatomy of lumbar spondylosis. *Clin Orthop* 193:20–37.

482. Schneiderman G, Flannigan B, Kingston S, Thomas J, Dillin WH, Watkins RG (1987): Magnetic resonance imaging in the diagnosis of disc degeneration: Correlation with discography. *Spine* 12:276–281.

483. Schonstrom N, Bolender NF, Spengler DM, Hansson TH (1984): Pressure changes within the cauda equina following constriction of the dural sac: An in vitro experimental study. *Spine* 9:604–607.

484. Schonstrom N, Lindahl S, Willen J, Hansson T (1989): Dynamic changes in the dimensions of the lumbar spinal canal: An experimental study in vitro. *J Orthop Res* 7:115–121.

485. Schreiber F, Rosenthal H (1952): Paraplegia from ruptured lumbar discs in achondroplastic dwarfs. *J Neurosurg* 9:648–651.

486. Schroth G, Thron A, Guhl L, Voigt K, Niendorf HP, Garces R-NL (1987): Magnetic resonance imaging of spinal meningiomas and neurinomas: Improvement of imaging by paramagnetic contrast enhancement. *J Neurosurg* 66:695–700.

487. Schwartz DA, Nair S, Hershey B, Winkelman AC, Finkelstein SD (1989): Vertebral arch hemangioma producing spinal cord compression in pregnancy. *Spine* 14:888–890.

488. Scoles PV, Linton AE, Latimer B, Levy ME, Digiovanni BF (1988): Vertebral body and posterior element morphology: The normal spine in middle life. *Spine* 13:1082–1086.

489. Scotti G, Scialfa G, Colombo N, Landoni L (1985): MR imaging of intradural extramedullary tumors of the cervical spine. *J Comput Assist Tomogr* 9:1037–1041.

490. Scotti G, Scialfa G, Pieralli S, Boccardi E, Valsecchi F, Tonon C (1983): Myelopathy and radiculopathy due to cervical spondylosis: Myelographic-CT correlations. *AJNR* 4:601–603.

491. Scoville WB (1966): Types of cervical disk lesions and their surgical approaches. *JAMA* 196:479–481.

492. Sebag GH, Moore SG (1990): Effect of trabecular bone on the appearance of marrow in gradient echo imaging of the appendicular skeleton. *Radiology* 174:855–859.

493. Sharif HS, Aideyan OA, Clark DC, Madkour MM, Aabed MY, Mattsson TA, Al-Deeb SM, Moutaery KR (1989): Brucellar and tuberculous spondylitis: Comparative imaging features. *Radiology* 171:419–425.

494. Sharif HS, Clark DC, Aabed MY, Haddad MC, Al Deeb SM, Yaqub B, Al Moutaery KR (1990): Granulomatous spinal infections: MR imaging. *Radiology* 177:101–107.

495. Shellock FG, Morisoli S, Kanal E (1993): MR procedures and biomedical implants, materials, and devices: 1993 update. *Radiology* 189:587–599.

496. Sherman JL, Barkovich AJ, Citrin CM (1987): The MR appearance of syringomyelia: New observations. *AJR* 148:381–391.

497. Sherman JL, Nassaux PY, Citrin CM (1990): Measurements of the normal cervical spinal cord on MR imaging. *AJNR* 11:369–372.

498. Sherry CS, Harms SE, McCroskey WK (1987): Spinal MR imaging: Multiplanar representation from a single high resolution 3D acquisition. *J Comput Assist Tomogr* 11:859–862.

499. Shirazi-Adl SA, Shrivastava SC, Admed AM (1984): Stress analysis of the lumbar disc-body unit in compression: A three-dimensional nonlinear finite element study. *Spine* 9:120–134.

500. Silbergleit R, Gebarski SS, Brunberg JA, McGillicudy J, Blaivas M (1990): Lumbar synovial cysts: Correlation of myelographic, CT, MR, and pathologic findings. *AJNR* 11:777–779.

501. Simmons Z, Biller J, Beck DW, Keyes W (1986): Painless compressive cervical myelopathy with false localizing sensory findings. *Spine* 11:869–872.

502. Simon JH, Szumowski J (1989): Chemical shift imaging with paramagnetic contrast material enhancement for improved lesion depiction. *Radiology* 171:539–543.

503. Sklar E, Quencer RM, Green BA, Montalvo BM, Post MJD (1989): Acquired spinal subarachnoid cysts: Evaluation with MR, CT myelography, and intraoperative sonography. *AJR* 153: 1057–1064.

504. Slasky BS, Bydder GM, Niendorf HP, Young IR (1987): MR imaging with gadolinium-DTPA in the differentiation of tumor, syrinx, and cyst of the spinal cord. *J Comput Assist Tomogr* 11:845–850.

505. Slone RM, Buck LL, Fitzsimmons JR (1986): Varying gradient angles and offsets to optimize imaging planes in MR. *Radiology* 158:531–536.

506. Smith AS, Blaser SI (1991): Infectious and inflammatory processes of the spine. *Radiol Clin North Am* 29:809–827.

507. Smith AS, Weinstein MA, Mizushima A, Coughlin B, Hayden SP, Lakin MM, Lanzieri CF (1989): MR imaging characteristics of tuberculous spondylitis vs vertebral osteomyelitis. *AJR* 153: 399–405.

508. Smith RV (1981): Intradural disc rupture. *J Neurosurg* 55:117–120.

509. Smith SR, Williams CE, Davies JM, Edwards RH (1989): Bone marrow disorders: Characterization with quantitative MR imaging. *Radiology* 172:805–810.

510. Smoker WRK, Godersky JC, Knutzon RK, Keyes WD, Norman D, Bergman W (1987): The role of MR imaging in evaluating metastatic spinal disease. *AJR* 149:1241–1248.

511. Sobel DF, Barkovich AJ, Munderloh SH (1984): Metrizamide myelography and postmyelographic computed tomography: Comparative adequacy in the cervical spine. *AJNR* 5:385–390.

512. Sobel DF, Zyroff J, Thorne RP (1987): Diskogenic vertebral sclerosis: MR imaging. *J Comput Assist Tomogr* 11:855–858.

513. Soitropoulos S, Chafetz NI, Lang P, et al (1989): Differentiation between postoperative scar and recurrent disk herniation: Prospective comparison of MR, CT, and contrast-enhanced CT. *AJNR* 10:639–643.

514. Solomon RA, Stein BM (1988): Unusual spinal cord enlargement related to intramedullary hemangioblastoma. *J Neurosurg* 68: 550–553.

515. Soloniuk DS, Pecoraro SR, Munschauer FE (1989): Myelopathy secondary to spinal epidural lipomatosis. *Spine* 14:119–122.

516. Sortland O, Magnaes B, Hauge T (1977): Functional myelography with metrizamide in the diagnosis of lumbar spinal stenosis. *Acta Radiol (Suppl)* 55:42–54.

517. Spencer DL, Irwin GS, Miller JJ (1983): Anatomy and significance of fixation of the lumbosacral nerve roots in sciatica. *Spine* 8:672–679.

518. Stambough JL, Cheeks ML, Keiper GL (1989): Nonglucocorticoid-induced lumbar epidural lipomatosis: A case report and review of literature. *J Spinal Disorders* 2:201–207.

519. Stanley JH, Schabel SI, Frey GD, Hungerford GD (1986): Quantitative analysis of the cervical spinal canal by computed tomography. *Neuroradiology* 28:139–143.

520. Stimac GK, Porter BA, Olson DO, Gerlach R, Genton M (1988): Gadolinium-DTPA-enhanced MR imaging of spinal neoplasms: Preliminary investigation and comparison with unenhanced spin-echo and STIR sequences. *AJR* 151:1185–1192.

521. Stoddard A, Osborn JF (1979): Scheuermann's disease or spinal osteochondrosis: Its frequency and relationship with spondylosis. *J Bone Joint Surg [Br]* 61:56–58.

522. Styf J, Lysell E (1987): Chronic compartment syndrome in the erector spinae muscle. *Spine* 12:680–682.

523. Sugimura K, Yamasaki K, Kitagaki H, Tanaka Y, Kono M (1987): Bone marrow diseases of the spine: Differentiation with T1 and T2 relaxation times in MR imaging. *Radiology* 165:541–544.

524. Suojanen J, Wang AM, Winston KR (1988): Pantopaque mimicking spinal lipoma: MR pitfall. *J Comput Assist Tomogr* 12: 346–348.

525. Suojanen JN, Lipson SJ (1989): Spinal cord compression secondary to ossified ligamentum flavum. *J Spinal Dis* 2:238–240.

526. Sward L, Hellstrom M, Jacobsson B, Nyman R, Peterson L (1991): Disc degeneration and associated abnormalities of the spine in elite gymnasts: A magnetic resonance imaging study. *Spine* 16:437–443.

527. Sze G, Abramson A, Krol G, Liu D, Amster J, Zimmerman RD, Deck MDF (1988): Gadolinium-DTPA in the evaluation of intradural extramedullary spinal disease. *AJR* 150:911–921.

528. Sze G, Brant-Zawadzki MN, Wilson CR, Norman D, Newton TH (1986): Pseudotumor of the craniovertebral junction associated with chronic subluxation: MR imaging studies. *Radiology* 161:391–394.

529. Sze G, Bravo S, Krol G (1989): Spinal lesions: Quantitative and qualitative temporal evolution of gadopentetate dimeglumine enhancement in MR imaging. *Radiology* 170:849–856.

530. Sze G, Krol G, Zimmerman RD, Deck MDF (1988): Intramedullary disease of the spine: Diagnosis using gadolinium-DTPA-enhanced MR imaging. *AJR* 151:1193–1204.

531. Sze G, Krol G, Zimmerman RD, Deck MDF (1988): Malignant extradural spinal tumors: MR imaging with gadolinium-DTPA. *Radiology* 167:217–223.

532. Sze G, Merriam M, Oshio K, Jolesz FA (1992): Fast spin-echo imaging in the evaluation of intradural disease of the spine. *AJNR* 13:1383–1392.

533. Szypryt EP, Gibson MJ, Mulholland RC, Worthington BS (1987): The long-term effect of chemonucleolysis on the intervertebral disc as assessed by magnetic resonance imaging. *Spine* 12: 707–711.

534. Szypryt EP, Twining P, Mulholland RC, Worthington BS (1989): The prevalence of disc degeneration associated with neural arch defects of the lumbar spine assessed by magnetic resonance imaging. *Spine* 14:977–981.

535. Szypryt EP, Twining P, Wilde GP, Mulholland RC, Worthington BS (1988): Diagnosis of lumbar disc protrusion: A comparison between magnetic resonance imaging and radiculography. *J Bone Joint Surg [Br]* 70:717–722.

536. Tajima N, Kawano K (1986): Cryomicrotomy of the lumbar spine. *Spine* 11:376–379.

537. Takahashi M, Yamashita Y, Sakamoto Y, Kojima R (1989): Chronic cervical cord compression: Clinical significance of increased signal intensity on MR images. *Radiology* 173:219–224.

538. Takata K, Inoue SI, Takahashi K, Ohtsuka Y (1988): Fracture of the posterior margin of a lumbar vertebral body. *J Bone Joint Surg [Am]* 70:589–594.

539. Tamura T (1989): Cranial symptoms after cervical injury: Aetiology and treatment of the Barré-Lieou syndrome. *J Bone Joint Surg [Br]* 71:283–287.

540. Taylor JR, Twomey LT (1986): Age changes in lumbar zygapophyseal joints: Observations on structure and function. *Spine* 11: 739–745.

541. Teitelbaum GP, Bradley WG Jr, Klein BD (1988): MR imaging artifacts, ferromagnetism, and magnetic torque of intravascular filters, stents, and coils. *Radiology* 166:657–664.

542. Teresi LM, Lufkin RB, Reicher MA, Moffit BJ, Vinuela FV, Wilson GM, Bentson JR, Hanafee WN (1987): Asymptomatic degenerative disk disease and spondylosis of the cervical spine: MR imaging. *Radiology* 164:83–88.

543. Teresi LM, Lufkin RL, Hanafee WN (1988): MRI of the cervical spine. *Appl Radiology* 17:31–44, 49.

544. Tervonen O, Koivukangas J (1989): Transabdominal ultrasound measurement of the lumbar spinal canal: Its value for evaluation of lumbar spinal stenosis. *Spine* 14:232–235.

545. Terwey B, Becker H, Thron AK, Vahldiek G (1989): Gadolinium-DTPA enhanced MR imaging of spinal dural arteriovenous fistulas. *J Comput Assist Tomogr* 13:30–37.

546. Thomas JE, Miller RH (1973): Lipomatous tumors of the spinal canal: A study of their clinical range. *Mayo Clin Proc* 48:393–400.

547. Thrush A, Enzmann D (1990): MR imaging of infectious spondylitis. *AJNR* 11:1171–1180.

548. Tien RD, Olson EM, Zee CS (1992): Diseases of the lumbar spine: Findings on fat-suppression MR imaging. *AJR* 159:95–99.

549. Torg JS, Pavlov H, Genuario SE, Sennett B, Wisneski RJ, Robie

BH, Jahre C (1986): Neurapraxia of the cervical spinal cord with transient quadriplegia. *J Bone Joint Surg [Am]* 68:1354–1370.

550. Toyone T, Takahashi K, Kitahara H, Yamagata M, Murakami M, Moriya H (1993): Visualisation of symptomatic nerve roots: Prospective study of contrast-enhanced MRI in patients with lumbar disc herniation. *J Bone Joint Surg [Br]* 75:529–533.

551. Tracy PT, Wright RM, Hanigan WC (1989): Magnetic resonance imaging of spinal injury. *Spine* 14:292–301.

552. Tsuruda JS, Norman D, Dillon W, Newton TH, Mills DG (1989): Three-dimensional gradient-recalled MR imaging as a screening tool for the diagnosis of cervical radiculopathy. *AJNR* 10:1263–1271.

553. Tsuruda JS, Remley K (1991): Effects of magnetic susceptibility artifacts and motion in evaluating the cervical neural foramina on 3DFT gradient-echo MR imaging. *AJNR* 12:237–241.

554. Uchida N, Sugimura K, Kajitani A, Yoshizako T, Ishida T (1993): MR imaging of vertebral metastases: Evaluation of fat saturation imaging. *Eur J Radiol* 17:91–94.

555. Uden A, Johnsson KE, Jonsson K, Pettersson H (1985): Myelography in the elderly and the diagnosis of spinal stenosis. *Spine* 10:171–174.

556. Ullrich CG (1989): Magnetic resonance imaging of the cervical spine and spinal cord. In: TCSRSE Committee, ed. *The cervical spine*. Philadelphia: Lippincott, p. 881.

557. Ullrich CG, Binet EF, Sanecki MG, Kieffer SA (1980): Quantitative assessment of the lumbar spinal canal by computed tomography. *Radiology* 134:137–143.

558. Urban JPG, McMullin JF (1988): Swelling pressure of the lumbar intervertebral discs: Influence of age, spinal level, composition and degeneration. *Spine* 13:179–187.

559. Valk J (1988): Gadolinium-DTPA in MR of spinal lesions. *AJR* 150:1163–1168.

560. Valk PE, Hale JD, Crooks LE, Kaufman L, Roos MS, Ortendahl DA, Higgins CB (1986): MRI of blood flow: Correlation of image appearance with spin-echo phase shift and signal intensity. *AJR* 146:931–939.

561. Van Schaik JP, Verbiest H, Van Schaik FD (1985): The orientation of laminae and facet joints in the lower lumbar spine. *Spine* 10:59–63.

562. VanDyke C, Ross JS, Tkach J, Masaryk TJ, Modic MT (1989): Gradient-echo MR imaging of the cervical spine: Evaluation of extradural disease. *AJR* 153:393–398.

563. Veidlinger OF, Colwill JC, Smyth HS, Turner D (1981): Cervical myelopathy and its relationship to cervical stenosis. *Spine* 6:550–552.

564. Verbiest H (1954): A radicular syndrome from the developmental narrowing of the lumbar vertebral canal. *J Bone Joint Surg [Br]* 36:230–237.

565. Verbiest H (1955): Further experiences on the pathological influence of a developmental narrowness of the bony lumbar vertebral canal. *J Bone Joint Surg [Br]* 37:576–583.

566. Verbiest H (1976): Fallacies of the present definition, nomenclature, and classification of the stenosis of the lumbar vertebral canal. *Spine* 1:217–225.

567. Verbiest H (1977): Results of surgical treatment of idiopathic developmental stenosis of the lumbar vertebral canal. *J Bone Joint Surg [Br]* 59:181–188.

568. Verbiest H (1979): The significance and principles of computerized axial tomography in idiopathic developmental stenosis of the bony lumbar vertebral canal. *Spine* 4:369–378.

569. Verbiest H (1983): Words, images, knowledge, and reality: Some reflections from the neurosurgical perspective. *Acta Neurochir* 69:163–193.

570. Viikari-Juntura E, Raininko R, Videman T, Porkka L (1989): Evaluation of cervical disc degeneration with ultralow field MRI and discography: An experimental study on cadavers. *Spine* 14:616–619.

571. Vinitski S, Griffey R, Fuka M, Matwiyoff N, Prost R (1987): Effect of the sampling rate on magnetic resonance imaging. *Magn Reson Med* 5:278–285.

572. Vogler JB III, Murphy WA (1988): Bone marrow imaging. *Radiology* 168:679–693.

573. Wallace CJ, Fong TC, MacRae ME (1992): Calcified herniations of the thoracic disk: Role of magnetic resonance imaging and computed tomography in surgical planning. *Can Assoc Radiol J* 43:52–54.

574. Waltz TA (1967): Physical factors in the production of the myelopathy of cervical spondylosis. *Brain* 90:395–404.

575. Watanabe AT, Teitelbaum GP, Lufkin RB, Tsuruda JS, Jinkins JR, Bradley WG Jr. (1990): Gradient-echo MR imaging of the lumbar spine: Comparison with spin-echo technique. *J Comput Assist Tomogr* 14:410–414.

576. Weinreb JC, Wolbarsht LB, Cohen JM, Brown CE, Maravilla KR (1989): Prevalence of lumbosacral intervertebral disk abnormalities on MR images in pregnant and asymptomatic nonpregnant women. *Radiology* 170:125–128.

577. Weinshel S, Maiman D (1989): Spinal subdural hematoma presenting as an epidural hematoma following gunshot wound: Report of a case. *J Spinal Disorders* 1:317–319.

578. Weinstein JN (1989): Spondylolisthesis. *Sem Spine Surg* 1:78–103.

579. Weinstein JN (1989): Surgical approach to spine tumors. *Orthopedics* 12:897–905.

580. Weisz GM (1983): Lumbar spinal canal stenosis in Paget's disease. *Spine* 8:192–198.

581. Whitecloud TS III, Seago RA (1987): Cervical discogenic syndrome: Results of operative intervention in patients with positive discography. *Spine* 12:313–316.

582. Wiesel SW, Tsourmas N, Feffer HL, Citrin CM, Patronas N (1984): A study of computer-assisted tomography: I. The incidence of positive CAT scans in an asymptomatic group of patients. *Spine* 9:549–551.

583. Wilberger JE Jr, Maroon JC, Prostko ER, Baghai P, Beckman I, Deeb Z (1987): Magnetic resonance imaging and intraoperative neurosonography in syringomyelia. *Neurosurgery* 20:599–605.

584. Wilkinson M (1960): The morbid anatomy of cervical spondylosis and myelopathy. *Brain* 83:589–617.

585. Williams AL, Haughton VM, Pojunas KW, Daniels DL, Kilgore DP (1987): Differentiation of intramedullary neoplasms and cysts by MR. *AJR* 149:159–164.

586. Williams MP, Cherryman GR, Husband JE (1989): Significance of thoracic disc herniation demonstrated by MR imaging. *J Comput Assist Tomogr* 13:211–214.

587. Wilson DA, Prince JR (1989): MR imaging determination of the location of the normal conus medullaris throughout childhood. *AJR* 152:1029–1032.

588. Wiltse L (1985): Far-out syndrome. In: Rothman SLG, Glenn Jr WV, eds. *Multiplanar CT of the spine*. Baltimore: University Park Press, pp. 384–393.

589. Wiltse LL, Guyer RD, Spencer CW, Glenn WV, Porter IS (1984): Alar transverse process impingement of the L5 spinal nerve: The far-out syndrome. *Spine* 9:31–41.

590. Wiltse LL, Widell EH Jr, Jackson DW (1975): Fatigue fracture: The basic lesion in isthmic spondylolisthesis. *J Bone Joint Surg [Am]* 57:17–22.

591. Winkler ML, Ortendahl DA, Mills TC, Crooks LE, Sheldon PE, Kaufman L, Kramer DM (1988): Characteristics of partial flip angle and gradient reversal MR imaging. *Radiology* 166:17–26.

592. Winston K, Rumbaugh C, Colucci V (1984): The vertebral canals in lumbar disc disease. *Spine* 9:414–417.

593. Wismer GL, Rosen BR, Buxton R, Stark DD, Brady TJ (1985): Chemical shift imaging of bone marrow: Preliminary experience. *AJR* 145:1031–1036.

594. Wolf BS, Khilnani M, Malis LI (1956): The sagittal diameter of the bony cervical spinal canal and its significance in cervical spondylosis. *J Mt Sinai Hosp NY* 23:283–292.

595. Wolfe BK, O'Keeffe D, Mitchell DM, Tchang SPK (1987): Rheumatoid arthritis of the cervical spine: Early and progressive radiographic features. *Radiology* 165:145–148.

596. Wynne AT, Southgate GW (1986): Discitis causing spondylolisthesis. *Spine* 11:970–972.

597. Xu GL, Haughton VM, Carrera GF (1990): Lumbar facet joint capsule: Appearance at MR imaging and CT. *Radiology* 177:415–420.

598. Yablon IG, Ordia J, Mortara R, Reed J, Spatz E (1989): Acute ascending myelopathy of the spine. *Spine* 14:1084–1089.

599. Yablon JS, Kasdon DL, Levine H (1988): Thoracic cord compression in Scheuermann's disease. *Spine* 13:896–898.

600. Yamamoto I, Matsumae M, Ikeda A, Shibuya N, Sato O, Nakamura K (1988): Thoracic spinal stenosis: Experience with seven cases. *J Neurosurg* 68:37–40.

601. Yamane T, Yoshida T, Mimatsu K (1993): Early diagnosis of lumbar spondylolysis by MRI. *J Bone Joint Surg [Br]* 75:764–768.

602. Yamashita Y, Takahashi M, Matsuno Y, Sakamoto Y, Yoshizumi K, Oguni T, Kojima R (1990): Spinal cord compression due to ossification of ligaments: MR imaging. *Radiology* 175:843–848.

603. Yang WC, Zappulla R, Malis L (1981): Case report: Neurolemmoma in lumbar intervertebral foramen. *J Comput Assist Tomogr* 5:904–908.

604. Yasuma T, Makino E, Saito S, Inui M (1986): Histological development of intervertebral disc herniation. *J Bone Joint Surg [Am]* 68:1066–1072.

605. Yasuma T, Ohno R, Yamauchi Y (1988): False-negative lumbar discograms. *J Bone Joint Surg [Am]* 70:1279–1290.

606. Yong-Hing K, Reilly J, Kirkaldy-Willis WH (1976): The ligamentum flavum. *Spine* 1:226–234.

607. Yousem DM, Atlas SW, Goldberg HI, Grossman RI (1991): Degenerative narrowing of the cervical spine neural foramina: Evaluation with high-resolution 3DFT gradient-echo MR imaging. *AJNR* 12:229–236.

608. Yu S, Haughton VM, Ho PSP, Sether LA, Wagner M, Ho KC (1988): Progressive and regressive changes in the nucleus pulposus: Part II. The adult. *Radiology* 169:93–97.

609. Yu S, Haughton VM, Sether LA, Ho KC, Wagner M (1989): Criteria for classifying normal and degenerated lumbar intervertebral disks. *Radiology* 170:523–526.

610. Yu S, Haughton VM, Sether LA, Wagner M (1988): Anulus fibrosus in bulging intervertebral disks. *Radiology* 169:761–763.

611. Yu S, Sether L, Haughton VM (1987): Facet joint menisci of the cervical spine: Correlative MR imaging and cryomicrotomy study. *Radiology* 164:79–82.

612. Yu SW, Sether LA, Ho PS, Wagner M, Haughton VM (1988): Tears of the anulus fibrosus: Correlation between MR and pathologic findings in cadavers. *AJNR* 9:367–370.

613. Yu YL, Stevens JM, Kendall B, de Boulay GH (1983): Cord shape and measurements in cervical spondylotic myelopathy and radiculopathy. *AJNR* 4:839–842.

614. Yuh WT, Zachar CK, Barloon TJ, Sato Y, Sickels WJ, Hawes DR (1989): Vertebral compression fractures: Distinction between benign and malignant causes with MR imaging. *Radiology* 172:215–218.

615. Zucherman J, Derby R, Hsu K, Picetti G, Kaiser J, Schofferman J, Goldthwaite N, White A (1988): Normal magnetic resonance imaging with abnormal discography. *Spine* 13:1355–1359.

The Adult Spine: Principles and Practice,
2nd edition, J.W. Frymoyer, Editor-in-Chief.
Lippincott-Raven Publishers, Philadelphia © 1997.

CHAPTER 30

Angiography of the Spine

Tony P. Smith and Andrew H. Cragg

Angiography can be used to study the vertebral column or spinal cord. This chapter deals with the former; however, one must have a thorough understanding of the vascular supply to the spinal cord prior to angiography if quality diagnostic studies of the vertebral column are to be achieved and complications avoided.

Historically, the study of blood supply to the spine (vertebral column and spinal cord) was based on cadaveric dissections performed in the late 1800s by such investigators as Adamkiewicz (1) and Kadyi (48). It was not until the advent of aortography and particularly selective angiography that the blood supply to the vertebral column and spinal cord was further elucidated.

Arteriovenous malformations (AVM) of the spinal cord were first reported in the 1950s from abdominal aortography and vertebral angiography (44,74). Djindjian et al. (21) reported what was probably the first systematic angiographic study for spinal cord AVM involving subtracted images, and DiChiro et al. (18) reported the first selective spinal angiogram in the 1960s. Since that time, most improvement has involved the development of better instruments (catheters, wires, etc.) and better imaging techniques (20). In addition, the use of

therapeutic embolization has become widespread since its introduction by Doppman et al. (28) and Newton and Adams in 1968 (69). Therapeutic embolization of vertebral column tumors has also found popularity since earlier cases were reported by Hilal and Michelsen in the mid-1970s (46).

Today, angiography of the spinal column is rarely performed solely for diagnostic purposes. The current indications are usually limited to:

definition of anatomy
determination of the degree of vascularity
determination of the suitability for embolization

Virtually all of these indications center around tumor mass(es), if hemangioma and arteriovenous malformations can be included in this broad category. Using less invasive imaging such as computed tomography (CT) and magnetic resonance imaging (MRI), a specific diagnosis is already highly suspected and the role of angiography is to plan therapy. When surgical resection is planned, the degree of vascularity must be known. Thus angiography may be indicated when a mass demonstrates marked enhancement on contrast CT or high blood flow areas on MRI, both suspicious for extensive vascularity. Before surgery, angiography may also be helpful to determine the radicular supply to the anterior spinal artery (ASA) and whether it arises from a vessel supplying the vascular mass as well as the location

   T. P. Smith, M.D.: Professor of Radiology, Duke University Medical Center, Durham, North Carolina 27710.
   A. H. Cragg, M.D.: Attending Radiologist, Fairview Riverside Medical Center, Minneapolis, Minnesota 55454.

of the ASA relative to the proposed surgical site. Finally, vascular masses may undergo selective embolization, usually preoperatively, which requires diagnostic angiography.

ANATOMY

Arterial Supply

Before performing spinal angiography, whether for the spinal cord or vertebral column, the angiographer must possess a thorough understanding of the anatomic blood supply. In the embryo, there are 62 segmental arteries, representing 31 paired structures, that penetrate the spine via the intervertebral foramina (24). At birth, the segmental arteries supply the vertebral column at each level and give a variable supply to the spinal cord, as there is a regression of the majority of the arteries to the

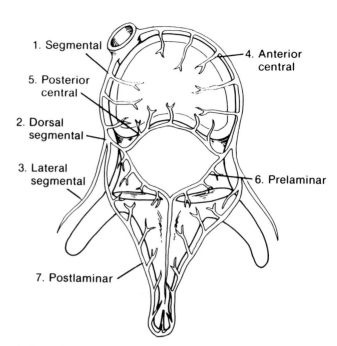

FIG. 2. Cross section of the spine demonstrating blood supply to the vertebral column. 1. Segmental artery. 2. Dorsal segmental artery. 3. Lateral segmental artery. 4. Anterior central arteries. 5. Posterior central artery. 6. Prelaminar artery. 7. Postlaminar artery.

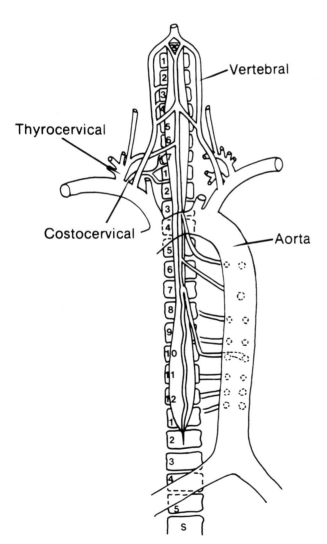

FIG. 1. Longitudinal view of the spinal cord with supply from the vertebral arteries, thyrocervical trunk, costocervical trunk, and aorta directly.

spinal cord at segmental levels (71). Segmental arteries originate as branches of the vertebral, subclavian, and hypogastric arteries and the aorta (Fig. 1). Each segmental artery initially divides into lateral and dorsal segments. The lateral segmental artery is totally somatic in its blood supply and is represented in the thorax and abdomen by the intercostal or lumbar arteries (Fig. 2). The dorsal segmental artery gives rise to four branches supplying the vertebral column: anterior central arteries, posterior central artery, prelaminar artery, and postlaminar artery (Fig. 3). The first and last of these branches originate outside the vertebral column; the other two arteries originate from the spinal branch inside the vertebral column. It is the spinal branch itself that gives rise to the posterior central and prelaminar arteries as well as an intermediate neural artery. The posterior central artery gives rise to caudal and cranial branches to supply the two adjacent vertebral bodies. The spinal cord and contents of the spinal canal receive their blood supply from the intermediate neural branch. Finally, at each segmental level small arterial branches originate to supply the nerve roots and nerve root ganglia (72).

The preceding description is typical for thoracic and lumbar vertebral bodies, but there is some deviation from this pattern in the sacral and cervical regions (71,87). In the sacral region, a significant arterial supply originates from the hypogastric arteries giving rise to the lateral sacral arteries, which anastomose with the middle sacral artery. From these arteries, the supply to the sacral

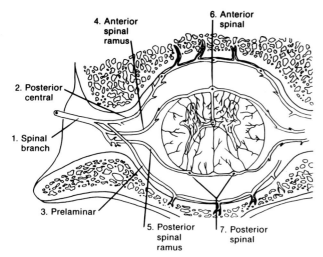

FIG. 3. Artery of the spinal cord in cross section. 1. Spinal branch. 2. Posterior central arteries. 3. Prelaminar arteries. 4. Anterior spinal ramus. 5. Posterior spinal ramus. 6. ASA. 7. PSA.

selective arteriographic study in this region (70). Overall, the vertebral arteries supply 77% of the cervical region but only 36% of the cervico-thoracic region (24). The remaining supply originates from branches of the subclavian and superior thoracic arch segmentals. The vertebral arteries can be viewed as the fusion of the original segmental vessels. The typical supply to the spine arises from the vertebral directly. As with the thoracic and lumbar regions, true spinal branches are at irregular levels.

Longitudinally, the blood supply to the spinal cord is composed of a single ASA and two smaller posterior spinal arteries (PSA) (23) (Fig. 3). The ASA courses continually from the medulla to the conus medullaris in the anterior median sulcus. Its cephalic origin is from the vertebral arteries just prior to their junction forming the basilar artery (Fig 4). These paired branches fuse after a

segments then is similar to that of the lumbar spine. In the cervical spine, there is significant variation (55). The lower cervical and upper thoracic regions are supplied in part by the thyrocervical and/or costocervical trunks. In addition, supply from the ascending pharyngeal artery contributes to the upper cervical spine and its contents. The most atypical arterial supply is to the atlanto-axial region; this should be reviewed before undertaking any

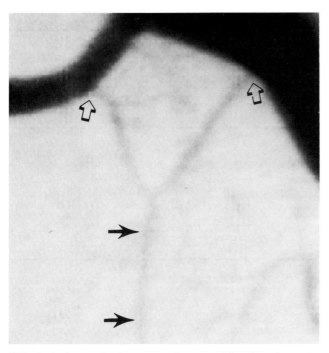

FIG. 4. Left vertebral artery angiogram with reflux down the right vertebral artery. Cervical ASA (arrows) originates from paired branches of the vertebral arteries (open arrows) before they join to form the basilar.

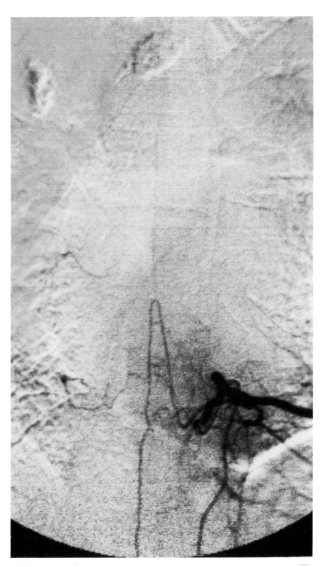

FIG. 5. Angiogram demonstrating the normal artery of Adamkiewicz. Note the smaller ascending branch and larger descending branch forming the ASA. This gives the characteristic "hairpin" configuration.

very short course to form a single ASA, which receives the variable segmental supply discussed above (Fig. 1). The PSAs are paired structures running posterolaterally along the entire length of the cord, although there may be noncontiguous areas. Each PSA is generally small, gaining only slightly in prominence at the conus medullaris. Like the ASA, the PSAs receive the segmental arterial supply along their length, but this supply is more numerous and smaller when compared to that of the ASA.

There are an average of eight ASA radicular arteries (range 2–17) and 12 paired PSA radicular arteries (range 6–25) (25). There are usually two to three originating from the vertebral arteries in the cervical region. The cervicothoracic region is supplied by branches of the costocervical trunk and/or the superior intercostal artery. The midthoracic (T4–T8) region represents the narrowest portion of the ASA and is often fed by a single radicular artery. The lower thoracic and upper lumbar regions are fed by one or more prominent arteries (57). It is in this region that the arteria radiculomedullaris magna (artery of Adamkiewicz) originates, usually from the left side (80% of the patients) and usually in the T9–T11 region, but ranging from T7 to L4 (23,26) (Fig. 5). This description constitutes the classic hairpin turn of the ASA composed of ascending and descending portions coupled with the feeding radicular branch. However, there may be more than one Adamkiewicz appearing vessel as this configuration of the ASA and its radicular supply can occur at more than one level, although not as prominently as in the lower thoracic region.

In cross section, the ASA supplies approximately the anterior two-thirds of the spinal cord and the PSAs supply the posterior one-third. Intramedullary arterial distribution is rather constant (26,42). Each artery gives off peripheral arteries, to supply the pia mater and white matter, and central arteries to supply gray matter and central white matter. Functionally, the PSAs usually supply the dorsal white columns and the posterior portions of the dorsal gray columns. The ASA supplies the remainder of the cord including the corticospinal tracts. There is of course variation and collateral supply is often unpredictable in the presence of vessel occlusion.

Venous Supply

The venous drainage of the entire spine is somewhat like the arterial supply (19), and the veins are variable in size, course, and distribution (71) (Fig. 6). Drainage consists of an external venous plexus and an internal venous plexus. The external venous plexus lies mostly anterior to the vertebral bodies, while the internal venous plexus is a series of valvulous epidural sinuses extending from the coccyx to the foramen magnum (4,7). Drainage

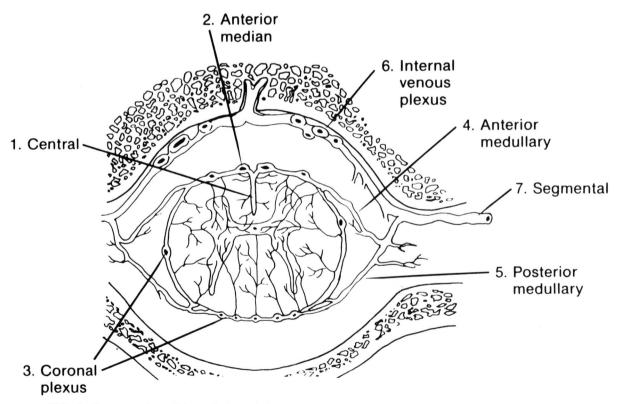

FIG. 6. Cross section of the spinal cord demonstrating venous drainage. 1. Central vein. 2. Anterior median spinal vein. 3. Coronal plexus. 4. Anterior medullary veins. 5. Posterior medullary veins. 6. Internal venous plexus. 7. Segmental vein.

from the cord can be thought of as involving two major systems (38). Anteriorly, the central vein receives blood from a large portion of the cord and this vein subsequently drains into the anterior median spinal veins, which run along the median sulcus. Laterally, posteriorly, and to a lesser extent anteriorly, smaller radial veins receive blood from the remainder of the cord and drain into the coronal plexus, which lies adjacent to the cord. Both systems drain via the medullary veins, which are somewhat variable in location (55).

There are anterior and posterior medullary veins and, as with the arterial supply, the posterior veins are often somewhat smaller and more numerous. At the level of the intervertebral foramina, the anterior and posterior medullary veins anastomose. It is at this site that segmental communicators from both the internal and external venous plexuses converge and drain into the paravertebral venous system. In the cervical region, the venous system is somewhat more variable but follows for the most part the distribution pattern identified for the more typical thoracic and lumbar regions (36).

TECHNIQUE

Before angiography, informed consent must be obtained from the patient. Because vertebral column angiography usually precedes embolization, the patient must also understand and consent for that procedure. Most angiography can be performed using mild sedation and local anesthesia. However, some clinical investigators have advocated the use of general anesthesia because some of these procedures can be long, tedious, and uncomfortable for the patient (93). In addition, patient motion can certainly degrade image quality, which is not an issue if general anesthesia is used. General anesthesia, however, precludes complete monitoring of neuromotor function until the patient has been awakened. Alternatively, the use of real time evoked potential monitoring may be used (5,40). Ultimately, the choice of anesthesia is based on the individual patient, and the anticipated complexity and duration of the procedure.

A useful procedure is to number the vertebral bodies in a consistent manner before angiography so that at film review the level(s) of abnormality can be easily determined and consistently discussed when planning therapy.

For most spinal angiography, a femoral artery approach is used; however, an axillary approach may be necessitated by the patient's arterial anatomy. At the site of arterial access, an introducer sheath should be placed to protect the artery during catheter exchanges that may be multiple in some cases. The aortogram is usually performed with a standard pigtail catheter. More selective catheterization can be accomplished with standard preshaped angiographic catheters. These catheters however

may not seat well enough into the vessel or be too large for subselective angiography or especially for subselective embolization. This is usually accomplished with coaxial systems. In these situations, a smaller catheter (usually 3 F) can be placed using small guidewires (<0.018") into very small vessels for subselective angiography or embolization. These catheters are easily placed in most situations and accept contrast injections and embolic material quite well. The standard angiographic catheter is acting as a guiding catheter in these situations and the entire coaxial complex is usually quite stable. The exact equipment and techniques utilized vary among intervention radiologists, but recent advances in devices have certainly made subselective angiography and embolization much more predictable.

Although there is some controversy about whether an aortogram is necessary, it is probably the best way to begin vertebral column angiography. It provides an excellent roadmap of the vessels and gives one an idea of the vascularity for proposed embolization. It also gives a direct comparison between pre- and postembolization in order to determine the degree of vessel occlusion and the degree of remaining vascularity. For the cervical and upper thoracic regions, aortography outlines the vertebral and subclavian arteries and in some instances their branches. For the thoracic and lumbar spine, the approximate location and number of segmental arteries are also outlined. However, in most situations, aortography is incomplete and selective angiography is mandatory.

Imaging studies, coupled with the aortogram, are used to guide the angiographer to the area of interest. When performing cervical spinal angiography, the vertebral arteries, costocervical and thyrocervical trunks, and external carotid arteries must be injected (Fig 7). For lower cervical lesions, the supreme and upper intercostal arteries should also be studied. For high thoracic lesions, the thyrocervical, costocervical, vertebral, external carotid (possibly subselective branches), and upper intercostal arteries should be injected. For thoracic and lumbar involvement, intercostal and lumbar arteries must be injected bilaterally. For lower lumbar and sacral involvement, the internal iliac arteries bilaterally should also be included as should the middle sacral artery. Thus a complete examination may be a very long process involving multiple catheters and a large volume of contrast material. In general, the segmental supply at the involved levels as well as at least one level above and below the abnormal areas should be selected. This means selective arterial catheterization should be carried out until normal arterial supply above and below the abnormality is demonstrated. In addition, depending upon the mode of therapy, the arterial supply to the cord in the region of interest may also need to be visualized, which would, of course, require additional angiography.

Digital subtraction angiography has proven to be a very useful modality for spinal arteriography (94). Al-

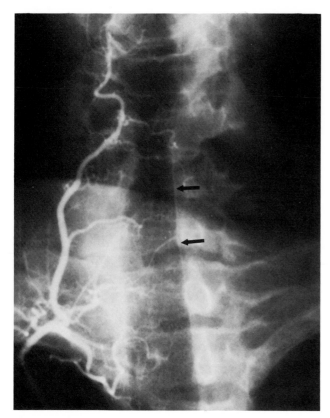

FIG. 7. Midcervical ASA (arrows) fills from selective injection of the costocervical artery on the right.

though initially intravenous injections were suggested as a screening technique, their widespread use has not materialized (32,59). Intra-arterial digital subtraction angiography, however, is in widespread use (29,32,94). Such angiography serves to reduce procedure time, contrast dosage, and film cost, and at the same time lessens patient discomfort.

TRANSCATHETER EMBOLIZATION

Catheters

When transcatheter embolization is to be undertaken, either as a therapeutic or preoperative measure, the techniques of diagnostic angiography are applied but with even greater care. Excellent preliminary films must be available and must provide a thorough delineation of normal and abnormal anatomy. Choice of catheters should be based on the lesion(s) to be embolized, arterial anatomy, and type of embolic agents. The catheter must be well seated into the site for embolization and must be adequate to accept the embolic agent of choice. As discussed in the preceding angiography section, coaxial catheter systems using newer smaller catheters and guidewires often allow relatively distal catheterization while being very stable for embolization. These catheters however do not have large luminal diameters. Although

this can be problematic in some situations, most vertebral column embolizations can be ideally performed using these systems.

Choice of Embolization Agents

Transcatheter embolization agents are usually divided on the basis of size and whether they are temporary or permanent. Larger agents occlude vessels more proximally and smaller agents occlude more distally, even to the capillary level. Proximal permanent agents consist of stainless steel coils and detachable balloons.

For most vertebral column embolizations, it is preferable to use a distal agent. If embolization is only performed proximally, the tumor will simply recruit vessels and remain highly vascular. The current principle therefore has been to use distal agents to occlude the smaller tumor vessels in the parenchyma such that embolization will be more effective and reduce the problem of vessel recruitment. More proximal agents are usually used once distal embolization has been performed to enhance thrombosis in the feeding vessel, hopefully allowing even better parenchymal vascular thrombosis. Proximal agents can also be used to prevent smaller agents from going into unwanted branches avoiding embolization of normal tissue.

If later definitive surgery is planned, embolotherapy can be performed with a temporary agent. The most common temporary agent is absorbable gelatin sponge (Gelfoam), which can be used either proximally or distally, depending on whether it is in a pledget or powder form. Gelatin sponge is absorbable, and some may begin absorption almost immediately, particularly when used as a proximal agent. However, in general, the gelatin sponges are thought to last at least several weeks, which should be long enough for surgery to be performed in most instances (3,31). At the present time, the most commonly used distal agent for vertebral column lesion embolization is polyvinyl alcohol (PVA) sponge (Ivalon). It is provided in particulate form in a range of sizes (75). PVA was once thought to be a permanent agent, but recently, there has been some question as to its long-term effects (41,67). Recurrence of symptoms and recanalization was reported to occur in one study (41) at an average of 5 months when PVA was used.

There are also liquid agents that can treat distal, small vessels effectively. There are a number of sclerosing agents for tumor embolization, the most popular of which has been absolute alcohol (12). Alcohol is easily and inexpensively obtained and can be easily injected through virtually any size catheter, including very small coaxial systems. Alcohol is usually rendered radiopaque by mixing with metrizamide powder. Alcohol causes severe endothelial damage resulting in permanent thrombosis (54). There are, however, several drawbacks with its use. It is often painful for the patient. In addition, because it is a liquid agent, it can easily reflux into vessels unintended for embolization and can of course flow through to the venous system if there is a significant degree of arteriovenous shunting. The latter problem has been more theoretical than real but the former can be quite problematic to those unaccustomed to using this embolic agent.

Cyanoacrylates (glue) permanently occlude by becoming solid (polymerization) in isotonic solution. Again because these are liquid agents, they can be placed through virtually any size catheter. However, because of the relatively slow flow of tumors, it has been quite difficult to control the polymerization times to make cyanoacrylates effective for vertebral column tumors. They have found greatest use in arteriovenous malformations.

Technique

Embolization should aim for complete obliteration of tumor vessels or for at least a significant decrease in vascularity. The decision to perform embolization must be based on the individual patient. The angiographer must be assured that there is no arterial supply to the spinal cord before undertaking embolization of a particular feeding vessel (Fig 8). Therefore, as stressed earlier, understanding the normal anatomy is essential. It is probably not necessary to characterize the blood supply to the spinal cord if good preliminary films of the region are obtained and no spinal cord supply is present. It is also probably wise not to attempt embolization if the ASA is supplied from the same pedicle (27). If such a supply is present and embolization is mandatory, identification of the collateral supply to the cord may still enable embolization to be performed safely. In addition, experience with superselective catheterization techniques often allows one to determine the degree of reflux into normal spinal arteries. Nowhere is this better demonstrated than in the cervical region with its vast anastomotic network of feeding vessels often originating from the vertebral artery. However, the feeding arteries may originate at arduous angles and be difficult to selectively catheterize. There may also be anastomoses with other branches of the vertebral artery. In high flow situations, such as AVM, some investigators have even advocated balloon occlusion of the vertebral artery during the embolization process (84).

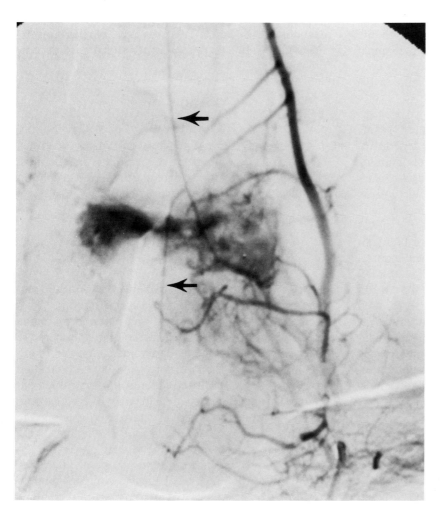

FIG. 8. Metastatic thyroid carcinoma to cervical vertebral body (C-4). Injection of costocervical artery shows ASA filling (*arrows*). Embolization of this branch should be avoided or more subselective catheterization performed beyond the origin of the radicular branch if possible.

Before embolization of a selected artery, provocative testing is recommended. Often called a spinal Wada, provocative testing is based upon the injection of either lidocaine or sodium amytal or both. The principles are like those of the traditional intracarotid injection in which neurologic testing is performed following injection of the agent (89). In general, lidocaine has been used in the external carotid system for peripheral nerve involvement, whereas sodium amytal has been advocated in the intracranial circulation. Because the cord in effect represents both central and peripheral circulation, many angiographers use both lidocaine and amytal before embolization. If neurologic changes are noted, then it can be concluded that neural tissues are at risk during embolization. It should be noted, however, that false-positive results can be obtained because provocative testing is performed with a liquid agent whereas most embolizations are performed with particles (49). Moreover, the liquid medication (amytal or lidocaine) spreads its effect throughout the network of capillaries whereas particles are believed to occlude before the capillary network, obviously depending on the particle size chosen. This characteristic may also result in an overestimation of the effects of embolization. Finally, it is often wise to reinject lidocaine and/or amytal after partial embolization of especially vascular masses to determine if the change in flow dynamics from embolization has altered the flow of embolic material, particularly to normal spinal branches. In such cases, embolization must be discontinued or the catheter position changed to a more favorable, safer location.

Somatosensory evoked potentials (SEP) have been advocated by some for use during embolization (47). This is especially true for patients who are under general anesthesia as there is no other way to effectively monitor neurologic function. SEP decrease when contrast material is injected into the ASA. There are also fluctuations during the injection of embolic material. Finally, there are definite changes following provocative testing should there be nervous system involvement. One must remember however that SEP are usually monitoring the dorsal columns which are supplied by the PSAs. Choi and Berenstein (13) suggest that they can recognize the ASA in greater than 80% of the cases. Berenstein et al. (5) used SEP during 33 therapeutic embolization procedures including 17 patients with spinal canal tumors and concluded SEP were a reliable method for electrophysiologic monitoring of spinal cord function and an important influence on the planning and execution of embolization.

Patient Selection

In patients with vertebral column abnormalities, it is obvious that the choice of treatment—surgery, embolization, or a combination of both—should be carefully individualized to the patient. As stated earlier, embolization of the vertebral column is usually done as a preoperative measure to decrease surgical blood loss. Preoperative embolization should be performed 24–48 hours before surgical intervention. This allows adequate time for more than one session if necessary and for additional thrombosis to occur. It is also often easy to briefly delay surgery since many patients have at least temporary improvement in their symptoms following embolization.

Embolization has also been performed to decrease pain and/or to relieve neurologic symptoms temporarily without surgery. Although embolization alone for vascular tumors has been successful, it is still mostly a preoperative measure (33,39,43,82). Relatively successful embolization of the lower lumbar spine for palliation of pain without surgery has been reported (82). Vertebral column embolization using chemotherapeutic agents has also been reported (16). Although these are attractive alternatives or adjuncts to surgery, only small clinical studies are available to date.

Although angiography is not usually indicated as a diagnostic tool for vertebral column abnormalities, it is performed occasionally following trauma or preoperatively for severe scoliosis to determine the arterial supply to the cord (9,45,85,91). It has also been performed to delineate the spinal cord arterial supply before thoracoabdominal aneurysm resection (51) or in planning extracavitary surgical approaches for spinal cord decompression and fusion (11).

VERTEBRAL COLUMN ABNORMALITIES

Angiography is most often indicated for suspected vascular lesions as a preoperative measure (22). The most common vascular lesions involving the vertebral column and the ones that will be discussed here are:

hemangiomas
aneurysmal bone cysts, giant cell tumors
metastatic tumors
arteriovenous malformations

Other vascular tumors such as angiosarcoma, angiolipoma, hemangiopericytoma, osteoid osteoma, pigmented villonodular synovitis, and neurofibrosarcoma are relatively rare in the vertebral column and therefore there is little data concerning the indications and findings from spinal angiography and/or embolization (14,15,53,60,62). However, if confronted with such patients, there is no reason to believe the principles concerning the more common lesions cannot be applied to these more unusual cases and of course individualized to a particular patient and his or her disease process.

Angiography for diagnostic purposes was attempted before the development of less invasive imaging modalities. In particular, there was an attempt to differentiate benign from malignant bone tumors (88). Benign tumors demonstrate vascular displacement, increased vascularity, a parenchymal stain, early venous drainage, and absence of tumor vessels. Malignant tumors, on the other hand, demonstrate these same findings as well as arteriovenous shunting, vascular lakes, neovascularization, and the presence of tumor vascularity. Tumor vascularity is characterized by vessels that are of irregular caliber, have a distorted course, and demonstrate abrupt angulations. Although the above findings are certainly characteristics of benign and malignant tumors, studies have demonstrated only an increase of approximately 20% in diagnostic accuracy when differentiating benign from malignant tumors based on the presence of tumor vascularity as demonstrated by angiography (88). In addition, these figures predate the further development of noninvasive imaging studies.

Hemangiomas

Among the more common tumors of the vertebral column are hemangiomas (Fig. 9). Autopsy studies have demonstrated an 11% incidence in the general population, although obviously very few become symptomatic (44). Hemangiomas occur most often in the lower thoracic and lumbar regions. The diagnosis can be made by the typical striated appearance on conventional roentgenograms.

Angiography is usually confined to a preoperative study for vascular anatomy and for possible preoperative embolization (33). Typically, the study demonstrates dense parenchymal staining with persistence of contrast in small pools often with an appearance of coalescence. There are, however, variances ranging from dense staining to virtually no staining, although the latter is quite rare. Even with dense persistent staining, there is little or no arteriovenous shunting. Draining veins when visualized, are not enlarged. Surgically it is important to demonstrate the supply to the hemangioma and particularly supply to the ASA if in an area where the ASA frequently originates such as the cervical and lower thoracic regions (63). It may also be clinically important to demonstrate the extra-osseous extent of the mass. This extent will be known from prior imaging, but its degree of vascularity and supply should be outlined.

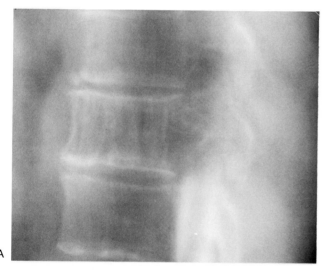

A

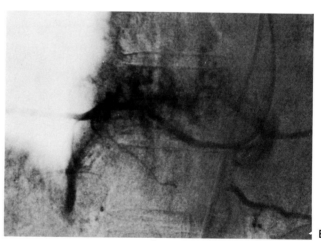

B

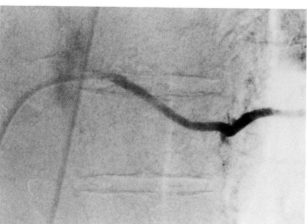

C

FIG. 9. A: Lateral view of the thoracic spine demonstrates the typical striated appearance of a vertebral hemangioma. B: Selective segmental arterial injection demonstrates the typical increased vascularity of the hemangioma. C: Embolization was performed using polyvinyl alcohol, and there is little remaining tumor stain. In this case the lateral segment (intercostal artery) remained patent. The embolization was a preoperative measure.

Embolization of hemangiomas has largely been a preoperative procedure. The data for embolization as the sole therapy consists of case reports. Raco et al. (73) have proposed that embolization alone may reduce the necessity for emergent laminectomy, and other investigators have reported lasting benefit from embolization as the sole therapy (39,43). Smith et al. (81) reported a group of 8 patients of whom 2 did not undergo later surgery; both had no symptomatic benefit from embolization. Most still believe the management of patients with progressive neurologic deficit should include preoperative angiography and embolization followed by decompressive surgery (35). Although based entirely on empirical data, the consensus of the literature is that embolization significantly decreases operative blood loss (2).

Aneurysmal Bone Cysts and Giant Cell Tumors

Aneurysmal bone cysts and giant cell tumors are basically indistinguishable by angiography (56,61,92). They

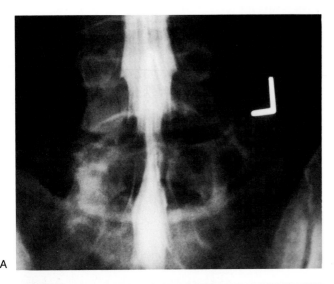

A

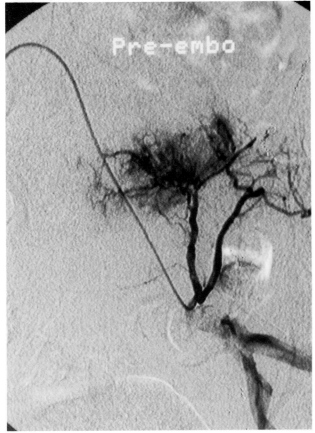

B

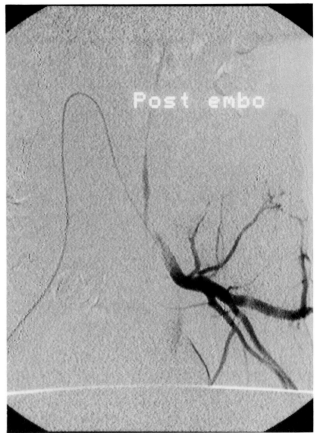

C

FIG. 10. A: Giant cell tumor of L5. Note the compression of the contrast-filled thecal sac. **B:** L5 segmental arterial injection demonstrates a somewhat hypervascular mass. **C:** Post-embolization study demonstrates good interruption of blood flow. Pathologic examination after tumor resection demonstrated a giant cell tumor with areas suggestive of aneurysmal bone cysts. Angiographically, it is probably best to treat these lesions as a continuum.

are probably best grouped together with a notation as to the degree of cystic change. The tumors are very vascular, usually at the periphery, with only small vessels centrally (Fig. 10). The feeding arteries are usually quite enlarged. Hypervascularity often extends into the paravertebral space. The parenchymal phase of the angiogram demonstrates multiloculated, vascular spaces (cysts) which demonstrate a degree of opacity throughout the entire cystic area. It is however patchy in distribution, therefore presenting a very uneven stain that is quite prolonged. This patchy appearance persists into the venous phase and is believed to represent contrast within the vascular lumina of the cysts. There is usually some degree of arteriovenous shunting. This description represents the typical angiographic appearance. Yaghmai (92) reviewed his findings with these tumors and noted that more than 50% of the cases failed to reveal cystic changes. In fact, these tumors were hypovascular or avascular in 12% of the cases, usually due to previous trauma, therapy, or spontaneous healing (92).

Most series of embolization of these tumors are very small or consist of case reports (17). There are several reports of successful definitive treatment with embolization (17,68,90), but most are preoperative with thus far promising results and low complications. However, the numbers reported are obviously very small.

Metastatic Disease

Vascular metastases demonstrate the typical changes of malignant tumors (Fig. 11). The feeding arteries are usually dilated. Overall there is an increased number of vessels which demonstrate an irregular caliber with abrupt angulations. The degree of vascularity varies from patient to patient and lesion to lesion, but often mimics the site of tumor origin (79,92). Tumor stains are seen early and there is irregular vascular persistence in a puddling appearance. There is usually a degree of arteriovenous shunting and in some tumors this may be quite ex-

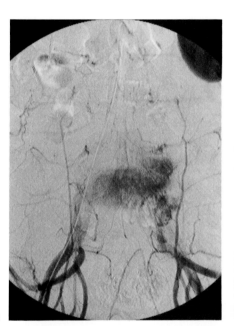

A

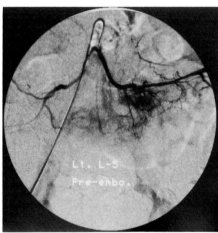

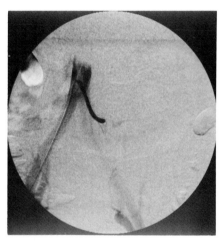

B,C

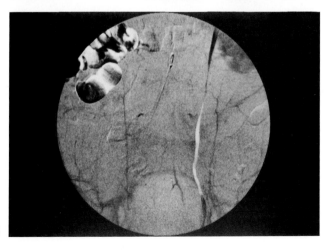

D

FIG. 11. A: Aortic flush angiogram demonstrates a hypervascular renal cell metastasis at the L5 level. **B:** Selective injections of the segmental arteries as well as branches of the internal iliac artery demonstrate hypervascularity. **C:** After embolization with polyvinyl alcohol, there is little remaining tumor stain. **D:** Follow-up flush angiogram at the termination of embolization demonstrates markedly reduced tumor blush. The embolization was a preoperative measure that markedly reduced the surgical blood loss.

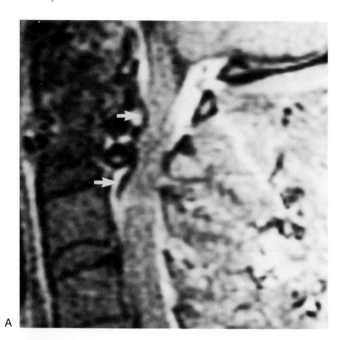

A

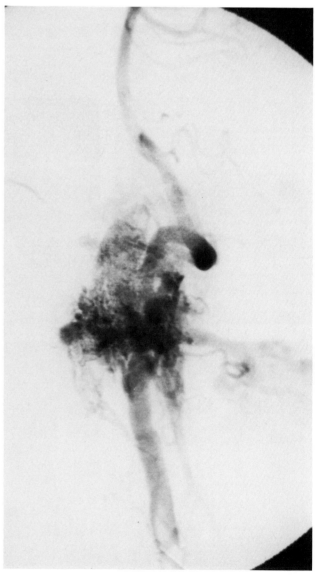

FIG. 12. Paraspinal AVM. **A:** MRI shows AVM with destruction of C-2 vertebral body. Draining veins are present within the spinal canal (arrows). **B:** Right vertebral and (**C**) left vertebral angiogram shows AVM with large draining veins. This AVM was embolized for pain as it was thought to be unresectable.

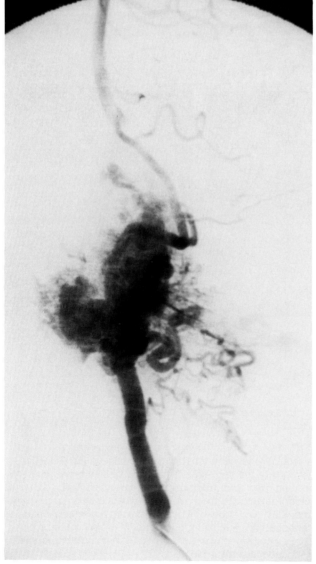

B

C

tensive. The most common vascular metastases to the spine which present for angiography are renal cell carcinoma, thyroid carcinoma, and melanoma. Breast and gastrointestinal adenocarcinoma among other metastatic lesions can also present with relatively vascular masses. Although the degree of vascularity can vary among these groups and within virtually any metastatic tumor, tumor vascularity and parenchymal staining are common. As with primary tumors, angiography is usually undertaken as a step before definitive surgical treatment.

There are reports of pain relief after embolization and this may occasionally be beneficial in patients who are not surgical candidates in whom there is difficulty controlling pain and/or progressive neurologic symptoms. However, the benefits from such embolization are probably not long lasting. Sundaresan et al. (83) reported successful embolization in 15 of 17 patients preoperatively for renal metastasis. No permanent complications were encountered. King et al. (52) reported 12 cases which had embolization before resection also for renal metastatic disease without complication and empirically felt there was evidence of decreased blood loss and operative times. These results are mirrored in other studies, all of which tend to be small series (6,8,78).

Arteriovenous Malformations

AVM represent an anomalous communication without an intervening capillary network. As with other spinal abnormalities the diagnosis of AVM is almost always made before angiography by imaging techniques (Fig. 12). Most AVM of the spine involve the spinal cord or its surrounding linings and present with appropriate neurologic findings. However, AVM may include the spinal column and paraspinal tissues either alone or in combination with the nervous system involvement. There are a number of classification systems for spinal AVM, but at present these are somewhat confusing and are still in a state of flux. Most classifications are focused on the anatomic location of the nidus relative to the spinal cord (77,80). The anatomic classification most easily understood is based on involvement of the vertebral column and consists of three main subgroups: intraspinal vascular malformations, paraspinal malformations, and disseminated and metameric AVM. It is usually the last two that may present for angiography based on findings referable to the vertebral column and surrounding soft tissues. Even with such an anatomic classification one should exercise caution. In a review of 150 cases, Merland et al. (66) found that one-third of their cases of spinal cord AVM had some extension outside the cord itself, representing a mixed type of AVM. Suffice it to say that when an AVM involves the vertebral column and paraspinal tissues, one must seek an intraspinal compo-

nent. This is often done by imaging studies, but this must be kept in mind during diagnostic angiography. The AVM itself may be situated outside the spinal canal, but have drainage within the canal. To that end, most of the vascularity visualized on imaging studies often consists of the enlarged draining vein or veins. There may be multiple levels of feeding arteries and quite commonly associated arterial or venous aneurysms. Paraspinal AVM are often very extensive and can cover several thoracic vertebral levels (76).

There are few reports in the literature concerning treatment of these malformations. Surgery can be notoriously difficult and embolization may be the only method of treatment (66). The principle of embolization is to occlude the nidus with a permanent agent such as cyanoacrylate. However, these lesions are often extensive and completely obliterating even the nidus may be impossible. In many cases, the goal of embolization is to decrease the symptoms referable to the AVM (10). In young patients, this may even be required to reduce cardiac failure from shunting (65).

LUMBAR EPIDURAL VENOGRAPHY

With the current imaging modalities of myelography, CT, and MRI, lumbar epidural venography is primarily of historic interest, and today is used only in highly selected patients.

Several interconnecting venous systems are of importance when performing epidural venography (37,86) (Fig. 13). The interosseous system drains the vertebral bodies into the epidural system (into a retrovertebral plexus), which has lateral and medial components. The lateral component consists of left and right singular veins that run the entire length of the vertebral column. The medial component is represented by multiple, somewhat irregular venous channels. The one variation in this pattern is found at the L5-S1 level, where the medial group lies more midline and further medial from the lateral group. At every segmental level, there are radicular veins (often both supra- and infrapedicular) that connect the epidural system to the paravertebral system. The paravertebral system is basically continuous, but is named for the region in which it is located: vertebral veins are contained within the neck, azygos and hemiazygos systems in the chest, ascending lumbar veins in the abdomen, and branches of the internal iliac veins (presacral veins) in the pelvis.

Epidural venography is usually performed by injecting contrast material into an ascending lumbar, presacral, or pedicular vein. As epidural venography can be somewhat uncomfortable, low osmolar contrast material has been advocated (64). The left femoral vein is usually the preferred access as it facilitates selective catheterization of the left ascending lumbar vein, which is the initial site of contrast injection (58).

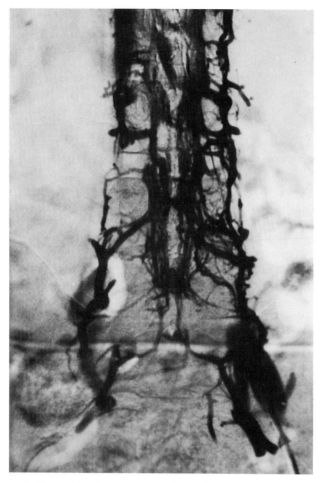

FIG. 13. Epidural venogram performed via the left ascending lumbar vein. Note the thinning at the L5-S1 level of the medial plexus, which is consistent with disc herniation at that level. This was confirmed surgically.

Epidural venography was most commonly used for the diagnosis of disc herniation (30). Such herniation appears as displacement or even obstruction of that portion of the epidural system in which the herniation occurs (Fig. 13). This technique has now been largely abandoned in favor of more recently developed imaging modalities, such as MRI. Another historic reason for performing epidural venography was spinal stenosis. Today the principal reason for performing epidural venography is probably the presence of an unusual epidural mass(es). Hopefully venography could supply additional information when other imaging modalities are technically limited and/or inconclusive. Before performing epidural venography, the angiographer should be well versed in the anatomy, techniques, and limitations of the study.

COMPLICATIONS OF ANGIOGRAPHY

There are a number of reports concerning the complications of spinal angiography. A recent study demon-

strates the frequency of neurologic complications to be 2.2%, which is within the range of neurologic complications reported for cerebral angiography (34). Some of the complications may be related to the process of catheterization such as thrombosis, embolization, or arterial spasm. However, spinal complications with aortic injections have also been reported (34). The mechanism of injury to the cord is unknown but has been hypothesized to be a direct neurotoxic effect of the contrast material. It is for this reason that newer, lower osmolality contrast materials are being used (50). Whether they will further reduce complications has not yet been established.

The direct complications of embolization in the studies reported to date have been very low, but these are small series and the data is obviously reflective of the numbers involved. More patients will be required before meaningful data can be generated.

Overall, it is clear that angiography and embolotherapy of the spine must be performed by someone who is knowledgeable in the field and experienced with catheter techniques. It is only with meticulous attention to detail that the lowest possible complication rates can be achieved.

REFERENCES

1. Adamkiewicz AA (1882): Die Blutgefasse des menschlichen Ruckenmarkes. I teil. Die Gefasse der Ruckenmarkssubstanz. Sitzungab. d.k. Akad. d. Wissensch. Math-Naturw Cl 3 abstr, Vienna 84: 469–502.
2. Bartels RHMA, Grotenhuis JA, Van Der Spek JAN (1991): Symptomatic vertebral hemangiomas. *J Neurosurg Sci* 35:187–192.
3. Barth KH, Strandberg JD, White RI Jr. (1977) Long term follow-up of transcatheter embolization with autologous clot, oxycel and gelfoam in domestic swine. *Invest Radiol* 12:273–280.
4. Batson OV (1940): The function of the vertebral veins and their role in the spread of metastases. *Ann Surg* 112:138–149.
5. Berenstein A, Young W, Ransohoff J, Benjamin V, Merkin H (1984): Somatosensory evoked potentials during spinal angiography and therapeutic transvascular embolization. *J Neurosurg* 60: 777–785.
6. Bhojraj SY, Dandawate AV, Ramakantan R (1992): Preoperative embolisation, transpedicular decompression and posterior stabilisation for metastatic disease of the thoracic spine causing paraplegia. *Paraplegia* 30:292–299.
7. Breschet G (1819): *Essai sur les veines der rachis.* Paris: Meguigon-Moruith.
8. Broaddus WC, Grady MS, Delashaw Jr JB, Ferguson RDG, Jane JA (1990): Preoperative superselective arteriolar embolization: A new approach to enhance resectability of spinal tumors. *Neurosurgery* 27(5):755–759.
9. Bussat P, Rossier AB, Djindjian R, Vasey H, Berney J (1973): Spinal cord angiography in dorsolumbar vertebral fractures with neurological involvement. *Radiology* 109:617–620.
10. Casasco AE, Houdart E, Gobin YP, Aymard A, Guichard JP, Rufenacht DA (1992): Embolization of spinal vascular malformations. *Neuroimag Clin North Am* 2(2):337–357.
11. Champlin AM, Benzel EC, Kesterson L, King JN, Orrison WW, Mirfakhraee M (1994): Preoperative spinal angiography for lateral extracavitary approach to thoracic and lumbar spine. *AJNR* 15: 73–77.
12. Choi IS, Berenstein A (1988): Surgical neuroangiography of the spine and spinal cord. *Radiol Clin North Am* 26:1131–1141.
13. Choi IS, Berenstein A (1990): Spinal angiography and embolization of tumors. In: Sundaresan N, Schmidek HH, Schiller AL, Ro-

senthal DI eds. *Tumors of the spine: diagnosis and clinical management.* Philadelphia: WB Saunders, pp. 52–62.

14. Clark LJP, McCormick PW, Domenico DR, Savory L (1993): Pigmented villonodular synovitis of the spine. *J Neurosurg* 79:456–459.

15. Coldwell DM (1989): Embolization of paraspinal masses. *Cardiovasc Intervent Radiol* 12:252–254.

16. Courtheoux P, Alachkar F, Casasco A, Adam Y, Derlon JM, Courtheoux F, L'Hirondel JL, Theron J (1985): Chemoembolization of lumbar spine metastases. *J Neuroradiol* 12:151–162.

17. DeRosa GP, Graziano GP, Scott J (1990): Arterial embolization of aneurysmal bone cyst of the lumbar spine. *J Bone Joint Surg* 72-A(5):777–780.

18. DiChiro G, Doppman J, Ommaya AK (1967): Selective arteriography of arteriovenous aneurysms of spinal cord. *Radiology* 88:1065–1077.

19. DiChiro G, Wener L (1973): Angiography of the spinal cord. A review of contemporary techniques and applications. *J Neurosurg* 39:1–29.

20. Djindjian R (1970): *Angiography of the spinal cord.* Baltimore: University Park Press, pp. 298–301.

21. Djindjian R, Dumesnil M, Faure C, LeFebvre J, Leveque B (1962): Etude angiographique d'un angiome intrarachidien. *Rev Neurol* [*Paris*] 106:278–285.

22. Djindjian R, Merland JJ, Djindjian M, Stoeter P (1981): *Angiography of spinal column and spinal cord tumors.* Stuttgart: Georg Thieme Verlag, pp. 3, 9–10.

23. Dommisse GF (1974): The blood supply of the spinal cord. A critical vascular zone in spinal surgery. *J Bone Joint Surg* [*Br*] 56:225–235.

24. Dommisse GF (1975): *The arteries and veins of the human spinal cord from birth.* Edinburgh: Churchill Livingstone, pp. 51–56.

25. Dommisse GF (1980): The arteries, arterioles, and capillaries of the spinal cord. Surgical guidelines in the prevention of postoperative paraplegia. *Ann Royal Coll Surg Engl* 62:369–376.

26. Doppman J, DiChiro G (1968): The arteria radicularis magna: Radiographic anatomy in the adult. *Br J Radiol* 41:40–45.

27. Doppman JL, DiChiro G, Oldfield EH (1985): Origin of spinal arteriovenous malformation and normal cord vasculature from a common segmental artery: Angiographic and therapeutic considerations. *Radiology* 154:687–689.

28. Doppman JL, DiChiro G, Ommaya A (1968): Obliteration of spinal-cord arteriovenous malformation by percutaneous embolisation. *Lancet* 1:477.

29. Doppman JL, Krudy AG, Miller DL, Oldfield E, DiChiro G (1983): Intraarterial digital subtraction angiography of spinal arteriovenous malformations. *AJNR* 4:1081–1085.

30. Drasin GF, Daffner RH, Sexton RF, Cheatham WC (1976): Epidural venography: Diagnosis of herniated lumbar intervertebral disc and other disease of the epidural space. *AJR* 126:1010–1016.

31. Ekelund L, Ek A, Forsberg L, Honkaas S, Henrikson H, Kalland T, Boijsen E. (1984): Occlusion of renal arterial tumor supply with absolute ethanol: Experience with 20 cases. *Acta Radiol* [*Diagn*] (*Stockh*) 25:195–201.

32. Enzmann DR, Brody WR, Djang WT, Riederer S, Keyes G, Collins W, Pelc N (1983): Intraarterial digital subtraction spinal angiography. *AJNR* 4:25–26.

33. Esparza J, Castro S, Portillo JM, Roger R (1978): Vertebral hemangiomas: Spinal angiography and preoperative embolization. *Surg Neurol* 10:171–173.

34. Forbes G, Nichols DA, Jack CR Jr, Ilstrup DM, Kispert DB, Piepgras DG, Wiebers DO, Earnest F IV, Axley PL (1988): Complications of spinal cord arteriography: Prospective assessment of risk for diagnostic procedures. *Radiology* 169:479–484.

35. Fox MW, Onofrio BM (1993): The natural history and management of symptomatic and asymptomatic vertebral hemangiomas. *J Neurosurg* 78:36–45.

36. Gabrielsen TO, Seeger JF, Crane JD (1972): Veins of the upper cervical spinal cord in vertebral angiography. *Acta Radiol* [*Diagn*] 13:801–807.

37. Gershater R, St Louis EL (1979): Lumbar epidural venography: Review of 1,200 cases. *Radiology* 131:409–421.

38. Gillilan LA (1970): Veins of the spinal cord. Anatomic details; suggested clinical applications. *Neurology* 20:860–868.

39. Gross CE, Hodge CH Jr, Binet EF, Kricheff II (1976): Relief of spinal block during embolization of a vertebral body hemangioma. *J Neurosurg* 45:327–330.

40. Hacke W (1985): Neuromonitoring during interventional neuroradiology. *Cent Nerv Syst Trauma* 2:123–136.

41. Hall WA, Oldfield EH, Doppman JL (1989): Recanalization of spinal arteriovenous malformations following embolization. *J Neurosurg* 70:714–720.

42. Hassler O (1966): Blood supply to human spinal cord. A microangiographic study. *Arch Neurol* 15:302–307.

43. Hekster RE, Luyendijk W, Tan TI (1972): Spinal-cord compression caused by vertebral haemangioma relieved by percutaneous catheter embolisation. *Neuroradiology* 3:160–164.

44. Henson RA, Croft PB (1956): Spontaneous spinal subarachnoid haemorrhage. *Q J Med* 25:53–66.

45. Hilal SK, Keim HA (1972): Selective spinal angiography in adolescent scoliosis. *Radiology* 102:349–359.

46. Hilal SK, Michelsen JW (1975): Therapeutic percutaneous embolization for extra-axial vascular lesions of the head, neck and spine. *J Neurosurg* 43:275–287.

47. John ER, Chabot RJ, Prichep LS, Ransohoff J, Epstein F, Berenstein A (1989): Real-time intraoperative monitoring during neurosurgical and neuroradiological procedures. *J Clin Neurophysiol* 6(2):125–158.

48. Kadyi H (1889): Uber die blutgefasse das menschlichen Ruschkenmarkes. Nach einer im XV. Bande der denkschriften d. math-naturw. Cl. d. Akad. d. Wissensch. In: *Krakav erschinen Monographie aus dem Polnishen ubersetzt vom Verfasser.* Lemberg: Gubrynowicz und Schmidt.

49. Katsuta T, Morioka T, Hasuo K, Miyahara S, Fukui M, Masuda K (1993): Discrepancy between provocative test and clinical results following endovascular obliteration of spinal arteriovenous malformation. *Surg Neurol* 40:142–145.

50. Kendall BE (1986): Spinal angiography with Iohexol. *Neuroradiology* 28:72–73.

51. Kieffer E, Richard T, Chiras J, Godet G, Cormier E (1989): Preoperative spinal cord arteriography in aneurysmal disease of the descending thoracic and thoracoabdominal aorta: Preliminary results in 45 patients. *Ann Vasc Surg* 3:34–46.

52. King GJ, Kostuik JP, McBroom RJ, Richardson W (1991): Surgical management of metastatic renal carcinoma of the spine. *Spine* 16(3):265–271.

53. Kuwabara H, Uda H, Nakashima H (1992): Pigmented villonodular synovitis (giant cell tumor of the synovium) occurring in the vertebral column. *Acta Pathol Jpn* 42(1):69–74.

54. Latschaw RF, Pearlman RL, Schaitkin BM, Griffith JW, Weidner WA. (1985) Intraarterial ethanol as a long-term occlusive agent in renal, hepatic, and gastrosplenic arteries in pigs. *Cardiovasc Intervent Radiol* 8:24–30.

55. Launay M, Chiras J, Bories J (1979): Angiography of the spinal cord: Venous phase. Normal features. Pathological application. *J Neuroradiol* 6:287–315.

56. Laurin S (1977): Angiography in giant cell tumors. *Radiologe* [*Berlin*] 17:118–123.

57. Lazorthes G, Gouaze A, Zadeh JO, Santini JJ, Lazorthes Y, Burdin P (1971): Arterial vascularization of the spinal cord. Recent studies of the anastomotic substitution pathways. *J Neurosurg* 35:253–262.

58. LePage JR (1974): Transfemoral ascending lumbar catheterization of the epidural veins. Exposition and technique. *Radiology* 111:337–339.

59. Levy JM, Hessel SJ, Christensen FK, Crowe JK (1983): Digital subtraction arteriography for spinal arteriovenous malformation. *AJNR* 4:1217–1218.

60. Lindbom A, Lindvall N, Soderberg G, Spjut H (1960): Angiography in osteoid osteoma. *Acta Radiol* 54:327–333.

61. Lindbom A, Soderberg G, Spjut HJ, Sunnqvist O (1961): Angiography of aneurysmal bone cyst. *Acta Radiol* 55:12–16.

62. MacLellan DI, Wilson Jr FC (1967): Osteoid osteoma of the spine. *J Bone Joint Surg* 49-A:111–121.

63. McAllister VL, Kendall BE, Bull JW (1975): Symptomatic vertebral hemangiomas. *Brain* 98:71–80.

64. Meijenhorst GC, deBruin JN (1980): Hexabrix (Ioxaglate), a new

low osmolality contrast agent for lumbar epidural double-catheter venography. *Neuroradiology* 20:29–32.

65. Merland JJ, Chiras J, Riche MC (1979): Arteriovenous malformations of the posterior wall of the thorax and abdomen. *J Neuroradiol* 6:221–229.

66. Merland JJ, Reizine D (1987): Treatment of arteriovenous spinal-cord malformations. *Semin Intervent Radiol* 4:281–290.

67. Morgan MK, Marsh WR (1989): Management of spinal dural arteriovenous malformations. *J Neurosurg* 70:832–836.

68. Murphy WA, Strecker WB, Schoenecker PL (1982): Transcatheter embolization therapy of an ischial aneurysmal bone cyst. *J Bone Joint Surg* 64-B(2):166–168.

69. Newton TH, Adams JE (1968): Angiographic demonstration and nonsurgical embolization of spinal cord angioma. *Radiology* 91:873–876.

70. Parke WW (1978): The vascular relations of the upper cervical vertebrae. *Orthop Clin North Am* 9:879–889.

71. Parke WW (1982): Applied anatomy of the spine. In: Rothman RH, Simeone FA, eds. *The spine, vol 1*. Philadelphia: WB Saunders, pp. 18–51.

72. Parke WW, Watanabe R (1985): The intrinsic vasculature of the lumbosacral spinal nerve roots. *Spine* 10:508–515.

73. Raco A, Ciappetta P, Artico M, Salvati M, Guidetti G, Guglielmi G (1990): Vertebral hemangiomas with cord compression: the role of embolization in five cases. *Surg Neurol* 34:164–168.

74. Rand RW, Rand CW (1960): *Intraspinal tumors of childhood*. Springfield: Charles C Thomas, pp. 281–284.

75. Repa I, Moradian GP, Dehner LP, Tadavarthy SM, Hunter DW, Castaneda-Zuniga WR, Wright GB, Katkov H, Johnson P, Chrenka B, Amplatz K (1989): Mortalities associated with use of a commercial suspension of polyvinyl alcohol. *Radiology* 170:395–399.

76. Riche MC, Merland JJ (1988): Embolization of vascular malformations. In: Mulliken JB, Young AE, eds. *Vascular birthmarks: hemangiomas and malformations*. Philadelphia: WB Saunders, pp. 436–453.

77. Riche MC, Reizine D, Melki JP, Merland JJ (1985): Classification of spinal cord vascular malformations. *Radiat Med* 3:17–24.

78. Roscoe MW, McBroom R, St Louis E, Grossman H, Perrin R (1989): Preoperative embolization in the treatment of osseous metastases from renal cell carcinoma. *Clin Orthop* 238:302–307.

79. Schobinger R (1958): The arteriographic picture of metastatic bone disease. *Cancer* 11:1264–1268.

80. Scialfa G, Cotti G, Biondi A, DeGrandi (1985): Embolization of vascular malformations of the spinal cord. *J Neurosurg Sci* 29:1–9.

81. Smith TP, Koci T, Mehringer CM, Tsai FY, Fraser KW, Dowd CF, Higashida RT, Halbach VV, Hieshima GB (1993): Transarterial embolization of vertebral hemangioma. *JVIR* 4:681–685.

82. Soo CS, Wallace S, Chuang VP, Carrasco CH, Phillies G (1982): Lumbar artery embolization in cancer patients. *Radiology* 145:655–659.

83. Sundaresan N, Choi IS, Hughes JEO, Sachdev VP, Berenstein A (1990): Treatment of spinal metastases from kidney cancer by presurgical embolization and resection. *J Neurosurg* 73:548–554.

84. Therom J, Cosgrove R, Melanson D, Ethier R (1986): Spinal arteriovenous malformations: Advances in therapeutic embolization. *Radiology* 158:163–169.

85. Therom J, Derlon JM, dePreux J (1978): Angiography of the spinal cord after vertebral trauma. *Neuroradiology* 15:201–212.

86. Therom J, Moret J (1978): *Spinal phlebography: Lumbar and cervical techniques*. Berlin: Springer-Verlag, pp. 27–31.

87. Turnbull IM, Brieg A, Hassler O (1966): Blood supply of cervical spinal cord in man. A microangiographic cadaver study. *J Neurosurg* 24:951–965.

88. Voegeli E, Fuchs WA (1976): Arteriography in bone tumours. *Br J Radiol* 49:407–415.

89. Wada J, Rasmussen T (1960): Intracarotid injection of sodium amytal for the lateralization of cerebral speech dominance. *J Neurosurg* 17:266–282.

90. Wallace S, Granmayeh M, DeSantos AL, Murray JA, Romsdahl MM, Bracken RB, Jonsson K (1979): Arterial occlusion of pelvic bone tumors. *Cancer* 43:322–328.

91. Wener L, DiChiro G, Gargour GW (1974): Angiography of cervical cord injuries. *Radiology* 112:597–604.

92. Yaghmai I (1979): *Angiography of bone and soft tissue lesions*. Berlin: Springer-Verlag, pp. 121–124.

93. Yasargil MG, Symon L, Teddy PJ (1984): Arteriovenous malformations of the spinal cord. *Adv Tech Stand Neurosurg* 11:61–102.

94. Yeates A, Drayer B, Heinz ER, Osborne D (1985): Intra-arterial digital subtraction angiography of the spinal cord. *Radiology* 155:387–390.

The Adult Spine: Principles and Practice,
2nd edition, J.W. Frymoyer, Editor-in-Chief.
Lippincott-Raven Publishers, Philadelphia © 1997.

CHAPTER 31

Nerve Root Injections

Mitsuo Hasue and Shinichi Kikuchi

HISTORICAL BACKGROUND

Although the idea of using local anesthetic agents in the paraspinal region for diagnostic purposes was already developed in the late 1940s (7,8,39), it was Macnab's milestone paper in 1971 (26) about nerve root injection that drew attention to this as a valuable diagnostic method. According to his later paper (5), he started to use the technique in 1967. He confirmed the position of his needle by injecting a small quantity of an oil-soluble iodine compound and analyzed a depicted outline of the nerve root. Furthermore, he confirmed the level of lesion by loss of symptoms following the injection of a local anesthetic solution. He did not refer to its therapeutic effect. One of us (MH) was quite impressed with his method when visiting him in 1969 and advised his junior colleagues to consider its use. Tajima et al. (34) reported their results in 1980 in which its therapeutic aspect was included. In the past two decades it has become popular in several centers around the world.

The modern development of imaging techniques such as magnetic resonance imaging (MRI) can help reveal the nerve root more clearly than before. Nerve root injection is, however, still the best method for depicting the nerve root silhouette along its intra- and extraspinal courses. Another drawback of all imaging modalities is their failure to correlate the morphologic abnormalities

with the patient's symptoms and signs. Morphologic abnormalities revealed by imaging modalities can exist without any symptoms and signs (1,13,14,40) and, therefore, their clinical significance should be questioned in many clinical cases. The enhanced MRI can show the symptomatic nerve root in the cases of lumbar disc herniation (35) but the sensitivity is rather low and the method is more difficult to interpret in patients with lumbar spinal stenosis, in which multilevel morphologic abnormalities frequently offer complicated problems with diagnostic levels. The functional or dynamic assessment of the nerve root can be achieved by nerve root injection and is most important for an accurate diagnosis of the symptomatic level. Combined contrast studies of myelography/peridurography and nerve root injection can be used for both morphologic and functional diagnostic purposes in lumbar spine disorders (19).

ANATOMIC BACKGROUND

When a contrast material is injected during the procedure, a serpentine or tubular figure of the nerve root is identified on the radiculogram, if correctly injected. This figure suggests that the injected material is localized to a single nerve root. In some cases, especially if the amount of the material is too much, the epidural space and/or the adjacent nerve root can be depicted simultaneously. On the other hand, if a sufficient amount of the material is injected into the epidural space as in the case of peridurography, it infiltrates through the intervertebral foramina and outlines the nerve roots very clearly. These

M. Hasue, M.D.: Department of Orthopedic Surgery, Japanese Red Cross Medical Center, Tokyo 150, Japan.
S. Kikuchi, M.D.: Professor, Department of Orthopaedic Surgery, Fukushima Medical College, Fukushima, 960-12 Japan.

clinical facts strongly suggest that there is a continuous membranous covering around the dura mater and nerve roots.

In the lumbar spinal canal a membranous structure called the extradural membrane (4) or epidural membrane (18) can be found between the dura mater and yellow ligament. Also in the intervertebral foramina there is a membranous covering, periradicular sheath (4), or epiradicular sheath (18), around the nerve root. It is formed by a lateral extension of the superficial layer of the posterior longitudinal ligament. These membranous structures blend into each other, forming a tubular sheath around the nervous tissues. The contrast material, if correctly injected, is located between the nerve root and the epiradicular sheath, depicting the nerve root in a tubular fashion. Normal variations in the connecting patterns of the ventral and dorsal roots and/or position of the dorsal root ganglia (10,22) can be related to variabilities in the depicted figures of the nerve roots and in the effect of the injected solutions.

PATHOPHYSIOLOGIC BACKGROUND

Nerve root injection is usually done at the extraspinal region distal to the usual site of lesion. Interestingly enough, radicular pain and its related signs can be abolished at least temporarily even in cases in which the injected local anesthetic is not presumed to infiltrate into the site of lesion. Not infrequently, the effect may persist for several months (20). On the other hand, sciatic or peroneal nerve blocks (17,44) are also effective for sciatica in several cases.

The pathomechanisms of radicular pain are not yet fully clarified. In 1930 Eccles and Sherrington (6) suggested in their elegant study of spinal reflex that summation of excitatory effects of a number of afferent nerve fibers may be necessary before a discharge is originated in the spinal cord. Recent basic and clinical studies (2,3,29,31,38,43) strongly suggest that an ectopic discharge and cross talk of the afferent nerve fibers at the site of lesion may result in sensitization of both the central and peripheral nervous systems, making a vicious circle (Fig. 1). The impulses from the periphery are suggested to be most critical in dynamically maintaining the mechanism of pain production. Blocking a large number of afferent impulses even at the site distal to the lesion can stop the critical impulses from the periphery, thus destroying a vicious circle in the nervous systems and making the second neurons in the spinal cord unable to discharge. Once a vicious circle is destroyed, it may take a long time for the nervous system to reconstruct the circle or a different type of pain transmission system may be formed. The exact mechanisms responsible for the effect of nerve root or peripheral nerve blocks are still to be proven.

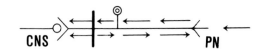

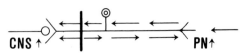

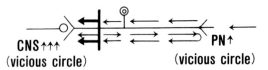

FIG. 1. Electrophysiologic abnormalities as related to the pathomechanisms of radicular pain. CNS, central nervous system; PN, peripheral nerve; ⊚, dorsal root ganglion; |: site of nerve root compression. (From Hasue M: Pain and the nerve root. *Spine* 1993;18:2053–2058.)

INDICATIONS AND CONTRAINDICATIONS

Nerve root injection is most frequently used in the lumbosacral region, although it can be applied to the cervicothoracic level. Radicular symptoms including radicular intermittent claudication can be investigated and/or treated by the procedure (5,11,15,23,33,34,36,37,42). It is mostly indicated for the cases for which operation is considered. The main indications may be divided into diagnostic and therapeutic ones.

Diagnostic Indications

A. Based on Symptoms and Signs

1. *Radicular pain and/or intermittent claudication without neurologic findings.* Although radicular pain patterns may suggest the involved nerve root, especially the L4 nerve root, they are not always conclusive. In patients without definite neurologic findings, particularly of equivocal imaging studies, nerve root injection is of considerable value.

2. *Atypical leg pain.* Sciatica may be accompanied by inguinal or anterior thigh pain or the distribution of leg pain is not segmental or vague. In these cases involvement of two/three nerve roots, existence of the furcal nerve at the involved level (21) or other causes should be distinguished. The functional assessment by nerve root injection is most significant for those cases.

3. *Multiple (two/three) nerve root signs.* Two or three nerve roots may be involved at one or two levels. Nerve root injection is useful for determining the symptomatic nerve roots and the site of the offending lesion.

4. *Radicular pain and/or intermittent claudication associated with other type of pain.* Lumbosacral radiculopathy may be associated with cervical or thoracic myelopathy, for example, as in cervicolumbar syndrome (27). It may also be accompanied by the hip joint disorders as in hip–spine syndrome (30) or by osteoarthritis of the knee joint (25). Nerve root injection and joint blocks can be used for the final diagnosis.

B. Based on Imaging Studies

1. *Multilevel abnormalities.* Cases of multilevel imaging abnormalities without definite neurologic findings should be investigated by nerve root injection (Fig. 2). Even when neurologic findings suggest the level of lesion, functional assessment of nerve roots is not infrequently necessary, especially in the cases of two/three nerve root signs or of the transitional vertebrae. In the latter cases

the anatomic level of the nerve root does not always coincide with the functional level (24).

2. *Discrepancy between imaging studies and clinical findings.* In those patients in whom routine imaging studies do not reveal unequivocal abnormalities or the morphologic abnormalities do not correspond to clinical findings, nerve root injection should be applied for detailed morphologic and functional assessments.

3. *Nerve root and/or spine anomalies.* The congenital root anomalies such as conjoined nerve roots (9,16,28) may offer a diagnostic problem. In patients with both nerve root and spine anomalies, it may be more difficult to determine the symptomatic nerve root and its site of lesion. Nerve root injection can be of considerable value in these cases.

4. *Failed back syndrome.* Since the imaging studies do not reveal definite symptom-related abnormalities in most of the cases, the functional assessment is of critical importance.

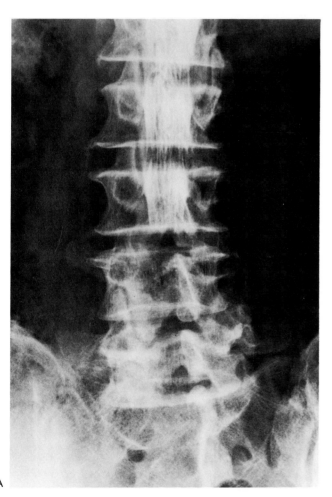

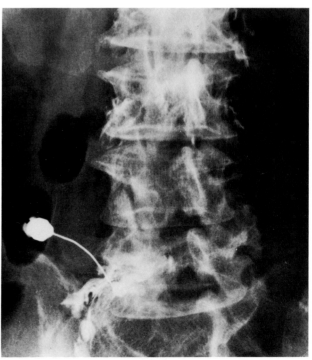

A

B

FIG. 2. A 65-year-old man complained of right sciatica. Only a slight sensory disturbance was detected on the lateral aspect of his right leg and foot. His pain was completely relieved by decompression of the right L5 nerve root. **A:** An anteroposterior myelogram showed a complete stop of the contrast material at the L3-4 level. **B:** A radiculogram suggested compression of the right L5 nerve root at the subarticular region. His radicular pain was reproduced by the injection and temporarily eliminated by local anesthetic block.

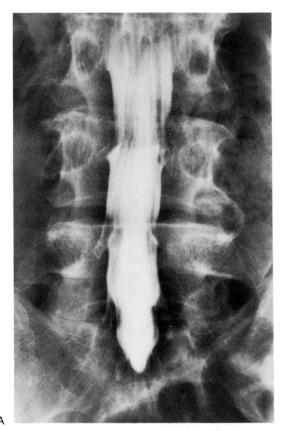

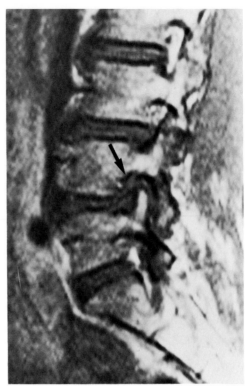

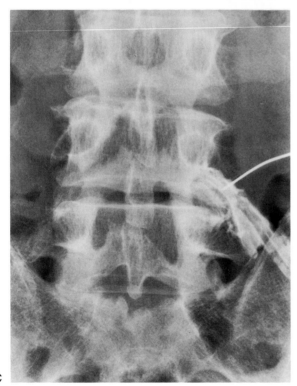

FIG. 3. A 57-year-old man complained of pain on the right anterior thigh and medial leg. Neurologic findings were not conclusive for the level diagnosis. **A:** An anteroposterior myelogram showed a slight defect of the right L5 nerve root. **B:** A parasagittal MRI showed an obstruction of the L4-5 intervertebral foramen (arrow). **C:** A radiculogram showed a transverse course of the right L4 nerve root, suggesting compression at the intraforaminal region. Reproduction and disappearance of his radicular pain by the procedure corfirmed the L4 nerve root to be symptomatic.

5. *Intra- and extraforaminal lesions.* In cases of foraminal encroachment (Fig. 3), pedicular kinking, or far-lateral syndrome (41) a clear view of the nerve root along its long course is necessary for detecting the site of lesion. Furthermore, the functional assessment is valuable in determining whether the investigated nerve root has related symptoms.

Therapeutic Indications

1. Severe radicular pain resistant to other therapeutic means.
2. Severe radicular pain for which operation is contraindicated.
3. Severe radicular pain for which the injection is anticipated empirically to be most effective.

Radicular intermittent claudication which is very disabling to the patient and resistant to other means may successfully be treated by nerve root injection.

Contraindications

Cases of disturbed consciousness, emotional instability, or lack of understanding the procedure are not good candidates for this type of investigation. In cases of iodine sensitivity the procedure with imaging studies is obviously contraindicated. In these cases the injection of local anesthetic and/or steroid solutions can be applied for diagnostic and/or therapeutic purposes, under the control of image intensifier.

TECHNIQUE

Several techniques of nerve root injection (5,11,12,15,23,32,33,36,37,42) have been reported; our current method is described here.

Before proceeding, the history should elicit allergic reactions, and an iodine test should be done prior to the investigation. Neither medication nor dietary control is necessary. Analgesic medication is not suitable because the patient's pain response is an important source of information for diagnostic purposes.

The procedure should be done in a radiology department equipped with an image intensifier. The patient is usually placed in the prone position. The lateral or oblique position can also be used, if necessary, especially in cases of failed back surgery. A pillow is inserted below the abdomen. The site of needle placement is chosen approximately 4 cm lateral to the upper margin of the lumbar spinous process.

Under an image intensifier, an 8-cm, 22-gauge needle is inserted perpendicular to the skin until it impinges upon the transverse process, anesthetizing the skin, fascia, and periosteum. Then the needle is pulled out slightly and then pushed in slightly medially and approximately 20° caudally so that it is advanced toward the intervertebral foramen, which is just inferior to the transverse process. At the S1 level the needle is placed approximately 3 cm lateral to the midline and advanced directly into the posterior sacral foramen. When the needle has struck the surface of the sacrum, it is advanced slightly medially and caudally into the foramen.

When the needle strikes the nerve root, a sharp pain radiating to the lower extremity is produced. It is useful at this stage to ask the patient whether or not this is his or her pain. The distribution of pain should be clarified as accurately as possible. After no blood or fluid is aspirated by suction, 1 ml of a water-soluble contrast medium is injected. The nerve root can then be depicted in a tubular or serpentine fashion. The anteroposterior roentgenogram is taken just afterward. Then 1 ml of 2% lidocaine is injected and thereafter subjective symptoms and objective findings of the patient are carefully checked. Disappearance of radicular and low back pain is questioned and spinal and neurologic findings are examined as precisely as possible and compared with those before the injection. If the blocked nerve root is symptomatic, painful limitation of the lumbar spine motion and tension signs such as positive straight-leg raising are markedly or totally improved. It must be stressed that the changes not only of symptoms but also of spinal and neurologic signs are critical for determining the blocked nerve root to be symptomatic. In cases of radicular intermittent claudication, the patient is asked to walk to check if a walking distance is markedly elongated after the procedure.

In cases in which a therapeutic effect is expected, a water-soluble corticosteroid mixed with a local anesthetic solution is injected. When nerve root injection is performed for the therapeutic purpose only, 3–5 ml of bupivacaine can be chosen for the cases without cardiac diseases.

Diagnostic Value

In our experience with more than 1,000 nerve root injections the reproducibility is excellent, if correctly performed, in its functional aspect: reproduction and disappearance of the patient's radicular pain (5,11,12,23,32, 33,36,37,42). However, the depicted image of the nerve root is not always the same, even when the contrast material is correctly injected. The main reason may be technical: the site of an inserted needle and the pressure of injecting the material might be different at each occasion. In addition, a normal variation in the connecting pattern of the ventral and dorsal nerve roots (22) may be related to some extent to variability of the depicted nerve root figure.

We investigated the results of 129 operated patients (158 nerve roots) with various degenerative lumbar spine disorders who presented with radicular pain and/or intermittent claudication. The false positives and negatives were determined at operation. The true positive, for example, means that compression of the symptomatic nerve root was found at operation and symptoms and signs were relieved by operation. The results of our investigation were as follows:

true positive: 116 cases, 137 roots
true negative: 12 cases, 12 roots
false positive: 9 cases, 9 roots
false negative: none

The causes for false positive were multiply operated back in 3 cases, psychiatric disease in 2, anomalous segmental innervation in 1, and unknown in 3. Therefore, the accuracy of nerve root injection is 94.3%, the sensitivity is 100%, and the positive predictive value is 92.8%. Since the number of true negatives in this series was only 12 roots and this invasive procedure cannot be applied to asymptomatic nerve roots in many cases, the true value of specificity is still to be questioned.

Advantages and Disadvantages

The advantages are twofold: morphologic and functional. The morphologic aspect is to be able to depict the nerve root figure more clearly in its intra- and extraspinal courses. It is useful for looking at the site of nerve root compression in a wide area. The functional aspect which is most characteristic of this procedure is the determination that the examined nerve root has related symptoms. Reproduction and disappearance of the patient's pain and related signs by the procedure are significant criteria for this purpose. The walking test after the block is also useful for cases of radicular intermittent claudication. Another advantage is to have a therapeutic effect decreasing the radicular pain/intermittent claudication. By injecting local anesthetic and corticosteroid solutions the aforementioned symptoms can be relieved for months or even years in several cases. Nerve root injection can therefore be employed as a therapeutic modality for radicular symptoms.

The main disadvantages are pain and irradiation to the patient, although both of them are indispensable for functional and morphologic aspects of the procedure. In order to lessen these drawbacks, the needle is slightly pulled back before injecting the contrast material and an anteroposterior roentgenogram only is taken in most cases.

The possible complications ascribed to the procedure are infection, nerve root irritation/injury, leakage of the cerebrospinal fluid, and perforation of the viscus (23,32,34). Actually, however, a transient increase of radicular pain and/or neural deficits has only rarely been reported. No serious complications have been encountered in our experience to date.

Diagnostic Limitations

Nerve root injection is not a purely objective method. Since reproduction and disappearance of radicular pain are important for the functional aspect of the procedure, accurate information must be given by the patient. In this regard the procedure is not suitable for patients who have difficulty expressing pain such as the very old or very young or those with emotional instability, disturbed consciousness, or mental retardation.

This technique cannot accurately locate the site of the irritation in a given nerve root. The site of irritation may be intra- or extraspinal, even if the nerve root is determined to be symptomatic. In cases of double crash lesion, for example, subarticular compression combined with extraspinal lesion, it is impossible by the procedure itself to decide if one or two sites are symptomatic. Furthermore, even when the site of the lesion is single, it may be at the lumbar spine, at the thoracolumbar region as in the case of spinal cord tumor, or at the sacrum as in the case of sacral tumor.

The procedure cannot offer an information on the pathology of the lesion. Other diagnostic modalities should be added for final pathologic diagnosis.

It is not useful for cases of paralysis without radicular pain. Cases of cauda equina syndrome without pain, for example, cannot be examined by the procedure.

Results of Nerve Root Injection

Nerve root injection which has usually been used as a diagnostic modality can be effective for radicular pain and/or intermittent claudication. It can be used once a week for 3 weeks. In our experience, about 25% of patients who have been admitted for possible operation have successfully been treated by injection and discharged without undergoing operation. Cases of lumbar spinal stenosis due to spondylosis or degenerative spondylolisthesis have benefited more than those of disc herniation and spondylolytic spondylolisthesis. Temporary relief of symptoms and signs within 2–3 hours after the procedure does not suggest a good outcome, whereas the effect continuing more than 24 hours is a good predictive sign for successful conservative treatment. Based on our clinical experience we believe that nerve root injection is useful and important for selected patients with radicular symptoms and signs as a therapeutic modality as described and only if indicated.

REFERENCES

1. Boden SD, Davis D, Dina TS, Patronas NJ, Wiesel SW (1990): Abnormal magnetic-resonance scans of the lumbar spine in

asymptomatic subjects: A prospective investigation. *J Bone Joint Surg* 72A:403–408.

2. Devor M (1988): Central changes mediating neruopathic pain. In: Dubner R, Gebhart GF, Bond MR eds. *Proceedings of the 5th Congress on Pain.* Amsterdam: Elsevier Science Publishers, pp 114–128.

3. Devor M (1991): Group report: Mechanisms of neuropathic pain following peripheral injury. In: Basbaum AL, Besson JM eds. *Towards a new pharmacology of pain.* New York: John Wiley & Sons, pp 417–440.

4. Dommisse GF (1975): Morphological aspect of the lumbar spine and lumbosacral region. *Orthop Clin North Am* 163–175.

5. Dooley JF, McBroom RJ, Taguchi T, Macnab I (1988): Nerve root infiltration in the diagnosis of radicular pain. *Spine* 13:79–83.

6. Eccles JC, Sherrington CS (1930): Reflex summation in ipsilateral spinal flexion reflex. *J Physiol* 69:1–28.

7. Falconer MA, Glasgow GI, Cole DS (1947): Sensory disturbances occurring in sciatica due to intervertebral disc protrusions; some observations on fifth and first sacral dermatomes. *J Neurol Neurosurg Psychiatry* 10:72–84.

8. Falconer MA, McGeorge M, Begg AC (1948): Observations on the cause and mechanism of symptom-production in sciatica and low back pain. *J Neurol Neurosurg Psychiatry* 11:13–26.

9. Hasue M, Kikuchi S, Sakuyama Y, Ito T (1983): Anatomic study of the interrelation between lumbosacral nerve roots and their surrounding tissues. *Spine* 8:50–58.

10. Hasue M, Kunogi J, Konno S, Kikuchi S (1989): Classification by position of dorsal root ganglion in the lumbosacral region. *Spine* 14:1261–1264.

11. Haueisen DC, Smith BS, Myers SR, Pryce ML (1985): The diagnostic accuracy of spinal nerve injection studies. Their role in the evaluation of recurrent sciatica. *Clin Orthop* 198:179–183.

12. Herron LD (1989): Selective nerve root block in patient selection for lumbar surgery: Surgical results. *J Spinal Dis* 2:75–79.

13. Hitselberger WE, Witten RM (1968): Abnormal myelograms in asymptomatic patients. *J Neurosurg* 28:204–206.

14. Holt Jr EP (1968): The question of lumbar discography. *J Bone Joint Surg* 50A:720–726.

15. Jonsson B, Stromqvist B, Annertz M, Holtas S, Sunden G (1988): Diagnostic lumbar nerve root block. *J Spinal Dis* 1:232–235.

16. Kadish LJ, Simmons EH (1984): Anomalies of the lumbosacral nerve roots. *J Bone Joint Surg* 66B:411–416.

17. Kibler RF, Nathan PW (1960): Relief of pain and paresthesiae by nerve block distal to a lesion. *J Neurol Neurosurg Psychiatry* 23:91–98.

18. Kikuchi S (1982): Anatomical and experimental studies of nerve root infiltration. *J Jpn Orthop Assoc* 56:605–614.

19. Kikuchi S, Hasue M (1988): Combined contrast studies in lumbar spine diseases: Myelography (peridurography) and nerve root infiltration. *Spine* 13:1327–1331.

20. Kikuchi S, Hasue M, Nishiyama K, Ito T (1984): Anatomic and clinical studies of radicular symptoms. *Spine* 9:23–30.

21. Kikuchi S, Hasue M, Nishiyama K, Ito T (1986): Anatomic features of the furcal nerve and its clinical significance. *Spine* 11:1002–1007.

22. Kikuchi S, Sato K, Konno S, Hasue M (1994): Anatomic and radiographic study of dorsal root ganglia. *Spine* 19:6–11.

23. Krempen JF, Smith BS (1974): Nerve-root injection. A method for evaluating the etiology of sciatica. *J Bone Joint Surg* 56A:1435–1444.

24. Kunogi J, Hasue M (1991): The functional level of lumbosacral. nerve root in the cases of transitional vertebrae. Presented at the 18th Annual Meeting of the International Society for the Study of the Lumbar Spine, Heidelberg, May 13, 1991.

25. Kunogi J, Hasue M, Miyoshi K (1992): Clinical significance of L4 nerve root involvement in degenerative lumbar spine diseases: An important cause of postoperative leg symptoms. Presented at the 19th Annual Meeting of the International Society for the Study of the Lumbar Spine, Chicago, May 22, 1992.

26. Macnab I (1971): Negative disc exploration. An analysis of the cause of nerve root involvement in sixty-eight patients. *J Bone Joint Surg* 53A:891–903.

27. Macnab I (1977): *Backache.* Baltimore: Williams & Wilkins, pp. 158–160.

28. Neidre A, Macnab I (1983): Anomalies of the lumbosacral nerve roots. *Spine* 8:294–299.

29. Nordin M, Nystrom B, Wallin U, Hagbarth K (1984): Ectopic sensory discharges and paresthesiae in patients with disorders of peripheral nerves, dorsal roots and dorsal columns. *Pain* 20:231–245.

30. Offierski CM, Macnab I (1983): Hip–spine syndrome. *Spine* 8:316–321.

31. Papir-Kricheli D, Devor M (1988): Abnormal impulse discharge in primary afferent axons injured in the peripheral versus the central nervous system. *Somatosens Mot Res* 6:63–77.

32. Schutz H, Lougheed WM, Wortzman G, Awerbuck BG (1973): Intervertebral nerve-root in the investigation of chronic lumbar disc disease. *Can J Surg* 16:217–221.

33. Stanley D, McLaren MI, Euinton EA, Getty CJM (1990): A prospective study of nerve root infiltration in the diagnosis of sciatica. A comparison with radiculography, computed tomography, and operative findings. *Spine* 15:540–543.

34. Tajima T, Furukawa K, Kuramochi E (1980): Selective lumbosacral radiculography and block. *Spine* 5:68–77.

35. Toyone T, Takahashi K, Kitahara H, Yamagata M, Murakami M, Moriya H (1993): Visualization of symptomatic nerve roots. *J Bone Joint Surg* 75B:529–533.

36. van Akkerveeken PF (1990): Pain patterns and diagnostic blocks. In: Weinstein JE, Wiesel SW, eds. *The lumbar spine.* Philadelphia: Saunders, pp 120–131.

37. van Akkerveeken PF (1993): The diagnostic value of nerve root sheath infiltration. *Acta Orthop Scand* (Suppl 251) 61–64.

38. Wall PD, Devor M (1983): Sensory afferent impulses originate from dorsal root ganglia as well as from the periphery in normal and nerve injured rats. *Pain* 17:321–339.

39. White JC, Gently RW (1944): Radiographic control for paravertebral injection of alcohol in angina pectoris. *J Neurosurg* 1:40–44.

40. Wiesel SW, Tsourmas N, Feffer HL, Citrin CM, Patronas N (1984): A study of computer-assisted tomography: 1. The incidence of positive CAT scans in an asymptomatic group of patients. *Spine* 9:549–551.

41. Wiltse LL, Guyer RD, Spencer CW, Glenn WV, Porter IS (1984): Alar transverse process impingement of the L5 spinal nerve: the far-out syndrome. *Spine* 9:31–41.

42. Wippula E, Jussila P (1977): Spinal nerve block. A diagnostic test in sciatica. *Acta Orthop Scand* 48:458–460.

43. Woolf CJ (1991): Generation of acute pain: central mechanisms. *Br Med Bull* 47:523–533.

44. Xavier AV, McDanal J, Kissin I (1988): Relief of sciatic radicular pain by sciatic nerve block. *Anesth Analg* 67:1177–1180.

The Adult Spine: Principles and Practice,
2nd edition, J.W. Frymoyer, Editor-in-Chief.
Lippincott-Raven Publishers, Philadelphia © 1997.

CHAPTER 32

Diagnostic Injections: An Overview of Discography, Facet Arthrography, and Nerve Root Infiltration

Pieter F. van Akkerveeken

This chapter presents a critical appraisal of diagnostic injections based on the literature and the documented experience of the author. Although these techniques have been used in the cervical and thoracic spine, this review is restricted to the lumbar spine.

To be useful in clinical practice a diagnostic test has to meet the following criteria: its reliability has to be established and its diagnostic value in terms of sensitivity, specificity, and predictive value has to be known, as presented in Chapter 20. These characteristics of discography, facet arthrography, and nerve root sheath infiltration will be discussed as far as the state of current knowledge allows. In addition, the rate of complications and the indications will be reviewed.

SYMPTOMATIC VERSUS ASYMPTOMATIC PATHOLOGY

Modern imaging techniques of the lumbar spine such as oil-based myelography, computed tomography (CT)

P. F. van Akkerveeken, M.D., Ph.D.: Orthopedic Surgeon, and Director Rugadviescentrum Nederland, Utrechtseweg 92, 3702 AD Zeist, The Netherlands.

(34), and magnetic resonance imaging (MRI) (4) have revealed in asymptomatic individuals findings similar to the morphology of disc protrusion and stenosis observed in symptomatic patients. The prevalence of these conditions correlates with age.

Similarly, degenerative changes of the lumbar spine are observed with equal prevalence in individuals with or without back pain and are more related to age than to symptoms. Therefore, the mere demonstration of radiographic changes, such as degeneration, disc protrusion, or stenosis, is not sufficient to prove that the observed pathology causes the symptoms of the patient.

How can we solve the diagnostic question "are the observed abnormalities the cause of symptoms or are they coincidental and unrelated to the patient's symptoms?" Theoretically, the probability of the observed imaging findings being symptomatic could be defined as data if the incidence of that pathology per age group is known. When similar findings have never been observed in asymptomatic people, the probability is that it is the cause of symptoms. At the other extreme, when the findings are occurring in every individual of the same age the probability is that it is asymptomatic.

To define whether the observed stenosis or disc protrusion is symptomatic, neurologic examination and neurophysiologic assessment are often helpful (Chapter 39), but sometimes they are not. Thus, precise determination of the symptomatic level in these patients is not possible on the basis of neurologic examination. In such cases techniques such as selective anesthetic blocks are then indicated.

The observed pathology is considered responsible for the patient's symptoms if they are relieved after infiltration with a local anesthetic. Steindler (27) postulated the following criteria:

- All symptoms of the patient, that is to say his or her typical pain pattern, must be reproduced by provocation. Provocation is the result of injection of small amounts of positive contrast medium or of hypertonic saline.
- Subsequently, complete relief of symptoms must be observed within 30 seconds after injection of a minimal amount of local anesthetic. The "minimal amount" relates to the reliability: large amounts of anesthetic will jeopardize the selectivity of the injection, as the fluid will diffuse into adjacent tissue, in particular in the area of the intervertebral foramen, where a number of significant structures are close to each other. One might consider adding adrenaline to decrease vascular transport of the anesthetic.
- Relief of symptoms must last at least 1 hour.

To Steindler's the following criteria must be added:

- Repetition of the test on another day must give the same response.
- The procedure must be radiographically controlled in two planes to make sure that the location of the needle tip is in close proximity to the lesion; in other words, the test has to be technically reliable.
- A positive response at one level has to be met by at least one negative response at a different level, because the response may be positive due to a placebo effect. This negative response is needed to enhance the internal validity of the test. When tests on different levels all yield a positive response, it is highly probable that the responses are positive due to a "placebo" effect.

Some reasonable criticisms remain despite these criteria: Kibler and Nathan (15) demonstrated that pain and paresthesia can be relieved by a nerve block distal to a lesion, and blocking a nerve innervating only part of a given region may relieve pain in the whole region. The postulate of Steindler seems also controversial in view of modern theories of the brain and spinal cord acting as a data processing and generating system. However, at this point there appears to be no better method available to define whether observed pathology is symptomatic or asymptomatic.

DISCOGRAPHY

Reliability of Technique

Posteroanterior and lateral radiographs after injection of the contrast medium have to be obtained by the examiner to assess reliably the location of the needle tip. These radiographs are also needed for documentation. As early as the late 1940s Lindblom (16), the initiator of discography, described false-positive images and pain provocation in patients due to annular injections of contrast medium. To avoid this the tip of the needle must be located in the center of the nucleus. A location close to the vertebral endplate is also incorrect, because with such an injection site one can provoke symptoms leading to a positive test result (false positive).

The lateral approach is widely accepted as the technique of choice (19). Only very rarely is a transdural approach indicated, i.e., in cases with the L5 disc space very deeply seated between the iliac crests.

To decrease the risk of infection the double needle technique (11) should be used: usually an 18-gauge needle is advanced to the outer annulus and then an inner needle (22–25 gauge) penetrates into the nucleus.

When the above precautions are met the reliability of the technique approaches 100%, because errors can be corrected during the procedure.

Reliability of Interpretation

Problems do not arise with the technique of discography but with the interpretation of the morphology on the images and of the pain response of the patient.

To make a comparison of the results of a diagnostic procedure possible, the same rating system has to be used by the various examiners. Because Adams and co-workers (2) correlated discography images to the stages of disc degeneration, their classification as modified by Simmons and co-workers (25) is recommended (Fig. 1). Their types 1 and 2 are normal discs, types 3 and 4 are discs with degenerative changes, and type 5 is a nondegenerative disc with a rupture in the annulus. Type 6 was added later and represents a nondegenerative disc with an endplate disruption. Unfortunately, the authors did not report the reliability of interpretation according to their classification. However, on a two-point scale ("normal" or "abnormal") this was done by Walsh and co-workers (32) from the University of Iowa Spine Center. They found a 96% "adjusted percent agreement" between five raters. Because the Adams classification is preferred from a morphologic point of view, further studies are needed to define the interobserver reliability.

The pain occurring on injection of the contrast medium is usually assessed in terms of "no pain," "atypical

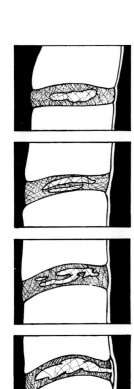

Cottonball
No signs of degeneration. Soft white amorphous nucleus.

Lobular
Mature disc with nucleus starting to coalesce into fibrous lumps.

Irregular
Degenerated disc with fissures and clefts in the nucleus and inner annulus.

Fissured
Degenerated disc with radial fissure leading to the outer edge of the annulus.

Ruptured
Disc has a complete radial fissure that allows injected fluid to escape. Can be in any state of degeneration.

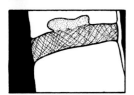

End Plate Fracture
Disruption of end plate.

FIG. 1. The six types of discograms and the stages of disc degeneration they represent. Adapted from Adams et al. (2).

pain," or "concordant pain." The last is pain recognized by the patient as "normal" pain. Often a further differentiation in total or partial reproduction of pain is used. Again, the only study on reliability is the Iowa study wherein Weinstein and his colleagues used the "pain thermometer" developed by Roland and Morris (24) which indicates levels of pain on a six-point scale (0 = no pain, 1 = minimum, 2 = moderate, 3 = bad, 4 = very bad, 5 = unbearable). They classified the pain response as positive when the intensity was 3 or more. Also, the provoked pain had to be similar to the typical pattern of the patient's pain. Furthermore, they assessed "pain-related behavior" by evaluating videotapes made of the patient during each discography procedure. They used a modified pain (26) behavior rating by Keefe (14), which

scores five types of pain-related behavior: guard/brace/withdraw, rubbing, grimacing, sighing, or verbalizing. When the patient demonstrated two or more of these expressions, pain-related behavior was considered to be present.

The reliability defined in terms of the interrater agreement between two independent examiners was very good for both intensity of pain and pain-related behavior (Pearson's r of 0.99 for the former and 0.93 for the latter).

For the overall result of discography, positive or negative, a 100% agreement was reached. The authors defined a discogram as positive when an abnormal disc morphology was observed in combination with reproduction of the typical pain with an intensity score of 3 or more.

In a position statement on discography, the executive committee of the North American Spine Society (23) emphasized proper technique, including multiple levels so as to evaluate the reliability of the pain response. They also declared, "The amount of resistance to the injection should be quantified," but the way to achieve that goal was not described.

On the basis of my clinical experience I emphasize the significance of time spent by the examiner for the assessment of pain reproduction: to perform the procedure well a relaxed patient is essential, and the observer has to be alert and cognizant of the time needed to obtain information from a patient under the threat of pain. One must adhere to a standard protocol and standard documentation.

To increase the internal validity of the test in a given patient, a negative test response on a different level decreases significantly the chances of the positive test result being misinterpreted.

Diagnostic Value

Radicular Syndrome

In the past lumbar discography had been used (8) instead of oil-based myelography to diagnose a disc protrusion, extrusion, or sequestration causing nerve root entrapment. This technique also proved in those days to be a useful tool, particularly as it relates to lateral disc herniations (1). Today there is general consensus that MRI is the imaging technique of choice for most patients with a lumbar radicular syndrome. For discussion and references see Chapter 28.

Degeneration

Although provocative discography remains controversial (22), it is nevertheless used in many centers around the world to assess whether degenerative changes in patients with low back pain with or without nonradicular pain are symptomatic or asymptomatic. To assess its diagnostic value a gold standard has to be employed. To that end the outcome of spinal fusion is often used. This remains suspect because it indicates a monofactorial relationship as to the origin of low back pain. That is obviously not correct; chronic back pain is a multifactorial phenomenon (31). Not only is it the symptomatic disc but other factors may be involved (18), i.e., trunk muscle condition and psychological processes such as somatization and operant conditioning. Thus, there are many problems in the use of the outcome of fusion as the gold standard. The fusion has to be solid. The current methods to define bony ankylosis of a lumbar spinal segment are still not 100% foolproof. Further, in a patient with bony ankylosis of an intertransverse fusion the disc may still generate nociceptive impulses and thus still be symptomatic (33). Therefore, the type of fusion, intercorporal versus intertransverse, has to be taken into account.

Although in biochemical research some progress has been made regarding the dilemma of symptomatic versus asymptomatic degeneration (10), there remains no reliable alternative to an anesthetic technique for use in daily clinical practice.

As noted, degenerative changes of the lumbar spine occur in many asymptomatic individuals (29) and their prevalence increases with age. To define, therefore, the false-positive rate for discography, data on the morphology of the disc in relation to age in asymptomatic individuals must be known, as well as data on the incidence of positive provocation of symptoms in a normal disc as well as in a degenerative disc in asymptomatic individuals. These data are as yet only partially available (32).

Many clinicians do not use lumbar discography as a diagnostic test on the basis of the study by Holt (12). However, this study remains controversial. Weinstein and his colleagues argue that some of Holt's statements were inconsistent with his data: in his text he reports 11 discs to be degenerate, and in those discs "usually severe pain was reported." However, he concludes "only 2 out of 9 degenerative discs were painful." Furthermore, the rate of false-positives was reported to be 36%. This was the ratio of the number of abnormal images to the number of technically correct injections. This means that Holt did not consider pain response as a criterion for a positive discogram: including the pain response, the false-positive rate would have been reported as 26%. Thirdly, as Holt also discusses, the contrast medium diatrizoate (Hypaque) is a known irritant to the nerve root, and therefore results should be excluded in patients with a ruptured disc because the dye leaking from the disc makes contact with the nerve root. Eliminating the 16 ruptured discs, the false-positive rate would be further reduced to only 4%.

But the most striking aspect is Holt's finding that 50% (15 of 30 individuals) had a pain-related response associated with at least one abnormal disc, indicating that half of the participants in the study had a positive discogram, whereas all of the participants were considered to be asymptomatic. On the basis of these data the authors question the effectiveness of the criteria that Holt used for characterizing individuals as asymptomatic. In particular, his data on having no history of pain in the back seem unreliable.

Therefore, the Iowa group repeated (32) Holt's study and found in 10 asymptomatic individuals, ranging in age from 18 to 32 years, that 5 (17%) of the 30 discs had abnormal morphology. This occurred in 5 of the 10 subjects. However, no positive pain response during injections in these subjects occurred. Therefore, the false-positive rate was 0 and the specificity 100% with a 95% confidence limit of 0.73–1.00, meaning that the specificity has a value between 73% and 100% with a probability of 95%. In the symptomatic group of 7 individuals with an age range of 26 to 60 years, 13 of 20 discs (65%) had abnormal morphology observed; thus, all 7 patients had abnormal discs at the previously operated level. Typical pain reproduction was reported in 8 discs in 6 patients. It was therefore concluded that the discogram was positive in 6 of the 7 patients. One annular injection was not included in the analysis. They mention that their study was not designed to define the false-negative rate (the sensitivity) of discography.

They concluded that the asymptomatic subjects had a lower percentage of positive discograms (0% versus 35%, $Z = 3.42$, $P < 0.0007$), a lower percentage of abnormal discographic morphology (17% versus 65%, $Z = 3.41$, $P < 0.0007$), a lower mean rating for intensity of pain, and on the average fewer pain-related behavioral signs. In comparing their results with the results of Holt's study the incidence of abnormal images in asymptomatic subjects was not significantly different; however, the false-positive rate was significantly lower. More studies using these methodologies and including larger numbers of individuals of all age groups need to be performed.

In the following section data on the diagnostic value of the outcome(s) of surgery, as a gold standard, will be discussed.

To define the sensitivity and the positive predictive value, Colhoun and co-workers of Oswestry (7) studied prospectively a group of patients with a solid bony ankylosis after anterior fusion for backache and pain referred to the lower limb in a nondermatomal pattern. Their criteria for assessing bony ankylosis were not clearly reported, although they observed, "Patients with a definite clear radiographic pseudarthrosis at the site of attempted fusion were excluded. A satisfactory clinical result was indicated by complete relief or significant subjective improvement in symptoms, resumption of work and/or normal duties and no intake of analgesics."

Assessing the discographic data, the sensitivity appeared to be 90% with the number of true positives 121 and false negatives 13. The positive predictive value was 88% on the basis of 121 true positives and 16 false positives. However, without taking the results of discography into account, 82%, 160 of 195 patients had a successful clinical result. This indicates that only a small improvement in prediction is achieved by the use of discography.

Reproduction of symptoms in normal discs in the Oswestry group was not a "feature," although "occasionally a patient had a mild backache or feeling of pressure." They also found a high rate of clinical success (93%) in patients with a morphologically abnormal but asymptomatic disc at the level adjacent to the symptomatic level, which therefore was not included in the fusion, indicating that the false-positive rate reported in the past is obviously far too high.

In a series of cases with major medicolegal implications, Milette and Melanson (20) reported reproduction of symptoms in 5% of 320 normal discs. Even if these examinations are valid, which is questionable due to the medicolegal situation, the false-positive rate of pain reproduction in normal subjects would not even be 2%. This corresponds to the findings of the Iowa group.

To the author it is obvious that there is a long way to go before the diagnostic value of discography is well defined. Nevertheless, discography appears to have some value in the armamentarium of diagnostic procedures.

Complications

The following early complications have been reported: disc space infection, retroperitoneal hemorrhage, allergic reactions and subarachnoid bleeding, nerve root sheath injuries, and annular or endplate injections due to incorrect needle placement resulting in a false-positive pain response. Ruling out faulty technique, only allergic reactions and the most serious complication, disc space infections, remain. Allergy to iodine can be prevented in the majority of patients, but discitis is a different issue.

Bernard (3) reported, out of 250 patients with 725 discs examined, only one case of disc space infection, an incidence of 0.13%. Fraser (11) found 2.7% of 222 patients acquired a disc space infection when an 18-gauge needle without a stilette was used, but this figure dropped to 0.7% in the 149 patients where a two-needle technique with stilettes was employed. In an additional experimental study, all contaminated discs demonstrated by 6 weeks the typical radiologic and histopathologic features of discitis, while most cultures were negative. This reported complication rate correlates with the author's experience; we have observed three cases of discitis in about 900 patients studied, or 2,600 levels of the lumbar spine.

Puncturing of the disc in and of itself could be harmful in the long run by causing early and progressive degeneration as a possible late complication. However, no evidence to support this speculation has been found in animal experiments or in human beings. On repeat discograms there have been no detrimental effects, although the size of the needle seems to be significant and must be small.

Indications

Reviewing the literature and our own experience, the author concludes that discography is indicated to define whether or not a degenerative lumbar segment is symptomatic.

The procedure seems to have a high specificity conditional on the fact that the test is technically performed correctly, including a proper assessment of pain provocation. The sensitivity and predictive value also seem high when discography performed at adjacent levels is negative. However, at this moment scientific proof is weak and needs to be strengthened.

In general terms a diagnostic procedure is indicated only when it bears consequences for treatment. This implies, in the case of discography, that the morbidity of the patient requires surgical management.

Discography is indicated in patients with severe incapacitating chronic (> 6 months) low back pain with or without "nonradicular" leg pain when all conservative measures have failed, the trunk muscle strength of the patient is normal, and psychological processes, in particular operant conditioning, are absent. Before surgical treatment is contemplated, these factors (often referred to as the *deconditioning syndrome* [18]) have to be treated. The following two conditions are possible:

1. Degeneration of one or more lumbar segments, without other pathology.
2. Nonspecific symptoms after lumbar decompression. This is of particular concern in patients after a wide decompression with denervation of the paraspinal muscles (17).

The indication for discography is minimal in patients with radicular symptoms unless the examination of choice, MRI, cannot be performed, and alternative methods such as CT scan or myelographically enhanced CT scan have yielded equivocal results. In cases of doubt neurophysiologic examination including evoked potentials is indicated. And in patients without neurologic disturbances, nerve root sheath infiltration can be of significant value (see below and Chapter 31).

FACET ARTHROGRAPHY

Reliability

No studies on the reliability of the technique and interpretation of facet arthrography have been published. However, many authors have stressed that the technique must include radiologic monitoring in anteroposterior and lateral projections to verify the correct intra-articular location of the needle tip. The easiest entrance to the joint in the majority of patients is the lower end, just distal to the articular processes. Because quantities of 2 to 3 ml of fluid can rupture the capsule (21), only very small volumes, to a maximum of 0.5 ml, should be used. That volume should include contrast medium and local anesthetic. Also, the injection should be performed slowly. As with discography, the typical pain of the patient should be reproduced by injection of contrast medium and relieved rapidly by intra-articular local anesthetic with that effect persisting at least 1 hour.

To increase the internal validity of the test, Aprill (see also Chapter 29) has advocated repeating the test on another day and addressed the significance of a negative test result on a different level to rule out the placebo effect. It is important that the patient be blinded to the level that is being injected.

In summary, the technique has been well described; however, the reliability of the technique and its interpretation have not.

Diagnostic Value

Many publications have described the therapeutic value; however, Jackson (13) and others have demonstrated that facet syndrome is not a distinct clinical entity, although the facet joint, like other synovial joints with a richly innervated capsule, can be a source of pain.

Regarding its diagnostic value no publications have been found which analyze the sensitivity and specificity of diagnostic facet joint blocks. But in one paper on the predictive value there was no significant correlation between the results of the facet joint block and the surgical outcome of fusion (9). Thus, the negative predictive value is unsatisfactory on the basis of this one paper.

The author does not argue that a facet joint, even a normal one, can be a source of pain. One could speculate that facet joints could be overloaded and a cause for pain in a patient with disc degeneration or with insufficient condition of trunk muscles.

Complications

No serious complications have been described. In particular, the rate of infection is apparently negligible.

Indications

Although the facet joint is an important source of back pain, a facet joint syndrome remains difficult to define, and facet joint blocks have not been proven to be predictive for the outcome of treatment, in particular fusion for a degenerative lumbar segment. Thus, today facet arthrography, as a diagnostic test, is a procedure in search of a cause.

Prospective, randomized studies for one level fusions are needed. These studies should control for other factors related to back pain, and a multifactorial design is necessary.

NERVE ROOT SHEATH INFILTRATION

Reliability of Technique

Hasue and Tajima (28) have reported that contrast medium injected into the epidural space may outline the nerve root and even the spinal nerve. Tajima argues that the contrast medium is "located between the nerve root and the epiradicular sheath depicting the nerve root in a tubular fashion." To the author it is not the image of the anatomy but the pain-response that is of significance: Castro and co-workers (5) have shown that the test is unreliable when large quantities of fluid, such as 1 ml or more, are used, because in the area of the spinal nerve outside the intervertebral foramen the upper proximal spinal nerve is often affected. Therefore, diffusion of a large quantity of local anesthetic will also block that spinal nerve, decreasing the selectivity of the test.

The experience of the author supports Castro's finding, and therefore the technique of choice is to use minimal amounts of fluid, preferably less than 0.5 ml, and not to rely on the anatomic image.

To obtain maximal technical reliability the needle tip should be located on anteroposterior and lateral views of the lumbar spine immediately below the pedicle on a line connecting the centers of two pedicles. No more than 0.5 to 0.7 ml, including contrast medium and local anesthetic, should be injected.

Reliability of Interpretation

On this topic no studies have been reported. In the experience of Hasue (see Chapter 31) and our own experience (6,30) however, it seems that the reproducibility and repeatability are high in experienced hands: "The examiner has to be experienced with the technique and even then has to take his time because the technique is demanding concentration from the examiner and patience and relaxation from the patient. This can be often hard under the threat of pain."

Diagnostic Value

Van Akkerveeken (6,30), being the first to define the sensitivity, specificity, and predictive value of this test, found 100% sensitivity, with a 95% confidence limit of

88–100%. In a series of 137 patients Hasue (see Chapter 31) had similar results. Due to the design of our study the specificity could not be established by us. At incidental observations in 23 patients, false positives were not observed. Hasue found a specificity of 57% (12 false positives out of 137 patients) in his study.

The predictive value for surgical decompression was 95% in our study, with a 95% confidence limit of 77–100%; Hasue found a similar figure of 93% in his population of 137 patients.

From two prospective studies it is concluded that the sensitivity and positive predictive value of the test are very high and that the test appears adequate to pinpoint the symptomatic level. However, not enough scientific data are available on the specificity of this test.

Complications

Temporary loss of neural function of the blocked nerve root may occur. Obviously this is not long-lasting and not an unexpected consequence. However, the patient has to be warned that it may happen. Also, temporary epidural anesthesia has been reported due to a needle tip located too far medially (30). Again, this generally lasts only a couple of hours. Significant and more serious complications have not been reported. However, incorrect interpretation may lead to operative treatment of the wrong level; this could be considered a major complication. For example, blocking the L4 nerve root at the L4 intervertebral foramen versus the L5 nerve root at the L5-S1 foramen. This may occur in particular, in inexperienced hands this may occur as radiologists are used to compression of the L5 nerve root by an L4-5 disc lesion. Therefore it is recommended to specify to the radiologist the specific nerve root at the specific intervertebral foramen to be examined.

Indications

As discussed for discography, this test is only indicated when surgical therapy is under consideration. The following indications have been reported:

1. Patients with intermittent claudication without canal stenosis but with signs of nerve root entrapment, usually due to degenerative changes, demonstrated with various imaging techniques.
2. Leg pain with signs of radiculopathy of more than one nerve root and/or roentgenographic evidence of nerve root entrapment. It is highly probable that only one nerve root is symptomatic, so that only that nerve root needs to be decompressed.
3. Patients with nerve root compression as demonstrated by a positive Lasègue test but without neurologic localizing signs and with radiologic observations inconsistent with the clinical presentation.
4. "Atypical" leg pain, no signs of nerve root compression, no radiculopathy, and radiologic signs of nerve root entrapment by degenerative changes of the lumbar spine.

If a roentgenographically entrapped nerve root proves to be symptomatic at nerve root sheath infiltration, unilateral interlaminar decompression of only that nerve root will yield a high chance (90%) of a successful outcome.

CONCLUSION

The reliability and diagnostic value of nerve root sheath infiltration are well studied and appear to be very good in experienced hands. It is indicated in diagnostic problems for patients who do not have localizing signs neurologically and/or neurophysiologically.

REFERENCES

1. Abdullah AF, Ditto EW, Byrd EB, Williams R (1974): Extremelateral lumbar disc herniations. Clinical syndrome and special problems of diagnosis. *J Neurosurg* 41:229–234.
2. Adams MA, Dolan P, Hutton WC (1986): The stages of disc degeneration as revealed by discograms. *J Bone Joint Surg* 68-B:36–41.
3. Bernard T (1990): Lumbar discography followed by computerized tomography: Refining the diagnosis of low back pain. *Spine* 15:690–707.
4. Boden S, Davis DO, Dina TS, Patronas NJ, Wiesel SW (1990): Abnormal magnetic resonance scans of the lumbar spine in asymptomatic subjects. *J Bone Joint Surg* 72A:403–408.
5. Castro WHM, Grönemeyer D, Jerosch J (1994): How reliable is lumbar nerve root sheath infiltration? *Eur Spine J* 3:255–257.
6. Castro WHM, Van Akkerveeken PF (1991): Der diagnostische Wert der selektiven lumbalen Nervenwurzelblockade. *Z Orthop* 129:374–379.
7. Colhoun E, McCall IW, Williams L, Cassar Publicino VN (1988): Provocation discography as a guide to planning operations on the spine. *J Bone Joint Surg* 70B:267–271.
8. Collis JS Jr, Gardner WJ (1962): Lumbar discography: An analysis of one thousand cases. *J Neurosurg* 19:452–461.
9. Esses SI, Moro JK (1993): The value of facet joint blocks in patient selection for lumbar fusion. *Spine* 18:185–190.
10. Franson RC, Saal JS, Saal JA (1992): Human disc phospholipase A2 is inflammatory. *Spine* 17:S129–132.
11. Fraser RD, Osti OL, Vernon-Roberts B (1987): Discitis after discography. *J Bone Joint Surg* 69B:26–35.
12. Holt EP Jr (1968): The question of lumbar discography. *J Bone Joint Surg* 50A:720–726.
13. Jackson RP (1992): The facet syndrome: Myth or reality? *Clin Orthop* 279:110–121.
14. Keefe FJ, Wilkins RH, Cook WA (1989): Direct observation of pain behaviour in low back pain patients during physical examination. *Pain* 20:59–68.
15. Kibler RF, Nathan PW (1960): Relief of pain and paraesthesiae by nerve block distal to a lesion. *J Neurosurg Psychiatry* 23:91–98.
16. Lindblom K (1948): Diagnostic puncture of intervertebral disks in sciatica. *Acta Orthop Scand* 17:231–239.
17. Macnab I, Cuthbert H, Godfrey CM (1977): The incidence of denervation of the sacrospinales muscles following spinal surgery. *Spine* 2:294–298.
18. Mayer TG, Gatchel RJ (1988): *Functional restoration for spinal disorders: The sports medicine approach.* Philadelphia: Lea & Febiger.

19. McCullogh JA, Waddell G (1978): Lateral lumbar discography. *Br J Radiol* 51:498–502.
20. Milette PC, Melanson D (1987): Lumbar discography. *Radiology* 163:828–829.
21. Moran R, O'Connell D, Walsh MG (1988): The diagnostic value of facet injections. *Spine* 13:1407–1410.
22. Nachemson A (1989): Editorial comment. Lumbar discography—where are we today? *Spine* 14:555–571.
23. North American Spine Society (1988): Position statement on discography. *Spine* 13:1343.
24. Roland M, Morris R (1983): A study of the natural history of back pain. Part 1. *Spine* 8:141–144.
25. Simmons JW, Emery SF, McMillin JN, Landa D, Kimmich SJ (1991): Awake discography. A comparison study with magnetic resonance imaging. *Spine* 16:S216–221.
26. Spratt KF, Lehmann TR, Weinstein JN, Sayze HA (1990): A new approach to the low back physical examination. Behavioral assessment of mechanical signs. *Spine* 15:96–102.
27. Steindler A (1940): Interpretation of sciatic radiation and syndrome of low back pain. *J Bone Joint Surg* 22A:28–34.
28. Tajima T, Furukawa K, Kuramochi E (1980): Selective lumbosacral radiculography and block. *Spine* 5:68–77.
29. Torgerson WR, Dotter WE (1976): Comparative roentgenographic study of the asymptomatic and symptomatic lumbar spine. *J Bone Joint Surg* 58A:850–853.
30. Van Akkerveeken PF (1989): *Lateral stenosis of the lumbar spine.* Thesis, Rijksuniversiteit Utrecht, the Netherlands.
31. Waddell G (1987): A new clinical model for the treatment of low back pain. *Spine* 12:632–644.
32. Walsh TR, Weinstein JN, Spratt KF, Lehmann TR, April C, Sayre H (1990): Lumbar discography in normal subjects. *J Bone Joint Surg* 72A:1081–1088.
33. Weatherly CR, Prickett CF, O'Brien JP (1986): Discogenic pain persisting despite solid posterior fusion. *J Bone Joint Surg* 68B:142–143.
34. Wiesel SW, Tsourmas N, Feffer HI, Citrin CM, Patronas N (1984): The incidence of positive CAT scans in an asymptomatic group of patients. *Spine* 9:549–551.

The Adult Spine: Principles and Practice,
2nd edition, J.W. Frymoyer, Editor-in-Chief.
Lippincott-Raven Publishers, Philadelphia © 1997.

CHAPTER 33

Other Diagnostic Studies: Electrodiagnosis

Russell H. Glantz and Scott Haldeman

The use of electrodiagnosis in the investigation of nerve root dysfunction is more than 35 years old (20,24). Initially, only needle electromyography was available for determining the presence of radiculopathy but in more recent times additional testing procedures have been developed. These tests include H reflexes, F responses, bulbocavernosus reflex responses, and somatosensory evoked responses. The purposes of these tests are not only to document the presence of radiculopathy, but also to determine its segmental level, and to have some estimate as to degree and chronicity of the nerve root dysfunction. After reviewing some anatomy and pathophysiology crucial to the understanding of electrodiagnosis, the different electrophysiologic procedures used will be discussed in detail. Following this, the benefits as well as pitfalls and limitations will be described.

ANATOMY

The spinal nerves are attached to the spinal cord by dorsal and ventral roots (Fig. 1). The majority of axons composing the ventral roots originate from cells in the anterior and lateral gray columns of the cord, whereas those composing the dorsal roots originate in the dorsal root ganglia. The dorsal root ganglia are situated distally along the dorsal roots near the point at which the latter join the anterior roots to form the spinal nerves. Hence, they are usually within the entrance of the bony intervertebral foramina (14). Immediately after exiting the intervertebral foramina, the spinal nerves terminate by dividing into anterior and posterior rami. The posterior rami innervate the paraspinal musculature and the anterior rami supply the limb muscles. The muscles sharing innervation from the same spinal cord segment and root constitute a myotome. Almost all muscles are constituents of more than one myotome, however, because they receive innervation from two or more contiguous roots (13). Needle electromyography is based entirely on finding abnormalities in these myotomal distributions. The cutaneous area served by fibers of a single root constitutes a dermatome. The territories of contiguous dermatomes overlap considerably. Many of the more recently introduced electrophysiologic techniques such as somatosensory testing assess the sensory component of the root by dermatomal stimulation (3).

PATHOPHYSIOLOGY

Spinal nerve root injury may be caused by a wide variety of mechanisms, although compression is the most common etiology. Other causes include stretch, infiltration, and even metabolic factors that may produce ra-

R. H. Glantz, M.D.: Associate Professor of Neurology, Department of Neurological Sciences, Rush Medical College, Rush-Presbyterian-St. Luke's Medical Center, Chicago, Illinois 60612.
S. Haldeman, M.D., Ph.D., F.R.C.P.: Associate Clinical Professor of Neurology, University of California, Irvine; and Los Angeles College of Chiropractic, Whittier, California 90609.

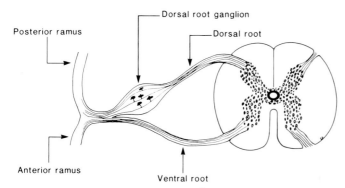

FIG. 1. Spinal nerve root anatomy. Note that the spinal nerves terminate by dividing into anterior and posterior rami.

diculopathy. Despite these possibilities, the nerve fiber itself only reacts to injury in two basic ways: (a) axon loss, resulting in the destruction of both the axon and its covering myelin sheath, and (b) those processes that affect only the myelin (focal demyelination), leaving the axons intact (11). Axonal degeneration is the usual end result of any severe focal nerve injury. Mild axon loss may produce few if any clinical abnormalities, but more severe axon loss is invariably associated with motor and/ or sensory dysfunction. The needle electromyography part of the examination is most frequently affected by axonal loss and this will be discussed subsequently.

With less severe focal nerve trauma, insufficient to cause axon loss, focal demyelination may occur. If the focal myelin loss is significant enough, muscle weakness will also be present, indistinguishable clinically from that due to axon loss. However, unlike the situation with axon loss, muscle atrophy does not occur and recovery is usually fairly rapid and complete once the compression is relieved and the myelin has had an opportunity to regenerate. As will be discussed, the needle electromyogram (EMG) examination in a pure myelin loss situation will be normal whereas some of the other electrodiagnostic parameters may show abnormality.

ELECTROPHYSIOLOGIC PROCEDURES USED IN THE DIAGNOSIS OF RADICULOPATHIES

Needle Electrode Examination (EMG)

EMG is still the most useful electrodiagnostic procedure in the evaluation of radiculopathies (9). A bipolar or monopolar needle electrode is inserted into a muscle and the electrical activity in the muscle is measured by oscilloscope under various functional conditions. A normally innervated muscle is quiet at rest and the oscilloscope shows a flat or straight line. If the muscle is denervated, as may occur in radiculopathy, there may be ongoing spontaneous activity at rest. The abnormal spontaneous waves may be in the form of fibrillation po-

tentials, positive sharp waves, or fasciculations. Examples of these abnormal potentials can be seen in Figure 2. Fibrillation potentials and positive sharp waves tend to develop in the muscles within the myotome in a proximal to distal sequence. Following onset of an acute lesion, they may be found after 6 or 7 days in the paraspinal muscles but require 5 to 6 weeks before appearing in the distal extremity muscles (20), although they may be seen by 3 weeks in the proximal extremity muscles. Examination of the paraspinal muscles as well as the limb muscles is important. Spontaneous activity in the paraspinal muscles indicates that the lesion affects the fibers of the posterior primary ramus and is therefore within or near the intraspinal canal (4).

Although the assessment of paraspinal muscles is of unquestioned benefit in the diagnosis of radiculopathies it does have limitations. The paraspinals may not show spontaneous activity with proven radiculopathies. This is because nerve fibers supplying them are spared due to incomplete root involvement, or the duration of the lesion is such that they have become reinnervated. Secondly, the presence of paraspinal spontaneous potentials is not synonymous with radiculopathy because they can result from such things as localized paraspinal muscle trauma, metastases to the posterior primary ramus, anterior horn cell disease, inflammatory and toxic myopathies, and diabetes mellitus. Thirdly, examination of the paraspinals may be more difficult than the limb muscles because satisfactory muscle relaxation can be difficult to achieve. Fourth, the extensive myotomal overlap makes it difficult to determine the particular root involved by the paraspinal evaluation alone. Finally, paraspinal muscle evaluation is of doubtful value in patients who have

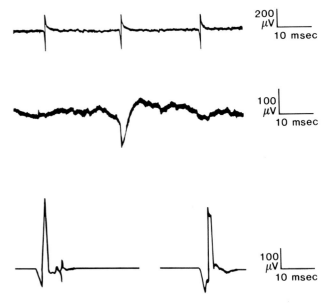

FIG. 2. Examples of abnormal potentials. Upper = fibrillations; middle = positive sharp wave; lower = fasciculations.

had previous spinal surgery, because any abnormality found could be related to damage to the posterior rami at the time of surgery. On the other hand, if these factors are taken into consideration, paraspinal abnormalities are extremely useful in the diagnosis of many radiculopathies. Whereas confirmation in myotomally equivalent extremity muscles is also sought, it is common clinical experience that the extremity finding may be minimal or negative with more prominent findings in the paraspinal musculature. In this situation, although the exact level of the radiculopathy cannot be stated because of the extensive myotomal overlap, a statement can at least be made that there was some dysfunction in the distribution of the posterior primary ramus.

After evaluation for the presence or absence of abnormal spontaneous activity, the patient is asked to contract the muscle that is being studied with minimal force, and at that time the morphology of a motor unit potential can be evaluated. The shape, amplitude, duration, and number of phases of the potential are determined and can be compared with motor unit potentials seen in a muscle that is healthy and has a normal nerve supply. After denervation, there will be an attempt to reinnervate muscle fibers with adjacent healthy neurons through sprouting of collateral axons, which then find their way and make synaptic connections with the denervated muscle fibers. This results in higher amplitude (giant) motor unit potentials with increased duration and number of phases (polyphasia) (Fig. 3). Lastly, the patient is asked to contract the muscle maximally and the nature of the increase in activity (recruitment pattern) and the number, duration, and amplitude of the electrical activity generated on maximal contraction (the interference pattern) are determined.

Therefore, a number of conclusions can be reached through EMG analysis. Firstly, the differentiation of acute from chronic denervation can be made. The acute changes result in the fibrillation potentials, positive sharp waves, and fasciculation during the resting phase, and the chronic changes result in the larger or giant motor unit potentials with polyphasia. Secondly, the severity of nerve dysfunction can also be estimated, although this is relatively crude. The quantity of denervation potentials allows some determination of the extent of the radiculopathy, but perhaps more important is the determination of the nature of the recruitment and degree to which a muscle is able to generate an interference pattern. A muscle that is affected only slightly may show abnormal potentials but still may be able to generate a full interference pattern. A more severely denervated muscle may be able to generate only weak interference patterns. Lastly, the level of a radicular injury can be determined within 1 or 2 segments by means of EMG. This is accomplished by testing multiple muscles in the extremity as well as paraspinal muscles and correlating the pattern of abnormality with the known anatomic distribution of each nerve root to the involved muscles.

As mentioned above, even when all facts are taken into account, needle electromyography remains the mainstay in the electrodiagnostic evaluation of radiculopathy. Aiello (1,2) report 71 to 100% true positive findings in patients with surgically documented disc herniation depending on the level of the involved intervertebral disc. Young et al (31) found that when needle EMG sampled multiplied muscles, it could correctly predict the level of radiculopathy in 84% of patients with clinical findings of nerve root pathology. In this study, the findings were negative in all patients without root pathology, but missed the level in 16% of cases.

H Reflex

The H reflex is a monosynaptic spinal reflex with both motor and sensory pathways traveling through the S1 nerve root by large diameter nerve fibers. The reflex is elicited by recording the electrical response generated by the soleus muscle on stimulation of the posterior tibial nerve in the popliteal fossa. A direct, early, or M-response resulting from the stimulation of the motor nerve is elicited. This is followed at approximately 23–32 ms following the stimulus (depending on age, leg length, and other factors) by a second contraction of the soleus muscle which is the H reflex response (Fig. 4). It first increases in amplitude with low stimulus intensities and then decreases in amplitude as the stimulus intensity increases. An absent H reflex correlates well with an S1 radiculopathy (24) and this in turn has been found to correlate well with an absent deep tendon reflex at the Achilles tendon. However, in milder S1 radiculopathies, the findings may not be as helpful in the diagnosis. One looks not only for latency changes (compared to the contralateral limb) but also for amplitude alterations. Fas-

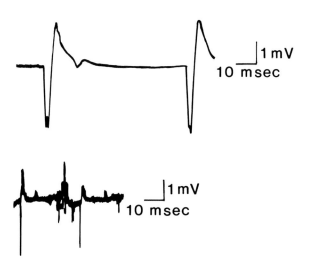

FIG. 3. Abnormal motor unit potentials. Upper = giant motor unit potentials; lower = polyphasic motor unit potential.

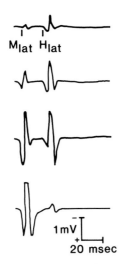

M_lat H_lat

1 mV

20 msec

FIG. 4. The H reflex.

tidious technique is always required and unless the electromyographer is experienced, subtle amplitude or latency changes may not permit a definitive diagnosis on the basis of the H reflex.

The other disadvantage of the H reflex is that it can only, under normal circumstances, be elicited in the soleus muscle, and is therefore of value only in studying S1 radiculopathies. Also, an abnormal H reflex is not synonymous with an S1 radiculopathy because it is mediated over a long pathway, which includes the tibial and sciatic nerves, sacral plexus, and spinal cord, as well as the S1 motor and sensory roots. Lesions at any of these levels can cause identical H reflex abnormalities. Additionally, once an H reflex is unelicitable because of S1 root compromise, it often remains so indefinitely. Thus, the procedure offers very little assistance in evaluating patients with prior S1 radiculopathies, particularly those who have undergone lumbar laminectomy. Finally, H reflexes are often absent bilaterally in patients with polyneuropathies and in persons over 60 years of age.

On the other hand, the H reflex has two advantages when added to EMG in the diagnosis of lumbar-sacral radiculopathies. It becomes abnormal immediately or shortly after an injury to the S1 nerve root, and it is abnormal in a strictly sensory S1 radiculopathy. In summary, therefore, the H reflex should be considered complementary to rather than replacing the EMG.

F Response

The F responses are late responses that can be recorded from a muscle after maximal stimulation of its nerve. The electrical stimulus that elicits the direct motor response also leads to an antidromic volley in the motor nerve and this activates a certain number of anterior horn cells in the spinal cord, causing orthodromic impulses to pass along the involved motor axons, thereby

generating F responses (22). The response is often inconsistent and of small amplitude when compared to the direct motor response and can show considerable variation in latency. For this reason it is necessary to elicit at least 10 responses for every tested nerve and to use the shortest or minimal latency. An example of an F response is illustrated in Figure 5.

The advantage of the F response is that it becomes abnormal immediately after an injury and may be the only early electrodiagnostic abnormality in patients with radiculopathy. It was hoped that the F wave response would be a valuable tool in the evaluation of patients with radiculopathies or other proximal nerve lesions. Initially high yields were claimed but subsequent experience has shown that F response studies are disappointing in patients with clinically unequivocal cervical and lumbar radiculopathies; frequently the studies are normal, and when abnormal, they are often redundant because EMG abnormalities are present as well. The reasons for this low sensitivity may be that F waves assess the functional integrity of only motor fibers. Secondly, many muscles from where this response is measured receive innervation from multiple nerve roots and the F response may be normal when only one of these nerve roots is damaged. Thirdly, because of the long motor pathway being assessed, even if focal slowing is present, the affected portion of the motor pathway is so small compared with the total pathway that any slowing may be obscured. Fourthly, even if an F response abnormality is present it is not diagnostic of radiculopathy. Similar to the H reflex, the F wave is mediated over a long pathway extending from the recorded muscle to the spinal cord and a motor fiber lesion at any level can cause an identi-

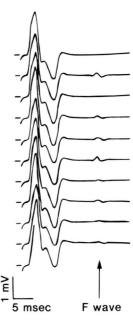

1 mV

5 msec   F wave

FIG. 5. The F wave or F response. Note that the response is inconsistent and of small amplitude.

cal F wave change. Lastly, the F response, like the H reflex, cannot distinguish between acute and chronic radiculopathies.

Conventional Motor and Sensory Nerve Conduction Studies

Motor and sensory nerve conduction studies are usually within normal limits with most single radiculopathies. Because of its physical location, the dorsal root ganglion is usually not traumatized by most causes of compressive radiculopathies. As a result, the sensory nerve action potentials are generally unaffected in the typical compressive radiculopathy, regardless of whether focal demyelination or axonal degeneration has occurred (5). This is true even in the presence of a significant clinical sensory deficit. This is because the lesion is proximal to the dorsal root ganglion and therefore has no effect on the dorsal root ganglion or its peripheral fibers. With a significant amount of axonal degeneration from radiculopathy, the amplitude of the compound muscle action potential may be reduced. Significantly low amplitude responses are seldom seen with partial single root lesions for two reasons. Firstly, the root compromise is incomplete and rarely do the majority of motor fibers degenerate. Secondly, another root also innervates the affected muscle, and its fibers are not involved (28). Therefore the amplitudes are likely to be low only in radiculopathies where the axonal degeneration has been very severe or when more than one root supplying the muscle has been affected. Even when radiculopathy is strongly suggested from the clinical point of view, it is still important to do at least one motor and sensory peripheral nerve conduction. Sometimes distal peripheral neuropathies coexist with radiculopathies and it is therefore good practice to screen the more distal aspects of the extremity.

Somatosensory Evoked Potentials (SEPs)

Electromyography and F responses have, as a primary shortcoming, the inability to detect either a spinal cord lesion or a purely sensory radiculopathy. With the development of relatively inexpensive electrodiagnostic instruments capable of computer averaging of small potentials, there has been a growing interest in the measurement of spinal and cortical potentials on stimulation of peripheral structures. These so-called somatosensory evoked potentials or responses can be divided into four basic categories. Although this topic is discussed in detail in Chapter 34, their discussion focuses on intraoperative monitoring and the detailed technical issues in spinal cord monitoring. Here we will focus on the use of these devices as diagnostic tools, which may be of use in the evaluation of spinal disorders.

Large Mixed Nerve SEPs

These potentials are measured over the proximal part of a peripheral nerve, the spinal cord, and the scalp on stimulation of the large mixed (motor and sensory) peripheral nerves (Fig. 6). The most common nerves stimulated are the posterior tibial and peroneal nerves in the lower extremities and the median and ulnar nerves in the upper extremities (7,19). It is, however, possible to obtain at least cortical evoked responses on stimulation of any nerve which is accessible to an electrode. It was initially hoped that these potentials would be able to detect sensory radiculopathies. However, the large mixed nerves carry fibers from multiple nerve roots so that a single level radiculopathy rarely causes any significant change in these potentials. This has virtually eliminated this test as a method of detecting nerve root lesions.

Mixed nerve evoked potentials, on the other hand, do have the ability to monitor certain spinal cord pathways and are quite sensitive in detecting certain types of spinal cord compromise. The use of these tests in the detection of spinal cord injuries, multiple sclerosis, spinal cord tumors, and cervical spondylodegenerative myelopathies has been widely documented and used. It must be remembered, however, that these potentials monitor only a portion of the spinal cord and a normal response does not exclude the possibility of a significant, usually motor, lesion in the spinal cord.

It is this property of mixed nerve SEPs that has led to their widespread use in monitoring the integrity of the spinal cord during scoliosis and decompressive surgery. The monitoring of these potentials after distractive or decompressive procedures can give useful information concerning the integrity of the spinal cord and has been demonstrated to be capable of reducing the incidence of

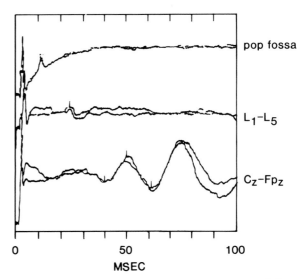

FIG. 6. An example of the mixed peripheral nerve SEPs on stimulation of the posterior tibial nerve.

postsurgical paralysis. The monitoring of these potentials, however, requires a knowledgeable and experienced clinician as the influence of anesthetics and interference from other equipment in the operating room can greatly alter the nature of an evoked response. This in turn can be misinterpreted as a disturbance caused by the surgery.

Small Sensory Nerve Evoked Potentials (SSEPs)

These potentials were initially studied in an attempt to isolate single level sensory radiculopathies (8). In the lower extremity the saphenous, superficial peroneal, cutaneous, and sural nerves are thought to reflect L4, L5, and S1 radiculopathies respectively. Stimulation of these small sensory nerves and recording the evoked cortical responses initially seemed to show a high correlation with documented radiculopathies. These responses have the additional advantage of being able to record a peripheral sensory nerve potential (SNAP) at the same time by recording over the nerve proximal to the stimulation site. This allows an internal control of the recording and helps to reduce the likelihood that poor electrode placement or an undetected peripheral neuropathy may be responsible for an abnormal response.

Unfortunately, some of the initial enthusiasm for this technique has not held up under greater scrutiny. These responses appear to be neither as sensitive nor as specific as initially hoped. They are, however, still of value as a complementary test to EMG and the reflex studies when a primary sensory nerve injury or radiculopathy is suspected.

Dermatomal Somatosensory Evoked Potentials (DSEPs)

An attempt to make the somatosensory evoked potentials more specific resulted in the direct stimulation of the skin and the recording of cortical responses (15,18,23). When applied to the skin representing a specific dermatome, the scalp potential obtained is called a dermatomal somatosensory evoked response or potential.

Cortical potentials can be obtained on stimulation of virtually any peripheral area of skin. The specificity of this test for a particular dermatome, therefore, is dependent upon the accuracy of placement of the stimulating electrodes and the likelihood that the particular area of skin is, in fact, innervated by a particular nerve root. Typically, lower extremity DSEPs are obtained by stimulating the lateral foot (S1), the skin over the dorsum of the big and second toes (L5), and the medial aspect of the calf just above the ankle (L4) (Fig. 7). Upper extremity DSEPs are obtained using ring electrodes to stimulate the thumb (C6), middle finger (C7), and little finger (C8).

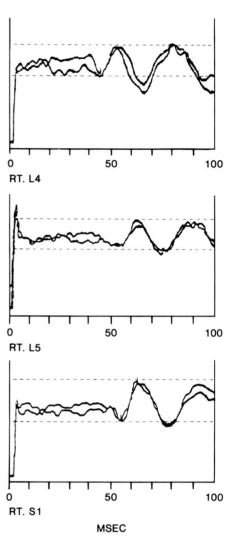

FIG. 7. Examples of normal DSEPs on stimulation of the L4, L5, and S1 nerve roots.

Any area of skin can, however, be stimulated and the test has been used to document such peripheral nerve disorders as meralgia parasthetica.

There have been a number of papers that have been very enthusiastic about the sensitivity of this test to sensory radiculopathies. Nonetheless DSEPs have not received universal acclaim. This is primarily due to excessive claims for sensitivity and the ease with which this test can be misinterpreted by an overzealous electrodiagnostician. The recording of DSEPs can also be technically demanding and requires an experienced and qualified technician in order to obtain a recording clear enough to read accurately. In patients with unilateral lumbosacral radiculopathy, one study showed a diagnostic yield of 25%, which is much lower than that of the EMG examination (3). However, when this technique is used in spinal stenosis, Snowden et al (27) demonstrated a sensitivity of 78% for multiple root disease and 93% for multiple plus single root disease.

Despite the problems with DSEPs, they appear to be

getting the greatest recognition for the documentation of sensory proximal lesions, including radiculopathy, that cannot be readily evaluated by peripheral nerve conduction studies. These studies, however, should be considered complementary to the clinical examination and electromyography. They do not, in any way, evaluate the motor component of a radiculopathy and have not been demonstrated to be as sensitive as electromyography in the diagnosis of nerve root lesions.

Magnetic stimulation of the spinal nerve roots is another technique for proximal stimulation (6). It is a painless test but does not consistently supramaximally stimulate the spinal nerves and may not detect abnormality (10,21).

Pudendal Evoked Responses (PERs)

All the tests listed so far in this chapter are used to evaluate the spinal cord, peripheral nerves, and nerve roots which innervate the upper and lower extremities. These tests, however, ignore the sacral nerve roots below S1. Lesions affecting these nerve roots can cause disturbances of bowel, bladder, and sexual function which can be incapacitating. Such disturbances are also often difficult to diagnose with confidence.

In order to fill this gap, attempts have been made to record spinal and cortical evoked responses on stimulation of organs innervated by the pudendal nerve (15,26). Cortical evoked responses have now been recorded in normal subjects and in patients with a variety of neurologic disorders. These evoked responses can be obtained by stimulating the dorsal nerve of the penis or clitoris using surface electrodes or by stimulating the urethra and anal sphincter using catheter electrodes. Spinal responses have only been recorded on stimulation of the dorsal nerve of the penis with ring electrodes. A recent modification allows for unilateral stimulation of the clitoral and penile nerves, which permits the documentation of neural deficits affecting only one pudendal nerve or only unilateral sacral nerve roots.

The major shortcoming of this test is the fact that only responses from sensory nerve fibers in the pudendal nerve are being recorded. In order to study the motor component of the pudendal nerve the bulbocavernosus reflex (BCR) can be recorded over the pelvic floor muscles on stimulation of the dorsal nerve of the penis or clitoris (26). Again, this can be accomplished on either unilateral or bilateral stimulation.

These tests have been correlated with cystometry, colonometry, and nocturnal tumescence in a variety of diseases (16,17). When these tests are used in a logical fashion and related to clinical symptoms, then a reasonable picture of the function of the sacral nerve roots and pudendal nerve can be obtained (11).

BENEFITS OF ELECTRODIAGNOSTIC EXAMINATIONS

The electrodiagnostic evaluation is the only laboratory study that directly assesses the physiologic integrity of the roots, thereby providing information of both diagnostic and prognostic relevance. Radiologic tests will not be helpful in patients with noncompressive radiculopathies and will also fail to indicate the severity or prognosis of compressive root lesions. Additionally, incidental radiographic abnormalities are common and electrophysiologic studies are important in determining whether anatomic abnormalities are of functional and clinical relevance. The electrodiagnostic study may also be abnormal when all other laboratory procedures, including radiographic ones, are unrevealing. Finally, electrophysiologic studies have low morbidity and can be used to follow the course of radiculopathies over time (29).

LIMITATIONS OF ELECTRODIAGNOSTIC EXAMINATIONS

Even with all of the new techniques included, electrodiagnosis does not detect all compressive radiculopathies. With some radiculopathies, although the clinical symptomatology may be prominent, the amount of actual axonal degeneration may be mild because only a few fibers are being compressed, and this makes the detection of radiculopathy difficult. The EMG examination is also very time-dependent. Studies may be falsely negative if they are performed too early or too late in the course of the radiculopathy. When the EMG is performed before sufficient time has elapsed for fibrillation potentials to develop fully throughout the myotome, the study may often be normal or inconclusive.

On the other hand, with chronic radiculopathies the EMG may be unrevealing, because muscles that had previously contained fibrillation potentials for a time after the onset of radiculopathy may have become completely reinnervated and therefore would not show any spontaneous activity. Even when changes consistent with radiculopathy are found on electrodiagnostic studies, some limitations are still present. The cause of the responsible process cannot be determined regardless of the electrodiagnostic procedure used in determining the radiculopathy. For example, similar findings may be obtained from nerve root compression by disc, tumor, or infarct. Although the root affected may have been determined, the anatomic site of the lesion, especially with regard to disc level, can only be estimated (18).

REFERENCES

1. Aiello I, Serra G, Migliore A, et al. (1983): Diagnostic use of H-reflex from vastus medialis muscle. *Electromyogr Clin Neurophysiol* 23:159–66.

2. Aiello I, Serra G, Tugnoli V, et al. (1984): Electrophysiological findings in patients with lumbar disc prolapse. *Electromyogr Clin Neurophysiol* 24(4):313–20.

3. Aminoff MJ (1986): Clinical electromyography. In: Aminoff MJ, ed. *Electrodiagnosis in clinical neurology,* 2nd ed. New York: Churchill Livingston, pp. 231–263.

4. Aminoff MJ, Goodin DS, Barbaro NM, et al (1985): Dermatomal somatosensory evoked potentials in unilateral lumbosacral radiculopathy. *Ann Neurol* 17:171–176.

5. Benecke R, Conrad B (1980): The distal sensory nerve action potential as a diagnostic tool for the differentiation of lesions in dorsal roots and peripheral nerves. *J Neurol* 223:231–239.

6. Chokroverty S, Sachdeo R, Dilullo J, Duvoisin RC (1989): Magnetic stimulation in the diagnosis of lumbosacral radiculopathy. *J Neurol Neurosurg Psychiatry* 52:767–772.

7. Dimitrijevic MR, Larsson LE, Lehmkuhl D, Sherwood A (1978): Evoked spinal cord and nerve root potentials in humans using a noninvasive recording technique. *EEG Clin Neurophysiol* 45:331–340.

8. Eisen A (1985): Electrodiagnosis of radiculopathies. *Neurol Clin* 3:495–510.

9. Eisen A, Hoirch M (1983): The electrodiagnostic evaluation of spinal root lesions. *Spine* 8:98–106.

10. Evans BA (1991): Magnetic stimulation of the peripheral nervous system. *J Clin Neurophysiol* 8:77–84.

11. Gilliatt R (1980): Acute compression block. In: Sumner A, ed. *The pathophysiology of peripheral nerve disease.* Philadelphia: Saunders, pp. 287–315.

12. Glick ME, Meshkinpour H, Haldeman S, Bhatia NN, Bradley WE (1982): Colonic dysfunction in multiple sclerosis. *Gastroenterology* 83:1002–1007.

13. Goodgold J, Eberstein A (1983): *Electrodiagnosis of neuromuscular diseases,* 3rd ed. Baltimore: Williams and Wilkins.

14. Goss CM, ed. (1973): *Gray's anatomy of the human body,* 29th ed. [American]. Philadelphia: Lea and Febiger, p. 1466.

15. Haldeman S (1984): The electrodiagnostic evaluation of nerve root function. *Spine* 9:42–48.

16. Haldeman S, Bradley WE, Bhatia N (1982): Evoked responses from the pudendal nerve. *J Urol* 128:974–980.

17. Haldeman S, Bradley WE, Bhatia NN, Glick ME, Ek A (1982): Neurologic evaluation of bladder, bowel and sexual disturbances in diabetic men. In: Goto Y, Horiuchi A, Kogure K, eds. *Diabetic neuropathy: Proceedings of the International Symposium on Diabetic Neuropathy and Its Treatment.* Tokyo, September 1981. Amsterdam: Excerpta Medica, pp. 298–301.

18. Haldeman S, Bradley WE, Bhatia NN, Johnson BK (1982): Pudendal evoked responses. *Arch Neurol* 39:280–283.

19. Jones SJ, Small DG (1978): Spinal and subcortical evoked potentials following stimulation of the posterior tibial nerve in man. *EEG Clin Neurophysiol* 44:299–306.

20. Lambert E (1973): Electromyography. In: Youmans J, ed. *Neurological surgery, vol. 1.* Philadelphia: Saunders, pp. 358–367.

21. McDonnell RAL, Cros D, Shahani BT (1992): Lumbosacral nerve stimulation comparing electrical with surface magnetic coil techniques. *Muscle Nerve* 15:885–890.

22. Panayiotopoulos CP (1979): F chronodispersion: A new electrophysiologic method. *Muscle Nerve* 2:68–72.

23. Scarff TB, Dallmann DE, Toleikis JR, et al (1981): Dermatomal somatosensory evoked potentials in the diagnosis of lumbar root entrapment. *Surg Forum* 32:489–491.

24. Schuchmann JA (1978): H reflex latency in radiculopathy. *Arch Phys Med Rehabil* 59:185–187.

25. Shea PA, Woods WW, Werden DH (1950): Electromyography in diagnosis of nerve root compression syndrome. *Arch Neurol Psychiatry* 64:93–104.

26. Siroky MB, Sax DS, Krane RJ (1979): Sacral signal tracing: The electrophysiology of the bulbocavernosus reflex. *J Urol* 122:661–664.

27. Snowden ML, Haselkorn JK, Kraft GH, Bronstein AD, Bigos SJ, Slimp JC, Stolov WC (1992): Dermatomal somatosensory evoked potentials in the diagnosis of lumbosacral spinal stenosis: Comparison with imaging studies. *Muscle Nerve* 15:1036–1044.

28. Wilbourn AJ (1982): The value and limitation of electromyographic examination and the diagnosis of lumbosacral radiculopathy. In: Hardy RW, ed. *Lumbar disc disease.* New York: Raven, pp. 65–109.

29. Wilbourn AJ, Aminoff MJ (1988): AAEE Minimonograph 32: The electrophysiologic examination in patients with radiculopathies. *Muscle Nerve* 11:1099–1114.

30. Wise CS, Ardizzone J (1954): Electromyography in intervertebral disc protrusions. *Arch Phys Med Rehabil* 35:442–446.

31. Young A, Getty J, Jackson A, Kirwan E, et al. (1983): Variations in the pattern of muscle innervation by the L5 and S1 nerve roots. *Spine* 8(6):616–24.

General Operative Considerations

The Adult Spine: Principles and Practice,
2nd edition, J.W. Frymoyer, Editor-in-Chief.
Lippincott-Raven Publishers, Philadelphia © 1997.

CHAPTER 34

Applications of Neurophysiological Measures During Surgery of the Spine

Jeffrey H. Owen and Tetsuya Tamaki

A complication associated with surgery of the spine is an intraoperatively induced postoperative neurological deficit. To detect the onset and possibly reverse the effects of a surgical complication, a variety of neurophysiological monitoring procedures can be employed. Based on the neural structures at risk, intraoperative neurophysiological procedures can be divided into two general categories: (a) methods for monitoring spinal cord function and (b) methods for monitoring nerve root function. The purpose of this chapter is to present information regarding the neurophysiological procedures administered during surgery that place the spinal cord or nerve roots at risk. Included will be developments of new monitoring techniques, as well as diagnostic and cost factors relating to these procedures. This chapter discusses currently available neurophysiological procedures, how the procedures are administered, and how the results can be applied to the patient, in order to assist the surgeon who

wishes to utilize neurophysiological monitoring during spine surgery.

BASIC ASSUMPTIONS OF INTRAOPERATIVE MONITORING

The primary purpose for intraoperative monitoring is to detect the onset of deleterious changes in the functional integrity of underlying neurological structures that result from either surgical or perisurgical variables. Secondary purposes for monitoring are to provide the surgeon with information regarding possible improvement in neurological function following surgical intervention and to determine the efficacy of salvaging techniques. To accomplish these purposes, a successful monitoring program must meet the following requirements: (a) the neurological pathways at risk must be at least partially intact; (b) the neurophysiological procedure must directly assess the functional integrity of these pathways; and (c) based on the neurophysiological data, the surgical technique can be modified.

A review of the literature reveals that many of the early neurophysiological techniques were only partially successful because they did not meet the basic requirements for monitoring. For example, while a postoperative sensory deficit should be avoided, the primary concern of

J. H. Owen, Ph.D.: Associate Professor, Department of Neurology, Johns Hopkins Medical Institutions, Baltimore, Maryland, 21287-7247.

T. Tamaki, M.D., Ph.D.: Professor and Chairman, Department of Orthopaedic Surgery, Wakayama Medical College, Wakayama, Japan, 641.

TABLE 1. *Neurophysiological monitoring procedures that can be administered during surgery that places the spinal cord at risk*

Posterior spinal fusion (PSF) below C6
    Posterior tibial nerve somatosensory evoked potentials (SEPs)
    Ulnar nerve SEPs
    Motor evoked potentials (MEPs)
Posterior spinal fusion at or above C6
    Posterior tibial nerve SEPs
    Median *and* ulnar nerve SEPs
    Motor evoked potentials
    Spontaneous and electrically triggered EMGs from upper extremity myotomes
Anterior spinal fusion below C6
    Posterior tibial nerve SEPs
    Ulnar nerve SEPs
    Femoral nerve SEPs (up-side leg)
    Peroneal nerve SEPs (down-side leg)
    Motor evoked potentials
Anterior spinal fusion at or above C6
    Posterior tibial nerve SEPs
    Median *and* ulnar nerve SEPs
    Motor evoked potentials
    Upper extremity EMGs

TABLE 2. *Neurophysiological procedures that can be administered during surgery that places nerve roots at risk*

Somatosensory evoked potentials
    Posterior tibial and ulnar nerve
    Dermatomal
Electromyographic (EMG) Recordings
    Mechanically elicited EMGs
    Electrically elicited EMGs

surgeons during surgery for the correction of a spinal deformity is a postoperative *motor* deficit. Originally, sensory-based somatosensory evoked potentials (SEPs) were used to monitor spinal cord function during these types of surgeries. The rationalization for using sensory-based potentials as opposed to a motor evoked potential, which is a direct measure of motor tract function, was based on the assumption that damage to spinal cord motor tracts also affects sensory tracts. However, because the SEP is sensory based, it did not meet the second requirement of a successful intraoperative monitoring technique; namely, it did not directly assess the functional integrity of the motor tracts. Consequently, there have been reports of false-negative SEP results relative to the presence of a postoperative motor deficit (5,13,53).

When determining which neurophysiological procedures should be administered, the neurophysiologist must ascertain the neurological structures at risk. Tables 1 and 2 list the procedures that should be chosen for pro-

cedures that place the neural structures at risk. Because their strengths and weaknesses vary, it is necessary to have an array of procedures available for use during surgery. To accomplish this type of testing, the monitoring instrumentation must be capable of simultaneously performing multiple procedures (47). By using a multimodality approach, the limitations of any individual procedure can be avoided, which will improve monitoring and reduce the incidence of postoperative neurological deficits.

SURGICAL MANEUVERS THAT AFFECT NEUROPHYSIOLOGICAL RESPONSES

Surgical maneuvers that affect the functional integrity of neural structures include overdistraction, compression, and derotation (translation) of the spinal column as well as direct mechanical forces applied to the nerve roots. From a neurophysiological perspective, these variables can be divided into two general categories: ischemic and mechanical. Table 3 lists the effects of ischemic and mechanical insults on evoked potentials. In general, ischemic insults have a slower onset of effect on the evoked potentials and appear to be more responsive to intervention than mechanical insults.

To appreciate the effects of ischemia and mechanical insults on the spinal cord, we performed anatomical studies on the spinal cord in pigs prior to and following ischemia and mechanical insults. To determine the effects of these maneuvers on spinal cord perfusion and

TABLE 3. *Neurophysiological "signature" of ischemic versus mechanical insults to underlying neural tissue*

	Ischemic	Mechanical
Time-to-onset of change in electrophysiological response	Slow	Rapid
Source of insult	Reduced spinal cord/nerve root perfusion from overdistraction (primary), hypotension (secondary)	Overdistraction, compression, derotation of the spinal cord, and/or nerve root irritation from transpedicular instrumentation
Typical spinal level of occurrence	More flexible segments of the spine	Spinal cord—more stiff segments Nerve roots—at any level
Responsiveness to intervention	Good	Poor
Effect on response characteristics	Latency—no significant change Amplitude—significantly reduced	Latency—significantly prolonged Amplitude—significantly reduced

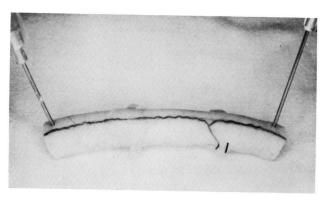
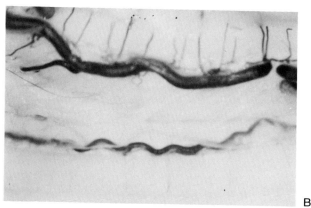

FIG. 1. Normal surface (**A**) and internal (**B**) perfusion in a pig's spinal cord under normal tension without any mechanical forces in place. (*Dark color* is blue silastic.)

anatomy, we injected the aorta with a blue silastic and allowed it to perfuse the spinal cord under normotension. Three groups of pigs were used: normal, animals administered ischemic maneuvers, and animals administered overdistraction. Figure 1 shows normal surface and normal internal perfusion of the spinal cord. To demonstrate ischemia, we overdistracted the spinal cord to an extent that a reduction in spinal cord perfusion occurred. Figure 2 shows a significant length of the spinal cord that was not being perfused on the surface or internally.

To demonstrate mechanical/structural changes to the spinal cord, we overdistracted the spinal cord from a pig to the point of anatomical disruption. Figure 3 depicts spinal cord perfusion and structure on the surface and internally following significant overdistraction. While this latter type of overdistraction is not typically administered during surgery, it does provide an indication of the effects of significant mechanical insult on spinal cord structure. As indicated in Figure 3, localized ischemia in the area of mechanical damage differed significantly from the ischemia depicted in Figure 2. Internally, the

spinal cord demonstrated structural changes that included mechanical disruption of the tissue as well as infiltration of blood into surrounding tissue.

A comparison of the effects of ischemia (Fig. 2) with the effects of mechanical insult (Fig. 3) showed that ischemia produces a multilevel reduction in spinal cord perfusion and a concomitant slow degradation in evoked potential response amplitude. There is little change in the latency of the evoked potential (33). Mechanical insult resulted in localized ischemia and structural damage, which are associated with a rapid degradation in the evoked potentials, which included an increase in response latency and a degradation in response amplitude (3,71).

OVERVIEW OF NEUROPHYSIOLOGICAL MONITORING

Neurophysiological procedures administered during spinal surgery must meet certain requirements, which vary as a function of surgery type. During surgeries for

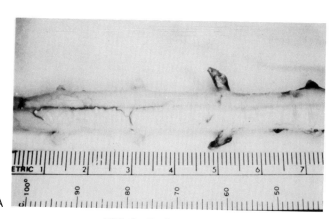
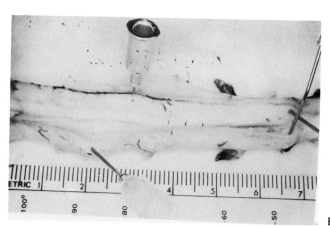

FIG. 2. Surface (**A**) and internal (**B**) ischemia in a pig's spinal cord following overdistraction.

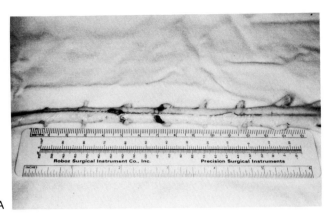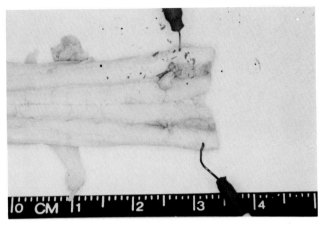

FIG. 3. Surface (**A**) and internal (**B**) ischemia and structural changes in a pig's spinal cord.

spinal deformities, it is necessary for the neurophysiological procedures to provide a direct measure of spinal cord sensory and motor tracts. However, during surgery for spinal degeneration, the neurophysiological procedures must be sensitive to individual nerve root function. A mixed nerve SEP would be an appropriate procedure to administer during surgery for spinal deformity; however, it would be inappropriate to use this procedure to monitor nerve root function.

MONITORING TO PROTECT THE SPINAL CORD

In order to monitor spinal cord function during surgery that places the spinal cord at risk, it is necessary that

appropriate neurophysiological procedures be administered. Traditionally, SEPs have been used to monitor during these surgeries. However, more recently, procedures that elicit motor evoked potentials (MEPs) have also been administered in conjunction with SEP-eliciting procedures. By recording both SEPs and MEPs, information regarding the spinal cord and sensory and motor tracts is obtained.

SEPs: Elicitation and Recording

To monitor the functional status of the sensory tracts within the spinal cord during surgery for spinal deformity, a mixed nerve SEP is used. Table 4 lists the primary sites for eliciting the SEP as a function of surgical level.

TABLE 4. *Acquisition parameters for eliciting and recording mixed-nerve somatosensory evoked potentials*

	Surgery above C6	Surgery at/below C6
Stimulation sites		
Primary	Median nerve, ulnar nerve, Posterior tibial nerve	Posterior tibial nerve (PSF, ASF) Peroneal nerve, femoral nerve, (ASF)
Secondary	Peroneal nerve, femoral nerve, axilla	Peroneal nerve
Recording sites		
Cortical	F_{pz}–C_{p3} F_{pz}–C_{pz} F_{pz}–C_{p4}	F_{pz}–C_{p1} F_{pz}–C_{pz} F_{pz}–C_{p2}
Cervical	Rostral to surgical level	F_{pz}—4th–5th cervical spine
Peripheral	Erb's point Popliteal fossa	Popliteal fossa
Filters		
Cortical	30–250 Hz	30–250 Hz
Cervical/peripheral	30–2000 Hz	30–2000 Hz
Stimulus rate	4.7/sec	4.7 sec
Time base	Upper extremity stim: 50 msec Lower extremity stim: 100 msec	
Intensity	Saturation level	
Sensitivity	Equivalent to a 10% rejection ratio	

PSF, posterior spinal fusion; ASF, anterior spinal fusion.

In general, during posterior spinal fusion (PSF) surgeries below C6, the primary site of stimulation is the posterior tibial nerve. During anterior spinal fusion (ASF), our protocol is to add femoral and peroneal nerve stimulation. When surgery is at or above C6, the primary stimulation sites include the median, ulnar, and posterior tibial nerves. To stimulate the median and ulnar nerves, the primary sites of stimulation are at the wrist. However, if these sites are not available (e.g., because of IV lines, etc.), alternative sites such as the antecubital fossa and ulnar groove can be used. As a last resort, the axilla can be stimulated, but the response loses its specificity as to which nerve is actually being stimulated (the median or the ulnar).

In some instances, it is not possible to stimulate at typical sites because of swollen or fractured ankles, peripheral neuropathies, and so on. In these instances, alternative stimulation sites such as the popliteal fossa should be considered. When stimulating at the popliteal fossa, the posterior nerve and the peroneal nerve are probably being stimulated. Although specificity of which nerve is being stimulated is lost, the response is more reliable and larger, and it still provides information regarding spinal cord function.

The neurophysiologist must ensure that the site of SEP elicitation is caudal to the level of surgery and that the recording sites are rostral. By doing so, the stimulus-elicited neurological activity will progress through the site of surgery. This assumption seems to be fairly basic; however, a review of the literature reveals instances in which this requirement was not met. In Lesser et al. (34), several case studies were reported in which the clinical utility of SEPs was investigated. The goal was to determine the occurrence of postoperative neurological deficits in patients who have "normal" intraoperative SEPs. A review of their cases indicates that in at least two instances, SEPs were elicited by stimulating the median nerve during a surgical procedure in which the operation was being performed at C7 and C8. Lesser et al. interpreted this as a weakness in SEP monitoring. However, this interpretation is not correct. By stimulating the median nerve, the SEP entered the spinal cord rostral to the level of surgery and did not travel through the surgical site. Not only did testing not provide the surgeon with any information regarding spinal cord function, but the false-negative results suggested that SEP monitoring was not useful as a measure of spinal cord function. The neurophysiologist must ensure that the sites of stimulation and recording relative to the levels of surgery are appropriate.

Regardless of the site of stimulation, it is necessary to use peripheral, cervical, and cortical recording sites to record the SEP. While the specific sites used will vary as a function of the level of surgery, multiple recording sites ensure that more reliable data are obtained. In a study by Owen et al. (54), SEPs were monitored during surgery for

neuromuscular scoliosis. When using a single-channel cortical recording site, the false-positive rate of the SEPs to posterior tibial nerve stimulation was 28%. These results agreed with those reported by Ashkenaze et al. (2) and Lubicky et al. (36). However, when a cervical recording site was added, the false-positive rate for SEPs decreased to 9%. Using a combination of cervical and cortical recording sites enabled monitoring of spinal cord function in patients who typically have demonstrated a high false-positive rate when only a single-channel cortical SEP was used.

As indicated in Table 4, an array of cortical, cervical, and peripheral sites are used to ensure that a reliable response is obtained. The use of a montage of three cortical recording sites is based on work by Nuwer (43), who reported that this improved the reliability and redundancy of the SEP. We have modified that technique somewhat so that the recording electrodes are placed primarily over the homuncular region of the somatosensory cortex that represents the anatomical sites of stimulation. For example, for surgeries below C7, we have found that by placing electrodes over the lower limb homunculus, SEPs elicited by posterior tibial nerve stimulation demonstrate superior redundancy and reliability as compared to either a single-channel cortical recording site or a recording site that uses different montages. Figure 4 depicts SEPs recorded cortically, cervically, and peripherally following right posterior nerve stimulation. As indicated in Figure 4, well-defined responses were present at the popliteal fossa, cervically, and at the three cortical sites. In addition to providing increased redundancy and reliability, multiple cortical recording sites demonstrate a paradoxical characteristic: responses recorded from the cor-

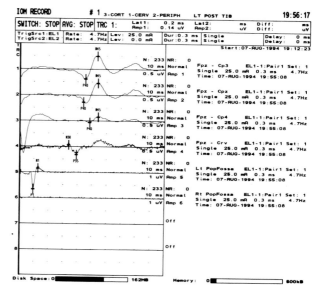

FIG. 4. Normal SEPs following posterior tibial nerve stimulation responses were recorded at C_{p1}, C_{pz}, C_{p2}, 4th-5th cervical vertebra, and the left popliteal fossa (*top to bottom*).

tex *ipsilateral* to the side of stimulation demonstrate a significantly larger amplitude than the responses recorded contralaterally (54).

When developing an intraoperative monitoring (IOM) program, there must be a reason to administer every aspect of the procedures. For example, there are two different reasons to record a peripheral and a cervical response. The peripheral response allows the examiner to determine if the stimulus has been neurologically encoded and has progressed rostrally. We routinely record the peripheral response during the collection of baseline data but do not typically record it during the entire surgery, because continuous recording of the peripheral response does not provide information regarding spinal cord function, which is the primary purpose for monitoring. Therefore, we collect a peripheral response during surgery only if there are any questions regarding neural encoding of the stimulus.

The cervical response is recorded because of its resistance to anesthetic agents. The cervical response, so called because of the site of its recording, originates within the brainstem and is smaller in amplitude and slightly more difficult to record than the cortical SEP. However, its resistance to anesthetic agents outweighs any limitations associated with it.

Figure 5 depicts SEPs elicited by stimulating at the left medial malleolus. In this figure, SEPs were recorded at the popliteal fossa, cervically, and cortically. During surgery, changes in anesthesia occurred that resulted in a degradation of the cortical component but no significant change in the cervical or peripheral component. These

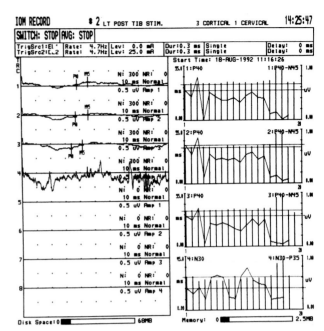

FIG. 6. SEPs demonstrating absent cortical and cervical responses following contact of a sublaminar wire with the spinal cord.

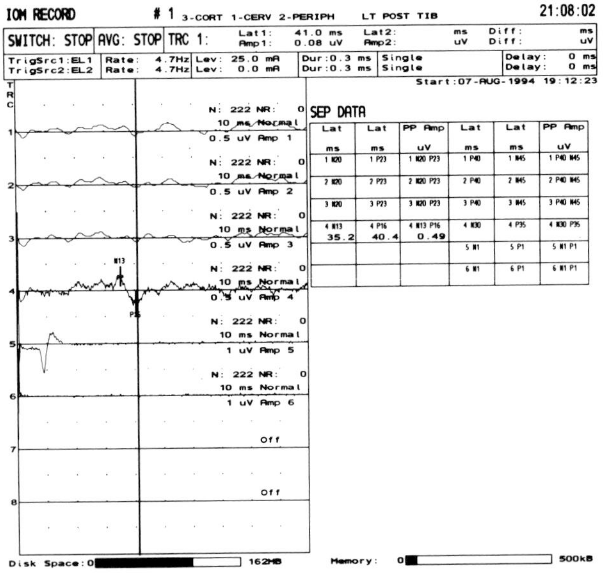

results were interpreted as indicating that the loss of cortical response resulted from anesthesia and it was not necessary to inform the surgeon of the degradation data. Figure 6 depicts a situation in which cortical as well as cervical data were lost, but the peripheral response remained present. In this figure, the baseline data were well formed and reliable. During the surgery, however, the spinal cord was mechanically irritated by the passage of a sublaminar wire that resulted in a nearly immediate degradation in the cortical and cervical response. Because both of these responses were lost, it was possible to determine that the changes resulted from a surgical insult. The surgeon was immediately informed and intervention strategy initiated.

To ensure that an SEP can be successfully recorded, certain conditions must be met. These conditions include the use of appropriate anesthesia, a technologist who is experienced and trained in the use of SEPs, and an effective method of troubleshooting.

Intervention

If SEPs are lost during surgery, the neurophysiologist should implement the following minimal steps to determine whether the loss of data has resulted from technical, perisurgical, or surgical variables: (a) Immediately re-perform the test and include a peripheral response to ensure that the eliciting stimulus is being neurologically encoded. (b) Conduct a visual and impedance check of all recording electrodes. (c) Ascertain from the anesthe-

FIG. 5. SEPs elicited by left posterior tibial nerve stimulation following introduction of inappropriate levels of nitrous oxide. Note diminution of responses on channels 1, 2, and 3 compared to data from the same patient in Figure 4.

siologist whether or not changes in the level of muscle relaxation or anesthetic have occurred. (d) Record a response following stimulation of a different limb (e.g., an upper extremity). (e) Contact the surgeon.

Prior to contacting the surgeon, it is imperative that the neurophysiologist rule out technical and perisurgical variables as being the source for the loss of data. If the peripheral, cervical, and cortical responses are absent, it is likely that a technical problem has occurred. If only the cervical or cortical response is lost, the cause(s) could be technical or perisurgical. Once the loss of data is determined to result from a surgical insult (e.g., both cervical and cortical data are lost in the presence of a peripheral nerve), the surgeon *must* be contacted. Some of the questions that the surgeon should ask pertaining to the loss of SEPs include: (a) What steps have been taken to rule out a technical loss of data? (b) How much have the data degraded? (c) When did the degradation begin relative to the last surgical maneuver (i.e., derotation, distraction, etc.)? Based on the answers to these questions, it is the surgeon's responsibility to determine if intervention needs to be initiated to reverse any possible damage. Intervention methods should be established prior to surgery and include increasing mean arterial pressure, removing corrective forces, removing hardware, or performing a Stagnara wake-up test.

Case Examples

To describe the relative strengths and weaknesses of SEPs, the following case examples are presented.

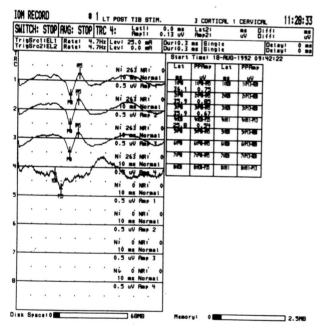

FIG. 7. Baseline SEPs in the same patient depicted in Figure 6, demonstrating the presence of reliable cortical (channels 1–3) and cervical (channel 4) data prior to spinal cord contact by the sublaminar wire.

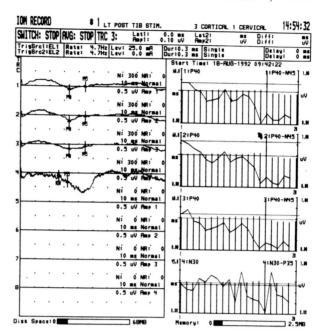

FIG. 8. Closing data from patient depicted in Figures 6 and 7. Note possible return of the cortical and subcortical responses following intervention.

Example 1: This 15-year-old boy underwent surgery for correction of neuromuscular scoliosis. Clinically, the patient demonstrated grossly normal motor and sensory function preoperatively. SEPs were elicited intraoperatively by stimulating the posterior tibial nerve at the ankle and were recorded peripherally, cervically, and cortically. Standard elicitation and recording parameters were used.

Figure 7 depicts baseline SEPs recorded from this patient intraoperatively. Reliable SEPs were present from all recording sites and remained unchanged until the surgeon started to pass sublaminar wires. At that time, the surgeon inadvertently irritated the spinal cord with a sublaminar wire, which resulted in an immediate degradation and subsequent loss of the SEPs (Figure 6). (It should be noted that MEPs were not being recorded from this patient.) The surgeon was immediately informed of the degraded data and intervention methodologies initiated. Intervention consisted of increasing the patient's mean arterial pressure to normal ranges and initiating a high-dose steroid protocol (6,7). Monitoring and the surgery continued, and the evoked potentials gradually improved (Fig. 8). At closure, the data had improved, but they were degraded relative to baseline. Following surgery, the patient demonstrated minor motor deficits in the lower extremities that resolved within 6 months.

This example demonstrates the following:

1. Mechanical insults (irritation of the spinal cord from the sublaminar wire) can immediately affect the SEP. Although MEPs were not recorded during this surgery, it is highly probable that they too would have been

deleteriously affected. Therefore, the assumption that SEPs will provide information regarding motor tract function following a mechanical insult to the spinal cord is probably correct.

2. The onset of evoked potential change was almost immediate, which is consistent with a mechanical injury to the spinal cord (3,52).

3. Continuous evoked potential monitoring can ensure the early detection of an insult and the earliest possible initiation of intervention strategies.

Example 2: This patient underwent a posterior spinal fusion of the cervical spine. The patient demonstrated preoperative cervical stenosis (Fig. 9) with minor upper extremity weaknesses and numbness. During surgery, only SEPs were used to monitor spinal cord function. MEPs were not monitored at the request of the surgeon because "this case was considered to be low risk." During surgery, the SEPs remained well formed and reliable and did not demonstrate any significant degradations. At closure, (Fig. 10), SEP data approximated baseline values. Upon awakening from anesthesia, the patient was quadriplegic, which resolved somewhat during the first 3 months postoperatively but continued to be present after 6 months. Based on vascular supply of the spinal cord and the origin of the SEPs, it appears that the patient's surgically induced postoperative quadriplegia resulted from ischemia of the spinal cord motor tracts and not from any mechanical damage to the spinal cord or ischemia of the sensory tracts.

Example 2 demonstrates that SEPs are not a direct

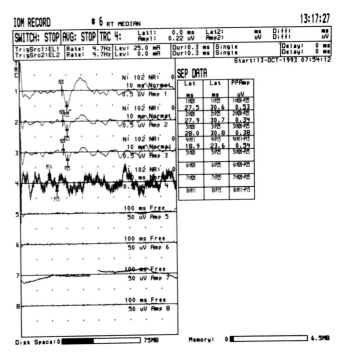

FIG. 10. Closing SEPs following right median nerve stimulation in the same patient depicted in Figure 9.

measure of motor tract function. Originally, it was assumed that because of the anatomical characteristics of the spinal cord, any damage to a motor tract would also affect the sensory tract and, therefore, degrade the SEP. Example 1 demonstrates that this assumption may be true for mechanical insults to the spinal cord. Example 2, however, indicates that this assumption may not be true in situations of spinal cord ischemia. To ensure that the spinal cord is being adequately protected during surgery for spinal deformity, it is necessary to record somatosensory *and* motor evoked potentials continuously throughout surgery. This is especially true because the type of spinal cord damage (i.e., mechanical versus ischemic) cannot be predicted.

APPLICATION OF MEPs TO PROTECT SPINAL CORD FUNCTION

The spinal cord consists of a series of parallel sensory and motor tracts. Because of their anatomical distribution as well as multiple sources of perfusion, it is necessary to monitor spinal cord function using both mixed-nerve SEPs and MEPs.

From an anatomical perspective, the primary motor tracts originate within the cortex, descend, and decussate within the brainstem. Originally called pyramidal and now known as corticospinal, these tracts proceed contralateral to their site of cortical origin and are located in the anterior lateral aspects of the spinal cord. Secondary (extrapyramidal) tracts descend the spinal cord ipsilat-

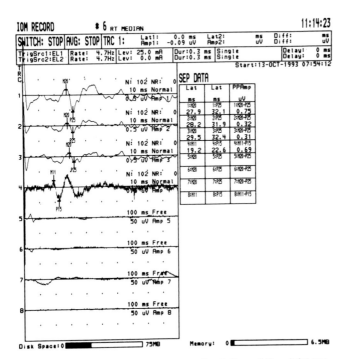

FIG. 9. Baseline SEPs following stimulation of the right median nerve during a cervical decompression surgery.

eral to their cortical site of origin, and decussate close to their point of termination. The corticospinal and extrapyramidal tracts synapse within the anterior horn, on the anterior horn cell. The axon of the lower motor neuron proceeds to the motor endplates.

It is generally assumed that the anterior two-thirds of the spinal cord is perfused by the anterior spinal artery, and the posterior one-third is perfused by a matrix of vessels originating from posterior radicular arteries. Because of these different sources of spinal cord perfusion, it is possible for spinal cord motor tracts to become ischemic, with subsequent postoperative motor deficits but without a significant change in the mixed-nerve SEP. Consequently, it is necessary to record a motor evoked potential and an SEP.

Methods for Eliciting and Recording Motor Evoked Potentials

MEPs can be elicited by stimulating either the cortical motor strip or the spinal cord. Effective stimuli include magnetic and electrical stimulation of the motor cortex, and electrical stimulation of the spinal cord (30).

In addition to the various sites and types of stimulation, it is possible to record two types of MEPs. One type is the compound muscle action potentials (CMAP), recorded on an electromyogram (EMG). The other type is the compound nerve action potential (CNAP), a neurogenic MEP (NMEP). As with any procedure, there are advantages and disadvantages to the various sites of stimulation, types of stimuli used, and the type of response recorded.

Motor Cortex Stimulation

Magnetic stimulation of the motor cortex was first reported by Merton and Morton (42). By using a circular coil placed over the motor cortex, it was possible to elicit peripheral EMG activity. The advantages of using magnetic stimulation to elicit a MEP include:

1. Magnetic stimuli are painless because there are no sensory receptors for this type of stimulus. While in an awake patient, magnetic stimulation of the motor cortex is somewhat uncomfortable because of severe muscle contraction of facial musculature, little sensation is associated with the actual stimulus.

2. Because magnetic stimulation is relatively painless, it is possible to obtain preoperative and postoperative information regarding the functional integrity of the motor system.

In 1989, Edmonds et al. (19) reported the results of using transcranial magnetic stimulation of the motor cortex to elicit myogenic motor evoked potentials (recorded on an EMG) from patients undergoing surgery for spinal deformity. In their study, EMGs were recorded from the anterior tibialis muscles from 11 neurologically normal patients with idiopathic scoliosis. Results indicated that a reliable response was obtained in 9 of the 11 cases.

In presenting their data, Edmonds et al. found that latency and amplitudes of the EMGs demonstrated a significant change during the duration of the surgery. Amplitudes demonstrated greater variance than response latency, even though all of the patients were neurologically intact following surgery. The sources for the fluctuation in the responses were ascribed to perisurgical variables. This study demonstrated that it was possible to record an EMG to magnetic stimulation of the motor cortex during surgery. However, because of the magnitude of the normal variance of response latency and amplitude, interpretative criteria must be based on presence versus absence of the response instead of a fixed percentage of change in amplitude or latency.

In two studies, Shields et al. (60) and Calancie et al. (10) investigated the use of intraoperative transcranial magnetic stimulation. In both of these studies, the authors reported that it was extremely difficult to record reliable EMG responses during surgery. In the Shields et al. study, MEPs were successfully recorded in only 8% of the patients. Additionally, it was not possible to discriminate between changes resulting from normal variability and those resulting from the onset of a neurological insult.

Thus, it appears that it is possible to record an EMG from peripheral musculature following magnetic stimulation of the motor cortex. Responses elicited from an individual who is awake and cooperative demonstrate high reliability in both amplitude and latency. However, following the onset of anesthesia, the reliability of these responses is significantly reduced, making it extremely difficult to determine whether the degradation results from the normal variability of the response or the onset of a surgically induced insult (49). Magnetic stimulation techniques have not gained widespread clinical use because of their many difficulties and the fact that the technique is not approved by the FDA for routine use.

An alternative method for eliciting MEPs is to stimulate the motor cortex electrically. In this methodology, fine needle electrodes are placed subdermally over the motor cortex (58). The typically recorded response is an EMG from peripheral muscles. Routine recording methodology (i.e., using surface electrodes, etc.) is used. It is also possible to record a descending motor potential that is neurogenic in origin directly from the spinal cord, as well as from a peripheral mixed nerve. To record the neurogenic response, either an electrode can be placed epidurally or needle electrodes can be placed in the immediate vicinity of the spine. In the periphery, it is possible to record the response over a peripheral mixed nerve by using subdermal needle electrodes. Typical recording sites from the periphery include the ulnar nerve, median nerve, and the popliteal fossa.

The stimulus used to stimulate the motor cortex is 0.2 msec in duration and is typically presented between 100 and 200 mA. The presentation rate is fairly low (i.e., 4.7/ sec) in order to avoid the elicitation of kindling activity on the patient's electroencephalogram (EEG). To eliminate a stimulus artifact, the ground electrode can be placed circumferentially around the head. This method of stimulation should be avoided in patients who have a history of seizure activity or who have had a previous craniotomy.

Patton and Amassian (55) have described the MEP recorded from the spine following electrical stimulation of the motor cortex in cats and monkeys. When anode stimulation is used to generate the descending potential, the response consists of a polyphasic series of action potentials that have been arbitrarily divided into two categories: direct (D) and indirect (I). The D wave was regarded as the action elicited by direct stimulation of the cortical spinal motor neuron. The I wave has been determined to be indirectly activated by repetitive synaptic bombardment of the pyramidal neurons through chains of cortical interneurons. The I wave is easily affected by anesthesia and asphyxia while the D wave is more resistant (1).

Interpretation of the MEP elicited following electrical stimulation of the brain is based on response latency and amplitude. Since the spinal cord evoked potential is very reproducible in morphology, Burke et al. (9) regarded an amplitude change of 20% to 30% as a warning to the surgeon of a significant change in spinal cord function. On the other hand, others have concluded that an amplitude attenuation of 50% should be regarded as meeting warning criteria (46,66,68). In a study by Forbes et al. (20), it was found that no patients who demonstrated amplitude reduction of 50% or less demonstrated any neurological sequelae. However, no postoperative neurological problems were demonstrated in 38% of the patients whose SEPs did drop more than 50%. In patients with a preexisting neurological condition, a different criterion should be selected. Every component of the electrically elicited MEP should be observed, and slight decrement in amplitude of 10% should be thought of as reaching a warning criterion (66). At the present time, there are no criteria for abnormality of the MEP recorded from the spine following electrical stimulation of the motor cortex. However, if amplitude of the response decreases by 50%, the neurophysiologist should be alert to any additional degradation. Subsequent degradations of 60% or more in response amplitude should be considered as meeting warning criteria and the surgeon should be informed immediately.

The advantage of electrical stimulation of the motor cortex compared to magnetic stimulation is that the electrically elicited MEPs are more reliable and less influenced by such perisurgical variables as anesthesia. However, just as with magnetic stimulation techniques, electrical elicitation of the motor cortex is affected by level of anesthesia (10,62). If inappropriate anesthetics are used, it is not possible to record a reliable potential. Additionally, electrical stimulation of the motor cortex is extremely painful and cannot be easily administered to an awake patient. In the United States, magnetic stimulation of the motor cortex has received more attention than electrical stimulation for eliciting an MEP. However, either methodology can be used for eliciting this response.

Spinal Cord Stimulation

An alternative to stimulating the motor cortex is to stimulate the spinal cord. While Machida et al. (37) have reported that it is possible to stimulate the spinal cord using magnetic stimulations, Konrad et al. (30) have reported conflicting data. Consequently, MEP techniques that stimulate the spinal cord use electrical rather than magnetic stimulation techniques.

In 1970, one of the authors (T.T.) was a Visiting Fellow at Rancho Los Amigos Hospital. At that time, because spine surgeons had started to perform the wedge osteotomy of the vertebral body anteriorly prior to placing posterior Harrington instrumentation, the need for intraoperative spinal cord monitoring was raised by Dr. Jacqueline Perry. Equipment limitations made it very difficult then to record a SEP under general anesthesia following peripheral mixed nerve stimulation. Because of the size and ease of recording spinal cord potentials, the author (T.T.) started to use a method that recorded these potentials from the subarachnoid space following direct stimulation of the spinal cord.

The main advantage of recording the signal in the subarachnoid space is the high amplitude of the evoked potentials, two to three times greater than if the recording electrode is placed in the epidural space, allowing rapid recognition and response even in the hostile electrical environment of the operating theater. Numerous basic and clinical studies on this spinal cord evoked potential (SCEP) have been performed, mainly in Japan (22,25, 26,31,32,39,65–69), not only in corrective surgery for spinal deformities but also during surgical procedures which manipulate the spinal cord directly.

Stimulation and recording are accomplished using specially made electrodes (Intermedics Co. Ltd., Japan) that consist of two helical platinum wires of 1 mm width attached to the end of a Teflon tube. The distance between the two metal contacts is approximately 15 mm (Fig. 11). The electrode is flexible so as to avoid injury to neural tissue in the subarachnoid space, but stiff enough that it can be advanced into the intrathecal or extradural space. The diameter of the electrode is 0.75 mm and it fits within the hole of an 18-gauge Tuohy needle. The same

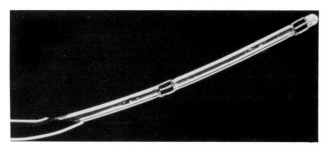

FIG. 11. Flexible tube-type electrode used to stimulate and record spinal cord evoked potentials.

type of electrode is used for both recording and stimulation.

The stimulating electrode for the spinal cord is introduced into the extra-dural space. The site used to stimulate the neural tissue should be selected to document the delivery of neural impulse at the level where the spinal cord may be at risk during surgery. According to the level monitored, the recording site is arbitrarily selected. For example, to monitor thoracic spinal cord, the recording electrode is placed at the level of the conus medullaris, and for the cervical spinal cord, the tip of the recording electrode is located at the rostral level of the thoracic spine.

The introduction of the recording electrode is preceded by lumbar puncture with an 18-gauge Tuohy's needle at the lower lumbar level (Fig. 12). The most frequently selected level is L5-S1 in scoliotic patients, as it is fairly rare to place a hook between L5-S1 and be able to avoid interfering with the operating field. Once the tip of a catheter-type electrode is introduced into the subarachnoid space, it can be advanced rostrally simply by

gently pushing it. For routine montage to pick up the SCEP elicited by the direct stimulation to the spinal cord, the tip of the electrode is placed at the lower thoracic level or close to the conus medullaris (Fig. 13).

It may seem wise to put 2 catheter-type electrodes into the subarachnoid space, and to use one of them as the stimulating electrode and the other as the recording electrode. However, this type of electrode setting is not practical as large electrical artifact interferes with the appropriate recording of the SCEP. Therefore, the stimulating electrode should be placed via a different route.

For the purpose of direct stimulation to the rostral spinal cord, the stimulating electrode is introduced into the epidural space using Tuohy's needle. This procedure can be carried out percutaneously or under direct vision intraoperatively after surgically exposing the laminae. Percutaneous insertion is preferred in cases with normal shape and alignment of the laminae of the spine and should be carried out on the alert patient prior to surgery. The insertion of Tuohy's needle into the epidural space is performed following the loss of resistance technique via the paramedian approach. Smooth advancement of the electrode and test stimulation with a tolerable amount of electrical stimulation signifies the entry of the electrode into the epidural space. If heparin is being used to prevent epidural hemorrhage, the electrode introduc-

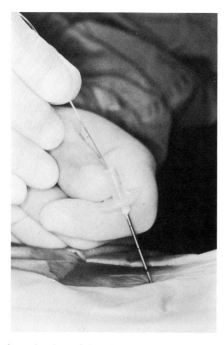

FIG. 12. Introduction of the electrode into the subarachnoid space at a lower lumbar level using a Tuohy needle.

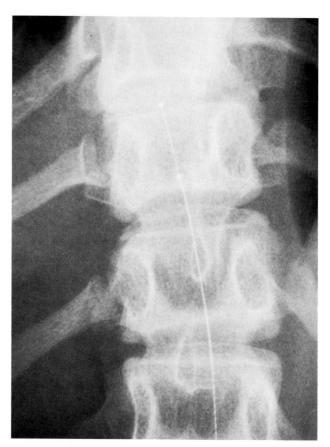

FIG. 13. The flexible electrode which was introduced intrathecally at the lower lumbar level and advanced to the lower thoracic spine.

tion should be carried out one day prior to the surgery and left in the epidural space for at least one day after the withdrawal of heparin.

Introduction under direct vision is performed after surgically exposing the laminae at least one level rostral to the hook placement or the surgical manipulation. For a case of scoliotic deformity, this direct insertion is suitable as the laminae are tilted and percutaneous epidural puncture is not always possible. Insertion can be carried out using an epidurally-placed Tuohy's needle with the technique of loss of resistance, or by confirming the epidural space by taking off a part of the interspinous ligament and the ligamentum flavum with a rongeur. Anchoring of the stimulating electrode is achieved by a stay suture to neighboring soft tissue close to the lamina and adhesive taping to the skin or the surgical drape. Care should be taken to avoid incidental movement and extraction of the electrode so as not to yield pseudo-positive information. Extraction of the electrode from the intrathecal space can be carried out simply by pulling it out. If multiple electrodes were inserted to record signals from multiple levels, pull them out one by one starting with the lastly-inserted electrode.

When the surgery involves some specific management after laminectomy, both stimulating and recording electrodes are introduced into the rostral and caudal epidural or subarachnoid spaces from the opened laminae or the dura mater. Such close placement of both electrodes is a "trick of the trade" to pick up very low amplitude-evoked potentials that travel through an injured spinal cord, although, it must be considered that the stimulation artifact can also be exaggerated. Furthermore, when both electrodes are located in the outside of the dura mater, leakage of the cerebro-spinal fluid (CSF) after opening the dura mater cause inefficient delivery of electric activity resulting in the decreased evoked potential. Accordingly, appropriate care should be taken to avoid false-positive judgment.

Once the electrodes are inserted in the appropriate position, it is easy to switch stimulation sites and recording sites as similar bipolar electrodes are used. The electrode placement allows us to record several kinds of evoked potentials if additional electrodes are used to stimulate the motor cortex and peripheral nerve trunks. Consequently, by using peripheral nerve stimulation, as well as electrical or magnetic stimulation of the motor cortex, various combinations of potentials can be recorded through electrodes placed at the spinal cord level. For example, following stimulation of a peripheral mixed nerve, it would be possible to record SSEP (spinal somatosensory evoked potential, Jones et al. 1983) from the subarachnoid space of the low spine and the epidural space of the high spine. By stimulating the motor cortex either electrically or magnetically, it is possible to record spinal MEP (spinal motor evoked potential, Levy et al. 1983, Matsuda 1987, 1989) at the rostral and caudal ends of the spinal cord. This kind of simultaneous re-

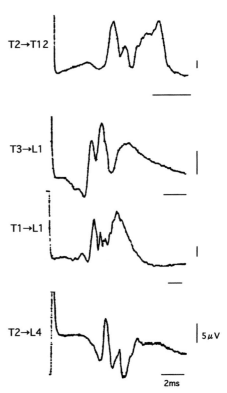

FIG. 14. SCEPs recorded from neurologically normal individuals. Notice the differences in wave configuration derived from delicate differences of electrode position in each case.

cording of multiple potentials to monitor the spinal cord functions is called multimodality spinal cord monitoring (Katayama 1986, Ben-David 1988, Burke 1992).

When electrically stimulating the spinal cord, the stimulus is typically 0.2–0.3 msec in duration. The intensity will range from 3 to 10 mAmps, and, a high/rapid presentation rate (i.e. 50Hz) can be used. To improve this signal-to-noise ratio, 50 to 100 responses are averaged. According to Tamaki (1981), a high rate of stimulation is preferred. For the past 25 years, the author (T.T.) has conducted more than 900 cases using this methodology without any serious complications caused by the electrical stimulation to the spinal cord. Whereas, Takakura et al. reported the hazards of continuous repetitive stimulation, even if the total amount of electric energy was comparable to interrupted train stimulation (Takakuwa et al. 1989). It appears, therefore, from these findings, that the free interval of 30–60 seconds between each run of 50–100 train stimulations is necessary.

Interpreting the SCEP

It is not possible to specify a standard wave pattern for SCEP; the wave configurations differ from patient to patient and are influenced by delicate differences of relation between the stimulating and recording electrodes (Fig. 14). The recorded SCEP basically consists of an initial sharp spike wave and following polyphasic waves. The initial sharp component has been recognized as the

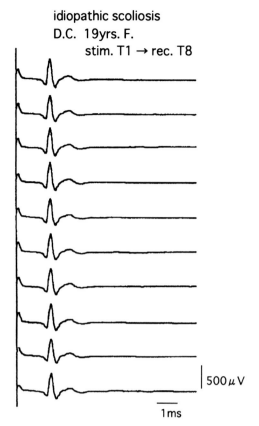

idiopathic scoliosis
D.C. 19yrs. F.
stim. T1 → rec. T8

500 μV

1ms

FIG. 15. Real-time monitoring once per second during sublaminar wiring, as described in Case Study 1.

summed electric activities of the large-diameter nerve fibers located in the posterolateral region of the spinal cord (26,31,70) and in all quadrants of the spinal cord (22,59). The dorsal column, where the fasciculus gracilis and the fasciculus cuneatus are located, was regarded to

be the conductor of the polyphasic waves. However, involvement of postsynaptically transmitted potentials in the polyphasic portion has been indicated by many researchers (17,61,65).

Therefore, the SCEP mainly reflects the action potentials traveling through the posterolateral and dorsal tracts of the spinal cord, though some electric activities related to the descending pathways are involved. Furthermore, one-to-one matching of these components of SCEP to the intricate function of the spinal cord has not been accomplished. The motor tracts can be selectively impaired by vascular compromise or direct manipulation to the spinal cord (24,64), so that a motor deficit can occur without associated dorsal column dysfunction detected by SCEP (5,24,38,64). Therefore, if any possibility of selective injury of the spinal tracts is anticipated, one should monitor as many tracts as possible using multimodality monitoring. For example, if a lesion to the anterior half of the cord is possible, concomitant monitoring of MEPs following motor cortex stimulation should be performed.

Interpretation of changes of the evoked potential must suffice to alert the surgeon before any adverse changes become irreversible. Because SCEPs are highly reproducible in nature, Burke et al. (9) suggested that an amplitude change of 20% to 30% is a sufficient indication to warn the surgeon. On the other hand, many researchers have empirically concluded that the alarm level should be around 50% attenuation of the amplitude in patients with intact spinal cord function (25,32,46,65,66,68). Interestingly, this level is a common standard in SEP (8) and MEP (29,73) and SSEP (27) as well. Prolonged latency can be also an alarm sign, although change of the latency may not be noticed immediately. Contrarily the

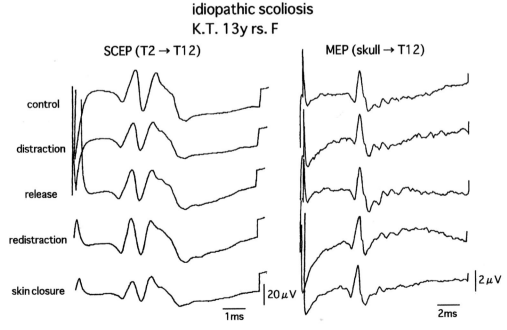

idiopathic scoliosis
K.T. 13y rs. F

SCEP (T2 → T12)   MEP (skull → T12)

control

distraction

release

redistraction

skin closure

20 μV   2 μV

1ms   2ms

FIG. 16. SCEPs and MEPs recorded at T12, as described in Case Study 2.

change of the amplitude is easily recognized instantaneously and its clinical relevance can be confirmed by prolonged latency. Therefore, we consider measurement of the latency as an adjunct to confirm an abnormality of the tracts transferring SCEPs. One exception is the effect of degraded body temperature which increases the latency of the SCEPs, sometimes without causing any change in the wave configuration.

In the clinical scene preoperative strategy for selecting methods to monitor intraoperative spinal cord function is fundamental to carry out effective and reliable monitoring. The best array of stimulation and recording sites to monitor the spinal cord should be arranged concerning the type of surgery and the neurological status of the spinal cord. In a patient with standard surgery for idiopathic scoliosis with possible injury to the global spinal cord, such as distraction or compression, single use of SCEP is frequently employed, although combined use of multiple methods is recommended. If any lesion to the anterior half of the spinal cord by compression or vascular compromise is expected, concomitant use of the MEP after stimulating the motor cortex should be performed. This multimodality monitoring paradigm is also mandatory to monitor intraparenchymal procedures for removal of intramedullary spinal cord tumor.

On a case which may have cauda equina injury, SSEP may be utilized after stimulating the nerve trunk in the lower extremity, although one must be aware that the

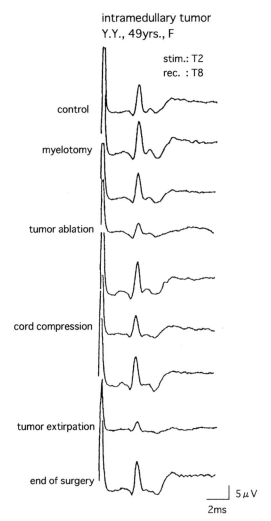

FIG. 18. SCEPs recorded at T8, after stimulating at T2, as described in Case Study 4.

SSEP is not sensitive enough to determine whether or not a particular cauda equina is damaged. SSEP travels into the spinal cord via multiple cauda equina or nerve roots, therefore, the SSEP may not be drastically influenced by lesioning any one of these nerves.

Case Studies

Case Study 1: Figure 15 depicts the SCEPs recorded from a neurologically normal 19-year-old woman undergoing surgery for the correction of scoliosis. The spinal cord was stimulated at T1 and the SCEP recorded at T8. The series of SCEPs was recorded at intervals of one second without averaging. This case shows that in neurologically normal cases the SCEPs are often large enough to be monitored without averaging, providing the surgeon with an essentially continuous and near real-time analysis of spinal cord function.

Case Study 2: Figure 16 depicts the SCEPs and MEPs recorded from a 13-year-old patient undergoing surgery for idiopathic scoliosis. Data were collected at baseline (control) and during various stages of the surgery. Fol-

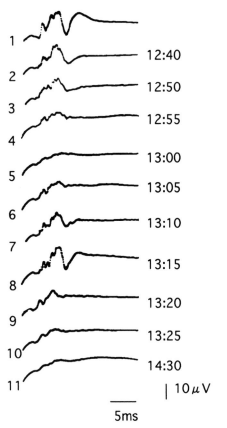

FIG. 17. SCEPs recorded at T11, following stimulation at T3, as described in Case Study 3.

lowing application of distraction to the spine, the initial spike component of SCEPs decreased to approximately 50% of control value. On the other hand, the "D" wave of MEPs maintained its amplitude and shape, while the following "I" waves demonstrated a gradual reduction. At the conclusion of the surgery, changes in the SCEP were determined to be the result of minor fine movement of the stimulating electrodes and/or alteration in impedance between the stimulating electrode and the spinal cord. However, changes in the potentials were seen only for the SCEP and not in the MEP. Consequently, the surgeon did not take intervention steps based upon the sole diminution and change in the morphological pattern of the SCEP. Upon awakening from anesthesia, the patient was neurologically normal. This case study indicates that the concomitant use of multimodality evoked potentials not only increases the sensitivity of monitoring two changes in spinal cord function but also helps eliminate false-positive and false-negative findings. It is strongly recommended that multimodality testing be administered to patients undergoing spinal surgery even in cases of idiopathic scoliosis.

Case Study 3: This patient underwent surgery for neurogenic scoliosis because of constriction of the dural tube from an unknown etiology (Fig. 17). During surgery there was a significant decrease of mean arterial pressure to 50 mm Hg. Blood transfusion was administered to reduce the hypovolemic situation and to increase blood pressure. During the periods of hypotension (at approximately 13:00 and from 13:20 to 14:20 in the figure) the SCEP demonstrated significant changes in morphology and amplitude. It should be noted that in this figure the basic morphology of the SCEP differs dramatically from that depicted in Fig. 15. Not only are the overall initial spike wave and the following polyphasic wave pattern different, but it is also difficult to discriminate the initial spike wave from the following polyphasic wave. With increases in blood pressure the SCEP recovered significantly. However, with further surgical manipulation (at approximately 13:25) the SCEPs continued to diminish.

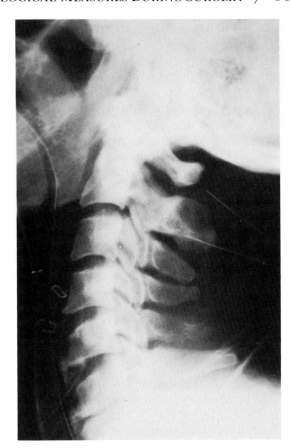

FIG. 20. X-ray of the percutaneous–percutaneous (P–P) electrodes placed in the cervical spine.

The surgeon was informed of this diminution, and intervention strategies were initiated. However, the patient woke up with a permanent paraplegia (47).

Case Study 4: Figure 18 depicts the SCEPs recorded from a patient undergoing surgery for removal of an intramedullary ependymoma. This case was monitored using only SCEPs during the removal of the tumor. The tumor was located primarily on the right side of the spinal cord at T5. The stimulating extradural electrode was placed within the epidural space at T2 and the recording electrode at T8 in the subarachnoid space. During various stages of the surgery, as indicated in Figure 18, significant alterations in the amplitude and morphology of the SCEP occurred. By the end of surgery, the SCEP had recovered significantly and no post-operative neurological deficits were expected. However, following surgery the patient had a prominent sensory disturbance and a Brown-Séquard type motor dysfunction.

It does appear that the monitoring was carried out on this case by observing mainly the functions of the preserved half of the spinal cord. Therefore, potentials traveled through the tracts of the compressed side were not well expressed in the evoked potentials during the monitoring.

If this assumption is accepted, it may be possible that this case is not a false negative case neurophysiologically since function of the preserved half of the spinal cord was

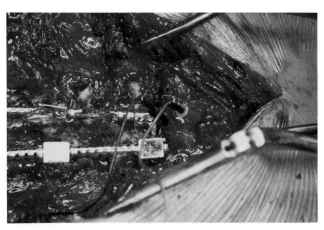

FIG. 19. Photograph of translaminar stimulating electrodes in place. Note: the anode electrode is rostral to the cathode.

well monitored. From the clinical point of view, however, this case was defined as a false negative case. Additionally post operative edema of the spinal cord, which was not monitored, might have contributed to the spinal cord disorders, therefore, one should be cautious in diagnosing false negative cases. Although this patient should be regarded as the case which indicates the necessity of multimodality monitoring as Maruyama (1982) and Ben-David (1988) pointed out, it should be remembered that one of the shortcomings of SCEP is inability to distinguish laterality of injury. This problem can be resolved by supplementing SSEPs after peripheral nerve trunk stimulation, or/and MEP elicited by transcranial electric stimulation.

Translaminar Stimulation

A second method for stimulating the spinal cord is the translaminar method, in which short, insulated, needle electrodes are placed into the cancellous bone of the spinous process within 1 cm of the spinal canal. The anode electrode is placed rostral to the cathode. Figure 19 depicts the placement of the translaminar stimulating electrodes. The advantages of using the translaminar stimulation technique are that a reliable response can be obtained at very low intensities, placement of electrodes

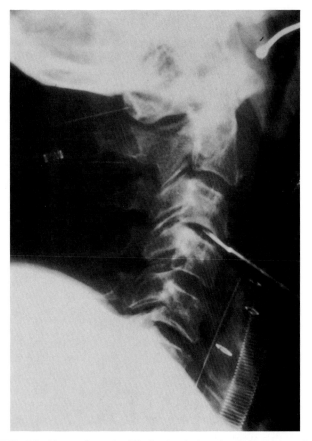

FIG. 21. X-ray of a pair of P–P stimulating electrodes, as well as a nasopharyngeal electrode (NP) used to stimulate the spinal cord.

is very easy, and it is possible to map the spinal cord in order to determine the level(s) of spinal cord involvement in the event data are lost.

The disadvantages of using translaminar placement include: (a) It is necessary for the surgeon to place the stimulating electrode in the surgical field; (b) If the electrodes get in the surgeon's way, the surgeon will typically remove them, which could occur at a critical time (i.e., during placement of instrumentation) and would leave the spinal cord motor tracts unprotected; and (c) It is possible for spinal instrumentation and fluids, near the stimulating electrodes, to shunt the electrical stimulus away from the spinal cord. This can be avoided if the electrodes are placed at least one segment away from the most rostral end of the spinal instrumentation. To avoid all of the limitations associated with transstimulation, two alternative stimulation techniques have been reported: percutaneous–percutaneous (P-P) and percutaneous–nasopharyngeal.

Percutaneous–Percutaneous

In 1992, Coe et al. (14) reported the development of a method for electrically stimulating the spinal cord using percutaneously placed stimulating electrodes. In this method, a pair of 60-mm EMG electrodes are placed percutaneously outside of the sterile field. Figure 20 depicts the placement of these electrodes. The advantage of using the P-P methodology is that it avoids the limitations associated with translaminar placement. Coe et al. (14) originally recommended that the electrodes be placed into the interspinous ligament. However, it may be safer to place the stimulating electrodes against the bone of the lamina at the base of the spinous process. When placed in this location, the danger associated with the possibility of an electrode being introduced into the spinal canal, via the interspinous ligament, is eliminated. We have found that the MEPs elicited by using P-P placement are reliable and provide data that are a direct measure of spinal cord motor tract function. The only limitation associated with the P-P placement is that in high cervical spine surgery, there may not be adequate space to place both stimulating electrodes. In this situation, we utilize a percutaneous EMG electrode in conjunction with a nasopharyngeal electrode.

Percutaneous–Nasopharyngeal Electrode Method

The nasopharyngeal electrode was originally developed to record EEGs; however, we now use this electrode as a stimulating electrode (Fig. 21). The nasopharyngeal electrode is introduced into the nasopharynx via the nose after the patient has been placed on the operating table. The nasopharyngeal electrode acts as the anode, and a percutaneously placed electrode acts as the cathode. When this methodology is used, a reliable response can be elicited in all of the extremities. There are essentially

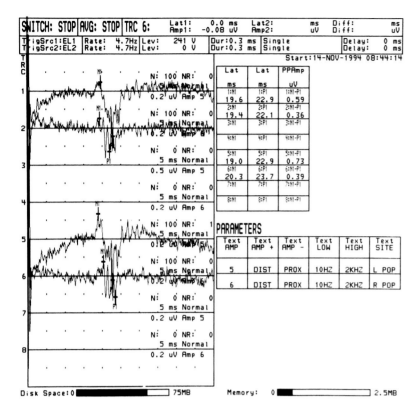

FIG. 22. Normal neurogenic MEPs recorded from a patient undergoing surgery. Data were recorded from the left and right popliteal fossa and two trials of data are depicted to demonstrate test–retest reliability.

no limitations associated with the percutaneous–nasopharyngeal methodology.

Neurogenic versus Myogenic Responses

MEPs can be recorded in two forms: as a compound nerve action potential (CNAP) or as a compound muscle action potential (CMAP). The CNAP is a neurogenic signal (neurogenic motor evoked potential, NMEP) that elicits the contraction in a muscle (Fig. 22). This is the neurological signal that originates rostral to the muscle

(i.e., within the motor tracts) and would result in the contraction of the muscle if complete muscle relaxation was not present. The CMAP is myogenic in origin (recorded on an electromyogram, EMG) and is the electrical activity associated with the actual contraction of a muscle (Fig. 23).

The advantage of recording an NMEP is that the response demonstrates a very reliable amplitude and latency. This high reliability improves the sensitivity of the response to the onset of a neurological deficit. Also, there is no patient "movement" resulting from the muscle contractions associated with the recording of an EMG.

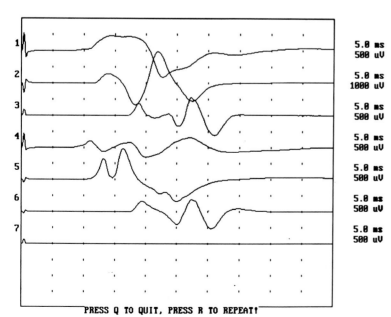

FIG. 23. Myogenic motor evoked potentials recorded from the following muscle groups after electrical stimulation of the spinal cord: *Traces 1 and 4* are from left and right quadriceps femoris muscles; *Traces 2 and 5* are from left and right tibialis anterior muscles; and *Traces 3 and 6* are responses from the left and right medial gastrocnemius muscles.

The disadvantage of the NMEP is that the response contains an orthodromic motor and antidromic sensory component (51). However, as it has been recently reported, it is possible to discriminate between these two components fairly easily within the response (21,51).

The advantage of recording an EMG motor evoked potential is that this response is a true MEP. While this response does contain the neurogenic component as well as an antidromic sensory component, the EMG component is of such large amplitude that these smaller components are not obvious. Even though the EMG response is a true MEP, it demonstrates several disadvantages: (a) The morphology and amplitude of the response are more unreliable especially in comparison to the NMEP. This requires that the interpretative criteria of the EMG be based upon the presence versus the absence of the response. By using a presence/absence interpretative criteria, the sensitivity of the response to the onset of a neurological deficit is reduced; and (b) To record the response, the patient's muscles must not be completely relaxed. Consequently, the patient will move on the operating table in response to stimulation when this type of response is recorded. Patient movement can be minimized by titrating the level of muscle relaxation to a twitch level of 2 to 3 twitches out of a train of 4. However, muscle blockage can affect the detectability of the EMG response.

Table 5 lists the parameters used for eliciting and recording MEPs according to whether a myogenic or neurogenic response is recorded. The acquisition parameters used to record a myogenic versus neurogenic MEP are

TABLE 5. *Acquisition parameters for eliciting and recording motor evoked potentials using spinal cord stimulation techniques*

	Myogenic responses	Neurogenic responses
Recording sites	Specific muscles	Popliteal fossa Ulnar groove Antecubital fossa
Filters	5–5000 Hz	30–2000 Hz
Stimulation rates	4–7/sec	4.7/sec
Time base	50 msec	50 msec
Intensity*	10% > threshold	10% > threshold
Sensitivity	10% rejection ratio	10% rejection ratio

* We utilize a constant voltage stimulus.

significantly different. Consequently, these parameters should be adjusted according to the response recorded.

We utilize an NMEP when information pertaining to the general function of an extremity is needed. For example, in a patient undergoing surgery for idiopathic scoliosis who is neurologically intact, we will record a NMEP. However, in a patient for whom information regarding specific muscle groups is requested by the surgeon, we record a myogenic MEP. For NMEPs, we use a warning criterion of 60% amplitude degradation and/or latency increases of 10%. Intervention criteria include a degradation of response amplitude of 80% or more. The intervention criterion for myogenic responses is all or none, meaning that response has to be completely gone before it is considered to be abnormal. There are no warning criteria for EMG responses.

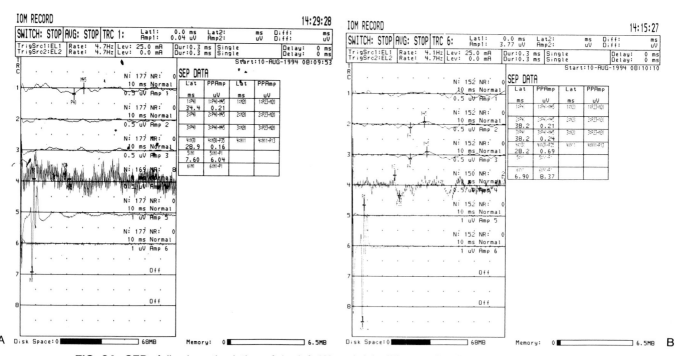

FIG. 24. SEPs following stimulation of the left (**A**) and right (**B**) posterior tibial nerve and described in Case Study 5.

Case Studies

The following case studies depict the relative sensitivity and specificity of the NMEP during surgery for spinal degeneration.

Case Study 5: A 15-year-old boy underwent surgery for kyphoscoliosis. The surgical approach consisted of an anterior spinal fusion for release of the thoracolumbar kyphotic curve and a posterior spinal fusion with Cotrel-Dubousset instrumentation. Preoperatively the patient was neurologically intact.

Somatosensory and neurogenic motor evoked potential procedures were administered. SEPs were elicited by stimulating the posterior tibial nerve at the ankle and recording the responses peripherally, cervically, and cortically (Fig. 24). MEPs were elicited by stimulating the spinal cord and recording the responses at each popliteal fossa (Fig. 25).

Somatosensory and motor evoked potentials remained well formed during the anterior spinal fusion phase of the surgery. The Stagnara wake-up test was not administered during the anterior spinal fusion. Following closure of the anterior spinal fusion, the patient was turned and posterior spinal fusion with instrumentation performed. During the posterior spinal fusion phase of the surgery, the MEPs demonstrated a significant degradation in response amplitude. SEPs did not demonstrate any significant changes. The surgeon was immediately informed of the degraded MEPs, and a Stagnara wake-up test was ordered. During the wake-up test, a pair of translaminar JO-5 stimulating electrodes (The Electrode Store, Enumclaw, WA) were handed to the surgeon so

that he could stimulate the spinal column at multiple sites along the spine. Starting caudally, the surgeon stimulated at approximately T12, T10, T8, and T4 (Fig. 26). When stimulating at or below T10, reliable and well-formed data were obtained. However, when stimulating rostral to T10, no reliable response could be obtained in the lower extremities. Based on these findings, it was concluded that there was damage to the spinal cord at approximately T10, which was at the apex of the kyphotic curve. Results from the Stagnara wake-up test were positive for paraplegia. The surgeon immediately closed the incision. During the next few days, the patient demonstrated some clinical improvement in the lower extremities. Two days later an attempt was made to complete the posterior spinal fusion.

During the second phase of the surgery, somatosensory and motor evoked potentials were administered. The MEPs enabled us to monitor the amount of corrective force applied to the spine. Whenever any changes in the MEPs occurred, the corrective force was reduced. The corrective forces were then released and MEPs recovered. By using this methodology, we were able to apply adequate correction to stabilize the spine without inducing neurological deficits. Upon awakening from anesthesia, the patient demonstrated grossly unchanged motor and sensory status.

This case study indicates that it is possible for SEPs to remain unchanged during a spinal surgery while the MEPs demonstrat a significant change. It should be noted that following the initial surgery, when the SEPs did not change and the MEPs did, the patient did not demonstrate a significant degradation of sensory function. However, the patient did demonstrate a significant reduction in motor function.

Case Study 6: This patient was a 31-year-old man undergoing surgery for spinal fusion. The patient demonstrated a Brown-Séquard syndrome in which the left lower extremity demonstrated normal motor function but reduced/absent sensory function, whereas the right lower extremity demonstrated reduced motor function but grossly normal sensory function. This case study demonstrates that NMEPs and SEPs are differentially sensitive to the functional status of motor and sensory tracts within the spinal cord.

SEPs were elicited by stimulating the posterior tibial nerve and recording peripherally, cervically, and cortically. NMEPs were recorded at the popliteal fossa following electrical stimulation of the spinal cord. Standard elicitation and recording parameters were used.

Baseline data, obtained following surgical incision, demonstrated poorly formed SEPs from the left lower extremity, while normal SEPs were recorded from the right (Fig. 27). MEPs were well formed when recorded from the left lower extremity but were essentially absent or significantly reduced when recorded from the right (Fig. 28). Data were maintained throughout surgery and did not demonstrate any significant changes. Upon

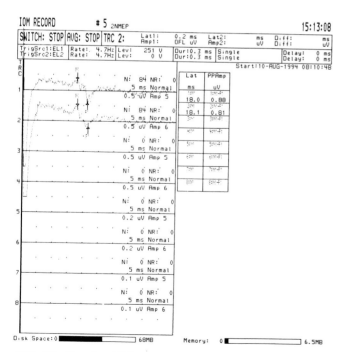

FIG. 25. Baseline NMEPs recorded in the patient described in Case Study 5.

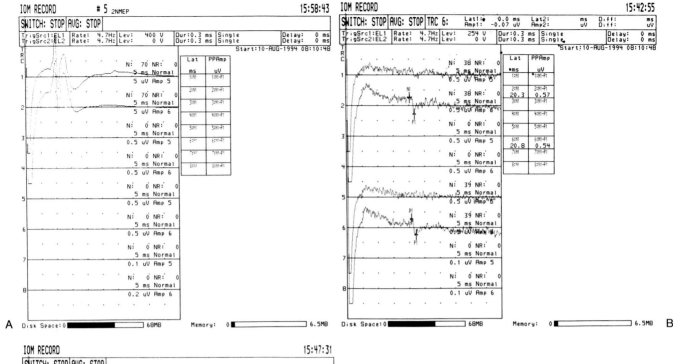

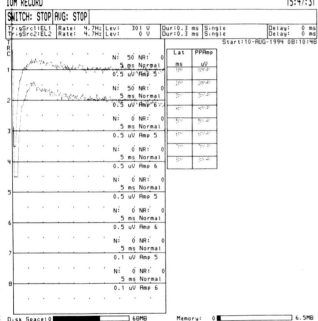

FIG. 26. NMEPs elicited by stimulating the spinal cord at approximately T12 (**A**) at T10 (**B**) and T6-7 (**C**) (Case Study 6).

awakening from anesthesia, the patient demonstrated grossly unchanged neurological function.

Case Study 7: This patient was a 13-year-old girl undergoing surgery for neuromuscular scoliosis. In addition, the patient demonstrated cerebral palsy and was an achondroplastic dwarf. Neurological function consisted of only motor function in the quadriceps femoris muscle groups in both lower extremities. There was no lower extremity sensory function nor were any of the remaining muscle groups functionally intact.

It was impossible to elicit and record an SEP, so we monitored spinal cord function using MEPs. MEPs were elicited by electrically stimulating the spinal cord and were recorded from the biceps femoris muscles bilater-

ally (Fig. 29). We used myogenic MEPs, instead of neurogenic, because only specific muscle groups were functionally intact. By using these potentials, we were able to maintain the functional integrity of these muscle groups throughout surgery. Upon awakening from anesthesia, the patient demonstrated grossly unchanged motor function in the lower extremities.

MONITORING TO PROTECT THE NERVE ROOTS

A second application for IOM is to protect nerve roots. At the present time, there are two types of neurophysiological procedures that can be used to monitor nerve root

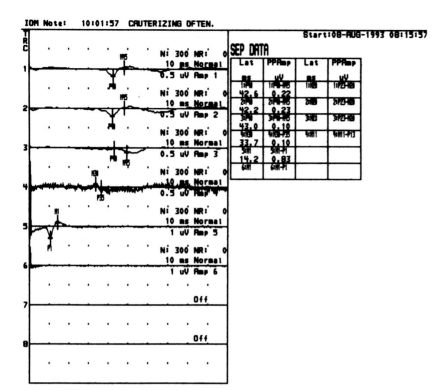

FIG. 27. SEPs recorded from patients demonstrating Brown-Séquard syndrome with abnormal left SEPs and normal right SEPs.

function: dermatomal SEPs (DSEPs) and EMGs (see Table 2). Unlike monitoring spinal cord function, neurophysiological procedures used for monitoring nerve root function must demonstrate certain characteristics, including specificity and sensitivity to instantaneous changes in individual nerve root function that can occur during surgery. Because of these two requirements, mixed-nerve SEPs are not appropriate for monitoring individual nerve root function.

Dermatomal SEPs

DSEPs are elicited by electrical stimulation of a peripheral dermatomal field. Investigation of these fields reveals variability among them. Consequently, when deciding on the specific site of stimulation, the examiner needs to determine which nerve root is at risk and where within the dermatomal field the response should be elicited. In a study by Cohen and Hultzenger (15), a very

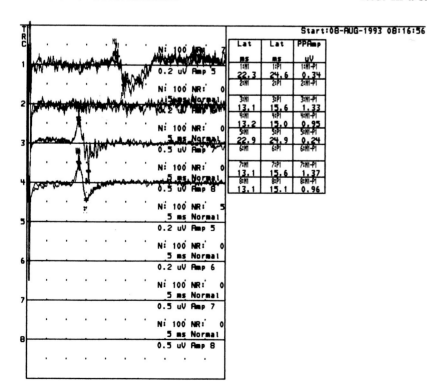

FIG. 28. NMEPs elicited by stimulating the spinal cord. *Trace 1* is a normal response from the left lower extremity and *Trace 2* is an abnormal response from the right lower extremity. *Traces 3 and 4* are NMEPs recorded from the femoral nerve (left/right) bilaterally.

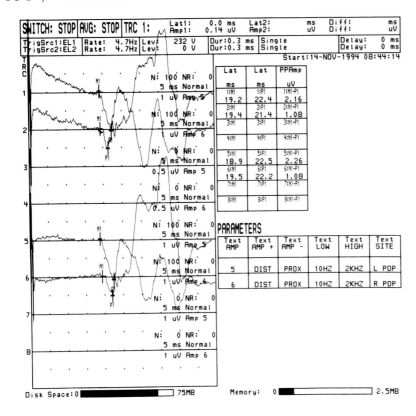

FIG. 29. EMGs recorded from the quadriceps femoris muscle groups (test–retest reliability) following electrical stimulation of the spinal cord. *Traces 1 and 3* are left leg responses and *Traces 2 and 4* are right leg responses (Case Study 7).

meticulous method for determining and preparing the site of dermatomal stimulation was described. In general, it is necessary to ensure that the stimulating electrodes are located well within the dermatomal field. Also, the intensity level of the stimulus must be adequate to stimulate peripheral nerve endings but avoid contraction of underlying muscles. In the diagnostic setting, an appropriate stimulation intensity is just below the patient's

tolerance. In the operating room, intensity levels of 25 mA are typically used (Table 6).

To record the DSEP, electrodes are placed over the homuncular region of the cerebral cortex that is representative of the site of stimulation. While responses can be elicited by stimulating cervical as well as lumbar and sacral dermatomal fields, the lumbar and sacral dermatomal stimulation sites are the most common. When re-

TABLE 6. *Parameters used to acquire DSEPs and EMGs*

	DSEPs	
Stimulation site:	Appropriate dermatomal fields	
Level of stimulation vs. recording site	Lower extremity	Upper extremity
	F_{pz}–C_{p1}	F_{pz}–C_{p3}
	F_{pz}–C_{pz}	F_{pz}–C_{p4}
	F_{pz}–C_{p2}	
Stimulus intensity	25 mA	
Stimulation rate	4.7/sec (slower if necessary)	
Filter setting	30–250 Hz	
Time base	100 msec	

	Spontaneous EMGs	Electrically elicited EMGs
Stimulation sites	N/A	Pedicle hole and pedicle screw
Recording sites	Appropriate myotomes	Appropriate myotomes
SIL*	N/A	20 V
Stimulation rate	N/A	2.2/sec
Filter setting	5–5000 H	5–5000 H
Time base	1 sec	50 sec

* SIL, search intensity level.

cording the response over the cerebral cortex, the morphology of the DSEP is essentially identical to that of the mixed-nerve SEP. The latency of the DSEP increases as a function of the distance between the stimulation and recording sites. In a very comprehensive study by Slimp et al. (62), the mean latencies and degree of variability of cervical, thoracic, lumbar, and sacral DSEPs were determined.

Interpretation of the DSEP is based primarily upon latency and to a lesser degree on response amplitude. However, latency is the primary interpretative criterion because of the effects of nerve root compression on the response. When a nerve root is compressed, the large diameter fibers typically are affected first. This compression results in a prolongation of response latency that

may be accompanied by a degradation in response amplitude. However, because the amplitude of the DSEP is unstable, especially in the operating room, latency is the primary interpretative criterion. Figure 30 depicts normal DSEPs recorded in the operating room.

The strength of the DSEP is that the response provides information regarding individual nerve root function. However, the DSEP has significant limitations in the operating room, especially when changes, such as in anesthetic regimen, occur. Because a reliable subcortical DSEP is difficult, if not impossible, to record, especially following stimulation of lumbar or sacral dermatomal fields, it is very difficult to determine if a change in the cortical DSEP is a result of perisurgical or surgical variables. When interpreting the DSEPs, the absolute latency

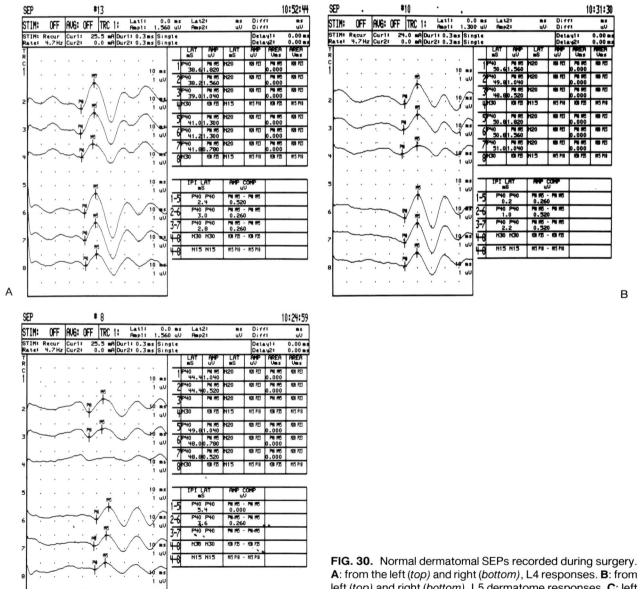

FIG. 30. Normal dermatomal SEPs recorded during surgery. **A**: from the left (*top*) and right (*bottom*), L4 responses. **B**: from left (*top*) and right (*bottom*), L5 dermatome responses. **C**: left (*top*) and right (*bottom*), S1 responses.

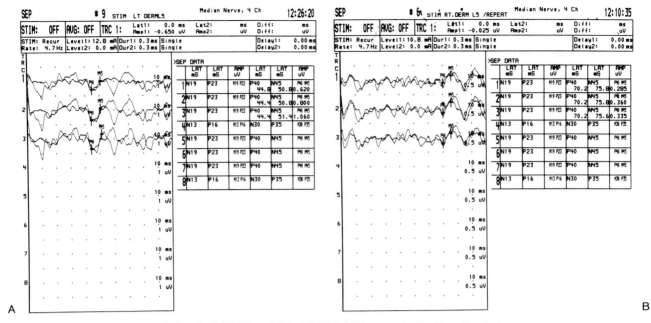

FIG. 31. Left L5 (**A**) and right L5 (**B**) DSEPs recorded in Case Study 8.

of the P40 response is compared within as well as between legs. There should be a gradual increase in the response latency of the P40 for responses elicited at more distal stimulation sites. For example, the L5 response should demonstrate a greater latency than L4 but a comparable latency to S1. Between-leg differences should not vary by more than 6 msec for responses following stimulation of the comparable nerve roots. For example, if the response of the right L5 demonstrates a latency 6 msec greater than that of the left L5, then the response with the longer latency should be considered pathologically prolonged.

Case Studies

The following case studies present information describing the use of DSEPs during surgeries for spinal degeneration.

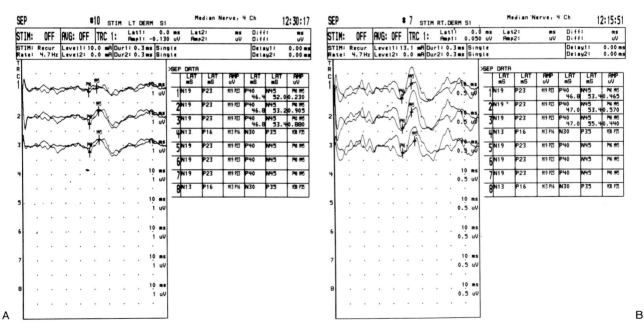

FIG. 32. Left S1 dermatomal SEPs (**A**) and right S1 dermatomal SEPs (**B**) recorded from the patient described in Case Study 8.

Case Study 8: This 50-year-old woman underwent surgery for spinal degeneration. The patient, who had had previous surgeries of the lumbar spine, and reported preoperative symptoms of low back pain and some radicular pain in both lower extremities. The surgery for nerve root decompression progressed uneventfully. EMGs were used to monitor nerve root function during the use of transpedicular instrumentation. No significant changes occurred in any data recorded during surgery.

Approximately 2 days following surgery, the patient reported numbness and eventually developed a foot drop in the right lower extremity. DSEPs were administered following the onset of the foot drop. Results demonstrated abnormal (Fig. 31) left and right L5 DSEPs, but essentially normal L4 and S1 data (Fig. 32), bilaterally. The pattern of postoperative DSEPs suggested that the fragment was more centrally located, which usually results in bilateral diminution of DSEPs at the same segmental level. Imaging studies were negative. Based on the DSEPs and the patient's symptoms, the patient was returned to the operating room and the surgical site was explored. It was found that a large bone fragment from the L5 pedicle hole was lying in the spinal canal. This fragment was clinically silent until the patient began to ambulate, at which time it demonstrated a compressive/irritant effect on the nerve roots.

Following removal of the fragment, repeated DSEP studies demonstrated a gradual improvement in nerve root function that coincided with the patient's improvement in clinical function. By using DSEPs, we were able to ascertain objectively the functional status of individual nerve roots in this patient and the effects of removing the pedicle wall fragment.

ELECTROMYOGRAPHIC RESPONSES: MECHANICALLY AND ELECTRICALLY ELICITED

An alternative to DSEPs for monitoring individual nerve root function during surgery, especially with the use of transpedicular instrumentation, is to record EMG responses. Responses are recorded from muscles that are innervated by nerve roots that are at surgical risk. EMGs can be elicited by either mechanical irritation (51) or electrical stimulation (11,12,18). These two methods provide information that is mutually exclusive. Therefore, both methods should be administered during surgery.

Mechanically Elicited EMGs

Mechanically, EMGs are elicited by irritation of the nerve roots. Irritation can occur following pedicle wall breakout resulting from a pedicle finder, a pedicle tap, or a pedicle screw, among other things. When controlling for the effects of perisurgical variables such as temperature of irrigating fluid or level of muscle relaxation, any EMG activity present is attributed to mechanical irritation of the nerve root. This is interpreted as indicating that whatever instrument was being used (e.g., pedicle finder, tap) has broken through the pedicle wall and is mechanically irritating the nerve root.

Procedures used to record mechanically elicited EMGs are administered continuously during the dynamic stages of surgery, those periods in which the surgeon is probing/tapping with the pedicle finder or actually placing a pedicle screw. To record the response, the signal averaging device is placed on "free run" and activity is continuously recorded; thus the testing is maximally sensitive to any type of mechanical irritation of the nerve root. Associated with the elicitation of an EMG is a popping sound that results from muscle contraction. This auditory feedback allows the surgeon to cease immediately any irritating maneuvers, further reducing the likelihood of a postoperative deficit.

Case Studies

The following case studies present information concerning the use of mechanically elicited EMGs during surgery for spinal degeneration that utilizes transpedicular instrumentation.

Case Study 9: The following case study presents information regarding mechanically elicited EMG activity as a function of surgical maneuver. In Figure 33, EMG activity was recorded following probing of the C6 foramen

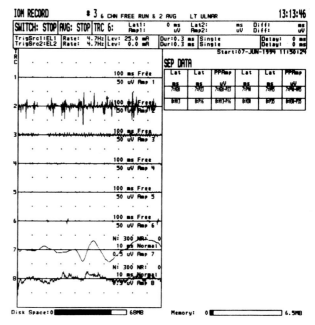

FIG. 33. Spontaneously elicited EMG activity recorded from a single muscle group following mechanical irritation of the nerve root, as described in Case Study 9.

after decompression. The surgeon used a small probe to ascertain the adequacy of decompression of the nerve root. During probing of the C6 foramen, mechanically elicited EMG data were recorded from the ipsilateral biceps femoris muscle. The surgeon was immediately informed that the foraminal probe was mechanically irritating the nerve root. The surgeon stopped the probing maneuver and further decompressed the nerve root. Upon re-probing the foramen, no elicited activity occurred and the surgeon stopped further decompression.

Case Study 10: This case study pertains to a patient undergoing surgery in the lumbosacral spine. While a pedicle finder was being used, no spontaneously elicited EMG activity occurred. However, during the use of the pedicle tap, EMG activity was elicited (Fig. 34). The surgeon was immediately informed of the elicited EMG activity and the orientation of the pedicle hole was inspected. It was found that the surgeon had directed the hole laterally, which resulted in mechanical irritation of an adjacent nerve root, causing the elicitation of EMG activity. By reorienting the pedicle hole, it was possible to avoid any additional nerve root irritation.

Electrically Elicited EMGs

Electrically elicited EMGs are administered during surgery for spinal degeneration, especially if transpedicular instrumentation is used. Following placement of the pedicle screw, the pedicle hole and pedicle screw are electrically stimulated using a cathodic stimulator. This methodology is based upon the work of Calancie et al. (11).

To conduct this procedure, the surgeon is handed a

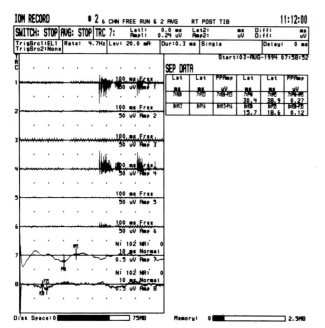

FIG. 34. EMG activity record from several muscle groups following mechanical irritation of nerve roots (Case Study 10).

stimulating probe that is attached to the cathode stimulator of the evoked potential instrument. The anode stimulating electrode, which is a 0.5-inch sterile subdermal needle electrode, is placed in the surgical field by the surgeon. who then stimulates either the pedicle hole or the pedicle screw. EMG activity in the peripheral musculature is recorded. The rationalization for this methodology is that the electrical insulating characteristics of an intact pedicle wall are adequate to prevent the spread of electrical current from the cathode electrode to the anode. However, if the pedicle wall has been fractured, the current will find the anode electrode through the path of least resistance (i.e., the fracture in the pedicle wall), which will result in stimulation of adjacent nerve roots.

When we use this method, we present the stimulus at a searching intensity level (SIL) of 20 V, whereas Calancie et al. recommend 6 mA. We use a constant voltage signal as opposed to constant current, because results can be obtained at lower intensities with greater resolution. The methodology we use consists of the following steps:

1. The stimulating electrodes (cathode and anode) are handed off to the surgeon. The anode needle is placed in the field and the cathode is used to stimulate.

2. A constant voltage signal is presented at 30 V.

3. The surgeon stimulates the bottom of the pedicle hole and halfway up the pedicle walls to determine if pedicle wall breakthrough has occurred. If the pedicle screw has already been placed, the head of the pedicle screw is stimulated prior to the attachment of any rods, crosslinks, etc.

4. If no response occurs at 30 V and if the pedicle screw or hole "feel good," no additional testing is warranted. If no response is obtained at 30 V, the pedicle hole/pedicle screw should be considered appropriate. If a response is obtained between 20 and 30 V, the surgeon can, using discretion, visually inspect the pedicle hole or screw.

5. If the response threshold is less than 20 V, some type of intervention needs to be initiated. Intervention can consist of repositioning/reorientating the pedicle hole, removing the pedicle screw, and retapping the pedicle with reinsertion of the screw, etc.

In a study by Darden et al. (18), the relationship between pedicle screw thresholds and the efficacy of intervention strategies during surgery that uses transpedicular instrumentation was investigated. Electrically elicited EMGs were recorded from 132 patients undergoing spinal arthrodesis with pedicle screw instrumentation. A total of 630 screw placements were evaluated. Based on the presence of EMG activity elicited at 20 V, results could be classified into two general categories: no response at 20 V (normal) or a response was present at less than 20 V (abnormal). A normal response was obtained in 90 patients (68%), and a response was obtained at less than 20 V in the remaining 42 patients (32%). After obtaining these initial responses, no intervention methods were administered to 50% of the patients with abnormal results and some type of intervention was administered to the other 50% of these patients. Intervention consisted of reorientating the pedicle hole, removing or repositioning the pedicle screw, and so forth. The pedicle hole/screw was retested until intervention resulted in the establishment of an EMG threshold of 20 V or more. Of the patients who demonstrated a response at less than 20 V and to whom no intervention was administered, 19% demonstrated a new surgically induced neurological deficit postoperatively. In the patients who demonstrated an initial EMG response at less than 20 V but were administered intervention, none demonstrated a new postoperative neurological change. These results indicate that intervention based on electrical stimulation techniques is effective and should be implemented in patients who demonstrate the presence of EMG activity at less than 20 V.

Case Study

Case Study 11: A 58-year-old man underwent posterior decompression with placement of transpedicular instrumentation at L4, L5, and S1, bilaterally. During placement of the left S1 screw, EMGs were elicited from mechanical irritation of the nerve root. Electrical stimulation of the screw (Fig. 35) revealed activity in the same muscle group. The screw was removed and reoriented. No additional EMG activity was noted.

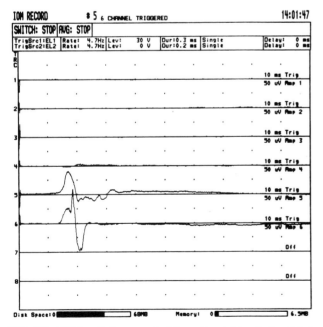

FIG. 35. EMG activity recorded from the right anterior tibialis (*Trace 5*) and right medial gastrocnemius muscle (*Trace 6*) following electrical stimulation of the right L5 and right S1 pedicle hole, respectively (Case Study 11).

DSEPs VERSUS EMGs: WHICH POTENTIAL TO USE?

Based on our experience, there are three reasons to monitor nerve roots during these types of surgeries: (a) to determine the level(s) of nerve root involvement, (b) to determine adequacy of nerve root decompression, and (c) to protect nerve roots during the use of transpedicular instrumentation and surgical manipulation.

To determine the level(s) of neural root involvement, the potential must demonstrate adequate nerve root specificity. The specificity of DSEPs has been investigated by a number of studies (15,49,50). The findings indicate that the specificity of the DSEPs varied as a function of segmental level. At more rostral levels (i.e., L3 and L4), specificity was not as great as at more caudal segmental levels. To determine the causes for the discrepancy between DSEPs and the level of nerve root involvement, Owen et al. (50) investigated the innervation patterns of lumbar and sacral nerve roots. They found that this discrepancy resulted from variations in the innervation patterns of the sensory nerve roots. These variations were comparable to those associated with motor fibers (56). Because of these variations in anatomy, DSEPs will never demonstrate 100% specificity in determining the level of nerve root involvement.

At the present time, no studies have investigated the specificity of EMG activity to levels of nerve root involvement. However, in a study by Phillips and Park (56), it was found that the variations in the innervation patterns of the anterior nerve roots were comparable to those of the dorsal (sensory) roots. Comparing the two methodologies, it appears that the DSEPs and EMGs demonstrate comparable specificity to level of nerve root involvement.

A second purpose for monitoring surgery for spinal degeneration is to determine the adequacy of nerve root decompression. In 1987, Herron et al. (23) investigated the effects of adequacy of nerve root decompression on intraoperatively recorded DSEPs. The purpose of their study was to determine if adequate decompression and postoperative pain relief were associated with improvement of intraoperative DSEPs. The authors reasoned that if adequate decompression of a nerve root was achieved, then the patient should demonstrate improved intraoperative DSEPs and less postoperative radicular pain. To ascertain adequacy of decompression, Herron et al. analyzed the amount of intraoperative improvement of the DSEP latency. Their results and those of Cohen et al. (16) support the use of the DSEP as a measure of adequacy of nerve root decompression. However, in a study by Owen et al. (53), it was found that the relationship between intraoperative improvement of DSEPs and adequacy of decompression was also affected by the duration of nerve root compression. If nerve root compression was of an acute nature (1 year or less), it was not unusual for DSEPs to improve during surgery following decompression. In this study, 82% of the patients demonstrated changes in the DSEP that correlated with postoperative pain relief. However, in the remaining 18%, the DSEP did not correlate with the alleviation of postoperative pain. At the present time, it does not appear that DSEPs provide information regarding adequacy of nerve root decompression in patients with chronic root compression. No studies have been published that attempt to correlate changes in EMGs with adequacy of decompression or postoperative pain relief.

The third reason for administering neurophysiological procedures during surgery for spinal degeneration is to protect nerve roots during the use of transpedicular instrumentation. As reported by Weinstein et al. (72), and Roberts and Bernhardt (57), the incidence of malpositioning of transpedicular screws ranged from 0% to 25%. Because damage to the nerve root results from pedicle wall breakthrough by the instrumentation, the neurophysiological procedures must be sensitive to *instantaneous* changes in nerve root function.

Comparing the sensitivity of DSEPs and EMGs to nerve root irritation from transpedicular instrumentation reveals significant differences. First, the DSEP is an averaged response. This means that before a response is available for interpretation, the peripheral dermatomal field must be stimulated at a certain rate (i.e., 4.7/sec) and an adequate number of responses (e.g., 300) recorded and averaged. This averaging process typically requires at least 1 minute before a response can be interpreted. Because of the time involved with averaging, changes in nerve root function can occur but not be immediately detected by the DSEP. Therefore, DSEPs do not meet the third requirement for monitoring during surgery that places nerve roots at risk. EMGs, however, provide the type of sensitivity needed to monitor nerve root function during the use of transpedicular instrumentation.

COST ANALYSIS OF OPERATIVE MONITORING

There are a variety of neurophysiological procedures that can be used to monitor surgery that places the spinal cord or nerve roots at risk. There are two costs associated with intraoperative monitoring: the professional fee and the technical fee. The professional fee relates to the charges associated with interpreting data. In the past, interpretation had been performed either while surgery was being performed or afterward. However, it is no longer considered appropriate to interpret data after the completion of surgery, because by then any neurological deficits will have already occurred.

The technical fee of the intraoperative monitoring charge pertains to the hospital costs associated with administering the program, which typically include the cost of the monitoring instruments and personnel, and which are added to the charge for use of the operating room.

In most testing facilities, the cost of intraoperative monitoring is based on an hourly rate. The exact amount charged per hour varies with the institution and with the geographic locale. Because of this variance, it is not possible to determine the relative cost-versus-benefit ratio for the entire United States. This is especially true because there is a lack of consistency in the neurophysiological procedures that are administered.

In reviewing the literature pertaining to spinal cord monitoring, the majority of monitoring programs in the United States utilize only mixed-nerve SEPs, not MEPs. While an argument can be made that mixed-nerve SEPs are adequate to detect the presence of a surgical insult to the spinal cord, there is literature that indicates that this is not the case. In a recent article by Nuwer et al. (44), it was found that the use of SEPs during surgery were influenced by several factors, including the experience of the surgeon and the monitoring personnel. If experience was adequate, the incidence of a major neurological deficit was 0.24%. From a cost perspective, Nuwer et al. reasoned that the average cost to monitor a surgery was $600 per case. If 200 surgeries were monitored, the cost for preventing one major persistent neurological deficit was $120,000, which is substantially less than the cost of providing medical care, physical therapy, and so forth for the duration of the patient's life. At Johns Hopkins Hospital, we routinely administer somatosensory and motor evoked potentials during all surgery that places the spinal cord at risk. Administering both procedures does not require a significant increase in the length of time needed to prepare the patient for testing, nor are there added costs to the monitoring charges. We have, however, always detected the onset of a surgically induced sensory or motor deficit. Since our false-negative rate is zero and the costs associated with administering both somatosensory and evoked potential procedures is low, it is strongly recommended that SEPs and MEPs be used during surgery that places the spinal cord at risk.

In reviewing the literature pertaining to monitoring during surgery for spinal degeneration, Calancie et al. (11,12) reported a 0% false-negative rate when using electrically elicited EMGs and a false-positive rate of 13%. This indicates that if pedicle wall breakthrough occurs, electrically elicited EMGs will always detect its presence. However, in 13% of the cases in which EMGs were positive for pedicle wall breakthrough, there was no indication of a new postoperative radiculopathy. This suggests that this method is extremely sensitive to the presence of pedicle wall breakthrough, but that the response is associated with an elevated false-positive rate. Because the false-negative rate is so low, this method should be considered for use.

Pertaining to mechanically elicited EMG activity, Owen et al. (51) reported a 0% false-negative rate and less than a 1% false-positive rate when discharges resulting from perisurgical variables were taken into consideration. Because of the high sensitivity to nerve root irritation, electrically and mechanically elicited EMG procedures are strongly recommended.

One final question that continues to be raised regarding neurophysiological monitoring is its clinical value. When neurophysiological procedures are administered appropriately, they have been found to significantly reduce postoperative neurological deficits resulting from either spinal cord or nerve root damage (44). However, a major limitation of most neurophysiological programs is the training and experience of the individuals administering and interpreting the various procedures. Although the American Board of Neurophysiological Monitoring is developing an examination process that will result in board certification for individuals involved with IOM, at the present time there are no guidelines, and until these examinations are developed, orthopedists and neurosurgeons who utilize IOM can expect variability in quality. By taking a more active role, the surgeon can improve the quality of monitoring and reduce postoperative neurological deficits.

SUMMARY AND CONCLUSIONS

The purpose of this chapter has been to provide information regarding the various methodologies available for monitoring spinal cord and nerve root function during surgery that places these anatomical structures at risk. For a successful program, appropriate instrumentation, personnel, and procedures must be available. When multimodality approaches are used, it is possible to demonstrate a significant reduction in postoperative deficit resulting from surgical and perisurgical insults. Intraoperative application of neurophysiological procedures has proven to be a cost-effective way to reduce the incidence of surgically induced postoperative neurological deficits.

REFERENCES

1. Amassian VE, Stewart M, Gregory J, Quirk BS, Rosenthal JL (1987): Physiological basis of motor effects of a transient stimulus to cerebral cortex. *Neurosurgery* 20(1):74–93.
2. Ashkenaze D, Mudiyan R, Boachie-Adjei O, Gilbert C (1993): Efficacy of spinal cord monitoring in neuromuscular scoliosis. *Spine* 18:1627–1633.
3. Been HD, Kalkman CJ, Traast HS, et al. (1994): Neurologic injury after insertion of laminar hooks during Cotrel-Dubousset instrumentation. *Spine* 19:1402–1405.
4. Ben-David B (1988): Spinal cord monitoring. *Orthop Clin North Am* 19(2):427–448.
5. Ben-David B, Haller G, Taylor P (1987): Anterior spinal fusion complicated by paraplegia: a case report of a false-negative somatosensory evoked potential. *Spine* 12:536–539.

6. Bracken MB, Shepard MJ, Collins WF, et al. (1990): A randomized controlled trial of methylprednisolone or naloxone in the treatment of acute spinal cord injury. *N Eng J Med* 322:1405–1411.
7. Bracken MB, Shepard MJ, Collins WF, et al. (1992): Methylprednisolone or naloxone treatment after acute spinal cord injury: one year follow-up data. *J Neurosurg* 76:23–31.
8. Brown RH, Nash CL (1979): Current status of spinal cord monitoring. *Spine* 4:466–470.
9. Burke D, Hicks R, Stephen J, Woodforth I, Crawford M (1992): Assessment of corticospinal and somatosensory conduction simultaneously during scoliosis surgery. *Electroencephalogr Clin Neurophysiol* 85:388–396.
10. Calancie B, Klose J, Baier S, et al. (1991): Isoflurane-induced attenuation of motor evoked potentials caused by electrical motor cortex stimulation during surgery. *J Neurosurg* 74:879–904.
11. Calancie BJ, Lebwohl N, Madsen P, Klose KJ (1992): Intraoperative evoked EMG monitoring in an animal model. *Spine* 17:1229–1235.
12. Calancie BJ, Madsen P, Lebwohl W (1994): Stimulus-evoked EMG monitoring during transpedicular lumbosacral spine instrumentation: initial clinical results. *Spine* 19:2780–2786.
13. Chatrian G, Berger MS, Wirch AL (1988): Discrepancy between intra-operative SSEPs and postoperative function. *J Neurosurg* 69:450–454.
14. Coe JD, Mongan PD, Chambers HG, Peterson RE (1992): *Spinal cord monitoring with neurogenic motor evoked potentials using percutaneously placed interspinous electrodes: a new technique for spinal cord stimulation.* Presented at the Scoliosis Research Society, Kansas City, MO.
15. Cohen BA, Hulzenger BA (1988): Dermatomal monitoring for surgical correction of spondylolisthesis: a case report. *Spine* 13:1125–1130.
16. Cohen BA, Major MR, Huizenga BA (1991): Predictability of adequacy of spinal cord decompression using evoked potentials. *Spine* 16:379–383.
17. Cracco RQ, Evans B (1978): Spinal evoked potentials in the cat: effects of asphyxia, strychnine, cord section and compression. *Electroencephalogr Clin Neurophysiol* 44:187–201.
18. Darden BJ, Wood KE, Skelly J, et al. (1993): *Evaluation of pedicle screw insertion monitored by intraoperative evoked electromyography.* Presented at North American Spine Society, San Diego, CA.
19. Edmonds HL, Paloheimo MP, Backman MH, et al. (1989): Transcranial magnetic motor evoked potentials (TCMEP) for functional monitoring of motor pathways during scoliosis surgery. *Spine* 14:683–686.
20. Forbes HJ, Allen PA, Waller CS, Jones SJ, Edgar MA, Webb PJ, Ransford AO (1991): Spinal cord monitoring in scoliosis surgery. *J Bone Joint Surg* 73B:487–491.
21. Haghighi SS, York DH, Gaines RW, Oro JJ (1994): Monitoring of motor tracts with spinal cord stimulation. *Spine* 19:1518–1524.
22. Harada Y (1983): Study on experimental spinal cord injuries by distraction using spinal cord evoked potentials. *J Jpn Orthop Assoc* 57:685–701.
23. Herron LD, Trippi AC, Gonyeau ML (1987): Intraoperative use of dermatomal somatosensory evoked potentials lumbar stenosis surgery. *Spine* 12:379–383.
24. Ihaya A, Morioka H, Noguchi H, et al. (1990): A case report of descending thoracic aortic aneurysm associated with anterior spinal artery syndrome descending thoracic aortic aneurysm associated with anterior spinal artery syndrome despite no marked ESP changes. *Kyoubugeka* 43(10):843–846.
25. Imai K (1988): A clinical study on intra-operative spinal cord monitoring with spinal evoked potential for scoliosis. *J Jpn Orthop Assoc* 62:511–521.
26. Imai T (1976): Human electrospinogram evoked by direct stimulation on the spinal cord through epidural space. *J Jpn Orthop Assoc* 55:1037–1056
27. Jones SJ, Edger MA, Ransford AO, Thomas NP (1983): A system for the electrophysiological monitoring of the spinal cord during operations for scoliosis. *J Bone Joint Surg* 65(B):134–139.
28. Katayama Y, Tsubokawa T, Sugitani M, Maejima S, Hirayama T, Yamamoto T (1986): Assessment of spinal cord injury with multimodality evoked spinal cord potentials, part I: localization of le-

sions in experimental spinal cord injury. *Neuroorthopedics* 1:130–141.

29. Kitagawa H, Itoh T, Takano H, Takakuwa K, Yamamoto N, Yamada H, Tsuji H (1989): Motor evoked potential monitoring during upper cervical spine surgery. *Spine* 14(10):1078–1083.

30. Konrad P, Owen JH, Bridwell KH (1994): Magnetic stimulation of the spine to produce lower extremity EMG responses: significance of coil position and the presence of bone. *Spine* 19:2812–2818.

31. Kurokawa T (1972): Spinal cord action potentials evoked by epidural stimulation of cord—a report of human and animal record. *Noha to Kindenzu* 1:64–66.

32. Kurokawa T (1979): Clinical application of the electrospinogram. *Shinkei Kenkyu no Shinpo* 23:409–420.

33. Laschinger JC, Owen JH, Rosenbloom M, et al. (1988): Direct non-invasive monitoring of spinal cord function during thoracic aortic occlusion: use of motor evoked potentials. *J Vasc Surg* 7:161–171.

34. Lesser RP, Raudzins P, Luders H, et al. (1986): Postoperative neurological deficits may occur despite unchanged intra-operative somatosensory evoked potentials. *Ann Neurol* 19:22–25.

35. Levy W, York D (1983): Evoked potentials from the motor tracts in humans. *Neurosurgery* 12(4):422–429.

36. Lubicky JP, Spadoro JA, Yuan HA, et al. (1989): Variability of somatosensory evoked potential monitoring during spinal surgery. *Spine* 14:790–798.

37. Machida M, Kimura J, Yanada T, Yarita M (1992): Magnetic coil stimulation of the spinal cord in the dog. *Spine* 17(11):1405–1408.

38. Machida M, Weinstein S, Yamada T, Kimura J (1985): Electrophysiological measures of sensory and motor function during spinal surgery. *Spine* 10(5):407–413.

39. Maruyama Y, Shimoji K, Shimizu H, Kuribayashi H, Fujioka H (1982): Human spinal cord potentials evoked by different sources of stimulation and conduction velocities along the cord. *J Neurophysiol* 48(5):1098–1107.

40. Matsuda H (1989): Intraoperative spinal cord monitoring using electric responses to stimulation of caudal spinal cord or motor cortex. In: Desmedt, ed. *Neuromonitoring in surgery.* Amsterdam: Elsevier, pp. 175–190.

41. Matsuda H, NN, Yasunami T, Yanai N, Funakoshi K, Nakamura H, Jou I, Yoshimura T, Shimazu A (1987): Descending evoked spinal cord potential and evoked peripheral nerve motor action potential elicited by tracscranial cerebral cortex stimulation. *Rinshounouha* 29(8):497–503.

42. Merton PA, Morton HB (1980): Electrical stimulation of human motor and visual cortex through the scalp. *J Physiol* 305:9014.

43. Nuwer MR (1986): *Evoked potential monitoring in the operating room.* New York: Raven Press, pp. 51–75.

44. Nuwer MR, Dawson EG, Carlson LG, Kanim LE, Sherman JE (1995): Somatosensory evoked potential monitoring reduces neurologic deficits after scoliosis surgery: results of a large multicenter survey. *Electroencephalogr Clin Neurophysiol* 96:6–11.

45. O'Brien MF, Lenke LG, Bridwell KH, et al. (1994): SSEP monitoring of upper extremity function during thoracic and lumbar deformity surgery: a prospective study. *J Spinal Disord* [in press].

46. Ohmi Y, Tohno S, Harada S, Nakano K (1984): Spinal cord monitoring using evoked potentials recorded from epidural space. In: Homma S, Tamaki T, eds. *Fundamentals and clinical application of spinal cord monitoring.* Tokyo, Japan: Saikon Press, pp. 203–210.

47. Owen JH (1993): Technology and equipment review: intraoperative monitoring equipment. *J Clin Neurophysiol* 10:526–539.

48. Owen JH (1993): Intraoperative stimulation of the spinal cord for prevention of spinal cord injury. In: Devinsky O, Beric V, Dogali J, eds. *Electrical and magnetic stimulation of the brain and spinal cord.* New York: Raven Press, pp. 271–288.

49. Owen JH, Bridwell KH, Grubb R, et al. (1991): The clinical application of neurogenic motor evoked potentials to monitor spinal cord function during surgery. *Spine* 16:S385–390.

50. Owen JH, Bridwell KH, Lenke LG (1993): Innervation pattern of dorsal roots and their effects on the specificity of dermatomal somatosensory evoked potentials. *Spine* 18:748–754.

51. Owen JH, Kostuik J, Gornet M, et al. (1994): The use of mechanically elicited EMGs to protect nerve roots during surgery for spinal degeneration. *Spine* 19:1704–1710.

52. Owen JH, Naito M, Bridwell KH (1990): Relationship among level of distraction, evoked potentials, spinal cord ischemia and integrity and clinical status in animals. *Spine* 15:852–857.

53. Owen JH, Padberg AM, Spahr-Holland L, et al. (1991): Clinical correlation between degenerative spine disease and dermatomal somatosensory evoked potentials in humans. *Spine* 16:201–205.

54. Owen JH, Sponseller PD, Szymanski J, et al. (1994): Efficacy of multimodality spinal cord monitoring during surgery for neuromuscular scoliosis. *Spine* 20:[in press].

55. Patton HD, Amassian VE (1954): Single and multiple unit analysis of cortical stage of pyramidal activation. *J Neurophysiol* 17:345–363.

56. Phillips LH, Park TS (1991): Electrophysiologic mapping of the segmental anatomy of the muscles of the lower extremities. *Muscle Nerve* 14:1213–1219.

57. Roberts RM, Bernhardt M (1992): *Accuracy of fluoroscopic guided pedicle screw placement in the lumbosacral spine.* Presented at the Scoliosis Research Society Meeting, Kansas City, MO.

58. Rossini PM (1988): The anatomic and physiologic bases of motor evoked potentials. *Neurol Clin* 6:751–769.

59. Satomi K, Nishimoto GI (1985): Comparison of evoked spinal potentials by stimulation of the sciatic nerve and the spinal cord. *Spine* 10:884–890.

60. Shields CB, Paloheimo MP, Backman MH, et al. (1988): Intraoperative transcranial magnetic motor evoked potentials are difficult to obtain during lumbar disc and spinal tumor operations. *Muscle Nerve* 11:993–998.

61. Shimizu H, Shimoji K, Maruyama Y, Sato Y, Harayama H, Tsubaki T (1979): Slow cord dorsum potentials elicited by descending volleys in man. *J Neurol Neurosurg Psychiatry* 42:242–246.

62. Slimp JC, Rubner DE, Snowden ML, et al. (1992): Dermatomal somatosensory evoked potentials: cervical, thoracic and lumbosacral levels. *Electroencephalogr Clin Neurophysiol* 84:55–70.

63. Takakuwa K, Tsuji H, Takano H, Kitagawa H (1989): Effects of epidural electrical stimulation modalities on spinal cord function and morphology in cats. *J Spinal Disord* 2:155–162.

64. Takano H, Takakuwa H, Kitagawa N, Yamamoto H, Tsuji H, Ueyama T (1991): Spinal cord monitoring in aortic aneurysm surgery. In: Shimoji K, ed. *Spinal cord monitoring and electrodiagnosis.* Berlin: Springer-Verlag, pp. 420–427.

65. Tamaki T, Kobayashi H, Yamase T, Egashira T, Tsuji H, Inoue S (1977): Clinical application of evoked spinal cord action potential (in Japanese). *Seikeigeka* 28:681–689.

66. Tamaki T, Noguchi T, Takano H, Tsuji H, Nakagawa T, Imai K, Inoue S (1984): Spinal cord monitoring as a clinical utilization of the spinal evoked potential. *Clin Orthop* 184:58–64.

67. Tamaki T, Takano H, Takakuwa H, Tsuji H, Nakagawa K, Imai, Inoue S (1985): An assessment of the use of spinal cord evoked potentials in prognosis estimation of injured spinal cord. In: Schramm J, Jones SJ, eds. *Spinal cord monitoring.* Berlin: Springer-Verlag, pp. 221–226.

68. Tamaki T, Tsuji H, Inoue S, Kobayashi H (1981): The prevention of iatrogenic spinal cord potential. *Int Orthop* 4:313–317.

69. Tamaki T, Yamashita T, Kobayashi H, Hirayama H (1972): Spinal cord monitoring [in Japanese] [abstract]. *Nouha to Kindenzu* 1:1969.

70. Tsuyama N, Tsuzuki N, Kurokawa T, Imai T (1978): Clinical application of spinal cord action potential measurement. *Int Orthop* 2:951–965.

71. Ueta T, Owen JH, Sugioka Y (1992): Effects of compression on physiologic integrity of the spinal cord, on circulation, and clinical status in four different directions of compression: posterior, anterior, circumferential, and lateral. *Spine* 17:217–226.

72. Weinstein JN, Sprah KF, Spengler D, et al. (1988): Spinal pedicle fixation: reliability and validity of roentgenogram-based assessment and surgical factors on successful screw placement. *Spine* 13:1012–1018.

73. Zentner J (1989): Noninvasive motor evoked potential monitoring during neurosurgical operations on the spinal cord. *Neourosurgery* 24:709–712.

The Adult Spine: Principles and Practice,
2nd edition, J.W. Frymoyer, Editor-in-Chief.
Lippincott-Raven Publishers, Philadelphia © 1997.

CHAPTER 35

Anesthesia, Positioning, and Postoperative Pain Management for Spine Surgery

Steven H. Rose, Beth A. Elliott, and Terese T. Horlocker

Providing anesthetic care for patients undergoing spine surgery poses interesting and challenging problems. Spine procedures and the patients who undergo them are a heterogeneous group. The patients may be in vigorous good health or have multiple medical problems, and they may vary in age from infants to the elderly. The procedures may be simple or complex, elective or emergent. In addition to the usual goal of providing an insensate patient, special consideration must be given to preoperative medical conditions, development of an appropriate anesthetic plan, and provision of postoperative pain relief.

S. H. Rose, M.D., Assistant Professor; B. A. Elliott, M.D., Assistant Professor; T. T. Horlocker, M.D., Assistant Professor: Department of Anesthesiology, Mayo Medical School, and Mayo Clinic, Rochester, Minnesota, 55905.

PREOPERATIVE CONSIDERATIONS

When performing a preanesthetic evaluation before spine surgery, many diverse factors must be considered. The evaluation should include the routine information sought before provision of anesthesia for any purpose, such as height and weight, blood pressure, medical and surgical history, a pertinent review of systems, medications, allergies, personal or family history of anesthetic or surgical problems, history of abnormal or excessive bleeding, and evaluation of the airway. Requirements for preoperative laboratory studies, a chest x-ray, and an electrocardiogram are determined by the age and health of the patient as well as by the scope of the procedure. The trend in recent years has been to decrease routine testing in many patients. Suggested screening tests in healthy patients are listed in Table 1.

TABLE 1. *Routine tests suggested before anesthesia and surgery** *

Age (yr)	CXR	EKG	Blood tests
<40	—	—	—
40–59	—	+	Creatinine, glucose
≥60	+	+	Creatinine, glucose, complete blood count

* Applicable only to patients in good general health. Other tests may be indicated by the patient's medical history, medications, physical examination, or scope of the procedure.
CXR, chest x-ray.

Airway evaluation is particularly important before spine surgery because of pathologic processes (including trauma) which may involve the cervical spine and at times render the cervical spinal cord susceptible to injury. Unfortunately, preoperative airway evaluation remains an inexact science. An excellent review of this issue that addresses preoperative recognition of the difficult airway by quantifying the relative tongue/pharyngeal size, degree of atlanto-occipital extension, and the size of the mandibular space was recently published by Benumof (6). Management of the difficult airway is addressed later in this chapter.

In addition to these universal concerns, particular attention should be directed toward issues related to the specific surgical procedure and the pathology that has made surgery necessary. Neuromuscular diseases, for example, may be associated with disorders of the spine and have important anesthetic implications. An appropriate neurologic evaluation should be performed and documented, especially if a deficit is present before surgery. During the physical examination, it is important to assess flexibility in anticipation of the proposed surgical position.

ANESTHETIC ISSUES SPECIFIC TO SCOLIOSIS

It is especially important to evaluate pulmonary and cardiac function before surgery for scoliosis. The heart and lungs may be directly affected (such as by mechanical pulmonary compromise), or they may be affected as part of a syndrome (such as Marfan's syndrome, which is associated with mitral valve prolapse, dilatation of the aortic root and aortic insufficiency). Most patients who present for surgical correction have sufficient myocardial and pulmonary reserve to tolerate the procedure. However, patients with more advanced disease or those with additional disease processes may require higher levels of perioperative support.

Monitoring must also be discussed with the patient preoperatively. If it is possible that a wake-up test will be required during surgery, the patient should be informed. It is important to reassure the patient that if this does occur, it is generally not associated with pain. It may also be useful to inform the patient of the importance of compliance with requests to move their extremities when asked to do so postoperatively in order to facilitate early neurologic evaluation.

Pulmonary Assessment in Scoliosis

As scoliosis progresses, it produces increasingly severe changes in pulmonary function. An important clinical determinant is assessment of the patient's exercise tolerance, which is one indicator of pulmonary reserve. The thoracic curvature compresses one hemithorax toward residual volume, while the other hemithorax increases toward total lung capacity. The resulting thoracic deformity causes a restrictive pattern of lung disease with decreases in total lung capacity, functional residual capacity, and residual volume. Decreasing lung volumes and corresponding increases in the work of breathing result in inefficient ventilation. Ventilation/perfusion mismatch leads to an increased alveolar–arterial oxygen difference and ultimately alveolar hypoventilation. The usual finding is a decrease in PaO_2 with a normal $PaCO_2$. As the disease progresses, hypercapnia may be seen, which is an indicator of severe pulmonary compromise.

In patients with idiopathic scoliosis, curvature of less than 65° is usually not associated with pulmonary compromise that necessitates postoperative mechanical ventilation. However, patients with neuromuscular disease, paralysis, or congenital scoliosis may show significant pulmonary compromise with lesser degrees of curvature. Scoliosis associated with neuromuscular disease has been shown to be accompanied by abnormalities in central respiratory control as well. If unchecked, pulmonary disease can progress to the point of irreversible pulmonary hypertension and cor pulmonale.

All patients with scoliosis should be asked to provide a pulmonary history preoperatively that includes an assessment of their exercise tolerance. Patients in whom significant pulmonary compromise is suspected should also undergo pulmonary function studies and have an arterial blood gas drawn. If the vital capacity is greater than 70% predicted, respiratory reserve should be sufficient. If the vital capacity is less than 40% predicted, postoperative mechanical ventilation will probably be required.

Cardiac Dysfunction in Scoliosis

In addition to pulmonary dysfunction, patients with scoliosis may have cardiovascular abnormalities. Cardiovascular abnormalities are most commonly caused by pulmonary hypertension (secondary to chronic hypoxia and/or hypercarbia). Right ventricular hypertrophy and cor pulmonale may develop as a result of the elevated pulmonary vascular resistance. Electrocardiographic changes associated with pulmonary hypertension and right atrial enlargement (P wave greater than 2.5 mm, R greater than S in V_1 and V_2) may be seen but are usually not evident until late in the disease process.

Scoliosis is also associated with congenital heart abnormalities, especially coarctation of the aorta and cyanotic disease. Mitral valve prolapse is common in patients with idiopathic scoliosis (a prevalence of about 25%). If a murmur is heard on physical exam, an echocardiogram is recommended. Patients with muscular dystrophies may have cardiac dysrhythmias and therefore warrant close perioperative monitoring. Marfan's syndrome and other similar abnormalities may be associated with mitral valve prolapse, dilatation of the aortic root, and aortic insufficiency. Agents that decrease myocardial contractility may be useful in these patients. Prophylaxis against infective endocarditis should be administered to patients who have mitral valve prolapse or other lesions resulting in disturbances of flow.

AIRWAY MANAGEMENT

The single most important aspect of anesthetic care is airway management. Airway management is a particular challenge if a difficult airway is encountered, or if concerns exist regarding the stability of the cervical spine. Any severely traumatized patient or any patient with a head injury should be assumed to have an unstable cervical spine until it is ruled out radiographically and clinically. Several methods may be used to intubate these patients. Awake fiberoptic intubation after topical anesthesia is applied to the upper airway is commonly used. If a fiberoptic bronchoscope is not available, awake intubation may be accomplished using a laryngoscope (after topical anesthesia) with the cervical spine stabilized. Blind or fiberoptic-guided nasal intubation may be used in patients who are breathing spontaneously, but this should be attempted only if there is no evidence of facial trauma or basilar skull fracture, to avoid neurologic injuries. Topical anesthesia and a vasoconstrictor (phenylephrine) may be administered as nasal sprays before nasal intubation to increase patient comfort and decrease bleeding. In an airway emergency, direct laryngoscopy and intubation may be necessary before cervical spine injury is excluded. In this instance, a second person should stabilize the cervical spine during the procedure to avoid, as much as possible, flexion or extension of the neck. Transtracheal jet ventilation through the cricothyroid membrane or tracheostomy may be necessary in some emergent situations.

MONITORING

Basic monitoring for patients undergoing spine surgery should follow established standards including blood pressure, heart rate, the electrocardiogram, pulse oximeter, temperature, and auscultation of breath and heart sounds via an esophageal stethoscope. A capnograph or mass spectrometer is useful for assessing adequacy of ventilation, as well as for detecting air embolus and malignant hyperthermia. Because of the duration of major spine surgical procedures and the potential for large volumes of fluid administration, an indwelling urinary catheter is routinely used to guide fluid management as well as to decompress the bladder. If the surgical wound is higher than the heart, a precordial Doppler may be used to detect venous air embolism. Decisions regarding the need for more invasive monitoring techniques should be made on a case by case basis with attention to preexisting medical conditions, the extent and duration of the planned surgical procedure, potential for blood loss, and access to the patient during surgery.

In most patients undergoing extensive spine surgery, an arterial catheter will be indicated. An arterial catheter provides a reliable minute-to-minute measure of arterial pressure and valuable access for blood sampling. Intraoperative arterial blood gas analysis, measurement of hematocrit and blood glucose, and coagulation tests are frequently used to follow the patient's metabolic status and help guide the rational use of blood and blood components.

Monitoring central venous pressure can also be useful in assessing intravascular volume and fluid status. While actual numerical values may not be of great benefit in a prone patient, following trends in central venous pressure can provide useful information to guide fluid replacement therapy. A central venous catheter has the added advantage of providing access to the central circulation for administration of pharmacologic agents and for volume administration. A central venous catheter can also be used for aspiration of air should venous air embolism occur. Patients with evidence of pulmonary hypertension or severe coexistent cardiovascular or pulmonary disease may require a pulmonary artery catheter for measurement of pulmonary artery and pulmonary artery occlusion pressures, determination of serial cardiac outputs, and calculation of pulmonary and systemic vascular resistance.

Spinal Cord Monitoring

Paraplegia is one of the most feared complications of spinal surgery. It is therefore essential that any intraoperative compromise of spinal cord function be detected as early as possible and reversed immediately. Methods developed for this purpose include the wake-up test and other types of neurophysiologic monitoring.

The Wake-up Test

The wake-up test consists of intraoperative awakening of patients after completion of spinal instrumentation. Ideally, the surgeon should notify the anesthesiologist 30 to 45 minutes in advance so that the patient may be gradually allowed to awaken. The patient is asked to move both hands and, after a positive response, both feet. If there is satisfactory movement of the hands, but not the feet, the distraction on the spine is reduced, and the wake-up test is repeated. Surgical manipulation should recommence only when the patient no longer responds to commands. Recall of the event occurs in 0% to 20% of patients and is only rarely viewed as unpleasant.

To date, there have been no false-negative wake-up test results; that is, no patient who was neurologically intact when awakened intraoperatively had a neurologic deficit upon completion of the procedure. However, certain hazards of the wake-up test exist and include recall, pain, air embolism, rod dislocation, accidental extubation, and accidental removal of intravenous and arterial catheters. In addition, the wake-up test requires patient cooperation and may be difficult to perform on young children or mentally handicapped individuals.

Neurophysiologic Monitoring

An adjunct or alternative to the wake-up test is neurophysiologic monitoring. Somatosensory evoked potentials (SSEPs), electromyography (EMG) and, more recently, motor evoked potentials (MEPs) are being used to detect early signs of spinal cord ischemia or insult. With SSEPs, cortical or subcortical response to a repetitive peripheral sensory stimulus is monitored. An electrical impulse is delivered to the posterior tibial nerve at the ankle and to the median nerve at the wrist. An insult to the spinal cord in the thoracolumbar area would affect only the posterior tibial response, whereas systemic events which can affect SSEPs would affect the impulse from both the posterior tibial and the median nerves. Systemic factors that can alter cortical responses with SSEPs include depth of anesthesia, hypercarbia, hypoxia, hypotension, and hypothermia. Subcortical responses, usually measured at the cervical spine, are generally more resistant to systemic factors. When SSEPs are acutely abnormal, spinal cord compromise should be assumed. Every attempt should be made to increase spinal cord blood flow and oxygen delivery and to decrease anesthetic depth. Arterial blood pressure should be returned to normal or slightly higher (20%), volatile anesthetics should be decreased or discontinued, and 100% oxygen should be administered. Arterial blood gas analysis may reveal a correctable metabolic abnormality or an unsuspected low hematocrit. If the SSEP abnormality continues despite correction of these factors, it may be necessary for the surgeon to release distraction on the cord and/or a wake-up test should be performed to rule out a false-positive test.

A significant drawback to using SSEPs alone when monitoring spinal cord integrity during surgery is that the vulnerable anterior motor tracts of the cord are left unmonitored. There are reports of patients who have awakened paraplegic after an apparently uneventful procedure with normal SSEPs. Motor evoked potentials (MEPs) have recently been introduced for use in selected cases considered at high risk for insult to the anterior spinal cord or its vascular supply. MEPs are elicited by activating motor pathways using transcranial electrical or magnetic stimulation or by electrical stimulation of the spinal cord. The true role of MEPs in spine surgery has yet to be determined.

Spinal cord monitoring is discussed further in Chapter 34.

POSITIONING

Proper positioning of patients for spine surgery can decrease blood loss, facilitate surgical exposure, and prevent position-related injury. All members of the patient care team share responsibility for positioning. A coordinated effort and adequate numbers of personnel are essential for optimal patient care.

The most common patient position for spine surgery is prone. Under usual conditions, induction of anesthesia precedes placement of invasive monitoring lines, intubation, and positioning. However, patients with an unstable spine may need to be positioned prior to the induction of anesthesia to allow for gross assessment of spinal cord integrity and insure patient comfort after prone positioning. Because access to the airway and intravascular access are quite limited in the prone position, they must be secured prior to transfer. Careful sedation is recommended during this period to increase patient comfort. A predetermined set of hand signals can be used to communicate with awake intubated patients.

One of the main goals when positioning patients in the prone position is to minimize pressure on the abdomen. Pressure on the abdomen displaces the abdominal contents, restricting diaphragmatic excursion and impairing ventilation. Concomitantly, pressure is increased within the epidural venous plexus, which can dramatically increase intraoperative bleeding (16,85).

A variety of devices are available to position patients prone. Longitudinal chest rolls placed from just below the clavicles to the iliac crests are perhaps the simplest to use (Fig. 1). The Walker frame, similar in function to longitudinal chest rolls, attaches to the operating table

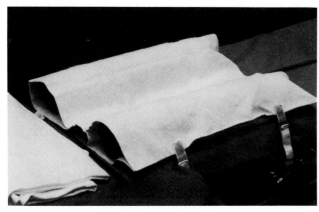

FIG. 1. Longitudinal support devices used in conjunction with a typical operating room table. Chest rolls. (From ref. 18.)

and markedly reduces lumbar lordosis (Fig. 2). The Tower table and the Relton frame are examples of pedestal-type systems, which support the patient's weight at the infraclavicular chest and the iliac crests (Fig. 3). Knees are flexed and weight-bearing. It is important to keep weight-bearing evenly distributed to decrease the likelihood of skin breakdown. Breasts should be directed medially to avoid injury (51). Male genitalia should be in a neutral midline position and free of compression.

Arm position may vary depending on the device used to achieve the position, the patient's body habitus, and operator preference. Arms tucked alongside the patient's body should be in an anatomical position and intravascular lines checked to assure patency. If an arm board is used, the arm should not be abducted more than 90°, to avoid brachial plexus injury, and the elbow should be flexed (92). Extra padding beneath the elbow will protect the ulnar nerve from compression. Some pedestal sup-

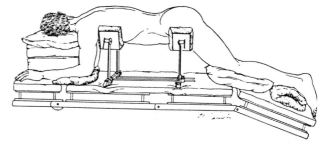

A

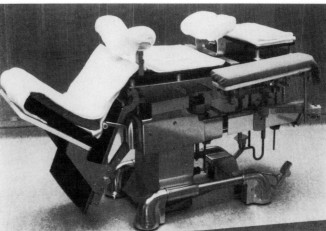

B

FIG. 3. Pedestal-type support device. **A:** Relton frame. (From ref. 85, with permission.) **B:** Tower table. (From ref. 18.)

port systems have an open space beneath the patient's abdomen into which the arms may be tucked. This is not recommended in obese patients as the weight of the pendulous abdomen can produce compartment syndromes in the forearm (R. A. Klassen, *personal communication*, 1991).

Head and neck range of motion should be thoroughly evaluated preoperatively. If patient mobility allows, the head is usually turned laterally. If only one arm is abducted, the head should face the abducted arm to avoid a stretch injury to the brachial plexus. Padding is placed beneath the forehead and chin to keep the dependent eye and ear free of pressure. If patient immobility or surgical needs dictate a neutral midline head position, a horseshoe head rest can be used to support the patient's head. Special attention should be paid to avoid pressure on the eyes with this device, as increased intraocular pressure can result in retinal ischemia and blindness. The eyes should be checked frequently during the procedure to assure that the head has not slipped from the original position. The use of pinions and halo head frame combinations to position the head is reserved for cases with a specific surgical indication.

Regardless of the method used to achieve the prone position, the legs are usually in a somewhat dependent position relative to the heart. Legs should be wrapped with lightly compressive dressings or stockings, or sequential compression devices should be used to prevent venous pooling.

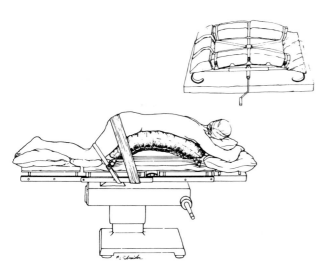

FIG. 2. Longitudinal support devices used in conjunction with a typical operating room table. Walker frame. (From ref. 50, with permission).

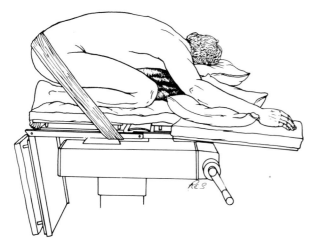

FIG. 4. Tuck position. (From ref. 85, with permission.)

In past years, the kneeling or tuck position was sometimes used for spine surgery (Fig. 4). The extreme degree of hip and knee flexion required to achieve this position is not feasible for many patients and can significantly compromise perfusion to the lower extremities, resulting in ischemia, thrombosis, compartment syndromes, and neurologic deficits (4,39). Few use this position today and it is not recommended.

Surgical procedures on the anterior aspect of the thoracic and lumbar spine are accomplished in the lateral decubitus position. The dependent arm is abducted and placed on an arm board. The upper arm can be placed on a padded over-arm board or sling, or it can be rested upon pillows. A chest roll or axillary roll is placed under the dependent chest wall just beneath the axilla to take pressure off the dependent shoulder and to prevent com-

pression of the neurovascular bundle by the humeral head. The head and cervical spine should be supported to maintain alignment of the central neuraxis and to free the dependent eye and ear from pressure. The dependent leg is typically flexed at the hip and knee while the uppermost leg is extended. Pillows are placed between the legs to avoid pressure injury from bony protuberances. The hips should be placed so the iliac crests lie over the kidney rest portion of the operating table. The kidney rest may be raised during anterior lumbar spine surgery to provide better surgical exposure. Placement of the kidney rest under the patient's flank or lower ribs jeop-

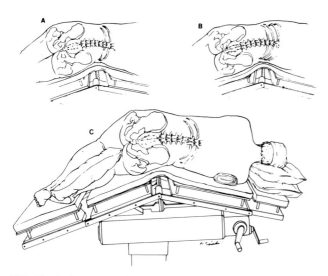

FIG. 5. A: Incorrect placement. **B:** Incorrect placement. **C:** Correct placement of the kidney rest beneath the iliac crest, resulting in the least interference with functions of the dependent lung and diaphragm. (From ref. 43, with permission.)

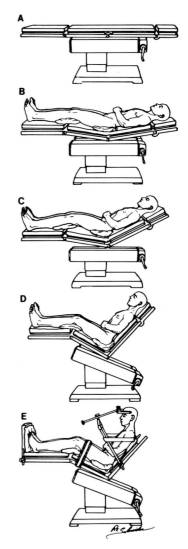

FIG. 6. Table manipulation sequence for establishment of the traditional sitting position. **A:** Initially flat table top. **B:** Top fully flexed and foot section depressed. **C:** Back section elevated as sustained perfusion permits. **D:** Chassis depressed as back section continues to be raised and legs are adjusted to heart level. **E:** Head holder and frame in place; head section of table removed; thigh strap and foot board added. Optional shoulder restraining tapes shown. Lateral padding to protect arms now shown for clarity. (From ref. 50, with permission.)

ardizes ventilation and risks vena caval obstruction (Fig. 5) (18).

The posterior cervical spine may be approached with the patient in the prone or sitting position. The sitting position has the advantage of providing a relatively bloodless surgical field and excellent surgical exposure. The primary disadvantage of the sitting position is the risk of venous air embolism (VAE). VAE can occur whenever the operative field is higher than the heart, allowing entrainment of air into open venous channels. VAE has been reported in the prone position as well but is less likely (52).

The operating table is prepared by placing several pillows in such a way that the patient's buttocks and legs are well supported with the knees flexed. After induction of anesthesia and placement of head pinions, the operating table is flexed and the upper back portion is raised to elevate the patient's head and torso into the sitting position. The lumbar spine should be snug against the operating table. At the same time, the table should be placed in a slight Trendelenburg position to bring the legs nearer to the level of the heart. The foot portion of the table is lowered to further flex the knees and the heels should be padded. When securing the final head position, care should be taken to avoid excessive neck flexion, as this can lead to impaired venous return from the head. Arms are flexed at the elbow and supported on the patient's lap (Fig. 6). Excessive hip flexion can lead to sciatic nerve injury and should be avoided (50).

ANESTHETIC TECHNIQUE

The choice of anesthetic technique is guided by the intraoperative neurophysiologic monitoring to be used, the anticipated need for an intraoperative wake-up test, the length and duration of surgery, and the patient's specific medical problems. Both general and regional anesthesia can be safely administered for lower thoracic and lumbar surgery. Some anesthesiologists and surgeons prefer spinal anesthesia for limited procedures; typically, a hypobaric solution is employed. Advocates of regional anesthesia maintain that it reduces blood loss and improves operating conditions by shrinking epidural veins. If regional anesthesia is used, a local anesthetic of sufficient duration must be selected or a catheter technique employed, because conversion to general anesthesia may be difficult or impossible. The majority of spine surgery, however, is performed under general anesthesia. General anesthesia is preferred for essentially all upper thoracic and cervical procedures because of the high dermatomal level that would be required with a regional technique. In addition, general anesthesia ensures airway access, is associated with greater patient acceptance, and may be preferred for lengthy operations.

Induction of anesthesia may be accomplished with any of the available induction agents. Sodium pentothal, 3 to 5 mg/kg IV, is used most often. Tracheal intubation is facilitated by administration of succinylcholine, 1 to 2 mg/kg IV (in the absence of preexisting neurologic deficit or other contraindication). Alternatively, if a nondepolarizing muscle relaxant is used, a relatively short-acting agent is preferred when EMG monitoring is planned so it is not delayed.

Anesthesia may be maintained with isoflurane, 0.25% to 1.0% inspired, or another volatile agent, 60% nitrous oxide, and a narcotic of choice. Some practitioners prefer a strict nitrous–narcotic anesthetic technique, thus completely avoiding the effect of inhalational agents on neurophysiologic monitoring. However, most practitioners prefer a balanced anesthetic technique using both narcotics and inhalational agents. The addition of an inhalational agent assists in providing hemodynamic stability and ensures lack of awareness during the surgical procedure. Should a wake-up test be required, the inhalational agent is easily discontinued and seldom delays neurologic testing.

SSEP monitoring is affected by all inhalational anesthetic agents. Signal amplitude diminishes and latency increases with increasing anesthetic depth. However, studies have shown and clinical practice has confirmed that SSEP monitoring can be accomplished when inhalational anesthetic levels remain relatively constant and do not exceed 0.75 minimal alveolar concentration (MAC) for isoflurane or 1.0 MAC for halothane and enflurane (each with 60% nitrous oxide). At these levels, subcortical signals remain relatively intact. Nitrous oxide can diminish the amplitude of the SSEP signal, but it is used routinely without major difficulty. Narcotics may increase the latency of cortical SSEPs but do not interfere significantly with subcortical signals.

Narcotics play a significant role in the anesthetic management of most patients undergoing spine surgery. The specific choice of narcotic is usually unimportant as long as sufficient doses are administered. Narcotic doses comparable to 10 mg morphine are listed in Table 2. Narcotics may be administered as a bolus or by continuous infusion. Longer acting narcotics (such as morphine or

TABLE 2. *Narcotic dosage with parenteral administration; comparable to 10 mg morphine*

Codeine phosphate	120–130 mg
Concentrated opium alkaloids, hydrochlorides	20 mg
Diacetylmorphine hydrochloride (heroin)	3–5.5 mg
Fentanyl citrate	200 μg
Hydromorphone hydrochloride	1.3–2 mg
Levorphanol tartrate	2–2.3 mg
Meperidine hydrochloride	75–100 mg
Methadone hydrochloride	8–10 mg
Oxymorphone hydrochloride	1–1.5 mg

Modified from McEvoy, ed. (52a).

oxymorphone) are usually administered as intermittent boluses. If a continuous infusion technique is chosen, a shorter acting drug is preferred (fentanyl 5 to 10 μg/kg IV bolus followed by an infusion of 5 to 10 μg/kg/hr). Fentanyl infusions should be discontinued 30 to 60 minutes before the end of the surgical procedure. Continuous narcotic infusion may reduce total narcotic requirement and results in a smoother and more rapidly achievable wake-up test. Excessive narcotic administration, which is more likely to occur with the intermittent bolus technique, may lead to prolonged ventilatory support and delay postoperative neurologic evaluation. An additional advantage of continuous narcotic infusion techniques is the elimination of bolus-induced variations in SSEPs, making it easier to interpret SSEP changes that occur during surgical manipulation.

Muscle relaxants should be avoided if intraoperative electromyography is monitored. Because of the low amplitude of SSEP signals, it is useful to use muscle relaxants when SSEPs alone are monitored in order to diminish electrical background noise from muscle activity. Muscle relaxants also decrease the possibility of patient movement during critical periods of the surgical procedure. Intermittent bolus injection is the most common method of administration, but continuous infusions of intermediate duration nondepolarizing relaxants such as atracurium or vecuronium can be used as well. In general, relaxants are administered to maintain T1 at 20% or more of baseline. A peripheral nerve stimulator should be used whenever muscle relaxants are administered.

Hypothermia

Patients undergoing spine surgery are at high risk for developing hypothermia because of the large volume of fluids administered, exposure of a large surgical wound to a cool operating room environment, prolonged ventilation with anesthetic gases, and altered thermoregulation resulting from anesthesia. Hypothermia may contribute to increased bleeding by interfering with platelet function. Peripheral vasoconstriction shifts intravascular volume centrally, resulting in overestimation of volume status based on measurement of central venous pressure. Prevention of hypothermia is more effective than treatment. Warming and humidification of inspired gases, forced-air warming devices, and maintaining a reasonable room temperature (19°C or higher) are the most effective means of preventing hypothermia.

One Lung Ventilation

Anterior approaches to the cervicothoracic and thoracolumbar spine may be necessary alone or in combination with a posterior fusion. Surgical access can at times be greatly facilitated by deflating the lung on the operative side. One lung ventilation (OLV) can be accomplished using either of two techniques. The most common involves a double lumen endotracheal tube (DLETT). A left DLETT is preferable because of the greater distance between the carina and the upper lobe bronchus on that side. The second technique involves the use of a bronchial blocker. The blocker is placed in the mainstem bronchus on the operative side using fiberoptic guidance. When lung deflation is desired, the cuff is inflated preventing further inspiratory gas flow. Since the blocker occludes expiratory flow as well, lung deflation can be facilitated by manual compression of the lung just before blocker cuff inflation. Advantages of DLETTs over bronchial blockers include greater access for suctioning and a provision of continuous positive airway pressure (CPAP) to the operative lung. OLV should be used only by experienced practitioners with sophisticated monitoring capability.

Venous Air Embolism

Though rare, VAE has been reported to occur in patients having spine surgery in the prone position. Positioning measures taken to decrease epidural venous pressure may exacerbate the gradient that exists between the surgical field and the heart. This factor, combined with a contracted blood volume or inadequate volume replacement, may increase the likelihood of VAE. Precordial Doppler monitoring is currently the most widely available sensitive device to detect the occurrence of VAE. It is not used routinely to monitor patients for spine surgery, but it should be considered for those patients with right-to-left intracardiac shunts who are at risk for paradoxical air embolism.

Postoperative Care

One of the goals of anesthetic management for patients having spine surgery is to have an awake, cooperative, and comfortable patient at the end of the procedure. Tests of gross neurologic function should be performed and documented on all patients before leaving the operating room.

Most spinal surgery patients, including those who undergo posterior fusion, can be extubated shortly after surgery if preoperative pulmonary function was acceptable. However, residual narcotics or muscle relaxants may lead to hypoventilation or apnea, especially in patients with an associated neuromuscular disease. Postoperative pneumothorax should be considered as a potential cause of respiratory distress as well. Aggressive postoperative pulmonary care, including incentive spirometry, is necessary to avoid atelectasis and pneumonia.

Continued hemorrhage remains a concern during the

postoperative period. Careful monitoring of blood pressure, central venous pressure, urine output, and wound drainage is essential. Neurologic status must also be monitored closely for early detection of a deficit.

BLOOD LOSS AND FLUID MANAGEMENT

Spine surgery can be associated with considerable blood loss and fluid changes, especially if the surgery involves multiple levels, or extensive decortication or instrumentation. Complications associated with homologous blood transfusion include acquired immunodeficiency syndrome (AIDS), hepatitis, and transfusion reactions. The use of autologous blood reduces these risks. Blood loss and transfusion requirements may also be reduced through the use of proper positioning, intraoperative blood salvage, induced hypotension, and intraoperative hemodilution.

Infectious Risks of Homologous Blood Transfusions

There has been an increased public awareness of the risks associated with transfusion of homologous blood and blood components in recent years, resulting in large part from concern regarding acquisition of the human immunodeficiency virus (HIV), which causes AIDS. Though less appreciated by the public, other transfusion-related infections, especially hepatitis, are far more common.

AIDS

Screening of blood for antibodies to HIV was initiated in 1985 (38,67). However, homologous blood that has been screened for HIV still poses some risk of infection. After an individual is initially exposed to HIV, a period of 6 to 14 weeks may transpire before antibodies to the virus can be detected (91). If blood is donated during this period, it may be infective but test negative.

Hepatitis

Hepatitis has remained the most common serious transfusion-related infection for many years. After testing was initiated for hepatitis B virus (HBV), the majority of cases have been caused by what was previously labeled non-A, non-B hepatitis, more recently designated hepatitis C (44). Hepatitis C is initially mild, with jaundice developing in less than 5% of those infected (36). However, up to half of these patients become chronic carriers, 10% of whom may develop serious complications (2).

Other Infectious Risks

Nearly any infectious disease can be transmitted by homologous transfusion (22,63,64,81,83). A particular concern is transfusion-related sepsis caused by bacterial contamination of blood or blood products (60,81). Platelets carry a higher risk of sepsis because they are stored at room temperature for up to 5 days, which may allow significant bacterial multiplication.

Transfusion Reactions

Hemolytic transfusion reactions are potentially fatal and in the vast majority of cases are caused by clerical errors resulting in transfusion of ABO-incompatible blood (62,63,81), although hemolytic reactions can occur with other red cell antigens as well. Hemolytic transfusion reactions result in hemodynamic instability, renal ischemia, and coagulation disorders (21,24). Treatment includes immediately discontinuing the transfusion, infusing crystalloid or colloid solutions, administration of furosemide, and alkalinization of the urine.

Transfusion-related acute lung injury (TRALI) is caused by immunologic activation initiated when a recipient leukocyte antibody interacts with a leukocyte antigen in transfused (donor) blood (71,72,90). The main consequence of this syndrome is pulmonary compromise with low-pressure pulmonary edema, hypoxia, bronchospasm, and an adult respiratory distress–like picture. Cardiovascular collapse may occur with this syndrome as well.

Other reactions include febrile and minor allergic reactions which are common but seldom of major clinical significance.

Transfusion of Blood

Oxygen transport is the primary function of transfused red blood cells. The point at which transfusion is necessary varies widely between patients based on a host of factors including age, myocardial reserve, blood viscosity, acuity of blood loss, and others. Although oxygen transport may be maximal at a hemoglobin of about 10 g% (46,58), in healthy patients transfusion may be unnecessary until a lower figure is reached. Regardless, the decision to transfuse red blood cells must be made after careful consideration of the entire clinical picture.

Massive Blood Loss

Spinal surgery can be associated with severe bleeding and require massive transfusion (transfusion of 1.5 times the blood volume or more). Massive transfusion may induce a coagulopathy, the most common cause of which is dilutional thrombocytopenia (59). However, it is difficult to determine when platelet transfusion is necessary. Some studies report series of patients receiving massive blood transfusion, in which only a relatively small percentage (less than 50%) develop significant coagulopathy despite receiving no component therapy (12,54,78). Similarly, it is difficult to predict when fresh frozen plasma (FFP) should be administered. FFP has not been shown to be effective prophylactically and is rarely clinically indicated (12). It appears that during massive transfusion, blood components should be administered based on the individual clinical circumstances and coagulation testing.

Coagulation Testing

The prothrombin time (PT) and activated partial thromboplastin time (aPTT) are not good indicators of the need for FFP (12,59,61,78). More useful tests to guide component therapy during massive transfusion include the platelet count, thromboelastogram (TEG), and fibrinogen level. If disseminated intravascular coagulation (DIC) is suspected, fibrin split products should also be measured.

Strategies to Diminish the Need for Homologous Blood Transfusion

Most blood loss in spinal instrumentation and fusion occurs with decortication, is proportional to the number of vertebral levels decorticated, and may necessitate perioperative transfusion. Surgical and anesthetic techniques that reduce the need for homologous blood transfusions result in fewer transfusion-related complications. Strategies to diminish the need for homologous blood transfusion are listed in Table 3.

Autologous Pre-donation

Autologous pre-donation of blood can be an effective method to decrease or eliminate the need for homologous blood transfusion. In a multi-institutional study of nearly 5,000 surgical patients (in tertiary care settings), about 68% of the patients who needed blood but did not

TABLE 3. *Strategies that may decrease homologous transfusion*

Autologous pre-donation
Wound infiltration with epinephrine
Norvolemic hemodilution
Intraoperative blood salvage
Postoperative blood salvage
Induced hypotension
Erythropoietin

pre-donate could have avoided homologous transfusion had they done so (88). Other studies have also shown high degrees of success with pre-donation (17,33,42). Despite concerns about cardiac reserve, older patients have been shown to be at low risk when they pre-donate blood (27,57,65,69).

Wound Infiltration with Epinephrine

Infiltration of the tissues with epinephrine before surgical incision is used by some surgeons to decrease the amount of incisional bleeding. It is extremely important that adequate communication between surgeon and anesthesiologist occur, that the dose of epinephrine be limited, and that its use be avoided when contraindicated [for example, in patients taking monoamine oxidase (MAO) inhibitors].

Normovolemic Hemodilution

Normovolemic hemodilution consists of acutely withdrawing autologous blood and replacing it with colloid or crystalloid shortly before surgery. The red cell mass is therefore decreased during surgical hemorrhage and can be returned to the patient thereafter. This technique has been shown to be efficacious during scoliosis surgery; in one study reducing homologous transfusion requirements from 4,370 mL to 750 mL (49). Concerns include maintenance of adequate oxygen transport to vital organs, particularly the kidneys, brain, and myocardium.

Intraoperative Blood Salvage

Intraoperative blood salvage is another technique used to avoid or minimize the need for homologous transfusion. A variety of devices are available for this purpose (14,56,95). Several are designed to spin salvaged blood in a centrifuge and simultaneously wash them with saline. Alternatively, blood can be passed through a filtration device which collects red blood cells. After filtration, the cells may or may not require washing before transfusion. A concern regarding any of these devices is their effect on coagulation. Unwashed RBCs may cause a coagulopathy resulting from activation of the coagulation cascade, formation of fibrin, and subsequent degradation of fibrin by fibrinolysis. Products of this degradation (fibrin split products) are known to interfere with platelet aggregation and adhesion and affect fibrin polymerization. Conversely, cell washing systems remove these degradation products but also remove coagulation factors and platelets and may contribute to coagulopathy in this way. Heparin is also present in small amounts when these systems are used.

Intraoperative blood salvage is seldom used when pus is present or spillage of bowel contents occurs. Despite these concerns, several studies have shown that clinical infections occur rarely, even if cultures of salvaged blood are positive (3,14,82). In general, sepsis has not been attributed to intraoperative salvage of blood, but such salvage remains not recommended in patients with sepsis except as a life-saving measure. Malignancy is another concern with intraoperative salvage and it is usually avoided in these patients. However, several studies have shown that the spread of cancer by this mechanism is suspect (10,30,34,41,80). Postoperative blood salvage has also been performed with success, most commonly after cardiac or thoracic procedures.

Induced Hypotension

Moderate induced hypotension [reduction of systolic blood pressure 20 mm Hg from baseline or lowering mean arterial pressure (MAP) to 65 mm Hg in the normotensive patient] has been shown to decrease blood loss, reduce transfusion requirements by up to 50%, and shorten operating times (47,55). However, induced hypotension is not without risk and has been reported to cause cord ischemia and neurologic deficits (31,32). Factors associated with an increased risk of spinal cord damage include preoperative hypertension, hypocapnia, intraoperative MAP less than 60 mm Hg, rapid decrease in blood pressure, and anemia (45). Patients with severe deformity, congenital scoliosis, or kyphosis may have an abnormal pattern of spinal cord blood supply that is more easily compromised during surgical distraction or compression. The purported benefits of deliberate hypotension must be weighed against the potential risk of acute neurologic complications.

Hypotension should be induced prior to surgical incision to prevent hemodilution and excess fluid administration. Blood pressure is slowly decreased to achieve an MAP of 60 to 70 mm Hg or a systolic blood pressure of 20 to 30 mm Hg less than preoperative systolic values (47,66). The various agents used to induce hypotension in scoliosis surgery include trimethaphan, nitroglycerine, sodium nitroprusside, halothane, enflurane, and isoflurane (66). The volatile agents provide anesthesia as well as hypotension. However, all volatile anesthetics produce a dose-dependent deterioration of SSEP waveforms. Sodium nitroprusside produces a reliable decrease in blood pressure and at least initially increases spinal cord blood flow, but it may be associated with tolerance, tachyphylaxis, toxicity, and rebound hypertension (20). Nitroglycerin maintains or increases spinal cord blood flow but may be ineffective in achieving target blood pressure (87,94). Pretreatment with a blocker such as propranolol or an angiotensin-converting enzyme inhibitor can prevent rebound hypertension and reflex tachycardia and reduce dose requirements and toxicity of intravenous hypotensive agents (73).

Erythropoietin

Erythropoietin has been shown to be effective at increasing RBC production after phlebotomy (19,25), though this is often unnecessary and is prohibitively expensive for general use.

Colloids and Crystalloids

Colloid and crystalloid infusions may be used to replace fluid loss due to evaporation, the production of urine, and "third spacing" during surgery. They may also be used to replace the loss of blood provided oxygen-carrying capacity remains adequate. Lactated Ringer's solution is the most commonly used crystalloid. Commonly used colloid solutions include albumin and hydroxyethyl starch. Both are free of infectious risks. Despite a large number of studies and reviews (15,70,89), the crystalloid versus colloid controversy remains largely unresolved.

SPINAL CORD INJURY

The consequences of spinal cord injury vary greatly depending on the level of the lesion and may involve several organ systems.

Autonomic Dysreflexia

Autonomic dysreflexia is a syndrome associated with chronic spinal cord injury. It is characterized by severe paroxysmal hypertension associated with bradycardia, ventricular ectopy, and various degrees of heart block. The stimulus of this event may be cutaneous, proprioceptive, or visceral (such as distention of a viscus like the bladder or the rectum). The syndrome does not generally occur if the lesion is below the T7 dermatome (40), but it does occur in about 85% of patients with complete cord transection above T5 (Table 4). The syndrome involves massive sympathetic outflow unopposed by the usual inhibition of higher centers. Consequently, pressure receptors are activated causing increased parasympathetic influence (via the vagus nerve). Cutaneous vasoconstriction is evident below the lesion, and cutaneous vasodilation is present above it (flushing).

TABLE 4. *Autonomic dysreflexia*

Severe paroxysmal hypertension associated with bradycardia, ventricular ectopy and heart block.
Stimulus may be cutaneous, proprioceptive or visceral.
Unusual if spinal cord lesion is below T7 dermatome.
Occurs in 85% of patients with complete spinal cord transection above T5.

Treatment involves removal of the noxious stimulus (e.g., bladder distention), increasing the level of anesthesia, and administration of direct-acting vasodilators. If left untreated, the syndrome may provoke a hypertensive crisis causing seizures, myocardial ischemia, or cerebral hemorrhage. Avoidance of this syndrome necessitates anesthesia for patients with spinal cord damage despite a lack of motor or sensory function in the area of the surgery. Either regional or general anesthesia may be used to prevent this phenomenon. Spinal anesthesia is preferred over epidural primarily because the presence of CSF that can be freely aspirated provides greater assurance of a successful block.

Respiratory Considerations

Ventilatory impairment increases with higher levels of spinal injury. Therefore, determination of the level of injury is crucial for assessing probable respiratory complications. A high cervical lesion that includes the diaphragmatic segments (C3-C5) will result in respiratory failure and death unless artificial pulmonary ventilation is instituted. Lesions between C5 and T7 cause significant alterations in respiratory function because of the loss of abdominal and intercostal support. The indrawing of flaccid thoracic muscles during inspiration produces paradoxical respirations resulting in a vital capacity reduction of 60%. Inability to cough and effectively clear secretions may result in atelectasis and infection. Paralytic ileus and gastric distension increase abdominal pressure, resulting in further compromise of diaphragmatic excursion. This effect can be reduced by placement of a nasogastric tube and attaching it to suction. It is also important not to overlook associated injuries such as pneumothorax or flail chest. Chronically, the incidence of pulmonary embolism is increased because of decreased muscle tone venodilatation.

Cardiovascular Considerations/Spinal Shock

During spinal shock, there is a loss of sympathetic vascular tone below the level of the injury. Bradycardia will occur if the cardioaccelerator fibers (T1-T4) are affected. The unopposed vagal tone associated with high lesions may lead to asystole during tracheal suctioning or laryngoscopy. Atropine may be administered to attenuate the vagal effects. Hemorrhagic shock is not accompanied by a compensatory tachycardia; heart rate may remain at 40 to 60 beats/min. The tendency to treat hypotension with fluids during spinal shock and the inability of the cardiovascular system to compensate in response to fluid loading may lead to the development of pulmonary edema. Pulmonary artery catheter placement is recommended for fluid management in patients with high cervical lesions (1). Autonomic instability should be treated with direct-acting vasoconstrictors, vasodilators, and positive and negative chronotropic drugs as needed. Indirect sympathetic agonists or antagonists should be avoided because of unpredictable clinical effects.

Maintaining Spinal Cord Integrity

All patients with spinal trauma should be considered to have spinal cord compromise, and an important component of anesthetic management is preservation of spinal cord blood flow. Blood pressure and intravascular volume should be maintained within normal levels to ensure adequate spinal cord perfusion pressure. Sustained hypotension may worsen neurologic deficits. Spinal cord blood flow parallels that of cerebral blood flow in both autoregulation and chemical regulation (35,48). Spinal cord blood flow autoregulates between mean arterial pressures of 60 and 150 mm Hg. Outside this range, flow is pressure dependent (29). Ischemia may occur if spinal cord perfusion pressure is maintained below autoregulatory limits. Likewise, spinal cord blood flow responds to arterial oxygen and carbon dioxide tensions in the same manner as cerebral blood flow (28). Hypocapnia decreases flow while hypercapnia and hypoxia result in vasodilation and increased flow. Acute administration of high-dose steroids has been advocated to reduce spinal cord swelling and improve neurologic outcome after spinal cord injury.

Electrolyte Abnormalities

Patients with motor deficits from spinal cord injuries may develop hyperkalemia after administration of succinylcholine (SCh). The amount of potassium released depends on the degree and acuity of paralysis. It is usually safe to administer SCh for the first 48 hours after injury. After that time, muscle cell membranes become supersensitive to depolarizing muscle relaxants. The increases in serum potassium are maximal between 4 weeks and 5 months after spinal injury (11). Serum potassium levels may increase from normal to as high as 14 mEq/L, causing ventricular fibrillation or cardiac arrest. Therefore, SCh should be avoided in all spinal cord injured patients after 48 hours. There are no contraindications to the nondepolarizing agents.

Hypercalcemia results from flaccid paralysis and immobilization, predisposing the patient to ventricular arrhythmias. In addition, the mobilization of bone calcium content may lead to osteoporosis, pathologic fractures, and renal calculi.

Temperature Control

Disruption of the sympathetic pathways carrying temperature sensation and subsequent loss of vasoconstriction below the level of injury cause spinal cord injured patients to be poikilothermic. Maintenance of normal temperature can be achieved by applying exogenous heat to the skin, increasing ambient air temperature, warming intravenous fluids, and humidifying gases.

POSTOPERATIVE PAIN MANAGEMENT

Adequate postoperative analgesia is increasingly recognized as an integral component of perioperative patient management. In addition to the humane desire to relieve pain and suffering, the desire to decrease the duration of hospitalization and the cost of surgery have been driving forces in the recent upsurge of interest in postoperative analgesia. There are a number of studies which demonstrate decreased patient morbidity and improved outcome as a result of improved postoperative pain management (74,96). Adequate analgesia to facilitate early ambulation and aggressive respiratory care and pulmonary toilet are key to achieving these goals.

Historically, postoperative pain management has been treated with standard orders for intramuscular opioids (see Table 2). Pharmacokinetic data have demonstrated that peak plasma levels of narcotics can vary fivefold from patient to patient after intramuscular administration. Time to peak levels will vary significantly as well (5). Busy postoperative nursing staffs, fears of addiction and overdose, and conservative interpretation of dose ranges, coupled with pharmacokinetic variability, have left many patients undertreated and experiencing significant pain (9).

Despite interpatient variability, the blood level at which a given patient experiences adequate pain relief is fairly constant (26). This level is referred to as the minimum effective concentration (MEC). The ideal postoperative pain management regimen would maintain MEC, and hence, patient comfort. This can be achieved to some degree with intravenous bolus dosing to patient comfort, followed by a continuous intravenous infusion to maintain that level. This technique works well in pediatric patients and others who may not be able to communicate their analgesic needs effectively. Patients receiving continuous infusions of opioids should be placed in a highly monitored setting because of the potential for relative overdose and respiratory depression.

One of the major drawbacks to the use of continuous infusions is that they do not take into account the variability of pain intensity. Patient-controlled analgesia (PCA) can allow the patient to anticipate painful stimuli such as ambulation and dressing changes, and to self-administer medication in anticipation of the increase in pain. A microcomputer processor is programmed to deliver a set dose of narcotic at a defined time interval when triggered by the patient. Some PCA devices can be programmed to provide a continuous background infusion

of narcotic in addition to what the patient triggers. This may help to avoid troughs in blood levels during periods of sleep, but it can also contribute to increased somnolence and respiratory depression (23,53,84). The most common mistake made when writing orders for PCA devices is to make the lockout period (the time interval between doses) too long. This interval should be short enough to allow the patient to rapidly titrate the dose to achieve MEC. PCA devices are designed to allow the patient to maintain a comfort level. For patients who have not yet achieved a comfort level, an initial bolus dose should be ordered in addition to the intermittent bolus dose. A 4-hour maximum dose is established to limit total drug use. Programming error leading to inadvertent overdose and interactions with concurrent medications remain concerns with PCA devices, but overall patient satisfaction with the technique is quite high (86).

Administration of narcotics via the central neuraxis (epidural or spinal) has achieved great success in patients who have undergone thoracic, major abdominal, and pelvic surgery (7,13). Selective nociception occurs as a result of the interaction between opioids and receptors within the dorsal horn of the spinal cord (93). Spinal opioids can be administered as single bolus injections or as continuous infusions. Initial concerns about the potential for life-threatening respiratory depression have been tempered with experience, and many centers routinely use epidural opioids on surgical wards (76). Judicious use of concomitant central nervous system depressants and assessment of level of consciousness as well as respiratory rate have proven useful in decreasing the risk of respiratory depression. Other commonly seen side effects include pruritus, nausea, vomiting, and urinary retention.

There is a growing body of literature supporting the use of epidural and spinal opioids for postoperative pain management in patients who have undergone spine surgery. Ross et al. (79) injected intrathecal preservative-free morphine (0.125 mg, 0.25 mg, or 0.5 mg) under direct vision using a #27 needle in 56 patients undergoing lumbar spine surgery. When compared to a control group receiving parenteral narcotics, the patients receiving intrathecal morphine had superior pain relief in a dose-dependent fashion. In addition, the patients receiving 0.25 and 0.50 mg of intrathecal morphine had significantly shorter hospital stays than the control group (5.6 days ± 0.4 and 5.7 days ± 0.6 versus 7.6 days ± 0.4, $p < 0.05$).

Epidural opioids can be administered through a catheter placed in the epidural space under direct vision at the time of surgery. As with intrathecal opioids, patients experience greater pain relief than those receiving parenteral narcotics (37). Side effects are similar to those seen with intrathecally administered opioids. Epidural administration has the advantage of not trespassing the dura. Rechtine and Love found that wound infiltration with local anesthetic did not provide additional pain relief in laminectomy patients who were receiving epidural morphine (77).

For those patients with a history of adverse reactions to opioids or for patients who have another reason to limit opioid use, ketorolac, a parenteral nonsteroidal anti-inflammatory drug (NSAID) has shown promise (75). Ketorolac is the only NSAID available for parenteral use in this country. It can be used alone or as an adjunct to opioids for the treatment of postoperative pain. Cataldo et al. found a 45% reduction in PCA morphine use in patients who were treated with ketorolac after extensive colon resections (8). Side effects include nausea, dyspepsia, abdominal pain, and edema. It should be used with caution in patients with impaired renal function (68).

Multiple studies have confirmed the importance of adequate postoperative pain control. Decreased patient morbidity, improved outcome, decreased length of hospital stays, and decreased expenditure of health care dollars can be attributed to advances in postoperative pain management. Many hospitals have established Acute Pain Services as a resource to provide consultation and management of the many modalities of acute pain therapy available today.

SUMMARY

Providing anesthetic care for spine surgery poses a variety of challenges. Patient care is optimized by a team approach that includes adequate preoperative evaluation and testing, development of an appropriate anesthetic plan, wisely selected monitoring, and the provision of postoperative pain management.

REFERENCES

1. Albin MS (1978): Resuscitation of the spinal cord. *Crit Care Med* 6:270–276.
2. Alter HJ (1985): Posttransfusion hepatitis: clinical features, risk and donor testing. *Prog Clin Biol Res* 182:47–61.
3. Andrews NJ, Bloor K (1983): Autologous blood collection in abdominal vascular surgery. Assessment of a low pressure blood salvage system with particular reference to the preservation of cellular elements, triglyceride, complement and bacterial content in the collected blood. *Clin Lab Haematol* 5:361–370.
4. Aschoff A, Steiner-Milz H, Steiner HH (1990): Lower limb compartment syndrome following lumbar discectomy in the knee-chest position. *Neurosurg Rev* 13:155–159.
5. Austin KL, Stapleton JV, Mather LE (1980): Multiple intramuscular injections: a major source of variability in analgesic response to meperidine. *Pain* 8:47–62.
6. Benumof JL (1991): Management of the difficult adult airway. *Anesthesiology* 75:1087–1110.
7. Benzon HT, Wong HY, Belavic AM, et al. (1993): A randomized double-blind comparison of epidural fentanyl infusion versus patient-controlled analgesia with morphine for postthoracotomy pain. *Anesth Analg* 76:316–322.
8. Cataldo PA, Senagore AJ, Kilbride MJ (1993): Ketorolac and patient controlled analgesia in the treatment of postoperative pain. *Surg Gynecol Obstet* 176:435–438.
9. Cohen FL (1980): Postsurgical pain relief: patients' status and nurses' medication choices. *Pain* 9:265–274.
10. Cole WH (1973): The mechanisms of spread of cancer. *Surg Gynecol Obstet* 137:853–871.
11. Cooperman LH (1970): Succinylcholine-induced hyperkalemia in neuromuscular disease. *JAMA* 213:1867–1871.
12. Counts RB, Haisch C, Simon TL, Maxwell NG, Heimbach DM, Carrico CJ (1979): Hemostasis in massively transfused trauma patients. *Ann Surg* 190:91–99.
13. Cullen ML, Staren ED, el-Ganzouri A, Logas WG, Ivankovich AD, Economou SG (1985): Continuous epidural infusion for analgesia after major abdominal operations: a randomized, prospective, double-blind study. *Surgery* 98:718–728.
14. Davies MJ, Cronin KC, Moran P, Mears L, Booth RJ (1987): Autologous blood transfusion for major vascular surgery using the Sorenson Receptal device. *Anaesth Intens Care* 15:282–288.
15. Dawidson I (1989): Fluid resuscitation of shock: current controversies. *Crit Care Med* 17:1078–1080.
16. DiStefano VJ, Klein KS, Nixon JE, Andrews ET (1974): Intraoperative analysis of the effects of body position and body habitus on surgery of the low back: a preliminary report. *Clin Orthop* 99:51–56.
17. Elawad AA, Fredin HO, Laurell M, Jonsson S (1991): Elderly patients' responses to preoperative autologous blood collection. *Med J Aust* 155:147–150.
18. Elliott BA (1993): Positioning and monitoring. In: Wedel DJ, ed. *Orthopedic anesthesia.* New York: Churchill-Livingstone, p. 99.
19. Eschbach JW, Kelly MR, Haley NR, Abels RI, Adamson JW (1989): Treatment of the anemia of progressive renal failure with recombinant human erythropoietin. *N Engl J Med* 321:158–163.
20. Fahmy NR, Mossad B, Milad M (1980): Spinal cord blood flow during induced hypotension: comparison of nitroprusside and trimethaphan. *Anesthesiology* 53:S87.
21. Faust RJ, Cucchiara RF, Messick JM Jr (1989): Transfusion medicine and cardiovascular anesthesia. In: Tarhan S, ed. *Cardiovascular anesthesia and postoperative care.* Chicago: Year Book Medical, p. 527.
22. Faust RJ, Warner MA (1990): Transfusion risks. *Int Anesthesiol Clin* 28:184–189.
23. Fleming BM, Coombs DW (1992): A survey of complications documented in a quality-control analysis of patient-controlled analgesia in the postoperative patient. *J Pain Symptom Management* 7:463–469.
24. Goldfinger D (1977): Acute hemolytic transfusion reactions—a fresh look at pathogenesis and considerations regarding therapy. *Transfusion* 17:85–98.
25. Goodnough LT, Rudnick S, Price TH et al. (1989): Increased preoperative collection of autologous blood with recombinant human erythropoietin therapy. *N Engl J Med* 321:1163–1168.
26. Gourlay GK, Kowalski SR, Plummer JL, Cousins MJ, Armstrong PJ (1988): Fentanyl blood concentration-analgesic response relationship in the treatment of postoperative pain. *Anesth Analg* 67:329–337.
27. Greenwalt TJ (1987): Autologous and aged blood donors [editorial]. *JAMA* 257:1220–1221.
28. Griffiths IR (1973): Spinal cord blood flow in dogs. 2. The effect of the blood gases. *J Neurol Neurosurg Psychiatry* 36:42–49.
29. Griffiths IR (1973): Spinal cord blood flow in dogs: the effect of blood pressure. *J Neurosurg Psychiatry* 36:914–920.
30. Griffiths JD, McKinna JA, Rowbotham HD, Tsolakadis P, Salsbury AJ (1973): Carcinoma of the colon and rectum: circulating malignant cells and five-year survival. *Cancer* 31:226–236.
31. Grundy BL, Nash CL, Brown RH (1981): Arterial pressure manipulation alters spinal cord function during correction of scoliosis. *Anesthesiology* 54:249–253.
32. Grundy BL, Nash CL, Brown RH (1982): Deliberate hypotension for spinal fusion: prospective randomized study with evoked potential monitoring. *Can Anaesth Soc J* 29:452–462.
33. Hansen HL (1989): A pre-operative autologous blood donation programme in a small hospital. *Arctic Med Res* 48:16–19.
34. Hart OJ III, Klimberg IW, Wajsman Z, Baker J (1989): Intraoperative autotransfusion in radical cystectomy for carcinoma of the bladder. *Surg Gynecol Obstet* 168:302–306.

The Adult Spine: Principles and Practice,
2nd edition, J.W. Frymoyer, Editor-in-Chief.
Lippincott-Raven Publishers, Philadelphia © 1997.

CHAPTER 36

Bone Grafts and Bone Graft Substitutes

Gary E. Friedlaender, Stephen L. Curtin, and Michael H. Huo

Bone has the unusual biologic capacity to regenerate following injury in contrast to the more common reparative events which end with scar tissue formation. Repair of the skeleton can often be further enhanced by the use of bone grafts, an approach that has been well recognized for centuries (10) and effectively practiced for more than 100 years (89,104). Bone grafts and other osteogenic materials have demonstrated usefulness in a wide variety of clinical circumstances including the replacement of major skeletal defects resulting from ablative surgery for bone tumors, restoration of bone stock in revision total joint arthroplasty, reconstruction of traumatic bone loss, and the filling of benign cystic defects as well as facilitating union in various forms of arthrodesis (46,55, 93,95,96). Much of the groundwork for our current confidence with and reliance upon bone grafts for enhancement of osteogenic potential and restoration of structural integrity of the skeleton was provided by the works

of Albee (1), Barth (7), Lexer (86), Phemister (109), and Senn (127) during the late nineteenth and early twentieth centuries. They also helped establish our fund of knowledge and scientific basis for the biology, banking, and widespread clinical applications of bone as a transplantable resource in orthopedic surgery (24).

Bone grafts can be obtained from several categories of donors (Table 1), each with distinct, inherent advantages and disadvantages. The majority of bone grafts used in clinical practice are autogenous (*autografts*), that is, tissue removed from one part of an individual and transferred to another location in the same individual. Autografts represent the maximum available biologic potential, pose no immunologic considerations, and obviate the concern for transfer of disease, especially infection, from donor to recipient. On the other hand, the availability of autografts is limited in terms of size, shape, and quantity and the potential exists for morbidity at the donor site. These considerations have prompted the search for alternative sources of osteogenic activity, including other types of bone graft as well as the use of synthetic implants and biosynthetic molecules with bone-inducing properties.

Allografts are tissues acquired from one member of a species and placed in another member of the same species. When obtained from cadaveric sources or incidental to an operative procedure, allografts circumvent most

G. E. Friedlaender, M.D.: Professor and Chairman, Department of Orthopaedics and Rehabilitation, Yale University School of Medicine, New Haven, Connecticut 06510.

S. L. Curtin, M.D.: Tucson Orthopaedic Institute, P.C., Tucson, Arizona 85712.

M. H. Huo, M.D.: Assistant Professor, Department of Orthopaedic Surgery, Johns Hopkins University School of Medicine, Baltimore, Maryland 21287.

TABLE 1. *Comparison of bone graft material*

Type of graft material	Advantages	Disadvantages
Autograft (same person)	Maximum biologic potential	Limited supply
	Histocompatible	Donor site morbidity
Allograft (same species)	Satisfactory biologic potential	Potential transfer of disease
	Abundant supply	Evokes immune response(s)
	No donor site morbidity	Requires rigorous banking methodology
Xenograft (different species)	Abundant supply	Evokes immune response(s)
	No donor site morbidity	Less biologic activity
		Requires processing and sterilization
		Anatomic parts not comparable to human
Synthetics	Abundant supply	Lacks mechanical strength
	No donor site morbidity	Not osteoinductive

disadvantages of autogenous sources, but simultaneously introduce concerns regarding their biologic efficacy, consequences of histocompatibility differences, and possible transfer of disease. Each of these potentially problematic areas has been sufficiently addressed to encourage the widespread use of bone allografts (55).

Tissues transplanted from one species to another are termed *xenografts*. To date, the use of osseous xenografts has proven less reliable than those from autogenous or allogenic sources, presumably based upon major histocompatibility differences and the nature of their processing for long-term storage. As our understanding of bone biology improves, opportunities to use xenografts more effectively may also materialize.

Synthetic preparations (65,67,83), particularly hydroxyapatite and tricalcium phosphate, alone or in combination with autogenous bone or bone marrow, and the use of aspirated bone marrow alone (34) represent other alternatives for promoting osseous repair or arthrodesis. These substances vary in their biologic and biomechanical properties, but can be manufactured in a variety of pore sizes and in large quantity.

Despite the wide use of these various forms of bone grafts and their synthetic substitutes, the precise mechanisms that control the biologic events of graft repair and remodeling are only partially understood. Furthermore, the surgical principles known to maximize bone graft incorporation and those circumstances that may contribute to its failure are often not fully appreciated by the clinicians using these reconstructive tissues. Many failures can be avoided or minimized by a better understanding of the nature of graft biology and biomechanics, the potential influence of surgical technique and postoperative care on osseous repair, as well as the consequences of various graft preservation methodologies (52).

BIOLOGY OF BONE GRAFTS

General Principles

Bone is unique in its ability to regenerate rather than heal by scar formation. Graft incorporation is at the end of the biologic spectrum of regeneration that begins with intact bone homeostasis and progresses through the events associated with fracture repair. The common denominator in these seemingly diverse activities is the bone remodeling cycle (Fig. 1), a circular sequence of events beginning with an activation signal(s), followed by a resorptive phase, and then new bone formation (6,20,113,114). Repetition of these cascading and synchronous events leads to repair, by regeneration and remodeling.

There is increasing information concerning the nature of molecular mediators and growth factors present at the site of fracture repair, and these same molecules are presumed important to bone graft incorporation as well. Nonetheless, the precise physiologic mechanisms that control graft incorporation are not clearly understood. The histologic stages of this complex process, however, are well described, predictable, and relatively consistent. Differences can be anticipated when comparing cortical to cancellous tissues (20,61,64) as well as variations induced by the size of graft particles, loads applied, the nature of the recipient site, age of the patient, and many other factors. Furthermore, the process varies if a blood supply is reestablished rapidly by microvascular anastomosis at the time of surgery or if the vascular pedicle to the transferred bone remains intact. This is in contrast to the conventional nonvascularized graft in which a slow

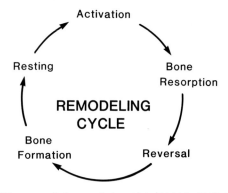

FIG. 1. The remodeling cycle is a circular sequence of events beginning with activation, followed by bone resorption, and then bone formation.

revascularization must occur from the host bed before proceeding with the remainder of the repair and incorporation process.

Nonvascularized Autogenous Bone Grafts

The initial events in the incorporation of nonvascularized autogenous cancellous and cortical grafts are similar. The process is characterized histologically, at the outset, by hemorrhage and followed by a nonspecific inflammatory response evoked by cell necrosis. The marrow space contains viable cells at the time of implantation, which rapidly become necrotic. Within a short period of time, the graft is invaded by fibrovascular tissue of host site origin that will eventually convey recipient-derived blood vessels and osteogenic cells into the graft. The few graft-derived cells that survive by diffusion may also contribute significantly to the incorporation process.

Two important characteristics of bone grafts are termed *osteoinduction* and *osteoconduction*. *Osteoinduction* is the process by which precursors of osteoblasts (osteoblastic stem cells and mesenchymal stomal cells) are actively induced to differentiate into mature bone-forming cells (phenotypic osteoblasts) (115,148). Autogenous bone graft is a storehouse of growth factors and osteoinductive agents which play a significant role in the local regulation of bone formation (8). The autocrine and paracrine functions of these growth factors are complex and not fully characterized. One subset of these factors, bone morphogenic proteins (BMPs), have been the focus of investigation for more than 25 years. They are a family of low-molecular-weight, noncollagenous proteins, termed BMP 1 through 7, which have been isolated from bone matrix (142,143,145–147) and some of which are now available through recombinant DNA synthesis (8, 149,157). *In vitro* studies suggest that BMP acts to stimulate bone formation by inducing undifferentiated cells to proliferate and differentiate to osteoblasts (30,82, 112,124,134).

BMPs 2 through 7 are related through amino acid homology to the supergene protein family of transforming growth factor-betas (TGF-β) (28). TGF-β appear to have synergistic effects with BMPs, but are incapable of initiating osteoinduction by themselves (9,26,28,149). Local factors, systemic hormones, and mechanical stresses may all play a role in the initiation and regulation of osteoinduction (8,98).

Osteoconduction is a passive characteristic of bone graft by which it acts as a scaffolding on which vascular invasion, resorption, and new-bone formation can occur. A graft or material's ability to "osteoconduct" is dependent on both structural and material properties including pore size (79) and porosity, surface texture, and affinity for osseous materials.

Cancellous graft incorporation differs from that of cortical grafts in the rate and completeness of repair. The more porous nature of cancellous tissue permits rapid ingrowth of host-derived blood vessels, which in turn are prerequisite to recruitment of osteoblasts followed by osteoclasts (20). New bone is initially deposited on the surfaces of preexisting trabeculae, but eventually the majority of implanted cancellous tissue is resorbed, replaced, and remodeled by the host. This is in contrast to less complete incorporation of cortical bone. This process of cancellous graft incorporation is usually complete within 6 months, but varies with the size of the implant (20).

Cortical graft incorporation differs from cancellous tissue in several ways. Vascular invasion usually occurs along preexisting haversian or Volkmann canals (Fig. 2). These channels are widened by the accompanying osteoclastic activity, and there is also prominent resorption along the periphery of the graft (Fig. 3). This resorptive phase results in a mechanically weaker graft during the initial several months of the incorporation process. Indeed, this significant increase in porosity may lead to mechanical failure and collapse of the cortical graft, prior to subsequent but adequate new-bone formation and remodeling, unless sufficient internal fixation and postoperative external protection are provided (52). Cortical grafts are usually not completely replaced by host bone. An admixture of viable and preexisting acellular bone can be demonstrated in large cortical grafts, but this circumstance is usually compatible with satisfactory biologic and biomechanical function of the graft (Fig. 4).

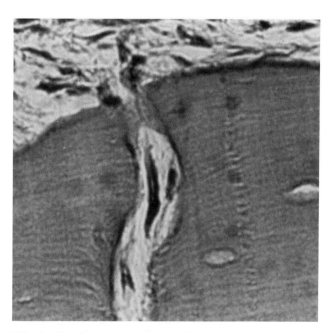

FIG. 2. Blood vessels and cells of host site origin invade the bone graft, often following preexisting Volkmann or haversian canals.

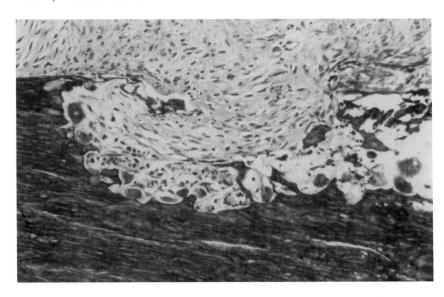

FIG. 3. Cortical grafts undergo intense osteoclastic resorption at their periphery. From AAOS, (4), with permission.

Cortical strut grafts from the iliac crest, fibula, or rib are often used in spine surgery for their mechanical properties, particularly load bearing. Structurally, cortical bone is more dense and compact than cancellous bone, and these properties are advantageous where strength is of primary importance. These same properties, however, will significantly slow the incorporation of the graft and again emphasize the need to plan an operative construct and postoperative program that will accommodate these biologic and biomechanical considerations.

Vascularized Autografts

Blood flow through cortical bone depends primarily on an intact medullary blood supply, whereas the contri-

bution from the periosteal vessels is normally less significant (118,138). Incorporation of vascularized grafts with an intact blood supply is characterized by minimal graft necrosis and a faster rate of repair (151). Indeed, the tissue repairs at either end of the transplanted segment by a process analogous to fracture healing. The use of a vascularized graft to bridge large bony defects began as early as 1905 (74). The application of this type of bone graft has increased substantially, especially with advances in microsurgery (19,152–154). The advantages of this technique include the short time to incorporation of the graft and the fact that the graft does not depend on vascular and cellular contributions from the local recipient bed. This is especially desirable in cases with a compromised host bed as occurs following radiation, sig-

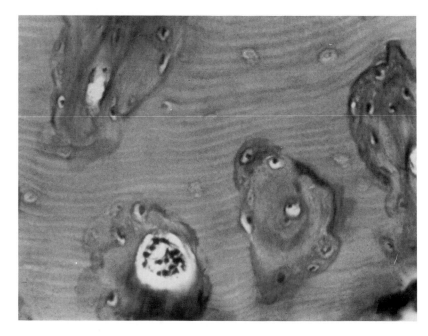

FIG. 4. Following resorption of preexisting cortical bone, osteons of new bone are created within a background of acellular bone graft material. From AAOS (4), with permission.

nificant trauma, or contamination. Limitations of vascularized grafts include the need for an adequate host-site blood supply, the lengthy operative time and expertise required to carry out the technique, as well as the constraints of a small number of potential donor sites. At this time, revascularized grafts are restricted to autogenous sources in humans which, for practical purposes, include fibula, rib, and iliac crest (151).

Allografts

The sequence of histologic events in the process of allograft incorporation is the same as that described for fresh autografts, but the pattern is slower to evolve and probably less complete (61). Once incorporated, however, allografts perform well with respect to their biologic and biomechanical functions.

Freeze-dried allografts are incorporated more slowly and less extensively than either autografts or deep-frozen allografts (52,55,64); however, both deep-freezing and freeze-drying, the two most commonly used preservation methods, have proven reliable in clinical practice (90,93). Causes of allograft failure are multifactorial, some of which may be immunologically mediated, and other adverse responses may reflect changes imparted by methods used for long-term preservation. Better understanding of these issues will no doubt enhance the clinical success of massive osteochondral allograft reconstruction in the future. Freeze-dried bone, for example, has inferior bending and torsional strength as compared to deep-frozen specimens of similar size. Compression testing parameters, however, are similar for both types of grafts (108). Irradiation in excess of 3 megarads, used for sterilization, is associated with significant weakening in torsion, compression, and bending strength of bone (107). The biomechanical properties of the graft must therefore be balanced against the type and magnitude of the load to which it will be subjected in the clinical setting.

Synthetic Materials

Autografts and allografts continue to be used extensively and effectively in orthopedic reconstructive procedures; however, limitations of quantity and potential donor site morbidity associated with autografts (155,159) and potential complications related to transmission of diseases from donor to recipient in the case of allografts (18,21) have prompted investigators to explore the use of synthetic bone substitutes (Table 2). In terms of spine surgery, synthetic graft material may be of value as a substitute for bone grafts, as adjuncts to "expand" limited amounts of graft material, or to act as a carrier for osteoinductive agents. These activities may be useful in de-

TABLE 2. *Synthetic graft materials*

Ceramics
  Hydroxyapatite (HA)
  Tricalcium phosphate (TCP)
Polylactic-polyglycolic acid polymers
Collagen
Bioactive molecules
  TGF-β
  BMP 1–7

TGF-β, transforming growth factor-beta; BMP, bone morphogenic proteins.

veloping a fusion mass or providing temporary structural support until bony fusion is attained.

Calcium Phosphate Ceramics

Various synthetic hydroxyapatite (HA) and tricalcium phosphate (TCP) crystalline or ceramic preparations have been manufactured with the intention of duplicating some of the biologic and biomechanical composition and responses attributable to bone. Hydroxyapatite preparations from sea coral, baked or sintered at high temperatures, and synthetic TCP are the most commonly used forms of bone substitutes. Pore sizes varying from 50 to 600 μm have been evaluated in a number of animal models and clinical circumstances. HA is not biodegradable, but TCP is slowly resorbed (16,49, 68,75,76,117). Varying the ratio of these two components will influence the speed and completeness of resorption of a given compound. These materials have been shown to be biocompatible, osteoconductive, nontoxic, and capable of creating intimate bonds with host bone because of their close similarity to the apatitic bone mineral component (16,17,25,36,66,67,75,129,141). Pore size, the ratio of HA to TCP, and the material structure are important variables in determining the osteoconductive nature (75,79), bioresorbability (49,68,75, 76,117), and mechanical properties (75) of these materials. Most authors agree that these biosynthetics possess little if any osteoinductive potential.

Biomechanically the calcium phosphate ceramics are extremely brittle and have low impact resistance and tensile strength (75). These properties have generally precluded their use as structural components in orthopedic surgery (35,128), although some investigators have reported variable success with ceramic HA in spinal surgery, either augmented with alumina ceramic (11), biodegradable polymers (158), or in block form (139). Currently, ceramics appear most efficacious as fillers of cancellous space voids (17), expanders of traditional bone grafts, and as potential vehicles or delivery systems for bone-inducing agents, including marrow-derived stem cells and bone morphogenic proteins (133,141).

In addition to the materials described above, a

nonceramic hydroxyapatite "cement" is being evaluated; it is characterized by its ability to be easily molded and extensively resorbed while retaining osteoconductive properties (38,78,129).

Polylactic-Polyglycolic Acid Polymers

Polylactic-polyglycolic acid polymers are biodegradable materials which have been used to construct a variety of bioimplants (65). In addition, these polymers have been used in conjunction with coralline HA to fill cranial defects in rabbits (5). However, these materials possess no osteoinductive nor osteoconductive properties, and their role as bone graft substitutes may be limited to acting as a vehicle for osteoinductive proteins (81,97,140).

Collagen

Collagen has proved useful in craniofacial surgery where its microfibrillar form has been added to autologous bone paste to provide substance and to enhance handling properties during surgery. Recently, collagen has been used as a graft expander in combination with HA and bone marrow (37) and as a carrier for osteoinductive proteins (e.g., BMP) (42,99,119).

Bioactive Molecules

One of the most exciting areas of investigation in bone biology has been the ability to manufacture bioactive molecules of the TGF-β superfamily which possess osteoinductive properties. Recombinant human BMP has been shown to induce bone formation in soft tissue sites in animals (149) and demineralized bone matrix as a carrier with recombinant human BMP (rhBMP-2) has demonstrated its ability to induce bone formation in rat femora (157). The results of recently initiated clinical trials are eagerly awaited.

Composites

Another promising area of recent investigation has been the development of bone graft substitutes that are composites of synthetic, osteoconductive carriers (e.g., HA) and biologically active osteoinductive matrix proteins (e.g., BMP). A number of animal models have been used to evaluate HA and BMP (42,69,105,125,140), HA and demineralized bone matrix (112), and sintered bovine bone and BMP (77); and these studies have demonstrated enhanced osteogenesis with the composite materials when compared to HA alone or controls (no graft). Polymers of polylactic-polyglycolic acid (81,97,140) and polydioxanone (103) have also been reported to serve as effective carriers of osteoinductive proteins.

In human clinical trial (37), a composite of HA/TCP beads, fibrillar collagen, and autogenous bone marrow was shown to be as efficacious as autologous bone graft in the treatment of acute long-bone fractures. Although this study has several limitations (including the absence of a nongrafted control group), it supported the safety associated with the use of this composite.

IMMUNOLOGIC CONSIDERATIONS

Efforts to define bone allograft antigenicity began in the early 1950s when clinical interest became aroused and newly developed immunologic concepts and methodology could be applied (12,22,29). In retrospect, it is important to keep in mind that the reported degree of recipient response may largely reflect the sensitivity and specificity of the methods employed for detection rather than an accurate representation of the cell-mediated and humoral immune responses being generated (51).

Animal Studies

Initial attempts to evaluate bone graft antigenicity were based upon histologic evaluation of the cellular infiltrate at the graft site. Although it is not possible to differentiate a nonspecific inflammatory reaction from that of a specific T cell–mediated immune response by this approach, these experiments were interpreted as support for the immunogenicity of fresh bone allografts, the presence of a detectable but reduced response to frozen bone, and markedly diminished or absent reactivity of grafts subjected to freeze-drying (12,29).

Using skin graft rejection patterns as a measure of cell-mediated immunity, investigators again concluded that freeze-dried bone failed to elicit a response (29,41). Frozen grafts caused a response, but less vigorous than fresh allografts. Reaction within lymph node draining sites of subcutaneous allograft implantation has also been observed and provided information similar to that reported using skin graft rejection patterns and histology (51).

In the mid 1970s, more sophisticated in vitro immunologic assays became available and were used in a variety of animal models. Muscolo and associates (101) have shown that both cell-mediated and humoral responses develop following transplantation of allogeneic but not syngeneic bone in rats. Langer and co-workers (84) demonstrated a positive lymphocyte migration assay following fresh allografts in rodents and suggested the existence of blocking factors that negated the adverse biologic consequences of sensitization. Rodrigo (122) has also provided evidence of suppressor T-cell activity in rat recipients of frozen bone allografts. Friedlaender and colleagues (56) reported the presence of detectable humoral and cell-mediated immune responses in rabbits using a sensitive microcytotoxicity assay. The intensive response associated with fresh allografts was reduced by deep-freezing and nearly undetectable after freeze-drying, consistent with most previous reports in animal models. More recently, Goldberg, Stevenson, and colleagues (59,60,132) demonstrated that frozen bone allografts exchanged between closely matched dogs were more successfully incorporated than exchanges across strong major histocompatibility complex (MHC) barriers, suggesting a relationship between graft immunogenicity and biologic fate of the bone grafts, and proposing an advantage to matching donors and recipients in terms of histocompatibility antigens. Whereas the presence of immune responses following bone allografts has been the subject of many studies, the nature of antigens responsible for sensitization has also been of interest.

The potential sources of bone-related immunogens are complex and diverse. Bone is a composite tissue consisting of cells, collagen, ground substance, and mineral. There is no evidence to suggest that hydroxyapatite crystals are immunogenic. Collagen can be a weak antigen under optimal circumstances (137). There is some evidence that proteoglycans can evoke a significant immune response (110,156). Cells, however, particularly those of bone marrow origin, have been shown to be the principal source of antigenic activity associated with fresh allogeneic bone (23). Rejection of soft tissue allografts is known to be mediated by host immunocompetent cells that recognize cell-surface alloantigens of the major histocompatibility complex. These alloantigens are then further processed by antigen presenting cells, most probably of the macrophage cell line, which in turn activate T cells to mount a specific alloreactive response mediated by lymphokines (41).

More recent studies by Horowitz and colleagues (71,72) have demonstrated that bone marrow–depleted bone was as immunogenic in an *in vitro* assay as bone marrow itself. Furthermore, MHC antigens specifically activated T cells of the killer/suppressor phenotype. It is hypothesized that this immune cell activation results in both direct effector cell responses as well as production of various cytokines [e.g., interleukin-1 and TNF(tumor necrosis factor)-α or TNF-β]. These cytokines or lymphokines are capable of activating osteoblasts, which can, in turn, through secretion of additional soluble factors result in osteoclast activation and bone (or bone graft) resorption.

Experience in Humans

In addition to studies in animals, a limited experience with bone allograft immunogenicity in humans is also available. Langer and co-workers (85) demonstrated humoral cytotoxic antibodies against fibroblasts derived from donor tissues when osteochondral allografts were used for reconstruction in unicompartmental degenera-

tive joint disease. Rodrigo and colleagues (121) found that 12 of 14 recipients of massive frozen bone allografts developed more humoral anti–human lymphocyte antigen (HLA) antibodies after surgery than individuals receiving multiple blood transfusions. Friedlaender and associates (57) evaluated 43 patients who received freeze-dried cortical and cortical-cancellous allografts, using a microcytotoxicity assay to assess the presence of anti-HLA antibodies in the recipients. Nine of these individuals (21%) developed donor graft–specific anti-HLA antibodies within 4 to 7 weeks after their surgical procedure. Sensitization, however, did not correlate with a poor clinical outcome. More recently, Muscolo et al. (100) was unable to establish a clear relationship between the pattern of histocompatibility responses and bone incorporation in 26 patients receiving massive osteochondral allografts.

Significance of Immune Responses

Despite their well-documented presence, the significance of bone graft–related immune responses with respect to graft biology is still unclear (54). The majority of assays used to assess bone allograft immunogenicity in the past have measured antibodies in the systemic circulation as opposed to T-cell activity. Graft rejection, in general, is a function of T cell–mediated responses. Investigators are currently involved in the characterization of alloantigen presentation and processing and the activation of T-cell subsets through mediators such as lymphokines (62,70,73). Monocytes and macrophages are major components of the immune cascade, and these immunocompetent cells share common precursors with cells of the bone remodeling system, most clearly osteoclasts (106). The newly defined and close interactions between cells of the immunologic and bone remodeling systems, and their cellular products, may provide better insight into the significance of bone allograft immunogenicity. Indeed, this immunologic activity may account for many of the clinical failures associated with these reconstructive tissues (92,93), and understanding the relationships between the immune system and bone remodeling may suggest ways to minimize adverse biologic responses and optimize clinical results.

BONE BANKING

The goal of bone banking is to assure a timely supply of safe bone allografts with predictable biologic and biomechanical properties, suitable for their intended clinical application. This requires a systematic approach to donor selection, tissue recovery, preservation techniques, and record keeping as delineated in the standards published by the American Association of Tissue Banks (2,43,50).

Donor Selection

Cadaveric donors are the major source of skeletal allografts, although femoral heads and rib can be acquired from living donors incidental to operative procedures. Authorization for donation must be obtained either antemortem from the individual or through permission granted by the appropriate next-of-kin following death. This process has been defined by the Uniform Anatomical Gift Act of 1969 (123).

Both living and cadaveric donors must be screened extensively for potentially harmful transmissible diseases to ensure the safety of recipients (Table 3) (27,87,130). A thorough medical history and the use of laboratory tests for evidence of hepatitis, venereal diseases, and infection with the human immunodeficiency virus (HIV) as well as microbial cultures are essential. Donors are excluded if the history or medical course suggests sepsis or infection of the tissues to be collected, or if the individual belongs to a high-risk group for HIV exposure. Other contraindications to donation include existence of a malignancy other than skin (or confined to the central nervous system), metabolic bone disease, chronic corticosteroid use, or the presence of toxic substances in potential harmful amounts within the body. Cultures should include screening for bacterial, viral, and fungal pathogens.

The AIDS epidemic has led to heightened awareness of and precautions for preventing the transmission of viral infections through transplantation of bone allografts. To date, there have been only two known cases of donors in the United States who failed to be recognized as infected with HIV during the screening process and subsequently transmitted the virus to a total of four recipients of musculoskeletal allografts. The first case began in 1984, prior to the routine availability of first generation serologic tests for detection of HIV in 1985. The donor, in this case, had a history of intravenous drug abuse that had not been elicited on initial screening (27). In the second case, the donor's serum tested negative for HIV antibody when organs and tissues were recovered at the time of his demise in 1985. However, when a recipient of a frozen allograft from this donor converted to an HIV-positive status, further testing of donor's stored lymphocytes several years later with more sensitive techniques revealed the presence of the HIV-1 virus. In this case, 3

of 4 recipients of fresh frozen allografts (2 femoral heads, 1 patella-tendon-tibial bone plug graft) became infected. One recipient of a fresh frozen femoral shaft which had been cleansed of its medullary contents at the time of surgery has remained HIV-negative. Twenty-five recipients of lyophilized and ethanol-treated bone graft from this same donor have also remained HIV-negative (131).

These two cases demonstrate that the HIV virus can be transmitted by frozen bone allograft, but also emphasize that the frequency of this event is extremely small. Furthermore, no additional cases have been reported since these donations, suggesting that contemporary serologic and history-based screening tests for HIV are very effective. In 1989, Buck and co-workers (18) estimated the risk of acquiring an infection with HIV from a bone graft to be rare (one in a million) if stringent screening and serologic tests were carried out. Using the blood bank experience, some authors have placed the risk of receiving HIV from blood that has tested negative for HIV antibody to be between 1/150,000 to 1/36,000, with most studies approximating 1/40,000 (21,33,40,80,150).

Guidelines have been established by the FDA (47,48) and adopted by the American Association of Tissue Banks (AATB) (3), requiring potential donors of tissue for transplantation to be identified by a distinct code, to be subjected to a comprehensive medical history review, including information regarding risk factors for HIV and hepatitis or signs and symptoms of these ailments, and documentation of serologic screening tests. Specifically, the donor must be tested at an FDA-certified laboratory for anti-HIV-1, anti-HIV-2, HB_sAg, and anti-HCV. Any information in the history or laboratory studies suggesting the presence or risk of HIV or hepatitis automatically excludes that individual from donating tissues for transplantation. It is in the best interests of orthopedic surgeons and their patients to obtain musculoskeletal tissues for transplantation from banks following the guidelines established by the FDA and AATB or similar independent certifying organizations.

Tissue Recovery

Tissue retrieval should be performed in a sterile environment, whenever possible, utilizing the same customary operative techniques used at the time of tissue transplantation. Nonsterile tissue recovery requires a method of secondary sterilization, such as the use of either high-dose irradiation or ethylene oxide (14,111).

Virtually any bone of potential usefulness as graft material can be recovered, and this is accomplished through standard longitudinal and extensile exposures made along the extremities and iliac crests. It is important to preserve capsular tissue, ligaments, and major muscle attachment sites, such as the greater and lesser trochanters and the rotator cuff, in order to facilitate subsequent

TABLE 3. *Contraindications to bone donation*

Infection (bacterial, fungal, viral)
High risk for AIDS
Malignancies (other than skin)
Long-term steroids
Metabolic bone disease
Toxic substances
Disease of unknown etiology

joint reconstruction. Dissection around the iliac crests should be done last because of the higher likelihood of contamination from the bowel flora.

Long-Term Preservation

Numerous approaches can be used for the long-term preservation of bone grafts. The most commonly applied methods are deep-freezing and freeze-drying (lyophilization). Freeze-drying equipment is relatively expensive and the process is both time-consuming and requires close monitoring (90). This preparation, however, offers the advantage of permitting storage for indefinite periods of time at room temperature in evacuated containers. Freeze-drying is not compatible with preserving articular cartilage, and it has been shown to cause structural changes leading to diminished torsional and bending strength (108).

Freezing is relatively simple and inexpensive and is compatible with cryopreservation of joint surfaces. This is accomplished by exposing the cartilage to dimethyl sulfoxide (DMSO) or glycerol prior to freezing (50,90). Biomechanical parameters of the allograft are not significantly affected by deep-freezing (108). It has also been shown that proteolytic enzymatic activity within the graft can be eliminated by using storage temperatures in the $-70°$ to $-80°$ C range (44). Grafts stored deep-frozen are usually wrapped in multiple layers of cloth, plastic, or both, or else in double glass jars (especially true for femoral heads) (135). Regardless of the method used for preservation, the packaging material must be a barrier to contamination and the integrity of the container material must not be affected by the storage conditions.

Record Keeping

The packages should be indelibly labeled with the donor identification code, date of tissue recovery, type and size of the graft, and preservation/storage approaches used. Other essential donor information that should be included in the records are age, sex, pertinent past medical history, and the results of the screening laboratory tests. If the graft was exposed to antibiotics during processing, this should be noted in order to avoid allergic reactions in hypersensitive recipients. Any known adverse circumstances related to use of this tissue should also be recorded and evaluated by the bank's medical director.

CLINICAL APPLICATIONS OF GRAFTS IN SPINE SURGERY

The stability of the spinal column is of paramount importance to the well-being of neurologic function. Stabilization of the injured spine can sometimes be achieved by various external support devices or may require direct internal fixation of the involved vertebral segments. Long-term success requires solid arthrodesis; and the use of bone graft, autogenous or allogeneic, is often prerequisite to establishing solid fusion.

Descriptions of specific surgical procedures and indications that involve the use of bone grafts in promoting fusion of the spine have been left to other authors. This discussion concentrates on those basic science principles that guide surgical technique and influence graft incorporation and, thereby, clinical results (52). Additional attention will also be focused on experience with allografts and bone graft substitutes in spinal fusions.

General Principles

Because incorporation is a partnership between the graft and its recipient site, adverse changes on either side of the graft–host interface can influence success. The recipient site, usually decorticated host bone and surrounding soft tissues (including muscle, fascia, subcutaneous fat), is the source of all new blood supply to the graft as well as the vast majority of osteogenic cell populations. Compromise of these local tissues may result from irradiation for control of malignancy, trauma, or infection, all of which may lead to a sclerotic or necrotic graft bed. The presence of local benign or malignant neoplasms, systemic metabolic bone disease, or the use of chemotherapeutic agents that reduce the pool of osteoprogenitor cells or the function of osteoblasts or osteoclasts (58) all have the potential to interfere with graft incorporation. Similarly, physical barriers placed between the graft and its host bed prevent successful revascularization and cell influx. Polymethylmethacrylate is particularly susceptible to misuse in this regard and will deprive bone grafts of required neovascularization and osteogenic cells if even a thin layer of cement is introduced or migrates between the graft and its otherwise supportive recipient site.

The bone graft itself contributes few, if any, cells to the incorporation process, but does play a crucial role in terms of its osteoconductive and osteoinductive properties. As discussed, these graft-derived characteristics may be influenced by approaches to graft preservation and sterilization, histocompatibility differences, and the manner in which the implants are mechanically loaded.

Most of the principles outlined above apply to bone grafts regardless of their source or pretreatment. Some potential issues, however, are intrinsic to nonautogenous grafts or graft substitutes, reflecting the nature of bone banking methodology or the consequences of immunogenicity.

Allografts

The biologic potential associated with autogenous grafts remains the benchmark against which allografts or bone substitutes are measured. The quantity of available bone autograft and potential donor site morbidity has prompted surgeons to seek alternatives (39,116). Properly screened and preserved bone allografts address many of these concerns and have been shown to be as effective in many clinical situations as autografts (55).

The most commonly reported uses of bone allograft in spinal fusions are for anterior cervical (Fig. 5) and posterior lumbar interbody arthrodeses. Many authors have demonstrated that the fusion rate was no different when allografts were compared with autogenous bone (15, 91,120,126). However, a more recent nonrandomized study of 87 consecutive patients undergoing one or two level anterior cervical discectomy and fusion found that those patients receiving allograft iliac crest bone had a higher incidence of radiographic nonunion (22% versus 8%) and graft collapse (30% versus 5%), when compared to those patients receiving autogenous iliac crest bone (160).

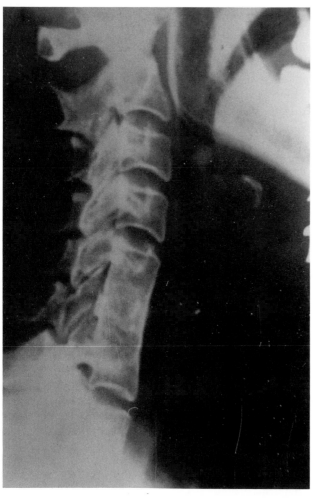

FIG. 5. Anterior cervical fusion using an autogenous graft at C5–C6 and freeze-dried allograft at C6–C7, both levels achieving comparable results. From Schneider and Bright (126), with permission.

Cloward (32) reported no added morbidity or infection with 187 gas-sterilized bone allografts used for posterior interbody fusion in 58 patients. Urist and Dawson (144) reported a pseudarthrosis rate of 12% in patients undergoing intertransverse process fusion with chemosterilized autolyzed antigen-extracted allografts (AAA) as compared to a pseudarthrosis rate of 8% in patients receiving autogenous grafts for the same purpose.

Vascularized rib autograft for the treatment of thoracic kyphosis has been described by Bradford (13). McBride and Bradford (94) subsequently reported a 100% fusion rate in six patients receiving both vascularized rib graft and frozen femoral head allograft for replacement of thoracic vertebral bodies. Allograft bone is particularly useful for fusions in patients with multiple-segment congenital or neuromuscular scoliosis (95). These patients are usually small in stature, and their iliac crests do not afford sufficient quantity or, at times, quality of autogenous graft material.

The incidence of infection has been reported to be no greater for allografts than autografts in spinal surgery (136). Most recently, a review of 90 patients receiving frozen allografts for anterior cervical spine fusion, with histologic examination of the fusion mass at the time of a second operative procedure, showed there was solid fusion, formation of viable lamellar bone within the graft, and no inflammation or foreign body reaction (102).

Synthetic Graft Materials

Methylmethacrylate (PMMA) has been used to supplement stabilization of severely compromised, bone stock deficient spinal columns (31,63). The biomechanical properties of methylmethacrylate are, however, inferior to that of a solid bony fusion. PMMA is also associated with a higher infection and wound dehiscence rate, especially in patients receiving adjunctive radiation therapy for local malignant disease. It should be used only in selected cases to supplement bony arthrodesis and internal fixation devices, particularly when only short-term stabilization is required for a terminally ill individual.

Studies of hydroxyapatite as graft material in a dog model have demonstrated a high rate of graft fracture and extrusion. Solid fusion was achieved, however, in those animals that did not extrude their graft (35).

SUMMARY

The biology of bone graft incorporation is crucial to a successful clinical outcome. The surgeon must keep in mind the temporal sequence of biologic events associated with graft repair and the complementary roles of the bone and its host site. Results may be compromised if these basic biologic principles are ignored or if alterations in graft biomechanics secondary to preservation methods are not recognized and addressed by the nature of the surgical procedure and postoperative care. Allograft bone serves as an attractive alternative to autogenous graft in spine surgery, having demonstrated both safety and efficacy. Currently, bone substitutes are more appropriate as adjuncts to autografts or allografts rather than useful as primary graft material in the spine, due primarily to their intrinsically poor biomechanical properties. The availability of biosynthetic molecules with osteogenic properties will add an important dimension to alternative approaches to bone grafting procedures in the future. No single bone graft material or implantation technique, however, is superior for all clinical applications. The biologic potential, biomechanical properties, and risks or complications associated with different osteogenic materials are vastly varied but largely predictable. Thus, the choice of graft and technique best suited to a specific set of circumstances reflects knowledge and understanding of bone and bone graft biology, the relationship of the graft to its recipient site, the biomechanical stresses to be experienced by the surgical construct over time, and the clinical goals of the operative procedure.

REFERENCES

1. Albee FH (1923): Fundamentals in bone transplantation: Experiences in three thousand bone graft operations. *JAMA* 81:1429–1432.
2. American Association of Tissue Banks (1987): *Standards for tissue banking.* Arlington, VA: American Association of Tissue Banks.
3. American Association of Tissue Banks *Information Alert,* vol. IV, no. 1, Feb. 22, 1994.
4. American Academy of Orthopaedic Surgeons: *Orthopaedic knowledge update III.* Rosemont, IL: AAOS, pp 167–175.
5. Antikainen T, Ruuskanen M, Tayrio R, Kallioinen M, Serlo W, Tormala P, Waris T (1992): Polylactide and polyglycolic acid-reinformed coralline hydroxyapatite for the reconstruction of cranial bone defects in the rabbit. *Acta Neurochirurgica* 117(1–2):59–62.
6. Baron R, Vignery A, Horowitz M (1984): Lymphocytes, macrophages and the regulation of bone remodeling. *Bone Miner Res* 2:175–243.
7. Barth A (1893): Ueber histologische Befunde nach Knochenimplantationen. *Arch Klin Chir* 46:409–417.
8. Baylink DJ, Finkelman RD, Mohan S (1993): Growth factors to stimulate bone formation. *J Bone Miner Res* 8(2):5565–5572.
9. Bentz H, Nathan RM, Rosen DM, Armstrong RM, Thompson QY, Segarini PR, Mathews MC, Dasch JR, Piez KA, Seyedin SM (1989): Purification and characterization of a unique osteoinductive factor from bovine bone. *J Biol Chem* 264:20805–20810.
10. Bick EM (1968): *Source book of orthopaedics,* 2nd ed. New York: Hafner.
11. Boker DK, Schultheiss R, Van Roost D, Osborn JF, Kaden B (1993): Anterior cervical discectomy and vertebral interbody fusion with hydroxy-apatite ceramic. Preliminary results. *Acta Neurochir* 121(3–4):191–195.
12. Bonfiglio M, Jeter WS, Smith CL (1955): The immune concept: its relation to bone transplantation. *Ann N Y Acad Sci* 59:417–433.
13. Bradford DS (1980): Anterior vascular pedicle bone grafting for the treatment of kyphosis. *Spine* 5:318–323.
14. Bright RW, Friedlaender GE, Sell KW (1977): Tissue banking: the United States Navy Tissue Bank. *Mil Med* 142:503–510.
15. Brown MD, Malinin TI, Davis PB (1976): A roentgenographic evaluation of frozen allografts versus autografts in anterior cervical spine fusions. *Clin Orthop* 119:231–236.
16. Bucholz RW, Carlton A, Holmes RE (1987): Hydroxyapatite and tricalcium phosphate bone graft substitutes. *Orthop Clin North Am* 18:323–334.
17. Bucholz RW, Carlton A, Holmes R (1989): Interporous hydroxyapatite as a bone graft substitute in tibial plateau fractures. *Clin Orthop* 240:53–62.
18. Buck BE, Malinin TI, Brown MD (1989): Bone transplantation and human immunodeficiency virus, an estimate of risk of acquired immunodeficiency syndrome (AIDS). *Clin Orthop* 240:129–136.
19. Buncke HJ, Furnas DW, Gordon L, Achauer BM (1977): Free osteocutaneous flap from a rib to the tibia. *Plast Reconstr Surg* 59:799–804.
20. Burchardt H (1987): Biology of bone transplantation. *Orthop Clin North Am* 18:187–196.
21. Busch M, Eble B, Heibron D, Vyas G (1990): Risk associated with transfusion of HIV antibody-negative blood [Letter]. *N Engl J Med* 322(12).
22. Burwell RG (1963): Studies in the transplantation of bone. V. The capacity of fresh and treated homografts of bone to evoke transplantation immunity. *J Bone Joint Surg [Br]* 45:386–401.
23. Burwell RG (1985): The function of bone marrow in the incorporation of bone graft. *Clin Orthop* 200:125–141.
24. Burwell RG, Friedlaender GE, Mankin HJ (1985): Current perspectives and future directions: the 1983 invitational conference on osteochondral allografts. *Clin Orthop* (197):141–157.
25. Cameron HU, MacNab I, Pilliar RM (1977): Evaluation of a biodegradable ceramic. *J Biomed Mater Res* 11:179–186.
26. Celeste AJ, Iannazzi JA, Taylor RC, Hewick RM, Rosen V, Wang EA, Wozney JM (1990): Identification of transforming growth factor β family members present in bone-inductive protein purified from bovine bone. *Proc Natl Acad Sci U S A* 87:9843–9847.
27. Centers for Disease Control (1988): Transmission of HIV through bone transplantation: case report and public health recommendations. *MMWR* 37:597–599.
28. Centrella M, McCarthy TL, Canalis E (1991): Current concepts review: transforming growth factor-beta and remodeling of bone. *J Bone Joint Surg [Am]* 73:1418–1428.
29. Chalmers J (1959): Transplantation immunity in bone homografting. *J Bone Joint Surg [Br]* 41:160–179.
30. Chen TL, Bates RL, Dudley A, Hammonds RG Jr, Amento EP (1991): Bone morphogenetic protein-2B stimulation of growth and osteogenic phenotypes in rat osteoblast-like cells: comparison with TGF-alpha 1. *J Bone Miner Res* 6:1387–1393.
31. Clark CR, Keggi KJ, Panjabi MM (1984): Methylmethacrylate stabilization of the cervical spine. *J Bone Joint Surg [Am]* 66:40–46.
32. Cloward RB (1980): Gas-sterilized cadaver bone grafts for spinal fusion operations. A simplified bone bank. *Spine* 5:4–10.
33. Cohen ND, Munoz A, Reitz BA, Ness PK, Frazier OH, Yawn DH, Lee H, Blattner W, Donahue JG, Nelson KE, Polk BF (1989): Transmission of retrovirus by transfusion of screened blood in patients undergoing cardiac surgery. *N Engl J Med* 320:1172–1176.
34. Connolly JF, Guse R, Tiedman J, Dehne R (1991): Autologous marrow injection as a substitute for operative grafting of tibial nonunions. *Clin Orthop* 266:259–270.
35. Cook SD, Reynolds MC, Whitecloud TS, Routman AS, Harding AF, Kay JF, Jarcho M (1986): Evaluation of hydroxyapatite graft materials in canine cervical spine fusions. *Spine* 11:305–309.
36. Cook SD, Thomas KA, Kay JF, Jarcho M (1988): Hydroxyapatite-coated titanium for orthopedic implant applications. *Clin Orthop* 232:225–243.
37. Cornell C, Lane J, Chapman M, Merkow R, Seligson D, Henry S, Gustillo R, Vincent K (1991): Multicenter trial of collograft as bone graft substitute. *J Orthop Trauma* 5(1):1–8.
38. Costantino PD, Friedman CD, Jones K, Chow LC, Sisson GA (1992): Experimental hydroxyapatite cement. *Cranioplasty Plast Reconstr Surg* 90(2):174–185; Discussion 186–191, 1992, Aug.

39. Coventry MB, Tapper EM (1972): Pelvic instability: a consequence of removing iliac bone for grafting. *J Bone Joint Surg [Am]* 54:83–101.

40. Cummings PD, Wallace EL, Schorr JB, Dodd RY (1989): Exposure of patients to human immunodeficiency virus through the transfusion of blood components that test antibody negative. *N Engl J Med* 321:941–946.

41. Czitrom AA, Axelrod T, Fernandes B (1985): Antigen presenting cells and bone allotransplantation. *Clin Orthop* 197:27–31.

42. Doll B, Towle H, Hollinger J, Reddi A, Mellonig J (1990): The osteogenic potential of two composite graft systems using osteogenin. *J Periodontol* 61(12):745–750.

43. Doppelt SH, Tomford WW, Lucas AD, Mankin HJ (1981): Operational and financial aspects of a hospital bone bank. *J Bone Joint Surg [Am]* 63:1472–1481.

44. Ehrlich MG, Lorenz J, Tomford WW, Mankin HJ (1983): Collagenase activity in banked bone. *Trans Orthop Res Soc* 8:166.

45. Elves MW (1974): Humoral immune response to allografts of bone. *Int Arch Allergy Appl Immunol* 47:708–715.

46. Enneking WF, Eady JL, Burchardt H (1980): Autogenous cortical bone grafts in the reconstruction of segmental skeletal defects. *J Bone Joint Surg [Am]* 62:1039–1058.

47. FDA Import Alerts No 57–08 12/17/93. *Banked human tissue for transplantation into other humans.*

48. *Federal Register* 1993 Dec 14; (53FR65514).

49. Ferraro JW (1979): Experimental evaluation of ceramic calcium phosphate as a substitute for bone grafts. *Plast Reconstr Surg* 63:634–640.

50. Friedlaender GE (1982): Bone-banking. *J Bone Joint Surg [Am]* 64:307–311.

51. Friedlaender GE (1983): Immune responses to osteochondral allografts. Current knowledge and future directions. *Clin Orthop* 174:58–68.

52. Friedlaender GE (1987): Bone grafts. The basic science rationale for clinical applications. *J Bone Joint Surg [Am]* 69:786–790.

53. Friedlaender GE (1990): Bone grafts. In: *Orthopaedic knowledge update 3: home study syllabus.* Park Ridge, IL: American Academy of Orthopaedic Surgeons, pp. 167–175.

54. Friedlaender GE: Bone allografts (1991): The biological consequences of immunological events [editorial]. *J Bone Joint Surg [Am]* 73:1119–1122.

55. Friedlaender GE, Mankin HJ, Sell KW (1983): *Osteochondral allografts: biology, banking, and clinical applications.* Boston: Little, Brown.

56. Friedlaender GE, Strong DM, Sell KW (1976): Studies on the antigenicity of bone. I. Freeze-dried and deep-frozen bone allografts in rabbits. *J Bone Joint Surg [Am]* 58:854–858.

57. Friedlaender GE, Strong DM, Sell KW (1984): Studies on the antigenicity of bone. II: Donor-specific anti-HLA antibodies in human recipients of freeze-dried allografts. *J Bone Joint Surg [Am]* 66:107–112.

58. Friedlaender GE, Tross RB, Doganis AC, Kirkwood JM, Baron R (1984): Effects of chemotherapeutic agents on bone. I. Short-term methotrexate and doxorubicin (Adriamycin) treatment in a rat model. *J Bone Joint Surg [Am]* 66:602–607.

59. Goldberg VM, Bos GD, Heiple KG, Zika JM, Powell AE (1984): Improved acceptance of frozen bone allografts in genetically mismatched dogs by immunosuppression. *J Bone Joint Surg [Am]* 66:937–950.

60. Goldberg VM, Powell A, Schaffer JW, Zika J, Bos GE, Heiple KG (1985): Bone grafting: role of histocompatibility in transplantation. *J Orthop Res* 3:389–404.

61. Goldberg VM, Stevenson S (1987): Natural history of autografts and allografts. *Clin Orthop* 225:7–16.

62. Gowen M, Beresford J, Gallagher DD (1983): Actions of interleukin 1 on bone metabolism in vitro. *Calcif Tissue Int* 35:642.

63. Harrington KD (1981): The use of methylmethacrylate for vertebral-body replacement and anterior stabilization of pathological fracture-dislocations of the spine due to metastatic malignant disease. *J Bone Joint Surg [Am]* 63:36–46.

64. Heiple KG, Chase SW, Herndon CH (1963): A comparative study of the healing process following different types of bone transplantation. *J Bone Joint Surg [Am]* 45:1593–1616.

65. Hollinger JO, Battistone GC (1986): Biodegradable bone repair materials. Synthetic polymers and ceramics. *Clin Orthop* 207:290.

66. Holmes RE (1979): Bone regeneration with a coralline hydroxyapatite implant. *Plast Reconstr Surg* 63:626–633.

67. Holmes RE, Bucholz RW, Mooney V (1987): Porous hydroxyapatite as a bone graft substitute in diaphyseal defects: a histometric study. *J Orthop Res* 5:114–121.

68. Hoogendoorn HA, Renooij W, Akkermans LM, Visser W, Witebol P (1984): Long-term study of large ceramic implants (porous hydroxyapatite) in dog femora. *Clin Orthop* 187:281–288.

69. Horisaka Y, Okamoto Y, Matsumoto N, Yoshimura Y, Kawada J, Yamashita K, Takagi T (1991): Subperiosteal implantátion of bone morphogenetic protein absorbed to hydroxyapatite. *Clin Orthop* 268:303–312.

70. Horowitz MC, Friedlaender GE (1987): Immunologic aspects of bone transplantation. A rationale for future studies. *Orthop Clin North Am* 18:227–233.

71. Horowitz MC, Friedlaender GE (1991): The immune response to bone cells. In Friedlaender GE, Goldberg VM (eds). *Bone and cartilage allografts: biology and clinical applications.* Park Ridge, IL: American Academy of Orthopaedic Surgeons, pp. 85–101.

72. Horowitz MC, Friedlaender GE (1991): Induction of specific T-cell responsiveness to allogeneic bone. *J Bone Joint Surg [Am]* 73:1157–1168.

73. Horowitz MC, Vignery A, Kaye J, Baron R (1986): A mechanism for the production of the bone resorbing lymphokines osteoclast activity factor by cloned helper T cells. *Bone Miner Res* 1:96.

74. Huntington TW (1905): Case of bone transference: use of a segment of fibula to supply a defect in the tibia. *Ann Surg* 41:249–251.

75. Jarcho M (1981): Calcium phosphate ceramics as hard tissue prosthetics. *Clin Orthop* 157:259–278.

76. Jarcho M, Kay JF, Gumaer KI, et al. (1977): Tissue, cellular and subcellular events at a bone-ceramic hydroxyapatite interface. *J Bioeng* 1:79–92.

77. Katoh T, Sato K, Kawamura M, Iwata H, Miura T (1993): Osteogenesis in sintered bone combined with bovine bone morphogenetic protein. *Clin Orthop* 287:266–275.

78. Kawakami T, Antoh M, Hasejawa H, Yamagishi T, Ito M, Eda S (1992): Experimental study on osteoconductive properties of a chitosan-bonded hydroxyapatite self-hardening paste. *Biomaterials* 12(11):759–763.

79. Klawitter JJ, Hulbert SF (1971): Application of porous ceramics for the attachment of load bearing orthopaedic applications. *J Biomed Mater Res* Symposium 2:161.

80. Kleinman S, Secord K (1988): Risk of human immunodeficiency virus (HIV) transmission by anti-HIV negative blood: estimates using the look back methodology. *Transfusion* 28:499–501.

81. Kleinschmidt JL, Marden LJ, Kent D, Quigley N, Hollinger JO (1993): A multiphase system bone implant for regenerating the calvaria. *Plast Reconstr Surg* 91(4):581–588.

82. Knutsen R, Mohan S, Wergedal J, Sampath K, Baylink DJ (1991): Osteogenic protein-1 stimulates proliferation and differentiation of human bone cells in vitro. *J Bone Miner Res* 6:231.

83. Lane JM, Cornell CN, Werntz JR, Sandu H (1991): Clinical applications of biosynthetics. In Friedlaender GE, Goldberg VM (eds). *Bone and cartilage allografts: biology and clinical applications.* Park Ridge, IL: American Academy of Orthopaedic Surgeons, pp. 279–294.

84. Langer F, Czitrom A, Pritzker KP, Gross AE (1975): The immunogenicity of fresh and frozen allogeneic bone. *J Bone Joint Surg [Am]* 57:216–220.

85. Langer F, Gross AE, West M, Urovitz EP (1978): The immunogenicity of allograft knee joint transplants. *Clin Orthop* 132:155–162.

86. Lexer E (1925): Joint transplantations and arthroplasty. *Surg Gynecol Obstet* 40:782–809.

87. Lord CF, Gebhardt MC, Tomford WW, Mankin HJ (1988): Infection in bone allografts. Incidence, nature, and treatment. *J Bone Joint Surg [Am]* 70:369–376.

88. Luyten FP, Yu YM, Yanagishita M, Vukicevic S, Hammonds RG, Reddi AH (1992): Natural bovine osteogenin and recombinant human bone morphogenetic protein-2B are equipotent in

the maintenance of proteoglycans in bovine articular cartilage explant cultures. *J Biol Chem* 267:3691–3695.

89. Macewen W (1881): Observations concerning transplantation of bone. Illustrated by a case of inter-human osseous transplantation whereby over two-thirds of the shaft of humerus was restored. *Proc R Soc London* 32:232–247.

90. Malinin TI, Martinez OV, Brown MD (1985): Banking of massive osteoarticular and intercalary bone allografts—12 years' experience. *Clin Orthop* 197:44–57.

91. Malinin TI, Rosomoff HL, Sutton CH (1977): Human cadaver femoral head homografts for anterior cervical spine fusions. *Surg Neurol* 7:249–251.

92. Mankin HJ, Doppelt SH, Sullivan TR, Tomford WW (1982): Osteoarticular and intercalary allograft transplantation in the management of malignant tumors of bone. *Cancer* 50:613–630.

93. Mankin HJ, Gebhardt MC, Tomford WW (1987): The use of frozen cadaveric allografts in the management of patients with bone tumors of the extremities. *Orthop Clin North Am* 18:275–289.

94. McBride GG, Bradford DS (1983): Vertebral body replacement with femoral neck allograft and vascularized rib strut graft. A technique for treating post-traumatic kyphosis with neurologic deficit. *Spine* 8:406–415.

95. McCarthy RE, Peek RD, Morrissy RT, Hough AJ Jr (1986): Allograft bone in spinal fusion for paralytic scoliosis. *J Bone Joint Surg [Am]* 68:370–375.

96. McGann W, Mankin HJ, Harris WH (1986): Massive allografting for severe failed total hip replacement. *J Bone Joint Surg [Am]* 68: 4–12.

97. Miyamoto S, Takaoka K, Okada T, Yoshikawa H, Hashimoto J, Suzuki S, Ono K (1992): Evaluation of polylactic acid homopolymers as carriers for bone morphogenetic protein. *Clin Orthop* 272:274–285.

98. Mohan S, Baylink DJ (1991): Bone growth factors. *Clin Orthop* 263:30–48.

99. Muschler G, Huber B, Ullman T, Barth R, Easley K, Otis J, Lane JM (1993): Evaluation of bone-grafting materials in a new canine segmental spinal fusion model. *J Orthop Res* 11(4):514–524.

100. Muscolo DL, Caletti E, Schajowicz F, Araujo ES, Makino A (1987): Tissue-typing in human massive allografts of frozen bone. *J Bone Joint Surg [Am]* 69:583–595.

101. Muscolo DL, Kawai S, Ray RD (1976): Cellular and humoral immune response analysis of bone-allografted rats. *J Bone Joint Surg [Am]* 58:826–832.

102. Nasca RJ, Whelchel JD (1987): Use of cryopreserved bone in spinal surgery. *Spine* 12:222–227.

103. Nichter LS, Yazdi M, Kosari K, Sridjaja R, Ebramzadeh E, Nimni ME (1992): Demineralized bone matrix polydioxanone composite as a substitute for bone graft: a comparative study in rats. *J Craniofac Surg* 3(2):63–69.

104. Ollier L (1867): *Traité experimental et clinique de la regeneration des os et de la production artificielle du tissu osseux*. Paris: Masson.

105. Ono I, Ohura T, Murata M, Yamaguchi H, Ohnuma Y, Kuboki Y (1992): A study on bone induction in hydroxyapatite combined with bone morphogenetic protein. *Plast Reconstr Surg* 90 (5): 870–879.

106. Osdoby P, Martini MC, Caplan AI (1982): Isolated osteoclasts and their presumed progenitor cells, the monocyte, in culture. *J Exp Zool* 224:331–344.

107. Pelker RR, Friedlaender GE (1987): Biomechanical aspects of bone autografts and allografts. *Orthop Clin North Am* 18:235–239.

108. Pelker RR, Friedlaender GE, Markham TC (1983): Biomechanical properties of bone allografts. *Clin Orthop* 174:54–57.

109. Phemister DB (1914): The fate of transplanted bone and regenerative power of its various constituents. *Surg Gynecol Obstet* 19: 303–333.

110. Poole AR, Reiner A, Choi H, Rosengberg LC (1979): Immunological studies of proteoglycan subunit from bovine and human cartilages. *Trans Orthop Res Soc* 4:55.

111. Prolo DJ, Pedrotti PW, White DH (1980): Ethylene oxide sterilization of bone, dura mater, and fascia lata for human transplantation. *Neurosurgery* 6:529–539.

112. Ragni P, Lindholm TS (1991): Interaction of allogeneic deminer-

113. Raisz LG (1988): Local and systemic factors in the pathogenesis of osteoporosis. *N Engl J Med* 318:818–828.

114. Raisz LG, Kream BE (1983): Regulation of bone formation. *N Engl J Med* 309:29–35, 83–89.

115. Reddi AH, Wientroub S, Muthukumaran N (1987): Biologic principles of bone induction. *Bone Grafting* 18:207.

116. Reid RL (1968): Hernia through an iliac bone-graft donor site. A case report. *J Bone Joint Surg [Am]* 50:757–760.

117. Rejda BV, Peelan JGJ, deGroot K (1977): Tricalcium phosphate as a bone substitute. *J Bioeng* 1:93.

118. Rhinelander FW (1973): Effects of medullary nailing on the normal blood supply of diaphyseal cortex. *Instr Course Lect* 22:161–187.

119. Ripamoni U, Ma S, Van den Heever B, Reddi A (1992): Osteogenins, a bone morphogenetic protein, absorbed on porous hydroxyapatite substrata, induces rapid bone differentiation in calvarial defects of adult primates. *Plast Reconstr Surg* 90(3):382–393.

120. Rish BL, McFadden JT, Penix JO (1976): Anterior cervical fusion using homologous bone grafts. A comparative study. *Surg Neurol* 5:119–121.

121. Rodrigo JJ, Fuller TC, Mankin HJ (1978): Cytotoxic HLA antibodies in patients with bone and cartilage allografts. *Trans Orthop Res Soc* 1:131.

122. Rodrigo JJ, Travis CR (1978): Suppressor T cell activity associated with distal femur allografts in rats. *Trans Orthop Res Soc* 3: 133.

123. Sadler AM Jr, Sadler BL, Stason EB, Stickel DL (1969): Transplantation: a case for consent. *N Engl J Med* 280:862–867.

124. Sampath TK, Maliakal JC, Hauschka PV, Jones WK, Sasak H, Tucker RF, White K, Coughlin JE, Tucker MM, Pang RHL, Corbett C, Ozkaynak E, Oppermann H, Rueger DC (1992): Recombinant human osteogenic protein induces new bone formation in vivo with specific activity comparable to natural bovine OP and stimulates osteoblast proliferation and differentiation in vitro. *J Biol Chem* 267:20352–20362.

125. Sato T, Kawumura M, Sato K, Iwata H, Miura T (1991): Bone morphogenesis of rabbit bone morphogenetic protein-bound hydroxyapatite-fibrin composites. *Clin Orthop* 263:254–262.

126. Schneider JR, Bright RW (1976): Anterior cervical fusion using preserved bone allografts. *Transpl Proc* 8(Suppl. 1):73–76.

127. Senn N (1889): On the healing of aseptic bone cavities by implantation of antiseptic decalcified bone. *Am J Med Sci* 98:219–243.

128. Shima T, Keller JT, Alvira MM, Mayfield FH, Dunsker SB (1979): Anterior cervical discectomy and interbody fusion. An experimental study using a synthetic tricalcium phosphate. *J Neurosurg* 51:533–538.

129. Shindo ML, Costantino PD, Friedman CD, Chow LC (1993): Facial skeletal augmentation using hydroxyapatite cement. *Arch Otolaryngol Head Neck Surg* 119:185–190.

130. Shutkin NM (1954): Homologous-serum hepatitis following use of a refrigerated bone-bank bone; report of a case. *J Bone Joint Surg [Am]* 36:160–162.

131. Simons RJ, Holmberg SD, Hurwitz RL, Coleman TR, Bottenfield S, Conley LJ, Kohlenberg SH, Castro KG, Dahan BA, Shable CA, Rayfield MA, Rogers MF (1992): Transmission of human immunodeficiency virus Type 1 from a seronegative organ and tissue donor. *N Engl J Med* 326(11):726–732.

132. Stevenson S, Li XQ, Martin B (1991): The fate of cancellous and cortical bone after transplantation of fresh and frozen tissue-antigen-matched and mismatched osteochondral allografts in dogs. *J Bone Joint Surg [Am]* 73:1143–1156.

133. Takaoka K, Nakahara H, Yosmikawa H, Masuhara K, Tsuda T, Ono K (1988): Ectopic bone induction on and in porous hydroxyapatite combined with collagen and bone morphogenetic protein. *Clin Orthop* 234:250–254.

134. Thies RS, Baudry M, Ashton BA, Kurtzberg L, Wozney JM, Rosen V (1992): Rocombinant human bone morphogenetic protein-2 induces osteoblastic differentiation in W-20-17 stoma cells. *Endocrinology* 130:1318–1324.

135. Tomford WW, Ploetz JE, Mankin HJ (1986): Bone allografts of

femoral heads: procurement and storage. *J Bone Joint Surg [Am]* 68:534–537.

136. Transfeldt E, Lonstein J, Winter R, Bradford D, Moe J, Mayfield J (1985): Wound infection in reconstructive spine surgery. *Orthop Trans* 9:128–129.

137. Trentham DE, Townes AS, Kang AH, David JR (1978): Humoral and cellular sensitivity to collagen in type II collagen-induced arthritis in rats. *J Clin Invest* 61:89–96.

138. Trueta J, Caladias AX (1964): A study of blood supply of the long bones. *Surg Gynecol Obstet* 118:485–498.

139. Tsuji H, Hirano N, Katoh Y, Ohsima H, Ishihara H, Matsui H, Hayasi Y (1990): Ceramic interspinous block (CISB) assisted anterior interbody fusion. *J Spinal Disord* 3(1):77–86.

140. Turk AE, Ishida K, Jensen JA, Wollmsn JS, Miller TA (1993): Enhanced healing of large cranial defects by an osteoinductive protein in rabbits. *Plast Reconstr Surg* 92(4):593–600; Discussion 601–602, 1993, Sept.

141. Uchida A, Nade S, McCartney E, Ching W (1985): Bone ingrowth into three different porous ceramics implanted into the tibia of rats and rabbits. *J Orthop Res* 3:65–77.

142. Urist MR: Bone formation by autoinduction (1965). *Science* 150:893.

143. Urist MR, Chang JJ, Lietze A, et al. (1987): Preparation and bioassay of bone morphogenetic hormone and polypeptide fragments. *Methods Enzymol* 146:294.

144. Urist MR, Dawson E (1981): Intertransverse process fusion with the aid of chemosterilized autolyzed antigen-extracted allogeneic (AAA) bone. *Clin Orthop* 254:97–113.

145. Urist MR, Delange RJ, Finerman GAM (1983): Bone cell differentiation and growth factors. *Science* 220:680.

146. Urist MR, Huoy K, Brownell AG, Hohl WM, Buyske J, Lietze A, Tempst P, Hunkapiller M, DeLange RJ (1984): Purification of bovine bone morphogenetic protein by hydroxyapatite chromatography. *Proc Natl Acad Sci U S A* 81:371–375.

147. Urist MR, Sato K, Brownell AG, Malinin TI, Lietze A, Huo YK, Prolo DJ, Oklund S, Finerman GA, DeLange RJ (1983): Human bone morphogenetic protein (hBMP). *Proc Soc Exper Biol Med* 173:194–199.

148. Urist MR, Silverman BF, Buring K, Dubuc FL, Rosenberg JM (1967): The bone induction principle. *Clin Orthop* 53:243–283.

149. Wang E, Rosen V, D'Alessandro J, Baudry M, Cordes P, Harada T, Israel D, Hewick R, Kerns K, LaPan P, Luxenberg D, McQuaid D, Moutsatsos I, Nove J, Wozney J (1990): Recombinant human bone morphogenetic protein induces bone formation. *Proc Natl Acad Sci U S A* 87:2220–2224.

150. Ward JW, Holmberg SD, Allen JR, et al. (1988): Transmission of human immunodeficiency virus (HIV) by blood transfusions screened as negative for HIV antibody. *N Engl J Med* 318:473–478.

151. Weiland AJ (1981): Current concepts review: vascularized free bone transplants. *J Bone Joint Surg [Am]* 63:166–169.

152. Weiland AJ, Daniel RK (1979): Microvascular anastomoses for bone grafts in the treatment of massive defects in bone. *J Bone Joint Surg [Am]* 61:98–104.

153. Weiland AJ, Daniel RK (1980): Congenital pseudoarthrosis of the tibia: treatment with vascularized autogenous fibular grafts. A preliminary report. *Johns Hopkins Med J* 147:89–95.

154. Weiland AJ, Moore JR, Daniel RK (1983): Vascularized bone autografts. Experience with 41 cases. *Clin Orthop* 174:87–95.

155. Whitecloud TS III (1978): Complications of anterior cervical fusion. *Instr Course Lect* 27:223–227.

156. Yablon IG, Brandt KD, Dellis RA (1977): The antigenic determinants of articular cartilage: their role in the homograft rejection. *Trans Orthop Res Soc* 1:90.

157. Yasko A, Lane J, Fellinger E, Rosen V, Wozney J, Wang E (1992): The healing of segmental bone defects, induced by recombinant human bone morphogenetic protein (rhBMP-2). *J Bone Joint Surg* 74:659–670.

158. Ylinen P, Kinnunen J, Laasonen EM, Lamminen A, Vainionpaa S, Raekallio M, Rokkanen P, Tormala P (1991): Lumbar spine interbody fusion with reinforced hydroxyapatite implants. *Arch Orthop Trauma Surg* 110(5):250–256.

159. Younger EM, Chapman MW (1989): Morbidity at bone graft donor sites. *J Orthop Trauma* 3:192–195.

160. Zdeblick TA, Ducker TB (1991): The use of freeze-dried allograft bone for anterior cervical fusions. *Spine* 16(7):726–729.

General and Degenerative Conditions

The Adult Spine: Principles and Practice,
2nd edition, J.W. Frymoyer, Editor-in-Chief.
Lippincott-Raven Publishers, Philadelphia © 1997.

CHAPTER 37

Spinal Degeneration: Pathogenesis and Medical Management

Robert D. Fraser, Jane F. Bleasel, and Roland W. Moskowitz

This chapter focuses on spinal degeneration as an important cause of symptoms as well as a normal part of the aging process. Degeneration is universal to all of the structures that comprise the functional spinal unit (FSU), including the intervertebral discs, facet joints, and connecting ligaments. In this chapter we will consider its macroscopic, biochemical, and physiologic features, as well as the general principles of nonsurgical treatment. Because much of our biochemical and physiologic information is derived from the lumbar spine, we have focused more on this anatomic region than the cervical and thoracic levels.

DISTRIBUTION OF DEGENERATIVE CHANGES WITHIN THE SPINE

The most complete information about the sites of spinal degeneration is derived from radiographic surveys. The usual criteria employed in these surveys are intervertebral disc narrowing and osteophyte formation, which are signs of advanced degeneration. Additional, less frequently used radiographic criteria are vertebral end-plate sclerosis, facet joint narrowing, osteophytes, and sclerosis (77). A far more sensitive imaging technique is magnetic resonance imaging, which permits a definition of the earlier stages of degeneration, including

R. D. Fraser, M.B., B.S., M.D., F.R.A.C.S.: Head of Spinal Unit, Department of Orthopaedics and Trauma, Royal Adelaide Hospital, North Terrace, Adelaide, South Australia.

J. F. Bleasel, M.B.B.S., F.R.A.C.P.: Department of Rheumatology, Rachel Forest Hospital, Sydney, New South Wales 2065, Australia.

R. W. Moskowitz, M.D.: Professor of Medicine, Case Western Reserve University School of Medicine; Director, Division of Rheumatic Diseases, University Hospitals of Cleveland, Cleveland, Ohio 44106.

some measures of disc physiology such as hydration (53,93,94,116), although Pearce et al. (115) have demonstrated that the brightness of the nuclear image correlates directly with the proteoglycan concentration, but not with the water or collagen content. To date, population-based statistics are not available for the entire spine using magnetic resonance imaging, although data are available for the lumbar spine (14).

All of the available radiographic data demonstrate consistency in the distributions of the degenerative lesions within the human spine (Fig. 1). The most advanced changes affect the midcervical and lower lumbar spine and the thoracolumbar junction. This pattern is thought to reflect the selective distribution of mechanical stresses, which result from human posture and function. In the cervical spine, the maximum motion occurs at the C5–C6 level, while in the lumbar spine the greatest torsional, shear, and compressive loads are seen at the L4–L5 and L5–S1 levels. Within the animal kingdom, the pattern of degeneration, although very different in distribution from humans, also occurs at areas of maximal mechanical stress. Animal models that simulate human bipedal posture result in redistribution of the sites of degeneration to a pattern more typical of humans (62).

It also seems evident that factors other than mechanical stresses promote spinal degeneration. Epidemiologic studies (70,71) reveal that an increased prevalence of neck pain occurs in subjects with low back pain. Radio-graphic surveys that demonstrate the presence of lumbar spine degeneration predict an increased risk for cervical degeneration (77). Lumbar spinal stenosis is frequently associated with cervical spondylosis. It is possible this last association may also be the result of genetically influenced or controlled spinal canal dimensions (60). Familial aggregations of spinal degeneration resulting in premature stenosis or an increased risk of lumbar disc herniation also point to genetic control mechanisms (81,148), as does a report of adolescent disc herniation in identical twins (57). Similar aggregations of advanced degeneration are also seen within the animal kingdom, such as in the sand rat and in chondrodystrophic canines. Environmental factors, such as cigarette smoking, also influence spinal degeneration.

DISTRIBUTION OF DEGENERATIVE CHANGES AT THE INDIVIDUAL SPINAL LEVEL

Historically, the greatest attention has been paid to the intervertebral disc as the site where spinal degeneration is initiated. Bywaters (25) proposed that primary degeneration of the disc results in secondary changes in the facet joints and ligaments as a result of load shifts from the discs to those structures. Experimental evidence in support of this view has been derived from animal models of disc degeneration. Lipson and Muir (84) produced anterior disc injuries in the rabbit which produced disc degeneration initially and facet degeneration as a later consequence. Another model of disc degeneration has been produced in dogs after intradiscal chymopapain injection (19). The initial disc space narrowing led to secondary facet degeneration as measured microscopically and chemically (52). The later restoration of disc height which then occurred was accompanied by biomechanical and macroscopic evidence of cartilage healing (52). Biomechanical experiments *in vitro* have also supported the concept of the intervertebral disc as the initiating structure in the degenerative process. Panjabi et al. (112) produced asymmetric disc injuries and measured the secondary effects on the kinematics of the functional spinal unit. Based on their results, they conceptualized a cascade of secondary changes affecting the facet joints as shown in Figure 2.

This concept of spinal degeneration has been challenged by others based on *in vivo* and *in vitro* morphologic, biomechanical, and biologic studies. Vanharanta (147) has shown that 20% of cervical and lumbar spine segments have macroscopic evidence of facet degeneration independent of any disc degeneration. Biomechanical analyses have shown that torsional stresses are the most potent cause of disc injury, which is more likely to occur when the facets are asymmetrically oriented at the same spinal level (44). Magnetic resonance imaging stud-

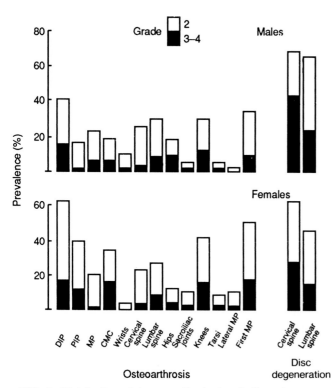

FIG. 1. Distribution of degenerative lesions in the spine compared to peripheral joints, as determined from epidemiologic radiographic surveys. From Kellgren (77) with permission.

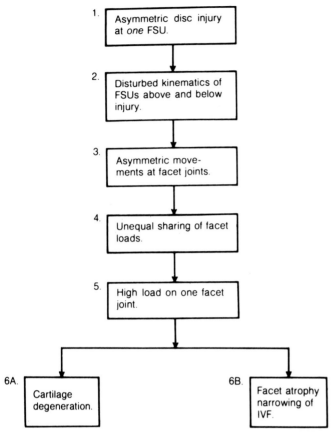

FIG. 2. The events that might follow injury to the disc and lead to more extensive degeneration at the motion segment. From Panjabi et al. (112) with permission.

been supported by recent MRI and CT studies, demonstrating no such relationship between facet tropism and degeneration of the annulus or nucleus (15,146).

The most dramatic association of facet degeneration with disc degeneration is the condition of degenerative spondylolisthesis, which itself is associated with facet joint angles greater than 45° as well as an increase in facet joint angles at other lumbar levels (15). The data from animal models is inconclusive. In these models attempts are made to simulate the effects of the facet joint pathology on the production of disc degeneration. The usual method is to remove the facets on opposite sides at the level above and below the disc of interest, resulting in torsional instability. Sullivan and Farfan (137) reported radiographic changes consistent with disc degeneration after this intervention. Cauchoix (26) refined his analysis of this animal model to include histochemical evaluation and showed that degeneration was accelerated. Yet in another study, destabilization did not cause biochemical changes consistent with degeneration, such as decreased water, decreased glucosaminoglycan concentrations, or increased collagen (136). Of importance was the observation that the initial instability was followed by restabilization over a 6-month interval. Similar observations have been made by Panjabi (113) in the canine cervical spine and by Latham et al. (80) in the ovine lumbar spine.

It is probably less important to debate the relative contribution of discs and facets in the initiation of the degenerative process and more important to conceptualize the functional spinal unit as a "three-joint complex" in which facets and discs are contributory. This conceptualization is also important to understanding the evolution of the degenerative process.

The three-joint concept was popularized by Kirkaldy-Willis (79) and forms the basis for the three stages of clinical/pathological evolution of spinal degeneration as shown in Figures 3 and 4. In stage I, subtle alterations in

ies have also suggested disc degeneration is more common in subjects with facet tropism (103). However, mathematical models dispute the importance of the facet joint and show that significant variations in the orientation of the facets have minimal effects on the stress distribution within the intervertebral disc (3). This view has

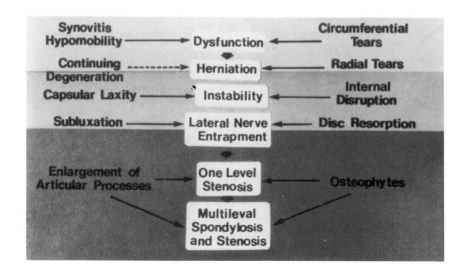

FIG. 3. The events that occur within the facet joints (left) and intervertebral discs (right) and their association with clinical syndromes. From Kirkaldy-Willis (79) with permission.

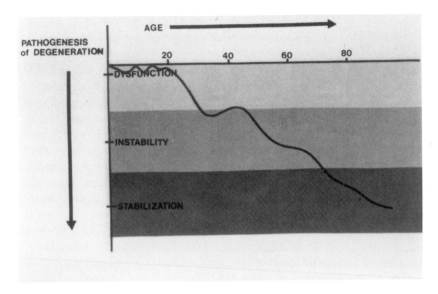

FIG. 4. The natural history of spinal degeneration in relation to age and the three proposed stages of degeneration. From Kirkaldy-Willis (79) with permission.

biochemistry, physiology, and biomechanics of the "three-joint complex" may result in clinical symptoms, although the precise cause of symptoms is only speculative. In stage II, these biochemical and biomechanical changes result in increased spinal mobility at the affected level(s); Kirkaldy-Willis (79) proposed that these events cause symptomatic instability. In stage III, the alterations in disc biochemistry, combined with the development of spinal osteophytes, causes increased stiffness of the functional spinal segment. These stabilization events may be accompanied by decreased symptoms other than spinal stiffness or may be associated with symptoms of spinal stenosis. When stenosis occurs, it is due to a narrowing of the spinal canal resulting from osteophytes impinging on spinal cord, nerve roots, or the cauda equina, in combination with bulging of the annulus fibrosus, and possibly buckling of the ligamentum flavum, although the importance of that ligament has been challenged by Schonstrom (130).

EVOLUTION OF THE DEGENERATIVE LESION

It must again be stressed that the macroscopic, microscopic, chemical, biomechanical, and radiographic changes observed in the various spinal structures are not specific to symptomatic degeneration, but are part of the normal aging process. As is emphasized throughout this book, separating normal aging from symptomatic degenerative lesions is one of the great challenges in the diagnosis and treatment of spinal pain. In a study that related lumbar spine pathology in cadavers to the known history of back pain, occupation, and physical loading, it was found that symmetric disc degeneration was associated with sedentary work, and vertebral osteophytosis was related to heavy work (151). It was found that the least pa-

thology stemmed from moderate or mixed physical loading, whereas the least back pain was associated with sedentary work.

INTERVERTEBRAL DISC

Gross Anatomic and Macroscopic Changes

The normal disc is comprised of the nucleus pulposus, which is embryologically derived from the notochord and the annulus fibrosus. Although it is common to think of the nucleus as anatomically distinct from the annulus, the two blend together at their junction (Figs. 5 and 6). Four anatomic subdivisions are made starting from the periphery: an outer layer of collagen fibrils, a thicker layer of fibrocartilage, a transitional zone between the fibrocartilaginous zone and the nucleus pulposus, and the nucleus itself. The nucleus contributes 50% of the entire surface area of the disc. The annulus can be separated into 60 or more distinct layers. Each layer is characterized by fibers oriented in opposite directions with a uniform angle of intersection (Fig. 7). A fifth important component is the vertebral end-plates. In the skeletally immature human, the end-plates are penetrated by the outer layer of collagen fibrils of the disc.

At birth, the boundary between the nucleus and the annulus is most distinct, because of the gelatinous composition of the disc. Vascular elements are also prominent and are at their greatest concentration in the posterior lamellae. Blood vessels are often identified which penetrate the annulus and even the nucleus from the adjacent vertebral end-plates (30,31).

During skeletal maturation, the notochordal cells gradually disappear from the nucleus, to be replaced by cells that resemble the chondrocytes. The gelatinous appearance of the nucleus slowly changes as more collagen

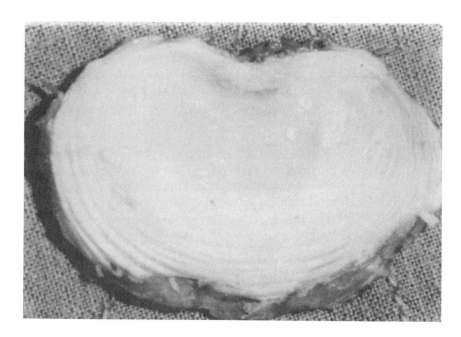

FIG. 5. The gross appearance of a young disc. Note the outer annular fibers are distinct, but the transition from annulus to nucleus is ill defined. From Frymoyer et al. (46) with permission.

is formed. At the same time the vascularity diminishes, such that by skeletal maturity the normal, uninjured disc is devoid of blood vessels except at its most peripheral layers. The adult discs, in aggregate, are the largest avascular structure in the human body.

After skeletal maturity, the concentration of collagen continues to increase and the discal water concentration decreases. The macroscopic appearance reflects these chemical changes. The nucleus becomes less glistening and lucent and the boundary between it and the surrounding annulus less distinct. The peripheral boundary of the vertebral body, which formed the growth center for the ring apophyses, disappears, and the peripheral hyaline cartilage is replaced by bone. The collagen fibrils

that initially penetrated this cartilage disappear and the peripheral annulus fibers become inserted directly into vertebral bone. Later in life these peripheral insertions are the common site of osteophyte formation.

As aging progresses, the nucleus becomes an even less distinct structure. Continued replacement of the nucleus by collagen is often accompanied by macroscopically apparent clefts and fissures. Microscopically, the chondrocyte population decreases in number and necrotic cells are usually identified. Disruption of annular fibers may also occur, and the clefts and fissures may extend into the periphery (Figs. 8 and 9). The entire disc appears yellowish, and focal areas of pyrophosphate deposition can be identified in 20 to 30% of specimens. Ultimately, the

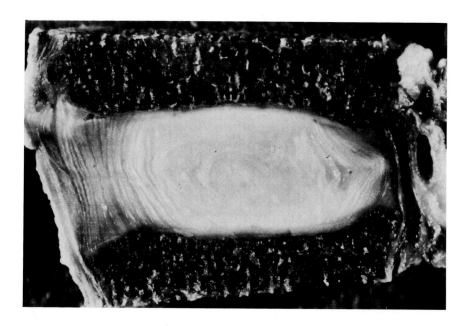

FIG. 6. The transition zone between the annulus fibrosus and the nucleus pulposus is apparent in this sagittal section of a young disc. Note the early cystic degeneration in the posterior transition zone with associated outfolding of the annular lamellae. From Osti et al. (108) with permission.

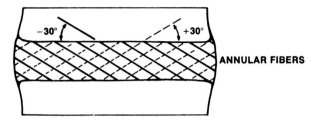

FIG. 7. A cut-away view of the disc demonstrating the alternating direction of the annular fibers. Approximately 60 individual lamellae comprise the adult nucleus. From White et al. (154) with permission.

entire disc assumes a somewhat disorganized appearance, the boundaries of the nucleus are completely obliterated, and large voids and fissures are often present. The radiologic corollary of this advanced state of degeneration is the vacuum sign. At the same time these events are occurring, the hyaline cartilage of the vertebral end-plates becomes thinner, particularly at their central portion. Depending on the magnitude of vertebral body osteoporosis, the disc may focally or diffusely bulge into the vertebral end-plates. The result is Schmorl's nodes or more diffuse disc "ballooning," which makes the disc height appear greater. Peripherally, osteophytes are formed at the annular insertion and are usually accompanied by concentric annular bulging. This concentric disc bulge found in most aging spines is to be differentiated from more focal bulges, which often are important to radiculopathies but are often unassociated with pain. Thirty to forty percent of pathologic specimens show these bulges consistent with the prevalence of focal herniations observed by CT and MRI studies in asymptomatic populations (14,155). This observation is of particular importance, as emphasized in other chapters of this book, because it tells us that not all disc bulges, or even frank herniations, produce symptoms. This evolution of anatomic changes forms the basis of grading scales for disc degeneration as measured by pathologic, radiologic, and magnetic resonance imaging criteria (Table 1 and Fig. 10).

Cellular Changes Accompanying Intervertebral Disc Degeneration and Aging

The cell composition of the disc includes notochordal cells (which disappear by skeletal maturity and are only rarely seen after age 10), chondrocytes, and fibrocytes (39). The overall mean cell density of the disc is 5,800 cells/gmL, but the cell density varies according to the structural divisions. The respective concentrations are 15,000 cells/gmL in the vertebral end-plates, which closely approximates the cell density of articular cartilage; 9,000 cells/gmL in the annulus; and 4,000 cells/gmL in the nucleus. The cell type also varies as a function of the location sampled in the disc. As might be expected,

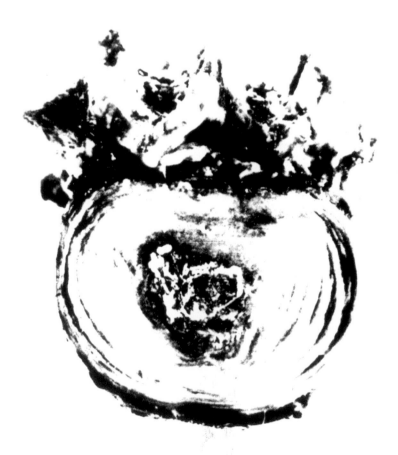

FIG. 8. Disc specimen injected with dye showing the migration of the nucleus asymmetrically toward the periphery, accompanied by the presence of radial tears in the annulus.

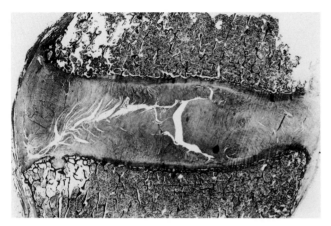

FIG. 9. This L4–L5 intervertebral disc of a 50-year-old man demonstrates a radial tear extending to the outer layers of the anterior annulus. Note the loss of demarcation between the annulus and the nucleus. From Osti et al. (108) with permission.

the annulus fibrosus is characterized by fibrocytes, whereas the nucleus pulposus is predominantly inhabited by chondrocytes. A mixture of chondrocytes and fibrocytes typifies the junctional zone between the annulus and nucleus. With aging, the cell population decreases as cellular necrosis occurs, particularly in the nucleus. The cellular ultrastructural changes that accompany the aging process have been reviewed in detail (39).

Disc Physiology

The discs taken collectively represent the largest avascular structure of the human body. Apart from blood vessels penetrating the outer annular fibers, no other vascular channels are observed in the adult disc unless injury has occurred. Thus, the nutrition of the disc is dependent on diffusion, which can be favorably or un-

TABLE 1. *Assessment of aging and degeneration of the human intervertebral disc*

Disc grade	Nucleus pulposus	Annulus fibrosus	End plate	Vertebral body
Assessment by gross morphology[a]				
I	Gel-like, bulging; blue-white	Discrete lamellae; white	Hyaline; uniform thickness	Margins rounded
II	Fibrous tissue band extending from the annulus fibrosus	Chondroid or mucinous material between lamellae	Irregular thickness of cartilage	Margins pointed
III	Consolidation of fibrous tissue	Extensive chondroid or mucinous material; loss of annulus–nucleus demarcation	Focal defects in cartilage	Early chondrophytes or osteophytes at margins
IV	Horizontal clefts parallel to end plate	Focal disruptions	Fibrocartilaginous tissue extending from subchondral bone; irregularity and focal sclerosis of subchondral bone	Osteophytes <2 mm
V	Clefts extending throughout	Clefts extending throughout	Diffuse sclerosis	Osteophytes >2 mm
Assessment by magnetic resonance imaging[b]				
I	Homogeneous; bright; demarcation distinct	Homogeneous; dark gray	Single dark line	Margins rounded
II	Horizontal dark bands extend across the annulus fibrosus centrally	Areas of increased signal intensity	Increase in central concavity	Tapering of margins
III	Signal intensity diminished; gray tone with dark and bright stippling	Indistinguishable from nucleus pulposus	Line less distinct	Small dark projections from margins
IV	Proportion of gray signal reduced; bright and dark regions larger	Indistinguishable from nucleus pulposus; some bright and dark signals contiguous with nucleus pulposus and annulus fibrosus	Focal defects in line	Projections <2 mm with same intensity as marrow
V	Gross loss of disc height; bright and dark signals dominant	Signals contiguous with nucleus pulposus	Defects and areas of thickening	Projections >2 mm with same intensity as marrow

From Frymoyer et al., ref. 46, with permission.
[a] Based on data from Vernon-Roberts (150).
[b] Using T2-weighted spin-echo images TR 2000 msec and TE 90 msec.

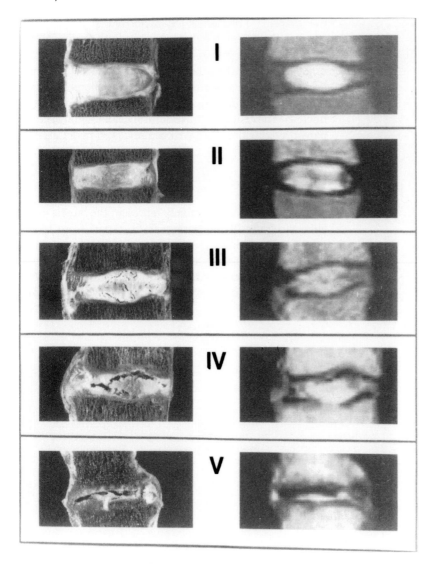

FIG. 10. The morphologic appearance of the disc, as correlated with MR images, forms the basis for commonly employed grading systems of disc degeneration. From Frymoyer et al. (46) with permission.

favorably affected by external and internal mechanical stresses, toxic substances, and the aging process.

Two nutritional pathways have been identified, based on radioisotope labeling studies (22). The first, and less important, is from the periphery by diffusion from the vessels penetrating the outer annulus. The second, and more important, is through the adjacent vertebral end-plates (104,142). It is also this latter route of nutrition which is at greatest risk (125). Terminal vascular buds are identified (Fig. 11) at the junction of the hyaline cartilage of the vertebral end-plate and the vertebral bone.

The concentration of these buds is greatest in the end-plate overlying the nucleus and progressively diminishes toward the periphery of the vertebra. This distribution of blood vessels parallels the selective permeability of the vertebral end-plates. In human specimens, 36% of the end-plate is permeable over the nucleus, diminishing to 11% at the vertebral periphery. A greater permeability has been calculated from *in vivo* canine experiments, where it approaches 80% in the region of the nucleus. In addition, Urban (143) has noted that nutrition of the disc is influenced by other factors such as solute partitions, matrix transport, and cellular demand.

Solute partitions are highly sensitive to matrix composition, charge, and solute size, similar to hyaline cartilage elsewhere in the body. Selective exclusion of anions and large solutes results in very low concentrations of these substances within the disc, whereas smaller cations are found in greater concentration in the disc than in the plasma. Furthermore, matrix composition, particularly that of the proteoglycan, is also of great importance. For example, the sulfate partition coefficient is low in the outer annulus (0.7 to 0.8), whereas in the nucleus the equivalent figure is 0.25 to 0.3. These differences correspond to the differing concentrations of proteoglycan between these two anatomic sites.

Matrix transport appears to occur primarily by diffusion rather than by an active pumping mechanism. Urban (144) has argued against a pumping mechanism based on the observation that the direction of fluid

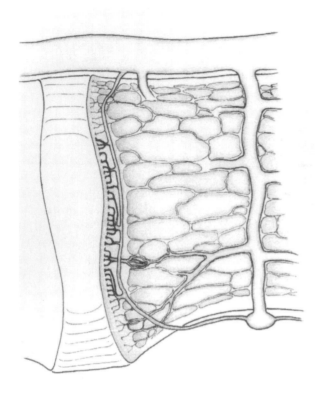

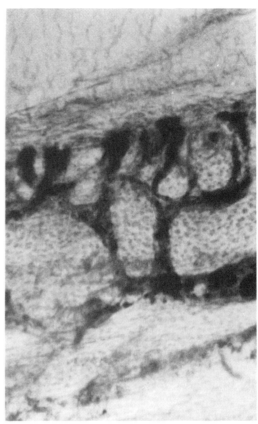

A

B

FIG. 11. The microvascular anatomy of the vertebral end-plates and their relationship to the disc. **A:** Schematic depiction. **B:** The actual morphologic appearance of the capillary tuft enhanced by ink–barium sulfate perfusion. From Frymoyer et al. (46) with permission.

transport is out of the disc three quarters of the day. She proposes that entrainment may be important for the movement of large solutes such as hormones, enzymes, and matrix breakdown products that have low diffusion. One of the major factors that does influence matrix transport is the cellular consumption of solutes. When there is a low metabolic requirement for a solute, the concentration gradients are quite flat, with the concentration at the center of the disc little different than at the surface. Thus, sulfate concentration at the disc center is 90% of that at the periphery. In comparison, solutes for which there is a high metabolic demand have steep gradients. Thus, the oxygen concentration at the periphery of the disc is 20 to 30 times greater than the concentration at the center of the nucleus. However, the availability of oxygen may be inadequate to meet the metabolic requirements, particularly in the nucleus, resulting in a greater reliance on anaerobic metabolism. These different metabolism requirements also result in significant variations in lactate concentration and pH as a function of the anatomic location within the disc. The lactate and pH profiles across the midsagittal line of the disc are shown in Figure 12. Similar observations are now being made in humans during percutaneous discectomy. Eyre (39) cites extensive references to this work.

Disc Nutrition

Effects of Environmental and Mechanical Stresses

Because the disc is so dependent on diffusion pathways for its nutrition, it is particularly sensitive to both environmental and mechanical stresses.

The effects of mechanical stresses have been studied both *in vitro* and *in vivo*. It has been suggested for some time that the average human loses an estimated one-half to one inch during the day. This height loss is then regained during the night by a process known as imbibition. More elegant measuring devices which control for postural changes that reduce height have confirmed an average height loss of 1 cm (121). The greatest contribution to this loss occurs in the lumbar spine. The average water loss is estimated to be 10% to 12% of the total disc fluid, but is increased in degenerate discs (4). Conversely, zero gravity environments halt or reverse this process. Astronauts have been found to have increased disc height after prolonged space flights.

In vitro measurements of human motion segments also demonstrate the mechanical effects of fluid loss. The application of compressive loads at a slow strain rate is followed by an initial phase of rapid deflection, followed

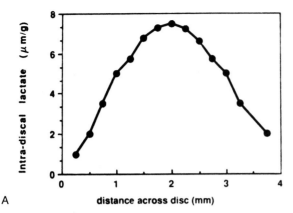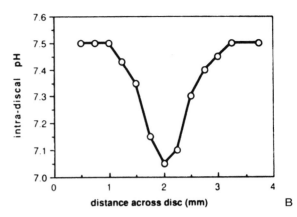

FIG. 12. The profiles of lactate concentration across the disc (**A**) and the pH profile (**B**). Note the expected inverse relationship between the two. From Holm (64) and Diamant et al. (34) with permission.

by a continuous, slower rate of disc deformation termed *creep* (Fig. 13) (76). As shown in Figure 13, this rate of creep is greater in degenerate than nondegenerate discs. If the load application is applied cyclically (vibration), the rate of deformation increases. This mechanical phenomenon is termed *vibrocreep*. Direct measurements of the effects of these mechanical loads on disc nutrition are now possible in animal models. Exposure of the pig to vibration results in decreased oxygen and sulfate transport and increased concentrations of lactate within the disc (69). These observations have particular relevance to spine disease, because vibration has been shown to be an important risk factor for neck and low back pain, as well as cervical and lumbar disc herniations. Conversely, absence of mechanical stress also appears to be an important factor in promoting spinal degeneration. The usual animal model to simulate immobilization is posterior spine fusion, which results in decreased disc nutrition and progressive degeneration (66).

Somewhere between mechanical overstress (vibration) and understress (immobilization) is an optimum mechanical environment. Although this optimum is not well understood in humans, animals trained in vigorous exercise demonstrate increased glycolysis and decreased lactate production (67). Some authorities have suggested

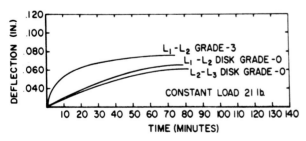

FIG. 13. The effects of continuous compression of an intervertebral disc for discs with varying degrees of degeneration. Note a rapid deflection, followed by slower continued deflections over time, termed *creep*. From Kazarian (76) with permission.

that 4 to 5 days of 30 minutes of vigorous aerobic exercise are adequate to optimize disc nutrition in the human (A. Nachemson, *personal communication,* 1989).

Nonmechanical factors are also relevant to disc nutrition. As the antithesis of aerobic conditioning, cigarette exposure has been shown to be a risk factor for both neck and low back pain, and cervical and lumbar disc herniations. Animal experiments demonstrate significant adverse effects of nicotine and cigarette smoke on disc nutrition, as measured by decreases in sulfate transport, oxygen diffusion, and increases in nuclear lactic acid concentration (68).

Other studies have shown that the presence of diabetes in animals adversely affects disc nutrition (65). How this observation relates to the human diabetic is uncertain, but association of diabetes with degenerative spondylolisthesis (127) and diffuse idiopathic skeletal hyperostosis suggests diabetes accelerates at least some forms of the degenerative process.

Finally, there is some indirect evidence that psychologic stress might also be a relevant factor. In World War II, increased disc space height was observed in the spinal radiographs of aviators returning from highly stressful combat missions. It was proposed this increase in disc height resulted in an increase in water imbibition possibly controlled by adrenocorticoids. Comparisons of stressed and unstressed rodents found significant increases in the disc water concentration of the stressed animals, but the effects on disc nutrition were not analyzed (132).

Effects of Degeneration

As the disc ages and degenerates, significant changes occur in its nutrition. In a sense this produces a "vicious cycle" where today's degeneration accelerates future, more severe, changes. With advancing age and disc degeneration, the permeability of the vertebral end-plates decreases. This process is initiated when the peripheral collagen fibrils, penetrating the end-plates, disappear at skeletal maturity and the peripheral cartilage becomes calcified. Later, degeneration may be accompanied by changes in the vertebral bone structure and marrow. The earlier stages of these changes are now evident in MRI (Fig. 14), and later apparent in radiographically visible vertebral end-plate sclerosis which accompanies advanced disc degeneration (33,95). Compromise of the end- plate route for disc nutrition may result in an even greater need for anaerobic metabolism, accompanied by increased lactic acid production and a decrease in pH. Although the conditions producing chondrocyte cell death are not fully understood, it is reasonable to suppose low pH and high lactic acid concentration create an environment that promotes cell death. Also, under these conditions the activity of degradative enzymes may increase, further promoting the loss of the proteoglycan cell matrix.

Biochemistry of the Intervertebral Disc

Comprehensive reviews and bibliographies of intervertebral disc biochemistry have been published (39). The major chemical constituents of the disc are water, which accounts for 70% of the wet weight, the extracellular matrix, and collagen. The chemical composition as determined by dry weight varies from annulus to nucleus. In the outer annulus, 60 to 70% is collagen, whereas in the central nucleus, collagen accounts for only 10 to 20%. Correspondingly, the extracellular matrix comprises the majority of the nucleus and the minority of the annulus.

Water Content

The movement of water in and out of the disc has already been presented in the previous section. With age

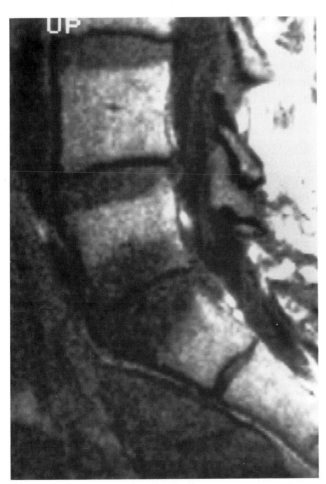
A

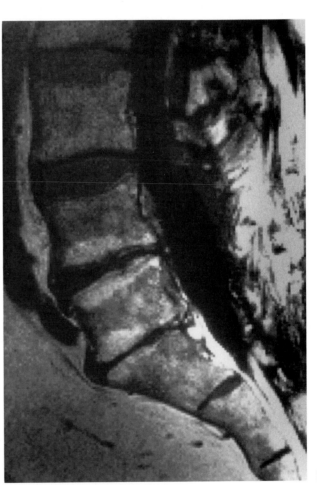
B

FIG. 14. Marrow changes accompanying degeneration have been classified by Modic et al. (95). Type 1 changes (**A**) are characterized by decreased signal intensity on T1-weighted images, as shown here, and increased signal intensity on T2-weighted images. Histologically they are characterized by fissuring and disruption of the end-plates with marrow replacement by vascularized fibrous tissue. Type 2 changes (**B**) show increased signal intensity on T1-weighted images, as shown here, and isodense or decreased signal intensity on T2-weighted images. Histologically, Type 2 changes are associated with yellow marrow replacement. Type 1 changes tend to progress to Type 2 over time, whereas Type 2 remains stable. From Modic et al. (95) with permission.

the water content decreases, particularly in the nucleus, corresponding to the changes in chemical composition that favor the production of collagen at the expense of matrix proteins.

Collagen

The collagen types and their normal distribution are given in Table 2. The majority of collagen is of types I and II, which are selectively distributed to the annulus (type I), and to the nucleus (type II). Review of Table 2 shows the remaining collagens are similarly distributed to the annulus or nucleus, with the exception of type IX. Of these remaining collagen types, type VI appears to be most abundant and is found at a concentration approximately one-fifth that of type II collagen. Each of the collagen subtypes is heavily cross-linked by an aldehyde-mediated mechanism. The turnover of collagen within the disc has eluded precise measurement to date, but it is estimated to be in excess of 100 years. As collagen ages, the more ancient fibrils covalently bond glucose residues. These products of glycosylation are thought to account for the yellowish discoloration commonly observed in the aging intervertebral disc.

The more important effect of aging is the alteration that occurs in collagen type and distribution. As part of the process of skeletal maturation and aging, type I collagen increases within the nucleus, which results in increased stiffness of that structure. Regional differences in these age-related trends have been established. The collagen content of the nucleus pulposus is highest in cervical discs and lowest in lumbar discs and increases with age in thoracic and lumbar discs (133). The high collagen levels in the cervical nucleus pulposus correlate with the greater ranges of torsional and shearing strains in the cervical spine. In addition to their potential effects on tissue

mechanical properties, glycation products may also stimulate cells, including chrondrocytes, to release cytokines and proteases that contribute to tissue degeneration (96). Recent work has suggested that in the degenerate annulus fibrosus, metalloproteinases (matrix-degrading enzymes) are induced in situ and local fibroblasts are activated to restore tissue integrity (74).

Proteoglycans

Chondroitin-6-sulfate, chondroitin-4-sulfate, and keratan sulfate are the predominant proteoglycans identified in the human intervertebral disc. The relative concentrations of these proteoglycans vary as a function of age and the location within the disc (Table 3). Some disc proteoglycans form large macromolecular aggregates with hyaluronic acid (aggregating proteoglycans), whereas others do not and are termed *nonaggregating proteoglycans*. Although it remains speculative, the current evidence favors differences between these two distinct subtypes with respect to the presence or absence of binding sites for hyaluronic acid, chondroitin sulfate, and keratan sulfate. In addition, link proteins have been identified as stabilizing the proteoglycan monomer–hyaluronate interaction.

Like the other chemical constituents, the distribution of these aggregating and nonaggregating proteoglycans also varies as a function of age and location within the disc. Also, it is found that the metabolic turnover is greater for the aggregating proteoglycans than for the nonaggregating proteoglycans, which, over time, results in an accumulation of the nonaggregating subtype. In degenerating and aging discs, proteoglycan degradation products are identified with increasing concentration, particularly in the nucleus pulposus. Thus, with increasing age the proportion of non-aggregated proteoglycans

TABLE 2. *Collagen types in the intervertebral disc*

Collagen type	Molecular formula	Tissue distribution	% of total collagen
Class 1: fibril-forming			
Type I	$[\alpha1(I)]_2\alpha2(I)$	Annulus fibrosus	Radial increase of 0 to 80% from transitional zone to outer rim
Type II	$[\alpha1(II)]_3$	Annulus fibrosus and nucleus pulposus	Radial increase of 0 to 80% from outer rim to transitional zone
Type III	$[\alpha1(III)]_3$	Possible traces in the nucleus and annulus fibrosus	—
Type V	$[\alpha1(V)]_2\alpha2(V)$ $1\alpha2\alpha3\alpha$ or	Annulus fibrosus	About 3%
Type XI	$[\alpha1(XI)\alpha2(XI)\alpha3(XI)]$	Nucleus pulposus	About 3%
Class 3: Short helix collagens			
Type VI	—	Annulus fibrosus	About 10%
		Nucleus pulposus	15% to 20%
Type IX	$[\alpha1(IX)]_2\alpha2(IX)]$	Annulus fibrosus and nucleus pulposus	1% to 2%

From Frymoyer et al., ref. 46, with permission.

TABLE 3. *Intervertebral disc glucosaminoglycans*

Tissue sample[a]	Ratios	
	Chondroitin sulfate to keratan sulfate[b]	Chondroitin-6-sulfate to chondroitin-4-sulfate[c]
3-week-old tissues		
Nucleus pulposus	2.15	2.40
Annulus fibrosus	2.00	2.47
Cartilage endplate	1.89	1.17
27-year-old tissues		
Nucleus pulposus	1.02	8.30
Annulus fibrosus	0.82	7.96
Cartilage endplate	0.68	6.30

From Frymoyer et al., ref. 46, with permission.

[a] Analysis of lyophilized A1 fraction from "associative" density gradient.

[b] Determined from peak areas after elution of chondroitinase ABC digests on Sephadex G50. Absorbance at 206 nm of the *N*-acetyl groups of the glucosaminoglycans was used to monitor the column fractions. Corrections were made for the contribution at 206 nm from peptides.

[c] Determined by high-performance liquid chromatography fractionation of unsaturated disaccharides after chondroitinase ABC digestion of proteoglycan samples.

progressively increases and the size of the proteoglycan molecules decreases markedly, especially in the nucleus pulposus (24)

These extensive alterations in proteoglycan structure begin early in life, years before the age-related changes in disc morphology, suggesting that this is one of the earliest events in the development of disc degeneration (23). The proteoglycans of the cartilaginous end-plate of the intervertebral disc also change after maturity (11), supporting the view that the cartilaginous end-plate participates in the process of aging and degeneration in the disc.

Effects of Aging and Degeneration on Proteoglycans

The changes described above in proteoglycan type and concentration, including possible changes in link proteins, and the increase in degradation products are associated with significant changes in water concentration and the mechanical properties of the disc. Alterations in the creep behavior and the increased stiffness observed in the aging and degenerate disc would appear to be significantly related to these chemical changes (Fig. 13).

DISC DEGENERATION AS A SOURCE OF SYMPTOMS

It has been emphasized up to this point that age-related changes in the morphology, biochemistry, and nutrition of the intervertebral disc cannot be differentiated from degenerative changes which caused symptoms. In clinical practice, this issue is of particular importance. To make a diagnosis of spine disease, the clinician relies upon clinical history, clinical signs, and imaging studies. The physician will often ascribe a clinical symptom of neck, thoracic, or low back pain to a degenerative condition based primarily on an imaging study, when in fact an age-related change is being observed. This risk is less when the clinical syndrome includes a mono- or polyradiculopathy. Here we will generally consider the disc as a source of symptoms. More specific descriptions of clinical syndromes follow in other chapters.

Disc Herniations

Taken together the age-related alterations in disc tissue following skeletal maturity appear to decrease the structural integrity of the disc and thereby contribute to changes in disc volume and shape and increase the probability of disc herniation (5). As already noted, lumbar disc herniations are identified in 30 to 40% of anatomic specimens, and an equivalent percentage of asymptomatic subjects, studied by myelography, CT scan, and MRI. Four subtypes of disc pathology are identified.

In stage I, diffuse bulging of the disc is observed, which is thought to represent nothing more than the loss of mechanical competence which accompanies the aging process. These changes are thought to be minimally relevant to spinal symptoms, except as they may contribute to symptoms in patients with congenital or acquired stenosis.

In stage II, focal bulges are identified. This stage is characterized macroscopically by radial fissures in the annulus and migration of nuclear material toward the periphery of the disc, commonly in the direction of the posterolateral corner (Fig. 8), which are thought to be promoted by torsional stresses. Application of static torsional stresses to human discs has been shown to cause posterolaterally distributed annular tears, which fits with the location predicted by mathematical models. In Kirkaldy-Willis' formulation, the radial tear may be the source of nonspecific spinal symptoms in stage I of symptomatic spinal degeneration.

In stage III, nuclear material becomes sequestered under the posterior longitudinal ligaments, but still remains in continuity with the disc, while in stage IV, a free fragment of nucleus escapes through the defect in the annulus. It is in this last stage that radicular symptoms are likely to be most severe, because the freed nucleus stimulates a local inflammatory response.

Spinal Stenosis

Degenerative spinal stenosis is usually a result of interactions between the disc, facet joints, and possibly spinal ligaments. The disc contributes to the loss of spinal canal dimensions by diffuse bulging, which is the mechanical consequence of alterations in the disc's structure and biochemistry.

Discogenic Pain

When nerve root symptoms are absent, it is difficult clinically to assess the role of the disc in the production of neck and back pain. A prevailing theory suggests that repetitive or acute compressive mechanical overloads cause disruption of the vertebral end-plates and are associated with changes in marrow (Fig. 14). This endplate disruption results in vascular ingrowth into the disc, possibly enzymatic degradation of the nucleus, and loss of mechanical competence. This accelerated focal degenerative process is then thought to cause pain, possibly through the production of neurogenic inflammatory mediators. This topic has been discussed in detail in Chapter 100.

Another theory is based on the common occurrence of back pain after an incident involving flexion and torsion that places the posterior annulus under stress. There is evidence suggesting the peripheral annulus tear to be of prime importance in the development of discogenic pain following such trauma (45). It has been demonstrated in an animal model that a peripheral annulus tear leads to inner annular failure and nuclear degeneration (107). Supporting this concept, a finite element model recently has suggested that the presence of discrete peripheral tears in the annulus fibrosus may have a role in the formation of concentric annular tears and in accelerating the degenerative process of the disc (101). From the postmortem histologic examination of 135 lumbar discs, it has been suggested that peripheral tears are due to trauma rather than biochemical degradation (108), with neurovascular ingrowth commonly occurring along the

margins of radiating clefts, circumferential tears, and rim lesions (149). Furthermore, a number of studies have revealed neuropeptide-immunoreactive nerves in the outermost parts of the annulus and adjacent peridiscal ligaments that may become sensitized when disc tissue is injured and which appear to be coupled to an alteration of neuropeptide pools in the nearby dorsal root ganglion (56). Finally, pain provocation during discography is associated with the presence of tears extending to the outer annulus (106). Another controversial mechanism of pain relates to the overall issues of segmental instability, which is discussed in Chapter 100.

FACET JOINTS

The apophyseal facet joints of the spine are typical diarthrodial joints. The anatomy of the facet joint is similar to that of peripheral joints, with hyaline articular cartilage overlying subchondral bone. These spinal joints undergo degenerative changes characteristic of osteoarthritis seen in other synovial articulations.

The gross anatomy of the facet joints varies by location within the spine. The most obvious feature is the change in orientation that occurs from the cervical to the lumbar spine (Fig. 15). These orientations relate to the principal planes of motion allowed at any spinal level and also influence the stresses placed on the disc. The close proximity of the facet joints to the nerve root canals also makes degeneration of these structures an important contributor to spinal stenosis.

Articular Cartilage Chemistry

Most of our knowledge of hyaline cartilage is derived from peripheral joints, but there is no reason to believe this information is not generalizable to the facets. Normal hyaline articular cartilage is comprised of four major constituents: chondrocytes, proteoglycans, collagens, and water. Chondrocytes, which make up only 5% of

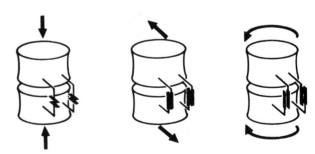

FIG. 15. The angle of the facet joints as they would best resist compressive shearing and torsional loads. The orientation shown for compression is representative of cervical vertebrae, while the orientation of those best resisting shear and torsion is representative of lower thoracic and lumbar vertebrae. From Owen et al. (109) with permission.

the volume of normal human cartilage, are metabolically active and the source of proteoglycan and collagen synthesis.

Approximately 75% of hyaline articular cartilage is water (88). Cartilage water, interacting with proteoglycans, is responsible for the mechanical property of cartilage compressibility. In addition, egress and ingress of water out of and into cartilage with joint activity is an essential component of joint nutrition and lubrication. Water content decreases only slightly with aging; in contrast, a 7 to 10% increase in water is an early and characteristic component of osteoarthritic change. Proteoglycans, which comprise almost 50% of the dry weight of cartilage, are complex chemical structures which exist in the form of monomer subunits and aggregates. Monomer subunits are comprised of a central protein core to which are attached long chain glucosaminoglycans, including primarily keratan sulfate and chondroitin sulfate.

Proteoglycan aggregates (Fig. 16) are made up of proteoglycan monomers attached to a long hyaluronic acid filament stabilized by link proteins. Studies have delineated the configuration of the proteoglycan monomer, showing that glycosaminoglycan chains are variably distributed along the protein core. In particular, few or no glycosaminoglycan chains are seen at the hyaluronate-binding region (HBR), the site of attachment to hyaluronic acid. Adjacent to the HBR is the keratan sulfate–rich segment containing primarily keratan sulfate moieties. The remainder of the chain consists of long chondroitin sulfate chains attached in clusters, together with a smaller number of shorter keratan sulfate chains.

Proteoglycan turnover is reasonably rapid, with some cartilage proteoglycans having a half-life as short as 8 days, and others exhibiting half-lives of 300 days or more (86). With aging, the concentration of chondroitin sulfate falls, with an associated increase in keratan sulfate (18,72,87). In patients with osteoarthritis, proteoglycan concentration decreases, glucosaminoglycan chains become shorter, and there is variable loss of proteoglycan aggregates. The concentration of keratan sulfate decreases, and there is an increased proportion of chondroitin-4-sulfate to chondroitin-6-sulfate.

Cartilage Collagen

The major collagen of articular cartilage is type II, which confers on cartilage its tensile strength. Collagen synthesis is more stable than that of proteoglycans in cartilage. More recently, the importance of so-called minor collagens, which make up 10 to 15% of cartilage collagens, has been emphasized (41). For example, type IX collagen, which is a composite of proteoglycan and collagen, is bound closely together with type II collagen in a hybrid structure (40,99,145). This interplay of proteoglycan and collagen appears to provide cartilage with a major component of its structural integrity (157,158). Fibronectin, a glycoprotein secreted by connective tissue cells, is increased in osteoarthritic cartilage. Fibronectin may also play a role in maintaining the fundamental integrity of the proteoglycan matrix.

Pathologic Changes in Degeneration

Pathologic responses in osteoarthritis are characterized by two major processes. One response is that of structural deterioration of cartilage, which leads to the development of focal and then diffuse erosions. Disease progression is associated with full thickness loss of cartilage down to the bone. Histopathologic findings reveal fibrillation of superficial cartilage layers and fissuring, which extends through various cartilage layers (Fig. 17). Chondrocyte response, in the early phase, reveals a general hypercellularity with increased numbers of chondrocytes, often in clusters. Later, as the disease progresses, decreased numbers of cells are identified. Alterations in proteoglycan matrix lead to loss of staining by metachromatic and orthochromatic stains. In contrast to these erosive changes, cartilage may also undergo a proliferative response characterized by the development of osteochondrophyte spurs, comprised of a central core of proliferating bone capped by hyaline and fibrocartilage. Additional pathologic changes noted include sclerosis of subchondral bone and subchondral bony cyst formation. All of these events are found in the facet joints.

Inflammation as a Component of the Degenerative Process

Synovial inflammation is a commonly seen component of the osteoarthritic process, particularly at later stages of the disease (49). Although inflammatory reactions in some patients may be associated with concurrent crystal deposition disease, such as calcium pyrophos-

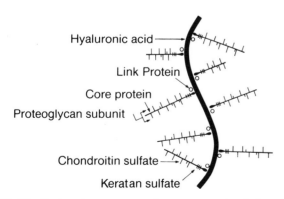

FIG. 16. Proteoglycan aggregates are comprised of proteoglycan monomers attached to a long hyaluronic acid filament stabilized by link proteins.

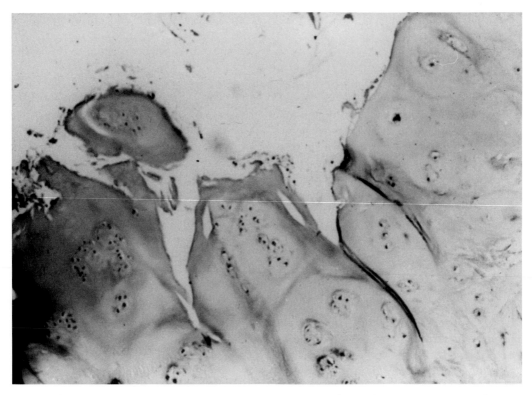

FIG. 17. Osteoarthritic histopathologic findings. Note the loss of superficial cartilage layers, fissuring, and proliferation of chondrocytes in clusters.

phate dihydrate or calcium apatite deposition, inflammatory reactions likely represent responses initiated by cartilage breakdown components in the synovial cavity interacting with synovial tissue. A role for immune completion is suggested by the observation that IgG and C3 complement are deposited in osteoarthritic joints, as demonstrated in humans and experimental animals (98). Cell-mediated immune responses to cartilage as an antigen have also been described (61).

Cartilage Degradation

An important role for enzymes capable of degrading proteoglycans and collagen has been suggested (90,118–120). Neutral metalloproteinases capable of degrading the protein core of proteoglycans and collagenolytic enzymes directed toward collagen are present in increased concentration in osteoarthritic cartilage. Tissue inhibitor of metalloproteases (TIMP), on the other hand, is increased, but to a lesser extent, so that increased hydrolytic activity of degrading enzymes is not sufficiently inhibited. Interleukin-1, derived from synovium or activated monocytes, can induce living, intact cartilage to release proteoglycanases and collagenases, and inhibit proteoglycan synthesis (Fig. 18) (35,128). These enzymes are released primarily in latent form; plasminogen activator released from chondrocytes may play a role in their activation. Cytokines involved in this process include

not only interleukin-1, but tumor necrosis factor as well. Both agents induce enzyme release and/or activation and suppress proteoglycan matrix synthesis.

Of recent interest is the concept that degradative breakdown by cytokines is counterbalanced by growth factors necessary to maintain synthetic repair responses. Growth factors such as insulin-like growth factor, fibroblast growth factor, and transforming growth factor-β act on cells to affect proteoglycan and collagen synthesis, cell proliferation, cell differentiation, and cell cycle regulation. Studies have demonstrated an increase in insulin and a decrease in insulin-like growth factor in clinical osteoarthritis (32).

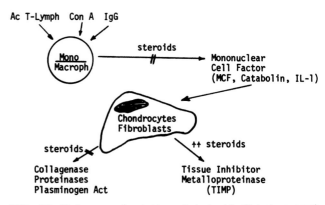

FIG. 18. Pathways of cytokines (interleukin-1) induce cartilage degradation.

Data from current and past investigations permit a schema (Fig. 19) to define the etiopathogenesis of osteoarthritis. Some unknown primary insult(s), which probably include biomechanical, biochemical, inflammatory, or immunological events, result in the release of proteolytic and collagenolytic enzymes from chondrocytes with degradation of cartilage matrix. Collagen fatigue and fracture occur with diminishing loads as the cartilage ages. Subchondral bone trabecular microfractures may then lead to increased bone stiffness and diminished shock-absorbing capacity. Cartilage attempts to repair itself through increases in matrix synthesis and cellular proliferation, but the failure of synthetic and proliferative responses to keep pace with degradative breakdown results in the clinical syndrome. Degenerative and inflammatory changes can be amplified by secondary humoral and cellular immune responses with release of inflammatory mediators.

Cartilage Nutrition

Effects of Activity and Inactivity in the Production of Degeneration

Because articular cartilage is avascular, nutrition is derived from noncartilaginous sources. In the adult mature cartilage, nutrition is derived primarily from synovial fluid, with minimal, if any, contribution from subchondral sources. The demonstration that fluid is expressed from the matrix of cartilage when the tissue is compressed and subsequently reabsorbed when the compressive force is released provides evidence for a pumping mechanism whereby nutrients are provided to chondrocytes. This pumping action augments transfer of nutrients from synovial fluid or other external sources related to simple diffusion. Accordingly, normal forces applied to cartilage in daily activities play an essential role in maintaining tissue nutrition.

On the other hand, excessive forces applied to cartilage and absolute immobilization have deleterious effects. Pathologic and metabolic changes similar to those identified in early osteoarthritis have been described in response to abnormal impact load (123,124). Radin and

his associates hypothesized that subchondral bone fractures which are caused by excessive activity result in stiffening of subchondral bone so that the overlying cartilage becomes exposed to additional stresses. In addition, collagen damage secondary to high shear stresses alters the collagen network, further promoting degenerative change. In the spine, evidence of subchondral microfractures adjacent to facets has been identified, which Farfan (43) proposed is important to the etiology of facet degeneration and spinal stenosis.

Conversely, degenerative cartilage changes occur with immobilization (38,58,138). Prolonged immobilization leads to restriction of motion with eventual intra-articular ankylosis. The events that lead to this ankylosis include proliferation of fibrous connective tissue and synovial hyperplasia. All of the histochemical and morphologic events that accompany the degenerative process may occur. The proposed mechanism by which immobilization leads to advanced degeneration is a reduction of cartilage nutrition associated with reduced synovial fluid diffusion, decreased pumping of nutrients into articular cartilage, and diminished synovial fluid production due to atrophy of the synovial membranes. Biochemical studies of cartilage from immobilized knees reveal increased water and decreased uronic acid content. Proteoglycan synthesis is markedly reduced and proteoglycan aggregates are lost. In the spine, immobilization produces these same effects on the facets. The models studied have included anterior interbody fusion (9), forcing a portion of the spine into a fixed posture (83), and the application of immobilizing spinal instruments (75).

The degenerative effects associated with immobilization may be compounded when compression is combined with joint disuse (129,139). Progressive cartilage degenerative changes represent a composite of findings associated with immobilization and additional effects due to compressive forces. In particular, cartilage becomes soft to the touch and focal lesions develop at sites of cartilage apposition. These findings are associated with the typical morphologic, histochemical, and biochemical events of osteoarthritis.

Pain in Osteoarthritis

Pain from osteoarthritic joints derives from a number of factors. Cartilage is aneural and insensitive to pain; accordingly, the pain must originate from nociceptors activated both within and surrounding the joints. Detailed clinical studies that involve injections of noxious stimuli into facet joints in the lumbar and cervical spine (17,63,82) clearly demonstrate this pain sensitivity, as well as the subjective distribution of pain which occurs at individual spinal levels. Detailed neuroanatomic studies (16,114,117,135) also demonstrate the rich innervation

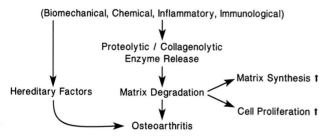

FIG. 19. Etiopathogenesis of osteoarthritis (current schematic concept).

of facet capsules by posterior primary rami. Both free nerve endings and mechanoreceptors have been identified. Elegant neurophysiologic studies suggest that mechanical stimuli activate nociceptor fibers (54). Possible mechanical factors that could activate these nociceptor mechanisms for pain production include pressure on exposed subchondral bone, intramedullary hypertension, trabecular microfractures, capsular distention, pinching of synovial villi, and periosteal elevations accompanying marginal bony spur formation. Inflammation of synovium and capsule secondary to the release of inflammatory mediators and immune responses, as previously noted, contributes further to pain.

FACET DEGENERATION AS A SOURCE OF SYMPTOMS

The facet syndrome has been a source of controversy for decades. Goldthwait (50), Putti (122), Ghormley (48), Mooney (97), and Bogduk (17) have promoted facets as a source of neck and low back pain. The clinical syndromes have usually included localized neck or back pain with radiation into upper or lower extremities consistent with the sclerotome represented by the individual facet. Relief of symptoms by local anesthetics has been reported as confirming that the facet was the source of pain (42), particularly when the duration of relief matches the expected responses to lignocaine and bupivacaine administered on separate occasions (131). Based on the results of such differential anesthetic blocks, Aprill and Bogduk (6,131) found the facet joint to be a more common source of symptoms in the neck than in the back. In the earlier phase of symptom production, radiographic changes are frequently absent. Eisenstein and Parry (37) identified histologic changes consistent with the pattern of early degeneration seen in chondromalacia. However, extensive studies of large patient cohorts suspected of "facet syndrome" have not revealed a consistent clinical pattern (73).

As facet degeneration progresses and radiographic changes are more visible, it is clear these joints are of importance to clinical conditions. Most dramatic is their contribution to spinal stenosis, affecting both the nerve root and central canals. A rarer cause of nerve root compression occurs in patients who develop synovial cysts in continuity with the joint capsule. Although these cysts are more common in the lumbar spine, they have also been reported in the cervical spine (105). It is likely, but less certain, that these joints are also an important source of pain in patients with focal and diffuse osteoarthritis affecting the entire spine.

LIGAMENTS

The spinal ligaments provide the connections between the adjacent vertebrae and serve as restraints to the extremes of motion in all planes. In this capacity the ligaments are predominantly, but not exclusively, subjected to tensile loads and absorb energy. Less well-known spinal ligaments are the transforaminal ligaments of Hoffman, which restrain movements of the lumbar nerve roots (51). In addition to these miningo-vertebral ligaments, more peripheral attachments within the intervertebral foramen, consisting of four distinct bands extending radially from a nerve root sleeve to the surrounding pedicle parts and facet joint capsule, have recently been described (55).

To date, there has been only minimal study of the chemical composition of spinal ligaments, although it is known they proportionally have a higher concentration of elastin (91). It is also known that with age the tensile properties of ligaments in general become reduced (36,100,111), and in nonspinal ligaments there is an increased concentration of collagen relative to elastin. This reduced concentration of elastin may result from enzymatic degradation by elastases, several of which have been identified in nonspinal ligaments. Structural, biochemical, and mechanical analyses of ligaments from anatomic sites other than the spine have given important insights into how mechanical stresses may favorably or adversely affect ligamentous integrity (91,134). When a joint is immobilized, macroscopic changes include (a) disorganization of ligament fibrillar and cellular alignment; (b) selective increases of collagen degradation over formation, resulting in a 10% loss within 12 weeks and the occurrence of reduced collagen cross-links; and (c) proteoglycan decreases with an associated loss of water, and resulting ligamentous weakening as measured by energy absorption to failure (91,134). These changes appear to be similar to the changes that accompany ligamentous aging. In comparison, mechanical stresses within the physiologic range appear to promote enhanced ligamentous strength, although this process takes a far longer exposure. The topic of soft tissue repair and response to activity and inactivity has been extensively reviewed by Woo and Buckwalter (156).

How the ligaments participate in the degenerative process is uncertain. As part of the aging process, the interspinal ligaments are often found to undergo macroscopic changes such as fraying, partial ruptures, necrosis, or cyst formation (25), and calcium pyrophosphate crystals are also identified. Recently the strength of the insertion of the anterior longitudinal ligament has been shown almost to halve during the aging years (102).

Focal symptoms that may result from these degenerative processes are thought to be the result of painful bursae, a condition termed Baastrup's disease (25). The ligaments, in particular the ligamentum flavum, have also been viewed as an important component of spinal stenosis. As degeneration occurs, the ligament has been thought to buckle and encroach posteriorly on the dura. This perspective has been challenged recently by more detailed anatomic and radiographic studies (130). A distinctive but rarer cause of spinal stenosis is calcification of spinal ligaments (140,141). This condition is found almost exclusively among East Asians, thus suggesting genetic or environmental factors are causative.

BONE

Degeneration of the discs, facets, and ligaments is accompanied by distinctive changes in bone. First, evolution of disc degeneration is accompanied by changes in the vertebral end-plates, including the loss of vascular channels during skeletal maturity. Later, ossification of the peripheral areas of the end-plate results in differential diffusion rates between the peripheral and central portions of the disc. With aging and degeneration, the increased bone formation adjacent to the end-plates reduces further the nutrition of the disc (10). The changes in MRI signal observed within bone in advanced degeneration may also be important to changes that occur in disc nutrition. Even later in the process, end-plate sclerosis is observed in anteroposterior and lateral spinal radiographs. This phenomenon is an expression of Wolff's law and is seen more commonly in spinal radiographs of heavy laborers (71,77). The mechanical effects of these changes are to increase the stiffness of the end-plates, which alters the mechanics of the adjacent disc. For example, this increase in end-plate stiffness reduces their contribution to energy absorption and shifts greater stresses to the disc. An extreme example of increased bone formation has been observed in a condition termed *idiopathic vertebral hyperostosis* (153). This condition is

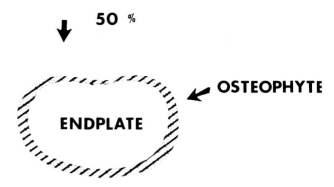

FIG. 21. The spinal osteophyte increases the surface area for load bearing and thus diminishes the force per unit area. Because the surface area increases as a squared function, modest changes have significant mechanical effects.

four times more common in females than males, has selective preference for the L4 vertebral body, and is associated with severe disc space narrowing and low back pain.

Subacute, traumatic failures in the end-plates are also thought to be a possible source of symptoms and to accelerate spinal degeneration. Anatomic studies reveal microfractures adjacent to the vertebral end-plates. It has been proposed that these microfractures, which are not visible on plain radiographs, may be one source of acute low back pain (59). More significant end-plate failures are radiographically visible as Schmorl's nodes. These occur with greater frequency in osteoporotic bone and spinal levels which are subjected to the greatest compressive loads (i.e., nonlordotic segments such as L3–L4, rather than lordotic segments such as L4–L5 and L5–S1) (44,150). The significance of these end-plate failures remains uncertain; Schmorl's nodes occur with equal frequency in patients with and without a history of back pain (47). Previously, we also noted that a possible mechanism of accelerated disc degeneration was vascular ingrowth into the disc following compression injury. This mechanism is thought to initiate "disc disruption syndrome," and in the cervical spine has been associated with the symptoms of "cervical angina."

The second area in which bone actively participates in the degenerative process is in the formation of peripheral osteophytes. The usual osteophyte, which Macnab (85) labeled the *claw spur*, occurs at the insertion of annular fibers adjacent to the disc (Fig. 20). Under compressive loads the disc bulges radially, placing increased tension on the annular fibers' insertions. Increased mechanical forces are also associated with osteophyte formation adjacent to the facet joints. However, spinal osteophytes are equally as common in patients with or without spinal pain (47). They are more frequently observed in the radiographs of individuals whose occupations have required heavy lifting (71,77). From a mechanical perspective, the presence of osteophytes may be beneficial because they increase the weight-bearing surface, thus decreasing the load per unit area (Fig. 21).

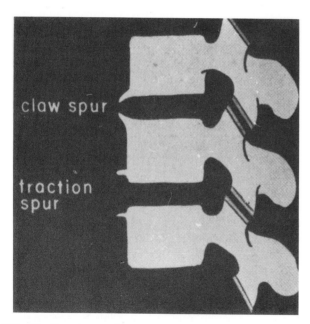

FIG. 20. Two types of spurs: the traction spur and the claw spur. The first is thought to be the result of abnormal shear loads and is proposed to be one sign of instability, while the second is proposed to arise from compressive loads and is a benign, age-related finding. From Macnab (85) with permission.

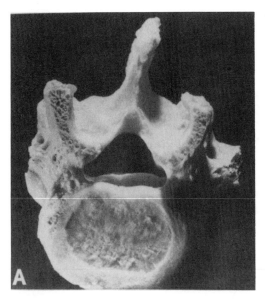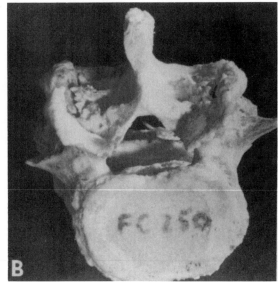

FIG. 22. A,B: Vertebral specimens are viewed from below, demonstrating torsional remodeling and deformity at the intervertebral level. From Farfan (43) with permission.

A third and more speculative role for bone is in the development of degenerative spondylolisthesis. Farfan (43) has proposed that applied repetitive torsional loads, particularly to the lumbar spine, may result in fatigue failures of the laminae adjacent to the facet joints. Over time these failures are associated with remodeling, which Farfan described as "buckling of the neural arch"; he proposed that these events cause rotatory deformities of the spinal canal and are important to the pathogenesis of stenosis (Fig. 22).

Lastly, spinal degeneration has been associated with increases in vertebral body and neural arch interosseous pressure (7). In other anatomic sites (such as the knee and hip) this measured increase in pressure has been correlated with dilated interosseous venous sinusoids. A speculative mechanism for osteoarthritic pain is that increased pressure activates perivascular nociceptors and results in the deep, boring pain often associated with severe osteoarthritis.

BASIC PRINCIPLES IN THE TREATMENT OF SPINAL DEGENERATION

Pain in patients with spinal degeneration is of multifactorial origin. In many patients, symptoms result primarily from mechanical factors such as nerve root compression, ligamentous distention, or muscle spasm. Less well recognized are the roles played by vascular, inflammatory, and immune responses in the causation of the patients' complaints. Disc degeneration may be associated with edema and increased vascularity of nerve roots, venous dilatation, and even thrombosis within the epidural venous plexuses. Autoimmune responses to nucleus pulposus tissue have been described (12,13). In ad-

dition, the facet joints play an important role in spinal pain. Accordingly, there is strong rationale for the use of nonsteroidal anti-inflammatory agents for analgesic and anti-inflammatory control of symptoms in patients with spinal degeneration.

Nonsteroidal Anti-inflammatory Drugs: Mechanisms of Action, Indications, and Complications

For many years aspirin and other salicylates were recommended for primary therapy as nonsteroidal anti-inflammatory agents in the treatment of various forms of musculoskeletal disease. They are relatively inexpensive and their effectiveness has been known for over a century. Over the past several decades, newer nonaspirin nonsteroidal anti-inflammatory agents have been introduced. These appear to have advantages over aspirin in terms of better patient tolerance and increased compliance because they require fewer tablets or capsules on a daily basis. Doses of aspirin required for treatment of acute back pain are less than those used for general systemic arthritides (such as rheumatoid arthritis), and doses of 640 mg four or five times daily are generally readily tolerated. Aspirin is best tolerated when taken with food or antacids. In certain patients with salicylate intolerance, enteric-coated aspirin or the use of aspirin with insoluble alkali may be helpful.

Patients with mild symptoms of salicylism characterized by tinnitus or decreased hearing can usually be managed by stopping the intake of salicylate for several days until symptoms clear, after which a lower total daily dose can be initiated. In addition to gastropathy and peptic ulcer disease, not infrequently associated with occult or gross bleeding, side reactions to the use of salicylates include severe bronchospastic reactions in patients with a history of asthma or nasal polyps, urticaria, angioedema, and in certain patients, hepatic abnormalities with elevated transaminase levels (8,126). Salicylate medications prepared without the acetyl radical, such as salicylsalicylic acid, choline salicylate, or choline magnesium trisalicylate have minimal or no effect on platelet aggregation. These nonacetylated salicylates are preparations of choice in patients with bleeding disorders or in whom bleeding may be a problem following procedures such as dental extraction or general surgery. These latter agents are also of value in that their use is associated with less gastrointestinal toxicity and minimal to absent renal effects.

The search for agents at least as effective as aspirin but with less overall toxicity and with increased ease of administration to improve compliance has led to development of a number of other nonsteroidal anti-inflammatory drugs (NSAIDs). Their introduction to the therapeutic spectrum has provided a major advance in agents available for use in treating musculoskeletal disorders. Agents currently available in the United States include indomethacin (Indocin), sulindac (Clinoril), tolmetin sodium (Tolectin), ibuprofen (Motrin), fenoprofen (Nalfon), naproxen (Naprosyn), meclofenamate sodium (Meclomen), piroxicam (Feldene), diflunisal (Dolobid), ketoprofen (Orudis), flurbiprofen (Ansaid), etodolac (Lodine), nabumetone (Relafen), oxaprozin (Daypro), and diclofenac (Voltaren).

The mechanisms of action whereby the newer nonsteroidal agents provide anti-inflammatory activity involve a number of different pathways. Initially, their ability to inhibit prostaglandin synthesis was considered to be the major mechanism explaining their anti-inflammatory activity. However, recent studies have demonstrated a more generalized effect of these agents on the inflammatory pathways (1,2). These drugs appear to inhibit leukocyte activation by mechanisms not related either to prostaglandins or leukotrienes (1,2). Studies, for example, have demonstrated an effect of NSAIDs on leukocyte aggregation, generation of superoxide ions, and secretion of lysosomal enzymes.

Mechanisms of action whereby these agents affect cartilage synthesis and catabolism are of particular interest in their use in the general management of musculoskeletal diseases (110). Nonsteroidal anti-inflammatory agents differ in their effect on proteoglycan synthesis: some agents decrease proteoglycan synthesis, some have no effect on synthesis, and some actually increase synthesis (20). Unloaded regions of cartilage appear to be more susceptible to inhibition of proteoglycan synthesis than are loaded regions from the same joints. In addition, inhibitory effects are markedly increased in osteoarthritic cartilage. Other studies have demonstrated an inhibitory effect of certain nonsteroidal anti-inflammatory agents on catabolic breakdown of

cartilage by cartilage-derived proteases (89). Accordingly, the overall effect of NSAIDs on cartilage represents an interplay of their effects on synthesis versus degradation. Although some studies suggest that NSAIDs accelerate the progression of osteoarthritis (29,92), overall clinical experience with these agents as used over a number of years and in many forms of arthritis is reassuring.

Toxic reactions seen with the various NSAIDs bear many similarities. They are, however, sufficiently different in their toxicity profiles to warrant individualization of use in given patients. General reactions include gastrointestinal upset and peptic ulcer formation, central nervous system reactions (including headaches, dizziness, and vertigo), and various forms of rashes. Fluid retention is not uncommon but generally is not a major problem. As with aspirin, patients with a history of any form of bronchospasm should be cautioned regarding their use, because there is demonstrated cross-reactive allergic reaction with salicylates.

Side reactions more unique to specific NSAIDs have been described. In patients receiving indomethacin, migraine-like headaches probably related to its serotonin-like effects may necessitate discontinuing treatment; this reaction is more likely to be seen in elderly patients. Ibuprofen administration has been associated with amblyopia and aseptic meningitis; the latter appears to be an unusual reaction seen mainly in patients with systemic lupus erythematosus and other inflammatory connective tissue disorders. Diarrhea is more commonly seen in patients receiving meclofenamate sodium. Although effects of NSAIDs on prothrombin time are usually minimal, prothrombin time determinations should be carefully monitored when the drugs are used in conjunction with coumarin derivatives. Furthermore, because gastritis accompanies all NSAIDs over time, use of NSAIDs is to be avoided if possible in all anticoagulated patients. In patients receiving sulindac, an unusual set of toxic reactions characterized by rash with desquamation, hepatomegaly, and jaundice has been described. Diclofenac has been associated with a slightly increased frequency of hepatic reactions.

Impairment of renal function secondary to NSAIDs has been described (21,27,28,78,152). This renal impairment may take several forms, including diminished creatinine clearance, particularly in patients whose renal function is already impaired, such as those with congestive heart failure or cirrhosis, acute oliguric renal failure, nephrotic syndrome, and interstitial nephritis. Allergic interstitial nephritis may be associated with a systemic reaction including fever, rash, and eosinophilia; this reaction has been seen more frequently in patients receiving fenoprofen therapy. Some studies suggest that sulindac may be associated with a decreased frequency of renal reactions (27). The renal abnormalities noted with NSAIDs are likely related to blocking of compensatory increases in renal prostaglandins involved in the autoregulation of renal blood flow and glomerular filtration.

Gastrointestinal intolerance to nonsteroidal anti-inflammatory agents may be relatively minor and characterized by abdominal cramping, pyrosis, and nausea. In other patients, gastropathy may be associated with major gastrointestinal bleeding, with or without peptic ulceration. Gastropathic changes characterized by mucosal erosions may be extensive in the absence of overt symptoms; conversely, symptoms of gastrointestinal intolerance are not infrequent despite absence of major gastric pathology. The use of agents that decrease gastric acidity and/or provide a mucosal cytoprotective effect may be helpful in managing patients taking these medications, particularly if the gastropathy is complicated by coincident primary peptic ulcer disease. Agents used in this regard include H2 blockers such as cimetidine (Tagamet), ranitidine (Zantac), famotidine (Pepcid), nizatidine (Axid), sucralfate (Carafate), or prostaglandin analogues such as misoprostol (Cytotec).

Although the new NSAIDs described above are not identical in terms of effectiveness and toxicity profiles, overall similarities in effectiveness and toxicity do not indicate that any one of these agents is distinctly advantageous for initial use in a given patient. In deciding which agent to use, the physician should evaluate such factors as drug cost, improved compliance to be anticipated with the need for only a few tablets daily, and experience with one or another of these preparations. Some patients tolerate certain of these agents better than others, and accordingly, certain of these agents may be better accepted by a given patient.

The newer NSAIDs represent a widely used class of pharmaceutical agents that are effective in relief of pain and inflammation in many forms of musculoskeletal disease. Judicious selection of these agents and appropriate monitoring of their use will allow physicians to take advantage of their benefits while minimizing toxic side reactions. Caution is particularly prudent in the elderly, who are at a greater risk of NSAID toxicity. Physical modalities and mild analgesics such as acetaminophen can often suffice.

SUMMARY AND CONCLUSIONS

This chapter has stressed that spinal degeneration and aging are identifiable pathologic processes, and that differentiation of clinically symptomatic disease from physiologic events is a difficult task. Certain features of the degenerative process seem apparent:

1. The lesions are distributed across the spine, corresponding to mechanical stresses produced by spinal motion and posture. The mechanical nature of the lesions is also substantiated by the increased frequency of spinal pain and disc herniations in heavy laborers and in animal models with selectively increased spinal stresses.

2. The development of spinal degeneration is also physiologically, and in some instances genetically, controlled. The precarious physiology of disc nutrition makes it susceptible to mechanical stresses and chemical exposures, in addition to aging.

3. The relationships between the biochemistry of discs, ligaments, and facet joints and their mechanical properties are now becoming understood. Perhaps the most important clinically applicable observation is the sensitivity of spinal structures to overstress, optimum stress, and understress. This leads to the conclusion that physiologic exercise is important to the maintenance of the spinal structures, and that prolonged immobilization is not effective and perhaps deleterious.

REFERENCES

1. Abramson S, Edelson H, Kaplan H, et al. (1983): Effects of conventional doses of non-steroidal anti-inflammatory agents (NSAIA) on the function of human neutrophils. *Arthritis Rheum* 26(Suppl):S43.
2. Abramson S, Korchak H, Kimmel S, et al. (1984): The cellular effects of nonsteroidal anti-inflammatory drugs (NSAID) cannot be due to inhibition of prostaglandin (PG) release. *Arthritis Rheum* 27(Suppl):S22.
3. Ahmed AM, Duncan NA, Burke DL (1988): The effect of facet geometry on the axial torque-rotation response of lumbar motion segments. *Trans Orthop Res Soc* 13:327.
4. Adams MA, Hutton WC (1983): The effect of posture on the fluid content of lumbar intervertebral discs. *Spine* 8:665–671.
5. Anderson GBJ (1993): Intervertebral disc: clinical aspects. In: Buckwalter JA, Goldberg BN, Woo SL-Y, eds. *Musculoskeletal soft tissue aging: impact on mobility*. Rosemont, Ill: American Academy of Orthopaedic Surgeons, pp. 331–347.
6. Aprill C, Bogduk N (1992): The prevalence of cervical zygapophyseal joint pain. A first approximation. *Spine* 17:744–777.
7. Arnoldi CC (1972): Intravertebral pressures in patients with lumbar pain: preliminary communication. *Acta Orthop Scand* 43:109–117.
8. Athreya BH, Moser G, Cecil HS, et al. (1975): Aspirin-induced hepatotoxicity in juvenile rheumatoid arthritis. A prospective study. *Arthritis Rheum* 18:347–352.
9. Baker WdeC, Thomas TG, Kirkaldy-Willis WH (1969): Changes in the cartilage of the posterior intervertebral joints after anterior fusion. *J Bone Joint Surg [Br]* 51:736–746.
10. Bernick S, Cailliet R (1982): Vertebral end-plate changes with aging of human vertebrae. *Spine* 7:97–102.
11. Bishop PB, Pearce RH (1993): The proteoglycans of the cartilaginous end-plate of the human intervertebral disc change after maturity. *J Orthop Res* 11:324–331.
12. Bisla RS, Marchisello PJ, Lockshin MD, Hart DM, Marcus RE, Granda J (1976): Auto-immunological basis of disk degeneration. *Clin Orthop* 121:205–211.
13. Bobechko WP, Hirsch C (1965): Auto-immune response to nucleus pulposus in the rabbit. *J Bone Joint Surg [Br]* 47:574–580.
14. Boden SD, Davis DO, Dina TS, Patronas NJ, Wiesel S (1990): Abnormal magnetic resonance scans of the lumbar spine in asymptomatic subjects. *J Bone Joint Surg [Am]* 72:403–408.
15. Boden SD, Riew KD, Yamaguchi K, Branch TP, Schellinger D, Wiesel SW (1994): *Lumbar facet joint tropism (asymmetry): defining "normal" and the relationship to disc disease*. Presented at the meeting of the International Society for the Study of the Lumbar Spine, Seattle, Washington.
16. Bogduk N (1983): The innervation of the lumbar spine. *Spine* 8:286–293.

17. Bogduk N, Marsland A (1988): The cervical zygapophysial joints as a source of neck pain. *Spine* 13:610–617.

18. Bollet AJ, Nance JL (1966): Biochemical findings in normal and osteoarthritic articular cartilage. II. Chondroitin sulfate concentration and chain length, water and ash content. *J Clin Invest* 45:1170–1177.

19. Bradford DS, Oegema TR Jr, Cooper KM, et al. (1984): Chymopapain, chemonucleolysis, and nucleus pulposus regeneration: a biochemical and biomechanical study. *Spine* 9:135–147.

20. Brandt KD (1987): Effects of nonsteroidal anti-inflammatory drugs on chondrocyte metabolism in vitro and in vivo. *Am J Med* 83(5A):29–34.

21. Brezin JH, Katz SM, Schwartz ÁB, Chinitz JL. (1979): Reversible renal failure and nephrotic syndrome associated with nonsteroidal anti-inflammatory drugs. *N Engl J Med* 301:1271–1273.

22. Brodin H (1955): Paths of nutrition in articular cartilage and intervertebral discs. *Acta Orthop Scand* 24:177–183.

23. Buckwalter JA (1995): Spine update. Aging and degeneration of the human intervertebral disc: structural and bio-chemical changes and mechanisms of aging. *Spine* 20:1307–1314.

24. Buckwalter JA, Ruffley PF, Rosemburg LC (1994): Age-related changes in cartilage proteoglycans: quantitated electron microscopic studies. *Micros Res Tech* 28:398–408.

25. Bywaters EGL (1982): The pathological anatomy of idiopathic low back pain. In: White AA III, Gordon SL, eds. *American Academy of Orthopaedic Surgeons symposium on idiopathic low back pain.* St. Louis: C. V. Mosby, pp. 144–177.

26. Cauchoix J, Yaacubi E, Romero CG, et al. (1984): An experimental model of lumbar degenerated discs in rabbits. Presented at the Tenth Meeting of the International Society for Study of the Lumbar Spine, Montreal, Canada.

27. Ciabattoni G, Cinotti GA, Pierucci A, et al. (1984): Effects of sulindac and ibuprofen in patients with chronic glomerular disease. *N Engl J Med* 310:279–283.

28. Clive DM, Stoff JS (1984): Renal syndromes associated with nonsteroidal anti-inflammatory drugs. *N Engl J Med* 310:563–572.

29. Coke H (1967): Long-term indomethacin therapy of coxarthrosis. *Ann Rheum Dis* 26:346–347.

30. Coventry MB (1969): Anatomy of the intervertebral disk. *Clin Orthop* 67:9–15.

31. Coventry MB, Ghormley RK, Kernohan JW (1945): The intervertebral disc: its microscopic anatomy and pathology: Part I. Anatomy, development, and physiology. *J Bone Joint Surg* 27:105–112.

32. Denko CW, Boja B, Moskowitz RW (1987): Serum levels of insulin and insulin-like growth factor (IGF-1) in osteoarthritis (OA). *Arthritis Rheum* 30(Suppl):S132.

33. de Roos A, Kressel H, Spritzer C, et al. (1987): MR imaging of marrow changes adjacent to end plates in degenerative lumbar disk disease. *AJR* 149:531–534.

34. Diamant B, Karlsson J, Nachemson A (1968): Correlation between lactate levels and pH in discs of patients with lumbar rhizopathies. *Experientia* 24:1195–1196.

35. Dingle JT (1984): The effect of synovial catabolin on cartilage synthetic activity. *Connect Tissue Res* 12:227–286.

36. Dumas GA, Beaudoin L, Drouin G (1987): In situ mechanical behavior of posterior spinal ligaments in the lumbar region: an in vitro study. *J Biomech* 20:301–310.

37. Eisenstein SM, Parry CR (1987): The lumbar facet arthrosis syndrome. Clinical presentation and articular surface changes. *J Bone Joint Surg [Br]* 69:3–7.

38. Engh GA, Chrisman OD (1977): Experimental arthritis in rabbit knees: a study of relief of pressure on one tibial plateau in immature and mature rabbits. *Clin Orthop* 125:221–226.

39. Eyre D (1989): Intervertebral disk. Basic science perspectives. In: Frymoyer JW, Gordon SL, eds. *New perspectives on low back pain.* Park Ridge, IL: American Academy of Orthopaedic Surgeons, pp. 147–207.

40. Eyre DR, Apon S, Wu J-J, Ericsson LH, Walsh KA (1987): Collagen type IX: evidence for covalent linkages to type II collagen in cartilage. *FEBS Lett* 220:337–341.

41. Eyre DR, Wu J-J, Apone E (1987): A growing family of collagens in articular cartilage: identification of 5 genetically distinct types. *J Rheumatol* 14(Spec No):25–27.

42. Fairbank JC, Park WM, McCall IW, et al. (1981): Apophyseal injection of local anesthetic as a diagnostic aid in primary low-back pain syndromes. *Spine* 6:598–605.

43. Farfan HF (1980): The pathological anatomy of degenerative spondylolisthesis. A cadaver study. *Spine* 5:412–418.

44. Farfan HF, Huberdeau RM, Dubow HI (1972): Lumbar intervertebral disc degeneration: the influence of geometrical features on the pattern of disc degeneration. A post mortem study. *J Bone Joint Surg [Am]* 54:492–510.

45. Fraser RD, Osti OL, Vernon-Roberts B (1993): Intervertebral disc degeneration. *Eur Spine J* 1:205–213.

46. Frymoyer JW, Gordon SL (1989): *New perspectives on low back pain.* Park Ridge, Illinois: American Academy of Orthopaedic Surgeons.

47. Frymoyer JW, Newberg A, Pope MH, Wilder DG, Clements J, MacPherson B (1984): Spine radiographs in patients with low-back pain. An epidemiological study in men. *J Bone Joint Surg [Am]* 66:1048–1055.

48. Ghormley RK (1933): Low back pain: with special reference to the articular facets, with presentation of an operative procedure. *JAMA* 101:1773–1777.

49. Goldenberg DL, Egan MS, Cohen AS (1982): Inflammatory synovitis in degenerative joint disease. *J Rheumatol* 9:204–209.

50. Goldthwait JE (1911): The lumbo-sacral articulation: an explanation of many cases of "lumbago," "sciatica" and paraplegia. *Boston Med Surg J* 164:365–372.

51. Golub BS, Silverman B (1969): Transforaminal ligaments of the lumbar spine. *J Bone Joint Surg [Am]* 51:947–956.

52. Gotfried Y, Bradford DS, Oegema TR Jr (1986): Facet joint changes after chemonucleolysis-induced disc space narrowing. *Spine* 11:944–950.

53. Grenier N, Kressel HY, Schiebler ML, et al. (1987): Normal and degenerative posterior spinal structures: MR imaging. *Radiology* 165:517–525.

54. Grigg P, Schaible HG, Schmidt RF (1986): Mechanical sensitivity of group III and IV afferents from posterior articular nerve in normal and inflamed cat knee. *J Neurophysiol* 55:635–643.

55. Grimes PF, Massie JB, Garfin SR (1994): Anatomic and biomechanical study of foraminal ligaments. Presented at the meeting of the International Society for the Study of the Lumbar Spine, Seattle, Washington.

56. Gromblad M, Weinstein JN, Santavirta S (1991): Immunohistochemical observations on spinal tissue innervation. A review of hypothetical mechanisms of back pain. *Acta Orthop Scand* 62:614–622.

57. Gunsburg R, Fraser RD, Fraser GA (1990): Lumbar intervertebral disc prolapse in teenage twins. *J Bone Joint Surg [Br]* 72:914–916.

58. Hall MC (1969): Cartilage changes after experimental relief of contact in knee joint of the mature rat. *Clin Orthop* 64:64–76.

59. Hansson T, Roos B (1981): Microcalluses of the trabeculae in lumbar vertebrae and their relation to the bone mineral content. *Spine* 6:375–380.

60. Heliövaara M, Vanharanta H, Korpi J, et al. (1988): Herniated lumbar disc syndrome and vertebral canals. In: Heliövaara M, ed. *Epidemiology of sciatica and herniated lumbar intervertebral disc.* Helsinki: Social Insurance Institution, Research Institute for Social Security, Rehabilitation Research Centre, pp. 433–435.

61. Herman JH, Houk JL, Dennis MV (1974): Cartilage antigen dependent lymphotoxin release. Immunopathological significance in articular destructive disorders. *Ann Rheum Dis* 33:446–452.

62. Higuchi M, Abe K, Kaneda K (1983): Changes in the nucleus pulposus of the intervertebral disk in bipedal mice. A light and electron microscopic study. *Clin Orthop* 175:251–257.

63. Hirsch C, Ingelmark B-E, Miller M (1963): The anatomical basis for low back pain: studies on the presence of sensory nerve endings in ligamentous, capsular and intervertebral disc structures in the human lumbar spine. *Acta Orthop Scand* 33:1–17.

64. Holm S (1989): *Does diabetes induce degenerative processes in the lumbar intervertebral disc?* Presented at the meeting of the International Society for the Study of the Lumbar Spine, Kyoto, Japan.

65. Holm S, Maroudas A, Urban JPG, et al. (1981): Nutrition of the

intervertebral disc: solute transport and metabolism. *Connect Tissue Res* 8:101–119.

66. Holm S, Nachemson A (1982): Nutritional change in the canine intervertebral disc after spinal fusion. *Clin Orthop* 169:243–258.

67. Holm S, Nachemson A (1983): Variations in the nutrition of the canine intervertebral disc induced by motion. *Spine* 8:866–874.

68. Holm S, Nachemson A (1984): Immediate effects of cigarette smoke on the nutrition of the intervertebral disc of the pig. *Orthop Trans* 8:380.

69. Holm S, Nachemson A (1985): Nutrition of the intervertebral disc: effects induced by vibrations. *Orthop Trans* 9:451.

70. Horal J (1969): The clinical appearance of low back disorders in the city of Gothenburg, Sweden: comparisons of incapacitated probands with matched controls. *Acta Orthop Scand* (Suppl) 118:1–109.

71. Hult L (1954): Cervical, dorsal and lumbar spinal syndromes. *Acta Orthop Scand* 24:174–175.

72. Inerot S, Heinegard D, Audell L, Olsson S-E (1978): Articular-cartilage proteoglycans in aging and osteoarthritis. *Biochem J* 169:143–156.

73. Jackson RP, Jacobs RR, Montesano PX (1988): 1988 Volvo Award In Clinical Sciences. Facet joint injection in low-back pain. A prospective statistical study. *Spine* 13:966–971.

74. Kääpä E, Wei W, Ervasti-Koivisto H, Konttinen Y, Poussa M, Vanharanta H (1994): Collagen chemistry in normal and degenerate human annulus fibrosus. Presented at the meeting of the International Society for the Study of the Lumbar Spine, Seattle, Washington.

75. Kahanovitz N, Arnoczky SP, Levine DB, et al. (1984): The effects of internal fixation on the articular cartilage of unfused canine facet joint cartilage. *Spine* 9:268–272.

76. Kazarian LE (1975): Creep characteristics of the human spinal column. *Orthop Clin North Am* 6:3–18.

77. Kellgren JH, Lawrence JS (1958): Osteo-arthrosis and disk degeneration in an urban population. *Ann Rheum Dis* 17:388–397.

78. Kimberly RP, Bowden RE, Keiser HR, Plotz H. (1978): Reduction of renal function by newer nonsteroidal anti-inflammatory drugs. *Am J Med* 64:804–807.

79. Kirkaldy-Willis WH (1983): *Managing low back pain*. New York: Churchill Livingstone.

80. Latham JM, Pearcy MJ, Costi JJ, Moore R, Fraser RD, Vernon-Roberts B (1994): Mechanical consequences of anular tears and subsequent intervertebral disc degeneration. *Clin Biochem* 9:211–219.

81. Lawrence JS (1977): *Rheumatism in populations*. London: Heinemann.

82. Lewis T, Kellgren JH (1939): Observations relating to referred pain, visceromotor reflexes and other associated phenomena. *Clin Sci* 4:47–71.

83. Lindblom K (1952): Experimental ruptures of intervertebral discs in rats' tails. A preliminary report. *J Bone Joint Surg* [*Am*] 34:123–128.

84. Lipson SJ, Muir H (1981): Experimental intervertebral disc degeneration: morphologic and proteoglycan changes over time. *Arthritis Rheum* 24:12–21.

85. Macnab I (1971): The traction spur: an indicator of segmental instability. *J Bone Joint Surg* [*Am*] 53:663–670.

86. Mankin HJ, Lippiello L (1969): The turnover of adult rabbit articular cartilage. *J Bone Joint Surg* [*Am*] 51:1591–1600.

87. Mankin HJ, Lippiello L (1970): Biochemical and metabolic abnormalities in articular cartilage from osteoarthritic human hips. *J Bone Joint Surg* [*Am*] 52:424–434.

88. Mankin HJ, Thrasher AZ (1975): Water content and binding in normal and osteoarthritic human cartilage. *J Bone Joint Surg* [*Am*] 57:76–80.

89. Martel-Pelletier J, Pelletier JP (1989): Molecular basis for the action of tiaprofenic acid on human osteoarthritic cartilage degradation. *Semin Arthritis Rheum* 18(Suppl):19–26.

90. Martel-Pelletier J, Pelletier JP, Cloutier JM, et al. (1984): Neutral proteases capable of proteoglycan digesting activity in osteoarthritic and normal human articular cartilage. *Arthritis Rheum* 27:305–312.

91. Miller EJ, Gay S (1987): The collagens: an overview and update. *Methods Enzymol* 144:3–41.

92. Milner JC (1973): Osteoarthritis of the hip and indomethacin. *J Bone Joint Surg* [*Br*] 54:752.

93. Modic MT, Masaryk TJ, Ross JS (1989): *Magnetic resonance imaging of the spine*. Chicago: Year Book Medical Publishers.

94. Modic MT, Pavlicek W, Weinstein MA, et al. (1984): Magnetic resonance imaging of intervertebral disk disease: clinical and pulse sequence considerations. *Radiology* 152:103–111.

95. Modic MT, Steinberg PM, Ross JS, et al. (1988): Degenerative disk disease: assessment of changes in vertebral body marrow with MR imaging. *Radiology* 166:193–199.

96. Monier VM, Sell DR, Hochfarmer J, Moskovitz R (1993): Post-translational protein modification by the Maillard reaction: relevance to aging of the extracellular matrix molecules. In: Buckwalter JA, Goldberg V, Woo SL-Y, eds. *Musculoskeletal soft tissue aging: impact on mobility*. Rosemont, IL: American Academy of Orthopaedic Surgeons, pp. 49–59.

97. Mooney V, Robertson J (1976): The facet syndrome. *Clin Orthop* 115:149–156.

98. Moskowitz RW, Kresina TF (1986): Immunofluorescent analysis of experimental osteoarthritic cartilage and synovium: evidence for selective deposition of immunoglobulin and complement in cartilaginous tissues. *J Rheumatol* 13:391–396.

99. Muller-Glauser W, Humbel B, Glatt M, Strauli P, Winterhalter KH, Bruckner P (1986): On the role of type IX collagen in the extracellular matrix of cartilage: type IX collagen is localized to intersections of collagen fibrils. *J Cell Biol* 102:1931–1939.

100. Nachemson AL, Evans JH (1968): Some mechanical properties of the third human lumbar interlaminar ligament (ligamentum flavum). *J Biomech* 1:211–220.

101. Natarajan RN, Ke JH, Andersson GBJ (1994): A model to study the disc degeneration process. *Spine* 19:259–265.

102. Neumann P, Ekstrom LA, Keller TS, Perry L, Hansson TH (1994): Aging, vertebral density, and disc degeneration alter the tensile stress-strain characteristics of the human anterior longitudinal ligament. *J Orthop Res* 12:103–112.

103. Noren R, Trafimow J, Andersson GBJ, Huckman M (1989): The importance of facet joint tropism and facet angle to the development of disc degeneration. *Spine* 16:530–532.

104. Ogata K, Whiteside LA (1981): 1980 Volvo Award winner in basic science. Nutritional pathways of the intervertebral disc. An experimental study using hydrogen washout technique. *Spine* 6:211–216.

105. Onofrio BM, Mih AD (1988): Synovial cysts of the spine. *Neurosurgery* 22:642–647.

106. Osti OL, Fraser RD (1992): MRI and discography of anular tears and intervertebral disc degeneration. A prospective clinical comparison. *J Bone Joint Surg* [*Br*] 74:431–435.

107. Osti OL, Vernon-Roberts B, Fraser RD (1990): Anulus tears and intervertebral disc degeneration. An experimental study using an animal model. *Spine* 15:762–767.

108. Osti OL, Vernon-Roberts B, Moore R, Fraser RD (1992): Anular tears and disc degeneration in the lumbar spine. A post mortem study of 135 discs. *J Bone Joint Surg* [*Br*] 74:678–682.

109. Owen R, Goodfellow J, Bullough P (1980): *Scientific foundations of orthopaedics and traumatology*. London: William Heinemann Medical Books Ltd.

110. Palmoski MJ, Brandt KD (1980): Effects of some nonsteroidal anti-inflammatory drugs on proteoglycan metabolism and organization in canine articular cartilage. *Arthritis Rheum* 23:1010–1020.

111. Panjabi MM, Goel VK, Takata K (1982): Volvo Award in biomechanics. Physiologic strains in the lumbar spinal ligaments: an in vitro biomechanical study. *Spine* 7:192–203.

112. Panjabi MM, Krag MH, Chung TQ (1984): Effects of disc injury on mechanical behavior of the human spine. *Spine* 9:707–713.

113. Panjabi MM, Pelker R, Crisco JJ, Thibodeau L, Yamamoto I (1988): Biomechanics of healing of posterior cervical spinal injuries in a canine model. *Spine* 13:803–807.

114. Paris SV (1983): Anatomy as related to function and pain. *Orthop Clin North Am* 14:475–489.

115. Pearce RJ, Thompson JP, Bebault GM, Flack B (1991): Magnetic resonance imaging reflects the chemical changes of aging degeneration in the human intervertebral disc. *J Rheumatol* (Suppl) 27:42–43.

116. Pech P, Haughton VM (1985): Lumbar intervertebral disk: correlative MR and anatomic study. *Radiology* 156:699–701.

117. Pedersen HE, Blunck CFJ, Gardner E (1956): The anatomy of lumbosacral posterior rami and meningeal branches of spinal nerves (sinu-vertebral nerves): with an experimental study of their functions. *J Bone Joint Surg [Am]* 38:377–391.

118. Pelletier JP, Martel-Pelletier J, Altman RD, et al. (1983): Collagenolytic activity and collagen matrix breakdown of the articular cartilage in the Pond-Nuki dog model of osteoarthritis. *Arthritis Rheum* 26:866–874.

119. Pelletier JP, Martel-Pelletier J, Ghandur-Mnaymneh L, et al. (1985): The role of synovial membrane inflammation in cartilage matrix breakdown in the Pond-Nuki model of osteoarthritis. *Arthritis Rheum* 28:554–561.

120. Pelletier JP, Martel-Pelletier J, Howell DS, et al. (1983): Collagenase and collagenolytic activity in human osteoarthritic cartilage. *Arthritis Rheum* 26:63–68.

121. Pope MH, Klingenstierna U (1986): Height changes due to autotraction. *Clin Biomech* 1:191–195.

122. Putti V (1927): New conceptions in the pathogenesis of sciatic pain. *Lancet* 2:53–60.

123. Radin EL, Ehrlich MG, Chernack R, et al. (1978): Effect of repetitive impulsive loading on the knee joints of rabbits. *Clin Orthop* 131:288–293.

124. Radin EL, Martin RB, Burr DB, Caterson B, Boyd RD, Goodwin C (1984): Effects of mechanical loading on the tissues of the rabbit knee. *J Orthop Res* 2:221–234.

125. Ratcliffe JF (1980): The arterial anatomy of the adult human lumbar vertebral body: a microarteriographic study. *J Anat* 131:57–79.

126. Rich RR, Johnson JS (1973): Salicylate hepatotoxicity in patients with juvenile rheumatoid arthritis. *Arthritis Rheum* 16:1–9.

127. Rosenberg NJ (1975): Degenerative spondylolisthesis. Predisposing factors. *J Bone Joint Surg [Am]* 57:467–474.

128. Saklatvala J (1981): Characterization of catabolin—the major product of pig synovial tissue that induces resorption of cartilage proteoglycan in vitro. *Biochem J* 199:705–714.

129. Salter RB, Field P (1960): The effects of continuous compression on living articular cartilage: an experimental investigation. *J Bone Joint Surg [Am]* 42:31–49.

130. Schonstrom N (1988): *The narrow lumbar spinal canal and the size of the cauda equina in man. A clinical and experimental study.* Göteborg, Sweden: Department of Orthopaedics, Gothenburg University, Sahlgren Hospital.

131. Schwarzer AC, Aprill CN, Derby R, Fortin J, Kine G, Bogduk N (1994): The relevant contributions of the disc and zygapophyseal joint in chronic low back pain. *Spine* 19:801–806.

132. Scott JC (1955): Stress factor in the disc syndrome. *J Bone Joint Surg [Br]* 37:107–111.

133. Scott JE, Bosworth TR, Cribb AM, Taylor JR (1994): The chemical morphology of age-related changes in human intervertebral disc glycosaminoglycans from cervical, thoracic and lumbar nucleus pulposus and annulus fibrosus. *J Anat.* 184:73–82.

134. Snyderman R, Koopman WJ, Prockop DJ (1987): Review of the National Arthritis Advisory Board Symposium, "Molecular biology: its potential for advancing rheumatology research." *Arthritis Rheum* 30:1191–1194.

135. Stilwell DL Jr (1956): The nerve supply of the vertebral column and its associated structures in the monkey. *Anat Rec* 125:139–169.

136. Stokes IA, Counts DF, Frymoyer JW (1989): Experimental instability in the rabbit lumbar spine. *Spine* 14:68–72.

137. Sullivan JD, Farfan HF, Kahn DS (1971): Pathologic changes with intervertebral joint rotational instability in the rabbit. *Can J Surg* 14:71–79.

138. Thompson RC Jr, Bassett CAL (1970): Histological observations on experimentally induced degeneration of articular cartilage. *J Bone Joint Surg [Am]* 52:435–443.

139. Trias A (1961): Effect of persistent pressure on the articular cartilage: an experimental study. *J Bone Joint Surg [Br]* 43:376–386.

140. Tsukimoto H (1960): On an autopsied case of compression myelopathy with a callus formation in the cervical spinal canal. *Nirongetahokan* 29:1003–1007.

141. Tsuyama N (1984): Ossification of the posterior longitudinal ligament of the spine. *Clin Orthop* 184:71–84.

142. Urban JPG, Holm S, Maroudas A (1978): Diffusion of small solutes into the intervertebral disc: an in vivo study. *Biorheology* 15:203–221.

143. Urban JPG, Holm S, Maroudas A, et al. (1982): Nutrition of the intervertebral disc: effect of fluid flow on solute transport. *Clin Orthop* 170:296–302.

144. Urban JPG, Maroudas A (1981): Diffusion coefficients of small solutes in the intervertebral disc. *Trans Orthop Res Soc* 6:125.

145. Van der Rest M, Mayne R (1988): Type IX collagen proteoglycan from cartilage is covalently cross-linked to type II collagen. *J Biol Chem* 263:1615–1618.

146. Vanharanta H, Floyd T, Ohnmeiss DD, Hochschuler SH, Guyer RD (1993): The relationship of facet tropism to degenerative disc disease. *Spine* 18:1000–1005.

147. Vanharanta H, Sachs BL, Spivey M, et al. (1988): A comparison of CT/discography, pain response and radiographic disc height. *Spine* 13:321–324.

148. Varlotta GP, Brown MD, Kelsey JL, Golden AL (1991): Familial predisposition for herniation of a lumbar disc in patients who are less than twenty-one years old. *J Bone Joint Surg* 73A:124–128.

149. Vernon-Roberts B (1992): Age related and degenerative pathology of intervertebral discs and apophyseal joints. In: Jayson MIV, ed. *The lumbar spine and back pain.* 4th ed. Edinburgh: Churchill Livingstone. Chapter 2:17–42.

150. Vernon-Roberts B, Pirie CJ (1973): Healing trabecular microfractures in the bodies of lumbar vertebrae. *Ann Rheum Dis* 32:406–412.

151. Videman T, Nurminen M, Troup JD (1990): Lumbar spinal pathology in cadaveric material in relation to history of back pain, occupation, and physical loading. *Spine* 15:728–740.

152. Wendland ML, Wagoner RD, Holley KE (1980): Renal failure associated with fenoprofen. *Mayo Clin Proc* 55:103–107.

153. White AA III, McBride ME, Wiltse LL, Jupiter JB (1986): The management of patients with back pain and idiopathic vertebral sclerosis. *Spine* 11:607–616.

154. White AA III, Panjabi MM (1978): *Clinical biomechanics of the spine.* Philadelphia: J. B. Lippincott, p. 3.

155. Wiesel SW, Tsourmas N, Feffer HL, et al. (1984): A study of computer-assisted tomography. I. The incidence of positive CAT scans. *Spine* 9:549–551.

156. Woo SL-Y, Buckwalter JA (1988): *Injury and repair of the musculoskeletal soft tissues.* Park Ridge, IL: American Academy of Orthopaedic Surgeons.

157. Wurster NB, Lust G (1982): Fibronectin in osteoarthritic canine articular cartilage. *Biochem Biophys Res Commun* 109:1094–1101.

158. Wurster NB, Lust G (1984): Synthesis of fibronectin in normal and osteoarthritic articular cartilage. *Biochem Biophys Acta* 800:52–58.

The Adult Spine: Principles and Practice,
2nd edition, J.W. Frymoyer, Editor-in-Chief.
Lippincott-Raven Publishers, Philadelphia © 1997.

CHAPTER **38**

Medical Management of Arthritis of the Spine

David Wright and Malcolm I.V. Jayson

Arthritis of the spine raises specific problems related to chronic pain management, immobility, and postural deformity in a patient who may also have significant peripheral joint involvement. Some patients develop radicular pain due to nerve root compression, while chronic inflammatory arthropathy may be complicated by osteoporotic vertebral collapse. Anxiety and depression are well recognized psychological consequences of chronic spinal pain that can impede rehabilitation and effective pain control, and the social and financial implications need also to be addressed. It is clear therefore that patients with arthritis involving the spine have multiple needs, and a detailed assessment of their functional impairment, disability and subsequent handicap is required. A multidisciplinary approach involving the physiotherapist, occupational therapist, social worker and other health professionals is essential.

The objectives of medical management are to treat symptoms such as pain and stiffness in order to maximize the spine's function and maintain normal posture. Pharmacotherapy has important roles both for symptomatic treatment and possibly for prevention of further joint damage (Table 1). At the same time, many of the commonly prescribed drugs have significant toxic effects, which require careful monitoring and remedial treatment in some cases. This chapter is concerned with the application of drug treatment for arthritis with specific reference to the spine. Other treatment modalities including local treatments, braces and appliances are dealt with elsewhere in this text.

PURE ANALGESICS

Pure analgesics have a central mechanism of action and virtually no peripheral anti-inflammatory activity (1). They are unlikely to provide effective symptom control in inflammatory arthritis when used alone, but may be complementary to nonsteroidal anti-inflammatory drugs (NSAIDs) when used intermittently or regularly. In osteoarthritis and other noninflammatory conditions, paracetamol (acetaminophen) may be as effective as NSAIDs and is unlikely to cause peptic ulceration or renal impairment. Simple analgesics may be preferred in elderly patients owing to lower risk of toxicity (2). Paracetamol is effective in doses of 500–1,000 mg given 4 to 6 hourly. It does, however, have a shallow dose response curve, and doses above 4,000 mg per day may cause hepatic damage (3). To achieve a greater analgesic effect, paracetamol may be given in combination with a weak opioid, for example, codeine or dextrapropoxyphene.

The use of morphine and other strong opioids in this context is controversial (4,5). Long-term use should be avoided wherever possible, although a few carefully selected patients with unremitting pain due to "burnt out" disease may benefit from a slow-release morphine formulation (6). Opiate-induced dependence, tolerance, and respiratory depression have probably been over-

D. Wright: M.B., Ch.B., B.Med. Sci., M.D., M.R.C.P.: Hunters Moor Rehabilitation Centre, Newcastle Upon Tyne, United Kingdom.
M. I. V. Jayson, M.D.: Professor of Rheumatology, University of Manchester, Hope Hospital, Salford M6 8HD, England.

TABLE 1. *Medical management of arthritis of the spine*

Symptomatic relief
  Simple analgesics
  Nonsteroidal anti-inflammatory drugs
  Psychotropics
  Anticonvulsants
  Muscle relaxants
Disease suppression
  Sulfasalazine
  Methotrexate
  Gold
  Azathioprine
  Antimalarials
  Penicillamine
  Corticosteroids
Disease complications
  Osteoporosis—estrogens, calcitonin, diphosphonates
  Vasculitis—cyclophosphamide, corticosteroids
  Anemia—iron, folic acid, erythropoietin
  Peptic ulceration—H2 blockers, misoprostol, omeprazole
  Depression—psychotropics

stated in patients with chronic nonmalignant pain (7,8). In acute back pain, opiates may be used for a limited term in order to promote mobilization after an initial short period of bed rest (9).

NONSTEROIDAL ANTI-INFLAMMATORY DRUGS (NSAIDS) (TABLES 2 AND 3)

NSAIDs are potent inhibitors of the inflammatory response due to inhibition of peripheral cyclooxygenase and prostaglandin synthesis, inhibition of neutrophil activation and aggregation, and inhibition of phospholipase C in mononuclear cells (10,11). They may also have central analgesic properties (12). They are of great importance in the management of ankylosing spondylitis (AS) and other inflammatory conditions affecting the spine but do not influence disease progression (13). Over 50 NSAIDs are available worldwide, but most patients can be effectively treated using a relatively small number of different drugs (14). The efficacy of the majority of NSAIDs appears to be similar to aspirin (15), but there are important differences in toxicity. Despite the introduction of newer agents, for example, nabumetone and etodolac, all NSAIDs cause adverse effects to a greater or lesser extent. They may be divided into groups with serum half-life less than 6 hours (for example ibuprofen, indomethacin, and diclofenac) or greater than 12 hours (piroxicam, naproxen, and nabumetone), but otherwise they share similar pharmacokinetics. Important interactions with warfarin, probenecid, lithium, and antihypertensive drugs are well recognized.

Gastrointestinal mucosal damage is the most commonly reported adverse effect, caused by interference with prostaglandin-mediated mucus production, mucosal blood flow, and bicarbonate production. A small number of deaths occur each year due to acute upper GI hemorrhage, but iron deficiency anemia is a more frequent presentation (16,17). Some NSAIDs are clearly more harmful to the gut than others, with ibuprofen

TABLE 2. *Dosage data and cost of NSAIDs available in 1994*

Generic name	Proprietary name	Largest unit dose (mg)	Half-life (hr)	Dosing frequency[a]	Monthly cost[b]
Aspirin	—	325	0.25	2 q4h	NA/$10
Diclofenac	Voltaren	75	2	bid	$84/NA
Diflunisal	Dolobid	500	10	bid	$90/$81
Etodolac	Lodine	300	6	qid	$134/NA
Fenoprofen	Nalfon	600	2–3	qid	$129/$67
Flurbiprofen	Ansaid	100	6	tid	$111/NA
Ibuprofen	Motrin	800	2	qid	$55/$29
Indomethacin	Indocin	50	4	tid	$101/$32
Ketoprofen	Orudis	75	3	tid	$118/$118
Ketorolac	Toradol	10	5	qid	$178/NA
Meclofenamate	Meclomen	100	2	tid	$126/$25
Nabumetone	Relafen	500	20–30	2 qd	$75/NA
Naproxen	Naprosyn	500	14	bid	$94/NA
Oxaprozin	Daypro	600	40–50	2 qd	$94/NA
Piroxicam	Feldene	20	30–86	qd	$96/$86
Salicylsalicylic acid	Disalcid	750	1	qid	$22/$22
Sodium salicylate	—	650	0.5	q4h	NA/$13
Sulindac	Clinoril	200	8–14	bid	$71/$71
Tolmetin	Tolectin	400	1–2	tid	$115/$88

[a] Dosage required for treatment of inflammation. Abbreviations: bid = twice a day; qd = each day; q4h = every 4 hours; qid = four times a day; tid = three times a day.

[b] Average wholesale price plus 40% pharmacy markup, expressed as price for proprietary drug/price for generic drug. (In some instances, the prices are the same because of the pricing strategies of the drug manufacturers.) NA = not applicable (because there is either no generic form or no proprietary form of the drug).

Reproduced with permission of: Nonsteroidal anti-inflammatory drugs. *J Am Acad Orthop Surg,* 256.

TABLE 3. *Adverse effects of nonsteroidal antiinflammatory drugs*

Organ system	Adverse effect	Association
Gastrointestinal (common)	Peptic ulceration	All NSAIDs, azapropazone, piroxicam and indomethacin highest risk
	Perforation	
	GI hemorrhage	
	Diarrhea	Indomethacin, diclofenac
	Small and large bowel ulceration	
Hepatic (rare)	Hepatitis	Azapropazone, diclofenac
	Cholestasis	
Renal (common)	Impaired renal perfusion	All NSAIDs
	Renal failure	Azapropazone, indomethacin,
	Interstitial nephritis	Fenoprofen
	Cystitis	Tiaprofenic acid
Hematogical (rare)	Thrombocytopenia	Phenylbutazone, indomethacin
	Neutropenia	Phenylbutazone, indomethacin
	Aplastic anemia	Phenylbutazone, indomethacin
	Hemolytic anemia	Mefenamic acid
Cutaneous (uncommon)	Photosensitivity	
	Erythema multiforme	Fenbufen
	Stevens-Johnson syndrome	
	Allergic skin rash	Azapropazone
Respiratory (rare)	Bronchospasm	All NSAIDs
CNS (uncommon)	Headache	Indomethacin, diclofenac
	Dizziness, drowsiness	
	Depression	
	Aseptic meningitis	
Cartilage (unknown)	Cartilage destruction?	Many NSAIDs

probably least toxic and azapropazone and piroxicam most toxic (18). Prophylactic ulcer-healing drugs should be considered in patients who require an NSAID and have other risk factors including previous peptic ulceration, age over 60 years, cigarette smoking, and concurrent use of anticoagulants or steroids (19). Ranitidine, an H2 receptor antagonist that suppresses gastric acid secretion, reduces gastric microbleeding induced by aspirin and prevents NSAID-associated duodenal ulceration (20). The synthetic prostaglandin analogue misoprostol is superior to ranitidine for prevention of NSAID-induced gastric ulceration, perhaps through its cytoprotective action (21). Little information is available about prophylactic use of acid pump blockers, though omeprazole is superior to ranitidine for gastric ulcer healing even when NSAID use is continued (22).

Other adverse effects of NSAIDs include renal impairment, hepatitis, blood dyscrasias, skin rashes, and CNS disturbance (23). All NSAIDs impair renal blood flow because of prostaglandin inhibition and may decrease renal function, whereas interstitial nephritis is probably idiosyncratic. Careful monitoring of renal function is important in the elderly, in patients with existing renal impairment, and in those receiving diuretic treatment (24). Sulindac is administered as a prodrug and appears to be less nephrotoxic (25).

The long-term effect of NSAIDs on articular cartilage is controversial, and recent experimental data suggests that indomethacin may accelerate progression of osteoarthritis, while there is a suggestion that tiaprofenic acid, diclofenac, and piroxicam are chondroprotective (26).

The variability of the patient's response to NSAIDs is well recognized (14), and several agents may be tried sequentially if no response occurs within 3 to 4 weeks of treatment. There is no advantage in using more than one NSAID at any time. Enteric coated oral preparations in once or twice daily dosage are preferable, though suppositories may produce less gastric irritation. Time of administration should coincide with the diurnal pattern of symptoms (23). Relatively few well-controlled studies have compared different NSAIDs in the rheumatic diseases, and choice of drug is often determined by prescriber and patient preference. Generally, the least toxic drug should be given at the lowest effective dose. Indomethacin (50 mg three times daily) may be the first choice for ankylosing spondylitis, being more effective than aspirin, though up to 50% of patients may develop adverse effects and 20% discontinue treatment (13,27). Phenylbutazone is unsuitable for long-term use owing to serious blood dyscrasias, but short courses may be given under careful medical supervision for severe ankylosing spondylitis (28). Ibuprofen (1,600–2,400 mg/day) produces fewer adverse reactions than indomethacin but has more modest anti-inflammatory activity. Naproxen and diclofenac are effective and well tolerated with a relatively low incidence of adverse effects.

PSYCHOTROPIC DRUGS

A substantial minority of patients with arthritis are clinically depressed, and in clinical trials both chronic pain and depression respond favorably to tricyclic anti-depressants (TCADs) (29). Agents with serotonergic and noradrenergic effects appear to have a separate analgesic effect, while controlled trials of selective serotonergic drugs show no significant difference between drug and placebo (30,31). Amitriptyline, imipramine, and dothiepin are effective analgesics for rheumatoid arthritis (RA), fibromyalgia, and chronic low back pain (32–34). In fibromyalgia, restoration of normal sleeping pattern is an important effect of sedative TCADs.

Amitriptyline 25 mg at night is a suitable initial treatment that may be slowly increased at weekly intervals. The onset of action in chronic pain states is more rapid than the usual antidepressant effect (3–7 days compared to 14–21 days), and a prolonged analgesic effect may occur (35). Maintenance treatment for several months or years may be possible, though some patients are intolerant of adverse effects, including drowsiness, dry mouth, postural hypotension, and urinary retention. In patients with cardiac conduction defects, TCADs are probably contraindicated (36). TCADs are also used for neuropathic pain and deafferentation syndromes which may follow spinal nerve root entrapment, having proven benefit in trigeminal and post-herpetic neuralgia.

ANTICONVULSANTS

Carbamazepine, phenytoin, or sodium valproate may be given for chronic radicular pain, particularly if the patient reports sharp shooting or electric shock–like components (dysesthesia). In resistant cases, a combination of a tricyclic antidepressent and an anticonvulsant may be tried, though some patients are unresponsive to all conservative measures. Monitoring of serum drug levels and periodic blood counts is advisable.

MUSCLE RELAXANTS

Muscle relaxants are sometimes given for acute low back pain when there is thought to be a major element of muscle spasms. However, muscle spasm cannot be reliably detected by clinical means, and it remains unclear whether increased muscle tone contributes to pain severity (37). Baclofen, chlormezanone, and diazepam act centrally, and in conventional doses frequently produce sedation as well as modest muscle relaxation. Baclofen (5mg three times daily) may be superior to placebo for severe back pain and may shorten the recovery period of acute episodes (38). Diazepam and other benzodiazepines may also help relaxation in the short term, but dependence is common among chronic back pain sufferers

and treatment should be restricted to a fixed time schedule.

SECOND LINE ANTIRHEUMATIC DRUGS (TABLE 4)

In rheumatoid arthritis, slow-acting antirheumatic drugs (SAARDs) such as gold, penicillamine, and sulfasalazine are given to prevent or restrict destruction of articular cartilage and adjacent bone, although there is little evidence to show that this effect is sustained for longer than 2 years. They have little direct anti-inflammatory effect and a therapeutic response may occur up to 3 months after starting treatment. A number of agents have proved to be beneficial in clinical trials, but no single drug is clearly superior. Methotrexate, injectable gold, D penicillamine, and sulfasalazine have similar efficacy, being significantly more effective than chloroquine and auranofin (39). Several were introduced by serendipity and their precise mode of action remains unclear. Long-term treatment requires careful monitoring and may be associated with severe adverse reactions necessitating withdrawal of the drug. There is no consensus about when SAARDs are introduced, though most clinicians would treat aggressively those patients whose symptoms are poorly controlled by NSAIDs alone in order to prevent joint damage. SAARDs are not routinely used for ankylosing spondylitis involving the spine, because the majority of patients have a good prognosis with an appropriate exercise program. The few with severe relentless disease would require effective disease modification, but drugs tested to date appear to have only marginal benefit for spinal involvement.

Sulfasalazine (SAS)

SAS is an established disease-suppressing agent in rheumatoid arthritis (RA) that was originally introduced in the 1930s as a combined analgesic and antimicrobial (40). There may be a link between the proposed enteropathic etiology of RA, and the antibacterial action of SAS. The drug is largely split into its constituents (5-aminosalicylic acid and sulfapyridine) in the colon by bacterial action. Sulfapyridine is well absorbed whereas intestinal absorption of 5-aminosalicylic acid is poor. Both constituents appear to be necessary for its disease-modifying effect though many adverse effects are sulfapyridine-related. Erosive changes may be suppressed though this has not yet been confirmed by long-term studies (41,42). In a meta-analysis, SAS was shown to produce modest improvement in ankylosing spondylitis (43), though other studies have failed to show any significant improvement in spinal involvement compared to placebo (44). In clinical practice, the drug is often reserved for peripheral arthritis in AS (45), and the

TABLE 4. *Slow acting antrheumatic drugs—monitoring and adverse effects*

Drug	Adverse effect	Management
Methotrexate	GI intolerance	Try lower dose, folate supplements
	Hepatic toxicity	Withdraw if ALT > twice normal
	Skin rash	Withdraw
	Pneumonitis	Withdraw
	Marrow suppression	Withdraw
Sulfasalazine	GI intolerance	May force withdrawal
	Oligospermia	Counseling
	Neutropenia	Withdraw, try lower dose
	Skin rash	Withdrawal in 50%
	Hepatitis	Withdraw if ALT > twice normal
Cold (sodium aurothiomalate)	Mouth ulcers, rash	Try lower dose? Withdraw
	Exfoliative dermatitis	Withdraw
	Proteinuria	Withdraw if >1 g/24 hours
	Thrombocytopenia	Withdraw, occasional steroids
	Neutropenia	Withdraw, use steroids
	Pneumonitis	Withdraw
	Hypogammaglobulinemia	Withdraw
Azathioprine	GI intolerance	Often forces withdrawal
	Neutropenia	Withdraw if WCC < 2.5, try lower dose
	Thrombocytopenia	Withdraw if plates < 80, try lower dose
	Marrow aplasia	Withdraw
	Hepatic toxicity	Withdraw
	Malignancy	Counseling
D-penicillamine	GI intolerance, taste distortion, mouth ulcers	Try lower dose, may force withdrawal
	Proteinuria > 0.5 g/day	Withdrawal preferable
	Glomerulonephritis	Withdraw, immunosuppression
	Blood dyscrasias	Withdraw
	Marrow asplasia	Withdrawal essential
	Pemphigus	Withdraw
	Autoimmune diseases	Withdraw, immunosuppression
Hydroxychloroquine	Retinopathy	Withdrawal essential
	GI intolerance	May force withdrawal
	Skin rash	
	Thrombocytopenia	

ALT, alanine aminotransferase; WCC, white blood cell count.

modest benefits need to be weighed against possible adverse effects and the need for regular monitoring. It can also be beneficial in psoriatic arthritis (46), but its efficacy in reactive arthritis is unproven.

SAS is given orally in enteric coated tablets, starting with 0.5 g daily and increasing to 1 g twice a day maintenance dose. Adverse effects, including nausea, abdominal pains, and dizziness, occur in up to 50% of patients and 70% of males develop reversible azoospermia (47). Two-thirds of adverse effects occur within 3 months of starting treatment, therefore clinical monitoring, blood counts, and liver biochemistry are required at fortnightly intervals during this period, followed by three monthly during maintenance treatment (48). Idiosyncratic reactions include thrombocytopenia and neutropenia, which are usually reversible, and serious bone marrow toxicity and pneumonitis, which are rare. Some patients develop biochemical features of hepatitis, though clinically significant liver disease is rare.

Methotrexate (MTX)

MTX has become a widely accepted treatment for RA because of its quicker onset of action compared to other SAARDs, and relatively low toxicity (49). It is a folate antagonist with anti-inflammatory and possible immunosuppressant actions though these may not explain it efficacy when used in low doses for RA (50). Its effects on joint inflammation are superior to auranofin and comparable to myocrisin, and onset occurs within 12 weeks in 80% of patients (51–53). The appearance of radiographic erosions may be delayed though further studies are needed (54,55). Long-term adverse effects are unknown and it remains unclear whether MTX should be used as early or later for RA. MTX is also used for psoriatic arthritis, although larger doses are required to control skin lesions (56). There are isolated reports of its use in AS (57).

For RA, weekly doses of 5–7.5 mg are often very

effective, although higher intravenous doses may improve resistant disease (58). Sulfamides and other folic acid antagonists should be avoided during treatment, and an interaction with NSAIDs is also recognized. Minor adverse effects including nausea and reversible changes in liver biochemistry are relatively common, particularly in patients with renal impairment, but are not an indication to stop treatment (39,59). Some evidence suggests that routine use of folic acid supplements improves gastrointestinal tolerance and does not diminish efficacy (60,61). Irreversible liver damage and pneumonitis occur rarely, but pretreatment chest x-ray and regular monitoring of liver biochemistry are mandatory. MTX may also cause severe septic complications and should be withdrawn before arthroplastic surgery.

OTHER SECOND LINE DRUGS

Sodium aurothiomalate has proven disease-modifying effect in RA (62) but no value in AS (63), and it is not routinely used for psoriatic arthritis owing to a very slow onset of action (64). Its long-term use is often restricted by a high incidence of adverse reactions which include skin rash, mouth ulceration, proteinuria and glomerulonephritis, marrow depression, and pneumonitis (58,59, 65). Auranofin is an oral formulation with weaker activity. Serious adverse reactions are unusual but up to 50% develop gastrointestinal intolerance (66).

Azathioprine is often reserved for patients with active disease who have failed to respond to other second line agents; it may also be a useful steroid-sparing drug. In doses of 1.5–2.5 mg/kg it is an effective disease-suppressing agent (67). Monthly blood counts and liver function testing are essential and long-term treatment is associated with a small increase in risk for lymphoma (68).

The antimalarial drugs chloroquine and hydroxychloroquine have mild disease-modifying effects in RA and systemic lupus erythematosus (SLE) but are not effective for AS. Ocular complications are rare when hydroxychloroquine is given in doses up to 200 mg daily, but annual ophthalmology checks for retinopathy and maculopathy are required (58). There is some evidence that they may be useful in combination with other second line agents (69). D Penicillamine is an effective agent for both RA and psoriatic arthritis but has no effect in AS. Its use is limited by a high incidence of adverse effects, and it is contraindicated in pregnancy due to teratogenicity (70). Cyclosporin A is effective for RA, possibly because of inhibition of interleukin-1 and interleukin-2, but invariably causes some reduction in renal function and a rise in blood pressure (71).

CORTICOSTEROIDS

Systemic corticosteroids produce dramatic relief of symptoms in inflammatory arthritis, but long-term use will inevitably lead to serious dose-related adverse effects in many patients. A rebound worsening of symptoms frequently follows withdrawal of steroids, so patients with RA may quickly become steroid-dependent (72). For these reasons, the use of long-term steroids should be restricted to patients who have vital organ involvement or who have proved resistant to other forms of treatment. Systemic corticosteroids are virtually contraindicated in AS, being of no proven value and likely to cause osteoporosis (73). Long-term steroids are indicted for systemic connective tissue diseases, vasculitides, and polymyalgia rheumatica.

Maintenance doses of prednisolone should always be kept as low as possible to minimize side effects, but steroid-induced osteoporosis may occur within 1 year even when doses below 10 mg daily are used (74,75). Prophylactic use of cyclical etidronate and calcium supplements or estrogen replacement in menopausal women may help to reduce bone loss in steroid-treated patients, although an effect on fractures has not yet been established (76). Deflazacort is said to have calcium-sparing qualities compared to prednisolone but is not widely available (77). Pulsed treatment with high-dose intravenous methylprednisolone (1 g) is often used to produce remission while slower acting agents take effect, but it is unclear whether long-term adverse effects are avoided (78). Intra-articular injection of long acting steroids (e.g., triamcinolone) is effective and remains a valuable treatment despite some concern about the late development of septic arthritis in the injected joint (79).

CONCLUSIONS

The causes and pathogenesis of the various forms of arthritis that affect the spine are unclear, and in the majority of cases curative treatment will not be possible. Therefore, all effective methods of ameliorating pain and disability should be pursued in each patient using a multidisciplinary approach. In AS and osteoarthritis few drugs seem to alter disease progression in the spine, and the role of medication is to ease symptoms to enable an effective exercise program. In the management of RA, the objective of drug treatment is to produce maximum suppression of synovitis without serious adverse effects. In all patients, the association of psychological distress and symptom perception should be recognized.

Patients who are likely to develop destructive arthritis of the spine may need to be treated aggressively at an early stage, but the long-term efficacy of existing disease-modifying agents is questionable. Over the coming years, several new antirheumatic treatments may emerge including monoclonal antibodies, cytokines, and cytokine inhibitors (80). Recently, encouraging short-term results were obtained in patients with RA using anti–tumor necrosis factor (81). Only long-term comparative trials using adequate numbers of patients will be able to define the true values of these newer agents.

REFERENCES

1. Flower RJ, Moncada S, Vane JR (1985): Analgesic-antipyretics and the anti-inflammatory agents: drugs employed in the treatment of gout. In: Gilman AG, et al, eds: *The pharmacological basis of therapeutics,* 7th ed. New York: Macmillan, pp 674–715.
2. McAlindon T, Dieppe P (1990): The medical management of osteoarthritis of the knee; An inflammatory issue? *Br J Rheumatol* 29:471–473.
3. Laska EM, Sunshine A, Meuller F, et al (1984): Caffeine as an analgesic adjuvant. *JAMA* 251:1771–1718.
4. Coniam SW (1989): Prescribing opioids for non malignant disease. In: Twycross RG, ed: *The Edinburgh symposium on pain control and medical education.* London: Royal Society of Medical Services, pp 205–210.
5. Brena SF, Sanders SH (1991): Opioids in non malignant pain: questions in search of answers. *Clin J Pain* 7:342–345.
6. Portenoy RK (1990): Chronic opioid therapy in chronic non malignant pain. *J Pain Symptom Management* 5(Suppl):S46–S62.
7. Portenoy RK, Foley KM (1986): Chronic use of opioid analgesics in non malignant pain: a report of 38 cases. *Pain* 25:171–186.
8. Taub A (1982): Opioid analgesics in the treatment of chronic intractable pain of non neoplastic origin. In: Kitahata LM, Collins JD, eds: *Narcotic analgesics in anaesthesiology.* Baltimore: Williams and Wilkins, pp 199–208.
9. Deyo RA, Diehl AK, Rosenthal M (1986): How many days of bed rest for acute low back pain? A randomised clinical trial. *N Engl J Med* 315:1064–1070.
10. Erickson N, Furst DE (1988): Mechanisms of action of NSAID. *Ther Drug Monit* 9:9–18.
11. Forest MJ, Brooks PM (1988): Mechanism of action of non steroidal anti-inflammatory drugs. *Baillieres Clin Rheumatol* 2:275–294.
12. Urqhart E (1993): Central analgesic activity of non steroidal anti-inflammatory drugs in animal and human pain models. *Semin Arthritis Rheum* 23(3):198–205.
13. Godfrey RG, Calabro JJ, Mills D, Maltz BA (1972): A double blind crossover trial of aspirin, indomethacin and phenylbutazone in ankylosing spondylitis (abstract). *Arthritis Rheum* 15:110.
14. Pincus T, Callaghan LF (1989): Clinical use of multiple non steroidal anti-inflammatory drug preparations within individual rheumatology private practices. *J Rheumatol* 16:1253–1258.
15. Heller LA, Ingelfinger JA, Goldman P (1985): Non steroidal anti-inflammatory drugs and aspirin: analyzing the scores. *Pharmacotherapy* 5:30–38.
16. Gabriel SE, Jakimainen L, Bombardier C (1991): Risk of serious gastrointestinal complications related to the use of NSAID's: a meta analysis. *Ann Intern Med* 114:257–263.
17. Langman MJS (1989): Epidemiologic evidence of the association between peptic ulceration and anti-inflammatory drug use. *Gastroenterology* 96 (Suppl 2) 640–646.
18. Garcia Rodriguez LA, Jick H (1994): Risk of upper gastrointestinal bleeding and perforation associated with individual non steroidal anti-inflammatory drugs. *Lancet* 343:769–772.
19. Fries JF, Williams CA, Bloch DA, Michel BA (1991): NSAID associated gastropathy: incidence and risk factor models. *Am J Med* 91:213–221.
20. Robinson MG, Griffin JW, Bowes J, et al (1989): Effect of ranitidine on gastroduodenal mucosal damage induced by NSAIDs. *Dig Dis Sci* 34:424–428.
21. Raskin J, White R, Jasewski R (1991): Double blind comparative study of the efficacy and safety of misoprostol and ranitidine in the prevention of NSAID induced gastric ulcers and upper GI symptoms: preliminary findings. *Digestion* 49 (Suppl 1): 50–51.
22. Walan A, Bader JP, Classen M, et al (1989): Effect of omeprazole and ranitidine on ulcer healing and relapse rates in patients with benign gastric ulcer. *N Engl J Med* 320:69–75.
23. Furst DE (1994): Are there differences among non steroidal anti inflammatory drugs? *Arthritis Rheum* 37:1–9.
24. Brookes PM, Day RO (1991): Non steroidal anti-inflammatory drugs: differences and similarities. *N Engl J Med* 324:1716–1725.
25. Ciabattoni G, Anotti GA, Pierucci A, et al (1984): Effects of sulindac and ibuprofen in patients with chronic glomerular disease. *N Engl J Med* 310:279–283.
26. Rashad S, Revell P, Hemingway A, et al (1989): Effect of non steroidal anti-inflammatory drugs on the course of osteoarthritis. *Lancet* ii:519–522.
27. Sunshine A, Olsen NZ (1993): Nonnarcotic analgesics. In *Textbook of Pain,* pp 923–942.
28. International Agranulocytosis and Aplastic Anaemia Study Group (1986): *JAMA* 256:1749–1757.
29. Puttini PS, Cazzola M, Boccasini L, et al (1988): A comparison of dothiepin versus placebo in the treatment of pain of rheumatoid arthritis and the association of pain with depression. *J Int Med Res* 16:331–337.
30. Frank RG, Kashani JH, Parker JC, et al (1988): Antidepressant analgesia in rheumatoid arthritis. *J Rheumatol* 15:1632–1638.
31. Onghena P, Van Haudenhove B (1992): Antidepressant induced analgesia in chronic non malignant pain: a meta analysis of 39 placebo controlled studies. *Pain* 49:205–219.
32. Goldenberg DL, Felson DT, Dinerman H (1986): A randomised controlled trial of amitriptyline and naproxen in the treatment of patients with fibromyalgia. *Arthritis Rheum* 29:1371–1377.
33. Caruso I, Sarzi Puttini PC, Boccassini L, et al. (1987): Double blind study of dothiepin versus placebo in the treatment of primary fibromyalgia syndrome. *J Int Med Res* 15:154–159.
34. Alcoff J, Jones E, Rust P, Newman R (1982): Controlled trial of imipramine for chronic low back pain. *J Fam Pract* 14:841–846.
35. Hameroff SR, Weiss JL, Lerman JC, et al (1984): Doxepin effects on chronic pain and depression: a controlled study. *J Clin Psychiatry* 45:45–52.
36. Glassman AH, Bigger JT (1981): Cardiovascular effects of therapeutic doses of tricyclic antidepressants. *Arch Gen Psychiatry* 36: 815–819.
37. Waddell G, Main CJ, Morris EW, et al (1982): Normality and reliability in the clinical assessment of backache. *Br Med J* 284:1519–1523.
38. Dapas F, Hartman SF, Martinez L, et al (1985): Baclofen for the treatment of acute low back pain syndrome: a double blind comparison with placebo. *Spine* 10:345–349.
39. Felson DT, Anderson JJ, Meenan RF (1990): The comparative efficacy and toxicity of second line drugs in rheumatoid arthritis: results of two meta analyses. *Arthritis Rheum* 33:1449–1461.
40. Svartz N (1942): Salazopyrin, a new sulfanilinamide preparation. *Acta Med Scand* 110:577–598.
41. Porter DR, Capell HA (1990): The use of sulphasalazine as a disease modifying antirheumatic drug. *Baillieres Clin Rheumatol* 4: 535–551.
42. Van der Heijde DM, van Riel PL, Nuver-Zwart IH, et al (1989): Effects of hydroxychloroquine and sulphasalazine on progression of joint damage in rheumatoid arthritis. *Lancet* i: 1036–1038.
43. Ferraz MB, Tugwell P, Goldsmith CH, Atra E (1990): Meta analysis of sulphasalazine in ankylosing spondylitis. *J Rheumatol* 17: 1482–1486.
44. Corkhill MM, Jobanputra J, Gibson T, MacFarlane DG (1990): A controlled trial of sulphasalazine treatment of chronic ankylosing spondylitis: failure to demonstrate a clinical effect. *Br J Rheumatol* 29:41–45.
45. Fraser SM, Sturrock RD (1990): Evaluation of sulphasalazine in ankylosing spondylitis—an interventional study. *Br J Rheumatol* 29:37–39.
46. Farr M, Kittas GD, Waterhouse L, et al (1990): Sulphasalazine in psoriatic arthritis: a double blind placebo controlled study. *Br J Rheumatol* 29:46–49.
47. Birnie G, McLeod T, Watkinson G (1981): Incidence of sulphasalazine induced male infertility. *Gut* 22:452–455.
48. Keisu M, Ekman E (1992): Sulfasalazine associated agranulocytosis in Sweden 1972–1989: clinical features, and estimation of its incidence. *Eur J Clin Pharmacol* 43:215–218.
49. Songiridej N, Furst DE (1990): Methotrexate—the rapidly acting drug. In *Slow acting antirheumatic drugs and immunosuppressives. Baillieres Clin Rheumatol* 4(3):575–593.
50. Denman AM, Brookes PM (1993): Antirheumatic therapy. In *Oxford Testbook of Rheumatology,* pp 329–349.
51. Fehlauer CS, et al (1989): Methotrexate therapy in rheumatoid arthritis: 2 years retrospective follow up study. *J Rheumatol* 16:307–312.
52. Morassut P, Goldstein R, Cyr M, et al (1989): Gold sodium thiomalate compared to low dose methotrexate in the treatment of

rheumatoid arthritis—a randomised, double blind 26 week trial. *J Rheumatol* 16:302–306.

53. Weinblatt ME, et al (1990): Low dose methotrexate compared with auranofin in adult rheumatoid arthritis: a 36 week, double blind trial. *Arthritis Rheum* 33:330—338.

54. Jeurissen MEC, Boerbooms AMTh, van der Putte LB, et al (1991): Influence of methotrexate and azathioprine on radiological progression in rheumatoid arthritis. *Ann Intern Med* 114:999–1004.

55. Sang J, Kaliski S, Couret M, Cuchacovich M, Daures JP (1990): Radiological progression during intramuscular methotrexate treatment of rheumatoid arthritis. *J Rheumatol* 17:1636–1641.

56. Black RL, O'Brien WM, Van Scott EJ, et al (1964): Methotaxate therapy in psoriatic arthritis. Double blind study on 21 patients. *JAMA* 189:743–747.

57. Handler RP (1989): Favourable results using methotrexate in the treatment of patients with ankylosing spondylitis (letter). *Arthritis Rheum* 32:234.

58. Gabriel S, Creagan E, O'Fallon WM, et al (1990): Treatment of rheumatoid arthritis with higher dose intravenous methotrexate. *J Rheumatol* 17:460–465.

59. Wolfe F, Hawley DG, Cathey MA (1990): Termination of slow acting antirheumatic therapy in rheumatoid arthritis: a 14 year prospective evaluation of 1017 consecutive starts. *J Rheumatol* 17:994–1002.

60. Morgan SL, et al (1990): The effect of folic acid supplementation on the toxicity of low dose methotrexate in patients with rheumatoid arthritis. *Arthritis Rheum* 33:9–18.

61. Buckley LM, Vacek PM, Cooper SM (1990): Administration of folinic acid after low dose methotrexate in patients with rheumatoid arthritis. *J Rheumatol* 17:1158–1161.

62. Epstein WV, Henke CJ, Yelin EH, Katz PP. (1991): Effects of parenterally administered gold therapy on the course of adult rheumatoid arthritis. *Ann Intern Med* 114:437–444.

63. Calabro JT (1986): Ankylosing spondylitis: a critical review of current management. *Adv Therapy* 3:20.

64. Dowart BB, Gall EP, Schumacher HR, Krauser RE. 1978 Chrysotherapy in psoriatic arthritis: efficacy and toxicity compared to rheumatoid arthritis. *Arthritis Rheum* 21:513–515.

65. Singh G, Fries JF, Williams CA, et al (1991): Toxicity profiles of disease modifying antirheumatic drugs in rheumatoid arthritis. *J Rheumatol* 18:188–194.

66. Williams HJ, et al (1988): One year experience in patients treated with auranofin following completion of parallel controlled trial comparing auranofin, gold sodium auromalate, and placebo. *Arthritis Rheum* 31:9–14.

67. Lugmani RA, Palmer RG, Bacon PA (1990): Azathioprine, cyclophosphamide and chlorambucil. *Baillieres Clin Rheumatol* 4:595–619.

68. Silman AJ, Petrie J, Hazelman B, Evans SJ (1988): Lymphoproliferative cancer and other malignancy in patients with rheumatoid arthritis treated with azathioprine: a 20 year follow up study. *Ann Rheum Dis* 47:988–992.

69. Scott DL, et al (1989): Combination therapy with gold and hydroxychloroquine in rheumatoid arthritis: a prospective placebo controlled study. British *J Rheumatol* 28:128–133.

70. Joyce DA (1990): D-Penicillamine. In *Slow acting antirheumatic drugs and immunosuppressives* (ed PM Brooks). *Baillieres Clin Rheumatol* 4(3):553–574. London: Bailliere Tindall.

71. Brookes PM. (1992): Current issues of methotrexate and cyclosporin. *Curr Opin Rheumatol* 4:309–313.

72. George E, Kirwan JR (1990): Corticosteroid therapy in rheumatoid arthritis. In: Brooks PM, ed. *Slow acting antirheumatic drugs and immunosuppressives. Baillieres Clin Rheumatol* 4(3): 621–647, London: Bailliere Tindall.

73. Wordsworth BP, Pearcy MJ, Mowat AG (1984): Inpatient regime for the treatment of ankylosing spondylitis: an appraisal of improvement in spinal mobility and the effects of corticotrophin. *Br J Rheumatol* 23:39–43.

74. Lubert BP, Raisz LG (1990): Glucocorticoid induced osteoporosis: pathogenesis and management. *Ann Intern Med* 112:352–364.

75. Loan RFJM, Van Riel PLCM, Van Erning LJ, et al. (1992): Vertebral osteoporosis in rheumatoid arthritis patients: effect of low dose prednisolone therapy. *Br J Rheumatol* 31:91–96.

76. Mulder H, Struys A. (1994): Intermittent cyclical etidronate in the prevention of corticosteroid induced bone loss. *Br J Rheumatol* 33:348–350.

77. Gray RE, Foherty SM, Galloway J, et al (1991): A double blind study of deflazacort and prednisolone in patients with chronic inflammatory disorders. *Arthritis Rheum* 34:466–476.

78. Smith MD, Ahern MJ, Roberts Thomson PJ (1990): Pulsed methyl prednisolone therapy in rheumatoid arthritis, unproved therapy, unjustified therapy or effective adjuvant treatment? *Ann Rheum Dis* 49:265–267.

79. Ostensson A, Geborek P (1991): Septic arthritis as a non surgical complication in rheumatoid arthritis: relation to disease severity and therapy. *Br J Rheumatol* 30:35–38.

80. Dayer JM, Fenner H (1992): The role of cytokines and their inhibitors in arthritis. *Baillieres Clin Rheumatol* 6:485–516.

81. Elliot MJ, Maini RN, Feldman M, et al (1993): Treatment of rheumatoid arthritis with chimeric monoclonal antibodies to tumor necrosis factor alpha. *Arthritis Rheum* 36:1681–1690.

The Adult Spine: Principles and Practice,
2nd edition, J.W. Frymoyer, Editor-in-Chief.
Lippincott-Raven Publishers, Philadelphia © 1997.

CHAPTER **39**

Spinal Stenosis: Development of the Lesion, Clinical Classification, and Presentation

J. Desmond O'Duffy

HISTORICAL BACKGROUND

In 1893 W. A. Lane (33) of Guy's Hospital, London, described the symptoms of lumbar stenosis and its surgical treatment. His patient had a well-defined cauda equina syndrome and complained of difficult gait and "weakness of her back and insecurity of her legs." Lane was able to diagnose coexistent spondylolisthesis intraoperatively, even excluding spondylolysis, without the use of x-ray.

"From the great density of the spinous process and lamina I concluded at once that there was no carious focus in the vicinity. On attempting to remove the lamina of the fifth lumbar vertebra, after cutting off its very prominent, largely developed and dense spinous process, it was found to be placed in the upper part of the sacral canal quite in front of its normal position. It was removed piecemeal with great difficulty. When the dura matral sheath of the cauda equina of the right side was seen to have been so severely compressed as not to expand then the bone pressing on it was removed" (33).

Early descriptions of neurogenic claudication and its relief by forward flexion were presented in 1889 (55) and 1911 (1). Hypertrophic changes in the lumbar spine were

stressed in the early reports. The concept of "congenital stricture of the spinal canal" was later proposed by Sarpyener (56). However, his series of 12 children presented with both upper and lower neuron disease. Verbiest (65), a Dutch surgeon, has championed the contribution of congenital narrowing, although a countryman of his, Van Gelderen (64), earlier proposed that a hypertrophied ligamentum flavum might be responsible. Nevertheless, Verbiest defined the clinical syndrome and, using Lipiodol as contrast agent, confirmed the spinal obstruction. Although Macnab (36) drew attention to "spondylolisthesis with an intact neural arch," he did not mention myelography or describe the neurogenic claudication that some of his patients may, in hindsight, be presumed to have had. Kirkaldy-Willis (31) reviewed the subject of lumbar stenosis in 1974, and underscored a spectrum of possible causes, including congenital narrowing and degenerative processes. The relative merits of congenital narrowing versus hypertrophic changes are still debated. In my opinion, those who espouse the latter make a stronger case.

The concept of cervical disc protrusion was proposed by Stookey in 1928 (59) and expanded in 1948 by Brain (8). These authors did not clearly distinguish cervical myelopathy from cervical disc disease. Later Pallis and coworkers (47) associated a myelopathy with cervical osteophytes and subluxation. Their descriptions were enlarged upon subsequently by the British neurologists Lees (34) and Nurick (44,45).

J. D. O'Duffy, M.B.: Professor, Department of Medicine, Mayo Medical School, Mayo Clinic, Rochester, Minnesota 55905.

LUMBAR STENOSIS

Definition

Although there is no accepted definition of lumbar stenosis, the term implies nondiscogenic compression of the cauda equina provoking a stereotyped symptom-complex including neurogenic claudication. Historically, evidence of myelographic obstruction to the flow of radiocontrast material in the spinal canal (17,20, 30,62) has been the confirmatory evidence. With new imaging techniques, measured reduction in the dimensions of the thecal sac due to extrinsic compressing structures is taken as confirmatory. Because the anteroposterior (AP) diameter of the canal varies in symptomatic patients from 10 to 15 mm, overlapping generously with asymptomatic individuals, there can be no definition based on arbitrarily defined intraspinal diameters (43,62).

The cardinal symptom of lumbar stenosis is neurogenic claudication (5,7,20,31,48,65,69). This is an intermittent pain and/or paresthesia in the legs brought on by walking and standing, and relieved by sitting or lying down. Confirmation of the diagnosis requires myelographic evidence of obstruction to distal flow of radiocontrast material or magnetic resonance imaging (MRI) or computed tomography (CT) confirmation. When indicated, compression of the caudal sac at laminectomy is yet another confirmation.

Development of the Lesion

Although a role for the disc in promoting canal stenosis has been proposed (39,43), its contribution, however, has been questioned (14), and even cast in some doubt (49). Frequently, there is neither radiologic evidence of disc space degeneration nor CT, MRI, nor myelographic evidence of disc protrusion.

Congenital narrowing of the canal has long been proposed (5,14,42,43,65). Developmentally, the lumbar canal reaches its full internal diameters in childhood. With growth it is the bony structures, not the lumen, that enlarge. The lumbar canal is normally narrowest at the level of L3 and L4 and indeed stenosis is most common at these sites. Before CT scanning, the normal AP diameter was generally regarded to be 12 to 15 mm when measured radiologically or intraoperatively (43).

Using dynamic CT–myelographic techniques, Penning and Wilmink (49) evaluated internal diameter and cross-sectional area of the caudal sac in 12 patients with myelographically proven lumbar stenosis and in control subjects. All measurements were done in flexion and extension and were corrected for radiologic enlargement by a factor of 35%. There was no significant difference between bony sagittal or interpedicular diameters be-

tween the two groups. However, a discrepancy in the area within the dura was significant; $66-105 \text{ mm}^2$ (range 70–138) in stenotics versus 145 mm^2 (range 86–230) in control subjects. They proposed that the key offender in stenosis was the enlarging apophyseal joints. By a series of diagrams the authors showed that the canal dimensions are greater in flexion, especially anteriorly, and reduced in extension. This observation can explain the clinical relief afforded by flexion as the lateral recesses at the anterolateral angles of the canal carrying the emerging nerve roots obtain the largest increase in area during flexion.

Table 1 lists contributing factors to lumbar stenosis. Figure 1 is a diagram of normal and pathologic lumbar vertebrae. Vertebra B is taken to represent the situation in congenital canal stenosis (or achondroplasia), but vertebra C with hypertrophic changes is the lesion most commonly encountered in patients with stenosis. The hypertrophy of the apophyseal joints and yellow ligament narrows the space available between the disc anteriorly and the superior articular facets posterolaterally (49). This pincer movement can be suspected on lumbar CT when the normal epidural fat is reduced. In some patients with the classic syndrome of neurogenic claudication an unexpected disc protrusion coexists (14,20, 49,69).

Gross features of canal stenosis are thickened laminae, facet hypertrophy, thickened ligamentum flavum, and narrow lateral recesses (43,48,69). At times, degenerative cysts arising from the apophyseal joints contribute. Does the ligamentum flavum contribute to stenosis? Some investigators have reported that it may be 7 to 8 mm thick instead of the usual 4 mm or less (31,69), but at times the ligament has a normal thickness (69). Rauschning (53), based on anatomic studies, has proposed that the ligament thickness is more apparent than real and is due to volume redistribution in a shortened spinal canal. Yoshida and colleagues (70), by CT and pathologic studies, have highlighted the role of the enthesis of a thickened ligamentum flavum in stenotics as compared to its size

TABLE 1. *Contributing factors to lumbar stenosis*

A. Degenerative changes
   1. Hypertrophy of apophyseal joints
   2. Ligamentum flavum hypertrophy
   3. Degenerative spondylolisthesis
   4. Calcium salt deposition
   5. Synovial cysts
   6. Scoliosis
B. Rheumatoid arthritis
   1. Spondylolisthesis
Less Common Causes
C. Congenital narrowing
D. Paget's disease of bone
E. Achondroplasia
F. Fluorosis

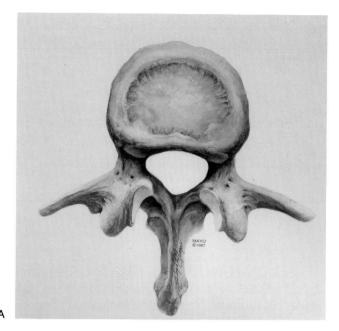

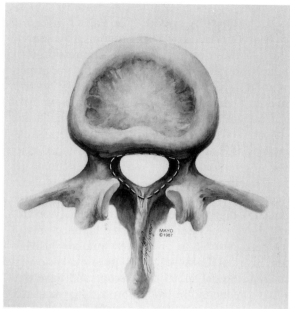

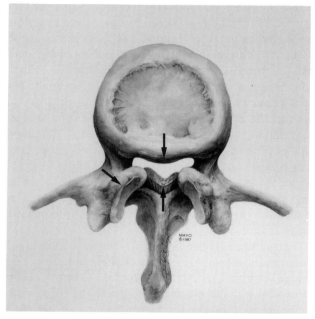

FIG. 1. A: Normal lumbar canal. **B:** Congenital narrowing of lumbar canal. **C:** Narrow lumbar canal due to enlarged apophyseal joints, ligamentum flavum, and prominent vertebral bossing (*arrows*). Floyd Hosmer, artist.

in patients with discogenic sciatica. Hypertrophy at that ligament's attachment to the apophyseal joint rather than at its interlaminar portion, and thickening of cartilage of the facets away from the joint at times with calcium crystal deposition and collagen degeneration, were associated with histologic changes that seem integral to osteoarthritis.

The degenerative process may also be associated with other structural deformities that contribute to or cause stenosis. Degenerative spondylolisthesis, especially of L4 on L5, is present in 25–35% of stenotics. Although failure of the sagittal to coronal orientation of the apophyseal joints as the lumbar spine descends is thought to pro-

mote listhesis, in one study this was not a feature in stenotics (19). Scoliosis in the lumbar spine appears to be another effect of degeneration of the apophyseal joints in the elderly (57). In degenerative joint disease, the lesions are loss of cartilage, increased bone formation, joint effusion, and ligamentous hypertrophy. Whether stenotics have an excess of osteoarthritis elsewhere has not been prospectively studied. There probably is an association with hip and knee degenerative joint disease (7,40). In one series, there was an inordinate number (10%) of patients with rheumatoid arthritis (30).

The less common causes include achondroplasts who have reduced canal volume, develop facet joint disease, and commonly are found to have either lumbar stenosis or cervical myelopathy or both (52). Paget's disease of bone may produce stenosis, and symptoms may respond either to calcitonin or to surgical decompression (66). Postspinal fusion stenosis, although thought to be important by some, is not discussed here. Metabolic diseases have seldom been incriminated, although calcium pyrophosphate crystals were detected in ligamentum flavum in some patients (11,16,18). Diffuse intervertebral skeletal hyperostosis (Forestier's disease) that produces bony bridging at multiple anterior vertebral junctions has been reported in association with lumbar stenosis (29).

Ischemia of nerve roots has been proposed as a cause of pain (5,43), but since the dura is not normally opened to allow nerve root inspection during laminectomy, it has not been possible to prove ischemia conclusively. Japanese investigators have studied gross blood flow intrathecally using the spinal myeloscope and have proposed that a reduction in blood flow can be visualized. Because the pain persists while standing still, it is unlikely that ischemia alone is causative. One of our patients died within 12 hours of three-level laminectomy. Autopsy examination of the excised cauda equina revealed segmental compression of the nerve roots with demyelination corresponding to the compressions of the roots at regular intervals (20). These demyelinated zones corresponded to the myelographic blocks, but there was no evidence of ischemia. This leads me to conclude that longstanding compression affecting the neural structures is the most significant causative factor.

Clinical Presentation

Most patients are men, although in some conditions, specifically degenerative spondylolisthesis and rheumatoid arthritis, women are more commonly affected. As the symptoms are difficult to correlate and signs are scarce or absent the patients have often been misdiagnosed. Typical misdiagnoses are psychoneurosis (31), osteoarthritis of the hip (7), fibrositis, and trochanteric bursitis. The cardinal symptom is pseudoclaudication (Table 2). This "neurogenic" claudication is usually bilateral and is reported as pain or weakness in the muscles of the thighs and calves provoked by both standing and walking, and relieved within minutes by sitting or lying down (5,20,31,48,65,69). Patients often report an accompanying numbness that may be described as a "rubbery" sensation or as "pins and needles" (5). In the extreme, giving away "drop episodes" may occur. Typically, the symptoms involve both lower extremities (20). Whereas other cauda equina diseases produce sphincteric disturbances, stenosis seldom does (5), and when present the symptoms are subtle. That they may at times be involved is evidenced by a patient who could only urinate when sitting (69). Sparing of the sacral roots

TABLE 2. *Symptoms of lumbar stenosis in 68 patients*

	Symptom	Prevalence (%)
Description	Pseudoclaudication	94
	Standing leg discomfort	94
	Pain	93
	Numbness	63
	Weakness	43
	Bilateral	69
	Accompanied by back pain	65
Site	Whole limb	78
	Above knee only	15
	Below knee only	7
	Radicular pain only	6

From Hall et al., ref. 20, with permission.

can be understood when one considers their central protected position in the lumbar canal. Absence of neurogenic claudication in patients operated for "stenosis" bodes ill for success of laminectomy (10).

If patients persist in walking they notice that their legs get weak and they may fall (20,31,48). All the symptoms reduce when the patient adopts a flexed position (Fig. 2). Patients achieve this by leaning on shopping carts, church pews, lawnmowers, or against walls. Patients avoid lines at supermarkets or shopping in malls and, when forced to stand for long, will shift weight from one foot to the other. One patient, when questioned about her walking and standing limits, responded "one block and one hymn!" In advanced cases, patients adopt a simian posture and, even in recumbency, must assume a flexed or fetal position to relieve symptoms. A restless legs syndrome termed "Vesper's curse" occurring in recumbency in stenotics appeared linked to congestive heart failure (32).

In true vascular claudication, by contrast, muscle pain is cramping, has no paresthetic quality, and is provoked by walking and relieved by standing. Whereas cycling provokes vascular claudication, it may be tolerated by stenotics as they are not weight-bearing in the flexed posture.

Patients usually recall no singular history of lumbar pains in early life and, unless spinal instability coexists, have surprisingly little back pain. Patients know their walking limits, which often may be less than 100 meters. When asked to show where the pain is, a standing patient may describe the radicular symptoms with a sweeping downward motion of the two hands from buttocks to heels. Valsalva maneuver will not provoke symptoms, whereas in discogenic sciatica it often does. Low back pain, when present, is mild and has a mechanical quality (20,48,69). In the series of Hall et al. at Mayo Clinic (20) less than 20% of patients could recall preexisting discogenic sciatica. This may be normal for a middle-aged cohort. Severe low-back pain in stenotics implies some degree of instability either due to listhesis or scoliosis (57).

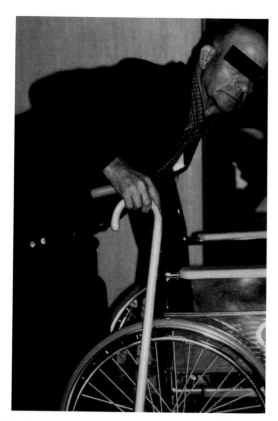

FIG. 2. Patient leaning on a wheelchair to get relief from neurogenic leg pain.

TABLE 3. *Neurologic signs of lumbar stenosis*

Reduced or absent ankle reflex	43%
Knee reflex decreased or absent	18%
Objective weakness	37%
Positive straight-leg raising test	10%
Electromyogram abnormal	92%

From Hall et al., ref. 20, with permission.

(5). When arthritis of a major weight-bearing joint, particularly the hip, is also present, an intra-articular injection of a local anesthetic can help weigh its contribution to the symptoms. However, successful arthroplasty in such patients sometimes is followed by the emergency of claudication, and two surgical procedures are eventually needed (40). The differential diagnosis of lumbar stenosis is shown in Table 4. Although there is no large epidemiologic study of the natural history, studies of the natural course of untreated lumbar stenosis by Johnsson (26,27) in 32 unoperated patients indicated that most patients were unchanged over 4 years of observation.

Diagnostic Tests

Radiographs of the lumbar spine show degenerative disc disease in 70% of this elderly patient population and osteoarthritis of the facet joints in 62% (20). Because these changes are common in the elderly not affected by stenosis, the diagnostic significance is minimal. If AP views of the lumbar spine show the apophyseal joints, this is a clue that can favor stenosis, as it suggests that the canal is sharply pitched like an A-frame roof and therefore not commodious. Patients may have one or more degenerative lumbar discs, i.e., spondylosis, but again the specificity of this finding is minimal. A degenerative spondylolisthesis, most often of grade I of L4 on L5, was seen in 35% of our series.

CT scans are commonly overinterpreted as showing evidence of lumbar stenosis. CT was predicted to become the leading diagnostic test (12,21,38) because it revealed the lateral recesses and the reduction of epidural fat. Advanced CT machines have provided high resolution but have lower specificity in the diagnosis of lumbar stenosis, in part because stenosis is present in those with-

Signs of stenosis are shown in Table 3. Few physical findings are present (9,20). The patient may be in a wheelchair or using a cane. If patients are observed standing or walking, they are soon seen to adopt a flexed posture. Reduced pedal pulses were noted in 9% of our series (20). In the same group of 68 patients, deep tendon reflexes were reduced at the ankles in 43% and at the quadriceps in 18%. The symptoms are shown in Table 2. Objective weakness was detected in 37%. Coexisting upper motor neuron lesions may at times occur since cervical myelopathies can coexist (20). Most patients can touch their toes while the knees are extended in standing. Therefore decreased range of lumbar motion is of little value in the diagnosis (20).

Nerve-root tension signs such as the straight-leg raising test of Lasègue are usually negative. When present, a tension sign suggests coexistent disc protrusion. Weakness, when present, is usually mild, can be unilateral or bilateral, and is usually in muscles innervated by L5 and S1 roots. This weakness can be evoked by attempts to walk on the heels or forefeet. When patients stand up for a few minutes they will seek a flexed position, as in leaning on the examining table. Walking nonstop for a few minutes will induce symptoms and may be a better test than any other. At times the deep tendon reflexes, when rechecked after exertion, may disappear or be reduced

TABLE 4. *Differential diagnosis of lumbar stenosis*

Vascular claudication—atherosclerotic
Osteoarthritis of hip or knees
Lumbar disc protrusion
Intraspinal tumor
Unrecognized neurologic disease
Arteriovenous malformation
Peripheral neuropathy

out symptoms. When CTs are read "blindly" in asymptomatic patients, there are abnormal results in 35%. Moreover, up to 9% of asymptomatic "normal" control subjects were thought to have spinal stenosis (67). In another study of patients surgically proven to have spinal stenosis, CT was diagnostically inferior to metrizamide myelography (2).

Besides false-positive results, the other difficulties with CT are technical difficulty and false-negative results (10,61,63). Window width differences can cause variation of measurements. Because the normal diameters of the lumbar canal vary between ethnic groups as well as between individuals, one cannot interpret diameters as absolute guidelines (15,51). In our series, 9% of patients had myelographic stenosis only at L1 or L2 or both, an area that is missed on conventional CT. Moreover, CT interpretation can miss a stenosis even within the area of viewing (20). Thus, it is my opinion that CT is best deferred until myelography. A postmyelogram CT enables the radiologist to view foramina at and below the level of blocks, sites that are missed in lateral recess stenosis (39).

MRI has an accuracy of 75–85% in diagnosis (4) and is considered by some to be adequate for diagnosis. Its false-positive rate for diagnosing stenosis in asymptomatic people varies from 7 to 21% (6,25). No single test is absolutely diagnostic. False-positive tests increase with age, as does the clinical entity.

In my opinion, myelography is the gold standard in diagnosis (14,20,51,65) and is essential when laminectomy is considered. The contrast material, usually injected with the patient in extension at L1 or L2, is blocked to caudal flow either completely or subtotally (20,31,65). Usually 10 to 15 ml contrast is needed (48,69), enough to fill the caudal subarachnoid space. Many neurosurgeons insist on tilting the table so that contrast can be allowed to flow cephalad. Otherwise, unsuspected high lesions are missed. Whereas pantopaque was formerly used (48,69), it is now preferable to use agents such as Iopamidol in order to avoid arachnoiditis (37,58). Flexion of the spine may allow blocked contrast material to flow distally (Fig. 3), thereby revealing if there are other blocks (14,62). The CT scan obtained after the myelogram allows measurement of the volume of the thecal sac and more precise imaging of nerve root relationships in the lateral recess.

Electromyography, in the hands of an expert, reveals one or more radiculopathies in 92% of patients (20). The most typical pattern is bilateral multiple radiculopathies with evidence of paraspinal muscle involvement. At times paraspinal denervation may not be elicited. The chronic neurogenic changes include increase in motor unit amplitude, and fibrillation potentials. Nerve root injections are discussed in other chapters.

Selection of patients for surgery depends on the severity of pain, presence or absence of serious concomitant disease, and a realistic expectation that good to excellent operative results may not exceed 75% (20).

CERVICAL CANAL STENOSIS

Although cervical spondylosis or disc degeneration is common and affects most people over 50, spondylotic cervical myelopathy is uncommon. Stenosis in the cervical spine is also less common than lumbar stenosis, but as the two can coexist, it is important to outline the

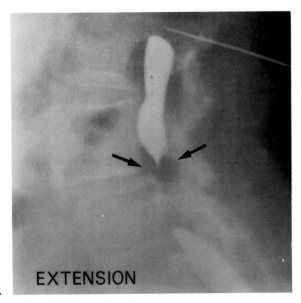
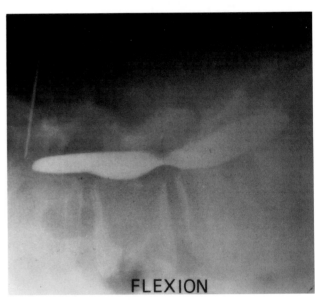

FIG. 3. Myelogram in lumbar stenosis. **A:** In extension: hour-glass deformity at L4–L5. Note grade I slip of L4 on L5. **B:** After flexion, radiocontrast passes below the block. From Dunsker (13) with permission.

symptoms of cervical disease (see Chapter 55). Spondylotic myelopathy is caused by constricting degenerative and hypertrophic changes in the cervical spine.

The early descriptions of both cervical disc protrusion and spondylotic myelopathy had overlapping features (59,68). One early report described "extradural ventral chondromas" as tumors pressing on the cervical cord (59) and another discussed the relative merits of disc protrusion versus a degenerative or neoplastic process in causing myelopathy (8).

Development of the Lesion

As the cervical cord AP diameter averages 10 mm and the internal spine diameter at C4 averages 17.7 mm, there is a large safety margin. The cervical discs, especially C5–C6 and C6–C7, degenerate in middle life showing signs of central dehydration (54). Spondylotic bars develop at the posterior margins of the vertebral bodies just above and below the disc. The "chondroma" described by Stookey (59) is a posterior bony exostosis and degenerated annulus fibrosus. This boss in front in combination with a hypertrophied ligamentum flavum and laminae behind compresses the cord (13,44,45,54). Subluxations of vertebrae can occur (44,45). The end result of the multilevel compression is an indented cervical cord (Fig. 5) similar to lumbar stenosis. Ischemia of the cord is not a likely contributor (13). A limited classification of cervical canal stenosis is shown in Table 5.

The corticospinal tracts are demyelinated below the level of compression whereas the ascending spinothalamic tracts are demyelinated above it (68). Ossification and/or hypertrophy of the posterior longitudinal ligament as a cause is mostly seen in Orientals (22). The cord may be deeply indented by spondylotic bars at several levels (Fig. 4). Cervical nerve roots can be compressed as the bars extend into the foramina. The nerve roots show compression of their dural sleeves (60). There is degeneration in the posterior and lateral white matter as well as the corticospinal tracts (3). Gliosis in gray matter and atrophy of nerve roots are seen.

The debate over the contribution of a congenitally narrow canal versus spondylotic changes parallels that for lumbar stenosis. Thus, the putative culprits incriminated again are internal osteophytes, subluxations, yellow ligament hypertrophy, and ischemia (44,45,54). Arguing against a constitutional narrowing are the findings by Nurick (44,45) of nearly equivalent internal spinal diameters in stenotics and control subjects. As deduced radiologically, the mean minimal AP diameter of stenotic cervical spines in myelopathic patients was 14.6 mm, whereas in controls it was 16.2 mm.

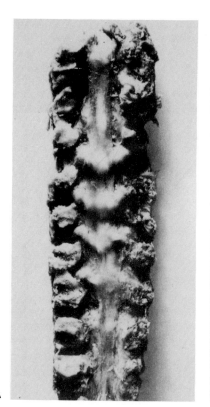
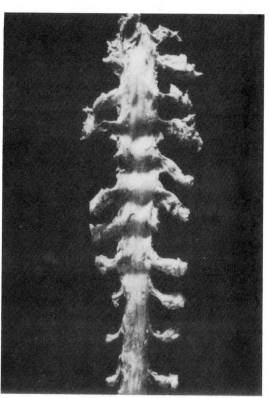

A

B

FIG. 4. A: Interior view of cervical canal showing transverse bars corresponding to **B,** indentations on stenotic cervical cord in same patient. From Penning et al. (50) with permission.

TABLE 5. *Nonmalignant causes of cervical stenosis with myelopathy*

Acquired	Cervical spondylosis
	Paget's disease, gout
	Fluorosis (ref. 41)
	Ossification of posterior longitudinal ligament
Congenital	Multiple hereditary exostoses (ref. 28)
	Maroteaux-Lamy syndrome
	Achondroplasia (ref. 52)

Clinical Presentation

Patients are usually 45 to 65 years old (34,44,45), with a 60 to 40 male to female ratio. Few patients with cervical spondylosis, even when followed for 6 years or more, develop myelopathy (34). Patients with myelopathy usually present with a disorder of gait and may have a history of cervical radiculopathy. Neck pain is often absent, and this adds to the difficulty in diagnosis. The most common clinical presentation is a spastic ataxic gait combined with weakness in the upper extremities (3,35) (Table 6). Depending on the site of the lesion, the upper extremities may have upper or lower motor neuron lesions or both (34,54,68). Babinski responses and increased knee and ankle jerks are expected. Coexistent peripheral neuropathy or lumbar stenosis modify the neurologic findings. In this case, leg reflexes may also be reduced. Involvement of spinothalamic tracts is usually revealed by a vague sensory level, and radicular involvement can give severe paresthesia and hypesthesia in the hands. Posterior column involvement is detected by reduced vibratory or joint sense in the lower extremities. Lhermitte's sign may be present. Frank bladder incontinence is uncommon, but sphincter disturbances are seen in half the patients (35,54).

Weakness and wasting of hand muscles, at times with

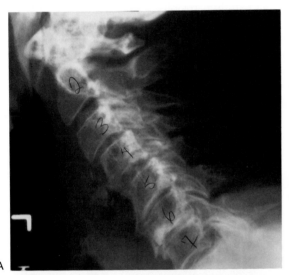

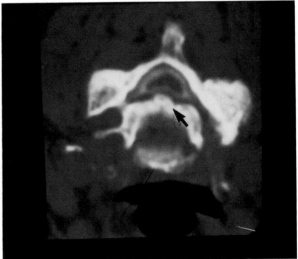

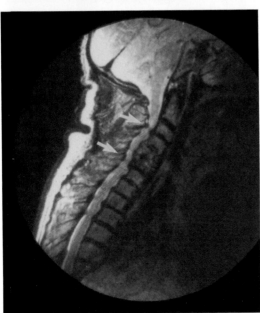

FIG. 5. A: Disc degeneration at C5–C6 and C6–C7, and subluxation at C3–C4. **B:** Spondylotic bar seen in CT–metrizamide myelogram protruding posteriorly compressing cord at C5–C6. **C:** MRI T2-weighted image with CSF appearing white, showing multilevel stenoses.

fasciculations, may occur (8). Cord compression at C6 is suspected when a patient presents with hyperactive triceps tendon jerks and absent biceps reflexes. Symmetry is not necessary as Brown-Sequard lesions can be mimicked (8).

A sudden worsening of all symptoms and signs may be produced by neck trauma (34), sometimes trivial, but the course of spondylotic myelopathy is usually indolent. In a careful, mostly prospective study, the natural history of cervical spondylotic myelopathy was observed (34). All patients had extensor plantar responses. Episodes of worsening preceded referral and they occurred at infrequent intervals over a period of 2 to 30 years. Of 51 controls, patients having spondylosis without myelopathy, none developed myelopathy during long observation. These authors recommended a conservative approach to the myelopathy (34). The differential diagnoses includes multiple sclerosis, cerebrovascular disease, low pressure hydrocephalus, cord tumor, and tabes dorsalis (3).

Radiologic Diagnosis

Cervical spine roentgenograms (Fig. 5A) reveal disc space degeneration at C5–C6 and C6–C7, and foraminal encroachment seen on oblique views is due to Luschka joint exostoses. As these changes are of spondylosis, they do not predict myelopathy. Likewise, CT reveals spondylosis (Fig. 5B) but does not prove myelopathy. The cord tends to be displaced posteriorly and can adapt to many shapes, including that of a banana (23,24,61). This configuration was the most likely to be causing myelopathy in the study of Houser et al. (23). In a study by Pen-

TABLE 7. *Differential diagnosis of cervical spondylotic myelopathy*

Cervical cord tumor
Syringomyelia
Cervical disc herniation
Arteriovenous malformation
Multiple sclerosis
Amyotrophic lateral sclerosis
Subacute combined degeneration
Neurosyphilis
Rheumatoid arthritis with subluxation

ning (50), CT when combined with myelography predicted that concentric compression of the cord in a narrowed canal would cause symptoms when the cord cross-sectional area was reduced to about 60 mm^2, i.e., by 30% from normal (50). Conventional myelography reveals obstruction to caudal contrast flow in neck extension (50). It may be supplemented with CT (Fig. 5B). If there is no block, then postmyelogram CT is probably unnecessary (50).

MRI can, when clinical findings are strongly suggestive, supplant myelography (37). The cervical canal on sagittal T2-weighted images shows multilevel stenosis (Fig. 5C). Moreover, MRI can rule out mimics, including intraspinal tumors and arteriovenous malformations. Cervical scoliosis makes MRI difficult to interpret. As with lumbar stenosis, the cerebrospinal fluid protein below the level of block is usually elevated. Cisternal myelography may be needed either when a block is not overcome by flexion or is multilevel, e.g., from C3–C6.

The differential diagnosis of cervical spondylotic myelopathy is shown in Table 7.

ACKNOWLEDGMENT. The author is deeply appreciative of the expert assistance provided by Ms. Jennifer Peterson in the preparation of this manuscript.

TABLE 6. *Symptoms and signs of myelopathy caused by spondylotic cervical myelopathy in 32 patients*

Type	Percent
Motor	
Hyperreflexia	87
Babinski sign	54
Spastic gait	54
Sphincter disturbance	49
Arm weakness	31
Paraparesis	21
Quadriparesis	10
Brown-Séquard	10
Hand atrophy	13
Fasciculation	13
Sensory	
Vague sensory level	41
Proprioceptive loss	39
Cervical dermatome sensory loss	33
Pain	
Radicular, arm	41
Cervical pain	26

From Lunsford et al., ref. 35, with permission.

REFERENCES

1. Bailey P, Casamajor L (1911): Osteoarthritis of the spine as a cause of compression of the spinal cord and its roots: with reports of 5 cases. *J Nerv Ment Dis* 38:588–609.
2. Bell GR, Rothman RH, Booth RE, et al (1984): A study of computer-assisted tomography. Comparison of metrizamide myelography and computed tomography in the diagnosis of herniated lumbar disc and spinal stenosis. *Spine* 9:552–556.
3. Bernhardt M, Hynes RA, Blume HW, White AA (1993): Current concepts review: cervical spondylotic myelopathy. *J Bone Joint Surg* 75A(1):119–128.
4. Bischoff RJ, Rodriguez RP, Gupta K, Righi R, Dalton JE, Whitecloud TS (1993): A comparison of computed tomography-myelography, magnetic resonance imaging, and myelography in the diagnosis of herniated nucleus pulposus and spinal stenosis. *J Spinal Dis* 6(4):289–295.
5. Blau JN, Logue V (1961): Intermittent claudication of the cauda equina. *Lancet* 1:1081–1086.
6. Boden SD, Davis DO, Dina TS, Patronas NJ, Wiesel SW (1990): Abnormal magnetic-resonance scans of the lumbar spine in asymptomatic subjects. *J Bone Joint Surg* 72A(3):403–408.

7. Bohl WR, Steffee AD (1979): Lumbar spinal stenosis: a cause of continued pain and disability in patients after total hip arthroplasty. *Spine* 4(2):168–173.

8. Brain WR, Knight GC, Bull JW (1948): Discussion on rupture of the intervertebral disc in the cervical region. *Proc R Soc Med* 41: 509–516.

9. Ciric I, Mikhael MA (1985): Lumbar spinal-lateral recess stenosis. *Neurol Clin* 3:417–423.

10. Deen HG, Zimmerman RS, Lyons MK, Wharen RE, Reimer R (1995): Analysis of early failures after lumbar decompressive laminectomy for spinal stenosis. *Mayo Clin Proc* 70:33–36.

11. Delamarter RB, Sherman JE, Carr J (1993): Lumbar spinal stenosis secondary to calcium pyrophosphate crystal deposition (pseudogout). *Clin Orthop* 289:127–130.

12. Dorwart RH, Volger JB 3d, Helms CA (1983): Spinal stenosis. *Radiol Clin North Am* 21:301–325.

13. Dunsker SB (1980): Cervical spondylotic myelopathy: pathogenesis and pathophysiology. In: Dunsker S, ed. *Seminars in neurological surgery. Cervical spondylosis.* New York: Raven Press, pp 119–134.

14. Ehni G (1969): Significance of the small lumbar spinal canal: cauda equina compression syndromes due to spondylosis. 1. Introduction. *J Neurosurg* 31:490–494.

15. Eisenstein S (1983): Lumbar vertebral canal morphometry for computerized tomography in spinal stenosis. *Spine* 8:187–191.

16. Ellman MH, Vazques LT, Brown NL, et al (1981): Calcium pyrophosphate dihydrate deposition in lumbar disc fibrocartilage. *J Rheum* 8(6):955–958.

17. Epstein JA, Epstein BS, Lavine L (1962): Nerve root compression associated with narrowing of the lumbar spinal canal. *J Neurol Neurosurg Psychiatry* 25:165–176.

18. Fukui K, Kataoka O, Sho T, Sumi M (1990): Pathomechanism, pathogenesis, and results of treatment in cervical spondylotic myelopathy caused by dynamic canal stenosis. *Spine* 15(11):1148–1152.

19. Grobler LJ, Robertson PA, Novotny JE, Pope MH (1993): Etiology of spondylolisthesis: assessment of the role played by lumbar facet joint morphology. *Spine* 18(1):80–91.

20. Hall S, Bartleson JD, Onofrio BM, et al (1985): Lumbar spinal stenosis. Clinical features, diagnostic procedures and results of surgical treatment in 68 patients. *Ann Intern Med* 103(2):271–275.

21. Hammerschlag SB, Wolpert SM, Carter BL (1976): Computed tomography of the spinal canal. *Radiology* 121:361–367.

22. Hase H, Hirasawa Y, Ogura S, Kusaka Y, Chatani K, Tanaka T, Kan T (1992): Severe cervical myopathy due to diffuse hypertrophy of the cervical posterior longitudinal ligament. *Spine* 17(11): 1417–1421.

23. Houser OW, Onofrio BM, Miller GM, Folger WN, Smith PL (1994): Cervical spondylotic stenosis and myelopathy: evaluation with computed tomographic myelography. *Mayo Clin Proc* 69: 557–563.

24. Houser OW, Onofrio BM, Miller GM, Folger WN, Smith PL, Kallman DA (1993): Cervical neural foraminal canal stenosis : computerized tomographic myelography diagnosis. *J Neurosurg* 79: 84–88.

25. Jensen MC, Brant-Zawadzki MN, Obuchowski N, Modic MT, Malkasian D, Ross JS (1994): Magnetic resonance imaging of the lumbar spine in people without back pain. *N Engl J Med* 331(2): 69–73.

26. Johnsson KE, Rosen I, Uden A (1992): The natural course of lumbar spinal stenosis. *Clin Orthop* 279:82–86.

27. Johnsson KE, Uden A, Rosen I (1991): The effect of decompression on the natural course of spinal stenosis. A comparison of surgically treated and untreated patients. *Spine* 16(6):615–619.

28. Johnston CE 2d, Sklar F (1988): Multiple hereditary exostoses with spinal cord compression. *Pediatr Orthoped* 11(8):1213–1216.

29. Karpman RR, Weinstein PR, Gall EP, et al (1982): Lumbar spinal stenosis in a patient with diffuse idiopathic skeletal hypertrophy syndrome. *Spine* 7(6):598–603.

30. Katz JN, Lipson SJ, Larson MG, McInnes JM, Fossel AH, Liang MH (1991): The outcome of decompressive laminectomy for degenerative lumbar stenosis. *J Bone Joint Surg* 73A(6):809–816.

31. Kirkaldy-Willis WH, Paine KW, Cauchoix J, et al (1974): Lumbar spinal stenosis. *Clin Orthop* 99:30–50.

32. LaBan MM, Viola SL, Femminineo AF, Taylor RS (1990): Restless legs syndrome associated with diminished cardiopulmonary compliance and lumbar spinal stenosis: a motor concomitant of "Vesper's curse". *Arch Phys Med Rehabil* 71:384–388.

33. Lane WA (1893): Case of spondylolisthesis associated with progressive paraplegia; laminectomy. *Lancet* 1:991.

34. Lees F, Turner JW (1963): Natural history and prognosis of cervical spondylosis. *Br Med J* 2:1607–1610.

35. Lunsford LD, Bissonette DJ, Zarub DS (1980): Anterior surgery for cervical disc disease. Part 2: treatment of cervical spondylotic myelopathy in 32 cases. *J Neurosurg* 53:12–19.

36. Macnab I (1950): Spondylolisthesis with an intact neural arch: the so-called pseudo-spondylolisthesis. *J Bone Joint Surg [Br]* 32(3): 325–333.

37. Masaryk TJ, Modic MT, Geisinger MA, et al (1986): Cervical myelopathy: a comparison of magnetic resonance and myelography. *J Comput Assist Tomogr* 10(2):184–194.

38. McAfee PC, Ullrich CG, Yuan HA, et al (1981): Computed tomography in degenerative spinal stenosis. *Clin Orthop* 161:221–234.

39. McIvor GW, Kirkaldy-Willis WH (1976): Pathological and myelographic changes in the major types of lumbar spinal stenosis. *Clin Orthop* 115:72–76.

40. McNamara MJ, Barrett KG, Christie MJ, Spengler DM (1993): Lumbar spinal stenosis and lower extremity arthroplasty. *J Arthro* 8(3):273–277.

41. Misra UK, Nag D, Husain M, Ray PK, et al (1988): Endemic fluorosis presenting as cervical cord compression. *Arch Environ Health* 43(1):18–21.

42. Nasca RJ (1987): Surgical management of lumbar spinal stenosis. *Spine* 12:809–816.

43. Naylor A (1979): Factors in the development of the spinal stenosis syndrome. *J Bone Joint Surg [Br]* 61(3):306–309.

44. Nurick S (1972): The natural history and the results of surgical treatment of the spinal cord disorder associated with cervical spondylosis. *Brain* 95:101–108.

45. Nurick S (1972): The pathogenesis of the spinal cord disorder associated with cervical spondylosis. *Brain* 95:87–100.

46. O'Duffy JD (1989): Spinal stenosis. In: McCarty DJ, ed. *Arthritis and allied conditions: a textbook of rheumatology,* 11th ed. Philadelphia: Lea and Febiger, pp. 1464–1472.

47. Pallis C, Jones AM, Spillane JD (1954): Cervical spondylosis. *Brain* 77:274–289.

48. Pennal GF, Schatzker J (1971): Stenosis of the lumbar spinal canal. *Clin Neurosurg* 18:86–105.

49. Penning L, Wilmink JT (1987): Posture-dependent bilateral compression of L4 or L5 nerve roots in facet hypertrophy. A dynamic CT–myelographic study. *Spine* 12:488–500.

50. Penning L, Wilmink JT, Van Woerden HH, et al (1986): CT myelographic findings in degenerative disorders of the cervical spine: clinical significance. *AJR* 146:793–801.

51. Postacchini F, Ripani M, Carpano S (1983): Morphometry of the lumbar vertebrae: an anatomic study in two caucasoid ethnic groups. *Clin Orthop* (172):296–303.

52. Pyeritz RE, Sack GH, Udvarhelyi GB (1980): Cervical and lumbar laminectomy for spinal stenosis in achondroplasia. *Johns Hopkins Med J* 146:203–206.

53. Rauschning W (1987): Normal and pathologic anatomy of the lumbar root canals. *Spine* 12:1008–1019.

54. Rowland LP (1984): Cervical spondylosis. In: Rowland LP, ed. *Merritt's textbook of neurology,* 7th ed. Philadelphia: Lea & Febiger, pp. 310–312.

55. Sachs B, Fraenkel J (1900): Progressive ankylotic rigidity of the spine (spondylose rhizomelique). *J Nerv Ment Dis* 27:1–15.

56. Sarpyener MA (1945): Congenital stricture of the spinal canal. *J Bone Joint Surg* 27:70–79.

57. Simmons ED, Simmons EH (1992): Spinal stenosis with scoliosis. *Spine* 17(6)(Suppl):S117–120.

58. Sortland O, Magnaes B, Haug T (1977): Functional myelography with metrizamide in the diagnosis of lumbar spinal stenosis. *Acta Radiol Suppl* 355:42–54.

59. Stookey B (1928): Compression of the spinal cord due to ventral extradural cervical chondromas. *Arch Neurol Psychiatry* 20:275–291.

60. Taylor AR (1953): Mechanism and treatment of spinal-cord disorders associated with cervical spondylosis. *Lancet* 1:717–720.

61. Thijssen HO, Keyser A, Horstink MW, et al (1979): Morphology of the cervical spinal cord in computed myelography. *Neuroradiology* 18(2):57–62.

62. Uden A, Johnsson KE, Jonsson K, et al (1985): Myelography in the elderly and the diagnosis of spinal stenosis. *Spine* 10(2):171–174.

63. Ullrich CG, Binet EF, Sanecki MG, et al (1980): Quantitative assessment of the lumbar spinal canal by computed tomography. *Radiology* 134:137–143.

64. Van Gelderen C (1948): Ein orthotisches (lordotisches) Kaudasyndrom. *Acta Psychiatr Neurol* 23:57–68.

65. Verbiest H (1954): A radicular syndrome from developmental narrowing of the lumbar vertebral canal. *J Bone Joint Surg* [*Br*] 36(2):230–237.

66. Weisz GM (1986): Lumbar canal stenosis in Paget's disease. *Clin Orthop* 206:223–227.

67. Wiesel SW, Tsourmas N, Feffer HL, et al (1984): A study of computer-assisted tomography. I. The incidence of positive CAT scans in an asymptomatic group of patients. *Spine* 9:549–551.

68. Wilkinson M (1971): In: Wilkinson M, ed. *Cervical spondylosis: its early diagnosis and treatment,* 2nd ed. Philadelphia: W.B. Saunders, pp 49–55.

69. Yamada H, Oya M, Okada T, et al (1972): Intermittent cauda equina compression due to narrow spinal canal. *J Neurosurg* 37:83–88.

70. Yoshida M, Shima K, Taniguchi Y, Tamaki T, Tanaka T (1992) Hypertrophied ligamentum flavum in lumbar spinal canal stenosis. Pathogenesis and morphologic and immunohistochemical observation. *Spine* 17(11):1353–1360.

Metabolic Disease

The Adult Spine: Principles and Practice,
2nd edition, J.W. Frymoyer, Editor-in-Chief.
Lippincott-Raven Publishers, Philadelphia © 1997.

CHAPTER 40

Metabolic Bone Disease of the Adult Spine

Jerome C. Hall and Thomas A. Einhorn

Back pain, spine deformity, and impaired spinal function can result from an alteration in vertebral bone metabolism. Although metabolic bone disease generally affects the entire skeletal system, the effects on spinal function are particularly profound and disabling. Osteoporosis, the most common nontumorous condition that affects the spinal column, can lead to vertebral compression fractures resulting in paraspinal, mid-, and low back pain, as well as kyphosis. In its most severe form, kyphosis can result in abnormal pressure on internal organs and even impair vena caval blood flow. Osteomalacia, a less common, but nevertheless prevalent disorder, may produce a similar clinical picture, although there are striking differences in the serologic findings. Paget's disease, another metabolic bone disorder, produces excessive amounts of poor-quality bone which, through direct expansion of bone, can lead to compression of the thecal sac and its neural elements. Because each of these conditions involves some alteration of bone formation or resorption, or the manner in which the individual constituents of bone tissue are organized, a detailed under-

standing of how bone metabolism affects spinal function is critical to the successful practice of spinal surgery. This chapter will review the basic biology of bone metabolism, discuss the diagnostic and treatment options for managing metabolic bone diseases of the spine, and offer specific recommendations to physicians who encounter these problems in their surgical practices.

BASIC BONE BIOLOGY

Bone differs from the other connective tissues in that it provides both structural and physiologic functions. These characteristics result from bone's unique composition, in which inorganic salts impregnate a well-organized collagen matrix. As a structural component, bone is responsible for protecting the vital organs and providing a rigid framework for the body's shape and locomotion. As an organ, bone serves as the primary site of hematopoiesis and acts as a reservoir for calcium ions, contributing directly to the regulation of extracellular fluid calcium concentrations. To provide these functions, bone is organized into two compartments: a cortical (compact bone) compartment, which provides strength and rigidity, particularly in torsional and bending modes; and a cancellous (trabecular bone) compartment, which serves both to resist compressive loads and to present a high surface-to-volume ratio of bone tissue to extracellular fluids. This latter function enhances

J. C. Hall, M.D.: Resident in Orthopedics, Department of Orthopedics, Mount Sinai Medical Center, New York, New York 10029-6574.

T. A. Einhorn, M.D.: Professor, Department of Orthopedics, School of Medicine, Mount Sinai Medical Center, New York, New York 10029-6574.

bone's metabolic activities and promotes bone remodeling in response to both physiologic as well as mechanical stimuli (1).

The ability of bone to be formed and remodeled and to adapt to its environment is dependent on the cells that regulate its functions. Osteoclasts, the predominant cell types responsible for bone resorption, are multinucleated giant cells found in cavities on bone surfaces called resorptive pits, or Howship's lacunae. They are characterized by a ruffled border, extensive membrane folding, and abundant mitochondria, rough endoplasmic reticulum, and Golgi complexes. Osteoclasts release protons by a carbonic anhydrase-dependent proton pump, which lowers local pH and thereby facilitates the action of specific acid proteases, which act upon mineral and degrade the extracellular matrix. They respond indirectly to numerous regulatory agents known to induce bone resorption, such as parathyroid hormone (PTH), 1,25 dihydroxyvitamin D (the active metabolite of vitamin D), osteoclast-activating cytokines (e.g., interleukin-1, interleukin-6), and prostaglandin E2. Because osteoclasts lack receptors for PTH or 1,25 dihydroxyvitamin D, their response is believed to be mediated by cells of the osteoblast lineage, which thereby act to influence the localization, induction, stimulation, and inhibition of osteoclastic resorption. Osteoclasts do have receptors for, and respond directly to, calcitonin, colchicine, and γ-interferon. Evidence supports the belief that osteoclasts are derived from mononuclear cells originating in bone marrow or other hematopoietic organs (1–3).

Osteoblasts are bone-forming cells that synthesize and secrete unmineralized bone matrix (osteoid), participate in bone calcification and resorption, and regulate the flux of calcium and phosphate in and out of bone. Osteoblasts contain intracellular organelles that are typical of cells engaged in protein synthesis; they are also characterized by their abundance of alkaline phosphatase and their ability to synthesize and secrete numerous matrix proteins, including type I collagen, osteocalcin, osteonectin, and specific receptor proteins such as PTH, 1,25 dihydroxyvitamin D, and others. They appear to play a key role in the activation of bone resorption by including osteoclasts. In this way, osteoblasts regulate bone remodeling through the control of both bone resorption and formation (1,2).

Once an osteoblast undergoes terminal cell division and is surrounded by a mineralized bone matrix, it becomes an osteocyte. Osteocytes are characterized by a higher nucleus-to-cytoplasm ratio, are arranged concentrically around the central lumen of an osteon and between lamellae, and are uniformly oriented with respect to the longitudinal and radial axes of the lamellae. Osteocytes have extensive cell processes that project through canaliculi, establishing communications with other osteocytes and with osteoblasts that line the surface of bone. Although the function of osteocytes is not clear at this time, several investigators have suggested that os-

teocytes mediate the transmission of mechanical signals through bone and may also participate in certain bone-resorptive activities (1,2).

The extracellular matrix of bone is an organic substance composed of collagen, noncollagenous proteins, and water. It imparts resilience and flexibility to the tissue. The inorganic component of bone is mineral consisting primarily of calcium and phosphate, mainly in the form of small hydroxyapatite crystals, with the composition $Ca_{10}(PO_4)_6(OH)_2$. It renders bone tissue hard and rigid and accounts for 65% to 70% of bone's dry weight (1–4).

Like other cells, bone cells exhibit a basal level of activity that is modified by systemic hormones and local factors. For example, PTH acts on bone and kidney and indirectly on the gut to increase the rates of calcium flow into the serum and extracellular space and to maintain the body's extracellular calcium concentration at nearly constant levels. The stimulus for PTH release is a drop in the serum ionized calcium concentration. Although the enhancing effect of PTH on bone resorption has been known for some time, it was surprising to learn that receptors for PTH are found only on osteoblasts and that osteoclasts do not respond to PTH directly (1,2). Parathyroid hormone causes cytoskeletal changes in the osteoblast resulting in rounding of the cell, such that it occupies less space on the bone surface. This configuration allows the osteoclast to gain access to bone surfaces. In addition, it may stimulate osteoblasts to produce factors that will stimulate osteoclasts or increase the recruitment of osteoclast progenitors. Both of these mechanisms will lead to enhanced bone resorption (1–3).

Vitamin D, a steroid hormone that is converted to $25(OH)D_3$ in the liver, then to its active form $1,25(OH)D_3$ in the kidney, plays a role in stimulating biosynthesis of the intestinal and renal calcium-binding proteins and enhances active calcium transport in the gut (5). How vitamin D is involved in mineralization is not yet known; however, its major role in enhancing intestinal calcium and phosphate absorption is critical to bone and mineral homeostasis. Its activation in the kidney is under the control of PTH, and thus a systemic regulatory control mechanism exists to maintain serum calcium levels (1,5).

Calcitonin, a peptide hormone, is secreted from the parafollicular cells of the thyroid gland in response to an acutely rising plasma calcium concentration. Calcitonin interacts with receptors on the osteoclast, leading to direct inhibition of this cell. The general physiologic role of calcitonin is uncertain, as it seems to play no role in steady-state calcium metabolism (6).

BONE METABOLISM IN RELATION TO SPINAL FUNCTION

The human skeleton is composed of cortical and trabecular bone in a volumetric ratio of 4:1 (7). Under normal physiologic conditions, the metabolic turnover rate of trabecular bone is eight times that of cortical bone, which turns over at a rate of only 3% per year (7). In the spine, however, the volumetric ratio of cortical to trabecular bone is 1:2 (8). It is thus evident that any imbalance in bone metabolism will have a greater effect on the spine than it will on other parts of the skeleton. Moreover, because the cortical shell makes only a 10% contribution to the compressive strength of each vertebra, any decrease in trabecular bone strength will have a major effect on spinal bone integrity (9).

The mechanism by which vertebral strength is lost is related, in part, to the architectural arrangement of the vertebral trabeculae. In this architectural arrangement, the cancellous portion of the vertebral body is oriented with vertical trabecular groups connected by horizontal trabecular struts to resist compressive forces. In osteopenic patients, the greatest loss of trabeculae occurs in the horizontal groups (10). As such, small incremental losses of bone mass in the spine can rapidly destabilize the ability of the vertebrae to support compressive loads because the mechanical affect of the interconnecting struts will be lost (Fig. 1).

By definition, osteopenia refers to reduced radiodensity and is a descriptive term rather than a diagnosis. Its presence in the spine can be detected on a routine lateral roentgenogram, which generally indicates at least a 30% reduction in total bone mass (7). Because the major function of the spinal column is to support compressive loads and, to a lesser extent, bending and torsional loads, any reduction in either the organic component (collagen and noncollagen protein) or the inorganic component (mineral) must be viewed in terms of its effects on load-bearing capacity. Burstein et al. (11) have shown that the elastic stiffness properties of bone are almost exclusively a function of collagen, independent of any mineral content. Bone strength, the most important mechanical property in terms of the development of clinical fractures, is dependent on both the mineral content and the distribution and organization of the mineral within the collagen framework (11). This suggests that the risk of fracture depends on both bone mineral content and the chemical and structural properties of the organic phase. In terms of spine mechanics, experiments have shown that measurements of bone mineral content provide reasonably good estimates of lumbar vertebral compressive strength (correlation coefficient = 0.86) (8). It is therefore possible to calculate the risk that an individual could sustain a vertebral fracture by measuring the spinal bone density.

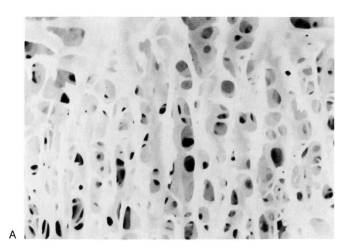

A

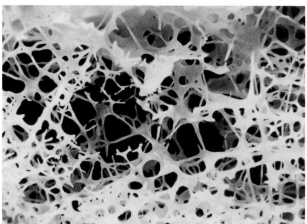

B

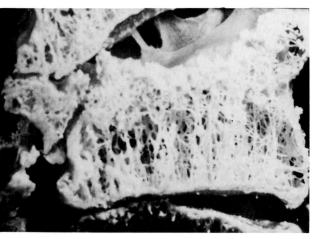

C

FIG. 1. **A:** Close-up view of the central portion of a T12 vertebral body from a normal 50-year-old woman who died in a motor vehicle accident. Note the extensive interconnections of the horizontal cross-ties in relation to the vertical columns. In addition, note that the architecture of this region of the anatomy consists of a combination of thickened trabeculae and bony plates. **B:** Close-up view of the central portion of a T12 vertebral body from a 75-year-old osteoporotic female. Note the loss of horizontal interconnections and the conversion of all architectural components into thin trabecular spicules. **C:** Sagittal section of a T10 vertebra with a wedge compression fracture. Note that the area of structural failure involves the central portion of the vertebral body.

THE CLINICAL SYNDROMES

Osteoporosis

Osteoporosis is a metabolic bone disorder character-ized by decreased amounts of normal-quality bone re-sulting in an increased susceptibility to fracture. Cur-rently, the condition is so prevalent that approximately 15 to 20 million people in the United States are afflicted, and the condition results in close to 1.5 million fractures per year (12).

All men and women lose bone as they age. However, not all patients have osteoporosis. To develop this syn-drome, certain risk factors must exist and systemic or environmental conditions must occur. One major risk factor in women is a sensitivity of the skeleton to estro-gen withdrawal, whether this happens as a result of a natural or surgically induced menopause (12). In other individuals, long-term calcium deficiency, secondary hy-perparathyroidism, or decreased physical activity have also been implicated (12,13). Other risk factors include a certain genetic predisposition (individuals who are fair skinned, slim, have hypermobile joints, are of Northern European ancestry, or who have scoliosis), cigarette smoking, or excessive alcohol intake (Table 1). Cigarette smokers show significantly increased incidences of bone loss and hip and vertebral fractures, and this may be due in part to the abnormal systemic handling of estrogen metabolites (14). Heavy alcohol users may develop os-teoporosis as a result of calcium diuresis or a direct de-pressive effect of alcohol on osteoblast function.

Osteoporosis can be divided into primary and second-ary forms (15). Primary osteoporosis, otherwise known as involutional or idiopathic osteoporosis, occurs in cer-tain individuals as they age or after they go through menopause. It is unrelated to any specific endocrinopa-thy or other disease state. Secondary osteoporosis is caused by an endocrinopathy, neoplastic disease, hema-tologic disorder, mechanical disorder, biochemical col-lagen disturbance, or nutritional aberration (Table 2) (15). These conditions must be eliminated before any at-tempt is made to alter a patient's bone metabolism therapeutically.

TABLE 1. *Osteoporosis risk factors*

Genetic and biological	Behaviorial and environmental
Caucasian race	Alcohol excess
Cigarette smoking	Inactivity
Fair skin and hair	Malnutrition
Northern European heredity	Caffeine use
Scoliosis	Exercise-induced amenorrhea
Osteogenesis imperfecta	
Early menopause	High-fiber diet
Slender body build	High-phosphate diet

TABLE 2. *Causes of secondary osteoporosis*

Thyroid excess
Parathyroid excess
Hypothalamic hypogonadism
Diabetes mellitus
Steroid exposure (endogenous, iatrogenic)
Multiple myeloma
Leukemia
Prolonged bed rest or inactivity.

Most individuals attain their level of "peak bone mass" between the ages of 16 and 25. This is the greatest amount of bone that individuals will ever have in their lifetime, and the higher this value is, the less chance that they will develop osteoporosis. The reason for this is that the ability of any specific rate of bone loss (from what-ever cause) to lead to a critically low level or fracture threshold is dependent on the amount of bone present before the bone loss begins. Men normally lose bone at a rate of 0.3% per year, whereas in women, the rate is as high as 0.5%. In the spine, because of the predominance of trabecular bone, there is an accelerated rate of bone loss, which may be as high as 6% per year in the years immediately after menopause (12). Riggs and Melton (12) introduced the term "fracture gradient of risk." Above a bone density of 1 g/cm^3, the prevalence of frac-tures is 32%; below 0.8 g/cm^3, it is approximately 50%. This accelerated rate of bone loss, which occurs at the rate of 2% to 3% per year, begins after natural or surgical menopause and may last from 6 to 10 years. Because it is women who are usually afflicted by this more rapid rate of bone loss, osteoporosis is much more common in females (12).

For the purposes of describing and understanding the disease, primary osteoporosis has been categorized into two distinct syndromes (16). Type I, known as post-menopausal osteoporosis, occurs most commonly in women within 5 to 10 years after menopause. It affects mostly trabecular bone and is clinically associated with vertebral crush, intertrochanteric hip, and distal radius fractures. Type II osteoporosis, known as senile osteopo-rosis, occurs in women and men older than 70, with a female to male ratio of 2:1. It affects cortical and trabec-ular bone equally and is associated with multiple verte-bral wedge, femoral neck, pelvic, proximal humeral, and proximal tibial fractures. Thus in Type I osteoporosis, estrogen deficiency plays a primary role whereas in Type II osteoporosis, aging and long-term calcium deficiency are more important (Table 3) (16).

In general, osteoporosis is a silent and progressive dis-order that comes to the attention of the patient or the physician only after an acute, painful fracture has oc-curred (Fig. 2). Occasionally, the condition may be rec-ognized by asymptomatic thoracic wedge or lumbar compression fractures on a routine lateral chest x-ray. However, there is a growing interest in prevention; phy-

TABLE 3. *Types of primary osteoporosis*

	Type I (postmenopausal)	Type II (senile)
Age (years)	51–75	>70
Sex ratio	6:1	2:1
Type of bone loss	Mainly trabecular	Trabecular and cortical
Fracture site	Vertebrae (crush)	Vertebrae (multiple wedge)
	Distal radius	Hip (mainly femoral neck)
	Hip (mainly intertrochanteric)	Proximal humerus Proximal tibia
Main causes	Factors related to menopause	Factors related to aging

Modified from ref. 15.

TABLE 4. *Differential diagnosis of spinal osteopenia*

Primary osteoporosis
  Type I, postmenopausal
  Type II, senile
Osteomalacia
  Impaired vitamin D metabolism
  Malabsorption
  Vitamin D-resistant rickets
  Aluminum intoxication (hemodialysis patients)
Endocrine disorders
  Cushing's disease
  Diabetes mellitus
  Estrogen deficiency
  Hyperparathyroidism
  Hypogonadism
  Iatrogenic glucocorticoid treatment
Disuse disorders
  Prolonged immobilization
  Paralysis
Neoplastic disorders
  Leukemia
  Multiple myeloma
Nutritional disorders
  Anorexia nervosa
  High-protein diet
  High-phosphate diet
  Low-calcium diet
  Alcoholism
Hematologic disorders
  Sickle cell anemia
  Thalassemia
Collagen disorders
  Homocystinuria
  Osteogenesis imperfecta

sicians are increasingly called upon to manage patients before fractures occur. The differential diagnosis of radiographic spinal osteopenia is extensive and involves metabolic, neoplastic, and a variety of other conditions (Table 4).

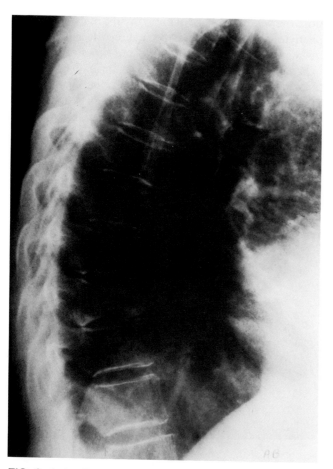

FIG. 2. Lateral radiograph of a portion of the vertebral column in a postmenopausal woman with a compression fracture of one of the lower thoracic vertebrae. Note the presence of decreased radiodensity as well as the wedge-shaped configuration of the compressed vertebrae.

Osteomalacia

Osteomalacia is a metabolic disorder involving inadequate mineralization of newly formed osteoid. It usually results from vitamin D deficiency, vitamin D resistance, intestinal malabsorption disorders, acquired or hereditary renal disorders, intoxication with heavy metals such as aluminum or iron, or other assorted etiologies (Table 5) (17). To make the correct diagnosis, one must consider all of these causes in an appropriate work-up. The childhood form of osteomalacia is termed rickets and it, too, has a multitude of causes. Rickets of the developing and growing skeleton due to dietary deficiency of vitamin D, however, has become rare since the widespread supplementation of dairy products with vitamin D.

The clinical diagnosis of osteomalacia is often difficult because patients usually have nonspecific complaints, such as muscle weakness or diffuse aches and pains. Radiographic evidence of osteomalacia can often mimic other disorders including osteoporosis. However, the presence of pseudofractures or Looser's transformation zones is good evidence that some degree of osteomalacia is present. (Looser's zones are radiolucent areas of bone resulting from multiple microstress fractures that heal by the formation of osteomalacic bone, which is not miner-

TABLE 5. *Causes of osteomalacia*

Vitamin D deficiency
  Dietary
  Malabsorption
    Intestinal disease
    Intestinal surgery
  Insufficient sunlight
Impaired vitamin D synthesis
  Liver disease
  Hepatic microsomal enzyme induction
  Dilantin
  Renal failure
Metabolic acidosis
Fanconi's syndrome (renal tubular defect)
Hypophosphatemia
  Malabsorption
  X-linked hypophosphatemic rickets
  Oncogenic
  Oral phosphate-binding antacid excess
Mineralization inhibition
  Disphosphonate
  Aluminum
  Fluoride
  Iron
Hypophosphatasia

to confirm the diagnosis of osteomalacia. The histologic hallmark of osteomalacia is an increase in the width and extent of osteoid seams with evidence of decreased rates of mineral apposition, as determined by tetracycline labeling (17,18). Unlike in normally mineralized bone, in which tetracycline labels show discrete uptake of tetracycline only at times when mineral is being deposited, in osteomalacic bone, the slow rate of mineralization prevents these labels from appearing separated in time and results in a "smudged" appearance (17) (Fig. 3).

Classic osteomalacia is caused by a decrease in the vitamin D content in the diet. These patients often maintain restrictive dietary habits such as vegetarianism or a diet extremely low in fat. However, osteomalacia is also common in patients who are elderly. It has been proposed that the "mild malabsorption" condition seen in some elderly individuals predisposes them to bone disease. This disorder is easily treated with vitamin D (17).

A variety of other conditions can cause osteomalacia (Table 5). Among the more common of these are gastrointestinal abnormalities such as "dumping syndrome," blind loops, malabsorption, or surgically induced malabsorption as a result of intestinal bypass surgery. In addition, the widespread use of anticonvulsant drugs such as phenytoin (Dilantin®) has been shown to cause osteomalacia by inducing the P-450 mixed-function oxidases in hepatic cells and thus converting vitamin D to inactive polar metabolites. This reduces the production of 25 hydroxyvitamin D and leads to insufficient quantities of the 25 hydroxyvitamin D substrate, which is required for renal conversion to the active 1,25 dihydroxyvitamin D metabolite (17). Less commonly, patients can present with osteomalacia as a result of metabolic acidosis, renal tubular dysfunction, hypophosphatemia, or exposure to environmental inhibitors of mineralization such as alu-

alized.) Looser lines are typically seen in the femoral neck, pelvic rami, and ribs (17). Biochemically, different forms of osteomalacia may present in different ways. However, the clinician can usually be alerted to the presence of this disease by an elevated serum alkaline phosphatase, low serum calcium, or low inorganic phosphorous level. Further investigation by ordering assays for specific vitamin D metabolites such as 25 hydroxyvitamin D or 1,25 dihydroxyvitamin D will further elucidate an abnormality.

In most patients, transiliac bone biopsy is necessary

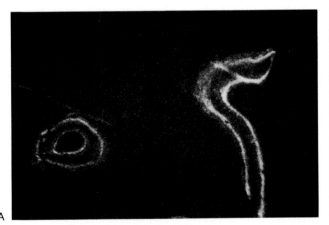 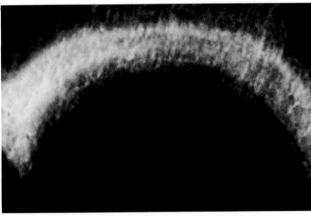

FIG. 3. A: High-power, unstained fluorescent photomicrograph of the mineralization front in normal bone. Note that there are two discrete fluorescent lines; these lines represent the two doses of tetracycline ingested by the patient before bone biopsy. The space between the lines represents the period of time between doses, when no tetracycline was ingested. **B:** High-power, unstained fluorescent photomicrograph of the mineralization front in the bone from a patient with osteomalacia. Note that although the patient adhered to the same tetracycline labeling protocol, slow and abnormal mineralization has caused the two lines to be indistinct and "smudged" together (× 100).

minum. Aluminum-associated osteomalacia, however, is not uncommon in patients receiving hemodialysis treatment (19).

Paget's Disease

Paget's disease is the second most common metabolic bone disturbance in the United States, after osteoporosis. It has an occurrence rate of approximately one in 1,000 persons and affects an estimated 3% of middle-aged and elderly individuals who are of Northern European ancestry (i.e., Britain, France, Germany, Australia, New Zealand). Not surprisingly, Paget's disease is more common in these countries. There is a slight geographic clustering in the prevalence of this disease, and people who have a family relative with Paget's disease are at increased risk of contracting it themselves. The male to female ratio is approximately equal. The disease has not been reported in identical twins (20).

Although any bone may be affected by Paget's disease, the vertebrae, pelvic bones, and femora are the most common (21). Bone scans show that approximately 60% of patients have involvement of the lumbar spine, 45% have involvement of the thoracic spine and sacrum, and only 15% have involvement of the cervical spine (21). The pathologic lesion is characterized by an excess of hyperactive osteoclasts and osteoblasts, with an intense increase in bone resorption, marrow replacement by hypervascular fibrous tissue, and a haphazard attempt by the body to regenerate bone (20–22). The new bone synthesized to replace the bone that has been lost appears as a disorganized woven bone tissue and is of poor quality (23).

The increased cellular activity and turnover of bone matrix in Paget's disease is evidenced by increased urinary output of collagen breakdown by-products (20). The excessive bone turnover is first characterized by a phase of increased osteoclastic resorption, followed by a phase of increased bone formation and eventually a "burnout" phase with little cellular activity. The poor tissue quality resulting from these cellular disturbances leads to the production of a brittle bone matrix which is susceptible to fracture.

The etiology of Paget's disease remains elusive despite evidence proposing a viral cause (24). Nuclear inclusion bodies have been demonstrated in the osteoclasts of patients with Paget's disease. The inclusion bodies were shown to be morphologically similar to the Paramyxovirus capsid (25). Despite this evidence, a viral cause is yet to be proven because no normal animal has been shown to develop Paget's disease as a result of experimental viral inoculation. Other proposed etiologies include inflammatory, endocrine, metabolic, and vascular causes.

Clinically, Paget's disease is manifested by a wide array of presentations. In some instances, a subclinical case is discovered when a patient has a radiograph taken or a serum alkaline phosphatase level measured for an unrelated reason. In other settings, a patient will present with an obvious bony deformity, pain, and extraskeletal involvement. In severe cases, high-output heart failure may result from an arteriovenous fistula that develops in the hypervascular pagetic bone. Back pain, a frequent cause of complaints in pagetic patients, has been reported to occur in 11% to 43% of patients who have Paget's disease involving the spine (26,27). However, the causal relationship between vertebral pagetic involvement and back pain has been disputed. There may be a compression fracture, central or lateral stenosis, a nonspecific syndrome of stiffness, or ache and fatigue due to arthritic changes in the facet joints. This may also lead to marked kyphosis of the spine. Pathologic fractures are uncommon; however, they can occur in either the osteolytic phase, because of decreased bone mass, or in the osteoblastic phase, because of loss of bone organization. Spinal complaints consist of a spectrum of ailments from deep, dull ache or pain in the back that is not relieved by rest, nonsteroidal anti-inflammatory drugs (NSAIDs), or anti-Paget's disease drugs, to neurologic radicular symptoms and spinal cord compression (27).

Although all areas of the spine may be involved by Paget's disease, the most common sites are the forth and fifth lumbar vertebrae (Fig. 4). When these vertebrae are severely affected, spinal stenosis is a common finding. Wyllie (28), in 1923, was the first to describe vertebral expansion in Paget's disease resulting in spinal stenosis. He noted that the stenosis may be lateral or central, or occur as a result of a combination of types leading to compression of the nerve roots and/or the spinal cord (Fig. 4). In addition to direct bony compression, other mechanisms have been implicated in the production of neural dysfunction. Neural ischemia produced by the so-called "arterial steal phenomenon," whereby hypervascular pagetic bone "steals" blood from the neural tissue, is also a possible etiology for the observed symptoms (29). Another proposed mechanism is direct compression of the vascular supply of the neural tissue (30,31).

Malignant degeneration occurs in 1% to 10% of patients with Paget's disease and is the most dreaded complication of this disorder. It generally presents as an acute increase in a patient's pain and is more common with polyostotic involvement (32,33). The most frequently occurring malignant tumor in pagetic bone is osteogenic sarcoma, followed by fibrosarcoma. Other less common tumors include chondrosarcoma, malignant fibrous histiocytoma, and reticulum-cell sarcoma. The most common site for pagetic tumor involvement is the femur, followed by the humerus, pelvis, and tibia. It is interesting that, in sharp contrast to uncomplicated Paget's disease, the incidence of malignant involvement of the spine is infrequent. Sarcomatous degeneration usually occurs after age 55 and always develops in a bone already affected

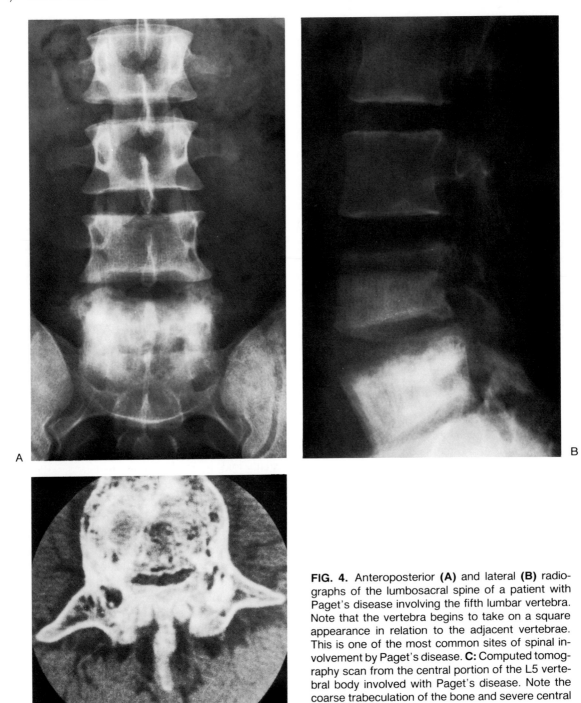

FIG. 4. Anteroposterior **(A)** and lateral **(B)** radiographs of the lumbosacral spine of a patient with Paget's disease involving the fifth lumbar vertebra. Note that the vertebra begins to take on a square appearance in relation to the adjacent vertebrae. This is one of the most common sites of spinal involvement by Paget's disease. **C:** Computed tomography scan from the central portion of the L5 vertebral body involved with Paget's disease. Note the coarse trabeculation of the bone and severe central and lateral stenosis of the spaces for the neural elements.

by Paget's disease (34). There have been several recent cases described in the literature of giant-cell tumors or giant-cell reparative granulomas in Paget's disease (35,36). These tumors are benign or low-grade malignancies with a tendency to spread to the adjacent soft tissues. Histologically, the tumors are filled with intracellular viral-like filamentous structures. The tumors may be partially sensitive to radiation treatment and/or chemo-

therapy. Of particular interest is that all patients in whom this particular giant-cell tumor develops appear to be of Italian descent, with ancestors originating from the province of Avellino (Fig. 5) (36,37). This phenomenon lends credence to a viral or genetic etiology for the disease.

The diagnosis of Paget's disease is based on history, physical examination, radiographic evaluation, and

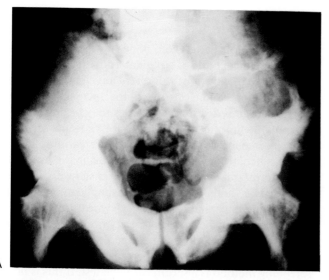

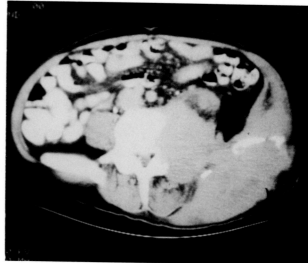

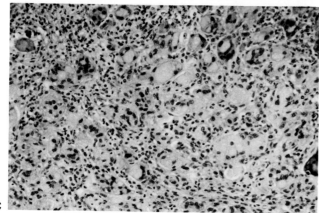

FIG. 5. A: Anteroposterior radiograph of the pelvis in a patient who has Paget's disease involving both proximal femora, the entire pelvis, and the lower lumbar vertebral bodies. Note severe destruction of the left hemipelvis by a neoplastic process. **B:** Computed tomography scan through the L5 vertebral body of this patient, showing severe destruction of the spinal elements as well as extra spinal soft-tissue extensions of this tumor mass. **C:** High-power photomicrograph of a biopsy specimen from this tumor showing extensive giant-cell formation mixed with abundant benign-appearing stromal cells. Some giant cells have peripheral nuclei, which are more typical of foreign-body giant cells (seen in reparative granulomata) than of osteoclasts. Vascular channels are also noted, indicating that this is a highly vascular tumor (hematoxylin and eosin, × 200).

measurement of biochemical markers. During the history and physical examination, the disease usually becomes apparent insidiously in a middle-aged or elderly person. Clinical symptoms such as an enlarging skull are recognized by an increase in hat size, headache, or progressive deafness. The lower extremities may be marked with a "saber shin," or anterior bowing of the tibia with overlying warm skin. Radiographically, the presentation is rarely ambiguous. The earliest evidence of the disease is often a flame-shaped, advancing osteolytic wedge seen in the mid-diaphysis of the long bones. One may also see well-demarcated round regions of decreased bone density. With subsequent compensatory osteoblastic bone formation, the bones become grossly enlarged and deformed with irregular, thickened cortices and coarsened trabeculae (20). The vertebrae show coarse trabeculae with thickened sclerotic cortices, and the shape of the vertebral body may become square (Fig. 4).

Serum and urine biochemical markers reflect the different phases of the disease and can also be used to characterize the effectiveness of therapeutic intervention. Historically, there is an elevated urinary excretion of hydroxyproline and hydroxylysine; both are degrada-

tion products of bone's organic matrix. Patients with Paget's disease can excrete up to 20 times more hydroxyproline than normal persons (20). However, because urinary measurement of hydroxyproline or hydroxylysine is expensive and cumbersome, the measurement of alkaline phosphatase is usually preferred. This enzyme is involved in the formation of bone; its elevation reflects the reactive osteoblastic phase of Paget's disease.

Recently, a urinary assay has been developed that measures the pyridinium derivatives hydroxylysylpyridinoline (HP) and lysylpyridinoline (LP), which are intermolecular cross-links of collagen collectively known as pyridinoline cross-links (38). In contrast to the wide distribution of type I and type II collagens, HP and LP are absent from skin, ligament, and fascia, and their major sources are bone and cartilage. Using a specific HP and LP assay, Uebelhart et al. (38) showed that the urine of patients with active Paget's disease had a 12-fold increase in pyridinolines compared with age-matched controls. Both HP and LP decrease significantly after treatment with aminopropylidene bisphosphonate (APB), a potent inhibitor of bone resorption, which indicates that urinary excretion of HP and LP reflects only collagen degradation occurring during osteoclastic resorption and not the degradation of newly synthesized collagen. As a result of these new assays for collagen breakdown, the need to measure hydroxyproline or hydroxylysine excretion has been reduced. Bone biopsy is rarely needed for diagnosis in a patient with Paget's disease except to determine whether malignant degeneration has occurred.

PATIENT EVALUATION

The work-up of the patient with metabolic bone disease is designed both to reach a diagnosis and to stage the disease for the purpose of planning and following treatment. The components of the work-up include the history, serum and urine biochemical tests, radiographic procedures, and, in the case of certain osteopenic conditions, bone density measurement and iliac crest bone biopsy. As will be discussed, some tests are provided to all patients, whereas others require certain indications. Bone biopsy, for example, is needed in the work-up of metabolic bone disease (including osteoporosis) only when all noninvasive tests have failed to produce an adequate diagnosis.

Medical History

The medical history in a patient with osteopenia is intended to document past and present illnesses, medications, surgeries, occupational exposures, nutrition, family history, and social habits, all of which are used to formulate an understanding of the patient's disease risk. Particular attention to specific risk factors (Table 1), causes of secondary osteoporosis (Table 2), and known causes of osteomalacia (Table 5) can be useful in directing further diagnostic tests. In addition, identification of certain iatrogenic conditions, such as drug-induced hyperthyroidism and steroid treatment, can lead to reappraisal of the patient, reduction in the use of particular pharmacologic agents, and improvement in bone mass.

Biochemical Tests

Serum and urine tests are done routinely to establish the biochemical basis of a patient's condition (Table 6). A complete blood count will reveal any hematologic disorders. Mineral and electrolyte imbalances and underlying, unrecognized systemic diseases may be detected on a simultaneous multiple analysis (SMA). Renal function can be screened by measuring serum creatinine levels, whereas hepatic function is assessed using the aspartate aminotransferase, alanine aminotransferase, alkaline phosphatase, and γ-glutamyl transpeptidase values. If the alkaline phosphatase level is elevated, fractionation of this enzyme is helpful, as isoenzymes are secreted by several tissues including bone, liver, kidney, and intestine. If malabsorption is suspected by history, a quick screening method is a serum carotene test. If this is positive, a more complete malabsorption work-up is indicated. The 24-hour urine collection is used to monitor bone resorption. As noted above, tests for pyridinoline cross-link assays are now important components of a bone resorption work-up. Calcium excretion remains an important way to determine the rate of bone loss, and the 24-hour urine collection is a means for determining calcium and phosphorus balance. If calcium excretion in the urine is increased, treatment may be indicated to augment total body calcium retention. Thiazide diuretics have been shown effective in maintaining total body calcium levels (39,40). If calcium excretion is low, there may be insufficient calcium ingestion, deficient calcium absorption, or vitamin D deficiency. Phosphorus excretion indicates the effects of PTH on the kidney and is usually elevated when the PTH activity is high.

Another important marker of bone turnover is the level of γ-carboxyglutamic acid in the serum or urine. This molecule, sometimes referred to as osteocalcin or β-glycerophosphatase (BGP), is a low-molecular-weight protein synthesized only by osteoblasts and secreted directly into the circulation. Although the osteocalcin bound to bone matrix is released from bone during bone

TABLE 6. *Laboratory tests*		
Routine	Special	Additional[a]
Complete blood count	25 (OH) vitamin D_3	Gastrointestinal (malabsorption)
Electrolytes, creatinine, blood urea nitrogen	1,25 (OH)$_2$ vitamin D_3	Serum carotene
Calcium, phosphorus, protein, albumin	Intact parathyroid hormone	Endocrine
Alkaline phosphatase, liver enzymes	Osteocalcin (bone Gla protein)	Thyroid function tests
24-hour urinary calcium	Urine pyridinium cross-links	Plasma cortisol
Serum protein electrophoresis		Dexamethasone suppression test
Thyroid function tests		Serum testosterone (men)
		Other
		Urine immunoelectrophoresis
		Bence Jones protein test

[a] Recommended panels for further work-up based on initial history.

resorption, measurement of the protein in serum or urine is indicative of bone formation. When levels are high, this suggests a metabolic disorder in which bone is being actively formed and degraded (e.g., high-turnover osteoporosis, renal osteodystrophy, Paget's disease). Measurements of specific osteotropic hormones such as PTH and the vitamin D metabolites are not necessarily standard components of the work-up for patients with metabolic bone disease. These more expensive tests should be reserved for those patients in whom a specific abnormality is suspected. To complete the biochemical evaluation, a serum protein electrophoresis is performed to rule out an occult lymphoproliferative malignancy such as myeloma. This condition is frequently a cause of spinal pain and bone loss and has been shown to mimic osteoporosis radiographically (Fig. 6). If there is an elevated γ-globulin region, serum immunoelectrophoresis is ordered to look for a monoclonal immunoglobulin spike. Urine immunoelectrophoresis may demonstrate the presence of a Bence-Jones protein to confirm a diagnosis of multiple myeloma (Table 6). (As an anecdote, the senior author [TAE] has diagnosed three patients with this malignancy who were originally referred for treatment of "routine osteoporosis".)

Radiologic Assessment

In the work-up of patients suspected of having metabolic bone disease, the orthopedist has available several radiologic diagnostic tools. Plain radiographs, radioisotopic studies, computed tomography (CT), magnetic resonance imaging (MRI), and bone densitometry techniques are all part of the diagnostic armamentarium. Because the vertebral bodies are the most common skeletal elements at risk for fracture, documentation of the status of the vertebrae at the onset of treatment establishes a baseline for assessing the clinical outcome of any given treatment protocol.

For the patient with osteoporosis, anteroposterior and lateral radiographs of the thoracic and lumbar spines are the first and often definitive radiologic studies. Using plain radiographs, Eastell et al. (41) proposed a vertebral fracture classification for osteopenic bone. Vertebral fractures were grouped according to fracture type (wedge, biconcavity, or compression) and by degree of deformity (Fig. 7). In a sample of 74 women suspected of having osteoporosis, 84% had vertebral fractures on plain x-ray, with an average of 3.3 fractures per person (41).

Magnetic resonance imaging may have an increasingly important role in the assessment of metabolic bone disease. Currently, it can be used to discriminate acute versus chronic fracture of the vertebrae and occult stress fractures of the proximal femur. These osteoporotic fractures demonstrate characteristic changes in the bone marrow, which distinguish them from other uninvolved parts of the skeleton and the adjacent vertebrae (Fig. 8) (42).

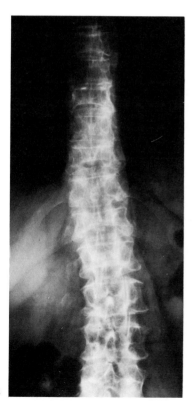
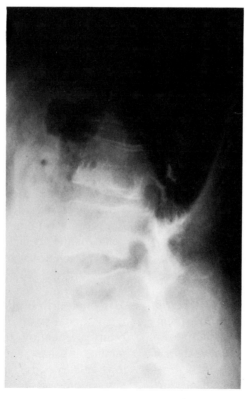

A,B

FIG. 6. Anteroposterior (A) and lateral (B) radiographs of the spine of a 58-year-old woman who was referred for work-up of "routine osteoporosis." The "moth-eaten" appearance of the vertebral bodies suggested a neoplastic process, and serum immunoelectrophoresis was ordered. An elevated gamma globulin region suggested a further work-up, and analysis of the urine by immunoelectrophoresis showed the presence of a Bence-Jones protein. A diagnosis of multiple myeloma was made.

CLASSIFICATION OF VERTEBRAL FRACTURES

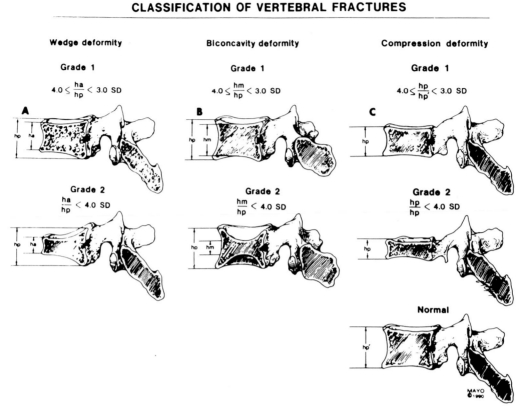

FIG. 7. Classification of vertebral fractures by type and grade. (Reprinted with permission from Eastell R, Cedel SL, Wahner HW, Riggs BL, Melton JL III [1991]: Classification of vertebral fractures. *J Bone Miner Res* 6:207–214.)

For Paget's disease, plain radiographs of the site in question are often definitive for making a diagnosis. These radiographs usually reveal a coarse trabeculation of the bone, with deformity and enlargement of the vertebra (Fig. 4). Upon polyphosphate-labeled isotopic scans in Paget's disease, bone will generally show increased uptake at the site of an active process. During the inactive phase, bone scans will demonstrate uptake only at the sites of fractures. Bone scans correlate well with serum alkaline phosphatase and hydroxyproline levels.

Scanning with CT is invaluable for assessing spinal involvement in Paget's disease, especially spinal stenosis associated with Paget's disease. The CT scan allows evaluation of facet hypertrophy, neural arch enlargement, and vertebral body expansion. Using the CT scan, a classification can be developed for spinal stenosis: Central stenosis is graded as mild if the encroachment is barely perceptible, moderate if the anteroposterior width of the spinal canal is reduced by 50%, and severe if there is greater than a 50% reduction in the width of the spinal canal. Lateral stenosis is diagnosed when the anteroposterior diameter of the lateral process measures less than 3 mm (43).

Perhaps the greatest advance in radiologic diagnostic technology in metabolic bone disease has been the development of bone densitometry (44). These methods, which measure the amount of bone mineral present at a given skeletal site, are accurate and noninvasive and can easily be repeated at 6- to 12-month intervals if necessary. At present, the most widely tested and clinically useful methods are single photon absorptiometry (SPA), dual energy quantitative computed tomography (QCT), and dual energy x-ray absorptiometry (DXA). The most important considerations in assessing the utility of each of these methods are the anatomical sites available for study, the radiation dose to the patient, and the precision and accuracy of the test. Precision is the coefficient of variation (standard deviation divided by the mean) for repeated measurements over a short period of time. Accuracy is the coefficient of variation for measurements in a specimen, the mineral content of which has been determined by other means (e.g., measurement of ash weight) (44).

In photon absorptiometry, a gamma ray source, a detector, and a system of electronics are used to measure beam attenuation through a section of bone. This method is usually applied to the radius with a relatively low radiation dose (10 to 20 mrem). For single photon absorptiometry, precision and accuracy are 1% to 3% and 5%, respectively (44,46).

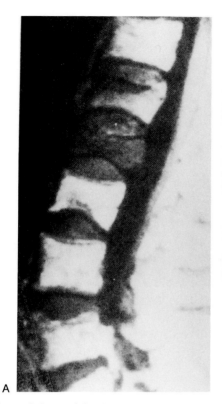
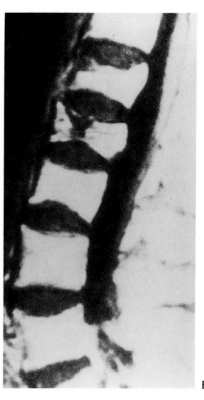

A   B

FIG. 8. Lateral views of the thoracolumbar spine showing acute and chronic vertebral fractures on sagittal T-1-weighted MRI. **A:** An acute fracture in which there is limited marrow activity, hence a weak signal. **B:** The same fracture 3 months later after normal marrow elements have begun to repopulate the trabecular spaces. The signal now appears bright. (Reprinted with permission from Majumdar S, Genant HK [1993]: QMR in assessment of trabecular bone mineral density and structure. Fourth International Symposium on Osteoporosis. Hong Kong, March 27-April 2.)

Quantitative computed tomography involves the use of a mineral calibration phantom in conjunction with a CT scanner. A lateral CT localizes the mid-plane of two to four lumbar vertebral bodies, and quantitative readings are then obtained from a region of trabecular bone in the anterior portion of the vertebra. The CT determination of density in the vertebra is then compared with known density readings of solutions in the phantoms. Measurements of the vertebrae are then averaged and used to calculate the density of trabecular bone, expressed as mineral equivalent of K_2HPO_4 (mg/cm^2). The radiation dose is 100 to 200 mrem, or approximately one-tenth of that used in a routine CT study (44,46). It has been shown that QCT measurements are fairly good at estimating vertebral strength as well as fracture risk (9). Precision and accuracy for QCT are 2% to 5% and 5% to 20%, respectively (45,46).

The most recent advance in bone densitometry technology is the use of DXA. In DXA, an x-ray tube emits an x-ray beam, the attenuation of which is detected by an energy-discriminating photon counter. This method is similar to photon densitometry except that it uses an x-ray beam as opposed to a photon beam, and it provides greater precision and accuracy and a lower radiation exposure (1 to 3 mrem). In addition, the average scan time for the spine is 5 minutes with DXA, compared with at least 20 minutes for QCT. Dual energy x-ray absorptiometry can be used to measure bone mass at the radius, calcaneus, hip, spine, or total body, and precision and accuracy are 0.5% to 2% and 3% to 5%, respectively (44,46).

The information obtained by a DXA scan shows the bone mineral density (BMD) of the patient and compares it with the normative BMD of other individuals of the same age and sex, as well as with that of younger individuals. These data are reported both as percentages and as points on a curve, allowing the physician to determine the degree to which the patient my deviate from the norm (Fig. 9). This information about the spine may help not only the physician, to manage the metabolic bone condition medically, but also the spinal surgeon, to decide whether there is sufficient bone mass to support metallic implants used during the process of spinal stabilization.

Bone Biopsy

An extremely useful test in certain metabolic bone disease evaluations is the transiliac bone biopsy. Although

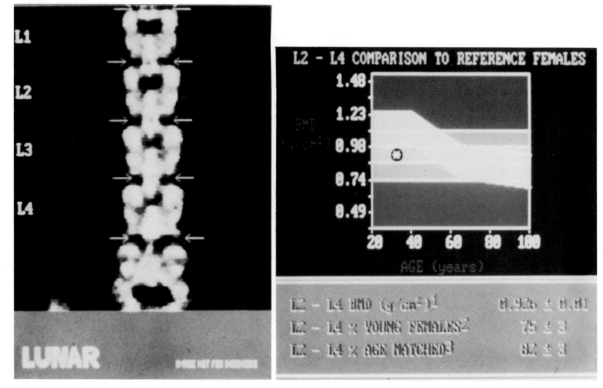

FIG. 9. Dual energy x-ray absorptiometry report on a patient with spinal instability who was referred for spinal stabilization. The patient is a 32-year-old woman whose bone mineral density is approximately 0.90 g/cm². This measurement is indicated as an asterisk on the graph shown on the right-hand side of the figure. Note that this graph has three types of shaded areas. The lightest area, which makes an angled path through the center of the graph, is the normal zone. The darkest areas on the top and bottom of the graph are the zones of abnormally increased or decreased densities, which are more than two standard deviations from the age-matched norm. The intermediate shaded area is one standard deviation from the norm. Note that the asterisk correlates with the bone density on the y axis and the patient's age on the x axis and falls within the intermediate shaded zone, indicating that the patient's bone density is low but within one standard deviation from the age-matched norm.

invasive, it is associated with minimal pain and inconvenience to the patient, can be performed on an ambulatory basis, and results in very few complications. It is indicated to establish a diagnosis in patients in whom osteomalacia or an occult malignancy is suspected, to distinguish between osteomalacia and osteitis fibrosa cystica in certain hemodialysis patients, or to elucidate the cause of severe osteopenia in patients whose blood and urine test results are insufficiently informative.

By convention, the biopsy is taken from a point 3 cm posterior and 3 cm inferior to the anterior superior iliac spine. The instrument used should produce a cylindrical specimen at least 6 mm in diameter, containing two cortices and an intervening marrow space. Once obtained, the specimen is embedded in methyl methacrylate and cut, processed, and stained using an undecalcified technique. Unstained sections are examined by fluorescence microscopy to determine the dynamic properties of bone. This is made possible by the presence of tetracycline labels (Fig. 3) (18). The cellular parameters of bone turnover are assessed by light microscopic examination of hematoxylin and eosin-stained sections. The technique involves preoperative administration of oral tetracycline in two doses that are separated by a specified number of days (e.g., tetracycline 250 mg orally three times a day for 3 days, off for 12 days, repeat for 3 more days, and biopsy between 3 and 7 days later).

Differentiation of mineralized from unmineralized osteoid is achieved using a salt stain such as Von Kossa, in which calcium and phosphorus salts appear dark, whereas unmineralized osteoid appears pale. Through the use of a computer-assisted calculating system, an optical drawing tube, and an integrated ocular eyepiece, a number of quantitative parameters of bone turnover are measured. This technique, known as "histomorphometry," enables the clinician to diagnose the disorder accurately and determine to what extent resorptive or blastic activities are influencing the disease. In patients with renal disease, special stains are used to identify the presence of aluminum in bone as a cause of osteomalacia.

This is particularly important because dramatic clinical improvements have been reported after removal of this metal from the bone (19).

TREATMENT

Osteoporosis

Preventive and treatment regimens for osteoporosis continue to evolve, as no single strategy is curative for this condition. This is particularly true for the treatment of primary osteoporosis, for which the etiology is not known. In secondary osteoporosis, however, an underlying cause of the disease can be identified and addressed before agents directed at correcting the skeletal lesion are introduced. Examples of conditions that are usually treatable include endogenous or iatrogenic hyperthyroidism, primary hyperparathyroidism, iatrogenic steroid-induced osteoporosis, and exercise-induced amenorrhea. In other cases, it is not possible to eliminate or reduce the effects of an instigating cause (e.g., steroid-induced osteoporosis), and treatment is extremely difficult. The recommendations offered in this section should be used as guidelines for treating patients with different types of osteoporosis. One must remember, however, that the responses of each patient to treatment may differ, necessitating alterations in management.

Medical treatment for osteoporosis can be broadly divided into anticatabolic and formation-stimulation therapies. Anticatabolic therapies include the use of drugs such as estrogen, calcitonin, and the bisphosphonates. These methods are aimed at producing a direct or indirect reduction in osteoclastic resorbing activity. The formation-stimulating therapies include sodium fluoride and PTH treatment.

The role of dietary calcium supplementation in the prophylactic treatment of osteoporosis appears to be most critical during the childhood and adolescent years, when peak bone mass is being built; today this is the cornerstone of prevention (47). An adequate dietary calcium intake is required at all times, however, to maintain normal skeletal health (Table 7). All patients being treated for osteoporosis should take 1.5 g of elemental calcium daily plus one or two multivitamins containing 400 units of vitamin D each. Patients who have or are at

TABLE 7. *Recommended dietary allowances of calcium (National Institutes of Health Advisory Panel, June 1994)*

Age	Elemental calcium (mg)
Birth–6 months	400
1–10 years	800–1200
11–24 years	1200–1500
25–50 years (women)[a]	1000
Postmenopausal years (women)[a]	1000–1500

[a] No information given for men who are older than 24 years.

risk for developing Type II osteoporosis should also follow this regimen (48). However, women at risk of developing Type I osteoporosis are not necessarily afforded protection by calcium supplementation alone (49). Although studies are in progress to determine the best preparation of oral calcium to use to enhance intestinal calcium absorption (e.g., calcium carbonate, calcium citrate, calcium citrate malate, etc.), it is clear that any calcium compound is best absorbed when taken with meals (50). At this time, the most effective treatment for most osteoporotic patients is estrogen. If the patient has no history of breast cancer or heart, thromboembolic, or endometrial disease, and if such therapy is indicated by her gynecologist, then estrogen is considered safe. The notion that estrogen therapy must begin within 5 years after menopause is no longer recognized as valid. As long as serum or urine biochemical tests, or bone biopsy, show that bone turnover (i.e., bone resorption) is still active, hormonal therapy will continue to be an effective form of therapy. The regimen used by the authors is: conjugated estrogen (0.625 mg/day) for days 1 to 25 of each month, progesterone (10 mg/day) for days 16 to 25, and neither medication from day 25 to the end of the month. A gynecologic examination is required at the onset of treatment, and an endometrial biopsy should be obtained 12 months after the initiation of therapy. If there is no unusual activity noted within the first year of treatment, no further biopsies are required. However, a yearly mammogram is strongly recommended.

Recently, the Food and Drug Administration approved two new drugs for the treatment of osteoporosis, Alendronate, a bisphosphonate compound, is the first non-hormonal drug approved for the treatment of this disease. Bisphosphonates are analogues of pyrophosphate that have been shown to have potent inhibitory effects on bone resorption. Alendronate is used in the dose of 10 mg per day, must be taken orally on an empty stomach, and the patient can only drink plain water (no other food or beverage) at the time of dosing. Because of the low bioavailability of this compound from the intestinal tract (approximately 0.7%) no food can be taken for at least thirty minutes after dosing. In addition, since some patients experience gastric side effects, the patient may not lie down for at least thirty minutes after dosing. Reports show that Alendronate prevents bone loss and is associated with gains in bone mass of up to 10% (51).

Calcitonin, a naturally occurring hormonal compound, has been approved by the FDA for several years in an injectable form. The approved dose of injectable salmon calcitonin is 100 units per day. Recently, the Food and Drug Administration approved a nasal spray formulation of this compound in a dose of 200 units per day. One spray to one nostril per day delivers this dose. Patients should alternate nostrils daily.

Although not yet approved for marketing by the Food and Drug Administration, a Food and Drug Administration Advisory Panel has recently recommended approval of a slow-release formulation of sodium fluoride. This drug has been shown to produce substantial increases in bone mass and a reduction in the incidence of new fractures (52).

Finally, if hypercalcuria accompanies the active osteoporotic state, one to two daily doses of thiazide are given to increase total body calcium retention.

Newer pharmacologic approaches aimed at increasing bone mass are now being investigated. These include PTH and the targeting of skeletal tissue with one of several growth factors identified as being active in bone. All of these approaches are highly experimental. Consequently, at present there are no well-established medical therapies for increasing bone mass.

Osteomalacia

Most osteomalacias respond to vitamin D therapy in doses of 50,000 units three to five times per week, combined with ample calcium intake (1500 mg/day). Certain forms in which hepatic, renal, or intestinal function is impaired require the addition of 25-hydroxyvitamin D_3 or phosphorus (17). When osteomalacia is caused by metabolic acidosis, a titrated dose of sodium bicarbonate is required (Table 8). To protect the patient from excess calcium absorption leading to renal calculus formation, urinary calcium excretion should be monitored every 3 months and maintained at less than 250 mg excreted per 24 hours. When aluminum or iron deposition has been identified in the bones of a patient with renal disease, removal of this metal with deferoxamine may be indicated (19).

Management of Osteopenic Spine Fractures and Rehabilitation

Symptomatic relief of spinal pain can be difficult to achieve in the treatment period of osteoporosis and osteomalacia. Although narcotic medications are some-

times effective, their use should be discouraged or at least limited because the abuse potential is high, given the prolonged period over which symptoms are expected to exist. In many instances, significant symptomatic relief can be achieved through physical therapy, rehabilitation, and bracing. External support in the form of a bivalved custom polypropylene body jacket is useful during the acute painful phase of a fracture, but should be discontinued when symptoms subside. In those patients who, after careful evaluation, are deemed able to withstand some low-level spinal stresses, a program of back extension and deep breathing exercises can be prescribed (53). In addition, counseling and instruction should be provided to all patients on the subjects of correct posture and body mechanics to prevent further pathologic fractures and the propensity to fall.

Spinal surgery is reserved for the patient who has a fracture that is causing gross deformity or neurologic impairment. The ability of the surgeon to obtain adequate purchase in bone is the main problem affecting any type of spinal fixation in osteopenic bone. Kostuik et al. (54) have reported the use of rods and screws inserted anteriorly into the vertebral body and have augmented these implants with polymethylmethacrylate, which was injected into enlarged drill holes. Kaneda et al. (55) described the use of anterior decompression and reconstruction with bioactive apatite-Wollastonite-containing glass ceramic vertebral prostheses. Recent developments in calcium phosphate-based ceramics research may lead to the availability of new materials such as fast-setting cements, which will ultimately be resorbed and replaced by bone. Such materials could be effective in enhancing both the fixation of spinal implants to mechanically impaired bone and the stability of spinal fixation systems (56).

Paget's Disease

The treatment of Paget's disease is based on the suppression of osteoclastic activity. Currently approved

TABLE 8. *Treatment of osteomalacia[a]*

Disorder	Vitamin D_2 (U)	25(OH)D_3 (μg)	1,25(OH)$_2D_3$ (μg)
Nutritional vitamin D deficiency	50,000 3–5 ×/week		
Malabsorption	50,000/day	20–200/day	
Anticonvulsant-induced osteomalacia (Dilantin[R])	50,000/day	20–100/day	
Renal osteomalacia[b]			1–2/day
Metabolic acidosis[c]	50,000/day		1–2/day
X-linked hypophosphatemia[d]			2–3/day until healing, then 0.5–1.0/day

With permission from Einhorn TA (1987): Evaluation and treatment methods for metabolic bone diseases. *Contemp Orthop* 14:21–34.
[a] All patients receive 1.5 g elemental calcium/day.
[b] Renal patients with bone aluminum may require deferoxamine.
[c] To correct acidosis, titrate blood pH with sodium bicarbonate.
[d] Add 1–2 g/day of phosphorus.

agents available in the United States include salmon and human calcitonin and etidronate disodium (Didronel®). Plicamycin (previously mithramycin), although not approved by the Food and Drug Administration for the treatment of Paget's disease, is available by prescription. The indication for treatment and the choice of therapeutic agent continue to be debated. Currently, the most widely followed indication for initiation of treatment is a serum alkaline phosphate level that is at least three times normal (20). Treatment is intended to alleviate patients' symptoms by suppressing osteoclastic activity. A decline in alkaline phosphatase or pyridinium cross-link levels of 50% or more can ameliorate symptoms in up to two-thirds of patients. Bone pain, headache, and low back pain are most likely to be relieved. Conversely, pain due to arthritic changes and bony deformity will not improve with medical treatment.

Human and salmon calcitonin are available in the United States as drugs that are administered by subcutaneous or intramuscular injection (calcitonin in the form of a nasal spray is currently undergoing clinical trials). Doses generally range from 50 units three times per week to between 100 and 200 units per day in severe cases. Symptoms may begin to improve over several weeks, and biochemical markers will begin to decline after 3 to 8 months. Decreasing effectiveness over time has been observed (57). Side effects are few and minimal, as noted above.

Etidronate disodium (Didronel®) is one of a family of agents known as the bisphosphonates, discussed previously in conjunction with their use in the treatment of osteoporosis. It is presently the only oral antiosteoclastic agent available, and it has been shown to have significant efficacy for the treatment of Paget's disease (20,57). It is commercially available in a 200- or 400-mg tablet. Although only a small amount of the drug is absorbed when ingested, more than two-thirds of patients will show improvement in their symptoms. The concern with etidronate is that, like some other bisphosphonates, at higher doses it inhibits not only bone resorption but also bone formation. For this reason, most patients are treated with cyclic regimens.

Plicamycin is a potent and toxic therapeutic modality that is indicated only for severe refractory cases, such as those involving spinal cord compression. It is administered intravenously and is infused every second to third day for five to ten infusions per cycle. Its action is to inhibit osteoclastic activity as well as reduce the hypervascularity associated with Paget's disease (20).

As noted, a variety of newer bisphosphonates are currently under study for the treatment of osteoporosis and Paget's disease. Pamidronate (Aredia®) has recently been approved for the treatment of hypercalcemia of malignancy and has been used to treat refractory Paget's disease. It is administered as an intravenous infusion, and its use requires careful medical monitoring. Other therapies, such as gallium nitrate, also have been used in experimental settings.

FINAL THOUGHTS

Current research in metabolic bone disease is directed toward improving noninvasive diagnostic tools, developing new and more effective pharmacologic and physical treatment modalities, and developing large-scale screening programs to identify high-risk groups in whom early prophylaxis should be started. While the pharmaceutical industry continues to develop better ways to control cellular function and the metabolic activity of bone, present management protocols must rely on existing knowledge. As spinal surgeons become more familiar with the metabolic pathways that govern spinal column function, their ability to manage some of the more challenging problems will improve. Intense efforts in the pharmaceutical industry are presently directed at improving drugs for treating bone loss. Recent evidence that osteoblasts possess estrogen receptors (58) may lead to the development of estrogen-like compounds that exert direct effects on bone cells without having oncogenic or atherogenic effects. New PTH-like peptides may be able to stimulate bone formation directly without increasing bone resorption. In the near future, a variety of bisphosphonates will appear on the market; these are touted as being more effective in preventing bone resorption than their antecedent analogues. These drugs will be used in the treatment of high-turnover osteoporosis, Paget's disease, and hyperparathyroidism.

Although the ability to actually "cure" existing osteoporosis by replacing lost trabeculae may seem farfetched, the current explosion of research and discovery in cellular and molecular biology suggests that this goal is attainable. As we learn more about cytokines, growth factors, proto-oncogenes, and cellular genes, perhaps it will become possible to alter the course of biology and reverse some of its flaws.

REFERENCES

1. Einhorn TA (1993): Bone metabolism and metabolic bone disease. In: Frymoyer JW, ed. Orthopaedic knowledge update 4 home study syllabus. Park Ridge, Illinois: *Am Acad Orthop Surg* 69–88.
2. Silver JJ, Majeska RJ, Einhorn TA (1995): An update on bone cell biology. *Curr Opin Orthop (in press)*.
3. Vaes G (1988): Cellular biology and biochemical mechanism of bone resorption: A review of recent developments on the formation, activation, and mode of action of osteoclasts. *Clin Orthop* 231:239–271.
4. Boskey AL (1989): Noncollagenous matrix proteins and their role in mineralization. *Bone Miner* 6:111–123.
5. Norman AW, Roth J, Orci L (1982): The vitamin D endocrine system: Steroid metabolism, hormone receptors and biological response. *Endocr Rev* 3:331–366.
6. Hurley DL, Tiegs RD, Wahner HW, Heath H (1987): Axial and appendicular bone mineral density in patients with long-term deficiency or excess of calcitonin. *N Engl J Med* 317:537–541.

7. Einhorn TA (1984): Osteoporosis and metabolic bone disease. *Adv Orthop Surg* 8:175–184.
8. Hansson T, Roos B, Nachemson A (1980): The bone mineral content and ultimate compressive strength of lumbar vertebrae. *Spine* 5:46–55.
9. McBroom RJ, Hayes WC, Edwards WT, Goldberg RP, White AA (1985): Prediction of vertebral body fracture using quantitative computed tomography. *J Bone Joint Surg* 67A:1206–1214.
10. Einhorn TA (1992): Bone strength: The bottom line. *Calcif Tissue Int* 51:333–339.
11. Burstein AH, Zilka HM, Heiple KG, Klein L (1975): Contributions of collagen and mineral to the elastic plastic properties of bone. *J Bone Joint Surg* 57A:956–961.
12. Riggs BL, Melton LJ III (1992): The prevention and treatment of osteoporosis. *N Engl J Med* 327:621–626.
13. Prince RL, Smith M, Dick IM, et al. (1991): Prevention of postmenopausal osteoporosis: A comparative study of exercise, calcium supplementation, and hormone-replacement therapy. *N Engl J Med* 325:1189–1195.
14. Jenson J, Christiansen C, Rodbro P (1985): Cigarette smoking, serum estrogens, and bone loss during hormone replacement therapy early after menopause. *N Engl J Med* 313:973–975.
15. Riggs BL, Melton LJ (1986): Involutional osteoporosis. *N Engl J Med* 314:1676–1686.
16. Riggs BL, Melton J (1983): Evidence for two distinct syndromes of involutional osteoporosis. *Am J Med* 309:899–901.
17. Frame B, Parfitt AM (1978): Osteomalacia: Current concepts. *Ann Intern Med* 89:966–982.
18. Frost HM (1969): Tetracycline-based histological analysis of bone remodeling. *Calcif Tissue Res* 3:211–236.
19. Malluche HH, Smith AJ, Abreo K, Faugere M-C (1984): The use of deferoxamine in the management of aluminum accumulation in bone in patients with renal failure. *N Engl J Med* 311:140–144.
20. Siris ES (1993): Paget's disease of bone. In: Favus MJ, ed. *ASBMR primer on metabolic bone diseases and disorders of mineral metabolism.* New York: Raven Press, pp. 375–384.
21. Meunier PJ, Slason D, Mathieu L, Chapuy MC, Delmas P, Alexandre C, Charhon S (1987): Skeletal distribution and biochemical parameters of Paget's disease. *Clin Orthop* 217:37–44.
22. Milgrom JW (1977): Radiographical and pathological assessment of the activity of Paget's disease of bone. *Clin Orthop* 127:43–54.
23. Meunier PJ, Coindre M, Edouard CM, Arlot ME (1980): Bone histomorphometry in Paget's disease. *Arthritis Rheum* 23:1095–1103.
24. Rebel A, Basle A, Pouplard A, Malkani K, Filmon R, Lepatezour A (1980): Bone tissue in Paget's disease of bone: Ultrastructure and immunocytology. *Arthritis Rheum* 23:1104–1114.
25. Basle MF, Rebel A, Fournier JG, Russell WC, Malkani K (1987): On the trail of Paramyxoviruses in Paget's disease of bone. *Clin Orthop* 217:9–15.
26. Altman RD, Brown M, Gargano F (1987): Low back pain in Paget's disease of bone. *Clin Orthop* 217:152–161.
27. Hadjipavlou A, Lander P (1991): Paget disease of the spine. *J Bone Joint Surg [AM]* 73:1376–1381.
28. Wyllie WG (1923): The occurrence in osteitis deformans of lesions of the central nervous system. *Brain* 46:336–351.
29. Herzberg L, Bayliss E (1980): Spinal cord syndrome due to noncompressive Paget's disease of bone: A spinal artery steal phenomenon reversible with calcitonin. *Lancet* 2:13–15.
30. Turner JWA (1940): The spinal complications of Paget's disease (osteitis deformans). *Brain* 63:321–349.
31. Schwartz GA, Reback S (1939): Compression of the spinal cord in osteitis deformans (Paget's disease) of the vertebrae. *AJR* 42:345–366.
32. Schajowicz F, Santini Araujo ES, Berenstein M (1983): Sarcoma complicating Paget's disease of bone. A clinicopathological study of 62 cases. *J Bone Joint Surg [Br]* 65:299–307.
33. Seret P, Basle MF, Rebel A, Reiner JC, Saint-Andre JP, Bertrans G, Audran M (1987): Sarcomatous degeneration in Paget's bone disease. *J Cancer Res Clin Oncol* 113:392–399.
34. Coley BL, Sharp GS (1931): Paget's disease predisposing factor to osteogenic sarcoma. *Arch Surg* 23:918.
35. Mirra JM, Bauer FCH, Grant TT (1981): Giant cell tumor with viral-like intranuclear inclusions associated with Paget's disease. *Clin Orthop* 158:243–251.
36. Jacobs TP, Michelson J, Polay JS, D'Adams AC, Canfield RE (1979): Giant cell tumor Paget's disease of bone: Familial and geographic clustering. *Cancer* 44:742–747.
37. Case Records of the Massachusetts General Hospital (1986): Weekly clinicopathological exercises. Case 1-1986 presentation of case. *N Engl J Med* 314:105–113.
38. Uebelhart D, Gineyts E, Chapuy MC, Delmas PD (1990): Urinary excretion of pyridinium crosslinks: A new marker of bone resorption in metabolic bone disease. *Bone Miner* 8:87–96.
39. Wasnich RD, Benfante RJ, Yano K, Heilbrun L, Vogel JM (1983): Thiazide effect on the mineral content of bone. *N Engl J Med* 309:344–347.
40. Morton DJ, Barrett-Connor EL, Edelstein SL (1994): Thiazides and bone mineral density in elderly men and women. *Am J Epidemiol* 139:1107–1115.
41. Eastell R, Cedel SI, Wahner HW, Riggs BL, Melton JL III (1991): Classification of vertebral fractures. *J Bone Miner Res* 6:207–214.
42. Majumdar S, Genant HK (1993): QMR in assessment of trabecular bone mineral density and structure. Fourth International Symposium on Osteoporosis. Hong Kong, March 27-April 2.
43. Zlatkin MB, Lander PH, Hadjipavlou AG, Levine JS (1986): Paget disease of the spine: CT with clinical correlation. *Radiology* 160:155–159.
44. Johnston CC Jr, Slemenda CW, Melton LJ (1991): Clinical use of bone densitometry. *N Engl J Med* 342:1105–1109.
45. Genant HK, Cann CE (1982): Quantitative computed tomography for assessing vertebral bone mineral. In: Genant HK, Chafetz N, Helms CA, eds. *Computed tomography of the lumbar spine.* Berkeley, California: University of California at San Francisco, University Press, pp. 289–314.
46. Genant HK, Block JE, Steiger P, Glueer CC, Ettinger B, Harris ST (1989): Advances in bone densitometry. In: *Osteoporosis including new diagnostic techniques.* ASBMR Workshop, Kelseyville. pp. 1–15.
47. Ott SM (1991): Bone density in adolescents. *N Engl J Med* 325:1646–1647.
48. Dawson-Hughes B, Dallal GE, Krall EA, Sadowski L, Sahyoun N, Tannenbaum S (1990): A controlled trial of the effect of calcium supplementation on bone density in postmenopausal women. *N Engl J Med* 323:878–883.
49. Riis B, Thomsen K, Christiansen C (1987): Does calcium supplementation prevent postmenopausal bone loss? A double-blind, controlled clinical study. *N Engl J Med* 316:173–177.
50. Recker RR (1985): Calcium absorption and achlorhydria. *N Engl J Med* 313:70–73.
51. Liberman UA, Weiss SR, Bröll J, Minne HW, Quan H, Bell NH, Rodriguez-Portales J, Downs RW, Dequeker J, Favus M, Seeman E, Recker RR, Capizzi T, Santora AC, Lombardi A, Shah RV, Hirsch LJ, Karpf DB (1995): Effect of Oral Alendronate on bone mineral density and the incidence of fractures in postmenopausal osteoporosis. *N Engl J Med* 333:1437–1443.
52. Pak CYC, Sakhaee K, Adams-Huet B, Piziak V, Peterson RD, Poindexter JR (1995): Treatment of postmenopausal osteoporosis with slow-release sodium fluoride. *Ann Intern Med* 123:401–408.
53. Sinaki M, Mikkelesen BA (1984): Postmenopausal spinal osteoporosis: Flexion versus extension exercises. *Arch Phys Med Rehabil* 65:593–596.
54. Kostuik JP, Errico TJ, Gleason TF (1986): Techniques of internal fixation for degenerative conditions of the lumbar spine. *Clin Orthop* 203:219–231.
55. Kaneda K, Asano S, Hashimoto T, Satoh S, Fujiya M (1992): The treatment of osteoporotic posttraumatic vertebral collapse using the Kaneda device and a bioactive ceramic vertebral prosthesis. *Spine* 17(8 Suppl):S295–303.
56. Lotz JC, Hu SS, Chiu FM, Glazer P, Poser RD, Contstantz BR (1995): In situ-setting hydroxyapatite augmentation of pedicle screw fixation in the lumbar spine: a cyclic study. *Trans Combin Orthop Res Soc* 2:241.
57. Kanis JA, Gray RE (1987): Long-term follow-up observations on treatment in Paget's disease of bone. *Clin Orthop* 217:99–125.
58. Eriksen EF, Colvard DS, Berg NJ, Graham ML, Mann KG, Spelsberg TC, Riggs BL (1988): Evidence of estrogen receptors in normal human osteoblast-like cells. *Science* 241:84–86.

Inflammatory Disorders

The Adult Spine: Principles and Practice,
2nd edition, J.W. Frymoyer, Editor-in-Chief.
Lippincott-Raven Publishers, Philadelphia © 1997.

CHAPTER 41

Differential Diagnosis and Conservative Treatment of Rheumatic Disorders

Louis Bessette, Jeffrey N. Katz, and Matthew H. Liang

This chapter discusses spine involvement in spondyloarthropathies, rheumatoid arthritis, and related disorders, with particular attention to ankylosing spondylitis and the rheumatoid cervical spine. Major emphasis is placed on pathogenesis, clinical features, diagnosis, prognosis, and conservative management.

L. Bessette, M.D., F.R.C.P.(C), M.S.: Laval University, Quebec, Canada; and Brigham and Women's Hospital, Boston, Massachusetts 02115.
J. N. Katz, M.D., M.S.: Assistant Professor, Harvard Medical School, Division of Rheumatology/Immunology, Brigham and Women's Hospital, Boston, Massachusetts 02115.
M. H. Liang, M.D., M.P.H.: Professor, Harvard Medical School, Robert Brigham Multipurpose Arthritis Center, Brigham and Women's Hospital, Boston, Massachusetts 02115.

SPONDYLOARTHROPATHIES

The spondyloarthropathies are a group of related disorders characterized by peripheral inflammatory arthritis, inflammation of sacroiliac joints, a tendency toward more diffuse spinal involvement, and sometimes extra-articular features including uveitis and conjunctivitis. Rheumatoid factor is usually absent. Pathologic changes in the spondyloarthropathies occur not only in joints but also in the entheses, attachments of ligaments into bone. Specific spondyloarthropathies include ankylosing spondylitis, psoriatic arthropathy, enteropathic arthropathy including Crohn's disease and ulcerative colitis, and reactive arthritis including Reiter's syndrome. Spine involvement may occur in all of the spondyloarthropathies but is especially common and severe in ankylosing spondylitis (AS). Ankylosing spondylitis is discussed in detail in this section, and the distinguishing features of other spondyloarthropathies are summarized.

ANKYLOSING SPONDYLITIS

Historical Aspects

Evidence of ankylosing spondylitis has been found in Egyptian mummies dating back to 2900 B.C. (32,155). Much later, clinical descriptions were presented by Bechterow and Marie and by Strumpell in the late 19th century (139). In the last 2 decades, it was distinguished from rheumatoid arthritis and linked with other spondyloarthropathies (6,135). The striking association between AS and the major histocompatibility antigen HLA-B27 (22,167) has provided a paradigm for understanding the role of genetic factors in the pathogenesis of rheumatic disease.

HLA-B27 and the Etiology of Ankylosing Spondylitis

The major histocompatibility complex (MHC), alternatively termed the HLA system, is a set of proteins encoded by genes on the sixth chromosome. The HLA antigens play critical roles in immune recognition of foreign molecules and tolerance to self. Dysfunction within the HLA system can lead to immunologic attack against the patient's own cells, the hallmark of autoimmunity (2).

HLA-B27 is found in 8% of American Caucasians but is present in more than 87.5% of American Caucasians with AS (93), which strongly suggests that HLA-B27 is important in the pathogenesis of AS. The last few years have brought important new insights into understanding the possible role of HLA-B27. Hammer et al. (89) have recently produced B27 transgenic rats. All rats in the line with very high gene copy numbers developed spontaneous inflammatory disease mimicking human spondyloarthropathy, with diarrhea, peripheral and axial arthritis, male genital tract inflammation, and psoriasiform skin and nail lesions. Despite these recent advances, the precise role of HLA-B27 remains unknown. It may resemble or serve as a receptor for an inciting antigen such as a virus (169). Alternatively, the genes encoding HLA-B27 may be linked closely with other genes that predispose to AS. The work of Hammer et al. argues for a more direct role. However, HLA-B27 is not the only factor predisposing to the disease, as only 2% of B27-positive whites have AS (107). In any case, AS is now viewed as an inflammatory disorder incited by infections and/or environmental agents in hosts rendered susceptible by HLA-B27 or related antigens (106,113).

Epidemiology

Estimates of the prevalence of AS vary considerably depending on the populations studied and the criteria used to identify cases (74). Population surveys from Rochester, Minnesota (38,40) and The Netherlands (186) indicated a prevalence of 0.1% to 0.2%, whereas smaller studies conducted in northern Norway and among blood donors at Stanford University pointed to a prevalence of 1% to 2% (36,75). The ratio of males to females also varies in these studies from 1:1 to 4:1. The prevalence may be underestimated, especially among women, who are less likely to receive pelvic radiographs and more likely to have less severe disease (73,104). Age at onset is usually between puberty and 45 years, peaking between 25 and 34 years. The incidence is much lower after the age of 55 (38).

It is also clear that the prevalence of AS varies directly with the prevalence of HLA-B27. For example, among American Caucasians, HLA-B27 is present in 8% and the prevalence of clinical disease is 0.1% to 0.2%. In comparison, HLA-B27 is present in 50% of Haida Indians, and their prevalence of AS is about 6% (93). Conversely, American Blacks have a 2% prevalence of HLA-B27, and the clinical disease prevalence of AS is approximately 75% of that seen in whites (10). The prevalence of AS and radiographic sacroiliitis among HLA-B27-positive Caucasians from different populations lies between 1% and 6.7% (111).

Pathology

The characteristic pathologic picture in AS is inflammation, bony erosion, and ankylosis. The inflammatory infiltrate is generally lymphocytic, and the target tissues include both joints and entheses. The latter are the sites where ligaments, tendons, and joint capsules attach to bone. In the axial skeleton, the sacroiliac, apophyseal, and costovertebral joints are generally involved and may eventually become ankylosed. Inflammation of the entheses, termed enthesopathy, is manifest in the axial skeleton by involvement of the junction of the annulus fibrosis and vertebral end plates. This leads to cortical erosions and the characteristic squaring of vertebral bodies often seen in spinal radiographs. Further inflammation and ossification of the annulus produce the bridging syndesmophytes (4,6,29) and the classic "bamboo" spine (Fig. 1). In the appendicular skeleton, arthritis of the knee and other diarthrodial joints is similar pathologically to rheumatoid arthritis. However, inflammation at the entheses may lead to bony erosions and spurs (6,29), often seen in the heel.

Clinical Manifestations

Axial Skeleton

Patients with AS usually present with insidious onset of low back pain and stiffness in the second and third decades. The location of pain varies from the trochanteric and gluteal regions to the thoracic spine. Buttock

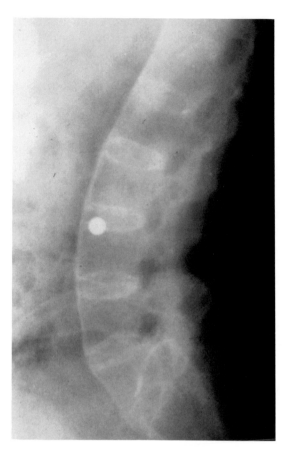

FIG. 1. Lateral radiograph of a 49-year-old male with long-standing ankylosing spondylitis. Note the complete ossification of anterior longitudinal ligaments and the preservation of disc spaces. The appearance is that of "bamboo" spine.

pain with radiation into the legs is common and may be confused with sciatica, but the pain from AS seldom radiates below the knee. Symptoms are usually worse in the morning and improve with exercise. This clinical feature helps distinguish AS from mechanical back pain, which generally is worse with activity and improves with rest. Patients with AS often complain of nocturnal pain, which interrupts sleep (104).

Patients with uncontrolled inflammation develop ankylosis of the lumbar, thoracic, and cervical spine. The disease generally progresses cephalad in a stepwise fashion (34). Patients assume a posture of lumbar flexion to transfer weight away from the inflamed apophyseal joints (175). Over time, thoracic kyphosis and limited cervical extension develop, resulting in a stooped posture. Pain from inflammation of the costovertebral joints inhibits chest expansion; eventual ankylosis of these joints may result in severe fixed limitations of chest expansion (104).

Complications

Spinal fracture is an uncommon but serious complication of advanced AS. The ankylosed spine has few mo-

bile segments. Thus, force applied perpendicular to the spine, as in a fall, must be absorbed by a rigid osteoporotic column. Fractures typically occur at C5 and C6 and through areas that were disc spaces before ankylosis, but can involve any spinal level. Fractures are often caused by minor trauma (95,137). Plain spinal radiographs often fail to visualize the fracture site, and tomography and bone scintigraphy may be required. Patients without neurologic deficits, or with stable neurologic deficits, are managed conservatively with immobilization. Progressive neurologic deficit is rare and is an indication for surgical decompression and fusion (71,95,137). Nonunion is a potential complication of conservative management and may lead to chronic pseudarthrosis, which is manifested radiographically by sclerosis of adjacent end plates, often with associated fractures of posterior elements. These lesions typically occur in the lumbar and lower thoracic spine and are sometimes extremely painful; they can be confused with infection or tumor (130).

Another complication of advanced AS is spondylodiscitis, which consists of focal, use-related pain accompanied by erosive sclerotic lesions in adjacent vertebral bodies. The levels most often involved are T8 through L2. It is not clear whether this lesion arises primarily from the inflammatory process or results from trauma. The radiologic appearances of spondylodiscitis, pseudarthrosis, and infectious discitis are similar. Anterior atlantoaxial subluxation is also described in AS patients. The prevalence of this complication is not known; it seems more common in those patients who have peripheral joint involvement and a long duration of disease, although in rare cases, it may be an early manifestation. Vertical, rotatory, and subaxial subluxations are extremely uncommon (94,180).

A rare neurologic complication of long-standing ankylosing spondylitis is the development of insidious damage to the lumbosacral nerve roots (cauda equina syndrome). Patients may present with pain in the distribution of the involved nerve roots, sensory loss, lower limb weakness, impotence, and bowel and bladder dysfunction. Radiologic evaluation usually shows enlargement of the caudal sac and multiple dorsal arachnoid diverticula, which may erode bone (94,127,182). Ossification of the posterior longitudinal ligament with myelopathy and spinal stenosis has also been described in AS (94).

Extraspinal Involvement

Peripheral arthritis occurs in more than one-third of patients with AS, sometimes as a presenting syndrome and more often as an associated event during a primary spinal syndrome. Hip involvement is common and is frequently bilateral, occurs early in the course of disease, and is a major cause of disability (52). Total hip replacement may be complicated by postoperative periarticular ossification and ankylosis (52). Indomethacin or irradiation administered in the perioperative period may prevent heterotopic bone formation (150). However, the results of hip replacement in AS seem comparable to those of other pathologic conditions. In a recent series of 150 total hip replacements in 87 patients with AS, only 9% required revision after an average follow-up of 7.5 years (35).

The most common sites of peripheral arthritis, in addition to the hip, are the shoulder, knee, wrist, metacarpal phalangeal joints, and metatarsal phalangeal joints (27,63). The arthritis is generally asymmetric, but may be symmetric and clinically indistinguishable from rheumatoid arthritis except for the absence of nodules and rheumatoid factor (63). Characteristic sites of peripheral enthesopathy include the ischial tuberosities, iliac crests, epicondyles of the elbows, shoulders, and insertions of the plantar fascia and Achilles tendon into the calcaneus (8,104).

Extraskeletal Features

The most common extraskeletal sites of involvement are the ocular, cardiac, and pulmonary systems. Nongranulomatous anterior uveitis occurs in 20% to 25% of patients. It is generally acute, unilateral, frequently recurrent, and manifested by pain and photophobia. Attacks subside in 4 to 8 weeks but may lead to visual impairment if not treated (157). Uveitis is also common in patients with the serologic findings of HLA-B27 who do not have the clinical features of AS; it is rare in HLA-B27-negative patients with AS. These observations suggest that uveitis may be an independent HLA-B27-related disease rather than a specific manifestation of AS (23,110,144).

Heart disease is a well-recognized complication of AS (13,26,179). The most prevalent lesions are aortic involvement and conduction defects. Autopsies in these patients reveal thickening and fibrosis of the aortic cusps and root, the ascending aorta, and the interventricular septum (26). Vascular disease and conduction disturbance each occur in 3% to 10% of patients (72) and may be fatal (179) or require a permanent pacemaker (13). Mitral valve disease, myocardial dysfunction, and pericarditis can also occur in AS.

Apical fibrobullous pulmonary disease develops insidiously in about 1% of patients with AS, with men at highest risk (158). Pulmonary function tests demonstrate restrictive physiology, and pathologic specimens reveal intra-alveolar and interstitial fibrosis. The lesions may cavitate and become infected by *Aspergillus*, mycobacteria, and other organisms; the infected cavities may invade blood vessels and cause hemoptysis (18,158). Although limited chest expansion due to costovertebral joint involvement is common, this complication alone rarely leads to significant respiratory compromise. Renal sediment abnormalities have been noted in AS (140), but renal dysfunction is rare and usually arises from secondary amyloidosis (104).

Women and Children

It has been postulated that AS has a different course in women than in men. Although there have been no well-designed and executed studies comparing AS in women and men, present knowledge indicates that there are no significant clinical or radiographic differences (73,98). "Skip lesions" of the cervical spine, occurring in the absence of lumbar or thoracic disease, were reported to be more common in females in one study (148) but not in other reports (19,55). However, the disease evolution is generally milder in women, as men show more severe and widespread radiographic changes (98). Patients with onset of AS before the age of 16 have a higher prevalence of peripheral arthritis and enthesopathy. These clinical manifestations may develop years before the onset of spinal symptoms or radiographic spine and sacroiliac involvement (28).

Natural History

Ankylosing spondylitis is a chronic disease with a highly variable course, most often characterized by spontaneous remissions and exacerbations (69). Although most patients present with relatively mild or self-limited disease and can maintain good functional capacity, AS may also be associated with significant disability and life-threatening complications. A study of 76 patients revealed that 30% were unable to work after 25 years of follow-up and 17% had to change jobs because of AS (125). Unfortunately, it is difficult to predict the prognosis in a single person. Patients with severe clinical disease in the first 10 years after onset are at greatest risk for subsequent disability (39). In a recent study, long-term disability was associated with cold working conditions and prolonged standing, whereas sedentary work, vocational counseling, and job training were favorable prognostic factors (84). Other risk factors for disability include peripheral arthritis, especially when the hip is involved (39).

The disease probably does not reduce life expectancy (38,40,100). Some series reported a decreased survival in AS patients, but these results are probably explained by selection bias, with higher mortality rates observed in patients with more severe disease (109,143). Patients who historically were treated with radiotherapy had decreased survival compared with age-matched normal subjects and also had a three-fold increased risk of leukemia (46,100).

Inflammatory Bowel Disease

Inflammatory bowel disease (IBD) is associated with spondyloarthropathy in about 15% to 20% of cases (79). The incidence is higher in Crohn's disease than in ulcerative colitis. In Crohn's disease, arthritis is more common in patients with colon involvement than in patients with involvement limited to the small intestine (79). Peripheral arthritis generally occurs acutely and concurrently with exacerbations of bowel disease. In contrast, spinal involvement progresses insidiously and independent of the bowel disease. About 5% of all patients with enteric arthropathy have HLA-B27, but the prevalence of HLA-B27 in patients with IBD and concomitant spine and sacroiliac involvement is 50% to 75%, indicating that HLA-B27 predisposes to spinal involvement (33,79).

Reactive Arthropathy (Reiter's Syndrome)

Reactive arthropathy refers to aseptic arthritides that develop during or soon after an infection elsewhere in the body (1). The arthritis may be accompanied by extraarticular features including conjunctivitis, iritis, urethritis, and mucocutaneous lesions. The triad of arthritis, urethritis, and ocular disease is referred to as Reiter's syndrome (197). The term "incomplete Reiter's" is often used if the entire triad is not present. The peripheral arthropathy is generally acute and oligoarticular, with a predilection for the lower extremities. Microbes implicated in HLA-B27 include the enteric pathogens Shigella, Salmonella, Yersinia, and Campylobacter, and venereally acquired Chlamydia. As with Reiter's syndrome, a relation between human immunodeficiency virus infection and spondyloarthropathies has been described in the last few years (30). An association with reactive arthritis has been postulated but not proven for *Clostridium difficile,* the gonococcus, β-hemolytic streptococci, and *Borrelia burgdorferi* (1,195). Sacroiliitis occurs in more than one-third of patients with Reiter's syndrome (61). Disability leading to unemployment or a change in job occurs in more than 25% of patients with Reiter's syndrome and is due primarily to calcaneal disease rather than spinal involvement (61).

The patterns of axial involvement in AS and IBD are clinically and radiographically indistinguishable and are quite distinct from the spondylitis associated with Reiter's syndrome and psoriasis (133). Sacroiliitis associated with AS and IBD is almost invariably bilateral and symmetric, whereas sacroiliitis may be unilateral or asymmetric in psoriatic and Reiter's spondyloarthropathy. Ossification of spinal ligaments and involvement of apophyseal and costovertebral joints is more pronounced in AS and enteric arthritis. Syndesmophytes develop in a stepwise cephalad progression in AS and IBD, whereas syndesmophyte formation is less prominent and more randomly distributed through the spine in Reiter's syndrome and psoriasis (133). Finally, patients with psoriatic and Reiter's spondyloarthropathy generally have better functional status than patients with AS or IBD, even when controlling for the extent of radiographic involvement. This difference has been attributed to the less prominent ligamentous and apophyseal joint involvement and the patchy distribution of syndesmophytes, which presumably allow greater spinal mobility (91).

SPINAL INVOLVEMENT IN RHEUMATOID ARTHRITIS

Epidemiology, Etiology, and Pathogenesis

Rheumatoid arthritis (RA) is a chronic systemic inflammatory disorder affecting multiple joints, including those of the cervical spine. The prevalence of RA is about 1%, with a peak incidence in the fourth through sixth decades. Females outnumber males at a ratio of approximately 2:1 (196). Although the etiology is unknown, it is postulated that RA develops after an environmental exposure, such as an infection, in genetically predisposed patients (174). Indeed, there is an association between RA and the Class II histocompatibility antigen HLA-DR4 (45). However, extensive searches for an infectious agent have proved fruitless to date.

Whereas the inciting cause of inflammation in RA is unknown, the inflammatory process itself has been well described. Initially, lymphocytes proliferate in the synovium, and polymorphonuclear leukocytes predominate in the synovial fluid. The polymorphonuclear leukocytes release hydrolytic enzymes, oxygen radicals, and arachidonic acid metabolites, which produce inflammation and cause tissue damage. Mononuclear cells produce lymphokines, which stimulate antibody production and the release of additional degradative products. The influx of fluid and the actions of inflammatory mediators produce the warmth, swelling, erythema, and pain that characterize rheumatoid synovitis (196).

A granulation tissue known as rheumatoid pannus is formed in the inflamed joint from proliferating fibroblasts and inflammatory cells. Pannus produces collagenase and other proteolytic enzymes capable of destroying adjacent cartilage, tendons, and bone. This destructive property leads to cartilage loss, bony erosions, tendon ruptures, and ligamentous laxity (196).

Clinical Features

Clinical manifestations of RA include arthritis, constitutional symptoms, and, in some patients, extraarticular involvement. Joint involvement is generally symmetric and polyarticular. The metacarpophalangeal and proximal interphalangeal joints, wrists, and knees are involved in more than 50% of cases. The neck, shoulders, elbows, hips, ankles, and talonavicular and metatarsal-phalangeal joints are also commonly affected. In general, joints that will ultimately develop severe destruction become symptomatic within the first year of disease onset (152).

Active inflammatory arthritis is usually accompanied by prominent morning stiffness and occasionally by low-grade fever. Fatigue is also common and may be disabling. It is not clear whether fatigue is largely a primary manifestation of inflammatory arthritis or a result of deconditioning (151).

Extra-articular manifestations are myriad and generally occur in patients with more severe arthritis and high titers of rheumatoid factor (96). Rheumatoid nodules arise in the subcutaneous tissue and have a predilection for pressure points over tendons and bone, such as the extensor surfaces of the arms. Ocular involvement includes keratoconjunctivitis sicca (Sjögren's syndrome), episcleritis and scleritis, and, rarely, scleromalacia perforans (59). Pericarditis is common and generally asymptomatic, whereas aortitis, myocarditis, and coronary vasculitis are rare and potentially fatal (78). Pleural effusions occur as well as rheumatoid pulmonary nodules, which are difficult to distinguish radiologically from malignancies. Felty's syndrome, characterized by splenomegaly and neutropenia, is often associated with other extra-articular features and with positive rheumatoid factor and may be complicated by pyogenic infections. Neurologic involvement includes compression neuropathies such as carpal tunnel syndrome, diffuse sensorimotor neuropathy, and mononeuritis multiplex arising from rheumatoid vasculitis. Inflammatory myopathy occurs in up to one-third of patients but is generally mild (88). Rheumatoid vasculitis affects small and medium-sized arteries and may be fatal (64). Mixed cryoglobulinemia and secondary amyloidosis occur rarely.

Diagnosis

The differential diagnosis of polyarthritis is extensive. Systemic lupus erythematosus, spondyloarthropathies, crystalline arthritis, acute hepatitis B, Lyme disease, and other disorders may be difficult to distinguish from RA, particularly early in the disease. Over months or years, these other self-limiting disorders usually resolve. The characteristic marginal erosions on radiographs also help distinguish RA from most other entities. The most helpful diagnostic findings for RA are symmetric swelling of several joints, particularly in the hand and wrist, accompanied by morning stiffness and fatigue.

Formal criteria for the classification of RA were established in 1958 (156). These criteria were modified by a

committee of the American College of Rheumatology, and the modified criteria were validated in a set of test patients in 1987 (3). The criteria are displayed in Table 6.

Therapy

The optimal care of the patient with RA requires a team approach incorporating internists, rheumatologists, orthopedists, and physical therapists along with social and psychological support. Medical therapy generally includes the administration of NSAIDs. Patients with ongoing inflammation or evidence of erosive disease despite adequate NSAID therapy are candidates for a slow-acting antirheumatic drug such as hydroxychloroquine, sulfasalazine, oral or intramuscular gold, penicillamine, azathioprine, cyclophosphamide, cyclosporine, or methotrexate. Slow-acting drugs are often termed remittive agents but have not been demonstrated conclusively to arrest the progression or promote healing of structural damage.

Methotrexate (MTX) has emerged in the last decade as among the more effective slow-acting drugs and is generally well tolerated (192). The probability of continuing MTX therapy at 7 years is between 46% and 72% (122,193). Its use is associated with side effects, mainly gastrointestinal, pulmonary, hematologic, cutaneous, and hepatic; toxicity represents the major reason for discontinuation of MTX (25). Monitoring liver disease with MTX has been a controversial subject for many years. Hepatic toxicity has been recognized for decades, but the experience in RA patients suggests that clinically serious liver disease is uncommon (190) and histologic changes are minimal (120,121). Recommendations for monitoring hepatic toxicity have been published recently (119). At present, routine surveillance liver biopsies are not recommended for RA patients receiving traditional doses of MTX, although this remains controversial. However, all

TABLE 6. *Proposed 1987 revised criteria for rheumatoid arthritis*

Four or more criteria must be present to diagnose rheumatoid arthritis:

1. Morning stiffness for at least 1 hour and present for at least 6 weeks.
2. Swelling of three or more joints for at least 6 weeks.
3. Swelling of wrist, metacarpophalangeal, or proximal interphalangeal joints for 6 or more weeks.
4. Symmetric joint swelling.
5. Hand roentgenogram changes typical of rheumatoid arthritis, which must include erosions or unequivocal bony decalcification.
6. Rheumatoid nodules.
7. Serum rheumatoid factor by a method positive in less than 5% of normals.

slow-acting drugs have potential toxic side effects even in experienced hands; thus, consultation with a rheumatologist experienced in their use is recommended.

Physical and occupational therapists attempt to maintain strength and range of motion, educate the patient about joint protection, and provide adaptive devices. End-stage joints may be managed surgically with arthrodesis or arthroplasty. Soft-tissue lesions, such as tendon rupture and refractory synovitis, may also require repair or synovectomy.

Prognosis

Age-adjusted mortality is about twofold greater in patients with RA than in population controls. Mortality is increased for specific causes such as infection, lymphoproliferative malignancy, and gastroenterologic disorders (199). Disability in work and home activities also may be considerable in patients with RA (53,173). The prognosis is variable, however, and a portion of patients will have mild disease without significant disability or excess mortality. Factors associated with increased disability, morbidity, and mortality include age, male sex, disease severity, functional impairment, education, nodules, joint count, rheumatoid factor, erythrocyte sedimentation rate, and prednisone use (199).

CERVICAL SPINE DISEASE IN RHEUMATOID ARTHRITIS

The cervical spine is among the most common sites involved in RA (15). Radiologic evidence of cervical spine disease has been noted in 19% to 88% of RA patients; the wide variation in reported prevalence is probably due to differences in disease severity, duration of disease, and radiologic criteria (15,87). The spine is particularly vulnerable in RA because it contains 32 synovial-lined joints, 2 atlanto-occipital, 1 atlanto-odontoid, 14 apophyseal, 10 uncovertebral, and 5 discovertebral (15).

Clinical Syndromes

Even in the absence of structural damage, inflammation in the cervical spine may cause substantial pain and stiffness. The pain is deep and aching in quality and varies in location according to the structures involved. Pain arising from the atlanto-occipital complex radiates to the occipital, retro-orbital, and temporal regions. Involvement of C3 and C4 causes pain that radiates to the side of the neck and clavicles, while C5 and C6 involvement causes pain that radiates to the deltoids. Pain may be accompanied by paravertebral muscle spasm.

Patients with persistent inflammation in the joints of the neck are at risk for structural damage, which produces several distinct syndromes. Subluxation is a consequence of cartilaginous damage, bone erosion, and ligamentous laxity. Classification of the principal types of subluxation is presented in Fig. 5. Each type of subluxation can occur alone or in combination. Consequently, it is always necessary to look for various combinations and phases of subluxations. Neurologic symptoms of cervical spine involvement are numerous and relate to the type and location of the lesion (Table 7). Unfortunately, the clinical manifestations of advanced RA, including weakness, atrophy, sensory neuropathy, ankylosis, and deformity, often seen in RA patients with cervical spine disease, may mask the neurologic signs.

Anterior Atlantoaxial Subluxations

Anterior atlantoaxial subluxation (AAS) is the most frequent radiologic spinal abnormality in RA, with a reported frequency of 19% to 70% (87). Normally C1 is prevented from sliding anteriorly with respect to C2 by the transverse ligament, which spans C1 posterior to the odontoid. The odontoid and the transverse ligament are separated by a synovial-lined space which may become inflamed, resulting in laxity of the transverse ligament. This allows anterior displacement of C1, particularly with neck flexion (see Fig. 6). Clinical manifestations of anterior AAS include occipital, retro-orbital, and temporal pain and a "clunking" sensation on neck flexion. An unusual but potentially disastrous complication of AAS is myelopathy resulting from compression of the spinal cord between the odontoid and the anteriorly displaced posterior arch of C1. Myelopathic findings are generally limited to hyperactive deep tendon reflexes, but may include incontinence, weakness, sensory loss, and paresis when involvement is severe.

Vertebrobasilar insufficiency is another complication of AAS. The vertebrobasilar arteries may become kinked around the anteriorly displaced C1. Symptoms include vertigo and, rarely, loss of consciousness or "drop attacks." Concomitant atherosclerosis may further contribute to the development of vertebrobasilar insufficiency (99).

Posterior C1-C2 Subluxation

Unlike anterior displacement, posterior C1-C2 subluxation is an extremely rare complication of rheumatoid cervical spine disease (87). In this syndrome, extensive erosion of the odontoid allows the arch of C1 to slip posteriorly, impinge on the spinal cord, and cause myelopathy. Defects in the arch of C1 may also allow posterior subluxation.

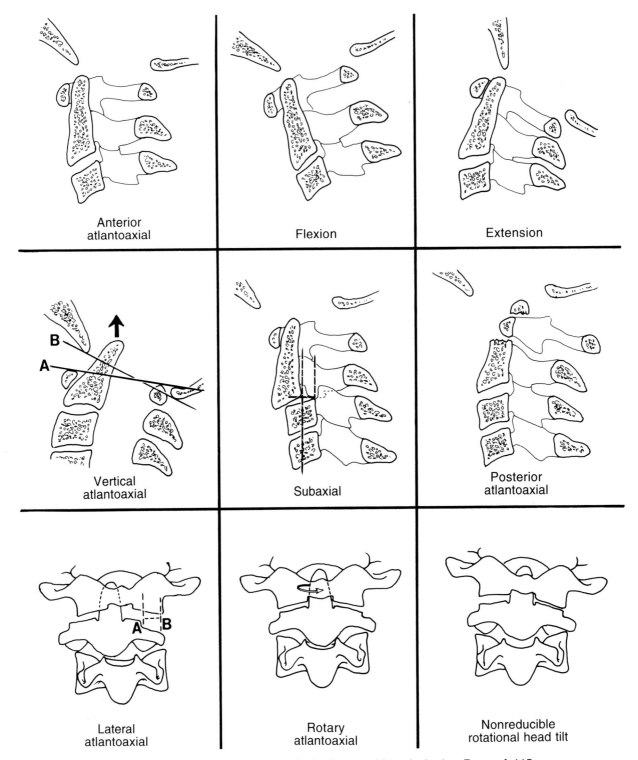

FIG. 5. Classification of subluxation in the rheumatoid cervical spine. From ref. 115.

TABLE 7. *Correlations between the types of rheumatoid cervical spine and the associated neurologic findings*

Rheumatoid changes	Area affected	Symptoms and signs
Anterior and posterior AAS	Occipital nerves	Occipitocervical pain
	Vertebrobasilar insufficiency	Ataxia, vertigo, dysarthria, nystagmus, drop attack
Vertical AAS	Brain stem	
	Cervical nerves, X, XI, XII	Dysphagia, dysphonia
	Cervical nerve VI	Diplopia
	Spinal nucleus of trigeminal nerve	Facial numbness, depressed corneal reflexes
Subaxial subluxation	Cervical nerves roots	Radicular pain, paresthesia, hyperesthesia; muscular weakness, atrophy; diminished tendon reflexes; diminished cutaneous sensibility
All forms	Pyramidal tract	Weakness, spasticity, paresis, Lhermitte's sign, increased tendon reflexes, diminished abdominal reflexes, extensor-plantar responses, incontinence
	Dorsal funiculus	Distal paresthesia, dissociated sensory loss
	Spinothalamic tract	Decreased pain sensation

Adapted from Santavirta et al. (162).

Vertical Subluxation

Vertical displacement of the odontoid into the foramen magnum is variously termed atlantoaxial impaction, vertical or cranial settling, or vertical subluxation. It is seen in 3% to 4% of the overall RA population and occurs in about 22% of RA patients with some type of cervical subluxation (42,194). This lesion is caused by progressive cartilage loss, bony erosion, and collapse of the articulations of the occipital condyles, lateral masses of the atlas, and particularly the lateral facet joints of C1-C2. As a result, the odontoid migrates vertically with respect to the occiput, entering the foramen magnum (see Figs. 7 and 8). The odontoid may compress the medulla oblongata, causing myelopathy and, rarely, death from brain stem compression (134,176).

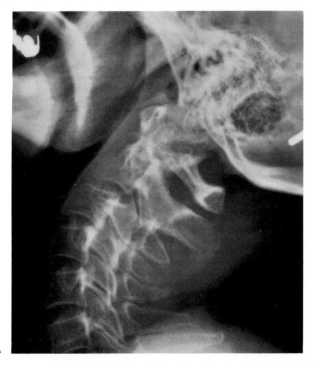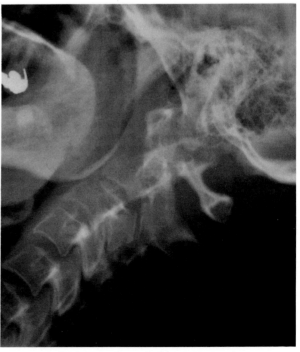

A   B

FIG. 6. Atlantoaxial subluxation in rheumatoid arthritis. **A:** With neck extension, the odontoid and the anterior arch of C1 are separated by just 1–2 mm. **B:** With neck flexion, the separation increases to 7 mm.

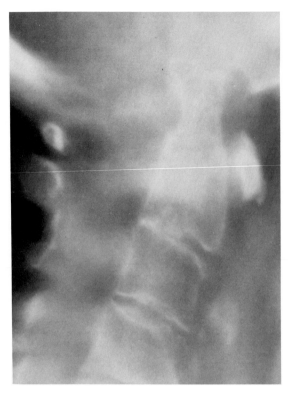

FIG. 7. Vertical subluxation in rheumatoid arthritis. Tomographic view reveals the odontoid entering the foramen magnum. Note that the anterior arch of C1 opposes the lower half of the odontoid rather than the upper half, as occurs normally.

Lateral and Rotation Subluxation

Asymmetric erosion and collapse of the lateral masses of C1 and C2 may result in lateral subluxation and rotation of C1 with respect to C2. The principal clinical finding is neck-shoulder pain and limited head rotation (86). In addition, some patients tilt the head in the direction of the most severely affected lateral facet joint (85,87). Nonreducible rotational head tilt in association with lateral mass collapse has been described in up to 10% of patients with advanced RA (85). Atlantoaxial (C1-C2) facet joint involvement is often associated with other types of subluxation (86).

Subaxial Subluxation and Spondylodiscitis

Subluxations below the second cervical vertebra occur in 7% to 29% of patients with RA, most commonly at the C2-C3 and C3-C4 levels. Serial cervical subluxations, producing a "staircase" appearance, are characteristic (Fig. 9). These lesions arise from laxity of the anterior and/or posterior longitudinal spinal ligaments and involvement of the facet joint. Myelopathy is uncommon, occurring only with severe dislocation or infiltration of

the spinal cord by pannus arising from the uncovertebral joints of Luschka (87,114).

Spondylodiscitis refers to extensive erosion of adjacent vertebral end plates, with disc space loss, in the absence of osteophytes. The pathogenesis of these lesions in RA is controversial. Some authors postulate a primary inflammatory process in the uncovertebral joints of Luschka (6), whereas others claim that these lesions are traumatic, arising from cervical instability (129,166). Spondylodiscitis is painful, may cause neurologic deficits, and is difficult to distinguish clinically from infection (87). If systemic features are prominent, aspiration may be indicated to exclude septic discitis.

Cervical Fusion: Juvenile Rheumatoid Arthritis

Cervical spine involvement occurs in 60% to 70% of patients with juvenile rheumatoid arthritis. These patients suffer the same spinal lesions as adults with RA and also have distinct abnormalities, including growth disturbances and zygapophyseal joint fusion. Cervical zygapophyseal fusion occurred in 52% of one series of referral patients (54). The C2-C3 segment was involved most frequently and was usually associated with ankylo-

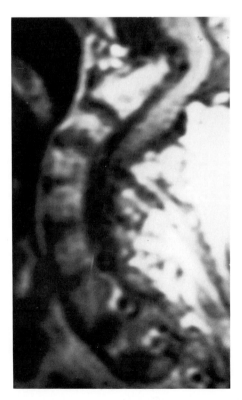

FIG. 8. T1-weighted magnetic resonance image of vertical subluxation in rheumatoid arthritis. The odontoid has projected into the foramen magnum, causing marked kinking of the spinal cord.

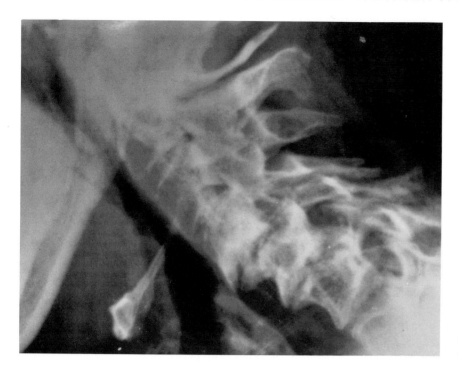

FIG. 9. Serial cervical subluxations (staircase subluxations) along with spondylodiscitis at C4–C5.

sis at lower levels. Cervical fusion was more common in patients with systemic or polyarticular involvement. Because zygapophyseal fusion frequently occurs during years of growth, hypoplastic vertebrae at the levels of fusion are common (54).

Diagnosis of Rheumatoid Cervical Spine Disease

History and Physical Examination

Persistent pain in the occipital, temporal, or retroorbital areas suggests pathology in the atlantoaxial complex. Vertigo is an extremely important historic finding because it suggests vertebral artery compression. On physical examination, hyper-reflexia and Babinski responses are the earliest clues to the presence of cervical spine compression. Sensory findings are not prominent in early cervical myelopathy and are more likely due to the generalized sensorimotor neuropathy commonly seen in advanced RA (96). The Sharp-Purser test has been suggested as a physical examination maneuver for the diagnosis of atlantoaxial subluxation. With the patient's head in slight flexion, the examiner places one index finger on the spinous process of C2 and attempts to slide the head posteriorly using the palm of the other hand on the forehead. If the head slides, the test is positive. In one series of 123 outpatients (183), the Sharp-Purser test had a sensitivity of 69% and a specificity of 96% for atlantoaxial subluxation compared with radiologic evidence of AAS. Nonetheless, it seems prudent to eschew any form of cervical manipulation in this setting.

Radiologic Diagnosis

Specific structural diagnosis of the rheumatoid cervical spine is made radiographically. Existing diagnostic criteria have been developed with conventional radiography and tomography, but CT and especially MRI have improved visualization of the rheumatoid spine and should be used to evaluate myelopathy.

Lateral, flexion, and extension views are used to diagnose atlantoaxial and posterior C1-C2 subluxation (see Fig. 6). Separation between the anterior odontoid and posteroinferior tubercle of C1 by more than 2.5 mm in women and 3.0 mm in men is indicative of AAS (114). This criterion is less valuable in the setting of vertical subluxation, wherein C1 articulates with the wider inferior aspect of the odontoid. This results in a deceptively small C1-odontoid distance despite reduction in the anteroposterior diameter of the spinal canal. Posterior subluxation is noted if the posterior aspect of the arch of C1 is aligned posterior to the anterior border of the body of C2 (194).

Several conventions have been employed to detect vertical subluxation on lateral radiographs (Table 8 and Fig. 10). The most widely used is McGregor's line. Projection of the odontoid greater than 4.5 mm superior to this line indicates vertical subluxation. The methods of McGregor, Chamberlain, and McRae have been criticized because the apex of the dens is often difficult to identify as a result of erosions and osteoporosis.

Ranawat's system assesses the collapse at the C1-C2 articulation (145). The Redlund-Johnell method detects

TABLE 8. *Lines used for the determination of cranial settling*

Names	Description	Normal value
McGregor	Most caudal point of the occipital curve of the skull to the dorsal margin of the hard palate	Odontoid tip <4.5 mm above this line
Chamberlain	Posterior lip of foramen magnum to dorsal margin of the hard palate	Odontoid tip <3 mm above this line
McRae	Posterior lip of foramen magnum to anterior border of foramen magnum	Odontoid tip below this line
Ranawat	Distance between the pedicle of the axis and the transverse axis of the atlas	Men: 17 ± 2 mm Women: 15 ± 2 mm
Redlung-Johnell	Distance between the lower end plate of C2 and McGregor line	Men: >34 mm Women: >29 mm

changes at both the occipitoatlantal and atlantoaxial joints (147). This system is adequate for follow-up but may be unsatisfactory for screening because it relies on the height of the odontoid, which varies widely between individuals. Kauppi et al. (101) recently described a new method for screening and grading vertical subluxation (not shown). This technique determines cranial settling by the presence of superior migration of the superior aspect of the body of C2 beyond a line drawn between the most inferior points of the anterior and posterior arches of C1.

Lateral subluxation is demonstrated on anteroposterior films if the lateral masses of C1 are displaced more than 2 mm lateral to the masses of C2 (194). Rotatory subluxation of C1-C2 is reflected in asymmetry in the size of the lateral masses of C1 and C2 (85). Subaxial subluxations characteristically are manifest by a serial "staircase" pattern of vertebral body subluxations on lateral x-rays, particularly at C2-C3 and C3-C4. These lesions may be reducible and visible only on flexion and extension views. Rheumatoid spondylodiscitis consists of disc-space narrowing, vertebral end-plate sclerosis,

and a paucity of osteophytes (114,129). These lesions are often best visualized with CT and MRI.

The radiographic degree of subluxation on plain radiographs does not reliably correspond to the development and extent of neurologic deficit (194,198). The risk of neurologic deficit appears to be increased with an anterior subluxation of >9 mm (194), the presence of atlantoaxial impaction (176), and a posterior atlanto-odontoid interval ≤13 mm (17).

CT is a more sensitive technique than conventional x-rays for detecting bony erosions and discriminating soft tissues, including the spinal canal (20). MRI is even more accurate in distinguishing soft tissues such as ligaments and pannus. It also visualizes the spinal cord and vertebral arteries without the use of intravenous or intrathecal contrast. Sagittal views may demonstrate alterations in the spinal cord such as kinking at the foramen magnum in cervical subluxations (51,171) (Fig. 8). MRI is now considered the preferred procedure in RA patients who have signs and symptoms of spinal cord or brain stem compression and vertebral artery compromise (118). A good correlation exists between neurologic symptoms

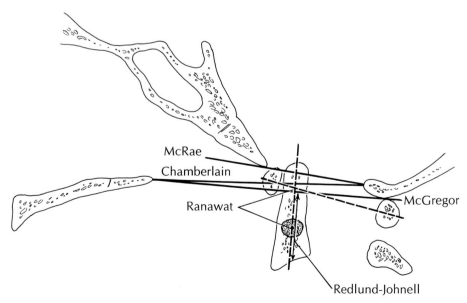

FIG. 10. Lines used for the determination of cranial settling.

and the degree of spinal cord compression on MRI (21,181). Functional MRI with flexion and extension has been recommended to identify spinal cord compression (51,154), but some studies have not shown any benefit compared with the combination of MRI in the neutral position and plain x-ray (124,142). Prolonged positioning of a patient who has severe AAS in cervical flexion may be fatal. In addition, the relatively high cost and long examination times of MRI limit its use.

Epidemiology and Natural History of Rheumatoid Cervical Spine Disease

The prevalence of structural deformities in the rheumatoid spine ranges from less than 10% to more than 80%, depending on the duration and severity of disease in the population under study. Cervical spine involvement may occur early in the course of disease. A prospective study of 100 RA patients with disease duration of less than 1 year at study entry revealed that within 5 years of follow-up, 12 had developed atlantoaxial subluxation, 20 had subaxial, and 3 had vertical subluxations (198). The major risk factor for the development of cervical subluxations is the severity of the underlying rheumatoid disease. Specifically, the presence of erosions, positive rheumatoid factor, and use of steroids are associated with a greater prevalence of cervical spine disease and increased progression over time (131,177).

The risk of neurologic deficits increases with greater C1-odontoid separation and with the presence of vertical subluxations (194). Not surprisingly, neurologic deficits are also more common in patients with seropositive, erosive, nodule-forming disease (131). Although up to 40% of patients with cervical subluxations may have abnormal neurologic examinations, the incidence of disabling neurologic damage is low. In one study of 130 patients with cervical subluxations followed for an average of 8 years, six patients developed symptomatic vertebrobasilar insufficiency and one developed tetraplegia (177). In two other studies of 76 (131) and 332 (97) patients followed for greater than 5 years, no disability or deaths related specifically to spinal cord compression were noted.

Although fatal neurologic events are rare, rheumatoid patients with cervical subluxations have greater mortality than RA controls and much greater mortality than age-matched population controls (165,177). It is well established that RA patients have higher mortality than the general population, that deaths are usually due to comorbid conditions or infections rather than direct complications of rheumatoid disease, and that disease severity is the major risk factor for mortality in RA (199). Hence, it appears that cervical spine disease is associated with high mortality because it is a marker of severe RA rather than a direct cause of death. This point has important therapeutic implications. Surgery may be life-saving in rare cases with rapid neurologic deterioration, but in general

surgery will not decrease the substantial mortality experienced by patients with cervical subluxations (165) due to other causes. Thus, prophylactic stabilization cannot be justified.

Therapy

The goals of therapy for RA cervical spine involvement include pain relief and stabilization of any progressive neurologic deficits. Patients with pain and stiffness primarily due to acute inflammation, rather than structural damage, often respond to treatment of the underlying disease with NSAIDs and slow-acting agents. Antiinflammatory medication cannot reverse structural damage.

Rigid or soft cervical collars are often offered to patients with neck pain associated with cervical subluxations. Soft collars only partially constrain cervical motion, but probably serve to remind patients to limit movement. Although they may ameliorate symptoms, collars do not arrest radiologic or neurologic progression of cervical subluxation (131,177). Range of motion and strengthening exercises; heat, cold, and ultrasound treatments; and the use of cervical support pillows are often prescribed as well. Although the efficacy of exercises and modalities has not been studied critically, these therapies appear to be beneficial (16).

Neck pain generally abates with the therapeutic measures outlined above, even in the presence of advanced subluxations. Resolution may require weeks to months. Persistent pain associated with significant apophyseal joint destruction may respond to corticosteroid injection of these joints. Patients with progressive neurologic deterioration are candidates for cervical fusion, as are patients with progressive vertebrobasilar insufficiency. The management of patients with stable, nondisabling neurologic deficits, such as hyperreflexia or Babinski responses, is less certain. Because neurologic deterioration is less common in the setting of mild subluxations, patients with radiographically mild AAS or vertical subluxation and stable neurologic deficits can be managed by careful observation (131). In more advanced subluxations, the threshold to operate should be lower, but it is still generally safe to observe the subluxation carefully if the neurologic examination is stable (131). Intractable neck pain in the setting of advanced cervical subluxations, even with a stable neurologic examination, may be approached surgically, often with substantial pain relief (163).

SPINAL INVOLVEMENT IN OTHER RHEUMATOLOGIC DISORDERS

Spinal involvement has been reported in crystalline arthropathies, metabolic disorders, and other inflammatory conditions.

Gout

Gout is an intermittent crystalline synovitis caused by monosodium urate deposition, typically involving single joints such as the first metatarsophalangeal joint, the ankle, wrist, and elbow. Chronic gout is characterized by more frequent attacks, occasional polyarticular involvement, and the appearance of tophi, which are deposits of monosodium urate in joints and periarticular tissues. There have been ten reported cases of neurologic syndromes arising from deposition of tophi in the spine. Patients with this complication generally have long-standing polyarticular tophaceous gout. Spinal column involvement has ranged from the C1 level to S1, including C1-C2 subluxation in three patients. All but one of the reported patients underwent laminectomy (187, 189). An indirect association also exists between elevations of serum uric acid and diffuse idiopathic skeletal hyperostosis (149). Neurologic syndromes associated with spinal tophi should be treated surgically if indicated and with antihyperuricemic drugs. Allopurinol is the drug most commonly used for the treatment of tophaceous gout. It decreases urate synthesis by inhibiting the xanthine oxidase enzyme (60). Patients with low urate excretion may be treated with uricosuric drugs (probenecid, sulfinpyrazone). NSAIDs are usually the treatment of choice during acute gouty attacks. Intra-articular glucocorticoids are also effective in acute gout limited to a single joint or bursa. Colchicine is a good alternative to NSAIDs, but its use is limited by its toxicity. The mechanism of action of colchicine is not fully understood. It appears to interfere with several steps of neutrophil action in the inflammatory response: decreased release of chemotactic factors, reduced leukocyte adhesion, and microtubule inhibition (43). It is also important in gouty patients to control possible precipitating factors, such as alcohol consumption and use of drugs (salicylates, diuretics).

Pseudogout

The syndrome of pseudogout refers to synovitis caused by deposition of calcium pyrophosphate crystals. Pseudogout occurs as an isolated disease or in association with Wilson's disease, hyperparathyroidism, hypothyroidism, hemochromatosis, hypomagnesemia, amyloidosis, osteoarthritis, and infection. Clinical manifestations are myriad and may include acute intermittent monoarthritis, particularly of the knee, and symmetric polyarthritis similar to RA. Calcium pyrophosphate deposition (CPPD) in the ligamentum flavum has been reported in 24 cases (5,24, 68,102,164) in the setting of myelopathy and spinal stenosis. Involvement of the cervical spine with radiculomyelopathy appears to be the most frequent neurologic manifestation (102), but lumbar spinal stenosis has also been

described in four cases (24,49). Treatment of CPPD involves correction of the associated metabolic disorders described above, if possible. However, no available therapy has proven effective to remove CPPD already present or to retard its deposition. NSAIDs and/or low doses of daily colchicine may provide symptom relief.

Ochronosis

Ochronosis is a rare autosomal recessive genetic defect caused by a deficiency of homogentisic oxidase, an enzyme involved in the metabolism of tyrosine and phenylalanine. Homogentisic acid accumulates and deposits preferentially in cartilage, skin, sclerae, and other sites. Homogentisic acid is oxidized to a dark pigmented product, which causes pigmentation of involved sites. It is believed that the pigment binds to collagen fibers in the joint, compromising the resiliency of articular cartilage and resulting in premature degenerative arthritis. Arthropathy usually develops in the third decade. Involvement of the lumbar spine is common and results in extensive disc degeneration and, occasionally, lumbar radiculopathy (70,168).

Acromegaly

Acromegaly arises from persistently elevated secretion of growth hormone and results in bony and soft-tissue changes, including widening of the vertebral bodies. These changes may, rarely, narrow the spinal canal, causing the syndrome of spinal stenosis (141). Endogenous or exogenous excess of glucocorticoids produces Cushing's syndrome, which has myriad manifestations including centripetal deposition of fat in the subcutaneous areas of the face, neck, and trunk. Two cases have been reported of epidural fat deposition in the lumbar spine, causing cauda equina compression and the spinal stenosis syndrome (126).

Amyloidosis

Amyloidosis is characterized by deposition of extracellular protein fibrils in target organs. Several distinct amyloidosis syndromes have been defined, as distinguished by the biochemical composition of the amyloid fibrils, the spectrum of associated diseases, and predilection for target organs. The most common musculoskeletal manifestation of amyloidosis is carpal tunnel syndrome (123). Five cases of spinal claudication due to amyloidosis have been reported, one of which was confirmed pathologically. Three of these patients had hereditary amyloidosis, and each had primary amyloidosis and amyloidosis associated with multiple myeloma (92). Amyloidosis may arise in the setting of long-term hemodialysis. The amyloid protein in these cases has been identified as B_2-microglobulin, which is inefficiently cleared by conventional dialysis membranes (184). Patients with dialysis-related amyloidosis have been noted to develop erosive spondyloarthropathy characterized by amyloid infiltration of the intervertebral discs and vertebral end plates (170). We have evaluated a patient in our institution with odontoid erosion and posterior C1-C2 subluxation due to the amyloidosis of hemodialysis (77). No treatment is available for this condition; the use of more permeable dialysis membranes has been recommended to enhance clearance of B_2-microglobulin (41). There is evidence that secondary hyperparathyroidism may also play a role in the spondyloarthropathy seen in long-term hemodialysis (132).

Systemic Lupus Erythematosus

Another important spinal manifestation of rheumatic disease is transverse myelitis due to systemic lupus erythematosus (SLE) (191). Approximately 30 cases have been reported in the literature, and most referral centers see a case every few years. This complication arises from inflammatory vascular lesions in the vessels supplying the spinal cord. Clinical findings include sensory loss at and below the level of the lesions and impaired sphincter control. Transverse myelitis has a grave prognosis in patients with SLE; one-third of patients die within 6 weeks of diagnosis and only 10% to 15% recover completely. High-dose corticosteroids, often with cytotoxic agents, have been used because of the dire nature of this complication, but the efficacy of treatment is not known. It is suggested that treatment should be initiated as early as possible (191).

Diffuse Idiopathic Skeletal Hyperostosis

Diffuse idiopathic skeletal hyperostosis (DISH) is an ossifying diathesis of unknown etiology that affects 5% to 10% of patients over 65 years of age (Fig. 11). DISH is characterized by flowing calcification and ossification of the anterolateral aspects of contiguous vertebral bodies, with frequent ossification of extraspinal sites as well (149). The diagnosis of DISH cannot be made in the presence of apophyseal joint erosions or radiographic sacroiliitis, and these must be excluded to avoid confusion of DISH with ankylosing spondylitis. DISH is often discovered incidentally, and symptoms are usually mild or nonexistent. However, dysphagia, cervical myelopathy, and lumbar spinal stenosis may result from the extensive calcification (80,149).

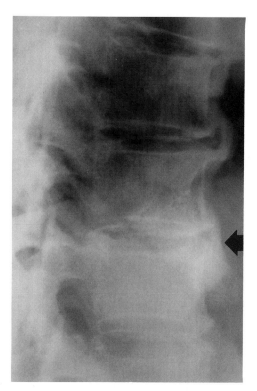
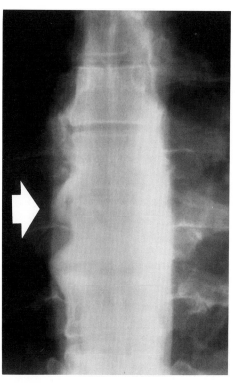

A   B

FIG. 11. A: Radiograph showing diffuse idiopathic skeletal hyperostosis (DISH). **B:** Anteroposterior radiograph of the same patient with DISH.

Fibromyalgia

Fibromyalgia, or fibrositis, is the final condition discussed in this chapter and probably the most prevalent. Originally described in the 19th century, fibromyalgia has been widely recognized only recently as a distinct clinical syndrome (66). Typical patients are female and aged 20 to 50 years. Their chief complaint is diffuse musculoskeletal pain, often most pronounced in the cervical spine and shoulder regions. The diagnosis should be entertained in patients with chronic musculoskeletal pain who have multiple tender points and no evidence of other systemic conditions. Additional common findings include fatigue, stiffness, sleep disturbance, and numbness. Classification criteria for fibromyalgia have been developed recently (200) (Table 9). Laboratory tests, radiographs, and muscle biopsies are generally unremark-able. In fact, despite extensive laboratory investigation, the mechanism of disease remains unknown. The most consistent objective finding is tenderness in specific characteristic spots. These points are bilateral and cluster in the trapezius, suboccipital muscle insertions, low cervical region, supraspinatus, second rib (costochondral junction), lateral epicondyle, gluteal region, greater trochanter, and the medial knee (Table 9).

Treatment is nonspecific. Controlled studies have demonstrated that cyclobenzaprine hydrochloride (Flexeril) at 10 to 40 mg/day (12) and amitriptyline 25 mg at night (67) decrease pain and tenderness and improve patients' sleep and overall well-being. Aerobic exercise is recommended as well (66). Although structural damage and excess mortality do not occur in fibromyalgia, the syndrome is usually chronic. Remissions are infrequent and usually transient (57).

Many patients have localized myofascial pain in the cervical or lumbar spine. Often these patients do not have the diffuse tenderness and sleep disturbance characteristic of the fibromyalgia syndrome. The management of localized myofascial pain should be individualized and may include muscle relaxants, heat, stretching exercises, and rest. Attention to ergonomic stressors, particularly in the workplace, is often useful. One potential mistake in treating fibromyalgia and localized myofascial pain syndromes is to undertake prolonged, expensive, and potentially invasive diagnostic evaluations. Another pitfall is to insist that patients comply with medical regimens, which may be minimally effective. Patients are often most satisfied with a thoughtful but focused evaluation and supportive care with an emphasis on reassurance rather than medication.

TABLE 9. *The American College of Rheumatology 1990 criteria for the classification of fibromyalgia[a]*

1. History of widespread pain.
   Definition. Pain is considered widespread when all of the following are present: pain in the left side of the body, pain in the right side of the body, pain above the waist, and pain below the waist. In addition, axial skeletal pain (cervical spine or anterior chest or thoracic spine or low back) must be present. In this definition, shoulder and buttock pain is considered as pain for each involved side. "Low back" pain is considered lower segment pain.
2. Pain in 11 of 18 tender point sites on digital palpation.
   Definition. Pain, on digital palpation, must be present in at least 11 of the following 18 tender point sites:
   Occiput: bilateral, at the suboccipital muscle insertions.
   Low cervical: bilateral, at the anterior aspects of the intertransverse spaces at C5–C7.
   Trapezius: bilateral, at the midpoint of the upper border.
   Supraspinatus: bilateral, at origins, above the scapula spine near the medial border.
   Second rib: bilateral, at the second costochondral junctions, just lateral to the junctions on upper surfaces.
   Lateral epicondyle: bilateral, 2 cm distal to the epicondyles.
   Gluteal: bilateral, in upper outer quadrants of buttocks in anterior fold of muscle.
   Greater trochanter: bilateral, posterior to the trochanteric prominence.
   Knee: bilateral, at the medial fat pad proximal to the joint line.
   Digital palpation should be performed with an approximate force of 4 kg.
   For a tender point to be considered "positive," the subject must state that the palpation was painful. "Tender" is not to be considered "painful."

Modified from Wolfe et al. (200).

[a] For classification purposes, patients will be said to have fibromyalgia if both criteria are satisfied. Widespread pain must have been present for at least 3 months. The presence of a second clinical disorder does not exclude the diagnosis of fibromyalgia.

ACKNOWLEDGMENT. We are grateful to Dr. Barbara Weissman for providing the radiographs and to Mrs. Jacqueline Mazzie for preparing the manuscript.

REFERENCES

1. Aho K (1989): Bowel infection predisposing to reactive arthritis. *Clin Rheumatol* 3:303–319.
2. Arnett FC (1987): Seronegative spondylarthropathies. *Bull Rheum Dis* 37:1–12.
3. Arnett FC, Edworthy SM, Bloch DA, et al. (1988): The American Rheumatism Association 1987 revised criteria for the classification of rheumatoid arthritis. *Arthritis Rheum* 31:315–324.
4. Aufdermaur M (1989): Pathogenesis of square bodies in ankylosing spondylitis. *Ann Rheum Dis* 48:628–631.
5. Baba H, Maezawa Y, Kawahara N, et al. (1993): Calcium crystal deposition in the ligamentum flavum of the cervical spine. *Spine* 18:2174–2181.
6. Ball J (1971): Enthesopathy of rheumatoid and ankylosing spondylitis. *Ann Rheum Dis* 30:213–223.
7. Baron M, Zendel I (1989): HLA-B27 testing in ankylosing spondylitis: An analysis of the pretesting assumptions. *J Rheumatol* 16:631–636.
8. Bartolome FJ (1986): Pedal radiographic manifestations of the seronegative spondyloarthritides. Part III: Ankylosing spondylitis. *J Am Podiat Med Assoc* 76:380–385.
9. Battafarano DF, West SG, Rak KM, et al. (1993): Comparison of bone scan, computed tomography, and magnetic resonance im-

aging in the diagnosis of active sacroiliitis. *Semin Arthritis Rheum* 23:161–176.

10. Baum J, Ziff M (1971): The rarity of ankylosing spondylitis in the Black race. *Arthritis Rheum* 14:12–18.

11. Bennett PH, Burch TA (1968): *Population studies in rheumatic diseases.* Amsterdam: Emedica Foundation, pp. 456–537.

12. Bennett RM, Gatter RA, Campbell SM, Andrews RP, Clark SR, Scarola JA (1988): A comparison of cyclobenzaprine and placebo in the management of fibrositis. *Arthritis Rheum* 31:1535–1542.

13. Bergfeldt L, Edhag O, Vedin L, Vallin H (1982): Ankylosing spondylitis: An important cause of severe disturbances of the cardiac conduction system. *Am J Med* 73:187–191.

14. Blackburn WD Jr, Alarcon GS, Ball GV (1988): Evaluation of patients with back pain of suspected inflammatory nature. *Am J Med* 85:766–770.

15. Bland JH (1974): Rheumatoid arthritis of the cervical spine. *J Rheumatol* 1:319–342.

16. Bland JH (1987): *Disorders of the cervical spine.* Philadelphia: W.B. Saunders, pp. 203–204.

17. Boden SD, Dodge LD, Bohlman HH, Rechtine GR (1993): Rheumatoid arthritis of the cervical spine: A long-term analysis with predictors of paralysis and recovery. *J Bone Joint Surg [Am]* 75:1282–1297.

18. Boushea DK, Sundstrom WR (1989): The pleuropulmonary manifestations of ankylosing spondylitis. *Semin Arthritis Rheum* 18:277–281.

19. Braunstein EM, Martel W, Moidel R (1982): Ankylosing spondylitis in men and women: A clinical radiographic comparison. *Radiology* 144:91–94.

20. Braunstein EM, Weissman BN, Seltzer SE, Sosman JL, Wang AM, Zamani A (1984): Computed tomography and conventional radiographs of the craniocervical region in rheumatoid arthritis. *Arthritis Rheum* 27:26–31.

21. Breedveld FC, Algra PR, Vielvoye CJ, Cats A (1987): Magnetic resonance imaging in the evaluation of patients with rheumatoid arthritis and subluxations of the cervical spine. *Arthritis Rheum* 30:624–629.

22. Brewerton DA, Hart FD, Nicholls A, et al. (1973): Ankylosing spondylitis and HL-A27. *Lancet* 1:904.

23. Brewerton DA, Nicholls A, Caffrey M, et al. (1973): Acute anterior uveitis and HLA27. *Lancet* 2:994–996.

24. Brown TR, Quinn SF, D'Agostino AN (1991): Deposition of calcium pyrophosphate dihydrate crystals in the ligamentum flavum: Evaluation with imaging and CT. *Radiology* 178:871–873.

25. Buchbinder R, Hall S, Sambrook PN, et al. (1993): Methotrexate therapy in rheumatoid arthritis: A life table review of 587 patients treated in community practice. *J Rheumatol* 20:639–644.

26. Bulkley BH, Roberts WC (1973): Ankylosing spondylitis and aortic regurgitation: Description of the characteristic cardiovascular lesion from study of eight necropsy patients. *Circulation* 48:1014–1027.

27. Burgos-Vargas R, Clark P (1989): Axial involvement in seronegative enthesopathy and arthropathy syndrome and its progression to ankylosing spondylitis. *J Rheumatol* 16:192–197.

28. Burgos-Vargas R, Naranjo A, Castillo J, Katona G (1989): Ankylosing spondylitis in the Mexican Metizo: Patterns of disease according to age at onset. *J Rheumatol* 16:189–191.

29. Bywaters EGL (1984): Pathology of the spondyloarthropathies. In: Calin A, ed. *Spondyloarthropathies.* Orlando, Florida: Grune and Stratton, pp. 43–68.

30. Calabrese LH (1993): Human immunodeficiency virus (HIV) infection and arthritis. *Rheum Dis North Am* 19:477–488.

31. Calabro JT (1986): Ankylosing spondylitis: A critical review of current management. *Adv Therapy* 3:1–20.

32. Calin A (1985): Ankylosing spondylitis. In: Kelley WN, Harris ED Jr, Ruddy Shaun, Sledge CB, eds. *Textbook of rheumatology, 2nd ed.* Philadelphia: W.B. Saunders, pp. 993–1006.

33. Calin A (1988): Ankylosing spondylitis and the spondyloarthropathies. In: Schumacher HR, ed. *Primer on rheumatic diseases,* 9th ed. Atlanta: Arthritis Foundation, pp. 142–147.

34. Calin A, Elswood J (1988): The relationship between pelvic, spinal and hip involvement in ankylosing spondylitis: One disease process or several? *Br J Rheumatol* 27:393–395.

35. Calin A, Elswood J (1989): The outcome of 138 total hip replace-

ments and 12 revisions in ankylosing spondylitis: High success rate after mean follow-up of 7.5 years. *J Rheumatol* 16:955–958.

36. Calin A, Fries JF (1975): The striking prevalence of ankylosing spondylitis in "healthy" W27 positive males and females. A controlled study. *N Engl J Med* 293:835–839.

37. Calin A, Porta J, Fries JF, Schurman DJ (1977): Clinical history as a screening test for ankylosing spondylitis. *JAMA* 237:2613–2614.

38. Carbone LD, Cooper C, Michet CJ, et al. (1992): Ankylosing spondylitis in Rochester, Minnesota, 1935–1989: Is the epidemiology changing? *Arthritis Rheum* 35:1476–1482.

39. Carette S, Graham D, Little H, Rubenstein J, Rosen P (1983): The natural disease course of ankylosing spondylitis. *Arthritis Rheum* 26:186–190.

40. Carter ET, McKenna CH, Brian DD, Kurland LT (1979): Epidemiology of ankylosing spondylitis in Rochester, Minnesota, 1935–1973. *Arthritis Rheum* 22:365–370.

41. Chanard J, LaVaud S, Toupance O, Roujouleh H, Melin JP (1986): Carpal tunnel syndrome and type of dialysis membrane used in patients undergoing long-term hemodialysis. *Arthritis Rheum* 29:1170–1171.

42. Chang DJ, Stephen AP (1993): Neurologic complications of rheumatoid arthritis. *Rheum Dis Clin North Am* 19:955–973.

43. Clements PJ, Paulus HE (1993): Nonsteroidal anti-inflammatory drugs (NSAIDs). In: Kelley WN, Harris ED Jr, Ruddy Shaun, Sledge CB, eds. *Textbook of rheumatology, 2nd ed.* Philadelphia: W.B. Saunders, pp. 700–730.

44. Corkill MM, Jobanputra J, Gibson T, Macfarlane DG (1990): A controlled trial of sulphasalazine treatment of chronic ankylosing spondylitis: Failure to demonstrate a clinical effect. *Br J Rheumatol* 29:41–45.

45. Cush JJ, Lipsky PE (1987): The immunopathogenesis of rheumatoid arthritis: The role of cytokines in chronic inflammation. *Clin Aspects Autoimmun* 1:2–13.

46. Darby SC, Doll R, Gill SK, Smith PG (1987): Long-term mortality after a single treatment course with x-rays in patients treated for ankylosing spondylitis. *Br J Cancer* 55:179–190.

47. Dougados M, van der Linden S, Juhlin R, et al. (1991): The European Spondylarthropathy Study Group preliminary criteria for the classification of spondylarthropathy. *Arthritis Rheum* 34:1218–1227.

48. Dougados M, Boumier P, Amor B (1986): Sulphasalazine in ankylosing spondylitis: A double blind controlled study in 60 patients. *Br Med J* 293:911–914.

49. Drouillard PJ, Mrstik LL (1988): Lumbar stenosis associated with hypertrophied ligamentum flavum and calcium pyrophosphate crystal deposition. *J Am Osteopath Assoc* 88:1019–1021.

50. Dunn NA, Mahida BH, Merrick MV, Nuki G (1984): Quantitative sacroiliac scinti-scanning: A sensitive and objective method for assessing efficacy of nonsteroidal antiinflammatory drugs in patients with sacroiliitis. *Ann Rheum Dis* 43:157–159.

51. Dvorak J, Grob D, Baumgartner H, Gschwend N, Grauer W, Larsson S (1989): Functional evaluation of the spinal cord by magnetic resonance imaging in patients with rheumatoid arthritis and instability of the upper cervical spine. *Spine* 14:1057–1064.

52. Dwosh IL, Resnick D, Becker MA (1976): Hip involvement in ankylosing spondylitis. *Arthritis Rheum* 19:683–692.

53. Erhardt CC, Mumford PA, Venables PJ, Maini RN (1989): Factors predicting a poor life prognosis in rheumatoid arthritis: An eight year prospective study. *Ann Rheum Dis* 48:7–13.

54. Espada G, Babini JC, Maldonado-Cocco JA, Garcia-Morteo O (1988): Radiologic review: The cervical spine in juvenile rheumatoid arthritis. *Semin Arthritis Rheum* 17:185–195.

55. Eustace S, Coughlan RJ, McCarthy C (1993): Ankylosing spondylitis. A comparison of clinical and radiographic features in men and women. *Ir Med J* 86:120–122.

56. Fam AG, Rubenstein JD, Chin-Sang H, Leung FY (1985): Computed tomography in the diagnosis of early ankylosing spondylitis. *Arthritis Rheum* 28:930–937.

57. Felson DT, Goldenberg DL (1986): The natural history of fibromyalgia. *Arthritis Rheum* 29:1522–1526.

58. Feltelius N, Hällgren R (1986): Sulphasalazine in ankylosing spondylitis. *Ann Rheum Dis* 45:396–399.

59. Ferry AP (1985): Ocular manifestations of rheumatic disease. In:

Kelley WN, Harris ED, Ruddy S, Sledge CB, eds. *Textbook of rheumatology.* Philadelphia: W.B. Saunders, pp. 511–532.

60. Fox IH (1993): Antihyperuricemic drugs. In: Kelley WN, Harris ED, Ruddy S, Sledge CB, eds. *Textbook of rheumatology.* Philadelphia: W.B. Saunders, pp. 822–831.

61. Fox R, Calin A, Gerber RC, Gibson D (1979): The chronicity of symptoms and disability in Reiter's syndrome: An analysis of 131 consecutive patients. *Ann Intern Med* 91:190–193.

62. Fraser SM, Sturrock RD (1990): Evaluation of sulphasalazine in ankylosing spondylitis—an interventional study. *Br J Rheumatol* 29:37–39.

63. Ginsburg WW, Cohen MD (1983): Peripheral arthritis in ankylosing spondylitis. *Mayo Clin Proc* 58:593–596.

64. Glass D, Soter NA, Schur PH (1976): Rheumatoid vasculitis. *Arthritis Rheum* 19:950–952.

65. Godfrey RG, Calabro JJ, Mills D, et al. (1972): A double-blind crossover trial of aspirin, indomethacin, and phenylbutazone in ankylosing spondylitis. *Arthritis Rheum* 15:110.

66. Goldenberg DL (1987): Fibromyalgia syndrome: An emerging but controversial condition. *JAMA* 257:2782–2787.

67. Goldenberg DL, Felson DT, Dinerman H (1986): A randomized, controlled trial of amitriptyline and naproxen in the treatment of patients with fibromyalgia. *Arthritis Rheum* 29:1371–1377.

68. Gomez H, Chou SM (1989): Myeloradiculopathy secondary to pseudogout in the cervical ligamentum flavum: Case report. *Neurosurgery* 25:298–302.

69. Goodacre JA, Mander M, Dick WC (1991): Patients with ankylosing spondylitis show individual patterns of variation in disease activity. *Br J Rheumatol* 30:336–338.

70. Gordon DA (1993): Alkaptonuria (ochronosis). In: Schumacher HR, ed. *Primer in the rheumatic diseases,* 10th ed. Atlanta: Arthritis Foundation, pp. 227–228.

71. Graham B, Van Peteghem PK (1989): Fractures of the spine in ankylosing spondylitis. *Spine* 14:803–807.

72. Graham DC, Smythe HA (1958): The carditis and aortitis of ankylosing spondylitis. *Bull Rheum Dis* 9:171–174.

73. Gran JT, Husby G (1990): Ankylosing spondylitis in women. *Semin Arthritis Rheum* 19:303–312.

74. Gran JT, Husby G (1993): The epidemiology of ankylosing spondylitis. *Semin Arthritis Rheum* 22:319–334.

75. Gran JT, Husby G, Hordvik M (1985): Prevalence of ankylosing spondylitis in males and females in a young middle-aged population of Tromso, northern Norway. *Ann Rheum Dis* 44:359–367.

76. Gran JT, Husby G, Hordvik M (1985): Spinal ankylosing spondylitis: A variant form of ankylosing spondylitis or a distinct disease entity? *Ann Rheum Dis* 44:368–371.

77. Gravallese EM, Baker N, Lester S, et al. (1992): Musculoskeletal manifestations in beta 2-microglobulin amyloidosis. Case discussion. *Arthritis Rheum* 35:592–602.

78. Gravallese EM, Corson JM, Coblyn JS, Pinkus GS, Weinblatt ME (1989): Rheumatoid arthritis: A rarely recognized but clinically significant entity. *Medicine* 68:95–106.

79. Gravallese EM, Kantrowitz FG (1988): Arthritic manifestations of inflammatory bowel disease. *Am J Gastroenterol* 83:703–709.

80. Griffiths ID, Fitzjohn TP (1987): Cervical myelopathy, ossification of the posterior longitudinal ligament, and diffuse idiopathic skeletal hyperostosis: Problems in investigation. *Ann Rheum Dis* 46:166–168.

81. Grill V, Smith M, Ahern M, Littlejohn G (1988): Local radiotherapy for pedal manifestations of HLA-B27-related arthropathy. *Br J Rheumatol* 27:390–392.

82. Gross M, Brandt KD (1981): Educational support groups for patients with ankylosing spondylitis: A preliminary report. *Pat Couns Health Educ* 3:6–12.

83. Guerra J, Resnick D (1984): Radiographic and scintigraphic abnormalities in seronegative spondyloarthropathies and juvenile chronic arthritis. In: Calin A, ed. *Spondyloarthropathies.* Orlando, Florida: Grune and Stratton, pp. 339–382.

84. Guillemin F, Briançon S, Pourel J, Gaucher A (1990): Long-term disability and prolonged sick leaves as outcome measurements in ankylosing spondylitis: Possible predictive factors. *Arthritis Rheum* 33:1001–1006.

85. Halla JT, Fallahi S, Hardin JG (1982): Nonreducible rotational head tilt and lateral mass collapse. *Arthritis Rheum* 25:1316–1324.

86. Halla JT, Hardin JG (1990): The spectrum of atlantoaxial facet joint involvement in rheumatoid arthritis. *Arthritis Rheum* 33:325–329.

87. Halla JT, Hardin JG, Vitek J, Alarcon GS (1989): Involvement of the cervical spine in rheumatoid arthritis. *Arthritis Rheum* 32:652–659.

88. Halla JT, Koopman WJ, Fallahi S, Oh SJ, Gay RE, Schrohenloher RE (1984): Rheumatoid myositis: Clinical and histologic features and possible pathogenesis. *Arthritis Rheum* 27:737–743.

89. Hammer RE, Maika SD, Richardson JA, Tang J-P, Taurog JD (1990): Spontaneous inflammatory disease in transgenic rats expressing HLA-B27 and human β_{2m}: An animal model of HLA-B27 associated disorders. *Cell* 163:1099–1112.

90. Handler RP (1989): Favorable results using methotrexate in the treatment of patients with ankylosing spondylitis (letter). *Arthritis Rheum* 32:234.

91. Hanly JG, Russell MI, Gladman DD (1988): Psoriatic spondyloarthropathy: A long-term prospective study. *Ann Rheum Dis* 47:386–393.

92. Harats N, Worth R, Benson MD (1989): Spinal claudication in systemic amyloidosis. *J Rheumatol* 16:1003–1006.

93. Hochberg M (1984): Epidemiology. In: Calin A, ed. *Spondyloarthropathies.* Orlando, Florida: Grune and Stratton, pp. 21–42.

94. Hunter T (1989): The spinal complications of ankylosing spondylitis. *Semin Arthritis Rheum* 19:172–182.

95. Hunter T, Dubo H (1978): Spinal fractures complicating ankylosing spondylitis. *Ann Intern Med* 88:546–549.

96. Hurd ER (1979): Extraarticular manifestations of rheumatoid arthritis. *Semin Arthritis Rheum* 8:151–176.

97. Isdale IC, Conlon PW (1971): Atlanto-axial subluxation: A six-year follow-up report. *Ann Rheum Dis* 30:387–389.

98. Jiménez-Balderas FJ, Mintz G (1993): Ankylosing spondylitis: Clinical course in women and men. *J Rheumatol* 20:2069–2072.

99. Jones MW, Kaufmann JC (1976): Vertebrobasilar artery insufficiency in rheumatoid atlanto-axial subluxation. *J Neurol Neurosurg Psychiatry* 39:122–128.

100. Karprove RE, Little AH, Graham DC, Rosen PS (1980): Ankylosing spondylitis: Survival in men with and without radiotherapy. *Arthritis Rheum* 23:57–61.

101. Kauppi M, Sakaguchi M, Konttinen YT, Hämäläinen M (1989): A new method of screening for vertical atlantoaxial dislocation. *J Rheumatol* 17:167–172.

102. Kawano N, Matsuno T, Miyazawa S, et al. (1988): Calcium pyrophosphate dihydrate crystal deposition disease in the cervical ligamentum flavum. *J Neurosurg* 68:613–620.

103. Kellgren JH, Jeffrey MR, Ball S (1963): *The epidemiology of chronic rheumatism,* vol I. Oxford: Blackwell Scientific, pp. 326–327.

104. Khan MA (1984): Ankylosing spondylitis. In: Calin A, ed. *Spondyloarthropathies.* Orlando, Florida: Grune and Stratton.

105. Khan MA (1987): A double blind comparison of diclofenac and indomethacin in the treatment of ankylosing spondylitis. *J Rheumatol* 14:118–123.

106. Khan MA (1988): Genetics of HLA-B27. *Br J Rheumatol* 27(suppl 2):6–11.

107. Khan MA (1992): An overview of clinical spectrum and heterogeneity of spondyloarthropathies. *Rheum Dis Clin North Am* 18:1–10.

108. Khan MA, Khan MK (1990): HLA-B27 as an aid to diagnosis of ankylosing spondylitis. *Spine* 4:617–625.

109. Khan MA, Khan MK, Kushner I (1981): Survival among patients with ankylosing spondylitis: A life table analysis. *J Rheumatol* 8:86–90.

110. Khan MA, Kushner I, Braun WE (1977): Comparison of clinical features in HLA-B27 positive and negative patients with ankylosing spondylitis. *Arthritis Rheum* 20:909–912.

111. Khan MA, van der Linden SM (1990): Ankylosing spondylitis and other spondyloarthropathies. *Rheum Dis Clin North Am* 16:551–579.

112. Kirwan J, Edwards A, Huitfeldt B, Thompson P, Currey H (1993): The course of established ankylosing spondylitis and the effects of sulphasalazine over 3 years. *Br J Rheumatol* 32:729–733.

113. Koivuranta-Vaara P, Repo H, Leirisalo M, et al. (1984): En-

hanced neutrophil migration in vivo in HLA-B27 positive subjects. *Ann Rheum Dis* 43:181–185.

114. Komusi T, Munro T, Harth M (1985): Radiologic review: The rheumatoid cervical spine. *Semin Arthritis Rheum* 14:187–195.

115. Konttinen Y, Santavirta S, Kauppi M, Moskovich R (1991): The rheumatoid cervical spine. *Curr Opin Rheumatol* 3:429–440.

116. Kozin F, Carrera GF, Ryan LM, Foley D, Lawson T (1981): Computed tomography in the diagnosis of sacroiliitis. *Arthritis Rheum* 24:1479–1485.

117. Kraag G, Stokes B, Groh J, et al. (1990): The effects of home physiotherapy and supervision on patients with ankylosing spondylitis—a randomized controlled trial. *J Rheumatol* 17:228–233.

118. Kramer J, Jolesz F, Kleefield J (1991): Rheumatoid arthritis of the cervical spine. *Rheum Dis Clin North Am* 17:757–772.

119. Kremer JM, Alarcón GS, Lightfoot RW, et al. (1994): Methotrexate for rheumatoid arthritis: Suggested guidelines for monitoring liver toxicity. *Arthritis Rheum* 37:316–328.

120. Kremer JM, Gordon IK (1989): Electron microscopic analysis of sequential liver biopsy samples from patients with rheumatoid arthritis: Correlation with light microscopic findings. *Arthritis Rheum* 32:1202–1213.

121. Kremer JM, Lee RG, Tolman KG (1989): Liver histology in rheumatoid arthritis patients receiving long-term methotrexate therapy. *Arthritis Rheum* 32:121–127.

122. Kremer JM, Phelps CT (1992): Long-term prospective study of the use of methotrexate in the treatment of rheumatoid arthritis: Update after a mean of 90 months. *Arthritis Rheum* 35:138–145.

123. Kyle RA, Greipp PR (1983): Amyloidosis (AL): Clinical and laboratory features in 229 cases. *Mayo Clin Proc* 58:665–683.

124. Larsson EM, Holtas S, Zygmunt S (1989): Pre- and postoperative MR imaging of the cranio-cervical junction in rheumatoid arthritis. *AJNR* 10:89–94.

125. Lehtinen K (1981): Working ability of 76 patients with ankylosing spondylitis. *Scand J Rheumatol* 10:263–265.

126. Lipson SJ, Naheedy MH, Kaplan MM, Bienfang DC (1980): Spinal stenosis caused by epidural lipomatosis in Cushing's syndrome. *N Engl J Med* 302:36.

127. Luken MG 3rd, Patel DV, Ellman MH (1982): Symptomatic spinal stenosis associated with ankylosing spondylitis. *Neurosurgery* 11:703–705.

128. Mander M, Simpson JM, McLellan A, Walker D, Goodacre JA, Dick WC (1987): Studies with an enthesis index as a method of clinical assessment in ankylosing spondylitis. *Ann Rheum Dis* 46:197–202.

129. Martel W (1977): Pathogenesis of cervical discovertebral destruction in rheumatoid arthritis. *Arthritis Rheum* 20:1217–1225.

130. Martel W (1978): Spinal pseudoarthrosis: A complication of ankylosing spondylitis. *Arthritis Rheum* 21:485–490.

131. Mathews JA (1974): Atlanto-axial subluxation in rheumatoid arthritis. A five-year follow-up study. *Ann Rheum Dis* 33:526–531.

132. McCarthy JT, Dahlberg PJ, Kriegshauser JS, et al. (1988): Erosive spondyloarthropathy in long-term dialysis patients: Relationship to severe hyperparathyroidism. *Mayo Clin Proc* 63:446–452.

133. McEwen C, DiTata D, Lingg C, Porini A, Good A, Rankin T (1971): Ankylosing spondylitis and spondylitis accompanying ulcerative colitis, regional enteritis, psoriasis and Reiter's disease: A comparative study. *Arthritis Rheum* 14:291–318.

134. Menezes AH, VanGilder JC, Clark CR, el-Khoury G (1985): Odontoid upward migration in rheumatoid arthritis. An analysis of 45 patients with "cranial settling." *J Neurosurg* 63:500–509.

135. Moll JM, Haslock I, MacRae IF, Wright V (1974): Associations between ankylosing spondylitis, psoriatic arthritis, Reiter's disease, the intestinal arthropathies and Behcet's syndrome. *Medicine* 53:343–364.

136. Murphey MD, Wetzel LH, Bramble JM, et al. (1991): Sacroiliitis: MR imaging findings. *Radiology* 180:239–244.

137. Murray GC, Persellin RH (1981): Cervical fracture complicating ankylosing spondylitis. A report of eight cases and review of the literature. *Am J Med* 70:1033–1041.

138. Nissila M, Lehtinen K, Leirisalo-Repo M, Luukkainen R, Mutru O, Yli-Kerttula U (1988): Sulfasalazine in the treatment of ankylosing spondylitis. *Arthritis Rheum* 31:1111–1116.

139. O'Connell D (1956): Ankylosing spondylitis: The literature to the close of the nineteenth century. *Ann Rheum Dis* 15:119–123.

140. Omdal R, Husby G (1987): Renal affection in patients with anky-

losing spondylitis and psoriatic arthritis. *Clin Rheumatol* 6:74–79.

141. Parikh M, Iyer K, Elias AN, Gwinup G (1987): Spinal stenosis in acromegaly. *Spine* 12:627–628.

142. Pettersson H, Larsson EM, Holtas S, et al. (1988): MR imaging of the cervical spine in rheumatoid arthritis. *AJNR* 9:573–577.

143. Radford EP, Doll R, Smith PG (1977): Mortality among patients with ankylosing spondylitis not given x-ray therapy. *N Engl J Med* 297:572–576.

144. Rahi AH (1979): HLA and eye disease. *Br J Ophthalmol* 63:283–292.

145. Ranawat CS, O'Leary P, Pellicci P, et al. (1979): Cervical spine fusion in rheumatoid arthritis. *J Bone Joint Surg [Am]* 61:1003–1010.

146. Rasmusseau JD, Hansen TM (1989): Physical training for patients with ankylosing spondylitis. *Arthritis Care Res* 2:25–27.

147. Redlund-Johnell I, Pettersson H (1984): Radiographic measurements of the cranio-vertebral region. *Acta Radiol* 25:23–28.

148. Resnick D, Dwosh IL, Goergen TG, et al. (1976): Clinical and radiographic abnormalities in ankylosing spondylitis: A comparison of men and women. *Radiology* 119:293–297.

149. Resnick D, Shapiro RF, Wiesner KB, Niwayama G, Utsinger PD, Shaul SR (1978): Diffuse idiopathic skeletal hyperostosis (DISH) [ankylosing hyperostosis of Forestier and Rotes-Querol]. *Semin Arthritis Rheum* 7:153–187.

150. Ritter MA, Sieber JM (1985): Prophylactic indomethacin for the prevention of heterotopic bone formation following total hip arthroplasty. *Clin Orthop* 196:217–225.

151. Robb-Nicholson LC, Daltroy L, Eaton H, et al. (1989): Effects of aerobic conditioning in lupus fatigue: A pilot study. *Br J Rheumatol* 28:500–505.

152. Roberts WN, Daltroy LH, Anderson RJ (1988): Stability of normal joint findings in persistent classic rheumatoid arthritis. *Arthritis Rheum* 31:267–271.

153. Roberts WN, Larson MG, Liang MH, Harrison RA, Barefoot J, Clarke AK (1989): Sensitivity of anthropometric techniques for clinical trials in ankylosing spondylitis. *Br J Rheumatol* 28:40–45.

154. Roca A, Bernreuter WK, Alarcón S (1993): Functional magnetic resonance imaging should be included in the evaluation of the cervical spine in patients with rheumatoid arthritis. *J Rheumatol* 20:1485–1488.

155. Rogers J, Watt I, Dieppe P (1985): Palaeopathology of spinal osteophytosis, vertebral ankylosis, ankylosing spondylitis, and vertebral hyperostosis. *Ann Rheum Dis* 44:113–120.

156. Ropes MW, Bennett GA, Cobb S, Jacox R, Jessar RA (1956): Proposed diagnostic criteria for rheumatoid arthritis. *Bull Rheum Dis* 7:121–124.

157. Rosenbaum JT (1992): Acute anterior uveitis and spondyloarthropathies. *Rheum Dis Clin North Am* 18:143–151.

158. Rosenow E, Strimlan CV, Muhm JR, Ferguson RH (1977): Pleuropulmonary manifestations of ankylosing spondylitis. *Mayo Clin Proc* 52:641–649.

159. Russel AS, Maksymowych W, LeClerq S (1981): Clinical examination of the sacroiliac joints: A prospective study. *Arthritis Rheum* 24:1575–1577.

160. Ryan LM, Carrera GF, Lightfoot RW Jr, Hoffman RG, Kozin F (1983): The radiographic diagnosis of sacroiliitis: A comparison of different views with computed tomograms of the sacroiliac joint. *Arthritis Rheum* 26:760–763.

161. Sadowska-Wronblewska M, Garwolinska H, Maczynska-Rusinack B (1986): A trial of cyclophosphamide in ankylosing spondylitis with involvement of peripheral joints and high disease activity. *Scand J Rheumatol* 15:259–264.

162. Santavirta S, Kankaanpää U, Sandelin J, et al. (1987): Evaluation of patients with rheumatoid cervical spine. *Scand J Rheumatol* 16:9–16.

163. Santavirta S, Slatis P, Kankaanpaa U, Sandelin J, Laasonen E (1988): Treatment of the cervical spine in rheumatoid arthritis. *J Bone Joint Surg [Am]* 70:658–667.

164. Sato R, Takahashi M, Yamashita Y, et al. (1992): Calcium crystal deposition in cervical ligamentum flavum: CT and MR findings. *J Comput Assist Tomogr* 16:352–355.

165. Saway PA, Blackburn WD, Halla JT, Alarcon GS (1989): Clinical characteristics affecting survival in patients with rheumatoid ar-

thritis undergoing cervical spine surgery: A controlled study. *J Rheumatol* 16:890–896.

166. Schils JP, Resnick D, Haghighi PN, Trudell D, Sartoris DJ (1989): Pathogenesis of discovertebral and manubriosternal joint abnormalities in rheumatoid arthritis: A cadaveric study. *J Rheumatol* 16:291–297.

167. Schlosstein L, Terasaki PI, Bluestone R, et al. (1973): High association of the HLA antigen, W-27, with ankylosing spondylitis. *N Engl J Med* 288:704–706.

168. Schumacher HR, Holdsworth DE (1977): Ochronotic arthropathy. I. Clinicopathologic studies. *Semin Arthritis Rheum* 6:207–246.

169. Schwimmbeck PL, Oldstone MB (1987): Molecular mimicry and auto-immune disease as the pathogenetic mechanism of ankylosing spondylitis and Reiter's syndrome. *Clin Res* 35:141A.

170. Sebert JL, Fardellone P, Marie A, et al. (1986): Destructive spondylarthropathy in hemodialyzed patients: Possible role of amyloidosis (letter). *Arthritis Rheum* 29:301–303.

171. Semble EL, Elster AD, Loeser RF, Laster DW, Challa VR, Pisko EJ (1988): Magnetic resonance imaging of the craniovertebral junction in rheumatoid arthritis. *J Rheumatol* 15:1367–1375.

172. Sheehan NJ, Slavin BM, Donovan MP, Mount JN, Mathews JA (1986): Lack of correlation between clinical disease activity and erythrocyte sedimentation rate, acute phase proteins or protease inhibitors in ankylosing spondylitis. *Br J Rheumatol* 25:171–174.

173. Sherrer YS, Bloch DA, Mitchell DM, Young DY, Fries JF (1986): The development of disability in rheumatoid arthritis. *Arthritis Rheum* 29:494–500.

174. Silman AJ (1989): Rheumatoid arthritis and infection: A population approach. *Ann Rheum Dis* 48:707–710.

175. Simkin PA, Downey DJ, Kilcoyne RF (1988): Apophyseal arthritis limits lumbar motion in patients with ankylosing spondylitis. *Arthritis Rheum* 31:798–802.

176. Slatis P, Santavirta S, Sandelin J, Konttinen YT (1989): Cranial subluxation of the odontoid process in rheumatoid arthritis. *J Bone Joint Surg [Am]* 71:189–195.

177. Smith PH, Benn RT, Sharp J (1972): Natural history of rheumatoid cervical luxations. *Ann Rheum Dis* 31:431–439.

178. Steven MM, Morrison M, Sturrock RD (1985): Penicillamine in ankylosing spondylitis. *J Rheumatol* 12:735–737.

179. Stewart SR, Robbins DL, Castles JJ (1978): Acute fulminant aortic and mitral insufficiency in ankylosing spondylitis. *N Engl J Med* 299:1448–1449.

180. Suarez-Almazor ME, Russell AS (1988): Anterior atlantoaxial subluxation in patients with spondyloarthropathies: Association with peripherial disease. *J Rheumatol* 15:973–975.

181. Takahashi M, Yamashita Y, Sakamoto Y, Kojima R (1989): Chronic cervical cord compression: Clinical significance of increased signal intensity on MR images. *Radiology* 173:219–224.

182. Tullous MW, Skerhut HEI, Story JL, et al. (1990): Cauda equina syndrome of long-standing ankylosing spondylitis: Case report and review of the literature. *J Neurosurg* 73:441–447.

183. Uitvlugt G, Indenbaum S (1988): Clinical assessment of atlantoaxial instability using the Sharp-Purser test. *Arthritis Rheum* 31:918–922.

184. Ullian ME, Hammond WS, Alfrey AC, Schultz A, Molitoris BA (1989): Beta-2-microglobulin-associated amyloidosis in chronic hemodialysis patients with carpal tunnel syndrome. *Medicine* 68:107–115.

185. Van der Linden S, Volkenburg HA, Cats A (1984): Evaluation of diagnostic criteria for ankylosing spondylitis. *Arthritis Rheum* 27:361–368.

186. Van der Linden SM, Valkenburg HA, de Jongh BM, Cats A (1984): The risk of developing ankylosing spondylitis in HLA-B27 positive individuals. *Arthritis Rheum* 27:241–249.

187. Varga J, Giampaolo C, Goldenberg DL (1985): Tophaceous gout of the spine in a patient with no peripheral tophi: Case report and review of the literature. *Arthritis Rheum* 28:1312–1315.

188. Vasey FB (1993): Psoriatic arthritis. In: Schumacher HR, ed. *Primer on the rheumatic diseases,* 10th ed. Atlanta: Arthritis Foundation, pp. 161–163.

189. Vervaeck M, De Keyser J, Pauwels P, et al. (1991): Sudden hypotonic paraparesis caused by tophaceous gout of the lumbar spine. *Clin Neurol Neurosurg* 93:233–236.

190. Walker AM, Funch D, Dreyer NA, Tolman KG (1993): Determinants of serious liver disease among patients receiving low-dose methotrexate for rheumatoid arthritis. *Arthritis Rheum* 36:329–335.

191. Warren RW, Kredich DW (1984): Transverse myelitis and acute central nervous system manifestations of systemic lupus erythematosus. *Arthritis Rheum* 27:1058–1060.

192. Weinblatt ME, Coblyn JS, Fox DA, Fraser PA, Holdsworth DE, Glass DN, Trentham DE (1985): Efficacy of low-dose methotrexate in rheumatoid arthritis. *N Engl J Med* 312:318–822.

193. Weinblatt ME, Weissman BN, Holdsworth DE, et al. (1992): Long-term prospective study of methotrexate in the treatment of rheumatoid arthritis. *Arthritis Rheum* 35:129–137.

194. Weissman BNW, Allabadi P, Weinfield MS, Thomas WH, Sosman JL (1982): Prognostic features of atlanto-axial subluxation in rheumatoid arthritis. *Radiology* 144:745–751.

195. Weyand CM, Goronzy JJ (1989): Immune responses to *Borrelia Burgdorferi* in patients with reactive arthritis. *Arthritis Rheum* 32:1057–1064.

196. Wilder RL (1993): Rheumatoid arthritis: epidemiology, pathology, and pathogenesis. In: Schumacher HR, ed. *Primer on the rheumatic diseases, ed 10.* Atlanta: Arthritis Foundation, pp. 86–89.

197. Willkens RF, Arnett FC, Bitter T, et al. (1981): Reiter's syndrome: evaluation of preliminary criteria for definitive disease. *Arthritis Rheum* 24:844–849.

198. Winfield J, Cooke D, Brook AS, Corbett M (1981): A prospective study of the radiologic changes in the cervical spine in early rheumatoid disease. *Ann Rheum Dis* 40:109–114.

199. Wolfe F, Mitchell DM, Sibley JT, et al. (1994): The mortality of rheumatoid arthritis. *Arthritis Rheum* 37:481–494.

200. Wolfe F, Smythe HA, Yunus MB, et al. (1990): The American College of Rheumatology 1990 Criteria for the Classification of Fibromyalgia. Report of the Multicenter Criteria Committee. *Arthritis Rheum* 33:160–172.

201. Wordsworth BP, Pearcy MJ, Mowat AG, (1984): Inpatient regime for the treatment of ankylosing spondylitis: an appraisal of improvement in spinal mobility and the effects of corticotrophin. *Br J Rheumatol* 23:39–43.

202. Wright V (1959): Rheumatism and psoriasis: a re-evaluation. *Am J Med* 27:454–462.

The Adult Spine: Principles and Practice,
2nd edition, J.W. Frymoyer, Editor-in-Chief.
Lippincott-Raven Publishers, Philadelphia © 1997.

CHAPTER 42

Rheumatoid Arthritis

Surgical Treatment

Richard B. Delamarter, Michael J. Bolesta, and Henry H. Bohlman

Abnormalities of the spine in patients with rheumatoid arthritis are the direct result of rheumatoid destruction of the supporting joints, ligaments, and bone, and are almost exclusively a clinical problem in the cervical area. These changes have been shown to be caused by the same array of inflammatory cells that cause damage in peripheral joints (40), where pannus causes articular cartilage destruction, ligament rupture, osteoporosis, synovial cyst formation, and osseous erosion. These same events cause cervical subluxation and instability. The instability produced, combined with proliferative synovitic tissue (pannus), may compress the spinal cord, nerve roots, and vertebral arteries, resulting in pain and neurologic abnormalities. Because there is a strong correlation between the severity of cervical disease and the degree of peripheral erosive disease, cervical subluxation is more likely in those patients with progressive peripheral periarticular erosions (83). Similarly, a history of corticosteroid therapy, seropositivity, the finding of rheumatoid subcutaneous nodules, and the presence of mutilating

peripheral articular disease are all factors indicating greater disease severity, and are predictive of greater progression of cervical instability and neural compression (17,30,76,77,80,83).

Over the past decade, improved imaging techniques (i.e., magnetic resonance imaging and computerized axial tomography) have greatly enhanced our understanding of the pathophysiologic changes that occur in the cervical spine of rheumatoid patients and have allowed improved management of these difficult and potentially lethal problems. The four abnormalities most commonly seen in rheumatoid cervical spine disease are (a) C1-C2 instability, (b) basilar invagination, (c) C1-C2 rotatory (lateral) subluxation, and (d) subaxial subluxation. A thorough understanding of the accompanying changes in bony architecture, soft tissue anatomy, and the central nervous system is critical to the management of these problems. In the lumbar spine, there is significant osteopenia, even in patients who have not received corticosteroids. This is most apparent in younger patients (15). For those receiving even low-dose steroids, osteoporosis is worsened. The spine appears to be more sensitive to this effect than the appendicular skeleton (36).

CLINICAL EVALUATION

Neurologic examination of rheumatoid patients may be difficult, as many of these patients have multiple joint involvement. The testing of muscle strength and tone as

R. B. Delamarter, M.D.: Associate Clinical Professor, Division of Orthopaedic Surgery, UCLA School of Medicine, Los Angeles, California 90024.

M. J. Bolesta, M.D., Assistant Professor, Department of Orthopaedic Surgery, University of Texas Southwestern Medical Center, Dallas, Texas 75235-8883.

H. H. Bohlman, M.D., F.A.C.S.: Professor, Department of Orthopaedic Surgery, Case Western Reserve University School of Medicine; Director, Reconstructive and Traumatic Spine Surgery Center, University Hospitals of Cleveland, Cleveland, Ohio 44106.

well as the elicitation of certain reflexes can be complicated by the loss of joint mobility and significant joint pain. Repeated careful neurologic evaluations are necessary to document any neurologic deterioration. If a rheumatoid patient presents with any neurologic signs or symptoms, neural compression of the cervical spine must be suspected, and the signs and symptoms should not simply be attributed to peripheral rheumatoid disease. Often, radiating pain and weakness are attributed to exacerbation of the systemic disease and not to cervical spine and spinal cord involvement. These patients may die unexpectedly with a clinical picture suggestive of a common condition such as cerebral vascular accident, myocardial infarction, or pulmonary embolism (7). Autopsies in these patients are infrequent, and even when an autopsy is performed, spinal cord compression is easily overlooked unless there is an analysis of the foramen magnum and upper cervical region. Consequently, autopsy reports probably underestimate the true frequency of death due to spinal cord compression and rheumatoid arthritis (3,22,26,51,57,60,78,79). A more complete autopsy study of 104 patients with rheumatoid arthritis revealed 11 with C1-C2 subluxation and cord compression (57). Seven of the 11 died suddenly, giving an estimated 10% rate of fatal medullary compression.

Recently, Delamarter and colleagues (26) performed postmortem analyses on 11 patients with paralysis secondary to rheumatoid arthritis of the cervical spine and found spinal cord compression to be the main cause of death in 10. This strongly suggests that once cervical myelopathy is established in patients with rheumatoid cervical spine disease, the natural history without surgical intervention is grave and mortality is more common than previously believed. In a report on 31 patients with rheumatoid arthritis and cervical myelopathy by Marks and Sharp (49), 19 of the 31 died, with 15 deaths occurring within 6 months of presentation. All who were untreated died, and 50% of those treated with a collar died. Only fusion provided a reasonable chance for survival.

We believe that fatalities in rheumatoid patients due to atlantoaxial subluxation have been underestimated as a result of the lack of clinical recognition of brain stem compression in these severely debilitated patients and inadequate postmortem examination of the foramen magnum and cervical spine. Sudden death associated with rheumatoid cervical spine disease appears to be the result of both ischemia and mechanical compression of the cardiorespiratory centers in the reticular formation of the medulla.

Boden and co-workers (29) studied 92 patients with rheumatoid involvement of the cervical spine and found 42 patients with paralysis secondary to the rheumatoid changes. Two variables were important: (a) The severity of paralysis rather than the duration of paralysis was the important factor in predicting the prognosis for neural recovery following surgery; and (b) the space available

for the cord (i.e., a posterior atlanto-odontoid interval or subaxial spinal canal of 13 mm or less) was the most accurate criterion for determining those patients at risk for myelopathy.

With this background, we will now present the pathoanatomy, clinical presentation, imaging studies, and treatment of the four main presentations of cervical spine involvement.

CERVICAL SPINE

Atlantoaxial Subluxation

Pathoanatomy

C1-C2 subluxation or atlantoaxial subluxation is the result of erosive rheumatoid synovitis in the atlantoaxial, atlanto-odontoid, and atlanto-occipital joints and in the synovial-lined bursa between C1, the odontoid, and the transverse ligament. Atlantoaxial instability is the most common cervical spine abnormality seen in patients with rheumatoid disease. It has been shown to be present in 19% to 71% of patients surveyed radiographically (5,11,17,27,50,52,74,77) and has been found in 11% to 46% of patients undergoing autopsy (2,30,51,60). Atlantoaxial stability depends on the transverse and alar ligaments and less so on the apical ligaments. An atlantoaxial distance measured on flexion/extension lateral x-rays of greater than 3.5 mm is considered abnormal in an adult, and subluxation of more than 10 to 12 mm implies destruction of the entire atlantoaxial ligamentous complex (32). Anterior atlantoaxial subluxation may result in compression of the cervical cord between the posterior arch of the atlas and the odontoid (Fig. 1). Even without significant abnormal motion on flexion/extension, exuberant pannus formation around the odontoid may be sufficient to cause cord compression (Fig. 2). During flexion of the neck, the spinal cord is particularly vulnerable to compression as the atlas slides forward in relation to the axis.

The clinical manifestations of C1-C2 instability are primarily due to compression upon the medulla, the upper portion of the cervical spinal cord, and occasionally the vertebral arteries. Compression may result in neural damage due to direct pressure on the spinal cord, diminution of the microvascular blood supply, or a combination of these factors (26,67). With compression of the spinal cord at the C1-C2 level, the ischemia may affect the anterior horn cells in more caudal portions of the cervical cord (Fig. 1). The corticospinal tracts, lateral sensory tracts, second cervical nerve roots, and spinal tract of the trigeminal nerve are at risk with C1-C2 subluxations.

Clinical Presentation

The most frequent symptom of C1-C2 subluxation is pain localized to the upper neck or radiating to the occi-

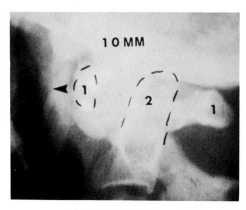
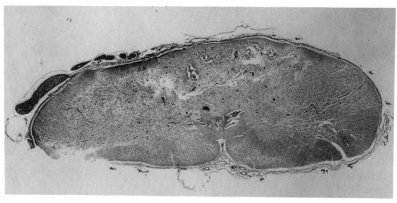

A

B

FIG. 1. This 65-year-old female with a 14-year history of rheumatoid arthritis was diagnosed with C1-C2 instability and treated for 3 years with medical therapy only. The surgeons were consulted only after the patient was brought by ambulance to the emergency room, quadriplegic with no history of trauma. The patient was immediately placed in skeletal tong traction, but died 3 hours later from cervical spinal cord compression. **A:** This lateral x-ray taken upon admission to the emergency room notes 10 mm of subluxation between the anterior arch of C1 and the odontoid, but of greater importance is only 8 mm of space available for the spinal cord measured from the posterior odontoid to the C1 laminae. **B:** This autopsy section at the level of compression at C1-C2 shows significant flattening of the spinal cord, vacuolization and gliosis of the spinal tracts, and atrophy of the spinal cord with thickening of the leptomeninges.

put, forehead, or eyes. Additionally, there may be paresthesias in the occipital area if the second cervical nerve roots are compressed. The pain associated with C1-C2 subluxation is generally increased with neck motion, particularly flexion and rotation, and occasionally these patients may complain of a clunking sensation or a feeling of the head falling forward (Sharp and Purser's sign) (74) with flexion and rotation motions. With advancing spinal cord or medullary compression, these patients may complain of weakness of the arms and/or legs, paresthesias, vertigo, gait abnormalities, incoordination of the hands (e.g., difficulty buttoning a shirt or handling small change), and rarely bowel or bladder problems. Flexion and rotation of the neck may induce an electrical shock sensation (Lhermitte's sign) into all four limbs, vertigo, or transient unconsciousness. Ataxia, nystagmus, bulbar signs, episodic unconsciousness, or even sudden death are indicative of involvement of the vertebral arteries and/or compression of the medulla.

A rare variant is posterior C1-C2 subluxation, generally a result of erosion and/or fracture of the odontoid process (45). It was noted in 6.7% of all C1-C2 subluxations in one large series (80) and may result in myelopathy secondary to spinal cord compression (45).

Treatment

The treatment of atlantoaxial subluxation must be based on a clear understanding of the patient's general health, the severity of symptoms, and the presence of neurologic findings. The indications for surgical management are severe or unremitting pain and neurologic abnormalities, and we believe surgery should be per-

formed as soon as neural dysfunction is recognized. The presence of C1-C2 subluxation in an asymptomatic patient is not an indication for surgical treatment unless space available for the cord as measured by the posterior atlanto-odontoid interval is 13 mm or less, since these patients are at risk for myelopathic changes (28).

The most common surgical procedure used for C1-C2 subluxation is stabilization by posterior arthrodesis (Fig. 2), which can be accomplished by a number of different techniques, most being variations of the Gallie procedure (14,31,38,42,57,68,81). Sometimes, if the C1-C2 subluxation is fixed and cannot be reduced by preoperative traction or extension of the neck at the time of posterior fusion, removal of the posterior arch of the atlas should be performed with extension of the fusion to the occiput. Postoperatively, these patients are treated in a rigid two-poster orthosis or halo vest for 2 to 3 months.

One technique of atlantoaxial arthrodesis uses posterior wiring and iliac crest strut grafts. A sublaminar loop is placed around C1 and a second wire through and around the base of the spinous process of C2, with both wires brought through iliac crest strut grafts on either side and tightened on top of the grafts. Recent reports of posterior cervical fusions with methylmethacrylate and wire mesh constructs (12,13,18) have noted high incidences of wound dehiscence and infection, and we have found these constructs to be neither necessary nor advisable in posterior cervical spine fusions. However, occasionally it may be necessary to use a halo apparatus to hold the atlantoaxial reduction while awaiting solid arthrodesis. Utilization of C1-C2 Magerl facet screws, although technically demanding, has improved fusion rates and made halo usage unnecessary in most cases (Fig. 3).

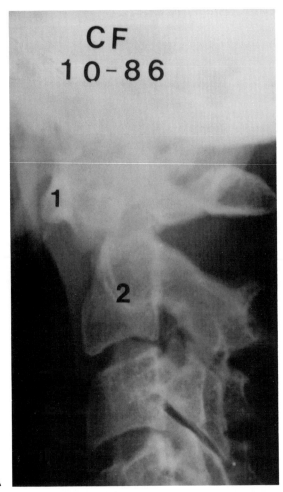
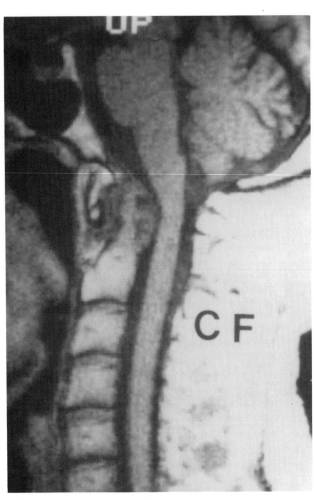

A

B

FIG. 2. This 50-year-old female with a several-year history of rheumatoid arthritis presented with severe progressive neck pain and a normal neurologic evaluation. **A:** This lateral x-ray reveals the C1-C2 subluxation. **B:** Sagittal MRI demonstrates the exuberant pannus around the partially eroded odontoid, causing partial cord compression. This pannus around the odontoid may cause cord compression in the absence of C1-C2 motion and can inhibit reduction of the C1-C2 instability.

Basilar Invagination

Pathoanatomy

Basilar invagination, also known as vertical subluxation, cranial settling, upward migration of the odontoid, and atlantoaxial impaction, occurs as a result of rheumatoid destruction of the bone, ligaments, and cartilage in the atlanto-occipital and atlantoaxial joints. In surveys of rheumatoid patients, basilar invagination has been found in 5% to 32% (27,61,65,69) and may be associated with C1-C2 subluxation.

In adults, the upper tip of the odontoid process normally lies 1 cm below the anterior margin of the foramen magnum. Vertical migration of the odontoid can be assessed radiographically by several methods (Fig. 4). Chamberlain's line is drawn from the posterior margin

of the hard palate to the posterior margin of the foramen magnum. McCray's line connects the anterior and posterior margins of the foramen magnum (basion to opisthion). The odontoid should not project above McCray's line. When Chamberlain's line is measured, the tip of the odontoid should not project more than 3 mm above; 6 mm is pathologic. The traditional measurement of basilar invagination has been McGregor's line, which connects the posterior margin of the hard palate to the most caudal point of the occiput. Because the margins of the foramen magnum are often difficult to precisely identify on plain x-rays, McCray's and Chamberlain's lines can be difficult to assess, and McGregor's line may be the most reliable. The tip of the odontoid should not project more than 4.5 mm above McGregor's line. All three of these measurements use the tip of the odontoid process as the key landmark. Patients with rheumatoid arthritis

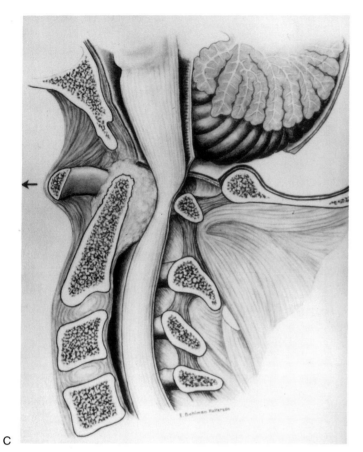

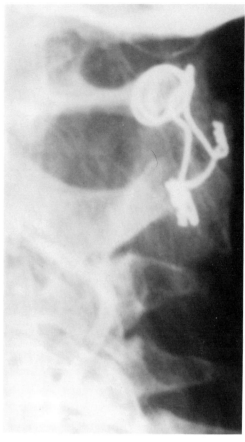

C

D

FIG. 2. (*Continued.*) **C:** An illustration of the MRI noted in Figure 2B revealing the spinal cord compression due to the C1-C2 instability and the pannus surrounding the odontoid tip. **D:** A close-up lateral x-ray of the C1-C2 posterior fusion 2 years postoperatively showing the rigid wire technique using iliac crest strut grafts. Two wires are used, one surrounding the C1 arch and the second wire through and around the C2 spinous process. Both wires are brought up through drill holes in the iliac crest grafts and tightened over the top of the bone. This patient had complete relief of the neck symptoms and remained with a normal neurologic examination at last follow-up 3 years after the fusion.

can have erosion or atrophy of the odontoid process. Additionally, the shadow of the tip of the odontoid process may be superimposed upon the base of the skull, and thus all three methods may prove difficult using plain x-rays. To overcome this difficulty, Ranawat (68) and Redlund-Johnell (70) have described new methods of measurement in which the tip of the odontoid process is not used as a landmark (see Fig. 4). Fishgold and Metzger (33) have also described a measurement on an open-mouth anteroposterior x-ray of the odontoid in which the tip of the odontoid should be 1 cm or more below the digastric line.

If basilar invagination is suspected on plain radiographs, newer imaging techniques such as magnetic resonance imaging, including flexion/extension magnetic resonance imaging (MRI), and sagittal reconstructions of computerized axial tomography are the best methods

of assessing vertical migration of odontoid C1-C2 instability and subsequent neural compression (25,54). We prefer to use plain tomograms, reconstructed computerized axial tomography, and magnetic resonance imaging studies for accurate diagnosis (Fig. 5). Breedveld et al. (8) have shown that distortion of the spinal cord on MRI evaluation correlates with the signs of myelopathy, and Bundschuh and co-workers (9) have shown that a brain stem cervicomedullary angle of less than 135° (normal 135° to 175°) on MRI also correlates with cervical myelopathy.

Clinical Presentation

Basilar invagination can be associated with all of the severe neurologic sequelae associated with C1-C2 sub-

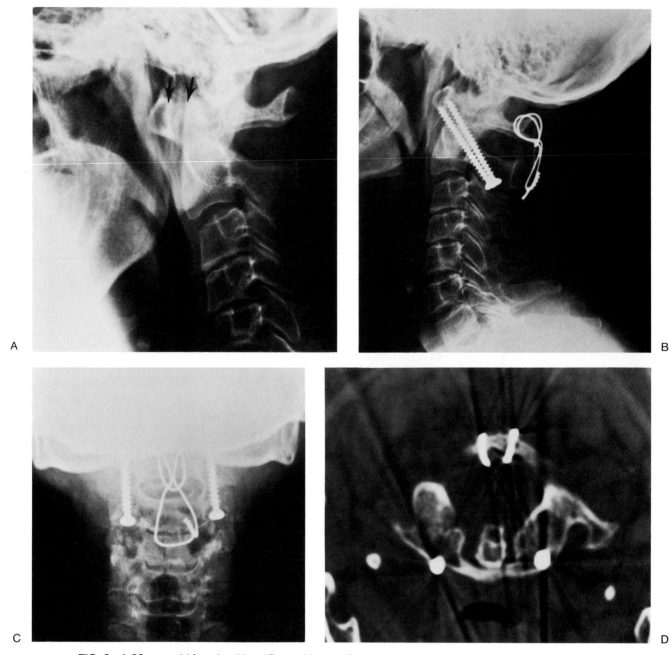

FIG. 3. A 62-year-old female with a 15-year history of rheumatoid arthritis presented with an 18-month history of increasing severe neck pain and tingling in the arms and legs. **A:** This lateral x-ray reveals a C1-C2 instability (*arrows*). **B:** Postoperative x-rays showing the C1-C2 facet screws and spinous process wiring with reduction of the C1-2 subluxation. **C:** AP x-ray revealing the C1-C2 facet screws and C1-C2 rigid wire technique. The bone graft was placed in the C1-C2 facet joints and between the arch of C1 and spinous process of C2. **D:** Postoperative CAT scan revealing the reduced odontoid. Note the tips of the C1-C2 screws just penetrating the anterior body of C1. Note the wire around the posterior arch of C1. Using the C1-C2 facet screw technique, these patients are kept in a Philadelphia collar for 6 weeks and excellent fusion rates can be expected.

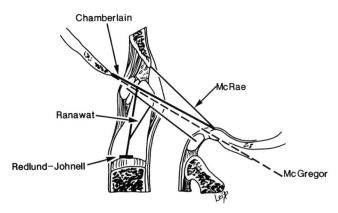

FIG. 4. Techniques to measure basilar invagination on lateral radiographs or tomograms.

luxation, including sudden death. When there are any neurologic signs or symptoms, particularly progressive quadriparesis, hospital admission is required for halo traction and surgical stabilization (Fig. 4). Conservative treatment of patients with basilar invagination accompanied by signs and symptoms of neural compression carries the risk of progressive neurologic impairment and sudden death, and in our opinion is contraindicated.

Treatment

Preoperative halo traction is used to reduce subluxations and pull the odontoid out of the foramen magnum. Posterior spinal fusion is the most common surgical procedure employed. Many techniques of occiput cervical fusion have been described. Perry and Nickel (66), as well as Newman and Sweetnam (62), have described an onlay graft technique and have reported a high fusion rate. Other techniques have included the use of various devices for internal fixation (12,13,18,71), methylmethacrylate (12), and anterior approaches (23). All these methods can be associated with serious complications and may require long periods of skeletal traction.

We prefer the technique of rigid wiring with iliac crest grafts described by Wertheim and Bohlman (81) (Fig. 6). With this technique, the skin is prepared with sterilizing iodine solution, and the subcutaneous tissue is injected with a 1:500,000 solution of epinephrine. A midline incision is made, extending from the external occipital protuberance to the fourth cervical level. The paraspinal muscles are sharply dissected subperiosteally with a scalpel and a periosteal elevator to expose the occiput and cervical laminae. Special care is taken to stay exactly in the midline in order to avoid the paramedian venous plexuses.

Just superior to the foramen magnum, the occipital bone is very thin, but at the external occipital protuberance it is thick, and the protuberance is the ideal location for the passage of wires without having to go through both tables of the skull. The transverse and superior sagittal sinuses are cephalad to the protuberance and thus are out of danger. At a point 2 cm above the rim of the foramen magnum, a high-speed diamond burr is used to create a trough on either side of the protuberance and thus make a ridge in the center. With a towel clip, a hole is then made in this ridge, through only the outer table of bone, and a 20-gauge wire is looped through the hole and around the ridge. Another 20-gauge wire is looped around the arch of the atlas, and a third is passed through a drill hole in the base of the spinous process of the axis and around the latter structure. Therefore, on each side of the spine there are three separate wires, which are utilized to secure the bone grafts (Fig. 6A).

The posterior part of the iliac crest is exposed and a thick, slightly curved graft of corticocancellous bone of measured length and width is obtained (Fig. 6B). This is then divided horizontally, and three drill holes are placed in each graft (Fig. 6C). The occiput is decorticated and the grafts are anchored in place on both sides of the spine by the wires (Fig. 6D). Additional cancellous bone is packed in between the two grafts. The wound is closed in layers over suction drains.

This rigid wiring technique allows immediate rigid internal fixation with minimal operative morbidity and permits early mobilization of the patient. It has resulted in successful fusion in all 13 patients reported to date with long-term follow-up (81). Using this technique we have had no complications of breakage of wires or loss of reduction.

Historically, postoperative mortality rates of 27% to 42% have been reported, although more recent studies have been encouraging with less than 10% mortality, most likely due to earlier surgical intervention and improved anesthetic and perioperative management (16,18,19,31,38,41,42,56,68,81).

As an alternative to posterior approaches, transoral decompression for irreducible basilar invagination and/or C1-C2 subluxation has been advocated by some, but its role remains unclear, and the techniques are associated with an extremely high morbidity and mortality rate (6,20,21,59,63). We have not found transoral decompression of the odontoid necessary or beneficial in most rheumatoid patients, but if considered we prefer excision of C2 and C1 to C3 fusion by the petropharyngeal approach to the base of the skull, C1, and C2 as reported by McAfee and others (53,55,75,82). Resection of the odontoid should always be accompanied by posterior fusion.

Successful surgical fusion predictably relieves pain (20,31,68,72,81), halts progression of neurologic dysfunction, and provides stability. Reports of neurologic improvement have been variable, although Wertheim and Bohlman, using the previously described technique of preoperative traction and occipital cervical fusion with rigid wiring technique and iliac crest strut grafts,

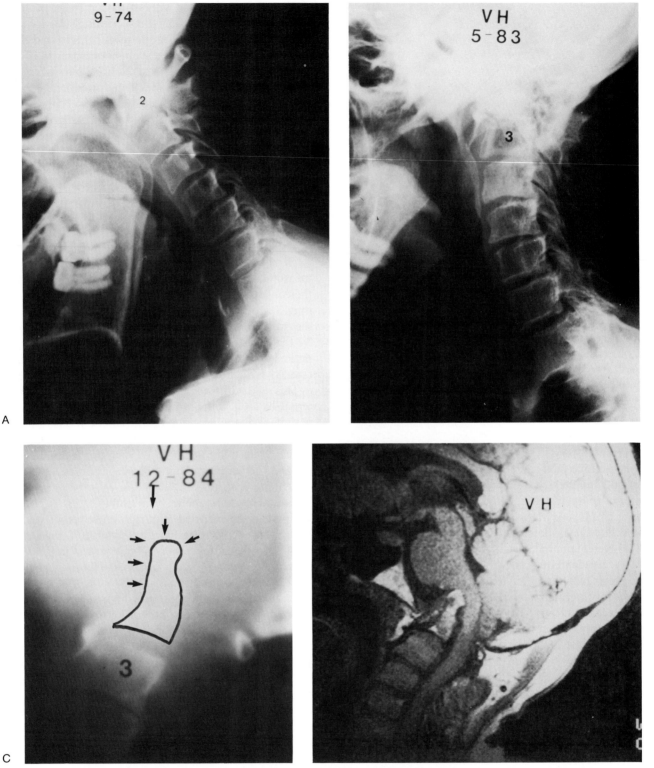

FIG. 5. This 68-year-old female had a 17-year history of rheumatoid arthritis. **A:** Lateral x-ray (1974) revealed a visible C2 vertebral body and minimal basilar invagination. Patient presented in 1983 with progressive neck pain and early myelopathy. **B:** Lateral x-ray (1983) showing severe basilar invagination with the C3 vertebra sitting at the base of the skull. The C2 vertebral body is not visible as it is completely invaginated into the foramen magnum. **C:** Lateral tomogram (1984). Note the severe basilar invagination with the entire odontoid cephalad to the base of the skull. **D:** Lateral MRI (1985). Note the proximal migration of the odonotoid into the foramen magnum with compression of the cervical medullary junction.

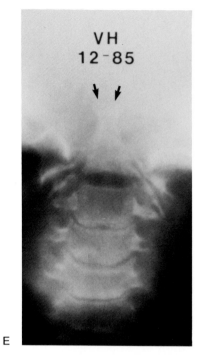
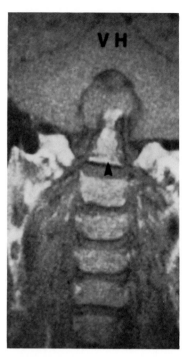
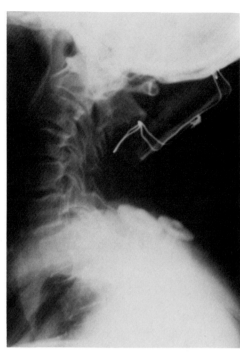

E

F,G

FIG. 5. (*Continued.*) **E:** AP tomogram (1985). Note the complete basilar invagination with the tip of the odontoid 3.5 cm above the base of the skull. **F:** Coronal MRI (1985) showing severe proximal migration of the odontoid with the base of the C2 vertebral body located at the base of the occiput. **G:** After 10 days of halo traction, a posterior fusion was performed. Lateral postoperative x-ray showing occipital to C4 fusion with iliac strut grafts and triple wire technique. This patient went on to solid fusion with complete resolution of symptoms.

found neurologic improvement in all 10 of the patients with preoperative myelopathy (81). Others have had less success, with neurologic improvement reported in 30% to 40% of patients (68).

Atlantoaxial Rotatory (Lateral) Subluxation

Pathoanatomy

Atlantoaxial rotatory subluxation, also known as lateral C1-C2 subluxation, occurs from the same destructive rheumatoid synovitis at the cervical-occipital and atlantoaxial joints, allowing rotation of the cranium on the cervical spine at either interval. This type of subluxation is progressive and may result in a fixed torticollis of the head and neck occurring over a 1- to 6-month period (Fig. 7). If not recognized and corrected, this deformity becomes permanent and painful.

Clinical Presentation

Cervical and occipital pain along with varying degrees of neurologic signs and symptoms are the usual clinical findings. Like Burry (10), we believe the incidence of C1-

C2 rotatory subluxation is underestimated, since it accounted for 21% of all atlantoaxial subluxations in one series (80), and nonreducible head tilt was found in 10% of a rheumatoid population in another series (37).

Atlantoaxial rotatory subluxation is defined as more than 2 mm of subluxation of the lateral masses of C1 on C2. This is always associated with a rotational deformity and can be best visualized on computerized axial tomography and plain tomography of the occipital C1-C2 complex.

Treatment

Treatment consists of halo ring traction at weights of 7 to 10 pounds. Over a period of 3 to 10 days the deformity, if not fixed, corrects and then an occiput-to-axis fusion can be performed to permanently hold the reduction (Fig. 8). Serial neurologic exams must be performed during correction by traction. Because of the severe osteoporosis in some rheumatoid patients, we prefer to use 6 to 8 pins when placing a halo ring, as this will improve the halo fixation and reduce pin loosening and pin complications. The posterior surgical technique is identical to that for C1-C2 subluxation. These patients are held in a halo vest for 10 to 12 weeks postoperatively and then placed in a soft collar for an additional 6 to 8 weeks.

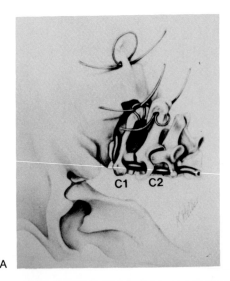

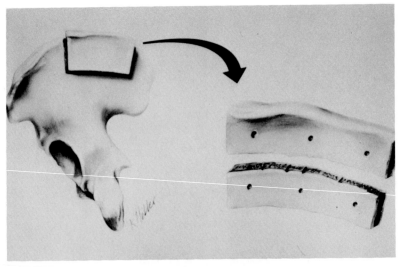

A

B

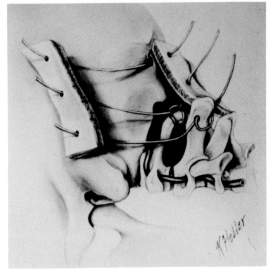

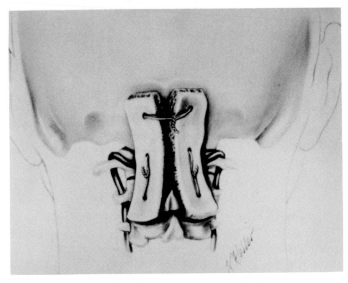

C

D

FIG. 6. **A:** A small burr is used to create a ridge at the external occipital protuberance and a hole is then made in this ridge. Wires are passed through the outer table of the occiput, under the arch of the atlas, and through the spinous process of the axis. **B:** Cortical cancellous bone graft is taken from the posterior part of the iliac crest, the graft is divided horizontally, and holes are placed in each graft. **C:** The bone grafts are placed on the wires. **D:** The grafts are wired into place. This rigid wiring technique with iliac crest bone grafts allows immediate rigid internal fixation with minimal operative morbidity, and permits early mobilization of the patient and results in successful fusion. It does not require the passage of wires through both cortices of the skull, and we have had no complications with breakage of wire or loss of reduction.

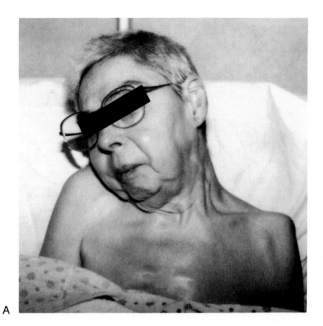

A

FIG. 7. This 63-year-old female with a 14-year history of rheumatoid arthritis—status post bilateral total shoulders, bilateral total knees, and bilateral total hips—presented with a painful nonmobile torticollis deformity of the head and neck. **A:** The patient was unable to move her head or neck as motion would incite painful neck spasms. Neurologic examination was normal. **B:** An open-mouth x-ray reveals asymmetry of the C1 lateral masses measuring 6 mm on the right (*closed arrows*) and 2 mm on the left (*open arrow*). Greater than 2 mm discrepancy of the lateral masses is diagnostic of C1-C2 rotatory (lateral) subluxation. **C:** A CT scan through the occipital C1-C2 complex notes the odontoid (*closed arrow*) subluxed and rotated from its normal central position (*open arrow*).

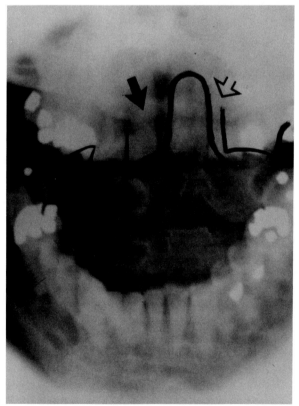

B

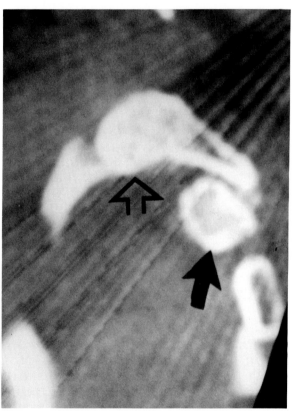

C

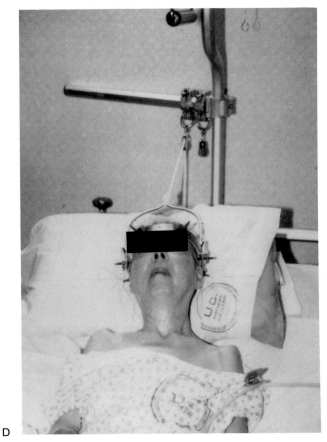

D

FIG. 7. (*Continued.*) **D:** Correction of the torticollis deformity was done with 10 pounds of halo traction over a 1-week period. An occipital to C2 fusion was done using the previously described technique. The patient was left in a halo for 3 months and in a soft collar for an additional 6 weeks. A solid fusion resulted in complete relief of her neck pain and deformity.

Subaxial Subluxations

Pathoanatomy

Subaxial subluxations of the cervical spine in patients with rheumatoid arthritis are the result of destructive rheumatoid changes in the facets, interspinous ligaments, and intervertebral discs (spondylodiscitis). Martel (50) has postulated that subaxial subluxation begins with destruction of the joints of Luschka, with erosion of the adjacent disc and bone allowing subluxation. Ball and Sharp (4) suggested that subaxial subluxation begins with primary facet arthritis and ligamentous laxity causing secondary chronic discal incompetency and destruction.

Clinical Presentation

The neurologic signs and symptoms of subaxial cervical subluxation range from neck and radicular arm pain with weakness to overt myelopathy. Subaxial subluxations often occur at multiple levels producing a "staircase" or "stepladder" deformity. The resultant deformity generally lacks osteophytes and most frequently occurs at the C2-C3 and C3-C4 segments, as well as below prior fusions (58,64). It is important to emphasize that the C7-T1 junction can sublux and is frequently misdiagnosed due to difficult visualization of this area by plain radiography (24). In addition to spinal cord compression from vertebral subluxation, rheumatoid inflammation of the dura mater has been reported in itself to compress the spinal cord (30,57).

Treatment

Partial reduction and stabilization with a posterior spinal fusion is the most common surgical procedure for subaxial subluxations (Fig. 9). If neurologic signs and symptoms progress or do not resolve, a second stage anterior discectomy and fusion may be indicated, but this is very rarely necessary. However, without prior posterior fusion, there is a tendency for anterior fusions to displace, resorb, and collapse. In one report of anterior fusion for subaxial subluxations, four out of five patients were unimproved and the procedure was not recommended (68). Laminectomy is contraindicated for treatment of subaxial subluxations and, if performed, should always be accompanied by fusion (46).

THORACOLUMBAR SPINE

Most physicians caring for individuals with rheumatoid arthritis are well aware of the cervical spine problems associated with this disease. Though rheumatoid arthritis is a systemic disorder, it does not often present as the etiology of thoracolumbar disease. In one radiographic series looking specifically for lumbar involvement, only 20 of 413 patients had findings that could be attributed to this disease process (43). Additionally, the early literature can be confusing in that a clear distinction was not always made between rheumatoid arthritis and ankylosing spondylitis. Both entities have been referred to as rheumatoid spondylitis. The clinical and radiographic courses of the two disorders are distinct, but the histopathology can be quite similar.

Baggenstoss et al. (1) performed an autopsy on an individual with rheumatoid arthritis. Radiographically, there had been a destruction of the T12 vertebral body with collapse. Histologically, there was granuloma infiltration of the marrow with destruction and necrosis, and around the central necrosis there were peripheral histiocytes and fibroblasts in both T12 and L1. These lesions were very similar to classic rheumatoid nodules found in the subcutaneous tissue and myocardium. The authors pointed out that this individual had widespread disease,

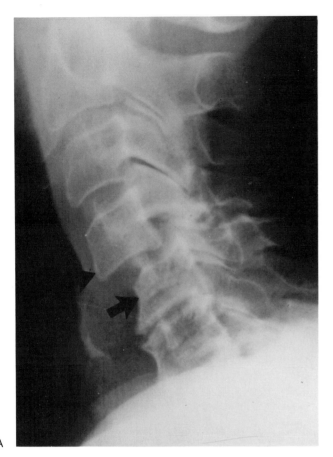 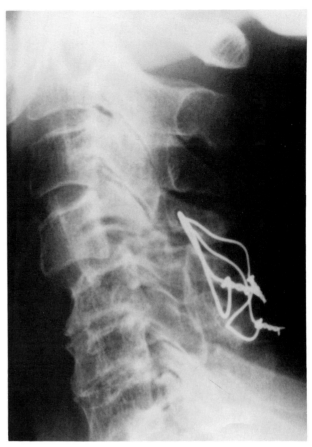

A

B

FIG. 8. This 55-year-old female with an 8-year history of rheumatoid arthritis presented with severe neck and bilateral shoulder pain. **A:** An AP x-ray revealed a subaxial subluxation at C4-C5. **B:** A posterior spinal fusion from C4-C6 with only slight reduction in the subluxation resulted in complete resolution of the neck and shoulder symptoms. A solid fusion is noted in this 2-year follow-up x-ray.

which might explain the thoracolumbar involvement. They also discussed three patients with similar radiographic lesions, but the films clearly showed that these individuals had ankylosing spondylitis, which has been noted by others (35).

Lorber et al. (47) described a 47-year-old with collapse of T7, T8, and T9. This man died and, like the patient of Baggenstoss et al. (1), had widely disseminated lesions of rheumatoid arthritis at necropsy. Histologically, there was infiltration of the T7, T8, and T9 vertebral bodies by rheumatoid granulation tissue. The authors related two other cases with similar radiographic findings, but the second case clearly had ankylosing spondylitis. The third case showed a T5 through T9 wedging, but probably had systemic lupus erythematosus, although there were some features of rheumatoid arthritis.

Glay and Rona (35) believed that vertebral body involvement began with formation of a rheumatoid nodule, leading to necrosis and collapse of the body, and that this was different from ankylosing spondylitis based on a study of one autopsy case with involvement of T12, L2,

and L3. Two clinical cases had similar radiographic findings, the first involving T12 and L1, the second T9, T10, T11, and T12. Review of the literature revealed only five reported cases of this in addition to their three (1,47,73).

Seaman and Wells (73) had a radiographic series of 13 patients, but 11 had ankylosing spondylitis; the remaining two had "peripheral rheumatoid arthritis," one associated with disc and vertebral erosion at C6-C7. The second had destruction at T8-T9 with a spontaneous anterior fusion. Both had the clinical and laboratory stigmata of rheumatoid arthritis. In all of these patients, the radiographic picture was of vertebral body collapse, sometimes accompanied by irregular erosions about the intervertebral disc.

Lawrence et al. (43) reviewed the lumbar radiographs on 413 patients with rheumatoid arthritis, only 20 of which had changes they attributed to rheumatoid arthritis, as compared to a control group. In the anterior column, they described disc narrowing with minimal formation of osteophytes. Vertebral subluxation was more

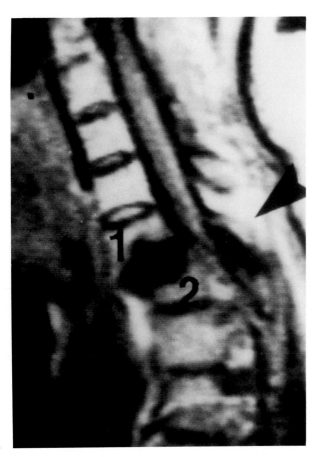
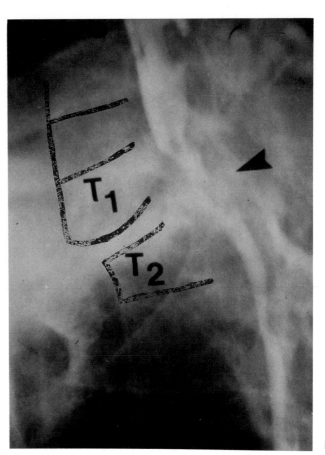

A

B

FIG. 9. This 59-year-old female with a 16-year history of rheumatoid arthritis presented with progressive lower extremity weakness, numbness, and tingling. **A:** A sagittal MRI showing T1 subluxed 50% anterior to T2 with spinal cord compression. **B:** A lateral myelogram revealing complete blockage of dye at the T1-T2 subluxation. A C7 to T2 laminectomy and fusion was performed. Postoperatively, the patient was maintained in a halo vest for 3 months. She had complete relief of symptoms at 2 years postoperative evaluation.

common in women and nonmanual laborers than in the control population. Osteopenia was a common finding. As compared to degenerative spondylosis, there were fewer osteophytes, less end-plate sclerosis, and little anterior wear of the bodies. It was difficult to see the facets well, but they identified erosive changes consistent with rheumatoid synovitis. They did not examine histologic material, but cited previous autopsy studies describing synovitis in the facet joints.

Involvement of diarthrodial joints is a hallmark of rheumatoid arthritis, so involvement of the apophyseal joints in the thoracolumbar spine is conceptually easy to accept. Though the disease is systemic and extra-articular manifestations such as rheumatoid nodules are well-known, involvement of fibrocartilaginous structures such as the intervertebral disc is controversial because of the nonspecific nature of the histologic changes. One school of thought holds that the destructive discovertebral lesions that are more commonly seen in the cervical spine are due to rheumatoid granulation tissue. Ball

(3) states that the uncovertebral joints are lined by synovium and provide this granulation tissue, which erodes the annulus, the annular attachments, and the subchondral bone. In support of this, he notes the rarity of such lesions in patients with juvenile rheumatoid arthritis, which generally occurs in individuals before formation of the uncovertebral joints. He contrasted the progressive ossification of ankylosing spondylitis with the instability of rheumatoid arthritis caused by destruction of both the apophyseal joints and the disc. Although instability could be seen throughout the spine, he felt frank dislocation was limited to the cervical spine because of the relative stability of the thoracic and lumbar regions. Because the lower portions of the spine lack uncovertebral joints, the disc changes were more nonspecific, such as disc degeneration, formation of Schmorl's nodes, and end-plate fractures.

Another school, typified by Martel (50), rejects the notion that fibrocartilaginous joints are involved with rheumatoid tissue, noting that the sternomanubrial articulation and the symphysis pubis were spared as distinct from the discs. Of 20 patients with rheumatoid arthritis and a minimum of 3 years' radiographic follow-up, he described progressive apophyseal arthritis and ligamentous laxity, and subsequent changes to the discs and vertebral bodies. He hypothesized that the instability engendered by the synovial facet joint involvement led to chronic trauma to the discovertebral joints by destroying the disc cartilage in the vertebral end-plates. Because other studies that included autopsies showed no inflammation or infection of the discovertebral joints, he believed that the granuloma formation described by others was not diagnostic of rheumatoid arthritis. He did admit that this was only a hypothesis inferred from his observations.

Involvement of the thoracolumbar disc and vertebral bodies appears to be uncommon, regardless of the exact mechanism. Facet synovitis is probably more common than anterior involvement. Instability of the thoracolumbar spine is quite uncommon. The few reported cases requiring surgery were all prompted by neural compression in the lumbar spine. Linquist and McDonnell (44) described a 52-year-old with longstanding rheumatoid arthritis with mild left quadriceps and extensor hallucis longus weakness. A subcutaneous mass was noted in the left lumbar region. Myelography revealed a large extradural defect that was left-sided, extending from the superior aspect of L3 to the midportion of L5. Pathologically, this was found to be a rheumatoid cyst arising from the left L3-L4 facet. There was extensive extraspinal extension through the musculature to the subcutaneous tissue, explaining the palpable mass. It also extended off the medial aspect of the joint into the spinal canal from L3 through L5. The cyst was not adherent to the dura and was easily removed at the time of laminectomy.

Friedman (34) treated a 42-year-old with a 7-year history of rheumatoid arthritis who presented with left buttock and posterolateral thigh pain. Myelography revealed left L4 and L5 dural compression. During exposure for laminectomy, a gray granular cyst was noted to invade the muscle at the L3 level. There was compression of the dura on the left from the upper aspect of L4 to the cranial aspect of S2. This too was a gray nodular mass compressing the left L5 and both S1 nerve roots. Measuring 3.5 x 2 x 3 cm, it was attached to the extraspinal cyst at the L3-L4 ligamentum flavum. Histologically, this was a solid mass showing fibrinoid necrosis and histiocytes, consistent with a rheumatoid nodule. It was easily removed from the spinal canal.

Magnaes (48) presented two patients with rheumatoid arthritis and neurogenic claudication. The clinical and radiographic picture was consistent with developmental lumbar spinal stenosis. Both had short, thick laminae, large facets, and thick capsule and ligamentum flavum. In addition, there was destruction of the facet cartilage

and infiltration of capsule, ligamentum flavum, facet joints, and laminae by granulation tissue consisting of lymphocytes, plasma cells, epithelioid cells, and fibrinoid necrosis, which appeared to be rheumatoid and infiltrative in nature.

Hauge et al. (39) described a 71-year-old with rheumatoid arthritis of 40 years' duration and only a short course of corticosteroids 5 years prior to presentation. Although she had had back pain for 2 years, 2 months before surgery she noticed a sudden increase in back and bilateral lower extremity pain with saddle anesthesia and difficulty voiding. Within 2 days, she had paresis of the left lower extremity. Radiographs demonstrated osteoporosis with narrowing of the L4-L5 disc and spondylolisthesis at L4-L5. There was a complete block at the L4-L5 level on myelogram, and laminectomies of L4 and L5 and a posterior interbody fusion were performed. The nucleus pulposus, annulus fibrosis, facet capsule, and ligamentum flavum were studied histologically, and all contained a highly vascular granulation tissue with lymphocytes, plasma cells, and fibrinoid necrosis, which they interpreted as rheumatoid granulation tissue. They mentioned five reported cases of cauda equina compression due to rheumatoid disease and summarized the four causes of neural compression as (a) epidural rheumatoid nodule, (b) intraspinal rheumatoid cyst from the facet joint, (c) infiltration of the facet, ligamentum flavum, facet joints, and laminae by rheumatoid granulation, and (d) destruction of the intervertebral joint complex by rheumatoid granulation leading to acute instability.

In summary, involvement of the facet joints in the thoracolumbar spine is probably common, but the clinical symptoms are mild or overshadowed by involvement in the cervical spine and appendicular skeleton. When there is wedging and vertebral body collapse, this may be due to rheumatoid involvement, low-grade instability due to facet disease, and the associated osteoporosis. Because these patients have an altered immune system and may be on immunosuppressive medication, the clinician must be sure that such lesions are not due to an infectious or neoplastic process. Rarely, rheumatoid involvement in the lower spine will lead to neural compression. Management should be tailored to the individual patient, adding arthrodesis to the decompression when instability is present.

REFERENCES

1. Baggenstoss AH, Bickel WH, Ward LE (1952): Rheumatoid granulomatous nodules as destructive lesions of vertebrae. *J Bone Joint Surg [Am]* 34:601–609.
2. Ball J (1958): Pathology of the rheumatoid cervical spine. *Ann Rheum Dis* 17:121.
3. Ball J (1971): Enthesopathy of rheumatoid and ankylosing spondylitis. *Ann Rheum Dis* 30:213–223.
4. Ball J, Sharp J (1971): Rheumatoid arthritis of the cervical spine. In: Hill AGS, ed. *Modern trends in rheumatology*, vol. 2. New York: Appleton-Century Crofts, pp. 117–138.

5. Bohlman HH (1978): Atlantoaxial dislocation in the arthritic patient: A report of 45 cases. *Orthop Trans* 2:197.
6. Brattstrom H, Elner A, Granholm L (1973): Case report: transoral surgery for myelopathy caused by rheumatoid arthritis of the cervical spine. *Ann Rheum Dis* 32:578–581.
7. Brattstrom H, Granholm L (1976): Atlanto-axial fusion in rheumatoid arthritis. *Acta Orthop Scand* 47:619–628.
8. Breedveld FC, Algra PR, Vielvoye CJ, Cats A (1987): Magnetic resonance imaging in the evaluation of patients with rheumatoid arthritis and subluxations of the cervical spine. *Arthritis Rheum* 30:624–629.
9. Bundschuh CV, Modic MT, Kearny F, et al (1988): Rheumatoid arthritis of the cervical spine; surface coil MR imaging. *Am J Neuro Rad* 9:565–571.
10. Burry HC, Tweed JM, Robinson RG, Howes R (1978): Lateral subluxation of the atlanto-axial joint in rheumatoid arthritis. *Ann Rheum Dis* 37:525–528.
11. Cabot A, Becker A (1978): The cervical spine in rheumatoid arthritis. *Clin Orthop* (131):130–140.
12. Cantore G, Ciappetta P, Delfini R (1984): New steel device for occipito-cervical fixation. Technical Note. *J Neurosurg* 60:1104–1106.
13. Castaing J, Gouaze A, Plisson JL (1963): Technique of cervico-occipital arthrodesis by iliac graft screwed into the occipital bone. *Rev Chir Orthop* 49:123–127.
14. Clark CR, Goetz DD, Menezes AH (1989): Arthrodesis of the cervical spine in rheumatoid arthritis. *J Bone Joint Surg* [*Am*] 71:381–392.
15. Compston JE, Crawley EO, Evans C, O'Sullivan MM (1988): Spinal trabecular bone mineral content in patients with non-steroid treated rheumatoid arthritis. *Ann Rheum Dis* 47:660–664.
16. Conaty JP, Morgan ES (1981): Cervical fusion in rheumatoid arthritis. *J Bone Joint Surg* [*Am*] 63:1218–1227.
17. Conlon PW, Isdale IC, Rose BS (1966): Rheumatoid arthritis of the cervical spine. An analysis of 333 cases. *Ann Rheum Dis* 25:120–126.
18. Cregan JCF (1966): Internal fixation of the unstable rheumatoid cervical spine. *Ann Rheum Dis* 25:242–252.
19. Crellin RQ, MacCabe JJ, Hamilton EBD (1970): Severe subluxation of the cervical spine in rheumatoid arthritis. *J Bone Joint Surg* [*Br*] 52:244–251.
20. Crockard HA, Essigman WK, Stevens JM, Pozo JL, Ransford AO, Kendall BE (1985): Surgical treatment of cervical cord compression in rheumatoid arthritis. *Ann Rheum Dis* 44:809–816.
21. Crockard HA, Pozo JL, Ransford AO, Kendall BE, Essigman WK (1986): Transoral decompression and posterior fusion for rheumatoid atlanto-axial subluxation. *J Bone Joint Surg* [*Br*] 68:350–356.
22. Davis FW Jr, Markley HE (1951): Rheumatoid arthritis with death from medullary compression. *Ann Intern Med* 35:451–454.
23. DeAndrade JR, Macnab I (1969): Anterior occipito-cervical fusion using an extra-pharyngeal exposure. *J Bone Joint Surg* [*Am*] 69:1621–1626.
24. Delamarter RB, Batzdorf U, Bohlman HH (1989): The C7–T1 junction: problems with diagnosis, visualization, instability and decompression. *Orthop Trans* 13:218.
25. Delamarter RB, Chafetz N, Lang P, Rothman SL, Sanny J, Rhodes ML (1989): Dynamic cine-MRI of the cervical spine. *Orthop Trans* 13:212.
26. Delamarter RB, Dodge L, Bohlman HH, Gambetti PL (1994): Postmortem neuropathologic analysis of eleven patients with paralysis secondary to rheumatoid arthritis of the cervical spine. *Spine* 19 (20):2267–2274.
27. Dirheimer Y (1977): *The craniovertebral region in chronic inflammatory rheumatic diseases.* Berlin: Springer-Verlag.
28. Dodge LD, Bohlman HH, Rechtine GR (1987): Paralysis secondary to rheumatoid arthritis—pathogenesis and results of treatment. *Orthop Trans* 11:473.
29. Boden S, Dodge LD, Bohlman HH, Rechtine GR (1993): Rheumatoid arthritis of the cervical spine: a long term analysis with predictors of paralysis and recovery. *J Bone Joint Surg* [*Am*] 75(9):1282–1297.
30. Eulderink F, Meijers KAE (1976): Pathology of the cervical spine in rheumatoid arthritis: a controlled study of 44 spines. *J Pathol* 120:91–108.
31. Ferlic DC, Clayton ML, Leidholt JD, Gamble WE (1975): Surgical treatment of the symptomatic unstable cervical spine in rheumatoid arthritis. *J Bone Joint Surg* [*Am*] 57:349–354.
32. Fielding JW, Cochran G van B, Lawsing JF 3rd, Hohl M (1974): Tears of the transverse ligament of the atlas. A clinical and biomechanical study. *J Bone Joint Surg* [*Am*] 56:1683–1691.
33. Fishgold H, Metzger J (1952): Etude radiographic de l'impression basilaire. *Rev Rheum* 19:261.
34. Friedman H (1970): Intraspinal rheumatoid nodule causing nerve root compression. Case report. *J Neurosurg* 32:689–691.
35. Glay A, Rona G (1965): Nodular rheumatoid vertebral lesions versus ankylosing spondylitis. *Am J Roentgenol* 94:631–638.
36. Hajiroussou VJ, Webley M (1984): Prolonged low-dose corticosteroid therapy and osteoporosis in rheumatoid arthritis. *Ann Rheum Dis* 43:24–27.
37. Halla JT, Fallahi S, Hardin JG (1982): Nonreducible rotational head tilt and lateral mass collapse. A prospective study of frequency, radiographic findings and clinical features in patients with rheumatoid arthritis. *Arthritis Rheum* 25:1316–1324.
38. Hamblen DL (1967): Occipito-cervical fusion. Indications, techniques and results. *J Bone Joint Surg* [*Br*] 49:33–45.
39. Hauge T, Magnaes B, Skullerud K (1980): Rheumatoid arthritis of the lumbar spine leading to anterior vertebral subluxation and compression of the cauda equina. *Scand J Rheumatol* 9:241–244.
40. Konttinnen Y, Santavirta S, Bergroth V, Sandelin J (1986): Inflammatory involvement of the cervical spine ligaments in rheumatoid arthritis. *Acta Orthop Scand* 57:587.
41. Lachiewicz PF, Inglis AE, Ranawat CS (1987): Methylmethacrylate augmentation for cervical spine arthrodesis in rheumatoid arthritis. *Orthop Trans* 11:7.
42. Larsson SE, Toolanen G (1986): Posterior fusion for atlanto-axial subluxation in rheumatoid arthritis. *Spine* 11:525–530.
43. Lawrence JS, Sharp J, Ball J, Bier F (1964): Rheumatoid arthritis of the lumbar spine. *Ann Rheum Dis* 23:205–217.
44. Linquist PR, McDonnell DE (1970): Rheumatoid cyst causing extradural compression. A case report. *J Bone Joint Surg* [*Am*] 52:1235–1240.
45. Lipson SJ (1985): Cervical myelopathy and posterior atlanto-axial subluxation in patients with rheumatoid arthritis. *J Bone Joint Surg* [*Am*] 67:593–597.
46. Lipson SJ (1989): Rheumatoid arthritis in the cervical spine. *Clin Orthop* 239:121–127.
47. Lorber A, Pearson CM, Rene RM (1961): Osteolytic vertebral lesions as a manifestation of rheumatoid arthritis and related disorders. *Arthritis Rheum* 4:514–532.
48. Magnaes B, Hauge T (1978): Rheumatoid arthritis contributing to lumbar spinal stenosis. *Scand J Rheum* 7:215–218.
49. Marks JS, Sharp J (1981): Rheumatoid cervical myelopathy. *Quart J Med* 50:307–319.
50. Martel W (1977): Pathogenesis of cervical discovertebral destruction in rheumatoid arthritis. *Arthritis Rheum* 20:1217–1225.
51. Martel W, Abell MR (1963): Fatal atlanto-axial luxation in rheumatoid arthritis. *Arthritis Rheum* 6:224–231.
52. Mathews JA (1969): Atlanto-axial subluxation in rheumatoid arthritis. *Ann Rheum Dis* 28:260–266.
53. McAfee PC, Bohlman HH, Ducker T, Eismont FJ (1986): Failure of stabilization of the spine with methylmethacrylate. A retrospective analysis of twenty-four cases. *J Bone Joint Surg* [*Am*] 68:1145–1157.
54. McAfee PC, Bohlman HH, Han JS, Salvagno RT (1986): Comparison of nuclear magnetic resonance imaging and computed tomography in the diagnosis of upper cervical spinal cord compression. *Spine* 11:295–304.
55. McAfee PC, Bohlman HH, Riley LH Jr, Robinson RA, Southwick WO, Nachlas NE (1987): The anterior retropharyngeal approach to the upper part of the cervical spine. *J Bone Joint Surg* [*Am*] 69:1371–1383.
56. Meijers KAE, Cats A, Kremer HPH, Luyendijk W, Onvlee GJ, Thomeer RTWM (1984): Cervical myelopathy in rheumatoid arthritis. *Clin Exp Rheumatol* 2:239–245.
57. Meijers KAE, Van Beusekom GT, Luyendijk W, Duijfjes F (1974): Dislocation of the cervical spine with cord compression in rheumatoid arthritis. *J Bone Joint Surg* [*Br*] 56:668–680.

58. Meikle JA, Wilkinson M (1971): Rheumatoid involvement of the cervical spine. *Ann Rheum Dis* 30:154–161.

59. Menezes AH, VanGilder JC, Clark CR, El-Khoury G (1985): Odontoid upward migration in rheumatoid arthritis. *J Neurosurg* 63:500–509.

60. Mikulowski P, Wollheim FA, Rotmil P, Olsen I (1975): Sudden death in rheumatoid arthritis with atlanto-axial dislocation. *Acta Med Scand* 198:445–451.

61. Morizono Y, Sakou T, Kawaida H (1987): Upper cervical involvement in rheumatoid arthritis. *Spine* 12:721–725.

62. Newman P, Sweetnam R (1969): Occipito-cervical fusion: an operative technique and its indications. *J Bone Joint Surg [Br]* 51:423–431.

63. Olerud S, Sjostrom L (1986): Dens resection in a case of vertical impression of the dens in the foramen magnum. *Acta Orthop Scand* 57:262.

64. Park WM, O'Neill M, McCall IW (1979): The radiology of rheumatoid involvement of the cervical spine. *Skeletal Radiol* 4:1–7.

65. Pellicci PM, Ranawat CS, Tsairis P, Bryan WJ (1981): A prospective study of the progression of rheumatoid arthritis of the cervical spine. *J Bone Joint Surg [Am]* 63:342–350.

66. Perry J, Nickel VL (1959): Total cervical spine fusion for neck paralysis. *J Bone Joint Surg [Am]* 41:37–60.

67. Rana NA, Hancock DO, Taylor AR, Hill AGS (1973): Upward translocation of the dens in rheumatoid arthritis. *J Bone Joint Surg [Br]* 55:471–477.

68. Ranawat CS, O'Leary P, Pellicci P, Tsairis P, Marchisello P, Dorr L (1979): Cervical spine fusion in rheumatoid arthritis. *J Bone Joint Surg [Am]* 61:1003–1010.

69. Rasker JJ, Cosh JA (1978): Radiological study of cervical spine and hand in patients with rheumatoid arthritis of 15 years' duration: an assessment of the effects of corticosteroid treatment. *Ann Rheum Dis* 37:529–535.

70. Redlund-Johnell I, Pettersson H (1984): Radiographic measurements of the cranio-vertebral region. *Acta Radiol Diagn* 25:23–28.

71. Sakou T, Kawaida H, Morizono Y, Matsunaga S, Fielding JW (1989): Occipitoatlantoaxial fusion utilizing a rectangular rod. *Clin Orthop* (239):136–144.

72. Santavirta S, Slatis P, Kankaanpaa U, Sandelin J, Laasonen E (1988): Treatment of the cervical spine in rheumatoid arthritis. *J Bone Joint Surg [Am]* 70:658–667.

73. Seaman WB, Wells J (1961): Destructive lesions of the vertebral bodies in rheumatoid disease. *Am J Roentgenol* 86:241–250.

74. Sharp J, Purser DW (1961): Spontaneous atlanto-axial dislocation in ankylosing spondylitis and rheumatoid arthritis. *Ann Rheum Dis* 20:47–77.

75. Simmons EH, du Toit G Jr (1978): Lateral atlantoaxial arthrodesis. *Orthop Clin North Am* 9:1101–1114.

76. Smith PH, Benn RT, Sharp J (1972): Natural history of rheumatoid cervical luxations. *Ann Rheumat Dis* 31:431–439.

77. Stevens JC, Cartlidge NE, Saunders M, Appleby A, Hall M, Shaw DA (1971): Atlanto-axial subluxation and cervical myelopathy in rheumatoid arthritis. *Quart J Med* 40:391–408.

78. Storey G (1958): Changes in the cervical spine in rheumatoid arthritis with compression of the cord. *Ann Phys Med* 4:216–218.

79. Webb FW, Hickman JA, Brew DS (1968): Death from vertebral artery thrombosis in rheumatoid arthritis. *Br Med J* 2:537–538.

80. Weissman BNW, Aliabadi P, Weinfeld MS, Thomas WH, Sosman JL (1982): Prognostic features of atlanto-axial subluxation in rheumatoid arthritis patients. *Radiology* 144:745–751.

81. Wertheim SB, Bohlman HH (1987): Occipitocervical fusion. Indications, technique, and long-term results in thirteen patients. *J Bone Joint Surg [Am]* 69:833–836.

82. Whitesides TE Jr, McDonald AP (1978): Lateral retropharyngeal approach to the upper cervical spine. *Orthop Clin North Am* 9(4):1115–1127.

83. Winfield J, Cooke D, Brook AS, Corbett M (1983): A prospective study of the radiological changes in the cervical spine in early rheumatoid arthritis. *Ann Rheum Dis* 42:613–618.

The Adult Spine: Principles and Practice,
2nd edition, J.W. Frymoyer, Editor-in-Chief.
Lippincott-Raven Publishers, Philadelphia © 1997.

CHAPTER **43**

Ankylosing Spondylitis: Surgical Treatment

John P. Kostuik

Historically, surgery for ankylosing spondylitis was rarely performed because of the high incidence of major complications. Today, corrective surgery can be considered for those patients with severe deformities. These include a loss of lumbar lordosis producing a flat back and thoracic kyphosis which may vary from mild to very severe. The patient's head and neck are thrust forward with increased flexion at the cervical thoracic junction, resulting in profound deformity and disability (Fig. 1). As a result of these severe deformities, the patient may be able to see only a few feet beyond his toes. In addition to functional disability, profound psychological disturbances and depression may ensue. Some patients become reclusive because of the markedly decreased visual field. In addition to these spinal deformities the hips may be involved, resulting in flexion contractures that further accentuate the loss of lumbar lordosis. Patients frequently have involvement of the temporomandibular joints, leading to inability to open their mouths, a challenge to intubation at the time of surgery. The upper extremities are rarely involved.

J. P. Kostuik, M.D., F.R.C.S.(C.): Professor, Department of Orthopaedic Surgery, Johns Hopkins University School of Medicine, Baltimore, Maryland 21287-0882.

HISTORY OF SURGICAL TREATMENT

Smith-Peterson and colleagues (28) performed the first spinal osteotomy for ankylosing spondylitis in 1945 and reported their results for six patients. Hyperextension of the lumbar spine was achieved and enabled the patient to see ahead. This pioneering effort was followed by subsequent reports from LaChapelle (10), Adams (1), Herbert (7), Law (11,12,14), McMaster (16), Goel (5), Emneus (4), and McMaster and Coventry (17,18).

The operative technique of Smith-Peterson and colleagues (28) has often been reported to involve a single lumbar vertebral level, but in fact two- and three-level osteotomies were done through the articular processes with resection of the spinous processes of L1, L2, and L3. They obtained correction of between 20° and 30° and were prepared to carry out a similar osteotomy at higher or lower levels as required. Postoperatively the patients were treated with plaster immobilization. Law (12) felt that 40° to 50° of correction could be achieved routinely at any level of the spine and as much as 80° to 90° could be gained without injury to the cauda equina or nerve roots.

LaChapelle (10) described a two-stage osteotomy. In his initial procedure, performed under local anesthesia, three spinous processes and the lamina of the second

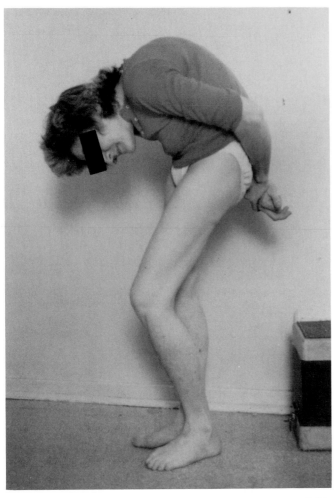
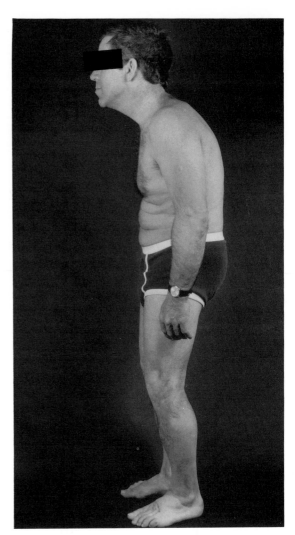

FIG. 1. A: Severe deformity of ankylosing spondylitis with loss of lumbar lordosis, thoracic kyphosis, and head and neck thrust. **B:** Less severe deformity.

lumbar vertebra and articular processes at L2–L3 were resected. Two weeks later an anterior osteotomy under general anesthetic was performed at the L2–L3 level, opening the disc space with bone blocks. Plaster immobilization was used.

Briggs and co-workers' (3) technique involved bilateral intervertebral foraminotomies, wherein a wedge was removed involving the superior articular processes of the fourth lumbar vertebra and some of the upper part of the pedicles. The pivot of angulation was at the posterior margin of the disc between the third and fourth lumbar vertebrae. These authors advocated the use of internal fixation and postoperative brace rather than plaster cast.

Herbert (7) described a two-stage procedure that involved resecting bone along the intervertebral lamina, including posterior resection over two levels, applicable to the lumbar and cervical spine (Figs. 2–5). Postoperatively, he positioned the patient on pillows which were

sequentially removed, allowing for some further correction of the deformity in the postoperative phase. The secondary anterior osteotomy was performed 2 or 3 weeks later, resecting the intervertebral disc at the level of the original posterior osteotomy. Again correction was obtained postoperatively over the subsequent 24 hours by positioning followed by application of a plaster jacket. In his reported 50 patients, some vascular complications occurred; there were three cases of nerve compression (two in the lumbar spine and one in the cervical spine), and four deaths. Deformity recurred in six patients, which Herbert thought was a result of an inadequate or insufficient degree of correction.

Law (12) has reported the greatest experience with osteotomies of the lumbar spine, detailing his results with 120 patients. He usually performed a single wedge osteotomy at L2–L3 as described by Smith-Peterson, and advocated the use of internal fixation and postoperative im-

loidosis), two with pneumonia, one with thrombosis of the spinal cord vessels, two with hemorrhagic shock, and one from unrelated causes. Recurrence of the deformity occurred only twice. A second osteotomy was carried out in these cases.

Scudese and Calabro (24) later described a modification of the Smith-Peterson osteotomy. Following posterior resection of the vertebral arch, the disc at the selected level together with the superior portion of the body was removed. The wedge was then closed. They felt this procedure was less likely to result in aortic or inferior vena cava obstruction (Fig. 6). Other authors, including Adams (1) and Lichtblau and Wilson (15), have also reported either rupture or obstruction of the aorta as a particular risk of anterior open wedge osteotomies.

The modern era for surgery in ankylosing spondylitis was led by Simmons (25). His major contribution to osteotomy of the cervical and lumbar spine was the use of local anesthesia, which allows continuous intraoperative monitoring of neurologic status (23). Prior to his report, almost all clinical analyses included a significant incidence of major complications with mortality ranging from 8% to 10%, whereas neurologic complications including paraplegia occurred in 30%. Other complications included rupture of the aorta, acute gastric dilation, superior mesenteric artery thrombosis, and psychological problems. However, with improved surgical techniques, the use of local anesthesia, and improved mobilization, morbidity, and mortality have markedly decreased.

GENERAL PRINCIPLES

Before operative intervention it is essential to assess specific problems that might result in intraoperative or perioperative complications. Because the spondyloarthropathies may be associated with ileitis or colitis, the nutritional status of the patient, as well as general bone density, should be evaluated. If significant osteopenia is present, fixation problems should be anticipated.

Respiratory function may be compromised by the kyphotic deformity, particularly if it is severe in the thoracic spine. Ankylosis of the ribs to the vertebral bodies often completely limits chest expansion. The patient should be forewarned of the possibility of postoperative respiratory problems including adult respiratory distress syndrome, particularly if there has been a history of smoking. The patient should be warned that postoperative pulmonary assistance may be needed, including a ventilator in major lumbar and thoracic cases.

Because ankylosis may occur at the temporomandibular joints and arytenoids, intubation may prove difficult. As a result of the impediment and because of the desire to monitor the patient's neurologic function intraoperatively, Simmons advocated the use of local anes-

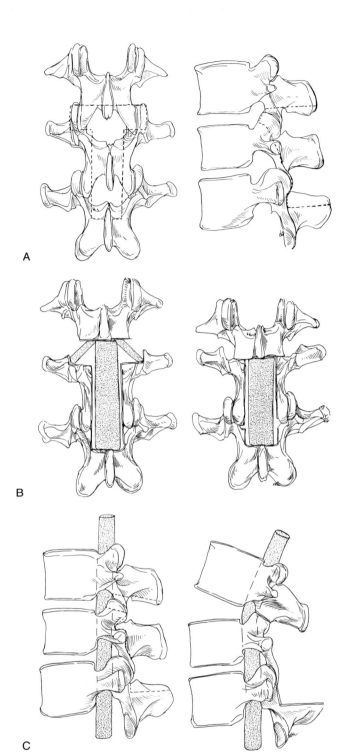

FIG. 2. **A:** Schematic drawing of vertebral osteotomy, showing outline of the bone block to be resected. **B:** Posterior view of vertebral osteotomy, showing outline after bone resection and after correction of the kyphosis. **C:** Lateral view of vertebral osteotomy, showing outline after bone resection and after correction of the kyphosis.

mobilization in plaster for 3 to 6 months followed by a spinal brace. In the early postoperative period 10 patients died: two with perforated gastric ulcers, two with high intestinal obstruction (one as the result of amy-

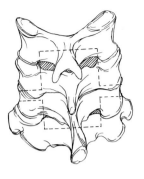

Posterior

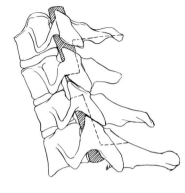

Lateral

FIG. 3. Schematic drawing of cervical osteotomy, showing outline of the bone block to be resected.

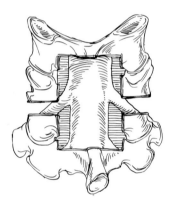

After Resection

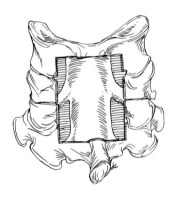

After Reduction of Kyphosis

FIG. 4. Posterior view of cervical osteotomy, showing outline after bone resection and after correction of the kyphosis.

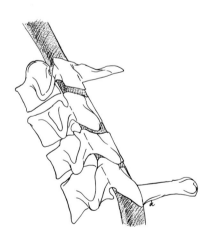

After Resection

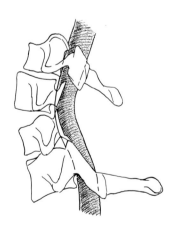

After Reduction of Kyphosis

FIG. 5. Lateral view of cervical osteotomy, showing outline after bone resection and after correction of the kyphosis.

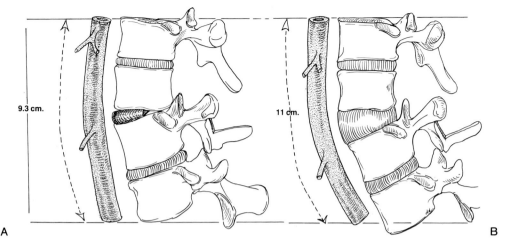

FIG. 6. A: No effective narrowing and stretching of the aorta when there is no appreciable lumbar lengthening. **B:** Narrowing and stretching of the aorta resulting from lumbar spine lengthening.

thesia. However, the majority of patients worldwide are still intubated and given a general anesthetic. This may necessitate intubating the patient awake either orally or nasally and in extreme cases even a tracheostomy may be required.

Careful attention should be given to clinical and radiologic examination of the hip joints. If there is decreased motion or ankylosis associated with a hip flexion deformity and loss of articular surface, total hip replacement should be performed before any surgical correction of the spinal deformity. If the hip involvement is bilateral, both hips should be done either concurrently or within a week or two of one another. If one hip arthroplasty is delayed after correction of the contralateral side, the first hip operated on may redevelop its hip flexion deformity.

Other musculoskeletal problems specific to the patient with ankylosing spondylitis are fractures, spinal instability, and spondylodiscitis. Fortunately, problems of subaxial subluxation and atlantoaxial instability are rare and unlike the significant risk in rheumatoid arthritis.

Because of the increased prevalence of aortic stenosis in these patients, a preoperative assessment should include, in addition to standard laboratory workup, pulmonary function studies, and evaluation of cardiac status.

Radiologic assessment should include routine chest, spine, and hip x-rays. For evaluation of the cervical spine, a flexion-extension view should be obtained to assess any possible level of instability. The chin-brow to vertical angle should be measured clinically with the neck in neutral position, and the measurements transposed to a lateral view of the spine. The amount of bone to be resected at each level can then be measured (Figs. 7 and 8). Similar films including flexion-extension views should be taken of the thoracic and lumbar spine.

FLEXION DEFORMITY OF THE SPINE

From an assessment of the clinical and radiographic evaluation, the site of the primary deformity should be determined. Ideally, the major surgical correction should be performed at that level. Because of the inherent problems of osteotomies in the thoracic spine, many surgeons

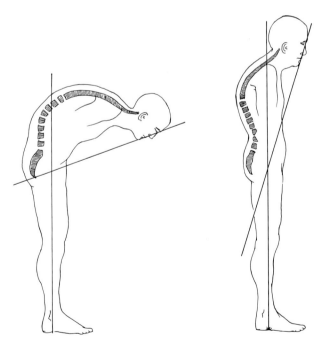

FIG. 7. Measurement of degree of flexion deformity of the spine in ankylosing spondylitis. The chin-brow to vertical angle is the angle measured from the brow to the chin to the vertical with the patient standing with the hips and knees extended and the neck in its fixed or neutral position.

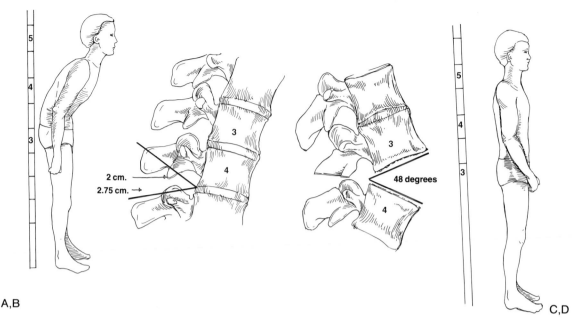

A,B   C,D

FIG. 8. A: Lateral view of patient standing with hips and knees extended. The patient's neck is still mobile and compensated by hyperextension. The chin-brow to vertical angle is measured with the neck in the neutral position (giving angle shown in B). **B:** The chin-brow to vertical angle measured with the patient's neck in the neutral position is transposed to a lateral view of the lumbar spine with the apex of the angle at the posterior margin of the L3–L4 disc space. The amount of bone to be resected at each level is indicated. **C:** Postoperative lateral view showing angle of correction obtained after closure of resected bone posteriorly with opening anterior osteoclasis at the L3–L4 level. **D:** Postoperative standing lateral view showing correction achieved after removal of the calculated wedge of bone as indicated by preoperative assessment.

have avoided surgery in this area. However, with improved techniques of internal fixation this area is now being attacked directly as well. Correction is achieved through multiple level anterior and posterior osteotomies, which are supplemented by posterior correction with segmental fixation (Fig. 9).

KYPHOTIC DEFORMITY OF THE LUMBAR SPINE

The objectives for performing a lumbar osteotomy in patients with ankylosing spondylitis include the following: (a) to enable the patient to assume a more erect posture; (b) to relieve compression of the abdominal viscera by the rib margin; (c) to improve diaphragmatic respiration which these patients frequently depend on because of ankylosis of the costovertebral margins; (d) to broaden the operative field required for upper abdominal surgery; and (e) to improve the patient's field of vision.

Operative Positioning and Anesthesia

In their original description, Smith-Peterson and colleagues (28) used general anesthesia with the patient lying in the prone position. Subsequent surgeons following

the work of Adams (1) preferred to perform the surgery with the patients lying on their sides. Because of the high neurologic morbidity and mortality rates, as noted, Simmons (26) favored correction of lumbar flexion deformities by resection extension osteotomy performed under local anesthesia and showed this technique to be safe, reliable, and practical.

With the advent of multiple level osteotomies distributing the corrective forces over multiple levels, most surgeons today prefer to perform lumbar and thoracic osteotomies with the patient prone, under general anesthesia. Spinal cord monitoring is routinely used. Postoperatively a nasogastric tube should be introduced because with extension osteotomies the superior mesenteric artery may be stretched over the third part of the duodenum resulting in gastric dilation.

Before the advent of rigid forms of internal fixation, plaster molds of the upper and lower halves of the body were prepared preoperatively. The upper half extended from the waist proximally, supporting the chest and head, and the lower half extended from the waist to the knees. These molds were used to support the patient postoperatively, so that they could be turned after correction.

Today, with the advent of improved internal fixation, particularly pedicle fixation or multiple level segmental fixation, plaster molds are rarely used postoperatively.

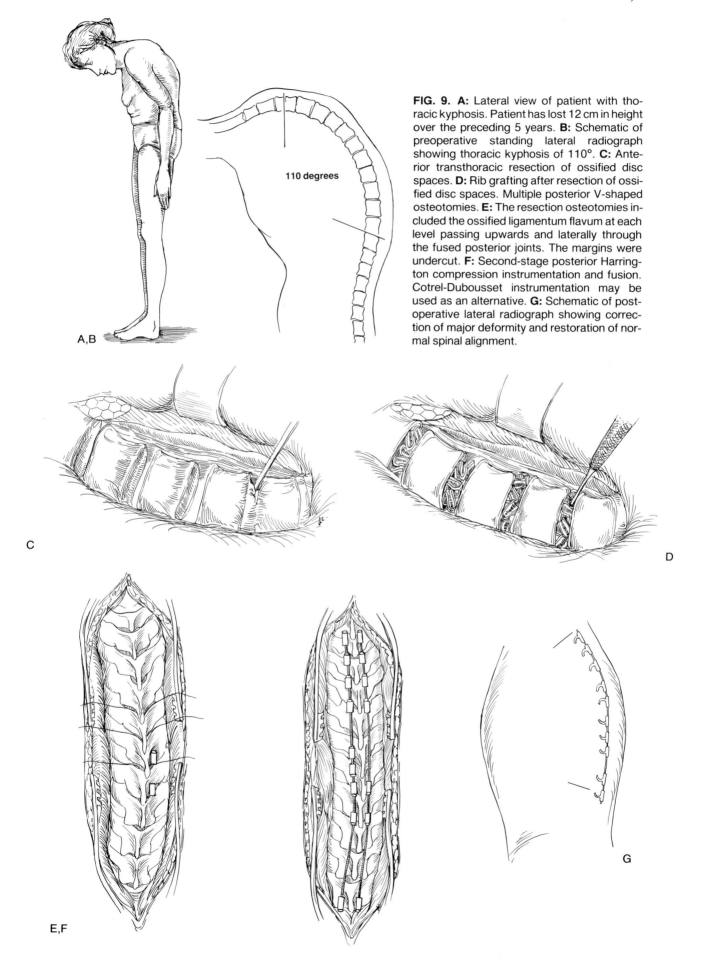

FIG. 9. A: Lateral view of patient with thoracic kyphosis. Patient has lost 12 cm in height over the preceding 5 years. **B:** Schematic of preoperative standing lateral radiograph showing thoracic kyphosis of 110°. **C:** Anterior transthoracic resection of ossified disc spaces. **D:** Rib grafting after resection of ossified disc spaces. Multiple posterior V-shaped osteotomies. **E:** The resection osteotomies included the ossified ligamentum flavum at each level passing upwards and laterally through the fused posterior joints. The margins were undercut. **F:** Second-stage posterior Harrington compression instrumentation and fusion. Cotrel-Dubousset instrumentation may be used as an alternative. **G:** Schematic of postoperative lateral radiograph showing correction of major deformity and restoration of normal spinal alignment.

110 degrees

A,B

C

D

E,F

G

The patients are allowed to ambulate within a few days and are usually fitted with a customized plastic orthosis which is worn for 6 months. For those few patients for whom plaster molds are required, a postoperative support is placed under the superior and inferior molds. The patients are nursed on a rotating bed which moves the patient from side to side. A well-molded posterior shell is then applied. This shell should be rigid and maintain the new contour of the spine with adequate support under the pelvis so that the thoracic kyphosis is not pushed forward in relationship to the lumbar spine. The patient lies in the supine position (Figs. 10–12). A posterior shell is necessary to support the patient in a supine position when the patient uses a bedpan and a trapdoor is removed on the bed.

Surgical Planning

A primary deformity in the lumbar spine is often associated with increased thoracic kyphosis. Balance is achieved by overcorrecting the lumbar deformity so the chin-brow to vertical angle is restored to as close to normal as possible. Simmons (26) has advocated that the level of correction be at the center of normal lumbar lordosis and below the spinal cord termination. The latter site is chosen to avoid possible damage to the spinal cord as the osteotomy is performed in the less dangerous area of the cauda equina. The amount of bone to be removed at a single level osteotomy is determined by measure-

ment of preoperative radiographs as advocated by Smith-Peterson (28) and subsequently by Simmons (26) (Figs. 8 and 13). Following bony resection and posterior closure, an opening wedge osteotomy is performed anteriorly resulting in deformity correction. Simmons stated that full correction or as close to full correction as possible should be obtained so that the line of weight-bearing is shifted posterior to the osteotomy line. In that position, gravity will help to maintain and possibly increase correction. Furthermore, Simmons (26) postulated that bony formation posteriorly across the osteotomy site was stimulated as a result of increased compressive forces at this point (see Fig. 8). To be certain the correction has been obtained, a radiolucent table facilitates the use of intraoperative x-rays.

Surgical Technique

A V-shaped wedge resection osteotomy is performed as recommended by Smith-Peterson (see Fig. 8). All bone removed at the site of osteotomy is kept for subsequent grafting purposes. A power burr or osteotome may be used. The dural sac is completely exposed bilaterally to the pedicles. The lamina must be undercut to avoid dural impingement during spine extension. In the presence of a small spinal canal, i.e., one that is stenotic and less than 20 mL in an anterior-posterior direction, it is particularly important that posterior decompression be generous, leaving an oval area open posteriorly. To de-

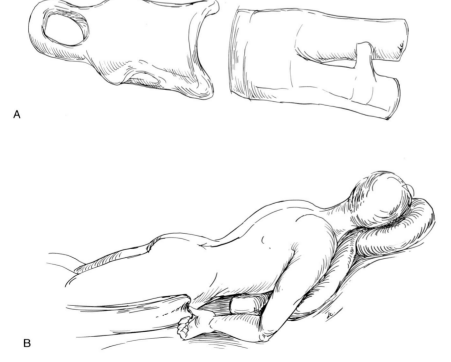

A

B

FIG. 10. A: Cephalad and caudad anterior mold made preoperatively. The cephalad mold supports the head and has an opening for the face. **B:** Postoperative view of patient with restored normal lordosis after correction of the deformity, lying in the prone position, in the anterior molds with a support under the upper mold.

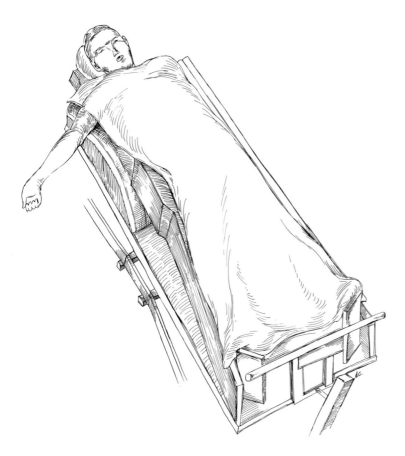

FIG. 11. Patient postoperatively in Roto-rest bed. The bed provides secure fixation with gentle side-to-side rotation avoiding the necessity to turn the patient from prone to supine positions. It facilitates and eases nursing care. It is important that the patient's spine be supported with a posterior shell so that on removal of the trap door for a bedpan, the spine is still supported.

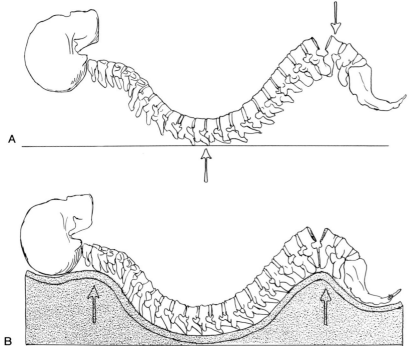

FIG. 12. A: Contour of corrected spine with patient lying with the spine unsupported. The dorsal projecting hump bears most of the weight with less support on the lumbar spine as well as below the osteotomy. **B:** With the patient supine in a well-molded rigid shell, there is equal distribution of weight throughout the spine with elimination of uneven contact points.

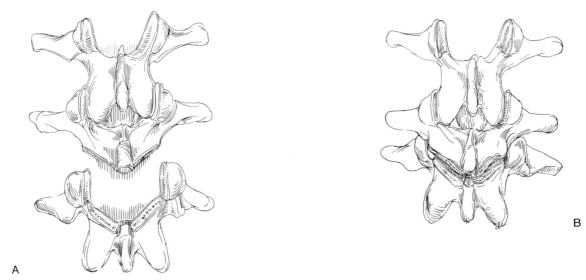

FIG. 13. A: Completion of fusion with resected bone placed posterolaterally on both sides creating an adequate autogenous fusion mass after V-shaped excision osteotomy. **B:** Closed V-shaped resection osteotomy with locking effect.

termine the dimensions of the osteotomy, Simmons advocated the use of careful intraoperative measurements in order to resect accurately the amount of bone determined by the preoperative radiologic assessment.

At the moment of anterior osteoclasis, Simmons (26) advocated the use of short-acting barbiturates supplemented with diazepam given just before the manipulation. The osteoclasis is achieved by extension of the hips and pelvis while posterior pressure is applied to the upper chest. The surgeon applies anterior pressure at the level of the osteotomy. Usually a distinct crack is heard. It is

usually not necessary to supplement the posterior arthrodesis with bone taken from sources other than the osteotomy site.

Other authors have reported that manual osteoclasis may be difficult to achieve. If this is the case then the dura can be gently moved to one side, a thin osteotome passed anteriorly, and an osteotomy carefully performed, first on one and then on the other side of the dural sac. Occasionally even this is not sufficient and an anterior open osteotomy must be performed at the level of the posterior osteotomy site. This can be easily

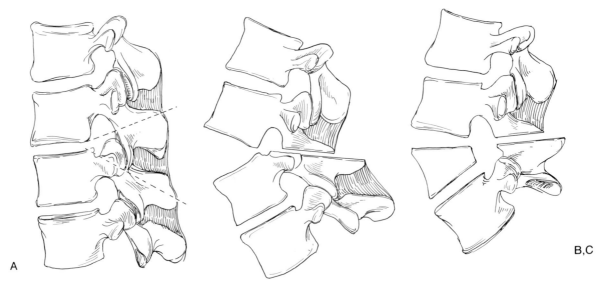

FIG. 14. A: Resected wedge marked with dotted lines. **B:** Wedge osteotomy with opening of the disc in front. **C:** Osteotomy with resection of wedge from behind and resection of the pedicles. The body is fractured with the wedging pointing backward.

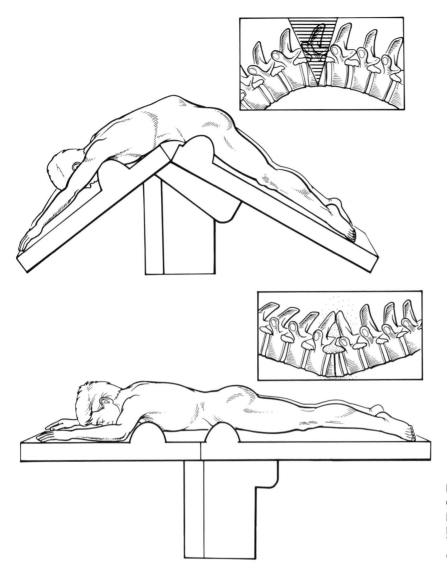

FIG. 15. Posterior lumbar vertebral body decancellization osteotomy. This may be performed at more than one level. Note the prone position before and after osteotomy. The operating room table assists in the correction.

achieved if the patient is lying on his side. If the patient is in the prone position, a supplemental posterolateral approach may be necessary with removal of the pedicle on the one side in order to weaken the anterior elements and allow for manual osteoclasis.

Most surgeons advocate the use of internal fixation, because it avoids risk of postoperative translation and allows for early postoperative mobilization. Initially this was achieved with either wires or Knodt rods. Later, Luque instrumentation together with Drummond buttons and wires were used. Today, most surgeons advocate the use of segmental fixation with screws or hooks in order to distribute load over several points of fixation.

Results

Correction of Deformity

Correction achieved by Simmons (26) ranged from 40° to 104° with an average of 56°. The preoperative chin-brow to vertical angle varied from 35° to 134° with an average of 60°, and the postoperative chin-brow to vertical angle ranged from −5° to +15° with an average of 5°.

Complications

Simmons (26) used single-level wedge osteotomy in 90 patients and noted that seven (8%) developed L3 or root cauda equina compression. This usually occurred 2 to 14 days after the operation and was more common in cases performed prior to the use of internal fixation for stabilization. This complication was thought to be secondary to slippage as the patient was turned postoperatively. Simmons also felt that decreased canal dimensions that occurred intraoperatively during the closure process of the posterior wedge might be a contributory cause. If the osteoclasis occurred through the body of the vertebra rather than through the disc space, the risks were greater.

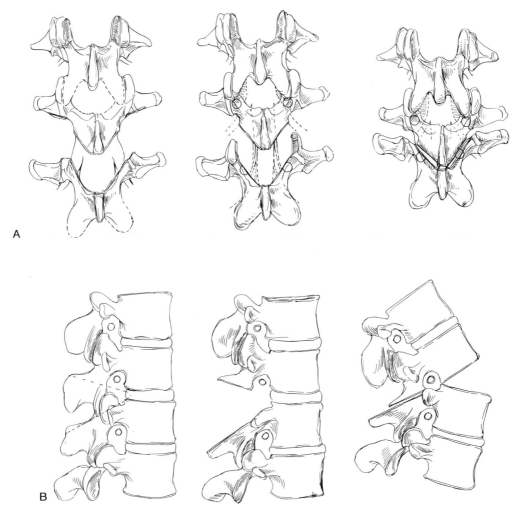

FIG. 16. Three stages of operation (**A,B**) showing the recommended technique for extension osteotomy of the lumbar spine.

He recommended anterior division of the disc at the appropriate level if ossification of the disc was believed to be greater than that of the vertebral body. In cases not stabilized, where neurologic problems occurred, Simmons recommended returning the patient to the operating room for stabilization following reduction of the deformity.

Modern Alternatives to Smith-Peterson Osteotomy

Many authors have advocated alternative techniques to the standard Smith-Peterson osteotomy. In 1985 Thomasen (32) recommended an osteotomy with resection of the lamina and transverse processes, usually at L2 (29). The pedicles are subsequently removed (Fig. 14) as is the upper part of the lamina of L3 and the articular processes of L2–L3. The dura and spinal nerves on either side are left lying free. After removal of the pedicles, a narrow rongeur is introduced to remove bone in the midpoint of the vertebral body. The side walls of the verte-

bral body and the immediate midline posterior aspect of the body are divided with a small osteotome, which may result in a good deal of hemorrhage. The patient is placed in the prone position and the wedge is slowly closed followed by internal fixation. Thomasen felt that by using this posterior compression of the vertebral body, no stretching of the cauda equina occurred and there was less potential for stretching the internal abdominal muscles and aorta.

In his series of 11 patients Thomasen had one patient with a neurologic complication due to translocation. The case occurred prior to the use of internal fixation devices. In none of his cases was the disc opened anteriorly. He did note a few patients who years later developed increased cervical kyphosis but this was not thought to be in any way attributable to lumbar surgery.

Thiranont and Netrawichien (31) and Jaffray et al. (9) have also independently described closing wedge osteotomies using transpedicular vertebral body decancellation together with internal fixation with good results (Fig. 15).

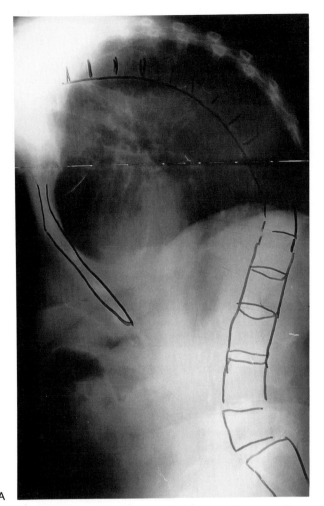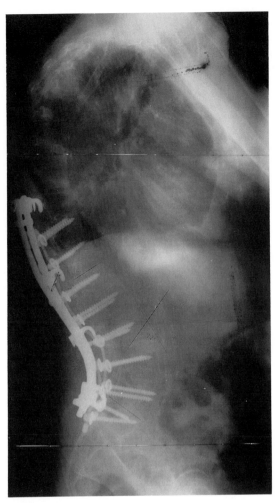

A

B

FIG. 17. A: A 57-year-old female with severe flexion deformity of the thoracic spine. **B:** Multiple level lumbar and thoracolumbar osteotomies with segmental fixation have restored the patient to the upright position, without performing surgery in the higher thoracic spine.

McMaster (17) developed a modified Smith-Peterson technique which was performed in 14 patients. He used a compression device that provided slow, finely controlled closure of the osteotomy and rigid internal fixation. All osteotomies were performed distal to the conus medullaris. The bony ends of the osteotomy defect should be parallel and 8 mm apart, depending on the angle of correction required. He recommended that the transverse axis of eventual closure about which correction would occur should lie anterior to the cauda equina, and that the osteotomy must extend anteriorly so that its apex lies at the anterior margin of the intervertebral canal and laterally to give good exposure of the nerve roots (Fig. 16). This position was thought to allow for relaxation of the cauda equina, as extension occurred when the osteotomy was closed. Enough bone must be removed from the pedicles above and below the intervertebral foramina to make sure that the nerve roots are not compromised on closure of the osteotomy. McMaster modified the 1,251 Harrington hooks by making a cut in the top of the hooks

to allow rod placement. He reported no neurologic complications, which he believed was due to the proper V-shaped osteotomy and slow closure of the osteotomy.

More recently Puschel and Zielke (22) recommended multiple wedge osteotomies at three or more levels of the lumbar spine in order to reproduce lumbar lordosis in kyphotic deformities associated with ankylosing spondylitis. Multiple laminectomies were done with extension across the pars interarticularis following the intervertebral foramina in a V-shaped fashion. They applied multiple pedicle screws to Zielke rods and closed the osteotomy site restoring lordosis. They reported that multiple V-shaped osteotomies together with the use of internal fixation allowed for a safer method of deformity reduction with minimal risk of neurologic complications as forces were dissipated over multiple levels (Figs. 17–20). Similarly, Roy-Camille et al. (23) has advocated internal fixation.

More recently we have adapted this technique and found it to be preferable to the single-stage osteotomy.

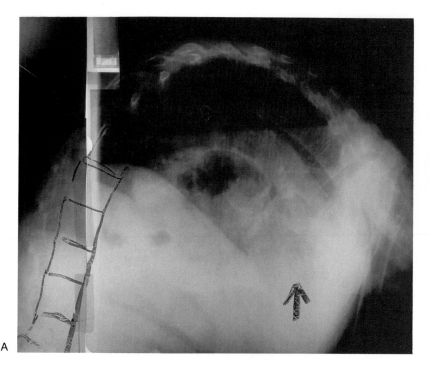

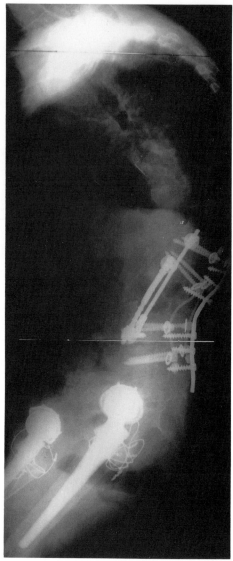

FIG. 18. A: A 53-year-old female (also shown in Fig. 1) with very severe thoracic deformity with flattening of the lumbar spine. Cervical lordosis was maintained. Bilateral hip flexion deformities of 30° were also present, requiring total hip replacement. **B:** Multiple level anterior (two) and posterior (four) osteotomies allowed for maximal compensating lumbar lordosis which, together with total hip replacements, allowed the patient to stand upright.

Using this technique now in ten cases, we have encountered no neurologic complications.

KYPHOTIC DEFORMITY OF THE THORACIC SPINE

Although kyphosis is always increased in the thoracic spine in ankylosing spondylitis, the deformity is rarely corrected at this level.

Simmons (26) identified two groups of patients with increased thoracic kyphosis in ankylosing spondylitis. In the first group the primary deformity was in the thoracic spine and was accompanied by loss of lumbar lordosis. If the increase in thoracic kyphosis was mild or moderate and the lumbar spine rigid and flattened, the overall deformity could be satisfactorily corrected by an osteotomy in the midlumbar spine. Compensation for the thoracic

kyphosis could be achieved, with restoration of spinal balance and a normal chin-brow to vertical angle. The second group had more severe thoracic kyphosis and normal cervical and lumbar lordosis. Simmons believed that these patients needed treatment of the primary thoracic deformity, which required multiple anterior and posterior intervertebral osteotomies with instrumentation and grafting (Fig. 21).

Simmons further identified subgroups in this second group of patients. The first subgroup had incomplete ossification of the thoracic spine or extensive areas of destructive spondylodiscitis. In these patients preliminary correction can be obtained by halo-dependent traction followed by multiple posterior resection osteotomies and instrumentation. A second stage consists of anterior resection of the discitis together with strut grafting.

In the second subgroup, patients had rigid thoracic ky-

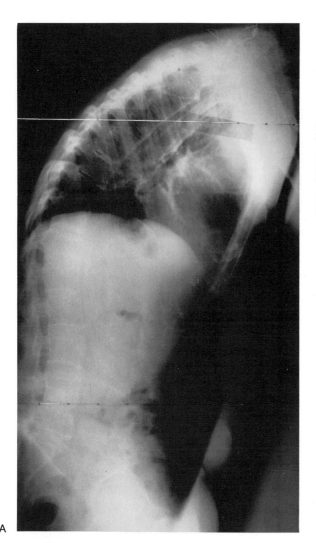
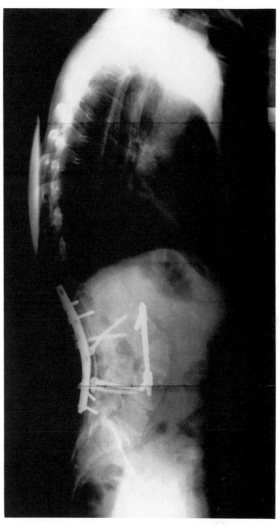

FIG. 19. **A:** A 50-year-old male with moderate deformity. A previous cervical osteotomy had been performed. **B:** Multiple level posterior osteotomies with segmental fixation were done. The opening wedge was so great that an anterior graft (bicortical iliac) and anterior Kostuik-Harrington instrumentation were added.

phosis but complete anterior ossification. In these patients, an anterior transthoracic approach is required first. The ossified disc spaces are completely resected back to the posterior annulus and filled with autogenous graft although surgeons have advocated the use of halo-dependent traction postoperatively. We have not done so and achieved equally satisfactory results. Ten days later, using a posterior approach, multiple V-shaped resection osteotomies are carried out at each level. The ossified ligamentum flavum and adjacent portions of the lamina are resected out through the foramina, removing enough bone to allow for adequate correction. This correction is achieved by bilateral compression instrumentation gradually closing the osteotomy sites (see Fig. 9).

Contrary to lumbar osteotomies and cervical osteotomies, thoracic osteotomies require general anesthesia for both procedures. Simmons recognized the hazard of this

approach and the possible necessity of performing a preoperative tracheostomy. The technique of multiple two-stage anterior-posterior osteotomies with posterior instrumentation has been used for primary thoracic deformity with normal cervical and lumbar lordosis, and was judged to be the procedure of choice by Simmons when a thoracolumbar deformity is greater than 40°. If the dorsal kyphosis is associated with reduced lumbar lordosis or if the thoracolumbar deformity is less than 40°, he advocated resection extension osteotomy in the midlumbar spine.

KYPHOTIC DEFORMITY
OF THE CERVICAL SPINE

The primary flexion deformity of the spine may occur in the cervical region or more particularly in the cervical

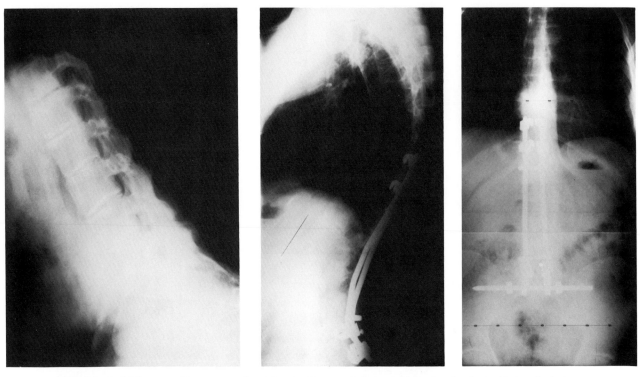

A
B,C

FIG. 20. A: Male, age 42, preoperative lateral with complete loss of lumbar lordosis. **B:** Lordosis has been restored by multiple wedge osteotomies. Note four points of fixation, two proximal, two distal. Hooks were used because of good bone quality, in place of pedicle screws. **C:** Sacral fixation using a modified Harrington sacral bar passed through Cotrel-Dubousset ring connectors.

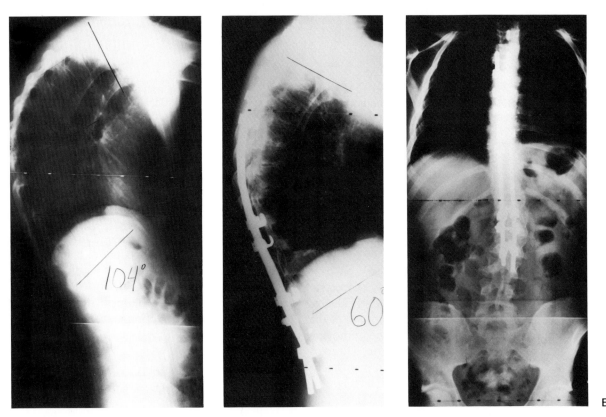

A
B,C

FIG. 21. A: Male, age 38 with a severe thoracic kyphosis measuring 104° T2–T12. **B–C:** An anterior release was performed from T2 to T12. The disc spaces were filled with morsellized autogenous rib graft. Under the same anesthetic, after turning the patient into the prone position. Multiple (six) posterior wedge osteotomies (3–4 mm wide) were done. Correction was obtained through segmental fixation.

thoracic region. This may be extremely disabling, with marked restriction of the field of vision, often combined with inability of or interference with mouth opening.

The objectives of cervical osteotomy are: (a) correction of deformity thus enabling the patient to see ahead more easily; (b) prevention of atlantoaxial subluxation dislocation which may result from the weight of the head being carried forward; (c) relief of tracheal and esophageal kinking accompanied by dyspnea or dysphagia; (d) relief of neurologic complications due to kinking of the spinal cord or undue traction of the nerve roots; and (e) prevention of deformity from cervical fracture. The last indication does not require cervical osteotomy if identified early enough, before a deformity is fixed.

Cervical Osteotomy Techniques

Urist (34) is credited with performing the first osteotomy of the cervical spine in 1958. In 1962 Law (13) made an extensive report of this technique.

Law stated that osteotomy could be performed at any

level below the second cervical vertebra and usually chose an osteotomy site between the third and fourth cervical or the sixth and seventh cervical levels. He thought that the level selected depended on the degree of ossification of the anterior longitudinal ligament and the severity of the deformity. This technique included grafting and internal fixation with wire or metal plates and postoperative immobilization in a plaster shell or Minerva or plaster jacket. An alternative method of immobilization was a halo cast, but he preferred to use internal fixation and insisted that the patient become ambulatory, thus decreasing nursing care. Law performed his cervical osteotomy under general anesthesia. In his first ten cases there was one death unrelated to the osteotomy. Subsequently he performed 100 cervical osteotomies with little morbidity, although others did not have this experience.

Because of possible hazards encountered with intubation and deformity correction under general anesthesia, Simmons (25) advocated the use of local anesthesia which he felt allowed for a consistent, satisfactory correction with relative safety. The procedure was performed under local anesthesia with the patient in the sitting po-

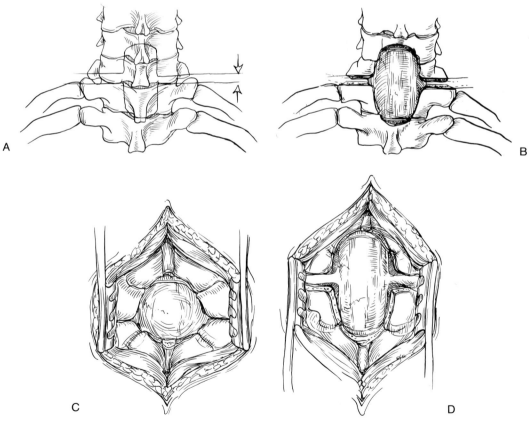

FIG. 22. A: Posterior cervical resection. The entire posterior arch of C7 is resected, the inferior half of the arch of C6, and the superior half of the arch of T1. **B:** Area of resection. The midline resection is beveled on the deep aspect to avoid impingement against the dura. The pedicles must also be undercut in a curved fashion to avoid impingement on the C8 nerve roots. **C:** Operative view: C8 nerve roots exposed. **D:** Operative view, after reduction.

sition. He believed that having the patient awake helped because the patient was able to indicate if paresthetic pain occurred along the distribution of the cervical roots. Unlike Law, he performed the osteotomy between the seventh cervical and the first thoracic vertebra (Fig. 22). The spinal canal is relatively wide at this level and the eighth cervical roots have reasonable mobility. He also believed that weakness caused by compromise of the eighth cervical root would cause less disability than other roots. Furthermore, there was less likelihood of damage to the vertebral artery and veins as these pass in front of the transverse process of the seventh cervical vertebra and enter the transverse foramina at the sixth vertebra (Fig. 23).

We prefer to perform the Simmons technique with the patient under local anesthesia in the sitting position, but advocate the use of internal fixation rather than halo cast immobilization. We have successfully used this technique in more than 25 cases. However, the surgeon should remember that the anatomic localization of the vertical arteries is not always consistent with entry at the sixth cervical vertebra.

Technique

A dental-type chair is used with the patient in the sitting position which allows for placement in the prone

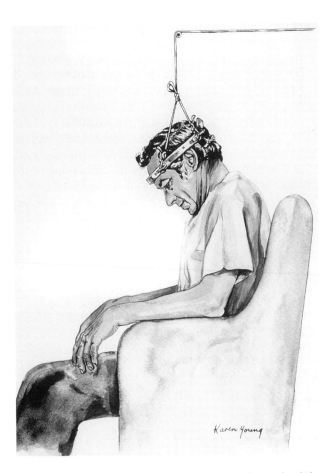

FIG. 24. Cervical deformity. Patient operated upon in sitting position with halo attached.

position if necessary (Fig. 24). Sedation is given preoperatively and supplementary analgesia may be used during the procedure if necessary, including such drugs as diazepam or fentanyl. Local anesthesia is used with epineph-

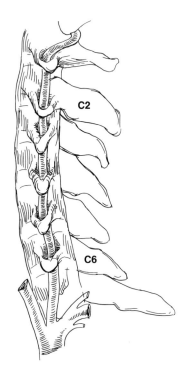

FIG. 23. Lateral view of cervical spine showing vertebral arteries and veins in front of the transverse process of the seventh vertebra and entering the transverse foramen at the sixth vertebra.

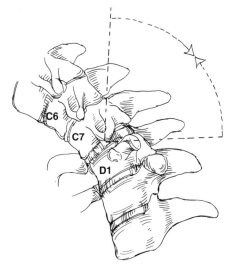

FIG. 25. Lateral diagrammatic outline of area of resection.

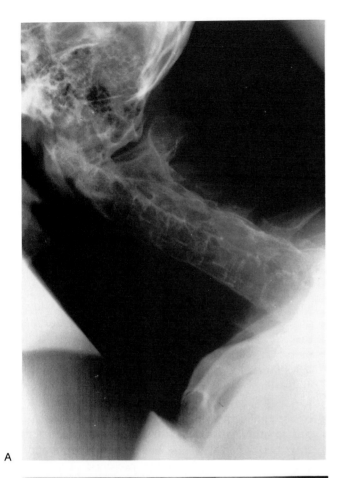

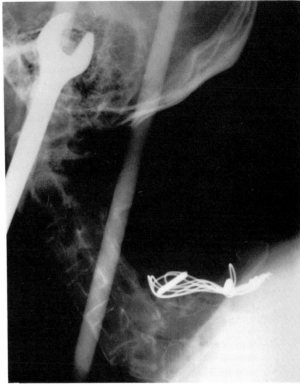

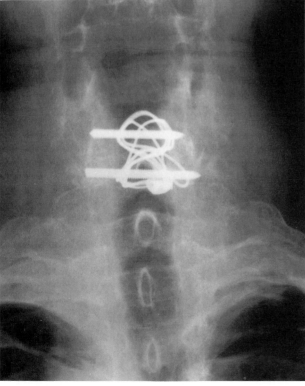

FIG. 26. A: Preoperative deformity. **B,C:** The osteotomy is held closed with threaded wires through the base of the spinous processes proximally and distally to the osteotomy. Wire is passed around the pins in order to hold the osteotomy closed.

rine in concentrations of 1 in 200,000. Usually no more than 20 cc of 1% local anesthesia is necessary. Patients should be monitored for possible air embolism with either Doppler apparatus or an esophageal stethoscope.

The amount of bone to be resected is determined from preoperative radiographs by the chin-brow to vertical angle. This angle is transposed to the lateral radiograph of the cervical spine at the apex of the posterior margin of C7 and T1 disc space. Tomograms may be necessary to show this clearly. The ideal position for the patient is one in which he is able to look ahead when walking and while working at a desk. Overcorrection must be avoided. To accomplish this accurately, the angle is centered over the posterior arch of C7 and the amount of bone that must be resected from the spinous processes and lamina is measured.

After exposure of the spine, the C7 spinous process and part of C6 and T1 are removed and preserved for grafting purposes. The entire posterior arch of C7 is removed including the inferior half of the arch of C6 and superior half of the arch of T1 (Fig. 25). Decompression is then carried out laterally beyond the spinal cord to the pedicles with undercutting of the lamina above and below in order to prevent impingement of the eighth cervical roots when the osteotomy is closed. The eighth cervical root canal is identified. A small amount of anesthesia may be necessary at this point on the nerve root in order to prevent painful paresthesia. The eighth nerve roots are decompressed completely by resecting bone laterally through the fused joints of C7–T1. The inferior aspects of the pedicles of C7 and the superior aspect of T1 are exposed. Bone from the pedicles may be removed (see Fig. 25). Thus, following extension no impingement of the eighth root will occur. The lateral masses must be resected so that no bone remains laterally to interfere with correction. More may be resected.

Simmons advocated sedation following decompression by the administration of a small dose of short-acting barbiturate. However, we have found that this is not necessary and have kept the patient awake during the procedure. The neck is extended by grasping the halo firmly and tilting the neck posteriorly, which results in a fracture. The lateral masses will come together posteriorly on either side.

After closure of the osteotomy site, Simmons grafted the lateral masses and closed the soft tissues. He then fixed the halo to the body cast, which was worn for 4 months. We prefer to apply internal fixation using the Dewar technique (Fig. 26), which consists of percutaneously passing threaded pins through the base of the spinous processes above and below the osteotomy site and then wiring these together. Supplemented by a graft, this technique eliminates the need for halo cast immobilization. Alternatively, we have used either plate fixation or compression hooks.

If adequate correction cannot be obtained at the time of surgery, internal fixation should not be used. Seven to ten days later and under sedation, the neck may be extended further and immobilization carried out with the halo cast or with internal fixation if the wound is reopened.

Results and Complications

In Simmons's series of 95 patients (25), there were four (3%) nonunions. Thirteen patients (12%) had transient C8 root weakness and five (5%) had persistent C8 deficits, one of which required further decompression with subsequent improvement. Other complications included Horner's syndrome in one patient and a mild transient cord syndrome in another.

The surgeon should also be aware of an increased incidence of gastric irritation and possible peptic ulceration. This may lead to intraabdominal or respiratory problems because patients with ankylosing spondylitis require their abdominal musculature for respiration. For these reasons, Simmons advocated placing all patients on prophylactic cimetidine pre- and postoperatively.

Mehdian and associates (19) have advocated the use of gradual halo traction starting with 2.25 kg and increasing to 4.5 kg slowly over a period of 3 weeks. This is followed by the application of a halo in order to maintain correction together with a posterior occipitocervical fusion was then performed 2 weeks later. They recommend this technique particularly in the presence of preexisting spontaneous fractures.

We think that this technique, though it has merit, is more costly than a direct surgical approach as advocated by Simmons and Law.

SPONDYLODISCITIS

Ankylosing spondylodiscitis is defined as an erosive and sclerotic process involving the intervertebral disc and adjacent vertebral bodies. The causes of this condition are not well understood, but some authors believe it is an expression of the inflammatory process encountered in ankylosing spondylitis. Others suggest spondylodiscitis is secondary to trauma resulting in a form of pseudarthrosis (8,18,20). Biopsies support the inflammatory etiology; however, lesions have been noted to occur in patients who have had an acute fracture that was not treated but only observed. The lesions are often found coincidentally on radiographic examination. They are often painful as a result of translational forces to the area, resulting in increased deformity; pain may be secondary to further bone destruction. If the deformity is not severe, anterior resection and grafting may be all that is indicated (Fig. 27).

If the spondylodiscitis occurs in the thoracolumbar area, Simmons and Duncan (27) advocates resection-extension osteotomy in the midlumbar spine to decrease

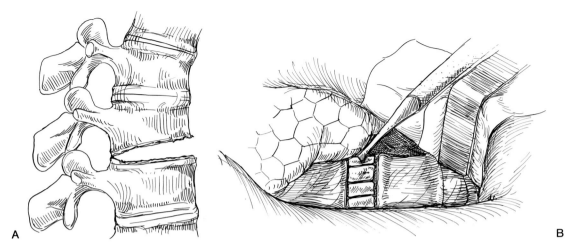

FIG. 27. A: Severe, painful spondylodiscitis showing destructive changes at the disc space with stress fracture of the fused posterior element. **B:** Operative view of spine following excision of spondylodiscitis and multiple fibular strut grafting.

stresses across the area of spondylodiscitis. This will place the lesion under more axial compression (Fig. 28) and may induce spontaneous healing.

FRACTURES

Fractures that occur in ankylosing spondylitis are potentially lethal. Although the majority of fractures occur in the low cervical spine, they may occur at all levels and often result in quadriplegia (2,6,21,28,30,33). Because of the chest's inability to move appropriately with respiration and because these patients rely entirely on diaphragmatic breathing, subsequent pulmonary compromise with pneumonia may occur, leading to death.

At the other extreme, the fractures may be unrecognized and the patient complains only of mild pain. If the

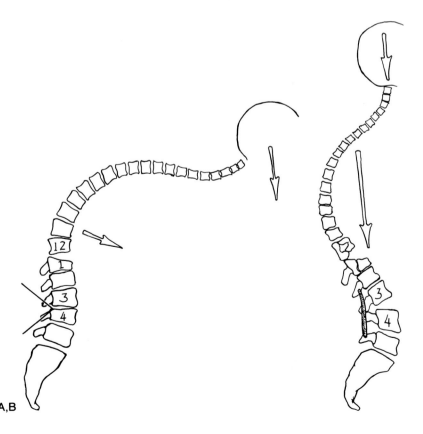

FIG. 28. A: Spondylodiscitis at the thoracolumbar junction subjected to shear stress. **B:** By correction of spinal deformity with lumbar osteotomy, the lesion will be under compression with resultant spontaneous healing.

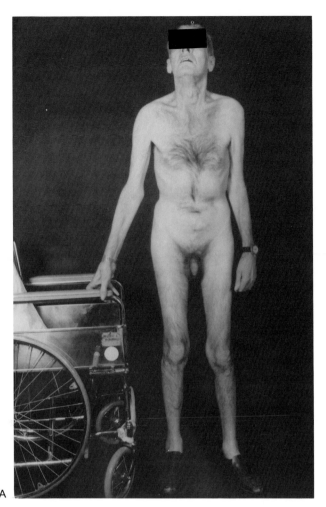

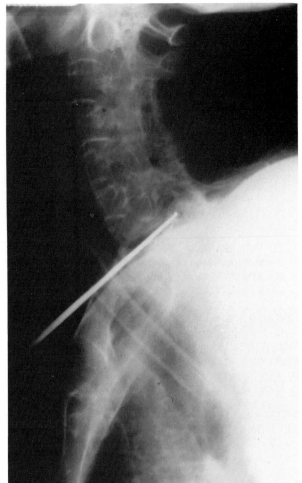

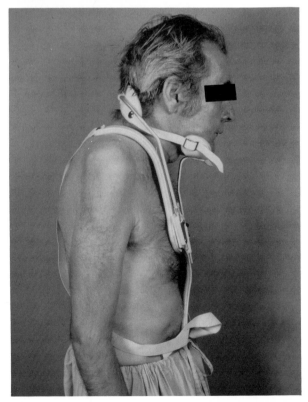

FIG. 29. A: A 52-year-old male with hyperextension deformity of the cervical spine secondary to cervical spine fracture. He was treated with traction and hyperextension on a Stryker turning bed. The patient could not see his feet and became a recluse. **B:** The deformity was corrected by an anterior and posterior C5–C6 osteotomy with **(C)** a good result.

patient sustains a traumatic incident, mild or otherwise, and subsequently develops a cervical deformity associated with pain, a fracture of the cervical spine must be assumed to be causative unless proven otherwise. Fractures occur in a transverse pattern and, therefore, are susceptible to stress forces and may translate easily. Fractures are often missed, particularly in the lower cervical spine where the shoulders may obscure the lesion. Tomography or swimmer's views or pillar views are often required. Simmons (25) noted that 36% of all patients who underwent cervical osteotomy had a history of preexisting cervical fracture which had been previously diagnosed in only 15%.

In the past, most surgeons have recommended the application of cranial halo traction for cervical fractures, positioning the head in a more functional position with subsequent immobilization with a halo cast. The latter is maintained for approximately 4 months. Care must be taken that the patient not be immobilized in hyperextension. This may lead to the opposite deformity, wherein the patient gazes at the sky only and cannot observe his or her feet (Fig. 29).

It is our policy to treat all acute fractures associated with ankylosing spondylitis as surgical emergencies, with open reduction and internal fixation. If there has been a preexisting deformity, the fracture may be used to help correct this in part, but care must be taken to avoid neurologic problems.

In the cervical spine, fractures may be treated by a posterior approach under local anesthesia. This avoids the necessity of intubation required when an anterior procedure is to be done. Similarly, fractures may be operated on in the thoracic and lumbar spine with local anesthesia and sedation if necessary. Preoperative computerized tomography or magnetic resonance imaging is important to rule out epidural hematomas which should be evacuated.

Less commonly, erosive fractures may occur posteriorly C1–C2 dislocation may present as a painful flexion deformity and may be associated with neurologic problems. Destructive changes may also occur at the atlantooccipital or atlantoaxial joints, resulting in flexion at these joints. A deformity of this type can often be corrected by the use of halo traction to restore the normal chin-brow to vertical angle. This should be followed by posterior stabilization under local anesthesia with an occipital cervical fusion and, if necessary, excision of the posterior arch of C1.

SURGICAL VERSUS NONSURGICAL TREATMENT

Graham and Van Peteghem (6) reported on 15 patients admitted to an acute spinal cord injury center who met the criteria of ankylosing spondylitis and acute frac-

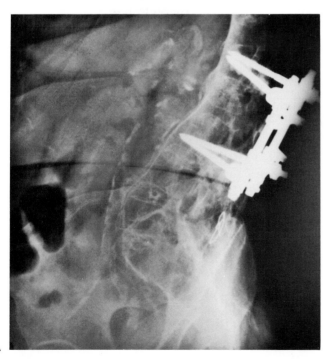
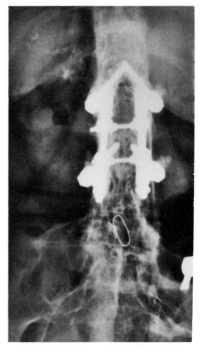

FIG. 30. A,B: This 62-year-old female sustained a lumbar fracture. No healing had occurred by 6 weeks. Internal fixation was used. Because of the severe osteopenia, bone cement was used in the pedicles.

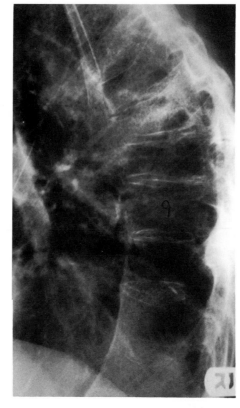

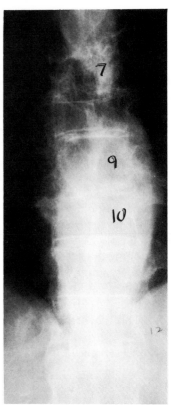

A,B

FIG. 31. A,B: Male, age 55, presented with severe paraparesis. The fracture was difficult to define on plain radiographs. C: MRI revealed prevertebral swelling and a posterior clot at T8–9. D,E: A laminectomy was performed to evacuate the hematoma. Rigid fixation was performed using pedicle fixation.

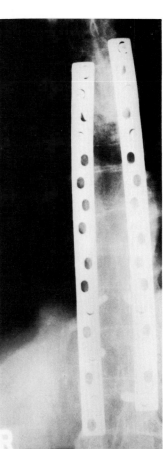

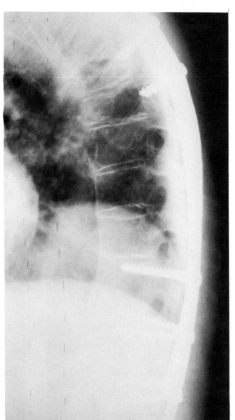

C

D,E

ture. All fractures occurred in the fused area of the spine. There were 12 injuries to the cervical spine, 10 of these in the midcervical spine; two injuries in the thoracic spine; and one in the lumbar spine. The mechanism of injury involved small forces in six cases with four of these involving falls from a standing position, and two from bed. Eleven of the 12 cervical cases had neurologic deficits although none were major. Thoracic spine injuries were associated with anterior cord syndrome in both cases; there was no neurologic injury in the single lumbar spine fracture. Radiographic assessment revealed several patterns of structural destruction including clear fracture lines through either the body or disc space. Displacement and angulation occurred in several instances, sometimes in association with severe comminution of the vertebral body. No compressive injuries were seen. Disruption of more than one site in the cervical spine was noted in two patients. In one case three distinct lesions were noted. All cervical and thoracic cases were treated nonoperatively, and all cases united. The treatment consisted of halo or skull-tong traction for 4 to 6 weeks followed by immobilization with a halo thoracic or Guilford brace. The average time of healing was 17 weeks. Injuries to the thoracic spine were treated by bed rest for 15 to 17 weeks. Subsequent immobilization was carried out with a brace. In the single lumbar case, advantage was taken of the fracture to perform an extension osteotomy. Two deaths occurred: one from myocardial infarction and pneumonia in a 90-year-old man, and one from airway obstruction followed by septic shock. Graham felt that the high rate of neurologic damage was due to either contusion or vascular insufficiency to the spinal cord secondary to traction within the rigid ankylosed spinal column at the time of injury. Displacement was usually associated with severe comminution of the vertebral elements and marked instability leading to difficulty in obtaining or maintaining closed reduction.

Controversy exists regarding the best method of management of these fractures either with or without neurologic injury (Figs. 30 and 31). Many reports emphasize conservative management. Other reports where surgical intervention has been the primary treatment have noted mortality rates as high as 50% versus 25% in nonoperated series. Graham and Van Peteghem (6) felt that operative indications included progressive neurologic lesion which in ankylosing spondylitis might be a result of epidural hemorrhage. Another indication for intervention was the failure of an incomplete neurologic lesion to improve. In Graham's series one patient developed a progressive neurologic lesion as a result of the difficulty to achieve and maintain reduction. The authors believed that nonoperative means could not control these inherently and that stable fractures and operative intervention were indicated. They felt laminectomy had no role to play. The mortality rate in Graham's series was 13%,

credited to the conservative management in a specific unit of these patients with spinal cord injury.

Given modern forms of internal fixation, in these inherently unstable fractures, stabilization is the preferred treatment method as it prevents prolonged bed rest and allows for earlier rehabilitation. This is particularly true concerning the already damaged spinal cord.

REFERENCES

1. Adams JC (1952): Technique, dangers and safeguards in osteotomy of spine. *J Bone Joint Surg [Br]* 34:226–232.
2. Amamilo SC (1989): Fractures of the cervical spine in patients with ankylosing spondylitis. *Orthop Rev* 18:339–344.
3. Briggs H, Keats S, Schlesinger PT (1947): Wedge osteotomy of the spine with bilateral intervertebral foraminotomy: correction of flexion deformity in five cases of ankylosing arthritis of the spine. *J Bone Joint Surg* 29:1075–1082.
4. Emneus H (1968): Wedge osteotomy of spine in ankylosing spondylitis. *Acta Orthop Scand* 39:321–326.
5. Goel MK (1968): Vertebral osteotomy for correction of fixed flexion deformity of the spine. *J Bone Joint Surg [Am]* 50:287–294.
6. Graham B, Van Peteghem PK (1989): Fractures of the spine in ankylosing spondylitis. Diagnosis, treatment, and complications. *Spine* 14(8):803–807.
7. Herbert JJ (1959): Vertebral osteotomy for kyphosis, especially in Marie-Strümpell arthritis. *J Bone Joint Surg [Am]* 41:291–302.
8. Huaux JP, Lokietek W, Vincent A, Nagant de Deuxchaisnes C (1986): Pace des traitements orthopédiques et chirurgicaux dans les ankyloses rachidiennes, les fractures et pseudarthroses vertebrales de la spondylarthrite ankylosante. *Acta Orthop Belg* 52:771–791.
9. Jaffray D, Becker V, Eisenstein S (1992): Closing wedge osteotomy with transpedicular fixation in ankylosing spondylitis. *Clin Orthop* 279:122–126.
10. LaChapelle EH (1946): Osteotomy of the lumbar spine for correction of kyphosis in a case of ankylosing spondylarthritis. *J Bone Joint Surg* 28:851–858.
11. Law WA (1952): Surgical treatment of the rheumatic diseases. *J Bone Joint Surg [Br]* 34:215–225.
12. Law WA (1959): Lumbar spinal osteotomy. *J Bone Joint Surg [Br]* 41:270–278.
13. Law WA (1962): Osteotomy of the spine. *J Bone Joint Surg [Am]* 44:1199–1206.
14. Law WA (1969): Osteotomy of the spine. *Clin Orthop* 66:70–76.
15. Lichtblau PO, Wilson PD (1956): Possible mechanism of aortic rupture in orthopaedic correction of rheumatoid spondylitis. *J Bone Joint Surg [Am]* 38:123–127.
16. McMaster PE (1962): Osteotomy of the spine for fixed flexion deformity. *J Bone Joint Surg [Am]* 44:1207–1216.
17. McMaster MJ (1985): A technique for lumbar spinal osteotomy in ankylosing spondylitis. *J Bone Joint Surg [Br]* 67:204–210.
18. McMaster MJ, Coventry MB (1973): Spinal osteotomy in ankylosing spondylitis. Technique, complications and long-term results. *Mayo Clin Proc* 48:476–486.
19. Mehdian H, Jaffray D, Eisenstein S (1992): Correction of severe cervical kyphosis in ankylosing spondylitis by traction. *Spine* 17(2):237–240.
20. Pastershank SP, Resnick D (1980): Pseudoarthrosis in ankylosing spondylitis. *J Can Assoc Radiol* 31:234–235.
21. Podolsky SM, Hoffman JR, Pietrafesa CA (1983): Neurologic complications following immobilization of cervical spine fracture in a patient with ankylosing spondylitis. *Ann Emerg Med* 12:578–580.
22. Puschel J, Zielke K (1982): Korrekturoperation bei Bechterew-Kyphose: Indikation, Technik, Ergebnisse. *Z Orthop* 120:338–342.
23. Roy-Camille R, Henry P, Saillant G, Doursounian L (1987): Chir-

urgie des grandes cyphoses vertébrales de la spondylarthrite ankylosante. *Rev Rhum* 54(3):261–267.

24. Scudese VA, Calabro JJ (1963): Vertebral wedge osteotomy. Correction of rheumatoid (ankylosing) spondylitis. *JAMA* 186:627–
631.

25. Simmons EH (1972): The surgical correction of flexion deformity
of the cervical spine in ankylosing spondylitis. *Clin Orthop* 86:132–
143.

26. Simmons EH (1977): Kyphotic deformity of the spine in ankylosing spondylitis. *Clin Orthop* 128:65–77.

27. Simmons EH, Duncan CP (1978): Fracture of the cervical spine
in ankylosing spondylitis—an analysis of its influence on severe
deformity presenting for spinal osteotomy. *Clin Orthop* 133:277.

28. Smith-Peterson MN, Larson CB, Aufranc OE (1945): Osteotomy
of the spine for correction of flexion deformity in rheumatoid arthritis. *J Bone Joint Surg* 27:1–11.

29. Styblo K, Bossers GTM, Slot GH (1985): Osteotomy for kyphosis
in ankylosing spondylitis. *Acta Orthop Scand* 56:294–297.

30. Surin VV (1980): Fractures of the cervical spine in patients with
ankylosing spondylitis. *Acta Orthop Scand* 51:79–84.

31. Thiranont N, Netrawichien P (1993): Transpedicular decancellation closed wedge vertebral osteotomy for treatment of fixed
flexion deformity of spine in ankylosing spondylitis. *Spine* 18(16):
2517–2522.

32. Thomasen E (1985): Vertebral osteotomy for correction of kyphosis in ankylosing spondylitis. *Clin Orthop* 194:142–146.

33. Thorngren KG, Liedberg E, Aspelin P (1981): Fractures of the thoracic and lumbar spine in ankylosing spondylitis. *Arch Orthop
Trauma Surg* 98:101–107.

34. Urist MR (1958): Osteotomy of the cervical spine: report of a case
of ankylosing rheumatoid spondylitis. *J Bone Joint Surg* [*Am*] 40:
833–843.

The Adult Spine: Principles and Practice,
2nd edition, J.W. Frymoyer, Editor-in-Chief.
Lippincott-Raven Publishers, Philadelphia © 1997.

CHAPTER **44**

Differential Diagnosis and Conservative Treatment of Infectious Diseases

Timothy L. Keenen and Daniel R. Benson

HISTORY

Osteomyelitis of the spine has been an affliction of mankind since before written history. Evidence of destruction of the spine by infection has been uncovered in Egyptian mummies. Hippocrates (400 BC) and Galen (150 AD) both described vertebral destruction caused by infection. Much later, the classic description of tuberculous spondylitis was given by Pott in 1779 (108). The first series of pyogenic spine infections reported was by Lannelongue in 1880 (78). Until relatively late in the twentieth century, the diagnosis had a lethal outcome in young patients. Mortality rates of over 70% for people under the age of 30 were reported (85). In 1936, Kulowski demonstrated an extravertebral site of origin for vertebral os-

teomyelitis from septic lesions of the skin (77). After 1940, improved diagnosis and treatment reduced the mortality rate to about 25%; the greatest improvements were among children. With the further development of antibiotics, the character of vertebral infections changed from a virulent disease affecting primarily children to a more chronic illness, seen more often in adults. Today, vertebral osteomyelitis is a relatively rare disorder and accounts for only 2% to 4% of all cases of osteomyelitis (120).

DEFINITIONS

The terminology used in describing spinal infections may be confusing. The adult disc space infection is most commonly a postoperative complication of posterior discectomy. If diagnosed and treated early, this condition does not progress to a true osteomyelitis.

The adult disc space infection is differentiated from discitis, which affects the pediatric population. Its cause

   T. L. Keenen, M.D.: Associate Professor, Department of Orthopaedics, Oregon Health Sciences University, School of Medicine, Portland, Oregon, 97201.
   D. R. Benson, M.D.: Professor of Orthopaedics, University of California, Davis, Sacramento, California, 95817.

is most commonly bacterial in nature, although it may also be viral. The source in most cases of discitis is hematogenous, and symptoms usually present early enough to prevent progression to vertebral osteomyelitis. Pediatric discitis responds to immobilization and antibiotics, and it rarely requires surgery (130).

Vertebral osteomyelitis develops when the infectious organism enters bone and, at least locally, overcomes the host immune system. The invading organism may be bacterial, viral, fungal, or parasitic. When the infection is bacterial, it is termed pyogenic osteomyelitis. When the invading organism is *Mycobacterium tuberculosis,* it is referred to as tuberculous spondylitis or Pott's disease.

Epidural abscesses may form adjacent to the area of osteomyelitis or, less commonly, occur *de novo.* Because most infections involve the anterior and middle columns, the most common site for an epidural abscess is adjacent to the posterior longitudinal ligament. Other epidural areas may become involved as a complication of posterior spinal surgery. Surgically, exact delineation of epidural abscess from osteomyelitis is not always possible because of the widespread bony destruction often present.

PATHOPHYSIOLOGY

Infections in the spine may affect the vertebral body, intervertebral disc, neural arch, or the posterior elements, but most commonly they involve anterior and middle columns (42,49,77,129). Batson (11,12) attributed this site of involvement to the venous plexus, which drains from the pelvis to the vertebral bodies. Wiley and Trueta (132) disputed the role of Batson's plexus, showing how small the branches are to the vertebral bodies. Furthermore, they showed that high pressures were required to fill the normally low- or even negative-pressure venous plexus. Using injection techniques, they showed a rich arterial system that supplies the vertebral bodies under physiologic arterial pressures. The richly vascular metaphyseal bone near the anterior longitudinal ligament correlates with the most common site of infections, thus implicating the arterial route for hematogenous osteomyelitis (133).

Change of the vascularity of the spine with aging may explain the frequency of the types of infections at different ages. Histologic analyses have confirmed that an endarteriolar supply to the disc is present during infancy and childhood and then is slowly obliterated in the first three decades of life (18,32,119). While the most common *de novo* infection in the child is discitis, the adult is at greater risk for anterior metaphyseal infections that begin near the endplate. Disc space infections that do occur in adults are usually associated with prior surgical disruption of the disc. Osteomyelitis involving the vertebral body can spread by direct extension to involve the neural arch and posterior elements. The infection can involve and cross cortical bone and longitudinal ligaments, leading to soft tissue abscesses. The more virulent organisms tend to violate fascial planes, leading to visceral involvement, while more indolent organisms tend to follow fascial planes.

CLASSIFICATION

The most functional way of classifying infections of the spine is by the causative organism. Disease outcome and treatment methods tend to be similar within each group. Pyogenic infections are caused by bacteria. Granulomatous disease refers to infections caused by organisms that result in granuloma formation in human tissue. These include all of the fungal infections and tuberculosis. Other organisms such as parasitic infections are rarely seen in the developed world.

PYOGENIC DISEASE

Presentation and History

Pyogenic infections may present acutely, sub-acutely, or chronically. The sub-acute or chronic presentation is most common. The acuteness and severity of the infection is determined by the level of virulence of the invading organism and the ability of the host response to subdue the infection. In general, a delay in diagnosis is the rule rather than the exception. The average time from onset of symptoms to definitive diagnosis has been reported to range from 8 weeks to 3 months (39,49,54, 129). The reasons for the delay in diagnosis vary from simple to complex. Often the patient ignores the symptoms until the infection has progressed significantly before seeking medical care. At other times the physician is not suspicious, so progressive symptoms and signs become relatively severe before the diagnosis is entertained. Another common error is to confuse the diagnosis with spinal tumor.

The onset is typically insidious, with back pain the most common symptom. The pain is localized at first to the level of the involved area, with a gradual increase in intensity. Most patients initially describe a relation of their pain to increased activity, with relief in recumbency. The pain eventually becomes so severe it is not relieved by complete bed rest. Usually neurological signs are not present until late in the disease course. Other symptoms variably present include chills, weight loss, dysuria, photophobia, and drainage from a wound or incision if there has been prior surgery.

The lumbar spine is most commonly involved, with cervical and thoracic sites less common (49,77,112). Lumbar disease can extend to the flank or groin region, resulting in a psoas abscess. Rarely, the abscesses will extend to such sites as a perirectal area or to the popliteal fossa. Abscesses may communicate with the skin, manifested by chronic, draining sinuses. Cervical involvement generally produces a retropharyngeal mass, which may cause dysphagia.

Of particular importance to the clinician who considers vertebral osteomyelitis as a possible diagnosis is the patient's prior history. Several pre-existing factors have an increased association with pyogenic spine disease. Patients with diabetes mellitus have a higher susceptibility to vertebral infections (29,42,49,129). As in other infectious processes that affect the diabetic, presentation tends to be delayed even longer than the norm for vertebral infections, because the patient may not show clinical manifestations of the inflammatory response.

The intravenous drug abuser is also at increased risk for spine infection (64,74,129). Bacteria probably infect the spine by direct hematogenous route; the patient's immune status may also be compromised. The commonly reported infectious agent in drug abusers is *Pseudomonas aeruginosa* (22,64,67,81,131).

Urinary tract manipulation or infection also results in an increased prevalence of the disease (4,36,45,57,60, 61,80,116). Presumably, hematogenous spread of bacteria is responsible for this association, although in a few cases the infection may be a direct extension. The organisms most commonly associated with urologic infections are *Escherichia coli*, *Proteus*, and *Pseudomonas*.

A patient who has had prior surgery of the spine is most susceptible to infection at the operated level. Because of the relative frequency of the surgical procedure, the most common presentation is after simple disc excision (105,123). Traumatic conditions such as stab wounds and gunshot wounds also predispose to pyogenic infections (58,65,96,111).

Recently an association of infections with non-operated thoracolumbar fractures has been reported (53,84,95). Again, delay in diagnosis is the rule because of focus on the original pathology rather than the possibility of a secondary infectious problem.

Other associations of medical problems with spine infections are sickle cell disease (43), immune deficiency states (including AIDS) (41), and preexisting paraplegia (129).

Physical Findings

Dramatic localized and regional pain exacerbated by motion or compression is the most common finding. Often a physician will mistake the symptoms as being exaggerated out of proportion to other physical findings. Most patients will present without the acute signs of sepsis. Nonetheless, the temperature should be checked. One report noted an elevated temperature over 100°F in only 33% of patients, and fever to 102°F in only two patients of 40 studied (49). In cases where the local process has spread, a local or remote fluctuant mass may be palpable. Muscle spasm may be detected in the posterior musculature. Limitation of motion is usually proportional to the level of pain. Occasionally an angular kyphos is seen when the process is chronic and advanced. The positive psoas sign may be an indication of a psoas abscess.

Laboratory Data

Numerous reports show the most consistent abnormal laboratory value at the time of diagnosis of pyogenic vertebral osteomyelitis has been the elevated erythrocyte sedimentation rate (ESR) (6,49,54,77). The ESR has an average value at diagnosis of 43 to 87 mm per hour (Westergren method) (49,54,112). Although it is a valuable aid in diagnosis of vertebral infection, the ESR is not particularly helpful in the differentiation of pyogenic from tuberculous infections. The ESR value may also be valuable as a marker for response to treatment.

White blood cell (WBC) count is a less reliable laboratory value, as it is commonly normal or only slightly elevated. The average WBC count at the time of diagnosis in our series of 38 patients was 11,800, with a range of 4,000 to 23,800 (normal, <10,800/mm^3). When the white count is elevated, it is usually associated with a "left shift" of increased band neutrophils (129).

Blood cultures can be an essential part in the diagnostic initial evaluation. A very high percentage of cultures obtained from a patient during a fever spike will be positive for the causative organism. However, during subacute or chronic phases, when fever spikes are absent, the yield is less.

Stone and Bonfiglio have reported high serum globulin values in 10 of 12 patients on whom they performed this test (122).

The Organism

Staphylococcus aureus is by far the most common pyogenic organism involved in spine infections. In most series, it is the primary organism in at least 50% of cases (19,49,54,77,129). There has been a relative increase in other organisms over the last 40 years, particularly the gram-negative organisms. *Escherichia coli* is associated with urinary tract and enteric causes of vertebral osteomyelitis. *Pseudomonas aeruginosa* infections are most often seen in the intravenous drug user or in patients who have received multiple antibiotics and have a decreased immune status. *Staphylococcus epidermidis*, *Streptococcus*, and *Proteus* species, along with a variety of others, have also been reported (9,13,25,26,40,51,66,83,101, 103,109,117). Multiple organism infections of the spine are relatively rare. In our series of 38 cases, we found none, and we were able to identify a single pathogen in all but eight cases (129).

Radiographic Studies

Radiographic evidence of a pyogenic spine infection not surprisingly shows up first where the infectious process involves the vertebral body. Spinal radiographs will show narrowing of the disc space, at the earliest within 2 or 3 weeks of infection (Fig. 1). The degree of narrowing does not seem to predict the subsequent course of the disease. Within 10 to 12 weeks, a second sign becomes visible: the adjacent endplates of the vertebral bodies at the involved level show an increased density. This occurs first in the subchondral bone and eventually affects the surrounding spongy bone of the vertebral body. The radiologic effect comes from both deposition of new bone on the existing trabeculae and from (sub)periosteal new bone (5,73).

Later, definition of the vertebral endplate becomes blurred (Fig. 2). Eventually, lytic changes occur in the endplates on each side of the disc. The borders of the bone may be ragged or smooth and scalloped out with a concavity towards the level of the infection. As the infection progresses, the radiologic appearance of increased surrounding vertebral bone density moves farther away from the disc space in both directions. This effect is partially from new inflammatory bone and partially from

the comparison to adjacent involved lytic bone (Figs. 3,4,5).

The subsequent radiologic appearance is quite variable. With time, the vertebrae may collapse, forming an acute kyphos at the level of involvement. Posterior elements are only rarely involved, and then usually only as a late complication of a longstanding anterior infection.

If the changes on plain radiographs are clear, further radiographic studies may not be warranted. However, the early changes are often subtle. Lateral tomograms are particularly useful at improving the definition of the image. Tomograms are most helpful in the thoracic spine, where high-definition plain films are hard to obtain. The tomograms may also delineate soft tissue abnormalities such as abscesses.

Computed tomography (CT) scans also have an important place in diagnosis. Early in the disease course, they show spongy bone erosion and rarefaction before plain radiographs do. They are valuable in showing the extent of vertebral destruction in transverse sections (1,20,72). The vertebral canal may be closely monitored for encroachment. CT scans have been shown to be particularly effective in assessing soft tissue abnormalities surrounding infections, including discs, abscesses, and paraspinal, subdural, and epidural spaces (23,52,90). Prior to CT scanning, the rate of soft tissue masses associated with pyogenic infections was thought to be 20%, although a more recent study using CT has shown this prevalence to be closer to 80% (79). The CT scan has

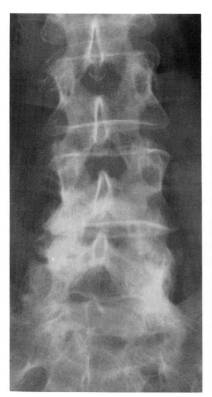

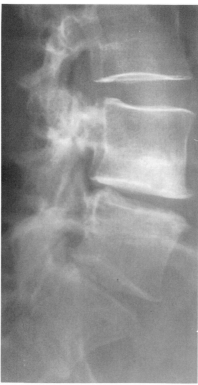

A,B

FIG. 1. Radiographic findings of infection may be subtle. A 59-year-old woman presented with a sudden increase in her chronic low back pain associated with chills. Erythrocyte sedimentation rate was 75 mm/hr and white blood cell count was 14,800/cu mm. She had had a *Pseudomonas aeruginosa* urinary tract infection 1 month prior. Anteroposterior (**A**) and lateral (**B**) radiographs show mild disc space loss and reactive bone formation at L4.

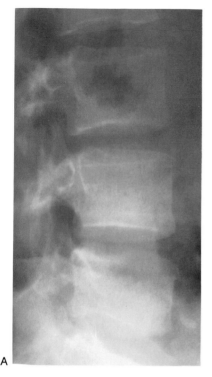

A

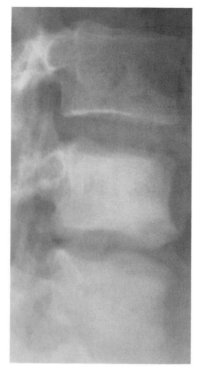

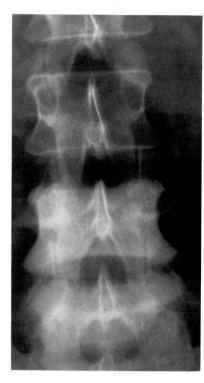

B,C

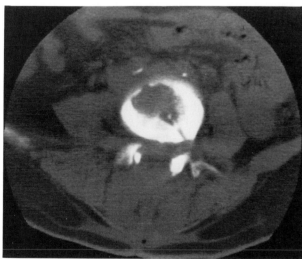

D

FIG. 2. A 35-year-old woman presented after a several-month history of low back pain. **A:** Lateral radiograph taken 1 year prior to presentation (taken for unrelated condition) showing normal structure. Lateral (**B**) and anteroposterior (**C**) radiographs demonstrate L4-L5 end-plate blurring and disc space height loss. **D:** CT scan shows the destructive lesion at L4. Cultures from biopsy grew *Staphylococcus epidermidis.*

also proven valuable in the distinction of infection from tumor in the spine, particularly when combined with the magnetic resonance imaging (MRI) scan (128).

The CT scan may also be used more directly in diagnosis by assisting with needle aspiration of a suspected lesion (31,90). Under light sedation, a spinal needle may be introduced from the posterior direction into the lumbar and thoracic spine under CT guidance. The yield of the needle biopsy in producing the infecting organism may be disappointingly low: previous reports have quoted rates as low as 50% (6). However, this rate may be acceptable if medical treatment will suffice and the larger anterior surgical exposure is avoided.

Myelography is often most helpful when used in combination with the CT scan. It is particularly useful for

visualization of the epidural or subdural spaces of the cervical and thoracic spine (90). The usual indication for myelography is the need for better definition to localize or define the extent of the compressive lesion when a neurological deficit is present. Myelography does carry the distinct disadvantage of being an invasive procedure that carries the risk of further spread (possibly subdurally) of the infection. For these reasons, the noninvasive MRI scan has become more the standard for evaluating the spinal canal.

Nuclear Studies

Nuclear scans are one of the most valuable tools in the diagnosis of vertebral osteomyelitis because of their high

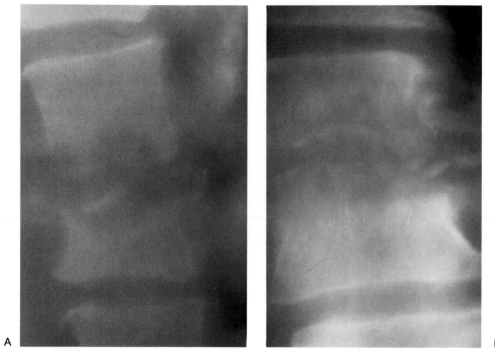

FIG. 3. A 63-year-old man presented to the emergency room after a fall with pain, with a temperature of 102°F and a white blood cell count of 15,100/mm³. Blood cultures later grew *Staphylococcus aureus*. Lateral (**A**) and anteroposterior (**B**) tomograms show classic lytic destruction of L3 and L4 endplates and the disc space between.

sensitivity, particularly early in the course of the illness (2) (Fig. 6). The technetium-99m bone scan was positive in all 19 patients in whom it was obtained in our series of confirmed pyogenic osteomyelitis of the spine (129). The bone scan is particularly valuable because it is very sensitive to inflammatory changes in the spine even before plain x-rays become positive for destructive changes. The nuclear scan may also be helpful at distinguishing tumor from infection, as in general the infection has a higher uptake of the radioisotope.

The indium-111-labeled leukocyte scan may be used in a similar manner to the bone scan for diagnosis of spinal infections. The indium-111 scan may actually be more specific and sensitive for the detection of low-grade osteomyelitis than sequential technetium–gallium scans (93), but a well-controlled trial evaluating specifically the spine has not yet been completed. The gallium scan alone may also be of use in the work-up, although its prolonged scanning time (up to 3 days) makes it less useful in the face of an acute infection, where treatment requirements are more urgent (59,63).

Magnetic Resonance Imaging

MRI has emerged as one of the most valuable tools in the evaluation of patients with possible spinal infections (71,99,107,113,118,121). The typical appearance using T1-weighted images is that of decreased signal intensity in the vertebral body and disc space, often with a loss of

distinction between the two. Using T2-weighted images, the vertebral body and disc space show increased signal intensity, with the disc having a streaky, linear appearance or absence of the intranuclear cleft (Figs. 7,8) (121). MRI is as sensitive or more sensitive than radionucleotide studies for the diagnosis of vertebral infection, with quoted rates of up to 96% (98). In addition, MRI is more specific (up to 93%) than combined plain radiographs and nuclear scans. Another advantage is its ability to provide anatomic information such as definition of the thecal sac, neural structures, psoas, and paravertebral muscles.

The MRI also may be helpful at distinguishing infection from tumor. In general, pyogenic infections will show destruction of contiguous endplates and the disc, whereas tumors characteristically destroy the anterior column with less crossing of the endplates. A recent review suggested that MRI in tuberculous infections may be more suggestive of tumor, with images showing less destruction of the endplate and disc (118). MRI in tuberculous infections also has demonstrated a higher rate of posterior element involvement, and T1-weighted images are less consistent at producing a decreased signal density in areas of involvement (118).

Patient Work-Up

Because every patient presents differently, seldom will two patient evaluations be exactly the same. Of course,

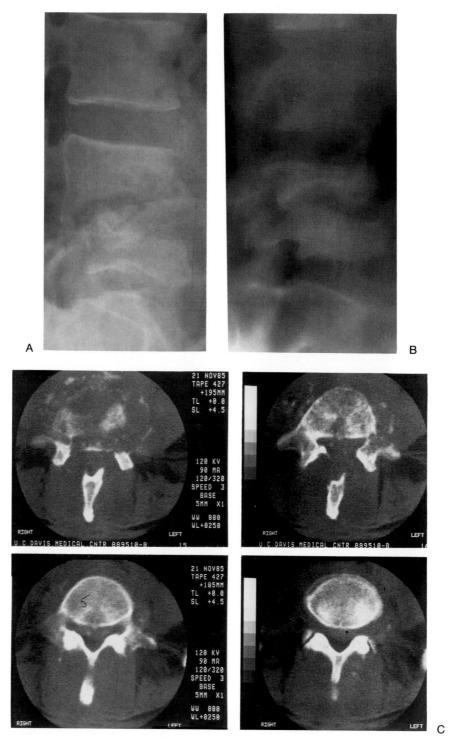

FIG. 4. A 69-year-old woman had progressive leg pain and sciatica, so an L4-L5 discectomy was performed. Two months later the pain had increased. **A:** Lateral radiographs show advanced destruction and collapse of L4 and L5. **B:** Lateral tomograms better delineate the amount of destruction. **C:** CT scan at L4-L5.

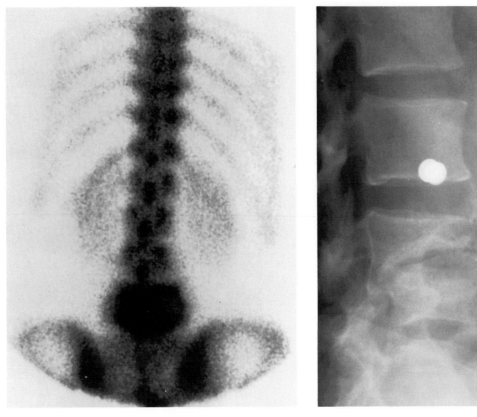

D   E

FIG. 4. *(Continued.)* **D:** Technetium 99m bone scan shows a high level of radioisotope uptake at L4-L5. Cultures grew *Staphylococcus aureus.* Patient was treated medically and with a brace because of her high operative risk. **E:** Lateral radiograph 5 months later.

most important in obtaining the correct diagnosis is a thorough history. Most patients will present with pain as the chief complaint. Many will have had x-rays that are at least suggestive of a destructive process anteriorly. A complete blood count with differential and an ESR are indicated. If the patient is febrile, blood cultures should be obtained, given the high rate of recovery for the causative organism of the infection. The nuclear scan is usually the next test that should be obtained. Given the high sensitivity rate, this test can almost rule out a significant vertebral infection if it is negative. The choice of the technetium-99m bone scan, indium-111-labeled WBC scan, or gallium-65 scan will depend on the acuteness of the presentation and the preference of the nuclear medicine specialist. Our preference is, in general, the technetium-99m bone scan, as it provides results quickly and has a very high sensitivity rate.

The MRI is an effective study early in the diagnostic evaluation. With sensitivity rates near those of the nuclear scans, its noninvasive nature makes the MRI an attractive screening tool. The MRI also has the benefit of defining the presence and extent of soft tissue masses and distinguishing infection from tumor.

In further work-up, particularly when surgery might be required, lateral tomograms are helpful at better

definition of the pathological involvement. As noted previously, we have found them to be especially useful in the thoracic spine, where definition of vertebral bodies on plain radiographs is obscured by overlying tissue.

The CT scan is best at definition of bony destruction and may also be useful in guiding a needle biopsy.

If the diagnosis is still in question after these tests, usually the differential includes spinal neoplasia. Even if the diagnosis is certain, often the causative organism remains in question. Thus a tissue specimen is indicated to guide appropriate antibiotic selection. In the cervical spine, this will usually require an operative anterior approach because of the high risk of perforating other structures with the needle. In the thoracic and lumbar spine, a posterior CT-guided needle biopsy may be a consideration. If more tissue is required, a posterior Craig needle biopsy may be done under regional or general anesthesia. The anterior thoracic spine can also be reached via a posterolateral costotransversectomy for the purpose of bacteriologic diagnosis and surgical treatment.

Principles of Non-Operative Treatment

The primary treatments of choice for pyogenic infections of the spine are rest and antibiotics. Immobiliza-

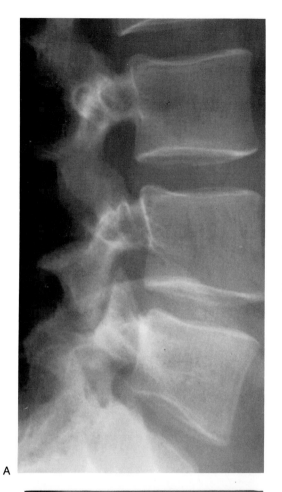

A

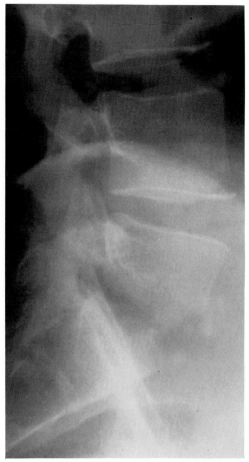

B

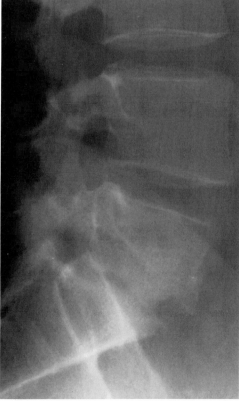

C

FIG. 5. A 25-year-old man received a closed head injury and pharyngeal lacerations in a motor vehicle accident. As he awoke from the head injury, he had symptoms of a herniated nucleus pulposus, confirmed on MRI, so an L5-S1 discectomy was performed. His back pain increased postoperatively, and the erythrocyte sedimentation rate was measured at 70 mm/hr. Within 9 days his lateral radiographs showed severe lytic destruction at L5-S1. Cultures from the discectomy grew *Branhamella catarrhalis,* presumably associated with his facial trauma. The patient was treated with body jacket immobilization and 6 weeks of ceftriaxone followed by oral antibiotics. **A:** Lateral radiographs taken preoperatively. **B:** Lateral radiographs 9 days postoperatively. **C:** Follow-up lateral radiograph, with a spontaneous anterior fusion mass at L5-S1.

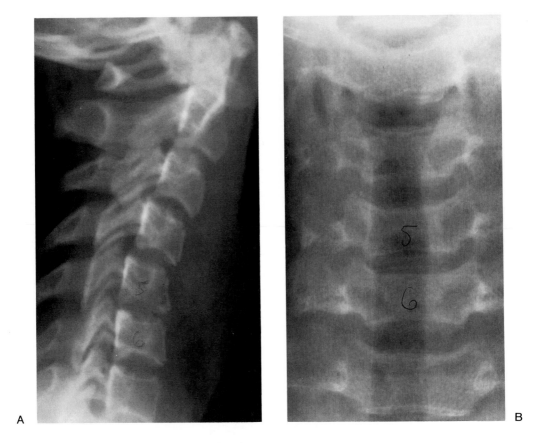

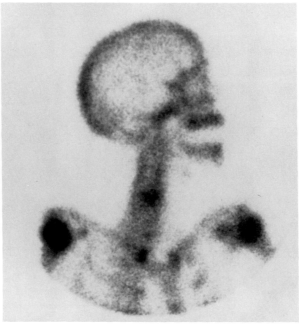

FIG. 6. A 14-year-old, mentally retarded girl presented with neck pain and torticollis. Lateral (**A**) and anteroposterior (**B**) radiographs show only mild bone lysis and possible early disc space narrowing. Technetium 99m bone scan (**C**) is clearly positive at C5-C6 level. Biopsy cultures grew *Staphylococcus aureus*. She was treated with antibiotics and a cervical orthosis because collapse was minimal.

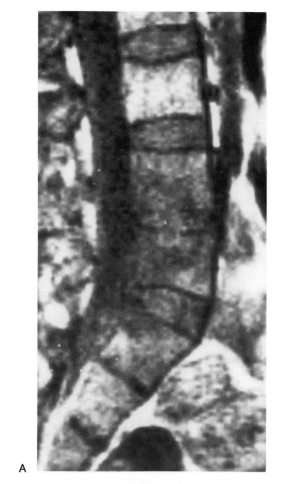

A

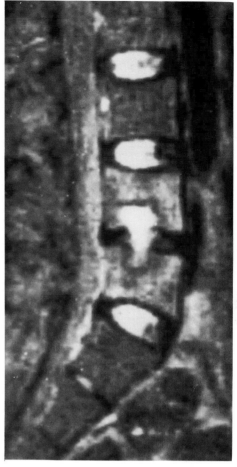

B

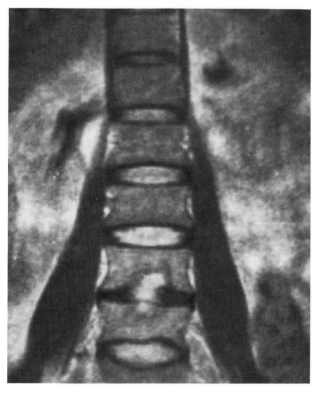

C

FIG. 7. A 23-year-old man presented with back pain 10 weeks after a rhinoplasty complicated by bacterial meningitis. The organism was *Klebsiella pneumoniae.* MRI scans proved useful in delineating the exact level of vertebral involvement. **A:** T1-weighted image. Note the low signal intensity of L4-L5 compared to adjacent uninvolved vertebral bodies. **B:** T2-weighted image. High signal density in the area of vertebral destruction with infection crossing the endplate and disc to involve the adjacent vertebral body. **C:** T2-weighted coronal image. (Courtesy of Michael Anselmo, M.D.)

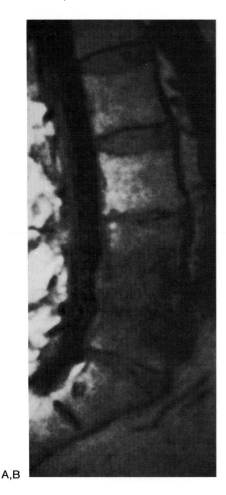
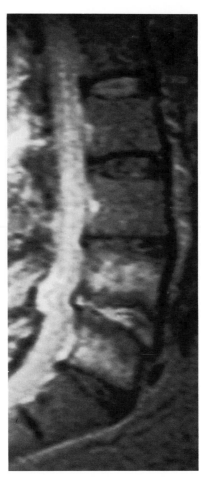

A,B

FIG. 8. A 79-year-old man underwent an L4-L5 discectomy for hip and leg pain. Six months later he complained of severe back pain, and he had an elevated erythrocyte sedimentation rate. He was treated with a prolonged course of intravenous antibiotics prior to debridement, and no organism was recovered. These MRI scans were obtained when he presented with back pain. **A:** T1-weighted image. Signal intensity is low in L4 and L5 bodies relative to adjacent vertebrae. **B:** T2-weighted image. Vertebral body and disc involvement has an increased signal intensity. (Courtesy of Michael Anselmo, M.D.)

tion is indicated when pain is a significant symptom, which is often the case. In the thoracic and lumbar spine, the immobilization method of choice is the thoracolumbosacral orthosis (TLSO). This plastic molded jacket is individualized to the body habitus of each patient. Often the immobilization offered by the TLSO will allow the patient to resume walking, which had previously been impossible because of pain. Immobilization in the cervical spine can be obtained using external braces of many different styles, or a halo vest if spinal instability is present.

The patient is also treated with a course of the appropriate intravenous antibiotic(s) as shown in Table 1. The length of treatment with antibiotics for a patient who is responding has generally been 6 weeks, although this length of time is somewhat arbitrary. This is then followed by another 6-week (or longer) period of oral antibiotics. The fine points of the long-term treatment course necessary to eradicate a spinal infection will usually warrant the assistance of an infectious disease specialist. The ESR is followed initially on a weekly basis to monitor the response to treatment. Typically, the fevers and any elevated WBC count will respond relatively soon after antibiotic therapy is started, whereas the ESR is slower to respond. Pain response after treatment is quite variable.

Should the ESR remain high in the face of appropriate antibiotics, consider that the disease process may have converted into a more sub-acute or chronic phase. Surgery may be indicated, particularly when ongoing vertebral destruction or instability are identified. The indications for surgical treatment for pyogenic infections will be presented in Chapter 45.

Spinal Epidural Abscess

The most salient feature of spinal epidural abscess is that most physicians will never see a case during their careers. It has an estimated prevalence of 0.000037% in primary care patients with back pain (37), and an incidence of two cases per 10,000 patients admitted to the hospital (10). The initial diagnosis for the presenting symptoms is unrelated to the spine in 68% of the cases reported in the literature (89). This offers an explanation for its characteristic delay in diagnosis of days to weeks, which can result in a poor outcome, as neurological symptoms usually do not reverse even with treatment. Early recognition and treatment are essential to a favorable outcome.

The literature to date includes case reports and series

TABLE 1. *Antibiotics of choice for pyogenic spinal infections*

| Organism | Parenteral | | Oral |
	Recommended	Alternative	
Staphylococcus aureus	Pencillinase-resistant synthetic penicillin (PRSP) (nafcillin, oxacillin)	Cephalosporin 1[a] Vancomycin	Dicloxacillin Cefuroxime axetil
Escherichia coli	Ceftazidime	Imipenem	Ciprofloxacin
Pseudomonas aeruginosa	Ceftazidime and tobramycin	Ticarcillin and tobramycin	Ciprofloxacin
Staphylococcus epidermidis	Vancomycin +/− gentamicin		
β-Hemolytic *Streptococcus*	Penicillin G	Multiple agents effective	Penicillin
Enterococci (group D strep)	Ampicillin and gentamicin	Vancomycin and gentamicin	Ampicillin
Bacteroides sp.	Metronidazole	Clindamycin	Metronidazole Clindamycin
Enterobacter sp.	Imipenem or ceftazidime +/− gentamicin	Ticarcillin clavulanate	Ciprofloxacin
Klebsiella sp.	Cephalosporin 3[b] (cefotaxime, ceftriaxone)	Gentamicin	Ciprofloxacin
Pasturella multocida	Penicillin G	Doxycycline	Penicillin V
Proteus mirabilis	Ampicillin	Trimethoprim/sulfamethoxazole	Ampicillin
Serratia marcescens	Amikacin or gentamicin	Cephalosporin 3[b]	Ciprofloxacin

From ref. 114.
[a] Cephalosporin 1, first generation.
[b] Cephalosporin 3, third generation.

totaling 398 cases (35,36,86,89,104). The most common presenting symptoms include spinal pain, extremity weakness, and a chief complaint of the patient's "worst pain ever." Reports of patients presenting without pain or with weakness only are documented (89). The only consistent laboratory finding is an elevated sedimentation rate, which has been reported in all series. *Staphylococcus aureus* is the most common pathogen, as it is in spinal column infections. The differential diagnosis for a patient presenting with back pain, fever, leukocytosis, and an elevated sedimentation rate includes spinal osteomyelitis, spinal epidural abscess, leukemia, bacteremia, and meningitis (89).

Predisposing conditions associated with spinal epidural abscess include osteomyelitis, discitis, degenerative joint disease, diabetes mellitus, intravenous drug use, and HIV infection. Potential sources of infection include previous surgery (especially spinal surgery), trauma, dental procedures, soft tissue infection, epidural injection (86), retropharyngeal abscess, and respiratory and sinus infections. No source of the infection is noted in 15% to 50% of the cases depending on the series, with the average rate of all published cases being about 20%.

The diagnostic study of choice is MRI and, if possible, with gadolinium (113). CT scans, myelography, and nuclear medicine studies are alternatives, but they have a lower sensitivity and do not outline the pathological anatomy as well.

Nonsurgical treatment has been recommended for (a) patients who are poor surgical candidates because of their medical condition, (b) an abscess that involves too long a length of the spinal column to consider surgical drainage, (c) absence of neurological deficit, and (d)

complete neurological deficit longer than 3 days (82). Abscess progression can occur despite culture- and sensitivity-appropriate antibiotics, indicating that nonsurgical treatment demands careful monitoring of the condition. In the face of a progressive neurological deficit, nonsurgical treatment alone should continue only if the patient's medical condition is a contraindication to an anesthetic and surgical treatment.

Surgical drainage of the abscess is the primary treatment, in association with initial intravenous antibiotics that are at a minimum specific for *Staphylococcus aureus*. If at all possible, cultures directly from the abscess should be obtained prior to initiating antibiotic treatment. Broader spectrum antibiotic coverage should be used while awaiting culture results in patients at risk for infection with organisms other than *Staphylococcus aureus*. Examples include patients that are immunosuppressed, have diabetes mellitus, or are actively using intravenous drugs. A posterior spinal approach is usually adequate for drainage. An anterior approach should be considered if it is evident on the preoperative diagnostic study that the abscess is not assessable from the posterior.

Complications of Conservative Treatment

The major risk in treating pyogenic infections of the spine conservatively is that the disease process may progress in spite of the treatment. This may then result in progressive spinal deformity, most typically anterior vertebral collapse as a result of structurally weak, infected bone of insufficient strength to be supported by a brace. With vertebral collapse, the risk of neurological compromise becomes greater (46). Neurological compromise may also occur when epidural abscesses grow in size, compressing the dura externally. After the process becomes more chronic, sinus tracts to the skin or other areas may also develop. A poorer neurological result has been associated with infections involving diabetes mellitus, rheumatoid arthritis, and a more cephalad level of the infection (42).

GRANULOMATOUS INFECTIONS OF THE VERTEBRAL COLUMN

The term *granulomatous* refers to organisms that produce an immune response that results in granuloma formation. Histologically this granuloma has a caseating central area of necrosis surrounded by a rim of Langhans giant cells. Worldwide, by far the most common granulomatous infection is tuberculosis, caused by the organism *Mycobacterium tuberculosis* (Fig. 9). Fungi may also cause a granulomatous infection. Fungal infections include coccidioidomycosis, blastomycosis, histoplasmosis, cryptococcosis, and sporotrichosis. In general, conservative management and surgical indications for each of these infections are similar, with the exception that antibiotic regimens differ as a function of the organism.

When granulomatous infections attack the skeleton, the vertebral column is often involved. For example, the spine is the most common site of osseous involvement in tuberculosis, with more than 50% of cases occurring there. As shown in pyogenic infections, the unique vascular anatomy of the spine may cause its propensity for granulomatous infection. The anterior metaphysis is well supplied with arterioles, particularly in the area of the anterior longitudinal ligament. This area is supplied by surface arterioles, as well as the main nutrient artery, which enters through the posterior vertebral nutrient foramen. The infection tends to spread quickly across the periphery of the disc, where anastomoses exist, to involve the metaphyses of the vertebrae above or below. The distribution of lesions within the vertebrae suggests spread through ascending and descending nutrient branches of the posterior spinal arteries.

Why tuberculous and other granulomatous diseases are particularly prone to infect the vertebral bodies, even in children, is not known. However, we do know that when the spine is affected, the onset is insidious, and massive destruction of the vertebral bodies, intervening discs, and ligaments occurs. When this proceeds unchecked by medical or surgical treatment, spinal column collapse and angulation result. This angulation, combined with the inflammatory debris and necrotic material, may compress the spinal cord or cauda equina, causing progressive paraplegia. An additional etiology of

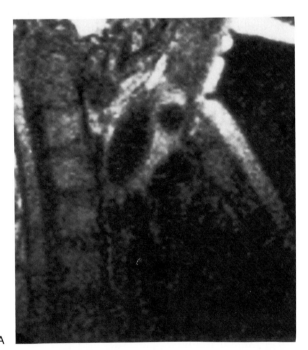
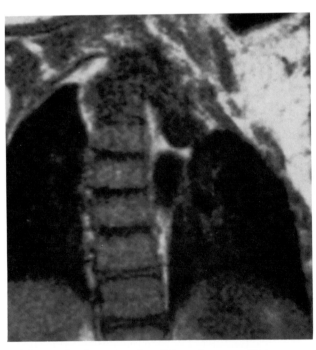

A

B

FIG. 9. A 12-year-old with tuberculous involvement of the cervicothoracic spine. When she presented (as a paraplegic), these MRI scans were obtained. **A:** Sagittal T1-weighted image. Note the step-off between cervical and thoracic vertebrae. **B:** Coronal T1-weighted image. Involved areas are less distinct than in pyogenic infections. In general, a bubbly area of decreased signal intensity is seen on T1-weighted images in tuberculosis.

paralysis is compression or inflammatory coagulation of the anterior spinal artery, causing a neurological deficit that is permanent and irreversible.

Therefore, it is critical in the treatment of granulomatous infection of the spine to make the diagnosis early so that antibiotic therapy and/or surgical debridement and fusion can be done before bony collapse and neurological compromise occur. Best results occur when treatment begins early in the disease process, whether that be medical or surgical.

Tuberculosis of the Spine (Pott's Disease)

Like any other osteoarticular lesion, spinal tuberculosis is the result of hematogenous dissemination from a primary infected visceral focus. The primary focus can be active or quiescent, apparent or obscure, and located in the lung, lymphatic system, kidney, or other viscus. In a typical lesion, the tuberculous bacilli find their way to the paradiscal area of two contiguous vertebrae, supporting the concept that the spread is via the arterial supply. The anterior extension of the lesion, with involvement of multiple vertebral bodies, is caused by extension of the abscess beneath the periosteum and anterior longitudinal ligament. The anterior and posterior longitudinal ligaments and periosteum are stripped from the vertebral bodies, resulting in loss of periosteal blood supply and destruction of the anterolateral surfaces of several contiguous vertebrae. Periosteal stripping, combined with arterial occlusion owing to endarteritis, causes ischemic infarction which in turn leads to necrosis of the involved bone. The body of the vertebra is thus mechanically weakened and yields to compressive forces.

The intervertebral disc is not involved primarily, because it is avascular. However, involvement of the paradiscal regions of the vertebra compromises nutrition of the disc. The disc may then be invaded by the infectious process and destroyed. Radiographically, it is typical to see more than one vertebra involved (average, 3.4 vertebrae) (62). The most common early findings are narrowing of the disc space and vertebral osteolysis. In more advanced disease, a paravertebral shadow is produced by extension of the tuberculous granulation tissue and the formation of an abscess in the paravertebral region. Later, vertebral collapse and angulation of the spine occur.

Treatment of tuberculous spinal disease basically involves rest of the involved area, chemotherapy using antituberculous medicines, and drainage of abscesses. There is some controversy as to whether or not more radical procedures (i.e., beyond simple incision and drainage) are indicated. Here we will review the experience and techniques of several authors in an attempt to address this area of controversy.

Treatment of Pott's Disease: Historical Background

In the past, tuberculosis was treated by resting the involved area, encouraging the patient to spend time in the fresh air, and relying on the natural recuperative powers of the patient (69). Abscesses were drained when necessary and the vertebral column debrided if the patient became paraplegic. In 1895, Menard (92) decompressed an abscess surrounding the spinal cord and was delighted to find that the patient recovered neurologically. This led him and other surgeons (24,115) to decompress the spinal cord through a variety of posterolateral and anterolateral approaches. In 1900, Menard reported on a series of successfully treated patients with Pott's disease (92). Others, including Albee (3), fused the spine to provide stability, thus "resting" the area. These were posterior fusion techniques and were not particularly advantageous in the patient with bony collapse and acute kyphotic angulation. Capener (24), Seddon (115), and others (62) further refined the techniques of surgical decompression and identified indications for operative intervention. The combination of rest, fusion, and debridement allowed the paraspinal abscesses to regress spontaneously (70). Some patients, however, did not improve but demonstrated progressive bony destruction, paralysis, and spread of the disease. Many patients died as the tuberculosis spread throughout their bodies.

Antituberculous drugs changed the surgical approach to treatment of spinal tuberculosis. It became obvious that patients could be cured not only of active disease, but also of paralysis, with drugs as the only treatment. Friedman (47) treated 64 patients without surgical fusion using antituberculous drugs, bed rest, and progressive ambulation with braces. The only surgical procedures were the evacuation of several large abscesses and decompressive laminectomies on several paraplegic patients. Of the eight patients with spinal cord involvement, four completely recovered and others showed degrees of recovery. The recommended therapy was 300 mg of isoniazid (INH) and 12 g of para-aminosalicylic acid (PAS) daily for 2.5 years (47). Friedman later described the newer regimens of chemotherapy in the treatment of bony tuberculosis (48).

Similarly, Tuli and colleagues, in India, used medical treatment alone for spinal tuberculosis (125). The only indications for surgery were Pott's paraplegia that did not resolve after 4 to 6 weeks of treatment, progressive or worsening paraplegia, or the development of spinal cord involvement where it had not previously been present. These authors did drain abscesses that were not clearing. In a later article, Tuli (124) described treatment by the "middle-path" regimen. Operative treatment was done for failure of drug therapy, recrudescence of disease, or if complications occurred. When patients were neurologically involved, only 38% recovered completely on drug treatment alone, whereas 69% had complete recovery after surgical decompression. Of the patients without neurological compromise, 94% had clinical healing of the lesion without surgery (124).

Konstam and Blesovsy, working in Nigeria, found surgery to be impractical and usually unnecessary (76). They treated patients basically as outpatients, with INH and PAS. Collapse of the spine was accepted as being inevitable and not necessarily undesirable. The only surgery was simple drainage for paraplegia. When a patient had paralysis, he was operated on only if unable to walk, and only 3 of 28 of these patients did not recover or died. It should be noted that they considered it necessary to treat patients this way because of hospital overload; they did not treat increased kyphosis (76).

Dickson, also of Nigeria, reviewed children with tuberculosis of the spine treated medically (38). Of 31 children, the gibbus worsened in all but four. He noted that the more severe the initial gibbus, the worse the final increase in angulation. Some of the less severely involved patients actually improved as growth occurred.

Martin looked at the results of treatment before and after the development of antituberculous drugs, and with and without surgical fusion (87). Of 227 patients treated without chemotherapy, bony ankylosis occurred within an average of 5.7 years. Those patients treated conservatively with chemotherapy fused in 4.9 years. Children treated without drugs took even longer to stabilize, averaging 9 years to bony ankylosis. His impression was that chemotherapy and surgical fusion produced a more stable spine within a shorter time. He reported a 96.2% fusion rate. In a later study of patients with Pott's paraplegia (120 of the 740 patients in his total series), Martin found that chemotherapy improved the patient's general condition and made the surgery safer (88). It did not, in his opinion, prevent paraplegia or promote recovery from it. He found that 24 of 50 patients (48%) recovered with chemotherapy alone, while 60% of patients who underwent surgical decompression recovered. He suggested that an early focal operation might prevent or abort the onset of paralysis.

Guirguis reported on 60 patients with Pott's paraplegia, of whom half were operated on and the other half treated conservatively (55). He found better results in the surgically treated patients, with 28 of 30 improving and many being completely cured of any neurological compromise. Many of the patients were relieved of their painful flexor spasms. Neville and Davis also studied patients treated with or without surgery, with emphasis on the fusion rate (102). In the nonsurgical group, 50% had an autofusion at an average of 15.2 months. The surgical group had a fusion rate of 92%. Arct found that elderly Polish people (older than 60 years) could tolerate and benefit from surgical fusion (8). Of 133 patients, 61 had conservative treatment, and 72 underwent surgical decompression with or without fusion. Only 13 of the conservatively treated patients returned to their regular life style; none was able to return to work as a farmer or laborer. Of the surgically treated patients, 41 of 72 had complete clinical and radiographic recovery, and 21 returned to agricultural work.

In summary, the medical treatment of tuberculosis has been amazingly effective in controlling spinal tuberculosis and even curing it. The newer drugs have been more effective in preventing recurrence of disease due to resistant organisms. However, for at least the first 6 months of chemotherapy, further bony destruction and collapse can occur, causing increased vertebral angulation and cord compression. This is particularly true if a significant degree of kyphotic angulation is already present when drug therapy is started. Without chemotherapy, there will be a progressive thinning of the intervertebral space, atrophy of osseous tissue, and decalcification, which can persist for an average of 2 to 3 years (55). It should be remembered that in properly selected patients, medical treatment is adequate and can be expected to yield a relatively high rate (up to 79% in one series) of solid bony fusion without surgical intervention (75).

Multidrug-Resistant Tuberculosis

Multidrug-resistant tuberculosis (MDR-TB) is gaining recognition as outbreaks are reported (17). The Center for Disease Control (CDC) has investigated outbreaks involving more than 300 cases (28). The salient features of MDR-TB are a high prevalence of HIV co-infection, rapid progression of the disease (median interval, 4 to 16 weeks), high fatality rates (up to 90%), prolonged time to organism identification and susceptibility testing, and significant rates of transmission to health care workers (126). Extrapulmonary involvement has been reported in about 50% of the cases, but specific rates of spinal column infection are not noted. We advise the prompt initiation of therapy with at least two drugs, after an aggressive attempt to obtain a specimen for culture. This initial empirical treatment should follow local institutional susceptibility reports based on organisms in previous outbreaks. In some institutions, this means initial treatment that include six or more drugs. At institutions where no outbreaks are known, a four-drug empirical regimen is advised (126). A radiometric culture system is encouraged in order to improve the availability of susceptibility testing (82).

Current Medical Recommendations

Medical recommendations for the treatment of acute tuberculosis of the spine include the following (114):

1. Isoniazid (INH): If given daily, 5 to 10 mg/kg per day p.o., up to 300 mg/day as 1 dose. If given twice weekly, 15 mg/kg, up to 900 mg/day maximum dose.

2. Rifampin: 10 mg/kg per day p.o., up to 600 mg/day q.d. as 1 dose.
3. Ethambutol: 25 mg/day p.o. for 2 months, and then 15 mg/kg per day q.d. as 1 dose.
4. Pyrazinamide: 25 mg/kg per day p.o. (maximum 2.5 gm/day) q.d. as 1 dose.
5. Streptomycin: 0.75 to 1.0 gm/day, IM initially for 60 to 90 days, then 1.0 gm 2 to 3 times per week q.d. as 1 dose.

Rifampicin and isoniazid are each administered for 12 months for extrapulmonary bone disease (114). Streptomycin (0.75 to 1.0 mg/day) may be given as a fifth drug, or in addition to any multidrug regimen. Antibiotic therapy is initiated prior to surgery and continued postoperatively. Ideally, the patient should receive the drug for 1 to 2 weeks before debridement of the vertebral column. In cases of acute paraplegia requiring emergency decompression, drug therapy should begin 24 hours before surgery.

Coccidioidomycosis

Coccidioidomycosis is caused by *Coccidioides immitis,* the most infectious of all fungi capable of producing systemic disease. The localized form is usually benign, but the disseminated form is progressive. Twenty percent of those with disseminated disease have osseous lesions. The fungus is endemic to the southwestern United States, Central America, and parts of South America. It is particularly prevalent in central California, where it carries the name of San Joaquin Valley fever (134) (Fig. 10).

Although the disease occurs in all ages, it is most prevalent in those 25 to 55 years of age, and dissemination is greater in men. The disseminated disease is 10 times more common in blacks than whites, and it is of even greater hazard to Filipinos (134).

If a patient in an endemic region develops respiratory symptoms and fever that last longer than 1 month, disseminated disease should be suspected. The organisms enter the body by way of the respiratory tract and are spread hematogenously.

In an endemic area, 50% to 84% of the population will have a positive coccidioidin skin test. It takes 3 to 6 weeks for an exposed patient to test positively. Owing to anergy, the test is unreliable when systemic disease is present. Immunodiffusion tests have recently become a key diagnostic test for coccidioidomycosis. A serologic

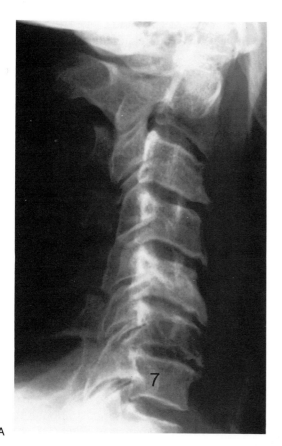
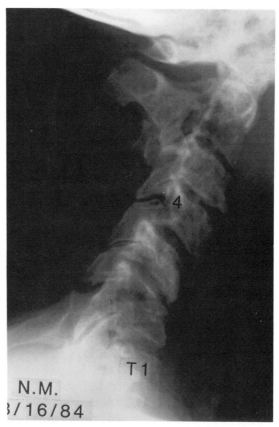

FIG. 10. A 51-year-old man presented with fatigue, night sweats, and a 25-pound weight loss. Biopsied skin lesions and cultures showed *Coccidioides immitis*. Later he developed neck pain. He was treated with systemic amphotericin B. **A:** Lateral radiograph when neck pain presented. **B:** Subsequent collapse within 6 months in spite of medical treatment. Anterior debridement and strut grafting were done.

complement fixation titer of 1:64 or higher is thought to be diagnostic of disseminated disease (134).

Most bony lesions are lytic in nature and indiscriminately involve the vertebrae. Often multiple spinal lesions are found. Although the discs are spared, paraspinal masses are seen with contiguous rib involvement (34).

Medical treatment of choice is fluconazole or itraconazole, with amphotericin B as an alternative drug (114). Surgery is reserved for patients with neurological compromise or those in need of structural support to prevent further deformity.

Blastomycosis

North American blastomycosis is caused by *Blastomyces dermatitidis*, a fungus causing chronic systemic infection which is respiratory in origin but capable of dissemination. It is endemic in the southeastern and midwestern United States. Men are affected nine times more frequently than women; all ages are affected, although there is a higher frequency in the third and fourth decades.

The disease usually begins as a mild respiratory infection, but as it disseminates hematogenously, generalized symptoms of fever, night sweats, anorexia, and weight loss develop. Skin tests are frequently negative early in the disease, but a culture of the skin or lesion will reveal budding yeast cells. Serologic tests may show a high titer only to *Histoplasma capsulatum.*

Osteomyelitis occurs frequently in disseminated blastomycosis and it has a greater tendency than coccidioidomycosis for fistula formation and erosion into joints. The disc cartilage is usually involved early, and large paravertebral masses involving ribs may be seen. Hilar adenopathy may be noted on the chest radiograph, as in tuberculosis (50).

Medical treatment consists of itraconazole, with ketonazole or amphotericin B as an alternative drug (114).

Cryptococcosis

Cryptococcosis is caused by *Cryptococcus neoformans* and is also a chronic systemic fungal disease originating in the respiratory tract. It affects all ages, but it is most prevalent between 40 and 60 years and is twice as common in men. This disease is commonly seen in patients with leukemia or Hodgkin's disease, or in those patients with sarcoidosis who have central nervous system involvement. The pulmonary disease is rarely symptomatic. The spread is by a hematogenous route and frequently results in a cryptococcal meningitis. Ten percent of the disseminated cases involve bone. The bony lesions are heralded by pain, swelling, and progressive loss of spine motion (33). Blood, spinal fluid culture, or cultures

from bony lesions may reveal the organism *C. neoformans.* The India-ink preparation may be helpful, particularly in evaluating spinal fluid.

Cryptococcus antibodies may be measured, and some authors believe their presence indicates a favorable prognosis. The radiographic findings are indistinguishable from coccidioidomycosis (33).

Treatment of choice is medical, with initial parenteral amphotericin B until the patient responds, discontinuing the amphotericin B and starting fluconazole p.o. (114).

Aspergillosis

Species of the fungus *Aspergillus* are widely found in our environment, in the soil, water, organic matter, and a variety of both wet and dry materials. Spores are light, resistant to desiccation, and easily spread through the air. Clinical infection with the ubiquitous fungus is most common in the immunocompromised population (21,100). Formation of "fungus balls" in the lung is most commonly seen with *Aspergillus fumigatus,* although several other species are also pathogenic. It is assumed that most spine infections are hematogenously spread from pulmonary lesions.

Radiographic appearance is similar to that of other granulomatous infections (Fig. 11). Lytic destruction of adjoining vertebral endplates may eventually progress to collapse, with severe pain and the risk of neurologic compromise (91). Diagnosis of *Aspergillus* infection is made by direct microscopic examination and culture of biopsy tissue, which will show characteristic branching hyphae. Serologic immunodiffusion tests can be helpful in diagnosis and speciation, particularly when tissue is difficult to obtain.

Medical treatment centers on amphotericin B or itraconazole (114). Prognosis of the disease is generally grave, although it is dependent upon the nutritional and immune status of the patient.

Surgery is not usually necessary, except for tissue diagnosis. Biopsy of the lesion will often be the crucial diagnostic factor. Surgery should be reserved for the relatively healthy patient who needs stabilization or neurological decompression with stabilization. This is best undertaken anteriorly, with strut grafting.

Medical Treatment of Fungal Spine Infections

Amphotericin B is the mainstay of treatment of the fungal infections. However, because of its toxic nature, care should be taken in its administration. A test dose of 1 mg in 20 ml of 5% dextrose in water (D5W) should be given intravenously over 20 minutes, followed by close observation of the vital signs over the next 4 hours. If no adverse reaction is seen, an initial dose of 0.25 mg/kg in D5W is given intravenously over 4 hours. The dose is

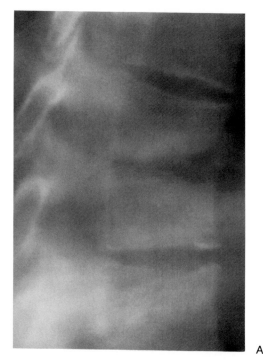

FIG. 11. A 46-year-old man presented with severe thoracic spine pain. Six months prior he had undergone anterior debridement and fusion for presumed *Staphylococcus epidermidis* infection at L1-L2. The patient had a history 10 years prior of intravenous drug use. Cultures from anterior debridement grew *Aspergillus.* **A:** Lateral tomograms are particularly valuable for definitions of thoracic lesions. **B,C:** Anterior debridement and strut grafting was performed, followed 2 weeks later by posterior stabilization with Moe rods and Wisconsin wiring. The patient was also treated with prolonged intravenous amphotericin B.

A

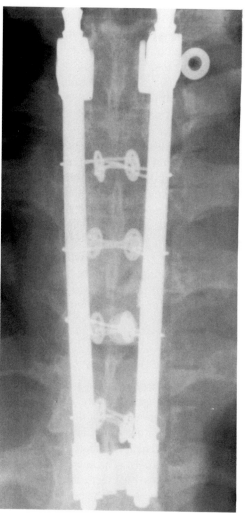

B

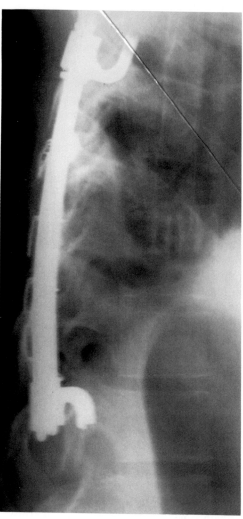

C

advanced slowly over 5 days to 0.5 mg/kg, which is then the maintenance dose. The goal should be to give the patient a total dosage of 30 mg/kg, which usually will take 6 to 10 weeks. For the more severe infections, a longer time interval may be required. If the dosing is stopped for more than 7 days because of adverse reactions, it should be restarted at 0.25 mg/kg and gradually increased again. Immunocompromised patients may require dosing up to 1 mg/kg per day. Dosing schedules may be changed to double doses every other day to minimize phlebitis if the patient can tolerate the higher doses.

If administered too rapidly, complications can include convulsions, anaphylaxis, hypotension, ventricular arrhythmias, and even cardiac arrest. Commonly reported side effects even with careful, slow dosing include fever, chills, phlebitis, nausea, vomiting, anorexia, abdominal pain, anemia, metallic taste, nephrotoxicity, and hypokalemia. The most common early difficulty is the febrile reaction, and the most common late problem is azotemia.

OTHER GRANULOMATOUS INFECTIONS

Brucellosis

Brucellosis is a systemic infectious disease caused by small, nonmotile, non-spore-forming, gram-negative rods of the genus *Brucella*. Farm animals, especially cattle, hogs, goats, sheep, and dogs are primary sources of infection, but many other animals can harbor the bacterium (135).

Human infection occurs primarily from ingestion of improperly prepared animal tissues or products, or from contamination of a skin wound by infected animal tissues. Infection via inoculation of the conjunctiva has been demonstrated, and there is some evidence that inhalation of aerosols can lead to the disease (14,15).

Brucella infections are often asymptomatic. Initial infection leads to further immunity in approximately 90% of cases (15,135). Men are affected more often than women, probably because of a higher rate of occupational exposure.

The usual incubation period is from 10 days to 3 weeks, depending on the size of the inoculum and host resistance. If the inoculum is small or early treatment is instituted, the body is able to contain the infection and granulomas do not form. If the host is overwhelmed, multisystem disease can occur with large, multiple granulomas.

Initial symptoms may include fever, sweats, weakness, weight loss, headache, myalgia, lymphadenopathy, and hepatosplenomegaly. Late complications are multisystemic and can include septic arthritis, central nervous system involvement, osteomyelitis, and spine involve-

ment (135). Of those patients with spinal brucellosis, approximately 12% will have some degree of spinal cord compromise.

A history of animal exposure or ingestion of unpasteurized or uncooked animal products should be carefully sought. *Brucella* can be cultured from the blood during a bacteremic episode, and from involved lymph nodes or granulomas later in the course of the disease. The organism is dangerous to laboratory personnel, and any suspected materials should be clearly identified. The *Brucella* agglutination test is quite reliable, and about 97% of infected individuals will become positive within 3 weeks of exposure. Brucellosis is a reportable disease.

Radiographic changes to the spine occur relatively late in the course of the disease, and they are similar to but less severe than those seen in tuberculosis (14,135). Technetium bone scans and gallium scans should be done early if spinal involvement is suspected but is not apparent on routine radiographs. If spinal cord compromise is suspected, CT scans, myelography, and perhaps MRI should be employed to determine the exact location and extent of the compression. A paravertebral abscess is not present (as in tuberculosis), and the usual site of spinal involvement is in the lumbar area (14,135).

The mainstay of treatment for brucellosis is antibiotic therapy, which includes doxycycline and gentamicin or doxycycline and rifampin (114). Surgical intervention is not usually necessary and should be reserved for tissue diagnosis. Stabilization of the spine, or decompression of the cord with stabilization, is determined by the clinical condition. The indications and techniques are identical to those proposed for treatment of the tuberculous spine. If there is spinal involvement but surgical intervention is not warranted, the spine should be protected until healing is complete, using recumbency followed by cast application or brace wear.

Brucellosis is a completely curable infection. The primary pitfall is a delay of more than 1 month in diagnosis and treatment (14,15,135), which can lead to multisystem involvement with severe sequelae. Antibiotic therapy should continue for at least 6 weeks, or until the sedimentation rate falls to normal.

Actinomycosis

The actinomycetes are a heterogeneous group; their morphology suggests they are a fungus, but they are classified as bacteria because of their small size (<1 micrometer), primitive nuclear organization, and cell wall composition. The usual infective organism in man is *Actinomyces israelii*. The bacteria are present in the oral cavity both in carious teeth and in tonsilar crypts. The pathological reaction of the body to *Actinomyces* is typically that of suppuration. Acute and chronic inflammatory tissues resemble those of staphylococcal infections.

Areas of infection are most characteristic for their gross appearance of "sulfur granules," which are actually collections of foamy macrophages.

The common sites of involvement are the face, the thorax, and the abdomen. Involvement in the spine is rare and usually associated with a thoracic infection (16,30,94). Diagnosis is made by direct culture of tissue. Standardized serologic tests are not routinely used, and skin tests have generally been equivocal. Medical treatment with penicillin is effective early in the course of the illness. This should include 6 weeks of intravenous therapy followed by 6 months of oral medication. Doxycycline and ceftriaxone are the alternative antibiotics, with clindamycin, erythromycin, and imipenem also effective (114).

Surgical debridement should be done for abscesses when there is a large amount of diseased tissue. Structural principles for bony destruction and collapse are the same as for other bacterial and fungal infections.

PARASITIC SPINE INFECTIONS

Echinococcosis

Echinococcosis is rarely seen in the United States. It is more commonly seen in the cattle- and sheep-raising areas of northern and southern Africa, South America, and occasionally Europe, Australia, Canada, and Alaska. The infecting organism is either *Echinococcus granulosus* or *E. multilocularis.* The eggs of the parasite are typically ingested by humans from water infected by cattle, sheep, or dog feces. After ingestion, embryos hatch from the eggs, traverse the intestine, and disseminate through venous and vascular channels. Cysts form in the viscera, typically the lungs and liver. In 1% to 2% of cases, the primary focus of invasion will be bone (68). The spine (50%) and pelvis are the most common sites (44). Patients typically present with pain and deformity. Large hydatid cysts may form, expanding the surrounding trabeculae. As the cyst expands, cysts may form in adjacent soft tissues.

The parasite will not elicit a large inflammatory reaction in bone as other infectious organisms do. It expands with irregular destruction of trabeculae and formation of daughter cysts. Cancellous bone is gradually weakened, with eventual collapse. Even after penetration of periosteum and invasion of soft tissues, there is no sharp demarcation between normal and diseased tissue.

Radiographs show an expansile lytic mass containing a few trabeculae, which may be confused with fibrous dysplasia, giant cell tumor, metastasis, or cartilage neoplasm. Diagnosis is made in patients at risk for this organism by a positive complement fixation test, positive hemagglutination test, and reaction to intradermal injection of hydatid fluid. Complications are common and include fracture or vertebral collapse through the cyst, secondary infection, rupture into the spinal cord with neurologic compromise, and compression of pelvic soft tissues and organs. The clinical course is often advanced when diagnosis is made because expansion typically progresses asymptomatically until a complication occurs.

Treatment should focus on surgical debridement. This should consist of complete removal of all affected bone and stabilization as needed, generally by the same techniques as discussed under pyogenic infections. In the past, formalin cyst wash-out has been used intraoperatively. This should not be used currently, as control of local tissue necrosis is poor, and anaphylaxis may result.

Reports of effective medical treatment with the antihelminthic mebendazole have brought promise to a previously dismal prognosis (26). Dosage has been recommended for 3 months, 100 mg orally 3 times daily, increasing up to 600 mg 3 times a day by the 7th day (27,44). Side effects include diarrhea, rash, neutropenia, and increased liver function tests, but these are relatively infrequent.

Results without treatment are poor, with a high rate of paraplegia (96,97,106,136). Because of the necessity of radical surgery due to progression of disease, surgical results in the past have been generally less than satisfactory (7,127). However, improved results are being reported with the use of mebendazole in combination with surgery (24,110,114).

REFERENCES

1. Abbey DM, Hosea SW (1989): Diagnosis of vertebral osteomyelitis in a community hospital by using computed tomography. *Arch Intern Med* 149:2029–2035.
2. Adatepe MH, Powell OM, Isaacs GH, Nichols K, Cefola R (1986): Hematogenous pyogenic vertebral osteomyelitis: diagnostic value of radionuclide bone imaging. *J Nucl Med* 27:1680–1685.
3. Albee BH (1919): *Orthopedic and reconstructive surgery.* Philadelphia: WB Saunders.
4. Adlerman EJ, Duff J (1952): Osteomyelitis of the cervical vertebrae as a complication of urinary tract disease. *JAMA* 148:283–285.
5. Allen EH, Cosgrove D, Millard FJ (1978): The radiological changes in infections of the spine and their diagnostic value. *Clin Radiol* 29:31–40.
6. Ambrose GB, Alpert M, Neer CS (1966): Vertebral osteomyelitis: a diagnostic problem. *JAMA* 197:619–622.
7. Apt WL, Fierro JL, Calderon C, Perez C, Mujica P (1976): Vertebral hydatid disease. *J Neurosurg* 44:72–76.
8. Arct W (1968): Operative treatment of tuberculosis of the spine in old people. *J Bone Joint Surg [Am]* 50:255–267.
9. Awad I, Bay JW, Petersen JM (1984): Nocardial osteomyelitis of the spine with epidural spinal cord compression. *Neurosurgery* 15:254–256.
10. Baker A, Ojemann R, Swartz M, Richardson E (1975): Spinal epidural abscess. *N Engl J Med* 293;463–468.
11. Batson OV (1940): The function of the vertebral veins and their role in the spread of metastases. *Ann Surg* 112:138–149.
12. Batson OV (1942): The vertebral vein system as a mechanism for the spread of metastases. *Am J Roentgenol Radium Ther* 48:715–718.
13. Beltrani VP, Echols RM, Vedder DK (1987): Vertebral osteomy-

elitis caused by Haemophilus influenzae. *J Infect Dis* 156:391–394.

14. Bennett JE (1985): Brucellosis. In: Wyngaarden JB, South LH, eds. *Cecil's textbook of medicine.* Philadelphia: WB Saunders, p. 1614.

15. Benson DR (1983): Orthopaedic disorders: the spine and neck. In: Gershwin ME, Robbins DL, eds. *Musculoskeletal diseases of children.* New York: Grune and Stratton, p. 494.

16. Birley HD, Teare EL, Utting JA (1989): Actinomycotic osteomyelitis of the thoracic spine in a penicillin-sensitive patient [letter]. *J Infect* 19:193–194.

17. Bloch A, Cauthen G, Onorato I, et al. (1994): Nationwide survey of drug resistant tuberculosis in the United States. *JAMA* 271;665–771.

18. Bohmig R (1929): Die Degenerationen der Wirbelbandscheiben und ihre Bedeutung fur die Klinik. *Munchener Med Wehnschr* 76:1318.

19. Bonfiglio M, Lange TA, Kim YM (1973): Pyogenic vertebral osteomyelitis. Disc space infections. *Clin Orthop* 96:234–247.

20. Brant-Zawadski M, Burke VD, Jeffrey RB (1983): CT in the evaluation of spine infection. *Spine* 8:358–364.

21. Brown DL, Musher DM, Taffet GE (1987): Hematogenously acquired *Aspergillus* vertebral osteomyelitis in seemingly immunocompetent drug addicts. *Western J Med* 147:84–85.

22. Bryan V, Franks L, Torres H (1973): *Pseudomonas aeruginosa* cervical diskitis with chondro-osteomyelitis in an intravenous drug abuser. *Surg Neurol* 1:142–144.

23. Burke DR, Brant-Zawadski M (1985): CT of pyogenic spine infection. *Neuroradiology* 27:131–137.

24. Capener N (1954): The evolution of lateral rhachotomy. *J Bone Joint Surg [Br]* 36:173–179.

25. Carvell JE, Maclarnon JC (1981): Chronic osteomyelitis of the thoracic spine due to *Salmonella typhi. Spine* 6:527–530.

26. Charles RW, Govender S, Naidoo KS (1988): Echinococcal infection of the spine with neural involvement. *Spine* 13:47–49.

27. Charles RW, Mody GM, Govender S (1989): Pyogenic infection of the lumbar vertebral spine due to gas-forming organisms. *Spine* 14:541–543.

28. Control CFD (1993): Outbreak of multidrug-resistant tuberculosis at a hospital—New York City, 1991. *Morb Mortal Wkly Rep* 42:427,433–434.

29. Cooppan R, Schoenbaum S, Younger MD, Friedberg S, D'Elia J (1976): Vertebral osteomyelitis in insulin-dependent diabetics. *S Afr Med J* 50:1993–1996.

30. Cope VZ (1951): Actinomycosis of bone with special reference to infection of the vertebral column. *J Bone Joint Surg [Br]* 33:205–214.

31. Cotty P, Fouquet B, Pleskof L, Audurier A, Cotty F, Goupille P, Valat JP, Alison D, Laffont J (1988): Vertebral osteomyelitis: value of percutaneous biopsy. *J Neuroradiol* 15:13–21.

32. Coventry MB, Ghormley RK, Kernohan JW (1945): The intervertebral disc, its microscopic anatomy and pathology. Part I: anatomy, development and physiology. *J Bone Joint Surg [Am]* 27:105–112.

33. Cowen NJ (1969): Cryptococcosis of bone: case report and review of the literature. *Clin Orthop* 66:174–182.

34. Dalinka MK, Dinnenberg S, Greendyk WH, Hopkins R (1971): Roentgenographic features of osseous coccidioidomycosis and differential diagnosis. *J Bone Joint Surg [Am]* 53:1157–1164.

35. Darouiche RO, Hamill R, Greenberg SB, Weathers S, Musher D (1992): Bacterial spinal epidural abscess. *Medicine* 71(6):369–385.

36. Deming CL, Zaff F (1943): Metastatic vertebral osteomyelitis complicating prostatic surgery. *Trans Am Assoc Genitourin Surg* 35:287–305.

37. Deyo R (1986): Early diagnostic evaluation of low back pain. *J Gen Intern Med* 1:328–338.

38. Dickson JA (1967): Spinal tuberculosis in Nigerian children. *J Bone Joint Surg [Br]* 49:682–694.

39. Digby JM, Kersley JB (1979): Pyogenic non-tuberculous spinal infection. *J Bone Joint Surg [Br]* 61:47–55.

40. Dolan SA, Everett ED, Harper MC (1987): *Salmonella* vertebral osteomyelitis treated with cefotaxime. *Arch Intern Med* 147:1667–1668.

41. Edwards JE Jr, Lehrer RI, Stiehm ER, Fischer TJ, Young LS (1978): Severe candidal infections. Clinical perspective, immune defense mechanisms, and current concepts of therapy. *Ann Intern Med* 89:91–106.

42. Eismont FJ, Bohlman HH, Soni PL, Goldberg VM, Freehafer AA (1983): Pyogenic and fungal vertebral osteomyelitis with paralysis. *J Bone Joint Surg [Am]* 65:19–29.

43. Engh CA, Hughes JL, Abrams RC, Bowerman JW (1971): Osteomyelitis in the patient with sickle-cell disease. *J Bone Joint Surg [Am]* 53:1–15.

44. Fitzpatrick SC (1965): Hydatid disease of the lumbar vertebrae. *J Bone Joint Surg [Br]* 47:286–291.

45. Frederickson B, Yuan H, Olans R (1978): Management and outcome of pyogenic vertebral osteomyelitis. *Clin Orthop* 131:160–167.

46. Freehafer AA, Furey JG, Pierce DS (1962): Pyogenic osteomyelitis of the spine resulting in spinal paralysis. *J Bone Joint Surg [Am]* 44:710–716.

47. Friedman B (1966): Chemotherapy of tuberculosis of the spine. *J Bone Joint Surg [Am]* 48:451–474.

48. Friedman B, Kapur VN (1973): Newer knowledge of chemotherapy in the treatment of tuberculosis of bones and joints. *Clin Orthop* 97:5–15.

49. Garcia A Jr, Grantham SA (1960): Hematogenous pyogenic vertebral osteomyelitis. *J Bone Joint Surg [Am]* 42:429–436.

50. Gehweiler JA, Capp MP, Chick EW (1970): Observations on the roentgen patterns in blastomycosis of bone. *Am J Roentgenol* 108:497–510.

51. Gelfand MS, Miller JH (1987): Pneumococcal vertebral osteomyelitis in an adult. *South Med J* 80:534–535.

52. Golimbu C, Firooznia H, Rafii M (1984): CT of osteomyelitis of the spine. *Am J Roentgenol* 142:159–163.

53. Govender S, Charles RW, Ballaram RS, Achary DM (1988): Vertebral osteomyelitis after a closed fracture of the spine. *S Afr Med J* 73:124–126.

54. Griffiths HE, Jones DM (1971): Pyogenic infection of the spine. A review of twenty-eight cases. *J Bone Joint Surg [Br]* 53:383–391.

55. Guirguis AR (1967): Pott's paraplegia. *J Bone Joint Surg [Br]* 49:658–667.

56. Guri JP (1946): Pyogenic osteomyelitis of the spine. *J Bone Joint Surg* 28:29–39.

57. Hale JE, Aichroth P (1974): Vertebral osteomyelitis: a complication of urological surgery. *Br J Surg* 61:867–872.

58. Harries TJ, Lichtman DM, Swafford AR (1981): Pyogenic vertebral osteomyelitis complicating abdominal stab wounds. *J Trauma* 21:75–79.

59. Harvey WC, Podoloff DA, Kapp DT (1975): [67]Gallium in 68 consecutive infection searches. *J Nucl Med* 16:2–4.

60. Henriques CQ (1958): Osteomyelitis as a complication in urology: with special reference to the paravertebral venous plexus. *Br J Surg* 46:19–28.

61. Henson SW Jr, Coventry MB (1956): Osteomyelitis of the vertebrae as the result of infection of the urinary tract. *Surg Gynecol Obstet* 102:207–214.

62. Hodgson AR, Stock FE (1960): Anterior spine fusion for the treatment of tuberculosis of the spine. *J Bone Joint Surg [Am]* 42:295–310.

63. Hoffer P (1980): Gallium and infection. *J Nucl Med* 21:484–488.

64. Holzman RS, Bishko F (1971): Osteomyelitis in heroin addicts. *Ann Intern Med* 75:693–696.

65. Horowitz MD, Dove DB, Eismont FJ, Green BA (1985): Impalement injuries. *J Trauma* 25:914–916.

66. Incavo SJ, Muller DL, Krag MH, Gump D (1988): Vertebral osteomyelitis caused by *Clostridium difficile. Spine* 13:111–113.

67. Jabbari B, Pierce JF (1977): Spinal cord compression due to *Pseudomonas* in a heroin addict. *Neurology* 27:1034–1037.

68. Jaffe HL (1972): *Metabolic, degenerative and inflammatory diseases of the bones and joints.* New York: Lea and Febiger, pp. 1072–1082.

69. Jones AR (1953): The influence of Hugh Owen Thomas on the evolution of treatment of skeletal tuberculosis. *J Bone Joint Surg [Br]* 35:309–319.

70. Karlen A (1959): Early drainage of paraspinal tuberculous abscesses in children. *J Bone Joint Surg* [Br] 41:491–498.

71. Karnaze MG, Gado MH, Sartor KJ, Hodges FJ 3d (1988): Comparison of MR and CT myelography in imaging the cervical and thoracic spine. *Am J Roentgenol* 150:397–403.

72. Kattapuram SV, Phillips WC, Boyd R (1983): CT in pyogenic osteomyelitis of the spine. *Am J Roentgenol* 140:1199–1201.

73. Kemp HB, Jackson JW, Jeremiah JD, Hall AJ (1973): Pyogenic infections occurring primarily in intervertebral discs. *J Bone Joint Surg* [Br] 55:698–714.

74. Kido D, Bryan D, Halpern M (1973): Hematogenous osteomyelitis in drug addicts. *Am J Roentgenol* 118:356–363.

75. King DM, Mayo KM (1973): Infective lesions of the vertebral column. *Clin Orthop* 96:248–253.

76. Konstam PG, Blesovsky A (1962): The ambulant treatment of spinal tuberculosis. *Br J Surg* 50:26–38.

77. Kulowski J (1936): Pyogenic osteomyelitis of the spine: an analysis and discussion of 102 cases. *J Bone Joint Surg* 18:343–364.

78. Lannelongue O (1880): *De l'osteomyelite aigue pendant la croissance.* Paris.

79. Larde D, Mathieu D, Frija J, Gaston A, Vasile N (1982): Vertebral osteomyelitis: disk hypodensity on CT. *Am J Roentgenol* 139:963–967.

80. Leigh TF, Kelly RP, Weens HS (1955): Spinal osteomyelitis associated with urinary tract infections. *Radiology* 65:334–342.

81. Lewis R, Gorbach S, Altner P (1972): Spinal *Pseudomonas* chondro-osteomyelitis in heroin users. *N Engl J Med* 286:1303.

82. Leys D, Lesoin F, Vicaud C, et al. (1985): Decreased morbidity from acute bacterial spinal epidural abscesses using computed tomography and non-surgical treatment in selected patients. *Ann Neurol* 17:350–355.

83. Liudahl KJ, Limbird TJ (1987): *Torulopsis glabrata* vertebral osteomyelitis. *Spine* 12:593–595.

84. Lowe J, Kaplan L, Liebergall M, Floman Y (1989): *Serratia* osteomyelitis causing neurological deterioration after spine fracture. *J Bone Joint Surg* [Br] 71:256–258.

85. Makins GH, Abbott FC (1896): On acute primary osteomyelitis of the vertebrae. *Ann Surg* 23:510–539.

86. Mamourian AC, Dickman C, Drayer B, Sonntag V (1993): Spinal epidural abscess: three cases following spinal epidural injection demonstrated with magnetic resonance imaging. *Anesthesiology* 78:204–207.

87. Martin NS (1970): Tuberculosis of the spine: a study of the results of treatment during the last 25 years. *J Bone Joint Surg* [Br] 52:613–628.

88. Martin NS (1971): Pott's paraplegia: a report on 120 cases. *J Bone Joint Surg* [Br] 53:596–608.

89. Maslen DR, Jones SR, Crislip MA, Bracis R, Dworkin RJ, Flemming JE (1993): Spinal epidural abscess. *Arch Intern Med* 153;1713–1720.

90. McGahan JP, Dublin AB (1985): Evaluation of spinal infections by plain radiographs, computed tomography, intrathecal metrizamide, and CT-guided biopsy. *Diagn Imaging Clin Med* 54:11–20.

91. McKee DF, Barr WM, Bryan CS, Lunceford EM Jr (1984): Primary Aspergillosis of the spine mimicking Pott's paraplegia. *J Bone Joint Surg* [Am] 66:1481–1483.

92. Menard V (1900): *Etude practique sur le mal de Pott.* Paris: Masson et Cie.

93. Merkel KD, Brown ML, Dewanjee MK, Fitzgerald RH Jr (1985): Comparison of Indium-labeled-leucocyte imaging with sequential Technetium-Gallium scanning in the diagnosis of low-grade musculoskeletal sepsis. *J Bone Joint Surg* [Am] 67:465–476.

94. Meyer M, Gall MB (1935): Mycosis of the vertebral column: a review of the literature. *J Bone Joint Surg* 17:857–866.

95. Milgram JW, Romine JS (1982): Spontaneous osteomyelitis complicating a compression fracture of the lumbar spine. *Spine* 7:179–182.

96. Miller BR, Schiller WR (1989): Pyogenic vertebral osteomyelitis after transcolonic gunshot wound. *Mil Med* 154:64–66.

97. Mills TJ (1956): Paraplegia due to hydatid disease. *J Bone Joint Surg* [Br] 38:884–891.

98. Modic MT, Feiglin DH, Piraino DW, Boumphrey F, et al. (1985): Vertebral osteomyelitis: assessment using MRI. *Radiology* 157:157–166.

99. Modic MT, Pflanze W, Feiglin DH, Belhobek G (1986): Magnetic resonance imaging of musculoskeletal infections. *Radiol Clin North Am* 24:247–258.

100. Morgenlander JC, Rossitch E Jr, Rawlings CE 3rd (1989): *Aspergillus* disc space infection. *Neurosurgery* 25:126–129.

101. Morrey BF, Kelly PJ, Nichols DR (1980): Viridans streptococcal osteomyelitis of the spine. *J Bone Joint Surg* [Am] 62:1009–1010.

102. Neville CH Jr, Davis WL (1971): Is surgical fusion still desirable in spinal tuberculosis? *Clin Orthop* 75:179–187.

103. Noble RC, Overman SB (1987): *Propionibacterium acnes* osteomyelitis. *J Clin Micro* 25:251–254.

104. Nussbaum ES, Rigamonti D, Standiford H, Numaguchi Y, Wolf A, Robinson W (1992): Spinal epidural abscess: a report of 40 cases and review. *Surg Neurol* 38;225–231.

105. Pilgaard S (1969): Discitis (closed space infection) following removal of lumbar intervertebral disc. *J Bone Joint Surg* [Am] 51:713–716.

106. Porat S, Robin GC, Wertheim G (1984): Hydatid disease of the spine causing paraplegia. *Spine* 9:648–653.

107. Post MJ, Quencer RM, Montalvo BM, Katz BH, et al. (1988): Spinal infection: evaluation with MR imaging and intraoperative US. *Radiology* 169:765–771.

108. Pott P (1779): *Remarks on that kind of palsy of the lower limbs which is frequently found to accompany a curvature of the spine and is supposed to be caused by it.* London.

109. Redfern RM, Cottam SN, Phillipson AP (1988): Proteus infection of the spine. *Spine* 13:439–441.

110. Robinson RG (1959): Hydatid disease of the spine and its neurological complications. *Br J Surg* 47:301–306.

111. Romanick PC, Smith TK, Kopaniky DR, Oldfield D (1985): Infection about the spine associated with low-velocity-missile injury to the abdomen. *J Bone Joint Surg* [Am] 67:1195–1201.

112. Ross PM, Fleming JL (1976): Vertebral body osteomyelitis. *Clin Orthop* 118:190–198.

113. Sadato N, Numaguchi Y, Digamonti D, Kodama T, Nussbaum E, Sato S, Rothman M (1994): Spinal epidural abscess with gadolinium-enhanced MRI: serial follow-up studies and clinical correlations. *Neuroradiology* 36:44–48.

114. Sanford JP (1995): *Guide to antimicrobial therapy,* 25th ed. Dallas: Antimicrobial Therapy.

115. Seddon HJ (1953): Pott's paraplegia and its operative treatment. *J Bone Joint Surg* [Br] 35:487.

116. Sierra MA, Luparello FJ, Lewin JR (1961): Vertebral osteomyelitis and urinary-tract infection. *Arch Intern Med* 108:128–131.

117. Sinnott JT 4th, Multhopp H, Leo J, Rechtine G (1989): *Yersinia enterocolitica* causing spinal osteomyelitis and empyema in a nonimmunocompromised host. *South Med J* 82:399–400.

118. Smith AS, Weinstein MA, Mizushima A, Coughlin B, et al. (1989): MR imaging characteristics of tuberculous spondylitis vs vertebral osteomyelitis. *Am J Roentgenol* 153:399–405.

119. Smith NR (1931): The intervertebral discs. *Br J Surg* 18:358–375.

120. Stauffer RN (1975): Pyogenic vertebral osteomyelitis. *Orthop Clin North Am* 6:1015–1027.

121. Steinmetz ND (1987): *MRI of the lumbar spine.* Thorofare, NJ: Slack, pp. 186–201.

122. Stone DB, Bonfiglio M (1963): Pyogenic vertebral osteomyelitis: a diagnostic pitfall for the internist. *Arch Intern Med* 112:491–500.

123. Sullivan CR, Bickel WH, Svien HJ (1958): Infections of vertebral interspaces after operations on intervertebral disks. *JAMA* 166:1973–1977.

124. Tuli SM (1975): Results of treatment of spinal tuberculosis by "middle-path" regime. *J Bone Joint Surg* [Br] 57:13–23.

125. Tuli SM, Srivastava TP, Varma BP, Sinha GP (1967): Tuberculosis of the spine. *Acta Orthop Scand* 38:445–458.

126. Turett GS, Telzak EE, Torian LV, Blum S, Alland D, Weisfuse I, Fazal B (1995): Improved outcomes for patients with multiresistant tuberculosis. *Clin Infect Dis* 21;1238–1244.

127. Turtas S, Viale ES, Pau A (1980): Long-term results of surgery for hydatid disease of the spine. *Surg Neurol* 13:468–470.

128. Van Lom KJ, Kellerhouse LE, Pathria MN, Moreland SI, et al.

(1988): Infection versus tumor in the spine: criteria for distinction with CT. *Radiology* 166:851–855.

129. Vincent KA, Benson DR, Voegeli TL (1988): Factors in the diagnosis of adult pyogenic vertebral osteomyelitis. *Orthop Trans* 12: 523–524.

130. Wenger DR, Bobechko WP, Gilday DL (1978): The spectrum of intervertebral disc-space infection in children. *J Bone Joint Surg* [*Am*] 60:100–108.

131. Wiesseman GJ, Wood VE, Kroll LL (1973): *Pseudomonas* vertebral osteomyelitis in heroin addicts. *J Bone Joint Surg* [*Am*] 55: 1416–1424.

132. Wiley AM, Trueta J (1959): The vascular anatomy of the spine and its relationship to pyogenic vertebral osteomyelitis. *J Bone Joint Surg* [*Br*] 41:796–809.

133. Willis TA (1949): Nutrient arteries of the vertebral bodies. *J Bone Joint Surg* [*Am*] 31:538–540.

134. Winter WG Jr, Larson RK, Honeggar MM, Jacobsen DT, Papagianis D, Huntington RW Jr (1975): Coccidioidal arthritis and its treatment. *J Bone Joint Surg* [*Am*] 57:1152–1157.

135. Wise RI (1980): Brucellosis in the United States. *JAMA* 244: 2318–2322.

136. Woodland LJ (1949): Hydatid disease of vertebrae. *Med J Aust* 2: 904–910.

The Adult Spine: Principles and Practice,
2nd edition, J.W. Frymoyer, Editor-in-Chief.
Lippincott-Raven Publishers, Philadelphia © 1997.

CHAPTER **45**

Infectious Diseases of the Spine

Surgical Treatment

Timothy L. Keenen and Daniel R. Benson

PYOGENIC DISEASE

Indications for Surgery

The general principles for the treatment of pyogenic spine infections are immobilization and antibiotics. Usually after 2 weeks of intravenous antibiotics, the infection has responded, as manifested by a more comfortable patient. Fevers, if present, should have subsided, the sedimentation rate should also have fallen, and the white blood cell count, if elevated before treatment, should also be normal. If this clinical response is not seen after 2 to 3 weeks, consideration should be given to operative debridement. In addition, other situations will require surgical debridement. Presence or progression of neurologic compromise may result from abscesses or vertebral collapse. When an abscess has formed, antibiotics are generally ineffective, and operative drainage is necessary.

Neurological deficits from significant anterior column failure are best treated with anterior debridement, decompression, and stabilization (40). The risk of neurological loss is greater in patients with diabetes, in those with rheumatoid arthritis, and in steroid users (8). The risk also increases as the vertebral level involved moves more cephalad, and as the age increases (8).

In patients with postoperative infections, the same principles of treatment with immobilization and antibiotics are recommended. Surgery is necessary only if these measures fail, or if vertebral collapse or neurological deficit develops. If surgical treatment is required soon after the original operation, the same incision can be used. Since the majority of these infections occur after posterior disc surgery, these patients usually can be debrided from a posterior approach: such patients are the one exception to the usual preferred anterior approach to infections. When significant vertebral collapse has occurred after posterior disc surgery, the anterior approach is definitely preferred.

As the infection becomes more chronic, other complications may require surgery. Draining sinus tracts to skin requires surgical excision, debridement of infected bone, and closure. Vertebral collapse may occur late in the

  T. L. Keenan, M.D.: Associate Professor, Department of Orthopaedics, Oregon Health Sciences University, Portland, Oregon, 97201.
  D. R. Benson, M.D.: Professor of Orthopaedics, University of California, Davis, Sacramento, California, 95817.

course of an infection despite adequate medical treatment, again warranting surgical care.

If possible, the patient should receive intravenous antibiotics for at least 2 weeks prior to debridement procedures. The amount of purulence and surrounding inflammation can be significantly diminished, tissue planes are better defined for surgical dissection, and the patient is less acutely ill and a better anesthetic risk.

General Principles of the Operative Approach

The involved vertebrae are exposed, usually from an anterior approach. Intraoperative radiographs are used to accurately localize the level if there is any question. Often the anterior longitudinal ligament is observed to be swollen, and the incision allows drainage of pus. In other patients, the infection will have destroyed enough anterior structures that the anterior longitudinal ligament is difficult to identify. After complete removal of necrotic tissue and debris, the cavity is irrigated with antibiotic solution. Intraoperative deep wound Gram stains and cultures are obtained but often are negative after antibiotics. At this juncture, a decision is made about further stabilization.

Bone grafts are not placed in the presence of purulence because of the risk of renewed infection. If the antibiotics have been effective, the swelling and purulence are usually minimal and primary bone grafting is possible. Specific surgical approaches are discussed later in the chapter.

TUBERCULOUS DISEASE: SURGICAL MANAGEMENT

Although chemotherapy has become a mainstay in the treatment of Pott's disease, some orthopedic surgeons continue to favor surgical debridement. Hodgson and Stock (19) proposed that the procedure be done as soon as possible after the diagnosis for the following reasons:

1. In the early stages of the disease, extirpation of the infected focus is easier and fusion without deformity is possible.
2. Secondary deformities occur as the disease progresses, impairing the vital organs.
3. The patient's general condition improves markedly after evacuation of the abscess.
4. The patient requires less extended hospitalization and can return to work earlier (i.e., within 4 to 6 months).
5. Late recurrence of the disease is less frequent.
6. Rapid progression of the abscess along the spine is prevented.
7. Surgical exploration of the tuberculous lesion is the only way to assure that the disease is indeed active or healed (19).

Hodgson and associates also confirmed that tuberculosis can penetrate the covering of the spinal cord (dura), causing irreversible paraplegia (18). Therefore, they emphasized an urgent need for surgical drainage to prevent this complication. In the first 100 patients whom they treated by early anterior debridement and fusion of the spine, there were four deaths and complications from inappropriate strut-grafting techniques. The fusion rate was 93%, and 26 of 35 patients with paraplegia recovered complete function. There was a close correlation between the preoperative duration of neurological symptoms and the time required to recover from paraplegia (19). Others have promoted the principles outlined by Hodgson (2,3,24,44). With tuberculosis, bone grafting is sage even in the presence of drainage (1,2).

Whereas anterior decompression and fusion of the spinal column seem effective in the neurologically compromised patient, posterior laminectomy is probably not, and it may lead to neurological deterioration (5). Infectious destruction is usually anterior, causing the involved vertebral body to collapse and angulate into kyphosis. Experience with trauma involving the anterior column supports the importance of anterior decompression. In acute injuries of the thoracic spine with incomplete paralysis, Bohlman and associates noted that 8 of 17 patients who had laminectomy lost neurological function or became completely paraplegic without recovery. On the other hand, no patient treated by anterior debridement and stabilization lost function (5). Another reason for anterior surgery is tissue diagnosis to identify the organism and determine sensitivity.

In tuberculosis and other granulomatous diseases, there is no question as to the superiority of the anterior approach (4,8). In children, Bailey and co-authors (4) noted that anterior tuberculous disease was almost always more widespread than demonstrated on radiographs. Of 100 children in their series, 43 had neural compression. Anterior debridement and fusion resulted in complete recovery in 37 children and partial recovery in the other six. Even late decompression (when symptoms have been present for an extended period) can produce neurological recovery in this disease. Bone graft is readily accepted in both children and adults, and it results in an acceptable fusion rate (2,23,24). Concerns have been expressed about progressive kyphosis in the immature spine, in spite of a solid fusion (13), because posterior growth may create further deformity (23). This issue was specifically addressed in a retrospective review of 33 children (less than age 10 years at operation) compared to 71 adults (greater than age 18 at operation), and no difference in progression of kyphosis could be identified (42). Progression of the kyphosis could be related only to loss of position of the bone graft. In children, combined anterior and posterior arthrodesis is not clearly necessary.

In a long-term, controlled trial comparing radical debridement and anterior fusion, simple debridement, and medical treatment alone, the Medical Research Council (7,11,14,37) showed radical debridement and fusion to be superior in the following ways:

1. Anterior bony fusion occurs earlier and in a higher percentage of patients (70% versus 20% and 26% at 5-year follow-up).
2. Kyphotic angulation was less common at 5 years (37).
3. At 10 years, kyphotic angulation increased in the simple debridement group, whereas it actually decreased in the radical debridement and fusion group (7).

Others have agreed with this philosophy (24,25,28, 36,39,44), although none have had the experience or stated their case so elegantly as the group from Hong Kong (13,19,20,21,23,46,47). Although the surgery is technically very demanding and risky, the alternative seems to be worse. Yau and Hodgson have reported on the penetration of the lung by vertebral abscesses (46) and on irreversible paraplegia from the tuberculous infection passing through the dura and directly involving the spinal cord (21,46).

The bony destruction, collapse, and angulation that can occur under medical treatment (29) are undesirable and preventable. Therefore, if proper facilities and expertise for surgical drainage and grafting of the infected vertebral column are available, surgical fusion is indicated.

Even late cases with severe kyphotic deformity can be candidates for surgery. Yau and associates have reported a series in which spinal osteotomy, halo-pelvic distraction, and anterior and posterior surgery have been used to correct these deformities. Although the complication rate from the use of the halo-pelvic traction and the multiple surgical procedures was high, the average amount of correction was 28.3% in 30 patients and, more important, further progression of the deformity was halted (47).

The major anatomic defect in all of the granulomatous diseases is failure of the anterior column. This is the area that usually needs to be drained or, if weakened by bony destruction, supported by grafting. Posterior procedures are in most cases supplemental to the anterior operation. When Pott's paraplegia exists, the choices of surgery include costotransversectomy, anterolateral decompression, and laminectomy. Arthrodesis of the spine is usually necessary to support the weakened anterior column. If a tense paravertebral abscess is present, the procedure of choice is a costotransversectomy. Strut grafting is difficult through this approach, suggesting that if it is necessary, an anterolateral operation would be better. When a tense abscess does not exist, an anterolateral approach is preferred. The pathology can be better identified and debrided and strut grafting accomplished using this approach. Only if posterior disease (rare) or spinal tumor syndrome (even rarer) exists, is a laminectomy indicated.

When anterior disease exists, posterior surgery further weakens the spinal column and potentially can cause further collapse and neurological deterioration (45). Each of these approaches will be described for the cervical, thoracic, and lumbar spine.

OTHER GRANULOMATOUS DISEASES: SURGICAL MANAGEMENT

The specific granulomatous diseases of the spine and their relative requirements for surgical debridement are discussed more in depth in Chapter 47. In general, less surgery is required for the granulomatous lesions than for pyogenic disease. This may be because the infectious process in granulomatous disease tends to be slower in forming, and collapse tends to be less commonly present at the time of diagnosis. However, the need for operative debridement of fungal and granulomatous infections arises, and the indications for surgical fusion and stabilization are similar to those for pyogenic disease.

SURGICAL PROCEDURES

Needle Biopsy (with Fluoroscopic or CT Guidance)

This technique may be used in the thoracic and lumbar spine, but it is generally too dangerous to attempt in the cervical spine because of surrounding structures (32).

After light sedation and with monitoring available, position the patient prone on the x-ray table or computed tomography (CT) gantry. Sterilely prepare and drape the area, and inject a subcutaneous anesthetic. Usually the anterior structures are the area of interest. If disc involvement is apparent, pass an 18-gauge spinal needle from the posterolateral direction, lateral to the dural sac, into the disc (Chapter 32). The patient may be examined fluoroscopically or scanned between needle adjustments for verification of the position of the needle. When proper placement is confirmed, aspirate the needle with a syringe. A small amount (1 cc) of saline may be injected for re-aspiration if necessary. If only bone appears to be involved and no disc, a pathway lateral to the facets is followed, similar to that of the posterior Craig needle biopsy. If posterior elements are involved, pass the needle directly into the area of infection under guidance of the fluoroscopy or CT scanner.

Drainage of Abscesses

Cervical Spine

In the cervical spine, an abscess may present retropharyngeally, in the posterior triangle of the neck, or in the supraclavicular area. Occasionally the abscess will extend under the prevertebral fascia into the mediastinum. Drainage of a retropharyngeal abscess should only be done in an absolute emergency (e.g., airway obstruction). Usually this can be done through an extraoral approach (30,33) (see Chapters 47 and 51). A 7-cm to 8-cm incision is made along the posterior border of the sternocleidomastoid muscle in the superior portion of the neck. After incising the superficial cervical fascia, look for the spinal accessory nerve, which goes through the sternocleidomastoid muscle and runs across the posterior triangle. Retract the sternocleidomastoid medially, or transversely cut it. Bluntly expose the levator scapulae and splenius muscles and displace the internal jugular vein anteriorly. The abscess should be palpable in front of the transverse processes and bodies of the infected vertebrae. Open and drain the abscess. A tracheostomy set should be available in case respiratory distress occurs during the postoperative recovery period.

The posterior triangle is drained through a similar incision, only slightly more caudal. Identify the scaleni muscles, and protect the phrenic nerve. Develop the plane between the scaleni muscles and the longus colli muscle obliquely into the paravertebral abscess, which is beneath the paravertebral fascia (33).

Thoracic Spine

In the thoracic spine, abscesses are generally drained through a costotransversectomy approach (Chapter 60). Make a midline spinal incision extending over two or three spinous processes. Reflect the muscle and soft tissues away from the spinous processes and the vertebral laminae on the side of the abscess. Widely expose the middle transverse process and resect it at its base. Reflect the periosteum from the contiguous rib, and resect the medial portion of the rib by dividing it 5 cm lateral to the tip of the transverse process. Do not enter the pleural cavity. By bluntly dissecting close to the vertebral body, the abscess can be reached. If necessary, remove more than one transverse process and rib to completely debride the abscess. The neurovascular bundle between the ribs will have to be dissected free, ligated, and sacrificed (6).

Seddon has described a similar approach (35). Make a semicircular incision lateral to the spine starting superior to the kyphotic deformity and ending inferior to it. Elevate the skin flap and muscles medially to expose the medial 8 cm of three or more ribs and their transverse processes. Subperiosteally resect the rib judged to be in the center of the abscess, being careful to stay outside the pleura. Remove the medial rib (at least 7 cm in the adult), freeing the medial end with an elevator. When the rib is teased free, pus should pour out of the gap created.

Explore and debride the abscess cavity. Remove the necrotic material and any sequestered bone, and thoroughly irrigate the cavity.

Lumbar Spine

Abscesses, both granulomatous and pyogenic, may present as externally palpable masses. In the lumbar spine, an abscess generally will follow the course of the psoas muscle, although it can also appear as a paravertebral mass. An abscess that migrates along the psoas is likely to present below Poupart's ligament on the anteromedial surface of the thigh (adductor region) or in the gluteal region. Occasionally an abscess will appear over the crest of the ilium in Petit's triangle.

Paravertebral Abscess

To drain a paravertebral mass, make an incision 4 cm to 8 cm lateral to the vertebral spinal processes in a line that is parallel to the spine. A dull instrument or even finger dissection can be used to bluntly dissect around the erector spinae muscles until the transverse processes of the vertebrae are reached. Usually the abscess is entered immediately. If not, puncture the thoracolumbar fascia that separates the quadratus lumborum muscle from the erector group. By working under the transverse process, the abscess can be located and drained (45).

After abscess drainage, close the tissues in layers, or pack the wounds open (20,24); this applies for all of the drainage procedures described below.

Psoas Abscess

Psoas abscesses are extraperitoneal and can be drained posterolaterally through Petit's triangle or anteriorly beneath Poupart's ligament. The sides of Petit's triangle are formed by the lateral margin of the latissimus dorsi muscle, the medial border of the external oblique abdominal muscle, and the base by the crest of the ilium. On the floor of the triangle is the internal oblique abdominal muscle. Make an incision 2.5 cm above the crest of the ilium in a line parallel with it. The incision should begin lateral to the erector spinae muscle group. Blunt dissection through the internal oblique muscle will provide access to the abscess cavity. The incision can also be made directly over the iliac crest, in which case the internal and external oblique muscles are detached and the inner surface of the ilium exposed. Palpate the abscess extraperitoneally, then open and drain.

Anterior drainage is accomplished by making an incision from the anterosuperior iliac spine and extending it distally and medially for approximately 6 cm. Identify the sartorius muscle and carry the dissection medial to it and to the level of the anteroinferior iliac spine. Protect the femoral nerve, artery, and vein, which lie just medial to this dissection. The abscess is found along the medial surface of the wing of the ilium, under Poupart's ligament (43,45).

A granulomatous psoas abscess can be completely excised through the above approach. This may require extension of the approach in each direction. Manually explore the retroperitoneal space fully. With more exposure, take care to visualize the ureter and ovarian vessels. A ureteral catheter can be placed pre- or intraoperatively to make localization easier. The inguinal ligament can be divided to facilitate exposure of the femoral canal if needed. If the abscess extends to the lesser trochanter or beyond, make a second incision over the femoral triangle to permit safer dissection along the femoral canal. After removing the entire sac of abscessed muscle and fascia, explore the vertebral bodies and remove any diseased bone or disc. If necessary, apply bone graft. For tuberculous abscesses, place antibiotics in the area of debridement. Close the wound over a suction drain and place interrupted absorbable sutures in each layer on the way out. Careful closure is particularly important with tuberculous abscesses, as wound dehiscence is a serious complication that is difficult to treat (41).

If the psoas abscess presents medially in the adductor region of the thigh, drainage can be accomplished through a Ludloff approach. Make a longitudinal incision on the medial aspect of the thigh, starting 2 cm to 3 cm below the pubic tubercle. The incision should be made in the interval between the adductor longus and brevis muscles anteriorly, and the gracilis and adductor magnus muscles posteriorly. Protect the posterior branch of the obturator nerve and the neurovascular bundle to the gracilis. The lesser trochanter (where the psoas muscle attaches) and the floor of the hip joint are located in the base of the wound. The abscess should be easily drained through this incision (45).

Drainage of a pelvic abscess is also possible through a coccygectomy approach. Excise the coccyx through a posterior incision and bluntly dissect up and anterior to the sacrum, where the abscess cavity should be located.

Vertebral Arthrodesis

In addition to evacuating the necrotic debris of the granulomatous infection, many authors have recommended immediate arthrodesis of the spine (1,2,19, 20,24,26). This usually requires a more formal approach than that for simple debridement. When neurologic compromise is present, the spinal cord or cauda equina may have to be decompressed by removing additional

bone or soft tissue. This is usually the result of bony collapse with the development of an acute gibbus.

The removal of diseased tissue is the same in all areas of the spine. Remove the debris, pus, sequestered bone, and disc using curettes and pituitary rongeurs. Some of this material can be removed using a large sucker tip. Remove the tissue across the entire breadth of the vertebral body. Remove diseased bone or areas where graft will be inserted using double-action rongeurs, a drill, or an osteotome. Expose the spinal canal for the entire length of the diseased area, decompressing the neural elements. Granulation tissue, fibrous tissue, or the posterior longitudinal ligament may require sharp incision to expose the dura mater. Remove the disc at each end of the cavity to expose the endplates of the vertebrae above and below. Scrape the cartilage off the endplates, revealing bleeding cancellous bone. Place the strut graft into the endplates, keying the grafts into mortises made with a drill or curette to prevent dislodgement. The strut graft should correct the deformity as much as possible and hold the vertebrae apart. The strut grafts should be strong yet osteogenic in nature; cortical or bicortical iliac crest grafts are ideal, but frequently the area to be grafted is too large for the iliac grafts to be sufficient. Longer struts can be obtained from the fibula or ribs. These should be supplemented with iliac bone, because the fibula is strong but mostly cortical bone (non-osteogenic), whereas the rib is osteogenic but relatively weak and will fail if stressed. The best source of bone is the patient's own ilium, but cadaver bank bone is a good second alternative. In the thoracic and lumbar spine, anterior struts should be supplemented with second-stage posterior instrumentation and fusion. With this technique, the rates of graft dislodgement and failure have decreased.

Decompression Techniques

Capener described a costotransversectomy approach for decompression, which is more complex than the same approach for abscess drainage (6). Make a curved incision starting 10 cm above the lesion in the midline, curving 7.5 cm laterally around it, and then returning to the midline, ending 10 cm below it. Reflect the skin and fascial layers medially as a flap. Reflect the trapezius muscle laterally after removing its origin from the spine, and divide the erector spinae muscles transversely over the rib to be removed. Dissect out the rib leading to the center of the abscess subperiosteally, then resect it from its angle to the transverse process of the vertebra. Separate the intercostal nerve from its accompanying artery and vein and divide it. The proximal end can be used to lead to the spinal cord during later dissection. Remove the medial end of the rib, the vertebral transverse pro-

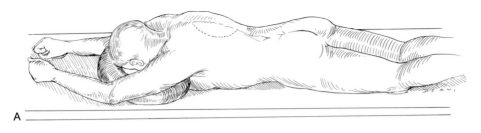

A

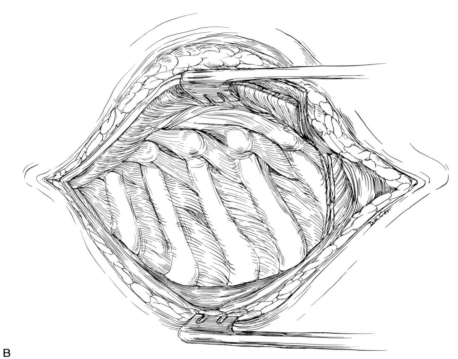

B

FIG. 1. This page. A: The incision for a costotransversectomy as described by Capener (6). With the patient in the prone position, a curved incision is started 10 cm above the lesion, curving 7.5 cm laterally and ending 10 cm below. **B:** The skin and fascial layers are reflected medially as a flap. **Opposite page. C:** A portion of the rib and the transverse process of the vertebra leading to the abscess cavity are removed, exposing the ribs and transverse process of several vertebrae. **D:** Working anterior and lateral to the vertebral body, the lateral surface can be elevated and debrided as well as possible. **E:** Decompression of the canal is possible if the pedicle and posterior surface of the vertebral body are removed. All debris is curetted or suctioned out of the cavity. It is difficult to insert a strut graft using this approach.

cess, and the pedicle using a double-action rongeur or a Kerison punch. Some surgeons prefer to use a motor-driven burr as they approach the dura. This exposes the dura and the posterior aspect of the vertebral body. In the area of disease, remove all tissue that appears to be compressing the vertebral canal (Fig. 1).

Seddon (35) describes a similar approach, except that three or four ribs are removed to provide greater access to the anterior spine. Push the pleura anteriorly and keep it intact, if possible. Follow the exposed neurovascular bundles into the spine, and the nerve into the neurofora-mina. Remove the bone laterally and anteriorly, but not posteriorly. A soft rubber catheter can be pushed along the canal above and below the decompression to assure that the spinal cord is not further affected beyond the debridement.

Anterior Approaches for Debridement and Fusion

Cervical Spine

Upper Cervical Spine

Infections involving C1 and C2 are relatively rare. Should anterior drainage be necessary, use the retropha-ryngeal (33,38) or transoral approach (10).

Anterior Triangle Approach

Most pyogenic infections of the cervical spine can be adequately reached through an anterior triangle approach. It allows excellent visualization of the anterior and lateral surfaces of the cervical vertebral bodies of C3 through C7 (22,27,33).

Place the patient in the supine position with a towel roll posteriorly between the scapulae to allow the shoulders to fall back. Use wide adhesive cloth tape to pull the shoulders caudally and attach the end of the tape to the operating table. This not only allows more room for the surgeon to operate, but it also results in better-quality intraoperative x-rays. Place Gardner-Wells tongs or a halter for cephalad traction. Tilt the head slightly away from the side to be approached. Prepare one of the iliac wings for a bone graft, then cover it with a drape that can be cut open later.

Debate has arisen over the best side from which to approach the cervical spine, because of both the course of the recurrent laryngeal nerve and the surgical ease of approach depending upon handedness of the surgeon. In general, the approach in infections should be chosen based on the side of maximal involvement. This will be determined by patient symptoms and signs, and by radiographic and nuclear studies.

The palpable anatomy of the neck will allow proper placement of the skin incision. The hyoid bone is level with C3, the thyroid cartilage is at C4 to C5, and the cricoid cartilage and carotid tubercle are at C6. Make a transverse incision in line with the skin creases of the neck. This will enable exposure of three bodies and two discs. If exposure of more area is anticipated, the less cosmetic longitudinal incision should be used, placed over the anterior border of the sternocleidomastoid. Split the platysma longitudinally, exposing fascia of sternocleidomastoid. Using finger dissection, pull the sternocleidomastoid laterally. A connecting vein between the anterior jugular vein and common facial vein may require ligation at this point for best exposure. Feel the pulse of the carotid artery and identify the carotid sheath without opening it. The carotid sheath contains the carotid artery medially, the internal jugular vein laterally, and the vagus nerve sandwiched between them. The superior and inferior thyroid arteries cross from lateral to midline structures and may limit proximal and distal exposure; ligate as necessary (Fig. 2).

Palpate the anterior surfaces of the cervical vertebral bodies after retracting the carotid sheath laterally and posteriorly, and the trachea and esophagus medially. Be certain that the esophagus is adequately retracted medially prior to placement of self-retaining Cloward retractors. This will help avoid esophageal perforation. Cut the longus colli muscle longitudinally in the midline and dissect it laterally by lifting subperiosteally beneath the anterior longitudinal ligament. With retraction beneath the longus colli, the recurrent laryngeal nerve is adequately protected. Avoid dissection too far laterally to avoid damage to the cervical sympathetic chain. Identify the level of exposure by placing a spinal needle in a disc space and taking a lateral x-ray.

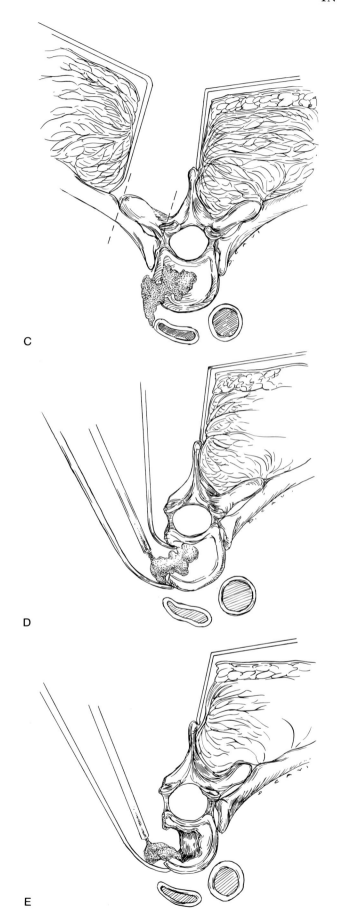

C

D

E

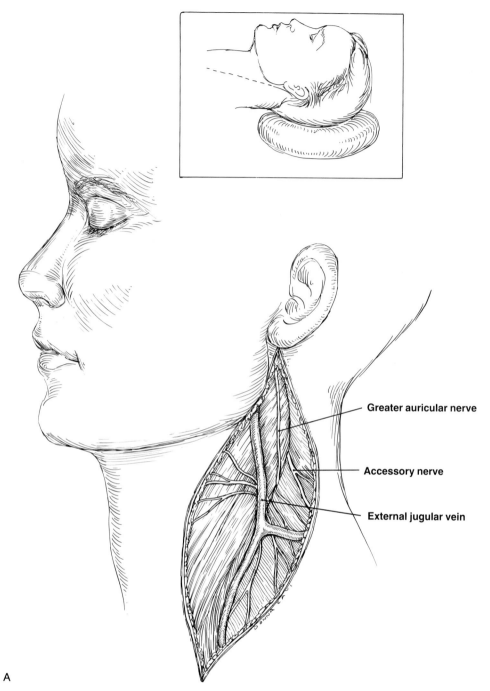

A

FIG. 2. A: For an anterior approach to the posterior triangle of C3 through C7, the patient is placed supine with a sandbag between the shoulders and the head turned away from the side to be operated. The incision can be made lateral to the collar line or along the posterior margin of the sternocleidomastoid muscle. After the skin, superficial fascia, and platysma are incised, the external jugular vein is located and ligated. The spinal accessory nerve, which goes through the sternocleidomastoid muscle and runs through the posterior triangle, must be protected. (Fig. 2,B–E follow.)

Greater auricular nerve

Accessory nerve

External jugular vein

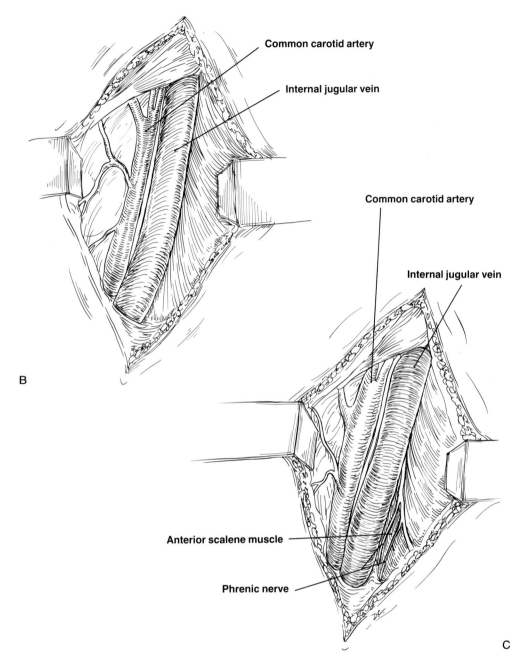

FIG. 2. (*Continued.*) **B:** The sternocleidomastoid muscle is retracted or cut transversely. **C:** The levator scapulae muscles are bluntly exposed and the internal jugular vein is displaced anteriorly. The anterior scalene will lie between the phrenic nerve and the anterolateral portion of the vertebral bodies. (Fig. 2,D–E follow.)

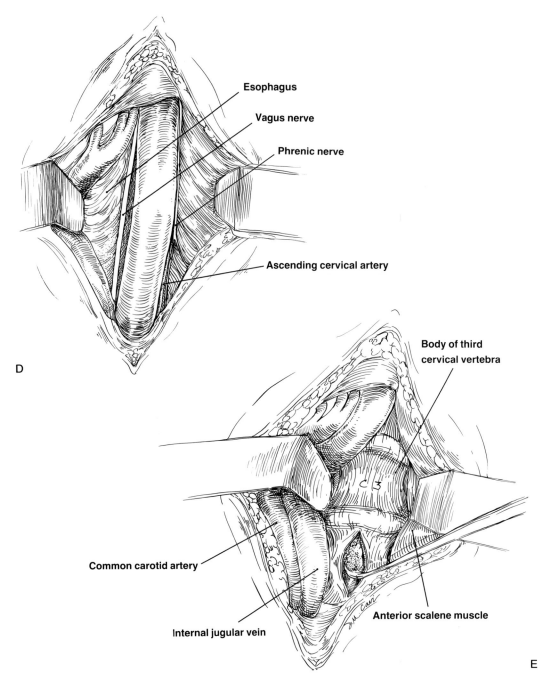

Esophagus

Vagus nerve

Phrenic nerve

Ascending cervical artery

D

Body of third cervical vertebra

Common carotid artery

Anterior scalene muscle

Internal jugular vein

E

FIG. 2. (*Continued.*) **D:** The vagus nerve will lie anteriorly along the posterior portion of the esophagus. **E:** The anterior scalene muscle is retracted posteriorly, protecting the phrenic nerve behind it. The abscess will be palpable in front of the transverse process over the bodies of the infected vertebrae. The fascia is opened and the abscess drained or debrided. Bone graft can be inserted to act as a strut for spinal fusion. A tracheostomy set should be available in case respiratory distress occurs in the postoperative period.

Clear the involved disc spaces and bone of granulation tissue and debris using curettes and pituitary rongeurs. Any necrotic bone should be removed to the posterior longitudinal ligament. If purulence is present, do not place bone graft acutely, but rather complete with a delayed procedure when the infection is better controlled. If no purulence is present, the ideal choice is a tricortical iliac crest bone graft. Approach the bone graft with a different sterile set of gown, gloves, and instruments, and by cutting through the prepared drape. After iliac wound closure and sterile covering, shape the graft to be keyed in to the defect created in the anterior spine. Spread the vertebrae with a lamina spreader, then gently impact the bone graft into place. Once in place, the lamina spreader and cervical traction can be released. Close the layer of platysma, and then the skin with a subcuticular stitch. Postoperatively, maintain the patient in a hard collar, four-poster brace, or halo vest, depending on the confidence in structural stability.

Posterior Triangle Approach

Infections, particularly abscesses, may present in the retropharyngeal posterior triangle of the neck. The tuberculous infection is most common in this area, although pyogenic infections may also present. In these cases, the posterior triangle approach will give best exposure for drainage, debridement, and bone grafting. The approach allows access to C3 through C7.

Place the patient in a supine position with a towel roll between the shoulders, and turn the head away from the side to be operated on (preferably the right side to avoid the thoracic duct). Make an incision parallel to the collar line, centering over the lesion to be drained. The incision should extend from the midline to the anterior border of the trapezius. The cricoid cartilage overlying the sixth cervical vertebra is a convenient surface landmark.

Cut through the skin, superficial fascia, and platysma. Ligate and divide the external jugular vein. Cut the sternocleidomastoid muscle in its distal third and retract the carotid sheath forward. Bluntly dissect the fat pad beneath this sheath to expose the prevertebral fascia that covers the cervical vertebral bodies. Try to leave intact the sympathetic chain, which runs laterally along the vertebral bodies. If seen, ligate and cut the artery to the sternocleidomastoid muscle. When the vertebral bodies are exposed, palpate them to locate the infected ones (20,24). Needle aspiration can be used to confirm the presence of pus. A lateral radiograph with the needle in place confirms the precise location.

Thoracic Spine

Right Thoracotomy C7 to T4

The standard approach to the upper thoracic spine is a right thoracotomy through the third rib bed. (If significant kyphosis is present, a costotransversectomy might be better.) Place the patient in a left lateral position with the right shoulder flexed to 120° and placed on an arm rest. Stand on the spinal side of the patient, tilting the table toward you to afford better visualization. Make a curved incision around the medial and inferior aspects of the scapula. After division of the parascapular muscles, retract the scapula forward and upward. Excise the third rib and enter the pleural cavity through its bed. To improve visualization, cut the insertion of the scalenus posterior muscle and remove the second rib. The level is decided by following the rib head into the vertebral body. The third rib head articulates with the junction between the second and third thoracic vertebral bodies (20).

If more cervical vertebrae are involved, a sternum-splitting operation may be indicated. The procedure is an extension of the exposure for the cervicothoracic junction. Extend the incision in the midline down the sternum to the xiphoid process. Clear the anterior mediastinal tissues by blunt dissection behind the manubrium, working distally from the suprasternal notch. Work proximally from the xiphoid process in the same manner. Divide the sternum with an oscillating saw and retract the two halves laterally. Using this approach, the vessels and midline structures can be retracted more widely. Mobilize the recurrent laryngeal nerve so that it will lie obliquely across the operative field. Protect it during the procedure with a moist sponge to prevent paralysis to the vocal cords.

Identify the vertebral artery behind the carotid sheath. It will pass upward and lateral to enter the foramen in the sixth cervical vertebra. It is best to approach the spine from the right because the innominate artery on that side takes off from the aorta at a lower level than the left subclavian vessels. In addition, the left innominate vein runs obliquely and distally to join the right innominate vein. The thoracic duct is also avoided. Anterior access to the distal cervical and proximal thoracic vertebrae is fairly good when the vessels are retracted.

After the vertebral work is complete, insert a suction drain and close the sternum with stainless steel wire or staples. If the pleura was opened, the chest should be drained with a large chest tube to underwater suction for at least 48 hours (24).

Approach to the Lower Thoracic Spine

The chest can be opened from either the left or the right side. In early disease, without kyphosis, the right side is best because fewer important structures are present. In more severe or chronic disease, when kyphosis is present, the left side is preferable because the vena cava or aorta can become incorporated in the infection. The side of the largest involvement or lung penetration may also determine the side of approach. Use a beanbag, which can be fixed in position by suction to hold the patient in a lateral decubitus position. The table should be flexed at the level of the lesion to facilitate exposure. Make an incision along the rib to be exposed. Additional ribs can be removed for better exposure. Divide muscle layers in line with the incision and resect the rib subperiosteally. Enter the pleural cavity and divide the adhesions (if present), freeing the lung as completely as possible (22) (Fig. 3).

In the case of tuberculous infections, thick adhesions between the lung and the abscess are often present. In this case, lung penetration is suggested. The lung abscess can then be opened and the caseous material removed (20). Close the cavity with absorbable suture.

When the parietal pleura covering the abscess is exposed, mobilize the aorta so an interval is developed between the two. Ligate and cut the segmental intercostal vessels traversing this segment. If a severe kyphosis exists, the aorta will be acutely angulated and the segmental vessels bunched together at the apex of the curve. After the aorta is mobilized and protected, open the abscess with a T-shaped incision. The transverse portion of the T-cut is made on the anterior portion of the vertebral body parallel to the aorta. Retract the triangular flaps created by the T-incision and attach them by stay sutures to the muscles at the wound edges.

Work from proximal and distal to the midportion of kyphosis, particularly if cord compression is present. Radically excise all bony sequestra, sequestered disc, granulation tissue, and avascular bone. The posterior longitudinal ligament forms the posterior limit of the abscess cavity and is just anterior to the spinal cord. Carefully incise the ligament and remove it with pituitary rongeurs. Allow the dura to slide or prolapse forward into the area vacated by the debridement. Debride the bone until bleeding cancellous bone surfaces are exposed. Cut or drill slots into the exposed cancellous bone. Posterior pressure on the kyphosis will open up the interval so it can be measured using a caliper. Place several ribs or an iliac bicortical graft into the slots and gently impact the graft into place. Release the posterior pressure on the spine and the grafts will be firmly held in compression. It is wise to supplement the impacted bone with additional struts, although these will not be under compression. Usually five to six ribs or two bicortical iliac crest grafts can be fitted into the thoracic spine (20,24).

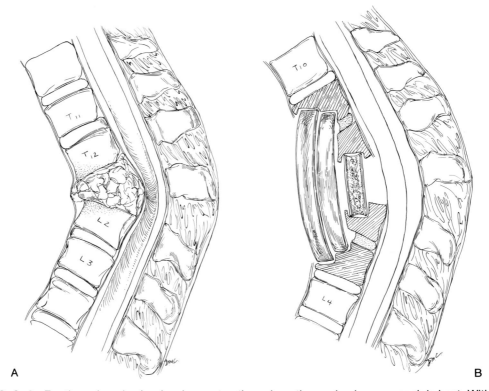

A   B

FIG. 3. A: For thoracic or lumbar involvement, a thoracic or thoracolumbar approach is best. With the patient in a lateral decubitus position, an incision over the rib just superior to the apex of the kyphos is made. The rib can be removed for use as a strut graft. The tuberculous debris, devascularized disc, and avascular vertebral body are removed by curettement or use of a power burr. B: If the cord is compressed, it is completely exposed anteriorly to remove any pressure. From good vertebrae to good vertebrae, strut grafts of bicortical ilium and rib or fibula are used to bridge the angular kyphosis. Sometimes correction of the kyphosis can be obtained during the grafting procedure. This anterior fusion may need anterior fusion with or without instrumentation to stabilize the spine to keep anterior strut grafts from displacing.

Complete closure of the abscess cavity flaps is not necessary.

Lumbar Spine

Retroperitoneal (Anterolateral) Approach

This approach allows access to L1 through S1. The approach is more difficult than midline transperitoneal incisions to reach the lumbosacral junction, but it offers the advantage of not contaminating the peritoneum with material drained from the infection (15,17,22,31,34,38).

Position the patient obliquely at 45° with the involved side up (left, if there is no preference), and hold the position with a beanbag. Make an oblique incision from the inferior border of the lowest rib, curving gently as the incision meets the lateral border of the rectus abdominis muscle. Divide the layers of the external oblique, internal oblique, and transversus abdominis along the line of the incision. The retroperitoneal fat can then be dissected away from the enveloping fascia of the psoas muscle using finger dissection. At this point, take care to identify the ureter, which can be retracted with the retroperitoneal fat anteromedially. If involvement of this plane of tissue with severe inflammation is anticipated, place a ureteral stent either pre- or intraoperatively to easily identify the ureter and avoid damaging it. The genitofemoral nerve lies on the anterior surface of the psoas muscle and should be protected. When a psoas abscess is present, open it longitudinally and follow the tract to the involved vertebral bodies. If a psoas abscess is not present, dissect medially over the anterior surface of the psoas muscle to localize the anterolateral border of the vertebrae. A segmental blood supply comes directly to each vertebra from the aorta and returns through the segmental veins to the vena cava. To mobilize the aorta and the vena cava as needed, each segmental vessel must be ligated. The vessels can then be retracted away from the anterior surfaces of the vertebral bodies. Now, using a sponge, the remaining soft tissue can be dissected away from the anterior longitudinal ligament. Take care to identify and retract (posterolaterally) the sympathetic chain as it runs along the lateral surface of the vertebral body just medial to the border of the psoas muscle. Window the anterior longitudinal ligament and enter the involved disc space. Confirm the proper level with a radiograph.

Debridement is completed with curettes and rongeurs. If debris is retropulsed posteriorly, clear out the area carefully until dura are exposed. If the area is clear of purulence, bone graft is then fashioned to strut the involved vertebrae. Our preference is generally two iliac crest tricortical pieces, although rib will be acceptable if stout enough. Fibula may also be used. Close each muscle layer separately with absorbable suture.

Results of treatment of pyogenic infections with anterior debridement and fusion with strut grafting are generally good (Fig. 4). A high rate of fusion and reduction of pain are seen. The recurrence rate of the infection is low and progressive kyphosis is prevented (9,36,40,41).

Posterior Procedures Combined with Anterior Debridement

If debridement has required the use of a strut graft, a second-stage posterior procedure is commonly planned. This is done to provide immediate stability, to support the strut anteriorly, and to prevent later collapse and angulation (12). In the cervical spine, this is a posterior wiring technique, whereas in the thoracolumbar spine, distraction instrumentation is most often used. In both cases, the instrumentation is combined with a posterolateral spinal fusion. In the cervical spine, the levels of the instrumentation extend from the first normal vertebra superiorly to the first normal vertebra inferiorly. In the thoracolumbar spine, it is important to include vertebrae at least two levels above and below the resected vertebral bodies (Figs. 5,6).

After the patient begins to recover, external immobilization is planned. A halo vest is used to control motion in the cervical spine, or a polypropylene fitted jacket does the same for the thoracolumbar area. External immobilization is continued for 3 months in the cervical spine and 6 months in the thoracolumbar spine. The patient may get out of bed as soon as the external immobilization device is applied and, if not paraplegic, may ambulate as early as tolerated.

Fusion is evaluated using radiographs and tomograms to confirm graft incorporation. The vertebral column is also monitored for any angulation or vertebral collapse during the later stages of recovery. Good nutrition and antibiotics complete the treatment program.

Complications of Anterior Procedures

Intraoperative Complications

The lungs can be penetrated during the operative procedure. This is usually of no special concern and can be ignored unless there is a significant air leak. This will generally scar and seal in time.

The dura can be opened accidentally during the decompression. Closure should be attempted; if unsuccessful, this error may result in a cerebrospinal fluid fistula. These eventually heal, but may persist for up to 3 or 4 months.

Injury to the sympathetic nerves in the cervical region will produce a Horner's syndrome, which usually is only temporary. In the lumbar area, the extremity of the operated side will be warmer. This too will usually resolve with time.

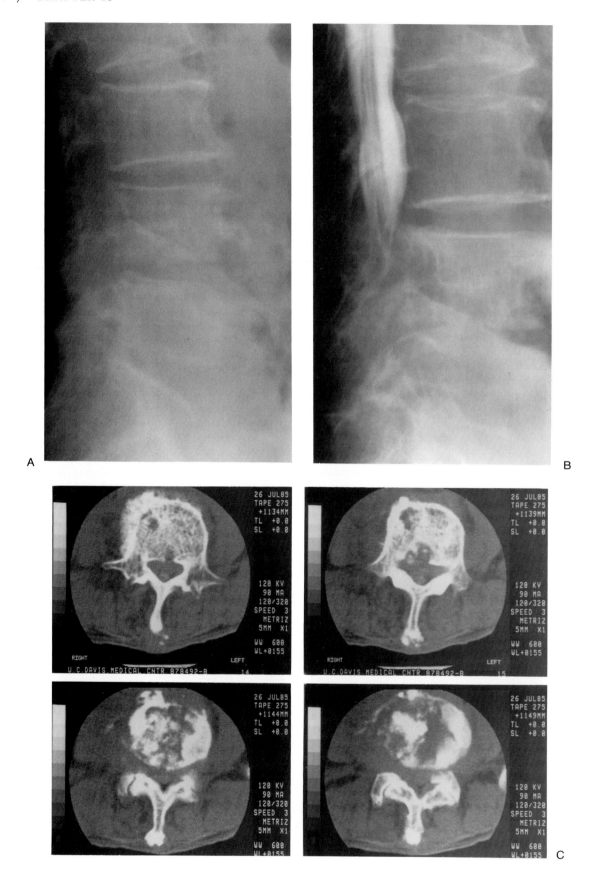

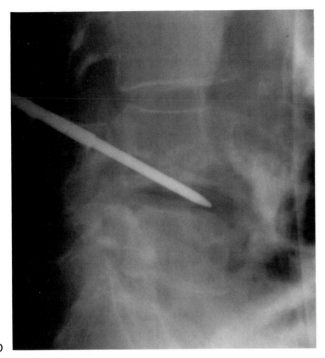
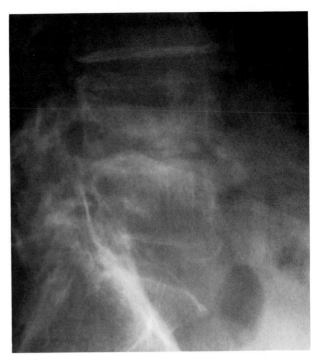

D

E

FIG. 4. A 72-year-old man presented with a 5-month history of low back pain and radicular radiation after bending down while gardening. Purified protein derivative (PPD) test was positive for 10 mm of induration. Cultures from his biopsy grew *Mycobacterium tuberculosis. Opposite page, top.* **A:** Lateral radiograph at presentation shows the lytic destruction of the vertebral bodies at L4 and L5. **B:** Myelogram, with canal compromise at the infected level. *Opposite page, bottom.* **C:** CT scan of L4-L5. Appearance of irregular cavitation is typical of tuberculosis. *This page.* **D:** Craig needle biopsy technique, as seen on intraoperative lateral radiograph. **E:** Anterior debridement and fusion followed by posterolateral fusion were done, as seen on the lateral radiograph 6 months postoperatively.

In cases where there is excessive retroperitoneal scarring, the ureter can be cut accidentally. If so, this must be recognized and reanastomosis performed. If preoperatively it is suspected that the ureter might be involved in the abscess, a stent can be placed onto the ureter on the side being operated on. This will make the ureter easier to palpate and therefore less likely to be cut. A stent with a fiberoptic light can even allow the ureter to be visualized among the debris and bleeding as the abscess is incised and cleaned out.

Occasionally the vena cava or aorta is cut or torn during mobilization of the great vessels. This is most likely at the lumbosacral junction, where the main structure preventing access and mobilization of the common iliac vessels is the iliolumbar vein. This vessel should be located before it is torn, and if it cannot be safely moved, it should be ligated and cut. If the vena cava or aorta is injured, vascular repair should be done. Usually a stitch or two will control the problem, but occasionally a friable vena cava will be impossible to repair and will need to be ligated.

Early Postoperative Complications

After anterior or even posterior spinal surgery in the thoracolumbar or lumbar area, a paralytic ileus is almost inevitable. The patient should not be fed until bowel sounds are present and active and the patient reports having noticed some flatus. Even fluids, if given too early, can aggravate the ileus and prolong final recovery.

Chest complications are also common, particularly after a thoracotomy. The most likely is atelectasis, which will respond to deep breathing, coughing, and use of the inspirometer. However, if left untreated, this can develop into pneumonia. If a chest tube is improperly placed or if it becomes blocked, pleural effusion or hemothorax can occur with lung collapse and subsequent pneumonia.

The most catastrophic complication is deterioration of the neurological status after anterior decompression. This probably is the result of excessive trauma to already jeopardized spinal cord. This is particularly true in cases where the paraparesis is of long duration and the surgical approach is difficult. This is likely to resolve, because the spinal cord in Pott's paraplegia is resilient and can stand a great deal of trauma without permanent damage. On the other hand, if worsening of the paraplegia is caused by spasm of the anterior spinal artery, then the prognosis for recovery is bleak. There is no good way to know which is the case, and treatment for either condition is not very effective. If the former is suspected, dexamethasone (Decadron) may be used to decrease the edema in

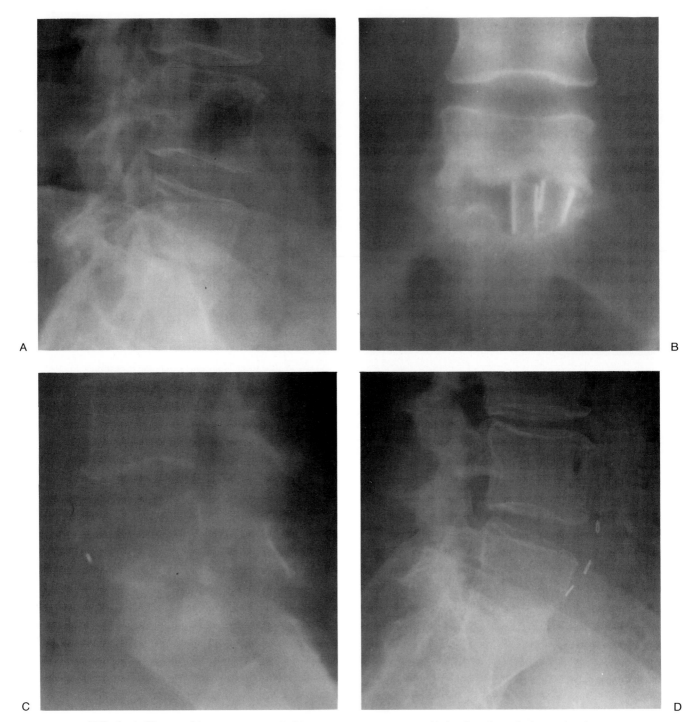

FIG. 5. A 49-year-old woman presented to an emergency room with back pain radiating to her lower abdomen after a chiropractic manipulation. She was treated initially for an *Escherichia coli* urinary tract infection, which resolved. However, 15 weeks later her back pain persisted. Lateral radiograph (**A**) shows disc height loss and endplate destruction. She was treated with anterior debridement and iliac tricortical strut grafting, as shown here on anteroposterior (**B**) and lateral (**C**) tomograms. Cultures grew *E. coli*. Long-term follow–up lateral radiograph (**D**) shows a solid fusion mass.

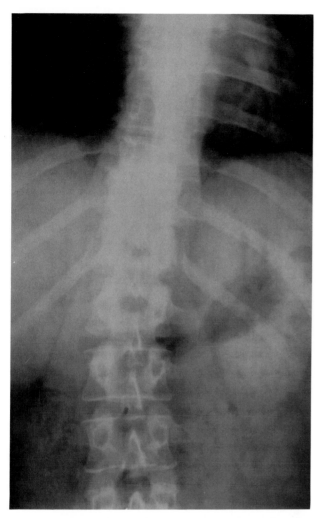
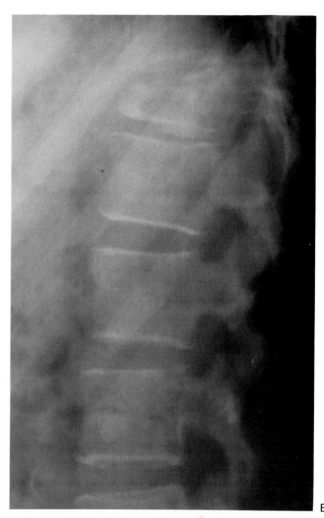

A   B

FIG. 6. These anteroposterior (**A**) and lateral (**B**) radiographs are of a 30-year-old baker who had back pain after stepping into a hole. He had an erythrocyte sedimentation rate of 1,200 mm/hour, a PPD which had 10 mm of induration, and a negative coccidioidomycosis titer. Note the loss of vertebral height and endplate destruction seen well on the lateral view. (Fig. 6,C–J follow.)

the area surrounding the exposed cord. The strut-grafted area should be radiographed or studied with a CT scan to assure that one of the grafts has not slipped posteriorly into the spinal cord. If this is suspected, the patient should be re-operated and the graft re-inserted into a firm bony bed so it will not impinge on the cord. Hematoma or abscess is unlikely to be causing compression, because the majority of the latter has been removed and the area around the debridement is not capable of containing the former.

Late Complications

If the inserted grafts become reabsorbed, it usually means that the infection is not being controlled by the antibiotics. This is usually evident 6 to 12 weeks after surgery, and culture and sensitivity reports will help in the modification of drug therapy. Usually the grafts do not have to be replaced, but if destruction is severe, re-operation should be considered.

Long grafts, particularly if cortical bone such as fibula is used, are subject to late fracture. These will occur 12 to 18 months after surgery when the bone is weakened by its resorption and replacement by new bone. These are like stress fractures and will heal with immobilization and rest. Fracture of the graft is best recognized using tomography in the sagittal (lateral) plane.

In some patients (7% to 8%), the spinal fusion will fail. If this is thought to be secondary to persistent, recurrent infection, it must be dealt with medically. When further spinal collapse and increase in the kyphosis occur, restabilization of the vertebral column is required. If the disease is judged to be quiescent, the kyphotic angle is stable, and the patient is asymptomatic, a non-union can be ignored. If symptoms do occur, an adjunct posterolateral fusion can be done.

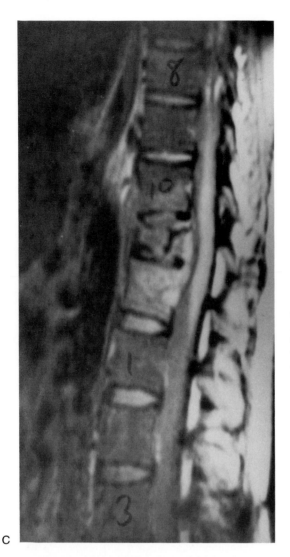

C

FIG. 6. (*Continued.*) Magnetic resonance imaging scan (T2-weighted) (**C**) demonstrates the amount of vertebral destruction and compression of the spinal cord. Because of the amount of vertebral body involvement, it was elected to debride and strut graft this lesion anteriorly and to fuse and stabilize the spine with instrumentation posteriorly. An anterolateral thoracic approach through the 10th rib was used to expose the 11th thoracic vertebra. This photograph (**D**) shows the abscess over the vertebral body expanding the parietal pleura. The aorta lies just anterior to the spinal column. (Fig. 6, E–J follow.)

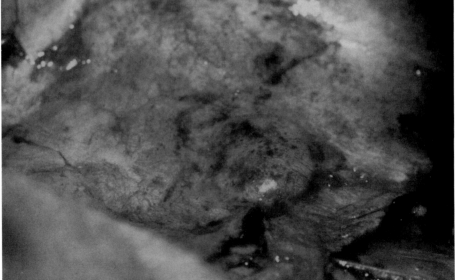

D

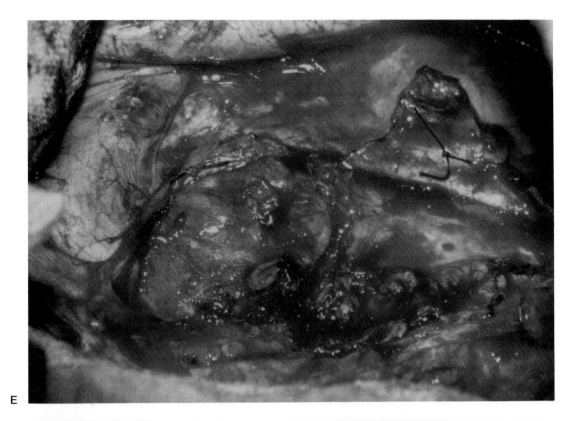

E

F

FIG. 6. *(Continued.)* A T-incision (**E**) is made along the lateral border of the spine to drain the abscess. Flaps of the T are elevated and anchored with stitches for later closure. Necrotic bone and debris are removed (**F**) by curettement or drilling using a high-speed burr. The involved bone, disc, and debris are removed until bleeding bone is located on each end of the lesion. If decompression of the spinal cord or cauda equina is needed, it is done at this time. (Fig. 6,G–J follow.)

FIG. 6. (*Continued.*) Bicortical bone can be removed from the ilium (**G**). This should be done using a separate draping and surgical set-up so as not to contaminate the graft site. The graft is measured before cutting to assure an adequate length to strut the defect. The strut is impacted into the defect created by the debridement (**H**), and the table, which had been previously flexed to provide access to the chest, is straightened, "locking" the graft into place. If an acute kyphosis is present, additional strut grafts may be needed to bridge the kyphosis completely. These are placed more anteriorly, and also they should be implanted into the bony portion of the vertebra. (Fig. 6, I–J follow.)

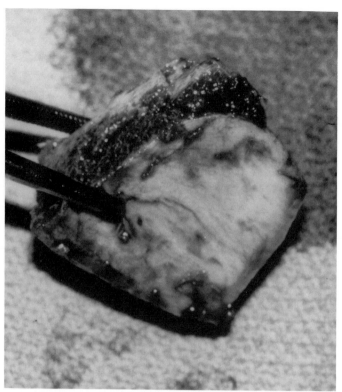

G

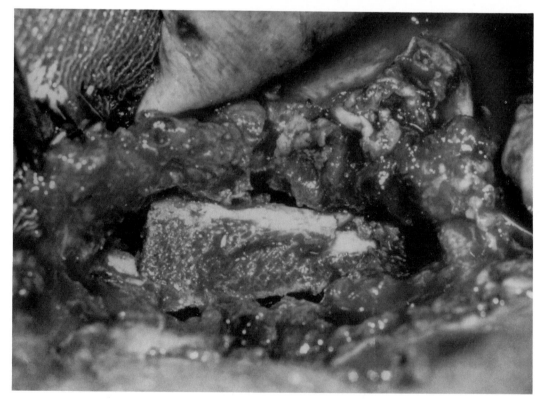

H

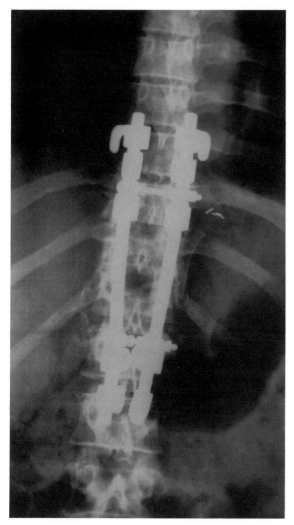
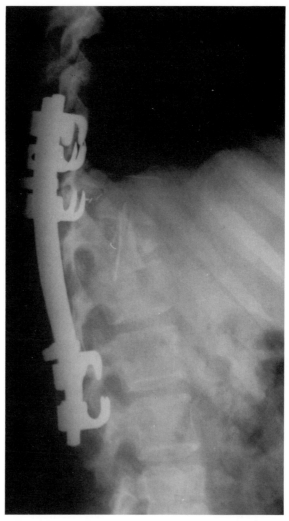

I   J

FIG. 6. (*Continued.*) Postoperative anteroposterior (**I**) and lateral (**J**) radiographs show that the iliac strut graft spans the infected level extending into the vertebrae above and below. Cotrel-Dubousset instrumentation extends an additional level above and below the 11th thoracic vertebra. A posterior fusion supplements this instrumentation. The patient was ambulatory, taking tuberculous medication, when he left the hospital 2 weeks after the second surgery. He will continue his medication for 1 year after surgery.

REFERENCES

1. Allen AR, Stevenson, AW (1957): The results of combined drug therapy and early fusion in bone tuberculosis. *J Bone Joint Surg* [*Am*] 39:32–42.
2. Allen AR, Stevenson, AW (1967): A ten-year follow-up of combined drug therapy and early fusion in bone tuberculosis. *J Bone Joint Surg* [*Am*] 49:1001–1003.
3. Arct W (1968): Operative treatment of tuberculosis of the spine in old people. *J Bone Joint Surg* [*Am*] 50:255–267.
4. Bailey HL, Gabriel M, Hodgson AR, Shin JS (1972): Tuberculosis of the spine in children. *J Bone Joint Surg* [*Am*] 54:1633–1657.
5. Bohlman HH, Freehafer A, Dejak J (1985): The results of treatment of acute injuries of the upper thoracic spine with paralysis. *J Bone Joint Surg* [*Am*] 67:360–369.
6. Capener N (1954): The evolution of lateral rhachotomy. *J Bone Joint Surg* [*Br*] 36:173–179.
7. Eighth report of the Medical Research Council (1982): A 10-year assessment of tuberculosis of the spine in patients in standard chemotherapy in Hong Kong. *J Bone Joint Surg* [*Br*] 64:393–398.
8. Eismont FJ, Bohlman HH, Soni PL, Goldberg VM, Freehafer AA (1983): Pyogenic and fungal vertebral osteomyelitis with paralysis. *J Bone Joint Surg* [*Am*] 65:19–29.
9. Emery SE, Chan DP, Woodward HR (1989): Treatment of hematogenous pyogenic vertebral osteomyelitis with anterior debridement and primary bone grafting. *Spine* 14:284–291.
10. Fang HS, Ong GB (1962): Direct anterior approach to the upper cervical spine. *J Bone Joint Surg* [*Am*] 44:1588–1604.
11. First report of the Medical Research Council Working Party on Tuberculosis of the Spine (1973): A controlled trial of ambulant out-patient treatment and in-patient rest in bed in the management of tuberculosis of the spine in young Korean patients on standard chemotherapy. A study in Masan, Korea. *J Bone Joint Surg* [*Br*] 55:678–697.
12. Fountain SS (1979): A single-stage combined surgical approach for vertebral resections. *J Bone Joint Surg* [*Am*] 61:1011–1017.
13. Fountain SS, Hsu LC, Yau AC, Hodgson AR (1975): Progressive kyphosis following solid anterior spine fusion in children with tuberculosis of the spine. *J Bone Joint Surg* [*Am*] 57:1104–1107.
14. Fourth report of the Medical Research Council Working Party on Tuberculosis of the Spine (1974): A controlled trial of anterior spi-

nal fusion and debridement in the surgical management of tuberculosis of the spine in patients on standard chemotherapy: a study in Hong Kong. *Br J Surg* 61:853–866.

15. Freebody D, Bendall R, Taylor RD (1971): Anterior transperitoneal lumbar fusion. *J Bone Joint Surg* [*Br*] 53:617–627.

16. Guri JP (1946): Pyogenic osteomyelitis of the spine. *J Bone Joint Surg* 28:29–39.

17. Hall JE (1972): The anterior approach to spinal deformities. *Orthop Clin North Am* 3:81–98.

18. Hodgson AR, Skinsnes OK, Leong CY (1967): The pathogenesis of Pott's paraplegia. *J Bone Joint Surg* [*Am*] 49:1147–1156.

19. Hodgson AR, Stock FE (1960): Anterior spine fusion for the treatment of tuberculosis of the spine. *J Bone Joint Surg* [*Am*] 42:295–310.

20. Hodgson AR, Stock FE, Fang HS, Ong GB (1960): Anterior spinal fusion: the operative approach and pathological findings in 412 patients with Pott's disease of the spine. *Br J Surg* 48:172–178.

21. Hodgson AR, Yau A, Kwon JS, Kim D (1964): A clinical study of 100 consecutive cases of Pott's paraplegia. *Clin Orthop* 36:128–150.

22. Hoppenfeld S, deBoer P (1985): *Surgical exposures in orthopaedics.* Philadelphia: Lippincott, pp. 232–280.

23. Jenkins DH, Hodgson AR, Yau AC, Dwyer AP, O'Mahoney G (1975): Stabilization of the spine in the surgical treatment of severe spinal tuberculosis in children. *Clin Orthop* 110:69–80.

24. Kemp HB, Jackson JW, Jeremiah JD, Cook J (1973): Anterior fusion of the spine for infective lesions in adults. *J Bone Joint Surg* [*Br*] 55:715–734.

25. Kirkaldy-Willis WH, Thomas TG (1965): Anterior approaches in the diagnosis and treatment of infections of the vertebral bodies. *J Bone Joint Surg* [*Am*] 47:87–110.

26. Kohli SB (1967): Radical surgical approach to spinal tuberculosis. *J Bone Joint Surg* [*Br*] 49:668–673.

27. Komisar A, Tabaddor K (1983): Extrapharyngeal (anterolateral) approach to the cervical spine. *Head Neck Surg* 6:600–604.

28. Kondo E, Yamada K (1957): End results of focal debridement in bone and joint tuberculosis and its indications. *J Bone Joint Surg* [*Am*] 39:27–31.

29. Konstam PG, Blesovsky A (1962): The ambulant treatment of spinal tuberculosis. *Br J Surg* 50:26–38.

30. McAfee PC, Bohlman HH, Riley LH, Robinson RA, et al. (1987): The anterior retropharyngeal approach to the upper part of the cervical spine. *J Bone Joint Surg* [*Am*] 69:1371–1383.

31. Mirbaha MM (1973): Anterior approach to the thoraco-lumbar junction of the spine by a retroperitoneal-extrapleural technic. *Clin Orthop* 91:41–47.

32. Ottolenghi CE (1969): Aspiration biopsy of the spine. *J Bone Joint Surg* [*Am*] 51:1531–1544.

33. Riley LH Jr (1973): Surgical approaches to the anterior structures of the cervical spine. *Clin Orthop* 91:16–20.

34. Riseborough EJ (1973): The anterior approach to the spine for the correction of deformities of the axial skeleton. *Clin Orthop* 93:207–214.

35. Seddon HJ (1953): Pott's paraplegia and its operative treatment. *J Bone Joint Surg* [*Br*] 35:487.

36. Shaw NE, Thomas TG (1963): Surgical treatment of chronic infective lesions of the spine. *Br Med J* 1(5324):162–164.

37. Sixth report of the Medical Research Council Working Party on Tuberculosis of the Spine (1978): Five-year assessments of controlled trials of ambulatory treatment, debridement and anterior spinal fusion in the management of tuberculosis of the spine: studies in Bulawayo (Rhodesia) and Hong Kong. *J Bone Joint Surg* [*Br*] 60:163–177.

38. Southwick WO, Robinson RA (1957): Surgical approaches to the vertebral bodies in the cervical and lumbar regions. *J Bone Joint Surg* [*Am*] 39:631–644.

39. Stern WE, Balch RE (1966): Surgical aspects of nonspecific inflammatory and suppurative disease of the vertebral column. *Am J Surg* 112:314–325.

40. Stone JL, Cybulski GR, Rodriguez J, Gryfinski ME, Kant R (1989): Anterior cervical debridement and strut-grafting for osteomyelitis of the cervical spine. *J Neurosurg* 70:879–883.

41. Tikhodeev SA (1988): [Results of the surgical treatment of patients with hematogenic osteomyelitis of the spine]. *Vestnik Khirurgii Imeni II Grekova* 140:42–46.

42. Upadhyay SS, Saji MJ, Sell P, Yau ACMC (1994): The effect of age on the change in deformity after radical resection and anterior arthrodesis for tuberculosis of the spine. *J Bone Joint Surg* 76A(5): 701–708.

43. Weinberg JA (1957): The surgical excision of the psoas abscesses resulting from spinal tuberculosis. *J Bone Joint Surg* [*Am*] 39:17–27.

44. Wiltberger BR (1952): Resection of vertebral bodies and bone-grafting for chronic osteomyelitis of the spine. *J Bone Joint Surg* [*Am*] 34:215–218.

45. Wood GW (1987): Infections of the spine. In: *Campbell's operative orthopaedics,* 7th ed. Crenshaw AH, ed. St. Louis: Mosby, pp. 3323–3345.

46. Yau AC, Hodgson AR (1968): Penetration of the lung by the paravertebral abscess in tuberculosis of the spine. *J Bone Joint Surg* [*Am*] 50:243–254.

47. Yau AC, Hsu LC, O'Brien JP, Hodgson AR (1974): Tuberculous kyphosis: correction with spinal osteotomy, halo-pelvic distraction, and anterior and posterior fusion. *J Bone Joint Surg* [*Am*] 56: 1419–1434.

Spinal Injury

The Adult Spine: Principles and Practice,
2nd edition, J.W. Frymoyer, Editor-in-Chief.
Lippincott-Raven Publishers, Philadelphia © 1997.

CHAPTER 46

Penetrating Injuries of the Spinal Cord: Stab and Gunshot Injuries

Robert L. Waters, Rodney H. Adkins, Serena S. Hu, Joy S. Yakura, and Ien H. Sie

EPIDEMIOLOGY

Penetrating injury is a major cause of spinal cord injury (SCI) among the United States civilian population, as well as in the military during armed conflict. Of 6,014 cases reported to the National Spinal Cord Injury Data Research Center by the various Regional SCI Systems between 1973 and 1981, approximately 14% were caused by penetrating injuries and 13% were the result of gunshot (69). In this series, gunshot injuries were the third leading cause of SCI after automobile accidents (38% of injuries) and falls (16%). All other penetrating injuries, predominantly stab wounds, accounted for less than 1% of the injuries.

The incidence of spinal cord injury resulting from penetrating injuries is higher in urban areas. In a prospective series conducted in Los Angeles on 148 patients admitted for SCI rehabilitation after penetrating injuries, 94% were men with an average age of 25 years. The ethnic distribution included 47% Black, 45% Hispanic, 4% White, and 4% miscellaneous (66). Of these 148 cases, 135 were the result of bullet injuries, 12 were due to stab wounds, and 1 was due to a fall from a scaffold onto a beam that penetrated the trunk. Other reported mechanisms (5,26) include acupuncture needles and glass.

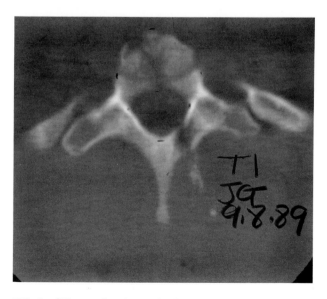

FIG. 1. CT scan showing path of the bullet through the spinal canal.

R. L. Waters, M.D.; R. H. Adkins, Ph.D.; S. S. Hu, M.D.; J. S. Yakura, M.S., P.T.; and I. H. Sie, M.S., P.T.: Rancho Los Amigos Medical Center, Downey, California 90242.

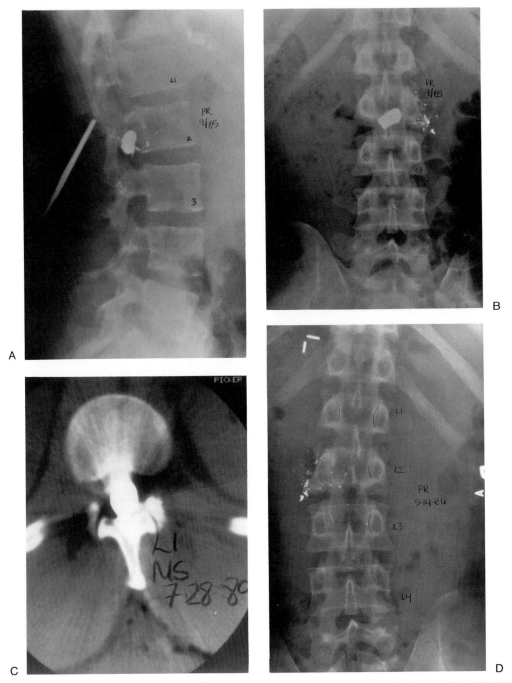

FIG. 2. Lateral (**A**) and anteroposterior (**B**) radiographs showing bullet lodged in the canal at L2. **C:** CT scan showing bullet lodged in the canal. **D:** Anteroposterior radiograph after bullet removal.

CHARACTERISTICS OF PENETRATING WOUNDS

For a stab wound to cause damage to the spinal cord, the tip of the penetrating instrument must enter the spinal canal. In contrast, a bullet does not have to come in contact with the spinal cord; the damage can result from concussive effects of the bullet (15). Nevertheless, in most cases the bullet passes through the spinal canal (Fig. 1) or remains lodged inside the canal (Fig. 2). In a group of 245 SCI patients admitted to Rancho Los Amigos Medical Center with injuries secondary to gunshot wounds, 96 patients were identified as having major bullet fragments lodged in the spinal canal (64). Thus, in this population, it can be expected that approximately one-third of the spinal cord injuries secondary to gunshot wounds will involve retention of bullet fragments in the spinal canal (28).

BALLISTICS

An understanding of the wounding potential of gunshot injuries requires a knowledge of ballistics. Based on the characteristics of the missile, such as composition, design, and velocity, a projectile will behave in a certain manner.

Bullets vary in size, with 22 to 45 caliber being the most common in civilian use. Caliber refers to the diameter of the bullet in hundredths of an inch. The shape of the bullet can be pointed, rounded, flat, or hollow, and these behave differently in air and in tissues. The more pointed a bullet's nose, the greater its ballistic coefficient, which determines the ability of the bullet to overcome air resistance (16). The hollow or dimpled bullet is often used by police. Its tip will flatten on impact, resulting in rapid deceleration so that the bullet is likely to remain in the target and is less likely to pass through and injure bystanders. Despite the rapid dissipation of energy by these bullets, they are not felt to result in greater wounding power (22).

Bullets are traditionally made of lead alloy because of its great density. However, lead has a low melting point and has a tendency to deform in the barrel when driven faster than 2,000 feet per second (fps). Jackets of copper, cupro-nickel, or soft steel are often used; this decreases the expansion of the lead and increases tissue penetration (15). According to international law (after the Geneva Convention), bullets for military use are required to be jacketed; however, civilian and hunting bullets are not so governed. Semi-jacketed bullets allow a mushrooming effect of the tip on impact (15).

A bullet is accelerated through a muzzle to a certain velocity that is limited by the weight of the bullet and the powder charge. A lighter bullet can be accelerated to higher velocities for a given charge. Low-velocity bullets are those that travel at less than 1,000 fps, medium velocity travel between 1,000 and 2,000 fps, and high velocity are those that travel faster than 2,000 fps. M-16 military rifles fire at 3,250 fps (15). Most civilian weapons are low velocity.

Once leaving its weapon source, a bullet is subject to certain destabilizing forces. These result in a deviation from the longitudinal axis of motion (yaw), as well as a circular deviation. Spin, which is imparted to the projectile by the barrel, stabilizes these effects in air to some extent. In water or soft tissues, the spin required to stabilize a bullet is considerably greater, and its inadequacy results in greater tumbling of bullets within tissues (25).

The damage created by a bullet injury is dependent upon the energy imparted to the tissues by the projectile. The maximal energy available is generally agreed to be the kinetic energy (15,16,25):

$$e = mv^2/2,$$

where m = mass of the projectile and v = velocity. Thus, doubling the velocity of a bullet quadruples the kinetic energy and therefore the wounding capacity, whereas doubling the mass of a bullet merely doubles the kinetic energy.

A bullet damages tissues by three mechanisms: (a) direct or crush injury, (b) shock waves, and (c) temporary cavitation (9,15,25,50). Crush is the main consideration for low-velocity injuries. The zone of crush widens as an expanding bullet passes through tissue (15). Entry wounds rely on the bullet's size and velocity as well as the distance from which it is fired and the specific gravity of the tissue it penetrates (7,16). Large entry wounds are found with close-range shotgun wounds or long-range rifle wounds. The former is due to the scatter of the pellets upon leaving the shotgun and is associated with contamination of the wound with wadding (generally paper, fiber, or felt). This signals a need for careful and wide debridement of wadding, skin edges, and accessible pellets (53). The latter is due to the decreased stability and increased tumbling in flight, resulting in a jagged wound (50). Even small entry wounds can belie severe underlying tissue destruction. Hollow point bullets, expanding bullets, small very high-velocity bullets, and some close-range shotgun wounds are all known to produce such patterns of damage (9,15,22,50,53). After penetration of the skin, fragments of soft tissue are ejected through the wound in what is called tail splash. Exit wounds will depend upon the tumbling of the bullet as it leaves the body and its shape or fragmentation.

When a projectile strikes tissue, the area compressed moves away as a shock wave. Shock waves are transmitted at high velocities and can be reflected in a fashion similar to sound waves. This results in pulsations of pressure and is significant for missiles at velocities greater than 500 fps (25,50). Air-containing viscera are more susceptible to shock waves than is bone or muscle. Above

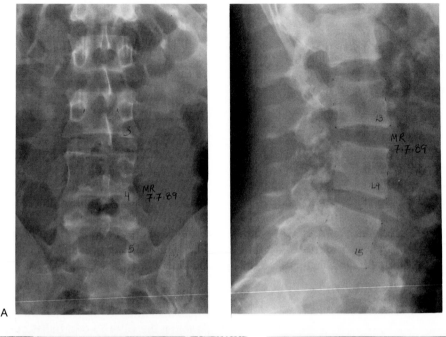

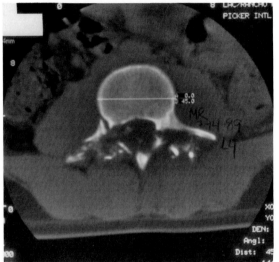

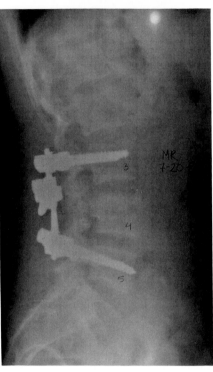

FIG. 3. A,B: Bullet entry via the flank, passing transversely through the spinal canal and posterior vertebral elements at L4. **C:** CT scan showing the bullet path that fractured the pedicle/facet bilaterally, causing acute spinal instability. **D:** Posterior spinal fusion with pedicle screw instrumentation performed to obtain spine stability.

1,000 fps, the phenomenon of temporary cavitation becomes important. The penetrating bullet accelerates the tissues around it both forward and sideways from the bullet tract. Because of inertia, the tissues will continue to move outward, producing the so-called temporary cavity. For nonexpanding bullets, the temporary cavity is conical in shape, being wider at the initiation of the bullet tract and then narrowing because of the progressive loss of velocity and energy. The size of the temporary cavity is proportional to the energy absorbed by the tissue and can reach up to 30 times the diameter of the missile (1,9,25). After the temporary cavity collapses, a narrower permanent cavity remains, as well as a zone of bruising that surrounds the bullet tract and corresponds to the temporary cavity (9,25). The region of bruising will become necrotic, and it is this region that requires debridement in higher-velocity, military-type injuries. There is an area of damage adjacent to this which has potential for recovery. With very high-velocity weapons (greater than 2,500 fps), formation of the temporary cavity can be so rapid that it appears explosive (25). With collapse of the temporary cavity, a negative pressure gradient is created, and air can be sucked in through entry and exit wounds.

The formation of a temporary cavity applies to bone as well. High-speed radiographs have shown fragmentation and expansion, but as the temporary cavity subsides, the supporting periosteum and soft tissues permit the comminuted bone to return to nearly its original configuration (25).

BULLET CALIBER

Reliable information on the caliber of bullets involved in civilian injuries is often difficult to obtain if the assailant is not apprehended. Nevertheless, based on radiographic examination, bullets can usually be grouped in three different sizes: large, 45 caliber; medium, 32 to 38, including 9-mm caliber; and small, 22 and 25 caliber. The most common type of gunshot injury is caused by medium-caliber bullets, followed by large (45 caliber) bullets and small-caliber bullet cases (66).

SPINE STABILITY

Little has been published to support the common belief that most gunshot wounds (GSW) are stable injuries. Meyer et al. (38) reported that of 1,300 GSW patients, none had demonstrated spinal instability.

However, we recently have observed both acute and chronic spine instability after gunshot wounds injuring the lumbar vertebrae (unpublished data). In all cases, the bullet passed transversely, fracturing both pedicles or facets. One patient had acute spine instability and underwent instrumentation and fusion in the immediate

post-injury period (Fig. 3). Another patient, originally believed to have a stable injury, complained of back pain and radicular symptoms 6 months after injury and had significant intervertebral translation on flexion/extension radiographs, requiring internal fixation and fusion. Spine instability has not been observed in cases in which one pedicle and facet remain intact.

It may be concluded that although spine instability resulting from civilian gunshot injuries is uncommon, the flight path of the bullet must be considered. Patients with flank entry wounds and fractures of both pedicles or facets in the lumbar region should be evaluated for spine stability. If stability is in question, appropriate studies such as flexion/extension views or computed tomography (CT) scan may be necessary.

NEUROLOGIC DEFINITIONS

The definitions recommended by the American Spinal Injury Association (ASIA) in the booklet, *Standards for Neurological and Functional Classification of Spinal Cord Injury* (2), adapted from Austin (4), provide an accurate method of communicating information on the extent of neurologic injury.

Manual muscle testing is performed using the standard six-grade scale: Absent = 0; trace = 1, visible or palpable contraction; poor = 2, active movement through range of motion with gravity eliminated; fair = 3, active movement through range of motion against gravity; good = 4, active movement through range of motion against resistance; and normal = 5.

The neurologic level of injury is defined as the most caudal segment that tests as intact for both sensory and motor functions on both sides of the body. By convention, if a muscle has at least a grade of "fair," it is considered intact. The motor level is defined as the level of the lowest key muscle having a grade of at least "fair," with the next most rostral key muscle required to test as "good" or "normal."

The term *incomplete SCI* denotes preservation of sensory and/or motor function below the neurologic level of injury and includes the lowest sacral segment. If there is no sensory or motor function in the lowest sacral segment, the injury is complete.

Because the most caudal normal sensory segment may not be the same as the most caudal normal motor segment, and the motor and sensory levels may not be the same on the right and left sides, it is possible to express the differences individually in a given patient. A patient with a complete C6 neurologic level of injury could have a right C6 sensory level and a C7 motor level, and a left C7 sensory and C8 motor level.

Numerically, the extent of motor function below the level of injury can be determined by the ASIA motor score. The strength of key muscles at each level from C5

TABLE 1. *ASIA motor index score[a]*

Grade on right		Muscle		Grade on left
0 to 5	C5	Deltoid and/or biceps	C5	0 to 5
0 to 5	C6	Wrist extensors	C6	0 to 5
0 to 5	C7	Triceps	C7	0 to 5
0 to 5	C8	Flexor profundus	C8	0 to 5
0 to 5	T1	Hand intrinsics	T1	0 to 5
0 to 5	L2	Iliopsoas	L2	0 to 5
0 to 5	L3	Quadriceps	L3	0 to 5
0 to 5	L4	Ankle dorsiflexors	L4	0 to 5
0 to 5	L5	Extensor hallucis longus	L5	0 to 5
0 to 5	S1	Gastrocnemius/soleus	S1	0 to 5
0 to 50				0 to 50

Source: Standards for neurological and functional classification of spinal cord injury (2).
[a] Highest possible score = 100.

through T1 and from L2 through S1 is determined using the numeric scale for motor strength described above. A total score of 100 is possible (Table 1).

The vertebral level of injury is the highest spinal level with radiographic evidence of vertebral injury due to bullet contact.

INITIAL INJURY

More than twice as many patients (40%) are shot in the back as in the front (19%). Also, more than twice as many patients are shot on the left side (27%) as on the right (66).

Table 2 provides the frequency distribution of the number of cases at each spinal level based on the level of vertebral injury and the neurologic level of injury (65). The cervical spine accounts for approximately 20%, the thoracic spine for 50%, and the thoracolumbar spine for 30% of all gunshot injuries causing spinal cord compromise.

In approximately 70% of injuries, the neurologic level is at least one level higher than the vertebral level; in 20%, the neurologic and vertebral levels are the same; and in 10%, the vertebral level is two levels lower than the neurologic level. Because of these differences, the distribution of the neurologic levels of injury is slightly different from the distribution of the vertebral levels of injury.

Table 3 is a cross-tabulation of the distribution of the neurologic and vertebral levels of injury for the cervical, thoracic, and thoracolumbar regions according to the completeness of SCI in 135 patients (65). Eight of the ten patients in whom the vertebral injury was above the neurologic level had thoracic injuries. In the majority of cases (>90%), the sensory level was below or equal to the motor level of injury.

More than half of all gunshot wounds resulting in SCI cause a complete neurologic lesion (66). The completeness of the spinal injury is related to the level of the vertebral injury and the bullet caliber. Table 4 shows how the completeness of injury is affected by the region of

injury. The percentage of complete SCI in the thoracic region is more than twice as great as in the thoracolumbar region (70% versus 33%). The percentage of patients with complete SCI increases with the size of the bullet, as follows: small, 47%; medium, 55%; and large, 61%.

On radiographic analysis, each bullet injury can be classified based on whether: (a) The bullet entered and remained within the spinal canal (30%); (b) the bullet entered and passed completely through the spinal canal (40%); or (c) the bullet did not enter the spinal canal (30%). When the bullet has not passed through the canal, radiographic inspection indicates in most cases that the lamina or pedicles are fractured from bullet impact (66).

TABLE 2. *Distribution of vertebral level of injury and neurologic level of injury*

	Vertebral		Neurologic	
	Frequency	Cumulative %	Frequency	Cumulative %
C2	2	1.5		
C3	1	2.2	5	3.7
C4	3	4.4	8	9.6
C5	4	7.4	9	16.3
C6	6	11.9	3	18.5
C7	10	19.3	4	21.5
T1	1	20.0	1	22.2
T2	8	25.9	10	29.6
T3	4	28.9	3	31.9
T4	9	35.6	12	40.7
T5	5	39.3	1	41.5
T6	5	43.0	11	49.6
T7	5	46.7	3	51.9
T8	5	50.4	7	57.0
T9	7	55.6	2	58.5
T10	13	65.2	17	71.1
T11	8	71.1	2	72.6
T12	5	74.8	23	89.6
L1	11	83.0	11	97.8
L2	12	91.1	2	99.3
L3	4	94.8	1	100.0
L4	3	97.0		
L5	2	98.5		
S1	2	100.0		

TABLE 3. *Neurologic level of injury minus vertebral level of injury*

	Incomplete SCI			Complete SCI		
	Cervical	Thoracic	Thoracolumbar	Cervical	Thoracic	Thoracolumbar
≤6			2		1	
−5			1		2	
−4			2		1	
−3			3	2	7	
−2	4	1	10	7	12	7
−1	3	6	6	1	11	4
0	1	7	2	4	10	2
+1	1	4		1		
+2		2			1	
+3	2	1			1	
+4					1	
+5					1	
≥6					1	

Few bullets that strike the vertebral body and do not enter or pass through the vertebral canal result in SCI.

The trajectory is significantly related to the completeness of SCI on initial examination (66). Seventy percent of cases in which the bullet passes completely through the spinal canal result in complete SCI. In contrast, approximately 50% of other GSW-related injuries result in complete SCI.

NEUROLOGIC RECOVERY

In terms of neurologic level (determined by the most caudally intact motor and sensory parameters), two-thirds of patients with complete lesions can be expected to make no additional improvement from initial to annual follow-up (65). An improvement of one level is evident in approximately 25% of patients with complete lesions.

Among patients with incomplete injuries, two-thirds will show no neurologic improvement between the time of initial injury and 1 year of follow-up. In the remaining cases, the amount of recovery can vary from one level to complete recovery.

There is a significant difference among the regions of injury, with cervical injuries showing the greatest improvement in the ASIA motor index score (17.8 ± 13.8); thoracolumbar injuries show the next greatest change (10.8 ± 9.5), and thoracic injuries show the least (4.8 ± 7.7). In addition, there is a significant difference in score improvement between complete (3.9 ± 6.0) and incom-

plete (16.0 ± 11.3) injuries. These two factors of region of injury and injury completeness combine to affect neurologic recovery.

Data regarding ambulatory status were available for 120 subjects (67). Twenty-four percent (29 cases) of individuals were able to ambulate at 1-year follow-up. Individuals with incomplete injuries were more likely to be ambulatory. Eighty-two percent of incomplete tetraplegics and 73% of incomplete paraplegics were ambulatory, whereas only 6% of complete paraplegics walked at follow-up. As expected, none of the complete tetraplegics were ambulatory.

STAB INJURIES

Stab wounds of the spine resulting in SCI are relatively rare outside of South Africa (33,42,61). A collaborative investigation was conducted among the Regional Model Spinal Cord Injury Systems, which are sponsored by the National Institute on Disability and Rehabilitation Research, to determine the nature of recovery in SCI caused by stab wounds. In cases of stab wounds or injury from other sharp weapons, 70% to 90% suffer an incomplete lesion, generally a form of Brown-Sequard (5,6,67). These incomplete lesions have a favorable prognosis for functional recovery. Complete lesions, as with other injury mechanisms, have a poorer prognosis for recovery.

In our experience, 60% of patients are ambulatory and

TABLE 4. *Vertebral region versus completeness of SCI*

	Complete SCI	Incomplete SCI
Cervical (C1–C7)	15	11
Thoracic (T1–T11)	49	21
Thoracolumbar (T12–L5)	13	26

TABLE 5. *ASIA motor score (AMS) changes from initial to annual follow-up: Stab wounds*

	N	AMS changes
Complete paraplegia	5	18.6 ± 13.6
Incomplete paraplegia	6	16.3 ± 5.1
Complete tetraplegia	2	6.0 ± 2.8
Incomplete tetraplegia	7	23.9 ± 12.9
Total	20	18.5 ± 11.3

50% demonstrate volitional bladder control at 1-year follow-up (67). The average increase in ASIA motor score is 18.5 ± 11.3 points; individuals with motor complete tetraplegia demonstrate the smallest increases in motor function (Table 5).

As will be discussed, delayed neurologic loss can result in a more severe deficit if a portion of a sharp object such as the tip of a knife blade is retained in the spinal canal, unlike bullet fragments which are smooth and usually cause no delayed neurologic injury (27,68). Therefore, surgical exploration is reserved for a retained weapon in the spinal canal or a cerebrospinal fluid (CSF) leak lasting longer than 3 to 4 days (6). If the latter occurs, accurate localization of a dural tear can be accomplished with myelography. It should be noted that metrizamide contrast is heavier than CSF, and detection of a dorsal laceration requires supine positioning of the patient (58).

ROLE OF SURGERY

There have been numerous reports discussing the various surgical aspects of penetrating wounds in which the injury involves the spinal canal and is associated with SCI. Many of these reports, particularly those based on wartime experience, favor removal of bullet fragments from the canal via laminectomy as mandatory for proper care (21,23,24,35–37,40,41,43,51,54,62,63). Others do not favor removal unless certain conditions are present, primarily progressive neurologic decline (20,30,34, 39,57,64). Those who favor laminectomy, wound debridement, and removal of bullet fragments indicate that this procedure prevents complications such as infection, CSF leak, lead toxicity, pain, and late neurologic decline.

Some consider laminectomy part of proper treatment of SCI regardless of whether bullet removal is a factor (11–13). Recent research indicates that laminectomy for the purpose of decompression alone is not effective in increasing neurologic recovery after SCI (4,8,10,20,39,57).

BULLET REMOVAL AND NEUROLOGIC RECOVERY

Clinically, whether a bullet fragment should be removed from the spinal canal, given stable neurologic status, remains a crucial surgical question surrounded by controversy. Investigation among the Regional Model Spinal Cord Injury Systems was undertaken in 1984 to answer this question (66). The primary purpose of this collaborative effort was to assess the influence of bullet removal from the spinal canal on neurologic outcome.

Serial motor and sensory examinations were conducted on patients with bullet fragments lodged in the spinal canal. The examinations were conducted on admission and at 1 year after injury. Patients were subdivided based on the location of the bullet within the spinal canal: cervical (C1-C7), thoracic (T1-T11), and lumbar (T12-L5). There were 14 patients with bullets in the cervical region, 32 with bullets in the thoracic spine, and 20 with bullets in the thoracolumbar spine. The number of cervical injuries was too small for statistical analysis and will not be discussed here. In examining the compiled results for all thoracic injuries, there was a difference between the scores of those who had the bullets removed versus those who did not. However, this difference was not statistically significant (Table 6). The apparent difference was due to the disparate distribution of bullet removal among those with incomplete injuries, coupled with the large average change for all incomplete thoracic lesions. In other words, as can be seen in Table 6, all incomplete injuries in this group improved substantially relative to complete injuries regardless of bullet removal, but a larger proportion of patients with incomplete lesions underwent bullet removal. Analyzing the complete and incomplete data separately suggests that removal of bullets lodged in the spinal canal in this region does not significantly affect motor change (Table 6).

Statistical analysis of the thoracolumbar injuries (T12 or below) demonstrated a highly significant difference

TABLE 6. *ASIA motor index score for T1–T10 injuries (Mean ± SD)*

	Initial	Annual	Difference	N
All thoracic injuries (T1–T10)				
Removed	45.4 ± 7.6	53.8 ± 14.4	8.8 ± 9.2	8
Not removed	47.9 ± 8.4	51.7 ± 13.0	3.8 ± 8.1	24
Total				32
Complete thoracic injuries (T1–T10)				
Removed	43.0 ± 6.5	46.0 ± 4.2	3.0 ± 4.2	5
Not removed	45.7 ± 5.0	47.2 ± 4.7	1.5 ± 3.7	21
Total				26
Incomplete thoracic injuries (T1–T10)				
Removed	49.3 ± 9.0	66.7 ± 17.0	17.3 ± 8.1	3
Not removed	64.7 ± 11.9	83.3 ± 2.9	19.7 ± 13.9	3
Total				6

Source: Waters et al. (66).

TABLE 7. *ASIA motor index score for T12–L4 injuries*

	Initial	Annual	Difference	N
All thoracolumbar injuries (T12–L4)				
Removed	58.5 ± 12.5	71.5 ± 14.0	12.9 ± 6.1	13
Not removed	52.9 ± 5.0	56.2 ± 7.3	3.3 ± 3.6	7
Total				20
Complete thoracolumbar injuries (T12–L4)				
Removed	56.0 ± 7.8	65.5 ± 13.0	9.5 ± 7.1	4
Not removed	50.0 ± 0.0	52.0 ± 4.0	2.0 ± 4.0	4
Total				8
Incomplete thoracolumbar injuries (T12–L4)				
Removed	59.7 ± 14.3	74.1 ± 14.3	14.4 ± 5.4	9
Not removed	56.7 ± 6.1	61.7 ± 7.5	5.0 ± 2.6	3
Total				12

Source: Waters and Adkins (65).

between the bullet-removed versus not-removed groups (Table 7). These trends held whether the group was sorted according to completeness of injury or analyzed as a whole.

Differences in the regional anatomy of the spinal cord and the greater susceptibility of the spinal cord to injury (compared with the spinal nerve roots) may account for the difference in the effects of bullet removal on neurologic recovery in the thoracic and thoracolumbar regions. In the thoracic spine above T12, the nerve roots exit the spinal canal just below the level from which they originate from the spinal cord. A bullet at this level can generally impinge only on the nerve roots emanating from one neurologic level. The effect of a gain of one thoracic nerve root (exclusive of T1) on function is clinically insignificant, and motor change in the thoracic region is not reflected in the ASIA motor score. On the other hand, in the lower thoracic spine, the spinal cord begins expanding at T10 to form the conus, which usually ends at the L1 and L2 junction (4). Lumbar nerve roots geneRally emerge from the conus at the T12 vertebral level, and sacral nerve roots emerge from the conus at the L1 vertebral level. These nerve roots may descend several vertebral levels before exiting the spinal canal (44,52). Therefore, a bullet in the spinal canal at T12 or below can impinge on many nerve roots that innervate the key muscles in the lower limbs, which is reflected in the ASIA motor score.

After SCI, which may damage cell bodies as well as axons, glial scar may form an impenetrable barrier to regenerating axons. After peripheral nerve injury, cell bodies are not usually damaged. There is also a relatively greater abundance of myelin surrounding the axon, and this means that there can be greater potential for recovery. Disintegration of a motor axon within a peripheral nerve due to local injury progresses proximally to the next node of Ranvier. In the region of the axonal degeneration, the Schwann cells proliferate and form neurilemmal tubules.

Growth from the central end of the damaged axon can be guided across the sites of trauma, allowing motor reinnervation over time. However, if the injury disrupts the Schwann cell layer and there is no longer continuity of the neurilemmal tubule, regeneration is possible but may result in only partial reinnervation, depending on the extent of injury.

To summarize, it is probable that patients with thoracolumbar injury have greater clinical improvement after bullet decompression because of the relatively large number of lumbar and sacral nerve roots that can be compressed by a bullet in this region, as well as the potential of axons to regenerate and promote recovery of neurologic function.

LATE NEUROLOGIC DECLINE

No cases of late neurologic deterioration have been observed by one of us (RLW) in following more than 1,000 patients with SCI secondary to GSW. However, there have been rare instances reported of delayed neurologic change secondary to retained bullet or weapon fragments. The delay from injury to onset of neurologic symptoms ranged up to 15 years (3,27,29,55,56,68). The symptoms varied and included radiating "electric shocks," low back pain, cauda equina symptoms, and Brown-Sequard neurologic loss. This last occurred in a patient who had a retained knife-tip blade in his spinal canal, which began to cause symptoms 8 years after injury (27).

The encroaching material can also be fibrous reactive tissue from bullet fragments remaining in a disc space or vertebral body (56,68). Improvement of symptoms followed excision of the reactive tissue and/or the foreign body. It appears that patients with retained bullet fragments in the spinal canal should be observed for development of neurologic symptoms, and the bullet or causative tissue should be excised if there is late development of symptoms or neurologic loss. Retained sharp objects such as the broken tip of a knife blade appear to have more potential for late complications and should probably be removed when injury occurs, particularly if the injury is incomplete.

INFECTION

Prevention of infection is commonly cited as a reason for bullet removal from the spinal canal when the bullet perforates the alimentary tract before spinal injury. Romanick et al. (49) reported 20 patients with low-velocity missile injuries to the abdomen associated with vertebral body fracture. Nine had SCI; 12 sustained a perforated viscus before the bullet entered the spinal column. Of eight patients with colon perforations, seven developed an infection. The authors concluded that bullet removal was indicated when the alimentary tract was perforated. However, most patients in this series received only a short course (2 to 4 days) of intravenous antibiotics.

Roffi et al. (48) recently reviewed 42 patients with SCI associated with perforation of the alimentary canal. Thirty-five of the 42 patients had bullet fragments lodged in the spinal canal, disc space, or vertebral body. Seventeen patients had debridement and bullet removal via laminectomy. No abscesses or signs of infection were found at operation surrounding the bullet fragments. Eighteen patients did not have the bullet fragments removed, and none of these developed spinal infection. Nine of these 18 had associated colon perforations and six had isolated stomach injuries. Unlike Romanick's sample (49), however, most of the patients in the latter series received a course of broad-spectrum intravenous antibiotics lasting 7 to 14 days. Roffi et al. attributed the absence of infection in patients in whom the bullet was left *in situ* to the longer course of prophylactic antibiotic therapy. They concluded that for civilian injuries, a 2-week course of broad-spectrum intravenous antibiotics is sufficient to prevent spinal infection caused by the introduction of bacteria by low-velocity bullets perforating the alimentary canal. Although the course and duration of antibiotic therapy were not specifically reviewed in the Regional Model Spinal Cord Injury Systems series, none of the 19 patients in whom the bullet perforated the alimentary canal developed infection, even though ten of the bullets were left in the spinal canal.

Among the differences between gunshot wounds sustained during wartime and those sustained by the civilian population, the primary difference is the velocity of missiles involved. Gunshot wounds sustained in warfare are usually the result of high-velocity missiles yielding more tissue destruction and greater probability of contamination. Thus, laminectomy, debridement, wound exploration, and removal of bullet fragments may be appropriate to prevent infection. Gunshot wounds sustained by the civilian population, on the other hand, are usually caused by low-velocity missiles fired from handguns. These cause considerably less tissue necrosis and have less potential for infection. Reports of late infection are extremely rare (60). Over a 12-year period, more than 1,000 cases of SCI due to GSW have been seen in the authors' service, and no patient has required treatment for delayed infection. We conclude that prophylactic removal of the bullet fragments from the canal in most civilian, low-velocity cases is not advisable.

GUNSHOT WOUND PAIN

Pain is a common problem in spinal cord-injured patients, but appears to have a higher incidence when the injury is secondary to a gunshot wound (45). Past authors have recommended removal of a retained bullet fragment to relieve pain. However, recent studies (46,47,65) have re-evaluated this approach and found that the incidence of post-injury pain was not affected by removal of the bullet. In fact, bullet removal appears to be associated with a higher incidence of deafferentation pain, which can be more difficult to treat (14).

LEAD TOXICITY

Lead from bullets is relatively insoluble and rarely causes significant effects when bullets are left in the body (17,59). Although there are isolated case reports of lead toxicity resulting from bullets lodged in the spine, this is extremely rare. In general, bullets become encapsulated by poorly vascularized fibrous tissue (59). This has been borne out by our experience when bullets are removed at least 3 to 4 weeks after injury; the encapsulated bullet does not communicate with the CSF.

However, the symptoms of lead poisoning (abdominal pain, anemia, headaches, memory loss, and muscle weakness) may occur if the lead object is in communication with synovial fluid, such as in a joint or pseudocyst (19,31,32,59). Better clinical results are obtained if medical treatment for lead intoxication is begun before surgical removal of the fragment. Chelation therapy, with EDTA (ethylenediaminetetra-acetic acid) or occasionally D-penicillamine or dimercaprol (BAL), is recommended for initial management of such patients (18).

SUMMARY

Penetrating injuries are becoming increasingly important causes of SCI. With gunshot wounds, significant neurologic injury can occur even if the projectile does not enter the spinal canal. Retained bullets rarely cause problems of delayed infection, delayed neurologic decline, or lead intoxication, obviating the need for prophylactic removal of bullet fragments. When the retained bullet is located at T12 or below, removal has been demonstrated to have a significantly favorable effect on neurologic recovery. In addition, retained sharp portions of knives, glass, and the like should be surgically removed, as they pose a greater hazard for significant, often irreversible neurologic damage.

Finally, comparing functional outcomes between these two forms of intentional violence, the outcome appears to be better in individuals with SCI due to stab wounds. Sixty percent of patients with stab wounds were able to ambulate at follow-up, compared with 24% of patients with SCI due to gunshot wounds.

ACKNOWLEDGMENT. This work was funded in part by the National Institute of Disability Rehabilitation Research, Field Initiated Grant Numbers G008435028 and H133G90115.

REFERENCES

1. Amato JL, Billy LJ, Lawson NS, et al. (1974): High velocity missile injury: An experimental study of the retentive forces of tissue. *Am J Surg* 127:454–459.
2. American Spinal Injury Association (1992): *Standards for neurological and functional classification of spinal cord injury.* ASIA, Chicago.
3. Arasil E, Tascioglu AO (1982): Spontaneous migration of an intracranial bullet to the cervical spinal canal causing Lhermitte's sign (case report). *J Neurosurg* 56:158–159.
4. Austin GM (1972): *The spinal cord: Basic aspects and surgical considerations,* 2nd ed. Springfield, Illinois: Charles C. Thomas.
5. Baghai P, Sheptak PE (1982): Penetrating spinal injury by a glass fragment: Case report and review. *Neurosurgery* 11:419–422.
6. [Editorial] (1978): Stab wounds of the spinal cord. *Br Med J* 1:1093–1094.
7. Callender GR, French RW (1978): Wound ballistics: Studies in mechanism of wound production by rifle bullets. *Milit Surg* 77:177–201.
8. Carey PD (1965): Neurosurgery and paraplegia. *Rehabilitation* (Jan-March):27–29.
9. Charters AC III, Charters AC (1976): Wounding mechanism of very high velocity projectiles. *J Trauma* 16:464–470.
10. Cloward RB (1963): Lesions of the intervertebral disks and their treatment by interbody fusion methods. The painful disk. *Clin Orthop* 27:51–77.
11. Comarr AE, Kaufman AA (1956): A survey of the neurological results of 858 spinal cord injuries: A comparison of patients treated with and without laminectomy. *J Neurosurg* 13:95–106.
12. Covalt DA, Cooper IS, Hoen TI, Rusk HA (1953): Early management of patients with spinal cord injury. *JAMA* 151:89–94.
13. Daniels JT (1946): Fractures and dislocations of the spine in warfare. *Am J Surg* 72:414–423.
14. Davidoff G, Roth E, Guarracini M, Sliwa J, Yarkony G (1987): Function-limiting dysesthetic pain syndrome among traumatic spinal cord injury patients: A cross-sectional study. *Pain* 29:39–48.
15. deMuth WE Jr (1966): Bullet velocity and design as determinants of wounding capability: An experimental study. *J Trauma* 6:222–232.
16. deMuth WE Jr (1969): Bullet velocity as applied to military rifle wounding capacity. *J Trauma* 9:27–38.
17. Dillman RO, Crumb CK, Lidsky MJ (1979): Lead poisoning from a gunshot wound. Report of a case and review of the literature. *Am J Med* 66:509–514.
18. Graef JW, Lovejoy FH (1987): Heavy metal poisoning. In: Braun-

wald E, et al., eds. *Harrison's principles of internal medicine,* 11th ed. New York: McGraw-Hill, p. 852.
19. Grogan DP, Bucholz RW (1981): Acute lead intoxication from a bullet in an intervertebral disc space. A case report. *J Bone Joint Surg [Am]* 63:1180–1182.
20. Guttmann L (1949): Surgical aspects of the treatment of traumatic paraplegia. *J Bone Joint Surg [Br]* 31:399–403.
21. Hagelstam L (1955): Late laminectomy in traumatic paraplegia. *Acta Chir Scand* 110:218–226.
22. Harrell JB (1979): Hollowpoint ammunition injuries: Experience in a police group. *J Trauma* 19:115–116.
23. Haynes WG (1946): Acute war wounds of the spinal cord. Analysis of 184 cases. *Am J Surg* 72:424–433.
24. Heiden JS, Weiss MH, Rosenberg AW, Kurze T, Apuzzo ML (1975): Penetrating gunshot wounds of the cervical spine in civilians. Review of 38 cases. *J Neurosurg* 42:575–579.
25. Hopkinson DA, Marshall TK (1967): Firearm injuries. *Br J Surg* 54:344–353.
26. Isu T, Iwasaki Y, Sasaki H, Abe H (1985): Spinal cord and root injuries due to glass fragments and acupuncture needles. *Surg Neurol* 23:255–260.
27. Jones FD, Woosley RE (1981): Delayed myelopathy secondary to retained intraspinal metallic fragment. *J Neurosurg* 55:979–982.
28. Kane T, Capen DA, Waters R, Zigler JE, Adkins RH (1991): Spinal cord injury from civilian gunshot wounds: The Rancho experience 1980–88. *J Spinal Disorders* 4:306–311.
29. Karim NO, Nabors MW, Golocovsky M, Cooney FD (1986): Spontaneous migration of a bullet in the spinal subarachnoid space causing delayed radicular symptoms. *Neurosurgery* 18:97–100.
30. Kuhn WG Jr (1947): The care and rehabilitation of patients with injuries of the spinal cord and cauda equina: Preliminary report on 113 cases. *J Neurosurg* 4:40–68.
31. Leonard MH (1969): The solution of lead by synovial fluid. *Clin Orthop* 64:255–261.
32. Linden MA, Manton WI, Stewart RM, Thal ER, Feit H (1982): Lead poisoning from retained bullets. Pathogenesis, diagnosis, and management. *Ann Surg* 195:305–313.
33. Lipschitz R (1976): Stab wounds of the spinal cord. In: Vinken PJ, Gruyn GW, eds. *Handbook of clinical neurology,* Vol. 25. North Holland Publ, pp. 197–207.
34. Lucas JT, Ducker TB (1979): Motor classification of spinal cord injuries with mobility, morbidity and recovery indices. *Am Surg* 45:151–158.
35. Matson DD (1948): *The treatment of acute compound injuries of the spinal cord due to missiles.* Springfield, Illinois: Charles C. Thomas.
36. McCravey A (1945): War wounds of the spinal cord. A plea for exploration of spinal cord and cauda equina injuries. *JAMA* 129:152–153.
37. Meirowsky AM (1963): Penetrating wounds of the spinal canal. Problems of paraplegia and notes on autonomic hyperreflexia and sympathetic blockade. *Clin Orthop* 27:90–110.
38. Meyer PR, Apple DF, Bohlman HH, Ferguson RL, Stauffer ES (1988): Symposium: Management of fractures of the thoracolumbar spine. *Contemp Orthop* 16:57–86.
39. Morgan TH, Wharton GW, Austin GW (1971): The results of laminectomy in patients with incomplete spinal cord injuries. *Paraplegia* 9:14–23.
40. Munro D (1952): *The treatment of injuries to the nervous system.* Philadelphia: W.B. Saunders.
41. Nino HE, Leppik IE, Lai CW, Martin S (1978): Progressive sensory loss one year after bullet injury of spinal cord. *JAMA* 240:1173–1174.
42. Peacock WJ, Shrosbree RD, Key AG (1977): A review of 450 stab-wounds of the spinal cord. *S Afr Med J* 51:961–964.
43. Pool JL (1945): Gunshot wounds of the spine. Observations from an evacuation hospital. *Surg Gynecol Obstet* 81:617–622.
44. Rauschning W (1985): Detailed sectional anatomy of the spine. In: Rothman SL, Glenn WV Jr, eds. *Multiplanar CT of the spine.* Baltimore: University Park Press, pp. 33–85.
45. Richards JS (1988): Pain secondary to gunshot wound during the initial rehabilitation process in spinal cord injury patients. *J Rehab Res Dev* 25(suppl):75.
46. Richards JS, Meredith RL, Nepomuceno C, Fine PR, Bennett G

(1980): Psycho-social aspects of chronic pain in spinal cord injury. *Pain* 8:355–366.

47. Richards JS, Stover SL, Jaworski T (1990): Effect of bullet removal on subsequent pain in persons with spinal cord injury secondary to gunshot wound. *J Neurosurg* 73:401–404.

48. Roffi RP, Waters RL, Adkins RH (1989): Gunshot wounds to the spine associated with a perforated viscus. *Spine* 14:808–811.

49. Romanick PC, Smith TK, Kopaniky DR, Oldfield D (1985): Infection about the spine associated with low-velocity-missile injury to the abdomen. *J Bone Joint Surg [Am]* 67:1195–1201.

50. Russotti GM, Sim FH (1985): Missile wounds of the extremities: A current concepts review. *Orthopedics* 8:1106–1116.

51. Scarff JE (1960): Injuries of the vertebral column and spinal cord. In: Brock S, ed. *Injuries of the brain and spinal cord and their coverings,* 4th ed. New York: Springer Publishing.

52. Shapiro R (1968): *Myelography,* 2nd ed. Chicago: Year Book Medical Publishers.

53. Shepard GH (1980): High energy, low velocity close-range shotgun wounds. *J Trauma* 20:1065–1067.

54. Shroyer RN, Fortson CH, Theodotou CB (1960): Delayed neurological sequelae of a retained foreign body (lead bullet) in the intervertebral disc space. *J Bone Joint Surg [Am]* 42:595–599.

55. Soges LJ, Kinnebrew GH, Limcaco OG (1988): Mobile intrathecal bullet causing relayed radicular symptoms. *AJNR* 9:610.

56. Staniforth P, Watt I (1982): Extradural 'plumboma.' A rare cause of acquired spinal stenosis. *Br J Radiol* 55:772–774.

57. Stauffer ES, Wood RW, Kelly EG (1979): Gunshot wounds of the spine: The effects of laminectomy. *J Bone Joint Surg [Am]* 61:389–392.

58. Sutton D, DeSilva RD (1984): Water-soluble contrast medium in the localisation of cord and dural stab wounds. *Clin Radiol* 35:483–484.

59. Switz DM, Elmorshidy ME, Deyerle WM (1976): Bullets, joints, and lead intoxication. A remarkable and instructive case. *Arch Intern Med* 136:939–941.

60. Tanguy A, Chabannes J, Deubelle A, Vanneuville G, Dalens B (1982): Intraspinal migration of a bullet with subsequent meningitis. A case report. *J Bone Joint Surg [Am]* 64:1244–1245.

61. Thakur RC, Khosia VK, Kak VK (1991): Non-missile penetrating injuries of the spine. *Acta Neurochir (Wien)* 113:144–148.

62. Tinsley M (1946): Compound injuries of the spinal cord. *J Neurosurg* 3:306–309.

63. Wannamaker GT (1954): Spinal cord injuries: A review of the early treatment in 300 consecutive cases during the Korean conflict. *J Neurosurg* 11:517–524.

64. Waters RL (1984): Gunshot wounds to the spine: The effects of bullet fragments in the spinal canal. *J Am Paraplegia Soc* 7:30–33.

65. Waters RL, Adkins RH (1991): The effects of removal of bullet fragments retained in the spinal canal: A collaborative study by the National Spinal Cord Injury Model Systems. *Spine* 16:934–939.

66. Waters RL, Adkins RH, Yakura J, Sie I (1991): Profiles of spinal cord injury and recovery after gunshot injury. *Clin Orthop* 267:14–21.

67. Waters RL, Adkins RH, Yakura J, Sie I (1995): Motor recovery following spinal cord injury caused by stab wounds: a multicenter study. *Paraplegia* 33:98–101.

68. Wu WQ (1986): Delayed effects of retained foreign bodies in the spine and spinal cord. *Surg Neurol* 25:214–218.

69. Young JS, Burns PE, Bowen AM, McCutchen R (1982): *Spinal cord injury statistics: Experience of the Regional Spinal Cord Injury Systems.* Phoenix, Arizona: Good Samaritan Medical Center.

The Adult Spine: Principles and Practice,
2nd edition, J.W. Frymoyer, Editor-in-Chief.
Lippincott-Raven Publishers, Philadelphia © 1997.

CHAPTER 47

Rehabilitation of the Patient with Traumatic Spinal Cord Injury

Christopher S. Formal and John F. Ditunno, Jr.

HISTORY AND SCOPE

An ancient anonymous Egyptian physician reviewed a case of complete tetraplegia and described it as "an ailment not to be treated" (33). A similar thought was expressed thousands of years later by Adolph Hanson, as he described his experience in World War I: "War wounds of the spine were particularly distressing. These injuries were so frequently associated with chest and abdominal wounds of a serious nature that one scarcely knew where to begin, if to begin at all" (30). Indeed it was possible, as recently as 1978, in a major American trauma center, for a young, otherwise healthy victim of traumatic tetraplegia to be allowed to die of respiratory failure. The ambivalence of physicians about the treatment of acute traumatic spinal cord injury (SCI) must have stemmed, in part, from concern about the quality of life of a person who survived the acute injury.

Acute management of traumatic SCI advanced, however, and in Great Britain there were approximately 700 survivors of SCI in World War II (29). In modern civilian trauma centers, 94% of victims survive the initial hospitalization (18).

A survivor of traumatic SCI faces a host of challenges. These overwhelmed the majority of survivors until approximately 50 years ago, when effective centers for the management of chronic SCI appeared. Sir Ludwig Guttmann presented the orientation of his Spinal Unit at Stoke Mandeville Hospital as follows:

> The basic principle of the new concept was the aim to provide for spinal paraplegics as well as tetraplegics a comprehensive service from the start of their injury or disease and throughout all stages involving all aspects of this multi-disciplinary subject of medicine—to rescue these men and women from the human scrap-heap and to return most of them, in spite of their profound disability, to the community as useful and respected citizens.

C. S. Formal, M.D.: Associate Professor, Magee Rehabilitation Hospital, Philadelphia, Pennsylvania, 19102.

J. F. Ditunno, Jr., M.D.: Professor, Department of Rehabilitation Medicine, Thomas Jefferson University Hospital, Philadelphia, Pennsylvania, 19107.

The chief object was not just to preserve the lives of paraplegics and tetraplegics, but to give them a purpose in life (29).

The comprehensive management espoused by Guttmann in England, Howard Rusk in the United States, and later by John Young encompassed the essential features of a Model Spinal Cord Injury System of Care. It goes beyond the traditional medical model and divides the problems encountered by a survivor of SCI into medical, functional, and psychosocial categories. These will serve as the primary divisions of this chapter. The breadth of the problems is beyond the scope of any single discipline, and thus patient management requires a team effort. Optimizing the medical, functional, and psychosocial status of the patient is the goal of rehabilitation.

Epidemiology

The following information applies to traumatic SCI occurring in the United States.

Patient Population

Traumatic SCI primarily afflicts young men. The mean age is 30.5 years, the median is 26, and the mode is 19; more than half of the victims are between the ages of 16 and 30. Over 80% are male. Non-Whites are disproportionately represented (15).

Mechanism of Injury

The most common cause of traumatic SCI is motor vehicle accidents (44.8%), followed by falls (21.7%), acts of violence (16%), and sports (13%). The most common act of violence causing SCI is shooting, and the most common sports activity causing SCI is diving (15). Traumatic SCI in people over 45 years is most commonly due to a fall. In non-Whites, the most common cause of traumatic SCI is an act of violence (55).

Time of Injury

The month with the highest number of cases of SCI is July; the nadir occurs in February. Saturday and Sunday account for 38.6% of injuries.

Level of Injury

The exact definition of "level" is discussed later in the section on neurologic assessment and classification. The level noted at discharge from the initial hospitalization will be considered.

The most common level is C5, followed by C4 and C6. For cases of paraplegia, the most frequent level is T12,

followed by L1 and T10. The majority of cases are symmetric, with the same level on each side (17). Tetraplegia is more common than paraplegia (55).

Completeness of Injury

A description of the American Spinal Injury Association (ASIA) Impairment Scale, which describes the degree of completeness of a spinal cord injury, is provided later in the section on neurologic assessment and classification. Admission ASIA grades will be considered.

The most common grade on admission is A (complete), involving 50.5% of cases. A grade of B (incomplete, preserved sensation only) applies to 13.2%; C (incomplete, preserved motor nonfunctional) applies to 12.9%, and D (incomplete, preserved motor functional) applies to 21.6%. Patients admitted with spinal fractures but no neurologic injury (and thus a grade of E) are not included (17).

Overall, cases of tetraplegia are more likely to be incomplete than complete, whereas cases of paraplegia are more commonly complete than incomplete. Older persons suffering traumatic SCI are far more likely to have tetraplegia than paraplegia, and a majority of these injuries are incomplete. This probably reflects a common mechanism of injury in the elderly in which a person with pre-existing cervical spinal stenosis due to degenerative arthritis suffers a fall (55). Evaluation of trends over time reveals an increase in the percentage of incomplete lesions compared with complete lesions; this may reflect improvement in emergency care (15).

Organization of Care

Victims of traumatic SCI face medical, functional, and psychosocial difficulties from the time of injury throughout the rest of their lives. Care can be divided into three phases: acute care, inpatient rehabilitation, and chronic care. Each phase of care may be delivered at a different setting.

Acute Care

This is delivered while the patient is on a surgical service. Surgical responsibilities include stabilization of the spine, provision of medication to foster neurologic recovery, and operative treatment, as well as primary supportive care.

Pharmacologic treatment may limit damaging processes that occur in the spinal cord in the hours or days after the initial injury. Treatment may also enhance the recovery process. Standard intervention is methylprednisolone given as a bolus of 30 mg/kg, followed by an infusion of 5.4 mg/kg/hour for 23 hours, beginning within 8 hours of injury (4,5). Treatment with tirilazad, gm-1 ganglioside, and a longer period of infusion of methylprednisolone are all under investigation (6, 26,27).

Operative treatment can optimize spinal alignment and stability, decreasing the risk of neurologic decline, spinal deformity, and pain. Surgery may also allow earlier mobilization of the patient, limiting the physiologic and psychological problems that would accompany prolonged bed rest. Hospital length of stay may also be shortened (27).

Functional concerns include maintenance of range of motion, strengthening, and establishment of bowel and bladder management programs. Psychosocial issues of adjustment, involving family as well as patient, are addressed, and discharge planning begins.

Inpatient Rehabilitation

This is delivered while the patient is on a rehabilitation service. Functional issues usually predominate, but this is a phase during which all problems presented by the case should be addressed in preparation for discharge to the community.

Chronic Care

This is provided while the patient is in the community. It is delivered through a combination of the rehabilitation outpatient system, the community medical system, and, where necessary, a visiting nursing agency.

Interaction of Sites of Care

Continuity of care between sites requires a high level of communication. Though the patient will ideally "flow in one direction" through the system, in reality interaction occurs in both directions. For example, a patient on a rehabilitation unit may have to return for surgical evaluation of spinal fusion, or a patient followed in the community may become ill and require acute-care hospitalization.

Organization of the Rehabilitation Team

The varied problems faced in the rehabilitation of traumatic SCI require the attention of several disciplines. These work as a team, ideally in a problem-oriented, interdisciplinary manner, in which all team members may contribute to solving each problem. The team is headed by a rehabilitation specialist or other physician with an interest in SCI. Medical problems are primarily addressed by the physician and nurse; functional problems are primarily addressed by the physical and occupational

therapists (the former managing problems of mobility and the latter, problems of activities of daily living), and psychosocial problems are primarily addressed by the psychologist and social worker. As noted, all team members are concerned with all problems.

Benefits of a System of Care

Patient outcome may be better if a patient is admitted early to a system of care dedicated to traumatic SCI (2). Hospital length of stay, cost, and incidence of pressure ulceration may be less than in patients not admitted early to such a system (14,52). "Coordinated systems of care that integrate treatment from the site of injury through long-term community follow-up are needed for mitigating the short-term effects of SCI and TBI and for reducing long-term disability" (47).

Hospital Length of Stay

This has decreased over time. In 1974, the average hospital length of stay was 149.6 days for tetraplegia and 122.3 days for paraplegia; in 1989 the figures had decreased to 92.4 and 74.9 days, respectively (15).

MEDICAL ISSUES

Neurologic Assessment and Classification

Introduction

Accurate neurologic assessment is required for proper management and prognostication. Standards have been developed by ASIA and endorsed by the International Society of Paraplegia (IMSOP) (1,19). The neurologic assessment is made entirely by physical examination; radiographic and other information does not contribute.

Tetraplegia (which is preferred to *quadriplegia*) refers to impairment of spinal cord function affecting the cervical or first thoracic segments; thus, function in all four extremities can be abnormal. *Paraplegia* refers to impairment of spinal cord function in the thoracic, lumbar, or sacral segments, but not the cervical and first thoracic segments; thus arm function is spared. The term can also be applied to other injuries occurring within the spinal canal, such as cauda equina injuries.

Sensory Examination

A key point is defined for 28 sensory levels, from C2 most rostrally through S4-5 (which are considered together) most caudally (Table 1, Fig. 1). Each point is assessed for pin sense, reflecting ventral tracts, and light touch, reflecting dorsal tracts. Sense is rated for each mo-

TABLE 1. *Key sensory points*

C2	Occipital protuberance
C3	Supraclavicular fossa
C4	Top of the acromioclavicular joint
C5	Lateral side of the antecubital fossa
C6	Thumb
C7	Middle finger
C8	Little finger
T1	Medial (ulnar) side of the antecubital fossa
T2	Apex of the axilla
T3	Third intercostal space (IS)
T4	Fourth IS (nipple line)
T5	Fifth IS (midway between T4 and T6)
T6	Sixth IS (level of xiphisternum)
T7	Seventh IS (midway between T6 and T8)
T8	Eighth IS (midway between T6 and T10)
T9	Ninth IS (midway between T8 and T10)
T10	Tenth IS (umbilicus)
T11	Eleventh IS (midway between T10 and T12)
T12	Inguinal ligament at mid-point
L1	Half the distance between T12 and L2
L2	Mid-anterior thigh
L3	Medial femoral condyle
L4	Medial malleolus
L5	Dorsum of the foot at the third metatarsal phalangeal joint
S1	Lateral heel
S2	Popliteal fossa in the midline
S3	Ischial tuberosity
S4–5	Perianal area (taken as one level)

From ref. 1.

dality as 2 (normal), 1 (impaired), or 0 (absent); if the pin is sensed as a touch without sharpness, the score is 0. The lower extremities may be assessed for proprioceptive sense. The perianal area must be examined for pin or touch sense, and rectal examination should be performed to detect deep rectal sensation.

Motor Examination

A key muscle is assigned for roots C5 through T1 and for L2 through S1 (Table 2). Each muscle is tested according to a six-point scale, scored 0 through 5. The score for each of the 20 muscles tested can be summed to give a total motor score, with a maximum score of 100. The motor score of the lower-extremity muscles can be considered alone in assessing the prognosis for ambulation; the maximum lower-extremity motor score is 50.

Level

The neurologic level is the most caudal level of the spinal cord with normal motor and sensory function. Levels can also be assigned for each side of the body and for motor and sensory function. Reflexes are not used in determining the level. Assigning a motor level is compli-

cated because most or all of the key muscles receive innervation from more than one root. For example, weakness in the triceps, which is the key muscle for the C7 root, does not necessarily indicate dysfunction of that root, because the triceps also receives innervation from C8. By convention, a root level may be considered normal if the key muscle is scored at least 3, provided that the next most rostral muscle is intact.

ASIA Impairment Scale

The ASIA impairment scale provides a description of the completeness of injury (Fig. 2). It evolved from the classic scale of Frankel et al. (23). Five grades, A through E, from most severe to least severe, are defined. An ASIA impairment scale grade of A refers to a complete lesion, without any sparing of sacral sensation or voluntary activity of the anal sphincter. A grade of B refers to sparing of sensation, including the sacral segments, but no sparing of motor function. A grade of C refers to sparing of motor activity, with the majority of the key muscles below the level of injury having a strength score of less than 3 out of 5. A grade of D refers to sparing of motor activity, with at least half of the key muscles below the level of injury scoring at least 3 out of 5. A grade of E refers to normal motor and sensory function.

Prognosis for Neurologic Recovery

Neurologic improvement can be assessed by change in the ASIA impairment scale grade and by change in level.

Prognosis Based on ASIA Impairment Scale Grade

Data for patients admitted to Model Systems centers within 24 hours are presented in Table 3. Admission and discharge grades are provided. A decline in grade is unusual. Improvement from a grade of A (complete) to a grade of D (preserved motor—functional) is also unusual. Overall, 27.6% of patients admitted with a grade of B (incomplete—preserved sensory) improved to D, as did 53.3% of those admitted with a grade of C (preserved motor—nonfunctional) (17). Prognostication is thus most difficult for those admitted with an ASIA grade of B or C. Other factors noted below can assist prognostication in these cases.

Prognosis for Change in Level

Generalization concerning a change in level is difficult with existing data. The question is most important for those admitted with a level of C4, C5, or C6 (the three most common admission levels) and discharged with

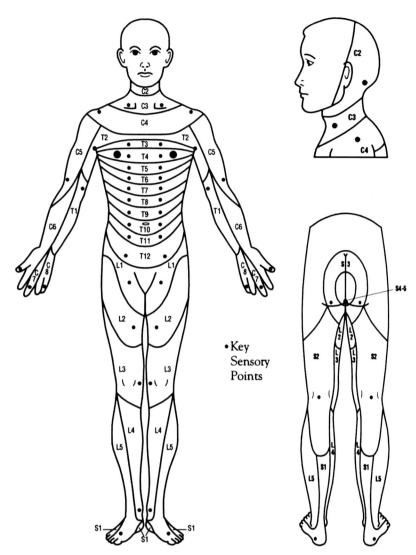

• Key
Sensory
Points

FIG. 1. Key sensory points (1).

motor complete (ASIA A and B) grades. It appears that these patients gain a motor level by the time of discharge. The sensory level (and thus the single neurologic level) usually does not change (17). For patients with cervical injuries, a change in motor level usually allows a significant improvement in function.

Prognosis Based on Other Factors

Preservation of pin sensation below the level of injury indicates a good prognosis for ambulation in those admitted with an ASIA grade of B (incomplete—preserved sensation); absence of pin sensation below the level of

TABLE 2. *Key muscles for levels C5 through T1 and L2 through S1*

C5	Elbow flexors (biceps, brachialis)
C6	Wrist extensors (extensor carpi radialis longus and brevis)
C7	Elbow extensors (triceps)
C8	Finger flexors (flexor digitorum profundus to the middle finger)
T1	Small finger abductors (abductor digiti minimi)
L2	Hip flexors (iliopsoas)
L3	Knee extensors (quadriceps)
L4	Ankle dorsiflexors (tibialis anterior)
L5	Long toe extensors (extensor hallucis longus)
S1	Ankle plantar flexors (gastrocnemius, soleus)

From ref. 1.

ASIA IMPAIRMENT SCALE

☐ **A = Complete:** No motor or sensory function is preserved in the sacral segments S4-S5.

☐ **B = Incomplete:** Sensory but not motor function is preserved below the neurological level and extends through the sacral segments S4-S5.

☐ **C = Incomplete:** Motor function is preserved below the neurological level, and the majority of key muscles below the neurological level have a muscle grade less than 3.

☐ **D = Incomplete:** Motor function is preserved below the neurological level, and the majority of key muscles below the neurological level have a muscle grade greater than or equal to 3.

☐ **E = Normal:** Motor and sensory function is normal.

FIG. 2. ASIA Impairment Scale (with permission from ref. 1).

injury in these patients indicates a poor prognosis for recovery (12). This may be due to the proximity of the motor tracts to the sensory tracts for pain sensation. Recovery of knee extensor function to greater than 3/5 strength on at least one side at 2 months indicates an excellent prognosis for ambulation in those admitted with an ASIA grade of C (11). Prognosis for ambulation is excellent for patients with the central cord pattern of injury if they are younger than 50; for those older than 50, the prognosis is much less certain (46). Patients with incomplete injuries and lower-extremity motor scores of 10 or above at 1 month are likely to ambulate with crutches and orthoses (57,58).

Aspects of Respiratory Management

Pathophysiology of Respiration After Traumatic SCI

The diaphragm, a muscle of inspiration, is innervated rostral to other muscles of respiration, such as the intercostals and abdominals, and may provide adequate ventilation by itself. However, loss of the muscles of active expiration, in particular the abdominals, may leave the patient with decreased vital capacity (the maximum volume that can be expired after a maximum inspiration) and weak or absent cough. Atelectasis, pneumonia,

ventilatory failure, and other problems can result, and some complication is likely in victims of more serious SCI (34). The left lung may be particularly vulnerable because of difficulty aspirating the left mainstem bronchus (21).

Early Interventions

Mobilization of secretions is critical. Medicinal and physical measures are employed. Medicinal measures include agents to thin secretions (guaifenisin, acetylcysteine, antibiotics when indicated) and agents to dilate airways (albuterol, aminophylline). Physical measures include "quad coughing," chest physical therapy, and suctioning (by bronchoscopy if necessary) (8).

Exercises to strengthen the diaphragm and accessory muscles should begin when tolerated. Incentive spirometry may be used. Later, placement of weights upon the abdomen for limited periods during supine breathing may provide further strengthening.

Patients lacking muscles of expiration may be assisted by an elastic abdominal binder, which is stretched as the diaphragm descends, and then recoils, providing a modest increase in expiratory force. Such patients may also breathe more easily while supine, as the abdominal contents are compressed when the diaphragm descends, and then provide a small increase in expiratory force when the diaphragm relaxes. These patients may develop ventilatory problems when taken from supine to sitting because of a decrease in vital capacity.

Ventilator Weaning

Ventilator weaning of tetraplegics appears best accomplished by serial trials off the ventilator rather than by intermittent mandatory ventilation (8,65). Brief periods free of the ventilator are begun while under constant supervision, with monitoring by pulse oximeter. The vital capacity is determined before and after weaning. If the patient remains clinically stable and the post-wean vital capacity remains within 25% of the pre-wean value, the weaning time is advanced.

TABLE 3. Admission and discharge ASIA impairment grades for patients admitted within 24 hours of injury, by percent[a]

Admission ASIA impairment grade	Discharge ASIA impairment grade				
	A	B	C	D	E
A	88.8	5.0	2.9	2.8	0
B	4.9	48.9	15.6	27.6	0.7
C	1.9	0.8	41.4	53.3	1.3
D	0.5	0.5	0.8	90.3	6.5

[a] Rows do not add to 100% because of unknown cases. (14).

Patients requiring a prolonged period for weaning may also benefit from the use of a cuffless tracheostomy tube. This allows air to pass over the vocal cords so that the patient can talk. Long-term complications of a cuffed tracheostomy tube may also be avoided.

Deep Venous Thrombosis and Pulmonary Embolus

Importance

Surveillance for and prophylaxis against deep venous thrombosis (DVT) and pulmonary embolus (PE) are among the most crucial medical issues after traumatic SCI. The reported incidence of these problems varies according to the surveillance method used; the incidence of DVT in the first 2 weeks may exceed 50% in cases of ASIA A, B, and C injuries (42). Recently, an incidence of over 80% was reported (25). PE is the third most frequent cause of death in the first year after injury; traumatic SCI increases the risk of dying from PE in the subsequent year by a factor of 210 (16).

Pathophysiology

Paralysis of lower-extremity muscles leads to a decreased pumping effect upon the lower-extremity venous system, causing venous stasis. Stasis is exacerbated by venous dilatation. A hypercoagulable state has also been demonstrated. A prophylactic regimen directed against both stasis and hypercoagulability may be preferable to a regimen targeted against only one of the factors (42).

Screening

Physical examination of the legs should be performed daily, and may reveal evidence of DVT. However, physical examination for DVT is neither sensitive nor specific. The high incidence of DVT shortly after SCI suggests that supplemental noninvasive testing, such as duplex ultrasonography, should be performed. It is reasonable to perform such studies weekly for the first 3 weeks after SCI and when otherwise clinically indicated, such as for evaluation of an edematous leg or in search of the source of a fever. Sensitivity is greater in patients with clinical signs (61).

Prophylaxis

There is no standard prophylactic regimen. An approach opposing both stasis and hypercoagulability may be the most effective. Compression boots applied during the first 2 weeks combat stasis; low-dose subcutaneous heparin or a low-molecular-weight heparin can combat hypercoagulability. Heparin should be continued for 3 months after injury (28).

Autonomic Hyperreflexia

Clinical Presentation

The combination of paroxysmal hypertension and agonizing headache is characteristic of autonomic hyperreflexia. The syndrome arises in patients with a spinal cord lesion above T6. If an episode does not abate, a variety of complications can result, including intracerebral hemorrhage, seizures, cardiac arrhythmias, and death (9).

Pathophysiology

An episode is triggered by a noxious stimulus originating below the level of injury. The stimulus elicits sympathetic activity within the spinal cord below the level. This causes responses including vasoconstriction and sweating, which are unmodified by supraspinal centers because of the spinal cord lesion. If the vasoconstriction includes the splanchnic bed (innervated by approximately T6 to L2), then hypertension and secondary headache result. If the splanchnic bed is not fully involved, then the vasoconstriction is usually not sufficient to cause hypertension; thus the syndrome is rare in those with lesions at T6 and below.

Acute Management

Acute management involves lowering the blood pressure and removing the inciting stimulus.

Generally, the patient should be placed sitting upright with the legs lowered to reduce intracranial blood pressure as much as possible. If medication is required, nifedipine 10 mg, sublingually or by "bite and swallow," may be effective, as are sublingual nitroglycerin, nitroglycerin ointment, or inhaled amyl nitrate. Other medications used during hypertensive emergencies may also be effective, with the exception of beta blockers, which should be avoided.

While the hypertension is being directly treated, a search is carried out for the responsible stimulus. A distended bladder is most commonly the cause, and placing or replacing a bladder catheter is a reasonable intervention in cases that do not respond promptly. Placement of anesthetic ointment on the catheter tip may provide protection against worsening the episode through catheter placement. Numerous other stimuli, including urologic procedures, bowel distention, urinary tract stones, ingrown toenails, and even sexual activity, can cause autonomic hyperreflexia. Occasionally, episodes are recurrent and investigation does not reveal a cause.

Prophylaxis

Proper management of bowel, bladder, skin, and extremities can prevent inciting stimuli. Several medications can be useful in prophylaxis of episodes, including ganglionic blockers such as mecamylamine, sympatholytics such as guanethidine, and alpha-blockers such as terazosin.

Reflex Sweating

Sweating, which is mediated by the sympathetic system, may occasionally be profuse in patients with SCI, in the absence of other signs of autonomic hyperreflexia. This can be severe enough to pose a cosmetic or medical problem. The responsible neurotransmitter is acetylcholine, and agents such as transdermal scopolamine are useful in prophylaxis (54).

Neurogenic Bladder

Pathophysiology

Bladder dysfunction after SCI is a complex problem that causes significant morbidity. Whatever the dysfunction, urine may drain from the bladder, but may do so in a manner that causes infection and renal injury.

A complete lower motor neuron injury (the bladder outflow is at chiefly S2-4) results in a flaccid, areflexic bladder. This type of bladder can fill to an abnormally high volume. At some point, urine will begin to leak in small amounts, frequently, and particularly with increases in intra-abdominal pressure, such as occur with coughing or straining. The post-void residual urine volume is elevated.

A complete upper motor neuron injury in the spinal cord can be followed by a prolonged period of bladder flaccidity. When local bladder and sphincter reflexes return, they will oppose each other because the center for coordinating bladder and sphincter function is located within the brainstem, and is isolated from the urinary tract by the SCI. This is termed *bladder-sphincter dyssynergia* (18). Voiding will be at unnaturally high intravesical pressure, which predisposes to complications (41).

Evaluation

Physical examination for sacral sensation and voluntary activity of the anal sphincter provides information about bladder and sphincter sensation and control. The anal wink and bulbocavernosus reflexes can provide information about the integrity of local reflex arcs. Measurement of the post-void residual urine volume (by catheterization or ultrasound) reflects the adequacy of bladder emptying. Urodynamic study provides the most detailed information, and in particular can measure the intravesical pressure required for bladder emptying.

Urinary Tract Complications

Urinary tract infection is among the most common complications of chronic SCI (10). Soft-tissue injury can be caused by drainage devices such as indwelling catheters and external collecting devices. Urinary tract stones can occur. High intravesical voiding pressures can lead to bladder changes and vesicoureteral reflux (Figs. 3 and 4).

Management

The goal of management is to establish a method of bladder drainage that is practical for the patient and that will minimize complications. Definitive management is usually determined during the rehabilitation phase of care. Management during the acute phase after injury can be by indwelling catheter.

Patients with adequate hand function can perform long-term intermittent catheterization. This involves limiting fluid intake and performing self-catheterization at regular intervals so that incontinence and bladder

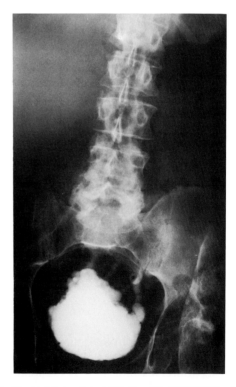

FIG. 3. Cystogram of a patient with paraplegia, showing multiple diverticula of the bladder wall.

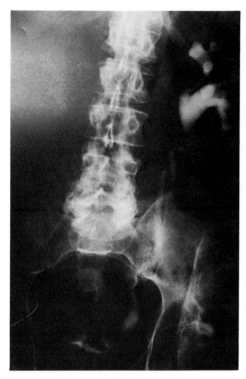

FIG. 4. Cystogram of a patient with paraplegia, showing reflux of contrast into the left ureter and renal pelvis.

overdistention are avoided. Reflex bladder contractions that cause incontinence can be treated with oxybutynin.

Men who cannot perform intermittent self-catheterization can often void by reflex into an external collecting device. The voiding may be under high pressure because of bladder-sphincter dyssynergia, and this can lead to problems over the long term (41). Voiding pressure can possibly be moderated by medications to decrease activity of the sphincters; if these are not effective, urologic surgery can defeat the sphincters and produce low-pressure voiding.

Women unable to perform intermittent self-catheterization can use an indwelling catheter on a chronic basis. This can lead to various complications, however. If adequate support is available, intermittent catheterization can be performed by others.

The frequency of problems related to the urinary tract makes regular surveillance appropriate. One protocol includes an annual cystogram to screen for stones, vesicoureteral reflux, and bladder changes, and an annual renal scan to evaluate renal function.

Heterotopic Ossification

Definition

Heterotopic ossification (HO) is the formation of new bone about a joint (or joints) in a person who has suffered traumatic SCI (or traumatic brain injury, or other neurologic damage). The pathophysiology is not known (22).

Clinical Presentation and Importance

The presentation varies. It typically develops in the months after SCI, most commonly about the hip, and does not occur in joints unaffected by the SCI. It may be an incidental finding on radiographs taken for some other cause and have no clinical significance. It can present as an edematous leg, and thus is included in the differential diagnosis of an edematous leg in a patient with SCI; it can be confused with (and can coexist with) problems such as DVT. It can present as loss of range of motion, often noted first by a therapist. This is clinically relevant as it impairs extremity function; severe cases progress to fusion.

Laboratory Findings

Radiographs can demonstrate HO; however, early in the course these may be negative, whereas triple-phase bone scanning is positive (Fig. 5). Serum alkaline phosphatase may be elevated.

Management

Goals of management include minimizing the amount of bone mass that forms and maintaining range of motion.

Disodium etidronate, nonsteroidal anti-inflammatory medications (NSAIDs), and irradiation have been used to minimize the amount of bone mass that forms. Disodium etidronate is administered in a dose of 20 mg/kg/day (given between meals) for 2 weeks, followed by 10 mg/kg/day for a period of 3 months or longer. Flaring of HO upon withdrawal of disodium etidronate has been observed; the risk of this may be minimized by prolongation of treatment and by tapering. Indomethacin and other NSAIDs are also thought helpful in minimizing bone mass formation. In severe cases, irradiation may be useful. None of these interventions are helpful after HO has matured; they are best used early in the course.

Range of motion is maintained by exercise and surgery. Despite concern that range-of-motion exercises might exacerbate HO, such exercises should be performed, and improve outcome. If range of motion becomes severely restricted, surgery can be performed to remove a wedge of bone, with the defect functioning as a crude joint (Fig. 6). Surgery must be deferred until the bone mass is judged to be mature (on the basis of stable radiographs and normal alkaline phosphatase). This may take more than 2 years. The surgery itself can be

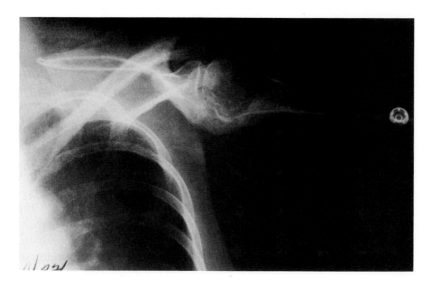

FIG. 5. Heterotopic ossification bridging the shoulder joint in a patient with quadriplegia.

difficult, with severe bleeding, and postoperative recurrence can occur (56).

Pressure Ulceration

Definition and Pathophysiology

A pressure ulcer occurs when necrosis of skin and other tissue has been caused by pressure. The pressure prevents normal capillary blood flow, and the resulting ischemia causes tissue death. Shear frequently contributes to the problem. Sitting at an angle in bed causes shear, as the sacrum is pulled inferiorly by gravity while the skin overlying the sacrum is fixed against the bed. The resulting tension between the sacrum and the tissues overlying it distorts blood vessels, causing tissue ischemia and an ulcer (49).

Clinical Importance

Pressure ulceration is one of the most frequent causes of morbidity after SCI (66). Specialized centers report an incidence of about 32% during acute care. Pressure ulceration can dramatically affect functional status; for example, a person with a deep ischial pressure ulcer should eliminate sitting. Pressure ulcers also contribute to mortality caused by septicemia.

Prophylaxis

Pressure ulcers develop from the application of pressure over a period of time; lesser pressures can be tolerated for greater time periods, and greater time periods can be tolerated with lesser pressures (36). Prophylaxis involves decreasing either the pressure or the time period over which pressure is applied (44). The former strategy is that used by specialized mattresses; the latter strategy

is used by rotating beds and alternating pressure mattresses. All patients suffering acute SCI should be nursed on a specialized bed or mattress to prevent pressure ulceration.

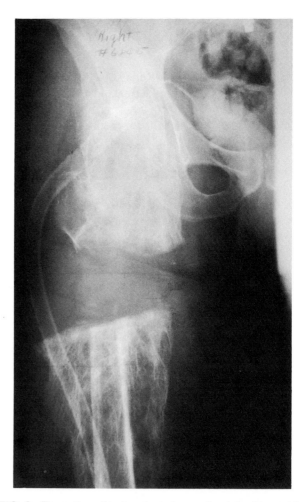

FIG. 6. Resection of heterotopic bone about the hip and femur of a patient with paraplegia.

Treatment

Treatment may include elimination of pressure, debridement, maintenance of an appropriate moisture level in the wound environment, control of infection, and surgery.

Pressure is decreased or eliminated by positioning and by specialized surfaces. A patient with a sacral ulcer should be positioned prone or side-lying. Specialized matresses include foam, static air, alternating air, gel, and water matresses (44). Foam, air, and gel wheelchair cushions are also available.

Debridement can be performed with scissors or scalpel. Occasionally, adherent necrotic tissue is difficult to debride with instruments, and chemical debridement with collagenase can be substituted.

Wounds may heal best in a moist rather than dry environment. Thus, occlusive or semiocclusive dressings may be preferable to gauze. Gauze is still appropriate for wounds that produce heavy secretions.

Topical antiseptics may slow healing and should be avoided in wounds that are not grossly infected. Topical antibiotics may control infection without inhibiting healing.

Some wounds require surgical closure, usually by myocutaneous flap. Surgical closure is usually required with ulcers that involve bone and with deep ischial ulcers. Several weeks of immobilization are required after surgery before sitting is allowed (18,66).

Morbidity and Mortality

Morbidity

SCI strongly predisposes a person to urinary tract infection and pressure ulceration, and a majority of patients experience these problems at some point (18). Other difficulties can also occur, including upper-extremity musculoskeletal syndromes from overuse, upper-extremity nerve entrapment syndromes, pneumonia, cholelithiasis, renal deterioration, urinary tract stones, pressure ulceration, osteoporosis with pathologic fracture, and ingrown toenails. Diagnosis can be delayed because SCI results in a lack of sensation of the problem by the patient.

Mortality

Death was the rule in cases of complete SCI before World War II, often due to infection from pressure sores or urinary tract infection (18). Death from renal failure (related to infection, problems with urinary tract drainage, and secondary amyloidosis caused by chronic infection) was also common. Outcome has improved, and life expectancy during the first 12 years after SCI is now 88%

of normal (13,15). Elderly people suffering severe SCI still do poorly. There has been some shift in the causes of death over time, with death due to renal failure becoming less frequent and causes of death becoming more similar to those of the general population (16).

The most common causes of death after traumatic SCI (for patients surviving more than 24 hours) are pneumonia and other respiratory diseases, followed by heart disease, then septicemia, then pulmonary embolus (16). Death from septicemia is commonly secondary to urinary tract infection, pressure ulceration, or pneumonia. If deaths occurring during the first year after traumatic SCI are considered, pneumonia and other pulmonary diseases remain most common, followed by heart disease and then pulmonary embolus.

Traumatic SCI particularly increases the risk of death due to septicemia, multiplying it by a factor of 64.2 above normal. The risk of death due to pulmonary embolus is increased by a factor of 47.1, and that due to pneumonia and other lung disease is increased by a factor of 40.1. If the first year after injury is considered, the risk of death from pulmonary embolus is found to increase by a factor of 210.

FUNCTIONAL ISSUES

Major Functional Areas of Concern

Function after SCI can be divided into aspects of mobility and self-care.

Bed mobility involves turning and sitting up on a bed or mat. Transfers involve changing from one surface to another; for example moving from sitting to standing. Other transfers include bed to wheelchair, wheelchair to automobile, floor to wheelchair, wheelchair to commode, wheelchair to tub, etc. Locomotion involves moving along a surface; thus traversing a room, whether by walking or by wheelchair, is an example of locomotion, as is management of stairs.

Self-care activities (also referred to as activities of daily living) include eating, grooming, bathing, dressing, toileting, and managing bowel and bladder function.

Evaluation of Functional Performance

Several scales are available for measuring functional capacity. The Functional Independence Measure (FIM) is the most widely used scale after SCI (Fig. 7).

The first factor considered by the FIM in assessing performance of an activity is whether the presence of another person is required; if not, then the score is 7 or 6, depending upon the necessity of using adaptive equipment. If the presence of another person is required, then the score is anywhere from 5 to 1, depending upon the relative contribution of the assisting person. The FIM

Functional Independence Measure (FIM)

L	7	Complete Independence (Timely, Safely)	No
E	6	Modified Independence (Device)	Helper
V		**Modified Dependence**	
E	5	Supervision	
L	4	Minimal Assist (Subject = 75%+)	
S	3	Moderate Assist (Subject = 50%+)	Helper
		Complete Dependence	
	2	Maximal Assist (Subject = 25%+)	
	1	Total Assist (Subject = 0%+)	

	ADMIT	DISCH
Self Care		
A. Eating	☐	☐
B. Grooming	☐	☐
C. Bathing	☐	☐
D. Dressing-Upper Body	☐	☐
E. Dressing-Lower Body	☐	☐
F. Toileting	☐	☐
Sphincter Control		
G. Bladder Management	☐	☐
H. Bowel Management	☐	☐
Mobility		
Transfer:		
I. Bed, Chair, Wheelchair	☐	☐
J. Toilet	☐	☐
K. Tub, Shower	☐	☐
Locomotion	W☐	W☐
L. Walk/wheelChair	C☐	C☐
M. Stairs	☐	☐
Communication	A☐	A☐
N. Comprehension	V☐	V☐
O. Expression	V☐	V☐
	N☐	N☐
Social Cognition		
P. Social Interaction	☐	☐
Q. Problem Solving	☐	☐
R. Memory	☐	☐
Total FIM	☐	☐

NOTE: Leave no blanks; enter 1 if patient not testable due to risk.

FIG. 7. Functional Independence Measure (1).

section involving communication and that involving social cognition may not be directly affected by SCI.

General Approach to Improving Function

This section surveys five aspects of fostering functional improvement. All are typically involved in rehabilitation after SCI. Examples are given without any attempt at comprehensiveness.

Maintenance of Range of Motion

Maintenance of joint range of motion is critical, as contractures can lessen extremity function as much as the loss of strength and sensation. Range is preserved by the regular performance of range-of-motion exercises and by the use of positioning devices. Wrist-hand splints,

for example, can prevent the development of contractures in patients with spasticity of the wrist and finger flexors; high-top sneakers or ankle splints can prevent the development of ankle plantar flexion contractures. Adequate hip and ankle range of motion is required for paraplegic standing. This is because the paraplegic stabilizes the hip joint by maintaining the body's center of gravity posterior to the joint, thereby using the force of gravity to lock the joint against the anterior ligaments about the hip. Such a posture is impossible in the presence of hip flexion or ankle plantar flexion contractures.

Increasing Strength

Muscular strength can improve by at least three mechanisms after SCI. A damaged motor neuron (upper or lower) can recover; a healthy lower motor neuron can take over denervated muscle fibers by peripheral sprouting; and muscle fibers in healthy motor units can hypertrophy through exercise. The last mechanism is the only one directly accessible to rehabilitation. Vigorous exercise should be used only with muscles that have greater than 3/5 strength; otherwise damage may occur. Spasticity can have either a beneficial or negative effect upon muscular strength; some patients are able to utilize spasticity whereas others are impaired by it. Thus, treatment of spasticity must be individualized.

Functional Retraining

Functional retraining involves teaching a patient to perform a task with a less than normal neuromuscular apparatus. Typically, the upper extremities are required to make up for lost lower-extremity function in activities such as transfers. Certain "tricks" can allow one muscle group to substitute for another. For example, if the hand is planted on a supporting surface, the elbow flexors can act as extensors. The wrist extensors can cause passive finger flexion, adequate for grasp, by passively tightening the finger flexors, in a person with, for example, C6 tetraplegia. This mechanism works better if the finger flexors have been allowed to shorten. In this situation, preservation of normal range of motion of the finger flexors may be detrimental.

Adaptive Equipment

If a patient lacks an adequate neuromuscular apparatus to perform a task, adaptive equipment may allow performance of the task without the assistance of another person. For example, a person with control of the shoulder and elbow but lacking control of the hand (as in tetraplegia with a level of C7) may use a splint to hold devices such as a toothbrush, eating utensil, or writing instrument. Bed rails may assist such a person with bed mobility, a transfer board with transfers, and a wheelchair with locomotion.

Family Training

If a patient cannot perform a task despite retraining and the use of adaptive equipment, then others must assist with the task. "Family training" usually occurs during the final period of inpatient rehabilitation.

Functional Improvement in the Acute Phase

Interventions to facilitate functional improvement should begin as soon as the patient enters the intensive care unit. Positioning devices should be used to prevent the development of ankle plantar flexion contractures and wrist contractures. Range-of-motion exercises can maintain other joints. The diaphragm can be strengthened by breathing exercises. These interventions can be applied by the nurse, physical therapist, and occupational therapist, who should be advised of any precautions. For example, shoulder range-of-motion exercises may be contraindicated by cervical instability, and hip exercises may be contraindicated by lumbar instability; DVT may contraindicate lower-extremity range-of-motion exercises.

Expected Functional Level According to Neurologic Level

Functional outcome depends upon many factors. Expected outcomes for selected levels for young patients with motor complete injuries are given in Table 4. There is less information correlating functional outcomes with ASIA motor scores. A total lower-extremity motor score of 30 or greater (out of the possible 50) corresponds to the ability to ambulate in the community (59).

Ambulation is regarded as one of the most important functional goals after SCI. However, though many paraplegic patients with levels above L2 are able to walk using equipment, the gait is too laborious to be functional, and most use a wheelchair. Gait training is beneficial for only a minority of such patients, who walk for exercise, or in selected situations.

Functional Electrical Stimulation

Electric current applied to paralyzed muscle can produce contraction. If several muscles are stimulated in a pattern, it is possible for them to perform a desired motor activity, either for exercise or for the performance of a task. This is functional electrical stimulation (FES). Because denervated muscle requires higher levels of stimu-

TABLE 4. *Typical functional outcomes for selected levels for young patients with motor complete spinal cord injuries (45).*

Motor level	Mobility	Self-care
C4	Independent in sip-and-puff or chin-controlled power wheelchair with power recliner May operate voice-controlled power bed Otherwise dependent	Drinks with long straw after setup
C7	Independent bed-to-chair transfers Independent in manual wheelchair in accessible environment Independent driving adapted vehicle	Independent dressing and bathing with equipment Independent management of bowel and bladder
T2–T10	Independent in manual wheelchair in accessible environment Ambulation, for exercise only, may be possible using knee-ankle-foot orthoses and walker	Independent
L3–S1	Independent ambulation in the community with ankle-foot orthoses and canes	Independent

lation, FES is used only with upper motor neuron paralysis (60). Though FES has been applied to the upper extremities after SCI (43), most work has been done with lower-extremity FES (35,40,60).

Paralyzed lower extremities can be stimulated so as to pedal a stationary "bicycle" apparatus. An exercise program using this mechanism can unquestionably improve the response of the paralyzed muscles to stimulation and produces other, more clinically relevant, effects, including cardiovascular conditioning and moderation of spasticity. Systems are commercially available for this, but are expensive and require the same degree of commitment as any long-term exercise program.

FES has been applied by various systems to achieve walking and standing. The systems vary in several ways. Some use orthoses and FES in combination ("hybrid" systems). Stimulating electrodes can be placed either externally or internally, or can be percutaneous. Control can be either open-loop, in which stimulation is applied according to a preset pattern, or closed-loop, in which a sensor detects, for example, joint position, and uses this to moderate stimulation. Food and Drug Administration approval and commercial funding may increase experience with the Parastep system, which provides stability in stance by stimulation of the quadriceps and provides swing by stimulation of the peroneal nerve (which elicits a flexor withdrawal response that brings about swing phase). Stimulation is controlled by a trigger in the handle of a walker.

Reconstructive Surgery of the Upper Extremity

Tetraplegic patients with stable neurologic status and adequate joint range of motion may be candidates for reconstructive surgery to improve upper-extremity function (38). They must be prepared to tolerate a decreased level of function during the postoperative period of immobilization. The major aims of the procedures are to provide active elbow extension and active grasp. Such procedures are not available for the lower extremity.

A tetraplegic person with a level of C5 or C6 may have excellent control of the shoulder and strong elbow flexion. However, if the arm is raised above the shoulder, the lack of active elbow extension causes the elbow to collapse; the hand falls and may strike the person in the face. This can be solved by using tendon to attach the posterior deltoid to the triceps.

A tetraplegic person with a level of C6 or C7 may have strong wrist extension but only weak or absent grasp. Stronger grasp can be provided by transfer of an available muscle, such as extensor carpi radialis longus, into the flexor digitorum profundus. Lateral key pinch of the thumb against the index finger can be provided by a tendon transfer to flexor pollicis longus; the interphalangeal joint of the thumb must be stabilized by fusion.

PSYCHOSOCIAL ISSUES

Adjustment

Long-Term Adjustment

Four recent reviews summarized research on long-term adjustment after traumatic SCI (18,24,45,48). Depression is definitely not universal, and quality of life and life satisfaction may remain good. Approximately 75% of persons who were spinal cord-injured for more than 20 years reported good or excellent quality of life (64). Adjustment appears to correlate less with the severity of injury than with other factors such as social integration, which is fortunate because the latter are more easily affected by the system of care. Even very severe injury is compatible with positive long-term life satisfaction and well-being (3).

Suicide

Although adjustment after traumatic SCI is better than might be expected, studies consistently find higher rates of suicide among those spinal cord-injured than among the general population (24). There is no clear correlation with severity of injury, though this finding is difficult to interpret because those more severely injured may be physically incapable of suicide. Suicide is more common in the early years after SCI than during later years. Health maintenance requires active participation after traumatic SCI, and some may passively commit suicide by allowing the development of pressure sores, pulmonary problems, and other complications.

Methodologic Issues

Depression, quality of life, and life satisfaction are used in evaluating adjustment. Measures of early adjustment may be affected by the acute medical status, by undiagnosed mild head injury, and by lack of realization of the severity or permanence of the injury. Measures of late adjustment may be affected by the culling effect of time; depressed patients may tend to die sooner, from suicide and other causes, and thus not be proportionally represented in a population of long-term survivors. Observers are unreliable in judging the adjustment of victims of traumatic SCI and tend to underestimate (3).

Marriage

Data are available reflecting the rates of marriage and divorce after traumatic SCI; the latter can be subdivided into rates of divorce for marriages occurring before and after traumatic SCI (24). The data are often contradictory and comparisons with figures for the general population are difficult to interpret, as those suffering traumatic SCI may not be a random subgroup of the general population. Traumatic SCI is followed by a lower rate of marriage than is seen in the general population. Persons with intact marriages at the time of traumatic SCI have a rate of divorce that is greater than that of the general population; however, a majority married at the time of injury are still married 5 years later. Data are contradictory regarding the relative durability of marriages occurring before traumatic SCI compared with those occurring after traumatic SCI.

Employment

A majority of victims of traumatic SCI are employed at the time of injury. This rate falls precipitously in the years immediately following traumatic SCI, but gradually increases to peak approximately 10 years after traumatic SCI, when nearly one-third are employed. The chance of employment correlates inversely with severity of injury and age at the time of injury; it correlates directly with pre-injury education and vocational experience (20).

Sexuality

Sexual Function in Men

Sexuality remains an important area of concern in men after traumatic SCI; in one study, subjects rated it more important than life areas such as employment, social life, and housing (63). The majority of men with upper motor neuron injury achieve reflex erections (but not psychogenic erections); these erections may or may not be sufficient for sexual activity. Ejaculation is very uncommon with complete upper motor neuron injury. Patients with complete cauda equina injury may retain the ability to have psychogenic erection, and some can ejaculate (51).

Sexual Function in Women

Sexual function after traumatic SCI is less studied in women than in men. This is probably due to the smaller number of women compared with men and the greater difficulty of studying female sexual response. Lubrication may parallel erection in the male, and uterine and vaginal contraction may parallel ejaculation (7).

Management of Erectile Dysfunction

A variety of interventions are available to augment erectile function after traumatic SCI. Implanted prostheses are generally not used because of the risk of erosion of the device through the penis. Injection of medication directly into the penis, such as prostaglandin E1, or the use of a vacuum tumescence device appears safer (7,32,40).

Sexual Satisfaction

Levels of sexual activity and sexual satisfaction decrease after traumatic SCI (7,63). However, sensations akin to those of orgasm can continue after traumatic SCI (52), and many subjects (and their partners) consider their sexual life to be satisfactory (37,50).

Fertility

Male Fertility

In the absence of intervention, complete traumatic SCI almost always results in male infertility. This is due to a combination of poor sperm quality and difficulty producing sperm. However, electroejaculation and other techniques have proven capable of producing sperm that can be used for artificial insemination (7,31). Repeated electroejaculation may improve sperm quality.

Female Fertility

Traumatic SCI is followed by a period of amenorrhea, but menses and fertility typically return. Pregnancy predisposes to problems such as pressure ulceration and urinary tract infection, and labor may not be detected by the patient because of lack of sensation. Thus, close observation is required as the pregnancy advances. Labor can be accompanied by autonomic hyperreflexia. Data suggest that patients with traumatic SCI can function effectively as parents (62).

Residence

The vast majority—over 90%—of victims of traumatic SCI who are discharged from rehabilitation enter private residences in the community (24). The risk of disposition to a nursing home correlates directly with age and severity of injury. As time from injury increases, the percentage living in the community increases slightly and the percentage residing in a nursing home declines.

ACKNOWLEDGMENTS

This manuscript was supported in part by awards from the National Institute on Disability and Rehabilitation Research to the Regional Spinal Cord Injury Center of Delaware Valley (G008535135) and the National Rehabilitation Research and Training Center in Spinal Cord Injury (H133B80017).

REFERENCES

1. American Spinal Injury Association, International Medical Society of Paraplegia (1992): *International standards for neurological and functional classification of spinal cord injury—revised 1992.* Chicago: American Spinal Injury Association.
2. Apple DF Jr, Hudson LM, eds (1990): *Spinal cord injury: The model. Proceedings of the national consensus conference on catastrophic illness and injury.* December 1989. Atlanta: The Georgia Regional Spinal Cord Injury Care System, Shepherd Center for Treatment of Spinal Injuries, Inc.
3. Bach JR, Tilton MC (1994): Life satisfaction and well-being measures in ventilator assisted individuals with traumatic tetraplegia. *Arch Phys Med Rehabil* 75:626–632.
4. Bracken MB, Shepard MJ, Collins WF Jr, et al. (1990): A randomized, controlled trial of methylprednisolone or naloxone in the treatment of acute spinal-cord injury. *N Engl J Med* 322:1405–1411.
5. Bracken MB, Shepard MJ, Collins WF Jr, et al. (1992): Methylprednisolone or naloxone treatment after acute spinal cord injury: 1-year follow-up data. *J Neurosurg* 76:23–31.
6. Bracken MB (1993): Pharmacological treatment of acute spinal cord injury: Current status and future prospects. *J Emerg Med* 11:43–48.

7. Cardenas DD, Farrell-Roberts L, Sipski M, Rubner D (1995): Management of gastrointestinal, genitourinary, and sexual function. In: Stover SL, Whiteneck G, DeLisa J, eds. *Model spinal cord injury systems: Two decades of managed care.* Gaithesburg, MD: Aspen Publishers, pp. 120–144.

8. Cohn JR (1993): Pulmonary management of the patient with spinal cord injury. *Traum Q* 9:65–71.

9. Colachis SC III (1992): Autonomic hyperreflexia with spinal cord injury. *J Am Paraplegia Soc* 15:171–186.

10. Consensus Panel of the Urinary Tract Infection Consensus Conference (1992): The prevention and management of urinary tract infections among people with spinal cord injuries. *J Am Paraplegia Soc* 15:194–207.

11. Crozier KS, Cheng LL, Graziani V, Zorn G, Herbison G, Ditunno JF Jr (1992): Spinal cord injury: Prognosis for ambulation based on quadriceps recovery. *Paraplegia* 30:762–767.

12. Crozier KS, Graziani V, Ditunno JF Jr, Herbison GJ (1991): Spinal cord injury: Prognosis for ambulation based on sensory examination in patients who are initially motor complete. *Arch Phys Med Rehabil* 72:119–121.

13. DeVivo MJ, Black KJ, Stover SL (1993): Causes of death during the first 12 years after spinal cord injury. *Arch Phys Med Rehabil* 74:248–254.

14. DeVivo MJ, Kartus PL, Stover SL, Fine PR (1990): Benefits of early admission to an organised spinal cord injury care system. *Paraplegia* 28:545–555.

15. DeVivo MJ, Richards JS, Stover SL, Go BK (1991): Spinal cord injury: Rehabilitation adds life to years. *West J Med* 154:602–606.

16. DeVivo MJ, Stover SL (1995): Long-term survival and causes of death. In: Stover SL, Whiteneck G, DeLisa J, eds. *Model spinal cord injury systems: Two decades of managed care.* Gaithesburg, MD: Aspen Publishers, pp. 289–310.

17. Ditunno JF Jr, Cohen ME, Formal C, Whiteneck G (in press): Functional outcomes. In: Stover SL, Whiteneck G, DeLisa J, eds. *Model spinal cord injury systems: Two decades of managed care.* Gaithesburg, MD: Aspen Publishers, pp. 170–184.

18. Ditunno JF Jr, Formal CS (1994): Chronic spinal cord injury. *N Engl J Med* 330:550–556.

19. Ditunno JF Jr, Young W, Donovan WH, Creasey G (1994): The international standards booklet for neurological and functional classification of spinal cord injury. *Paraplegia* 32:70–80.

20. Donovan WH (1994): Operative and nonoperative management of spinal cord injury. A review. *Paraplegia* 32:375–388.

21. Fishburn MJ, Marino RJ, Ditunno JF Jr (1990): Atelectasis and pneumonia in acute spinal cord injury. *Arch Phys Med Rehabil* 71:197–200.

22. Formal C (1992): Metabolic and neurologic changes after spinal cord injury. *Phys Med Rehabil Clin North Am* 3:783–795.

23. Frankel HL, Hancock DO, Hyslop G, et al. (1969): The value of postural reduction in the initial management of closed injuries of the spine with paraplegia and tetraplegia. *Paraplegia* 7:179–192.

24. Gans BM, Gordon WA (1995): The aftermath of spinal cord injury. In: Stover SL, Whiteneck G, DeLisa J, eds. *Model spinal cord injury systems: Two decades of managed care.* Gaithesburg, MD: Aspen Publishers, pp. 185–212.

25. Geerts WH, Code KI, Jay RM, Chen E, Szalai JP (1995): A prospective study of venous thromboembolism after major trauma. *N Engl J Med* 331:1601–1606.

26. Geisler FH, Dorsey FC, Coleman WP (1991): Recovery of motor function after spinal-cord injury—A randomized, placebo controlled trial with GM-1 ganglioside. *N Engl J Med* 324:1829–1838.

27. Geisler FH (1993): GM-1 ganglioside and motor recovery following human spinal cord injury. *J Emerg Med* 11:49–55.

28. Green D, Hull RD, Mammen EF, Merli GJ, Weingarden SI, Yao JST (1992): Deep vein thrombosis in spinal cord injury. Summary and recommendations. *Chest* 102:633S–635S.

29. Guttmann L (1976): *Spinal cord injuries: Comprehensive management and research,* 2nd ed. London: Blackwell Scientific Publications.

30. Hanson AM (1927): Management of gunshot wounds of the head and spine in forward hospital, American expeditionary forces. In: Ireland MW, ed. *The medical department of the United States Army in the world war.* Washington, DC: Government Printing Office, 11:776–794.

31. Hirsch IH, Seager SWJ, Sedor J, King L, Staas WE Jr (1990): Electroejaculatory stimulation of a quadriplegic man resulting in pregnancy. *Arch Phys Med Rehabil* 71:54–57.

32. Hirsch IH, Smith RL, Chancellor MB, Bagley DH, Carsello J, Staas WE Jr (1994): Use of intracavernous injection of prostaglandin E1 for neuropathic erectile dysfunction. *Paraplegia* 32:661–664.

33. Hughes JT (1988): The Edwin Smith surgical papyrus: An analysis of the first case reports of spinal cord injuries. *Paraplegia* 26:71–82.

34. Jackson AB, Groomes TE (1994): Incidence of respiratory complications following spinal cord injury. *Arch Phys Med Rehabil* 75:270–275.

35. Jaeger RJ (1992): Lower extremity applications of functional neuromuscular stimulation. *Assist Technol* 4:19–30.

36. Kosiak M (1961): Etiology of decubitus ulcers. *Arch Phys Med Rehabil* 42:19–29.

37. Kreuter M, Sullivan M, Siösteen A (1994): Sexual adjustment after spinal cord injury (sci) focusing on partner experiences. *Paraplegia* 28:225–235.

38. Lamb DW (1991): Reconstructive surgery for the upper limb and hand in traumatic tetraplegia. In: Lee BY, Ostrander LE, Cochran GVB, Shaw WW, eds. *The spinal cord injured patient, comprehensive management.* Philadelphia: W.B. Saunders, pp. 231–243.

39. Linsenmeyer TA (1991): Evaluation and treatment of erectile dysfunction following spinal cord injury: A review. *J Am Paraplegia Soc* 14:43–51.

40. Marsolais EB, Kobetic R, Chizeck HJ, Jacobs JL (1991): Orthoses and electrical stimulation for walking in complete paraplegia. *J Neurol Rehab* 5:13–22.

41. McGuire EJ, Woodside JR, Borden TA, Weiss RM (1981): The prognostic significance of urodynamic testing in myelodysplastic patients. *J Urol* 126:205–209.

42. Merli GJ, Crabbe S, Palluzzi RG, Fritz D (1993): Etiology, incidence, and prevention of deep vein thrombosis in acute spinal cord injury. *Arch Phys Med Rehabil* 74:1199–1205.

43. Mulcahey MJ, Smith BT, Betz RR, Triolo RJ, Peckham PH (1994): Functional neuromuscular stimulation: Outcomes in young people with tetraplegia. *J Am Paraplegia Soc* 17:20–35.

44. Panel for the Prediction and Prevention of Pressure Ulcers in Adults (1992): *Pressure ulcers in adults: Prediction and prevention. Clinical practice guideline, number 3, AHCPR publication no. 92-0047.* Rockville, Maryland: Agency for Health Care Policy and Research, Public Health Service, U.S. Department of Health and Human Services.

45. Patterson DR, Miller-Perrin C, McCormick TR, Hudson LD (1993): When life support is questioned early in the care of patients with cervical level quadriplegia. *N Engl J Med* 328:506–509.

46. Penrod LE, Hegde SK, Ditunno JF Jr (1990): Age effect on prognosis for functional recovery in acute, traumatic central cord syndrome. *Arch Phys Med Rehabil* 71:963–968.

47. Pope AM, Tarlov AR, eds (1991): *Disability in America: Toward a national agenda for prevention.* Washington, DC: National Academy Press.

48. Ragnarsson KT, Gordon WA (1992): Rehabilitation after spinal cord injury. The team approach. *Phys Med Rehabil Clin North Am* 3:853–878.

49. Reichel SM (1958): Shearing force as a factor in decubitus ulcer in paraplegics. *JAMA* 166:762–763.

50. Siösteen A, Lundqvist C, Blomstrand C, Sullivan L, Sullivan M (1990): Sexual ability, activity, attitudes and satisfaction as part of adjustment in spinal cord-injured subjects. *Paraplegia* 28:285–295.

51. Sipski ML (1991): Spinal cord injury: What is the effect on sexual response. *J Am Paraplegia Soc* 14:40–43.

52. Staas WE Jr, Ditunno JF Jr (1991): A system of spinal cord injury care. *Phys Med Rehabil Clin North Am* 3:893–902.

53. Staas WE Jr, Formal CS, Gershkoff AM, et al. (1993): Rehabilitation of the spinal cord-injured patient. In: DeLisa JA, Gans BM, eds. *Rehabilitation medicine: Principles and practice,* 2nd ed. Philadelphia: J.B. Lippincott, pp. 886–915.

54. Staas WE Jr, Nemunaitis G (1989): Management of reflex sweating in spinal cord injured patients. *Arch Phys Med Rehabil* 70:544–546.

55. Stover SL, Fine PR, eds (1986): *Spinal cord injury: The facts and figures.* Birmingham, Alabama: The University of Alabama at Birmingham.

56. Stover S, Niemann KMW, Tulloss JR (1991): Experience with surgical resection of heterotopic bone in spinal cord injury patients. *Clin Orthop* 263:71–77.

57. Waters RL, Adkins RH, Yakura JS, Sie I (1994): Motor and sensory recovery following incomplete paraplegia. *Arch Phys Med Rehabil* 75:67–72.

58. Waters RL, Adkins RH, Yakura JS, Sie I (1994): Motor and sensory recovery following incomplete tetraplegia. *Arch Phys Med Rehabil* 75:306–311.

59. Waters RL, Adkins R, Yakura J, Vigil D (1994): Prediction of ambulatory performance based on motor scores derived from standards of the American Spinal Injury Association. *Arch Phys Med Rehabil* 75:756–760.

60. Weber RJ (1993): Functional neuromuscular stimulation. In: DeLisa JA, Gans BM, eds. *Rehabilitation medicine: Principles and practice,* 2nd ed. Philadelphia: J.B. Lippincott, pp. 886–915.

61. Weinmann EE, Salzman EW (1994): Deep-vein thrombosis. *N Engl J Med* 331:1630–1641.

62. Westgren N, Levi R (1994): Motherhood after traumatic spinal cord injury. *Paraplegia* 32:517–523.

63. White MJ, Rintala DH, Hart KA, Young ME, Fuhrer MJ (1992): Sexual activities, concerns, and interests in men with spinal cord injury. *Am J Phys Med Rehabil* 71:225–231.

64. Whiteneck GG, Charlifue SW, Frankel HL, et al. (1992): Mortality, morbidity, and psychosocial outcomes of persons spinal cord injured more than 20 years ago. *Paraplegia* 30:617–630.

65. Wicks AB (1989): Ventilator weaning. In: Whiteneck G, Lammertse DP, Manley S, Menter R, eds. *The management of high quadriplegia.* New York: Demos Publications, pp. 141–147.

66. Yarkony GM, Heinemann AW (1995): Pressure ulcers. In: Stover SL, Whiteneck G, DeLisa J, eds. *Model spinal cord injury systems: Two decades of managed care.* Gaithesburg, MD: Aspen Publishers, pp. 100–119.

Spinal Neoplasms and
Vascular Malformations

The Adult Spine: Principles and Practice,
2nd edition, J.W. Frymoyer, Editor-in-Chief.
Lippincott-Raven Publishers, Philadelphia © 1997.

CHAPTER 48

Differential Diagnosis and Surgical Treatment of Primary Benign and Malignant Neoplasms

Stefano Boriani and James N. Weinstein

The diagnosis and treatment of primary spine tumors have evolved dramatically over the past 3 decades. Significant improvements in both the short- and long-term outcomes have been obtained by extending to these le-

S. Boriani, M.D.: Modulo Di Chirurgia Vertebrale, 5ᵃ Divisione, Instituto Ortopedico Rizzoli Institute, Bologna 40136, Italy.

J. N. Weinstein, D.O., M.S.: Division of Orthopedics and Neurosurgery, Senior Faculty Member, Center for Clinical Evaluative Sciences, Dartmouth Medical School, Dartmouth Hitchcock Medical Center, Hanover, NH 03755.

sions the same criteria adopted for limb tumors (e.g., the application of an oncologic staging system), by careful surgical planning (requiring a specific preoperative work-up), and by using various adjuvant therapies (chemotherapy, radiation therapy, cryotherapy, selective arterial embolization). The tremendous progress in radiologic imaging techniques has made careful preoperative planning possible for newer surgical techniques. Despite these technologic advancements, there has been no uniform approach to the diagnosis and treatment in these patients and little uniformity in reporting outcome. This makes comparison of treatment protocols difficult and conclusions regarding definitive management somewhat tenuous. In all patients afflicted by a primary bone tumor of the spine, surgical treatment (sometimes correctly associated with adjuvants) now offers a reasonable likelihood of functional improvement and pain relief, and in selected cases, cure of the disease can be expected. Some primary tumors, however (e.g., aneurysmal bone cyst or plasmacytoma), rarely require surgery and must be submitted to a careful cost/benefit evaluation as to the difficulty and possible risk of a surgical procedure versus an effective nonsurgical treatment.

Because of the opportunity to provide patients with such significant improvements, it is more imperative than ever that the treating physician appreciate the symptoms and characteristics of spinal neoplasias, and that the principles of tumor staging and management be followed closely whenever such a lesion is suspected. The correct approach should include: (a) complete clinical and imaging work-up before biopsy; (b) the correct biopsy technique; (c) appropriate surgical, medical, and possible adjuvant treatment according to the tumor oncologic stage and the patient's overall conditions; (d) surgery planned according to a standardized surgical staging of the tumor extent; (e) maximum effort to preserve neurologic function; and (f) maintenance of spinal column stability. Although the treatment of patients with spine tumors must be individualized, specific principles should be observed for managing tumors in general and for specific tumor types in order to meet these goals.

SPINAL NEOPLASMS IN GENERAL

Neoplastic disease of the spine may arise from local lesions developing within or adjacent to the spinal column or from distant malignancies spreading to the spine or paraspinous tissues by hematogenous or lymphatic routes. Local involvement of the spine may result from primary tumors of bone, primary lesions arising in the spinal cord or its coverings, or contiguous spread of tumors of the paraspinous soft tissues and lymphatics. Regional or distant spread of metastatic disease to the spine may occur with almost any of the solid tumors of the body, with osseous malignancies of the appendicular skeleton, and with systemic lymphoreticular malignancies such as multiple myeloma and lymphoma. The likelihood that any one of these tumors will account for any given lesion depends on intrinsic patient-related and tumor-related characteristics. Understanding these relationships allows the surgeon faced with an unknown spinal lesion to formulate a useful differential diagnosis and appropriately direct subsequent examinations. Such a directed approach allows the physician to quickly establish a definitive diagnosis and treatment plan.

Epidemiology

Although both metastatic and primary tumors can be found in all age groups and at all levels of the spinal column, metastatic tumors are far more common than primary lesions (see Chapter 49). Metastatic carcinoma accounts for skeletal lesions in 40 times as many patients as are affected by all other forms of bone cancer combined. It has been estimated that between 50% and 70% of patients with carcinoma will develop skeletal metastases before death, and this number may be as high as 85% for women with breast carcinoma (50). Primary tumors of the spine are very rare, and for the most part their relative incidence reflects that of the skeleton in general. Certain tumors (chordoma, osteoblastoma) do show a predilection for the spinal column, but these still make up a very small proportion of all spinal tumors. This chapter addresses primary tumors of the spine. However, in many instances, information regarding metastatic spine tumors is applicable, and in those instances the crossover will be mentioned briefly.

Presentation

The interval between the onset of symptoms and presentation to the physician has both diagnostic and prognostic significance. Although tumors of the spinal column may remain asymptomatic for some time, when symptoms do develop, they are usually a consequence of one or more of the following: (a) expansion of the cortex of the vertebral body by tumor mass, with fracture and invasion of paravertebral soft tissues; (b) compression or invasion of adjacent nerve roots; (c) pathologic fracture due to vertebral destruction; (d) development of spinal instability; and/or (e) compression of the spinal cord. Obviously, rapidly progressive symptoms of pain or neurologic compromise will be associated with the more malignant, rapidly destructive tumors, whereas patients who present with symptoms that have progressed slowly over the years will typically have slowly growing tumors with a better long-term prognosis. The caveat to this point is that slowly growing, locally aggressive tumors that might be easily managed in the extremities may prove inexorable and lethal when extensively established in the spine.

Patient's Age

The age of the patient at diagnosis is an important prognosticator, in that age is highly correlated with malignancy in both primary and metastatic disease. The relationship between age and metastatic disease is well known, as most carcinomas demonstrate a peak incidence in the fourth, fifth, and sixth decades of life. Systemic diseases such as myeloma and lymphoma are also predominant in the fifth and sixth decades of life. Primary spinal neoplasms also show a strong correlation between age and malignancy, though the breakpoint is somewhat lower. In patients older than 21 years of age, more than 70% of primary tumors will prove to be malignant, whereas benign lesions produce the majority of lesions in patients less than 21 years. Clearly, in a patient presenting in middle age with an undiagnosed lesion of the spine, the suspicion of malignancy must be very high (113).

Location

Location of the lesion within the vertebra is another important prognosticator for benign or malignant disease. The majority of malignant tumors, both primary and metastatic, will originate anteriorly, involving the vertebral body and possibly one or both pedicles. Strictly posterior localization, even when more than one level is involved, is far more typical of benign lesions.

DIAGNOSIS

In a review of 82 primary neoplasms of the spine, pain and weakness were the most common presenting complaints (Table 1) (113); pain was present in nearly 85% of these patients, including 20% who reported radicular symptoms. At the time of initial evaluation, more than 40% of patients had subjective complaints of weakness; objective neurologic deficits could be identified in 35% of patients with benign tumors and 55% of patients with malignancies. A palpable mass was detectable in only 16% of patients. The series of 323 primary tumors of the spine treated at Rizzoli Institute has been specifically reviewed; 40 cases of primary malignant tumors (46%) and 18 cases of benign (7.6%) tumors presented with cord or cauda compression, provoking complete or incomplete

TABLE 1. *Patterns of presenting symptoms*

Presenting symptom	Number	Percent
Back pain	25	30.5
Radicular pain	8	9.75
Weakness	7	8.5
Back pain and weakness	15	18.3
Radicular pain and weakness	8	9.75
Mass	4	4.9
Pain and mass	9	11.0
Pain, weakness, and bowel and bladder dysfunction	4	4.9
Asymptomatic	2	2.4
Total	82	100

paralysis. A palpable mass was observed in 47% of primary malignant tumors and in only 6% of benign (aneurysmal bone cyst and exostosis). The clinical presentation usually provides clues that alert the physician to the presence of a spinal neoplasm.

Symptoms

The most consistent complaint of patients affected by spine tumor is pain. Although back pain is an exceedingly common and nonspecific complaint, pain associated with neoplasia tends to be progressive and unrelenting, and does not have the association with activity as seen with mechanical back pain. Pain at night is particularly worrisome. Pain symptoms may localize to a specific spinal segment and may be reproduced by pressure or percussion over the involved segment. Radicular symptoms are less common but are frequently seen in patients with cervical or lumbar involvement. Radicular pain in the thoracic region may result in "girdle" pain, forming a belt of dysesthesias and paresthesias circumferentially from the level of vertebral involvement.

Pain usually arises from one of several causes. Local tumor growth will produce expansion of the cortex of the vertebral body, resulting initially in thinning and remodeling of the cortex and later in pathologic fracture and invasion of paravertebral soft tissues. As the cortex expands, the overlying periosteum is distorted and stretched, stimulating pain receptors in that tissue. Local extension of tumor tissue from a paravertebral mass or following fracture may produce compression of adjacent nerve roots, resulting in radicular symptoms of pain or paresthesias. Pathologic fracture may result from the extensive bone loss associated with vertebral body destruction, producing acute pain symptoms similar to those seen in traumatic compression fractures and frequently leading to the development of spinal instability. Finally, in any case, pain may be associated with acute or slow compression of the spinal cord, resulting in focal and radicular symptoms of pain, paraparesis, or paraplegia (37). Radicular symptoms similar to those seen with a herniated nucleus pulposus may be caused by either benign or malignant spine tumors, leading to confusion in diagnosis and treatment. Sim et al. (96) reviewed 38 cases of bone tumors simulating lumbar disc herniation and 23 patients with lumbar or sacral neoplasms. He noted that the pain associated with these lesions was usually unremitting and progressive and was not relieved by rest or recumbency. Spinal deformity may also be associated with the onset of pain, and usually results from paraspinous muscular spasm. Scoliosis is frequently associated with osteoid osteoma (51) (sometimes with osteoblastoma) and typically presents with localized nightly paravertebral pain, paravertebral muscle spasm, and limitation of motion (1). The onset of such a scoliosis may be rapid. The tumor is usually found on the concave side of the deformity and usually at the apex of the curve (54). Although these deformities usually disappear after tumor excision, curves neglected for prolonged periods will become structural. The bone scan is highly sensitive to foci consistent with osteoid osteoma and can significantly improve the efficiency of treatment by providing an earlier diagnosis and accurate localization of the tumor (13,111).

Neurologic deficits can be fairly common in patients presenting with spinal tumors; they are seen most often in rapidly expanding malignant lesions, but any slowly progressive, expansile neoplasm may produce a deficit if left alone long enough. Weakness, usually in the lower extremities, may become apparent months or years after the onset of pain and is rarely the first symptom seen. Nonetheless, as many as 70% of patients will manifest clinical weakness by the time the correct diagnosis is made. This should emphasize the importance of maintaining a high index of suspicion when following patients with persistent back or radicular pain, and particularly those with a history of systemic malignancies (98). Bowel and bladder dysfunction may develop before diagnosis in as many as half of patients with cord compression. Patients with compression at the level of the conus medullaris may present with isolated sphincter dysfunction, but it is far more common to see associated lower-extremity impairments. The neurologic assessment in these patients must be thorough and should include an evaluation of bladder function if any deficits are suspected.

Imaging Techniques

Plain Films

Plain roentgenograms should be obtained in any case when a neoplasm is suspected. Anteroposterior (AP) and lateral views of the involved vertebra can provide considerable information about the nature and behavior of the lesion and may be sufficient to identify some characteristic tumor types. Even when the specific tumor type is not identified, the benign or malignant nature of the lesion may be deduced from the pattern of bony destruction. Geographic patterns of bone destruction suggest a slowly expanding lesion, typically benign, whereas more rapidly growing tumors produce a moth-eaten appearance, and highly malignant, aggressive lesions produce a permeative pattern of destruction (58). Early on, however, a vertebral lesion may be difficult to detect, as radiographic evidence of bone destruction is not apparent until between 30% and 50% of the trabecular bone has been destroyed. The most classic early sign of vertebral

involvement is the "winking owl" sign seen on the AP view. The loss of the pedicle ring unilaterally results from destruction of the cortex of the pedicle, usually by the tumor invading from the vertebral body proper. Vertebral collapse secondary to erosion of bone by the tumor is another common radiographic finding. A pathologic compression fracture may be difficult to differentiate from a traumatic injury, particularly in patients with osteoporosis, but a periosteal reaction that seems too old for the acute trauma, or the presence of a soft-tissue mass or soft-tissue calcifications, should alert the physician to obtain more definitive diagnostic tests. Distinguishing neoplastic vertebral destruction from that of pyogenic osteomyelitis may also prove difficult; the differential diagnosis is based on the preservation of the intervertebral disc in patients with neoplasms. The disc is highly resistant to tumor invasion and will usually maintain its height even after extensive collapse of the vertebral body. In the presence of infection, the disc is frequently destroyed along with the adjacent vertebral body.

Bone Scan

A sensitive test for neoplastic disease of the spine is the 99m technetium bone scan. Technetium scans are sensitive to any area of increased osteoid formation and will detect lesions as small as 2 mm, whether in trabecular or cortical bone, provided there is some osteoblastic response in the surrounding bone. When an isolated lesion is detected by scintigraphy, the differential diagnosis must include fracture, infection, neoplasm, or local soft-tissue inflammation, and further evaluation with plain films or tomography is necessary to make a diagnosis. Although scans have a high incidence of false-positive findings, their sensitivity makes them a valuable tool in assessing symptomatic patients with negative or equivocal radiographs or in determining the extent of dissemination in those patients with systemic disease (16,111). Although bone scans lack specificity, patterns of uptake showing multiple areas of skeletal involvement are virtually diagnostic for metastatic disease in the patient with a known primary malignancy. In patients in whom a primary malignancy has not been identified, such a pattern is still very suggestive and will enable the surgeon to choose the most accessible lesion for biopsy. One should remember, however, that even in patients with a known malignancy, a solitary abnormality on bone scan may prove falsely positive in one third of all cases. The most common source of false-positive scans is osteoarthritis, frequently present in the older population, most commonly seen with metastatic disease (19). Finally, the observation that some neoplastic conditions (e.g., myeloma or chordoma) frequently do not provoke any uptake can be useful in the process of differential diagnosis.

Computed Tomography Imaging

Computed tomography (CT) scanning offers improved sensitivity in the detection of spinal neoplasms. CT has proven highly sensitive to alterations in bone mineralization and is able to demonstrate neoplastic involvement far more reliably than plain radiographs. Lesions may be visualized at an earlier time in their development, before extensive bony destruction or intramedullary extension has occurred and before cortical erosion has progressed to the point of impending fracture. For surgical staging and planning, CT often remains the most helpful imaging device (7,11,112,113,115).

Myelography

Once the only reliable way to assess spinal cord and nerve root compression, myelography has now given way to magnetic resonance imaging (MRI) in most cases. In combination with CT, however, it remains extremely helpful in detecting cord compression due to fracture and bony soft-tissue impingement. It can be less precise in the presence of stainless-steel devices producing metal artifacts (scatter), thus preventing early detection of recurrences. Myelography with a water-soluble contrast agent also provides some dynamic information. A complete block on myelography often conclusively demonstrates pressure on the neural structures, evidence that can only be inferred from MRI. Cerebrospinal fluid can be removed at the time of examination and may be submitted for cytologic examination and determination of protein and glucose levels. There are drawbacks to myelography. The procedure is invasive and uncomfortable, and can lead to unpleasant and, rarely, devastating complications. In cases of complete myelographic block, a second injection of contrast may be necessary to demonstrate the proximal extent of the tumor.

Magnetic Resonance Imaging

MRI has proven useful in evaluating a variety of spinal diseases and is well tolerated, noninvasive, and safe. The ability to quantify tumor growth in T2-weighted images, the superior soft-tissue detail provided, and the ability to obtain multiplanar images enhance the diagnostic and treatment-planning capabilities of the surgeon considerably. MRI often provides better delineation than CT of soft-tissue tumor extension and adherence or invasion of paravertebral structures. Direct sagittal and coronal images are for some lesions superior to current reconstructions available through CT, and unlike CT, MRI is able to depict the spinal cord without the aid of intrathecal contrast material.

Biopsy Techniques

Once a biopsy incision has been made, there are very few choices left in planning the definitive tumor removal. When the surgeon selects an approach for biopsy, he or she is often committed to that approach from there on. For instance, if a posterolateral incision has been made for the biopsy, tumor excision must be completed through that incision, and the incision excised with the tumor; it would not be possible to switch to a posterior approach for the definitive excision without violating the principles of good tumor surgical technique (11,64). The importance of a carefully planned biopsy cannot be overemphasized. To date, the issues of biopsy and tumor surgery of the spine have been ignored. The hazards of biopsy seen in musculoskeletal tumors of the extremities may be even more apparent in the axial skeleton. The incidence of inadequate or inappropriate extremity biopsy that significantly alters a patient's care is greater than one in three overall (64), and this may be even higher in lesions of the spine. This risk can be reduced significantly when the biopsy is performed by the treating, rather than the referring physician.

Three traditional forms of spinal biopsy are available to the surgeon: excisional, incisional, and needle biopsy. On occasion, a posteriorly located lesion may prove suitable for an excisional biopsy, but most lesions of the spinal column require the incisional or needle biopsy technique. Needle biopsies are subject to sampling errors and provide small specimens for evaluation; better results can be achieved by trocar under CT scan control (Fig. 1). The primary role of needle or trocar biopsy is confirmation of metastatic disease, of recurrence of a known lesion, or of sarcomatous histology in an otherwise classic clinicoradiologic presentation of osteosarcoma (71). Culture results may also be obtained to rule out infection. When the differential diagnosis is narrow and limited to lesions that are easily distinguished histologically, a needle biopsy may be ideal. In more complex lesions and those with a more subtle differential diagnosis, the specimen obtained will most often prove inadequate (98). The incisional biopsy should be the last step in staging the patient, performed just before the definitive surgical resection. Both procedures may be performed under the same anesthetic if proper preoperative staging has been completed and the frozen section provides a clear diagnosis. The surgical technique used during biopsy influences both the yield of the procedure and the risk of postoperative complications.

A number of basic principles should be observed when performing the biopsy. The biopsy incision should be placed so that it may be excised with the tumor during the definitive procedure. Unlike limb tumors, this has not been the standard for spine tumor surgery. Transverse incisions and flaps should be avoided; the tu-

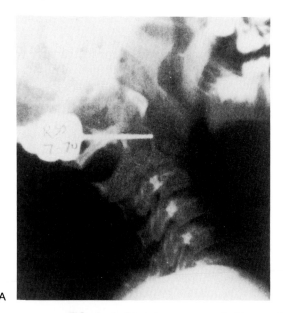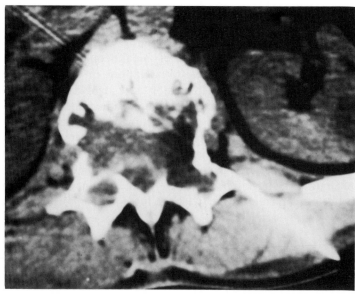

A
B

FIG. 1. A: Percutaneous needle biopsy of C2 osteoblastoma. **B:** CT scan-directed trocar biopsy of L1 giant cell tumor.

mor should be approached in the most direct manner possible. Tissues should be handled carefully, and hemostasis should be meticulous. Bone should not be removed or windowed unless absolutely necessary. Bleeding from exposed bone or from uncauterized vessels and injured muscle will form a postoperative hematoma that may carry tumor cells beyond the margins of the intended excision and contaminate tissues far proximal or distal to the primary lesion. As in limb surgery, tissue contaminated during the biopsy or by hematoma must be excised if surgical control is expected. Even a moderate-sized hematoma may make this impractical

(98). Once the tumor is exposed, an adequate sample of tissue must be obtained.

The specimen obtained should be large enough to allow histologic and ultrastructural analysis as well as immunologic stains. The margin of the soft-tissue mass is often the most helpful to biopsy, as central portions are frequently necrotic. The surgeon should take care not to crush or distort the specimen, so as to maintain its architecture. If a soft-tissue component exists, a frozen section should be obtained. Finally, if the definitive excision is to follow the biopsy under the same anesthetic, it is essential that all instruments used during the biopsy be dis-

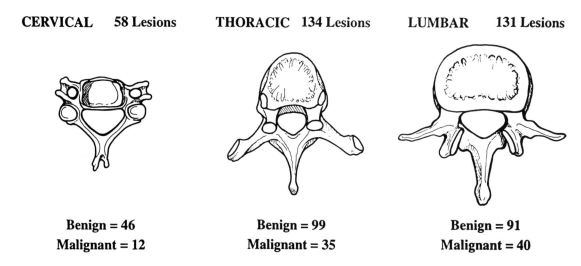

FIG. 2. Primary spine tumors by location (series from Rizzoli Institute).

carded. The field should be redraped, and the surgeons should change gowns and gloves before the excision is begun. If fusion is planned, bone graft should be taken through a separate incision using a separate surgical setup.

There are times when biopsies are not indicated for primary spine tumors. Radiographic and other staging procedures often allow the surgeon to perform the definitive surgical procedure at one sitting (e.g., in the case of osteoid osteoma). In many cases, this avoids the many hazards of biopsy and at the same time enhances the opportunity for employing good tumor surgery principles.

PRIMARY TUMORS OF THE SPINE

Primary tumors arising in the spine are uncommon. Review of 323 primary neoplasms of the spine seen over a 50-year period at Rizzoli Institute identified 236 benign and 87 malignant lesions, representing 13 benign and 5 malignant tumor types (Fig. 2). Plasmacytoma and lymphomas were excluded. Malignant tumors arose almost

exclusively from the body (85%), whereas the prevalence of benign tumors from the body dropped to 70%. Of the benign tumors, 58.7% arose in the first 2 decades of life, versus 27.6% of malignant neoplasms. The review by Bohlman et al. (4) of 23 patients with primary neoplasms of the cervical spine also showed a marked difference in tumor type with patient age. In that series, all patients less than 21 years old had benign tumors, whereas 10 of 14 (71%) patients over age 21 had a malignancy. Five-year survival was reported as 86% in patients with benign tumors and 24% in patients with malignancies (113).

BENIGN TUMORS

Osteochondroma (Exostosis)

Multiple osteochondromatosis is the most common of the skeletal dysplasias. Exostosis, either single or multiple, is among the most common lesions of bone (12,63,76). Vertebral involvement occurs in approximately 7% of these patients, but neurologic compromise

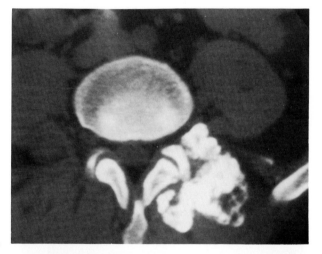

A

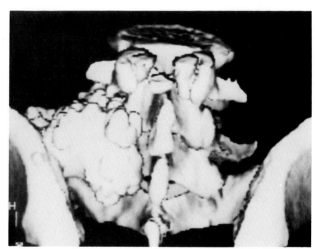

B

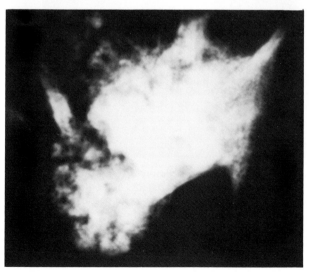

C

FIG. 3. CT scan **(A)** and three-dimensional CT scan **(B)** of osteochondroma arising from the transverse process of L5. **C:** Radiogram of the resected specimen.

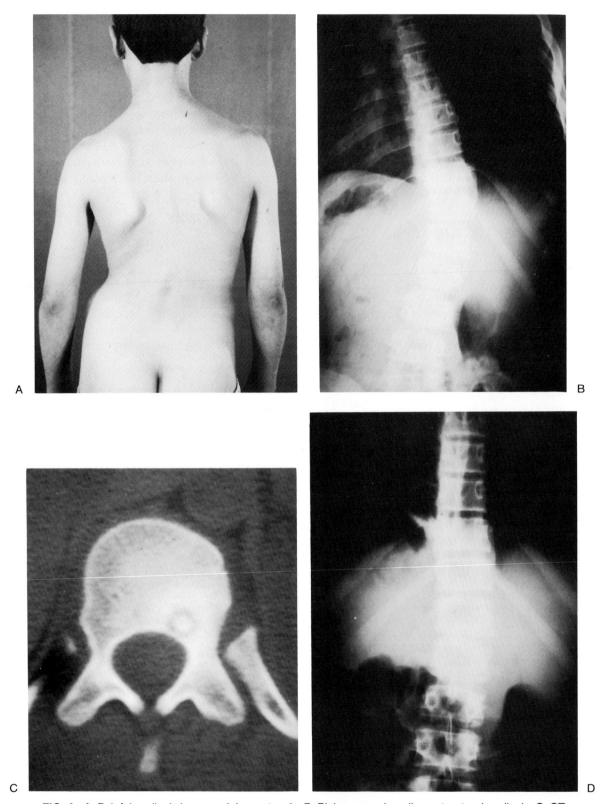

FIG. 4. A: Painful scoliosis in a preadolescent male. **B:** Plain x-rays describe a structural scoliosis. **C:** CT scan (performed at the level of isotope scan "hot point") shows a typical aspect of osteoid osteoma with the cancellous bone of the T10 body. **D:** After tumor excision, the patient had complete relief of the pain, and the scoliosis almost completely disappeared.

is rarely seen (60). When symptoms of cord compression do occur, routine imaging studies may not be adequate. Tomography will outline the bony lesion and establish its point of origin, but the radiolucent cartilage cap, which causes the compressive symptoms, may not be visualized without CT, myelography, or MRI. Sixteen cases of osteochondroma have been reported with symptomatic cord compression. More than 60% of lesions arose in the cervical spine, and another 19% arose in the thoracic spine at or above the T6 level (15,52,63,97). Although 14 patients (88%) experienced good neurologic recovery after decompression, the other two died because of cervical cord compression and respiratory failure. One of these experienced sudden death from an odontoid lesion, and the other manifested symptoms of compression months before dying from C1 compression by a lesion of the foramen magnum. Because of the very slow progression of the compressive cord lesion, excision of the tumor provides excellent recovery of neurologic function. The rate of recurrence is related to the oncologic stage, evaluated grossly by the depth of the cartilaginous cap. Exostosis is generally included in stage 1 (latent) or 2 (active) lesions and therefore can be submitted to piecemeal excision. Larger tumors can sometimes include areas diagnosed subsequently by the pathologist as grade 1 chondrosarcoma. These cases should be resected en bloc (Fig. 3).

Osteoblastoma and Osteoid Osteoma

Osteoblastoma and osteoid osteoma are osteoblastic lesions differentiated primarily by size. These benign lesions show a propensity for spinal involvement, usually involving the posterior elements. In one review of 36 patients with osteoid osteoma, nine cases (25%) occurred in the spine, all located in the posterior elements (54).

Forty-seven osteoid osteomas of the spine were observed at Rizzoli Institute among 465 cases observed in 50 years; 30% of them were located in the vertebral body. Osteoblastoma shows an even greater propensity for the spine. In a review of 197 osteoblastomas, Marsh et al. (65) noted that 41% were located in the spine and that these lesions always originated in the posterior elements. In our series of 28 cases (30% of the osteoblastomas observed at Rizzoli Institute), 25% arose from the vertebral body, mostly asymmetrically. Patients usually present in their second or third decade of life, and the most common complaint is of back pain. The pain is typically persistent and unrelated to activity, and often is most noticeable at night. Although aspirin classically provides dramatic relief of symptoms, this is not universal. Lack of a response to aspirin does not rule out the diagnosis. No case of osteoid osteoma was observed at Rizzoli in patients over the age of 30, whereas 20% of osteoblastomas arose after the third decade. The clinical onset is quite different: osteoid osteoma of the thoracic and lumbar spine manifests in 80% of the cases as a painful scoliosis (Fig. 4A,B) or with a painful muscle spasm in the cervical spine. Scoliosis is reported in only 40% of thoracic and lumbar osteoblastomas; the remaining patients complain only of night pain. In Marsh's review, scoliosis was present in approximately 50% of the patients whose tumor arose from the thoracolumbar spine or from the ribs, and Pettine and Klassen (78) reported that of 41 patients with osteoid osteoma or osteoblastoma of the spine, 63% had a significant scoliosis. Nearly all patients in that series had improvement or resolution of their scoliosis when the tumor was removed within 15 months of the onset of symptoms, but only 1 patient out of 11 had any improvement when symptoms had been present for more than 15 months (78). Ransford et al. (82) saw similar results in 15 patients with scoliosis, but noted that skeletally mature patients did not develop a structural

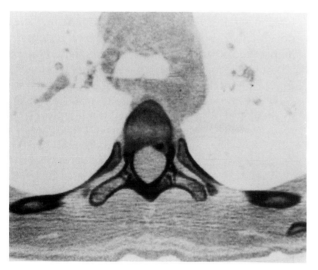

A

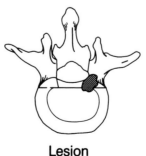

Lesion

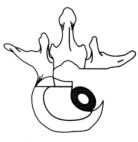

Resection with
Rib Graft

B

FIG. 5. **A:** CT scan of T4 osteoid osteoma. **B:** Resection and rib grafting.

scoliosis even when the duration of symptoms was more than 2 years.

Radiographic demonstration of osteoid osteoma is difficult. The lesion by definition is less than 2.0 cm in diameter and is easily obscured by the overlapping shadows of the vertebral column. CT demonstrates the lesion very well (Fig. 4C), but if the cuts are at the wrong level or too wide, the tumor may be missed completely. The most sensitive method of locating an osteoid osteoma is bone scan. The technetium bone scan provides accurate localization of the lesion, decreasing the average duration of symptoms by providing an early diagnosis and allowing prompt treatment (78).

Osteoblastomas are considerably larger than osteoid osteomas and may be quite apparent on plain radiographs. In stage 2 lesions, the tumor is characterized radiographically by expansion of the cortical bone, maintaining a thin rim of reactive bone between the lesion and the surrounding soft tissue. There is often a rim of reactive bone separating the tumor from the rest of the medullary bone. Although the tumor may show stippling in some cases, there is rarely a lobulated or soap-bubble appearance to these lesions (65); ossifications can be found within the tumor mass. Stage 3 osteoblastomas can invade precociously the epidural space; four cases of cord compression (14%) have been observed in our series.

The treatment of osteoid osteoma is intralesional excision. This does not require removal of the perilesional sclerotic reaction, but the tumor must be completely removed (Fig. 5); only one recurrence was observed in the 47 cases of Rizzoli Institute, due to incomplete removal of the tumor. Excision provides reliable pain relief, and the spinal deformity is improved or disappears in the majority of patients (Fig. 4) (54).

For the treatment of osteoblastoma, curettage was advocated in the past as the treatment of choice (38,65); in our view, osteoblastomas must be treated according to their oncologic staging. Intralesional excision is adequate for stage 2 lesions, even if it does not prevent recurrence (one recurrence followed 14 intralesional excisions in our experience) (Figs. 6 and 7). Radiotherapy as an adjuvant to excision is required in stage 3 lesions (no recurrences in six cases) because intralesional excision is not adequate (two recurrences in seven cases). Marginal resection, when feasible, is the safest oncologic option. Some authors have advocated instrumentation and posterior spine fusion for large scoliotic curves present for 2 years or more, but this need not be done at the time of excision (1).

Aneurysmal Bone Cyst

The spine is the preferred site of occurrence of this pseudotumoral condition (12), found most commonly in the thoracolumbar spine and involving the posterior elements approximately 60% of the time. Forty cases were observed at Rizzoli Institute, three of them presenting at the onset with cord compression syndrome, seven with a palpable mass as a prominent clinical finding, and six provoking pathologic fracture of the affected vertebra. Ten cases were located in the cervical spine, 20 in the thoracic. Thirty-two cases (80%) arose in the first 2 decades and only one (2.5%) in a patient over 50. These lesions have a tendency to involve adjacent vertebrae (43) and may involve three or more vertebrae in sequence (Fig. 8). Radiographs typically demonstrate an expansile, osteolytic cavity with strands of bone forming a bubbly appearance. The cortex is often eggshell thin and blown out. The CT scan demonstrates different tissues (Fig. 9A) because of the different densities within the tumor itself (blood and membranes).

The role of radiation therapy has been overestimated in the past (in the 1970s, one patient in our series died from local compression despite two courses of radiation therapy), and the risk of radiation-induced sarcoma is growing. Surgery, however, does not necessarily prevent recurrences, which developed in 13% of cases in the review by Hay et al. (43), all successfully treated by a second curettage or excision. For the past few years, selective arterial embolization has become, in our experience, the first advised approach, capable of healing or involuting the cyst (Fig. 9B,C) or at the least reducing intraoperative bleeding.

Hemangioma

Vertebral angiodysplasias are common lesions, found at autopsy in approximately 10% of all people; hemangiomas are frequently diagnosed (latent stage 1 lesions) and are rarely symptomatic or of clinical importance. Reports of deformity or pain associated with vertebral hemangiomas are uncommon, but cases of soft-tissue extension with nerve root and cord compression have been documented (Fig. 10). The diagnosis of vertebral body hemangioma can usually be made on plain radiographs, although CT or MRI imaging will provide more information about thecal impingement. Plain films classically show prominent vertical striations produced by the abnormally thickened trabeculae of the involved vertebral body. Stage 1 conditions do not require any kind of treatment, unless a pathologic fracture requires stabilization. When symptomatic, these lesions frequently respond to radiotherapy alone, but selective arterial embolization seems a safer and more effective treatment. Angiography of the spinal cord is mandatory for lesions of the thoracolumbar area to identify the primary vascular supply to the cord (the artery of Adamkiewitz). Surgical excision may be made difficult by the vascularity of the condition itself and may be further complicated by a consumptive

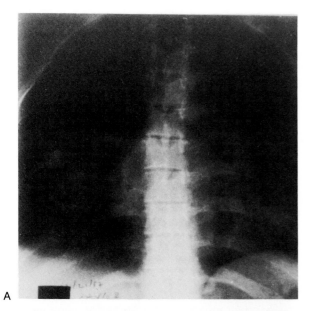

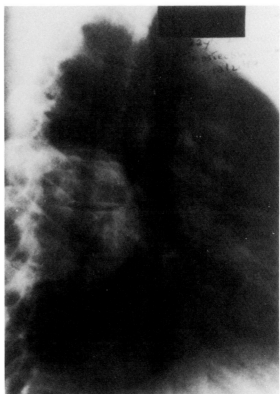

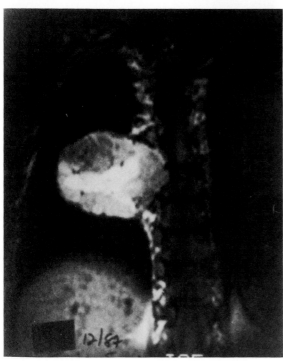

FIG. 6. T7 osteoblastoma. **A:** Anterior radiograph shows the expansile lesion from the body of T7, including and up to the body of T6; the ribs of T7 and T8 are clearly involved. Some calcification of the lesion is apparent. **B:** Lateral image shows a large expansile mass in the area of T6, T7, and T8, with some calcification. **C:** Coronal MR image shows growth of a large osteoblastoma off the vertebral bodies of T6 and T7 with some central calcification.

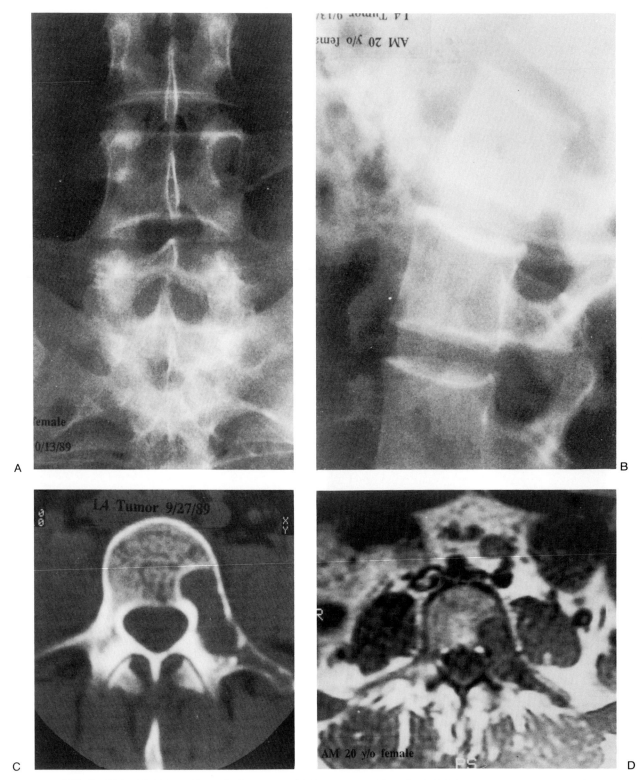

FIG. 7. Plain AP **(A)** and lateral **(B)** x-rays of L4 tumor involving the left L4 transverse process and pedicle. Diagnosis: osteoblastoma/aneurysmal bone cyst/solid ABC. CT scan **(C)** and MR image **(D)** of the lesion preoperatively. Diagnosis: stage 2 osteoblastoma occupying the locations 8 to 10, layers B and C. Locations and layers are depicted in Fig. 17.

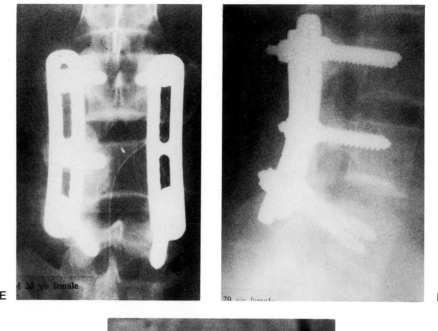

E

F

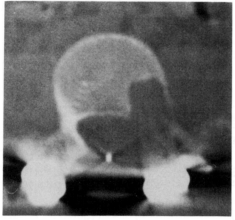

G

FIG. 7. *(Continued.)* AP **(E)** and lateral **(F)** x-rays after excision of the tumor. **G:** Axial CT image after excision of radiating zones 8 to 12.

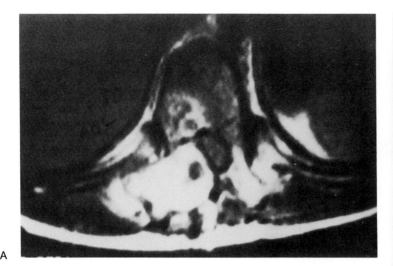

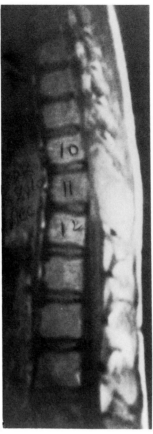

FIG. 8. Aneurysmal bone cyst of the posterior elements of T10, T11, and T12 of an 8-year-old girl. **A:** Axial MR image shows a large aneurysmal bone cyst involving the posterior elements of T10, part of the vertebral body of T10, and the rib on the right of T10, and compressing the spinal cord to the left. **B:** Sagittal MR image of the same patient shows the extent of the posterior aneurysmal bone cyst from T10 to T12 with cord compression.

coagulopathy, occasionally encountered in cavernous hemangiomata (61). When cord compression develops (2 of 16 cases treated) and surgical treatment is considered, embolization or operative ligation (9,23) must be performed before the curettage.

Giant Cell Tumor

Giant cell tumor is a benign tumor, usually presenting as stage 2 or 3, but is sometimes unpredictable. Spinal involvement is usually seen in patients in the third and fourth decades of life, and symptoms may exist for many months before the patient sees a physician. Of the 29 cases observed (4 in the cervical spine, 14 in the thoracic, 11 in the lumbar), 18 arose in the third decade (62%) and the others were equally distributed up to the 70s. Pain was the constant complaint, together with cord compression syndrome in nine cases (31%). Plain radiographs usually demonstrate an area of focal rarification, though some have a more geographic lytic appearance and marginal sclerosis. Giant cell tumors are most commonly found in the vertebral body and may expand the surrounding cortical bone extensively as the tumor enlarges.

CT is especially important in the evaluation of these tumors preoperatively because complete resection is very important to the eradication of local disease. CT is also crucial in the early identification of recurrences and should be used in postoperative follow-up on a routine basis (Fig. 11).

Many series have been published with contrasting and confusing conclusions because of the lack of homogeneity of the cases considered. Prolonged disease-free survivals have been reported after resection or curettage and radiotherapy, although some patients required two or three additional procedures because of local recurrence (115). In the Iowa series, giant cell tumors involving the spine had a particularly bad prognosis because of their locally invasive nature (115). Two-fifths of those patients died as a result of recurrent and invasive local disease (113). Dahlin (22) reported better results and has even suggested that lesions of the spine are less aggressive than those in the extremities.

In the series from Rizzoli Institute, radiation therapy, apart from being highly risky (72), was not so effective even in stage 2 lesions (one recurrence in three cases), whereas complete intralesional excision gave good results in stage 2 lesions (no recurrences in three cases) and

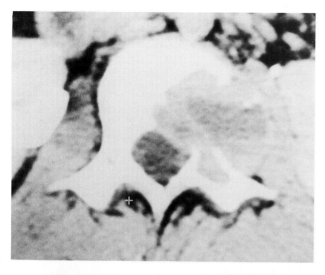

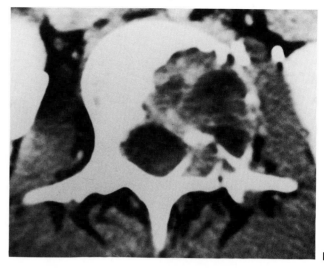

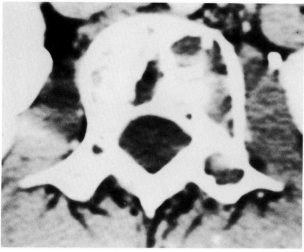

FIG. 9. Aneurysmal bone cyst at L3. **A:** Blood and membranes contained within the lesion form the typical levels. **B:** Three months after selective arterial embolization, showing mass reduction and initial peripheral ossification. **C:** Two years later, showing ossification of the cyst.

in stage 3 lesions, if combined with sequential radiotherapy (no recurrences in 12 cases). En bloc resection should be the treatment of choice in stage 3 lesions (no recurrences in four cases), completely avoiding the risks of radiation therapy (87) (Fig. 12). Stener and Johnsen (101) described a resection of three adjacent vertebrae in a young woman with a giant cell tumor of the 12th thoracic vertebra. This kind of procedure requires great care to perform an en bloc resection to achieve a marginal or at best a wide margin, the only possibility in preventing recurrence. Lubicky et al. (62) described a two-stage vertebrectomy for an L4 giant cell tumor, with the anterior vertebrectomy performed 1 week after laminectomy, biopsy, and posterior stabilization with Harrington rods and methylmethacrylate. Unfortunately, the rods were quite short and did not supply adequate stabilization, so that when the anterior iliac crest grafts were placed without further anterior stabilization, they collapsed into

moderate lateral tilt and mild kyphosis. Nonetheless, the graft united and the patient had no evidence of recurrence at early 1-year follow-up (62). These reports emphasize the technical demands of vertebrectomy and stabilization, but even more important the need for oncologic and surgical staging to allow correct surgical planning.

Eosinophilic Granuloma

This is a process of unproven etiology that produces focal destruction of bone (49); it is benign and sometimes self-limiting when isolated, and sometimes evolves into disseminated and/or multisystemic conditions, known as Hand-Schuller-Christian disease (multifocal, chronic, and disseminated form) or Letterer-Siwe's disease (acute disseminated or infantile form) (32,73). Eosinophilic

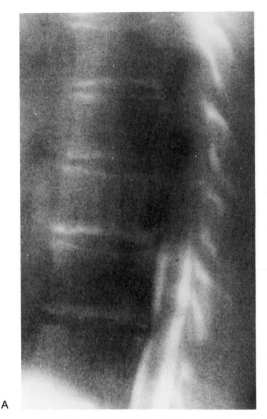

A

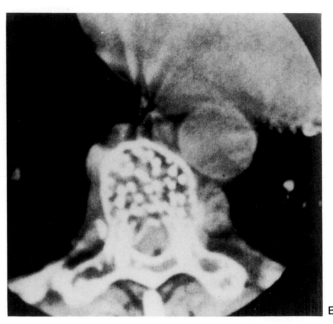

B

FIG. 10. A: Lateral thoracic myelogram demonstrating obstruction of contrast flow. Diagnosis: hemangioma at T8 with soft-tissue extension. **B:** CT scan of T8 hemangioma with extradural extension.

granuloma is most commonly seen in children before the age of 10 years (65% of 52 lesions observed at Rizzoli Institute). Lesions of the skull are most common, but any bone may be affected; vertebral involvement occurs in approximately 10% to 15% of cases. The vertebral body is typically involved, usually in the thoracic or lumbar spine; only six cases (11%) in the series of Rizzoli Institute arose in the cervical spine.

The ensuing bony destruction may produce cavitation, partial vertebral collapse, and the classic "vertebra plana" following complete collapse of the vertebral body. Only seldom does the vertebral collapse produce pain and focal spasm, whereas torticollis is common in cervical lesions. Mild to moderate kyphosis is frequently observed. Neurologic symptoms may develop with or without associated vertebral collapse. As long as treatment is instituted without delay, recovery of neurologic function is usually excellent. Early in the disease process, radiographs show a central lytic lesion with poorly defined margins and permeative bone destruction. At this point, the lesion may produce a marked periosteal reaction, and distinguishing it from osteomyelitis or a high-grade sarcoma may be impossible. An outstanding feature is the small amount of pathologic tissue found on

CT scan compared with the masses detected early in round cell sarcomas. As the vertebral body collapses and settles, radiographs demonstrate the flattened disc of dense cortical bone retained between the two intact intervertebral discs (18,92). This "coin on end" appearance of vertebra plana is a classic finding in eosinophilic granuloma but is not pathognomonic; a similar appearance can be produced by either infection or Ewing's sarcoma. The finding of abscess or a huge mass of neoplastic tissue orients the diagnosis; however, with such a broad differential, the importance of obtaining an adequate biopsy specimen before beginning treatment cannot be overstated. Open biopsy is preferable, to assure an adequate specimen and to allow definitive treatment at the same procedure (18,32,37) if the diagnosis of eosinophilic granuloma is confirmed.

The treatment of eosinophilic granuloma is somewhat controversial, but it is clear that many patients will heal their lesions without any treatment, at least other than biopsy. Low-dose radiotherapy (500–1000 rads) has been advocated in the past, but this may be avoided in most patients as it could affect the vertebral height reconstitution. Local corticosteroid injection after frozen-section biopsy seems to be the treatment of choice.

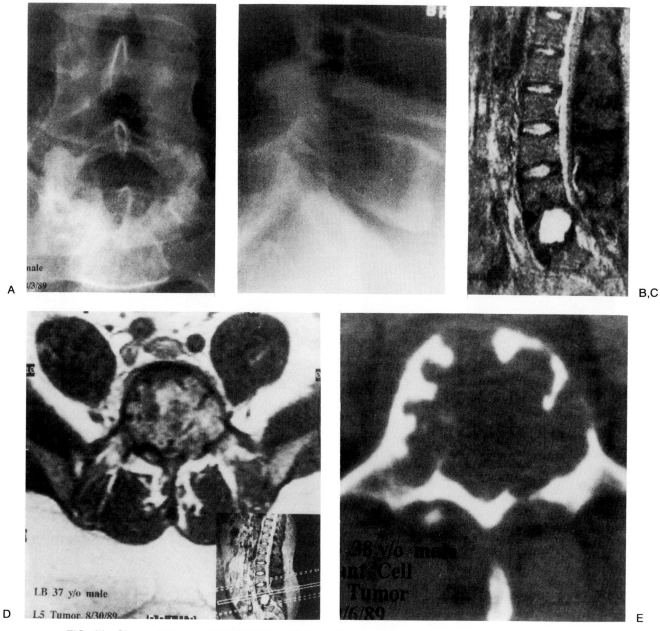

FIG. 11. Giant cell tumor at L5. AP **(A)** and lateral **(B)** roentgenograms, T2-weighted sagittal **(C)** and axial **(D)** MR images, and axial CT image **(E)**.

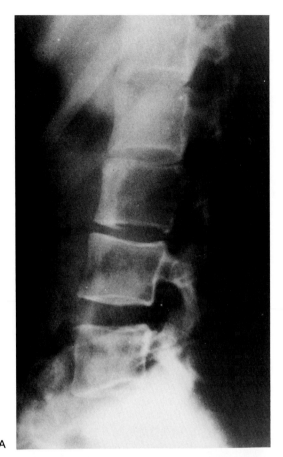

A

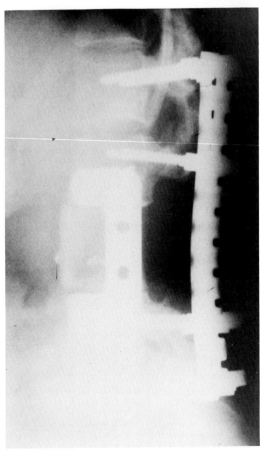

E

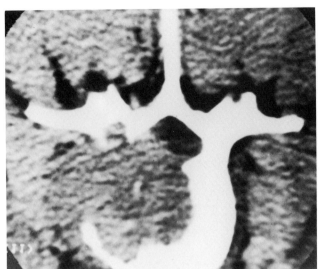

B

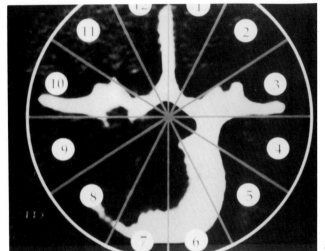

C

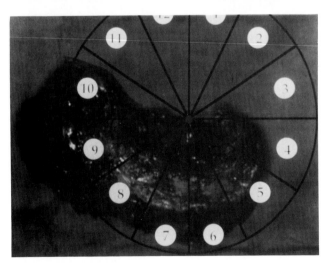

D

FIG. 12. Giant cell tumor at L2. Plain x-ray **(A)** and axial CT **(B)** describing a stage 3 lesion. **C:** According to the WBB surgical staging, the lesion occupies the radiating zones 6 to 10, layers A to D. **D:** Resected specimen after en bloc resection of the vertebral body (marginal margin) by double approach vertebrectomy. Reconstruction was achieved by posterior pedicular plates, anterior plate, and allograft. **E:** No recurrence 36 months later.

Surgical decompression must be included in the rare cases of cord compression. Courses of chemotherapy are indicated in disseminated disease.

MALIGNANT TUMORS

Malignant Multiple Myeloma and Solitary Plasmacytoma

These conditions probably deserve some discussion here, as most authors today would consider multiple myeloma and solitary plasmacytoma as two manifestations in a continuum of B-cell lymphoproliferative diseases, quite far from the concept of primary disease of bone. Because the natural histories of these two lesions differ so significantly, the clinical distinction between solitary plasmacytoma and multiple myeloma remains pertinent.

Multiple myeloma is an uncommon neoplastic process with an incidence of two to three cases per 100,000 people among the general population. True solitary plasmacytoma is a rare entity representing only 3% of all plasma cell neoplasms (20). Patients with solitary and multiple myeloma differ in terms of age and sex distributions and survival (3). Though the course of multiple myeloma is usually rapidly progressive and lethal, patients with solitary plasmacytoma may have prolonged survival despite eventual progression. The treatment of solitary plasmacytoma must, therefore, be considered somewhat differently than the treatment of a spinal focus of multiple myeloma.

Solitary plasmacytoma is an isolated lesion, the treatment of which may provide long-term disease-free survival or cure. The spinal lesion in multiple myeloma represents a metastasis in a progressive, systemic disease that commonly results in death within 2 to 3 years despite local or systemic treatment. Both the overall survival and the 5-year survival in solitary plasmacytoma of the spine are significantly increased when compared with those of multiple myeloma (68). The prognosis for survival of patients with disseminated myeloma is poor, with a 5-year survival of 18% and a median survival of 28 months. In cases involving the spinal column, the outcome is even worse. Valderrama and Bullough (108) reported that 76% of such patients were dead within a year of their diagnosis, and all were dead within 4 years. The prognosis is significantly better for patients with solitary plasmacytoma of the spine. Bergsagel and Rider (3) reported a 35% disease-free 5-year survival for patients with solitary plasmacytoma of bone, with a median survival of 48 months (3). The 5-year disease-free survival in 84 cases of spinal solitary plasmacytoma was roughly 60%, with a median survival of 92 months (Table 2). Survival of 20 years and more was seen both in our group and in previous case reports (68,88,113).

The treatment of choice of the affected vertebra in solitary plasmacytoma and in multiple myeloma is radiation. Because of the radiosensitivity of this tumor, surgical treatment has less influence in determining outcome than it does in other tumor types. Hoping to prevent vertebral body collapse and cord compression, some reviewers have recommended prophylactic laminectomy and stabilization before radiotherapy. We have not seen any case of onset or progression of neurologic deficit during radiotherapy and do not recommend surgical intervention unless cord compromise or spinal instability is present. If cord compromise is the presenting sign, there is no previous history of myeloma, and rapid decompression is indicated, the lesion may be treated similarly to metastatic disease, with decompression and stabilization with metal-reinforced methylmethacrylate. Dissemination of myeloma may occur after many years of disease-free survival, and routine follow-up is indicated for an indefinite period. Serum protein immunoelectrophoresis has proven the most accurate indicator of dissemination and should be followed closely after therapy is introduced. If dissemination does occur, systemic chemotherapy should be instituted.

Primary Osteosarcoma

This is a high-grade tumor typical of those most active in the metaphysis of long bones (knee and shoulder) in the adolescent. Long-term survival has dramatically im-

TABLE 2. *Characteristics and survival of patients with multiple myeloma, solitary plasmacytoma of bone, and solitary plasmacytoma of the spine*

	Percent male	Age at presentation	Disease-free interval (months)	Overall survival (months)	Percent 5-year survival
Multiple myeloma	51	M = 60 F = 61		24	18
Solitary plasmacytoma (bone)	68	M = 50 F = 55	78	86	35
Solitary plasmacytoma (spine)	74	M = 51 F = 57	76	92	60

From ref. 68.

proved, and it is now possible to perform limb salvage surgery thanks to the protocols of preoperative intra-arterial multiple drug chemotherapy. This treatment has yet to be performed effectively in the spine, the site of occurrence of approximately 2% of all osteogenic sarcomas. An oncologically correct treatment of these lesions in the spinal column is difficult, as en bloc resection without preoperative chemotherapy is frequently impossible; therefore, the outcome in these tumors remains very poor. In a review of 27 cases of osteosarcoma of the spine, median survival was 10 months from the time of diagnosis; only seven patients survived more than 1 year, and one patient survived over 5 years (93). Similar results were seen by Barwick et al. (2), who reported a median survival of 6 months for ten patients.

Vertebral osteosarcoma arises from the anterior elements in more than 95% of cases. The radiographic findings include both lytic and sclerotic lesions, with cortical destruction, ossifications within the tumoral mass, and collapse in advanced cases. CT demonstrates intraspinal and paraspinal soft-tissue masses more clearly, allowing more accurate preoperative planning. As happens with high-grade malignancies, cord compression is frequent (9 of the 12 cases treated at the Rizzoli Institute).

Traditionally, therapy has consisted of limited tumor excision, chemotherapy, and radiotherapy (even if the radiosensitivity has not been proved). As noted above, the outcomes associated with this approach have been poor (two 5-year survivors in 12 cases). In the hope of improving survival in this and other spinal malignancies, some authors have advocated a more aggressive surgical approach (106,113), performed in the more recent cases. In reviewing treatment results in a larger group of patients, Sundaresan et al. (106) reported seven cases undergoing wide resection or vertebral body resection combined with radiotherapy. Although three of these patients died of their disease at a mean of 11 months after their operation, four others were still alive and three had no evidence of disease at a mean survival of 52 months. Although the early indication is that en bloc resection of the tumor may result in longer survival, especially if combined with chemotherapy, longer follow-up is needed before assumptions can be made about our ability to cure these tumors.

Secondary Osteosarcoma

This subgroup of the osteosarcoma tumor type arises secondarily in pagetoid or previously irradiated bone. Patients presenting with secondary osteosarcomas are significantly older than those with primary osteosarcoma; of the osteosarcomas of bone in patients over the age of 60, more than 60% were secondary lesions (48). The majority of patients with post-irradiation sarcoma present in the fourth or fifth decade of life, whereas those with Paget's sarcoma are usually in their sixth decade. Although secondary lesions account for between 3.6% and 5.5% of all intramedullary osteosarcomas (22,47), these patients represent approximately 30% of all osteosarcomas of the spine (2,93). Most patients with Paget's disease who develop an osteosarcoma have polyostotic disease. Tumors typically arise in diseased pagetoid bone and progress rapidly. They are aggressive lesions, producing extensive bony destruction and metastasizing early. These lesions are typically very anaplastic. The prognosis for long-term survival in patients with sarcomatous transformation of Paget's disease is dismal, with less than 5% of patients having long-term survival (81).

The association between irradiation and osteosarcoma has been appreciated for many years (10,72). Although it is sometimes reported in patients with low levels of radiation exposure, most patients who develop a post-irradiation sarcoma have received in excess of 5000 rads. Many demonstrate radiographic evidence of radiation ostitis. The majority of these patients were originally irradiated for nonosseous disease, such as Hodgkin's lymphoma, breast carcinoma, and cervical carcinoma. Of those receiving irradiation for skeletal disease, the most common underlying neoplasms are giant cell tumors and Ewing's sarcoma. The survival in these patients is only slightly better than for those with Paget's disease; the 5-year disease-free survival is approximately 17%. Even though most victims are older, post-irradiation osteosarcoma has been reported in childhood, occurring in a 14-year-old who had undergone previous radiation for a cervical astrocytoma and later posterior fusion to correct a progressive scoliosis. This case was typical in the long latency (11 years) between irradiation and presentation of the tumor and in the rapid progression of the lesion, resulting in paraplegia and death 3 weeks after the onset of symptoms (26). Sundaresan et al. (105) have reported a case of post-irradiation osteosarcoma occurring in a woman 31 years after treatment for Hodgkin's disease. Progression was rapid and there was limited response to chemotherapy. Considering the prolonged latency between exposure and the development of disease, patients with a history of irradiation or of Paget's disease warrant added vigilance in the evaluation of acute back pain or spinal pathology.

Ewing's Sarcoma

This is a round cell malignant tumor typical of the first three decades. Approximately 3.5% of all Ewing's tumors arise in the spinal column, with the majority originating in the sacrum (117). The thoracic spine is more frequently involved in the mobile spine (15 of 29 cases). Though prognosis is generally poorer than for those with extremity lesions, long-term survivals are reported (86). Neurologic compromise is common in the presentation of either primary or metastatic Ewing's sarcoma (10 of 29 cases treated at Rizzoli Institute). Pilepich et al. (79) reported 22 cases of primary vertebral Ewing's and noted that 14 of these patients had neurologic deficits at the time of diagnosis. The permeative appearance of Ewing's tumors on radiographs can make diagnosis difficult, even in advanced disease, and collapse of the vertebral body may produce a vertebra plana difficult to differentiate from that seen in eosinophilic granuloma (80). Metastatic Ewing's sarcoma arising in the spinal epidural space, without bony involvement, is a rare but documented phenomenon (88,91).

The treatment of choice for Ewing's sarcoma involves multiagent chemotherapy and high-dose radiotherapy. The primary role of surgery is to perform en bloc resections; these procedures sometimes become feasible after chemo- and radiotherapy. At times, a few courses of chemotherapy are able to reduce the mass dramatically and to produce an almost complete necrosis. Even if wide resection will be done, it is wise to perform radiation therapy. With current regimens of therapy, excellent local control and encouraging disease-free survivals are obtainable in the spine, though the long-term outlook for most patients remains grim (55).

Chordoma

Chordoma is a low-grade malignant tumor typically arising from the clivus and the spine as it originates from the remnants of the notochord (51,70) (Fig. 13). It occurs predominantly in the fifth or sixth decade of life. Although this tumor is characterized by its slow but relentless local spread, it is a fully malignant lesion capable of distant metastases. Initial symptoms are usually mild and progress slowly as the tumor expands. Chordomas may reach a considerable size before metastasizing, and symptoms of dyspnea, constipation, urinary frequency, or nerve root compression may appear before patients present to their physician. In a review of 21 cases of chordoma of the mobile spine (5 in the cervical, 2 in the thoracic, 14 in the lumbar spine), 11 cases had cord compression as the presenting symptom (6).

Chordoma is not sensitive to any chemotherapeutic drug, and only high-dose radiotherapy seems to slow the evolution of the disease without eradicating the tumor. Intralesional excision is not effective in preventing progression or recurrence of the chordoma, even if associated with conventional high-dose radiotherapy (6). The only curative procedure seems to be en bloc wide-margin resection, which means maintaining a cuff of normal tissue over the tumor. Biopsy should not be performed until all appropriate staging studies have been evaluated, after which a CT scan-guided trocar biopsy is the best

option to avoid tumor contamination of the healthy tissues. The biopsy incision must be excised en bloc with the tumor at the time of the definitive resection. Local recurrence of a chordoma is a grim prognostic sign, dramatically reducing the likelihood of cure. Kaiser et al. (51) demonstrated that simply exposing the tumor during resection increased the recurrence rate of this tenacious lesion from 28% to 64%. The feasibility of wide resection is more frequent in sacrococcygeal chordoma (100) even if high sacral lesions may necessitate a colostomy and functionally important nerve roots will be sacrificed; in such cases significant morbidity should be expected. Surprisingly little morbidity or functional loss is referred providing the S2 roots can be spared bilaterally (34,83). In the mobile spine, the huge myxoid masses found at presentation and the surgically inaccessible sites (such as the high cervical vertebrae) make resection difficult or impossible to perform. In cases like these, intralesional excision as completely as possible is the only possible treatment, combined with neutron-beam radiation therapy (103).

Chondrosarcoma

Approximately 10% of chondrosarcomas arise in the spinal column. These conditions grow slowly, sometimes manifesting at the onset with signs of cord compression (9 of 19 cases observed at the Rizzoli Institute). These tumors are resistant to radiotherapy and chemotherapy, and because of the difficulties in performing wide-margin resections, lesions of the vertebral column have a poor prognosis independent of the histologic grade. Long-term survivals have been reported in low-grade chondrosarcomas in patients who have been treated with repeated inadequate excisions of recurrent disease, but few lesions can be managed this way with any success (46,94). Radiographically, chondrosarcoma has a fairly characteristic appearance. In advanced disease there is a large area of bone destruction, an associated soft-tissue mass, and flocculent calcifications of the soft-tissue mass. If there is no soft-tissue mass, the vertebral lesion may be primarily lytic, with sclerotic margins and with no mottled calcification (45). CT scanning is invaluable in demonstrating the extent of the lesion and evaluating cord compromise. A complete surgical excision is required to cure the patient with chondrosarcoma, though this is sometimes impossible to obtain. In some vertebral locations, this requires difficult and long procedures via a combined anterior and posterior approach (Fig. 14). Stener (102) has described a thoracic vertebrectomy for chondrosarcoma with en bloc excision of the T6-T8 vertebral bodies for a large T7 tumor. This combined anterior and posterior procedure produced good postoperative stability, without evidence of recurrent disease at 15 months.

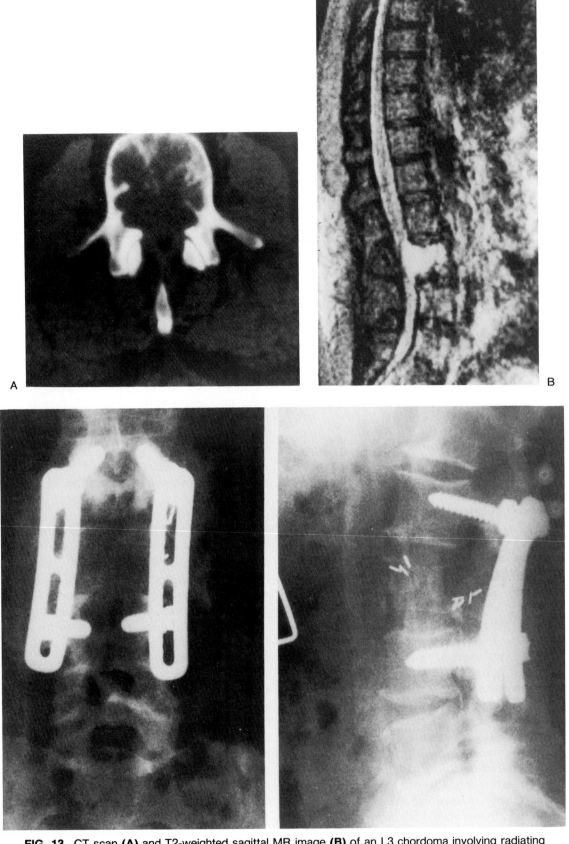

FIG. 13. CT scan **(A)** and T2-weighted sagittal MR image **(B)** of an L3 chordoma involving radiating zones 4 to 9, layers B, C, and D. Standard x-ray AP **(C)** and lateral **(D)** view 3 years postoperatively, with no signs of recurrence to date.

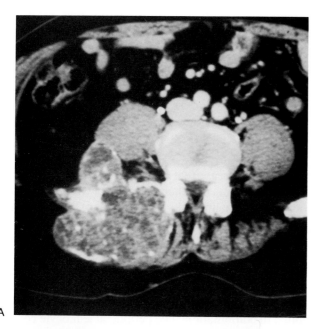

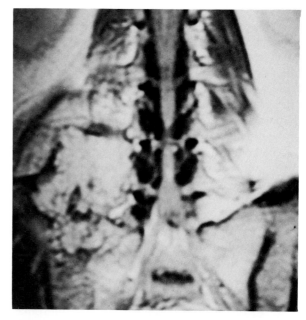

A

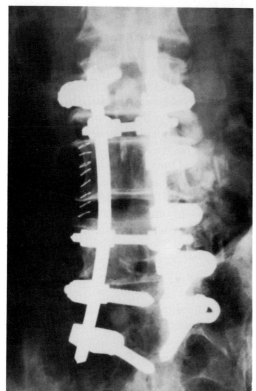

B

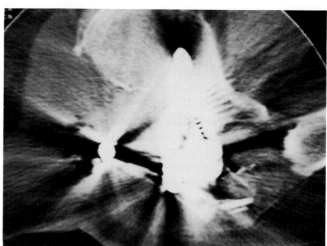

FIG. 14. A: Chondrosarcoma arising from the transverse process of L5, invading asymmetrically L4 and the sacroiliac joint, radiating zones 9 to 11, layers A to C. B: Submitted to en bloc sagittal resection by double combined surgical approach, according to the planning showed in Fig. 18B. Margin achieved: wide.

Lymphoma

Lymphoma may present as a systemic disease with skeletal manifestations or as an isolated bony tumor, referred to in the past as a reticulum cell sarcoma. It is not consistently included in reviews of primary bone tumors

as the treatment of this disease is pertinent to the oncologist, being that the condition is sensitive to radiation and chemotherapy. The surgical treatment of lymphoma of the spine is palliative, aiming to prevent, maintain, or reconstruct the spinal neurologic dysfunction and any associated instability.

SPINAL TUMORS IN CHILDREN

Although this book is dedicated to the adult spine, a spine surgeon dealing with spine tumors must be familiar with the diagnosis and treatment of tumors seen in children (88,114). Spinal tumors are uncommon in children, but the problems they present to the spine surgeon include both short-term and long-term challenges. Aside from the usual complexities of treating the neoplasm itself—whether it is benign but locally aggressive, primarily malignant, or a metastasis from another malignancy that will require systemic therapy—the added dimension in the care of children's tumors is the management of spinal deformities that may develop as a result of treatment. Tumors of the immature spine differ from those seen in adults, particularly in terms of the malignant lesions. Nearly 70% of primary bone tumors seen in children are benign. Eosinophilic granulomas are almost exclusively seen in the pediatric age group; together with osteoid osteomas, osteoblastomas, osteochondromas, and aneurysmal bone cysts, they account for more than 40% of all primary spinal lesions seen in pediatric patients.

Ewing's sarcoma is the most common primary malignancy (Table 3) (113). Although the metastatic lesions of adulthood are generally absent, metastasis or contiguous invasion from neuroblastoma, embryonal carcinoma, and various sarcomas predominates. These highly aggressive lesions have a poor prognosis regardless of treatment. Ewing's sarcoma may arise primarily in the spine, but is more commonly a metastatic lesion. If intramedullary spinal cord tumors are excluded, 37% of the spinal lesions in Tachdjian and Matson's series were malignant (107). Neuroblastoma alone accounted for 20% of the lesions seen in this series. In the review by Fraser et al. (33) of 40 pediatric spine tumors, neuroblastoma accounted for nearly 30% of all tumors, and in Leeson's review of metastatic tumors, neuroblastoma accounted for 41% of the lesions. Nearly 70% of the patients in Tachdjian's series (107) had been misdiagnosed originally, and treatment delay played a major factor in their survival and deformities associated with treatment.

Leukemia

Another disease that enters the differential diagnosis in these patients is leukemia. In 6% of children with leukemia, back pain and vertebral collapse are the initial findings at presentation. During the course of the disease, 10% will sustain a pathologic vertebral fracture, sometimes involving multiple levels. When first seen, these children manifest a variety of nonspecific constitutional symptoms, and the correct diagnosis is often hard to make. Lethargy, anemia, and fever occur commonly and often in combination. The peripheral leukocyte count is elevated in 60% of patients, and the erythrocyte sedimentation rate is also increased. Radiographs may not demonstrate any focal abnormality, or they may show focal lytic lesions, occasional sclerotic lesions, or isolated periosteal reactions. It is important to keep in mind that radionuclide scans are unreliable in patients with leukemia, in some cases showing no uptake in areas of obvious bony destruction (17). These symptoms and signs mimic those seen in patients with osteomyelitis or joint sepsis, and this misdiagnosis is common. Keys to making the correct diagnosis in these confusing presentations are the identification of anemia, the recognition of those 40% of patients who are leukopenic at presentation, the presence of inconsistent bone scan results, and a high index of suspicion on the part of the examining physician.

Spinal Deformity

Progressive deformity may occur for any of a number of reasons after treatment of pediatric spinal tumors. As in adults, deformity may result from structural deficiencies caused by the erosion of bone by tumor or by aggressive surgical resection. These deformities may be more severe or progressive in children, however, particularly in the case of post-laminectomy kyphosis and in the thoracic spine. The younger the child at the time of laminectomy, the more severe the eventual deformity is likely to be (33). Irradiation and rib resection are well-known factors in the development of iatrogenic scoliosis. Deformity after congenital or acquired paraplegia is also common and tends to be more severe in children with earlier onset of paralysis and higher levels of cord injury. Surgical management of these patients must anticipate the later development of deformity and seek to minimize it. Patients with deformity that is certain to progress must

TABLE 3. *Primary bone tumors found in the spinal column in 31 patients less than 18 years of age*

Tumor	Number (percent)
Benign	
Osteoblastoma	4
Osteochondroma	4
Aneurysmal bone cyst	4
Giant cell tumor	3
Eosinophilic granuloma	2
Osteoid osteoma	2
Hemangioma	1
Angiolipoma	1
Malignant	
Ewing's sarcoma	3
Chordoma	1
Osteosarcoma	1
Malignant giant cell tumor	1
Chondrosarcoma	1
Others	3
Total	31

be identified early on and treatment instituted to halt this progression.

CERVICAL SPINE TUMORS

In a review of 20 cases of cervical spine tumors treated by anterior vertebrectomy and bone grafting, there were no cases of graft failure, either through collapse or extrusion. Iliac crest, fibular, and tibial grafts were all used, and posterior fusions were used in 13 cases to augment stability. In patients with primary benign tumors, anterior resection and grafting eliminated symptoms in each case, and there were no recurrences. In primary malignancies and in metastatic lesions there was excellent stability, with resolution of neurologic symptoms and pain. Quality of life and longevity were improved in these patients. Because a recurring tumor is likely to involve the vertebrae above and below the site of previous excision, it is recommended that the posterior fusion span two levels above and below the site of fusion (29). In a review of 13 benign and 10 malignant primary neoplasms of the cervical spine, anterior excision with iliac crest autograft, supplemented with posterior grafting in some cases, proved to be reliable in relieving pain and neurologic symptoms, providing stability, and improving the overall quality of life. Large tumors involving anterior, lateral, and posterior elements of the vertebral body were excised through staged anterior and posterior approaches. An intralesional margin was obtained in all

malignant tumors. Only two patients with malignancy had survived more than 3 years (4,110). A serious criticism must be explored about the validity of such reviews from an oncologic point of view. Too little importance was given to the main problem of primary tumors, that is, the oncologically appropriate surgery as proposed by the Enneking staging system (27) and planned according to the Weinstein-Boriani-Biagini (WBB) surgical staging (Fig. 17). In the future, this will provide a more reliable means of assessing treatment and outcome.

THE TREATMENT OF SPINE PRIMARY TUMORS BASED ON ONCOLOGIC STAGING AND ANATOMIC EXTENT OF LESION

It has been proposed that some pseudotumoral conditions require specific treatments: Localized eosinophilic granuloma heals after corticosteroid injection; many aneurysmal bone cysts heal after one or repeated embolizations. Attempts at surgical extirpation of primary tumors of the spine without following the oncologic criteria (27) are fruitless and should not be attempted (4). The ability to resect the primary tumor completely plays a role in overall patient survival and in recovery and maintenance of neurologic function (101,102,112).

The vertebral body, anterior and posterior longitudinal ligaments, the intervertebral discs, and the dura may all be resected. Neural, muscular, and vascular structures may all be sacrificed to obtain a surgical margin appro-

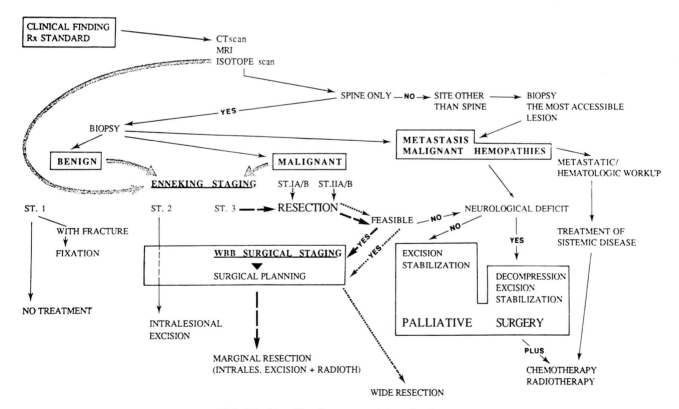

FIG. 15. Algorithm for approach to spine tumors.

priate to the biologic aggressiveness of the tumor. Such an approach has been responsible for excellent results in the treatment of bone tumors in the limb, based on staging tumors according to histologic grading and anatomic extension. This system, proposed by Enneking et al. (27), resulted in the ability to describe the boundaries of the tumor and the normal tissue reaction before and after chemotherapy, and has been helpful in choosing the best surgical margin to minimize recurrences. The surgical planning for bone tumors of the spine requires a system able to describe the anatomic extent of the tumor, in order to decide how to perform a surgical procedure to obtain the best possible margin (Fig. 15).

The oncologic staging of Enneking et al. (27)—widely accepted for the study and treatment of bone tumors of the limbs—was not originally conceived for the spine and does not consider the anatomic specificity of the vertebral column. It has been applied to the spine (5,6,11) and has proven useful in understanding the biologic activity of the tumor and in determining the appropriate surgical margin.[1] This staging system divides benign tumors into three stages and malignant tumors into six stages (Fig. 16). This classification is based on clinical features, radiographic pattern, CT/MRI data, and histo-

---

[1] intralesional: within the tumor mass; marginal: en bloc resection along the pseudocapsule; wide: en bloc resection outside the pseudocapsule; radical: en bloc resection of the whole compartment (impossible in the spine unless sectioning the dural sac and its contents).

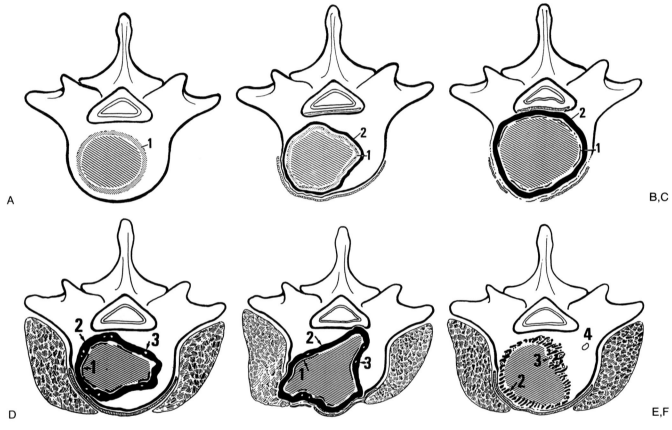

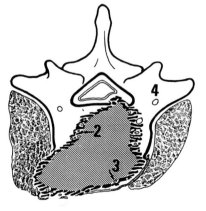

FIG. 16. **A:** Benign tumors, stage 1: The tumor is inactive and contained within its capsule **(1)**. **B:** Benign tumors, stage 2: The tumor is growing; the capsule **(1)** is thin and bordered by a pseudocapsule of reactive tissue **(2)**. **C:** Benign tumors, stage 3: The aggressiveness of these tumors is witnessed by the wide reaction of healthy tissue **(2)**, whereas the capsule **(1)** is very thin and discontinued. **D:** Malignant tumors, stage IA. The capsule **(1)**, if any, is very thin; the pseudocapsule **(2)** is wide and contains islands of tumor **(3)**. **E:** Malignant tumors, stage IB. The capsule **(1)**, if any, is very thin; the pseudocapsule **(2)** is wide and contains islands of tumor **(3)**. The tumoral mass is growing outside the compartment of occurrence. **F:** Malignant tumors, stage IIA. The pseudocapsule **(2)** is infiltrated by tumor **(3)**; an island of tumor can be found far from the main tumoral mass (skip metastasis—**4**). **G:** Malignant tumors, stage IIB. The pseudocapsule **(2)** is infiltrated by tumor **(3)**, which is growing outside the vertebra; an island of tumor can be found far from the main tumoral mass (skip metastasis—**4**).

logic findings preferably obtained by CT scan-guided biopsy, a technique to minimize tumoral contamination of surrounding tissues.

Benign Tumors

The first stage of benign tumors (S1) includes latent and asymptomatic lesions bordered by a true capsule. A well-defined margin all around the circumference of the lesion is seen even on plain radiograms. These tumors do not grow, or grow very slowly. No treatment is required unless palliative surgery is needed for decompression or stabilization.

In the second stage, the benign tumors (S2) are active lesions, growing slowly. A thin capsule and a layer of reactive tissue are demonstrated on plain radiograms as an enlargement of the tumor outline, better pointed out by MRI. Bone scan is positive. An intralesional excision (curettage) can be performed with a low rate of recurrences (5). The incidence of recurrences can be lowered further by local adjuvants (cryotherapy, embolization, radiation therapy).

The third stage of benign tumors (S3) includes rapidly growing benign tumors that are locally aggressive; the capsule is very thin, discontinued, or absent. The tumor invades neighboring compartments, and a reactive hypervascularized tissue (pseudocapsule) is often found. Bone scan is highly positive; fuzzy limits are seen on plain x-rays, CT scan shows compartmental extension, and MRI clearly defines a pseudocapsule and its relationship to the neurologic structures. Intralesional curettage, even if augmented by radiation, can be associated with a significant rate of recurrence (5). A marginal resection is the appropriate treatment.

Malignant Tumors

Low-grade malignant tumors are included in stage I, which is subdivided into IA (the tumor remains inside the vertebra) and IB (the tumor invades paravertebral compartments). No true capsule is associated with these lesions, but a thick pseudocapsule of reactive tissue permeated by small microscopic islands of tumor is seen. A resection performed along the pseudocapsule often leaves residual foci of active tumor; high-dose radiation can be added to reduce the risk of recurrence (6,103). The treatment of choice if feasible is a wide resection.

High-grade malignant tumors are defined as IIA and IIB. The neoplastic growth is so rapid that the host has no time to form a continuous reactive tissue. There is continuous seeding with neoplastic nodules (satellites). Moreover, these tumors can have neoplastic nodules at some distance from the main tumor mass (skip metastases). These malignancies are generally seen on plain radiograms as radiolucent and destructive, and in many

cases are associated with a pathologic fracture. CT and MRI give details regarding the transverse and longitudinal extent of these tumors and may confirm the absence of reactive tissue. Invasion of the epidural space is rapid in stage B, particularly in small cell tumors (Ewing's sarcoma, lymphomas) characterized by semifluid tissue, able to occupy the epidural space after infiltrating the cortical border of the vertebra.

The margin of the resection must be wide (it is not possible in the spine to achieve a "radical" margin), and courses of radiation and chemotherapy (according to the tumor type) must be considered for local control and the avoidance of distant spread.

SURGICAL STAGING

A surgical staging system describing the anatomic extent of a spine tumor is needed to provide a uniform classification to communicate data within and across institutions, but, more important, it is necessary to plan a surgical procedure aimed at obtaining the appropriate surgical margin advised by the Enneking staging system. Such a surgical staging was introduced by Weinstein (112), subsequently modified (7,114), submitted to clinical evaluation (6,115) and now called WBB staging system. On the transverse plane, the vertebra is divided into 12 radiating zones (numbered 1 to 12 in a clockwise order) and into 5 layers (A to E from the prevertebral to the dural involvement). The longitudinal extent of the tumor is also recorded (Fig. 17).

Some commonly used terms, *vertebrectomy* (removal of all the elements of the vertebra), *corpectomy,* and *somectomy* (removal of the vertebral body), have no significance from an oncologic viewpoint of outcome if they are not specified according to the oncologic terminology: *Excision* is the piecemeal removal of the tumor. *Resection* is the en bloc removal of the tumor. This can be performed along the pseudocapsule *(marginal resection)* or outside the pseudocapsule, removing the tumor with a continuous shell of healthy tissues *(wide resection)*. *Palliation* is a surgical procedure aimed at a functional purpose (cord decompression, fracture stabilization) with or without partial (piecemeal) removal of the tumor.

In the authors' experience, there are three ways to perform an en bloc resection in the thoracolumbar spine: *vertebrectomy, hemivertebrectomy,* and *resection of the posterior arch.*

Vertebrectomy (Marginal/Wide Resection of the Vertebral Body)

A resection of the vertebral body can be performed if the tumor is confined to zones 4 to 8 or 5 to 9 (centrally located and at least one pedicle free from the tumor).

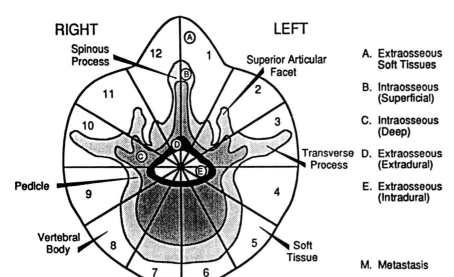

RIGHT   LEFT

Spinous Process

Superior Articular Facet

Transverse Process

Pedicle

Vertebral Body

Soft Tissue

A. Extraosseous Soft Tissues

B. Intraosseous (Superficial)

C. Intraosseous (Deep)

D. Extraosseous (Extradural)

E. Extraosseous (Intradural)

M. Metastasis

FIG. 17. Anatomic extent of spine tumors by radiating zones (locations) and layers.

An en bloc resection must be performed in two stages (Fig. 18A).

The posterior approach (patient supine) allows excision of posterior elements, which then enables section of the annulus fibrosus and of the posterior longitudinal ligament and hemostasis of the epidural venous plexus.

The anterior approach (transpleural thoracotomy, retroperitoneal, thoracoabdominal) allows ligature of segmental vessels (at the lesional level, above and below), proximal and distal discectomies, and en bloc removal of the vertebral body.

Hemivertebrectomy (Marginal/Wide Sagittal Resection of the Vertebra)

A tumor occupying zones 3 to 5 (or 8 to 10) means that it arises eccentrically within the body, the pedicle, or the transverse process (Fig. 18B). In these cases, a resec-

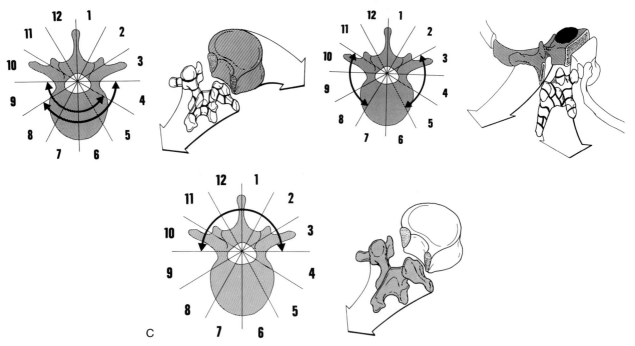

FIG. 18. A: Indication for vertebral body en bloc resection: tumor confined to locations 4 to 8 or 5 to 9. The resection is achieved by combined double approach (vertebrectomy). **B:** Indication for sagittal en bloc vertebral body and arch resection (hemivertebrectomy): tumor confined to locations 3 to 5 (or 8 to 10). The resection is achieved by a combined double approach. **C:** Indication for en bloc arch resection: tumor confined to locations 10 to 3. The resection is achieved by a posterior approach.

tion of even more than one level can be performed. If necessary, this may include one or more ribs and is performed in a single stage, allowing a 300° view of a thoracolumbar vertebra.

The patient is placed in a lateral decubitus position. A "T" incision is performed; in the thoracic spine, a midline posterior incision combined with an oblique thoracotomic incision on the rib of the affected level, and in the lumbar spine, the lateral branch is the classic retroperitoneal approach. The posterior healthy structures are removed, including the pedicle (to make room for the dural displacement). The nerve root(s) of the affected segment is (are) ligated, if necessary. The vertebra is cut by chisel or osteotome far from the tumor (at least one zone free from tumor) after protecting the major vessel (isolated by the anterior approach), obtaining an en bloc resection.

Marginal/Wide Resection of the Posterior Arch

When the tumor is located between zones 10 and 3, en bloc resection can be performed by a simple posterior approach (Fig. 18C). To achieve this result, a wide laminectomy must expose the dural sac above and below the tumor. Lateral dissection must expose the pedicles, which are sectioned by osteotome or Gigli saw.

BIOMECHANICS OF SPINE TUMOR RECONSTRUCTION

A number of different surgical situations requiring reconstruction may be encountered. These range from the posterior stabilization used in the palliative surgery of anterior tumors requiring radiotherapy (combined or not with laminectomy) to the more complex reconstructions required after vertebrectomy, when the muscles sacrificed must also be considered. Sometimes no reconstruction is required; this is the case with benign lesions such as osteoid osteomas, which must be treated by simple nidus excision, leaving in place the reactive bone; or anterior or posterior lesions, in which the stability is seldom affected by such a simple procedure. Eosinophilic granuloma, especially in the younger child, only rarely requires reconstruction; curettage and injection of corticosteroid are usually followed by spontaneous reconstruction. Posterior excision of some osteoblastomas or aneurysmal bone cysts performed without interruption of both posterior columns has been successful. In the recent past, reconstruction was not performed in some cases at particular risk of recurrence to allow a careful follow-up study. Nowadays, titanium devices are used that are MRI compatible, and no major artifacts are seen. This allows prompt detection of pathologic tissue, that is, recurrence (Fig. 19).

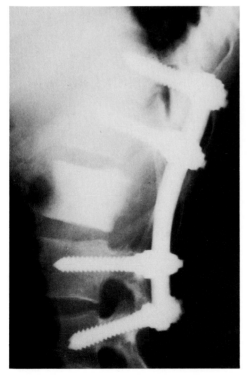
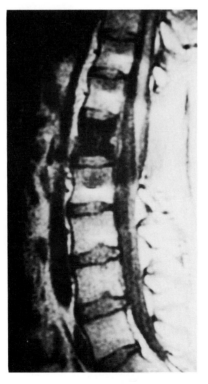

FIG. 19. Postoperative x-ray **(A)** and MR image **(B)** of decompression and stabilization performed by titanium VSP plates in a case of unresectable Ewing's sarcoma. The titanium plates do not cause any major artifact and do not prevent careful study of the tumor after radiotherapy and chemotherapy, so it can be considered for resection.

A,B

Harrington distraction and compression rods have been used for many years to stabilize lesions of the thoracic and lumbar spine. This system, especially if combined with sublaminar wiring, is still appropriate even if both the anterior and middle columns are involved, as is seen in extensive vertebral metastases. However, these devices cannot counter the excessive bending and tension loads and are at risk for late failure (35,116) from the bony effects of radiotherapy. Moreover, although the Harrington system can restore proper alignment and in some cases restore appropriate vertebral height to the spinal elements, retropulsed vertebral fragments responsible for cord impingement often are left unreduced. Even with an intact annulus and posterior longitudinal ligament, reduction of a fracture can be associated with a residual stenosis in 25% (119). In cases of extensive vertebral involvement and cord compression, Harrington distraction rods should not be used without anterior decompression, anterior grafting, and fixation. Stabilization with Luque instrumentation and sublaminar wiring has been successful in cervical, thoracic, and lumbar segments. Although there are risks involved in passing sublaminar wires, this technique may provide better fixation in soft bone than the Harrington system. After lam-

inectomy, the fixation should be carried three levels above and two to three levels below the laminectomized segments. Wires may be passed at all levels above and below and also over the transverse processes or through the neural foramina at operated segments (31). Newer instrumentation systems for posterior stabilization have been applied in specific situations with good short-term results. Although the indications for the use of the Cotrel-Dubousset instrumentation system (21) and the variety of pedicle fixation systems (85,99) have been established for scoliosis, segmental instability, and trauma, published experience with these systems in tumor care is limited (112). Regardless of the technique used, posterior instrumentation alone cannot provide a stable construct in all cases. When the anterior and middle columns of the spine have already been compromised by extensive vertebral collapse (24), laminectomy is likely to result in severe postoperative instability. These patients are placed at high risk for iatrogenic cord injury and paraplegia (30). Even when fusion and stabilization are obtained posteriorly, excessive motion of the anterior elements still may occur if there is no attempt to reconstruct the anterior and middle columns. It has been shown that even when the posterior elements are rigidly fixed, there

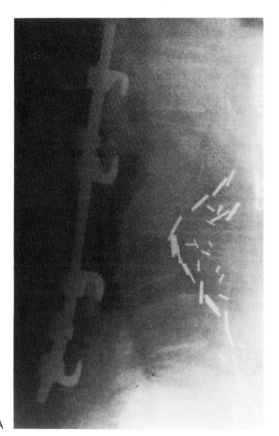

A

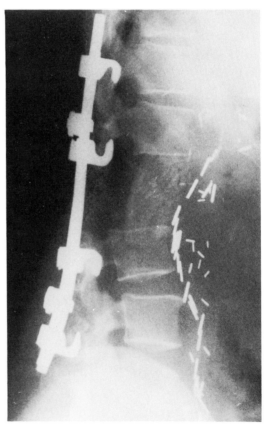

B

FIG. 20. A: Three-month postoperative "flexion" roentgenogram after resection of L2 metastatic testicular carcinoma. **B:** "Extension" roentgenogram demonstrating abnormal motion after resection bone grafting and inadequate fixation for this resection.

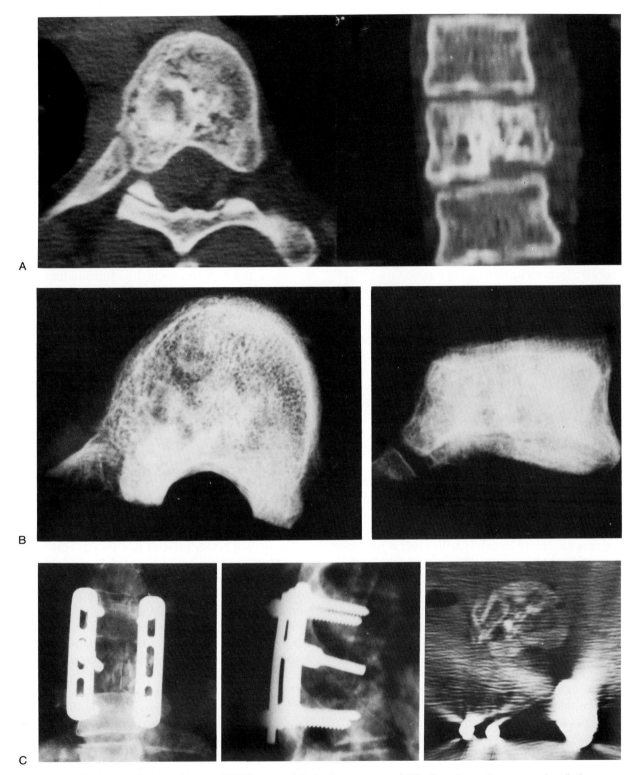

FIG. 21. A: Axial and coronal CT image of Ewing's sarcoma of T7 after chemotherapy and radiation therapy, reducing the tumor to the locations 5 to 8. **B:** Specimen x-ray of the tumor after en bloc resection (wide margin) by double approach vertebrectomy. **C:** Reconstruction achieved by VSP plates and carbon prosthesis to bridge the intervertebral space.

can be significant motion anteriorly in response to physiologic compression and bending loads (Fig. 20) (116). To deal with this dilemma, a number of techniques of anterior stabilization have been developed, some depending on methylmethacrylate (at best associated with wires, screws, or mesh to improve stability) or other synthetic spacers (carbon-fiber prosthesis) (Fig. 21), and others using bone graft in anticipation of a solid arthrodesis. Some authors have advocated use of autogenous or allograft bone, with or without internal fixation, to fill even very large postoperative defects (53,101,102). Such an approach is clearly favored in the treatment of benign or slowly growing tumors, for which patient survival is expected to be measured in years.

When a resection is performed for the treatment of a primary tumor and a good prognosis is expected, the goal is not only the immediate recovery of functional activity but also long-term spine stability. A three-column reconstruction must be performed, combining metallic devices with grafting.

Even when associated radiotherapy is required postoperatively, incorporation of the graft can be expected. In metastatic lesions, bone graft is commonly augmented by internal fixation and a methylmethacrylate construct. The methacrylate functions well as a spacer, but is prone to displacement. The hardware functions to restore the height lost during excision of the vertebral body and fix the methacrylate construct in place. When considering radiation in the setting of bone grafting, it is recommended to postpone radiation treatment for as long as possible, preferably until wounds are healed and/or for an additional period of 6 to 12 weeks.

Spinal reconstruction using methylmethacrylate remains somewhat controversial. If arthrodesis is not obtained, it may be only a matter of time before the methacrylate construct fails; only patients with a limited life expectancy should be indicated for methacrylate fixation without bone grafting (28). The way in which methylmethacrylate is used also determines the likelihood of failure. Cement used as an adjunct to posterior stabilization is loaded in tension, where it is weakest and more susceptible to fatigue failure. Methylmethacrylate is strongest in compression. It proves quite resilient and dependable for anterior vertebral reconstructions where, functioning as a spacer, it is primarily exposed to compressive loads (116). Reinforcing methylmethacrylate with wire or wire mesh increases its tensile strength and improves its ability to withstand bending loads, particularly when used in posterior stabilization procedures. Longitudinal Steinmann pins may be used anteriorly to enhance both the bending resistance of the construct and its fixation to the adjacent vertebral bodies. Sundaresan et al. (104) have used this technique with good results, inserting two or more Steinmann pins, 1 to 5 mm in diameter, into the adjacent vertebral bodies before instilling liquid cement into the defect. Seigal has advocated

the use of Harrington distraction rods and, more recently, Moe sacral hooks and threaded rods to obtain anterior purchase. Harrington (42) has used Knodt rods for several years to the same purpose.

Reconstruction of the vertebral body with methylmethacrylate requires care to avoid contact of the cement with the dural sac posteriorly. Although studies have indicated that even with direct contact, thermal injury to the cord is unlikely, reports of postoperative dural compression due to cement impingement have suggested that some space must be maintained between the cement mass and the posterior longitudinal ligament. Cement used in the dough phase allows better control of placement, and interposing a sheet of gel foam or fat anterior to the dural elements will further shield them (25). During polymerization, a steady flow of saline irrigation will minimize the heat transmitted to surrounding tissues. Because of problems with fixation and cord impingement, some authors have recommended against the use of methylmethacrylate in patients with a life expectancy greater than 1 year (67). On the other hand, biomechanical studies in postmortem specimens have shown excellent stability in the cervical spine as long as 7 years after fixation with methacrylate (77). These reports emphasize that the key to longevity of fixation using methylmethacrylate is augmentation with an adequate autogenous bone graft.

PROGNOSIS

Benign Tumors

The overall 5-year survival rate for patients with benign tumors of the spine reported by Weinstein and McLain (113) was 86%. In that series, there was no significant relationship between the extent of initial excision and either survival or recurrence rate, except in the case of benign giant cell tumors. When compared with other benign lesions, giant cell tumors demonstrated an aggressive tendency toward local recurrence, with two of the five patients eventually dying from their extensive recurrences and cord compromise. Aside from those with giant cell tumor, the only patient to die from a benign spinal neoplasm presented with a massive sacral osteoblastoma, which was unresectable. Local recurrence was seen in 21% of patients undergoing surgical treatment of their lesions, and half of these recurrences were in the giant cell tumor group. Sixty-six percent of local recurrences were apparent within the first year. One patient with a benign giant cell tumor suffered a malignant transformation after biopsy and irradiation. In the series of the Rizzoli Institute, a patient died of renal complications due to the growth of an aneurysmal bone cyst of L2, which proved insensitive to radiation therapy and repeated excisions. Another patient died in the postoperative course of an incomplete excision of a very vascularized cervical osteoblastoma. Today, routine preoperative selective arterial embolization may have prevented such a lethal outcome.

Malignant Tumors

Among the patients with malignant lesions, survival varied with the tumor type and the extent of the initial surgical excision (113). Slow-growing, locally aggressive tumors were associated with greater mean and overall survival rates when compared with the rapidly progressive, early-metastasizing lesions. Overall survival was greatest in the solitary plasmacytoma group (Table 4) and was least for those patients with osteosarcoma and lymphoma. The only patient group with greater than a 50% 5-year survival was the solitary plasmacytoma group. To eliminate any bias introduced by the relatively few long-term survivors in each group, survival data were truncated to a maximum of 60 months when survival exceeded 60 months. No statistically significant difference was seen among the various tumor groups, though the group of patients with solitary plasmacytoma showed a strong trend toward longer survival. There was a significant correlation between survival and the extent of the initial surgical excision (Table 5). Among patients who underwent surgical treatment for their spinal lesion, the mean survival was 17 months (survival truncated to 60 months), with only 15% of the cases surviving 5 years. For those having a surgical biopsy but no further attempt at tumor removal, the mean survival was 33.5 months and the 5-year survival was 33%. These patients tended to do better than those who had curettage or incomplete resection of their tumors, groups with 17.5- and 23.2-month mean survivals, respectively. There were no 5-year survivors in the curettage group. The best results obtained in patients with malignant spinal tumors were in patients undergoing complete excision of their lesion at their initial surgery. These patients had a mean survival of 48.4 months and a 5-year survival rate of 75%. This was a significantly better result than that obtained

TABLE 4. *Survival in patients with malignancy by tumor type[a]*

Tumor type	Number of patients	Mean survival
Solitary plasmacytoma	15	38.27
Chondrosarcoma	4	28.00
Chordoma	11	27.73
Ewing's sarcoma	4	27.50
Osteogenic sarcoma	3	18.33
Lymphoma	5	13.40
Others	4	36.25
Total	46	

[a] Survival scores truncated to 60 months.

TABLE 5. *Survival in patients with malignancy by surgical excision[a]*

Type of surgical treatment	Number of patients	Mean survival (months)	5-year survival
None	5	17.00	15%
Curettage	4	17.50	0%
Incomplete resection	17	23.18	18.7%
Biopsy only	10	33.50	33%
Complete excision	10	48.40	75%
Total	46		

[a] Survival scores truncated to 60 months.

by either curettage or incomplete excision. The group of patients with solitary plasmacytomas had the greatest mean survival regardless of surgical treatment (68,113). This was thought to be due to the lesion's unique radiosensitivity. To determine what bias, if any, this patient group might have introduced into our results, mean and 5-year survivals were calculated excluding patients with this diagnosis. There was no significant change in the relative outcomes among surgical groups, and complete excision demonstrated a significantly improved survival when compared with the other treatment groups. Local recurrence occurred in 11 patients (21%) with malignant tumors. Recurrence was clearly associated with specific tumor types: 6 of 11 chordoma patients, 2 of 4 chondrosarcoma patients, and 1 patient with malignant giant cell tumor developed a local recurrence. Of all recurrent lesions, 70% were apparent within the first 2 years after surgery.

Extradural Tumors

Extradural, extraosseous tumors are very uncommon. The majority are benign soft-tissue lesions that expand slowly and have little invasive potential.

Epidural Hemangioma

Epidural hemangiomas represent approximately 4% of all epidural tumors and 12% of all intraspinal hemangiomas (75). They are almost always located in the upper thoracic spine and are characterized by slowly progressive spinal cord compression, usually present for some months before presentation. Acute progression and increase in symptoms may be precipitated if hemorrhage occurs and an epidural hematoma forms.

Epidural Lipoma

Epidural lipomas are an unusual cause of spinal cord compression, but their occurrence is well documented and the increased risk in patients with Cushing's syndrome should be appreciated. Failure to appreciate the extensive nature of these benign tumors can lead to inadequate excision and can be disastrous (36). Steroid-induced lipomatosis usually involves the thoracic spine. Signs of cord compression can appear acutely, though the process has usually been ongoing for many months. Patients may present with rapidly progressive weakness and a myelographic block that involves the entire thoracic canal. Lesions have been misdiagnosed as epidural abscesses or as vertebral metastases, and some patients have even undergone irradiation, with a dismal outcome (34). MRI has proven useful in demonstrating the full extent and character of these lesions, the severity of cord compression, and the relative tumor location anteriorly or posteriorly in the canal (44,118). Although regression of lipomatosis may occur after decreasing or discontinuing steroid medications, laminectomy with surgical decompression is the treatment of choice in progressive lesions, providing neurologic improvement in 90% of cases (39).

Extradural Meningioma

Extradural meningiomas represent approximately 7% of meningiomas treated. These are rare tumors almost always associated with an intradural component, even though a communication between the two cannot always be demonstrated (57). The extradural lesions tend to be vascular and may erode bone, giving an appearance of an extradural metastasis. When excised, these tumors have a tendency to recur, but neurologic recovery is usually satisfactory after decompression. Whenever an extradural meningioma is encountered, an intradural lesion must be ruled out, possibly through intradural exploration.

Neurofibroma

Neurofibromas are a relatively common spinal cord tumor, accounting for approximately one quarter of all spinal tumors. Although 80% are intradural lesions, approximately 10% will be entirely extradural and another 10% will have both intradural and extradural components. The tumors are usually solitary but may be multiple, and usually arise from the spinal nerve root. They are the most common cause of an hourglass or dumbbell tumor, though other neoplasms can produce this appearance. Because 20% of these lesions may undergo malignant degeneration and produce significant cord compression, excision is indicated. Whenever an extradural neurofibroma is encountered, intradural exploration to rule out an intradural tumor should be strongly considered.

Lymphoma

The most common malignancy found in the epidural space is lymphoma. Although extension from para-

spinous nodes or from the vertebral body is thought to account for most lymphomas of the spinal canal, there have been a number of cases of primary lymphoma reported to arise within the epidural space (14). Plain radiographs may show some bony erosion in these cases or may be completely normal. Myelography has traditionally been most reliable for demonstrating the presence and extent of the lesion. Surgical decompression usually involves laminectomy, and neurologic improvement depends to a great extent on the preoperative grade of neurologic deficit.

SUMMARY

The prognosis for survival has improved dramatically for cancer patients over the past 3 decades. New approaches to treating systemic disease have prolonged survival even in those who cannot be cured. As survival has increased, the importance of managing spinal column disease and protecting the spinal cord has also increased. Any patient presenting with some residual neurologic function and enough physical reserve to withstand an operation will often benefit from a stable spine, relief of pain, and spinal cord decompression; there are very few exceptions. Advances in surgical techniques and materials have not only improved survival and functional outcome, but also have limited many of the postoperative complications that plagued earlier treatment techniques. This is true for metastatic lesions of the spine as well as for conditions such as lymphomas and plasmacytoma. The approach to most rare primary tumors is quite different: First, achieve the diagnosis; second, stage the lesion and decide the adequate margin; and third, plan surgery according to these criteria. An oncologic and surgical staging system is required. The main aim must be oncologically adequate treatment of the lesion. To this purpose, the development of techniques of surgical en bloc resection not only for the limbs, but also for the mobile spine, has proven essential and is made possible by a surgical planning system that informs the surgeon of the objectives to achieve. Stability of the spine and neurologic problems are solved as a consequence, but they are not the first objective of the treatment. Treating these problems before achieving the correct diagnosis will prevent one from reaching the correct treatment paradigm and expose patients to the potential risks of recurrence and dissemination of their disease.

ACKNOWLEDGMENT. Special thanks go to Mario Campanacci, M.D.; Michael Bonfiglio, M.D.; Bertil Stener, M.D.; Henk Verbiest, M.D.; and Jody Buckwalter, M.D. for their leadership and tutelage.

Dedicated to Mike Bonfiglio, "Teacher, Scientist, Surgeon, and Friend."

REFERENCES

1. Akbarnia BA, Rooholamini SA (1981): Scoliosis caused by benign osteoblastoma of the thoracic or lumbar spine. *J Bone Joint Surg* [*Am*] 63:1146–1155.

2. Barwick KW, Huvos AG, Smith J (1980): Primary osteogenic sarcoma of the vertebral column: A clinicopathologic correlation of ten patients. *Cancer* 46:595–604.

3. Bergsagel DE, Rider WD (1985): Plasma cell neoplasms in cancer. In: De Vita VT, Hellman S, Rosenberg SA, eds. *Principles and practice of oncology,* 2nd ed. Philadelphia: J.B. Lippincott.

4. Bohlman HH, Sachs BL, Carter JR, Riley L, Robinson RA (1986): Primary neoplasms of the cervical spine. Diagnosis and treatment of twenty-three patients. *J Bone Joint Surg* [*Am*] 68:483–494.

5. Boriani S, Capanna R, Donati D, Levine A, Picci P, Savini R (1992): Osteoblastoma of the spine. *Clin Orthop* 278:37–45.

6. Boriani S, Chevalley F, Weinstein JN, Campanacci L, DeIure F, Biagini R (1996): Chordoma of the spine above sacrum—Treatment and outcome in 21 cases. *Spine* (in press).

7. Boriani S, Weinstein JN, Biagini R (1996): A surgical staging system for therapeutic planning of primary bone tumors of the spine: A contribution to a common terminology. *Spine* (in press).

8. Brice J, McKissock W (1965): Surgical treatment of malignant extradural spinal tumours. *BMJ* 1:1341–1344.

9. Bucknill T, Jackson JW, Kemp HB, Kendall BE (1973): Haemangioma of a vertebral body treated by ligation of the segmental arteries. Report of a case. *J Bone Joint Surg* [*Br*] 55:534–539.

10. Cahan WG, Woodward HQ, Higinbotham NL, Stewart FW, Coley BL (1948): Sarcoma arising in irradiated bone; Report of 11 cases. *Cancer* 1:3–29.

11. Campanacci M, Boriani S, Savini R (1983): Staging, biopsy, surgical planning of primary spine tumors. *Chir Organi Mov* 75:99–103.

12. Campanacci M (1990): *Bone and soft tissue tumors.* New York: Springer Verlag.

13. Capanna R, Boriani S, Mabit CH, Donati D, Savini R (1991): Osteoid osteoma of the spine. *Rev Chir Orthop* 77:545–550.

14. Cappellani G, Giuffre F, Tropea R, Guarnera F, Augello G, Chiaramonte I, Mancuso P (1986): Primary spinal epidural lymphomas. Report of ten cases. *J Neurosurg Sci* 30:147–151.

15. Chiurco AA (1970): Multiple exostoses of bone with fatal spinal cord compression: Report of a case and brief review of the literature. *Neurology* 20:275–278.

16. Citrin DL, Bessent RG, Greig WR (1977): A comparison of sensitivity and accuracy of the 99m-Tc phosphate bone scan and skeletal radiograph in the diagnosis of bone metastases. *Clin Radiol* 28:107–117.

17. Clausen N, Gotze H, Pedersen A, Riis-Petersen J, Tjalve E (1983): Skeletal scintigraphy and radiography at onset of acute lymphocytic leukemia in children. *Med Pediatr Oncol* 11:291–296.

18. Compere EL, Johnson WE, Coventry MB (1954): Vertebra plana (Calve's disease) due to eosinophilic granuloma. *J Bone Joint Surg* [*Am*] 36:969–980.

19. Corcoran RJ, Thrall JH, Kyle RW, Kaminski RJ, Johnson MC (1976): Solitary abnormalities in bone scans of patients with extraosseous malignancies. *Radiology* 121:663–667.

20. Corwin J, Lindberg RD (1979): Solitary plasmacytoma of bone vs. extramedullary plasmacytoma and their relationship to multiple myeloma. *Cancer* 43:1007–1013.

21. Cotrel Y, Dubousset J, Guillaumat M (1988): New universal instrumentation in spinal surgery. *Clin Orthop* 227:10–23.

22. Dahlin DC (1977): Giant-cell tumor of vertebrae above the sacrum: A review of 31 cases. *Cancer* 39:1350–1356.

23. DeCristofaro R, Biagini R, Boriani S, Ricci S, Ruggieri P, Rossi G, Fabbri N, Roversi R (1992): Selective arterial embolization in the treatment of aneurysmal bone cyst and angioma of bone. *Skeletal Radiol* 21:523–527.

24. Denis F (1983): The three column spine and its significance in the classification of acute thoracolumbar spinal injuries. *Spine* 8:817–831.

25. Dolin MG (1989): Acute massive dural compression secondary to methyl methacrylate replacement of a tumorous lumbar vertebral body. *Spine* 14:108–110.

26. Dowdle JA Jr, Winter RB, Dehner LP (1977): Postradiation osteosarcoma of the cervical spine in childhood. A case report. *J Bone Joint Surg* [*Am*] 59:969–971.

27. Enneking WF, Spanier SS, Goodmann MA (1980): A system for surgical staging of musculoskeletal sarcoma. *Clin Orthop* 153:106–120.

28. Fidler MW (1985): Pathologic fractures of the cervical spine. *J Bone Joint Surg* [*Br*] 67:352–357.

29. Fielding JW, Pyle RN Jr, Fietti VG Jr (1979): Anterior cervical vertebral body resection and bone-grafting for benign and malignant tumors. A survey under the auspices of the Cervical Spine Research Society. *J Bone Joint Surg* [*Am*] 61:251–253.

30. Findlay GF (1987): The role of vertebral body collapse in the management of malignant spinal cord compression. *J Neurol Neurosurg Psychiatry* 50:151–154.

31. Flatley TJ, Anderson MH, Anast GT (1984): Spinal instability due to malignant disease. Treatment by segmental spinal stabilization. *J Bone Joint Surg* [*Am*] 66:47–52.

32. Fowles JV, Bobechko WP (1970): Solitary eosinophilic granuloma in bone. *J Bone Joint Surg* [*Br*] 52:238–243.

33. Fraser RD, Paterson DC, Simpson DA (1977): Orthopaedic aspects of spinal tumors in children. *J Bone Joint Surg* [*Br*] 59:143–151.

34. Gennari L, Azzarelli A, Quagliuolo V (1987): A posterior approach for the excision of sacral chordoma. *J Bone Joint Surg* [*Br*] 69:565–568.

35. Gertzbein SD, MacMichael D, Tile M (1982): Harrington instrumentation as a method of fixation in fractures of the spine. *J Bone Joint Surg* [*Br*] 64:526–529.

36. Goyal RN (1980): Epidural lipoma causing compression of the spinal cord. *Surg Neurol* 14:77–79.

37. Green NE, Robertson WW Jr, Kilroy AW (1980): Eosinophilic granuloma of the spine with associated neural deficit. Report of three cases. *J Bone Joint Surg* [*Am*] 62:1198–1202.

38. Griffin JB (1978): Benign osteoblastoma of the thoracic spine. Case report with fifteen-year follow-up. *J Bone Joint Surg* [*Am*] 60:833–835.

39. Haid RW Jr, Kaufman HH, Schochet SS Jr, Marano GD (1987): Epidural lipomatosis simulating an epidural abscess: Case report and literature review. *Neurosurgery* 21:744–747.

40. Hall AJ, MacKay NN (1973): The results of laminectomy for compression of the cord or cauda equina by extradural malignant tumour. *J Bone Joint Surg* [*Br*] 55:497–505.

41. Harrington KD, Sim FH, Enis JE, Johnston JO, Diok HM, Gristina AG (1976): Methylmethacrylate as an adjunct in internal fixation of pathological fractures. Experience with three hundred and seventy-five cases. *J Bone Joint Surg* [*Am*] 58:1047–1055.

42. Harrington KD (1981): The use of methylmethacrylate for vertebral-body replacement and anterior stabilization of pathological fracture-dislocations of the spine due to metastatic malignant disease. *J Bone Joint Surg* [*Am*] 63:36–46.

43. Hay MC, Paterson D, Taylor TK (1978): Aneurysmal bone cysts of the spine. *J Bone Joint Surg* [*Br*] 60:406–411.

44. Healy ME, Hesselink JR, Ostrup RC, Alksne JF (1987): Demonstration by magnetic resonance of symptomatic spinal epidural lipomatosis. *Neurosurgery* 21:414–415.

45. Hermann G, Sacher M, Lanzieri CF, Anderson PJ, Rabinowitz JG (1985): Chondrosarcoma of the spine: An unusual radiographic presentation. *Skeletal Radiol* 14:178–183.

46. Hirsh LF, Thanki A, Spector HB (1984): Primary spinal chondrosarcoma with eighteen-year follow-up: Case report and literature review. *Neurosurgery* 14:747–749.

47. Huvos AG, Woodward HQ, Cahan WG, Higinbotham NL (1985): Post-radiation osteogenic sarcoma of bone and soft tissues. A clinicopathologic study of 66 patients. *Cancer* 55:1244–1255.

48. Huvos AG (1986): Osteogenic sarcoma of bones and soft tissues in older persons. A clinicopathologic analysis of 117 patients older than 60 years. *Cancer* 57:1442–1449.

49. Ippolito E, Farsetti P, Tudisco C (1984): Vertebra plana. Long term follow-up in five patients. *J Bone Joint Surg* [*Am*] 66:1364–1368.

50. Jaffe HL (1958): *Tumors and tumorous conditions of the bones and joints.* Philadelphia: Lea and Febiger.

51. Kaiser TE, Pritchard DJ, Unni KK (1984): Clinicopathologic study of sacrococcygeal chordoma. *Cancer* 54:2574–2578.

52. Kak VK, Prabhakar S, Khosla VK, Banerjee AK (1985): Solitary osteochondroma of spine causing spinal cord compression. *Clin Neurol Neurosurg* 87:135–138.

53. Kaneda K, Abumi K, Fujiya M (1984): Burst fractures with neurologic deficits of the thoracolumbar-lumbar spine. Results of anterior decompression and stabilization with anterior instrumentation. *Spine* 9:788–795.

54. Keim HA, Reina EG (1975): Osteoid-osteoma as a cause of scoliosis. *J Bone Joint Surg [Am]* 57:159–163.

55. Kornberg M (1986): Primary Ewing's sarcoma of the spine. A review and case report. *Spine* 11:54–57.

56. Kostuik JP (1983): Anterior spinal cord decompression for lesions of the thoracic and lumbar spine, techniques, new methods of internal fixation results. *Spine* 8:512–531.

57. Levy WJ, Latchaw J, Hahn JF, Sawhny B, Bay J, Dohn DF (1986): Spinal neurofibromas: A report of 66 cases and a comparison with meningiomas. *Neurosurgery* 18:331–334.

58. Lodwick GS, Wilson AJ, Farrell C (1980): Determining growth rates of focal lesions of bone from radiographs. *Radiology* 134:577–583.

59. Loftus CM, Michelsen CB, Rapoport F, Antunes JL (1983): Management of plasmacytomas of the spine. *Neurosurgery* 13:30–36.

60. Loftus CM, Rozario RA, Prager R, Scott RM (1980): Solitary osteochondroma of T4 with thoracic cord compression. *Surg Neurol* 13:355–357.

61. Lozman J, Holmblad J (1976): Cavernous hemangiomas associated with scoliosis and a localized consumptive coagulopathy. A case report. *J Bone Joint Surg [Am]* 58:1021–1024.

62. Lubicky JP, Patel NS, DeWald RL (1983): Two-stage spondylectomy for giant cell tumor of L4. A case report. *Spine* 8:112–115.

63. Malat J, Virapongse C, Levine A (1986): Solitary osteochondroma of the spine. *Spine* 11:625–628.

64. Mankin HJ, Lange TA, Spanier SS (1982): The hazards of biopsy in patients with malignant primary bone and soft-tissue tumors. *J Bone Joint Surg [Am]* 64:1121–1127.

65. Marsh BW, Bonfiglio M, Brady LP, Enneking WF (1975): Benign osteoblastoma: Range of manifestations. *J Bone Joint Surg [Am]* 57:1–9.

66. Martin NS, Williamson J (1970): The role of surgery in the treatment of malignant tumours of the spine. *J Bone Joint Surg [Br]* 52:227–237.

67. McAfee PC, Bohlman HH, Ducker T, Eismont FJ (1986): Failure of stabilization of the spine with methylmethacrylate. A retrospective analysis of twenty-four cases. *J Bone Joint Surg [Am]* 68:1145–1157.

68. McLain RF, Weinstein JN (1989): Solitary plasmacytomas of the spine: A review of 84 cases. *J Spinal Disorders* 2:69–74.

69. Meissner WA, Warren S (1966): In: Anderson WAD, ed. *Neoplasms in pathology*, Vol. 1, 5th ed. St. Louis: C.V. Mosby, pp. 534–540.

70. Mindell ER (1981): Chordoma. *J Bone Joint Surg [Am]* 63:501–505.

71. Mirra JM, Gold RH, Picci P (1989): In: Mirra JM, ed. *Osseous tumors of intramedullary origin in bone tumors: Clinical, radiologic and pathologic considerations.* Philadelphia: Lea & Febiger, pp. 31–33.

72. Mirra JM, Gold RH, Picci P (1989): In: Mirra JM, ed. *Osseous tumors of intramedullary origin in bone tumors: Clinical, radiologic and pathologic considerations.* Philadelphia: Lea & Febiger, pp. 350–358.

73. Nesbit ME, Kieffer S, D'Angio GJ (1969): Reconstitution of vertebral height in histiocytosis X: A long-term follow-up. *J Bone Joint Surg [Am]* 51:1360–1368.

74. Nicholls PJ, Jarecky TW (1985): The value of posterior decompression by laminectomy for malignant tumors of the spine. *Clin Orthop* 201:210–213.

75. Padovani R, Poppi M, Pozzati E, Tognetti F, Querzola C (1981): Spinal epidural hemangiomas. *Spine* 6:336–340.

76. Palmer FJ, Blum PW (1980): Osteochondroma with spinal cord compression: A report of three cases. *J Neurosurg* 52:842–845.

77. Panjabi MM, Goel VK, Clark CR, Keggi KJ, Southwick WO (1985): Biomechanical study of cervical spine stabilization with methylmethacrylate. *Spine* 10:198–203.

78. Pettine KA, Klassen RA (1986): Osteoid-osteoma and osteoblastoma of the spine. *J Bone Joint Surg [Am]* 68:354–361.

79. Pilepich MV, Vietti TJ, Nesbit ME, Tefft M, Kissane J, Burgert O, Pritchard D, Gehan EA (1981): Ewing's sarcoma of the vertebral column. *Int J Radiat Oncol Biol Phys* 7:27–31.

80. Poulsen JO, Jensen JT, Thommesen P (1975): Ewing's sarcoma simulating vertebra plana. *Acta Orthop Scand* 46:211–215.

81. Price CH, Goldie W (1969): Paget's sarcoma of bone: A study of 80 cases from the Bristol and the Leeds bone tumour registries. *J Bone Joint Surg [Br]* 51:205–224.

82. Ransford AO, Pozo JL, Hutton PA, Kirwan EO (1984): The behaviour pattern of the scoliosis associated with osteoid osteoma or osteoblastoma of the spine. *J Bone Joint Surg [Br]* 66:16–20.

83. Rich TA, Schiller A, Suit HD, Mankin HJ (1985): Clinical and pathologic review of 48 cases of chordoma. *Cancer* 56:182–187.

84. Rogalsky RJ, Black GB, Reed MH (1986): Orthopaedic manifestations of leukemia in children. *J Bone Joint Surg [Am]* 68:494–501.

85. Roy-Camille R, Saillant G, Mazel C (1986): Internal fixation of the lumbar spine with pedicle screw plating. *Clin Orthop* 203:7–17.

86. Russin LA, Robinson MJ, Engle HA, Sonni A (1982): Ewing's sarcoma of the lumbar spine: A case report of long-term survival. *Clin Orthop* 164:126–129.

87. Savini R, Gherlinzoni F, Morandi M, Neff JR, Picci P (1983): Surgical treatment of giant-cell tumor of the spine. The experience at the Istituto Ortopedico Rizzoli. *J Bone Joint Surg [Am]* 65:1283–1289.

88. Savini R, Giunti A, Boriani S (1995): Benign and malignant spinal tumor. In: Bradford DS, Hensinger RM, eds. *The pediatric spine.* New York: Thieme Inc.

89. Savitz MH, Goldstein HB, Jaffrey IS, Rothschild EJ, Bobroff LM (1988): Ewing's sarcoma arising in the sacral epidural space: Case report. *Mt Sinai J Med* 55:339–342.

90. Schajowicz F (1981): *Tumors, and tumor-like lesions of bone and joints.* New York: Springer-Verlag, pp. 281–302.

91. Sharma BS, Khosla VK, Banerjee AK (1986): Primary spinal epidural Ewing's sarcoma. *Clin Neurol Neurosurg* 88:299–302.

92. Sherk HH, Nicholson JT, Nixon JE (1978): Vertebra plana and eosinophilic granuloma of the cervical spine in children. *Spine* 3:116–121.

93. Shives TC, Dahlin DC, Sim FH, Pritchard DJ, Earle JD (1986): Osteosarcoma of the spine. *J Bone Joint Surg [Am]* 68:660–668.

94. Shives TC, McLeod RA, Unni KK, Schray MF (1989): Chondrosarcoma of the spine. *J Bone Joint Surg [Br]* 71:1158–1165.

95. Siegal T, Siegal T (1989): Current considerations in the management of neoplastic spinal cord compression. *Spine* 14:223–228.

96. Sim FH, Dahlin DC, Stauffer RN, Laws ER (1977): Primary bone tumors simulating lumbar disc syndrome. *Spine* 2:65–74.

97. Slepian A, Hamby WB (1951): Neurologic complications associated with hereditary deforming chondrodysplasia; review of literature and report on 2 cases occurring in the same family. *J Neurosurg* 8:529–535.

98. Springfield DS, Enneking WF, Neff JR, Makley JT (1984): *Principles of tumor management.* Instructional Course Lectures 33:1–25.

99. Steffee AD, Biscup RS, Sitkowski DJ (1986): Segmental spine plates with pedicle screw fixation: A new internal fixation device for disorders of the lumbar and thoracolumbar spine. *Clin Orthop* 203:45–53.

100. Stener B, Gunterberg B (1978): High amputation of the sacrum for extirpation of tumors. Principles and technique. *Spine* 3:351–366.

101. Stener B, Johnsen OE (1971): Complete removal of three vertebrae for giant-cell tumour. *J Bone Joint Surg [Br]* 53:278–287.

102. Stener B (1971): Total spondylectomy in chondrosarcoma arising from the seventh thoracic vertebra. *J Bone Joint Surg [Br]* 53:288–295.

103. Suit HD, Goiten M, Munzenreider J, et al. (1992): Definitive radiation therapy for chordoma and chondrosarcoma of base of skull and cervical spine. *J Neurosurg* 56:377–385.

104. Sundaresan N, Galicich JH, Lane JM, Bains MS, McCormack P (1985): Treatment of neoplastic epidural cord compression by vertebra 1 body resection and stabilization. *J Neurosurg* 63:676–684.

105. Sundaresan N, Huvos AG, Rosen G, Lane JM (1986): Postradia-

tion osteosarcoma of the spine following treatment of Hodgkin's disease. *Spine* 11:90–92.

106. Sundaresan N, Rosen G, Huvos AG, Krol G (1988): Combined treatment of osteosarcoma of the spine. *Neurosurgery* 23:714–719.

107. Tachdjian MO, Matson DD (1965): Orthopaedic aspects of intraspinal tumors in infants and children. *J Bone Joint Surg [Am]* 47:223–248.

108. Valderrama JA, Bullough PG (1968): Solitary myeloma of the spine. *J Bone Joint Surg [Br]* 50:82–90.

109. Verbiest H (1969): Anterolateral operations for fractures and dislocations in the middle and lower parts of the cervical spine. Report of a series of forty-seven cases. *J Bone Joint Surg [Am]* 51:1489–1530.

110. Verbiest H (1978): Lesions of the cervical spine: A critical review. In: Carrea R, ed. *Neurological surgery.* International Congress series 433. Amsterdam: Excerpta Medica, pp. 374–383.

111. Waxman AD (1981): Bone scans are of sufficient accuracy and sensitivity to be part of the routine work up prior to definitive surgical treatment of cancer. In: Van Scoy-Mosher MB, ed. *Medical oncology: Current controversies in cancer treatment.* Boston: G.K. Hall Medical Publishers, pp. 69–76.

112. Weinstein JN (1989): Surgical approach to spine tumors. *Orthopedics* 12:897–905.

113. Weinstein JN, McLain RF (1987): Primary tumors of the spine. *Spine* 12:843–851.

114. Weinstein JN (1994): Primary tumors. In: Weinstein S, ed. *The pediatric spine.* New York: Raven Press.

115. Weinstein J, Hart R, Boriani S, Biagini R, Currier B (1994): *Spine tumors: Surgical staging and clinical outcome.* Application to Giant Cell Tumors of the Spine. 21st ISSLS Annual Meeting, Seattle.

116. White AA III, Panjabi MM (1978): Surgical constructs employing methylmethacrylate. In: *Clinical biomechanics of the spine.* Philadelphia: J.B. Lippincott, pp. 423–431.

117. Whitehouse GH, Griffiths GJ (1976): Roentgenologic aspects of spinal involvement by primary and metastatic Ewing's tumor. *Can Assoc Radiol J* 27:290–297.

118. Wiedemayer H, Nau HE, Reinhardt V, Hebestreit HP (1987): Spinal cord compression by extensive epidural lipoma. A case report. *Eur Neurol* 27:46–50.

119. Willen J, Lindahl S, Irstam L, Nordwall A (1984): Unstable thoracolumbar fractures: A study by CT and conventional roentgenology of the reduction effect of Harrington instrumentation. *Spine* 9:214–219.

The Adult Spine: Principles and Practice,
2nd edition, J.W. Frymoyer, Editor-in-Chief.
Lippincott-Raven Publishers, Philadelphia © 1997.

CHAPTER 49

Differential Diagnosis and Surgical Treatment of Metastatic Spine Tumors

John P. Kostuik

In recent years there has been an increasing interest in the care of patients presenting with metastatic disease to the spine. As a result of the availability of improved imaging techniques, diagnosis has become more accurate. Significant advances have also occurred in the surgical treatment of patients with metastatic disease with or without neurologic involvement.

Metastases are by far the most common skeletal tumors seen by the orthopedist, and the spine is the most common site of skeletal involvement (15). Skeletal metastases are produced by almost all forms of malignant disease but are usually secondary to carcinomas of the breast, lung, or prostate, and less frequently to renal, thyroid, or gastrointestinal carcinomas (Table 1) (4,31, 33,39,53–55). Breast cancer is the principal source of bony metastasis in females; between 65% and 85% of women with breast cancer develop skeletal disease prior to death (78). Among men, bronchogenic and prostatic carcinomas occur with the greatest frequency. Multiple myeloma and lymphoma are the most common sources of disseminated skeletal lesions, though whether they are classified as metastatic or primary lesions has varied from author to author, making an accurate assessment of their relative importance difficult.

In the spinal column metastatic disease most commonly arises from carcinoma of bronchogenic or breast origin, or from the lymphoreticular malignancies, lymphoma and myeloma. Metastases from these tumor types account for approximately half of the spinal lesions seen in most clinical studies. However, the relative prevalence of specific primary tumors varies significantly among published reports (Table 2) (4,17,20,36,57,60). When only the solid tumors are considered, breast, lung,

J. P. Kostuik, M.D.: Professor, Department of Orthopaedic Surgery, Johns Hopkins University School of Medicine, Baltimore, Maryland 21287-0882.

TABLE 1. Location of primary neoplasms producing metastatic lesions of bone (summary of 5,006 cases)

Primary	Number	Percent
Breast	2,020	40
Lung	646	13
Prostate	296	6
Kidney	284	6
Gastrointestinal	255	5
Thyroid	110	2
Bladder	160	3
Other		25
Total	5,006	100

and prostate carcinomas comprise the majority of spinal metastases, followed by renal, gastrointestinal, and thyroid carcinomas. Although rarely mentioned in reviews of metastatic disease, tumors of the gastrointestinal system result in significantly more spinal metastases (and skeletal metastases in general) than do thyroid carcinomas, which are more often included in the "textbook" differential diagnosis.

Estimating the prevalence of metastasis for each tumor type varies depending on whether one looks at autopsy studies of clinically significant metastasis or data available from clinical reviews. Moreover, the clinical behavior of the primary tumor will determine the perceived prevalence and ultimately determine the clinical importance of that lesion for each patient. For example, patients with breast and prostate carcinoma frequently survive long enough to require treatment of their spinal metastasis, whereas patients with pulmonary malignancies often succumb so rapidly that little more than supportive care is required. Because gastrointestinal carcinoma tends to involve the liver and lungs long before it involves the spine, these patients often die before their spinal lesion becomes clinically apparent.

PATHOPHYSIOLOGY

The distribution of metastatic disease in the skeleton is influenced by three factors. First, tumor emboli enter the bloodstream and tend to arrest in the natural filters of the vascular tree—the capillary beds of the liver, lungs, and bone marrow (71). To become established in the medullary canals of the spine, tumor emboli first must go through the capillary beds of the liver and lungs, often establishing a metastasis at these locations. Alternatively the tumor emboli may circumvent these filters and reach the medulla sinusoids by an entirely different route. Tumors of the lung may seed the vertebral column directly through the segmental arteries, whereas carcinomas of the breast and prostate are thought to reach the vertebral system through communications with the paravertebral venous plexus originally described by Batson (2). Venous

drainage from the breast by the azygos veins communicates with the paravertebral venous plexus in the thoracic region, whereas the prostate drains through the pelvic plexus, which communicates in the lumbar region. Retrograde flow through Batson's plexus has been shown to occur during the Valsalva maneuver and may allow implantation of tumor cells in the vascular sinusoids of the vertebral body without passing through the usual capillary networks.

A second factor thought to be important in tumor distribution involves the tissue receptivity to embolic neoplasms. Certain tissues probably provide a more favorable environment for the survival of the tumor embolus. This "seed and soil" theory postulates that the red marrow of bone provides a biochemically and hemodynamically suitable environment for implantation and proliferation of tumor cells. Because the capillary network of the vertebral red marrow is particularly susceptible to tumor implantation and invasion, tumor cells find it easier to escape from the circulation and multiply within the fine network of cancellous bone (36).

Finally, there are intrinsic factors inherent to the tumor cells that may give one cell line a particular advantage in surviving and growing in the medullary space. Specifically, the elaboration of prostaglandins and the stimulation of osteoclast activating factors by breast cancer cells have been associated with the establishment of lytic metastases in bone (28,61). These cells may also produce a protective fibrin sheath that further isolates them within the marrow, once a metastatic nidus is established.

BIOLOGY

The inherent nature of specific primary and metastatic neoplasms determines their biologic behavior, dictating which will have slow or rapid growth, which will be invasive, and which will produce metastases. Although metastatic lesions usually demonstrate behavior similar to their parent lesions, this is not always true; some metas-

TABLE 2. Location of primary tumors producing metastatic disease of the spinal column (summary of 2,748 cases)

Primary neoplasm	Number	Percent
Breast	576	21.0
Lung	377	14.0
Prostate	211	7.5
Thyroid	73	2.5
Kidney	154	5.5
Lymphoma	180	9.0
Gastrointestinal	134	5.0
Other		35.5
Total	2,748	100.0

tases may be far more invasive or rapidly growing than the primary lesion of origin. It is this biologic behavior of the primary or metastatic lesion that determines the likelihood and rate of spinal cord compression. Rapid tumor expansion may produce vertebral erosion, fracture, and result in acute cord compression with a poorer prognosis for improvement. Understanding the tumor types and its biology allows the surgeon to reasonably predict when and if a specific lesion will endanger neurologic structures.

DIAGNOSIS

The first and most universal symptom of osseous metastasis is pain, which usually begins insidiously, progresses relentlessly, and persists despite the patient's attempts to limit activities and rest. It is usually localized, rather than diffuse spinal pain, at least initially, and often seems worse at night. Patients may associate the onset of symptoms with some minor trauma, but the temporal relationship is usually tenuous and inconsistent. Because of the relatively high prevalence of back pain in the general population, patients are frequently treated empirically for arthritis or "rheumatism" and may see a number of physicians before the correct diagnosis becomes evident. In most patients the primary cancer has been diagnosed months or years before symptoms of spinal involvement become apparent.

In Gilbert and associates' (30) review of 130 patients with spinal cord compression, only 10 patients (8%) presented with neurologic involvement as the first symptom of cancer. Similarly, Siegal et al. (67,68) reported that 16 of 113 patients (14%) with cord compression presented with primary neurologic involvement. Patients may present with back symptoms many years after the treatment of their primary disease, particularly when breast carcinoma is the primary tumor (30). Regardless of how remote the history of malignancy may be, metastatic disease must be considered whenever unexplained spinal pain develops in a patient with a known primary cancer.

Helweg-Larsen and Sorensen (40) reviewed the signs and symptoms in metastatic spinal cord compression with a view to the progression from first symptom until diagnosis in 153 patients. Radicular pain was predominant in the lumbar area. Seventy of the patients with motor symptoms were positively correlated with thoracic metastases. The most common initial symptom was radicular pain followed, with decreasing frequency, by motor weakness, sensory complaints, and bladder dysfunction. The progression of motor weakness influenced the probability of establishing the diagnosis of spinal cord compression.

The medical evaluation of patients with spinal metastases may be more complicated than that for patients with isolated malignancies. Patients with metastatic disease are by definition systemically ill. The extent of this illness is variable and may not become apparent until a detailed clinical examination is completed. Patients with advanced disease usually are cachectic, anemic, and often have little respiratory reserve as well as disturbances of gastrointestinal function. Those receiving chemotherapy may be immunosuppressed and thrombocytopenic. Patients who have been irradiated previously may have regions of skin unsuitable for surgical incision. In addition, renal function may be compromised and hypercalcemia associated with malignancies may be present. If a surgical intervention is to be considered, chemical and nutritional abnormalities should be corrected and the patient's medical fitness maximized if possible. In patients with widespread malignancy and other comorbidities, the risk of surgical mortality must be weighed carefully against the risks of incapacitating pain, paralysis, and a shortened life expectancy if surgical treatment is withheld.

Radiologic Evaluation

Plain radiographs are mandatory. They may show an absent pedicle, vertebral body collapse, or soft tissue mass (Fig. 1). Historically, skeletal scintigraphy has been the gold standard in assessment of metastatic disease of the spine but the advent of improved imaging techniques, such as CT and MRI, has greatly enhanced our ability to accurately assess these lesions.

Colletti et al. (12) correlated skeletal scintigraphy with spinal MRI and suspected metastasis in 64 patients with suspected spinal metastatic disease and spinal cord compression. Spinal lesions were confirmed by radiography, CT, myelography, or MRI, and radionuclide imaging (skeletal scintigraphy) in 56 patients (88%). MRI detected 11 lesions not identified on skeletal scintigraphy while the latter detected two lesions not reported on MRI. A retrospective review of the skeletal scintigraphy detected six lesions not previously reported and retrospectively MRI showed all lesions. Those lesions seen on scintigraphy were rather subtle when reviewed retrospectively. In general, lesions not well seen on scintigraphy had relatively more bone marrow abnormality and less cortical bone involvement and in some cases MRI showed spinal marrow lesions not well seen on planar scintigraphy. Masaryk (51) concluded that MRI was the single most effective modality for evaluationing spinal neoplasms because of its ability to visualize the spinal cord directly and noninvasively at a high level of sensitivity. He also reported that intravenous paramagnetic contrast enhancement was a useful adjunct in further delineating lesions.

Algra et al. (1) has also compared MRI and bone scintigraphy in a double blind prospective analysis of 71 pa-

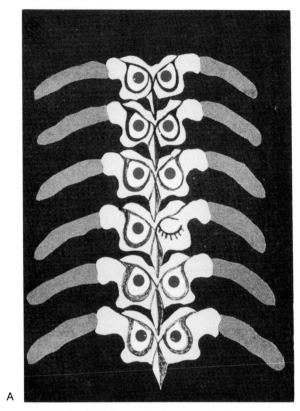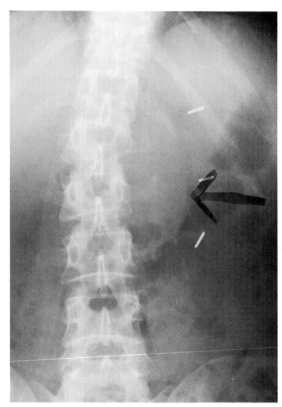

FIG. 1. A: Schematic diagram of missing pedicle "winking owl sign." **B:** At L1, the pedicle is absent together with some vertebral body collapse and soft tissue swelling.

tients with histologically proven skeletal metastases. They discovered that MRI was far more sensitive in the detection of metastases by almost 50%. Chadwick et al. (10) evaluated MRI with particular reference to metastatic disease secondary to urologic malignancy. They found MRI to be more specific than isotope bone scans or plain radiographs and detected lesions in 7 of 66 patients with no other imaging evidence of disease.

Sze (73) noted MRI was not only the most sensitive technique for detection of tumors in the vertebral bodies but for defining the extent of the tumor in the extramedullary space. MRI was as accurate as myelography and postmyelography CT with the added benefit of being noninvasive. He concluded that in the intramedullary space MRI was unquestionably the procedure of choice in the evaluation of suspected cord tumors.

Van der Sande et al. (77) did a prospective study on patients suspected of having spinal epidural metastases using total lumbar and thoracic myelography. Fifty-four of 106 myelograms showed at least one epidural metastasis. Twelve showed two separate lesions while 4 showed three separate lesions. In all 16 cases, at least one of the lesions was asymptomatic. He concluded that multiple spinal epidural metastases are a common occurrence and occur in one-third of cases. Additionally, the findings may have important clinical implications and evaluation of the spinal canal from epidural metastases

should not be confined to the clinically suspected area but should include all possible areas of the spinal canal.

Others have evaluated the roles of myelography and of CT in detecting spinal metastases. Boesen et al. (5) evaluated the use of CT in patients with intraspinal metastasis causing complete block on myelography. Eighty-eight percent of patients with complete block on myelography had sufficient proximal leakage of the contrast medium to allow determination of the cranial limit of the metastasis on CT scan. He concluded that a postmyelographic spine CT scan can replace a supplementary cervical myelogram in the majority of patients with epidural metastasis causing a complete myelographic block.

In the authors' opinion MRI is of value in detecting subtle lesions and assessing canal compromise; however, in planning surgical management CT is an important test because of its greater sensitivity to the degree of bone destruction and is often combined with angiography. Myelography has a minimal role.

Biopsy

Ghelman et al. (29) evaluated percutaneous CT-guided biopsy of the thoracic and lumbar spine in 76 patients with thoracic and lumbar spinal lesions. Prebiopsy evaluation included radiographs, bone scans, CT, and MRI. Histologic diagnosis confirmed the clinical suspicion and adequate material for diagnosis obtained on the first biopsy attempt in 86% of cases. Of the 76 patients, 45 were diagnosed as having metastatic lesions, 11 infection and 12 had primary bone tumors. He concluded that biopsy has a high probability of producing a histologic diagnosis when there is a sound basis for clinical suspicion. Depending on an institution's experience, obtaining a diagnosis may be quite variable.

A variety of approaches may be considered for the biopsy. Renfrew et al. (62) have recommended CT-guided percutaneous transpedicular biopsy of the spine for cases where the location of the lesion does not allow easy access by means of the posterolateral approach. In this author's opinion this technique may be safe to use but the posterolateral approach to all lesions in the thoracic and lumbar spine is possible and preferable. An anterolateral approach to cervical spine vertebral bodies, of course, can be safely done. The authors prefer a core biopsy using a trephine varying in diameter from that of a lead pencil to one-half that rather than a free needle biopsy. If closed biopsy fails, then an open biopsy may be necessary especially if a primary malignancy is suspected. If a primary malignancy is part of the differential diagnosis, then the site of the biopsy must be carefully planned in order to avoid extra excisional tissue contamination regardless of which technique is used.

Although it causes little morbidity, closed percutaneous biopsy is not always indicated. For example, it is not required in obviously known metastases, whereas an unknown diagnosis especially with no evidence of other distant lesions will require a tissue diagnosis.

In cases requiring emergent neurologic decompression obviously time does not permit a biopsy.

Vascular Embolization

If surgical intervention is contemplated, vascular embolization should be considered as a significant adjunct prior to surgical resection for highly vascular vertebral metastases, particularly renal cell carcinoma. Broaddus et al. (8) reported on the supraselective arteriolar embolization. They felt the key factor in their technique was the use of microfibrillar collagen, which allows occlusion of tumor vessels as small as 20 μm. The types of tumors treated were metastatic renal cell carcinoma, metastatic thyroid carcinoma, metastatic melanoma, and primary giant cell tumors of the sacrum. Estimated blood loss in 7 of the 9 procedures performed on 6 patients ranged from 300 to 800 cc. Two cases of extensive resection required postoperative transfusion. No significant complications occurred either at surgery or embolization.

King et al. (42), in a review of surgical management of metastatic renal carcinoma of the spine, noted that preoperative embolization was beneficial. In their series of 31 patients, 2 patients had to have surgery terminated because of excessive blood loss where embolization was not used. Subsequent embolization allowed for repeat surgery (Fig. 2).

Preoperative angiography may also be useful without embolization. For example, Champlin et al. (11) reviewed 61 patients as to safety, efficacy, and value of preoperative angiography. Only two minor hematomas occurred.

In 17 of 22 patients, the arterial supply to the spinal cord was in the region of planned surgery, thus dictating an alternative surgical approach than originally contemplated.

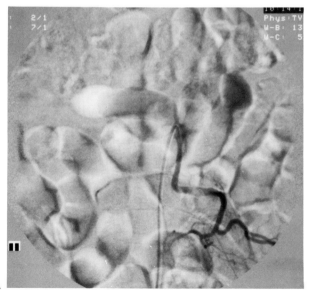

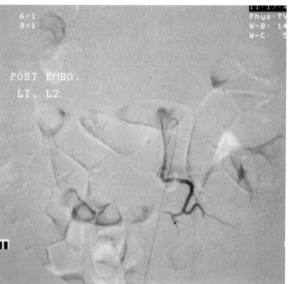

FIG. 2. A: Pre-embolization in a case of suspected renal cell metastasis reveals a very vascular tumor. Dynamic flow picture. **B:** Post-embolization reveals a marked decrease in blood flow. There was little blood loss at the time of surgery. This is a static flow, i.e., no circulation.

DETERMINANTS OF SURGICAL APPROACH: INDICATIONS AND ALTERNATIVES

Neurologic Status

The pretreatment neurologic status clearly correlates with post-treatment outcome as measured by the likelihood and extent of recovery, the ability to maintain or regain ambulation, and the preservation or loss of bowel and bladder function. Depending on the patient population surveyed, between 60% and 95% of the patients who can walk at the time of diagnosis of a spinal metastasis will retain that ability following treatment. Only 35% to 65% of the patients presenting with paraparesis will regain their ability to walk, and less than 30% of paraplegic patients will regain ambulation (4,22,34,37,38,44, 47,57).

The rate of progression of the neurologic deficit also has clear prognostic significance. If a patient progresses from the earliest onset of symptoms to a major deficit in less than 24 hours, the prognosis for recovery is poor irrespective of treatment. Conversely, slow progression of neurologic involvement has a favorable prognosis for neurologic recovery following treatment (36). All these factors plus the surgical approach determine the eventual return of neurologic function, which in favorable cases can be dramatic.

Patients who present with a "complete" neurologic loss, that is complete paraplegia or quadriplegia, regardless of etiology, generally are not candidates for decompression. Patients with metastatic carcinoma of the lung, particularly those with oat cell carcinoma who show widespread metastases, also must be seriously considered as nonoperative candidates as many of these patients have a survival of less than 2 to 3 months.

Radiation Therapy and Laminectomy

Radiation therapy has been the traditional standard of treatment for cord impingement, particularly in metastatic disease. Surgical decompression in the past has usually consisted of a laminectomy with removal of whatever tumor could be reached laterally in the spinal canal or through the pedicle. Laminectomy was sometimes combined with posterior stabilization, and frequently combined with radiotherapy. Unfortunately, the results of laminectomy were often no better than radiotherapy alone, and posterior decompression often resulted in postoperative acquired instability (30,36,66). Constans et al. (13) reported that 46% of his patients treated with decompressive laminectomy and radiotherapy had significant neurologic improvement compared to 39% of patients treated with radiotherapy. Similarly, Gilbert et al. (30) reported that satisfactory results were obtained in 46% of patients treated with laminectomy and radiotherapy alone. Others have noted that less than half the patients treated by either radiotherapy or laminectomy obtained a satisfactory result in terms of retaining or regaining their neurologic function (65). Today, the results of surgical decompression through the anterior approach are more favorable and offer a genuine improvement over the results obtained with radiotherapy alone. Table 3 shows published data that compares anterior and posterior decompressions. How one approaches these tumors is, therefore, determined by a number of the following factors.

Tumor Location

Location of the neoplasm within the vertebral body or spinal canal determines the symptoms and signs pro-

TABLE 3. *Maintenance and recovery of neurologic function in patients treated surgically (anterior versus posterior decompression) for cord compression due to metastatic or primary spinal tumor*

Reference	Number of patients	% Improvement	% Satisfactory outcome
Anterior decompression			
Sundaresan (72)	160	80	78
Siegal (67,68)	75	80	80
Fidler (23)	17	73	78
Harrington (35–39)	77	84	73
Kostuik (43–44)	70	73	84
Manabe (47)	28	82	89
Total patients	427	Average 78	Average 80
Posterior Decompression			
Wright (80)	86	35	33
White (79)	226	38	37
Hall (34)	126	30	29
Gilbert (30)	65	45	46
Nather (57)	42	13	29
Siegal (67–68)	25	39	39
Sherman (66)	149	27	48
Kostuik (43–44)	30	36	37
Total patients	746	Average 33	Average 37

duced, and, in part, dictates the surgical approach required for treatment. In metastatic and primary spinal malignancies, the vertebral body initially is most commonly involved. When tumor from an anterior vertebral lesion encroaches on the spinal cord, the anterior columns of the spinal cord are usually compressed first. This leads to early loss of motor function, and progressive loss of sensory function as the cord is pressed back against the lamina. Cord compression occurs most commonly in the thoracic region of the spine, where the cord is relatively large with respect to the vertebral canal.

Stability in Metastatic Disease

The mechanical demands on the vertebral elements differ between anterior and posterior columns. Location also has value in predicting which lesions will develop vertebral collapse and segmental instability. For both these reasons, tumors involving the anterior and middle columns are associated with more frequent and more profound neurologic injury. As noted, this is particularly true in the thoracic spine because the room available for the spinal cord is more limited than elsewhere in the canal. Thus, the cervical, thoracic, and lumbar spinal regions differ in the propensity for cord compression. Although considerable thought has been expressed as to a good definition of stability in the presence of metastatic disease, currently there is no clear consensus.

Kostuik et al. (44) have attempted to base stability on the column structure of the spine. In contrast to that for standard fractures classification, the spine is divided into an anterior and posterior column (Figs. 3 and 4). The anterior column consists of the vertebral body including the anterior and posterior cortex, while the posterior column consists of the pedicles, laminae, and spinous processes. The anterior and posterior columns are divided into right and left halves. The anterior column is further divided into four segments: anterior right, anterior left, middle right, and middle left. In a retrospective analysis attempting to define this schema in relationship to instability, the following definitions were formulated. If no more than one or two of the six columns is destroyed, then it is felt that the patient is probably stable. If three or four of the columns are destroyed, then it is an unstable lesion. When more than four are involved, it is markedly unstable. Additionally, angulatory deformity greater than 20° was considered as a sign of instability. The definitions of stability do not take into account soft tissue extension or epidural spread. One must be careful in defining instability both in terms of columns involved and the different tumor types. Further study of mechanical properties for a particular tumor type is needed.

Pain and Metastasis

Operative intervention for pain alone must be considered, although symptoms can often be controlled by drugs. Significant levels of drug intake may result in profound psychological disturbances or somnolence, rendering nursing care difficult and having significant psychosocial impact upon family members. Frequently doses as high as 100 mg of morphine given intravenously every few hours preoperatively may be completely stopped following decompression and surgical stabilization.

Analysis of pain following surgical intervention is difficult to perform. Patients with metastatic disease often have residual pain that may be unrelated to the spine. An analysis of pain following surgical decompression revealed that 81% of patients with metastatic disease in subjective reports had good or excellent relief of their pain. Thirteen percent of the patients reported moderate relief and only 4% reported poor relief of their preoperative symptoms. The results are not as good as those noted in primary malignant or benign tumors of the spine where most patients report relief of pain.

Function

The factors most important to the patient are preservation and/or restoration of ambulation as well as preservation and restoration of bowel and bladder function. On this basis patients may be divided into three groups: (a) those who are normal with no subjective or objective neurologic complaints, (b) those with minimal or no radiologic evidence of neural impingement, and (c) those with neurologic impairment severe enough to prevent

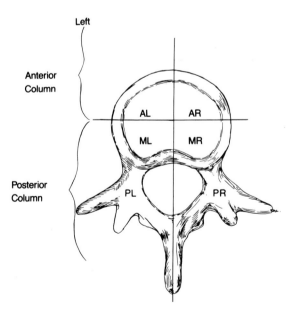

FIG 3. An axial CT scan of the lesion is divided into six columns. The lesion is stable if only two columns are destroyed, unstable if three or four columns are destroyed, and markedly unstable if five or six columns are affected.

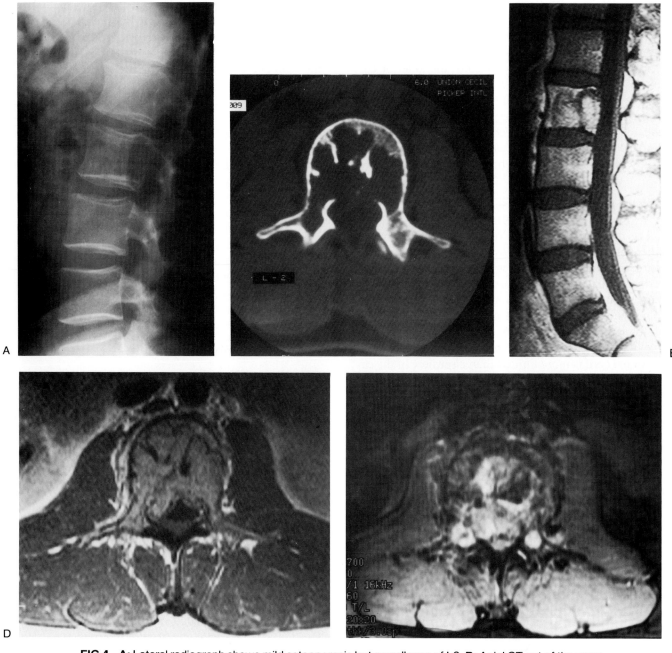

FIG 4. A: Lateral radiograph shows mild osteoporosis but no collapse of L2. **B:** Axial CT cut of the same lesion done at the same time as plain radiographs shows that five columns are affected. **C:** MRI of the lesion taken at the same time demonstrates the lesion in the body of L2. There is no evidence of dural compression. **D:** Axial MRI cut shows vertebral body damage but no dural compression.

unaided ambulation or cause impaired bowel and bladder function. Treatment considered to be significant is that which allows return of ambulation, bowel or bladder function, or complete recovery of a minor deficit. More complete documentation of bowel and bladder function should include urodynamic studies of bladder function. Frequently, this is not possible because of time constraints and, therefore, has generally not been analyzed. We will now look at the specific issues that dictate neurologic involvement and treatment.

Spinal Cord Compression

Spinal cord compression is reported to occur in between 5% and 20% of patients with widespread cancer of all types (5,67,68). In all, spinal cord compression may result from one of four types of pathologic process: (a) direct compression from an enlarging soft tissue mass, (b) pressure due to fracture and retropulsion of bony fragments into the canal, (c) severe kyphosis following vertebral collapse, and (d) pressure due to intradural me-

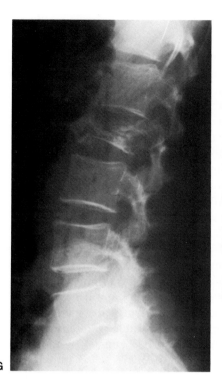
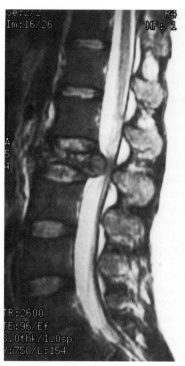

F,G

FIG. 4. (Continued.) E,F: One week later the body of L2 has collapsed. Neurologic compromise resulted. This could have been avoided by earlier intervention. G: Sagittal MRI indicates marked dural compression.

tastases. The most common cause of cord compression is mechanical pressure from tumor tissue or bone extruded from the collapsing vertebral body (36). Because of the flexion moment acting on the vertebrae of the thoracic spine, erosion of the vertebral body tends to produce collapse into kyphosis, extruding tumor as well as the posterior cortex of the vertebral body dorsally into the spinal canal. Direct compression of the cord may occur without vertebral erosion if the tumor expands directly into the canal. Fortunately, the spinal cord is well protected by the dura, which is quite resistant to tumor infiltration. In the presence of an epidural metastasis the dura is often found to be considerably thickened. Occasionally, compression of the spinal cord or a nerve root may result from extension of a paraspinal tumor through the intervertebral foramen. Intradural metastases are very rare though they have been reported (39).

Although the pathology responsible for the spinal cord compression may vary, the symptoms of compression remain constant (34). The early recognition of these symptoms is crucial to providing early intervention and preventing progressive and permanent neurologic injury. In order of appearance the most prominent symptoms are back pain, radicular or "girdle" pain, weakness in the lower limbs, sensory loss, and loss of sphincter control. Although nearly all patients experience some localized back pain, patients with cervical and lumbosacral lesions are also likely to experience radicular pain. Patients with thoracic lesions occasionally experience bilateral radicular pain, producing a segmental band or "girdle" of pain (30). Localized back pain that persists or

progresses and radicular pain are the most useful warning symptoms of impending spinal cord compression, but may precede actual cord compromise by days or years (4). Although bowel and bladder dysfunction are not commonly seen at initial presentation, they are almost never isolated findings. When autonomic dysfunction occurs in the absence of motor or sensory loss, the lesion is usually located between the T10 and T12 vertebral bodies.

Some of the important factors in determining the prognosis for neurologic outcome include tumor biology, pretreatment neurologic status, and tumor location within the spinal canal (67,68).

PROGNOSIS

Survival and outcome in metastatic disease are dependent on several interrelated factors. Probably the most important determinant is the tumor type. Although sex, age, location of metastases, and interval between diagnosis of disease and appearance of metastases have all been correlated with differences in outcome, none of these variables are independent of tumor type. For instance, women as a group may be expected to have a better survival and a greater percentage of satisfactory treatment results than men, but this is because breast carcinoma in women has a more favorable prognosis, whereas pulmonary carcinoma predominates in men and has a less favorable prognosis. Again, since thoracic metastases frequently arise from pulmonary tumors in men and breast tumors in women, men with thoracic spine metastases will have a significantly worse outcome than women with thoracic disease but gender is not the determinant (66).

The evaluation of patients with metastatic spinal disease is difficult in terms of providing some reasonable prognosis of outcome. Tokuhashi et al. (74) have developed a scoring system for the preoperative evaluation of metastatic spine tumor prognosis. Six parameters were used in the assessment system, including the general condition, the number of extraspinal bone metastasis, the number of metastasis in the vertebral body, metastasis to major internal organs (lungs, liver, kidneys, and brain), the primary site of the cancer, and the severity of spinal cord involvement. The parameter received a score from zero to two points. The total score obtained for each patient was correlated with the prognosis. They found the prognosis could not be predicted from a single parameter. They felt that surgery could be performed in those cases that scored above nine points while palliative operations were indicated for those who scored under five points.

A recent analysis of 60 patients using the Tokuhashi scoring system, by the author has substantiated this evaluation scoring system. Patients with metastatic disease to the spine from lung carcinoma fared poorly and might have been spared surgery since their longevity was in the majority of cases measured in weeks.

TREATMENT OPTIONS

Surgery

O'Neil et al. (59) reviewed the treatment of 33 patients with metastatic lesions to the thoracic and lumbar spine. He found that 94% had good to excellent pain relief. Of 24 patients unable to walk preoperatively, postoperatively 75% regained the ability to walk independently. Kostuik et al. (44) analyzed 71 metastatic lesions of the cervical, thoracic, and lumbar spine. Both anterior and posterior surgical approaches were used and stabilization was augmented with methylmethacrylate. Good to excellent pain relief was obtained in 81%. Significant improvement of neurologic deficits was obtained in 40% of patients with posterior decompression and 71% of patients decompressed anteriorly. Overall survival averaged 11.3 months. In a series reported by Harrington (36,38), 72 of 77 patients (94%) treated by anterior decompression and stabilization experienced good to excellent pain relief. Sixty-two of these patients had a major neurologic impairment preoperatively and 42 (68%) made significant improvement after surgery; 26 had a complete recovery and 16 others had a significant functional improvement after decompression.

Radiotherapy

Despite the fact that favorable results are obtained by surgical decompression, radiotherapy historically has been the treatment of choice for spinal osseous metastases and still remains the most reasonable treatment option for many patients. Particularly, patients with spinal pain and occasionally patients with neurologic compromise without vertebral collapse will receive significant benefit from radiotherapy alone. As with surgery, the preoperative neurologic status of the patient dictates the likely outcome. Although 70% of the patients who are ambulatory will retain that functional ability after radiotherapy, rarely will patients who have lost this ability regain it after radiation alone (76). The nature of the metastasis is also important to the outcome following radiotherapy because of the significant difference in radiosensitivity between tumor types and between different clones of the same tumor type. Prostatic and lymphoreticular tumors are usually quite radiosensitive and excellent clinical results can be obtained by radiation alone in most patients (9,56,76). Metastases from breast carcinoma are usually responsive to irradiation, but as many as 30% of the patients treated may be unresponsive to radiation alone (32,76). Gastrointestinal and renal tumors usually are quite resistant to radiotherapy.

The value of radiotherapy versus surgery or as an adjunct to surgery remains controversial. Certain tumors that are radiosensitive, such as metastatic carcinoma of the breast, are often best treated with radiation even in the presence of mild cord compression. Tumors that are obviously not radiosensitive are best treated surgically.

Maranzano et al. (48) evaluated the radiation therapy in metastatic spinal cord compression in a prospective review of 105 consecutive patients. Steroids were administered and radiotherapy commenced within 24 hours. They felt the surgery should precede radiotherapy where diagnosis was in doubt or stabilization was necessary. Chemotherapy or hormonal therapy was added as well. Surgery plus radiotherapy was administered to 9.2% of patients, whereas 90.8% of patients received radiotherapy alone. In patients receiving radiotherapy alone, back pain was improved in 80%; of those with motor dysfunction, 48.6% improved; and there was no deterioration in 31.4% without motor disability. Forty percent of patients with autonomic dysfunction responded to radiotherapy. Median survival time was 7 months with a 36% probability of survival for 1 year. Median duration of improvement was 8 months. The most important prognostic factor was early diagnosis. They felt the radiosensitivity of tumors was only important in paraparetic patients with response to radiotherapy. A complete myelographic block significantly diminished the response to radiotherapy but vertebral body collapse did not influence response or survival.

In these authors' opinion, the response of motor dysfunction to radiotherapy shows no particular benefits over past reported results. In this series, 48.6% improved, which is approximately the same as past reports. This is similar to posterior decompression together with stabilization but considerably less than anterior decompression where neurologic improvement has been reported to be as high as 80% of cases.

Braces

The halo vest is an important option for neurologically intact patients with cervical metastasis, who have instability and/or pain. Used in conjunction with appropriate radiotherapy, symptomatic relief is reasonably good and bony healing of the lesion will occur in many cases. Most importantly, neurologic injury can be prevented by the halo vest while medical therapy is instituted. In patients with metastatic prostate carcinoma Danzig et al. (16) reported good maintenance of neurologic function and no morbidity using the halo vest. However, these patients wore the halo for roughly a third of their remaining lives. Braces such as the thoracolumbar sacral orthosis (TLSO) are likewise viable and important tools in the management of thoracolumbar and sacral lesions, but we believe their use is indicated only as an adjunct to treatment, rather than as the primary treatment modality.

INDICATIONS FOR SURGICAL TREATMENT

Assuming the patient's overall status permits and there is a likelihood for survival, the broad indications for surgical treatment have been outlined by a number of different authors. Gilbert (30) suggested that decompressive laminectomy was indicated in metastatic disease when: (a) the nature of the primary tumor was not known or the diagnosis was in doubt, (b) relapse of tumor occurred following maximal radiotherapy to that segment, and (c) symptoms progressed inexorably during radiotherapy. With the acceptance of more aggressive surgical treatments, these indications have been expanded. Recent publications have recommended surgical intervention in instances of an isolated primary and some isolated metastatic lesions or a solitary site of relapse; pathologic fracture or deformity producing neurologic symptoms or pain; radioresistant tumors, metastatic or primary; and segmental instability following radiotherapy (18,26,27,36,44,47). All of these authors presume a patient who is healthy enough to survive surgery, but it is not incumbent to expect a long survival. Any patient with expectations of surviving 6 weeks or longer who is not hopelessly bedridden may be given consideration for surgery.

The dignity of a person with metastatic disease must also be considered in a shared decision-making process. Because the average longevity for someone with spinal metastasis is probably 1 year following surgical treatment, it is important that these unfortunate patients be given every chance to lead a life with as little pain as possible and with preservation of neurologic function. It is the authors' opinion that any patient who presents with an impending fracture or marked gibbus (kyphosis), even in the absence of neurologic problems, be considered for a surgical approach, using scientifically based shared decision making and informed consent, particularly if the tumor is not radiosensitive. It is the authors' opinion that the morbidity currently experienced from a surgical approach is low enough to justify considering surgical intervention in hopes of restoring or preserving neurologic function and preventing possible bowel and bladder incontinence and other sequelae of paraplegia.

A particular subset of patients may present with paraparesis or quadriparesis as an emergency with no known history of a primary malignant tumor. Radiologic investigations reveal evidence of neurocompression. In our opinion, it is best to deal with these patients on an emergency basis. Attempts to improve the microvasculature should be carried out with the addition of corticosteroids, and decompression, usually anterior, is performed. Often stabilization is performed with a methylmethacrylate spacer.

Such a procedure is often performed without knowing the tumor type that caused the vertebral collapse and neurologic problem. Later the histologic evaluation may reveal myeloma or lymphoma, which may respond well to appropriate oncologic treatment. If a formal fusion was not carried out as part of the initial emergent treatment, later fusion may be considered. We have had the opportunity of doing this second-stage procedure on a number of patients who have had emergent decompression either for multiple myeloma or for a lymphoma and who have at 1 year postoperatively responded well to oncologic treatment. Because it is anticipated that they may live many years to come, it is felt that the metal-reinforced methylmethacrylate construct may not survive the lifespan of the patient.

SURGICAL APPROACHES

A number of different surgical approaches are available to the spine surgeon and variations of each have been described (Table 4). Choosing the correct approach for any given situation is perhaps the most important technical step in treating metastatic malignancies. In general, below the level of T2 anterior approaches may be used to restore stability, while above T2 posterior stabilization is usually indicated. Laminectomy should be

TABLE 4. *Surgical approaches to spinal neoplasms*

Level	Anterior	Posterior
Cervical (C1–C2)	Transoral	Midline posterior
(C1–T2)	Anterolateral	Posterolateral
	Trans-sternal	
Thoracic	Thoracotomy	Midline posterior
		Costotransversectomy
Thoracolumbar (T11–L2)	Thoracoabdominal—10th–12th rib resection, detachment of diaphragm	Midline posterior
		Posterolateral
Lumbar	Retroperitoneal	Midline posterior
	Transabdominal	

restricted to those rare cases where the site of compression has been shown to be strictly posterior (22).

In lesions of the cervical spine above the level of C3, a posterior approach is advocated. But if the dens is preserved and the body of C2 destroyed, an anterior approach may be used, fixing the dens to C3 or C4 with metal-reinforced methylmethacrylate. In a series of 11 patients with high cervical metastases, posterior decompression and stabilization provided good to excellent pain relief in all patients but was not adequate to prevent collapse in one case with severe anterior vertebral destruction (22). In metastatic lesions below C3, an anterior approach with decompression and methylmethacrylate stabilization has been advocated. Some surgeons, however, prefer the posterolateral approach to lesions involving multiple adjacent cervical levels. Below C3, a single nerve root may need to be sacrificed to allow adequate anterior decompression by this approach. Stabilization following a posterolateral decompression may be accomplished by segmental fixation and sublaminar wiring augmented with methylmethacrylate as needed (43,44).

Anterior Versus Posterior Decompression

The selection of anterior decompression versus posterior decompression depends to some degree on the extent of involvement of the spine and the presence or absence of skip lesions and the degree of epidural tumor. A careful analysis of preoperative plain radiographs, CT scans combined with myelography, and/or MRI will help to define the extent of destruction and epidural spread. MRI sometimes has limits in defining the extent of the tumor. Therefore, myelography with CT is often necessary and may provide the best preoperative evaluation.

Anterior compression in the presence of epidural tumor over five or six levels generally will not respond well to anterior vertebrectomy alone. Generally the selection of anterior decompression is restricted to patients with metastatic disease ideally limited to one to two adjacent vertebral segments or where significant kyphosis exists in conjunction with vertebral body destruction. Skip lesions with single-level anterior destruction can be treated anteriorly but one must consider the possible morbidity to the patient. Ideally, multiple level lesions are best treated by a posterior approach (Fig. 5).

The use of costotransversectomy for debulking of metastatic tumors combined with posterior, segmental stabilization has been reported, but the results have not been as good as with the anterior approach. Only 1 of 5 patients regained the ability to walk with assistance, and survival was limited to a mean of 5 months (17). Somewhat better results have been reported through a modified costotransversectomy approach with anterolateral decompression, but access to the tumor is always limited anteriorly and results are still inferior to those obtained by a formal anterior approach.

Posterior Laminectomy

In an uncontrolled, retrospective review of 38 patients treated by laminectomy, only 24% of patients demonstrated any improvement in neurologic function (58). Whether laminectomy provides any significant benefit to patients with cord compression beyond that provided by radiotherapy is debatable. Although Constans et al. (13) showed some improvement in results using laminectomy with radiotherapy, Gilbert and associates' (30) results showed very little difference between patients treated with radiotherapy alone and those treated with both laminectomy and radiation. The proportion of satisfactory outcomes was less than 50% in each case.

Livingston and Perrin (45) in 1978 reviewed the results of 100 extensive laminectomies for neurologic deficits in metastatic disease. They defined satisfactory results as the ability to walk, retention of urinary continence, and survival of 6 months or longer. This was achieved in 40% of the patients; however, they did not differentiate between those who were ambulatory pre- and postoperatively. Doppman and Girton (19) in 1976 reported the results of laminectomies in anterior epidural masses in an angiographic study in 16 rhesus monkeys. They concluded that an anterior epidural mass of greater than 4 mm in diameter could not be adequately decompressed with posterior laminectomy.

A,B
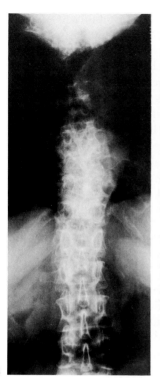
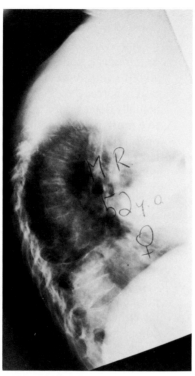
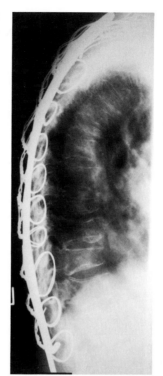
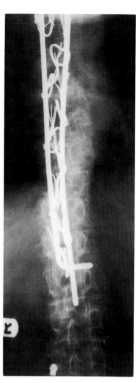
C,D

FIG. 5. A,B: Anterior posterior and lateral radiographs demonstrate osteopenia, kyphosis, and bone destruction in a 52-year-old female with metastatic breast cancer and paraparesis spread over multiple levels. **C,D:** Posterolateral decompression over multiple levels, together with posterior segmental stabilization (Luque technique, inexpensive, rapid, effective) with rods, sublaminar wires, and cement resulted in effective functional pain-reduced outcome.

A number of authors have reported their results in cases of cord or cauda equina compression treated by posterior decompression, in which most deficits and outcomes were graded according to the classification of Brice and McKissock (7). This classification, based on mild, moderate, and severe neurologic deficits, defined satisfactory outcome as restoration and maintenance of ambulation and bowel and bladder function. It is not directly comparable to the more objective Frankel classification widely used today. This lack of continuity makes comparison of data for anterior and posterior approaches more difficult, but the trend seen in comparison is still quite clear (Table 3). Of 746 reported cases treated by posterior decompression, only 37% of patients had a satisfactory neurologic outcome, and only 33% with neurologic deficit showed significant improvement (30,34,44,57,66–68,79,80). Although the addition of stabilization significantly improved the pain relief and maintenance of neurologic function relative to laminectomy alone, the overall results were still somewhat disappointing.

It is evident, therefore, that laminectomy does not provide adequate decompression in all lesions and may, in fact, increase instability. The spinal cord is also endangered during laminectomy, especially in the thoracic region, because of the narrowness of the canal and the need

to manipulate the cord to reach anterior or anterolateral tumor tissue (50). In certain cases laminectomy may be distinctly detrimental to neurologic outcome in patients with cord compression. Findlay (25) reviewed the results of laminectomy in patients with and without vertebral collapse and noted a poorer rate of recovery and twice the rate of postoperative paraplegia in patients with collapse. Laminectomy fails in these patients for two reasons. First, often inadequate decompression of the cord is obtained. Second, the resulting destabilization of the spinal column puts these patients at high risk of postoperative cord compression and paraplegia. Combining a destabilizing posterior decompression with an already unstable anterior column is clearly unwise.

If in metastatic disease the process is at more than two adjacent levels and is essentially posterior where there is extensive epidural spread as shown by MRI, myelography, or enhanced CT scanning, decompression can be performed posterolaterally on the most affected side (Fig. 5). In the thoracic spine, one or more roots may be sacrificed. Stabilization is then achieved with segmental fixation and the liberal use of methylmethacrylate bone cement.

Occasionally a posterolateral approach can be done if the tumor is anterior, there are multiple lesions, and extensive stabilization is necessary. The costotransversectomy approach combined with posterior instrumentation has been advocated. In our opinion this is a satisfactory approach for multiple level problems with the epidural spread. In the thoracic spine, nerve roots can be sacrificed and the dural sac rotated slightly to allow for anterior evacuation of tumor without morbidity, which should be done from one side only in order to minimize vascular compromise to the cord.

SURGICAL STABILIZATION

The specific types of stabilization depend upon the specific tumor type and anticipated response to treatment as well as the extent of destruction of the anterior and posterior columns, the general condition of the patient, and the expected survival time.

Posterior Stabilization

Because of the increased incidence of infection and wound breakdown associated with posterior instrumentation, Harrington (37) has recommended posterior stabilization only when: (a) combined anterior and posterior decompression is necessary, (b) lengthy anterior fixation is inadequate to restore stability, (c) posterior instability is produced by tumor lysis of posterior elements, and/or (d) with lesions either anteriorly or posteriorly distal to the L3 vertebral body. Posterior stabilization should be used wherever posterior decompression is required or considered.

Anterior Stabilization

Anterior decompression has been successfully used in treating cord compression caused by a variety of different lesions. Johnson et al. (41) described 25 cases of spinal cord compression treated with anterior surgery, including cases of fracture, neoplasm, infection, and congenital deformity. Improvement in neurologic function was obtained in all groups but was most dramatic in those with acute compression due to fracture, infection, and tumor. Of the 25 patients reviewed, 17 had a partial recovery and 5 had a complete recovery from their neurologic deficits. Patients with early intervention had the best outcome with respect to neurologic recovery. This has reinforced previously reported observations of significant neurologic improvement in patients decompressed anteriorly for metastatic disease (Fig. 6) (23,36).

In one of the few prospective studies, Siegal and Siegal (67,68) chose an anterior vertebrectomy approach for decompression in patients with metastatic lesions located anterior to the cord, and a posterior laminectomy approach for lesions located posterior to the cord. If patients did not satisfy these indications, they were treated with radiotherapy alone. Only 30% of patients treated

with radiotherapy alone regained the ability to walk, as opposed to 40% of the laminectomy patients and 80% of the anteriorly decompressed vertebrectomy patients. Of 13 paraplegic patients treated by anterior vertebrectomy, all but 1 improved at least one grade in neurologic function, whereas 5 of 25 patients treated with laminectomy actually deteriorated as a result of treatment. The operative mortality was similar for both approaches, but postoperative complications were far more frequent in the laminectomy group. This was commonly the result of poor wound healing following operations performed through irradiated tissue. In 4 of 27 cases following anterior decompression in which objective grading of neurologic recovery was reported, 79% had a significant improvement, and overall 77% obtained a satisfactory outcome, i.e., independent ambulation and intact autonomic function.

Eleven of 17 patients reviewed by DeWald et al. (17) presented with severe paraparesis or paraplegia. Following either combined anterior and posterior procedures or combined costotransversectomy and posterior procedures, 5 of 11 had significant neurologic improvement and 6 were unchanged. Good to excellent pain relief was obtained in 11 of 17 patients. Intraoperative blood loss and surgical time vary from report to report. Harrington (35) reported blood loss of between 200 and 550 cc for anterior decompressions, depending on the level. The mean blood loss for combined anterior and posterior procedures was considerably greater and averaged 2,250 cc. Operative time for Harrington's patients was just less than $2\frac{1}{2}$ hours for cervical lesions and just under 4 hours for thoracic and thoracolumbar lesions.

Loquet et al. (46) in a review of 31 patients noted pain reduction in 78%, and 70% underwent neurologic improvement together with improved quality of life. All were treated anteriorly. Rompe et al. (63) in a review of 43 patients, 37 of whom were treated by posterior methods, noted amelioration of neurologic function in 58%. After surgery life expectancy was 11 months. All patients were neurologically impaired prospectively.

Cooper et al. (14) in a review of 33 patients noted that 94% of patients had either improvement or stabilization of their function. Average mean survival was 10.2 months. They advocated the anterior approach whenever possible. If the posterior elements were destroyed as well as the anterior elements, they advocated anterior and posterior approaches with stabilization anteriorly and posteriorly.

Specific Surgical Stabilization Techniques

Cervical Spine

Stabilization depends upon the location of the tumor. The use of methylmethacrylate reinforced bone cement has generally been reserved for patients with a life expec-

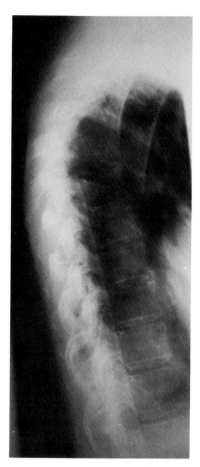
A

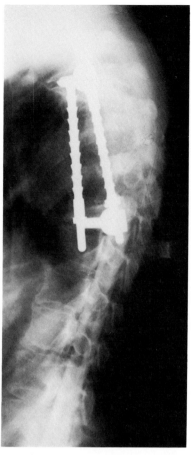

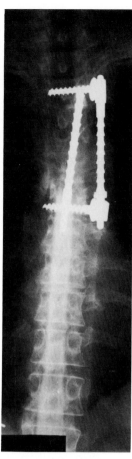
B,C

FIG. 6. A: Lateral radiograph of a 56-year-old patient who presented with sudden paraparesis (Frankel Grade B) of unknown etiology. **B,C:** Emergent anterior decompression and stabilization with metal and cement with correction of kyphosis was done with complete resolution of the paraparesis. The tumor proved to be a myeloma. One year later, this healthy woman underwent a formal posterior arthrodesis. She is alive and well 5 years from the time of her first operative intervention.

tancy of less than 1 year. In such cases, if the disease is limited to the anterior column, an anterior resection and stabilization with reinforced methylmethacrylate (Figs. 7 and 8) can safely be done.

Anterior approaches can safely be done up to and including the odontoid. If the odontoid is destroyed, then posterior stabilization from C1 distally will be necessary. If, however, the odontoid is preserved and only the body of C2 is destroyed, anterior stabilization alone may suffice. The metal construct is inserted into an evacuated odontoid, which is filled with methylmethacrylate.

For a metastatic lesion in the upper cervical spine, a right-sided longitudinal sternocleidomastoid approach is often used. With lesions located in the mid or distal cervical spine a left-sided approach is often used in an attempt to decrease the incidence of neurologic deficit involving the recurrent laryngeal nerve.

In the authors' experience, if the disease is limited to one or two levels, no posterior reinforcement is necessary. If the disease is more extensive or if more involvement is noted in the posterior column, posterior rein-

forcement is necessary (Figs. 9 and 10). If the disease is primarily posterior, a posterior approach may be done with posterior stabilization using metal reinforced with methylmethacrylate.

In anterior cervical reconstruction following decompression, careful assessment of the quality of the vertebral bodies proximally and distally must be made to ensure there is no major tumor involvement that might have been overlooked in the preoperative imaging studies. One stabilizing technique involves using an angled curette; a hole is made in the vertebral body proximally and distally. A heavy threaded Steinmann pin or a small-diameter rod can be inserted by first passing the pin/rod proximally, then driving it distally. If the next most proximal disc can be transgressed, this aids in stabilization. The pin/rod is then removed and the hole packed with cement. The rod or rods are then reintroduced with cement, which is then packed around the rod. Newer plate designs as well as various types of vertebral spacers are also available.

In an analysis by Kostuik et al. (44) of 35 patients who

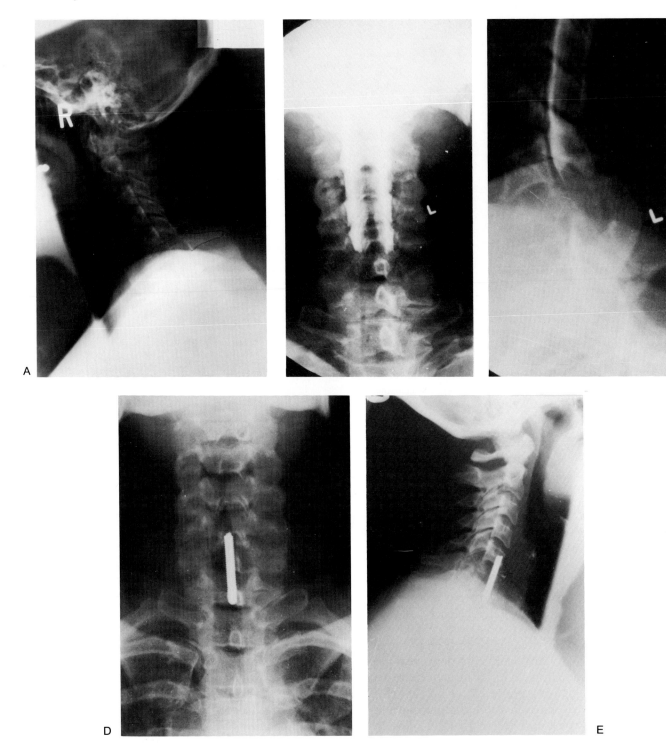

FIG. 7. A: Metastatic lesion C6 in a 56-year-old with complete collapse and quadriparesis. **B,C:** Myelogram demonstrates a complete block. **D,E:** Anterior decompression with cement-metal-reinforced, intervertebral construction was done (inexpensive, simple, effective) with resolution of the quadriparesis.

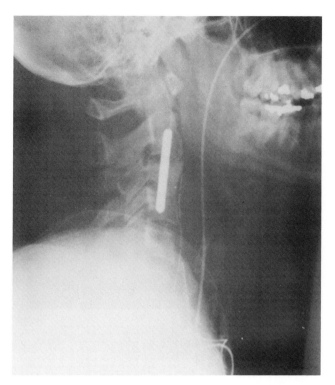

FIG. 8. Postoperative lateral view demonstrates fixation following anterior decompression at C3.

underwent procedures for metastatic disease in the cervical spine, 16 underwent anterior decompression and stabilization with reinforced methylmethacrylate. A similar number underwent posterior stabilization with reinforced methylmethacrylate following decompression. Three patients had posterior stabilization alone.

Fielding et al. (24) reviewed 20 cases of cervical spine tumors treated by anterior vertebrectomy and bone grafting. There were no cases of graft failure, either through collapse or extrusion. Iliac crest, fibular, and tibial grafts were all used, and posterior fusions were used in 13 cases to augment stability. In patients with primary benign tumors, anterior resection and grafting eliminated symptoms in each case and there were no recurrences. In primary malignancies and in metastatic lesions there was excellent stability, with resolution of neurologic symptoms and pain. Quality of life and longevity were improved in these patients.

For posterior cervical stabilization a variety of constructs have been used including Luque loops with sublaminar wires or the passage of threaded Steinmann pins through the base of normal spinous processes proximal and distal to the decompression. If the spinous processes are used, a minimum of two proximal and two distal should be incorporated in the construct. Wires are then passed around the threaded pins. Cement is then added producing a reinforced cement construct (Fig. 9).

Tumor recurrence often involves the vertebrae above and below the site of previous resection. Therefore, it is recommended that the posterior fusion span two levels above and below the site of recurrence (24). In a review of 13 benign and 10 malignant primary neoplasms of the cervical spine, anterior excision with iliac crest autograft (supplemented with posterior grafting in some cases) proved to be reliable in relieving pain and neurologic symptoms, providing stability, and a better quality of life. Large tumors involving anterior, lateral, and posterior elements of the vertebral body were excised through staged anterior and posterior approaches. An intralesional margin was obtained in all malignant tumors. Only two such patients with malignancy survived more than 3 years (6,78).

Approaches to the cervical thoracic spine are difficult (21,49). The upper thoracic spine can be approached through either a transthoracic or retropleural approach through the fourth rib. Occasionally, inadequate exposure is obtained and the scapula is mobilized by detaching it posteriorly, allowing it to rotate up and then doing a costotransversectomy approach to the upper ribs (Fig. 10). Birch et al. (3) have described a novel approach in the lower cervical and upper thoracic spine exposing the brachial plexus and related vessels. This method involves elevation of the medial corner of the manubrium, the sternoclavicular joint, and the medial half of the clavicle on a pedicle of the sternomastoid muscle. They employed this in 17 cases with few complications but pointed out the necessity of high standards of anesthesia,

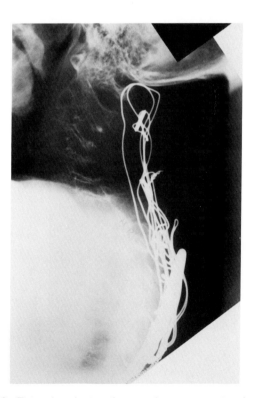

FIG. 9. Extensive destruction requires more extensive decompression and stabilization with wire-reinforced cement. This woman also had extensive thoracic disease.

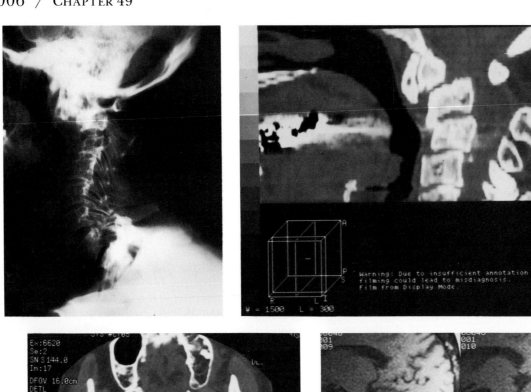

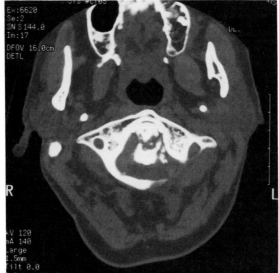

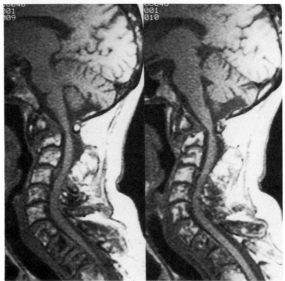

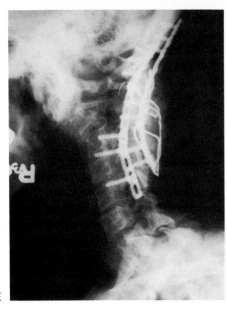

FIG. 10. A: Lateral view of cervical spine reveals a generalized moth-eaten appearance as well as a pathologic fracture of the odontoid with anterior displacement. **B,C:** This is confirmed on CT. **D:** MRI reveals some cord compression. **E:** Occipitocervical stabilization with plates, wire, and cement. This patient has had no problems for 2 years to date.

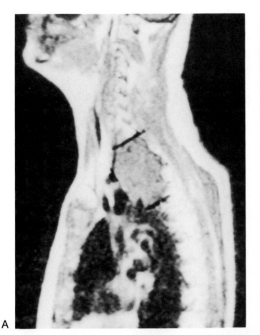

A

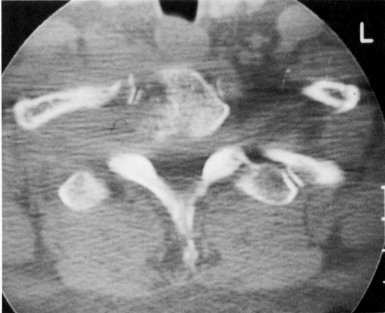

L

B

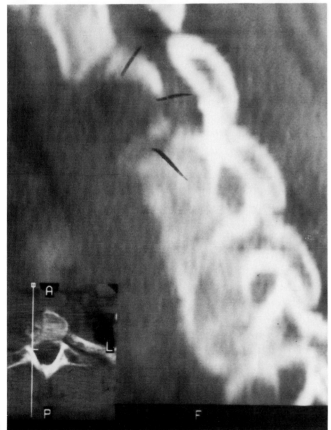

C

FIG. 11. A: MRI of a 31-year-old male with carcinoma of the lung, paraparesis, and brachial plexus involvement (Pancoast tumor) with destruction primarily at T1–T2. **B,C:** CT scan axial and saggital reconstruction demonstrates bone destruction.

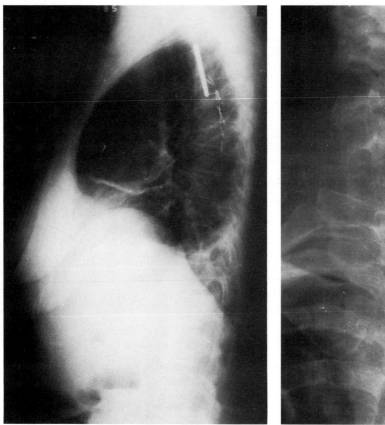
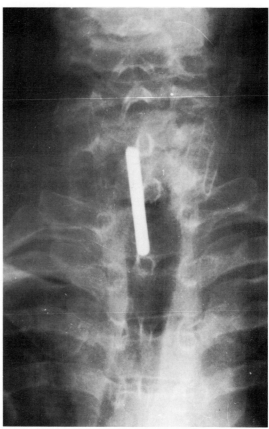

D

E

FIG. 11. (*Continued.*) **D,E:** Through a scapular mobilization and thoracotomy, the lung tumor was resected, the cord and brachial plexus decompressed and the spine stabilized. The patient is alive and well 1 to 5 years later.

surgical technique, and postoperative care. In the authors' opinion all this may be of value in certain specific cases. A thoracotomy, either extrapleural or intrapleural, provides access to the upper thoracic spine satisfactorily and can be combined with anterolateral approach to the cervical spine at the same time if necessary to approach the lower cervical spine.

Sjostrom et al. (69) have stabilized the odontoid with the use of screws and methylmethacrylate combination for pathologic fractures of the odontoid. No external support was used postoperatively. In such a case it is necessary that the body of C2 be reasonable.

Thoracic and Lumbar Spine

In an analysis of 75 patients with metastatic disease involving the thoracic and lumbar regions, 23 patients underwent anterior decompression and stabilization and 26 had posterior procedures. The remaining 26 patients had combined anterior and posterior procedures. In general, single-level disease may be treated by anterior decompression and stabilization (Fig. 11).

Three distinct types of posterior instrumentation were employed: two posterior Harrington rods generally reinforced with methylmethacrylate; posterior segmental in-

strumentation using either Luque one quarter inch rods; or Harrington rods with sublaminar wires, which was the most commonly used construct. A small number of cases had pedicle fixation in which either Luque rods were wired to the screws or plates were utilized. Most of the stabilization devices were reinforced with methylmethacrylate.

In contrast to the cervical spine, anterior stabilization of the thoracic or lumbar spine is based on multiple segmental rods reinforced with methylmethacrylate. As many as four levels of anterior decompression have been used without reinforcement posteriorly, but generally anterior decompression without posterior stabilization has been limited to two levels (Figs. 12 and 13).

Today we prefer the pedicle bone screw fixation to sublaminar wires, if there is significant osteopenia involving the levels proximal and distal to the decompression or where there is involvement of the posterior lamina with tumor where the pedicles are preserved.

Lumbosacral Region

In metastatic disease of the lumbosacral junction, laminectomy alone may suffice for neural decompression. If there is extensive destruction, then anterior stabilization

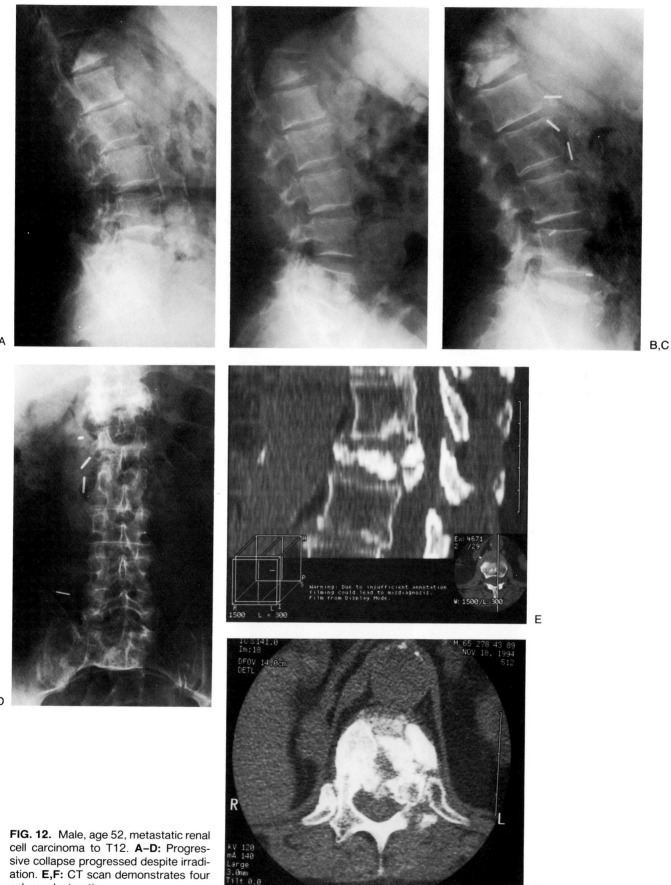

FIG. 12. Male, age 52, metastatic renal cell carcinoma to T12. **A–D:** Progressive collapse progressed despite irradiation. **E,F:** CT scan demonstrates four column destruction.

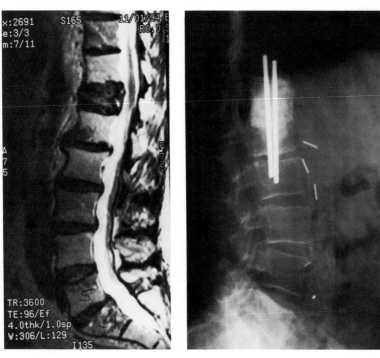
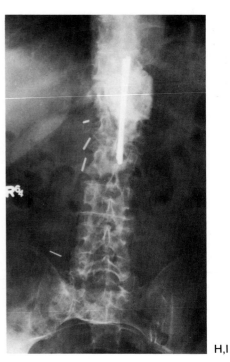

FIG. 12. (Continued.) **G:** MRI demonstrates neurologic compression. **H,I:** Postoperative stabilization and decompression. Note two rods. In the cervical and upper thoracic spine, one rod is used. In the distal lumbar spine, three rods can be used (Fig. 12).

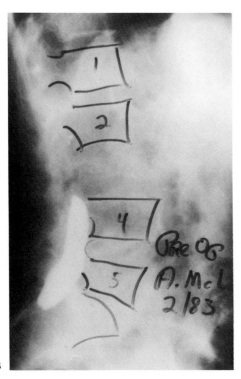
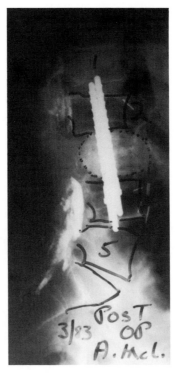

FIG. 13. Metastatic renal cell carcinoma to L3 with a marked cauda equina lesion (Frankel grade B). Following vascular embolization, decompression, and stabilization (note the three rods in the lumbar spine), the patient recovered neurologic function (Frankel grade D), including bowel and bladder function, but died 1 year later.

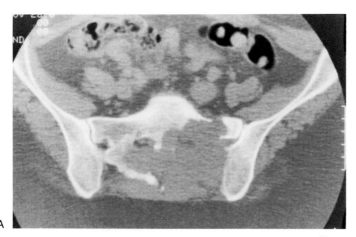

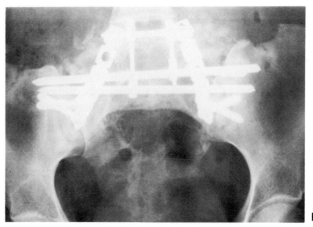

FIG. 14. Multiple myeloma. **A:** Note marked sacral destruction involving both sacroiliac joints and cauda equina compression. The tumor was debulked. **B:** The lumbosacral–pelvic area was stabilized with two Harrington sacral bars, plates from L5 to the pelvis. A cross bar from right to left at L5 was used with linkage to the sacral bars producing a rigid quadrilateral frame. Bone graft was used between L5 and the pelvis. Cement was used to reinforce the screws in the pelvis. The patient is 4 years post-surgery.

may be necessary. Because of the large vascular and autonomic structures anterior to the lumbar and sacral vertebrae, anterior reconstruction may be difficult, particularly when the vessels are involved in the disease tumor. Whenever possible, posterior stabilization is preferred using pedicle fixation with metal reinforced with methylmethacrylate cement. The choice of the surgical alternatives depends to some degree on whether or not adequate screw fixation can be obtained in the sacrum and whether or not the sacrum is involved in the disease process.

Stabilization of the lumbosacral junction may be indicated if there is: (a) an associated destruction of all the sacral iliac joints, (b) the iliolumbar ligamentous complex is disrupted, and/or (c) if there is extensive destruction of the posterior lumbosacral joints together with anterior L5 or S1 destruction (Fig. 14).

SPECIAL PROBLEMS

Renal Cell Carcinoma

Renal tumors present special challenges to the surgical oncologist. Patients frequently present with osseous metastases at the time of initial diagnosis, and demonstrate a highly variable course in terms of survival (64,70). Renal cell carcinoma is notoriously radioresistant and unresponsive to chemotherapy. Consideration has been given to wide resection as a possible curative procedure or as a consideration in the prevention of local recurrences.

Sundaresan et al. (72) reported on 43 patients with renal cell carcinoma. Thirty-two underwent anterior resec-

tion for cord compression and 11 had radiation only. The mean survival of the surgical group was 13 months, compared to 3 months for those treated with radiation alone. Patients undergoing complete resection of tumor anteriorly had a 37% survival at 2 years while none of those treated with radiotherapy alone survived 2 years. Significant neurologic improvement was seen in 70% of surgical patients compared to 45% of radiated patients. Other authors have reported survival rates of 30% or more at 5 years following aggressive resection of solitary renal metastases (75). Stener et al. (71) have advocated an approach to metastatic renal cell carcinoma similar to that for primary malignant tumors, that is, radical en bloc resection including, if necessary, the dura. He felt this aggressive surgical approach might lead to better long-term results. This approach may be indicated if the disease appears to be limited to one area of the spine with no other evidence of skeletal involvement. We have adopted Stener's approach but feel a prospective study should be done to validate this philosophy.

A recent analysis by King et al. (42) of 33 patients with renal cell metastatic disease of the spine has shown that approximately 50% of those patients had local recurrence of their tumor following decompression. It occurred more frequently in those patients whose involvement was more posterior than anterior. Those patients all underwent repeat decompression with similar improvement of their neurologic status as had occurred at the time of their first decompression. Six patients underwent decompression more than two times, again, with generally beneficial but limited results.

Renal cell carcinoma that has metastasized to the skeleton also has been noted to be notoriously vascular. Because of this potentially life-threatening problem, angiography should be performed preoperatively, if possible.

In acute paraplegia, this study is sometimes difficult to obtain. The blood loss has been compared in patients who underwent angiography preoperatively with embolization compared to those who were not embolized. The blood loss was similar in both patient groups. However, two patients who had their tumors approached posteriorly had to have surgery prematurely abandoned because of significant blood loss. Both patients were subsequently embolized and decompression was then possible. On the basis of this experience, we would advocate preoperative angiography for the assessment of vascularity with embolization if possible, despite the fact that it may influence the outcome in only a few patients. A contraindication to embolization is when the major feeder to the tumor is also a major source of blood to the spinal cord.

COMPLICATIONS

A number of published reports have implicated iatrogenic instability and deformity as a reason for lack of neurologic improvement and occasional progression of neurologic dysfunction. Therefore, prevention of postoperative kyphotic deformity and instability is important to the maintenance of neurologic integrity. Instability may result from inadequate reconstruction or stabilization at the time of initial surgery or from the late failure of fixation caused by progression of disease or implant failure. Attention to the mechanics of reconstruction must always be considered. In this example a different construct may have avoided this serious complication. In Harrington and associates' (39) series of 77 patients treated with posterior stabilization and methylmethacrylate, five patients suffered loss of fixation and required restabilization. In addition, six patients subsequently developed spinal instability due to metastatic disease at other levels of the spine.

There is a higher complication rate when methylmethacrylate is used, particularly in posterior stabilization constructs. Of 24 complications reported by McAfee et al. (52), only five occurred after anterior stabilization using methylmethacrylate. Of the 19 patients with posterior methylmethacrylate stabilization, 15 suffered loss of fixation, and a number of these subsequently developed a significant kyphosis. Six patients developed deep infections, three of whom suffered associated, significant neurologic deterioration. It is important to always supplement the methylmethacrylate with internal fixation as described earlier.

One hundred patients analyzed by Kostuik et al. (44) showed three cases of instrumentation failure. One failure occurred in a patient who had an anterior reinforced methylmethacrylate construct for metastatic disease in the cervical spine, because it was not recognized that the disease extended into the proximal vertebral body, which had been used for insertion of the stabilization construct.

A second procedure was successful. Two other major failures occurred. Both were in the thoracic spine, and both were associated with the use of posterior Harrington instrumentation without the use of sublaminar wires. The proximal hooks pulled out in one patient 1 week postoperatively in whom a dual Harrington distraction rod construct had been reinforced with methylmethacrylate bone cement. The second patient had a construct utilizing bilateral heavy Harrington compression rods reinforced with methylmethacrylate cement. The lower thoracic hooks pulled out after several months. Both patients underwent reconstruction with sequelae.

Up to the present time 125 anterior constructs have been done using reinforced metal rods passed into the vertebral bodies proximally and distally, reinforced by methylmethacrylate. These constructs have lasted for as long as 4 years, and to date only one failure has occurred.

Although it appears that methylmethacrylate can last over a long interval, it should not be used in isolation but only with metal reinforcement. Some authors have advocated that if the expected longevity of the patient is greater than 1 year, a bone graft should be performed using either the patient's own bone or an allograft. In our experience this additional bone grafting has not been necessary since the methylmethacrylate/metal implant constructs have lasted for as long as 4 years. Not everyone agrees with this philosophy. Unlike other reports, the incidence of infection is low using methylmethacrylate constructs and occurred in only three patients. None of these three patients underwent failure of the construct and the wounds were debrided and allowed to heal by secondary intention accompanied by antibiotic coverage. All three patients subsequently died as a result of their tumor disease, rather than as a complication of infection.

Finally, surgery in the patient with metastatic disease must be considered in the face of all other options. It should not, however, be considered only as the final alternative. In fact, in many select cases surgery offers the more conservative approach and may be less morbid to the patient than either chemotherapy, radiation, or high-dose narcotics. The surgical oncologist of the spine should be consulted early and often as the decision tree grows in these difficult cases.

REFERENCES

1. Algra PR, Bloem JL, Tissing H, Falke TH, Arndt JW, Verboon LJ (1991): Detection of vertebral metastases: comparison between MR imaging and bone scintigraphy. *Radiographics* 11:219–232.
2. Batson OV (1942): The role of the vertebral veins in metastatic processes. *Ann Intern Med* 16:38–45.
3. Birch R, Bonney G, Marshall RW (1990): A surgical approach to the cervicothoracic spine. *J Bone Joint Surg [Br]* 72:904–907.
4. Black P (1979): Spinal metastasis: current status and recommended guidelines for management. *Neurosurgery* 5(6):726–746.
5. Boesen J, Johnsen A, Helweg-Larsen S, Sorensen PS (1991): Diag-

nostic value of spinal computer tomography in patients with intraspinal metastases causing complete block on myelopathy. *Acta Radiol* 32:1–2.

6. Bohlman HH, Sachs BL, Carter JR, Rile L, Robinson RA (1986): Primary neoplasms of the cervical spine. *J Bone Joint Surg [Am]* 68:483–494.

7. Brice J, McKissock W (1965): Surgical treatment of malignant extradural spinal tumors. *Br Med J [Clin Res]* 1:1341–1344.

8. Broaddus WC, Grady MS, Delashaw JB Jr, Ferguson RD, Jane JA (1990): Preoperative superselective arteriolar embolization: a new approach to enhance resectability of spinal tumours. *Neurosurgery* 27:755–759.

9. Bruckman JE, Bloomer WD (1978): Management of spinal cord compression. *Semin Oncol* 5:135–140.

10. Chadwick DJ, Gillatt DA, Mukerjee A, Penry JB, Gingell JC (1991): Magnetic resonance imaging of spinal metastases. *J R Soc Med* 84:196–200.

11. Champlin AM, Rael J, Benzel EC, Kesterson L, King JN, Orrison WW, Mirfakhraee M (1994): Preoperative spinal angiography for lateral extracavitary approach to thoracic and lumbar spine. *Am J Neuroradiol* 15(1):73–77.

12. Colletti PM, Dang HT, Deseran MW, Kerr RM, Boswell WD, Ralls PW (1991): Spinal MR imaging in suspected metastases: correlation with skeletal scintigraphy. *Magn Reson Imaging* 9(3):349–355.

13. Constans JP, de Divitiis E, Donzelli R, Spaziante R, Meder JF, Haye C (1983): Spinal metastases with neurological manifestations: review of 600 cases. *J Neurosurg* 59:111–118.

14. Cooper PR, Errico TJ, Martin R, Crawford B, DiBartolo T (1993): A systematic approach to spinal reconstruction after anterior decompression for neoplastic disease of the thoracic and lumbar spine. *Neurosurgery* 32(1):1–8.

15. Dahlin DC (1978): *Bone tumors: general aspects and data on 6,221 cases.* 3rd ed. Springfield: Charles C Thomas.

16. Danzig LA, Resnick D, Akeson WH (1980): The treatment of cervical spine metastasis from the prostate with a halo cast. *Spine* 5:395–398.

17. DeWald RL, Bridwell KH, Prodromas C, Rodts MF (1985): Reconstructive spinal surgery as palliation for metastatic malignancies of the spine. *Spine* 10:21–26.

18. Dolin MG (1989): Acute massive dural compression secondary to methylmethacrylate replacement of a tumourous lumbar vertebral body. *Spine* 14:108–110.

19. Doppman JL, Girton M (1976): Angiographic study of the effect of laminectomy in the presence of acute anterior epidural masses. *J Neurosurg* 45:195–202.

20. Drury AB, Palmer PH, Highman WJ (1964): Carcinomatous metastasis to the vertebral bodies. *J Clin Pathol* 17:448–457.

21. Fessler RG, Dietze DD Jr, Millan MM, Peace D (1991): Lateral parascapular extrapleural approach to the upper thoracic spine. *J Neurosurg* 75(3):349–355.

22. Fidler MW (1985): Pathological fractures of the cervical spine. *J Bone Joint Surg [Br]* 67(3):352–357.

23. Fidler MW (1986):Anterior decompression and stabilization of metastatic spinal fractures. *J Bone Joint Surg [Br]* 68:83–90.

24. Fielding JW, Pyle RN Jr, Fietti VG Jr (1979): Anterior cervical vertebral body resection and bone-grafting for benign and malignant tumors. *J Bone Joint Surg [Am]* 61(2):251–253.

25. Findlay GF (1987): The role of vertebral body collapse in the management of malignant spinal cord compression. *J Neurol Neurosurg Psychiatry* 50:151–154.

26. Flatley TJ, Anderson MH, Anast GT (1984): Spinal instability due to malignant disease. Treatment by segmental spinal stabilization. *J Bone Joint Surg [Am]* 66:47–52.

27. Fraser RD, Paterson DC, Simpson DA (1977): Orthopaedic aspects of spinal tumors in children. *J Bone Joint Surg [Br]* 59(2):143–151.

28. Galasko CS (1981): The development of skeletal metastases. In: Weiss L, Gilbert HA, eds. *Bone metastases.* Boston: GK Hall Medical.

29. Ghelman B, Lospinuso MF, Levine DB, O'Leary PF, Burke SW (1991): Percutaneous computed tomography guided biopsy of the thoracic and lumbar spine. *Spine* 16:736–739.

30. Gilbert RW, Kim JH, Posner JB (1978): Epidural spinal cord com-

pression from metastatic tumor: diagnosis and treatment. *Ann Neurol* 3(1):40–51.

31. Graham WD (1966): Metastatic cancer to bone. In: *Bone tumours.* London: Butterworth, pp. 94–100.

32. Greenberg HS, Kim JH, Posner JB (1980): Epidural spinal cord compression from metastatic tumor. *Ann Neurol* 8:361–366.

33. Habermann ET, Sachs R, Stern RE, Hirsh DM, Anderson WJ Jr (1982): The pathology and treatment of metastatic disease of the femur. *Clin Orthop* 169:70–82.

34. Hall AJ, MacKay NN (1973): The results of laminectomy from compression of the cord or cauda equina by extradural malignant tumour. *J Bone Joint Surg [Br]* 55(3):497–505.

35. Harrington KD (1981): The use of methylmethacrylate for vertebral-body replacement and anterior stabilization of pathologic fracture-dislocations of the spine due to metastatic malignant disease. *J Bone Joint Surg [Am]* 63:36–46.

36. Harrington KD (1986): Metastatic disease of the spine. *J Bone Joint Surg [Am]* 68(7):1110–1115.

37. Harrington KD (1988): Anterior decompression and stabilization of the spine as a treatment for vertebral collapse and spinal cord compression from metastatic malignancy. *Clin Orthop* 233:177–194.

38. Harrington KD (1988): Metastatic disease of the spine. In: Harrington KD, ed. *Orthopaedic management of metastatic bone disease.* St. Louis: CV Mosby, pp. 309–383.

39. Harrington KD, Sim FH, Enis JE, Johnston JO, Diok HM, Gristina AG (1976): Methylmethacrylate as an adjunct in internal fixation of pathological fractures. *J Bone Joint Surg [Am]* 58:1047–1055

40. Helweg-Larsen S, Sorensen PS (1994). Symptoms and signs in metastatic spinal cord compression: a study of progression from first symptom until diagnosis in 153 patients. *Eur J Cancer* 30A(3):396–398.

41. Johnson JR, Leatherman KD, Holt RT (1983): Anterior decompression of the spinal cord for neurological deficit. *Spine* 8(4):396–405.

42. King GJ, Kostuik JP, McBroom RJ, Richardson W (1991): Surgical management of metastatic renal carcinoma of the spine. *Spine* 16:265–271.

43. Kostuik JP (1983): Anterior spinal cord decompression for lesions of the thoracic and lumbar spine, techniques, new methods of internal fixation results. *Spine* 8:512–531.

44. Kostuik JP, Errico TJ, Gleason TF, Errico CC (1988): Spinal stabilization of vertebral column tumors. *Spine* 13(3):250–256.

45. Livingston KE, Perrin RG (1978): The neurosurgical management of spinal metastases causing cord and cauda equina compression. *J Neurosurg* 49:839–843.

46. Loquet E, Thibaut R, Thibaut H, Hendrick M (1993): Surgical treatment of spinal metastases. *Acta Orthop Belg* 59 (Suppl. 1):79–82.

47. Manabe S, Tateishi A, Abe M, Ohno T (1989): Surgical treatment of metastatic tumors of the spine. *Spine* 14:41–57.

48. Maranzano E, Latini P, Checcaglini F, Ricci S, Panizza BM, Aristei C (1991): Radiation therapy in metastatic spinal cord compression: a prospective analysis of 105 consecutive patients. *Cancer* 67:1311–1317.

49. Marchesis DG, Boos N, Aebi M (1993): Surgical treatment of tumors of the cervical spine and first two thoracic vertebrae. *J Spinal Disord* 6(6):489–496.

50. Martin NS, Williamson J (1970): The role of surgery in the treatment of malignant tumours of the spine. *J Bone Joint Surg [Br]* 52(2):227–237.

51. Masaryk TJ (1991): Neoplastic disease of the spine. *Radiol Clin North Am* 29:829–845.

52. McAfee PC, Bohlman HH, Ducker T, Eismont FJ (1986): Failure of stabilization of the spine with methylmethacrylate. *J Bone Joint Surg [Am]* 68:1145–1157.

53. McLain RF, Weinstein JN (1989): Solitary plasmacytomas of the spine: a review of 84 cases. *J Spinal Disord* 2(2):69–74.

54. Meissner WA, Warren S (1966): Neoplasms. In: Anderson WAD, ed. *Pathology, vol. I,* 5th ed. St. Louis: CV Mosby, pp. 435–540.

55. Milch RA, Changus GW (1956): Response of bone to tumor invasion. *Cancer* 9(2):340–351.

56. Millburn L, Hibbs GC, Hendrickson FR (1968): Treatment of spi-

nal cord compression from metastatic carcinoma. *Cancer* 21:447–452.

57. Nather A, Bose K (1982): The results of decompression of cord or cauda equina compression from metastatic extradural tumors. *Clin Orthop* 169:103–108.

58. Nicholls PJ, Jarecky TW (1985): The value of posterior decompression by laminectomy for malignant tumors of the spine. *Clin Orthop* 201:210–213.

59. O'Neil J, Garner V, Armstrong G (1988): Treatment of tumors of the thoracic and lumbar spinal column. *Clin Orthop* 227:103–112.

60. Perrin RG, McBroom RJ (1987): Anterior versus posterior decompression for symptomatic spinal metastasis. *Can J Neurol Sci* 14:75–80.

61. Powles TJ, Dowsett M, Easty GC, et al. (1976): Breast-cancer osteolysis, bone metastases, and the anti-osteolytic effect of aspirin. *Lancet* 1:608–610.

62. Renfrew DL, Whitten CG, Wiese JA, El-Khoury GY, Harris KG (1991): CT-guided percutaneous transpedicular biopsy of the spine. *Radiology* 180:574–576.

63. Rompe JD, Eysel P, Hopf C, Heine J (1993). Metastatic spinal cord compression: options for surgical treatment. *Acta Neurochir* 123(3–4):135–140.

64. Saitoh H, Hida M, Nakamura K, et al. (1982): Metastatic processes and potential indication of treatment for metastatic lesions of renal adenocarcinoma. *J Urol* 128:916–918.

65. Shaw MD, Rose JE, Paterson A (1980): Metastatic extradural malignancy of the spine. *Acta Neurochir* (Wien) 52:113–120.

66. Sherman RM, Waddell JP (1986): Laminectomy for metastatic epidural spinal cord tumors. *Clin Orthop* 207:55–63.

67. Siegal T, Siegal T (1985): Surgical decompression of anterior and posterior malignant epidural tumors compressing the spinal cord. *Neurosurg* 17:424–430.

68. Siegal T, Tiqva P, Siegal T (1985): Vertebral body resection for epidural compression by malignant tumors. *J Bone Joint Surg* [*Am*] 67:375–382.

69. Sjostrom L, Olerud S, Karlstrom G, Hamberg M, Jonsson H (1990): Anterior stabilization of pathologic dens fractures. *Acta Orthop Scand* 61:391–393.

70. Skinner DG, Colvin RB, Vermillion CD, et al. (1971): Diagnosis and management of renal cell carcinoma. *Cancer* 28:1165–1177.

71. Stener B, Henriksson C, Johansson S, et al. (1984): Surgical removal of bone and muscle metastases of renal cancer. *Acta Orthop Scand* 55(5):491–500.

72. Sundaresan N, Scher H, DiGiacinto GV, Yagoda A, Whitmore W, Choi IS (1986): Surgical treatment of spinal cord compression in kidney cancer. *J Clin Oncol* 4:1851–1856.

73. Sze G (1991): Magnetic resonance imaging in the evaluation of spinal tumors. *Cancer* 67:1229–1241.

74. Tokuhashi Y, Matsuzaki H, Toriyama S, Kawano H, Ohsaka S (1990): Scoring system for the preoperative evaluation of metastatic spine tumor prognosis. *Spine* 15:1110–1113.

75. Tolia BM, Whitmore WF Jr (1975): Solitary metastasis from renal cell carcinoma. *J Urol* 114:836–838.

76. Tomita T, Galicich JH, Sundaresan N (1983): Radiation therapy for spinal epidural metastases with complete block. *Acta Radiol* 22:135–143.

77. Van Der Sande JJ, Kroger R, Boogerd W (1990): Multiple spinal epidural metastases; an unexpectedly frequent finding. *J Neurol Neurosurg Psychiatry* 53:1001–1003.

78. Verbiest H (1978): Lesions of the cervical spine: a critical review. In: Carrea R, ed. *Neurological surgery*. International Congress series 433. Amsterdam-Oxford: Excerpta Medica, pp. 374–383.

79. White AA III, Panjabi MM, eds. (1978): Surgical constructs employing methylmethacrylate. In: *Clinical biomechanics of the spine*. Philadelphia: JB Lippincott, pp. 423–431.

80. Wright RL (1963): Malignant tumors in the spinal extradural space: results of surgical treatment. *Ann Surg* 157(2):227–231.

The Adult Spine: Principles and Practice,
2nd edition, J.W. Frymoyer, Editor-in-Chief.
Lippincott-Raven Publishers, Philadelphia © 1997.

CHAPTER **50**

Intradural Tumors

John R. Cassidy, Thomas B. Ducker, and Elizabeth A. Dienes

The first report of a successful operation for a spinal cord tumor is credited to Victor Horsley. He described an operation performed on a profoundly paraparetic British naval captain for an intradural-extramedullary fibrosarcoma. The lesion was completely removed, and the patient made a nearly complete recovery. This initial success prompted Horsley to advocate surgical removal of spinal cord tumors as their preferred treatment (12). Subsequent reports of individual operations for spinal cord tumors were sporadic until Elsberg published his classic surgical monograph in 1916 (8). Careful review of this paper reveals that the surgical successes were not as great as Horsley's first case suggested they might be. The techniques of that era were not well suited to intradural spinal surgery. Greenwood's technical advances in microneurosurgery, including the introduction of bipolar cautery and the use of magnifying loupes, heralded a new era of spinal surgery. His series of six patients published in 1954 demonstrated for the first time that aggressive surgical removal of intramedullary lesions could be performed safely (14).

J. R. Cassidy, M.D.: Neurological Associates, Sarasota, Florida 34239.

T. B. Ducker, M.D.: Professor of Surgery, Johns Hopkins Medical Institutions, Baltimore, Maryland 21205.

E. A. Dienes, M.D.: Medical Director, MRI, Venice Hospital, Venice, Florida 34285.

EPIDEMIOLOGY

Primary spinal tumors are much less common than brain tumors. A population-based study in Olmstead County, Minnesota, estimated the annual incidence of primary spinal tumors to be 2.5 per 100,000 and the prevalence to be 12.9 per 100,000. In the same study, primary brain tumors were estimated to be approximately four times more common than spinal neoplasms (16).

The patient's signs and symptoms, the radiologic features of a spinal cord tumor, and the surgical approach to the tumor relate more to the anatomic compartment that the lesion occupies than to its histology. Hence, discussion of spinal cord tumors is customarily organized according to their intramedullary, extramedullary-intradural, or extradural location. We will follow this convention by dividing the discussion between intramedullary tumors and extramedullary-intradural tumors (32).

INTRAMEDULLARY TUMORS

Intramedullary tumors represent at most only one third of intradural tumors (19,28), of which astrocytomas are the most common. If one includes glioblastomas, oligodendrogliomas, and other less differentiated but glial-derived tumors, this category accounts for approximately 50% of all lesions (16,28,34). Ependymo-

TABLE 1. *Types of intramedullary tumors*[a]

Histology	Frequency
Astrocytoma, oligodendroglioma	50%
Ependymoma	30%
Hemangioblastoma	5–10%
Lipomas	<5%
Dermoids	<5%
Teratomas	<5%
Cavernous angioma	<5%

[a] Intramedullary tumors represent one-third of intradural tumors.

mas are the second most common intramedullary tumor and constitute roughly 30% of these lesions. The remaining 20% are divided among several different tumor types, but hemangioblastomas are probably the most common, followed by lipomas and dermoids (Table 1).

Epidemiology

Intramedullary ependymomas and astrocytomas have no particular predilection for any given age or sex. An intramedullary tumor discovered in a younger patient, however, should raise the suspicion of hemangioblastoma or teratoma.

Anatomic Location

Greenwood's review of intramedullary lesions indicated that 17.5% were located in the cervical cord, 37.5% in the thoracic region, and 47.5% in the lumbar region (13). Ependymomas are more heavily represented in the lumbar region because of their association with the filum terminale, and are usually fungating lesions that are primarily outside the substance of the spinal cord. A review of the published series on hemangioblastomas suggests that they tend to be located in the cervicothoracic region (15,38). Astrocytomas are almost invariably completely intramedullary, as are the more rostrally located ependymomas.

Clinical Findings

Compared with extradural tumors, intradural tumors have a less rapid progression of symptoms, which frequently results in a significant delay in diagnosis. One exception to this rule is hemangioblastoma, in which a hemorrhage can present acutely. Pain is the most common presenting symptom. The pain is generally not radicular, although a local band of dysesthesia or hyperpathia, similar to that seen in syringomyelia, may mimic radiculopathy. Furthermore, as in syringomyelia, the

sensory loss may be dissociated, as pain and temperature are disproportionately affected. Other common features associated with cord dysfunction may be seen, including spastic gait, hand weakness, and Brown-Sequard syndrome. However, these often occur late in the course of the disease.

Physical examination tends to parallel the symptoms. Motor and sensory function are more severely affected at the level of the lesion than distally.

Radiologic Findings

Plain Roentgenograms

Owing to their slow growth and fusiform expansion of the spinal cord, intramedullary tumors most commonly show widening of the spinal canal on plain x-rays. This is best seen in the anteroposterior (AP) projection as widening of the interpedicular distance and is sometimes associated with erosion and thinning of the pedicles (Fig. 1). Lateral projections are often normal, although one can occasionally see flattening or increased scalloping of the vertebral bodies at the involved levels (Fig. 2).

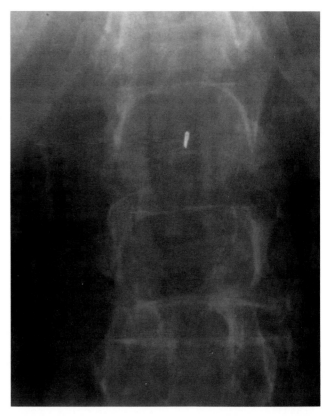

FIG. 1. AP L1 and L2 spinal x-ray in a patient with a long-standing conus tumor. In this picture, the tumor was originally biopsied and continued to grow. The AP diameter of the canal was widened, as demonstrated on these x-rays.

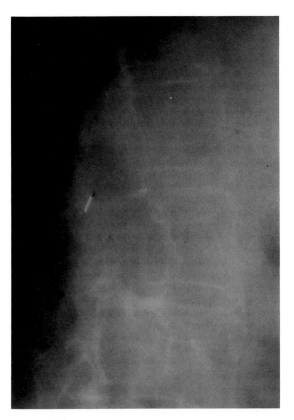

FIG. 2. Lateral lumbar spine in the same patient as in Fig. 1 with a long-standing intradural spinal tumor. In this picture, there is scalloping even of the vertebral bones.

Computed Tomography-Myelography

The distinction between intramedullary, extramedullary-intradural, and extradural lesions can usually be made easily by myelography (Fig. 3). The diffuse symmetric expansion of the cord characteristic of intramedullary tumors is readily seen. Since the advent of water-based contrast media, complete myelographic block is very uncommon. If there is an apparent block on myelography, computed tomography (CT) scanning above the level of the block will frequently reveal contrast medium and allow adequate imaging of the lesion, thereby obviating the need for a C1-C2 puncture (Figs. 4 and 5). CT scanning is also helpful in that any significant concentration of intramedullary contrast should raise the question of syringomyelia. Before the introduction of magnetic resonance imaging (MRI), delayed CT was often the only means of identifying a syrinx. A bit of caution should be taken in diagnosing an intramedullary lesion based on myelography alone. A ventral extradural lesion can splay the cord against the dura in such a way that the AP projection often will falsely suggest diffuse expansion of the spinal cord. Again, post-myelography CT scanning and lateral myelographic projections will differentiate intradural from extradural lesions.

Angiography

Certain vascular cord tumors necessitate angiographic imaging. The hemangioblastoma poses a unique problem because of its extreme vascularity. Myelographically, blood vessels and varices on the surface of the spinal cord are occasionally seen, and the possibility of arteriovenous malformation (AVM) should be considered. Yasargil notes that the cord is not usually expanded by AVM, whereas this is typically the case with hemangioblastomas. If the diagnosis remains uncertain, angiography may be indicated. The hemangioblastoma usually demonstrates a dense homogeneous stain lasting from the early arterial phase to the late venous phase. Individual vessels are not readily visualized. Early draining veins or dilated feeding arteries suggest the diagnosis of a spinal cord AVM.

Magnetic Resonance Imaging

MRI has revolutionized imaging of intramedullary spinal lesions and essentially supplanted CT myelography. As a rule, intramedullary tumors cause a fusiform enlargement of the spinal cord, with the tumor demon-

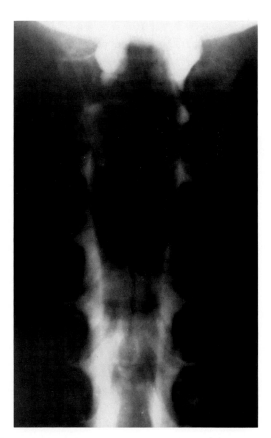

FIG. 3. Myelogram in patient with a cervical intramedullary ependymoma. In this picture, there is diffuse widening of the spinal cord in both AP and lateral views.

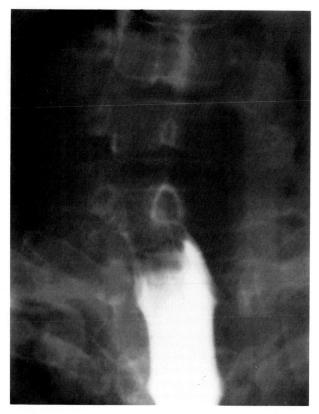

FIG. 4. Myelogram of a patient with an intradural and extramedullary lesion. Note that the contrast material is distorted around the lesion. This has to be appreciated in the myelographic block so that one rules out a lesion not in the spinal cord itself. This particular patient had a meningioma.

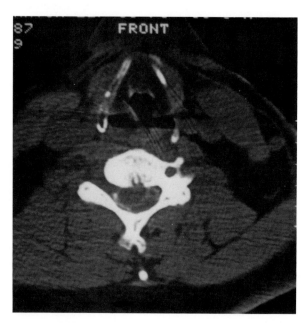

FIG. 5. Post-myelographic CT scan demonstrates the spinal cord and the tumor, both of which are in the dural sac. In this particular patient, the tumor was a meningioma.

strating isointense or slightly decreased intensity on T1-weighted imaging (Fig. 6). T2-weighted images show generally increased signal intensity with respect to the spinal cord, although the borders of the tumor are frequently difficult to delineate. The surrounding edema in the spinal cord also shows increased signal intensity on T2-weighted imaging. Consequently, the borders of the tumor are not well defined and the entire spinal cord may appear involved. Attempting to predict whether a lesion is an astrocytoma or ependymoma remains difficult despite the advances of MR imaging. Ependymomas are supposed to enhance with generally better-defined borders than astrocytomas. Astrocytomas are somewhat more likely to have associated necrosis or cyst formation. Nevertheless, the overlap is great, and frequently no distinctive features are evident.

Myxopapillary ependymomas are a separate category of ependymoma and are more characteristic in their MR imaging. These tumors are found in the conus medullaris or filum terminale and have much better-defined borders with respect to the neuropil. They are frequently lobulated and can have prominent vascularity, as evidenced

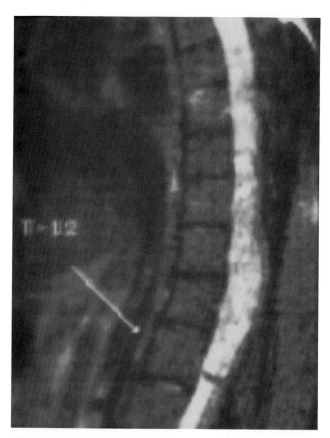

FIG. 6. MRI scan of a patient with long-standing intramedullary ependymoma over many segments of the thoracic spinal cord. In this patient, the lesion had grown quite large before she sought medical help. The MRI scan clearly delineates the extent of the lesion. Axial cuts of the same patient show that the lesion was intra-axial, in this case an ependymoma.

by flow voids in or around the tumor. These tumors are more prone to hemorrhage than are other glial tumors, and their enhancement may be more heterogeneous because of their vascularity.

Hemangioblastoma is another intramedullary lesion that can frequently be distinguished from the glial tumors. It has a much more typical appearance, with prominent vascularity and serpiginous flow voids that can be so impressive as to sometimes suggest an AVM. Obviously, when associated with Von Hippel-Lindau disease, these can be multicentric. It is not uncommon to see a very large cystic component associated with hemangioblastomas; in fact, the tumor may be seen only as a small mural nodule, in a manner analogous to intracranial hemangioblastomas. The nodule is usually isointense or slightly increased in signal intensity on T1-weighted imaging and has variable characteristics on T2-weighted imaging. The cystic portion has decreased signal intensity on T1-weighted imaging and increased signal intensity on T2-weighted imaging. The nodule usually enhances prominently with gadolinium, whereas the cyst does not.

Intramedullary metastases are being recognized with increasing frequency, probably in part because of the sensitivity of MRI. They generally cause fusiform enlargement of the spinal cord, although tumors with extramedullary nodular excrescence can be seen as well. Their features are not particularly distinguishing from other intramedullary tumors. With respect to the spinal cord, they are isointense to hypointense on T1-weighted imaging and slightly increased in signal intensity on T2-weighted imaging. Again, the borders of the tumor are not generally well defined, secondary to the edema of the spinal cord, showing similar increased signal intensity on T2-weighted imaging. These tumors enhance in an uncharacteristic fashion with gadolinium (30).

If hemorrhage is suspected in or around a tumor, as evidenced by sudden clinical deterioration or lack of enhancement with gadolinium on MR imaging, spin echo (SE) sequences or gradient echo (GE) sequences can be done to confirm the presence of blood products. The changes in signal intensity associated with blood products as they age are not as well established in the spinal cord as in the brain; however, one should remember that increased signal intensity on T1-weighted imaging is seen almost exclusively in hemorrhage and fatty tissue. Very low signal intensity is generally deoxyhemoglobin.

Intramedullary dermoids and teratomas do not have a consistent appearance on either T1- or T2-weighted imaging, perhaps because of their inherently heterogeneous makeup and the variability of their cholesterol content.

One of the more important issues in evaluating intramedullary lesions is whether there are cysts associated with the tumor or if the lesion is a benign syrinx. If this is a concern, the cervicomedullary junction should be imaged to exclude a Chiari malformation. Syrinxes are usu-

ally larger and have smooth borders. Enhancement of any portion of the wall with gadolinium strongly supports the diagnosis of tumor. Finally, dynamic imaging techniques are being developed that can sometimes demonstrate cerebrospinal fluid (CSF) flow within the cavity. This would certainly be more likely to occur in a syrinx than in a tumor-associated cyst (9).

A final word of caution regarding MR imaging of spinal cord lesions. MRI is so sensitive to spinal cord pathology that many lesions are discovered that have increased signal intensity on unenhanced T1 and T2 images. These lesions are not necessarily tumors. A tumor should both enhance with gadolinium and enlarge the axial dimension of the spinal cord. The absence of either of these characteristics should seriously raise the question that the lesion may not be a tumor. Sarcoid, multiple sclerosis, foix-Alajouanine, and subacute necrotizing myelopathy all are nonsurgical disease processes that can mimic a tumor on MRI. If there is doubt as to the diagnosis, the patient should be followed closely both clinically and radiographically until a more certain conclusion can be reached.

Surgical Technique

Once the rostral and caudal extents of the tumor have been defined roentgenographically, a laminectomy can be planned that will completely encompass the lesion. Thoracic and lumbar tumors are usually operated on in the prone position, although Malis (26) advocates a semilateral position. He believes that this provides a more comfortable position for the surgeon while using the operating microscope. For cervical operations, some authors (24) use the sitting position although many, because of the risk of air embolus, prefer to position the patient prone. In many patients with cervical involvement, awake fiberoptic intubation is necessary to confirm preservation of neurologic function before positioning the patient on the operating table.

Spinal cord monitoring has been found to be of limited use once the intradural portion of the procedure commences. There is frequent marked diminution in the evoked responses, even when the surgeon feels that there is not excessive manipulation of the spinal cord. Conventional somatosensory evoked potentials rely on the dorsal columns for transmission of their signals, and complete loss of the wave form is common if a midline myelotomy is required for an intramedullary tumor. In the future, we may find motor evoked potentials to be more predictive of postoperative motor function than somatosensory evoked potentials. At this time, however, several authors feel that reliance on spinal cord monitoring for intradural surgery is misleading and that its principal usefulness is in positioning the patient, as the signals can exhibit a marked decline in amplitude if the patient's neck is placed in maximal flexion. These changes are corrected once the position is relaxed.

Extreme flexion of the neck should be avoided for several reasons. The vascularity of the underlying spinal cord may be already compromised, and the ventral aspect of the cord and its anterior spinal artery can be affected further in the presence of a ventral osteophyte. Second, extreme flexion causes venous distention. Not only is this troublesome in controlling epidural venous bleeding, but it may also cause venous engorgement of the tumor and surrounding spinal cord, making it more difficult to handle and causing edematous neural tissue. By modest flexion of the head downward using three-point Mayfield pin fixation, the table can be rotated in a reverse Trendelenburg angle such that when the neck is parallel to the floor, it is safely above the level of the heart.

A careful laminectomy must be taken as far lateral as is necessary to allow the dura to be opened widely. The underlying spinal cord must be assumed to be already compromised; consequently, this portion of the procedure must be performed gently so as to minimize downward forces on the dura.

Osteoplastic laminotomies are favored over laminectomy in some surgeon's hands, and in particular in managing pediatric tumors (7,10). Several factors predispose these patients to postoperative spinal deformity, the most important being: (a) a skeletally immature spine, (b) pre-existing deformity, (c) profound preoperative neurologic deficit, (d) a large number of levels requiring laminectomy, and (e) involvement of the cervical spine. As a rule, in the adult population, if there is no pre-existing spinal deformity, a standard laminectomy is a simple, safe, and adequate approach to exposing these tumors.

Throughout the exposure, meticulous attention must be paid to hemostasis; blood running down into the surgical field once the dura is opened is unacceptable. Bone wax is applied to the bone edges, and moist cotton strips are draped over the adjoining muscle edges. The operating microscope is often introduced at this stage of the procedure. The dura is opened and tacking sutures are placed. The arachnoid may be adherent to underlying vessels, which can be avulsed if the dura is reflected before the vessels are freed. If a cyst or syrinx is anticipated, it is probably advisable to drain it at this time. However, the surgeon must resist the temptation to empty the cyst or syrinx completely, as it may be more difficult to locate later. This cavity will in part define the direction and extent of the myelotomy. If the location of the cyst is uncertain, ultrasound may be of some value. If there is no cyst present, then a brief review of the appearance of the spinal cord is in order. The cord should be inspected at its lateral and ventral aspects to exclude an extra-axial lesion or exophytic portion of an intramedullary lesion. Usually these will not be evident.

The myelotomy should be performed at or near the midline, at a point where the normal neurologic tissue appears most thinned. Frequently there is a midline vein, and the pial incision should be made adjacent to it. Numerous small branches will arise at right angles to the parent vessel, and these will need to be sacrificed. As the myelotomy is lengthened and deepened, the tumor will be encountered. It is frequently advantageous to extend the pial incision well above and below the rostral/caudal extent of the lesion. Pial tacking sutures can then be placed easily and tied to the dura. As the myelotomy is performed, the normal spinal tissue tends to retract laterally to join the pia, and the interface between the spinal cord and tumor can be addressed with less manipulation of normal neural tissue.

If an astrocytoma is suspected, a biopsy is useful at this time to confirm the diagnosis. Pool (29) states that morphologically, an astrocytoma characteristically has a whitish-yellow, stringy, tough edematous stroma (Figs. 7 and 8). Astrocytomas frequently do not have a clear plane of dissection between the tumor and normal spinal cord, which is not true of most other intramedullary tumors. The pathologic report on the biopsy will be very helpful in directing the surgery. The surgical approach to intramedullary astrocytomas has historically been somewhat controversial; some authors recommend biopsy alone and radiation therapy, whereas others are much more aggressive with the initial surgical therapy. There appears to be an emerging consensus, however, that anaplastic or malignant astrocytomas do not benefit from radical surgery and that in fact, efforts to remove these tumors completely are almost uniformly associated with significant postoperative morbidity (2,6,7,10). Biopsy of these lesions followed by radiation and treatment is a reasonable approach, although it appears that these tumors have a uniformly poor prognosis regardless of the treatment (4).

The surgical management of grade I and II astrocytomas has also become more clearly defined in recent years. Many of these tumors have well-defined cleavage planes and can be dissected successfully from surrounding neural tissue. It is interesting that their histology is generally that of a more fibrillary astrocytoma with adjacent cystic components. One might liken them to juvenile pilocystic astrocytomas, and it appears that safe resection and long-term disease-free survival can be expected (7,10). There are, however, spinal astrocytomas of low grade that do not appear as easily dissected. The interface between tumor and spinal cord is uncertain and, in fact, analysis of pathologic specimens has revealed normal axons and neurons intermingled with tumor cells (6). This has led Cooper (6) to conclude that attempts at radical resection of difficult, low-grade astrocytomas in the spinal cord do not yield improvement in long-term outcome. Other papers seem to confirm this opinion, although Epstein has reported successful radical excision in virtually all of his patients with adult intramedullary astrocytomas. Seventeen patients survived;

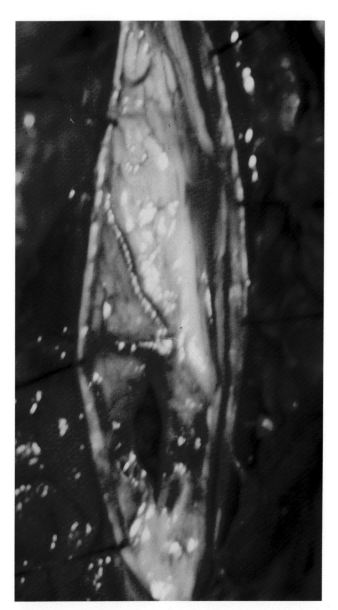

FIG. 7. Intramedullary astrocytoma. This is a nonresectable tumor, and the prognosis is very poor.

two had clinical evidence of tumor recurrence. Small residual neoplasms were identified without subsequent radiologic progression.

Different approaches are used in resecting these tumors. Sometimes this can be done with bipolar coagulation and conventional microsurgical instrumentation. After gutting the center of the tumor and coagulating the periphery, the tissue frequently retracts, serving to expose the fine bridging vessels and gliotic tumor border. Removal of the central portion of the tumor can be accomplished with a Cavitron ultrasonic surgical aspirator as well. The CO_2 laser can be used successfully to vaporize the tumor in fine layers, which is particularly helpful as one approaches the gliotic border or normal white matter of the spinal cord (18).

Low-grade astrocytomas pose one of the more tedious surgical challenges; yet every effort should be made to achieve as complete a resection as can safely be accomplished. Subsequent tumor recurrence can be difficult to treat through surgical re-exploration. The dura is invariably adherent to the underlying cord, and opening and reflecting it is not a benign part of the procedure. Furthermore, the tumor plane will be obscured by scar, greatly increasing the risk attendant to radical excision.

Ependymomas almost always have a discrete dissection plane that allows complete surgical excision (27). They frequently have a striking bluish-purple appearance, which distinguishes them from the surrounding

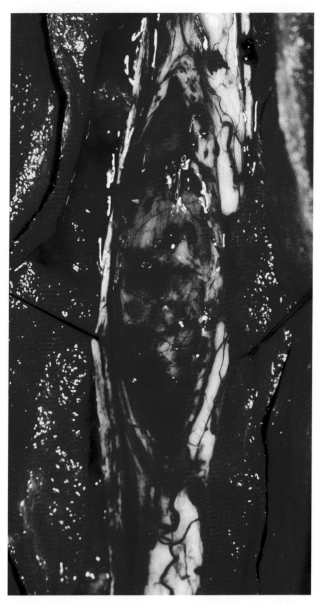

FIG. 8. Intramedullary astrocytoma clearly showing ependymoma feature with well-defined border. The tumor was totally resected over seven spinal cord segments, but because it has clear glioma features, the prognosis is not good.

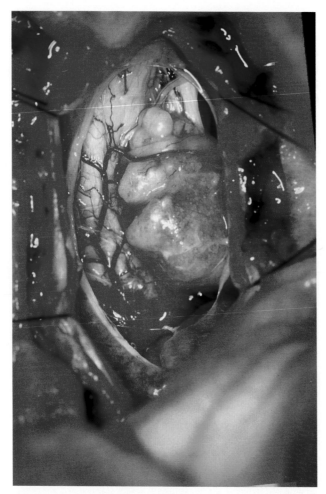

FIG. 9. Intramedullary ependymoma that was totally removed, with no postoperative radiation. The patient has done well for 3 years. This is a cervical lesion, and the patient uses his hands easily for computer work.

spinal cord (Figs. 9 and 10). The same microsurgical techniques are employed for their removal as are used with astrocytomas. It should be emphasized that debulking the core of the tumor may be necessary to define the edges of the lesion without manipulating neural tissue. The vast majority of these should be amenable to complete surgical resection. Evidence to date suggests that the likelihood of recurrence in these patients is quite small if the resection is performed en bloc, whereas incompletely resected ependymomas are likely to progress; even piecemeal-resected tumors may recur.

Hemangioblastomas appear similar to cavernous angiomas at the time of surgery. The lesion consists of a tightly packed collection of blood vessels. Nevertheless, the intraoperative behavior can be quite different. The tumor substance of a hemangioblastoma can be exceedingly bloody, in contrast to the cavernous angioma. If a hemangioblastoma is strongly suspected by preoperative MRI characteristics, a biopsy of the lesion or an attempt at centrally debulking the tumor is relatively contraindi-

cated. These lesions should be handled in a manner similar to AVMs, in which the nidus of vessels is dissected within the gliotic plane and special attention is devoted to coagulating and dividing the arterial input before sacrificing the venous outflow. In many of these tumors, however, the afferent and efferent vessels appear intermediate in nature between arterial and venous, and a distinction cannot possibly be made. As is the case with ependymomas, a clear plane of dissection is the rule, and a surgical cure is a reasonable and achievable goal.

Intramedullary lipomas are uncommon lesions, although review of the literature seems to suggest that complete surgical removal of these is very difficult and probably dangerous. Bipolar cautery should be used to shrink the volume of the fat, and a discrete cleavage plane is usually not found.

Finally, at the end of any tumor resection, if the dura cannot be easily closed in a watertight fashion, a dural patch should be used. Freeze-dried dura and tensor fascia lata are the most widely available dural substitutes. The importance of a nonconstricting dural closure that allows expansion and room for spinal fluid flow is particu-

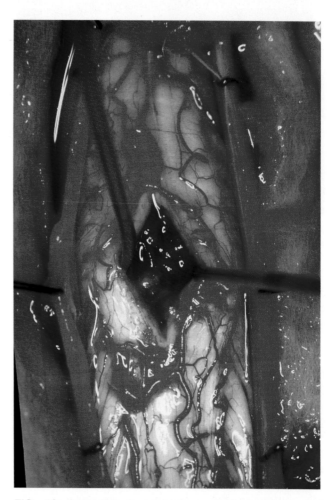

FIG. 10. Anterolateral meningioma displacing the spinal cord. It can be removed by first debulking the tumor.

larly relevant to surgery on any tumor that might recur. Late neurologic deterioration from arachnoidal adhesions has been observed, and this likelihood might be minimized if normal pathways of CSF flow are maintained.

Surgical Outcome

Even after the most careful resection of an intramedullary spinal tumor, significant postoperative morbidity may result. Patients with relatively intact motor function may have great difficulty in ambulation because of the disturbance of the dorsal columns. For obvious anatomic reasons, the legs are more likely to be affected than the arms, and the loss of position sense alone is sufficient to render a patient ambulatory only with assistive devices. Central spinal cord pain is another postoperative sequela that can cause significant functional impairment. This syndrome can occur after any spinal cord insult and is characteristically identified as a burning, dysesthetic pain that involves the trunk and extremities distal to the lesion. As is the case with central cord pain after trauma, medical treatment is often unsatisfactory, and this problem can contribute greatly to the patient's long-term disability.

It is widely held that the greater the neurologic deficit preoperatively, the more likely that the patient will be worse postoperatively. Most of the immediate postoperative deficit can be expected to improve in the ensuing months; however, recovery cannot be said to be complete until a year or 18 months has elapsed.

Most patients see no deterioration in their neurologic performance as compared with their preoperative status once their recovery is complete. A significant minority suffer long-term impairment as a result of surgery, and overall improvement in neurologic performance occurs in an even smaller minority of patients. This has been reported in a number of studies, and its implications for informed surgical consent cannot be ignored. These patients must be told that this surgery is being done to prevent future neurologic decline and that they should be thankful if their neurologic deficit can be stabilized by the surgery. Furthermore, recovery from the surgery may be difficult and protracted.

Prognosis

The prognosis for spinal cord astrocytomas is clearly not as good as it is for other intramedullary tumors. Guidetti et al. (16) compiled a large series of astrocytomas, but statistical methods were difficult to apply given the variability of follow-up. Nevertheless, they concluded that aggressive resection of these lesions might forestall the progression of disease for approximately 5 years. High-grade astrocytomas were felt to have a poorer prognosis than low-grade tumors. Cooper (6) has found higher-grade astrocytomas to be more aggressive, with no 2-year survivors of histologically graded malignant astrocytomas. Similar results have been published on malignant astrocytomas in the pediatric population (3). Several surgeons have reported that no improvement in outcome could be demonstrated in their patients who had more aggressive resections for astrocytomas (5,16,17). The authors proposed that radical excision appears to prolong the time to recurrence for low-grade astrocytomas. There is no statistical evidence to support this conclusion, in part because of the indolent nature of these lesions. Virtually all investigators now agree that malignant astrocytomas cannot be helped by surgery.

On the other hand, review of the literature strongly suggests that patients who have had complete excision of other intramedullary tumors fare better than those who have undergone partial resections. One can usually expect long-term tumor-free survival after the total removal of hemangioblastomas and ependymomas.

Adjunctive Therapies

Radiation therapy is frequently considered in the postoperative management of intramedullary spinal tumors. Whether the lesion is an ependymoma or astrocytoma, if there is complete excision the consensus is that radiation is not required. These patients should be followed with serial MRI, and if recurrence develops, either repeat surgery or radiation therapy should be considered. There is some evidence to suggest that even if an ependymoma is completely excised, if the resection was done in a piecemeal fashion rather than en bloc, recurrence is more likely. It is interesting that these are not necessarily local recurrences; there seems to be some possibility of subarachnoid seeding from the piecemeal removal with distant tumor recurrence. In fact, in those instances in which en bloc resection of an ependymoma is impossible, and in particular if only subtotal resection was achieved, radiation should be strongly considered. Current recommendations for postoperative irradiation are to use wide fields to prevent distant recurrence, as described above (36,37).

Malignant astrocytomas are generally not surgically resectable, and postoperative irradiation is usually recommended for these. As mentioned previously, these tumors have a uniformly poor prognosis, and there are no studies demonstrating clearly that life expectancy is prolonged by postoperative radiotherapy. The customary protocol for radiation of the spinal cord is 4500 cGy distributed over a 5-week period, at 200 cGy per treatment session (23). Routine irradiation of low-grade astrocytomas, particularly those that are completely resected, is probably not warranted. MRI is now so sensitive in detecting recurrence that there is very little loss in following these patients with MR imaging.

Adjuvant chemotherapy in the management of intra-medullary spinal cord tumors is considered experimental at this time.

EXTRAMEDULLARY-INTRADURAL TUMORS

Epidemiology

The two most common extramedullary-intradural tumors are meningiomas and neurofibromas, which occur with equal frequency. Together they represent approximately 70% of all extramedullary-intradural tumors. Sarcomas are probably the third most common tumor in this compartment, accounting for roughly 10% of the total (28). Other less common tumors include dermoids, epidermoids, angiomas, and, rarely, lymphomas or metastatic deposits.

Meningiomas, neurofibromas, and sarcomas tend to occur in middle-aged or elderly patients. Neurofibromas and sarcomas occur with equal frequency in men and women. Meningiomas, on the other hand, are generally reported to occur with disproportionate frequency (80%) in women (28).

Anatomic Location

Meningiomas are found most frequently (80%) in the thoracic region (Fig. 10) (33). Lumbar and cervical lesions are far less common. Neurofibromas are more evenly distributed (28), although some believe that the thoracic region is more common than the lumbar, which is more common than the cervical. Diagnostic lumbar punctures performed before the advent of styletted needles have been implicated in the formation of dermoid tumors, hence these are most frequently located in the lumbar region as well (35).

One third of neurofibromas are extradural and two thirds are intradural. Some small fraction of these, however, are actually found in both compartments. Meningiomas are more frequently found in an intradural location; only 15% are partly or completely extradural (31).

Neurofibromas originate more commonly from the dorsal root than the ventral root (80%) (Figs. 11 and 12). Fortunately, meningiomas also occur more frequently in a dorsal or lateral location. It has been reported that they may have a predilection for originating in the region of the dentate ligament (22).

Clinical Findings

Meningiomas and neurofibromas are both benign, slow-growing tumors. They are more likely to present with radicular pain than are intramedullary tumors and less likely to be associated with central cord pain. Night

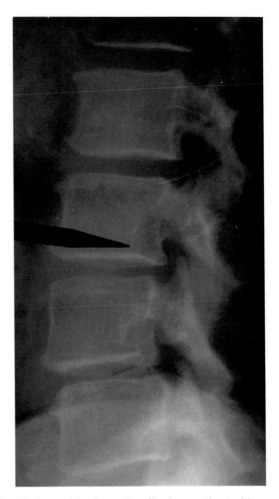

FIG. 11. Lateral lumbar spine film in a patient with neurofibroma. Note the scalloping and enlargement of the neural foramen with the changes in the vertebral body and the adjacent pedicle.

pain is frequently mentioned with these lesions, although the physiology behind this phenomenon is uncertain. Pain is often the only symptom when the lesion is located in the lumbar theca. Involvement of more than the attached nerve root occurs late and is almost invariably associated with a myelographic block. Cervical and thoracic lesions tend to produce asymmetric motor deficits more so than intramedullary tumors, hence a Brown-Sequard syndrome should suggest an intradural extramedullary tumor.

Finally, the diagnosis of foramen magnum meningioma is notoriously elusive. This is the one anatomic region in the nervous system in which unusual combinations of extremity involvement can be seen; for example, right arm and left leg, or all extremities except one arm. Complaints of nausea, vomiting, dizziness, dysphagia, and clumsiness may be elicited. Because of the slow growth of this lesion and its unusual constellation of symptoms, it is occasionally misdiagnosed as multiple sclerosis.

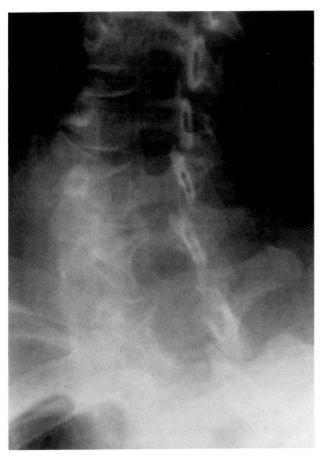

FIG. 12. Oblique cervical spine x-ray in a patient with neurofibroma. Note the enlargement of the neural foramen, which is completely destroyed with the expansion of the tumor.

Radiologic Findings

Plain X-Rays

Plain films are usually normal in patients harboring meningiomas. Neurofibromas frequently show widening of the intervertebral foramen of the involved nerve root. This is particularly common with the dumbbell lesions. The bony margins are smooth because of the slow process of remodeling (Figs. 11 and 12). Erosion of the bone or pedicle suggests malignancy.

Ependymomas of the lumbar theca may show widening of the interpediculate distance. This is most likely to occur in the younger age groups.

Computed Tomography-Myelography

Typically, the spinal cord is shifted to one side of the canal, as evidenced by tapering of the myelographic column on that side (Fig. 5). On the opposite side, the subarachnoid space is widened (Fig. 13). The contrast agent then outlines the adjacent aspect of the tumor, which is usually smoothly rounded in the case of a neurofibroma. A meningioma may be situated in an en plaque fashion

over the lateral aspect of the dura, and the appearance may not be as smooth as in the case of a neurofibroma. Similarly, sarcomas are less regular lesions. Special attention should be paid to the patient's physical findings, as both of these tumors may be found in multiple locations in the neuraxis. Neurofibromatosis is not always immediately clinically evident, and the finding of an isolated neurofibroma is often the first step in making the diagnosis. If there is any uncertainty that the demonstrated lesion completely accounts for the patient's deficits, further imaging or pan-myelography may be indicated.

Magnetic Resonance Imaging

MRI is now the imaging modality of choice for extramedullary-intradural lesions. Characteristics that allow one to distinguish neurofibromas from meningiomas are subtle but have some predictive value. Neurofibromas tend to be well-circumscribed tumors. On T1-weighted imaging, they are isointense or mildly hypointense with respect to the spinal cord. On T2-weighted imaging, they

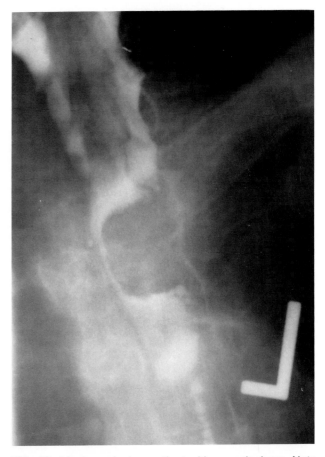

FIG. 13. Myelography in a patient with a meningioma. Note that this type of diagnostic study is still useful in delineating the exact extent of the lesion. The spinal cord can be visualized as well as the tumor.

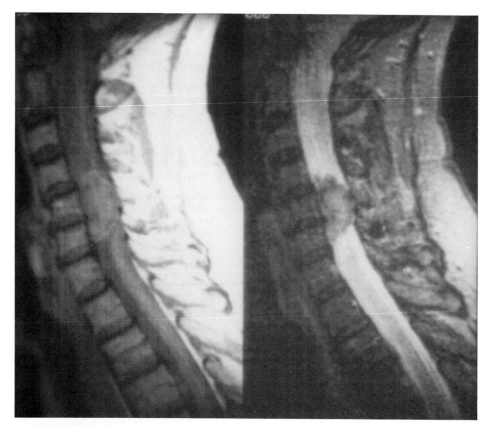

FIG. 14. Sagittal MRI in a patient with a neurofibroma. The standard MRI techniques often will delineate the neurofibroma on the T1- and T2-weighted images.

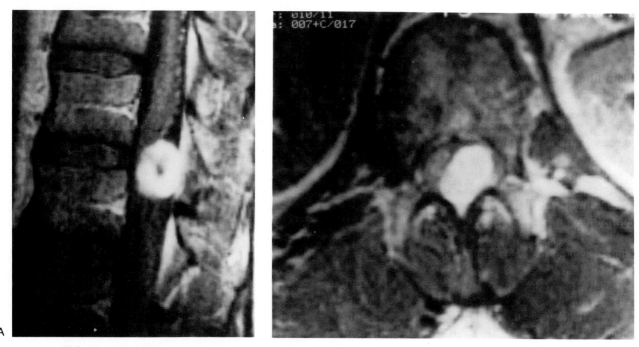

FIG. 15. A,B: MRI scans enhanced with gadolinium will more clearly define intradural extra-axial lesions. In this case, a small discrete neurofibroma is clearly depicted. The spinal cord can be seen. The gadolinium enhancement clearly defines the lesion.

are variably hyperintense and rarely hypointense (Fig. 14). Hypointensity on T2-weighted imaging is more suggestive of meningioma. The neurofibromas and meningiomas do not tend to incite the edema in the spinal cord that is seen with intramedullary lesions. Hence, the spinal cord does not show the increased signal intensity on T2-weighted imaging that occurs with intramedullary lesions. Gadolinium enhancement of neurofibromas can be homogeneous or heterogeneous. Meningiomas are more likely to enhance homogeneously. Enhancement only on the periphery, even when the tumor is noncystic, is strongly suggestive of neurofibroma (Fig. 15). Cystic cavitation of these tumors is more common in the spine than in the brain. On T1-weighted imaging, the cyst is generally hypointense, with signal almost as low as that of CSF; signal intensity increases on T2-weighted imaging almost to the degree of CSF again. Sometimes a central hypointense region can be seen on T2-weighted sequences that is thought to correspond histologically to the dense fibrous component of the tumor.

Meningiomas are particularly common in the thoracic spine. They are well circumscribed, discrete, and very isointense with the spinal cord. The most consistent distinguishing characteristic between meningiomas and neurofibromas is the tendency for meningiomas to remain isointense or even become hypointense on T2-weighted imaging. Furthermore, they can be surprisingly bright on proton density sequences as compared with the spinal cord, and this finding also suggests meningioma. Meningiomas tend to enhance intensely and homogeneously, and supposedly earlier in the administration of contrast media or dynamic imaging. Meningiomas usually do not incite the bony changes that can be seen with their intracranial counterparts. Calcium deposits are infrequently seen within the tumor, again in contrast to meningiomas in the brain.

Paragangliomas are another uncommon intradural tumor, which generally occur in the cauda equina but are also reported in the thoracic spine. They also have very prominent vessels and may have cystic components. As is true with intradural tumors, they tend to be isointense on T1-weighted imaging and slightly hyperintense on T2-weighted imaging. They enhance prominently and serpiginous flow voids may be seen, making these lesions difficult to distinguish from hemangioblastomas or myxopapillary ependymomas.

Epidermoid tumors are generally well-circumscribed lesions. They are homogeneous and isointense to CSF on T1-weighted imaging sequences; on T2-weighted imaging, they can again be isointense to CSF. This is a very distinguishing characteristic, and except for occasional confusion with arachnoid cysts, these tumors can be strongly predicted histologically by MRI. Generally the epidermoids do not enhance, but a thin rim of enhancement can sometimes be appreciated.

Intradural lipomas also have characteristic imaging patterns. On T1-weighted imaging they are very bright, and on T2-weighted imaging the signal fades. This is typical of any fatty deposit on MRI. The bright T1-weighted signal is the indicator that this is fat, although subacute hemorrhage must be considered. Certainly, if there are changes in the soft tissues suggestive of spinal dysraphism, one can be confident that the lesion is a benign lipoma.

Surgical Technique

For lesions that are confined to the spinal canal, a routine midline approach and laminectomy are preferred. The dura is opened in the midline to an extent that the most superior and inferior aspects of the tumor can easily be seen. We prefer to use a microscope for all of these lesions. Once the dura is open, care is taken to place large cotton balls above and below the lesion to obliterate the large subarachnoid space that surrounds the spinal cord. This effectively prevents blood from tracking up or down the spinal column in the subarachnoid space. Frequently, once the dura is open, the neurofibroma is immediately visualized in a dorsolateral position. The lesions are always well encapsulated and there is little, if any, associated scarring. Microsurgical technique usually allows quick and precise mobilization of the capsule from the adjacent spinal cord (Fig. 16). The surgeon is occasionally tempted to remove a neurofibroma in one piece. However, this is usually not practical and should never be done if spinal cord retraction is required to deliver the lesion. Instead, the capsule should be coagulated and incised and its contents removed with either a curette or cavitron. If the neurofibroma originates from a sensory radical, we prefer to take the root with the lesion (Fig. 17). This is based on the histologic knowledge of these lesions, in which the fibers of the root are splayed and widely distributed throughout the substance of the lesion. Fortunately, there is little appreciable deficit in sacrificing the root (20). It has been hypothesized that growth of the lesion and gradual disruption of that nerve root may allow function to be transferred to adjacent roots. An occasional large, ventrally situated lesion will pose more of a technical challenge. Adjoining uninvolved nerve roots may be draped over the lesion, as they exist in a dorsolaterally displaced spinal cord. Again, when confronted with this situation, one must gut the lesion to the point of nearly complete intracapsular removal. We have always found that in virgin lesions, the capsule is then separable from the normal neural elements.

The large dumbbell lesion merits special consideration. When approached via laminectomy, it frequently cannot be removed completely (Fig. 17). Attempting to follow it out the foramen without adequate visualization can result in unnecessary disruption of a penetrating seg-

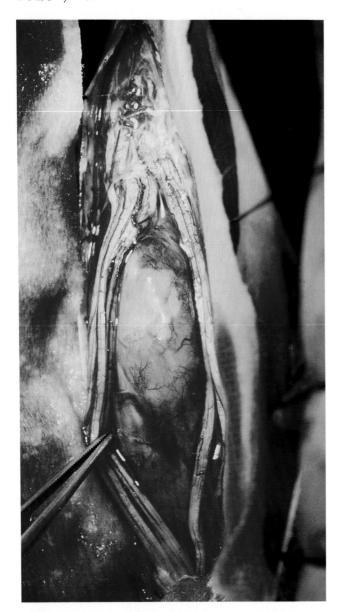

FIG. 16. Conus medullaris/cauda equina tumor. These can be ependymomas or neurofibromas, or even on occasion hemangiomas or other lesions. Removal without increasing deficit is a reasonable goal. This is a neurofibroma.

mental vessel. Obviously, a facet joint must be sacrificed to afford wider lateral visualization of the lesion, providing the midline skin incision is long enough. This sometimes allows the surgeon to circumscribe the lesion. In the thoracic spine, this is well tolerated, but in the cervical or lumbar spine, the resultant destabilization may necessitate fusion. Most frequently, when we cannot remove a lesion from the midline approach, we mark the lateral boundary of the surgical resection with gelfoam or a patch of freeze-dried dura. Because patients are usually operated on for myelopathy, removal of the portion of tumor within the spinal canal results in adequate resolution of the spinal cord compression, and symptoms resolve. The patient can then be followed with serial MRI.

If, however, the remaining extradural tumor is felt to cause symptoms, it can be excised in a second procedure through a more lateral or anterior approach. The patch of freeze-dried dura serves as a marker for the medial extent of the resection. Over time, these lesions do not appear to erode through the dural substitute, although they will stretch it medially if their regrowth begins to encroach again on the canal. It is noteworthy that in the past, some authors have recommended marking the borders of the surgical resection with Weck clips, which are metallic. Given the current trend to use MRI to follow these lesions, we have chosen to avoid this practice.

The meningioma is approached in a similar fashion. Defining the rostral and caudal extents of the lesion is the

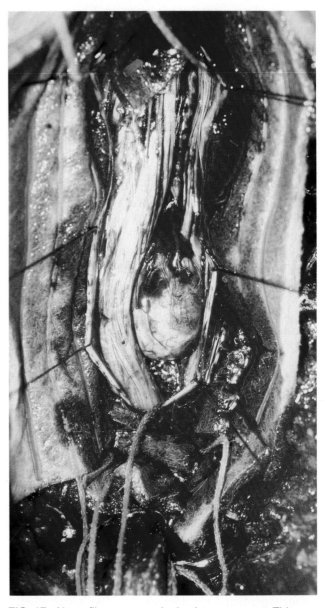

FIG. 17. Neurofibroma on major lumbar nerve root. This was both intramedullary in the neural foramen and extended down the nerve root. These tumors can be removed with a very good prognosis.

first and simplest task. A meningioma that is adherent to the spinal cord may not be as easily dissected as a neurofibroma. The cavitron can prove very helpful in removing the dorsal or lateral aspect of the tumor from the vertebral structures before addressing the tumor-spinal cord interface. This will allow some room to retract the tumor gently rather than the spinal cord when developing the proper plane of dissection. These tumors are invariably removed in a piecemeal fashion; hence meticulous attention must be paid to the margins if one is to achieve a complete resection.

Prognosis

It is generally felt that complete excision of a neurofibroma or meningioma is curative, although there are few published data to confirm this belief. Similarly, angiomas and dermoids are not expected to recur if they are completely resected. There is always concern in approaching a dermoid or epidermoid that if the capsule is violated and its contents spilled, the lesion will recur (1). Re-exploration for these lesions is certainly only palliative. However, recent data have suggested that the long-term prognosis for incompletely resected lesions may be quite good (25). The behavior of sarcomas, on the other hand, is no less aggressive in this location than in any other, and adjunctive therapy is recommended.

REFERENCES

1. Baily IC (1970): Dermoid tumors of the spinal cord. *J Neurosurg* 33:676–681.
2. Brotchi J, Desvitte O, Levivier M, et al. (1991): A survey of 65 tumors within the spinal cord: Surgical results and importance of preoperative magnetic resonance imaging. *Neurosurgery* 29:651–657.
3. Chigasaki H, Pennybacker JB (1968): A long follow-up study of 128 cases of intramedullary spinal cord tumours. *Neurol Med Chir (Tokyo)* 10:25–66.
4. Ciapetta P, Salvati M, Capoccia G, et al. (1991): Spinal glioblastomas: Report of seven cases and review of the literature. *Neurosurgery* 28:302–306.
5. Cohen AR, Wisoff JH, Allen JC, Epstein F (1989): Malignant astrocytomas of the spinal cord. *J Neurosurg* 70:50–54.
6. Cooper PR (1989): Outcome after operative treatment of intramedullary spinal cord tumors in adults: Intermediate and long-term results in 51 patients. *Neurosurgery* 25:855–859.
7. Cristante L, Herrmann HS (1994): Surgical management of intramedullary spinal cord tumors: Functional outcome and sources of morbidity. *Neurosurgery* 35:69–76.
8. Elsberg CA (1916): *Diagnosis and treatment of surgical diseases of the spinal cord and its membranes.* Philadelphia: W.B. Saunders.
9. Enzmann DR, O'Donohue J, Rubin JB, et al. (1987): CSF pulsations within non-neoplastic spinal cord cysts. *AJR* 149:149–157.
10. Epstein FJ, Farmer JP, Freed D (1992): Adult intramedullary astrocytomas of the spinal cord. *J Neurosurg* 77:355–359.
11. Garrido E, Stein BM (1977): Microsurgical removal of intramedullary spinal cord tumors. *Surg Neurol* 7:215–219.
12. Gowers WR, Horsley V (1888): A case of tumour of the spinal cord: Removal, recovery. *Med-Chir Trans (London)* 71:377–430.
13. Greenwood J Jr (1963): Intramedullary tumors of the spinal cord.
A follow-up study after total surgical removal. *J Neurosurg* 20:665–668.
14. Greenwood J Jr (1954): Total removal of intramedullary tumors. *J Neurosurg* 11:616–621.
15. Guidetti B, Fortuna A (1967): Surgical treatment of intramedullary hemangioblastoma of the spinal cord. Report of six cases. *J Neurosurg* 27:530–540.
16. Guidetti B, Mercuri S, Vagnozzi R (1981): Long-term results of the surgical treatment of 129 intramedullary spinal gliomas. *J Neurosurg* 54:323–330.
17. Hardison HH, Packer RJ, Rorke LB, Schut L, Sutton LN (1987): Outcome of children with primary intramedullary spinal cord tumors. *Childs Nerv Syst* 3:89–92.
18. Herrmann HS, Neuss M, Winkler D (1988): Intramedullary spinal cord tumors resected with CO2 laser microsurgical technique: Recent experience: Fifteen patients. *Neurosurgery* 22:518–522.
19. Kernohan JW, Sayre GP (1952): *Tumors of the central nervous system. Fascicle 35.* Washington, DC: Armed Forces Institute of Pathology, pp. 1–129.
20. Kim P, Ebersold MJ, Onofrio BM, Quast LM (1989): Surgery of spinal nerve schwannoma. Risk of neurological deficit after resection of involved root. *J Neurosurg* 71:810–814.
21. Kurland LT (1958): The frequency of intracranial and intraspinal neoplasms in the resident population of Rochester, Minnesota. *J Neurosurg* 15:627–641.
22. Levine E, Huntrakoon M, Wetzel LH (1987): Malignant nerve-sheath neoplasms in neurofibromatosis: Distinction from benign tumors by using imaging techniques. *AJR* 149:1059–1064.
23. Lindstadt DE, Wara WM, Leibel SA, et al. (1989): Post-operative radiotherapy of primary spinal cord tumors. *Int J Radiat Oncol Biol Phys* 20:781–786.
24. Long DM (1983): Cervical cord tumors. In: Baily RW, ed. *The cervical spine* (The Cervical Spine Research Society). Philadelphia: J.B. Lippincott, pp. 323–335.
25. Lunardi P, Missori P, Gagliardi FM, Fortuna A (1989): Long-term results of the surgical treatment of spinal dermoid and epidermoid tumors. *Neurosurgery* 25:860–864.
26. Malis LI (1978): Intramedullary spinal cord tumors. *Clin Neurosurg* 25:512–539.
27. McCormick PC, Torres R, Post KD, Stein BM (1990): Intramedullary ependymoma of the spinal cord. *J Neurosurg* 72:523–532.
28. Nittner K (1976): Spinal meningiomas, neurinomas and neurofibromas-hourglass tumors. In: Vinken PJ, Bruyn GW, eds. *Handbook of clinical neurology,* Vol. 20. New York: Elsevier, pp. 177–322.
29. Pool JL (1970): The surgery of spinal cord tumors. *Clin Neurosurg* 17:310–330.
30. Post JM, Quencer RM, Green BA, et al. (1987): Intramedullary spinal cord metastases, mainly of non-neurogenic origin. *AJR* 148:1015–1022.
31. Russell DS, Rubinstein LJ (1977): *Pathology of tumours of the nervous system.* London: E.A. Pall.
32. Shapiro R (1984): Tumors. In: Shapiro R, ed. *Myelography.* Chicago: Yearbook Medical Publishers, pp. 345–421.
33. Simeone FA, Lawner PM (1982): Intraspinal neoplasms. In: Rothman RH, Simeone FA, eds. *The spine.* Philadelphia: W.B. Saunders, pp. 1041–1054.
34. Slooff JL, Kernohan JW, MacCarty CS (1964): *Primary intramedullary tumors of the spinal cord and filum terminale.* Philadelphia: W.B. Saunders.
35. Van Gilder JC, Schwartz HG (1967): Growth of dermoids from skin implants to the nervous system and surrounding spaces of the newborn rat. *J Neurosurg* 26:14–20.
36. Wen B-C, Hussey DH, Hitchon WP, et al. (1991): The role of radiation therapy in the management of ependymomas of the spinal cord. *Int J Radiat Oncol Biol Phys* 20:781–786.
37. Whitaker SJ, Bensell EM, Ashley SE, et al. (1991): Postoperative radiotherapy in the management of spinal cord ependymoma. *J Neurosurg* 74:720–728.
38. Yasargil MG, Antic J, Laciga R, DePreux J, Fideler RW, Boone SC (1976): The microsurgical removal of intramedullary spinal hemangioblastomas: Report of twelve cases and a review of the literature. *Surg Neurol* 3:141–148.
39. Yasargil MG (1970): Surgery of vascular lesions of the spinal cord with the microsurgical technique. *Clin Neurosurg* 17:257–265.

The Adult Spine: Principles and Practice,
2nd edition, J.W. Frymoyer, Editor-in-Chief.
Lippincott-Raven Publishers, Philadelphia © 1997.

CHAPTER 51

Vascular Anomalies of the Spinal Cord

David Rothbart, Gregory R. Criscuolo, and Donlin M. Long

Since Gaupp's (39) original description of a spinal arteriovenous malformation (AVM), much has been learned about this heterogeneous group of vascular anomalies. Technical advances such as selective spinal arteriography (3,22,23,29,31,54,64,79) and microvascular Doppler ultrasonography (40,47) have allowed the classification of spinal AVMs to evolve into one that is based upon both anatomic and pathophysiologic detail. It is now recognized that the vast majority of these lesions are dural arteriovenous (AV) fistulas. Clinical awareness of these lesions is important because they frequently cause myelopathy that is potentially reversible. Appropriate therapy is directed by establishing an accurate diagnosis and by understanding the pathophysiologic mechanisms

at play in a particular type of lesion. Evaluation has been enhanced by neuroradiologic advances in computed tomography (CT) scanning, magnetic resonance imaging (MRI), and selective spinal arteriography. Treatment options include endovascular obliteration with cyanoacrylate glue or latex balloons and surgical resection. Improved outcome relates to a more precise definition of pathophysiologic mechanisms (19,40,47,88), the introduction and advancement of microneurosurgical methodology (67,78,94,107,108), the refinement of interventional neuroradiologic technique, and the availability of agents that can permanently occlude AVM vessels.

HISTORIC PERSPECTIVE

Gaupp (39) is credited with the first documentation of a spinal AVM in his report of "hemorrhoids of the pia mater" in 1888. The first description of a dural arteriovenous fistula was by Brasch (14) in 1900. Although Krause (57) described the first surgical exposure of a spinal AVM in 1910, the patient's outcome was poor. The

  D. Rothbart, M.D. Clinical Assistant Professor; G. R. Criscuolo, M.D., Assistant Professor: Division of Neurosurgery, Yale University School of Medicine, New Haven, Connecticut, 06510.
  D. M. Long, M.D., Ph.D.: Professor and Director, Department of Neurosurgery, Johns Hopkins Medical Institutions, Baltimore, Maryland, 21205.

first successful operation for "enlarged varicose veins of the spinal cord" was performed by Charles Elsberg (35) in 1914. At surgery, he ligated and resected an engorged posterior spinal vein adjacent to the eighth thoracic spinal nerve as it penetrated the dura. His patient's paraparesis and sensory deficit completely resolved after the procedure. In 1925, Sargent (90) reviewed the cases of 21 previously reported spinal AVMs and concluded that the majority of these lesions were venous in origin. The first myelographic description of a spinal AVM was by Perthes (81) in 1926. In the same year, Foix and Alajouanine (37) described the syndrome of "subacute necrotic myelopathy" with paraplegia evolving in a progressive fashion and resulting in death. Lhermitte et al. (63), in 1931, recognized the association of this process with an AVM of the spinal cord. Later, Wyburn-Mason (105) and Flament et al. (36) reaffirmed the association between rapidly progressive myelopathy, vascular thrombosis, and abnormal spinal cord vasculature. Pia and Vogelsang (82) concluded that Foix-Alajouanine disease was not a distinct entity but a complication of spinal AVMs that was caused by thrombosis within the abnormal vessels of the spinal cord. In 1970, Wirth et al. (103) agreed with this view of the pathophysiology of this syndrome and first described a patient in whom chronic clinical deterioration was correlated with these intraoperative findings of an extensively thrombosed AVM and spinal cord atrophy. They discouraged surgical intervention in these patients because they felt this to be an end-stage, irreversible process from which neurologic improvement could not be expected. A recent reconsideration of the pathogenetic mechanisms at play in patients with dural AV fistulas who present with the Foix-Alajouanine syndrome has suggested that the progressive myelopathy in these cases may be caused by venous congestion and not necessarily by thrombosis. This conclusion was based upon five patients who presented in this manner and subsequently improved after embolic and surgical intervention. Therefore, recognition of this clinical entity and aggressive surgical therapy are extremely important because what appears to be irreversible cord injury can potentially be improved (19,77). The MRI appearance and intraoperative findings in a patient with Foix-Alajouanine syndrome have been reported recently (83).

In the 1960s and 1970s, DiChiro et al. (23,24), Doppman (31,34), Ommaya et al. (79), Djindjian (28–30), Kendall and Logue (54), Logue (3–5,64), and others (58,65,103,107) advanced the technique of selective spinal arteriography, which aided in the understanding of AVM pathophysiology. This insight allowed a classification scheme based upon vascular anatomy, location, and flow pattern. The modern era of treatment of spinal AVMs began with the introduction of microneurosurgical methodology (64,67,78,94,107,108). The first embolization of a spinal dural arteriovenous fistula (AVF) was performed by Doppman, in which he introduced 3-mm stainless-steel pellets into the feeding artery of the lesion. Since then, interventional neuroradiologic techniques and materials have been tremendously refined and have become a major component of the therapeutic approach to spinal vascular malformations. Hassler et al. (47) and Giller et al. (40) reported results from studies using intraoperative microvascular Doppler ultrasonography to document the hemodynamics in dural AVFs, which served to reaffirm the validity of these theories.

NORMAL SPINAL VASCULAR ANATOMY

The arterial circulation of the spinal cord is derived primarily from branches of the vertebral arteries and multiple radicular arteries arising from segmental vessels at various levels (i.e., ascending and deep cervical, intercostal, lumbar, and sacral arteries). The vertebral arteries give rise to the upper segments of the anterior spinal artery and contribute to the paired posterior spinal arteries. The anterior spinal artery descends in a midline course from the foramen magnum to the filum terminale, narrowing significantly in the midthoracic region. It gives rise to sulcal branches that perfuse the anterior two-thirds of the spinal cord, including the anterior horns and the spinothalamic and corticospinal tracts. The paired posterior spinal arteries traverse the spinal cord medial to the dorsal roots. These vessels form two plexiform channels on the posterolateral spinal cord surface that supply the posterior third of the cord, including the posterior columns and, to a lesser extent, the corticospinal tracts. At the level of the conus medullaris, there is a constant anastomotic loop uniting the distal anterior spinal and the two posterior spinal arteries to form the cruciate anastomosis (41,60,66,97).

The anterior spinal artery and the two posterior spinal arteries are dependent upon anastomoses along their lengths with branches from the spinal arteries. At each segmental level, these spinal arteries arise as dorsal rami from the vertebral, subclavian, or thoracic and lumbar intercostal arteries. After entering the intervertebral foramina at each level, the spinal artery penetrates the outer surface of the dura and divides, thus giving rise to: (a) a dural artery, which supplies the nerve root sleeve and spinal dura; and (b) a radicular artery, which penetrates the subarachnoid space to supply the anterior and posterior nerve roots. In addition, with moderate variability, a spinal artery will give rise to (c) a medullary artery, which, upon entering the subarachnoid space, will join an anterior or posterior spinal artery. In the developing fetus, these medullary arteries anastomose with the anterior and posterior spinal arteries at each segmental level. The majority of these vessels will regress by 6 months' gestation. Hence, the total number of medullary arteries contributing to the anterior spinal artery is commonly between six and ten. The artery of Adamkiewicz

(arteria radicularis magna) is the principal medullary artery providing blood supply to the lower half of the spinal cord. It originates from an intercostal artery between T9 and T12 in 75% of cases, but may range from T5 to L4. In 80% of cases, it is found on the left side. Portions of the thoracic and upper lumbar spinal cord are extremely vulnerable to ischemic compromise, as there is minimal collateral supply to the spinal cord between the junction of the artery of Adamkiewicz and the anterior spinal artery.

The venous drainage pattern of the spinal cord closely parallels that of the spinal arteries. The definitive description of the anatomic detail of the spinal venous system was provided by Gillian in 1970 (42). He stressed the significance of two principal sets of intrinsic radial draining veins. A central group provides venous return from the anterior horns and surrounding white matter. These, in turn, drain into the central veins in the anterior median fissure that ultimately form the anterior median spinal vein. The second group is a discrete collection of small valveless radial veins that originate from a capillary plexus and drain the peripheral dorsal and lateral cord tissue through centrifugal flow. These vessels empty into

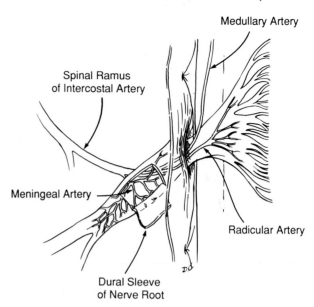

FIG. 2. Normal branching of spinal intercostal arteries. The vessel enters the dura adjacent to the nerve root ganglion, after which it ascends and joins an anterior or posterolateral spinal artery to supply the cord parenchyma. [Reprinted from Criscuolo and Rothbart (20), with permission.]

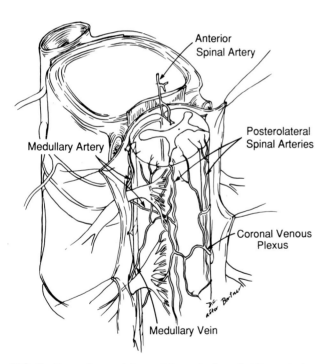

FIG. 1. Normal vasculature of the spinal cord. After entering the intervertebral foramina at each level, the spinal artery penetrates the outer surface of the dura and divides, thus giving rise to: (a) a dural artery, which supplies the nerve root sleeve and spinal dura; and (b) a radicular artery, which penetrates into the subarachnoid space to supply the anterior and posterior nerve roots. In addition, with moderate variability, a spinal artery will give rise to (c) a medullary artery, which, upon entering the subarachnoid space, will join an anterior or posterior spinal artery. [Reprinted from Criscuolo and Rothbart (20), with permission.]

the coronal venous plexus, a plexiform network of valveless interconnecting vessels on the cord surface. Venous blood passes from the intradural coronal plexus to the epidural venous plexus of Batson through spinal medullary veins. These medullary veins pierce the dura adjacent to, but distinct from, the dural penetration of the nerve roots. Despite the lack of functional anatomic valves at each segmental level, there remains some segregation of the epidural from intradural venous systems because of a normally occurring constriction in the vein at its dural transition, which prevents reflux into the medullary venous system. The epidural venous plexus ultimately communicates with the superior and inferior cavae, azygos and hemiazygos veins, as well as the cerebral veins and dural venous sinuses (Figs. 1 and 2).

CLASSIFICATION OF SPINAL VASCULAR ANOMALIES

The initial categorization of spinal AVMs was predicated upon pathologic descriptions (35–37). Sargent (90) originally proposed a venous origin for the majority of AVMs. However, in 1943, Wyburn-Mason's (105) landmark series of 110 patients identified two predominant types of spinal vascular anomalies: arteriovenous angiomas, which occurred in 32%, and purely venous angiomas, which affected 68%. Thus, the early histologic investigations of spinal cord AVMs indicated that most had predominantly venous elements, which most commonly involved the dorsal surface of the spinal cord.

TABLE 1. *Classification of spinal arteriovenous malformations*

A. Dural arteriovenous fistulas (Type I)
B. Intradural arteriovenous malformation
   1. Glomus AVMs (Type II)
   2. Juvenile AVMs (Type III)
   3. Direct perimedullary arteriovenous fistulas (Type IV)

DiChiro and associates' (23) introduction of selective spinal arteriography in the mid-1960s provided impetus for the evolution of the classification of spinal AVMs into one based upon the vascular anatomy, location, and direction of blood flow. This led to the identification of three varieties: single coiled vessel (Type I spinal AVM), glomus (Type II spinal AVM), and juvenile (Type III spinal AVM). In 1977, Kendall and Logue (54) reported a series of nine patients in whom the site of the AV fistula was on or adjacent to the dural sleeve of the proximal portion of a spinal root. Despite the associated congestion and tortuosity of the coronal venous plexus on the dorsal cord surface (the "single coiled vessels"), these patients improved neurologically after excision of the nidus of the dural AV fistula. Therefore, the previously described "single coiled vessel" and "venous angiomas on the cord surface" are actually constituents of the normal venous drainage of the spinal cord that have undergone arterialization secondary to the reception of blood from the dural AV fistula (76–78,94,106).

Present insight into the anatomic and pathophysiologic characteristics of spinal AVMs has impelled the evolution of a four-category system, which includes one dural and three intradural types (Table 1).

Dural Arteriovenous Fistulas (Type I)

Original nomenclature such as *angioma racemosum venosum, single coiled vessel malformation, malformation retromedullaire,* and *long dorsal arteriovenous malformation* reflect the previously held belief that the nidus of these spinal AVMs was the engorged coronal venous plexus. Since the elucidation of the actual site of the nidus within the nerve root sleeve dura, the appropriately descriptive term *dural arteriovenous fistula* has been adopted.

Dural AV fistulas account for 80% to 85% of spinal AVMs. The dural branch of the spinal ramus of an intercostal or lumbar artery supplies one, or, rarely, more than one, feeding vessel to the dural AV fistula (Fig. 3). This malformation is almost invariably located in the lower thoracic or lumbar region. Selective spinal arteriography reveals the nidus of the fistula within the intervertebral foramen and the adjacent lateral aspect of the

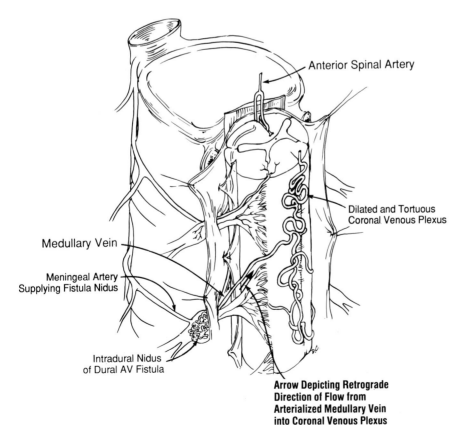

Anterior Spinal Artery

Dilated and Tortuous Coronal Venous Plexus

Medullary Vein

Meningeal Artery Supplying Fistula Nidus

Intradural Nidus of Dural AV Fistula

Arrow Depicting Retrograde Direction of Flow from Arterialized Medullary Vein into Coronal Venous Plexus

FIG. 3. The dural AV fistula (Type I spinal AVM) is supplied by a dural artery and is drained by a medullary vein, which carries blood retrograde to the normal direction of venous drainage to the coronal venous plexus. The coronal venous plexus becomes elongated, tortuous, thickened, and dilated by the increased venous pressure, which is in turn transmitted to the cord tissue and causes myelopathy. [Reprinted from Criscuolo and Rothbart (20), with permission.]

spinal canal. Medullary veins drain the fistula in a retrograde manner into the dilated, tortuous coronal venous plexus on the dorsal pial surface of the spinal cord. Characteristically, these are low-flow lesions that induce increased pressure in the arterialized venous system.

Approximately 15% of patients with a spinal dural AV fistula will present with an acute or subacute progression of myelopathy without evidence of hemorrhage (Foix-Alajouanine syndrome). Unless prompt therapeutic intervention is initiated, progression to irreversible paraplegia or quadriplegia is inevitable (20,36,37,103).

Intradural Arteriovenous Malformations

This group represents 10% to 15% of spinal AVMs and includes the glomus AVMs (Type II spinal AVM), juvenile AVMs (Type III spinal AVM), and direct spinal AV fistulas (Type IV spinal AVM). Various characteristics distinguish these lesions from the dural AV fistulas.

The glomus AVM involves the substance of the spinal cord (Fig. 4) and is distributed equally along the entire longitudinal axis of the spinal cord. The blood supply is derived from medullary arteries and is usually situated in an anterior, intramedullary location. The nidus is a tightly coiled mass of blood vessels confined to a short segment of the spinal cord. Outflow is orthograde into a dilated coronal venous plexus. These arterialized vessels differ from those of a dural AV fistula in that they are typically far more complex and engorged. Apoplectic deterioration commonly occurs secondary to subarachnoid or intramedullary hemorrhage (88).

The juvenile AVM is analogous to the intracranial AVMs, with multiple vessels feeding a capacious nidus. The blood supply derives from medullary arteries originating from the anterior and posterior spinal arteries (Fig. 5). The nidus is large, sometimes involving several vertebral segments, the subdural and epidural space, and the adjacent soft tissues and bone. At times, a spinal bruit may be auscultated. These patients can present with hemorrhage or progressive neurologic decline.

Finally, the direct perimedullary AV fistula (Fig. 6) is an intradural perimedullary lesion that represents a direct connection between the intrinsic blood supply to the spinal cord (usually the anterior spinal artery) and a draining spinal vein (spinal medullary vein or coronal plexus). Consequently, these lesions induce aneurysmal dilatation of the venous system without any intervening small vessel network. Initially described by Djindjian et al. in 1977 (27), they were later added to the classification scheme by Heros et al. (48) as Type IV lesions. Although they may be located throughout the spinal cord, they are most often found at the level of the conus medullaris (6). Onset of symptomatology is usually insidious and the clinical course tends to be progressive, although subarachnoid hemorrhage may occur.

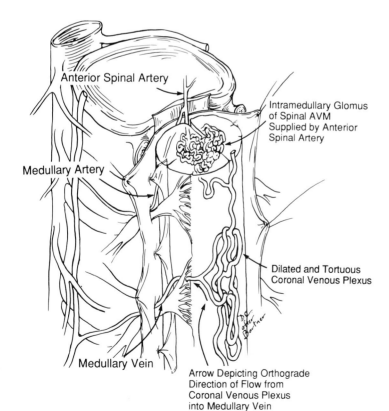

Anterior Spinal Artery

Intramedullary Glomus of Spinal AVM Supplied by Anterior Spinal Artery

Medullary Artery

Dilated and Tortuous Coronal Venous Plexus

Medullary Vein

Arrow Depicting Orthograde Direction of Flow from Coronal Venous Plexus into Medullary Vein

FIG. 4. The nidus of a glomus AVM (Type II spinal AVM) is a tightly packed, localized collection of abnormal blood vessels that receives its supply from a single medullary artery. Venous drainage is orthograde. [Reprinted from Criscuolo and Rothbart (20), with permission.]

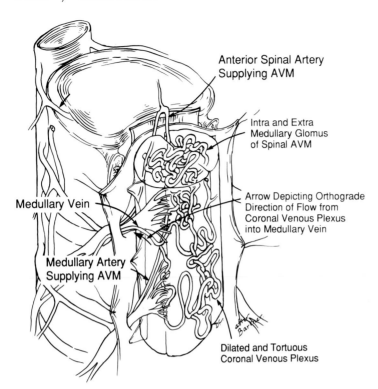

Anterior Spinal Artery
Supplying AVM

Intra and Extra
Medullary Glomus
of Spinal AVM

Medullary Vein

Arrow Depicting Orthograde
Direction of Flow from
Coronal Venous Plexus
into Medullary Vein

Medullary Artery
Supplying AVM

Dilated and Tortuous
Coronal Venous Plexus

FIG. 5. The juvenile type of intramedullary AVM (Type III spinal AVM) is supplied by multiple medullary arteries. The nidus is large, often fills the spinal canal at involved levels, and contains neural parenchyma within the nidus of the AVM. Venous drainage is orthograde. [Reprinted from Criscuolo and Rothbart (20), with permission.]

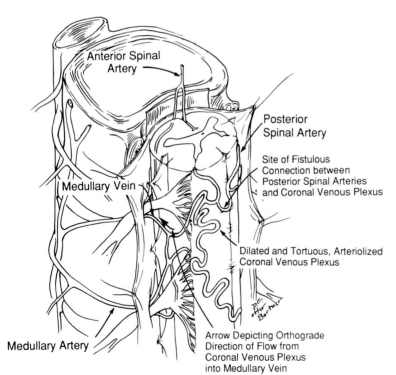

Anterior Spinal
Artery

Posterior
Spinal Artery

Site of Fistulous
Connection between
Posterior Spinal Arteries
and Coronal Venous Plexus

Medullary Vein

Dilated and Tortuous, Arteriolized
Coronal Venous Plexus

Medullary Artery

Arrow Depicting Orthograde
Direction of Flow from
Coronal Venous Plexus
into Medullary Vein

FIG. 6. A direct perimedullary AV fistula (Type IV spinal AVM) located on the pial surface and fed by a medullary artery. Venous drainage is orthograde. [Reprinted from Criscuolo and Rothbart (20), with permission.]

CLINICAL FEATURES OF SPINAL ARTERIOVENOUS MALFORMATIONS

Case Reports

Case 1

A 43-year-old male was admitted to the Johns Hopkins Hospital with a 2-year history of progressively worsening distal paresthesias in the lower extremities and weakness and atrophy in both calves. He initially developed a limp, which subsequently progressed to a paraparesis. The numbness and paresthesias were worse on the right side, where they extended from the knee into the lateral calf and foot. The patient denied any pain or changes in bowel and bladder function. Motor examination revealed bilateral 4/5 weakness in the gluteal, psoas, hamstring, quadriceps, gastrocnemius, invertor and evertor muscle groups; right-sided 3+/5 plantar and dorsiflexor weakness; and 0/5 weakness in the right extensor hallucis longus. Mild atrophy was evident throughout the lower extremities. Sensory examination demonstrated decreased pinprick, light touch, temperature, and vibration sense along the right lateral calf, dorsum of the right foot, and extending over the great toe. Deep tendon reflexes were diminished on the right knee and ankle, but tone was normal. Plantar reflexes were flexor bilaterally. The patient was unable to perform tandem walk, and his gait had a mildly widened base with a list to the right. He was unable to walk on his toes but could perform this task on his heels. Proprioception was impaired bilaterally, and consequently he exhibited a positive Rhomberg sign. Sphincter tone and abdominal and cremasteric reflexes were normal. There was no evidence of a hemangioma or paraspinal bruit. Diagnostic evaluation included a lumbar CT/myelogram, which was unremarkable. MRI revealed widening of the conus medullaris, increased signal intensity on T2-weighted images, and slight enhancement with gadolinium (Fig. 7). The MRI was repeated 2 months later and demonstrated no significant changes. The diagnosis at that time was felt to be an intramedullary tumor such as an ependymoma, and the patient underwent an exploratory laminectomy from T12 to L2. Intradural exposure revealed a tangled mass of engorged, tortuous blood vessels on the dorsal pial surface. Because there was no evidence of tumor or hemorrhage, it was elected to abort the procedure at that time.

Postoperatively, the patient was neurologically unchanged, and selective spinal arteriography was scheduled. This showed a laterally situated dural AV fistula nidus on the left side at the T6 level (Fig. 8). The malformation was embolized with bucrylate glue mixed with Pantopaque® and tantalum powder. The patient improved within several days after this procedure. How-

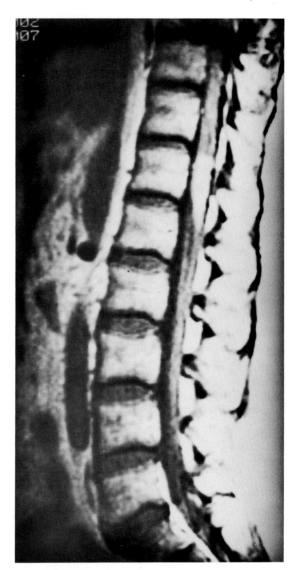

FIG. 7. MRI reveals increased signal intensity and widening on T2-weighted images in the lower thoracic spinal cord extending caudally to the conus medullaris. Minimal enhancement was observed on gadolinium studies. Note that the upper extent of the area of increased signal appears as a linear border or cut-off characteristic of vascular processes.

ever, a follow-up angiogram 3 months later revealed recanalization of the nidus and dorsal draining veins. The patient was clinically stable and underwent a T5-T8 laminectomy. A mass of arterialized, serpentine veins was noted at the T6 level, and the radiculomeningeal shunt vein had become intertwined with the sixth thoracic dorsal nerve root (Fig. 9). After coagulation and clipping of the shunt vessel, the coronal venous plexus shrank rapidly and, concomitantly, the color of its contents changed from red to blue. The patient's neurologic examination improved postoperatively, and a repeat angiogram before discharge failed to demonstrate any residual fistula or abnormal draining veins.

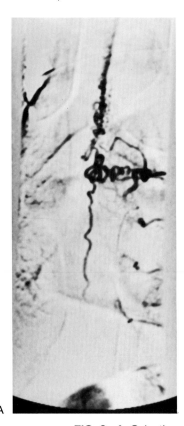

A

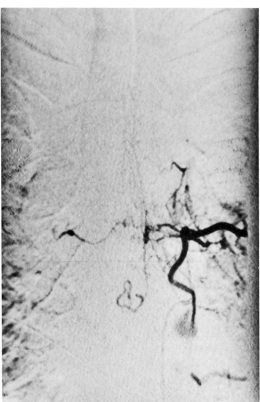

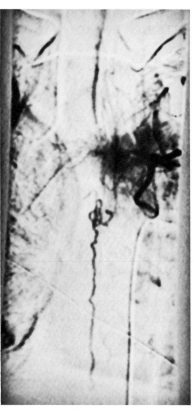

B,C

FIG. 8. A: Selective spinal arteriography of the patient in case 1 reveals the nidus in the intervertebral foramen of the sixth thoracic nerve root on the left. The engorged serpentine coronal venous plexus is well demonstrated. **B:** Complete obliteration of the fistula after embolization. **C:** A follow-up arteriogram 3 months post-embolization revealed recanalization of the nidus and dorsal draining veins.

Case 2

A 67-year-old male was admitted to Yale-New Haven Hospital with an 18-month history of progressive lower-extremity dysfunction beginning with progressive numbness, which had increased in severity and ascended to the abdominal region. In addition, he was experiencing increasingly severe weakness, which was more pronounced on the left side and had caused him to fall several times. He also complained of difficulty in maintaining his balance when closing his eyes while in the shower or when entering a dark or dimly illuminated room. Two months before admission, he began having difficulty initiating micturition. Pain was absent. Motor examination revealed bilateral weakness and spasticity, with the left leg exhibiting 3+/5 strength proximally and 4+/5 distally. The right leg was slightly stronger, at 4−/5. There was a marked decrease in his ability to perform rapid alternating movements in his toes bilaterally. Sensory examination demonstrated diminished pinprick below the level of T8 and decreased vibration and proprioception, with the left side being more affected than the right. Knee and ankle jerks were diminished, plantar reflexes were extensor, and unsustained clonus was present bilaterally. He walked with a spastic paraparetic gait

and exhibited a positive Rhomberg sign. MRI with gadolinium showed a prominent dorsal coronal venous plexus and increased signal intensity on T2-weighted images in the dorsal half of the spinal cord (Fig. 10). Myelography confirmed this finding by demonstrating serpentine filling defects in the dye column along the dorsal spinal cord surface (Fig. 11).

The patient was diagnosed as having a dural AV fistula and underwent selective spinal arteriography. This revealed the nidus to be located on the right side at the T11 level (Fig. 12). Obliteration of the fistula was accomplished with n-butyl-2-cyanoacrylate (NBCA). Within the first 24 hours after the procedure, the patient demonstrated remarkable improvement in his neurologic condition, with almost complete reversal of his myelopathy (20).

Clinical Features

Various characteristics help differentiate among the various spinal vascular malformations, as summarized in Table 2 (1–4,17,19,20,48,64,65,84,87,94). With dural AVMs, there is a strong male predilection (85%), whereas for intradural AVMs, the incidence is distrib-

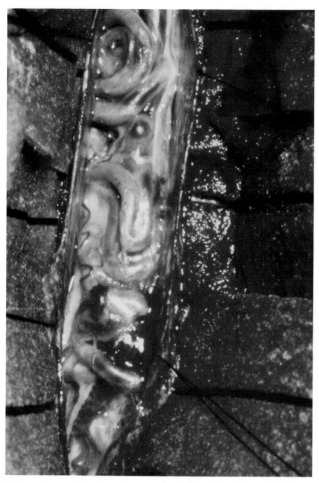

FIG. 9. Intraoperative photograph depicting extensive dilatation, elongation, and tortuosity of the coronal venous plexus.

uted more evenly between the sexes. Intradural AVMs tend to occur at a younger age. In the National Institutes of Health (NIH) series (88), the mean age of patients with symptoms from dural AV fistulas was 49 years, and only one patient was younger than 25. In contrast, 65% of patients with intradural AVMs were younger than 25 years of age, with a mean age of 27. Dural AV fistulas are thought to be acquired lesions because of their presentation in an older age range, their predominance in the lower half of the spine, and their lack of association with other vascular anomalies. The occurrence of intramedullary AVMs in both children and young adults, equal distribution among males and females, uniform distribution along the entire longitudinal axis of the spinal cord, and the 20% incidence of associated vascular anomalies (Table 3) support a congenital origin for these lesions. Further support for this tenet derives from a recent case report documenting the association of a chylous abnormality with an intradural AVM (56). Intramedullary AVMs are thought to be caused by dysvasculogenesis in embryonic development (77,78,87). These observations suggest that dural AV fistulas are probably acquired, whereas intramedullary AVMs are congenital in nature.

The initial clinical symptoms associated with spinal AVMs include paresis, pain, sensory abnormalities, and sphincter disturbances (4,62,64,78,88,94,99). The most common presenting symptom in patients with dural AV fistulas in the NIH series was paresis (44%) (88). Pain may be present in various forms. Paresthesias or hyperpathia in a radicular distribution is a common mode of presentation. In addition, pain may take the form of low back pain or neurogenic claudication. If subarachnoid hemorrhage occurs, then the typical triad of severe headache, photophobia, and meningism may be present. Sensory disturbances consist of numbness, hyperesthesia, dysesthesia, dissociated sensory loss, or decreased proprioception and vibration. Bowel, bladder, and sexual dysfunction are often accompanying symptoms.

Neurologic symptoms experienced by patients with dural fistulas may not be static and may manifest marked variability. Many patients note a specific inciting factor that exacerbates their symptoms. Dejerine (21) initially described an "intermittent claudication of the spinal cord." This condition is characteristic of dural AVMs and describes exercise-induced exacerbation of pain and paresis. Exercise or certain postures that temporarily induce systemic or venous hypertension exacerbated the symptoms in 42% to 70% of patients with a diagnosis of spinal dural AV fistula (87,94). Other reported aggravating factors are trauma, surgery, angiography, lumbar puncture, pregnancy, and menses (10,47,55,70,88, 94,102).

By the time a diagnosis of spinal AVM is ascertained, most patients have signs of sensory and motor deficits. Motor deficits affecting the upper extremities are more likely with intradural AVMs because of their incidence in the cervical spinal cord (88). Dural AVMs typically affect only the lower extremities. Findings include a combination of upper and lower motor neuron signs that may take the form of paraparesis, sciatica, or the cauda equina syndrome. Myelopathic signs such as hyperreflexia, spasticity, clonus, extensor plantar responses, and abnormal abdominal, anal, bulbocavernosus, and cremasteric reflexes are frequently present. Although a distinct sensory level can be elicited in most instances, no sensory findings may be appreciable or they may involve only a radicular distribution. Precise clinical localization may be difficult because of the propensity for venous hypertension to induce symptoms beyond the actual site of the fistula and occasionally quite remote from the nidus (80). Spinal bruits or cutaneous stigmata are extremely unusual findings, but, if present, will correspond to the metameric level of the malformation. Meningismus is indicative of subarachnoid hemorrhage, which occurs most frequently with the intramedullary lesions. Postural changes such as kyphosis, scoliosis, and lordosis,

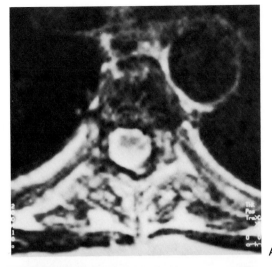

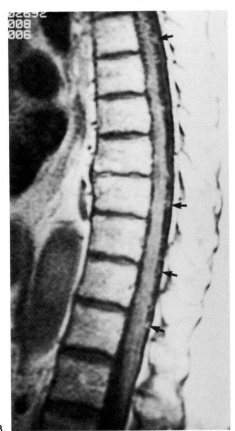

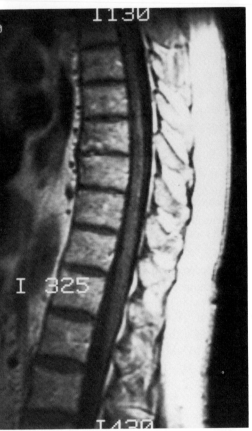

FIG. 10. MRI of the patient in case 2. **A:** Axial T2-weighted image demonstrates increased signal intensity in the dorsal half of the spinal cord. **B:** Sagittal image with gadolinium. Arrows indicate venous coils of dilated coronal venous plexus. **C:** Sagittal image with gadolinium 2 months after embolization, demonstrating absence of venous coils. (Reprinted from Criscuolo and Rothbart (20), with permission.]

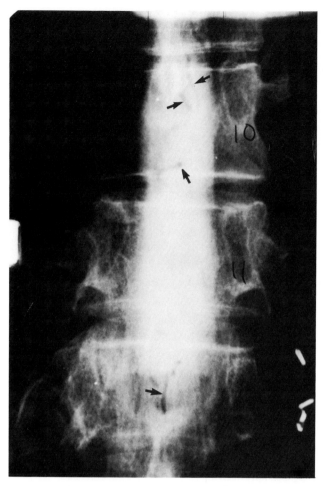

FIG. 11. Myelography imaged with the patient in the supine position revealed the characteristic serpentine filling defects (noted by arrows) in the dye column along the dorsal spinal cord surface. [Reprinted from Criscuolo and Rothbart (20), with permission.]

which are known to occur with other intraparenchymal lesions, may also be present.

The clinical progression of neurologic deterioration ranges from apoplectic to a chronic course. Sudden vascular catastrophes such as subarachnoid or intramedullary hemorrhage will lead to an apoplectic presentation. These events occur almost exclusively in the setting of intradural AVMs, in part because of the known association (44%) with aneurysms and varices. Subacute deterioration in the absence of hemorrhage (Foix-Alajouanine syndrome) is more likely with dural AVMs. This is due to venous congestion and stasis, resulting in spinal cord edema and progressive vascular thrombosis (19,20,36, 37,51,76,78,88,103). The most common course is one of gradual onset and chronic progression of neurologic deterioration. This is experienced by the vast majority of patients with dural AVMs and by many patients with intramedullary malformations. Factors contributing to this slowly evolving myelopathy include: (a) partially

compensated venous hypertension, (b) ischemia from vascular steal, or (c) dilatation of vascular structures leading to spinal cord compression. In a manner similar to that of demyelinating diseases, symptoms may worsen during a febrile illness (4). The interesting phenomenon of spinal myoclonus has been associated with these lesions. It may be induced by iodinated contrast dye, Valsalva maneuvers, or forced exhalation after a deep breath, or may occur spontaneously. The episodes consist of sudden, involuntary contractions of muscles innervated by a limited segment of the spinal cord. The most consistent therapeutic results in attempting to suppress spinal myoclonus have been achieved with serotonergic agents, including clonazepam and L-5-hydroxytryptophan in combination with carbidopa (2,62,91, 99,100).

In summary, distinguishing clinical features between dural AV fistulas and intradural spinal AVMs may help in the differential diagnosis. Intradural malformations should be suspected when a patient is less than 30 years old, with an acute onset of symptoms and the presence of subarachnoid hemorrhage or a spinal bruit, and with symptoms affecting the upper extremities. In contrast, patients with dural AVMs are usually older than 40 years, have an insidious onset and progressive worsening of symptoms, and experience exacerbation of symptoms with activity. The dural lesions are almost invariably located in the lower spinal cord segments and, therefore, typically affect only the lower extremities (88).

DIFFERENTIAL DIAGNOSIS

Because of the lack of pathognomonic symptoms and signs associated with spinal AVMs, the differential diagnosis is extremely important because the associated progressive myelopathy may be confused with other, more common, neurologic conditions. Spinal AVMs are quite rare; Table 4 outlines some of the more likely pathologic processes associated with myelopathy. Within this group, several conditions tend to create greater diagnostic dilemmas. Lumbar spondylosis is generally the initial diagnosis considered when a patient presents with a history of neurogenic claudication. Differentiation between these entities becomes even more confounded when pain is the major complaint and there are a paucity of long tract findings. However, urinary complaints and significant weakness tend to occur only late in the course of lumbar spondylosis and may provide an important diagnostic clue. In patients whose course is highlighted by remissions and exacerbations, the diagnosis of demyelinating disease may be entertained. Demographic differences may provide some guidance for the clinician. Spinal AVMs have a strong male predilection and tend to occur in an older age range. In addition, pain is not a usual accompaniment of demyelinating diseases. The of-

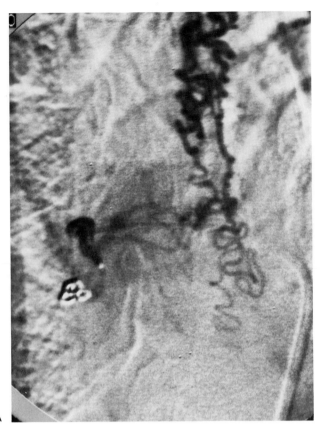
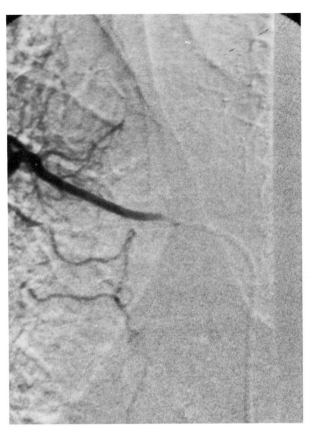

A   B

FIG. 12. A: Selective spinal arteriography demonstrates the nidus on the right at the T11 level. Note the prominent medullary vein and extensively transfigured coronal venous plexus, which is flowing retrograde in a primarily rostral direction. **B:** After injection of the distal intercostal artery and AV fistula nidus with an NBCA glue-tantalum suspension, anomalous retrograde flow from the AV fistula into the coronal venous plexus is no longer demonstrable. [Reprinted from Criscuolo and Rothbart (20), with permission.]

TABLE 2. *Characteristics differentiating dural AV fistulas and intradural AVMs*

Feature	Dural AV fistula	Intradural AVM
Percentage of AVMs	85–90%	10–15%
Demographics		
Gender (male)	85–95%	50%
Age range	22–72	4–58 (65% <25)
Mean age	49	27
Clinical features		
Acute onset	10–15%	50%
Chronic progression	85–95%	50%
Hemorrhage	None	50–70%
Other vascular anomalies	None	20%
Exacerbation with activity	Yes (70–80%)	No
Foix-Alajouanine syndrome	15%	None
Anatomic spinal level	Lower thoracolumbar	Diffuse
Arteriographic features		
Number of feeding vessels	1 or 2	Multiple
Type of artery	Dural (100%), shared Medullary (15%)	Medullary (100%)
Flow rate	Slow	Fast
Location of nidus	Dura lateral to spinal cord	Parenchyma/pial surface
Venous drainage	Retrograde; rostral (rarely both rostral and caudal)	Orthograde; rostral and caudal

Reprinted from Criscuolo and Rothbart (20), with permission.

TABLE 3. *Conditions associated with intradural spinal AVMs*

Cerebral aneurysms
Chylous malformations
Multiple cutaneous nevi
Wyburn-Mason syndrome
von Hippel-Lindau disease
Vascular agenesis/hypoplasia
Rendu-Osler-Weber syndrome
Sturge-Kalischer-Weber syndrome
Arteriovenous anomalies located elsewhere

ten similar presentations of spinal neoplasms may present yet another diagnostic challenge.

Diagnostic Evaluation

Although our currently available diagnostic armamentarium is vast, the history and physical examination remain paramount in narrowing the differential diagnosis. This, in concert with the physician's clinical acumen, will serve to direct a focused diagnostic evaluation.

Initial radiographic studies usually include plain spine x-rays and MRI. The results will dictate the need for further neuroradiologic evaluation such as myelography, selective spinal arteriography, or brain MRI. The latter may detect a lesion that can mimic a spinal cord process, such as a parasagittal tumor, foramen magnum tumor, syringobulbia, multiple sclerosis plaques, or a tentorial dural AV fistula. Along with the usual hematologic screening panel (complete blood count, electrolytes, liver function studies, and coagulation times), additional studies that may prove useful include: serum vitamin B_{12}, red blood cell folate levels, viral titers (hepatitis, human immunodeficiency virus (HIV), cytomegalovirus, Epstein-Barr), blood cultures, and serum electrophoresis. If lumbar puncture is performed, cerebrospinal fluid (CSF) should be sent for differential cell count, protein, glucose, cytopathology, Gram stain, culture and sensitivity, viral titers, cryptococcal antigen, india ink prep, myelin basic protein, immunoglobulin G index, and oligoclonal banding. Neurophysiologic testing such as pattern-reversed visual evoked responses, brainstem auditory evoked responses, and somatosensory evoked potentials (SSEPs) may provide support in diagnosing demyelinating disease. In addition, electromyography, nerve-conduction velocities, and the H-reflex and F-response latencies may provide extremely useful data in ruling out peripheral neuropathy as a diagnosis and in localizing the lesion within the cord (1).

Neuroradiologic Evaluation

In recent years, MRI has supplanted myelography as the initial procedure of choice for evaluating myelopathy because the former is noninvasive and allows evaluation of the spinal cord, including the detection of intrinsic damage such as edema, infarction, and hemorrhage. Doppman and associates' review (32) of 12 patients with spinal AVMs helped define the role of MRI by reaching the following conclusions. The pathologically induced anatomic changes are best visualized on T1-weighted sagittal images. The characteristically rapid flow rates associated with intradural AVMs generate intramedullary signal voids on both T1- and T2-weighted images. Enlarged draining veins in the subarachnoid space are visualized as serpentine filling defects, which are best demonstrated with T2 weighting whereby CSF provides a high signal contrast, especially when thin slices and surface coils are used. Dural AVMs are associated with vascular extravasation and spinal cord edema and swelling. These findings, when demonstrated by increased signal on T2-weighted images, are believed to be secondary to increased water content from venous congestion. MRI can demonstrate resolution of these changes after surgical interruption or embolization. In addition, it may be helpful in identifying postoperative thrombosis or embolic obliteration of the nidus (43). By identifying a major intramedullary component, MRI may distinguish intramedullary from extramedullary lesions. In doing so, it helps assess the indication for spinal arteriography and

TABLE 4. *Differential diagnosis of myelopathy*

Degenerative
  Spinal spondylosis
  Intervertebral disc disease
Neoplastic
  Metastatic carcinoma (prostate, lung, breast, colon,
    myeloma, renal, thyroid)
  Spinal cord tumor (glioma, ependymoma,
    hemangioblastoma, neurofibroma, meningioma)
  Paraneoplastic (acute necrotic myelopathy secondary to
    systemic carcinoma)
Infectious
  Epidural abscess
  Acute disseminated encephalomyelitis
  Infectious arteritis (chronic meningovascular syphilis)
  Tuberculous osteomyelitis of the spine (Pott's disease)
  Transverse myelitis (mumps, rabies, vaccinia, variola,
    varicella, HIV)
Traumatic
  Blunt
  Penetrating
Neurodengenerative (autoimmune, nutritional)
  Demyelinating disease (Devic's neuromyelitis optica)
  Amyotrophic lateral sclerosis (motor neuron disease)
  Subacute combined degeneration (vitamin B_{12} deficiency)
Developmental
  Syringomyelia
  Arachnoid cyst
  Meningomyelocele
  Chiari malformation
  Spinal arteriovenous malformation
  Intracranial dural arteriovenous fistula

guide the angiographic procedure. Furthermore, MRI may discriminate these lesions from vascular neoplasms such as hemangioblastomas, which may resemble an intramedullary AVM on myelography. Hemangioblastomas characteristically demonstrate low signal intensity on T1-weighted images but increased signal intensity on T2-weighted images.

Isu et al. (51) added further perspective in our understanding of the clinical utility of MRI by reporting two cases of spinal dural AV fistula. The authors confirmed the difficulty of visualizing the small, intraforaminal nidus via MRI. However, they did note that increased intramedullary signal intensity seen on T2 weighting was most prominent at the level where a delay in venous circulation was demonstrated on angiography. They also reported a significant postoperative diminution of intramedullary signal changes, which coincided with the neurologic improvement in their patients. From these observations, they concluded that MRI provides a simple method of delineating the parenchymal changes known to occur with dural AV fistulas. This information can in turn be useful to correlate with clinical responses after therapeutic intervention. In evaluating these lesions, one must remember that small AVMs, like dural AVFs or small intradural perimedullary AVFs, may be difficult to detect by standard spin-echo MRI techniques. However, recent advances in magnetic resonance angiography (MRA) have revealed this modality to be quite useful in both the pre- and postoperative evaluation of spinal AVMs (71). Nonetheless, it may still be necessary to pursue additional studies in the setting of an unexplained myelopathy and inconclusive MRI findings. In addition, a recent report emphasized the occasional need to consider the craniocervical and cervical sites when a patient presents with unexplained lumbar myelopathy (104) or subarachnoid hemorrhage (86,102).

Despite the rapid evolution of neuroradiologic investigations, myelography remains an extremely sensitive method of determining the diagnosis of a spinal AVM. The sensitivity when combining this procedure with CT approaches 100%. Therefore, normal results from a technically acceptable study performed with the patient in the supine position may negate the need for arteriography. However, a positive result yields little specific anatomic detail and requires further delineation of the vascular supply to the spinal cord and AVM.

Selective spinal arteriography plays a crucial role in the radiographic evaluation of spinal AVMs (23,24). The precise location of the AVM and delineation of the feeding vessels, extension, hemodynamic characteristics, and drainage pattern must be accurately defined before surgery or embolization (8). In a large group of 81 patients, Rosenblum et al. (88) reported a number of pertinent angiographic criteria to distinguish dural from intradural AVMs. They observed that intradural AVMs were located throughout the length of the spinal cord, whereas

dural AVMs were located almost exclusively in the lower thoracolumbar levels, with a peak incidence from T7 to T12. Although most dural AVFs are found in the thoracolumbar regions, the shunt can occasionally be located anywhere from the posterior fossa to the sacrum (38,94,102). The nidus of dural AVMs was universally situated in the lateral spinal canal, within the intervertebral foramen. Blood supply was via the dural branch of a spinal artery in all cases and was supplemented by a medullary artery in 15% of cases. Intradural AVMs were predominantly intramedullary (80%), with the remainder being distributed on the dorsal cord surface (9%) or ventral to the spinal cord (11%). A medullary artery was the feeding vessel in 100% of cases. Associated aneurysms were present in 44% of intradural AVMs, but were never present in conjunction with dural AV fistulas. In addition, the lesions could be distinguished by hemodynamic characteristics. Dural AVMs were noted to have slow flow in 100% of cases, in contrast to intrathecal lesions, which had rapid flow in 80% of cases. Whereas intradural malformations demonstrated orthograde drainage in the cranial (81%) and caudal (72%) directions, dural fistulas exhibited retrograde flow in a predominantly cranial direction (100%), and bidirectional flow was the exception (4%).

The series of Mourier et al. (73) of 35 cases of intradural perimedullary AVFs revealed these lesions to range in size from small fistulas, fed by a thin anterior spinal artery, to large AVFs fed by multiple, enormously dilated anterior and posterior spinal arteries draining into a giant venous ectasia embedded in the spinal cord. The majority of the AVFs (62%) fell into the latter category. The small to medium-size AVFs were found at the level of the conus medullaris or on the initial portion of the filum terminale. This was in contrast to the large perimedullary lesions, which were found exclusively in the cervical or thoracic region. Finally, the hemodynamic features of the small lesions were similar to those of dural AVFs, and the large lesions were closer to those of intramedullary AVMs.

PATHOPHYSIOLOGY OF SPINAL ARTERIOVENOUS MALFORMATIONS

Dural AV Fistulas

Early investigations into the pathophysiology of spinal AVMs relied upon clinical observations, gross intraoperative findings, and postmortem investigations. However, the evolution of neuroradiologic studies and surgical tools such as the operating microscope and microvascular Doppler ultrasonography have provided substantial insight into the mechanistic processes involved in these lesions. Various pathophysiologic mechanisms have been identified as playing a role in spinal cord dysfunction related to spinal vascular anomalies (Table 5). The most salient of these include the following: (a) venous hypertension with secondary congestive myelopathy; (b) venous thrombosis attributed to end-stage venous congestion; (c) hemorrhage with consequent ischemia, cord compression, or delayed scarring from arachnoiditis; (d) mass effect from varices or aneurysms; and (e) vascular steal leading to ischemia (2,3,13,15,25,26,40,44,47,51, 64,76–78,103,104).

The most common clinical course of a dural AV fistula is characterized by a slow onset of symptoms and progressive spinal cord dysfunction. It is rare for these patients to suffer an acute deterioration induced by subarachnoid hemorrhage, an observation most likely attributable to the low flow associated with these anomalies. This was evident in the NIH series, which did not report any patients presenting in this manner (88). However, 15% of patients with a dural AV fistula will present with an acute or subacute deterioration in the absence of hemorrhage. "Subacute necrotic myelopathy" was originally described by Foix and Alajouanine (37) in 1926 in two patients as a progressive thrombotic disorder involving the spinal cord, which ultimately resulted in fatal complications. The etiology was ascribed to a vascular mechanism because of the enlarged, serpentine, thickened vessels identified on the pial surface. Further investigation revealed extensive intramedullary necrosis. Since the initial description, other investigators have documented the association between spinal dural AV fistulas, vascular sclerosis, thrombosis, and the Foix-Alajouanine syndrome (19,20,36,82,103). Recent evidence suggests that early in the course, venous congestion, and not thrombosis, is responsible for the rapid neurologic decline. Thus, if therapeutic intervention is initiated before thrombotic sequelae, neurologic deficits may be reversible (19,20).

Dural AV fistulas consist of an anomalous communication between a dural branch of the spinal ramus of a spinal intercostal or lumbar artery and a medullary vein. These lesions are low-flow shunts and drain in a retrograde fashion into an engorged, tortuous coronal venous plexus on the dorsal cord surface. Because there are no valves between the coronal venous plexus and the radial veins draining the spinal cord, the increased pressure is transmitted directly to the cord tissue, and myelopathy

TABLE 5. *Pathophysiology of myeloradiculopathy associated with spinal AVMs*

Hemorrhage
Arachnoiditis
Vascular thrombosis
Ischemia secondary to venous congestion
Ischemia secondary to vascular steal phenomenon
Mass effect secondary to tangle of abnormal vessels or
  aneurysmal dilatations

results. The implication of venous hypertension as a primary pathophysiologic mechanism of spinal dural AVMs is based upon the data of several different studies. Selective spinal arteriography provided the initial information that identified the site of the fistula in the spinal nerve root dural sleeve, the low-flow shunt, and the retrograde drainage in a predominantly rostral direction. These observations imply a coexisting defect in the normal spinal venous drainage (23,24,26,27,33,76–78,87,88). Several authors have suggested that an angiographic pattern showing a lack of normal draining radicular veins at the thoracolumbar levels with delayed emptying of the medullary venous system strongly suggests venous hypertension (80,95). Investigations incorporating MRI as a diagnostic modality have also supported this concept. By using T2-weighted images, investigators documented intramedullary changes such as increased signal intensity and cord swelling in the region of the AV fistula. After obliteration of the nidus, these intramedullary changes and spinal cord swelling were remarkably diminished. With these findings, it became evident that these T2 signal changes represent spinal cord edema caused by venous hypertension, which in turn was induced by delayed drainage of the spinal veins. Furthermore, the authors felt that this demonstrated the potentially reversible nature of the process. If treatment is delayed, however, irreversible spinal cord damage will predictably ensue (32,51,95).

The advent of microvascular Doppler ultrasonography provided further characterization of the flow-related changes in dural AVMs. Using these techniques, Giller et al. (40) documented the hemodynamics of a single dural AV fistula. By examining the results of altering systemic mean arterial blood pressure and pCO_2 upon the blood flow in the venous system, they were able to document impaired autoregulation and lack of CO_2 reactivity, and confirm retrograde venous outflow. In addition, changes in the Doppler signals as the draining vein was clipped were dramatic and immediate. The previously pulsatile signal from the coronal venous plexus vanished, as did the the signal deep within the cord. This supports the presence of significant venous hypertension arising from dural AV fistulas. Moreover, the signal over the nerve root persisted after the draining vein was clipped and did not diminish until the nidus was eradicated, thus emphasizing the necessity to obliterate the nidus. Hassler et al. (47) conducted a similar study involving nine cases to elucidate further the hemodynamic conditions of these malformations. Using Doppler ultrasonography, they documented insightful results. Venous hypertension was quantified, with mean pressures in the perimedullary draining veins ranging between 60% to 87.5% of the mean systemic arterial pressure and decreasing by 16.4% to 64.3% of the previous values after interruption of the fistula. The transfiguration of the coronal venous plexus into the characteristic serpentine appearance was ascribed to these elevated pressures. After the authors occluded the nidus, Doppler sonographic examination of the large draining veins showed no detectable flow signal. Although the diameter of the draining veins decreased slightly, they did not collapse because of the remaining pressure in the venous system. This supports the concept that blood flow from the shunt enters the normal venous outflow pathways. Vascular steal phenomena did not appear to have an impact, as medullary arteries supplying the cord parenchyma were not involved.

The NIH study (88) likewise discounted vascular steal as a plausible mechanism by revealing that only 15% of dural AV fistulas were supplied by a medullary artery that also supplied the spinal cord. Although impairment of venous drainage was most pronounced at the level of the fistula, venous hypertension was demonstrable for large distances in the rostral and caudal directions. Therefore, localization of the lesion according to the site of clinical symptoms is unreliable because of the potential for spinal cord dysfunction at sites distant from the fistula. Furthermore, elevation of the mean systemic arterial pressure induced increased venous pressure in the perimedullary draining vein and decreased flow in the deep parenchymal veins. This important observation may explain the known exacerbation of symptoms that accompanies physical activity. In contrast to the findings of Giller et al. (40) and unlike cerebral AVMs, CO_2 vasomotor responses were found to be undisturbed. Because spinal venous pressure is normally controlled by venous drainage from medullary veins into epidural veins, the paucity of available normal draining veins may further exacerbate the induced venous hypertension. The typical cranial direction of venous drainage, which is commonly observed in these malformations, as opposed to the cranial and caudal venous drainage of intradural AVMs, supports this concept. Kuroda et al. (59) described the postmortem findings of a patient presenting with Foix-Alajouanine syndrome. Pathologic findings were consistent with venous congestion and included marked pallor of the cord parenchyma, spongiform changes, thinning of the myelin sheath, axonal enlargement, and perivascular infiltration of phagocytes.

Several interesting pathophysiologic parallels can be drawn between cerebral and spinal dural AV fistulas. Hurst et al. (50) reported a patient with an intracranial dural AVM who presented with left hemiparesis and mental status abnormalities. Angiography revealed a dural AVM involving the right transverse occipital sinus. The lesion was fed almost entirely from external carotid branches supplying the dura, and only a minimal supply originated from pial vessels. Therefore, the absence of a significant cortical arterial supply allows elimination of a vascular steal phenomenon as an explanation for the clinical symptoms at a site remote from the malformation. Moreover, the hemiparesis and cognitive changes resolved completely after embolization of the AVM.

Thus, it was postulated that the patient's symptoms were secondary to passive congestion of veins draining distant normal tissue. In a histopathologic study, Sakaki et al. (89) provided evidence that thrombosis may be an epiphenomenon involved in the clinical progression, as well as an etiologic factor in dural AVMs. Therefore, certain parallels may be drawn between cranial and spinal AVFs: (a) All dural AVFs are likely to be acquired lesions, (b) clinical symptoms are primarily related to venous congestion, (c) both lesions rarely present with hemorrhages, and (d) thrombosis may play a role in both the genesis and progression of these anomalies (15, 49,74,89).

Enough data now exist to explain the pathogenesis of spinal cord dysfunction related to spinal dural AV fistulas. Venous congestion is created by the altered hemodynamics induced by the AV shunt. This congestion is presumably compounded by a diminished venous outflow. Consequently, ischemia arises from the venous hypertension, increased tissue pressure, and the subsequent diminution of the AV pressure gradient. Untreated, this process will result in myelopathy and eventual spinal cord necrosis and atrophy (19,83).

Intradural AVMs

In contrast to dural AV fistulas, with intramedullary AVMs approximately 50% of patients will initially present in an apoplectic fashion resulting from subarachnoid or intramedullary hemorrhage. The nidus of these lesions is found in an intraparenchymal location and is distributed throughout the longitudinal axis of the spinal cord. Therefore, the upper extremities may be involved. Intradural AVMs share a common blood supply with the spinal cord and are usually fed by an enlarged medullary artery originating from the anterior spinal artery. These high-flow shunts are commonly supplied by multiple feeding arteries (26). The characteristically turbulent flow dynamics may explain the high incidence of associated varices and aneurysms (44%) and the occasional finding, most commonly with the juvenile type, of an audible bruit (6%) at the level of maximal shunting (88). These malformations may also present with fluctuating symptoms or a progressive myelopathy. In addition, the vast majority of intradural perimedullary AVFs present with a progressive conus medullaris and cauda equina syndrome (73). The pathophysiologic mechanism in these cases remains to be elucidated, as it is unclear whether ischemia or venous hypertension plays a role. Thus, intradural AVMs may induce myelopathy via thrombosis, venous congestion, compression from the nidus or associated vascular anomalies such as aneurysms and varices, or ischemia secondary to vascular steal. Although this latter mechanism has been proposed for many years, this finding has never been documented (Table 6).

TABLE 6. *Types of myelopathy associated with spinal vascular anomalies*

Congestive myelopathy
  Dural AV fistula
  Direct perimedullary AV fistula
Ischemic myelopathy
  Glomus AVM
  Juvenile AVM
Compressive myelopathy
  Glomus AVM
  Juvenile AVM
  Epidural varicose veins
  Cavernous malformations
Thrombotic myelopathy
  Dural AV fistula
  Juvenile AVM

MANAGEMENT OF SPINAL ARTERIOVENOUS MALFORMATIONS

General Principles of Surgical Management

Because the goals and the techniques of treatment of the individual types of spinal AVMs differ, the initial stage in their successful management involves diagnosing the distinct type of AVM with which an individual patient is afflicted and assessing the neurologic condition of the patient. Neuroradiologic studies should demonstrate the presence and precise location of the vascular nidus of the AVM, define the angioarchitecture, determine the operability of the malformation, and aid in the safe obliteration of the lesion by defining the vascular anatomy of the malformation and the normal spinal cord. In addition, it is imperative to recognize that the pathogenetic mechanisms differ in the various AVM types and that the goals of intervention should be modified accordingly. However, certain generalizations concerning the treatment of all spinal AVMs can be applied (8,17,20,58,64,65,67,76–78,94,106).

The patient is positioned prone on chest rolls, a Wilson frame, or an Andrews frame. The latter is particularly helpful because it provides maximum protection from the transmission of intra-abdominal pressure to the spinal vasculature. Induced hypotension is occasionally beneficial in large lesions with rapid flow.

The lamina of the neural arches one level above and below are removed widely. The dura is incised in the midline, being careful to maintain the arachnoid intact so that tearing of the delicate underlying vessels is avoided. This is especially important when a subarachnoid hemorrhage has occurred, wherein the underlying vessels may be tenaciously adherent to the arachnoid. Consequently, it is recommended to postpone surgery in patients with recent subarachnoid hemorrhage so that lysis of the clot may occur. If adhesions are not present, traction sutures are placed to retract the dura and arachnoid laterally. The operating microscope and appropriate microsurgical instrumentation and technique allow optimal exposure and identification of the anatomy of the AVM and adjacent neural tissue. It is essential to correlate the intraoperative findings with the vascular anatomy as defined by preoperative studies. Throughout the dissection, meticulous hemostatic principles must be followed, as blood-stained pia will interfere with visualization of anatomic details. Microdissection with the tips of the bipolar forceps or microdissectors should establish a plane in the gliotic tissue between the intramedullary malformation and surrounding cord tissue. This allows dissection of the malformation from the spinal cord and gradual control of any ventrally located vessels involved in the nidus. Prudent use of bipolar coagulation facilitates dissection by progressively shrinking the nidus, diminishing friability of the periphery, and reducing tumescence in the AVM. Use of irrigating bipolar forceps prevents coagulated vessel walls from adhering to the tips of the forceps. Patency is preserved in at least one of the major draining veins until completion of the circumferential dissection and occlusion of all arterial feeding vessels. Metallic clips are rarely needed and should be avoided, as they interfere with postoperative imaging.

Before a watertight dural closure is made, hemostasis is reassessed. Intraoperative angiography may be a useful adjunct in assessing parent-vessel patency and complete obliteration of the lesion (11). The utility of evoked potentials in monitoring risk to the spinal cord has not yet been clearly defined. Because 85% of spinal AVMs are dural AV fistulas located on the dorsal surface, and the commonly used SSEPs primarily monitor dorsal column sensation, the utility of these data remains indeterminate.

The decision to implement therapeutic intervention, which may involve considerable risk of permanent loss of neurologic function, must take into account the natural history of these vascular anomalies. Aminoff and Logue (2–5) reported the dismal prognosis associated with untreated AVMs. Recognition of dural AV fistulas was not evident at the time of their investigations. As a result, differentiation between the natural histories of dural and intradural malformations cannot be determined from that study. However, because dural AV fistulas account for at least 80% of all spinal AVMs, it is probable that their conclusions are mainly indicative of the natural history of these anomalies. Six months after the onset of neurologic dysfunction, 19% of their patients were unable to ambulate unassisted or were confined to bed. This number increased to 91% if left untreated for 3 years. Therefore, an aggressive approach to the treatment of symptomatic dural AV fistulas must be advocated. In contrast, the natural history of intradural AVMs is less certain. Minimally symptomatic lesions are therapeutic dilemmas because of the significant risk associated with treating these lesions.

TREATMENT OF INDIVIDUAL TYPES OF SPINAL ARTERIOVENOUS MALFORMATIONS

Dural AV Fistula

The first operation for "enlarged varicose veins" of the spinal cord was reported by Elsberg (35) in 1916. Retrospectively, we now know that this was, in fact, a dural AV fistula. By ligating and excising a dilated posterior spinal vein as it entered the dura adjacent to the eighth thoracic nerve root, the physician successfully reversed the patient's severe myelopathy.

When spinal arteriography was initially introduced, the tiny vascular connections from the substance of the spinal cord to the transfigured coronal venous plexus were considered to be the actual site of shunting. These dilated pial vessels, which drain blood from the cord parenchyma into the coronal venous plexus, were thought to be the nidus of the AVM. Thus, early therapy was directed at interrupting these vessels. It is now well recognized that the actual site of the fistula is the dural nerve root sleeve and adjacent spinal dura.

The goal of treatment of dural AV fistulas is eradication of spinal venous hypertension. This is achieved by interrupting the arterialized veins that drain blood from the nidus into the dilated coronal venous plexus and obliterating the AV fistula completely. This may be accomplished by endovascular or direct surgical intervention. As these lesions are supplied by a dural branch of the spinal ramus of an intercostal or lumbar artery, the intrinsic blood supply to the spinal cord does not typically participate in the fistula. Consequently, several investigators have recommended that dural AVMs be initially treated with embolization because the risk to normal cord parenchyma is minimal (16,72).

Embolization can prove particularly helpful in patients who present with the Foix-Alajouanine syndrome by inducing an immediate reduction in venous congestion, as visualized at arteriography. This allows neurologic function to recover and, at least temporarily, prevents the progression of spinal cord damage. It had previously been felt that the Foix-Alajouanine syndrome was a thrombotic process with a uniformly dismal outcome. However, it has been demonstrated that some patients with this entity may manifest a remarkable resolution of their neurologic deficits when embolization is used alone or in concert with surgical resection (19). However, endovascular approaches are not without inherent disadvantages and risks. Several reports have demonstrated a significant incidence of recanalization when polyvinyl alcohol (PVA) particles were used as the embolic material (46,70,72). The advent of cyanoacrylate glues as embolic agents has greatly decreased the risk of recanalization. An appropriate embolization will occlude the distal feeding vessel, the fistula itself, and the proximal portion of the efferent vein. If the occlusion is too proximal, recruitment of new feeding vessels may occur. In addition, neurologic deterioration may result if the occlusion is too distal in the venous drainage system. Finally, it must be remembered that 10% to 15% of patients with dural AVFs share a common blood supply with the spinal cord; embolization is contraindicated in these cases. Therefore, because of the low surgical morbidity associated with these lesions and the diminished risk of recanalization, surgery may be regarded as a first-line treatment in medically suitable patients (6,8,77, 78,88,94).

Exposure is accomplished by laminectomy, foraminotomy, and a midline dural opening. Intradural exploration should identify the draining medullary vein in proximity to the site of dural penetration of the nerve root. The proximal intradural portion of this vein is then divided. After interruption of the draining vein, the arterialized coronal venous plexus loses its turgidity and reverts to its normal blue color. However, to avoid recurrence, the definitive treatment of choice is to excise directly the portion of dura containing the fistula or to obliterate it with bipolar coagulation or the Nd:YAG laser (93). For patients in whom the same intercostal artery also supplies a medullary artery to the spinal cord (e.g., the artery of Adamkiewicz), obliteration of the fistula by excision or coagulation can lead to spinal cord infarction. In the past, treatment consisted of stripping the dilated coronal venous plexus from the pial surface. This practice is no longer advocated because it fails to address the pathogenetic mechanism involved. Moreover, it may induce further cord damage by impairing venous drainage from the removal of the normal, albeit arterialized, coronal venous plexus. In addition, an extensive laminectomy may be required, as these transfigured veins have a propensity to ascend many levels (19,20,76–78).

Glomus AVMs

These lesions are tightly coiled masses of blood vessels confined to a short segment of the spinal cord. They typically occur in the anterior half of the spinal cord and are supplied by spinal medullary arteries. Rarely, this type of malformation will have a partially extramedullary component, or it may be situated on the pial surface. Glomus AVMs located in the cervical region are particularly amenable to excision because of the inferior and superior collateral contributions to the anterior spinal artery. Lesions in the thoracic and lumbar region pose greater hazards because of the limited collateral blood supply, which reaches the spinal cord in a rostral direction only. Endovascular techniques, as both the sole treatment and as an adjunct to surgery, have been used increasingly to treat these lesions. Williams et al. (101) reported the successful resection of a ventrally located thoracic glomus AVM via an anterolateral transthoracic approach. These lesions must be evaluated on an individual basis to determine the most appropriate therapeutic course, be it endovascular, surgical, or a combined approach.

Juvenile AVMs

These voluminous AVMs are complex collections of abnormal vessels that typically contain cord parenchyma within the nidus. Because these lesions are supplied by medullary arteries, which also provide blood to the spinal cord, juvenile AVMs are typically viewed as unresectable lesions. Embolization is merely palliative and is recommended only when there is hemorrhage or deteriorating neurologic function. Two cases of juvenile AVMs have been treated successfully by a combination of embolization and surgery (92,96). Touho et al. (96) reported intraoperative embolization with isobutyl-2-cyanoacrylate (IBCA) after cannulation of the posterior spinal artery in combination with surgical resection in a patient with a thoracic juvenile AVM. Postoperatively, the patient demonstrated slight neurologic improvement; spinal angiography revealed no residual AVM and preservation of the anterior spinal artery.

Intradural Perimedullary AVFs

Several varieties of direct spinal AV fistulas have been reported in the literature. These lesions are situated in an intradural, perimedullary position. They are direct fistulas between the intrinsic blood supply to the spinal cord, either the anterior spinal artery or a combination of the anterior and posterior spinal arteries, and the coronal venous plexus or spinal medullary veins. The result is a dilatation of the venous drainage system that ranges in size from slightly dilated to a giant venous ectasia. Because of the relative lack of clinical experience with direct AV fistulas, little is known concerning their prognosis or natural history. The therapeutic goal of interrupting the fistula may be accomplished in several ways, depending upon the vascular anatomy of the lesion in question. If the arterial feeding vessel consists of a single, small-caliber anterior spinal artery, then the fistula is surgically eliminated because of the inherent risk of occluding the normal anterior spinal artery at the time of embolization. Surgical excision often requires an anterior approach for adequate exposure of the lesion. However, if the vascular anomaly is intermediate in size and composed of an enlarged anterior spinal artery and a venous varix, then alternatives include embolization, surgery, or a combination of both modalities. Surgery may be assisted by the use of temporary balloon occlusion of the anterior spinal artery. The most difficult of these lesions are the large, multipedicled fistulas consisting of a high-flow shunt and consequent massive venous ectasias. The hemodynamics often preclude safe emboliza-

tion or surgical excision, and these lesions therefore may be amenable only to intraluminal balloon occlusion (73).

ENDOVASCULAR INTERVENTION AND MATERIALS

Reestablishing normal spinal cord hemodynamics by permanently obliterating the AVM nidus while preserving normal spinal cord parenchyma and intrinsic blood supply is the ultimate therapeutic goal in treating spinal AVMs. Treatment must be individualized to the specific type of AVM and the associated pathophysiologic mechanism. For those lesions that pose a significant risk from surgical intervention, embolization is the treatment of choice (12,33,46,73,85). Technical advances in arteriographic catheter design and digital subtraction techniques have facilitated endovascular intervention. Embolic agents that have been used are summarized in Table 7. Embolic occlusion may reduce vascular steal and resultant ischemia of the cord, decrease the potential risk of hemorrhage, and relieve venous hypertension (7,13,26,34). Thus, patients may exhibit dramatic improvement after the procedure. As previously stated, however, the improvement may be only transient. In many patients undergoing embolization with PVA or Gelfoam®, recanalization of the nidus occurs and collateral vessels subsequently develop, thereby reestablishing blood flow to the AVM (46,70,72). This problem was eradicated with the development of IBCA, a permanent embolic glue that prohibits recanalization. However, the polymerization characteristics of IBCA occasionally led to technical difficulties, such as the angiographic catheter being glued *in situ*. Furthermore, in lesions requiring surgical intervention after embolization with IBCA, intraoperative problems arose because of its rigid nature. Consequently, IBCA has been replaced at many centers with NBCA because of its more pliable quality and decreased risk of intravascular adherence to the angiographic catheter.

CAVERNOUS MALFORMATIONS

Until recently, spinal cord cavernous malformations (CMs) were not considered in the differential diagnosis

TABLE 7. *Materials used for embolization of spinal AVMs*

Gelfoam
Clotted blood
Metallic pellets
Lyophilized dura
Muscle fragments
Detachable balloon
Microfibrillar collagen
Polyvinyl alcohol (PVA)
Silicone (spheres, fluid)
Isobutyl-2-cyanoacrylate (IBCA)
n-Butyl-2-cyanoacrylate (NBCA)

of patients with myelopathic syndromes. Aminoff stated that spinal cord CMs are extremely rare and usually of little clinical significance (2). Jellinger estimated that CMs account for 5% to 12% of spinal vascular malformations, but most of the referenced lesions arose from the vertebrae or the epidural compartment (53). However, as a result of MRI, CMs are being diagnosed with increasing frequency throughout the central nervous system and are now being recognized as rare but treatable causes of myelopathy (9,18,68,69,75).

The age at presentation can be quite variable, but most patients tend to become symptomatic in the fourth decade of life (75). Females are affected approximately twice as often. Spinal CMs are most common in the thoracic region but have been reported from the upper cervical cord to the cauda equina (7,69). Although exophytic lesions have been described, the vast majority are entirely intramedullary (18,69). Familial occurrence and coexistence of intracranial CMs, multiple intramedullary CMs, and associated cutaneous vascular nevi have been described (9,61,68).

Ogilvy et al. (75) reviewed 36 patients who demonstrated several patterns of sensorimotor symptom progression ranging from acute to progressive to episodic. The acute presentation, seen in approximately one-third of patients, is most likely attributable to hemorrhage. The hemorrhage may be confined within the sinusoidal cavities of the CM, resulting in acute expansion of the lesion, or frank hematomyelia may occur. Although the onset of pain and neurologic deficit is sudden, evolution of symptoms may continue for several hours to a few days. This is distinct from the acute presentation of maximal neurologic deficit associated with hematomyelia secondary to intramedullary AVMs. Although a complete and permanent paralysis may be the final result, most patients presenting with CMs experience an incomplete deficit followed by some degree of recovery. Pain is present in about 50% of the cases (68). Rebleeding has been reported, but the annualized risk of recurrent hemorrhage associated with spinal CMs remains unknown. It is interesting that subarachnoid hemorrhage has not been reported from an intramedullary CM, but has been seen in lesions involving the spinal nerve roots (98). One-third of patients have a course characterized by episodic deteriorations that may mimic a demyelinating process. This may be the result of continued micro-hemorrhages or sinusoidal thrombosis resulting in a lesser parenchymal injury.

Several pathophysiologic explanations have been proposed for the progressive course seen in the remaining one-third of patients. This type of clinical decline may be due to enlargement of the lesion through ongoing angiogenesis, repeated hemorrhage followed by organization and recanalization, compromise of the surrounding microcirculation, or a neurotoxic effect of hemosiderin deposition (68,75).

Pathologically, CMs are characterized by lobulated, thin sinusoidal vascular spaces arranged in a honeycomb pattern without intervening neural tissue. They are typically well circumscribed and clearly demarcated from the surrounding hemosiderin-stained parenchyma. Their gross appearance has been likened to that of a mulberry because of their dark red or purple lobulated configuration.

MRI has vastly improved our ability to diagnose intramedullary pathology and is consequently the procedure of choice for evaluating CMs. The findings are usually diagnostic, and typically consist of a central core of mixed signal intensity from various stages of red blood cell degradation surrounded by a hypointense hemosiderin ring. However, not all lesions will exhibit this typical appearance. Occasionally, surrounding edema, cyst formation, or homogeneous signal from within the lesion may obscure the diagnosis. In addition, resolving hematoma from any etiology may mimic the MRI appearance of a CM (9,69,75). Myelography and CT are much less sensitive, although they may show evidence of spinal cord widening suggestive of an intramedullary process. Arteriography is not helpful because CMs are angiographically occult lesions.

In most cases, the optimal treatment of symptomatic patients with intramedullary CMs consists of surgical resection. Gross total removal should be the surgical goal (68,69,75). The technique for removal is similar to that of an intramedullary neoplasm and has been described by McCormick and Stein. Often the lesion can be visualized as an area of discoloration beneath the dorsal surface of the cord and thus guide the placement of a small myelotomy. If the lesion is not visualized, then the preoperative MRI will guide the placement of a myelotomy in the midline or over the dorsal root entry zone. Despite the absence of a true capsule, a glial plane can usually be identified between the lesion and the spinal cord. If a hematoma is present, the walls of the hematomyelic cavity must be carefully inspected under high magnification to avoid missing small residual portions. In most cases reported in the literature, intramedullary CMs could be resected safely and completely (9,18,68,69,75). Because of the rarity of these lesions, the natural history of spinal CMs is poorly understood, and no treatment is currently advised for asymptomatic lesions.

EPIDURAL VARICES

Spinal epidural varices are extremely rare causes of isolated nerve root compression syndromes such as sciatica (0.5% to 1.3% prevalence) (45,109) or the cauda equina syndrome (radicular pain, lower motor neuron weakness, and urinary dysfunction) (25,52). These lesions have been ascribed to both congenital and acquired etiologies. Dysraphia and spinal anomalies are reported in up to 75% of patients with epidural varicosities. However, mechanical factors such as trauma, disc herniation, obesity, and pregnancy may also play a role. Patients with these rare low-flow lesions may present with either myelopathy or radicular signs secondary to compression. A case report of a myelopathy secondary to an epidural varicose vein located at the cervicothoracic junction provides evidence of the potential for these anomalies to cause significant neurologic dysfunction (25). Obliteration is accomplished by laminectomy, bipolar cautery, and simple surgical excision.

CONCLUSION

Spinal AVMs consist of a heterogeneous group of non-neoplastic vascular lesions. Therapeutic options consist of surgical excision and embolization. Selection of the appropriate treatment is based upon accurate studies to establish the diagnosis and a thorough understanding of the involved pathophysiology. Improved microsurgical and interventional methodologies, as well as technical advances in neuroradiologic imaging and embolization materials, have allowed the current abilities to diagnose precisely and to influence therapeutically spinal vascular anomalies.

REFERENCES

1. Case records of the Massachusetts General Hospital (1992): Weekly clinicopathological exercises. Case 12—1992. A 64-year-old woman with the abrupt onset of paraparesis after 10 months of increasing episodic leg weakness. *N Engl J Med* 326:816–824.
2. Aminoff M (1976): In: *Spinal angiomas.* Oxford, England: Blackwell Scientific, pp. 32–37, 82–96, 101–106, 166–168.
3. Aminoff MJ, Barnard RO, Logue V (1974): The pathophysiology of spinal vascular malformations. *J Neurol Sci* 23:255–263.
4. Aminoff MJ, Logue V (1974): Clinical features of spinal vascular malformations. *Brain* 97:197–210.
5. Aminoff MJ, Logue V (1974): The prognosis of patients with spinal vascular malformations. *Brain* 97:211–218.
6. Anson JA, Spetzler RF (1992): Classification of spinal arteriovenous malformations and implications for treatment. *BNI Quarterly* 8:2–8.
7. Anson JA, Spetzler RF (1992): Interventional radiology for spinal pathology. *Clin Neurosurg* 39:388–417.
8. Anson JA, Spetzler RF (1992): Spinal dural arteriovenous malformations. In: Awad IA, Barrow DL, eds. *Dural arteriovenous malformations.* Park Ridge, Illinois: American Association of Neurological Surgeons, pp. 175–191.
9. Anson JA, Spetzler RF (1993): Surgical resection of intramedullary spinal cord cavernous malformations. *J Neurosurg* 78:446–451.
10. Awad IA, Barnett GH (1990): Neurological deterioration in a patient with a spinal arteriovenous malformation following lumbar puncture. Case report. *J Neurosurg* 72:650–653.
11. Barrow DL, Boyer KL, Joseph GJ (1992): Intraoperative angiography in the management of neurovascular disorders. *Neurosurgery* 30:153–159.
12. Berenstein A, Young W, Ransohoff J, Benjamin V, Merkin H (1984): Somatosensory evoked potentials during spinal angiography and therapeutic transvascular embolization. *J Neurosurg* 60:777–785.
13. Brainen M, Samec P (1983): Venous hemodynamics of arteriove-
nous meningeal fistulas in the posterior cranial fossa. *Neuroradiology* 25:161–169.
14. Brasch F (1900): Ueber einen schweren spinalen Symptomencomplex bedingt durch eine aneurysma-serpentinumartige Veränderung eines Theils der Ruckenmarksgefässe. *Berl Klin Wochenschr* 37:1210–1213.
15. Chaudhary M, Sachdev V, Cho S (1982): Dural arteriovenous malformations of the major venous sinuses: An acquired lesion. *AJNR* 3:13–19.
16. Choi IS, Berenstein A (1988): Surgical neuroangiography of the spine and spinal cord. *Radiol Clin North Am* 26:1131–1141.
17. Cogen P, Stein BM (1983): Spinal cord arteriovenous malformations with significant intramedullary components. *J Neurosurg* 59:471–478.
18. Cosgrove GR, Bertrand G, Fontaine S, Robitaille Y, Melanson D (1988): Cavernous angiomas of the spinal cord. *J Neurosurg* 68:31–36.
19. Criscuolo G, Oldfield E, Doppman JL (1989): Reversible acute and subacute myelopathy in patients with dural arteriovenous fistulas: Foix-Alajouanine syndrome reconsidered. *J Neurosurg* 70:354–359.
20. Criscuolo GR, Rothbart D (1992): Vascular malformations of the spinal cord: Pathophysiology, diagnosis, and management. *Neurosurg Quarterly* 2:77–98.
21. Dejerine J (1906): Sur la claudication intermittente de la moelle epiniere. *Rev Neurol* 14:341–350.
22. DiChiro G (1972): Development of spinal cord angiography. *Acta Radiol (Stockh)* 13:767–770.
23. DiChiro G, Doppman J, Ommaya A (1967): Selective arteriography of arteriovenous aneurysms of the spinal cord. *Radiology* 88:1065–1077.
24. DiChiro G, Rieth KG, Oldfield EH, Tievsky AL, Doppman JL, Davis DO (1982): Digital subtraction angiography and dynamic computed tomography in the evaluation of arteriovenous malformations and hemangioblastomas of the spinal cord. *J Comput Assist Tomogr* 6:655–670.
25. Dickman C, Zabramski J, Sonntag V, Coons S (1988): Myelopathy due to epidural varicose veins of the cervicothoracic junction. Case report. *J Neurosurg* 69:940–941.
26. Djindjian M, Djindjian R, Hurth M, Houdart R, Rey A (1978): Steal phenomena in spinal arteriovenous malformations. *J Neuroradiol* 5:187–201.
27. Djindjian M, Djindjian R, Rey A, Hurth M, Houdart R (1977): Intradural extramedullary spinal arterio-venous malformations fed by the anterior spinal artery. *Surg Neurol* 8:85–93.
28. Djindjian R (1969): Arteriography of the spinal cord. *Am J Roentgenol Radium Ther Nucl Med* 107:461–478.
29. Djindjian R, Houdart R, Hurth M (1969): Angiography of the spinal cord. *Acta Radiol* 9:707–726.
30. Djindjian R, Hurth M, Houdart R (1972): Angiography of the spinal cord. Yield and orientation of the research after 10-years' experience. *Acta Radiol* 13:771–791.
31. Doppman JL (1972): Arteriography of the spinal cord. *Semin Roentgenol* 7:231–239.
32. Doppman JL, Di CG, Dwyer AJ, Frank JL, Oldfield EH (1987): Magnetic resonance imaging of spinal arteriovenous malformations. *J Neurosurg* 66:830–834.
33. Doppman JL, Di CG, Oldfield EH (1985): Origin of spinal arteriovenous malformation and normal cord vasculature from a common segmental artery: Angiographic and therapeutic considerations. *Radiology* 154:687–689.
34. Doppman JL, Di CG, Ommaya AK (1971): Percutaneous embolization of spinal cord arteriovenous malformations. *J Neurosurg* 34:48–55.
35. Elsberg C (1916): In: *Diagnosis and treatment of surgical diseases of the spinal cord and its membranes.* Philadelphia: W.B. Saunders, pp. 194–204.
36. Flament J, Vicente A, Coers C, Gauzzi G (1960): La myelomalacie angiodygenetique (Foix-Alajouanine) et sa differenciation des necroses spinales sur angiomatose intra-medullaire. *Rev Neurol* 103:12–29.
37. Foix C, Alajouanine T (1926): La myelite necrotique subaique. *Rev Neurol* 2:1–42.
38. Friedman AH, Gray L (1992): Clinical and radiological findings

of spinal dural arteriovenous fistula. In: Barrow DL, ed. *Perspectives in neurological surgery.* St. Louis: Quality Medical Publishing, pp. 1–15.

39. Gaupp J (1888): Hamorrhoiden der Pia mater spinalis im Gebiet des Lendenmarksss. *Beitr Pathol* 2:516–518.

40. Giller CA, Meyer YJ, Batjer HH (1989): Hemodynamic assessment of the spinal cord arteriovenous malformation with intraoperative microvascular Doppler ultrasound: Case report. *Neurosurgery* 25:270–275.

41. Gillian L (1958): The arterial supply of the human spinal cord. *J Comp Neurol* 110:75–103.

42. Gillian L (1970): Veins of the spinal cord. Anatomical details; suggested clinical applications. *Neurology* 20:860–868.

43. Gray L, Brothers M, Friedman AH, et al. (1991): MRI—New gold standard for identifying a spinal dural venous fistula. *AJNR* 12:27–32.

44. Greenberg J (1970): Spontaneous arteriovenous malformations in the cervical area. *J Neurol Neurosurg Psychiatry* 33:303–309.

45. Gumbel U, Pia H, Vogelsang H (1969): Lumbrosacrale gefassanomalien als ursache vov ischialgien. *Acta Neurochir (Wien)* 20:131–151.

46. Hall WA, Oldfield EH, Doppman JL (1989): Recanalization of spinal arteriovenous malformations following embolization. *J Neurosurg* 70:714–720.

47. Hassler W, Thron A, Grote E (1989): Hemodynamics of spinal dural arteriovenous fistulas. An intraoperative study. *J Neurosurg* 70:360–370.

48. Heros RC, Debrun GM, Ojemann RG, Lasjaunias PL, Naessens PJ (1986): Direct spinal arteriovenous fistula: A new type of spinal AVM. Case report. *J Neurosurg* 64:134–139.

49. Houser O, Campbell J, Campbell R, Sundt T (1979): Arteriovenous malformation affecting the transverse dural venous sinus—An acquired lesion. *Mayo Clin Proc* 54:651–661.

50. Hurst R, Hackney D, Goldberg H, Davis R (1992): Reversible arteriovenous malformation-induced venous hypertension as a cause of neurological deficits. *Neurosurgery* 30:422–425.

51. Isu T, Iwasaki Y, Akino M, Koyanagi I, Abe H (1989): Magnetic resonance imaging in cases of spinal dural arteriovenous malformation. *Neurosurgery* 24:919–923.

52. Ivanovici F (1970): Urine retention: An isolated sign in some spinal cord disorders. *J Urol* 104:284–286.

53. Jellinger K (1975): The morphology of centrally situated angiomas. In: Pia HW, Gleave JRW, Grote E, Zierski J, eds. *Cerebral angiomas: Advances in diagnosis and therapy.* New York: Springer-Verlag.

54. Kendall BE, Logue V (1977): Spinal epidural angiomatous malformations draining into intrathecal veins. *Neuroradiology* 13:181–189.

55. Kim D, Choi I, Berenstein A (1991): A sacral dural arteriovenous fistula presenting with an intermittent myelopathy aggravated by menstruation. *J Neurosurg* 75:947–949.

56. Kraus GE, Bucholz RD, Weber TR (1990): Spinal cord arteriovenous malformation with an associated lymphatic anomaly. Case report. *J Neurosurg* 73:768–773.

57. Krause F (1911): In: *Chirurgie des Gehirns and Ruckenmarks nach eigenen Erfahrungen.* Berlin: Urban & Schwarzenberg, pp. 775–776.

58. Krayenbuhl H (1971): Microsurgical approach to cerebrospinal lesions. *J R Coll Surg Edinb* 16:38–51.

59. Kuroda S, Hayashi Y, Ishizu H, Oda T, Kuyama K, Otsuki S (1991): An autopsy case of spinal arteriovenous malformation (Foix-Alajouanine syndrome). *Acta Med Okayama* 45:451–456.

60. Lazorthes G, Gouaze A, Zadeh JO, Santini JJ, Burdin P (1971): Arterial vascularization of the spinal cord. Recent studies of the anastomotic pathways. *J Neurosurg* 35:253–262.

61. Lee KS, Spetzler RF (1990): Spinal cord cavernous malformation in a patient with familial intracranial cavernous malformations. *Neurosurgery* 26:877–880.

62. Levy R, Plassche W, Riggs J, Shoulson I (1983): Spinal myoclonus related to an arteriovenous malformation. Response to clonazepam therapy. *Arch Neurol* 40:254–255.

63. Lhermitte J, Fribourg-Blanc A, Kyriaco N (1931): La gliose angeiohypertrophique de la moelle epiniere (myelite necrotique de Foix-Alajouanine). *Rev Neurol* 2:37–53.

64. Logue V (1979): Angiomas of the spinal cord: Review of the pathogenesis, clinical features and results of surgery. *J Neurol Neurosurg Psychiatry* 42:1–11.

65. Luessenhop AJ, Cruz TD (1969): The surgical excision of spinal intradural vascular malformations. *J Neurosurg* 30:552–559.

66. Luyendijk W (1979): The arterial supply of the spinal cord. *Surg Neurol* 11:369–372.

67. Malis LI (1979): Microsurgery for spinal cord arteriovenous malformations. *Clin Neurosurg* 26:543–555.

68. McCormick PC, Michelsen WJ, Post KD, Carmel PW, Stein BM (1988): Cavernous malformations of the spinal cord. *Neurosurgery* 23:459–463.

69. McCormick PC, Stein BM (1993): Spinal cavernous malformations. In: Awad IA, Barrow DL, eds. *Cavernous malformations.* Park Ridge, Illinois: American Association of Neurological Surgeons, pp. 145–150.

70. Morgan MK, Marsh WR (1989): Management of spinal dural arteriovenous malformations. *J Neurosurg* 70:832–836.

71. Mourier KL, Gelbert F, Reizine D, et al. (1993): Phase contrast magnetic resonance of the spinal cord. Preliminary results in spinal cord arterio-venous malformations. *Acta Neurochir* 123:57–63.

72. Mourier KL, Gelbert F, Rey A, et al. (1989): Spinal dural arteriovenous malformations with perimedullary drainage. Indications and results of surgery in 30 cases. *Acta Neurochir (Wien)* 100:136–141.

73. Mourier KL, Gobin YP, George B, Lot G, Merland JJ (1993): Intradural perimedullary arteriovenous fistulae: Results of surgical and endovascular treatment in a series of 35 cases. *Neurosurgery* 32:885–891.

74. Nishijima M, Takaku A, Endo S, et al. (1992): Etiological evaluations of dural arteriovenous malformations of the lateral and sigmoid sinuses based on histopathological examinations. *J Neurosurg* 76:600–606.

75. Ogilvy CS, Louis DN, Ojemann RG (1992): Intramedullary cavernous malformations of the spinal cord: Clinical presentation, pathological features, and surgical management. *Neurosurgery* 31:219–230.

76. Oldfield E, Criscuolo G (1989): Spinal arteriovenous malformations. In: Tindall GT, ed. *Contemporary neurosurgery.* Baltimore: Williams and Wilkins, pp. 1–6.

77. Oldfield EH, Di CG, Quindlen EA, Rieth KG, Doppman JL (1983): Successful treatment of a group of spinal cord arteriovenous malformations by interruption of dural fistula. *J Neurosurg* 59:1019–1030.

78. Oldfield EH, Doppman JL (1988): Spinal arteriovenous malformations. *Clin Neurosurg* 34:161–183.

79. Ommaya AK, Di CG, Doppman J (1969): Ligation of arterial supply in the treatment of spinal cord arteriovenous malformations. *J Neurosurg* 30:679–692.

80. Partington MD, Rufenacht DA, Marsh WR, Piepgras DG (1992): Cranial and sacral dural arteriovenous fistulas as a cause of myelopathy. *J Neurosurg* 76:615–622.

81. Perthes G (1927): Uber das Rankenangiom der weichen Haute des Gehirns und Uuckenmarks. *Dtsch Ztschr Chir* 203–204:93–103.

82. Pia H, Vogelsang H (1965): Diagnosie und therapie spinaler angiome. *Dtsch Z Nervenhelik* 187:74–96.

83. Renowden SA, Molyneux AJ (1993): Case report: Spontaneous thrombosis of a spinal dural AVM (Foix-Alajouanine syndrome)—Magnetic resonance appearance. *Clin Radiol* 47:134–136.

84. Report of the joint committee for stroke facilities. IX. Strokes in children (1973): *Stroke* 4:1007–1052.

85. Riche MC, Modenesi FJ, Djindjian M, Merland JJ (1982): Arteriovenous malformations (AVM) of the spinal cord in children. A review of 38 cases. *Neuroradiology* 22:171–180.

86. Rinkel GJE, van Gijn J, Wijdicks EFM (1993): Subarachnoid hemorrhage without detectable cause. *Stroke* 24:1403–1409.

87. Rosenblum B, Bonner R, Oldfield E (1987): Intraoperative measurement of cortical blood flow adjacent to cerebral AVM using laser Doppler velocimetry. *J Neurosurg* 66:396–399.

88. Rosenblum B, Oldfield EH, Doppman JL, Di CG (1987): Spinal arteriovenous malformations: A comparison of dural arteriove-

nous fistulas and intradural AVMs in 81 patients. *J Neurosurg* 67: 795–802.

89. Sakaki S, Furuta S, Fujita M, Kohno K (1991): Dural arteriovenous malformation of the transverse and sigmoid sinus with special reference to its pathological features. *Br J Neurosurg* 5:87–92.

90. Sargent P (1925): Hemangioma of the pia mater causing compression paraplegia. *Brain* 48:259–267.

91. Shivapour E, Teasdall R (1980): Spinal myoclonus with vacuolar degeneration of anterior horn cells. *Arch Neurol* 37:451–453.

92. Spetzler RF, Zabramski JM, Flom RA (1989): Management of juvenile spinal AVMs by embolization and operative excision. Case report. *J Neurosurg* 70:628–632.

93. Strugar J, Chyatte D (1992): In situ photocoagulation of spinal dural arteriovenous malformations using the Nd:YAG laser. *J Neurosurg* 77:571–574.

94. Symon L, Kuyama H, Kendall B (1984): Dural arteriovenous malformations of the spine. Clinical features and surgical results in 55 cases. *J Neurosurg* 60:238–247.

95. Tomlinson FH, Rufenacht DA, Sundt TM, Nichols DA, Fode NC (1993): Arteriovenous fistulas of the brain and spinal cord. *J Neurosurg* 79:16–27.

96. Touho H, Karasawa J, Shishido H, Yamada K, Shibamoto K (1991): Successful excision of a juvenile-type spinal arteriovenous malformation following intraoperative embolization. Case report. *J Neurosurg* 75:647–651.

97. Turnbull I (1971): Microvasculature of the human spinal cord. *J Neurosurg* 35:141–147.

98. Ueda S, Saito A, Inomori S, Kim I (1987): Cavernous angioma of the cauda equina producing a subarachnoid hemorrhage: Case report. *J Neurosurg* 66:134–136.

99. Uhl GR, Martinez CR, Brooks BR (1981): Spinal seizures following intravenous contrast in a patients with a cord AVM (letter). *Ann Neurol* 10:580–581.

100. Van Woert M, Hwang E (1978): Biochemistry and pharmacology of myoclonus. In: Klawans H, ed. *Clinical neuropharmacology.* New York: Raven Press, pp. 167–184.

101. Williams FC, Zabramski JM, Spetzler RF, Rekate HL (1991): Anterolateral transthoracic transvertebral resection of an intramedullary spinal arteriovenous malformation. Case report. *J Neurosurg* 74:1004–1008.

102. Willinsky R, TerBrugge K, Lasjaunias P, Montanera W (1990): The variable presentations of craniocervical and cervical dural arteriovenous malformations. *Surg Neurol* 34:118–123.

103. Wirth F Jr, Post K, DiChiro G, Doppman J, Ommaya A (1970): Foix-Alajouanine disease. Spontaneous thrombosis of spinal cord arteriovenous malformation: A case report. *Neurology* 20:1114–1118.

104. Wrobel C, Oldfield E, DiChiro G, Tarlov E, Baker R, Doppman J (1988): Myelopathy due to intracranial dural arteriovenous fistulas draining intrathecally into spinal medullary veins. Report of three cases. *J Neurosurg* 69:934–939.

105. Wyburn-Mason R (1943): *The vascular abnormalities and tumours of the spinal cord and its membranes.* London: H. Kimpton.

106. Yasargil M, DeLong W, Guarnaschelli J (1975): Arteriovenous malformations of the spinal cord. In: Symon L, ed. *Advances and technical standards in neurosurgery.* Vienna: Springer-Verlag, pp. 61–102.

107. Yasargil MG, DeLong WB, Guarnaschelli JJ (1975): Complete microsurgical excision of cervical craniocervical and intramedullary vascular malformations. *Surg Neurol* 4:211–224.

108. Yasargil MG, Symon L, Teddy PJ (1984): Arteriovenous malformations of the spinal cord. *Adv Tech Stand Neurosurg* 11:61–102.

109. Zarski S, Styczynski T (1978): Zylakowatosc dolnego odcinka kanalu kregowego. *Neurol Neurochir Pol* 12:67–72.

PART III

CERVICAL SPINE

Editor: Thomas S. Whitecloud III

The Adult Spine: Principles and Practice,
2nd edition, J.W. Frymoyer, Editor-in-Chief.
Lippincott-Raven Publishers, Philadelphia © 1997.

CHAPTER 52

Anatomy and Pathology of the Cervical Spine

Wolfgang Rauschning

Increasingly detailed studies of the anatomy of the spine have been necessitated both by the development of new surgical techniques and improved instrumentations, as well as by the advent of computerized imaging techniques, especially computed tomography (CT) and magnetic resonance (MR) tomography (2–4,11,13–18).

The classical descriptive gross anatomy, systematized into categories such as osteology, myology, syndesmology, angiology, and so forth is necessary for the elementary understanding of structures, their function, and of basic designative terms. For the clinician, diagnostician, and surgeon alike, topographic relational and clinical anatomy are of greater value. Topographic relationships in two dimensions, such as displayed in computerized tomograms, are extremely difficult to interpret and comprehend in their three-dimensional context.

These recent developments have prompted surgeons and radiologists (and a few anatomists) to study various aspects of clinical and imaging anatomy (2,7,11,13–18). New techniques, such as plastination, casting, cryodissection, and injection molding, have been developed. The images in the current chapter have been created with the Uppsala Cryoplaning Technique, which allows detailed assessment of bone and soft tissue relationships in frozen and undecalcified specimens (14).

In this chapter the running text briefly alludes to some clinically significant anatomic features of the cervical spine. The normal and imaging correlation anatomy has been described elsewhere and in greater detail (15). Anatomy can neither be taught ex cathedra nor be verbalized in writing; it can only be seen and explored hands-on. This chapter contains only a small selection from a database of more than 30,000 images from more than 100 cervical spinal cadaveric studies. Along with illustrations of some normal anatomic relationships, examples of clinically relevant pathologic anatomy are presented.

Figures 1–3 are from the upper cervical spine and craniocervical junction. The unique atlantoaxial motion segment was formed by the assimilation of the bodies of C1 and C2. In these two segments roughly half of the rotatory movement of the entire cervical spine occurs (8). The atlantoaxial articulation (similar to the shoulder joint) lacks bony congruity and stability. Only ligaments and joint capsules resist excessive motion. A true synovial joint is located between the lateral masses of the atlas and axis and between the anterior arch of the atlas and the odontoid process (6). Another synovial joint is found between the transverse ligament (strictly speaking: the transverse portion of the cruciate ligament) and the dens

W. Rauschning, M.D., Ph.D.: Professor of Clinical Anatomy, Department of Orthopaedic Surgery, Uppsala University Academic Hospital, Uppsala, S-75185 Sweden; and the Swedish Medical Research Council.

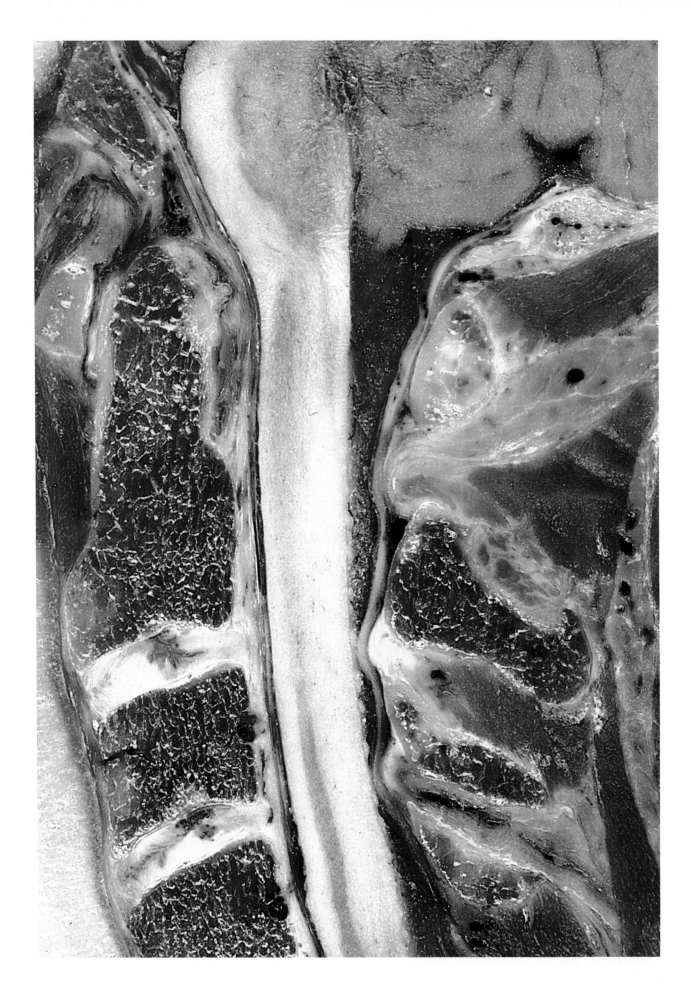

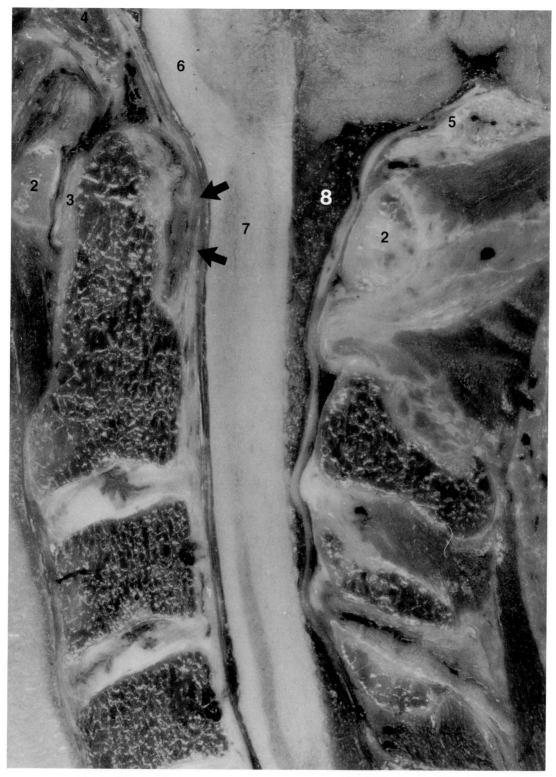

FIG. 1. Mid-sagittal section through the upper cervical spine of a 34-year-old man. The odontoid process (*1*) is the most prominent structure. Only that and the posterior arch (*2*) are seen. The true synovial joint between the anterior arch (*3*) of the atlas and the dens is degenerated in this specimen. Arrows indicate the transverse portion of the cruciate ligament which holds the odontoid process posteriorly. The "transverse ligament" is covered by the tectorial membrane which constitutes a reinforcement of a parietal blade of the dura mater and which is continuous with the dura mater of the skull (pachymeninx). In addition, the thin apical ligament of the dens directly anchors the tip of the dens to the clivus portion (*4*) of the foramen magnum. Posteriorly, the thin atlanto-occipital membrane connects the posterior arch of the atlas (*5*) with the rim of the foramen magnum. In the angle between the pons (*6*), the medulla oblongata (*7*), the cerebellar tonsils the posterior wall of the vertebral canal the cisterna magna is located (*8*).

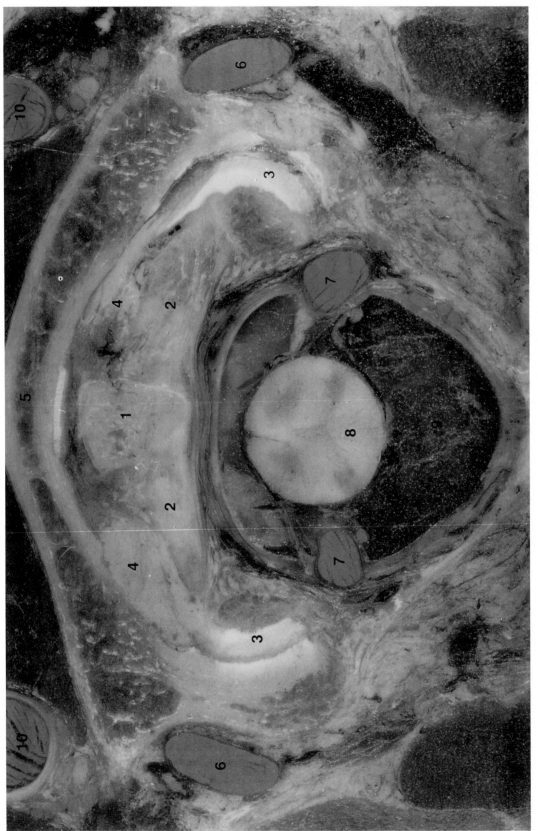

FIG. 2. Axial section through the superior portion of the atlas at the level of the tip of the odontoid process (*1*) lateral of which the strong alar ligaments (*2*) insert into notches at the anterior-inferior aspect of the occipital condyles (*3*). Richly vascularized areolar fat tissue (*4*) occupies the angles between the dens and the anterior arch of the atlas (*5*). Laterally the vertebral arteries (*6*) present as they curve posteriorly immediately after having left the transverse foramina of the atlas. A few millimeters cranial to this section the vertebral arteries (*7*) have pierced the atlanto-occipital membrane into the vertebral canal and are also traversing the thecal sac to become the intrathecal constituents of the basilar artery which forms by merging of these arteries anterior to the medulla oblongata in the midline. Posterior to the round lower medulla oblongata (*8*) the CSF compartment of the cisterna magna expands (*9*). Small intrathecal rootlets are located lateral to the medulla, thicker posterior rootlets are separated from thinner anterior root filaments by the suspensory dentate ligament. Anterior to the atlas lies the longus colli muscle. At their lateral aspect lie the internal carotid arteries (*10*) posterior to which the vagus nerve and the sympathetic trunk are located.

1060

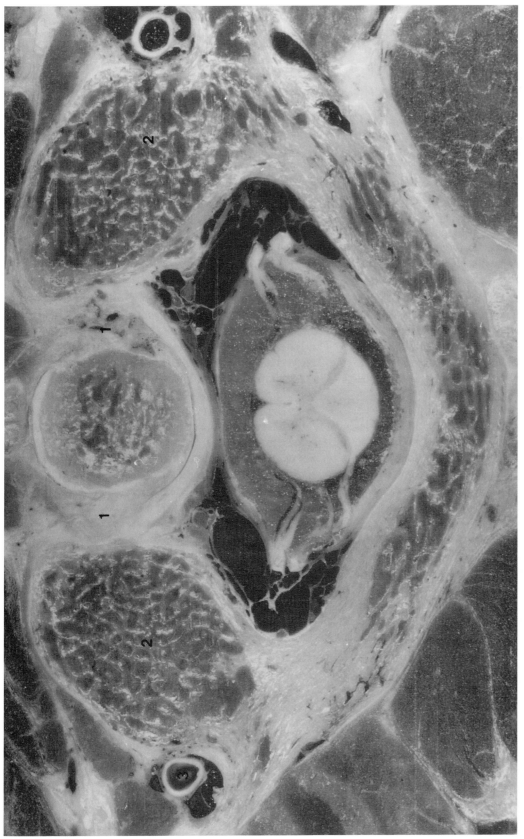

FIG. 3. Axial section of the atlas at the level of the lateral masses and the posterior arch and immediately inferior to the anterior arch. The mid-portion of the odontoid process displays articular cartilage anteriorly and also posteriorly where it articulates with the transverse ligament. Lateral to the dens loose areolar tissue with a rich supply of blood vessels and lymphatics is located (1). The lateral masses (2) are composed of strong cancellous bone whereas the arches contain more cortical bone. The vertebral arteries (3) are about to enter the transverse foramina of the atlas. They are surrounded by a rete of veins which is continuous with the venous sinusoids which surround the nerve roots in the root canals (periradicular venous plexus) and with the wide sinusoids which surround the thecal sac (epidural veins, internal vertebral venous plexus). These venous compartments display black on cadaveric sections because they are filled with cruor mortis. Note that these epidural veins constitute wide vascular compartments with relatively few septa rather than a serpiginous rete of veins. The thecal sac is oval and renders ample space for the spinal cord which clearly displays the anterior median fissure and the posterior median sulcus. A great number of rootlet filaments emerging from the anterolateral and posterolateral sulcus stepwise merge intrathecally to larger dorsal and ventral roots. The butterfly configuration of the gray matter is clearly outlined.

(Figs. 1 and 3). Far thicker than the transverse ligament and probably more important are the alar ligaments (Fig. 2). In addition, the tectorial membrane anchors the odontoid process directly to the skull base (foramen magnum).

The tip of the odontoid process abuts the lower pons and the medulla oblongata (Fig. 1). Posteriorly, the wide cisterna magna provides spatial reserve for a translatory posterior movement of the dens. The posterior soft tissue elements of the cervical spine are comparatively thin and resilient. These include the interlaminar ligamentum flavum, sparse strands of interspinous process ligament, and the flaccid joint capsules.

The spinous processes of the cervical spine are short and carry bifid tips. Contrary to textbook descriptions there is no supraspinous ligament. A complex suspensory system comprises a midsagittal septum of fibrous strands extending posteriorly in the midline and attaching to the strong elastic yellow ligamentum nuchae, which is continuous with the superficial layers of the thoracic aponeurosis and stretches from the spinous process of C7 to the occipital tubercle. In the neutral position, the ligamentum flavum bulges slightly anteriorly. This bulge is more pronounced in extension and disappears in flexion.

The anterior wall of the cervical vertebral canal is perfectly straight in normal specimens (Fig. 1). In extension, this wall displays no bulge from the discs but a segmental "shingling," which is caused by the retrolisthesis of the upper vertebra in relation to the lower vertebra. This retrolisthesis is caused by the obliquity of the facet joints (Figs. 4 and 5) which induces this translatory movement through coupled motion.

The cervical intervertebral discs allow this sagittal translation, whereas the uncinate processes effectively resist lateral movement that could have deleterious effect on the vertebral artery (2,6,7,9). The artery is tightly held in the costotransverse foramina of C3 to C6 and then runs through a knee-shaped, bony tunnel in the lateral mass of the axis and finally curves around the lateral aspect of the atlantoaxial joint (10). Instability at this level and/or osteoarthrotic lipping of the joint surfaces may erode the vertebral artery or cause arterial thrombosis (Figs. 6 and 7).

Figure 5 also displays meniscoid synovial folds in the facet joints of the midcervical spine. Little is known about their function and their potential role in post-traumatic, degenerative, and inflammatory neck pain (6,12,15). The author has observed significant post-traumatic changes, such as fresh ruptures, entrapment, and late fibrosis in these meniscoids (16,18).

In the cervical spine below C2, the segmental nerves have to transgress a distance of about 2 cm from the piercing of the thecal sac to the tubercles of the transverse process. Whereas the lumbar nerves invariably curve around the inner, inferior border of the pedicle of the upper vertebra of the motion segment, the cervical nerves run over the upper border of the pedicles and slope laterally and anteroinferiorly along the upper surface of the composite transverse process, which is formed by the transverse process proper posteriorly and the anterior assimilated rib equivalent (Anlage in German). Both bony processes are connected by the distally convex intertransverse bar that forms the lateral border of the costotransverse foramen. The cervical spinal nerves exit their root canals through a musculotendinous slit between the scalenus muscles/tendons that insert into the tubercles of the transverse process and the rib anlage process (4,9,12,15).

Figure 4 also shows the topographic relationships in a C5-C6 motion segment of a spine which had been frozen *in situ* in moderate flexion. The epidural veins of the cervical spine are not a rete or convolute of veins but a system of wide communicating sinusoids that can fill and empty rapidly. This hydraulic system facilitates the swift and considerable volume variations of the osseoligamentous conduits that occur during the movements of the highly mobile cervical spine (15).

Extension decreases the sagittal diameter of the cervical vertebral canal. Retrolisthesis of the upper vertebra of the motion segment pushes its lower end-plate toward the spinal cord, which is bound anterolaterally by the roots that in turn are attached to the walls of the root canals. This does not occur in the more rigid thoracic spine (Fig. 8).

Extension allows the ligamentum flavum to retract and thicken by volume redistribution and relaxation of its pretension. This thickening occurs underneath the lamina. This dynamic effect of extension is even more accentuated in the root canals because the posterior movement of the lower end-plate of the suprajacent vertebra compresses the neural bundle against the anterior surface of the superior articular process.

The "root" is a complex structure composed of structurally and neurophysiologically highly dissimilar elements: the root sleeve, housing intrathecal motor and sensory roots, the highly vascularized and pressure-sensitive dorsal root ganglion, which at this level is still separate from the motor root, and finally the postganglionic composite spinal nerve. Pressure exerted on the "root" may trigger different neurodysfunctional phenomena, depending on which of the components of the root is compromised. Even though the term *root* is short, concise, and established, its complex composition of structural and neurophysiologically dissimilar elements may be better designated by terms such as *root complex* or *root bundle*.

In its long course through the root canal, the root sleeve, ganglion, and nerve cannot yield superiorly because the root lies in a deep oblique furrow at the anterior aspect of the superior articular process (Fig. 5). In degenerative conditions such as spondylosis and uncovertebral arthrosis, the uncinate process becomes sclerotic and hypertrophic (Fig. 7) and sometimes curves posteriorly.

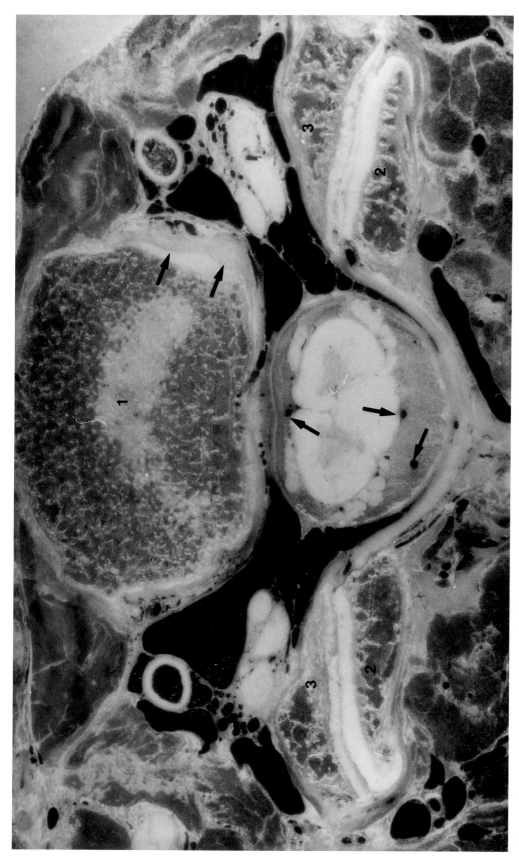

FIG. 4. Axial section through the C5–C6 motion segment of a normal cervical spine which was positioned and frozen in situ in moderate flexion. The osseous elements are the lower endplate of C5 (*1*) which on the right also displays the uncovertebral cleft (*arrows*), the inferior articular processes of C5 (*2*), and the upper articular processes of C6 (*3*). The oblique orientation of the articular facets of the cervical spine (see Fig. 5) causes a translatory anterior movement of C5 in relation to C6, considerably widening the sagittal diameter of the vertebral canal as well as the long osseoligamentous intervertebral conduits which commonly are referred to as neuroforamina but which rather constitute radicular or root canals of more than 2 cm length from the offset of the root sleeve from the dura to the tubercles of the transverse process. The thecal sac, the root sleeves, and the vertebral arteries are surrounded by one large continuous venous compartment which is subdivided only by a few thin membranes and septa. The thecal sac is almost round, posteriorly bordered by (but not attached to) the arcade of the interlaminar ligamentum flavum. Anteriorly the dura is firmly affixed to the posterior longitudinal ligament which "fans out" as it approaches the endplates and the disc, firmly attaching the dura anteriorly at each motion segment. The flexion causes the spinal cord to move anteriorly in the thecal sac. Tension variations of the roots in various postures and the denticulate ligament control the movements of the spinal cord. Note the anterior and posterior spinal arteries and veins on the surface of the spinal cord and a free artery in the subarachnoid space (*arrow*).

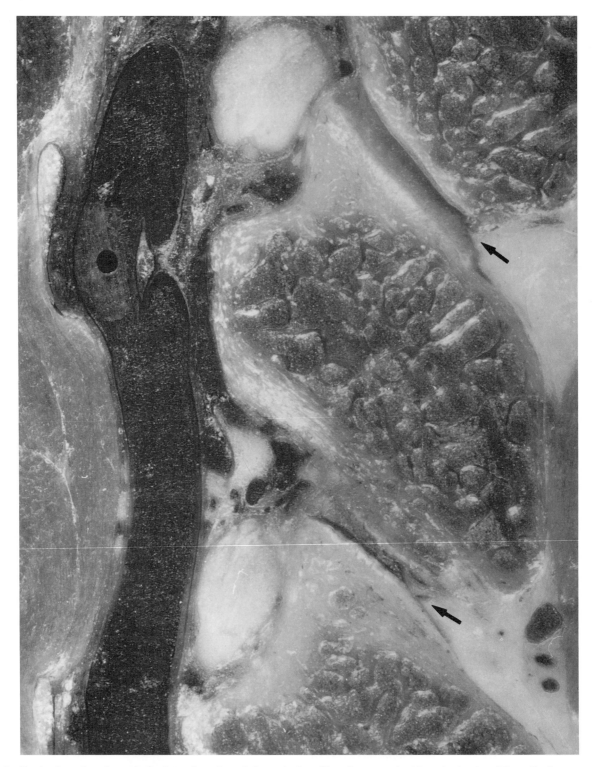

FIG. 5. Sagittal section through the lateral portion of the articular pillar of a normal midcervical spine. The articular masses are roughly rhomboid and carry obliquely sloping articular facets dorso-superiorly and ventro-inferiorly into which circumferential meniscoid synovial folds (tags) project (*arrows*). Anterior to the upper articular process deep notches accommodate the root sleeve, ganglion portion of the root, and the postganglionic cervical spinal nerve. This section also displays the vertebral artery (here *black*) running through the transverse foramina of the vertebrae. Anteriorly the artery is bounded by the thin bony shell of the rib anlage portion of the composite transverse process (see text).

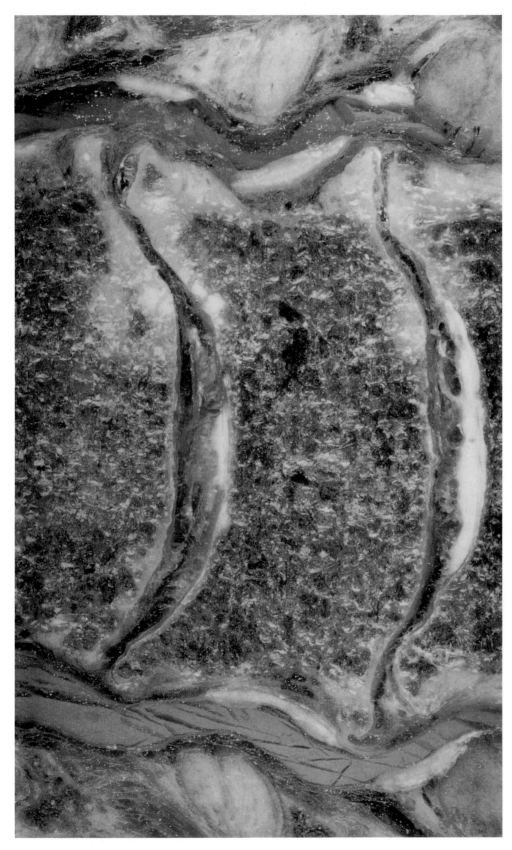

FIG. 6. Coronal section through a severely degenerated lower cervical spine of a 70-year-old woman who had neck pain but no history of radiculopathy or vertebral artery insufficiency. The spondylosis (degeneration between the vertebral bodies, i.e., the "disc joint") encompasses severe degeneration of the intervertebral discs and endplate sclerosis especially in the uncovertebral pseudojoints at which reactive degenerative bone apposition entails ridging which segmentally displaces the vertebral arteries laterally, causing them to take an undulating serpiginous course. On both sides the segmental nerves emerge behind the vertebral artery (see Fig. 5).

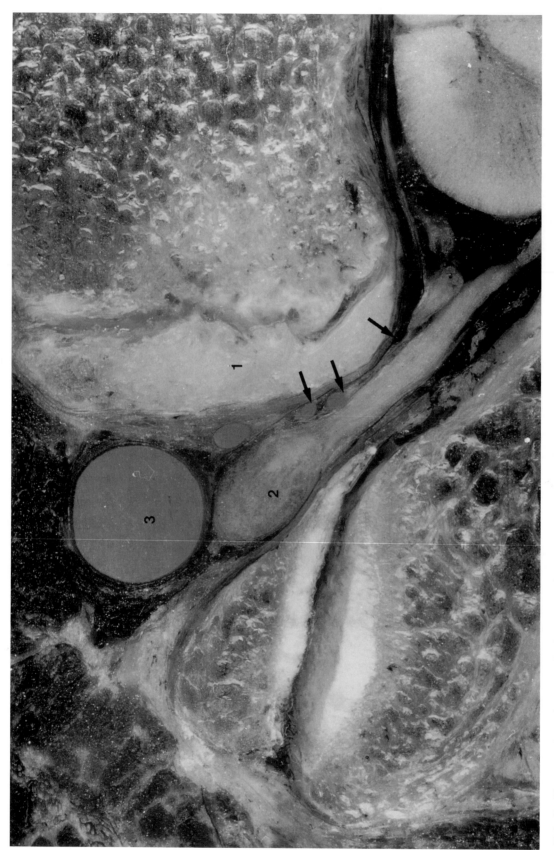

FIG. 7. Close-up view of a severely degenerated upper cervical spinal motion segment in axial section displaying advanced uncovertebral spondylosis and slight facet joint arthrosis. The uncinate process (*1*) has a sagittal orientation and is sclerotic and thickened, projecting laterally towards the vertebral artery (see also Fig. 6) and posteriorly into the root canal (foramen). Medially in the canal the motor root and the radicular arteries are compressed (*arrows*). The cylindrical and darker dorsal root ganglion (*2*) is buttressed against the superior articular process and its notch (see Fig. 6). Note the location of the vertebral artery (*3*) immediately anterior to the ganglion. The epidural and periradicular veins are small in this specimen. The orientation of the uncinate process and its relationships to the radicular structures and its contribution to neurovascular compromise is essential for the surgical strategy in decompressive procedures such as unco-foraminotomy. Most degenerated specimens displayed significant "anterior" encroachment emanating from the uncovertebral region. Facet joint osteophytes were usually small and rarely projected into the root canals.

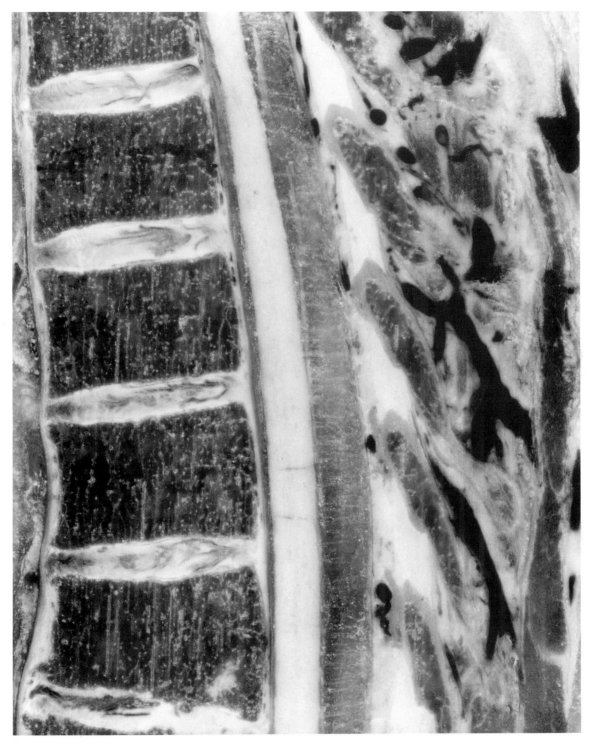

FIG. 8. Mid-sagittal section through the midthoracic spine of a 64-year-old female cadaver. The spine portion had been frozen in situ during routine autopsy in the supine position. The veins posterior to the spine are engorged as a result of rigor mortis; yet the spinal cord closely follows the vertebral bodies. All discs show degenerative changes, the disc between T9 and T10 is completely resorbed, and the cartilaginous endplates have fused. In the most spondylotic segments the anterior longitudinal ligament is thicker than in the less degenerated segments. Normally, thoracic discs have a perfectly straight posterior margin, even in extension they do not bulge into the vertebral canal. Of particular surgical interest is the relationship of the laminae to the intervening ligamentum flavum. The long slender spinous processes as well as the flat wide laminae overlap like obliquely sloping shingles, completely hiding the ligamentum flavum. The latter attaches to the adjacent laminae in a consistent fashion: It inserts into the anteriorly and slightly inferiorly directed surface of the suprajacent lamina and into the upper rim (margin) of the infrajacent lamina. Viewed from the spinal canal (anteriorly) only a narrow band of bone is visible; the posterior wall of the spinal canal thus is predominantly elastic-ligamentous, yet shielded by the "hidden" lamina portion. Note that the veins behind the dura (belonging to the posterior internal venous plexus) are invariably located at the level of the bony lamina, not the ligamentum flavum.

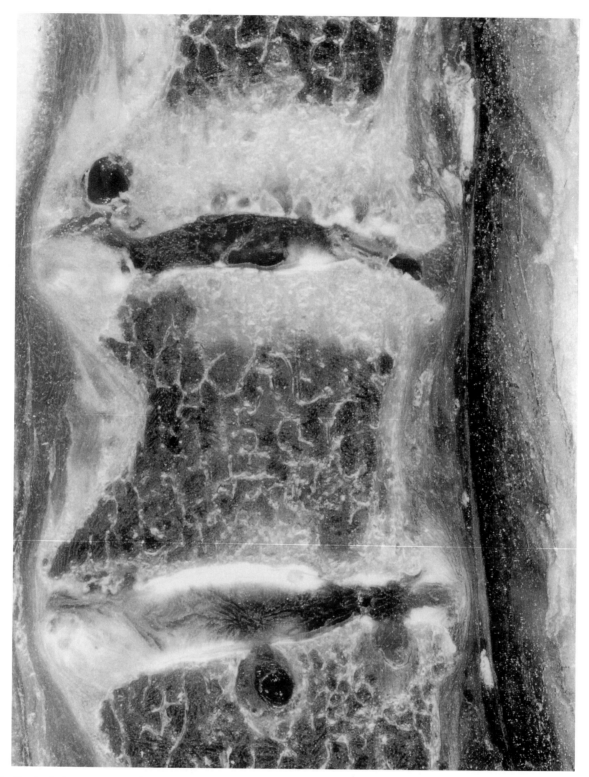

FIG. 9. Sagittal close-up view of two severely degenerated cervical spinal segments (C4–C5 and C5–C6) from a middle-aged woman who had suffered a significant "whiplash" injury 12 years before she died. All other discs had a normal appearance. At C4–C5, the disc is completely resorbed and the endplates are sclerotic. The disc space is occupied by gelatinous slightly hemorrhagic tissue. Posteriorly, endplate ridges project into the spinal canal. At the C5–C6 level, the anterior portion of the disc is reasonably intact whereas the central and posterior portions are liquified. In the upper endplate of C6 two large Schmorl's nodes communicate through defects of the bony endplate with the disc space. Note also the anterior endplate flanges which render the normally trapezoid sagittal cross-section of the cervical spinal vertebra an hourglass-shape. This close-up section shows the arrangement of the cancellous bony trabeculae and the dark gray bone marrow compartments.

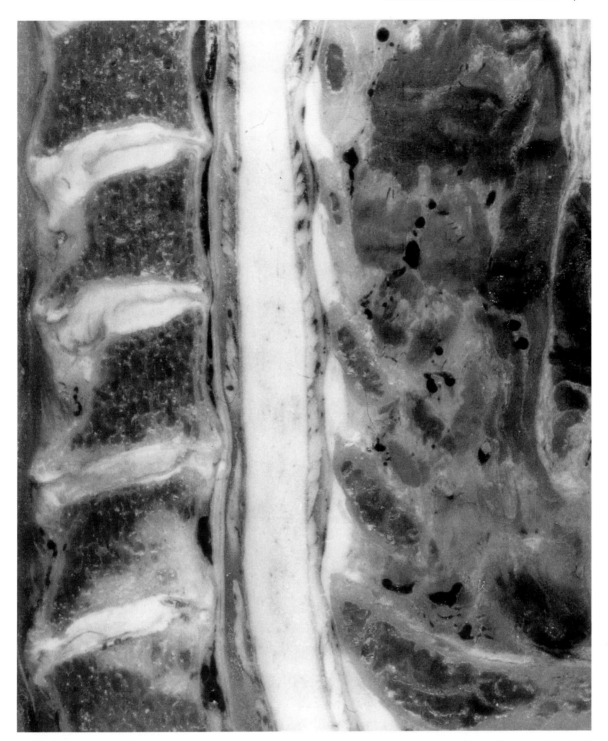

FIG. 10. Mid-sagittal section through the "sub-axial" cervical spine (from C3 to T1) of an elderly deceased who had a history of occasional neck pain but no neurological symptoms. At C5–C6, and even more pronounced at C6–C7, there are severe spondylotic changes. Anteriorly, the circumferential flanges present as a "spur" on this sectional image. At C5–C6 these flanges are ridging anteriorly and have almost fused by ossification of the anterior annulus fibrosus. The dark texture in most vertebral bodies represents cancellous bone with normal hematopoetic bone marrow. This contrasts to the lighter portions posteriorly in the bodies of C6 and C7 which represent eburnation (sclerosis) of the cancellous bone. The posterior ridging of the endplates renders a waist shape to the vertebrae and also entails a thickening of the anterior wall of the dura mater in the degenerated segments. Note that the dura in normal segments (e.g., C7–T1) is barely discernible. Since the height of the discs in this specimen is reasonably preserved, there is no infolding of the ligamentum flavum. The segmental narrowing caused by this multilevel spondylosis is an almost exclusively anterior phenomenon where "beaks" formed by the sclerotic endplate flanges and the intervening hard remnant of the posterior annulus segmentally indent the dura. Motion between these "beaks" and the thecal sac probably accounts for the reactive thickening of the dura. This thickening is a common observation during surgery in spondylotic spines.

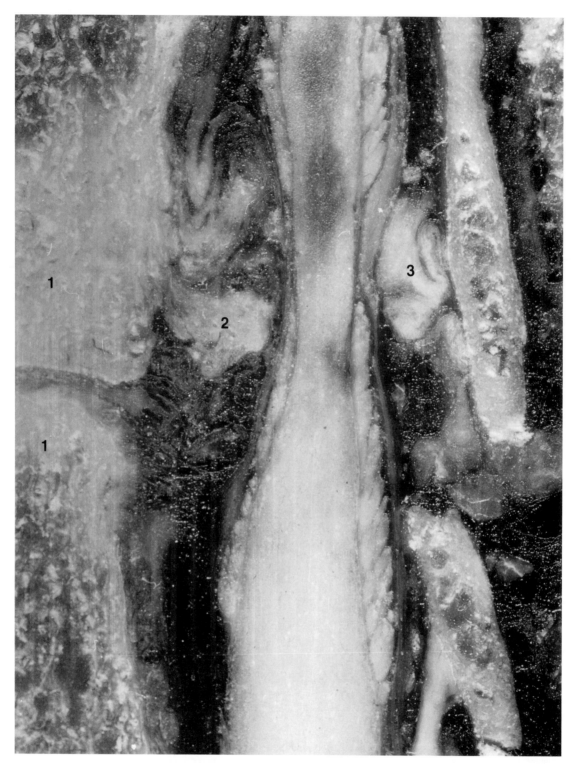

FIG. 11. A 63-year-old man was rendered tetraplegic after a traffic accident. He was operated on a C5–C6 fracture dislocation with posterior wiring and bone grafting but without anterior decompression and died two weeks post-operatively from respiratory and cardiovascular collapse. This paramedian sagittal close-up section shows sclerosis of the upper and lower endplate at the fracture level (*1*) and marked compression of the lateral portion of the spinal cord and the anterolateral and posterolateral intrathecal root filaments. Note the inveterated intramedullary hematoma. Spinal cord compression is caused anteriorly by a more than 2 cm wide spondylosis ridge (*2*) which is firmly attached to the vertebra by periosteum and peripheral annulus fibrosus lamellae. Posteriorly, the ruptured ligamentum flavum has retracted and is curled up under the lamina, abutting the anterior osseous compression by the bony flange (*3*). Especially the anterior bone fragment may be overlooked. If it cannot be removed, a hemicorpectomy or vertebrectomy may become necessary. Behind the lamina the wound hematoma and a bone graft are seen.

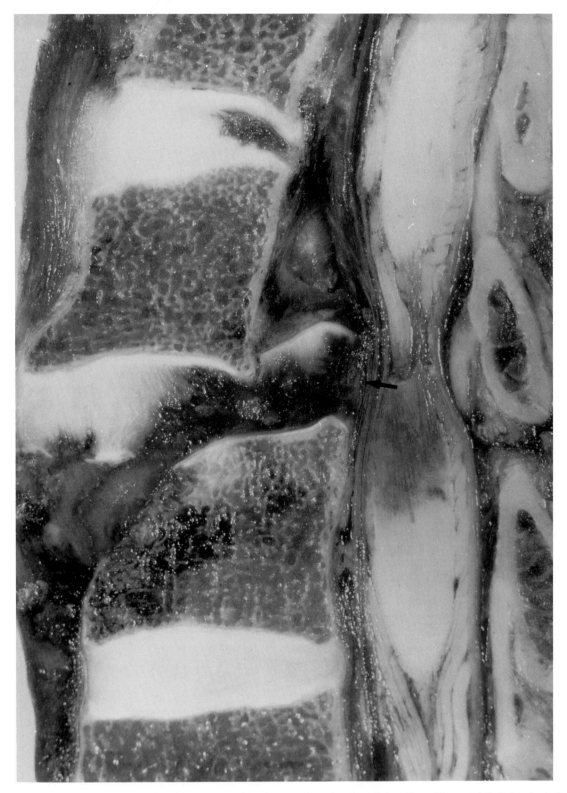

FIG. 12. Lower cervical spine of a young man who sustained a complete fracture dislocation with complete tetraplegia in a motor vehicle accident. He died after several closed reduction attempts from aspiration of massive stress ulcus hemorrhage. This paramedian sagittal section shows the anterior subluxation of the upper vertebra from which the annulus fibrosus and the periosteum and posterior longitudinal ligaments are stripped along the entire posterior surface of the vertebra, forming a triangular pouch into which large hinged disc fragments are dislodged. A small triangular ridge from the lower posterior endplate of the upper vertebra (*arrow*) effectively traps the disc fragments. Axial traction obviously would increase the compression of the cord. Note also the hemorrhage posteriorly in the disc above the fracture and the complete rupture of the interlaminar ligamentum flavum.

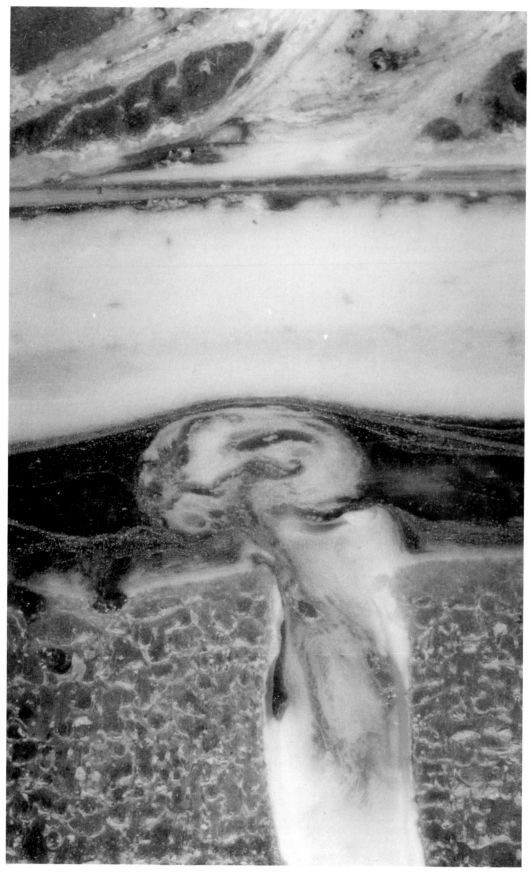

FIG. 13. Sagittal close-up view of a fresh, traumatic disc herniation in the cervical spine of a 23-year-old man who was run over by a car. During forensic autopsy, severe fractures of the facial skeleton as well as a fracture of the skull base were found, but no lesions of the cervical spine were seen. Plain AP, lateral, and oblique x-rays of the specimen were perfectly normal. Cryoplaning revealed a large herniation of the nucleus pulposus through a wide transverse rupture of the posterior annulus at its insertion into the apophyseal ring of C5. The herniation extended from the center of the spinal canal to the left side. Above and below the pedunculated disc fragment the venous sinuses are enlarged and engorged. The thecal sac at the level of the disc herniation is emptied of CSF and pushed posterior against the lamina. The anterior aspects of the dura and of the spinal cord are indented. The discs above and below this level both showed small ruptures of the posterior annulus fibrosus.

This immobilizes and encases the root bundle from anteriorly and superiorly. Compromise of the vertebral canal size and compression of the spinal cord have been observed when the lower end-plate carries spondylotic spurs and ridges, especially when the spine is extended and when ossification of the posterior longitudinal ligament is present (7–10,12,15,16) (Figs. 9 and 10).

Numerous fractures and traumatic soft tissue injuries of the cervical spine have been studied in great detail (1,5). A few pathomorphologic features in fracture dislocations of the elderly are shown in Figure 11. The clinical, diagnostic, and pathoanatomic data of the case presented in Figure 12 have been previously reported in detail (17). A traumatic disc herniation is shown in Figure 13. Our recent investigations include systematic assessment of cervical spinal injuries associated with skull fractures and detailed examinations of fractures and metastases of the cervical spine in which surgical decompression and/or stabilization had been conducted (11–13,16,18).

Only the diligent examination of spines of deceased patients in which surgery had been performed can render the immediate and vital feedback to the clinician that is necessary for both improvement of surgical techniques and the improvements of accuracy and specificity of the expensive computerized imaging modalities.

ACKNOWLEDGMENTS. The author wishes to thank the Swedish Medical Research Council, the Swedish Cancer Research Foundation, and the Trygg Hansa Insurance Company, Stockholm.

Halldór Jónsson, Jr., M.D., contributed Figure 13 in this chapter.

REFERENCES

1. Bohlman HH, Eismont FJ (1981): Surgical techniques of anterior decompression and fusion for spinal cord injuries. *Clin Orthop* (154):57–67.

2. Flannigan BD, Lufkin RB, McGlade C, Winter J, Batzdorf U, Wilson GH, Rauschning W, Bradley WG (1987): MR imaging of the cervical spine: neurovascular anatomy. *Am J Neuroradiol* 8:27–32.

3. Ghoshaajra K, Rao KC (1980): CT in spinal trauma. *J Comput Tomogr* 4:309–318.

4. Gonsalves CG, Hudson AR, Horsey WJ, Tucker WS (1978): Computed tomography of the cervical spine and spinal cord. *Comput Tomogr* 2:279–293.

5. Green BA, Callahan RA, Klose KJ, De La Torre J (1981): Acute spinal cord injury: current concepts. *Clin Orthop* (154):125–135.

6. Grieve GP (1981): *Common vertebral joint problems.* New York: Churchill Livingstone.

7. Hadley LA (1961): Anatomico-roentgenographic studies of the posterior spinal articulations. *Am J Roentgenol* 86:270–276.

8. Hohl M, Baker HR (1964): The atlanto-axial joint. Roentgenographic and anatomical study of normal and abnormal motion. *J Bone Joint Surg [Am]* 46:1739–1752.

9. Holt S, Yates PO (1966): Cervical spondylosis and nerve root lesions. Incidence at routine necropsy. *J Bone Joint Surg [Br]* 48:407–423.

10. Jones RT (1966): Vascular changes occurring in the cervical musculoskeletal system. *S Afr Med J* 40:388–390.

11. Jónsson H, Rauschning W, Petrén-Mallmin M, Andréasson I (1988): Pathoanatomy of cervical spine tumors and fractures studies with surface cryoplaning and correlations with CT and MRI. Cervical Spine Research Society Annual Meeting, Marseilles. *Orthop Trans* 12:454.

12. Payne EE, Spillane JD (1957): The cervical spine. An anatomico-pathological study of 70 specimens (using a special technique) with particular reference to the problem of cervical spondylosis. *Brain* 80:571–596.

13. Petrén-Mallmin M, Jónsson H Jr, Bring G, Sahlstedt B, Rauschning W (1989): Occult cervical spinal lesions in craniocerebral trauma. 75th Meeting of the Radiological Society of North America, Chicago. *Radiology* 173 (Suppl):29.

14. Rauschning W (1983): Computed tomography and cryomicrotomy of lumbar spine specimens. A new technique for multiplanar anatomic correlation. *Spine* 8:170–180.

15. Rauschning W (1985): Detailed sectional anatomy of the spine. In: SLG Rothman, WV Glenn, eds. *Multiplanar CT of the spine.* Baltimore: University Park Press, pp. 33–85.

16. Rauschning W, Jónsson H Jr, McAfee P (1989): Pathoanatomical and surgical findings in cervical spinal injuries. *J Spinal Dis* 2:213–222.

17. Rauschning W, Sahlstedt B, Wigren A (1980): Irreponible Luxationsfraktur der unteren Halswirbelsäule. Eine pathologisch-anatomische Studie mit der Gefrierschneidemethode. *Chirurg* 51:529–533.

18. Sahlstedt B, Bring G, Rauschning W, Jónsson H (1989): Radiographically occult cervical spinal lesions in fatal head injuries. *Acta Orthop Scand* (Suppl. 231) 60:41.

The Adult Spine: Principles and Practice,
2nd edition, J.W. Frymoyer, Editor-in-Chief.
Lippincott-Raven Publishers, Philadelphia © 1997.

CHAPTER 53

Biomechanics of the Cervical Spine

I. General Trauma

Martin H. Krag

Knowledge of the biomechanics of the cervical spine provides an essential framework for understanding the consequences of injury and other disorders, as well as intelligent planning for operative procedures and conservative treatment with orthoses. In this chapter, the anatomy of the cervical spine will be reviewed from the biomechanical perspective, including the issues of kinematics and instability. The biomechanics and classification of cervical injury then will be reviewed, followed by analysis of surgical constructs and orthoses.

SPINAL COMPONENT BIOMECHANICS

Vertebrae

Lower Cervical

The lower cervical vertebrae are usually considered to include C3 through C7, although T1 and even T2 to some extent function largely as if they were cervical.

M. H. Krag, M.D.: Department of Orthopaedics & Rehabilitation, McClure Musculoskeletal Research Center and Vermont Rehabilitation Engineering Center, University of Vermont, Burlington, Vermont 05405. `

Careful three-dimensional (3D) measurements of major features have been reported by Panjabi et al. (108). Each vertebra basically is made up of a cylindrical body with a group of posterior elements attached by means of the pedicles (Fig. 1). The body primarily serves as a compressive load-bearing element, and it is significantly smaller than that of the thoracic or lumbar vertebrae. For example the anteroposterior diameter of the body of C4 is slightly less than half that of L4 (8), which reflects the smaller loads imposed on the cervical vertebrae. The uncus or uncinate process (68), also known as the neurocentral lip (58), serves to modify the basic cylindrical shape of the body. It consists of a ridge oriented anteroposteriorly and slightly curved along each side of the upper endplate and is present from C3 to T1 (18). This functions as a rail (18) to provide resistance to lateral shifting, which would tend to happen with lateral loading of the superjacent vertebra. The region between the uncinate process and the superjacent vertebra is referred to as the uncovertebral joint or neurocentral joint of Luschka (74). Although there is some argument to the contrary, it does not seem to be a synovial joint (51,68,102,120,150).

The posterior elements function primarily as handles or levers for producing and controlling the vertebral mo-

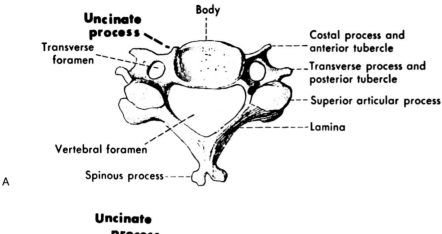

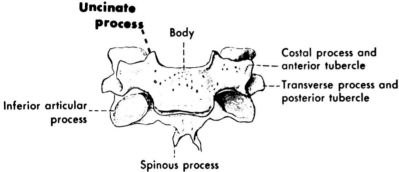

FIG. 1. Typical vertebra between C3 and C7. **A:** Superior view. **B:** Anterior view.

tion. Various muscles attach to each of the individual processes; virtually the only site at which muscles do not attach to the vertebrae is the anterior part of the body. This absence has clinical utility. During the anterior approach to the cervical spine, the nonmuscular gap between right and left longus colli muscles is a helpful landmark.

The increase in length of the spinous processes between C3 and T1 or T2 is consistent with the increase in torque along the spine needed to resist a given load on the head (Fig. 2). The longer the spinous process, the greater the leverage that the attached muscle has available to produce torque. However, if the spinous processes protruded too far posteriorly in the midline, adjacent ones would hit each other during extension of the neck. Because the spinous processes of the central cervical vertebrae are bifid, these processes "nest" together in extension, which allows a greater range of motion than would otherwise be possible (Fig. 2).

The articular processes, which make up the facet (or apophyseal) joints, provide major resistance to anterior shifting (translation) of each vertebra on its subjacent vertebra. Additional resistance is also provided by muscles whose orientation results in a component of anteroposterior pull. The facet joint is a major determinant of the intervertebral motion (53), although by no means is it the only one. Indeed, the concept that the facet joints control the motion is an oversimplification and will be discussed further in the section on kinematics.

The orientation of the articular surfaces is different in the cervical region than in either the thoracic or the lumbar region, and it also differs within the cervical region itself (Fig. 3). Detailed 3D measurements are provided by Panjabi et al. (113). The articular plane is almost transverse at C1-C2, but at C2-C3 it abruptly steepens to 55° to 60° above the plane of the inferior endplate, or 45° to the longitudinal axis of the spinal canal (18,34,76). It then remains approximately constant to C7-T1. At and below C3-C4, the facet joint planes are perpendicular to the sagittal plane, which allows easy visualization of the articular space by lateral view x-ray. At C2-C3, however, the joint planes also slope anterolaterally by 10° to 20° (18) and thus normally are not as clearly seen on lateral view x-ray. The transitional nature of C2-C3 (i.e., between C1-C2 and C3-C4) has been detailed by Mestdagh (91).

The transverse processes provide an important basis for attachment of various neck muscles, both anteriorly and posteriorly. The vertebral arteries pass through the foramina of the transverse processes. The C7 transverse process typically has neither foramen nor any scalene muscle origination.

The foramina, formed between adjacent pedicles and continuing anterolaterally by the transverse processes on each side, are all oriented approximately parallel when the neck is in the neutral position. The orientation of the foramina is anterolaterally 45° and anterocaudad 15°. Either axial rotation of the head relative to the thorax or

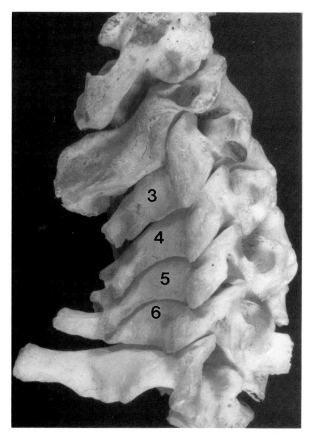

FIG. 2. Spinous process length gradually increases caudally. Synovial joint orientation at C1-C2 is transverse, whereas below this it is oblique. Bifid spinous processes "nest" together to allow extension without decrease in spinous process length.

Upper Cervical

The occipito-atlanto-axial (or Oc-C1-C2) complex is a highly specialized articulation to provide a relatively large range of motion between the head and torso. The special nature of this region (Fig. 4) is reflected by the absence of any intervertebral discs. All the articulations are synovial joints. For this reason, the majority of cervical spine problems caused by rheumatoid arthritis are in this upper region, most commonly C1-C2 subluxation or Oc-C1 settling (10). The complexity of this structure requires quite elaborate embryologic development (142), including the "theft" of the C1 vertebral body by C2 to form the odontoid. Not surprisingly, a variety of abnormalities can occur (74), such as various degrees of hypoplasia of the posterior arch of C1 or of the odontoid. An extensive treatise on this region has been published by Von Torklus and Gehle (154).

The basic structure of the Oc-C1-C2 complex is a biconcave ring (C1) interposed between two convex structures: the occipital (Oc) condyles from above and the upper facets of the C2 lateral masses from below. In addition, the odontoid (or dens) projects upwards from C2 to provide a post to which are anchored both the C1 ring and the occiput. The major ligamentous connec-

shifting of the head forward (capital protraction) will cause the foraminal axes to be no longer parallel. These relationships have particular importance when cervical radiographs are obtained. If oblique films are obtained with the x-ray source located posteriorly and the patient upright (central beam 45° medially, 15° caudad; plate perpendicular to central beam), there is a tendency for both axial rotation and capital protraction to occur, resulting in poor visualization of the foramina. If instead the oblique films are taken with the X-ray source anteriorly (central beam 45° medially, 15° cephalad), there is less tendency for these malpositions to occur.

Anterior oblique films may be accomplished either with the patient upright, which allows the cassette easily to be perpendicular to the central beam and thus gridded, or with the patient supine and the cassette horizontal at 45° to the central beam and thus nongridded. The supine technique is particularly useful in assessing the traumatized patient, since no movement is needed. The absence of a grid and the "smearing out" from cassette angulation present minimal problems in film interpretation.

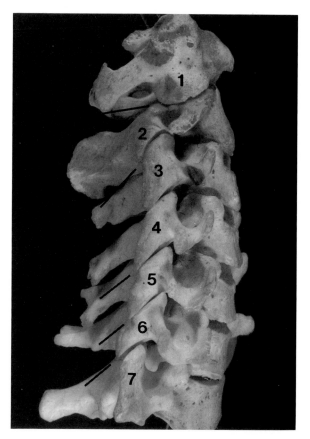

FIG. 3. The facet orientation and its change at different anatomic levels.

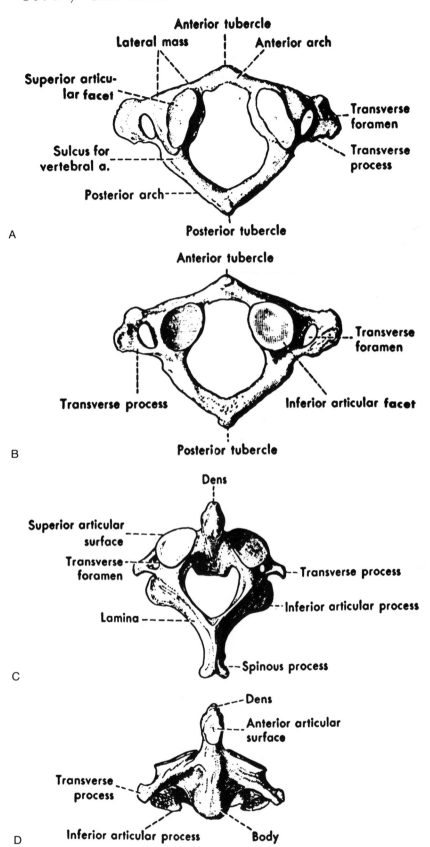

FIG. 4. C1 and C2 vertebrae. **A:** C1 superior. **B:** C1 inferior. **C:** C2 superior. **D:** C2 anterior.

tions of the Oc are not to C1 but instead directly to C2, as detailed below. The Oc condyles are oriented approximately anteroposteriorly but converge somewhat anteriorly, and fit into corresponding concavities on the upper surface of the C1 lateral masses. The right and left portions of this joint are similar to miniature versions of the medial and lateral portions of the knee joint. The C1-C2 articulation consists of three joints: one between the odontoid and C1 anterior arch, and two (right and left) between the lateral masses of C1 and of C2.

Discs

As mentioned previously, there is no disc between the occiput and C1 or between C1 and C2. The discs from C2-C3 and below are very similar in structure, consisting of an outer fibrous ring (annulus fibrosus) and a central semisolid core (nucleus pulposus). One characteristic of this specialized structure appears to be its ability to transmit compressive loads throughout a range of motion and yet to prevent excessive stress concentration from occurring. This seems to be accomplished by posterior shifting of the nucleus with flexion and anterior shifting during extension (78,79) in the lumbar spine; presumably the same mechanism occurs in the cervical spine. Similar to those in the lumbar spine, herniations of the cervical nucleus pulposus tend to occur posterolaterally, where the rate of curvature of the annulus fibrosus is the greatest. This leads to stress concentration and fiber breakdown (160), which weaken the annulus and may allow herniation to occur. Unfortunately, the very site where herniations occur most often is the site at which the nerve root is the most closely applied to the annulus, setting the stage for the clinical problem of cervical radiculopathy from either disc herniation or osteophyte formation.

Ligaments

Ligaments may be considered as spanning across either multiple motions segments or only a single motion segment. The only significant ligament in the first category is the ligamentum nuchae, which usually is a dense, fibrous, posterior midline band that runs from the external occipital protuberance to the spinous process of C7; the attachments to C2-C6 are much less substantial (72). Perhaps this is the reason why "clay shoveler's" fractures (139) (avulsion of the spinous process) typically occur at C7. This structure is generally considered to provide a major constraint to excessive cervical flexion (19,21,23), although Halliday et al. (62) and Johnson et al. (75) have found this not always to be the case. Ligaments spanning across individual motion segments may be considered in two groups.

Lower Cervical

The major ligaments from front to back are the anterior longitudinal ligament (ALL), intertransverse process ligaments, posterior longitudinal ligament (PLL), facet joint capsules, ligamentum flavum, interspinous ligament, and supraspinous ligament (SL). Although the ALL, PLL, and SL span multiple levels, they attach at each individual vertebra, unlike the ligamentum nuchae. Careful and clinically relevant anatomic descriptions have been reported by various authors, for example Johnson et al. (75). Quantitative 3D descriptions are reported by Panjabi et al. (112). Biomechanical testing (static and dynamic) of isolated bone–ligament–bone preparations of ALL and of ligamentum flavum has been reported by Yoganandan et al. (164). The rich innervation of facet joint capsules has been described by Wyke (163) who infers from this a possible proprioceptive role for the capsule. The effect of ligament damage on motion segment behavior is described later in the section on hyperflexibility.

Upper Cervical

As mentioned previously, the odontoid of C2 provides a sturdy post to which are anchored both the Oc and the ring of C1. The Oc is attached directly, without intermediate C1 attachment, to the odontoid (Fig. 5) by the alar ligaments (50) and the much less substantial apical ligament and the upper arm of the cruciform ligament. The C1 ring is attached to the odontoid by the quite sturdy transverse ligament (or transverse arms of the cruciform ligament) as well as the accessory C1-C2 ligaments (or C1-C2 portion of the alar ligament) (47) and C1-C2 facet capsules. Panjabi et al. (111) measured the lengths and 3D orientations of the apical, transverse, and alar ligaments. Dvořák et al. (50) showed that the tensile strength of the transverse ligament was almost twice as strong (350 newtons) as that of the alar ligaments (200 N). The connection between the Oc and C1 is less substantial and is really limited just to the facet joint capsules.

Careful study of cadaveric Oc-C1 and C1-C2 motion before and after alar or C1-C2 capsular ligaments has been performed (35,36,99,106,107). Increases in axial rotation of C1-C2 produced by a 1.5 Nm torque to the right were as follows: 1° from cutting the left C1-C2 capsular ligament, 2° from cutting left and right C1-C2 capsular ligaments, 1.9° from cutting the left alar ligament, and 2.4° from cutting left and right alar ligaments. Cutting of the left alar ligament allows increases in not only right, but also left axial rotation, contrary to what has often been assumed (35,36,107). The clinical significance of these results obtained using such a small torque as 1.5 Nm remains to be established.

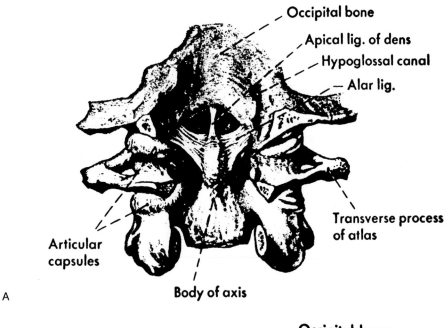

Occipital bone
Apical lig. of dens
Hypoglossal canal
— Alar lig.
Transverse process of atlas
Body of axis
Articular capsules

A

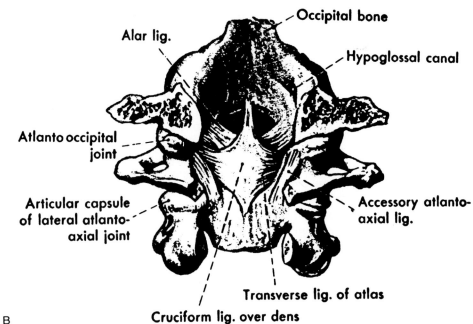

Occipital bone
Hypoglossal canal
Alar lig.
Atlanto occipital joint
Articular capsule of lateral atlanto-axial joint
Accessory atlanto-axial lig.
Transverse lig. of atlas
Cruciform lig. over dens

B

FIG. 5. Ligaments between occiput, C1, and C2 seen from the dorsal aspect. **A:** After removal of posterior elements and posterior longitudinal ligament. **B:** After removal of the cruciform ligament.

Muscles and Tendons

The role of muscles and tendons in the neck is to produce motion and control position of the head relative to the thorax. The passive elements (bone, disc, ligaments, joints) exert important control over translations, as well as the location of the centers of rotation. However, the angles of rotation are controlled almost totally by the muscles, except perhaps at the end of the range of motion when ligaments dominate. The spinal column certainly does not function as a stiff rod that can support itself upright, but rather it functions as a series of ball and socket joints which require muscle action to prevent buckling collapse (158).

The general structure of these tissues in the neck is similar to that throughout the multisegmented axial skeleton in that there are some gross-function muscles that span across many or a few motion segments, and other fine-function muscles that cross just one or two segments. The gross-function muscles anteriorly are the longus colli, longus capitis, and scalenes which originate from either the vertebral bodies or the transverse processes. The fine-function anterior muscles are the intertransversarii, which span just one segment. Posteriorly, the gross-function muscles attached to the spinous processes are the splenius capitis and semispinalis cervices; attached to the transverse processes are longissimus cervices and iliocostalis cervices. The posterior fine-function muscles are either between spinousprocesses (interspinals), between transverse processes (intertransversarii), or cross from spinous to transverse processes (long and short rotatores).

Another general feature of the neck muscles is the large extent to which their orientation is angulated off-axis, or away from the longitudinal axis of the spine. Muscles oriented parallel to the longitudinal axis can efficiently produce the head rotations of flexion, extension, or lateral bendings, but it is the off-axis muscles that are needed to efficiently produce shifting (translation) of the head anteriorly, posteriorly, or laterally, as well as rotation about the longitudinal axis. For example, rotation of the head and upper cervical spine toward the right is caused by contraction of the right sternocleidomastoid and upper trapezius muscles as well as the left splenius capitis and longissimus capitis muscles. Quantitative detail of muscle-site attachments and muscle forces *in vivo* and *in vitro* have been determined for purposes of neck biomechanical models (39,94,97). A recent functionally oriented review of muscle structure has also been reported by Parke and Sherk (119). Interesting work has been done by Ashton-Miller et al. (9) about the activity of various neck muscles during controlled, noxious stimulation of the sternocleidomastoid muscle by localized, hypertonic saline injection.

Muscle bulk in the neck is notably more massive posteriorly than anteriorly. This is related to the general tendency for the head to be positioned in such a way that its center of gravity is positioned anteriorly to the vertical support provided by the spinal column. This feature is obviously the case for quadrupeds, but it is also true for bipeds. This feature, plus the much more extensive muscular attachment to the spinous processes than to the anterior aspect of the vertebral body, typically requires more muscular disruption during posterior surgical approaches than during anterior approaches.

The extent to which tendons are used within the cervical spine is fairly limited. Some of the small, fine-function muscles have a tendinous insertion to small attachment sites, such as the rotatores to the spinous processes. The role of tendons to allow a change in muscle direction around a pulley-like structure is encountered in the neck only with the omohyoid, the superior and inferior bellies of which are typically separated by a tendinous portion that passes through a fascial sling to the clavicle (81).

Cord, Dura, and Nerve Roots

Three major topics will be discussed, each of which has direct clinical relevance.

Effect of Neck Motion

Because the spinal cord is situated posteriorly to the centers of rotation for vertebral flexion and extension, it becomes longer and thinner with flexion, and shorter and thicker with extension. Breig (19–23,25) has written extensively about this phenomenon. He performed dissections of cadavers and studied dynamic air myelograms of patients, and he observed overall spinal cord length changes of 45 to 75 mm. More recently, this phenomenon has been demonstrated by magnetic resonance scanning (32). An associated phenomenon is the longitudinal motion of the cord produced during flexion-extension relative to each vertebra. The "neutral point" at which no relative motion occurs between cord and vertebrae is at C5 [for humans (127)] or C4 [for primates (145)]. Maximum relative shifting of up to 18 mm occurred in the upper thoracic region (127).

Tensile forces in the neural elements produced by cervical flexion are carried primarily by the dura (19,152) and the pia–arachnoid (153) rather than the cord and nerve roots, and they are balanced by tensile forces not from the filum terminale but rather from the nerve roots (145). These forces are transmitted to the cord predominantly by the dentate ligaments rather than the roots and rootlets themselves (19,127,153).

The effect of these mechanical changes on clinical findings or neurophysiologic function was investigated extensively by Breig (19–25), who described patients with spondylitic myelopathy, acute trauma, or multiple sclerosis in whom flexion worsened the neurologic deficits or produced Lhermitte's sign (26,84). Because he observed a decrease in anteroposterior compression of the cord with flexion (decreased cord diameter and increased canal diameter), he reasoned by exclusion that the increased neurologic deficits resulted from increased contact pressure against the anterior aspect of the cord, caused by forward shifting of the cord resulting from the flexion–induced tension. For cervical trauma or spondylosis, the contacting object is outside the cord (disc or endplate spurs); for multiple sclerosis it is within the cord (sclerotic lesion). The biomechanical result is essentially the same for both (20). This same author developed a surgical technique ("cervicolordodesis") that involved a connective tissue graft in the posterior aspect of the neck to limit flexion, and he reported favorable results in 21 patients (22,23). For acute trauma management, Breig (25) recommended avoidance of flexion not only to prevent abnormal intervertebral motion, but also to prevent increased cord tension, which might cause or worsen neural damage.

Spinal Cord's Internal Stress/Strain

The relationship between internal stresses and strains and spinal cord injury production was investigated early on by McVeigh (90) who noted that axial compressibility was greater for the central gray matter than for the peripheral white matter. This topic is also contained in Ommaya's review of earlier literature (101). It has also been noted (27,86,136,137) that external cord compression causes greater tissue damage centrally than peripherally. The connection between these findings is the stress distribution that develops within spinal cord models, which has been reviewed and illustrated by Panjabi and White (115). Also related to this stress distribution is the viscoelastic behavior of the cord (140).

Experimental Cord Trauma

An experimental technique important for understanding the pathophysiology and improving the treatment of cord trauma is the creation of known, carefully controlled cord trauma. Allen's method (2) from 1911 was used for decades (42,44), but it was flawed from a biomechanical viewpoint (44). Using a more appropriate measure for the mechanical injuring input (impulse rather than the Allen method of mass multiplied by drop distance), Dohrmann and Panjabi (43) were able to establish a direct correlation between mechanical input and cord lesion volume. The experimental technique (105) also measured impact force over time and isolated cord deflection from thoracic deflection. Hung et al. (69) have also used a standardized impact load, and Somerson and Stokes (146) have developed an electromechanical injuring device. Most recently, Panjabi and Wrathall (118) have reported on the strong correlation between carefully controlled biomechanical input and *in vivo* functional outcome.

SPINAL COMPOSITE BIOMECHANICS

The components described above are the building blocks for the cervical spine. The manner in which they function together in the cervical spine has many different aspects. Three aspects that are particularly relevant clinically will be discussed here.

Kinematics

The motion or kinematics of the cervical spine is not determined solely by the passive elements (facets, disc, ligaments, bone) but is also influenced by the active elements (muscles and tendons). An obvious example is forward flexion of the head relative to the thorax. For any specified position of the head, there is an infinite number of different postures that may be assumed by the cervical vertebrae, each produced by different amounts of contraction of the various cervical muscles. A less obvious example is that even with forward flexion of a single motion segment, subtle variations in anteroposterior or axial rotational position may occur. Resulting abnormal motion of the facet joints may be one cause of snapping noises in the neck. Because muscle action can affect the kinematics, interpretation of cadaveric biomechanical studies must be performed carefully, especially when multivertebral specimens are used.

To define the motion of an object in 3D space requires six independent numbers, for example three coordinates (along the x, y, and z axes) to specify the translation or shifting of the object and three angles (about the x, y, and z axes) to specify the rotation of the object. Such motion is thus said to have six degrees of freedom. For two-dimensional space such as a cervical flexion–extension radiograph, only three independent numbers are needed to specify the motion of an object such as the image of a vertebra. In this circumstance only three degrees of freedom exist. Choosing which three independent numbers to use is a matter of convenience. One choice (Fig. 6A) would be to use the x and y components of translation of point 1 and the rotation angle A. The value of A will be the same regardless of where on the object it is measured; however, the x and y components will be different for each point (unless A = 0). Another choice (Fig. 6B) for these three independent numbers would be to use the x and y location of the center of rotation (CR), and again the angle A, which will be the same for the CR as for any other point on the object. The CR may be thought of as that one special point that has no translation (131).

Lower Cervical

A useful approximation of the range of motion at each motion segment between C2-C3 and C7-T1 is 10° for each of the following: total excursion from flexed to extended, axial rotation to each side, and lateral bending to each side. There is a tendency for flexion–extension and

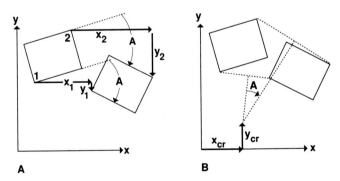

FIG. 6. Two different descriptions of planar vertebral motion, each of which requires three independent numbers. **A:** Motion x_1, y_1 of vertebral point 1 and vertebral rotation angle A. Note that motion x_2, y_2 at any other point 2 will be different from that at point 1. **B:** Location x_{cr}, y_{cr} of center of rotation and vertebral rotation angle A. Note that only a single center of rotation occurs, and that the rotation angle is still A.

axial rotation to be greatest in the mid-cervical region (decreasing both above and below this), and for lateral bending to be greatest at C2-C3, then to gradually decrease down the cervical spine (91). Also, there are fairly large variations in the values reported in the literature (55,85,157,158) and reviewed thoroughly by Dimnet et al. (40). Nonetheless, the above approximation is valid.

A number of recent motion studies have been performed. For rotations about all three axes, Ålund and Larsson (6) studied head versus thorax motion by five serially arranged goniometers in normal subjects. Intervertebral motion was measured by stereoradiography for normal subjects without implanted metallic markers (92), for cadavers with spinous process pins (134), and with implanted metallic point markers (83). Flexion-extension in normals was investigated by Dvorák et al. (49) [using a method (45) in which the examiner manually applies gentle force to the head].

For flexion-extension, the location of the CR for each pair of vertebrae is generally located within the body of the lower vertebra, but at progressively lower cervical levels it gradually shifts from a position in the lower dorsal quadrant (of C3 for C2-C3 motion) to the middle of the upper endplate (of C7 for C6-C7 motion) (18,121). The CR is also approximately at the center of the circle passing through the articular surface of the facet joint. Although the CR may move between steps of motion throughout the flexion-extension range, this motion (the tracing of which is known as the centrode) is relatively small compared to that in the lumbar spine (40). As flexion occurs, the amount of overlap or contact between the facets gradually decreases to the point that subluxation or actual dislocation can occur. Flexion-extension also causes changes in neural foramina and spinal canal dimensions. Yoo et al. (167) measured the former and showed a 10% increase from 0° to 30° flexion and a 13% decrease from 0° to 30° extension. Farmer and Wisneski (52) showed that neck extension increased intraforaminal pressure and that this was relieved by shoulder abduction. The spinal canal anteroposterior diameter was shown by Chen et al. (29) to be decreased from the flexed to the extended posture by 10.8% due to disc bulging and by 24.3% due to ligamentum flavum bulging.

For lateral bending, the CR for each pair of vertebrae is located not in the lower vertebral body but rather in the upper one, because of the constraints imposed by the uncinate processes. For axial rotation, both the uncinate processes and the facet joints constrain the motion. Because the facet joint planes are perpendicular to the sagittal plane, these joints must either open up sightly (e.g., right joint opens with right axial rotation), or some lateral bending must occur. Probably it is the latter that most typically happens. The combination of these two movements is really equivalent to rotation of the neck about a vertical axis with the neck in a forward inclined position (121). This movement is very commonly used

and allows minimal constraint to motion by the facet joints. In this circumstance, the rotation axis is perpendicular to the articular plane, therefore the articular processes need only slide along and not separate from each other.

To date, abnormal kinematics have not been well characterized for cases in which obvious fracture or dislocation is absent, despite various efforts to accomplish this goal as reviewed by Dimnet et al. (40). The measurements are somewhat tedious and prone to error, and both inter- and intrasubject variability are problems. To control for this variability, comparison between the level above and level below the one in question is probably quite important. Widely accepted standards of abnormality for voluntarily produced movements have not yet been developed.

Abnormally large or small rotations are perhaps the most obvious and easily measured kinematic abnormalities, but they are not the only ones possible. Because planar motion (such as flexion-extension) has three degrees of freedom as described earlier, rotation angle measurement of the CR is also needed. If only the rotation is measured, a kinematic abnormality consisting of an abnormal CR location will be missed.

Upper Cervical

The basic motion pattern here is flexion-extension to some extent at both Oc-C1 and C1-C2, axial rotation at C1-C2 alone, and lateral bend only slightly at Oc-C1 alone (Table 1). This could be predicted from the arrangement of articular surfaces and ligamentous connections. Flexion-extension for Oc-C1 occurs about a CR approximately at the center of curvature of the Oc condyles. Flexion-extension for C1-C2 entails motion of the anterior arch of C1 cephalad and slightly posteriorly, facilitated by the curved anterior surface of the odontoid.

Axial rotation for Oc-C1 requires one Oc condyle to slide anteriorly on C1 and the contralateral one to slide posteriorly. The relatively deep fit of the condyles into the C1 upper articular concavity substantially limits this motion (122). In contrast, the fairly flat C1 and C2 lateral mass articular surfaces allow almost half of the entire cervical axial rotational range to occur at this joint (122,155,157,158). Furthermore, within the central portion of neck axial rotation, almost all the rotation is at C1-C2 (18,66). As C1 rotates toward the right, the

TABLE 1. *Cervical motion*

	Oc-C1	C1-C2	C3-C7
Flexion-extension	Some	Some	Major
Axial rotation	No	Major	Some
Lateral bend	Slight	No	Major

No = none to slight.

anteromedial-most portion of the right lateral articular mass shifts posteriorly and laterally, while that of the left lateral articular mass shifts anteriorly and medially (the CR is posterior to these portions of the articular surfaces). An anteroposterior open-mouth x-ray will erroneously suggest subluxation laterally of C1 on C2. Careful neutral positioning of both head and torso for x-ray exposure will prevent this misleading radiographic image.

Lateral bending occurs only to a small extent at Oc-C1. The strong alar ligaments force the rotation to be about the tip of the odontoid. This is allowed to occur by some lateral shifting of the C1 ring (18), which in turn requires some stretching out of the transverse ligament (transverse portion of the cruciform ligament). Lateral bending at C1-C2 is negligible.

Abnormal kinematics of the Oc-C1-C2 region is probably best illustrated by the C1-C2 subluxation, which can occur by means of rheumatoid arthritic damage to the transverse ligament. This allows an abnormally large anterior translation of C1 on C2. Even though there may be no angular hypermobility, the CR can clearly be seen to be abnormally located. Abnormal kinematics can also occur with posttraumatic rotatory hypermobility (instability). This condition is probably underdiagnosed, especially in the adult, and it has been elegantly studied with functional CT scanning by Dvorák and co-workers (46,48), and by Penning et al. (122). Also, stereoroentgenography has been used by Iai et al. (71).

Instability

The most common mechanical definition of this term is that an abnormally or unexpectedly large motion occurs in response to an applied load. This may be illustrated by a simple example. If an average-sized individual (the load) sits on the edge of an unstable boat, it will tip by a large amount compared to a more stable boat, for which only a minimal tip occurs with the same load. A second, closely related yet really very different meaning of instability is that any further load application beyond a certain critical load leads to increasing motion even without additional load increase. Subsequently, even if the load is removed, the system does not return to its initial position but remains in a new stable position. An example is a catamaran that is allowed to tip just a bit too far: even though the load is not increased, the boat will continue to tip more and more, flip over, and tend to remain in a new stable position.

In both of these examples it can be seen that assessment of stability depends on knowing not only the motion but also the loads involved. The problem is that in a clinical setting the loads acting upon the vertebrae are not known. Even when the external load on the neck is

known (e.g., longitudinal traction as in the stretch test) (117,135,158), the internal loads on the vertebrae or ligaments are not known. This is because there is loadsharing between these components and the muscles, and the loads taken by the muscles are not quantified.

Application of the term *stability* to spinal problems can thus be quite difficult. Loads are important in the true mechanical definition of stability, and muscles are important in producing these loads, yet the magnitude of these loads is difficult to measure. Thus, the lack to date of an explicit, quantitative, agreed-upon definition of instability in the clinical literature is understandable.

Rather than continuing to struggle with this difficulty, perhaps the term *mechanical insufficiency* has a vagueness that accurately conveys the imprecision of our current knowledge, and *instability* as it is typically used clinically is often misleading and goes beyond today's knowledge. *Mechanical insufficiency* also has a breadth of meaning which could encompass various subtypes as our knowledge expands and terms become more precise. For example, *spinal dyskinesia* could be used to mean any abnormal motion even though the forces are not known, and *spinal segmental hypermobility* could mean a special type of dyskinesia, namely abnormally large motion at a single motion segment. *Hyperflexibility* (discussed below) could be used to describe situations both in which the loads and the displacements are known, as would result from use of the stretch test (117,135), and in which the displacements are large relative to the corresponding loads.

Instability could then be used in its true engineering sense, as in the catamaran example above. After all, the usual decision that needs to be made in a clinical setting is not really whether the spinal segment in question is stable, but rather whether treatment of a particular type (e.g., internal fixation and grafting) will be helpful. Use of a less specific term such as *mechanical insufficiency* may allow a clearer focus on this clinical decision, without the distraction of imprecisely or unmeasurably defined instabilities.

Hyperflexibility

Flexibility has to do with the ratio between loads and displacements. Strictly speaking, flexibility is the load required to produce a given displacement, whereas stiffness is the displacement produced from a given load. Panjabi et al. (114) tested human cadaveric motion segments from C2-C3 through C6-C7; they used a full array of force types (anterior and posterior, right and left lateral, and tension and compression), and they measured all six displacement components, i.e., translation along and rotation about each of the three axes. They defined a neutral zone in the load-displacement curves within which displacements occurred with very little load change.

Flexibility testing *in vivo* has been done only to a limited extent. Measurements of the effect of cervical traction have been done by various investigators. Goldie and Reichmann (61) used 150 N longitudinal distraction force and showed no disc widening in 47 of 54 discs in 15 normal subjects. Seven of 54 widened from 0.4 to 0.7 mm, but this was unrelated to other radiographic features or to clinical findings. Schlicke et al. (135) applied traction equal to one third of body weight to normal volunteers in order to establish normal values for a diagnostic stretch test. They found that the mean disc height increased 0.70 mm (SD, 0.50) and the segmental extension angle increased 0.9° (SD, 2.4). Some variation with vertebral level occurred (largest at C3-C4 and C4-C5, intermediate at C5-C6, and smallest at C2-C3).

The effect of deliberately produced structural abnormalities on flexibility has been investigated using cadaveric specimens, of course. Panjabi et al. (116) investigated the response of human motion segments to an anteriorly directed force as ligaments were sequentially transected either from back to front or front to back. Eventually they reached a "pre-failure state," after which cutting one more ligament would produce complete dislocation. For this pre-failure state, the average amount of flexion was 11° more than that present before any ligaments were cut. The average amount of anterior translation was 3.5 mm as measured at the inferior dorsal corner of the upper body relative to the superior dorsal corner of the lower body. Interestingly, this value is very close to the 3.5 mm mean maximum anterior displacement seen in intact cadaveric specimens subjected to an anteriorly directed force, as described above. Further ligament transection work was done by Moroney et al. (93) who subjected degenerated specimens and specimens with posterior elements removed to not only flexion–extension, but also to lateral bending and axial rotation.

The relationship of these ligament transection results to *in vivo* abnormal kinematics is far from clear, for at least two reasons. The pattern of ligament disruption leading to abnormal motion *in vivo* is probably very different from sequential total transection of each ligament. In addition, the force distribution *in vivo* is not known and may be very different from that used in cadaveric testing. Thus, use of these values for clinical decision-making remains to be validated.

Similar cadaveric work has been done using longitudinal traction instead of an anteriorly directed force (117) to help establish a normal basis for a clinical stretch test. One third body weight was applied, and ligaments were cut from front to back. The increased anterior disc height just prior to failure was 3.3 mm and the increase in extension angle was 3.8°. For the posterior to anterior cutting sequence, spinous process spread increase was 27 mm and the increase in flexion angle was 30°. Here again, the relation between these data and *in vivo* clinical problems has not been tested and remains to be established.

Wetzel et al. performed a corresponding study on rabbit spines (156), that demonstrated both important similarities to and differences from the human spine specimen results. They also documented for the first time in the cervical spine the time course of healing after experimentally produced injuries (interspinous ligament sectioning, laminectomy, laminectomy and facet capsule excision, and sham operation).

The effect of removal of various amounts of facet joint structures has been investigated by a number of authors. Raynor et al. (126) compared a partial medial facetectomy of 50% to that of 70%: under shear loadings, the latter failed much more often by articular process fracture than did the former. Nowinski et al. (98) showed that 25% partial facetectomy increased specimen flexibility significantly compared to intact, whereas laminoplasty did not. Zdeblick et al. showed, in response to flexion loading, significant increased flexibility versus intact for 75% but not 50% partial medial facetectomy (168) or for partial facet capsulectomy (169). No comparative *in vivo* studies appear to have been done to establish clinical relevance of these studies.

TRAUMA

To facilitate communication about the wide variety of injuries that can occur in the cervical spine, various injury types have been defined and various classification schemes proposed. We will focus here only on the indirect injuries, defined as those produced by forces applied to the head either by contact with another object (e.g., diving into shallow water) or by acceleration or deceleration (whiplash). Direct injuries such as gunshot or knife wounds are excluded here and are discussed in Chapter 49. Two basically different approaches to the naming and classification of indirect injuries have been followed: (a) radiographic appearance (16), or (b) mechanistic (3,18,63,64,130), according to the direction or location of the force presumed to have caused the damage.

The first approach has the advantage of being very direct: the bony structural damage or malposition can be visualized by x-ray and the associated ligamentous structural damage can be reasonably well inferred. The injury type is derived directly from the radiographic appearance. Since treatment largely involves repairing or compensating for the structural damage, only a small step is needed to go from diagnosis to treatment. For example, if the radiograph shows a bilateral facet subluxation, one infers a torn interspinous ligament and facet joint capsules, and one may treat this by replacing the torn interspinous ligament with a wire loop for temporary stabilization and by bone graft for permanent fusion. One major problem, of course, is that the radiograph shows only the residual displacement and not the maximal displacement during injury production, which may have been much worse. For example, Chang et al. (28) showed that during experimental impact loading, the spinal canal diameter was transiently reduced down to 37% of that present after injury production.

The disadvantage of this radiographic approach to classification is that the biomechanics get "lost." Mechanically important relationships between injury types are not clearly apparent within the classification. Very different structurally defined injuries may be caused by the same force. For example, both Jefferson fractures and burst fractures of C5 are caused by a compressive force with the neck in the neutral position. The reverse situation can also occur; that is, similar structural damage may be caused by very different forces. For example, bilateral C5 laminar fractures may be caused by forward flexion (in association with C4-C5 interspinous ligament failure and C5-C6 bilateral facet capsule failure), or they may be caused by a compressive force acting on an already extended neck (causing the C4 inferior articular processes to be forced downward and the C5 lamina to fracture in hyperextension). As another example, Crowell et al. (37) loaded some cadaveric specimens with a pure flexion moment and others with combined flexion and compression: the structural damage in the two groups was similar. As a result of the complex relation between load type and injury type, radiographic appearance does not readily convey full information about mechanical damage or instability, as noted by many authors (77,109).

To overcome these and other related disadvantages, the mechanistic approach to naming and classification has been used by a number of authors. An early method was that of Roaf (130), who proposed to classify injuries as flexion, compression, extension, lateral bend, and rotation. As a more detailed understanding of injury subtypes has evolved and a wider range of treatment options has been developed, this classification scheme has become too simple for many purposes. Largely because of a gradually improved understanding of injury biomechanics, more useful classification schemes are now available.

Such a scheme for the lower cervical spine was described by Allen et al. (3,4) and represents a major advance. The scheme consists of six categories: compressive flexion, vertical compression, distractive flexion, compressive extension, distractive extension, and lateral flexion. These terms, however, present certain problems. First, flexion is always associated with some compression of anterior elements and distraction of posterior elements. Thus compressive flexion and distractive flexion are not specific to traumatic situations. This same problem is presented by the terms *compressive extension* and *distractive extension.* Second, by *distractive flexion,* the authors really mean flexion without any external compressive loads, but that absence does not really constitute distraction. Third, *spinal compression* usually is considered to mean a force acting downward along the longitudinal axis of the spine. In this context *vertical compression* is confusingly redundant.

In an effort to build on the substantial conceptual advance of this system and also to clarify the terminology, a modified system has been developed (Table 2). There is a growing body of experimental data that show the influence of neck posture on resulting damage, even for the same applied force (5,89,100,104,109,110,143,147, 165,166). Thus, in this classification system, each injury category is defined by two items: the force type that is applied to the head, named for the dominant motion

TABLE 2. *Injuries categorized by force types and neck postures*

Load type	Neck posture				
	Flexed	Neutral	Extended	Axially rotated	Laterally bent

Flexing	Dens
	Spinous process
	Bilateral facet
	  dislocation
				Unilateral facet
				  dislocation
					Unilateral facet
					  dislocation

Compressing	Wedge
	Tear drop
		Jefferson
		Split
		Burst
			Spinous process
			Hyperextension
			  fracture/dislocation
					Lateral wedge
					Articular
					  compression
					Horizontal facet

Extending			Dens Avulsion		
Distracting			Hangman's		
Lateral bending					Lateral wedge Articular compression Horizontal facet

that that force tends to produce, and the posture of the neck at the instant structural failure occurs. There are five force types (flexing, compressing, extending, distracting, and lateral bending) and five neck postures (flexed, neutral, extended, axially rotated, and laterally bent). The interaction between force type and neck posture is illustrated in Fig. 7.

Many of the 25 possible combinations need not be considered. Some combinations do not occur because neck postural change is produced before significant damage; e.g., a flexing force will move the neck from an extended or a neutral posture to the flexed posture before significant injury occurs. By similar reasoning, the combinations of extending and flexed, extending and neutral,

or lateral bending and neutral also do not occur. Distraction in any posture other than extended does not occur because a distracting force can be applied to the head only anteriorly, that is, to the mandible (except in the special case of hanging). Other combinations probably do not result in clinically distinct injuries: compressing and axially rotated; extending and axially rotated or laterally bent; and lateral bending and flexed, extended, or axially rotated.

After excluding these types from the 25 possible combinations, only ten remain. These can be used to classify the full range of both upper and lower cervical injuries in a mechanistically clear manner. These are presented below, in the same order as they appear in Table 2.

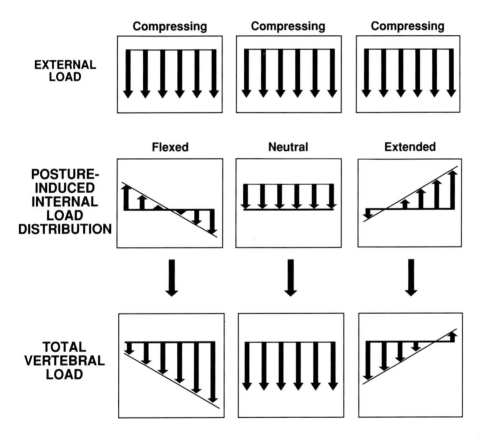

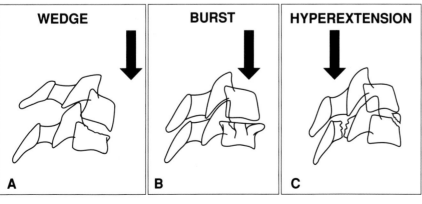

FIG. 7. Effect of neck posture on total vertebral loads during compression injuries. **A:** Compressing/flexed: Anteriorly, large compressive loads are present, which cause vertebral compression. Posteriorly, the loads are also compressive, which prevents tensile failures. **B:** Compressing/neutral: Uniform load distribution results in a burst fracture. **C:** Compressing/extended: Anteriorly, only slight tensile loads occur, causing an avulsion fracture. Posteriorly, the compressive loads cause laminar fractures.

Flexing/Flexed

A variety of radiographically different injuries are all produced in the flexing/flexed (FF) manner. Oc-C1 dislocations are usually anterior (63,124,158) and apparently involve a flexing force, although the exact mechanism is not known. Usually these injuries are fatal and involve high energy input by contact with the head or are associated with multiple other injuries that make assessment difficult. Myers et al. (96) showed that an applied axial torque produced Oc-C1 dislocation but no injury below C1; however, such a loading mechanism (a torque rather than a force) probably seldom occurs *in vivo.*

There are no typical C1 fractures known to be produced by this mechanism, although Mouradian et al. (95) found that an anteriorly directed pull on the occiput resulted in bilateral posterior arch fractures in 2 of 15 cadaveric specimens.

Acute traumatic C1-C2 subluxations presumably are produced by this same mechanism but are usually fatal (56) and thus are not encountered often in clinical practice. Fielding et al. (56) found that the atlanto–dens interval was 3 to 5 mm just prior to failure from an anterior pull on C1 with C2 fixed. Thus, subluxation forward of more than 5 mm provides a strong argument for ligamentous disruption when there is a history of trauma in an otherwise normal patient. Oda et al. (100) found in cadaveric specimens injured by a dropped-weight technique (110) that the altanto–dens interval during application of a modest flexion moment was 3 mm or more if the transverse ligament was disrupted but less than 3 mm if it was intact.

Unilateral or rotatory dislocations apparently may occur by this FF mechanism (18) or may occur in a flexing/axially rotated (FA) or flexing/laterally bent (FL) manner.

Dens fractures have been conjectured to be caused by this mechanism, and Mouradian et al. (95) produced cadaveric specimen fractures in this manner. However, as will be discussed later in the section on compressing/flexed injury mechanisms, it appears more likely that some significant compressing component is needed as well.

Bilateral pars interarticular fractures of C2 (so-called hangman's fracture: see the section on extending/extended injury mechanisms) are more frequently reported to be caused with the neck extended, but FF injury mechanisms have also been described (38,149) based on the history and associated occipital scalp injuries. This probably is an uncommon occurrence.

In the lower cervical spine, spinous process fractures may occur. These may belong in the FF injury category but may also be caused by an extending/extended (EE) mechanism. There has also been conjecture that these injuries may be caused by a lateral pull (158).

Also occurring in the lower cervical spine, bilateral facet subluxations or dislocations seem to be in this FF category. Bauze and Ardran (11) have produced this injury with anteriorly offset axial compression alone. However, the spinal specimen was immobilized in a manner somewhat different from usual, which raises some questions as to the clinical relevance of their result.

Various patterns of structural damage can occur. For example, a C4-C5 bilateral facet dislocation can occur either by failure of the C4-C5 interspinous ligament or by failure of the C3-C4 interspinous ligament plus bilateral laminar fractures of C4. Which of these occurs may well be influenced by subtle variations in the relative strength of the two different interspinous ligaments, rather than by the details of the force applied to the head.

Flexing/Axially Rotated, and Flexing/Laterally Bent

The FA and FL categories probably may be combined because they do not seem to produce clinically distinguishable spinal damage. Both involve asymmetric loading and can result in unilateral facet fracture subluxation or dislocation on the side opposite to that toward which the axial rotation or lateral bending occurred.

Presumably, a unilateral facet dislocation could also occur even without any asymmetric forces. For this to happen there must be sufficient asymmetry in facet joint capsular strength and the injuring force must be strong enough to tear the weaker but not the stronger facet capsule. In these circumstances, the upper vertebra flexes forward and axially rotates about the stronger facet joint as the weaker facet joint dislocates. Thus, it is possible for a unilateral facet dislocation to be produced by loads other than an applied axial torque.

Compressing

Four injury categories are grouped together here. The force type for each is the same (compressing), but the neck posture for each is different. One special feature of this group of injury categories is that the injuring force almost always results from contact between the head and some object. Forces arising from momentum of the head during deceleration are usually not great enough to produce such injuries. Another special feature is that the injuring force passes along the spine close to or directly through the injury site. This is in contrast to all the other force types, which generally lie approximately in the transverse plane of the head and thus are relatively far from a mid- or lower-cervical injury site. Thus, even a small change from the neutral position into flexion, extension, or lateral bending will cause the compressing force vector to fall anteriorly, posteriorly, or laterally to the vertebral bodies. Each of these postures will in turn result in structurally quite different injuries (Fig. 7) (100,109,110,166).

This effect of neck posture on injury pattern produced by compressive loading has been shown by various investigators (5,89,100,104,109,110,147,165,166) who have studied experimental injuries in cadaveric spine specimens. An anterior movement of the upper cervical spine of only 1 cm was enough to convert the buckling pattern from extension to flexion in axially compressed cadaveric specimens (89).

To understand this effect, it may be helpful to consider separately the externally applied force (compressing) and the internally derived forces resulting from neck posture (Fig. 7). For example, the flexed posture produces compression at the front of the vertebral body and tension posteriorly (Fig. 7A). A superimposed compressing force will further increase the compressive loads anteriorly, but it will neutralize and reverse the posterior tensile loads to produce small compressive loads posteriorly. As a result, no tensile failure occurs posteriorly and compressive failure is worst anteriorly (wedge fracture).

Compressing/Flexed

In the upper cervical spine, dens fractures can be caused either by compressing/flexed, compressing/extended, or compressing/laterally bent space mechanisms. These three mechanisms of injury have been demonstrated by Althoff (5) in carefully performed impact loadings of cadaveric specimens. The key feature is the presence of a compressing force passing near to the dens. Without this, neither Althoff (5) nor Blockley and Purser (14) were able to produce dens fractures in whole cadavers [although Mouradian et al. (95) and Doherty et al. (41) were able to do so in isolated C2 vertebrae].

Indirect evidence in support of these experimentally based compression mechanisms is the clinical observation that forceful contact with the head is required. Momentum of the head alone during decelerations (e.g., FF or EE) is not sufficient to produce this injury (7,31,70,103).

Both compressing/flexed and compressing/extended seem to be more common causes than the compression/laterally bent mechanism. Of the 25 cases of dens fractures in which the mechanism of injury seemed fairly clear, Mouradian et al. (95) found that 16 of 20 were struck from behind, while 4 of 20 were struck from the front. Corresponding values in the review by Blockey and Purser (14) were 8 of 51 and 6 of 51 (with 37 of 51 not clear). White and Panjabi (158) state that an extension mechanism is more common, but no supportive data are provided.

It should be kept in mind that the residual displacement for an injury as hypermobile as a dens fracture may be very different from, even opposite in direction to, the displacement at the instant of injury. For example, even though a dens fracture may be caused by an extending

force resulting in transient posterior displacement, the initial x-ray may show anterior residual displacement. Although anterior residual displacement is clearly more common than posterior displacement (14,31,70), the injury mechanism cannot necessarily be inferred from this observation.

It is not clear what determines whether an anteriorly directed force will produce a transverse ligament tear or a dens fracture. Only the former were produced by anterior loading applied to the ring of C1 (56), while both injury types (nine specimens with dens fractures, three with ligament tears) were produced by anterior loading applied to the occiput (95). This probably is an example of the way in which subtle relative variations in strength determine injury pattern: if the dens is slightly weaker than the transverse ligament, a fracture will occur, and *vice versa,* even though the force direction and magnitude are constant (77).

In the lower cervical region, the combination of the external compressing force and the internal force distribution from the flexed posture tends to produce a wedge fracture at lower loads (Fig. 7A), and a tear-drop fracture (with its typical sagittal plane component) if the compressing force is large enough. The rate of load application may also be important in determining which of these injuries occurs. The name *tear drop* is vague and has meant very different things to different authors. Harris (63) summarizes the major literature and uses the terms *flexion tear-drop fracture–dislocation* and *extension tear-drop fracture* to distinguish between these two very different types of tear drop. The former designation is that originally described by Schneider and Kahn (137) and used by others (1,12,13,59,60,123,130,132), and it also has been referred to as a three-part, two-plane fracture (151). This generally is a very unstable injury. The extension tear-drop fracture (Fig. 8) involves avulsion of the anteroinferior corner of the vertebral body (67,125,133).

The displacement associated with a minor or moderate wedge fracture is not usually sufficient to cause severe

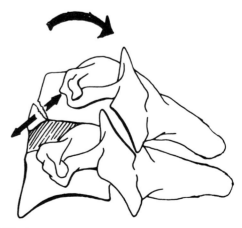

FIG. 8. Extension tear-drop fracture mechanism.

disruption of the interspinous ligament or facet capsules. In addition, the posterior body height is usually maintained and the inferior endplate is intact. The more severe flexion tear-drop fracture–dislocation involves both anteriorly and posteriorly, and often bilateral, facet subluxation as well. The interspinous ligament may also be torn.

Compressing/Neutral

In the upper cervical spine, the compressing/neutral (CN) combination results in a Jefferson fracture as shown experimentally by Panjabi et al. (128). Jefferson's contribution (73) was to call attention to two features of this injury: it is by no means necessarily fatal, and the mechanism of injury is tensile failure of the C1 ring, produced by an axial compressive force acting on the wedge-shaped lateral masses. It is interesting that none of Jefferson's own four cases and only three of the 25 cases described in his comprehensive literature review had four-part fractures (most were two-part fractures). Furthermore, Jefferson did not attach any special significance to the number of fractured parts of the C1 ring. Thus *Jefferson fracture* should refer not only to four-part, but also to two- or three-part, C1 fractures. Landells and Van Peteghem (80) have described a classification of these injuries. Panjabi et al. (110), using a dropped-weight technique on cadaveric Oc-C3 specimens, produced two-, three-, and four-part Jefferson fractures.

If the resulting spread between the two lateral masses becomes too great, the transverse portion of the cruciform ligament will become torn, allowing anterior subluxation of C1 on C2. Spence et al. (148) tested ten cadaveric Oc-C1-C2 specimens and showed that transverse ligament rupture, produced by quasistatic loading, occurred at a mean of 6.3 mm (range, 4.8 to 7.6 mm) of increased C1 lateral diameter. The strength of this ligament is quite great: 350 N for loading along the ligament (right to left) (50) and 690 N for loading transverse to it (posterior to anterior) (65).

In the lower cervical spine, this CN injury mechanism produces a force distribution across the superior endplate that is fairly uniform (Fig. 6B). Because the uncinate processes support the inferior endplate along its lateral edges, vertebral body failure may occur along the sagittal plane where the stresses are highest. This may be the explanation for the vertical compression fracture (15,18,82,128,132), which is also one component of the true tear-drop fracture–dislocation described above.

With higher forces, burst fractures occur typically with extensive fragmentation of the entire vertebral body but typically without much disruption to the facet capsules. Bozic et al. (17), using a fine-mesh finite element mathematical model, predicted that failure from a uniformly applied axial compressive load would begin with central vertebral body cancellous failure.

There is no consensus on the relation of burst fractures to tear-drop fracture–dislocation. Some authors have regarded these terms to mean significantly different injuries (30,60,63,123,130,137), while others have considered the tear drop to be a specific type of burst or to be synonymous with burst (12,13,67,132). Until the definitions are made more explicit and the mechanical characteristics of each are established, it is not clear whether this distinction is important.

Compressing/Extended

Jefferson fractures can be produced in this manner at lower loads than for the CN mechanism (110), although the clinical relevance of this is not clear. This mechanism can also produce dens fractures (as discussed in the section on compressing/flexed mechanisms above) and bilateral pars interarticularis fracture of C2, as suggested by Cornish (33). The latter may occur, for example, to an inadequately restrained driver in a deceleration automobile accident whose forehead strikes against the windshield with the upper neck in extension. This same injury can also be caused by the EE and FF mechanisms. Williams (161) emphasized the difference between these mechanisms and those occurring in a judicial hanging in which distraction is also present.

In the lower cervical spine, the extended posture results in compression along the posterior annulus and tension along the anterior annulus. Even with a superimposed compressing force, small tensile forces may remain anteriorly, with large compressive forces occurring posteriorly. In the lower cervical spine, the resulting injury does not have a widely agreed-upon name but has been described by Forsyth (57) as a hyperextension fracture–dislocation, and even more clearly by Allen et al. (3,4) as a subtype of a compressive extension injury. The injury includes tensile failure anteriorly and bending failure posteriorly of lateral masses or laminae, or both, or of the spinous process.

Compressing/Laterally Bent, and Lateral Bending/Laterally Bent

Clear separation between the compressing/laterally bent (CL) and lateral bending/laterally bent (LL) injury mechanisms is not presently feasible in terms of the structural damage produced. Dens fractures were produced by Althoff (5) by this mechanism, as discussed in the section on compressing/flexed mechanisms). In the lower cervical spine, lateral wedge fractures involve asymmetric collapse of the upper endplate. Unilateral articular process compression may produce a triangular rather than diamond-shaped lateral mass (159) seen on lateral x-ray, or it may fracture the pedicle and lamina which allows the entire lateral mass to rotate (57). Brachial plexus injuries are often associated with these injuries (129).

Extending/Extended

Occipital dislocations in the posterior direction are placed into the EE category, although these occur more commonly in an anterior direction. Bilateral C1 laminar fractures, either in isolation or in combination with a C2 bilateral pars interarticularis fracture, probably result from an extension mechanism (54,158), although the details are not clear and this injury certainly can be produced experimentally by an FF injury mechanism (95). Perhaps the Oc-C1 joint is extended enough so that the capsular ligaments of these joints force the C1 arch down against the C2 spinous process. Alternatively, since the Oc-C1 joint extends posteriorly to the C1-C2 joint, perhaps instead it is a downward and backward thrust of the Oc condyles that causes the C1-C2 hyperextension. Another speculation is that the compression of the C1 arch between the occiput and C2 arch during hyperextension is the cause (144). White and Panjabi (158) conjecture that the hyperextending occiput may push downward on the arch of C1, while C1-C2 motion is blocked.

Dens fractures appear to require a compressing force component for their causation either in the extended, flexed, or laterally bent postures (discussed above). The major point to be made here is that these can be very unstable injuries and the method of reduction is determined by the residual displacement, not necessarily by the mechanism of injury.

Bilateral pars interarticularis fractures of C2 can be caused by an EE mechanism, but also by FF, compressing/extended, or distracting/extended mechanisms as discussed further in the respective sections. Various authors report injuries involving force applied to the face or chin without apparent compressing or distracting force (87,138,149). There appear to be no well-documented reports concerning frequency of these different injuring mechanisms, but those involving an extended posture of the upper cervical spine seem to be more common.

In the lower cervical spine, bony failure may occur in the form of an avulsion injury of the anteroinferior part of the body (88) (Fig. 8), or by bending failure of a spinous process resulting from its striking the one below it. Typically, the spinous process fragment remains slightly tipped up (159), which distinguishes this injury from a clay shoveler's fracture (FF injury type). Extension sufficient to cause substantial cord damage may occur even when there is no spinous process fracture or any other apparent spinal column disruption (125). This

cord injury can result from shortening and inward bulging of the ligamentum flavum and shortening and thickening of the cord itself, since both of these structures are located behind the center of rotation (see the section on spinal cord, dura, and nerve roots).

Distracting/Extended

Cervical spine injuries do not often occur in the distracting/extended (DE) manner because it is only under very special circumstances that a longitudinal distracting force can be applied to the neck. This mechanism has been investigated in cadaveric specimens by Shea et al. (141) who refer to it, somewhat ambiguously, as hyperextension. (Hyperextension could be caused in many different ways, such as by a distracting force anteriorly, a pure torque, or a posterior force on the forehead.) An upward blow to the chin can produce quite forceful extension but only a modest longitudinal force. Backward motion of the head tends to cause loss of further contact with the injuring object, preventing further distraction. The obvious exception is judicial hanging (with the knot under the chin) in which the circumferential noose allows application of substantial distracting force as well as extension. The resulting injury is a bilateral pars interarticularis fracture, or so-called hangman's fracture (162). Because the name so vividly conveys the sense of a distracting force, and because none of the other causes of this injury involve significant distraction (i.e., FF, compressing/extended, EE), the name *hangman's fracture* should be reserved for injuries resulting from this one very special mechanism.

SUMMARY

The cervical spine is structurally quite complex, yet knowledge of its anatomy is very important for correctly dealing with clinical problems. Easy availability of computed tomography or magnetic resonance imaging scans can aid, but not substitute for, this knowledge. Continued efforts by the clinician to learn and use correctly the concepts and language of the biomechanician will help to improve, through better communication and research, the quality of patient care.

REFERENCES

1. Alem NM, Nusholtz GS, Melvin JW (1984): *Head and neck response to axial impacts.* Proceedings of the 28th STAPP Car Crash Conference, Society of Automotive Engineers, Warrendale, Pennsylvania.
2. Allen AR (1911): Surgery of experimental lesion of spinal cord equivalent to crush injury of fracture dislocation of spinal column: preliminary report. *JAMA* 57:878–880.
3. Allen BJ Jr (1989): Recognition of injuries to the lower cervical

spine. In: Sherk HH, et al., eds. *The cervical spine,* 2nd ed., Philadelphia: JB Lippincott, pp. 286–298.

4. Allen BJ Jr, Ferguson RL, Lehmann TR, O'Brien RP (1982): A mechanistic classification of closed, indirect fractures and dislocations of the lower cervical spine. *Spine* 7:1–27.

5. Althoff B (1979): Fracture of the odontoid process. *Acta Orthop Scand Suppl* 177:1–95.

6. Ǎlund M, Larsson S-E (1990): Three dimensional analysis of neck motion: a clinical method. *Spine* 15:87–91.

7. Anderson LD, D'Alonzo RT (1974): Fractures of the odontoid process of the axis. *J Bone Joint Surg* 56A:1163–1174.

8. Anderson RJ (1883): Observations on diameters of human vertebrae in different regions. *J Anat* 17:341–344.

9. Ashton-Miller JA, McGlashen KM, Herzenberg JE (1989): A study of cervical muscle response to experientally-induced muscle pain. *J Biomech* 22(10):982.

10. Bailey RW (1983): *Dislocations of the cervical spine.* In: Bailey RW, Sherk HH, et al., eds. *The cervical spine,* 2nd ed. Philadelphia: JB Lippincott, pp. 362–387.

11. Bauze RJ, Ardran GM (1978): Experimental production of forward dislocation in the human cervical spine. *J Bone Joint Surg [Br]* 60:239–245.

12. Beatson TR (1963): Fractures and dislocation of the cervical spine. *J Bone Joint Surg [Br]* 45:21–35.

13. Bedbrook GM (1971): Stability of spinal fractures and fracture-dislocations. *Paraplegia* 9:23–32.

14. Blockey NJ, Purser DW (1956): Fractures of the odontoid process of the axis. *J Bone Joint Surg [Br]* 38:794–817.

15. Blumensaat C (1953): Zum Problem der sagittalen Langsbrüche der Halswirbelkörper. *Chirurg* 24:193–195.

16. Bohlman HH, Boada E (1989): Fractures and dislocations of the lower cervical spine. In: *The cervical spine,* 2nd ed. Baily RW, Sherk HH, et al., eds. Philadelphia: JB Lippincott, pp. 368–373.

17. Bozic KJ, Keyak JH, Skinner HB, Bueff U, Bradford BS (1994): Three-dimensional finite element modeling of a cervical vertebra: an investigation of burst fracture mechanism. *J Spinal Disord* 7(2):102–10.

18. Braakman R, Penning L (1971): *Injuries of the cervical spine.* Amsterdam: EMedica Publ., pp. 1–262.

19. Breig A (1960): *Biomechanics of the central nervous system. Some basic normal and pathological phenomena concerning spine, discs and cord.* Stockholm: Almqvist & Wiksell.

20. Breig A (1970): Overstretching of and circumscribed pathological tension on the spinal cord: a basic cause of symptoms in cord disorders. *J Biomech* 3:7–9.

21. Breig A (1972): The therapeutic possibilities of surgical bioengineering in incomplete spinal cord lesions. *Paraplegia* 9:173–182.

22. Breig A (1973): Pathological stress in the pons-cord-tissue tract and its alleviation by neurosurgical means. *Clin Neurosurg* 20: 85–94.

23. Breig A (1978): *Adverse mechanical tension in the central nervous system.* Stockholm: Almqvist & Wiksell.

24. Breig A (1989): *Skull traction and cervical cord injury.* Berlin: Springer-Verlag, pp. 1–84

25. Breig A, El-Nadi AP (1966): Biomechanics of the cervical spinal cord. Relief of contact pressure on and overstretching of the spinal cord. *Acta Radiol Diagn [Stockh]* 4:602–624.

26. Brody IA, Wilkins RH (1969): Lhermitte's sign. *Arch Neurol* 21: 338–340.

27. Bucy PC, Heimburger RF, Oberhill HRO (1948): Compression of the cervical spinal cord by herniated intervertebral discs. *J Neurosurg* 5:471–492.

28. Chang DG, Tencer AF, Ching RP, Treece B, Senft D, Anderson PA (1994): Geometric changes in the cervical spinal canal during impact. *Spine* 19(8):973–980.

29. Chen IH, Vasavada A, Panjabi MM (1994): Kinematics of the cervical spine canal: changes with sagittal plane loads. *J Spinal Disord* 7(2):93–101.

30. Cheshire DJE (1969): The stability of the cervical spine following the conservative treatment of fractures and fracture-dislocations. *Paraplegia* 7:193–203.

31. Clark CR, White AA III (1985): Fractures of the dens: a multicenter study. *J Bone Joint Surg [Am]* 67:1340–1348.

32. Condon BR, Hadley DM (1988): Quantification of cord deformation and dynamics during flexion and extension of the cervical spine using MR imaging. *J Comput Assist Tomogr* 12:947–955.

33. Cornish BL (1968): Traumatic spondylolisthesis of the axis. *J Bone Joint Surg* 50:31–43.

34. Crellin RQ, MacCabe JJ, Hamilton EBD (1970): Severe subluxation of the cervical spine in rheumatoid arthritis. *J Bone Joint Surg [Br]* 52:244–251.

35. Crisco JJ III, Oda T, Panjabi MM, Bueff HU, Dvořák J, Grob D (1991): Transections of the C1-C2 joint capsular ligaments in the cadaveric spine. *Spine* 16(S10):S474–479.

36. Crisco JJ III, Panjabi MM, Dvořák J (1991): A model of the alar ligaments of the upper cervical spine in axial rotation. *J Biomech* 24(7):607–614.

37. Crowell RR, Shea M, Edwards WT, Clothiaux PL, White AA III, Hayes WC (1993): Cervical injuries under flexion and compression loading. *J Spinal Disord* 6(2):175–81.

38. De Lorme TL (1967): Axis-pedicle fractures. *J Bone Joint Surg [Am]* 49:1472.

39. Deng YC, Goldsmith W (1987): Response of a human head/neck/upper torso replica to dynamic loading. II. Analytical/numerical model. *J Biomech* 20:487–497.

40. Dimnet J, Pasquet A, Krag MH, Panjabi MM (1982): Cervical spine motion in the sagittal plane: Kinematics and geometric parameters. *J Biomech* 15:959–969.

41. Doherty JB, Heggeness MH, Esses SI (1993): A biomechanical study of odontoid fractures and fracture fixation. *Spine* 18:178–84.

42. Dohrmann GJ (1972): Experimental spinal cord trauma: a historical review. *Arch Neurol* 27:468–473.

43. Dohrmann GJ, Panjabi MM (1976): "Standardized" spinal cord trauma: biomechanical parameters and lesion volume. *Surg Neurol* 6:263–267.

44. Dohrmann GJ, Panjabi MM, Banks D (1978): Biomechanics of experimental spinal cord trauma. *J Neurosurg* 48:993–1001.

45. Dvořák J, Froehlich D, Penning L, Baumgaertner H, Panjabi MM (1988): Functional radiographic diagnosis of the cervical spine: flexion/extension. *Spine* 13:748–755.

46. Dvořák J, Hayek J, Zehnder R (1987): CT-functional diagnostics of the rotatory instability of the upper cervical spine. II. An evaluation on healthy adults and patients with suspected instability. *Spine* 12:726–731.

47. Dvořák J, Panjabi M (1987): Functional anatomy of the alar ligaments. *Spine* 12:183–189.

48. Dvořák J, Panjabi M, Gerber M, Wichmann W (1987): CT-functional diagnostics of the rotary instability of upper cervical spine. I. An experimental study on cadavers. *Spine* 12:197–205.

49. Dvořák J, Panjabi MM, Novotny JE, Antinnes JA (1991): In vivo flexion/extension of the normal cervical spine. *J Orthop Res* 9(6): 828–834.

50. Dvořák J, Schneider E, Saldinger P, Rahn B (1988): Biomechanics of the craniocervical region: the alar and transverse ligaments. *J Orthop Res* 6:452–461.

51. Ecklin U (1960): *Die Alterveränderungen der Halswirbelsäule.* Berlin: Springer-Verlag.

52. Farmer JC, Wisneski RJ (1994): Cervical spine nerve root compression: an analysis of neuroforaminal pressures with varying head and arm positions. *Spine* 19(16):1850–1855.

53. Fick R (1904-1912): *Handbuch der Anatomie und Mechanik der Gelenke unter Berücksichtigung der bewegenden Muskeln.* Jena: G Fischer, pp. 1904–1912.

54. Fielding JW (1983): The atlanto axial joint. In: Evarts CM, ed. *Surgery of the musculoskeletal system,* vol. 2. New York: Churchill Livingston.

55. Fielding JW (1964): Normal and selected abnormal motion of the cervical spine from the second cervical vertebra to the seventh cervical vertebra based on cineroentgenography. *J Bone Joint Surg [Am]* 46:1779–1781.

56. Fielding JW, Cochran GVB, Lawsing JF III, Hohl M (1974): Tears of the transverse ligament of the atlas: a clinical and biomechanical study. *J Bone Joint Surg [Am]* 56:1683–1691.

57. Forsyth HF (1964): Extension injuries of the cervical spine. *J Bone Joint Surg [Am]* 46:1792–1797.

58. Frazer JE (1958): In: Breathnach AS, ed. *Anatomy of the human skeleton,* 5th ed. London: JA Churchill, p. 22.

59. Fuentes JM, Blancourt J, Vlahovitch B, Castan P (1983): Tear drop fractures. Contribution to the study of its mechanism and os osteo-disco-ligamentous lesions. *Neurochirurgie* 29:129–134.

60. Garber WN, Fisher RG, Holfman HW (1969): Vertebrectomy and fusion for "tear-drop" fracture of the cervical spine. *J Trauma* 9:887–893.

61. Goldie IF, Reichmann S (1977): The biomechanical influence of traction on the cervical spine. *Scand J Rehabil Med* 9:31–94.

62. Halliday DR, Sullivan UR, Hollinshead WH, Bahn RC (1964): Torn cervical ligaments: necropsy examination of normal cervical region. *J Trauma* 4:219–232.

63. Harris JH Jr (1978): *The radiology of acute cervical spine trauma.* Baltimore: Williams & Wilkins, pp. 1–116.

64. Harris JH Jr, Edeiken-Monroe B, Kopaniky OR (1986): A practical classification of acute cervical spine injuries. *Orthop Clin North Am* 17:15–30.

65. Heller JG, Amrani J, Hutton WC (1993): Transverse ligament failure: a biomechanical study. *J Spinal Disord* 6:162–165.

66. Hohl M, Baker HR (1964): The atlanto-axial joint, roentgenographic and anatomical study of normal and abnormal motion. *J Bone Joint Surg [Am]* 46:1739–1752.

67. Holdsworth FW (1963): Fractures, dislocations and fracture-dislocations of the spine. *J Bone Joint Surg [Br]* 45:6–20.

68. Hollinshead WH (1969): The back. In: *Anatomy for surgeons, vol. III: The back and limbs,* 2nd ed. New York: Harper & Row, pp. 79–206.

69. Hung TK, Lin HS, Albin MS, Bunegin L, Jannetta PJ (1979): The standardization of experimental impact injury to the spinal cord. *Surg Neurol* 11:470–477.

70. Husby J, Sorensen KH (1974): Fractures of the odontoid process of the axis. *Acta Orthop Scand* 45:182–192.

71. Iai H, Moriya H, Goto S, Takahashi K, Yamagata M, Tamaki T (1993): Three-dimensional motion analysis of the upper cervical spine during axial rotation. *Spine* 18(16):2388–2392.

72. Janes JM, Hooshmand H (1965): Severe extension-flexion injuries of the cervical spine. *Mayo Clin Proc* 40:353–369.

73. Jefferson G (1920): Fracture of the atlas vertebra: report of 4 cases and a review of those previously recorded. *Br J Surg* 7:407–422.

74. Jeffreys E (1980): *Disorders of the cervical spine.* London: Butterworth, pp. 1–147.

75. Johnson RM, Crelin ES, White AA III, Panjabi MM, Southwick WO (1975): Some new observations on the functional anatomy of the lower cervical spine. *Clin Orthop* 111:192–200.

76. Johnson RM, Southwick WO (1975): Surgical approaches to the spine. In: RH Rothman, FA Simeone, eds. *The spine.* Philadelphia: WB Saunders, pp. 98–103.

77. Krag MH, Pope MH, Wilder DG (1986): Mechanisms of spine trauma and features of spinal fixation methods. Mechanisms of injury. In: *Spinal cord injury medical engineering.* Ghista D, ed. Springfield, IL: Charles C Thomas.

78. Krag MH, Seroussi RE, Wilder DG, Pope MH (1987): Internal displacement distribution from in vitro loading of human lumbar spinal motion segments: experimental results and theoretical predictions. *Spine* 12:1001–1007.

79. Krag MH, Trausch I, Wilder DG, Pope MH (1983): *Internal strain and nuclear movements of the intervertebral disc.* Proceedings International Society Study Lumbar Spine 10th Ann Mtg, Cambridge, England.

80. Landells CD, Van Peteghem PK (1988): Fractures of the atlas: classification, treatment and morbidity. *Spine* 13:451–452.

81. Langsam CL (1941): M. omohyoideus in American whites and Negroes. *Am J Phys Anthropol* 28:249–259.

82. Lee C, Kim KS, Rogers LF (1982): Sagittal fractures of the cervical vertebral body. *Am J Roentgenol* 139(1):55–60.

83. Lee S, Harris KG, Nassif J, Goel VK, Clark CR (1993): In vivo kinematics of the cervical spine. Part I: Development of a roentgen stereophotogrammetric technique using metallic markers and assessment of its accuracy. *J Spinal Disord* 6(6):522–534.

84. Lhermitte J (1929): Multiple sclerosis: the sensation of an electric discharge as an early symptom. *Arch Neurol Psych* 22:5–8.

85. Lysell E (1969): Motion in the cervical spine. *Acta Orthop Scand (Suppl)* 123:1–61.

86. Mair WGP, Druckman R (1953): The pathology of spinal cord lesions and their relation to the clinical features in protrusion of cervical intervertebral discs. *Brain* 76:70–91.

87. Marar BC (1975): Fractures of the axis arch. *Clin Orthop* 106: 155–165.

88. Marar BC (1974): Hyperextension injuries of the cervical spine: the pathogenesis of damage to the spinal cord. *J Bone Joint Surg [Am]* 56:1655–1662.

89. McElhaney JH, Paver JG, McCrackin HJ, Maxwell GM (1983): *Cervical spine compression responses.* Proceedings 27th STAPP Car Crash Conference, Soc Automotive Engineers, Warrendale, Pennsylvania, pp. 163–177.

90. McVeigh JF (1923): Experimental cord crushes; with a special reference to the mechanical factors involved and subsequent changes in the areas of the cord affected. *Arch Surg* 7:573–600.

91. Mestdagh H (1976): Morphological aspects and biomechanical properties of the vertebroaxial joint (C2-C3). *Acta Morphol Neerl Scand* 14:19–30.

92. Mimura M, Moriya H, Watanabe T, Takahashi K, Yamagata M, Tamaki T (1989): Three-dimensional motion analysis of the cervical spine with special reference to the axial rotation. *Spine* 14: 1135–1139.

93. Moroney SP, Schultz AB, Miller JAA (1988): Analysis and measurement of neck loads. *J Orthop Res* 6:713–720.

94. Moroney SP, Schultz AB, Miller JAA, Andersson GBJ (1988): Load-displacement properties of lower cervical spine motion segments. *J Biomech* 9:769–779.

95. Mouradian WH, Fietti VG Jr, Cochran GV, Fielding JW, Young J (1978): Fractures of the odontoid: A laboratory and clinical study of mechanisms. *Orthop Clin North Am* 9:985–1001.

96. Myers BS, McElhaney JH, Doherty BJ, Paver JG, Gray L (1991): The role of torsion in cervical spine trauma. *Spine* 16:870–874.

97. Nolan JP Jr, Sherk HH (1988): Biomechanical evaluation of the extensor musculature of the cervical spine. *Spine* 13:9–11.

98. Nowinski GP, Visarius H, Nolte LP, Herkowitz HN (1993): A biomechanical comparison of cervical laminaplasty and cervical laminectomy with progressive facetectomy. *Spine* 18(4):1995–2004.

99. Oda T, Panjabi MM, Crisco JJ III (1991): Three-dimensional translational movements of the upper cervical spine. *J Spinal Disord* 4(4):411–419.

100. Oda T, Panjabi MM, Crisco JJ III, Oxland TR, Katz L, Nolte L-P (1991): Experimental study of atlas injuries. II: Relevance to clinical diagnosis and treatment. *Spine* 16(10):S466–473.

101. Ommaya AK (1968): Mechanical properties of tissues of the nervous system. *J Biomech* 1:127–138.

102. Orofino C, Sherman MS, Schechter D (1960): Luschka's joint: a degenerative phenomenon. *J Bone Joint Surg [Am]* 42:853–858.

103. Osgood RB, Lund CC (1928): Fractures of the odontoid process. *N Engl J Med* 198:61–72.

104. Oxland TR, Panjabi MM, Southern EP, Duranceau JS (1991): An anatomic basis for spinal instability: a porcine trauma model. *J Orthop Res* 9:452–462.

105. Panjabi MM, Dicker DB, Dohrmann GJ (1977): Biomechanical quantification of experimental spinal cord trauma. *J Biomech* 10: 681–687.

106. Panjabi MM, Dvorák J, Crisco JJ III, Oda T, Hilibrand A, Grob D (1991): Flexion, extension, and lateral bending of the upper cervical spine in response to alar ligament transections. *J Spinal Disord* 4(2):157–167.

107. Panjabi MM, Dvorák J, Crisco JJ III, Oda T, Wang P, Grob D (1991): Effects of alar ligament transection on upper cervical spine rotation. *J Orthop Res* 9:584–593.

108. Panjabi MM, Duranceau J, Goel V, Oxland T, Takata K (1991): Cervical human vertebrae: Quantitative three-dimensional anatomy of the middle and lower regions. *Spine* 16(8):861–869.

109. Panjabi MM, Duranceau JS, Oxland TR, Bowen CE (1989): Multidirectional instabilities of traumatic cervical spine injuries in a porcine model. *Spine* 14:1111–1115.

110. Panjabi MM, Oda T, Crisco JJ III, Oxland TR, Katz L, Nolte L-P (1991): Experimental study of atlas injuries. I: Biomechanical

analysis of their mechanisms and fracture patterns. *Spine* 16(10): S460–465.

111. Panjabi MM, Oxland TR, Parks EH (1991): Quantitative anatomy of cervical spine ligaments. Part I. Upper cervical spine. *J Spinal Disord* 4(3):270–276.

112. Panjabi MM, Oxland TR, Parks EH (1991): Quantitative anatomy of cervical spine ligaments. Part II. Middle and lower cervical spine. *J Spinal Disord* 4(3):277–85.

113. Panjabi MM, Oxland T, Takata K, Goel VJ, Duranceau J, Krag M (1993): Articular facets of human spine: Quantitative three-dimensional anatomy. *Spine* 18:1297–1310.

114. Panjabi MM, Summer DJ, Pelker RR, Videman T, Friedlander GE, Southwick WO (1986): Three-dimensional load-displacement curves due to forces on the cervical spine. *J Orthop Res* 4: 152–161.

115. Panjabi MM, White AA III (1989): Biomechanics of nonacute cervical spinal cord trauma. In: Sherk HH, et al., eds. *The cervical spine*, 2nd ed. Philadelphia: JB Lippincott, pp. 91–96.

116. Panjabi MM, White AA III, Johnson RM (1975): Cervical spine biomechanics as a function of transection of components. *J Biomech* 8:327–336.

117. Panjabi MM, White AA III, Keller D, Southwick WO, Friedlaender G (1978): Stability of the cervical spine under tension. *J Biomech* 11:189–197.

118. Panjabi MM, Wrathall JR (1988): Biomechanical analysis of experimental spinal cord injury and functional loss. *Spine* 13:1365–1370.

119. Parke WW, Sherk HH (1989): Normal adult anatomy. In: Bailey RW, Sherk HH, et al., eds. *The cervical spine*, 2nd ed. Philadelphia: JB Lippincott, pp. 15–18.

120. Payne EE, Spillane JD (1957): The cervical spine. An anatomico-pathological study of 70 specimens (using a special technique) with particular reference to the problem of cervical spondylosis. *Brain* 80:571–596.

121. Penning L (1989): Functional anatomy of joints and discs. In: Bailey RW, Sherk HH, et al., eds. *The cervical spine*, 2nd ed. Philadelphia: JB Lippincott, pp. 33–56.

122. Penning L, Wilmink JT (1987): Rotation of the cervical spine: a CT study on normal subjects. *Spine* 12:732–738.

123. Petrie JG (1964): Flexion injuries of the cervical spine. *J Bone Joint Surg [Am]* 46:1800–1806.

124. Powers B, Miller MD, Kramer RS, Martinez S, Gehweiler JA Jr (1979): Traumatic anterior atlanto-occipital dislocation. *Neurosurgery* 4:12–17.

125. Rand RW, Crandall PH (1962): Central spinal cord syndrome in hyperextension injuries of the cervical spine. *J Bone Joint Surg [Am]* 44:1415–1422.

126. Raynor RB, Push J, Shapiro I (1963): Cervical facetectomy and its effect on spine strength. *J Neurosurg* 63:278–282.

127. Reid JD (1960): Effects of flexion-extension movements of the head and spine upon the spinal cord and nerve roots. *J Neurol Neurosurg Psychiatry* 23:214–221.

128. Richman S, Friedman RL (1954): Vertical fractures of the cervical vertebral bodies. *Radiology* 62:536–543.

129. Roaf R (1963): Lateral flexion injuries of the cervical spine. *J Bone Joint Surg [Br]* 45:36–38.

130. Roaf R (1960): A study of the mechanics of spinal injuries. *J Bone Joint Surg [Br]* 42:810–823.

131. Rodrigues O (1840): Des lois géométriques qui régissent les déplacements d'un système solide dans l'espace, et de la variation des coordonées provenant de ces déplacements considérés indépendamment des causes qui peuvent les produire. *J Math Pures Appl* 5:380–440.

132. Rothman RH, Simeone FA, eds. (1975): *The spine.* Philadelphia: WB Saunders, pp. 1–922.

133. Roy-Camille R, Saillant G, Mazel C (1989): Internal fixation of the unstable cervical spine by a posterior osteosynthesis with plates and screws. In: Sherk HH, et al., eds. *The cervical spine*, 2nd ed. Philadelphia: JB Lippincott, pp. 390–403.

134. Ruston SA (1984): *Movements of the cervical spine measured by biplanar photogrammetry.* Thesis (M.Sc.), University of Strathclyde, Scotland.

135. Schlicke LH, White AA III, Panjabi MM, Pratt A, Kier L (1979): A quantitative study of vertebral displacement and angulation in

the normal cervical spine under axial load. *Clin Orthop* 140:47–49.

136. Schneider RC, Cherry G, Pantek H (1954): Syndrome of acute central cervical spinal cord injury with special reference to the mechanism involved in hyperextension injuries of the cervical spine. *J Neurosurg* 11:546–577.

137. Schneider RC, Kahn EA (1956): Chronic neurologic sequelae of acute trauma to the spine and spinal cord. Part I. The significance of the acute-flexion or "tear-drop" fracture-dislocation of the cervical spine. *J Bone Joint Surg [Am]* 38:985–997.

138. Schneider RC, Livingston KE, Cave AJE, Hamilton G (1965): "Hangman's fracture" of the cervical spine. *J Neurosurg* 22:141–154.

139. Schultz RJ (1972): *The language of fractures.* Malabar, FL: RE Krieger, pp. 298–299.

140. Scull ER (1979): The dynamic mechanical response characteristics of spinal cord tissue: a preliminary report. *Paraplegia* 17:222–232.

141. Shea M, Wittenberg RH, Edwards WT, White AA III (1992): In vitro hyperextension injuries in the human cadaveric cervical spine. *J Ortho Res* 10:911–916.

142. Sherk HH, Parke WW (1989): Developmental anatomy. In: Sherk HH, et al., eds. *The cervical spine*, 2nd ed. Philadelphia: JB Lippincott, pp. 1–10.

143. Shono Y, McAfee PC, Cunningham BW (1993): The pathomechanics of compression injuries in the cervical spine: nondestructive and destructive investigative methods. *Spine* 18(14):2009–2019.

144. Sinbert SE, Berman MS (1940): Fracture of the posterior arch of the atlas. *JAMA* 114:1996–1998.

145. Smith CG (1956): Changes in length and position of the segments of the spinal cord with changes in posture in the monkey. *Radiology* 66:259–266.

146. Somerson SK, Stokes BT (1987): Functional analysis of an electromechanical spinal cord injury device. *Exp Neurol* 96:82–96.

147. Southern EP, Oxland TR, Panjabi MM, Duranceau JS (1990): Cervical spine injury patterns in three modes of high-speed trauma: a biomechanical porcine model. *J Spinal Disord* 3(4): 316–328.

148. Spence KF, Decker S, Sell KW (1970): Bursting atlantal fracture associated with rupture of the transverse ligament. *J Bone Joint Surg [Am]* 52:543–549.

149. Termansen NB (1974): Hangman's fracture. *Acta Orthop Scand* 45:529–539.

150. Töndury G (1959): The cervical spine: its development and changes during life. *Acta Orthop Belg* 25:602–626.

151. Torg JS, Pavlov H, O'Neill MJ, Nichols CE Jr, Sennett B (1991): The axial load teardrop fracture. A biomechanical, clinical and roentgenographic analysis. *Amer J Sports Med* 19(4):355–364.

152. Tunturi AR (1977): Elasticity of the spinal cord dura in the dog. *J Neurosurg* 47:391–396.

153. Tunturi AR (1978): Elasticity of the spinal cord, pia and denticulate ligament in the dog. *J Neurosurg* 48:975–979.

154. Von Torklus D, Gehle W (1972): *The upper cervical spine: regional anatomy, pathology and traumatology. A systematic radiological atlas and textbook.* (Translated by LS Michaelis.) New York: Grune & Stratton.

155. Werne S (1957): Studies in spontaneous atlas dislocation. *Acta Orthop Scand (Suppl)* 23:1–150.

156. Wetzel FT, Panjabi MM, Pelker RR (1989): Temporal biomechanics of posterior cervical spine injuries in vivo in a rabbit model. *J Orthop Res* 7:728–731.

157. White AA III, Panjabi MM (1978): The basic kinematics of the human spine. *Spine* 3:12–20.

158. White AA III, Panjabi MM (1990): *Clinical biomechanics of the spine,* 2nd ed. Philadelphia: JB Lippincott.

159. Whitley JF, Forsyth HF (1960): Classification of cervical spine injuries. *Am J Roentgenol* 83:633–644.

160. Wilder DG, Pope MH, Frymoyer JW (1988): The biomechanics of lumbar disc herniation and the effect of overload and instability. *J Spinal Disord* 1:16–32.

161. Williams TG (1975): Hangman's fracture. *J Bone Joint Surg* 57: 82–88.

162. Wood-Jones F (1913): The ideal lesion produced by judicial hanging. *Lancet* 1:53.
163. Wyke B (1978): Clinical significance of articular receptor systems. *Ann R Coll Surg Engl* 60:137.
164. Yoganandan N, Pintar F, Butler J, Reinartz J, Sances A Jr, Larson SJ (1989): Dynamic response of human cervical spine ligaments. *Spine* 14:1102–1110.
165. Yoganandan N, Pintar FA, Sances A Jr, Reinartz J, Larson SJ (1991): Strength and kinematic response of dynamic cervical spine injuries. *Spine* 16(10):S511–517.
166. Yoganandan N, Sances A Jr, Maiman DJ, Myklebust JB, Pech P, Larson SJ (1986): Experimental spinal injuries with vertical impact. *Spine* 11:855–860.
167. Yoo JU, Zou D, Edwards WT, Bayley J, Yuan HA (1992): Effect of cervical spine motion on the neuroforaminal dimensions of human cervical spine. *Spine* 17(10):1131–1136.
168. Zdeblick TA, Abitbol JJ, Kunz DN, McCabe RP, Garfin S (1993): Cervical stability after sequential capsule resection. *Spine* 18(14):2005–2008.
169. Zdeblick TA, Zou D, Warden KE, McCabe R, Kunz D, Vanderby R (1992): Cervical stability after foraminotomy. *J Bone Joint Surg.*

The Adult Spine: Principles and Practice,
2nd edition, J.W. Frymoyer, Editor-in-Chief.
Lippincott-Raven Publishers, Philadelphia © 1996.

Biomechanics of the Cervical Spine

II. Internal Fixation

Martin H. Krag

Development of surgically implanted devices for mechanical support of the cervical spine extends back almost a century to Hadra's use of posterior spinous process wiring in 1891 (75,76) and has continued to the present at an increasingly rapid rate. Along with internal fixation, bone graft has come to be used almost universally as well, based on the recognition that over time, implant loosening is highly likely without solid bone fusion. It is almost prophetic that in Hadra's original case, in which no bone graft was used, the wire slipped "after some weeks" and reoperation was performed. Thus, very few recent series have been reported in which bone graft was not used, although there certainly have been some, for trauma (44,54,88,96,114,126,146,163,178), rheumatoid arthritic upper cervical spine subluxation (17,96), and spinal tumors (see section on polymethylmethacrylate below).

An integral factor in spinal implant development has been an improved understanding of spinal and implant biomechanics. Summaries of this topic are contained in various recent works (187,188).

One of the major rationales for use of internal fixation is the rapid mobilization after spinal trauma that it allows, compared to nonoperative treatment. As reported by Murphy et al. (123) early internal fixation for traumatic quadriplegia resulted in 21 days' shorter hospital stay, 40 days' sooner leave of absence from primary re-

habilitation, and no decrease in functional status at final follow-up. Cotler et al. (34) showed a 30% reduction in hospital charges and 60% reduction in length of stay by internal fixation for traumatic cervical dislocations. Lower morbidity was seen with internal fixation performed before, versus 72 hours after, injury for quadriplegics (103). Not all studies, however, have reported a significant effect from operative treatment (43).

UPPER CERVICAL SPINE

Wires

Wiring of C1-C2 has been attempted through a wide variety of posterior techniques. The forerunner of these was the use by Mixter and Osgood (116) of a "stout braided silk . . . passed about [the C1] posterior arch . . . [and] firmly anchored by tying the silk band about the [C2] spinous process. . . ." Willard and Nicholson (193) used a strip of fascia lata, both ends of which were pulled through a loop passed around the arch of C1 (Fig. 1A). Although this pattern is widely attributed to Gallie, neither of Gallie's early works (61,62) make any mention of vertebral levels or the wiring pattern used. Although at least one standard textbook (36) refers to Mixter and Osgood (116) for the method, those authors used only a single strand of silk suture passed once around the C1 lamina and under the C2 spinous process. Rogers (140), who really popularized wire fixation for trauma management, described two cases involving C1. In both cases, only a single strand of wire was passed around the C1 arch. Thus it appears that the Gallie wiring pattern should really be attributed to Willard and Nicholson (Fig. 1A).

In response to a fairly high non-union rate with these previous wiring patterns, a number of other techniques were developed in the last 20 years that were intended to provide improved motion control. A bone graft was incorporated under the single loop of wire by McGraw and Rusch (113) (Fig. 1B). Variations of this technique were described by a number of authors (4,39,57,107, 139,195). Two separate grafts (one on each side) contoured to fit between the laminae were wired into place using either one loop (21,166) (Fig. 1C) or two loops (72) of wire on each side (Fig. 1D). Presumably because of the improved motion control gained by the latter two methods, fusion rates of 94% and 97%, respectively, were achieved.

In order to obtain or maintain reduction of a C1 anterior subluxation, a posteriorly directed force would be the most effective. None of the C1-C2 wiring and grafting techniques described above are particularly strong in this regard because the graft and wire can flex forward by rotating about the lamina of C2. To overcome this, Forsyth et al. (58) used rib allograft anchored by circumlaminar wires at C2 and at C3 (Fig. 1E). The C1 wire is thus able to provide anterior–posterior position control in a more secure manner, but it also incorporates an additional vertebra into the fusion. The effectiveness of this compared to other techniques is hard to judge because most reports of C1-C2 techniques do not describe the residual subluxation after graft healing.

Instead of C2 and C3, another alternative is to use C2 and the occiput for provision of the two anchor points for anterior–posterior control of C1. A variety of wiring methods for this technique exist and have been reviewed elsewhere (38,70,148). In the first of these, occipital holes for wire fixation were used as described in 1960 (138). Various graft patterns have been used, such as a single unicortical iliac plate (38,148) or bilateral bicortical iliac strips (70).

Because of the greater mobility at Oc-C1 than at C2-C3 and because of the greater difficulty in attaching to the occiput than to C3, the C1-C2-C3 method seems preferable to the Oc-C1-C2 method. Crellin et al. (35) refer to persistent symptoms if the Oc-C1 joint is not included (with rheumatoid arthritis patients), but many studies have had good results by fusing only C1-C2 without including the occiput. There have been no studies comparing these various techniques.

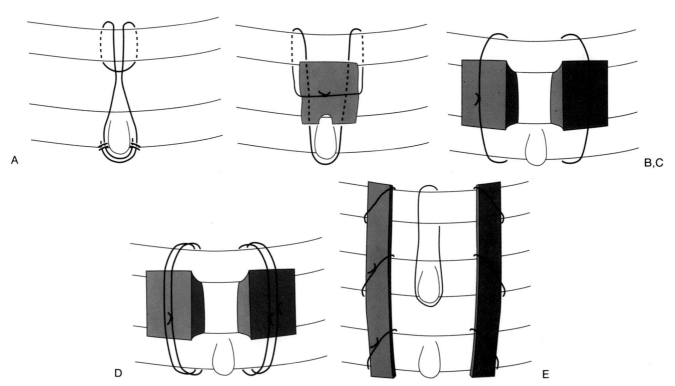

FIG. 1. Posterior wiring and bone graft methods for C1-C2. **A:** Willard and Nicholson, 1941 (193), the so-called Gallie. **B:** McGraw and Rusch, 1973 (113). **C:** Brooks and Jenkins, 1978 (21). **D:** Griswold et al., 1978 (72). **E:** Forsyth et al., 1959 (58).

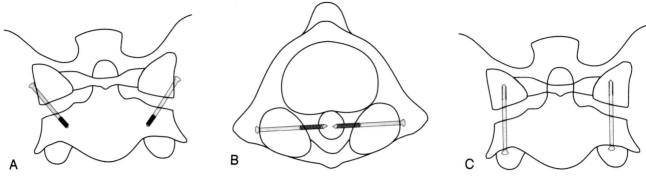

FIG. 2. Screw fixation of C1-C2. **A,B:** Barbour, 1971 (8), anterior and cephalad views. **C:** Magerl and Seeman, 1987 (109).

Screws

The attachment of C1 to C2 by posterior wires is prevented if the C1 lamina is hypoplastic, fractured, or surgically removed. To handle such cases, screws may be placed across the C1-C2 articular surfaces on each side. This can be accomplished using two screws oriented approximately in the coronal plane, inserted using a lateral approach on each side of C1 (8,46,162) as shown in Figures 2A and 2B; however, this gives a very limited exposure. An alternative, from the anterior aspect, is to place the screws somewhat similarly to those for dens fracture fixation (see below), except to enter C2 more laterally and to direct the screw more dorsally and slightly laterally, across the C1-C2 articular facets [illustrated in Dickman et al. (40), along with a number of other superb illustrations of screw fixation techniques]. A clinical series apparently has not yet been published. Magerl and Seeman (109) described another method used through a single posterior incision (Fig. 2C), which has become more widely used. Each screw enters one of the C2 inferior articular processes from below, angles upward and forward across the C1-C2 joint, crosses the lateral mass

of C1 obliquely, and just penetrates through its anterior cortex. This Magerl technique is significantly stronger and stiffer than the so-called Gallie wiring, as shown by mechanical testing of cadaveric spine specimens (37,81). Supplemental posterior wiring can be done in combination with the screws. Magerl and coworkers, in two different reports (90,109) have reported 100% union and maintenance of alignment with this technique. Grob et al. (74) reported 99.4% union. None of these three techniques is simple, however, and one should have a solid understanding of the anatomic details before attempting them (see Chapters 55 and 58).

A fractured dens can be reattached to the C2 body by means of one or two screws placed from below (Fig. 3). This method apparently was first reported in 1982 (12,124) and has been used by others since then (2,52,67,183). Knöringer (98) devised a screw which has no head, but rather a second short segment of somewhat larger diameter threads, in an effort to reduce soft tissue irritation or C2-C3 disc damage. A similar effort using Herbert screws has been reported (29). Despite the general presence of a hypodense region of trabecular bone just below the dens (83), cut-out of properly placed

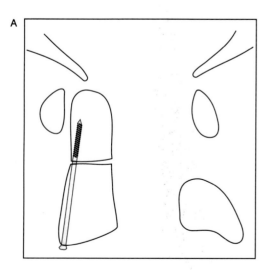

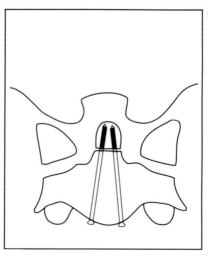

FIG. 3. Screw fixation of dens fracture according to Böhler, 1982 (12). **A:** Lateral. **B:** Anterior.

screws has not been a significant problem. *In vitro* testing (41) shows that a single 3.5-mm cortical screw across an experimentally produced dens fracture reconstitutes 50% of the pre-fracture dens strength. Also, no biomechanical difference resulted from use of one versus two screws (71,152). Clinical results have been encouraging (for example, 29,51,52,92,183): fusion rates have been high, complications relatively low, and C1-C2 mobility good (92). Some problems at C2-C3 do occur: decreased mobility in 11 and fusion in 2 of 18 patients (183). Important instrumentation improvements have occurred recently, but this still is a technically demanding close-tolerance procedure, and its risk–benefit ratio relative to that of other methods of treating dens mechanical insufficiency is not yet well established.

Plates and Rods

To improve on the security of wired-in bone grafts for fusions between the occiput and the upper cervical spine (78), a number of posterior metallic implants have been developed: Luque rods (48,89,173), Luque rectangles (19,111,132,134), and Harrington rods (122) have been attached to the cranium and laminae by wires. Various plate and screw systems have also been described (55,73,86,146). Opinions vary as to whether the occipital screws should penetrate the inner cortex (146) or not (86).

For C1-C2 fusions, various types of clamp and rod systems have been described, such as the Halifax clamp (88,121,178) and others (56,115,141). The Halifax clamp, like a Gallie or interspinous process wire, functions largely as a two-point fixation system: anterior translation can still occur (101). To create a three-point fixation system, a load-bearing bone graft can be placed between the Halifax clamp and the C2 lamina (121) (Fig. 4) or an L-shaped rod can be used (56). Anterior plates in the upper cervical region have a fairly limited application: Schmelzle and Harms (155) and Jeszenszky et al. (93) describe anterior plating for Oc-C1 rotatory subluxation. Streli (168–170) describes a "T" or cruciate plate for C1-C2-C3 fixation of dens fractures. And Tuite et al. (179) describe C2-C3 Caspar plating for severe C2 bilateral pars interarticular fractures.

LOWER CERVICAL SPINE

Spinous Process and Laminar Wires

As mentioned previously, Hadra (75,76) appears to have performed the earliest cervical wiring. Details of the method are not given except that the wire was passed "four to five times around [the C6-C7 spinous processes] in a figure of 8." Details of the revision, after the wire slipped off, are not given. Gallie (61,62) also gives no de-

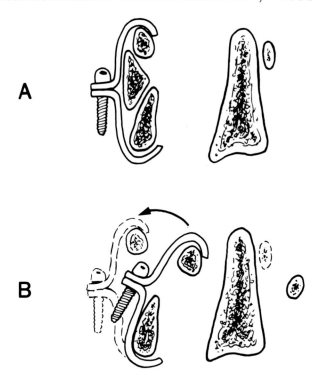

FIG. 4. Halifax clamp. **A:** Bone graft between clamp and C2 lamina resists anterior shifting of C1 on C2. **B:** Without such a bone graft, the clamp functions similarly to a wire around the laminae of C1 and C2. [Used with permission from Moskovich and Crockard (121).]

tails of his method except that "the spines of the two vertebrae involved" were fastened "together with fine steel wire." Details were first presented by Ryerson and Christopher (147) in their case report. At first the wire went through the middle of the spinous process of C6 and of C7 in a simple loop and no bone graft was used. After the C6 spinous process fractured at 9 weeks, the wire was repositioned around the C6 lamina and under the C7 spinous process; this time a bone graft was used.

The first series of patients was reported by Rogers (140). Forsyth et al. (58) simplified and strengthened the wiring pattern by placing it under the entirety of the lower spinous process and through the upper spinous process, in particular "near the top of [its] base," thereby decreasing the likelihood of spinous process failure. Bohlman (14) and Weiland and McAfee (186) modified the Rogers technique by adding two additional transverse wires to hold unicortical bone graft plates against the spinous processes. Other methods have also been reported (154,158,174).

No clear differences between these wiring methods have been shown in terms of clinical outcome. The Forsyth pattern is probably the simplest to perform and has the largest amount of the upper spinous process enclosed within the wire loop. The additional neurologic risks of wire passage around the lamina instead of the spinous processes (15,53) seem unnecessary and ill advised unless spinous process fractures are present.

Various wire sizes, number of strands, and materials have been tried. For years, single-strand stainless steel wires were used: Rogers (140) used 24-gauge, Forsyth et al. (58) used 20-gauge, and Bohlman's group (14,112,186) used a combination of gauges. To reduce flexural rigidity, yet maintain adequate tensile strength, two strands of 24- or 26-gauge wire were twisted together by Robinson and Southwick (137). Carrying this further, Songer et al. (165) (Fig. 5) described 49-stranded stainless steel cable and showed that this had 6 to 22 times greater fatigue life than single-strand wire of similar tensile strength. They reported no wire breakage, although this has been described as a cause of cord injury by Blacklock (9). Titanium wire has recently been used: it has less magnetic resonance imaging (MRI) artefact than stainless steel or cobalt chrome but significantly less fatigue life (157).

Concerning wire fastening techniques, Wang et al. (184) showed knotting was stronger than twisting, although the ease, adjustability, and low failure rate makes the latter the most widely used technique. Recently available multistrand cables are usually secured by a special collar which is crimped into place.

Articular Process (Facet) Wires

Wires passed through the inferior articular process (perpendicular to the articular surface) provide a useful vertebral attachment when the laminae are absent (e.g., fractured or excised). Robinson and Southwick (138) first described the method in which multiple laminectomized vertebrae are tethered to a lower cervical spinous process. This was later modified (26) so that the

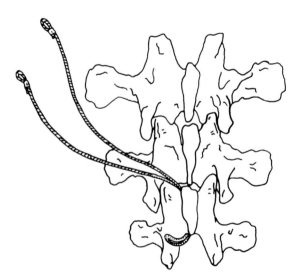

FIG. 5. Songer cable. [Used with permission from Songer et al. (165).]

articular process wires were tied around a longitudinal tricortical iliac graft on each side. Recently, others have tied these wires around Harrington compression rods instead (63,122). This construct has been shown (69) *in vitro* to restrict cervical spine motion to approximately 20% of that seen in the intact spine. This technique is safe and effective for dealing with difficult multilevel laminectomies. Although it may not provide as much rigidity as posterior plates, the graft bed is not obstructed as much and the risk of screw penetration through the anterior cortex of the lateral mass is entirely eliminated.

Articular process wires are also useful for dealing with superior articular process fractures (25). The wire passes obliquely from the intact inferior articular process of the superjacent vertebra, down and around the spinous process of the fractured vertebra. This provides a de-rotating force to prevent axial rotation and unilateral forward subluxation. This may be reinforced by an additional wire around both spinous processes. Articular process oblique wiring alone is useful even if the spinous process or lamina of the upper vertebra is fractured or excised.

Hooks and Rods

In 1963 Tucker (178) began using an implant very much like a miniature Harrington compression rod. The hooks were shaped to fit around the upper or lower laminar edges, and were connected by a threaded bolt. A large clinical series of trauma patients was reported by Holness et al. (88) from Halifax. In neither series was bone graft used. Although in two of the 51 patients, the clamp slipped soon after surgery, there were no late failures. Patients were followed 1 to 10 years, and spontaneous bone fusion was reported to be present in all 32 of the patients who were followed for longer than 4 years.

Mechanical comparisons between Halifax clamps and other fixation methods are described below. Clinical comparisons appear not to have been reported. Soft-tissue irritation may be more of a problem from the clamp, because of its greater bulk, than from a spinous process wire.

Load-Bearing Bone Grafts

Although not strictly implants, anterior interbody grafts do function in a load-bearing capacity. An inlay graft was first used in 1952 at the University of Michigan (7). This graft was 1/2 inch wide and 3/16 inch deep and thus did not have large load-bearing capacity. In 1954 Robinson and Smith (136) at Johns Hopkins University began the use of a tricortical or "horseshoe" graft placed between adjacent vertebrae. A smaller loss of interbody height was noted when the endplates were left intact than when they were removed. Emery et al. (49) also noted this, although Brodke et al. (20) did not. Cloward in 1956 began the use of a unicortical, dowel-shaped graft (31). Simmons and Bhalla used a trapezoidal tricortical "keystone" graft (160,161), and Whitecloud and La Rocca (189) used a fibular graft.

Testing with the grafts implanted between vertebrae (187) showed that the dowel graft is 82% and the inlay graft is only 64% as strong as the tricortical graft in compression testing. Failure occurred mainly by the graft sinking into the upper or lower vertebra. Thus the tricortical construct graft was stronger primarily because the endplates were left intact. Testing of various graft types alone (194) showed that the compressive strength of each was quite high.

To try to obtain improved compressive strength, Bloom and Raney (10) suggested placement of a tricortical graft in a reversed position (noncortical border of graft placed anteriorly). In 55 patients with 81 such grafts, Geibel et al. (66) described anterior fragmentation of four grafts and extrusion (followed by reoperation) of one graft. In a similar series, Brodke et al. (20) used a Caspar vertebral body unicortical pin distractor and endplate decortication and had no extrusion.

Because of the tricortical graft extrusion problem in some series (e.g., 66,94), a "double mortise and tenon" graft (Fig. 6) has been reported (167). In a series of 92 patients with 106 interbody grafts (102) no graft extrusions occurred. Another strategy to prevent graft extrusion is the use of one or more anteroposteriorly oriented screws placed along the graft–endplate interface. Graft

pull-out force *in vitro* was significantly improved (196). Graft dislodgement at 1 week *in vivo* in sheep was 80% without and 30% with the screws (182).

Anterior displacement of the graft has occasionally been a problem, both for the Cloward (95) and the tricortical patterns (94). One solution to this problem is to use a double mortise and tenon graft (167), the upper and lower tabs of which prevent displacement (Fig. 6).

Posterior Plates

These have been used since the 1950s, according to Roy-Camille and Saillant (142), who have developed an extensive set of flat plates (Fig. 7) for use throughout the cervical spine (143–146). The screws are placed through holes 13 mm apart, enter the middle of the lateral mass at the most dorsally prominent location, and are directed 10° laterally to avoid the vertebral artery. Because spontaneous fusion was seen to occur, Roy-Camille does not use a bone graft (145,146). There was no postoperative displacement in 85%, up to 5° in 9%, and 5° to 20° in 6% of 221 patients. Details of follow-up and measurement method are not given. Other authors (33,42,47,153) report favorable experience with this method, and additional information on other systems is also available (6,54,106,125,150).

A "hook plate" was described by Magerl et al. (108) and Weidner (185) (Fig. 8), the lower end of which hooks

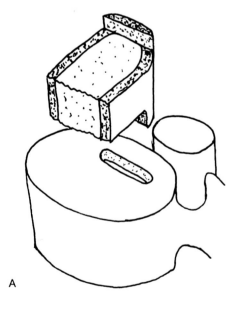

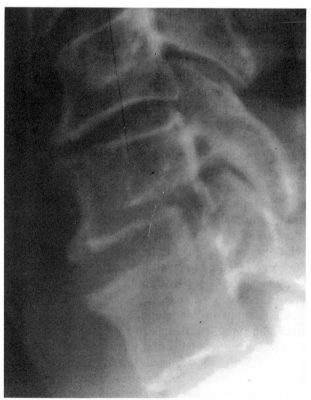

FIG. 6. A: Displacement prevented by mortise and tenon graft. **B:** Lateral x-ray of mortise and tenon graft.

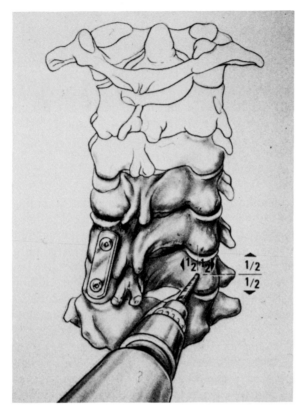

FIG. 7. Roy-Camille lower cervical plate (*left*) and drill entry site (*right*). [Used with permission from Roy-Camille et al. (145).]

ence clearly is needed to establish whether the risks of this method outweigh the benefits.

Anterior Plates

Initial efforts began in 1964 (11) and used plates that were not specifically designed for the cervical spine (18,85). In 1971 the first specially designed plates began to be used, both by Senegas and Gauzere [described by Lesoin et al. (104)] and by Oroszco and Tapies [described by Böhler and Gaudernak (13)]. Both early designs have apparently evolved to a virtually identical five-hole "H" plate in use since 1975 (13). Other plate designs have also evolved, including those by Caspar (27), Oliveira (127),

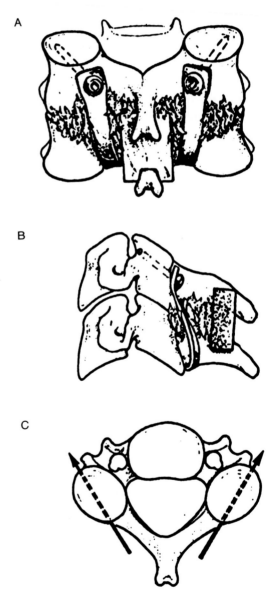

FIG. 8. Hook plate. **A:** Posterior. **B:** Lateral. **C:** Screw orientation in axial view. [Used with permission from Magerl et al. (108).]

under the lamina, just medial to the facet joint. The upper end is attached by a screw oriented parallel to the facet joint (Fig. 8B) and anterolaterally (Fig. 8C) and placed through the anterior cortex of the lateral mass. The advantages of this system are that there are two fewer drill holes to be made and the screws are oriented obliquely upward and through the anterior cortex of the lateral mass, which strengthens (see below) the screw attachment. Good clinical experience has been reported (91).

The Roy-Camille and Magerl methods for lateral mass screw placement are different: the former is 0° anterocephalad and 10° anterolateral, and the latter is parallel to the articular facet and approximately 30° anterolateral. Comparative mechanical *in vitro* tests (50,118) show a greater strength and stiffness of the Magerl method. Mock-up screw placement in human cadavers (84) shows the Magerl method to result in less frequent facet damage (2% versus 23% for Roy-Camille) but more frequent threatened nerve root damage (27% versus 11% for Roy-Camille). Based upon an anatomic study, An et al. (5) recommend an anterolateral angle of 33°.

A preliminary recent report (1) describes screws placed anteromedially through the lateral masses into the pedicles to attach posterior plates for treatment of acute trauma in a small number of patients. Further experi-

TABLE 1. *Use of plates: study results*

Reference	Posterior cortex	Plate type	Postoperative bracing	Patients (N)	Percent of patients with		
					Increased deficit	Screws loose	Non-union
Bohler (13)	Through	Oroszco "H"	No casts	21	0	0	0
Caspar (27)	Through	Caspar	None	50	0	8 (4/50)	0
Tippets (175)	Through	Caspar	None	28	0	0	0
Oliviera (127)	Through	Oporto "H"	Collar	40	0	0	?
				139		2.9%	
Lesoin (104)	14 mm	Senegas "H"	Collar	145	0	1 (2/145)	?
Brown (22)	Not into	Oroszco "H"	Minerva	13	0	15 (2/13)	0
Cabanela (24)	To, not through	Oroszco "H"	Halo vest	8	0	0	0
				166		2.4%	
Gassman (65)	?	Oroszco "H"	Various	13	0	8 (1/13)	0
Weidner (185)	?	Oroszco "H"	None	62	0	5 (3/62)	10 (6/62)
				75		5.3%	

Fuentes et al. (59), and Streli (169). Some of these have been reviewed elsewhere (185).

One of the big concerns regarding use of these plates is screw loosening and resultant esophageal damage or loss of fixation. The rate of screw loosening with the early plate designs, which allowed only one screw per vertebra, was higher according to Weidner (185) than the new plates which allow two screws per vertebra. A summary of results from reports on the latter is in Table 1: the overall loosening rate is 3%, which is quite low. Irritation from the plate itself has not been reported. Cadaveric testing by Sandor and Antal (149,151) showed that screw torque fall-off with 10,000 flexion–extension cycles was quite small, which is consistent with the clinical experience.

How important is it to insert the screw through the posterior cortex? As shown in Table 1, the overall loosening rate for screws not through the posterior cortex (22,24,104) is 2.4% (4 of 166 patients). For screws that do penetrate the posterior cortex (13,27,127,175), the rate is a virtually identical 2.9% (4 of 139). Thus, penetrating the posterior cortex does not seem to provide an advantage. This comparison should be made only cautiously, however, because these studies varied in patient diagnosis, postoperative bracing regimen, and follow-up length. Biomechanical comparisons of screws placed to versus through the posterior cortex show no difference for screw pull-out (110) but do show significantly greater strength of the through-cortex screws for flexion–extension fatigue loading (60).

In order to further reduce the screw loosening, modified screws have been designed. Lesoin et al. (105) developed an "expansion screw," the diameter of the dorsal end of which could be increased by a set screw. Morscher et al. (120) have taken a similar approach (Fig. 9), although the set screw expands the ventral end of the screw against the hole in the plate, rather than the dorsal end against bone. Fenestration of these screws to allow bony

ingrowth resulted in breakage of a number of screws and significant reduction in fatigue life (87). The solid screws have not had this problem (3,99,135,171,176).

The other big concern with these plates is spinal cord damage by drill bit or screw, especially if the posterior cortex is deliberately penetrated. Drill guides and image intensifiers should be used very carefully to prevent overpenetration. It is encouraging that in none of the reported 318 patients (Table 1) was there any apparent cord damage.

Although the exact role that these plates have in cervical spine surgery remains to be further defined, they clearly can be useful for high-grade mechanical insufficiency, and they may prevent the need for a second posterior procedure. The reported non-union rate of 0% (Table 1) is a bit difficult to completely believe, but if

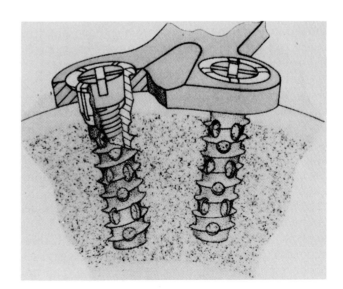

FIG. 9. Anterior cervical locking plate manufactured by Synthes: close up of lower end of plate, showing locking screw inside of bone screw. [Used with permission from Kostuik et al. (99).]

true, it is certainly an improvement over nonplated anterior graftings. In addition, graft extrusions have been virtually eliminated because the plate prevents anterior shifting, and the screw into the graft prevents posterior shifting. The most recent clinical studies (3,64,99, 117,135,171) show very satisfactory results, even for high-grade trauma without any supplemental posterior fixation (64,117,135), although some biomechanical testing (32,150,164,172,180) suggests concern for this construct, as discussed below.

COMPARATIVE MECHANICAL TESTING

A number of studies have been done recently that compare two or more fixation devices *in vitro*. Useful as these studies are, they are limited by the usual factors affecting *in vitro* studies such as absence of muscles, lack of knowledge of *in vivo* load values, unknown relevance of the experimental "injury" to *in vivo* injuries, and absence of any healing processes. These limitations must be kept clearly in mind for accurate interpretation of these studies, and caution should be exercised to prevent overinterpretation.

Crisco et al. (37) compared various C1-C2 fixation methods: Magerl, Halifax clamp, Brooks, and Gallie. For axial loading, there were no significant differences between constructs in neutral zone parameters. For anteroposterior shear loading, the only significant differences were between Magerl and Gallie.

Hajek et al. (77) showed for C1-C2 specimens that the axial rotational stiffness of Halifax clamps was greater than that of Gallie wiring. The anterior translational stiffness of Halifax and Brooks were equal and both greater than that of Gallie wiring.

Hanley and Havell (79), also studying C1-C2 fixation, showed that addition of an interlaminar bone graft to a Gallie wiring produced no significant stiffening effect, but that Brooks was significantly stiffer than Gallie.

Gill et al. (68) compared interspinous process wiring (Forsyth pattern), Halifax clamps, 1/3 semitubular posterior plates with unicortical screws, and these same plates with bicortical screws. Individual intact motion segments were tested in flexion or extension using one at a time of each of three different implants per specimen. There was no statistically significant difference among any of the four implants.

Ulrich et al. (180,181) studied a posterior injury model at C5-C6 using an anterior "H" plate, a Magerl posterior hook plate, circumlaminar wiring, and various combinations of these, and found that the hook plates gave superior results, although their loading method (pull upward on the upper spinous process) may not be very relevant for the *in vivo* situation. Similar testing (150) compared posterior Roy-Camille type plates to combined anterior and posterior plating, and found little

difference in terms of screw torque fall-off with 10,000 flexion–extension cycles.

Coe et al. (32) compared intact specimens to those with extensive posterior damage by cutting all connective tissue from posteriorly up through the dorsal half of the disc. The specimens were instrumented sequentially with the following: (a) circumlaminar wires, (b) Rogers spinous process wiring, (c) Bohlman triple wiring, (d) Roy-Camille posterior plates, (e) Magerl posterior hook plate, (f) Magerl posterior hook plate and Caspar anterior plate, and (g) Caspar anterior plate alone. Six specimens were tested using each of five different load or displacement types. Quite low load values were used in order to prevent specimen damage, so multiple devices could be tested on each specimen. The major findings were the following: (a) there were no significant differences between implants for many of the outcome measures; (b) circumlaminar wires were no better than spinous process wires; and (c) the anterior plate alone provided significantly less resistance than all other implants for compression- or flexion-induced posterior strain. A related study on bovine specimens was done by Sutterlin et al. (172).

In contrast, using a more realistic C5 fracture model, Traynelis et al. (177) showed that anterior plating provided greater stiffness not only for extension and lateral bending, but also for flexion (although the latter was not significant).

Polymethylmethacrylate

Broadly speaking, three approaches have evolved for the use of polymethylmethacrylate (PMMA) since its initial application to spinal problems (97). The most controversial of these is to use PMMA without bone graft in patients who do not have a short life expectancy. Kelly and co-workers (16,96,163) have reported a very favorable experience in treating otherwise healthy trauma patients with circumlaminar wires and PMMA, with follow-up of up to 9 years. Duff (44) described the use of lateral mass bicortical screws linked longitudinally by PMMA in 26 trauma patients, eight of whom were followed for 5 years. A noteworthy report is that by Whitehill et al. (191). Twenty posttraumatic patients treated by posterior wiring and PMMA alone had their surgeries performed by the Department of Neurosurgery and their follow-ups performed by the Department of Orthopaedics. Eleven were found by x-ray not to be solid; four of these underwent further "stabilizing" surgery.

The second approach is to use PMMA in combination with bone grafting for those situations in which additional strength is believed to be desirable, such as to forego postoperative bracing in a patient with severe rheumatoid arthritis. Brattström and Granholm (17) performed Oc-C1-C2 surgery for rheumatoid C1-C2 subluxation. They placed PMMA over the Oc-C1-C2 wire on one side and bone graft on the other side. In 28 patients there were two infections, two C2 spinous process fractures, and two broken wires. Bryan et al. (23) used a similar approach for 11 patients with complex rheumatoid deformities. They reported four instances of wound dehiscence, two of which were infected.

The third approach has been to use PMMA as a stop-gap measure in patients with very short life expectancies. The rationale is that death will occur before the potential long-term benefit of a solid bony fusion can be achieved, and thus the morbidity of bone graft harvest and the inconvenience of orthosis wear are not worth incurring. Scoville et al. (156) first used PMMA in this fashion to supplement occipito-cervical wiring for upper cervical metastases. Dunn (45) collected cases among members of the Cervical Spine Research Society and reported on 24 cases, all but four of whom were able to be mobilized by the third postoperative day with either no or minimal orthosis wear. A more recent series (100) of 18 patients has also demonstrated the utility of this approach, as have a number of other reports, some of which have also described use of bone graft with PMMA (28,30,80,82, 133). Various technical details concerning PMMA placement have been described, including use of a metal spacer and a mold for PMMA containment (128).

There is fairly strong consensus concerning this third approach, less so for the second, and much less so for the first. The basic argument against the first approach (PMMA and no bone graft in normal life expectancy patients) is that the bone–PMMA (or bone–metal–PMMA) interface will eventually weaken and lead to problems, either because of inadequate connective or bony tissue healing, or because of irritation to surrounding tissue resulting from motion. In addition, there is concern over an increased rate of infection, either postoperatively or from late hematogenous seeding. These concerns have been highlighted by a report of 24 cases (112) in which significant complications were encountered with the use of PMMA without bone grafting: 15 (14 cervical) for trauma and nine (eight cervical) for metastatic disease. The most common complication was loss of fixation, which occurred at a mean of 208 days (range, 1 to 730 days), all instances of which were in posterior constructs. There were six deep wound infections, three of which occurred at more than 4 months postoperatively, one of which clearly occurred by hematogenous seeding after a dental procedure.

Pelker et al. (131) showed *in vitro* that addition of PMMA substantially stiffened cadaveric human spine specimens instrumented in various ways. However, Whitehill et al. (190,192), studying PMMA fusions in dogs at various time points, clearly showed the ingrowth between PMMA and bone of a fibrous layer which weakened the overall construct during the first month postop-

eratively. In contrast, the bone-grafted spines by two months postoperatively were stronger than normal spines. The postmortem mechanical testing by Panjabi et al. (129,130) is consistent with these experimental observations.

SUMMARY

The rapid evolution of spinal implants in the past one to two decades has resulted in a tremendous improvement in patient care and has developed because of thorough and ongoing collaboration between bioengineers and clinicians. However, much remains to be learned concerning the relationship between laboratory biomechanical results and their clinical implications.

REFERENCES

1. Abumi K, Itoh H, Taneichi H, Kaneda K (1994): Transpedicular screw fixation for traumatic lesions of the middle and lower cervical spine: description of the techniques and preliminary report. *J Spinal Disord* 7(1):19–28.
2. Aebi M, Etter C, Coscis M (1989): Fractures of the odontoid process: treatment with anterior screw fixation. *Spine* 14:1065–1070.
3. Aebi M, Zuber K, Marchesi D (1991): Treatment of cervical spine injuries with anterior plating: indications, techniques, and results. *Spine* 16(3S):S38–45.
4. Althoff B, Goldie F (1980): Cervical collars in rheumatoid atlantoaxial subluxation: a radiographic comparison. *Ann Rheum Dis* 39:485–489.
5. An HS, Gordin R, Renner K (1991): Anatomic considerations for plate-screw fixation of the cervical spine. *Spine* 16(10):S548–551.
6. Anderson PA, Henley MB, Grady MS, Montesano PX, Winn HR (1991): Posterior cervical arthrodesis with AO reconstruction plates and bone graft. *Spine* 16(3S):S72–79.
7. Bailey RW, Badgley CE (1960): Stabilization of the cervical spine by anterior fusion. *J Bone Joint Surg [Am]* 42:565–594.
8. Barbour JR (1971): Screw fixation in fractures of the odontoid process. *South Austr Clin* 5(1):20–24.
9. Blacklock JB (1994): Fracture of a sublaminar stainless steel cable in the upper cervical spine with neurological injury. Case report. *J Neurosurg* 81(6):932–933.
10. Bloom MH, Raney FL (1981): Anterior intervertebral fusion of the cervical spine: a technical note. *J Bone Joint Surg* 63A:842.
11. Böhler J (1967): Sofort- und Frühbehandlung traumatischer Querschnittlähmungen. *Zeitschr Orthopäd Grenzgebiete* 103:512–528.
12. Böhler J (1982): Anterior stabilization for acute fractures and non-unions of the dens. *J Bone Joint Surg [Am]* 64:18–27.
13. Böhler J, Gaudernak T (1980): Anterior plate stabilization for fracture-dislocations of the lower cervical spine. *J Trauma* 20:203–205.
14. Bohlman HH (1985): Surgical management of cervical spine fractures and dislocations. *Am Acad Orthop Surg Instr Course Lect* 34:163–186.
15. Braakman R, Penning L (1971): *Injuries of the cervical spine.* Amsterdam: Excerpta Medica Publ., pp. 1–262.
16. Branch CL Jr, Kelly DL Jr (1987): Failure of stabilization of the spine with methylmethacrylate. A retrospective analysis of twenty-four cases (*letter*). *J Bone Joint Surg [Am]* 69:1108–1110.
17. Brattström H, Granholm L (1976): Atlanto-axial fusion in rheumatoid arthritis: a new method of fixation with wire and bone cement. *Acta Orthop Scand* 47:619–628.
18. Bremer AM, Nguyen TQ (1983): Internal metal plate fixation combined with anterior interbody fusion in cases of cervical spine injury. *Neurosurgery* 12:649–653.

19. Bridwell KH (1986): Treatment of a markedly displaced hangman's fracture with a Luque rectangle and a posterior fusion in a 71 year old man. Case report. *Spine* 11:49–52.

20. Brodke DS, Zdeblick TA (1992): Modified Smith-Robinson procedure for anterior cervical discectomy and fusion. *Spine* 17:S427–430.

21. Brooks AL, Jenkins EB (1978): Atlanto-axial arthrodesis by the wedge compression method. *J Bone Joint Surg [Am]* 60:279–284.

22. Brown JA, Havel P, Ebraheim N, Greenblatt SH, Jackson WT (1988): Cervical stabilization by plate and bone fusion. *Spine* 13:236–240.

23. Bryan WJ, Inglis AE, Sculco TP, Ranawat CS (1982): Methylmethacrylate stabilization for enhancement of posterior cervical arthrodesis in rheumatoid arthritis. *J Bone Joint Surg [Am]* 64:1045–1050.

24. Cabanela ME, Ebersold MJ (1988): Anterior plate stabilization for bursting teardrop fractures of the cervical spine. *Spine* 13:888–891.

25. Cahill DW, Bellesarrisue R, Ducker TB (1983): Bilateral facet to spinous process fusion: a new technique for posterior spinal fusion after trauma. *Neurosurgery* 13:1–4.

26. Callahan RA, Johnson RM, Margolis RN, Keggi KJ, Albright JA, Southwick WO (1977): Cervical facet fusion for control of instability following laminectomy. *J Bone Joint Surg [Am]* 59:991–1002.

27. Caspar W (1987): Anterior stabilization with the trapezial osteosynthetic plate technique in cervical spine injuries. In: Kehr P, Weidner A, eds. *Cervical spine,* I. New York: Springer-Verlag, pp. 198–204.

28. Chadduck WM, Boop WC Jr (1983): Acrylic stabilization of the cervical spine for neoplastic disease: evolution of a technique for vertebral body replacement. *Neurosurgery* 13:23–29.

29. Chang KW, Liu YW, Cheng PG, Chang L, Suen KL, Chung WL, Chen UL, Liang PL (1994): One Herbert double-threaded compression screw fixation of displaced type II odontoid fractures. *J Spinal Disord* 7(1):62–69.

30. Clark CR, Keggi KJ, Panjabi MM (1984): Methylmethacrylate stabilization of the cervical spine. *J Bone Joint Surg [Am]* 66:40–46.

31. Cloward RB (1958): The anterior approach for removal of ruptured cervical disks. *J Neurosurg* 15:602–617.

32. Coe JD, Warden KE, Sutterlin CE III, McAfee PC (1989): Biomechanical evaluation of cervical spinal stabilization methods in a human cadaveric model. *Spine* 14:1122–1131.

33. Cooper PR, Cohen A, Rosiello A, Koslow M (1988): Posterior stabilization of cervical spine fractures and subluxations using plates and screws. *Neurosurgery* 23:300–306.

34. Cotler HB, Cotler JM, Alden ME, Sparks G, Biggs CA (1990): Medical and economic impact of closed cervical spine dislocations. *Spine* 15:448–452.

35. Crellin RQ, MacCabe JJ, Hamilton EBD (1970): Severe subluxation of the cervical spine in rheumatoid arthritis. *J Bone Joint Surg [Br]* 52:244–251.

36. Crenshaw AH (1971): *Campbell's operative orthopaedics,* 5th ed. St. Louis: CV Mosby, p. 628.

37. Crisco JJ, Panjabi MM, Oda T, Grob D, Dvorák J (1991): Bone graft translation of four upper cervical spine techniques in a cadaveric model. *J Orthop Res* 9(6):835–846.

38. de Groote W, Vercauteren M, Uyttendaele D (1981): Occipitocervical fusion in rheumatoid arthritis. *Acta Orthop Belg* 47:685–698.

39. de los Reyes RA, Malik GM, Wu KK, Ausman JI (1981): A new surgical approach to stabilizing C1-2 subluxation in rheumatoid arthritis. *Henry Ford Hosp Med J* 29:127–130.

40. Dickman CA, Sonntag VKH, Marcotte PJ (1992): Techniques of screw fixation of the cervical spine. *Barrows Neurol Inst Quarterly* 8:9–26.

41. Doherty BJ, Heggeness MH, Esses SI (1993): A biomechanical study of odontoid fractures and fracture fixation. *Spine* 18(2):178–184.

42. Domenella G, Berlanda P, Bassi G (1982): Posterior-approach osteosynthesis of the lower cervical spine by the R. Roy-Camille technique. (Indications and first results). *Ital J Orthop Traumatol* 8:235–244.

43. Donovan WH (1994): Operative and nonoperative management of spinal cord injury. A review. *Paraplegia* 32(6):375–388.

44. Duff TA (1986): Surgical stabilization of traumatic cervical spine dislocation using methylmethacrylate: long term results in 26 patients. *J Neurosurg* 64:39–44.

45. Dunn EJ (1977): Role of methylmethacrylate in the stabilization and replacement of tumors of the cervical spine: a project of the Cervical Spine Research Society. *Spine* 2:15–24.

46. Dutoit G (1976): Lateral atlantoaxial arthrodesis: a screw fixation technique. *South Afr J Surg* 14:9–12.

47. Ebraheim NA, An HS, Jackson WT, Brown JA (1989): Internal fixation of the unstable cervical spine using posterior Roy-Camille plates: preliminary report. *J Orthop Trauma* 3:23–28.

48. Ellis PM, Findlay JM (1994): Craniocervical fusion with contoured Luque rod and autogeneic bone graft. *Can J Surg* 37(1):50–54.

49. Emery SE, Banks M, Bolesta MJ, Bohlman HH (1991): Robinson anterior cervical fusion: a comparison of the standard versus modified technique. Proc Cervical Spine Society Annual Meeting, 1990; In: *Orthop Trans* 15:678.

50. Errico T, Uhl R, Cooper P, Casar R, McHenry T (1992): Pullout strength comparison of two methods of orienting screw insertion in the lateral masses of the bovine cervical spine. *J Spinal Disord* 5(4):459–463.

51. Esses SI, Bednar DA (1991): Screw fixation of odontoid fractures and nonunions. *Spine* 16(10S):S483–485.

52. Etter C, Coscia M, Ganz R, Aebi M (1989): Bone screw osteosynthesis of dens fractures. Technical surgical aspects and results. *Unfallchirurg* 92:220–226.

53. Fairbank TJ (1971): Spinal fusion after laminectomy for cervical myelopathy. *Proc Soc Med* 64:634–636.

54. Fehlings MG, Cooper PR, Errico TJ (1994): Posterior plates in the management of cervical instability: Long-term results in 44 patients. *J Neurosurg* 81(3):341–349.

55. Fidler MW (1986): Posterior instrumentation of the spine: an experimental comparison of various possible techniques. *Spine* 11:367–372.

56. Fidler MW, Valentine NW, Rahmatalla AT (1994): Posterior atlantoaxial fusion. A new internal fixation device. *Spine* 19(12):1397–1401.

57. Fielding JW, Hawkins RJ, Ratzan SA (1976): Spine fusion for atlanto-axial instability. *J Bone Joint Surg [Am]* 58:400–407.

58. Forsyth HF, Alexander EA, Davis CH, Underdal RG (1959): Advantages of early spine fusion in the treatment of fracture-dislocations of the cervical spine. *J Bone Joint Surg [Am]* 41:17–36.

59. Fuentes JM, Blancourt J, Vlahovitch B, Castan P (1983): Tear drop fractures. Contribution to the study of its mechanism and os osteo-disco-ligamentous lesions. *Neurochirurgie* 29:129–134.

60. Gallagher MR, Maiman DJ, Reinartz J, Pintar F, Yoganandan N (1993): Biomechanical evaluation of Caspar cervical screws: comparative stability under cyclical loading. *Neurosurgery* 33(6):1045–1050.

61. Gallie WE (1937): Skeletal traction in the treatment of fractures and dislocations of the cervical spine. *Ann Surg* 106:770–776.

62. Gallie WE (1939): Fractures and dislocations of the cervical spine. *Am J Surg* 46:495–499.

63. Garfin SR, Moore MR, Marshall LF (1988): A modified technique of cervical facet fusions. *Clin Orthop* 230:149–153.

64. Garvey TA, Eismont FJ, Roberti LJ (1992): Anterior decompression, structural bone grafting, and Caspar plate stabilization for unstable cervical spine fractures and/or dislocations. *Spine* 17(10):S431–435.

65. Gassman J, Seligson D (1983): Anterior cervical plate. *Spine* 8:700–707.

66. Geibel PT, Whitecloud TS III, Olive PM, Levet B (1990): Anterior cervical fusion using a reversed Robinson-Smith graft. *Orthop Trans* 14:3.

67. Geisler FH, Cheng C, Poka A, Brumback RJ (1989): Anterior screw fixation of posteriorly displaced Type II odontoid fractures. *Neurosurgery* 25:30–38.

68. Gill K, Paschal S, Corin J, Ashman R, Bucholz RW (1988): Posterior plating of the cervical spine: a biomechanical comparison of different posterior fusion techniques. *Spine* 13:813–816.

69. Goel VK, Clark CR, Harris KG, Schulte KR (1988): Kinematics of the cervical spine: effects of multiple total laminectomy and facet wiring. *J Orthop Res* 6:611–619.

70. Grantham SA, Dick HM, Thompson RC Jr, Stinchfield FE (1969): Occipitocervical arthrodesis, indications, technique and results. *Clin Orthop* 65:118–129.

71. Graziano G, Jaggers C, Lee M, Lynch W (1993): A comparative study of fixation techniques for type II fractures of the odontoid process. *Spine* 18(16):2383–2387.

72. Griswold DM, Albright JA, Schiffman E, Johnson R, Southwick WO (1978): Atlanto-axial fusion for instability. *J Bone Joint Surg [Am]* 60:285–292.

73. Grob D, Dvorák J, Panjabi M, Froehlich M, Hayek J (1991): Posterior occipitocervical fusion: a preliminary report of a new technique. *Spine* 16(3):S17–24.

74. Grob D, Jeanneret B, Aebi M, Markwalder TM (1991): Atlanto-axial fusion with transarticular screw fixation. *J Bone Joint Surg* 73B:972–976.

75. Hadra BE (1981): Wiring of the spinous process in injury and Potts' disease. *Trans Am Orthop Assoc* 4:206.

76. Hadra BE (1975): The classic: wiring of the vertebrae as a means of immobilization in fractures and Potts' disease. *Clin Orthop* 112:4–8.

77. Hajek PD, Lipka J, Hartline P, Saha S, Albright JA (1993): Biomechanical study of C1-C2 posterior arthrodesis techniques. *Spine* 18(2):173–177.

78. Hamblen DL (1967): Occipital-cervical fusion, indications, technique and results. *J Bone Joint Surg* 49B:33–45.

79. Hanley EN Jr, Harvell JC Jr (1992): Immediate postoperative stability of the atlanto axial articulation: a biomechanical study comparing single midline wiring, and the Gallie and Brooks procedures. *J Spinal Disord* 5:306–310.

80. Hansebout RR, Blomquist GA Jr (1980): Acrylic spine fusion: a 20 year clinical series and technical note. *J Neurosurg* 53:606–612.

81. Hanson P, Sharkey N, Montesano PX (1988): Anatomic and biomechanical study of C1-C2 posterior arthrodesis techniques. Proceedings Cervical Spine Research Society 16th Annual Meeting, Key Biscayne, FL, pp. 100–101.

82. Harrington KD (1981): The use of methylmethacrylate for vertebral-body replacement and anterior stabilization of pathologic fracture dislocation of the spine due to metastatic malignant disease. *J Bone Joint Surg [Am]* 63:36–46.

83. Heggeness MH, Doherty BJ (1993): The trabecular anatomy of the axis. *Spine* 18(14):1945–1949.

84. Heller JG, Carlson GD, Abitbol JJ, Garfin SR (1991): Anatomic comparison of the Roy-Camille and Magerl techniques for screw placement in the lower cervical spine. *Spine* 16(10):S552–557.

85. Herrmann HD (1975): Metal plate fixation after anterior fusion of unstable fracture dislocations of the cervical spine. *Acta Neurochir (Wien)* 32:101–111.

86. Heywood AWB, Learmonth ID, Thomas M (1988): Internal fixation for occipito-cervical fusion. *J Bone Joint Surg [Br]* 70:708–711.

87. Hollowell JP, Reinartz J, Pintar FA, Morgese V, Maiman DJ (1994): Failure of synthes anterior cervical fixation device by fracture of Morscher screws: a biomechanical study. *J Spinal Disord* 7(2):120–125.

88. Holness RO, Huestis WS, Howes WJ, Langille RA (1984): Posterior stabilization with an interlaminar clamp in cervical injuries: technical note and review of the long term experience with the method. *Neurosurgery* 14:318–322.

89. Itoh T, Tsuji H, Katoh Y, Yonezawa T, Kitagawa H (1988): Occipitocervical fusion reinforced by Luque's segmental spinal instrumentation for rheumatoid diseases. *Spine* 13:1234–1238.

90. Jeanneret B, Magerl F (1992): Primary posterior fusion C1/2 in odontoid fractures: indications, technique, and results of transarticular screw fixation. *J Spinal Disord* 5(4):464–475.

91. Jeanneret B, Magerl F, Ward EH, Ward J-CH (1991): Posterior stabilization of the cervical spine with hook plates. *Spine* 16(3)S56–63.

92. Jeanneret B, Vernet O, Frei S, Magerl F (1991): Altantoaxial mobility after screw fixation of the odontoid: a computed tomographic study. *J Spinal Disord* 4(2):203–211.

93. Jeszenszky D, Beele B, Harms J, Stoltze D (1995): Surgical treatment of old rotation luxation injuries of C1-C2. Proceedings European Cervical Spine Society Annual Meeting, Erlangen, Germany, June 7-10, p. 51.

94. Johnson RM, Southwick WO (1975): Surgical approaches to the spine. In: RH Rothman, FA Simeone, eds. *The spine.* Philadelphia: WB Saunders, pp. 98–103.

95. Keblish PA, Keggi KJ (1967): Mechanical problems of the dowel graft in anterior cervical fusion. *J Bone Joint Surg [Am]* 49:198.

96. Kelly DL Jr, Alexander E Jr, Davis CH Jr, Smith JM (1972): Acrylic fixation of atlanto-axial dislocations. Technical note. *J Neurosurg* 36:366–371.

97. Knight G (1959): Paraspinal acrylic inlays in treatment of cervical and lumbar spondylolysis and other conditions. *Lancet* 2:147–149.

98. Knöringer P (1987): Double-threaded compression screws in osteosynthesis of acute fractures of the odontoid process. In: Voth D, Glees O, eds. *Disease in the cranio-cervical junction.* New York: de Gruyter, p. 217.

99. Kostuik JP, Connolly PJ, Esses SI, Suh P (1993): Anterior cervical plate fixations with the titanium hollow screw plate system. *Spine* 18(10):1273–1278.

100. Kostuik JP, Errico TJ, Gleason TF, Errico CC (1988): Spinal stabilization of vertebral column tumors. *Spine* 13:250–256.

101. Krag MH (1991): Biomechanics of thoracolumbar spinal fixation (8902.0). *Spine* 16(3S):S84–99.

102. Krag MH, Robertson PA, Johnson CC, Stein A (1995): Anterior cervical fusion using a modified tricortical bone graft: a radiographical analysis of outcome. *Spine (submitted).*

103. Krengel III WF, Anderson PA, Yuan H (1992): Early versus delayed stabilization after cervical spinal cord injury. Proceedings of North American Spine Society, 7th Annual Meeting, Boston, MA, July 9-11, p. 89.

104. Lesoin F, Cama A, Lozes G, Servato R, Kabbag K, Jomin M (1982): Anterior approach and plates in lower cervical posttraumatic lesions. *Surg Neurol* 21:581–587.

105. Lesoin F, Jomin M, Viaud C (1983): Expanding bolt for anterior cervical spine osteosynthesis: technical note. *Neurosurgery* 12:458–459.

106. Louis R (1982): *Posterior vertebral bone plates.* Paris: Ceprime.

107. Louis R (1983): Surgery of the spine: surgical anatomy and operative approaches. New York: Springer-Verlag.

108. Magerl F, Grob D, Seemann P (1987): Stable dorsal fusion of the cervical spine (C2-T1) using hook plates. In: Kehr P, Weidner A, eds. *Cervical Spine I,* New York: Springer-Verlag, pp. 217–221.

109. Magerl F, Seeman P-S (1987): Stable posterior fusion of the atlas and axis by transarticular screw fixation. In: Kehr P, Weidner A, eds. *Cervical Spine I,* New York: Springer-Verlag, pp. 322–327.

110. Maiman DJ, Pintar FA, Yoganandan N, Reinartz J, Toselli R, Woodward E, Haid R (1992): Pull-out strength of Caspar cervical screws. *Neurosurgery* 31(6):1097–1101.

111. Matsunaga S, Sakou T, Morizono Y, Yone K (1988): Occipito-atlanto-axial fusion utilizing a rectangular rod. Proceedings Cervical Spine Research Society 16th Annual Meeting, Key Biscayne, FL, pp. 106–107.

112. McAfee PC, Bohlman HH, Ducker T, Eismont FJ (1986): Failure of stabilization of the spine with methylmethacrylate. *J Bone Joint Surg [Am]* 68:1145–1157.

113. McGraw RW, Rusch RM (1973): Atlanto-axial arthrodesis. *J Bone Joint Surg [Br]* 55:482–489.

114. McLaurin RL, Vernal R, Salmon JH (1972): Treatment of fractures of the atlas and axis by wiring without fusion. *J Neurosurg* 36:773–780.

115. Mitsui H (1984): A new operation for atlanto-axial arthrodesis. *J Bone Joint Surg [Br]* 66:442–445.

116. Mixter SJ, Osgood RB (1910): Traumatic lesion of the atlas and axis. *Ann Surg* 51:193–207.

117. Moerman J, Harth A, Van Trimpont I, Uyttendaele D, et al. (1994): Treatment of unstable fractures, dislocations and fracture-dislocations of the cervical spine with Senegas plate fixation. *Acta Orthop Belg* 60(1):30–35.

118. Montesano PX, Juach E (1988): Anatomic and biomechanical study of posterior cervical spine plate arthrodesis. Proceedings

Cervical Spine Research Society Annual Meeting, Key Biscayne, FL, pp. 39–40.

119. Montesano PX, Juach E, Jonsson H Jr (1992): Anatomic and biomechanical study of posterior cervical spine plate arthrodesis: an evaluation of two different techniques of screw placement. *J Spinal Disord* 5:301–305.

120. Morscher E, Sutter F, Jenny H, Ölerud S (1986): Die vordere Verplattung der Halswirbelsäule mit dem Hohlschrauben-Plattensystem aus Titanium. *Chirurg* 57:702–707.

121. Moskovich R, Crockard HA (1992): Atlantoaxial arthrodesis using interlaminar clamps: an improved technique. *Spine* 17:261–267.

122. Murphy MJ, Daniaux H, Southwick WO (1986): Posterior cervical fusion with rigid internal fixation. *Orthop Clin North Am* 17:55–65.

123. Murphy KP, Opitz JL, Cabanela ME, Ebersold MJ (1990): Cervical fractures and spinal cord injury: outcome of surgical and nonsurgical management. *Mayo Clin Proc* 65(7):949–959.

124. Nakanishi T, Sasaki T, Tokita N, Hirabayashi K (1982): Internal fixation for the odontoid fracture. *Orthop Trans* 6:176.

125. Nazarian SM, Louis RP (1991): Posterior internal fixation with screw plates in traumatic lesions of the cervical spine. *Spine* 16(3S):S64–71.

126. Nielsen CF, Annertz M, Persson L, Wingstrand H, Säveland H, Brandt L (1991): Posterior wiring without bony fusion in traumatic distractive flexion injuries of the mid and lower cervical spine: long-term follow-up in 30 patients. *Spine* 16:467–472.

127. Oliveira JC (1987): Anterior plate fixation of traumatic lesions of the lower cervical spine. *Spine* 12:324–329.

128. Ono K, Tada K (1975): Metal prosthesis of the cervical vertebra. *J Neurosurg* 42:562–566.

129. Panjabi MM, Dicker DB, Dohrmann GJ (1977): Biomechanical quantification of experimental spinal cord trauma. *J Biomech* 10:681–687.

130. Panjabi MM, Goel VK, Clark CR, Keggi KJ, Southwick WO (1985): Biomechanical study of cervical spine stabilization with methylmethacrylate. *Spine* 10:198–203.

131. Pelker RR, Duranceau JS, Panjabi M (1991): Cervical spine stabilization: a three-dimensional, biomechanical evaluation of rotational stability, strength, and failure mechanisms. *Spine* 16:117–122.

132. Ransford AO, Crockard HA, Pozo JL, Thomas NP, Nelson IW (1986): Craniocervical instability treated by contoured loop fixation. *J Bone Joint Surg [Br]* 68:173–177.

133. Raycroft JF, Hockman RP, Southwick WO (1978): Metastatic tumors involving the cervical vertebrae: surgical palliation. *J Bone Joint Surg [Am]* 60:763–768.

134. Rea GL, Mullin BB, Mervis LJ, Miller CL (1993): Occipitocervical fixation in nontraumatic upper cervical spine instability. *Surg Neurol* 40(3):255–261.

135. Ripa DR, Kowall MG, Meyer PR, Rusin JJ (1991): Series of ninety-two traumatic cervical spine injuries stabilized with anterior ASIF plate fusion technique. *Spine* 16(3S):S46–55.

136. Robinson RA, Smith GW (1955): Anterolateal cervical disc removal and interbody fusion for cervical disc syndrome. *Bull Johns Hopkins Hosp* 96:223–224.

137. Robinson RA, Southwick WO (1960): Indications and techniques for early stabilization of the neck in some fracture-dislocations of the cervical spine. *South Med J* 53:565–579.

138. Robinson RA, Southwick WO (1960): Surgical approaches to the cervical spine. *Am Acad Orthop Surg Instr Course Lect* 27:299–316.

139. Rodrigues FAC, Hodgson BF, Craig JB (1991): Posterior atlantoaxial arthrodesis: a simplified method. *Spine* 16(8):878–880.

140. Rogers WA (1942): Treatment of fracture-dislocation of the cervical spine. *J Bone Joint Surg* 24:245–258.

141. Roosen K, Travschel A, Grote W (1982): Posterior atlanto-axial fusions: a new compression clamp for laminar osteosynthesis. *Arch Orthop Trauma Surg* 100:27–31.

142. Roy-Camille R, Saillant G (1972): Chirurgie du rachis cervical. 1. Généralités. Luxations pures des articulaires. *Nouv Presse Med* 1(33):2330–2332.

143. Roy-Camille R, Saillant G (1972): Chirurgie du rachis cervical. 2. Luxation-fracture des articulaires. *Nouv Presse Med* 1(37):2484–2485.

144. Roy-Camille R, Saillant G (1972): Chirurgie du rachis cervical. 3. Fractures complexes du rachis cervical inferieur; tetraplegies. *Nouv Presse Med* 1(40):2707–2709.

145. Roy-Camille R, Saillant G, Laville C, Benazet JP (1992): Treatment of lower cervical spinal injuries—C3 to C7. *Spine* 17(10S):S442–446.

146. Roy-Camille R, Saillant G, Mazel C (1989): Internal fixation of the unstable cervical spine by a posterior osteosynthesis with plates and screws. In: *The cervical spine*, 2nd ed. Bailey RW, Sherk HH, et al., eds. Philadelphia: JB Lippincott, pp. 390–403.

147. Ryerson EW, Christopher F (1937): Dislocation of cervical vertebrae: operative correction. *JAMA* 108:468–470.

148. Sadeghpour E, Noer HR, Mahinpour S (1981): Skull-C2 fusion in rheumatoid patients with atlanto-axial subluxation. *Orthopaedics* 4:1369–1374.

149. Sandor L (1985): Primary stability of AO-plate osteosynthesis of the lower cervical spinal column. II. Anterior spondylodesis with H-plate osteosynthesis. *Z Exp Chir Transplant Kunstliche Organe* 18:93–101.

150. Sandor L (1985): Primary stability of AO-plate osteosynthesis of the lower cervical spinal column. III. Posterior and combined spondylodesis. Conclusions. *Z Exp Chir Transplant Kunstliche Organe* 18:102–110.

151. Sandor L, Antal A (1985): Primary stability of AO-plate osteosynthesis of the lower cervical spinal column. I. Load-bearing capacity of the cervical vertebrae. *Z Exp Chir Transplant Kunstliche Organe* 18:87–92.

152. Sasso R, Doherty BJ, Crawford MJ, Heggeness MH (1993): Biomechanics of odontoid fracture fixation: Comparison of the one- and two-screw technique. *Spine* 18(14):1950–1953.

153. Savini R, Parisini P, Cevellati S (1987): Surgical treatment of late instability of flexion rotation injuries in the lower cervical spine. *Spine* 12:178–182.

154. Schlicke LH, Schulak DJ (1981): Wiring of the cervical spinous process. *Clin Orthop* 154:319–320.

155. Schmelzle R, Harms J (1987): Craniocervical junction—diseases, diagnostic application of imaging procedures, surgical techniques (translated from German). *Fortschritte der Kiefer-und Gesichts-Chirurgie* 32:206–208.

156. Scoville WB, Palmer AH, Samra K, Chong G (1967): The use of acrylic plastic for vertebral replacement or fixation in metastatic disease of the spine: technical note. *J Neurosurg* 27:274–279.

157. Scuderi GJ, Greenberg SS, Cohen DS, Latta LL, Eismont FJ (1993): A biomechanical evaluation of magnetic resonance imaging-compatible wire in cervical spine fixation. *Spine* 18(14):1991–1994.

158. Segal D, Whitelaw GP, Gumbs V, Pick RY (1981): Tension band fixation of acute cervical spine fractures. *Clin Orthop* 159:211–222.

159. Sherk HH, Parke WW (1989): Developmental anatomy. In: Sherk HH, et al., eds. *The cervical spine*, 2nd ed., Philadelphia: JB Lippincott, pp. 1–7.

160. Simmons EH, Bailey SI, Light KI, Simmons ED, Maguire JK (1991): Anterior cervical discectomy and fusion with the keystone technique: a long-term evaluation. Proc Cerv Sp Res Soc Ann Mtg 1990. *Orthop Trans* 15:678.

161. Simmons EH, Bhalla SK (1969): Anterior cervical discectomy and fusion. Clinical and biomechanical study with 8 year follow-up. *J Bone Joint Surg [Br]* 51:225–237.

162. Simmons EH, Dutoit G (1978): Lateral atlanto-axial arthrodesis. *Orthop Clin North Am* 9:1101–1114.

163. Six E, Kelly DL Jr (1981): Technique for C1, C2 and C3 fixation in cases of odontoid fracture. *Neurosurgery* 8:374–376.

164. Smith SA, Lindsey RW, Doherty BJ, Alexander JW, Dickson JH (1992): In-vitro biomechanical testing of the cervical spine locking plate. Proceedings North American Spine Society, 7th Annual Meeting, Boston, MA, pp. 127–128.

165. Songer MN, Spencer DL, Meyer PR, Jayaraman G (1991): The use of sublaminar cables to replace Luque wires. *Spine* 16(8S):S418–421.

166. Sorenson KH, Husby J, Hein O (1978): Interlaminar atlanto-axial fusion for instability. *Acta Orthop Scand* 49:341–349.

167. Stein A, Krag MH, Hugus J (1987): Anterior cervical interbody fusion: description of a new technique with clinical follow-up of the first 20 patients. Proceedings 15th Annual Meeting Cervical Spine Research Society, Washington, DC.

168. Streli R (1981): Kompressionsosteosynthese bei Frakturen und Pseudarthrosen des Dens epistrophei. *Zeitschr Orthop* 119:675–676.

169. Streli R (1987): Dens transfixation plate. In: Kehr P, Weidner A, eds. *Cervical spine I*, New York: Springer-Verlag, pp. 239–243.

170. Streli R (1987): Double hole plate fixation of the lower cervical spine. In: Kehr P, Weidner A, eds. *Cervical spine I*. New York: Springer-Verlag, pp. 175–179.

171. Suh PB, Kostuik JP, Esses SI (1990): Anterior cervical plate fixation with the titanium hollow screw plate system: a preliminary report. *Spine* 15:1079–1081.

172. Sutterlin CE III, McAfee PC, Warden KE, Rey RM Jr, Farey ID (1988): A biomechanical evaluation of cervical spine stabilization methods in a bovine model: static and cyclical loading. *Spine* 13:795–802.

173. Suzuki N, Mitani T (1984): A new method of skull-trunk fixation. Proceedings Scoliosis Research Society.

174. Taddonio RF, Israelski RH (1992): The use of interspinous srummond wiring instrumentation in cervical spine instability. Proceedings North American Spine Society 7th Annual Meeting, Boston, MA, p. 125.

175. Tippets RH, Apfelbaum RI (1988): Anterior cervical fusion with the Caspar instrumentation system. *Neurosurgery* 22:1008–1013.

176. Tominaga T, Koshu K, Mizoi K, Yoshimoto T (1994): Anterior cervical fixation with the titanium locking screw-plate: a preliminary report. *Surg Neurol* 42(5):408–413.

177. Traynelis VC, Donaher PA, Roach RM, Kojimoto H, Goel VK (1993): Biomechanical comparison of anterior Caspar plate and three-level posterior fixation techniques in a human cadaveric model. *J Neurosurg* 79(1):96–103.

178. Tucker HH (1975): Technical report: method of fixation of subluxed or dislocated cervical spine below C1-C2. *Can J Neurol Sci* 2:381–382.

179. Tuite GF, Papadopoulos SM, Sonntag VKH, Hadley MN, Klara PM (1992): Caspar plate fixation for the treatment of complex hangman's fractures. *Neurosurgery* 30(5):761–765.

180. Ulrich C, Wörsdorfer O, Claes L, Magerl F (1987): Comparative study of the stability of anterior and posterior cervical spine fixation procedures. *Arch Orthop Trauma Surg* 106:226–231.

181. Ulrich C, Wörsdorfer O, Kalff R, Claes L, Wilke HJ (1991): Biomechanics of fixation systems to the cervical spine. *Spine* 16(3):S4–9.

182. Vazquez-Seoane P, Yoo J, Zou D, Fay LA, Frederickson JG, Handal JG, Yuan HA, Edwards WT (1993): Interference screw fixation of cervical grafts: a combined in vitro biomechanical and in vivo animal study. *Spine* 18:946–954.

183. Verheggen R, Jansen J (1994): Fractures of odontoid process: analysis of the functional results after surgery. *Eur Spine J* 3:146–150.

184. Wang GJ, Reger SI, Jennings RL, McLaurin CA, Stamp WG (1981): Variable strengths of wire fixation. *Orthopaedics* 5:435–436.

185. Weidner A (1989): Internal fixation with metal plates and screws. In: Sherk HH, et al., eds. *The cervical spine*, 2nd ed. Philadelphia: JB Lippincott, pp. 404–421.

186. Weiland DJ, McAfee PC (1991): Posterior cervical fusion with triple-wire strut graft technique: one hundred consecutive patients. *J Spinal Disord* 4(1):15–21.

187. White AA III (1989): Clinical biomechanics of cervical spine implants. *Spine* 14:1040–1045.

188. White AA III, Panjabi MM (1990): *Clinical biomechanics of the spine,* 2nd ed. Philadelphia: JB Lippincott.

189. Whitecloud TS III, La Rocca H (1976): Fibula strut graft in reconstructive surgery of the cervical spine. *Spine* 1:33–43.

190. Whitehill R, Barry JC (1985): The evolution of stability in cervical spinal constructs using either autogenous bone graft or methylmethacrylate cement: a follow-up report on a canine in vivo model. *Spine* 10:32–41.

191. Whitehill R, Cicoria AD, Hooper WE, Maggio WW, Jane JA (1988): Posterior cervical reconstruction with methylmethacrylate cement and wire: a clinical review. *J Neurosurg* 68:576–584.

192. Whitehill R, Stowers SF, Fechner RE, Ruch WW, Drucker S, Gibson LR, McKernan DJ, Widweyer JH (1987): Posterior cervical fusions using cerclage wires, methylmethacrylate cement and autogenous bone graft: an experimental study of a canine model. *Spine* 12:12–22.

193. Willard D, Nicholson JT (1941): Dislocation of the first cervical vertebra. *Ann Surg* 113:464–475.

194. Wittenberg RH, Moeller J, Shea M, White III AA, Hayes WC (1990): Compressive strength of autologous and allogenous bone grafts for thoracolumbar and cervical spine fusion. *Spine* 15(10):1073–1078.

195. Wu KK, Malik G, Guise ER (1982): Atlanto-axial arthrodesis: a clinical analysis of 22 cases treated at Henry Ford Hospital. *Orthopaedics* 5:865–871.

196. Zou D, Woo J, Ordway N, Wu S-S, Handal JA, Fredrickson BE, Bayley JC, Yuan HA, Edwards WT (1991): Interference screw fixation of cervical grafts: a biomechanical study of a new method of cervical fixation. *J Spinal Disord* 4(2):168–176.

The Adult Spine: Principles and Practice,
2nd edition, J.W. Frymoyer, Editor-in-Chief.
Lippincott-Raven Publishers, Philadelphia © 1996.

Biomechanics of the Cervical Spine

III. Orthoses

Martin H. Krag

Orthoses are used either as a stand-alone treatment method or in combination with internal fixation. Surprisingly little research has been done in this area, and most of that has been biomechanical and not clinical. Comparative, data-based treatment recommendations are very few.

MECHANICAL SUPPORT BY ORTHOSES

A wide variety of designs have evolved and various classifications (18,24,25,59) for describing these orthoses have been suggested. Many of the terms have been based on certain structural characteristics (e.g., 4-poster) or place of origin (e.g., Philadelphia collar), which unfortunately convey little meaning about the actual or intended function. Orthoses for the limbs have come to be named by the body parts they contact or immobilize; the same method is also useful for the spine. Wolf and Johnson (59) use the categories of cervical, head-cervical, head-cervical-thoracic, and halo devices. A somewhat different system (Table 1) is used here because (a) the term *head* covers too wide a range and is too nonspecific, and (b) *halo devices* gets right back to using structural features for naming the device and thus departs from the principle of using the involved body parts for classifying the orthosis.

Certain basic principles should be kept in mind regarding orthoses and evaluations of their function. First, voluntarily produced neck motion (whether by normal or patient volunteers) is not necessarily the same as the motion occurring during activities of daily living. For example, soft foam rubber collars can easily be deformed through almost a full normal range of motion (24), yet patients wearing a collar often actually move far less than this allowable range. Another example involves the halo vest: cervical spine flexion–extension motion was found to be significantly larger between lying down and sitting up (29,31,35,36,51) than between voluntarily produced flexed and extended postures in seated volunteers (7,24,39).

A second principle is that the relationship between motions and loads (forces or moments) in the neck is quite complex. Radiographic measures of motion alone do not give a full understanding of the load distributions, and ultimately it is the latter that produces, for example, a loss of reduction or undesired intervertebral motion.

A third principle is that muscle forces probably are important in determining outcomes with orthoses (56). This is illustrated by the observation that patients seem to seldom "hang" on their orthoses, even halo vests (16). Its importance remains to be studied.

A final principle is that short-term biomechanical performance outcomes are not necessarily the same as longer term clinical outcomes, such as maintaining reduction, obtaining fusion, or preventing neurologic deficit increase. No randomized comparative clinical studies appear to have been done.

TABLE 1. *Cervical orthoses*

Category	Example
Cervical	Collar
Occipito-mandibular-cervical	Collar and chin piece
	Queen Anne collar
Occipito-mandibular-high thoracic	Philadelphia
	4-poster
Occipito-mandibular-low thoracic	Extended Philadelphia
	SOMI
Cranio-thoracic	Minerva
	Halo vest

CATEGORIES OF UPPER SPINAL ORTHOSES

Cervical

These orthoses (Fig. 1), commonly referred to as neck collars, derive little or no support from either the occiput or mandible above, or from the thorax below. They are made of various materials, ranging from soft foam rubber to fairly noncompressible polyethylene. Probably more than any other orthoses, these devices function as reminders to restrict motion, rather than actually mechanically prevent or block motion (1,11,24).

Occipito-Mandibular-Cervical

These orthoses extend cephalad to contact and restrict motion of the mandible (especially the chin) or the occiput to a greater or lesser extent depending on the material stiffness. The thorax is not gripped to a significant extent. Examples of these (Fig. 2) are the collar with chin piece and the Queen Anne collar, motion restriction by which was reported by Colachis et al. (11).

Occipito-Mandibular-High Thoracic

These extend caudally to the upper portion of the sternum and interscapular region. Addition of a chin cup restricts axial motion as well as flexion. Examples include the semirigid Philadelphia collar (Fig. 3) and the much stiffer 4-poster (24), also known as an adjustable Thomas collar (45). The straps connecting front and back halves on both of these designs are flexible. Some other more recent orthoses of this type are illustrated in Plaiser et al. (43).

Pressure sores near the edges of a collar can occur, especially at the upper edge of a hard collar as it crosses over the occiput (34,43), although these can occur over the angle of the mandible (21). Higher skin pressures (over occiput, mandible body, and chin) have been measured in those orthoses that were also rated as less comfortable (43). Out of concern that intracranial pressure may be elevated in head-injured patients, Ferguson et al. (14) described the skin pressures at multiple sites on the neck for various collars: those collars that contacted the mandible, base of skull, and shoulder girdle had the lowest pressures and also (based on the work of others) the best immobilization effect. Kuhnigk et al. (32) monitored intracranial pressure directly in head-injured patients and showed no increase after placement of either of two collars [collars different from those studied by Ferguson et al. (14)].

Occipito-Mandibular-Low Thoracic

These extend along the length of the sternum anteriorly and along much or all of the thoracic spine posteriorly. The extended Philadelphia collar, Yale brace (23), SOMI (sternal occipital mandibular immobilizer), and cervico-thoracic orthosis (18,24) are examples (Fig. 4).

Cranio-Thoracic

The cephalad attachment for these includes (or in the case of the halo vest is limited to) the cranium. The Minerva cast contacts almost the entirety of the head, including occiput and mandible. The thermoplastic Minerva jacket (7,39) is not clearly described in terms of occipital or mandibular contact but includes a circumferential head band. To prevent obstruction of mandibular motion (to allow emergency airway management) and yet maintain good cranial control, Rubin et al. (46) designed a Minerva-like device that uses pads under and in front of both zygomatic arches.

The vest portion of the halo vest originally was made of plaster (40,42) (Fig. 5). In the 1970s, it was made from

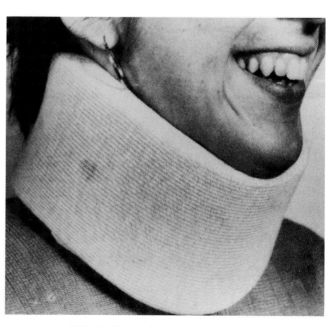

FIG. 1. Cervical orthosis (soft collar).

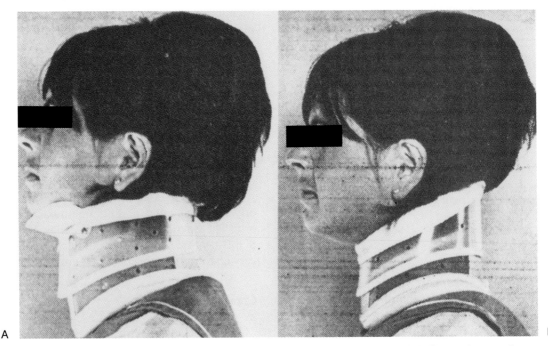

FIG. 2. Occipito-mandibular-cervical orthoses. **A:** Collar with chin extension. **B:** Queen Anne collar.

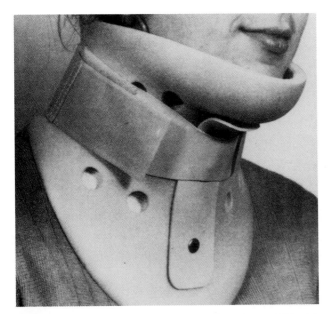

FIG. 3. Occipito-mandibular-high thoracic orthoses. Philadelphia collar.

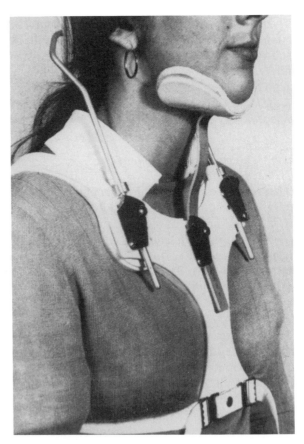

FIG. 4. Occipito-mandibular-low thoracic orthoses. Sternal-occipital-mandibular immobilizer (SOMI).

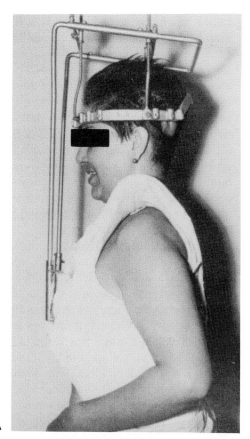

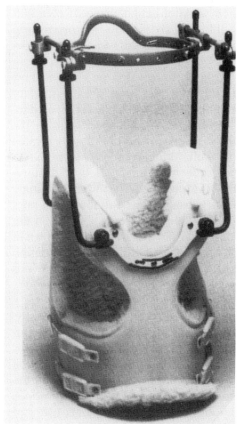

A

B

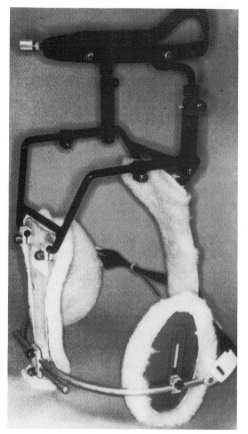

C

FIG. 5. Cranio-thoracic orthoses. **A:** Original halo vest made from plaster. Note absence of contact between over-the-shoulder straps and top of shoulders. Also note absence of contact with upper thoracic spine and presence of contact with abdomen. **B:** Traditional plastic halo vest. This provided a major advance in terms of skin care and access for hygiene. Vest design was basically unchanged. **C:** Four-pad halo vest. Total absence of contact with shoulders and epigastrium avoids undesired force application by these structures. Contact with upper thoracic spine and multidirectional adjustability provides improved grip on thorax.

plastic, but without a major design change. Recently it has undergone substantial redesign to improve its grip on the thorax (6,16,30,47,51), as shown in Fig. 6 and described further below.

Recent research has also focussed on the pin. Low placement on the forehead improves pin–skull interface rigidity (4). Wong and Haynes (61) suggest computed tomographic (CT) scanning before pin placement in patients less than 11 years of age to avoid variably located thin regions of the skull. Although an increase from 6 to 8 in-lbs of pin torque was supported by a history-controlled study (8), a prospective, randomized study (44) showed no difference for these two torques in rates of pin loosening or infection. However, for a given pin torque, disturbingly wide variations have been shown in pin–skull compression force. At 8 in-lbs, the variation across different halo types in two different studies was 51% [pin on skull (58)] and 71% [pin on load cell (28)], and after lock nut placement it was 353% (28)!

MRI compatibility has also been investigated recently. Clayman et al. (10) briefly studied five occipito-mandibulo-thoracic and four cranio-thoracic orthoses and focussed attention on not only the connecting rod material but also electrically conductive loops and the strong artefact from titanium pins. Deflection of various halo vests (and a wide range of other implants) (48) and heating of a single vest by MRI magnetic fields (49) were shown by Shellock et al. to be negligible. A carefully performed comparison of different vest types by Ballock et al. (5) showed significantly more image artefact from components of stainless steel than of aluminum, graphite composite, or titanium.

QUANTITATIVE EVALUATION OF ORTHOTIC FUNCTION

Some of the earlier studies used cineradiography to visualize cervical motion within an orthosis (19,26). However, the difficulty in quantifying cineradiography has restricted the usefulness of these reports.

Colachis et al. (11) had normal subjects forcibly flex and extend while wearing no orthosis, a soft collar, a collar with chin piece, then a Queen Anne collar. Lateral view flexion–extension radiographs were taken to assess motion. They noted that the soft collar only slightly restricted extension and that the chin piece and occipital extension restricted flexion and extension, respectively, to a moderate extent. No statistical analysis was provided.

Fisher et al. (15) studied more rigid devices, namely the polyethylene collar with chin and occipital pads, Philadelphia collar, 4-poster, and SOMI. They also used normal subjects and voluntarily produced maximum flexion and extension efforts. Important methodologic

improvements consisted of standardizing the pressure under chin or occiput during flexion and extension, respectively, and statistical analyses of their results. They showed that: (a) for C3-C4 to C6-C7, the Philadelphia and polyethylene collars reduced motion to approximately two thirds of normal, whereas the SOMI and 4-poster reduced motion to approximately one third of normal, a statistically significant difference; (b) for C2-C3, all four designs restricted motion almost totally; and (c) for Oc to C2, all four designs produced "paradoxical" motion; that is, with forward rotation of the head and neck, local extension occurred at the upper cervical spine, more so for the Philadelphia and polyethylene collars than for the other two orthoses.

Althoff and Goldie (1) examined rheumatoid arthritis patients in each of the following: soft collar, Philadelphia collar, SOMI, and 4-poster. Lateral x-rays were used to assess flex–extension range at C1-C2 and C2-C4 as well as the atlanto–dens interval (ADI) in the flexed and extended positions. The major findings are: (a) the C1-C2 flexion–extension range was restricted only from between 20% (soft collar) and approximately 45% (4-poster), and (b) ADI increase with flexion was restricted only slightly compared to unbraced (4% by the soft collar up to approximately 20% by the 4-poster).

In the most thorough works on this topic, Johnson and co-workers (23,24) studied both flexion–extension and lateral bend radiographically, as well as axial rotation photographically. Orthoses tested were the cervical collar, Philadelphia collar, Philadelphia collar with rigid extensions (Yale brace), SOMI, 4-poster, a cervico-thoracic orthosis, and halo vests. All were tested on normal volunteers except the halo vest, which was used on patients. The major results from the study are the following: (a) the longer and stiffer devices generally do a better job at immobilization; (b) the nonhalo devices are quite varied in their restriction of flexion–extension (13% to 74% of normal range) and lateral bending (18% to 83%), but none of them do a very good job for axial rotation (51% to 92%); (c) the simple-to-fabricate Yale brace functions very much like the more complex cervico-thoracic orthosis or 4-poster; (d) the upper cervical spine is not well immobilized by any of the nonhalo devices; (e) even the typical halo vest allows motion in the lower cervical spine comparable to that seen with the 4-poster or cervico-thoracic orthosis; and (f) although clearly superior in the upper cervical spine, the typical halo vest still allows approximately 20% of the normal range of flexion–extension motion at both Oc-C1 and C1-C2, some of which is a "paradoxical" or "snaking" motion (upper cervical extension with lower cervical flexion and vice versa). The authors emphasize that performance of orthoses on normal volunteers may not be directly applicable to patients.

To try to obtain a more repeatable motion task, some

studies (22,37) have used a modest force applied to the relaxed subject's head to produce the desired neck motion during wear of various occipito-mandibulo-thoracic orthoses. The work by Lunsford et al. (37) showed that the most restrictive of the four orthoses studied reduced motion down to approximately half of the normal range but also that it was the least comfortable.

Benzel et al. (7) compared the thermoplastic Minerva orthosis described by Millington et al. (39) to a standard halo vest by means of flexion–extension lateral x-rays of ten patients. They found identical overall motion (occiput to C6 or to C7) with both orthoses: 5.2°. The Minerva, however, allowed less "snaking" (upper cervical flexion with lower cervical extension, and vice versa), as measured by adding together the absolute values of the motion at each motion segment, the mean value of which was 23.4° for the halo vest but only 14.8° for the Minerva. Since cervical "snaking" is produced by capital protraction and retraction, its prevention requires control of anteroposterior motion between the orthosis and thorax. Differences in this feature between the halo vest and the Minerva orthosis probably explain the results. Unfortunately, no details concerning this are described or discussed by the authors.

Although halo vests represent a major step forward for cervical orthoses, there remain certain problems with the traditional halo vest [reviewed more thoroughly elsewhere (30)]. The first problem is the surprisingly large amount of motion that can occur. Koch and Nickel (29) found 31% of the normal cervical range of motion occurring during various activities of daily living in patients fitted with Ace halo vests. Using basically the same vest design and a larger number of activities of daily living, Lind et al. (35,36) found greater motion occurring: approximately 70% of the full normal range. Wang et al. (55) using a modified vest apparently found even more motion than did Lind et al., although Anderson et al. (2) found less. These are all in contrast to Johnson et al. (24) who report only 4% of the normal flexion–extension motion. However, the latter study involved voluntary flexion/extension efforts in normal subjects rather than activities of daily living in patients.

The second problem is the loss of reduction during halo vest wear, which has been reported by various authors (9,12,20,24,27,33,50,53,57). Bucci et al. (9) and Whitehill et al. (57) have described this problem particularly clearly. Despite this, it should be kept in mind that excellent results have been reported with halo vest treatment of cervical spine trauma (30,35,36).

The third problem is that surprisingly high loads may be applied unintentionally by the wearer to the vest, and thus through the uprights to the neck. Koch and Nickel (29) measured peak distraction forces (mean ± SD) of 75 ± 40 N (16.8 ± 9.0 lbs) during flexion, and 65 ± 66 N (14.5 ± 14.8 lbs) during shoulder shrug. Ersmark et al.

(13) reported distraction forces up to 50 N (11.2 lbs) during coughing. Lind et al. (35,36) showed much larger distraction forces (mean ± SD) of 159.6 ± 72.4 N (35.9 ± 16.3 lbs) during shoulder shrug and 122.9 ± 40.5 N (27.6 ± 9.1 lbs) during deep inspiration. Walker et al. (54) studied anterior–posterior and medial–lateral forces as well, and found the former comparable in magnitude to the distraction–compression forces.

The fourth problem is that the vest clearly contributes to pressure-sore development (by covering over the scapulae) and may contribute to cranial pin loosening by allowing shoulder and abdominal motion to transmit undesired forces to the pins through the vest and uprights (30,40,41,54,60).

Finally, by covering a large portion of the thorax and abdomen, the vest can be uncomfortably warm, and dressing or washing underneath is difficult. In addition, it results in substantial pulmonary function reduction (though this apparently is not clinically significant) (38).

In response to one or more of these problems, various halo vest modifications have been investigated. Appleby et al. (3) replaced the vest with a skeletal fixation framework attached by screws to the clavicles and scapulae. Movement of the clavicle and scapula with respect to the thorax and the cervical spine remained a predictable major and insurmountable problem. Garfin et al. (17) designed and tested a variety of skull pin tips in the laboratory, in an effort to decrease loosening. Wang et al. (55) in normal subjects and Triggs et al. (52) in cadavers studied the effect of vest length on cervical motion: the shorter vests worked about as well as the longer ones.

Krag and Beynnon (30) reported the rationale and initial biomechanical test results of a fundamentally different four-pad vest design (6,47) (Fig. 6), which avoids contact with the shoulder girdle or abdomen and provides thorough adjustability to allow close fitting to the relatively nonmobile portions of the thorax. The initial testing compared the mobility of each of seven standard and one experimental vest designs on each of four normal volunteers in response to each of nine load types. The mean rank order values (across load types and subjects) varied from 6.77 (most mobile) for the DePuy vest down to 3.22 (least mobile) for the experimental vest. Analysis of clinical experience from 1986 to 1992 showed equal or better clinical outcomes and substantial reduction in cervical motion compared to standard vests (51), and also that control of anterior–posterior motion of the head (relative to thorax) is important for control of cervical segmental flexion–extension (by way of reduced "shaking") (31). In a recent, comparative, biomechanical test of three different vests on each of ten subjects (16), strains between the halo and the vest were measured during a variety of activities of daily living (ADL) and of test tasks. Substantially lower forces were seen in almost all ADL tasks in the four-pad vest. Further investigation

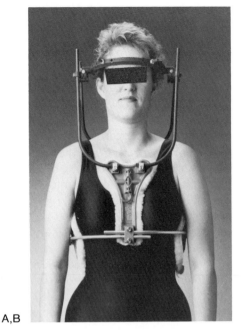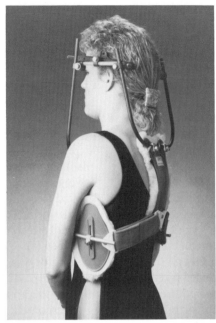

A,B

FIG. 6. Four-pad halo vest. **A:** Front view. **B:** Posterolateral view. [Used with permission from Schneiderman et al. (47).]

will examine the clinical relevance of this and other results from this study.

SUMMARY

Much remains to be established concerning optimal cervical orthosis use. Almost no comparative clinical studies have been done. In spite of the widespread use in laboratory studies of maximum voluntary cervical range of motion (without or with some sort of force application to the head), clinical relevance of such results has not been established. Although many advances have been in design and application of cranio-thoracic orthoses, very little is known about forces between pin and skull or halo and vest and about how these affect maintenance of cervical alignment or pin loosening.

REFERENCES

1. Althoff B, Goldie F (1980): Cervical collars in rheumatoid atlanto-axial subluxation: a radiographic comparison. *Ann Rheum Dis* 39:485–489.
2. Anderson PA, Budorick TE, Easton KB, Henley MB, Salciccioli GG (1991): Failure of halo vest to prevent in vivo motion in patients with injured cervical spines. *Spine* 16(S10):S501–505.
3. Appleby DM, Fu FH, Mears DC (1984): Halo-clavicle traction. *J Trauma* 24:452–455.
4. Ballock RT, Lee TQ, Triggs KJ, Woo SL, Garfin SR (1990): The effect of pin location on the rigidity of the halo pin–bone interface. *Neurosurgery* 26(2):238–241.
5. Ballock RT, Hajek PC, Byrne TP, Garfin SR (1989): The quality of magnetic resonance imaging, as affected by the composition of the halo orthosis. *J Bone Joint Surg* 71A:431–434.
6. Barr JS Jr, Krag MH, Pierce DS (1989): Cranial traction and the halo orthosis. In: Bailey RW, Sherk HH, et al., eds. *The cervical spine*, 2nd ed, Philadelphia, JB Lippincott, pp. 299–311.
7. Benzel EC, Hadden TA, Saulsbery CM (1989): A comparison of the Minerva and halo jackets for stabilization of the cervical spine. *J Neurosurg* 70:411–414.
8. Botte MJ, Byrne TP, Garfin SR (1987): Application of the halo device for immobilization of the cervical spine utilizing an increased torque pressure. *J Bone Joint Surg* 69A:750–752.
9. Bucci MN, Dauser RC, Maynard FA, Hoff JT (1988): Management of post-traumatic cervical spine instability: operative fusion versus halo vest immobilization. Analysis of 49 cases. *J Trauma* 28:1001–1006.
10. Clayman DA, Murakami ME, Vines FS (1990): Compatibility of cervical spine braces with MR imaging: a study of nine nonferrous devices. *Am J Neuroradiol* 11:385–390.
11. Colachis SC Jr, Strohm BR, Ganter EL (1973): Cervical spine motion in normal women: radiography study of effect of cervical collars. *Arch Phys Med Rehabil* 54:161–169.
12. Ekong CEV, Schwartz ML, Tator CH, Rowed DW, Edmonds VE (1981): Odontoid fracture: management with early mobilization using the halo device. *Neurosurgery* 9:631–637.
13. Ersmark H, Kalen R, Löwenhielm P (1988): A methodical study of force measurements in three patients with odontoid fractures treated with a strain gauge-equipped halo-vest. *Spine* 13:433–455.
14. Ferguson J, Mardel SN, Beattie TF, Wytch R (1993): Cervical collars: a potential risk to the head-injured patient. *Injury* 24(7):454–456.
15. Fisher SV, Bowar JF, Awad EA, Gullickson G Jr (1977): Cervical orthoses' effect on cervical spine motion: roentgenographic and goniometric method of study. *Arch Phys Med Rehabil* 58:109–115.
16. Fukui Y, Krag M, Huston D, Ambrose T, Vaccaro A, Brennan M, Conant A, Tranowski J (1994): 3-D dynamic halovest loads: full crossover comparison of 3 vest types. Proceedings Cervical Spine Research Society 22nd Annual Meeting, Baltimore, MD, Dec., pp. 131–133.
17. Garfin SR, Lee TQ, Roux RD, et al. (1986): Structural behavior of the halo orthosis pin-bone interface: biomechanical evaluation of standard and newly designed stainless steel halo fixation pins. *Spine* 11:977–981.
18. Hart DL, Johnson RM, Simmons EF, Owen J (1978): Review of cervical orthoses. *Phys Ther* 58:857–860.
19. Hartman JT, Palumbo F, Hill BJ (1975): Cineradiography of the braced normal cervical spine: a comparative study of five commonly used cervical orthoses. *Clin Orthop* 109:97–102.

20. Haw DW (1982): Collapse of cervical spine treated by Down's Ace mark III halo assembly. *Br Med J* 285:410.
21. Hewitt S (1994): Skin necrosis caused by a semi-rigid cervical collar in a ventilated patient with multiple injuries. *Injury* 25:323–324.
22. Hovis WD, Limbird TJ (1994): An evaluation of cervical orthoses in limiting hyperextension and lateral flexion in football. *Med Sci Sports Exerc* 26(7):872–876.
23. Johnson RM, Hart DL, Owen JR, Lerner E, Chapin W, Zeleznik R (1978): The Yale cervical orthosis: an evaluation of its effectiveness in restricting cervical motion in normal subjects and a comparison with other cervical orthoses. *Phys Ther* 58:865–871.
24. Johnson RM, Hart DL, Simmons EF, Ramsby GR, Southwick WO (1977): Cervical orthoses: a study comparing their effectiveness in restricting cervical motion in normal subjects. *J Bone Joint Surg [Am]* 59:332–339.
25. Johnson RM, Owen JR, Hart DL, Callahan RA (1981): Cervical orthoses: a guide to their selection and use. *Clin Orthop* 154:34–45.
26. Jones MD (1960): Cineradiographic studies of the collar-immobilized cervical spine. *J Neurosurg* 17:633–637.
27. Kelly EG (1981): Loss of reduction in cervical fracture-dislocations managed in the halo cast. *Proceedings American Academy Orthopedic Surgeons Annual Meeting.*
28. Kerwin GA, Chou KL, White DB, Shen KL, Salciccioli GG, Yang KH (1994): Investigation of how different halos influence pin forces. *Spine* 19:1078–1081.
29. Koch RA, Nickel VL (1978): The halo vest: an evaluation of motion and forces across the neck. *Spine* 3:103–107.
30. Krag MH, Beynnon BD (1988): A new halo-vest: rationale, design and biomechanical comparison to standard halo-vest designs. *Spine* 13:228–235.
31. Krag MH, Tomonaga T, Novotny JE (1995): Pattern of cervical motion segment rotations from positive change during wear of adjustable 4-pad halo vest. *Spine (submitted).*
32. Kuhnigk H, Bomke S, Sefrin P (1993): Effect of external cervical spine immobilization on intracranial pressure. *Aktuelle Traumatologie* 23(8):350–353.
33. Levine AM, Edwards CC (1985): The management of traumatic spondylolisthesis of the axis. *J Bone Joint Surg [Am]* 67:217–226.
34. Liew SC, Hill DA (1994): Complication of hard cervical collars in multi-trauma patients. *Aust N Z J Surg* 64(2):139–140.
35. Lind B, Sihlbom H, Nordwall A (1988): Forces and motions across the neck in patients treated with halo vest. *Spine* 13:162–167.
36. Lind B, Sihlbom H, Nordwall A (1988): Halovest treatment of unstable traumatic cervical spine injuries. *Spine* 13:425–432.
37. Lunsford TR, Davidson M, Lunsford BR (1994): Effectiveness of four contemporary cervical orthoses in restricting cervical motion. *J Prosth Orthop* 6:93–99.
38. Maeda CJ, Baydur A, Waters RL, Adkins RH (1990): The effect of the halovest and body position on pulmonary function in quadriplegia. *J Spinal Disord* 3:47–51.
39. Millington PJ, Ellingsen JM, Hauswirth BE, Fabian PJ (1987): Thermoplastic Minerva body jacket: a practical alternative to current methods of cervical spine stabilization. A clinical report. *Phys Ther* 67:223–225.
40. Nickel VH, Perry J, Garrett A, Heppenstall M (1968): The halo. A spinal skeleton traction fixation device. *J Bone Joint Surg [Am]* 50:1400–1409.
41. Perry J (1972): Halo in spinal abnormalities: practical factors and avoidance of complications. *Orthop Clin North Am* 3:69–80.
42. Perry J, Nickel VL (1959): Total cervical spine fusion for neck paralysis. *J Bone Joint Surg [Am]* 41:37–60.
43. Plaiser B, Gabram SG, Schwartz RJ, Jacobs LM (1994): Prospective evaluation of craniofacial pressure in four different cervical orthoses. *J Trauma* 37(5):714–720.
44. Rizzolo SJ, Piazza MR, Cotler JM, Hume EL, Cautilli G, O'Neill DK (1993): Effect of torque pressure on halo pin complication rates: a randomized, prospective study. *Spine* 18:2163–2166.
45. Rogers WA (1942): Treatment of fracture-dislocation of the cervical spine. *J Bone Joint Surg* 24:245–258.
46. Rubin G, Dixon M, Bernknopf J (1978): An occipito-zygomatic cervical orthosis designed for emergency use: a preliminary report. *Bull Prosth Res,* Spring, pp. 10–29.
47. Schneiderman GA, Hambly M (1993): Spinal orthoses. In: Hochschuler SH, Cotler HB, Guyer RD, eds. *Rehabilitation of the Spine—Science and Practice,* St. Louis: Mosby, pp. 213–222.
48. Shellock FG, Morisoli S, Kanal E (1993): MR procedures and biomedical implants, materials, and devices: 1993 update. *Radiology* 189(2):587–599.
49. Shellock FG, Slimp G (1990): Halo vest for cervical spine fixation during MR imaging. *Am J Roentgenol* 154:631–632.
50. Smith MD, Phillips WA, Hensinger RN (1991): Complications of fusion to the upper cervical spine. *Spine* 16(7):702–706.
51. Tomonaga T, Krag MH, Novotny J (1993): 4-Pad halo-vest: clinical and X-ray experience 1986-92. *Proceedings Cervical Spine Research Society 21st Annual Meeting.* New York, Dec. 2–3, pp. 53–55.
52. Triggs KJ, Ballock RT, Byrne T, Garfin SR (1993): Length dependence of a halo orthosis on cervical immobilization. *J Spinal Disord* 6:34–37.
53. Van Peteghem PK, Schweigel JF (1979): The fractured cervical spine rendered unstable by anterior cervical fusion. *J Trauma* 19:110–114.
54. Walker PS, Lamser D, Hussey RW, Rossier AB, Farberov A, Dietz J (1984): Forces in the halo-vest apparatus. *Spine* 9:773–777.
55. Wang GJ, Moskal JT, Albert T, Pritts ROT, Schuch CM, Stamp WG (1988): The effect of halo-vest length on stability of the cervical spine. *J Bone Joint Surg [Am]* 70:357–360.
56. White AA III, Southwick WO, Panjabi MM (1976): Clinical instability in the lower cervical spine: a review of past and current concepts. *Spine* 1:15–27.
57. Whitehill R, Richman JA, Glaser JA (1986): Failure of immobilization of the cervical spine by the halo vest. A report of five cases. *J Bone Joint Surg [Am]* 68:326–332.
58. Whitesides TE, Mehserle WL, Hutton WC (1992): The force exerted by the halo pin. *Spine* 17(10S):S413–417.
59. Wolf JW Jr, Johnson RM (1989): Cervical Orthoses. In: Sherk HH, et al., eds. *The cervical spine,* 2nd ed. Philadelphia: JB Lippincott, pp. 97–105.
60. Wolf JW, Jones HC (1980): Comparison of immobilization of the cervical spine by halocasts versus plastic jackets. *Proceedings Cervical Spine Research Society Annual Meeting,* Palm Beach.
61. Wong WB, Haynes RJ (1994): Osteology of the pediatric skull: considersations of halo pin placement. *Spine* 19(13):1451–1454.

The Adult Spine: Principles and Practice,
2nd edition, J.W. Frymoyer, Editor-in-Chief.
Lippincott-Raven Publishers, Philadelphia © 1997.

CHAPTER **54**

Internal Fixation of the Cervical Spine

Paul A. Anderson and John C. Steinmann

Internal fixation of the cervical spine was first described in 1891 when Hadra (38) reported on the use of an interspinous wire technique in the management of a cervical spine fracture. In this case the internal fixation failed presumably because a fusion was not performed. In 1911 Hibbs (43) and Albee (3) separately reported on the use of bone graft to achieve spinal fusions. Rogers, in 1942 (62,63), reported experience with a technique of posterior spinous process wiring and fusion in the treatment of cervical spine fractures. However, it was not until 1953 that Holdsworth and Hardy (45) popularized the combination of internal fixation and fusion in the treatment of spinal fracture dislocations.

More recently, alternatives to the use of wire internal fixations have been popularized. An anterior cervical plate and screw to support an anterior cervical fusion was used by Bohler in 1964 (8). This procedure was refined

and modified a few years later by Orozco and others (22,29,58,59). These initial plates required bicortical purchase in the vertebral body for adequate biomechanical strength. Plate loosening with screw backout was occasionally encountered. The plates that have evolved and are available today appear to provide adequate strength with unicortical fixation and have mechanisms that lock the screws to the plate to avoid screw backout (2,56,75).

Roy-Camille, in 1970 (64,66,68–70), proposed the use of a posterior plate with screws into the articular processes as a means of rigid internal fixation. Magerl modified this technique with a posterior hook plate (36). Current posterior plates have the advantage of greater freedom in screw placement and are made of titanium to allow for improved postoperative imaging (7). Other techniques of screw fixation of the odontoid process or atlantoaxial articulation have been popularized in Europe and are rapidly gaining acceptance in North America (9,36). Finally, occipitocervical fusion using plate fixation to the occiput and cervical articular masses was developed by Roy-Camille in 1983 (65) with modifications by Grob in 1991 (35) and Smith and Anderson in 1993 (71).

P. A. Anderson, M.D.: Clinical Associate Professor, Department of Orthopaedic Surgery, University of Washington, Harborview Medical Center, Seattle, Washington 98122.
J. C. Steinmann, D.O.: Clinical Professor, Department of Orthopedic Surgery, Loma Linda University, Loma Linda, California 92354.

INDICATIONS AND ALTERNATIVES TO INTERNAL FIXATION

The intact cervical spine provides protection to the spinal cord, holds the head upright and allows for painless motion. Instability indicates an inability of the spine to provide these functions under physiologic loads. White, Southwick, and Panjabi (80,81) have defined clinical instability as loss of the ability of the spine under physiologic loads to maintain relationships in such a way that there is neither damage nor subsequent irritation to the spinal cord or nerve roots and, in addition, there is no development of incapacitating deformity or pain due to structural changes.

Factors important in determining instability include assessment of the integrity of the vertebral body and posterior elements, the sagittal plane translation and angulation, and neurologic function. White and Panjabi (79) have developed objective parameters for cervical spine instability. This experimental work has resulted in a checklist for the diagnosis of clinical instability in the lower cervical spine. Although no such checklist exists for the upper cervical spine, the same principles would seem to apply.

The pathologic causes of cervical spine instability include traumatic, infectious, neoplastic congenital, rheumatologic, iatrogenic, and degenerative disorders. The clinical management goal in patients with documented cervical spine instability is to restore and maintain anatomic alignment during the period of healing or fusion while providing for early mobilization.

Despite recent advances in internal fixation, these goals can often be achieved with a brace or halo vest. The halo vest, in particular, effectively stabilizes the cervical spine in most cases. Johnson et al. (48) have compared the effectiveness of different cervical orthoses in restricting cervical motion in normal subjects. Although the halo vest, first proposed by Perry and Nickel in 1959 (60), has been reported to be the most stable orthosis (15,48), it is not without significant complications and failures (7,14,20,27,31,49,51,83).

The particular benefit of successful internal fixation is that it effectively maintains sagittal plane alignment and allows early patient mobilization. Furthermore, with rigid internal fixation, a halo vest can often be avoided. Internal fixation of the cervical spine, therefore, is indicated when (a) a halo vest or brace immobilization will not reliably maintain satisfactory alignment during healing, (b) a brace or halo vest is contraindicated due to other injuries, (c) a posterior or extensive multilevel anterior fusion is planned, or (d) an open reduction or neural decompression of an unstable motion segment is required.

The purpose of this chapter is to review the indications and various techniques for internal fixation in the treatment of cervical spine instability.

OCCIPITAL CERVICAL ARTHRODESIS

Indications

Occipital cervical instability can result from traumatic ligament injuries, congenital malformations, rheumatologic disorders, infections, and neoplastic disease. Techniques for achieving occipital cervical fusion have been described using only bone graft (20,25,57), bone graft with adjunctive methylmethacrylate (13,20,53,82), and bone graft with internal fixation using wire or plate fixation (33,34,40,44,47,73,78,84).

Occipital cervical fusion with only bone graft is successful, especially in children (50), but this technique requires prolonged traction or halo immobilization. Disadvantages of this simple method include failure to maintain occipitocervical alignment and the addition of distraction forces imparted by the halo vest. Though distraction may benefit certain rheumatologic conditions, this is potentially dangerous in post-traumatic ligamentous instabilities of the occipitocervical junction.

The use of adjunctive methylmethacrylate has been advocated for patients with severe osteoporosis and patients with extensive bone loss due to inflammatory or neoplastic destruction. Methylmethacrylate, however, has been shown to be associated with increased infection rate, especially when placed under tension (53). Animal studies have shown loosening of the acrylic from the bone structure and wire within 4 to 6 weeks (82). This construct cannot reliably achieve long lasting stability and therefore should be considered a last resort or salvage procedure only, particularly in patients with a predictably limited lifespan.

Internal fixation using wire or bone plates offers more reliable fixation, improved rate of fusion, and often eliminates the need for postoperative halo immobilization. A thorough knowledge of the neural, vascular, and bony anatomy of the occipitocervical junction is essential for safe, effective internal fixation.

Wire Fixation

Wire can be used to provide stabilization of the occipital atlantoaxial axial complex as well as to secure bone grafts in an attempt to improve the fusion rate. Many techniques have been advocated, including: (a) wiring of tricortical iliac crest graft to the occiput, lamina, and spinous processes of the upper cervical spine (19,78); (b) wire passed through the occiput and looped around spinous processes; (c) wire securing metallic implants such as Hartshill-Ransford loop, contoured Steinmann pin, or contoured Luque rod (47,71,73,77).

Wertheim and Bohlman (78) have described a technique of occipital cervical arthrodesis using thick plates of iliac crest bone grafts wired to the occiput and cervical lamina. Their technique avoids intracranial wire passage by creating an interosseous tunnel between two grooves placed on either side of the external occipital protuberance. Thirteen patients were studied an average of 3.6 years following this procedure. All 13 were considered to have a solid arthrodesis and relief of neck pain. All 10 myelopathic patients demonstrated an improvement in their neurologic function.

Bohlman Technique of Occipital Cervical Fusion

General anesthesia is recommended. In cases in which this is not medically advisable, local anesthesia may be used. Patient positioning is dependent upon the underlying condition. Traction is not advised for traumatic atlanto-occipital dislocations. Position in these patients can be maintained intraoperatively with a halo vest or Mayfield skull pins. Conversely, in patients with basilar invagination, maintenance of intraoperative traction using a Mayfield headrest and Gardner-Wells tongs is advisable. It is essential to obtain a preoperative lateral roentgenogram following positioning to confirm appropriate relationship of the occiput to the atlas.

Following a sterile preparation and draping, the subcutaneous tissue is injected with a 1:500,000 epinephrine solution. A midline incision is made from the external occipital protuberance to the fourth cervical vertebrae. The posterior elements are subperiostally exposed. A 5- to 7-mm hole is placed on either side of the external occipital protuberance approximately 2 cm above the foramen magnum (Fig. 1A). A tunnel is created under the outer cortex between the two holes using angled curettes and a Lewin clamp. In most cases this tunnel can be created between the two cranial cortices, which avoids intracranial passage of wires. A 20-gauge wire is double looped through this hole. A separate 20-gauge wire is passed around the arch of the atlas and a third wire is placed through the spinous process of the axis (Fig. 1B). In patients with a fixed atlantoaxial subluxation, or where a large pannus is present, the sublaminar wire at C1 should be avoided.

The posterior iliac crest is exposed, and an appropriate length of corticocancellous bone is harvested. The graft must be 7–10 mm thick to provide sufficient strength. This graft is divided horizontally and three drill holes are placed in each graft (Fig. 1C). Additional cancellous bone is harvested. The occiput, arch of C1, and lamina of C2 are decorticated with a high-speed burr. The wires are passed through the bone graft and tightened (Fig. 1D,E). Additional cancellous bone is packed between the two grafts. Extension below C2 into the subaxial spine is possible with further spinous process wires fixing the tricortical iliac crest bone graft. The wound is then closed in layers.

Postoperative immobilization is dictated by the degree of preoperative instability and an assessment of intraoperative fixation strength. Traumatic occipital cervical dislocations should be protected for 12 weeks in a halo vest. Occipital cervical fusion for tumors, congenital anomalies, and rheumatologic conditions can generally be treated postoperatively in a cervical thoracic orthosis for 12 weeks providing intraoperative fixation is deemed to be secure at the completion of the operative procedure.

Occipitocervical Plate Fixation

Plate and screw fixation offers many advantages over wire fixation for occipital cervical fusion. The main advantage is a more rigid construct, thus decreasing the need for postoperative immobilization. Except at C1, plate fixation avoids the passage of wires through the foramen magnum or spinal canal. Plate fixation can be easily extended caudad for subaxial and even cervical thoracic fixation (71). Plate and screw fixation can be modified to achieve rigid internal fixation, even in cases with significant bone loss or following extensive decompression (4). Finally, with plate and screw fixation, the construct is not dependent on the strength, and size, of the iliac crest graft, thus allowing for fusion with a less extensive harvest of autogenous graft.

Plate and screw fixation techniques utilize bicortical purchase at two or more sites in the occiput. Fixation to C1 is achieved either with a wire passed around the arch of the atlas (71) or by a C1-C2 transarticular screw, providing fixation to both the atlas and the axis (35). Fixation to the axis is achieved either by a transarticular screw as mentioned above (35), or by a C2 pedicle screw (71). Subaxial fixation is achieved by screws directed obliquely cephalad and laterally within the lateral masses as described by Anderson (7).

Occipital cervical fixation has been described using a single plate (35,44), or more commonly two parallel plates (67,71). Some plates are prebent (67), but most require intraoperative bending to achieve a contour congruent to the bony anatomy of the occipital atlantoaxial spine. The contouring creates an acute bend caudal to the occiput that can be strengthened if necessary by stacking the plates in this region. Titanium plates are available for occipital cervical fixation allowing for improved postoperative imaging.

Smith et al. (71) reported on 14 patients treated by occipital cervical arthrodesis using AO reconstruction plates with a 1-year follow-up. All patients demonstrated radiographic evidence of fusion. No neurovascular injuries, cerebral spinal fluid fistula, or wound infections occurred. Grob (35) reported 14 patients following occipital cervical fixation using an inverted Y plate. All patients demonstrated radiographic evidence of osseous union. Neurologic improvement occurred in all six patients who had a preoperative neurologic deficit. One

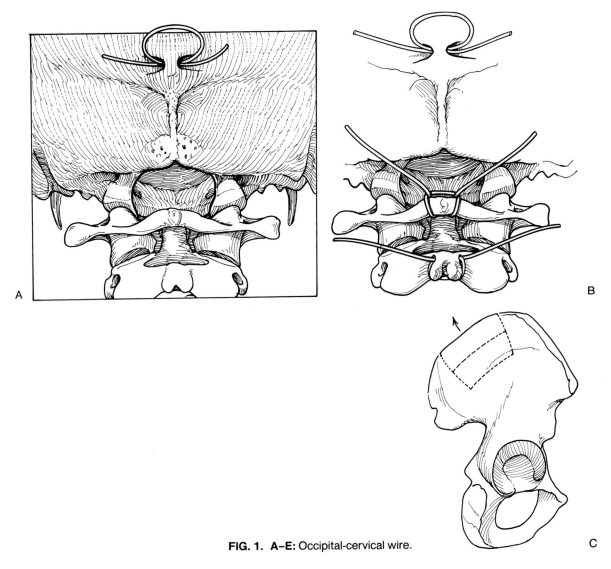

A

B

C

FIG. 1. A–E: Occipital-cervical wire.

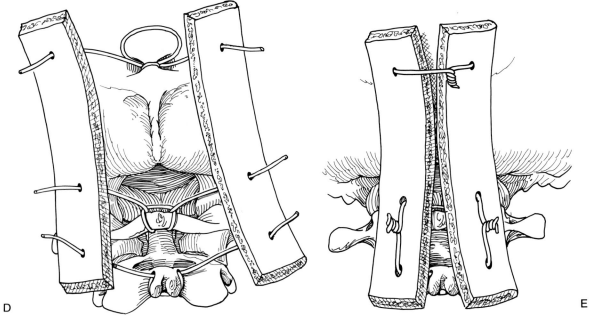

D

E

case of uneventful screw loosening and no postoperative wound infections were reported.

Technique of Occipital–Cervical Fusion with AO Plates

The anesthetic technique and patient positioning is as previously described. The skin is prepared in a sterile fashion and the subcutaneous tissue is infiltrated with a 1:500,000 epinephrine solution. A midline incision is extended from the inion to the lower level of anticipated fusion. All midline ligamentous structures anterior to the superspinous ligament are preserved and the occiput, arch of C1, and lamina of C2 are subperiostally exposed. Exposure of the occiput to a width of 5 cm is required.

A malleable plate template is contoured to the occiput and lateral masses of the cervical vertebrae. At least two and preferably three occiput screws per plate are required. A 2.7 or 3.5 mm AO reconstruction plate of appropriate length is contoured to match the template.

The C2 pedicle screw is drilled and placed first, followed by the subaxial lateral mass screws, and lastly the occipital screws. For placement of the C2 pedicle screw, the pedicle should be visualized and palpated using a curette and Penfield elevator (Fig. 2A). The pedicle will be located by careful dissection along the superior edge of the lamina. The starting point for drilling is located 5 mm. above the C2,3 facet joint just medial to the mid part of the facet. Using an adjustable drill guide, a 2-mm K-wire is sequentially advanced into the pedicle at an angle of 10–20° medially and 25° cranially (Fig. 2B,C). Palpation of the pilot hole periodically with a 1-mm K-wire and direct inspection of the pedicle will ensure that inadvertent penetration of the pedicle has not occurred. Under normal circumstances the vertebral artery passes from anterior to posterior within the superior lateral quadrant of the C2 lateral mass. The above described technique of screw placement should take place in a safe medial and posterior position relative to the vertebral artery. However, anomalies of the vertebral artery are frequent and each patient's CT scan should be carefully evaluated in order to ensure that screws can be safely placed.

Pilot holes in the C2 pedicle are drilled to an average depth of 20–22 mm and are then tapped with a 3.5 mm tap. The plate is fixed to C2 with appropriate length 3.5 cortical screws. If necessary, subaxial lateral mass screws can then be drilled and placed through the plate using the technique described in the section on posterior subaxial cervical plating (Fig. 3).

The adjustable drill guide is initially set at 8 mm and a 2-mm K-wire is used to create pilot holes for the occipital screws. Alternatively a 2-mm diamond burr may be used as a drill. Two or three screws are placed through the plate and into the occiput (Fig. 3). No screw should be placed cranial to the inion to avoid entrance into the intracranial venous sinuses. Bicortical purchase is necessary and generally requires an 8 to 10 mm screw. If cerebral spinal fluid is encountered after drilling, the hole should be sealed with bone wax and the screw placed. In our experience, persistence of cerebral spinal fluid leak has not been encountered.

All exposed bone of the occipit, C1, and lamina of remaining cervical vertebrae is decorticated and autogenous cortical cancellous strips are placed to span the occipital cervical junction. Long struts of corticocancellous grafts can be wired at the occiput and C2 if desired. If subaxial extension of the plate is to be performed, all involved facet joints are decorticated and packed with cancellous bone before applying the plate.

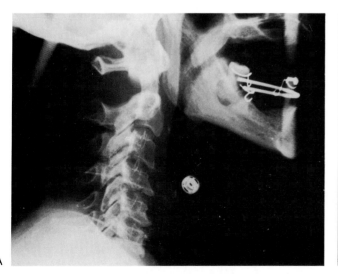
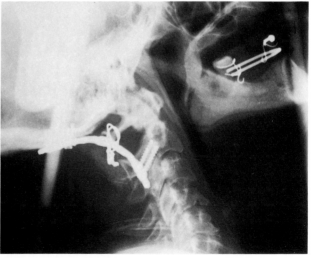

A   B

FIG. 2. A: Occipito-atlantoaxial instability demonstrated in a 43-year-old female following a motor vehicle accident. **B:** Stabilization using a contoured 3.5 reconstruction plate with screw fixation in the occiput and C2 pedicle and wire fixation around the arch of the atlas.

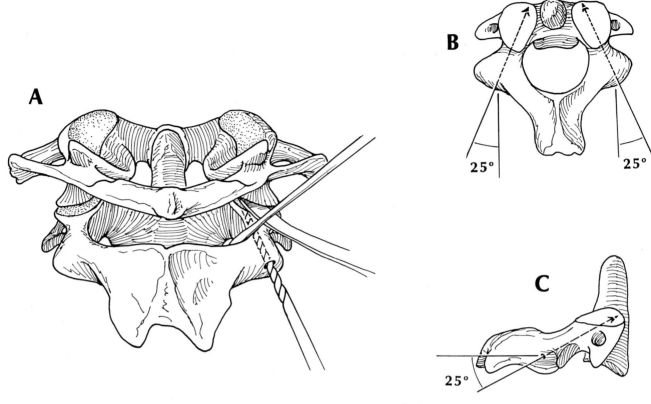

FIG. 3. **A–C:** C2 pedicle screw technique.

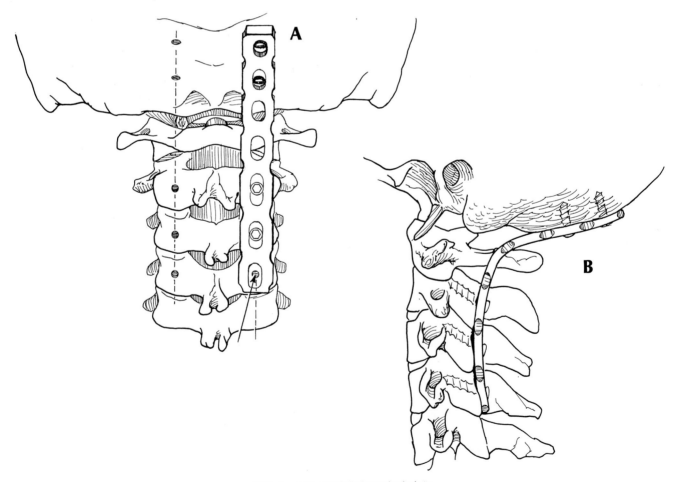

FIG. 4. **A,B:** Occipital cervical plate.

The wound is closed in layers with or without a suction drain based on the surgeon's experience and preference. Postoperatively, patients are immobilized in a hard collar or cervical thoracic brace for 8–12 weeks depending upon the degree of preoperative instability and the intraoperative assessment of fixation strength (Fig. 4).

ATLANTOAXIAL FIXATION

Indications

Atlantoaxial instability may result from congenital, traumatic, rheumatologic, infectious, or neoplastic disorders. Common congenital causes include odontoid hypoplasia, aplasia, or os odontoideum. Traumatic conditions of atlantoaxial instability include transverse ligament ruptures and more commonly odontoid fractures. Systemic disorders such as rheumatoid arthritis can lead to bone or ligamentous erosion with resultant ligamentous laxity or rupture. Occasionally, severe osteoarthritis of the atlantoaxial articulations can lead to a painful condition requiring atlantoaxial fusion. Finally, tumors and infection can lead to significant bone and ligamentous destruction, leading to atlantoaxial instability. Thus, atlantoaxial arthrodesis is indicated in patients with demonstrated atlantoaxial instability that would not be expected to heal with closed treatment, and in whom the surgical risks are tolerable (Fig. 5).

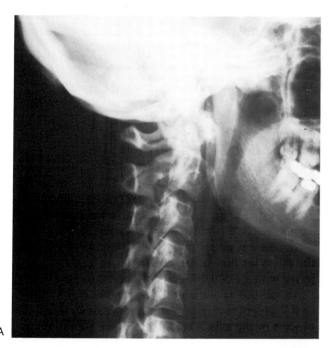

A

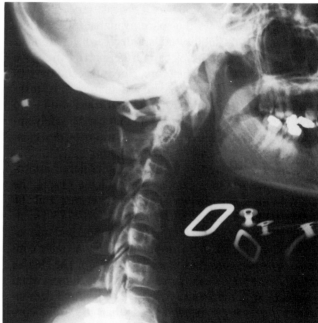

B

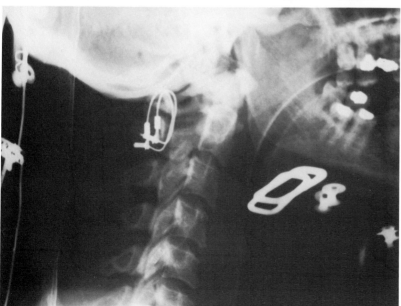

C

FIG. 5. A: Slightly widened atlanto–dens interval in a 37-year-old female following a motor vehicle accident. **B:** Significantly increased atlanto–dens interval developed within 1 week of closed treatment in a cervicothoracic brace. **C:** Stabilization of atlantoaxial instability using titanium cables and a Brooks arthrodesis technique.

Atlantoaxial arthrodesis can be accomplished using bone graft alone, with halo vest stabilization, bone graft with methylmethacrylate augmentation, or bone graft with wire (12,26), screw (52), or interlaminar clamp fixation (46). Patients with severe osteopenia or an incompetent arch of the atlas will require fixation through the articular facets at C1,C2 or extension of the arthrodesis to the occiput. Though anterior fusion and bilateral lateral transarticular screw fixation techniques have been described, posterior grafting and stabilization is the most common method of achieving atlantoaxial arthrodesis.

Biomechanics

The normal atlantoaxial axial articulation is responsible for approximately 50% of cervical spine rotation. This rotation narrows the space available for the cord at C1 and C2. Instability adds a degree of freedom in translational motion which can further narrow the space available for the cord. Therefore, constructs and devices used to stabilize the atlantoaxial articulation must principally be able to control rotation and translation. The most appropriate construct is one that can be safely applied, is not technically demanding, and provides satisfactory control of rotation and translation.

Biomechanical studies of atlantoaxial posterior arthrodesis techniques have evaluated the Gallie fusion, the Brooks fusion, the Halifax intralaminar clamp, and the Magerl transarticular facet screw fixation. Hajek (39) studied 15 embalmed cervical spines for rotational and translational strength after stabilization with either a Gallie construct, a Brooks construct, or a Halifax clamp. The Halifax clamp showed significantly greater rotational stiffness when compared with the Brooks construct, which itself demonstrated significantly greater stiffness than the Gallie construct. In translation, the Halifax and Brooks constructs

were not significantly different, but were both significantly superior to the Gallie construct.

Grob (33) studied the four different posterior atlantoaxial fixation techniques. Ten fresh human cadaveric cervical spines were tested intact, injured, and stabilized with (a) wire and single supralaminar graft (Gallie), (b) wire and two interlaminar grafts (Brooks), (c) two bilateral intralaminar clamps (Halifax), and (d) posterior transarticular facet screw fixation (Magerl). Spines were subjected to flexion extension axial rotation and lateral bending forces. The Brooks, Halifax, and Magerl constructs were not significantly different. The Gallie construct, however, showed significantly more motion in flexion extension, lateral bending, and rotation.

Montesano et al. (55) compared the Gallie construct to the Magerl transarticular screw technique. Again, the Magerl technique was found to be stiffer in rotation and allowed no anterior–posterior translation.

Techniques of Posterior Atlantoaxial Fusion

Awake intubation and positioning is safest and allows continual assessment of neurologic function. Intraoperative somatosensory evoked potentials may be indicated if further reduction is anticipated during the procedure, when the patient is anesthetized. The patient is positioned prone, with or without traction, in a Stryker bed or a Mayfield headrest. Preoperative lateral roentgenograms are obtained to assess sagittal alignment. The operative field is prepared and draped, including access to the posterior iliac crest. The subcutaneous tissue is injected with a 1:500,000 epinephrine solution.

An incision is made from the occiput to C3. The nuchal ligament is divided vertically to expose the spinous process of the axis. The spinous process and lamina of the axis are exposed by subperiosteal dissection with care

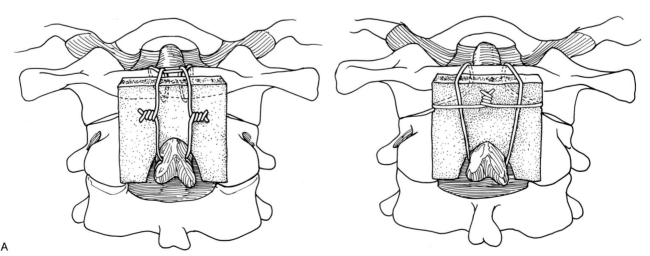

A

B

FIG. 6. A,B: Gallie technique of atlantoaxial fusion.

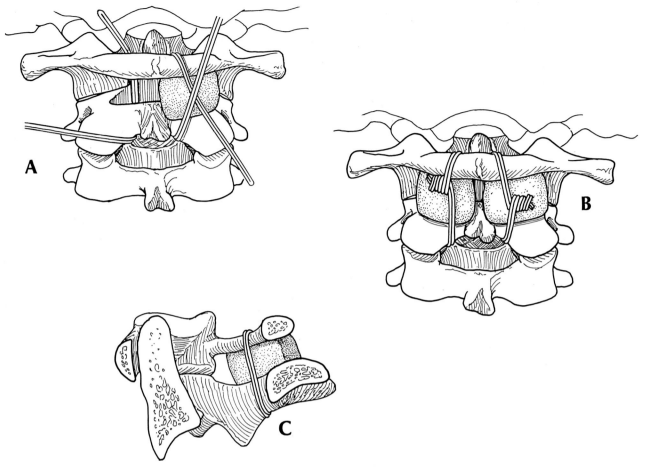

FIG. 7. A–C: Brooks technique of atlantoaxial fusion.

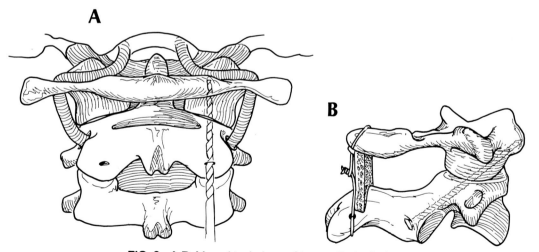

FIG. 8. A,B: Magerl technique of transarticular fusion.

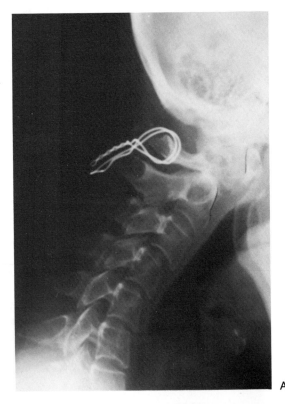

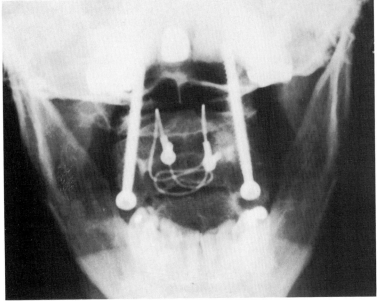

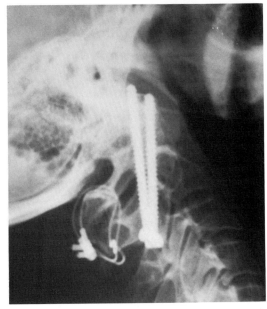

FIG. 9. A: Flexion x-rays in a 39-year-old female demonstrating nonunion of a Gallie fusion. Anteroposterior (**B**) and lateral (**C**) x-rays following Brooks fusion with titanium cable and Magerl transarticular facet screws.

to avoid injury to the C2,3 facet joints. The posterior arch of the atlas is subperiosteally exposed. Exposure of the atlas should extend only 1.5 cm lateral to the midline to avoid injury to the vertebral arteries and greater occipital nerves.

Gallie Technique

A single block of corticocancellous bone graft measuring approximately 1.5 cm by 3 cm is harvested from the posterior iliac crest. This graft is then notched inferiorally to accept the spinous process of C2. The arch of the atlas and lamina of the axis are then decorticated. A 20-gauge wire is looped around the arch of C1. A separate 20-gauge wire is looped through the spinous process of the axis. The wires are then tightened over the bone graft, securing the bone graft to the arch of C1 and lamina of C2 (Fig. 6A). Alternative wire configurations have been described (Fig. 6B).

Brooks Technique

Two large cortical cancellous trapezoidal shaped grafts are harvested, each measuring approximately 1.5 cm by 2 cm. The arch of the atlas and lamina of the axis are decorticated. The superior portion of the C2 lamina is fashioned to accept the rectangular block of intralaminar bone graft. To prevent posterior translation, it is essential that the bone graft wedge between the laminae of C1 and C2 as the wires are tightened.

Heavy sutures are passed under the lamina of C1 and C2 aided by a suture carrier or passer (Fig. 7A). Two 20-gauge wires on each side are tied to the sutures and passed from caudal to cranial under the lamina of C2. The process is repeated at C1. The trapezoidal bone blocks are placed between the arch of C1 and lamina of C2 and secured in place by tightening the wires over the bone graft (Fig. 7B,C). Alternatively, a titanium cable system (72) or Halifax intralaminar clamp may be utilized to replace the 20-gauge wire used in the above constructs.

C1-C2 Transarticular Screw Fixation—Magerl Technique

To allow easier access for screw insertion, the head must be flexed as much as possible while maintaining C1-C2 reduction. The head is best controlled with Mayfield skull pins. After prone positioning the reduction is checked with C-arm fluoroscopy or radiography.

If anterior subluxation is present, the head can be lifted upwards while maintaining flexion of the upper cervical spine. This will facilitate screw orientation.

A midline exposure of C1 and C2 posterior elements is performed. Dissection with a curette is carried out along the superior laminar ridge of C2 until the atlantoaxial joints are exposed. The capsule can be dissected free and retracted cranially with the greater occipital nerve, which is located medial and passes superficial to the C1-C2 articulation. Venous bleeding is frequently encountered and is best controlled with bipolar cautery or packing with Gelfoam sponges. If desired, decortication and bone grafting of the articular cartilage with a high-speed burr or curette can be performed. By dissection medially, the isthmus or pedicle of C2 is exposed. This defines the medial border for screw passage. If the posterior arch of C1 is present, 20-gauge wires or cables are passed sublaminarly. Additionally a 3-mm hole is placed in the base of the spinous process of C2 and a second wire is double looped around the spinous process. These wires will be used to secure a posterior Gallie type bone graft. If persistent malalignment is still present, then pressure can be applied to the C2 spinous process using a Kocher clamp until the desired position is achieved.

The starting point for screw insertion is located along the inferior edge of the lamina of C2 and 2–3 mm lateral to the medial edge of the C2 inferior facet (Fig. 8A). This corresponds to a point on the sagittal line that passes through the C2 pedicle. Under biplanar fluoroscopic control, a 2.5-mm drill is advanced forward in the sagittal plane aiming cranial toward the upper half of the C1 anterior arch (Fig. 8B). To achieve the proper angle required, the drill with drill sleeve can be percutaneously placed at about C7. Alternatively, the skin incision can be carried down to this level. During advancement the drill should be able to be visualized as it passes through the C1-C2 articulation. Drilling is complete when it penetrates the far cortex. The depth is checked and the pilot hole is tapped with a 3.5-mm cortical tap. To prevent redislocation, the drill can be left in place while the process is repeated on the contralateral side. Fully threaded 3.5-mm cortical screws are inserted. Alternatively, a cannulated technique with 3.5 or 4.0 mm screws could be used. A corticocancellous H-shaped graft is harvested and is placed on the lamina of C1 and C2 and secured by tightening the previously placed wires. The wound is closed in layers. Postoperatively the patients are immobilized in a hard collar for 10 weeks (Fig. 9). A technique of lateral transarticular screw fixation of the atlantoaxial joint, described by DuToit (23) requires two incisions, and possibly a third, for posterior arthrodesis and therefore is unnecessarily more extensive than the single approach described by Magerl.

ODONTOID SCREW FIXATION

Anatomy/Biomechanics

The atlantoaxial articulation is stabilized by the unique arrangement of the anterior arch of the atlas, the odontoid process, and the transverse ligament. Fracture of the odontoid process is a common injury and can result in spinal cord injury in 5–10% of cases. Anderson and D'Alonzo (5) have classified odontoid fractures based on anatomic location of the fracture. This classification is useful in predicting union and in directing clinical management of odontoid fractures.

Type I fractures are avulsion fractures of the tip of the odontoid. This is a rare injury and stability of the atlantoaxial complex is generally not affected. Theoretically the ipsilateral alar ligament may be compromised with the potential for occipitocervical instability. Type II fractures are located at the base of the odontoid and carry a significant risk for nonunion. Stability of the atlantoaxial articulation is compromised with a type II fracture. Closed treatment of type II odontoid fractures has resulted in a recorded nonunion rate varying from 5% to 80%. Factors increasing the likelihood of nonunion include age greater than 40 and initial displacement greater than 4 mm, as well as untreated type II odontoid fractures and those treated with traction.

In a multicenter study by the Cervical Spine Research Society, Clark (20) reported no cases of successful nonoperative treatment of a type II fracture treated in any orthosis other than the halo vest, whereas surgical treatment was successful. In his study, Clark reported a 96% union rate in type II odontoid fractures treated by posterior C1-C2 fusion.

Type III fractures occur through the body of C2. The stability of the atlantoaxial articulation is compromised with this fracture, however, stable union predictably occurs with proper closed treatment. Clark reported an 86% union rate for type III odontoid fractures treated closed, which conforms to the 92% union rate reported by Anderson and D'Alonzo (5).

Excessive flexion applied to the atlantoaxial articulation leads to rupture of the transverse ligament. Odontoid fractures therefore occur as a result of extension forces and lateral bending forces applied to the atlantoaxial articulation. More specifically, it has been repeatedly shown that pure extension forces typically result in a fracture of the odontoid that extends down into the body of C2 (type III). Lateral bending forces typically result in a fracture through the base of the odontoid (type II).

Indications for Odontoid Screw Fixation

Type I fractures of the odontoid are typically stable and will heal with closed treatment in a collar or a brace. Type III fractures of the odontoid also predictably heal with closed treatment. Halo vest immobilization is recommended for a period of 3 to 4 months in treatment of type III odontoid fractures. Management alternatives for patients with type II fractures include halo vest immobi-

lization, posterior atlantoaxial arthrodesis, or anterior odontoid screw fixation.

Closed treatment of type II odontoid fractures is appropriate providing reasonable alignment can be obtained and maintained in a halo vest. Many studies have demonstrated significant intersegmental and fracture site motion within the halo vest (6). Supine and upright lateral roentgenograms, therefore, are essential to confirm maintenance of satisfactory reduction.

Operative treatment is indicated for situations in which a patient refuses halo vest immobilization, has significant contraindications to halo immobilization, or in cases where fracture alignment cannot be maintained in a halo vest. Operative treatment is also indicated in those fractures with a predicted significant risk of nonunion. These include type II fractures in patients greater than 40 years of age, and those fractures with initial displacement greater than 4 mm. Specific contraindications to halo vest management include significant head trauma, chest wall trauma, and polytraumatized patients with multiple long bone fractures.

The operative treatment of type II odontoid fractures is generally a posterior Gallie or Brooks type fusion. The Gallie fusion should be protected postoperatively with a halo vest, whereas a Brooks type fusion can be satisfactorily protected in a cervicothoracic brace. When the arch of the atlas is fractured, a posterior Gallie or Brooks type fusion is not possible. In this situation a posterior C1-C2 transarticular facet screw as described by Magerl or an anterior odontoid screw fixation can be used. The anterior odontoid screw fixation has the advantage of maintaining atlantoaxial motion (Fig. 10).

Before performing anterior odontoid screw fixation, it is essential to obtain a reduction of the fracture. A CT scan should be performed to assess both the cross-sectional diameter of the odontoid as well as the relative bone density of the C2 vertebral body. Type II fractures that are transverse or inclined posteriorly are suitable for anterior odontoid screw fixation, whereas fractures with an anterior inclination may require an alternative form of stabilization.

Technique of Anterior Odontoid Screw Fixation

The technique can be used for the placement of one or two odontoid screws. A single screw has proven to produce adequate biomechanical strength, however, two screws provide improved rotational control. The decision to use one or two screws should be determined by an assessment of the space available within the odontoid and the need for rotational control (41).

Anesthesia is administered by means of an awake nasotracheal intubation with a radiolucent endotracheal tube. The patient is positioned in the supine position on the operating table and the head is securely held with

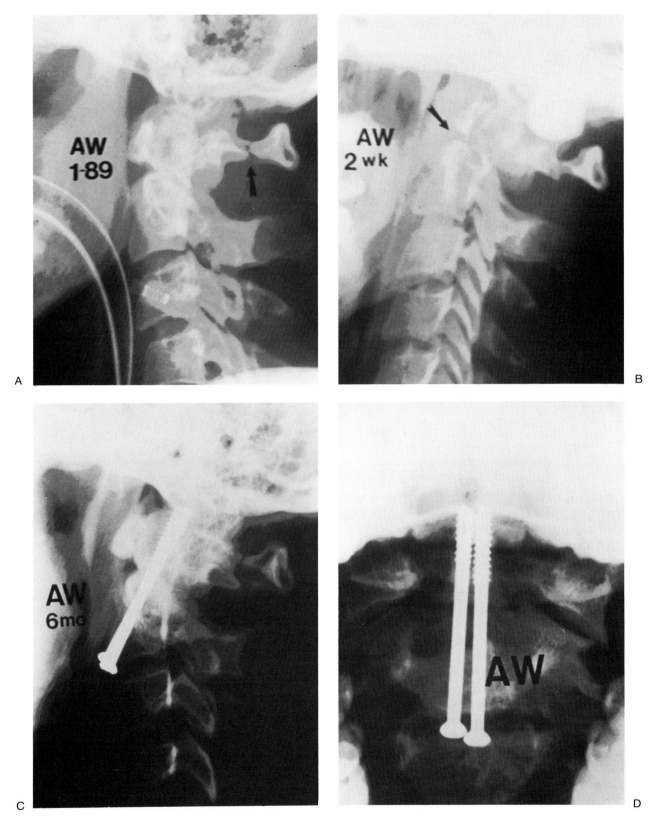

FIG. 10. A: A 28-year-old male following a motor vehicle accident presents with a nondisplaced type II odontoid fracture and fracture of the arch of the atlas *(arrow)*. **B:** Upright radiographs in a halo demonstrate considerable instability of the odontoid fracture *(arrow)*. Anteroposterior **(C)** and lateral **(D)** roentgenogram following odontoid screw fixation and removal of the halo vest.

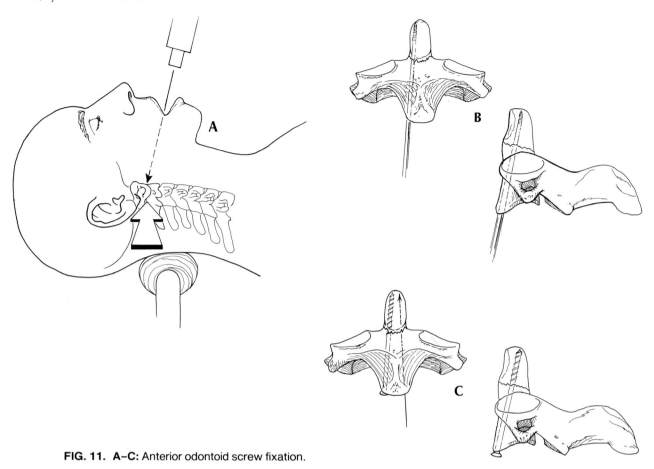

FIG. 11. A–C: Anterior odontoid screw fixation.

skull pins in the Mayfield attachment. Positioning must allow anteroposterior and lateral fluoroscopic imaging. The A-frame attachment to the Mayfield headrest allows anteroposterior visualization by eliminating a midline attachment. The large radiolucent bite block is placed between the upper and lower teeth on one side of the patient's mouth to obtain the open mouth view of the odontoid. A separate C-arm image intensifier should be positioned to obtain both high-quality open mouth and lateral images of C2 (Fig. 11A).

Adjustments are often required under image intensification to obtain a near anatomic reduction of the type II odontoid fracture. An accurate reduction must be made prior to screw placement. The subaxial spine, which is suspended, often requires an anteriorly directed force to achieve this reduction. For this purpose we have modified and padded a crutch that is placed from the floor to the neck and acts as a radiolucent neck roll. It is very important that adequate extension at the cervicothoracic junction be obtained in order to allow for the appropriate sagittal direction of the drill and guide pins. Patients with a large barrel chest, or fixed kyphosis at the cervicothoracic junction may not be candidates for anterior odontoid screw fixation. Additionally, patients with narrow spondylitic spinal canals cannot tolerate the cervical extension required.

A standard anterior Smith-Robinson approach to the cervical spine, via a transverse skin incision, is made at approximately the C4-C5 interspace. Dissection is carried out between the carotid sheath laterally and the trachea and esophagus medially. The anterior longitudinal ligament of the cervical spine is identified and followed up to the C2,3 disc space. The anterior annulus of the C2-C3 disc is divided to allow access to the inferior endplate of C2. A cannulated screw system allows the surgeon to safely and accurately position one or two small threaded guidepins into the tip of the odontoid under biplanar fluoroscopy. The starting point for the guidepin insertion is the anterior-most portion of the inferior end-plate of C2 (Fig. 11B). It is important to avoid the error of starting the guidepin in the anterior cortex of the body of C2, for this greatly increases the potential for screw cut-out. When two odontoid screws are to be placed, each guidepin is started 3 to 4 mm lateral to midline and angled medially so as to nearly converge at the tip of the odontoid. Following placement of both guidepins, each is then overdrilled with a 2.5 mm cannulated drill bit. It is extremely important to continuously observe the tip of the guidepin during drilling. Incarceration of the guidepin within the drill can lead to propagation of the guidepin through the tip of the odontoid and into the brainstem. The guidepin should be originally placed just beyond the tip of the odontoid and drilling should take place short of the tip of the guidepin. A measurement of the drill is then performed and a 3.5-mm cannulated, partially threaded cortical screw of appropriate length is then inserted over one guidepin after tapping the pilot hole (Fig. 11C). Again, continuous observation of the guidepin is necessary during placement of the screw. The adjacent screw is then placed in a similar fashion.

Postoperatively, providing stable internal fixation has been achieved, the patient is placed into a hard cervical collar for 6 to 8 weeks.

LOWER CERVICAL SPINE

General Concepts of Stability

The definition of clinical instability has been previously discussed. This definition is applied appropriately to a clinical situation only after a comprehensive evaluation of the structural integrity of the spine and the neurologic examination of the patient have been completed. White and Panjabi (79) have proposed objective criteria for the diagnosis of subaxial cervical spine instability (Table 1).

Instability of the lower cervical spine most commonly occurs as a result of trauma. Neoplasms, infections, rheumatoid arthritis, and wide laminectomies can also render the spine incapable of performing its structural and protective functions under physiologic loads. Stability can be recovered by closed or surgical methods depending upon the etiology and need for early mobilization of the patient.

Surgical Techniques

The goals of surgical stabilization of the subaxial spine are to obtain and maintain satisfactory alignment, pro-

TABLE 1. *Checklist for the diagnosis of clinical instability in the lower spine[a]*

Element	Point value
Anterior elements destroyed or unable to function	2
Posterior elements destroyed or unable to function	2
Relative sagittal plane translation > 3.5 mm[b]	2
Relative sagittal plane rotation > 11°	2
Positive stretch test	2
Medullary (cord) damage	2
Root damage	1
Abnormal disc narrowing	1
Dangerous loading anticipated	1

[a] Total of 5 or more = unstable.
[b] Tube-plate distance at 180 cm.

mote fusion, and allow for safe early mobilization. Since 1891 when Hadra (38) first applied internal fixation to an unstable cervical spine, many techniques have been developed in an attempt to achieve these goals. Techniques differ in safety, ease of application, cost, biomechanical strength, and requirements of postoperative immobilization. Each technique has advantages and disadvantages, and techniques familiar to the surgeon and appropriate for the patient s pathoanatomy should be chosen. Rogers popularized the cervical wiring and fusion in 1957 (63). Multiple techniques have since been proposed for achieving internal fixation of the cervical spine including variations of interspinous wiring (54), facet wiring (61), oblique facet wiring (24), and wires attached to threaded and smooth rods. Rigid segmental instrumentation, through the use of anterior and posterior cervical plates, has more recently been developed (7,18,21,30,37,69).

Biomechanics

Internal fixation of the subaxial cervical spine will be subjected to varying degrees of compression, distraction, and rotation. Posterior wiring techniques serve as tension bands that satisfactorily resist distraction and can resist flexion provided an intact anterior column exists. Posterior wiring techniques by themselves cannot resist bending forces, compressive forces, or rotational forces. Posterior and anterior plate fixation has been developed to provide improved resistance to compressive and rotational forces applied to the unstable cervical spine.

Sutterlin et al. (76) tested the biomechanical strengths of C4,5 functional spinal units stabilized with Rogers wiring method (Fig. 12), Bohlman's triple wire technique (Fig. 13), sublaminar wiring, anterior cervical plate instrumentation, and posterior hook plate stabilization. This study found the posterior hook plate to be biomechanically the most rigid, effectively reducing posterior and anterior strain. Interestingly this study failed to identify any biomechanical advantage of the anterior cervical plate in comparison to conventional wiring techniques.

Gill et al. (30) compared four different posterior fixation constructs. These included Rogers intraspinous wiring, Halifax interlaminar clamp, bilateral one-third tubular plates using unicortical screws, and bilateral one-third tubular plates using bicortical screws. Lateral mass plates secured with bicortical screws provided the highest mean stiffness.

Technique of Interspinous Wiring

The triple wire technique described by Bohlman (54) provides fixation that reliably resists tension and secures

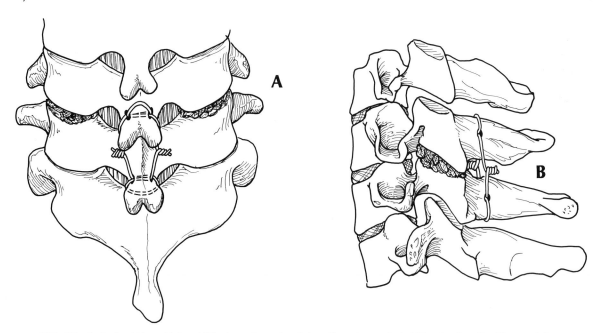

FIG. 12. Anterior (**A**) and lateral (**B**) view of a subaxial motion sigment stabilized using the Rogers interspinous wiring technique.

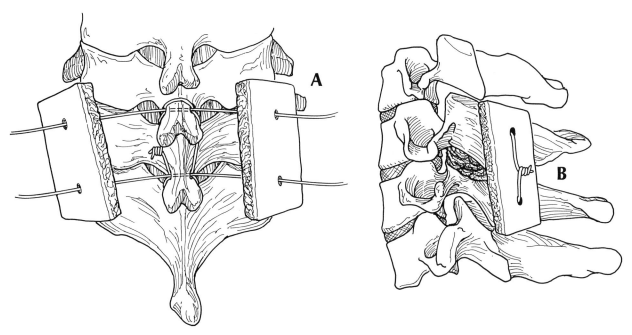

FIG. 13. A,B: Bohlman triple wire technique.

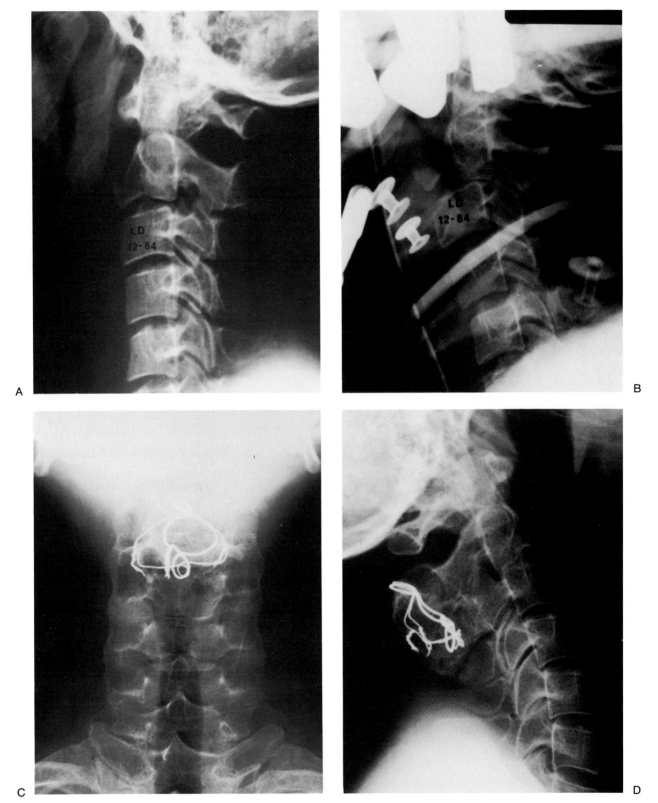

FIG. 14. A: A 24-year-old male with an extension injury at C2,3. **B:** Significant instability demonstrated on upright x-ray in a halo vest. Anteroposterior (**C**) and lateral (**D**) x-rays demonstrating a healed posterior C2-C3 fusion using a Bohlman triple wire technique.

bone graft to the posterior elements (Fig. 13). The authors prefer this technique for posterior wiring with appropriate indications. Posterior ligamentous ruptures and facet dislocations can be satisfactorily stabilized with this technique providing adequate anterior column support exists.

Somatosensory evoked potential monitoring is used in patients with intact or incomplete spinal cord function when further intraoperative reduction or decompression of high-grade stenosis is planned. Maintenance of neurologic function can be assessed with the use of awake intubation and positioning.

Following induction of anesthesia, a lateral cervical roentgenogram is obtained to confirm appropriate sagittal plane alignment. A routine sterile preparation and draping is followed by a standard posterior approach with subperiosteal exposure of the spinous processes and laminae of the intended fusion. A localizing radiograph is obtained. Care is taken to avoid extension of exposure beyond segments intended for fusion. A 3-mm burr is used to create a hole at the base of the spinous process on each side. A towel clip or Lewin clamp enlarges this hole and allows the passage of 18- or 20-gauge wires. One wire is initially placed through the intraspinous ligament above the uppermost spinous process and looped back through the hole created in the spinous process. One end of the wire is passed beneath the caudal spinous process, again looped around its inferior edge and passed back through the hole. Next, 22-gauge wire is passed through and around the cranial spinous process. A third wire (22-gauge) is similarly passed through the caudal spinous process.

Corticocancellous bone grafts of appropriate length are harvested from the posterior iliac crest and drill holes are placed through them to accept the wires. Further cancellous bone is harvested as well.

The posterior one-half of the facet joints are decorticated and packed with cancellous bone. The initial wire is then tightened, creating a tension band effect, applying compression to the posterior elements and facet joints. The remaining wires are passed through the cortical cancellous bone grafts, which are then tightened down to the exposed decorticated lamina. Additional cancellous bone is packed around these grafts (Fig. 14).

Postoperative immobilization should be maintained for 6 to 8 weeks using either a cervicothoracic brace or halo vest, depending on the degree of preoperative instability.

The strength of the triple wire technique is superior to the standard Rogers spinous wiring technique in cyclical flexion and torsion. Bohlman (10) reported a 100% fusion rate at 2-year follow-up in 72 patients treated with this technique. Subsequently, McAfee (54) also reported a 100% fusion rate in 100 patients treated with triple wire technique.

Facet Wiring Techniques

Spinous process wiring techniques require intact spinous processes and lamina. In conditions such as postlaminectomy instability and fractures involving the spinous process and lamina, alternative procedures are required to provide stable internal fixation. Some facet wiring techniques allow stable internal fixation of the cervical spine without requiring fixation to the spinous process.

Robinson and Southwick in 1960 (61) described a facet wiring technique for patients with absent or compromised posterior elements. Fixation is accomplished by looping a wire through the inferior articular facet in the sagittal plane at each level of intended fusion. These wires are then tightened over a cortical cancellous graft to provide fixation (Fig. 15).

Modifications of the facet wiring technique have been proposed. Edwards (24) proposed an oblique wire technique that passed the facet wire additionally around the caudal spinous process to control rotation in unilateral facet fracture dislocations (Fig. 16). Callahan et al. (16) looped the facet wires around a smooth U-shaped Luque rod. Garfin et al. (28) looped the facet wires around a threaded Harrington rod to improve stability between the wires and the rod.

Facet Wiring Technique—Edwards Oblique Wire

Facet wiring requires full exposure of the lateral masses out to the far edge. The joint capsules are removed and a Freer elevator is placed into the facet joint. Using a 3-mm high speed burr, a drill hole is placed in the inferior facet of the cranial vertebrae exiting into the facet joint. The starting point is just caudal to the next cranial facet joint and is aimed directly downward passing into the facet joint. The Freer elevator acts as a backstop and aiming device. A 20-gauge wire or twisted 22-gauge cable is passed through the hole and looped around the caudal spinous process and tightened. This construct can be augmented by a simple Rogers interspinous wire (Fig. 17). Bone graft is placed along the spinous process and lamina. For postlaminectomy defects, multiple facet wires can be passed in a similar manner and tightened over a long corticocancellous or graft or metallic implant.

Posterior Cervical Plate Fixation

Anatomy

Posterior cervical plate fixation is indicated in conditions of subaxial cervical spine instability that cannot be satisfactorily stabilized with posterior intraspinous wire

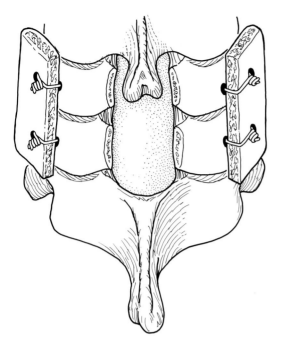

FIG. 15. Facet wiring technique.

technique (Fig. 18). The plate is segmentally fixed to the cervical spine with screws inserted into the lateral masses. Lateral mass fixation does not require intact lamina or spinous processes and therefore can be used when they are fractured or missing. In some cases this may shorten the overall fusion length. Additional indications for lateral mass fixation are multilevel instabilities, rotational instability, especially when fractures of the facets are present, extension translational injuries, and where fixation is required to extend to either the occiput or the thoracic spine (7).

A thorough knowledge and understanding of the anatomy anterior to the lateral mass is essential to the safe application of this technique. When viewed dorsally the lateral mass is square or rectangular shaped. The four borders must be completely exposed and identified. The medial boundary is an easily perceptible valley at the junction of the lamina and facet. The lateral boundary is the far edge of the facet. The superior and inferior boundaries are the cranial and caudal facet joints.

The vertebral artery lies directly anterior to the medial border of the lateral mass at the junction of the lamina and lateral mass. Screw starting point and angulation should therefore begin lateral to this valley and angle outward to avoid injury to the vertebral artery or cervical nerve root. It is essential to review the CT scan preoperatively for the relationship of the lateral mass to the neural foramina and vertebral artery.

Techniques for screw placement have been described by Roy-Camille and Magerl. Roy-Camille (70) recommends starting the screw at the exact center of the lateral

mass and angling straight forward and 10° outward. Magerl (52) recommends that screws start 1–2 mm medial and cranial to the center of the lateral mass and angle parallel to the articular facet and 20° laterally. An (4) recommends starting the screw 1 mm medial to the center of the lateral mass and angling 15° cranial and 30° laterally. These techniques have been investigated for safety and biomechanical strength. Heller (42) found that the Roy-Camille has less risk to the exiting nerve root than the Magerl technique, but frequently crossed the caudad facet joint. The vertebral artery or spinal cord were not at risk with either technique. To increase the safety of screw placement into the lateral masses, Anderson (7) introduced the use of an adjustable drill guide that prevents inadvertent overpenetration of the drill.

Montesano (55) compared pullout strength of screws placed by the Roy-Camille and Magerl methods. He found that significantly longer screws could be safely placed with the Magerl technique and that the Magerl screws had a significantly increased pullout strength. Gill (30) compared lateral mass screws with unicortical to bicortical purchase and found a significant increase in strength with the bicortical screws.

Technique of Posterior Cervical Plate Fixation with AO Reconstruction Plates

The patient is positioned prone on the Stryker wedge turning frame with maintenance of cervical traction using Gardner-Wells tongs. A preoperative lateral roent-

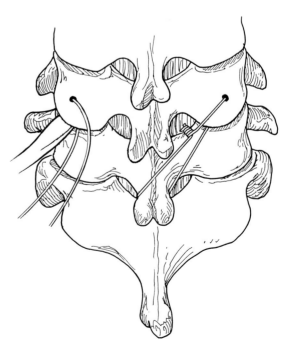

FIG. 16. Edwards oblique wiring technique.

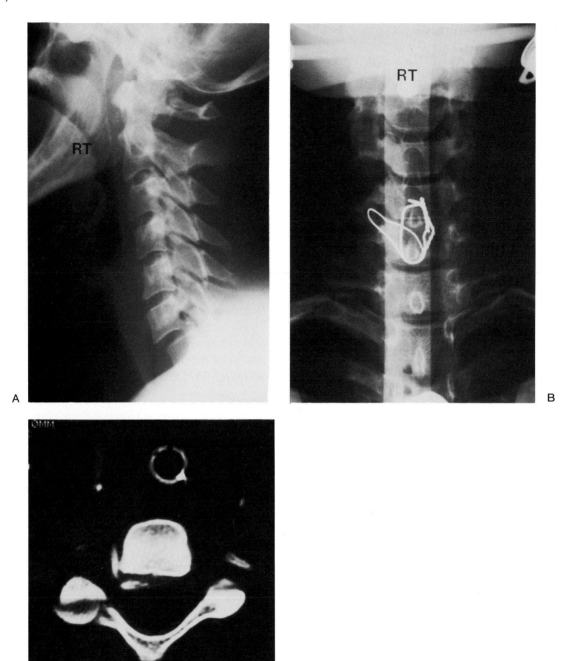

FIG. 17. Stabilization using an oblique wiring technique (courtesy of S. Garfin, M.D.).

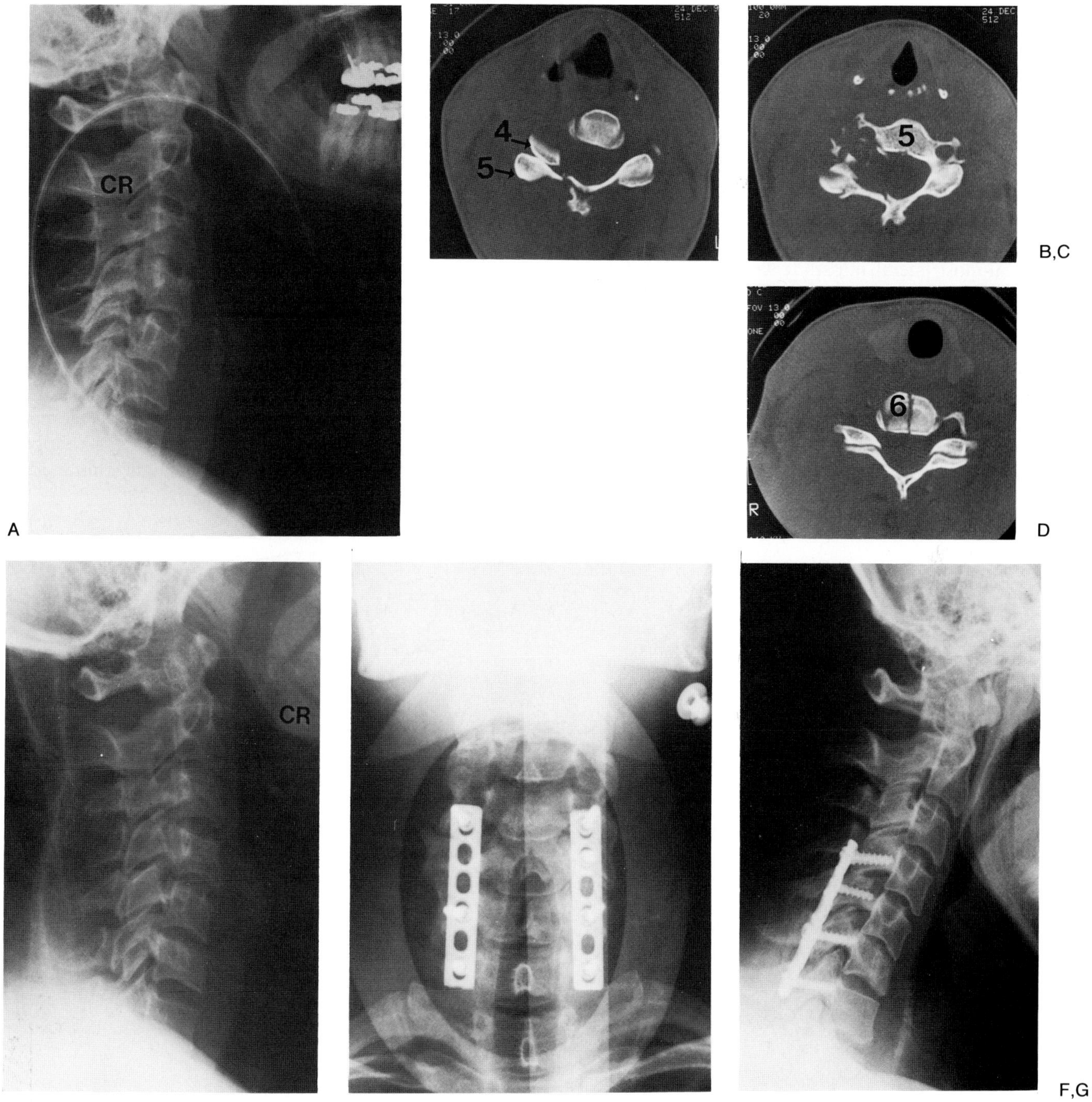

FIG. 18. A 26-year-old female after a motor vehicle accident presented with weakness and dysesthesia in the right C5 and C6 distribution. **A:** Lateral roentgenograms upon admission. **B:** Right C4-C5 facet dislocation. **C:** C5 comminuted pedicle and lamina fracture. **D:** C6 body fracture. **E:** Closed reduction using Gardner-Wells tongs. Anterior (**F**) and lateral (**G**) roentgenograms following posterior stabilization using lateral mass plates.

genogram is obtained to confirm satisfactory sagittal plane alignment and fracture reduction. A routine preparation and draping is followed by a standard posterior approach to the dorsal elements of the cervical spine. The vertebrae intended for fusion are subperiosteally exposed out to the far edge of the lateral mass. The lateral mass is defined medially at the junction with the lamina, superiorly and inferiorly at the facet joints. The far edge of the articular mass creates the lateral boundary.

Initially, pilot holes are drilled in the cranial and caudal-most lateral masses to be included in the construct. The authors' preference is a modified Magerl technique for screw insertion (7). The starting point is located 1 mm medial to the center of the lateral mass (Fig. 19). A 2-mm K-wire or drill is then directed 30–40° cranial (parallel to facet joints) and 10–20° laterally. An adjustable drill guide is initially set at 14 mm and advanced in 2-mm increments until the anterior surface of the lateral mass is penetrated. Following each successive drilling, a 1-mm K-wire is used to probe and palpate the pilot hole to check for far cortex penetration. Using AO/ASIF screws, the length of screw is selected 1 to 2 mm longer than the length of K-wire needed to penetrate the far cortex. This accounts for plate thickness and ensures bicortical screw purchase. In young patients with good bone stock, only unicortical purchase is needed. Screw length averages 16 to 18 mm for subaxial lateral masses. The dorsal cortex is tapped with a 3.5-mm cancellous tap.

The dorsal half of the facet joints intended for arthrodesis are decorticated with a high-speed burr and packed with autogenous cancellous bone graft. Patients will differ in the distances between the lateral masses and therefore plates with different hole spacings are required. AO titanium reconstruction plates have 8- and 12-mm hole spacings. A malleable template is used to determine hole spacing, length and contour of the plate. The appropriate length posterior cervical plate is then contoured to

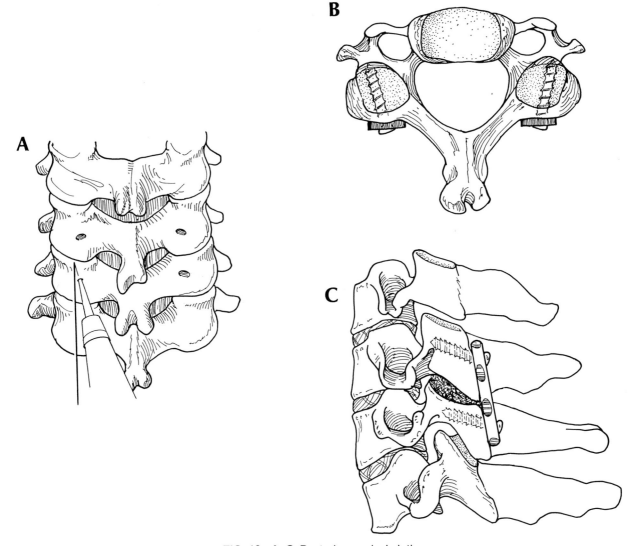

FIG. 19. A–C: Posterior cervical plating.

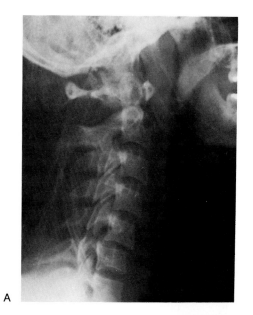

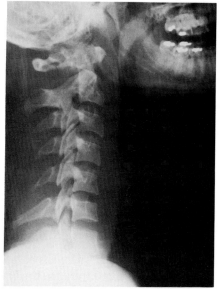

A

B

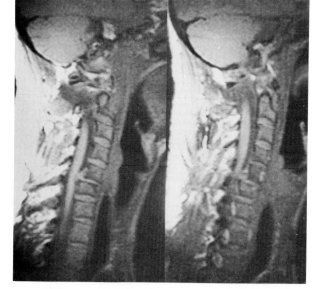

FIG. 20. Anterior cervical plate. **A:** This 31-year-old female sustained a C5-C6 facet fracture, subluxation in a motor vehicle accident. She is neurologically intact. **B:** Reduction using Gardner-Wells tongs. **C:** Post-reduction, preoperative MRI scan reveals a C5-C6 disc rupture. **D,E:** Decompression and stabilization achieved by means of an anterior cervical discectomy and fusion using an anterior cervical plate.

C

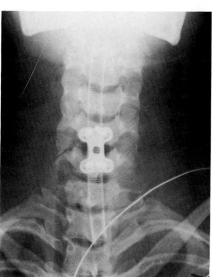

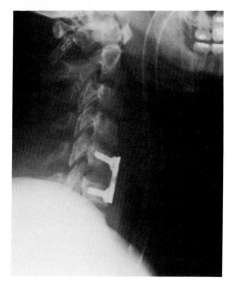

D

E

the cervical lordosis and fixed to the lateral mass with the appropriate length 3.5 cortical screws. Fixation at the remaining intervening lateral masses is performed through the available holes in the plate using the adjustable drill guide and the angulation described above. Lateral radiographs are obtained to confirm appropriate plate position and sagittal alignment. Additional cortical cancellous bone is placed medial and lateral to the plate after decortication of the exposed bone.

Postoperatively, patients are immobilized in a hard cervical collar or cervicothoracic brace for 8 weeks. Flexion and extension lateral roentgenograms are obtained before weaning out of the cervical collar or brace.

Anderson and Grady (32) have reported on 102 patients who have been stabilized with this technique. Fusions have been documented by flexion extension radiographs in all 102 patients. There has been no documented hardware breakage or injury to vertebral artery. Two patients had transient postoperative radiculopathy. Although plain radiographs and CT demonstrated proper screw placement the root injury was most likely secondary to the screw drilling and placement. This indicates the need for caution and meticulous technique when placing lateral mass screws.

Anterior Cervical Plate Fixation

The anterior cervical approach allows for decompression of the central aspect of the spinal cord and nerve roots. Reconstruction is performed by iliac crest or fibula strut grafts. Anterior grafts placed in the presence of posterior ligamentous instability are potentially unstable and may displace or angulate even in the presence of halo vest immobilization (74). Additionally, nonunion of these grafts has been reported to occur in 11% of cases, more so in multilevel fusions (11). Anterior cervical plates have been developed to provide rigid internal fixation to the anterior cervical spine and increase fusion success (Fig. 20). Anterior cervical plates have been biomechanically compared to posterior cervical plates and conventional wiring techniques (76). These in vitro biomechanical studies have found that the anterior cervical plate systems satisfactorily resist extension, yet demonstrate very poor resistance to flexion bending moments. Contrary, clinical investigations, however, have reported excellent results with few fixation failures using anterior cervical plates in the treatment of unstable cervical spine injuries even in the presence of posterior injury.

Bohler first used anterior cervical plate fixation in 1964 (8). Orozco in 1970 (59) developed an H plate specifically for anterior spine fixation. Many authors have subsequently demonstrated satisfactory results with the use of this plate in anterior cervical fusions (22,29).

Caspar (17) developed a slotted trapezoidal shaped plate fixed to the spine through 3.5-mm screws (Fig. 21). In the Caspar and Orozco techniques the screws are not fixed rigidly to the plate. Therefore, these both require bicortical purchase through the anterior and posterior vertebral body cortex of the cervical spine to lessen the incidence of screw loosening. Complications, including screw compression of the neural elements and loosening with the threat of esophageal perforation, have been reported (Fig. 22).

Morscher (56) introduced a titanium anterior cervical plate system with a mechanism that allows the locking

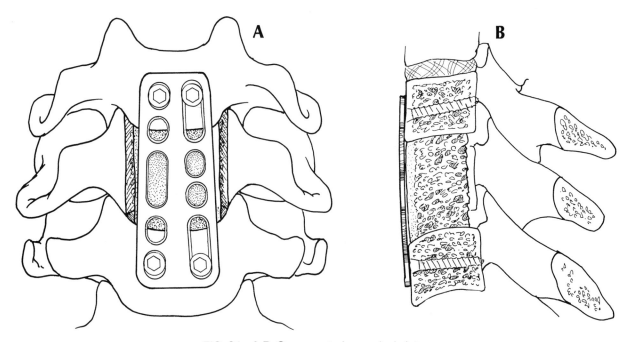

FIG. 21. A,B: Caspar anterior cervical plate.

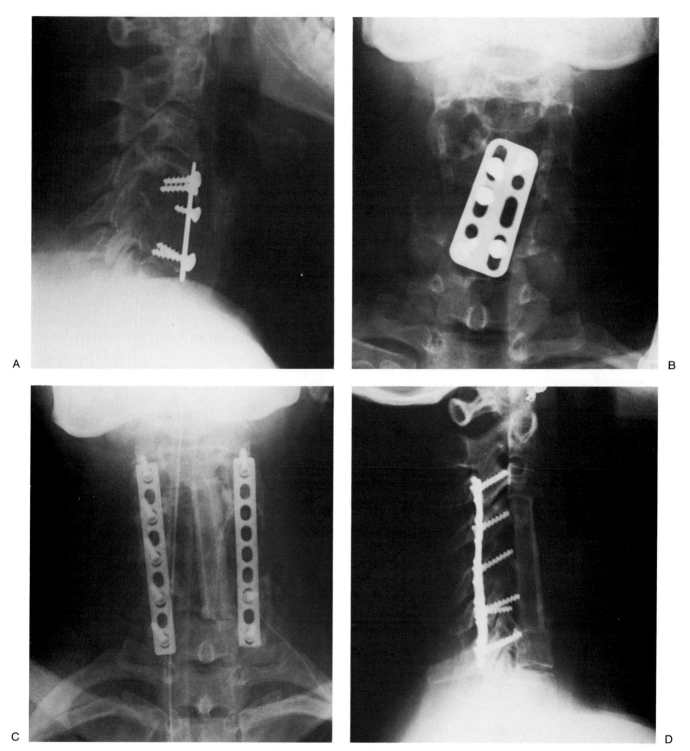

FIG. 22. A 28-year-old female 1 year after C5 corpectomy and Caspar plating for aneurysmal bone cyst at C5, presented with recurrence of tumor, loose plate, and significant C5 and C6 weakness. Lateral (**A**) and anteroposterior (**B**) roentgenogram upon presentation. Anterorposterior (**C**) and lateral (**D**) roentgenogram after removal of loose plate corpectomy and tumor resection C4-C6 and stabilization using autologous fibular graft and posterior cervical plating.

of the screws to the plate (Fig. 23). Due to this locking mechanism and the direction and size of the screws, bicortical purchase is not necessary for biomechanical strength. Biomechanical studies have demonstrated no significant difference between the Morscher plate and the Caspar plate fixed with bicortical screws (1).

Technique—Anterior Cervical Plate Stabilization with the Morscher Plate

The patient is positioned awake in the supine position with cervical spine traction applied through Gardner-Wells tongs. An awake nasotracheal intubation is carried out. After routine preparation and draping, the anterior approach is used to expose the anterior surface of the vertebral body. Lateral radiographs are obtained for localization purposes. In the case of a burst fracture or tumor, a corpectomy is performed after first removing the adjacent discs back to the posterior longitudinal ligament. Removal of the vertebral body is performed with the use

of high-speed burrs until only a thin posterior center remains. This can then be removed by curettes or the diamond burr. The decompression is carried out laterally until the dura and posterior longitudinal ligament appear slightly convex in shape.

Tricortical iliac crest graft of appropriate length is harvested. The end-plates at the intended arthrodesis levels are prepared by removing all end-plate cartilage and decorticating with a high-speed burr. The end-plates should be slightly concave to allow notching of the ends of the bone graft. The autogenous tricortical iliac crest bone graft is then placed between the end-plates. Temporary distraction by pulling on the Gardner-Wells tongs will facilitate graft placement. Alternatively, 14-mm Caspar pins may be placed in the vertebral bodies above and below and distraction performed with the Caspar invertebral disc distractor. An appropriate length anterior plate is selected and placed in position. Confirmation of proper length and positioning of the screw holes is obtained by a lateral roentgenogram (Fig. 24). Plates spanning greater than one level generally require contouring

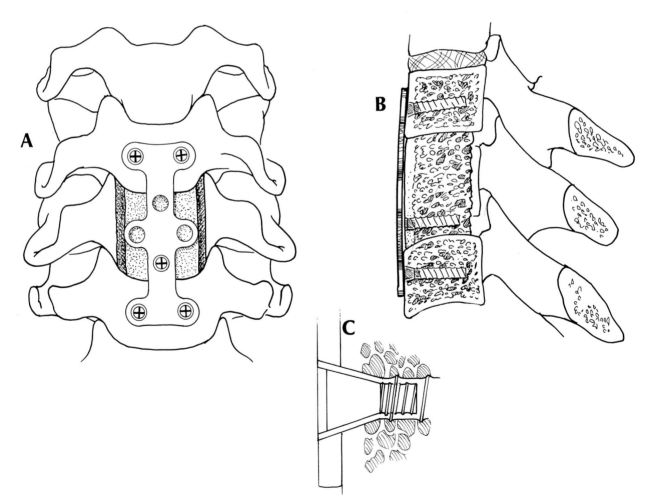

FIG. 23. Mërscher anterior cervical locking plate. Anteroposterior (**A**) and lateral (**B**) diagram of the Mërscher cervical locking plate. **C:** A small screw is inserted into the head of the main screw, spreading and locking it into place.

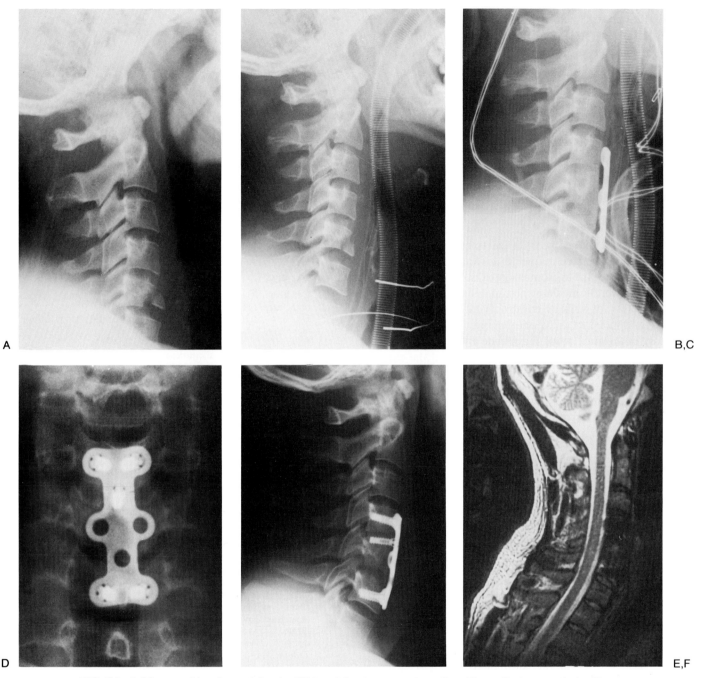

A

B,C

D

E,F

FIG. 24. A 28-year-old male sustained a C5 burst fracture snowboarding. The patient presented with incomplete C5 quadriplegia. **A:** Initial lateral cervical spine roentgenogram. **B:** Reduction in Gardner-Wells tongs. **C:** Intraoperative x-ray confirming the proper length of the anterior cervical plate. Anteroposterior (**D**) and lateral (**E**) roentgenogram following stabilization with an anterior cervical plate. **F:** Postoperative MR image showing the ability to image the cord when titanium is used.

for the cervical lordosis. With the plate secure against the anterior vertebral bodies, 3.5-mm holes are drilled to the 14-mm depth using the stopped drill guide. These holes are tapped and a solid 4.0-mm screw is placed loosely into the vertebral body. All screws are placed before final tightening is performed. The small set screws are then inserted. A lateral radiograph is taken to assure correct alignment and implant position.

Postoperatively, the patient is immobilized in a cervical thoracic brace or hard cervical collar for 8 weeks.

CONCLUSION

Many powerful techniques and implants are available to the spinal surgeon for the treatment of cervical spine instability. Each technique has advantages and disadvantages with regard to biomechanical strength and safety of application. Biomechanical studies have helped to define the ability of various constructs to control pathologic forces applied to the cervical spine. A thorough knowledge of the anticipated magnitude and direction of loads placed on the unstable cervical spine, and the capacity of various implants to resist these pathologic forces, is essential to the appropriate choice of stabilization technique.

REFERENCES

1. Abitbol JJ, Zdeblick T, Kunz R, McCabe R, Cooke M: *Biomechanical analysis of modern anterior and posterior cervical stabilization technique.* Read at the XX annual meeting of the Cervical Spine Research Society, Palm Desert, CA, Dec. 3–5, 1992.
2. Aebi M, Zuber K, Marchesi D (1991): Treatment of cervical spine injuries with anterior plating: indications, techniques, and results. *Spine* 16:S38–45.
3. Albee FH (1911): Transplantation of a portion of the tibia into the spine for Pott's disease: a preliminary report. *JAMA* 57:885.
4. An H (1992): Internal fixation of the posterior cervical spine. *Semin Spine Surg* 4:142–151.
5. Anderson LD, D Alonzo RT (1974): Fractures of the odontoid process of the axis. *J Bone Joint Surg* 56A:1663–1674.
6. Anderson PA, Budorick TE, Easton KB, Henley MB, Salciccioli GG (1991): Failure of halo vest to prevent in vivo motion in patients with injured cervical spines. *Spine* S501–505.
7. Anderson PA, Henley MB, Grady MS, et al. (1991): Posterior cervical arthrodesis with AO reconstruction plates and bone graft. *Spine* 16:S72–79.
8. Bohler J (1967): Sofort- und Frühbehandlung traumatischer Querschnittlahmungen. *Zeitschr Orthopäd Grenzgebiete* 103:512–528.
9. Bohler J (1982): Anterior stabilization for acute fractures and non-unions of the dens. *J Bone Joint Surg* 64A:18–27.
10. Bohlman HH (1979): Acute fractures and dislocations of the cervical spine: an analysis of three hundred hospitalized patients and review of the literature. *J Bone Joint Surg* 61A:1119–1142.
11. Bohlman HH (1993): Anterior cervical discectomy and arthrodesis for cervical radiculopathy: long term follow up of 122 patients. *J Bone Joint Surg* 75A:1298–1307.
12. Brooks AL, Jenkins EB (1978): Atlanto-axial arthrodesis by the wedge compression method. *J Bone Joint Surg* 60A:279–284.
13. Bryan WJ, Inglis AE, Sculco TP, Ranawat CS (1982): Methylmethacrylate stabilization for enhancement of posterior cervical arthrodesis in rheumatoid arthritis. *J Bone Joint Surg* 64A:1045–1050.
14. Bucholz RW, Burkhead WZ (1979): The pathological anatomy of fatal atlanto-occipital dislocations. *J Bone Joint Surg* 61A:248–250.
15. Budorick TE, Anderson PA, Rivara FP, Cohen W (1991): Flexion-distraction fracture of the cervical spine. *J Bone Joint Surg* 73A:1097–1100.
16. Callahan RA, Margolis RN, Keggi KJ, Albright JA, Southwick WO (1977): Cervical facet fusion for control of instability following laminectomy. *J Bone Joint Surg* 59A:991–1002.
17. Caspar W, Barbier D, Klara P (1989): Anterior cervical fusion and Caspar plate stabilization for cervical trauma. *Neurosurgery* 25:491–502.
18. Chapman JR, Anderson PA (1991): Internal fixation techniques for the treatment of injuries in the lower cervical spine. *Orthop Trauma* 1:204–219.
19. Clark CR, Goetz DD, Menezes AH (1989): Arthrodesis of the cervical spine in rheumatoid arthritis. *J Bone Joint Surg* 71A:381–392.
20. Clark CR, White AA III (1985): Fractures of the dens. *J Bone Joint Surg* 67A:1340–1348.
21. Cooper PR (1988): Posterior stabilization of the cervical spine using Roy-Camille plates: a North American experience. *Trans Orthop* 12:43.
22. De Olivera JC (1987): Anterior plate fixation of traumatic lesions of the lower cervical spine. *Spine* 12:324–329.
23. DuToit G (1976): Lateral atlanto-axial arthrodesis: a screw fixation technique. *S Afr J Surg* 14:9–12.
24. Edwards CC, Matz SO, Levine AM (1985): The oblique wiring technique for rotational injuries of the cervical spine. *Trans Orthop* 9:142.
25. Fielding JW (1983): Rheumatoid arthritis of the cervical spine. *Instr Course Lect* 32:114–131.
26. Gallie WE (1939): Fractures and dislocations of the cervical spine. *Am J Surg* 46:495–499.
27. Garfin SR, Botte MJ, Waters RL, Nickel VL (1986): Complications in the use of the halo fixation device. *J Bone Joint Surg* 68A:320–325.
28. Garfin SR, Moore MR, Marshall LF (1988): A modified technique for cervical facet fusions. *Clin Orthop* 230:149–153.
29. Gassman J, Seligson D (1983): The anterior cervical plate. *Spine* 8:700–707.
30. Gill K, Paschal S, Corin J, Ashman R, Bucholz R (1988): Posterior plating of the cervical spine: a biomechanical comparison of different posterior fusion techniques. *Spine* 13:813–816.
31. Glaser JA (1986): Complications associated with the halo vest. *J Neurosurg* 65:762–769.
32. Grady MS, Anderson PA (1991): Management of cervical spine injuries. *Contemp Neurosurg* 13:1–6.
33. Grob D, Crisco JJ, Panjabi M, Wang P, Dvorak J (1992): Biomechanical evaluation of four different posterior atlantoaxial fixation techniques. *Spine* 17:480–490.
34. Grob D, Dvorak J, Gschwend N, Froehlick M (1990): Posterior occipital cervical fusion and rheumatoid arthritis. *Arch Orthop Trauma Surg* 110:38–44.
35. Grob D, Dvorak J, Panjabi M, Froehlich M, Hayek J (1991): Posterior occipitocervical fusion: a preliminary report of a new technique. *Spine* 16:S17–24.
36. Grob D, Magerl F (1987): Dorsal spondylosis of the cervical spine using a hooked plate. *Orthopäde* 16:55–61.
37. Grob D, Magerl F (1987): Surgical stabilization of C1 and C2 fractures. *Orthopäde* 16:46–54.
38. Hadra BE (1891): Wiring the vertebrae as a means of immobilization in fractures and Pott's disease. *Trans Am Orthop Assoc* 4:206. In *Clin Orthop* 112:4–8, 1975.
39. Hajek PD, Lipka J, Hartline P, Saha S, Albright J (1993): Biomechanical study of C1-C2 posterior arthrodesis techniques. *Spine* 18:173–177.
40. Hamblin DL (1967): Occipito-cervical fusion: indications, technique and results. *J Bone Joint Surg* 49B:33–45.
41. Heller JG, Alson MD, Schaffler MB, Garfin SR: Quantitative internal dens morphology. *Spine* 17: 861–866, 1992.
42. Heller JG, Carlson GD, Abitbol J, Garfin SR (1991): Anatomic comparison of the Roy-Camille and Magerl techniques for screw placement in the lower cervical spine. *Spine* 16:S552–557.

43. Hibbs PA (1911): An operation for progressive deformities. *NY State J Med* 93:1013.

44. Heywood AWB, Learmonth ID, Thomas M (1988): Internal fixation for occipito-cervical fusion. *J Bone Joint Surg* 70B:708–711.

45. Holdsworth FW, Hardy A (1953): Early treatment of paraplegia from fractures of the thoraco-lumbar spine. *J Bone Joint Surg* 35B:540–550.

46. Holness RO, Huestis W, Howes WJ, Langille RA (1984): Posterior stabilization with an interlaminar clamp in cervical injuries: technical note and review of the long term experience with the method. *Neurosurgery* 14:318–322.

47. Itoh T, Tsuji H, Katoh Y, Yonezawa T, Kitagawa H (1988): Occipito-cervical fusion reinforced by Luque's segmental spinal instrumentation for rheumatoid diseases. *Spine* 13:1234–1238.

48. Johnson RM, Hart DL, Simmons EF, Ramsby GR, Southwick WO (1977): Cervical orthoses: a study comparing their effectiveness in restricting cervical motion in normal subjects. *J Bone Joint Surg* 59A:332–339.

49. Koch RA, Nickel VL (1978): The halo vest: an evaluation of motion and forces across the neck. *Spine* 3:103–107.

50. Letts M, Slutsky D (1990): Occipitocervical arthrodesis in children. *J Bone Joint Surg* 72A:1166–1170.

51. Lind B, Sihlbom H, Nordwall A (1988): Forces and motions across the neck in patients treated with halo vest. *Spine* 13:162–167.

52. Magerl F, Seemann P (1985): Stable posterior fusion of the atlas and axis by transarticular screw fixation. In: Kehr P, Weidner A, eds. *Cervical spine I.* Wien: Springer-Verlag, pp. 322–327.

53. McAfee PC, Bohlman HH, Ducker T, Eismont FJ (1986): Failure of stabilization of the spine with methylmethacrylate: a retrospective analysis of twenty-four cases. *J Bone Joint Surg* 68A:1145–1157.

54. McAfee PC, Bohlman HH, Wilson WL (1985): The triple wire fixation technique for stabilization of acute cervical fracture-dislocations: a biomechanical analysis. *Trans Orthop* 9:142.

55. Montesano PX, Juach EC, Anderson PA, Benson DR, Hanson PB (1991): Biomechanics of cervical spine internal fixation. *Spine* 16:S1016.

56. Morscher E, Sutter F, Jennis M, Olerud S (1986): Die vordere Verplattung der Halswirbelsäule mit dem Hohlschrauben-Plattensystem. *Chirurg* 57:702–707.

57. Newman P, Sweetnam R (1969): Occcipito-cervical fusion: an operative technique and its indications. *J Bone Joint Surg* 51B:423–431.

58. Orozco R (1971): Osteosintesis en las lesiones traumáticas y degenerativas de la coluna cervical. *Rev Traumatol Cirurg Rehabil* 1:42–52.

59. Orozco DR, Llovet TJ (1970): Osteosintesis en las fracturas de raquis cervical. Nota de technica. *Rev Ortop Traumatol* 14:285–288.

60. Perry J, Nickel VL (1959): Total cervical-spine fusion for neck paralysis. *J Bone Joint Surg* 41A:37–60.

61. Robinson RA, Southwick WO (1960): Indications and technics for early stabilization of the neck in some fracture dislocations of the cervical spine. *South Med J* 53:565–579.

62. Rogers WA (1942): Treatment of fracture-dislocation of the cervical spine. *J Bone Joint Surg* 24A:245–258.

63. Rogers WA (1957): Fractures and dislocations of the cervical spine: an end-result study. *J Bone Joint Surg* 39A:341–376.

64. Roy-Camille R (1984): Arguments en faveur de la voie posterieure dans la chirurgie traumatique du rachis cervical. *Rev Chir Orthop* 70:550–557.

65. Roy-Camille R, Camus JB, Saillant GD, Conlon Y (1983): Luxation atloidoaxiodenne avec impression basilaire et signes medul-laries du cours d'un rhumatisme inflammatoire chronique. *Rev Chir Orthop* 69:81–83.

66. Roy-Camille R, Mazel C, Saillant G (1987): Treatment of cervical spine injuries by a posterior osteosynthesis with plates and screws. In: Kehr P, Weidner A, eds. *Cervical spine I.* New York: Springer-Verlag, pp. 163.

67. Roy-Camille R, Mazel C, Saillant G, Benazet JP (1991): Rationale and techniques of internal fixation in trauma of the cervical spine. In: Errico J, Bauer RD, Waugh T, ed. *Spinal trauma.* Philadelphia: JB Lippincott, pp. 163–191.

68. Roy-Camille R, Saillant G (1970): Actualités de chirurgie orthopédique de l Hôpital Raymond-Poincaré. In: Judet R, ed. *Fractures du rachis cervical,* vol. 8. Paris: Masson & Cie, pp. 175–195.

69. Roy-Camille R, Saillant G, Berteaux D, Serge MA (1979): Early management of spinal injuries. In: McKibbin B, ed. *Recent advances in orthopaedics.* Edinburgh: Churchill-Livingstone, pp. 57–87.

70. Roy-Camille R, Saillant G, Mazel C (1989): Internal fixation of the unstable cervical spine by a posterior osteosynthesis with plates and screws. In: Sherk HH, ed. *The cervical spine.* 2nd ed. Philadelphia: Lippincott, pp. 390–403.

71. Smith MD, Anderson P, Grady MS (1993): Occipitocervical arthrodesis using contoured plate fixation: an early report on a versatile fixation technique. *Spine* 18: 1984–1990.

72. Songer MN, Spencer DL, Meyer PR, Jayaraman G (1991): The use of sublaminar cables to replace Luque wires. *Spine* 16:S418–421.

73. Stambough JL, Balderston RA, Grey S (1990): Technique for occipito-cervical fusion in osteopenic patients. *J Spinal Dis* 3:404–407.

74. Stauffer ES; Kelly EG: Fracture dislocation of the cervical spine: instability and recurrent deformity following treatment by anterior interbody fusion. *J Bone Joint Surg* 59:45–48, 1977.

75. Suh P, Kostuik JP, Esses SI (1990): Anterior cervical plate fixation with the titanium hollow screw plate system: a preliminary report. *Spine* 15:1079–1081.

76. Sutterlin CE, McAfee PC, Warden KE, Rey RM, Farey ID (1988): A biomechanical evaluation of cervical spinal stabilization methods in a bovine model: static and cyclical loading. *Spine* 13:795–802.

77. Van Peteghem PK, Schweigel JF (1979): The fractured cervical spine rendeied unstable by anterior cervical fusion. *J Trauma* 19:110–114.

78. Wertheim SB, Bohlman HH (1987): Occipitocervical fusion: indications, technique, and long-term results in thirteen patients. *J Bone Joint Surg* 69A:833–836.

79. White AA, Panjabi MM (1978): *Clinical biomechanics of the spine.* Philadelphia: JB Lippincott, pp. 191–235.

80. White AA, Southwick WO, Panjabi MM (1971): An experimental study of the immediate load bearing capacity of three surgical constructions for anterior spine fusions. *Clin Orthop* 91:21–28.

81. White AA, Southwick WO, Panjabi MM (1976): Clinical instability of the lower cervical spine. A review of past and current concepts. *Spine* 1:5–27.

82. Whitehill R, Reger SI, Fox E, et al. (1984): The use of methylmethacrylate cement as an instantaneous fusion mass in posterior cervical fusions. *Spine* 9:246–252.

83. Whitehill R, Richman JA, Glaser JA (1986): Failure of immobilization of the cervical spine by the halo vest. *J Boint Joint Surg* 68A:326–332.

84. Zoma A, Sturrock RD, Fisher WD, Freeman PA, Hamblen DL (1987): Surgical stabilisation of the rheumatoid cervical spine. *J Bone Joint Surg* 69B:8–12.

The Adult Spine: Principles and Practice,
2nd edition, J.W. Frymoyer, Editor-in-Chief.
Lippincott-Raven Publishers, Philadelphia © 1997.

CHAPTER **55**

Surgical Approaches to the Craniocervical Junction

Arnold H. Menezes

The first anatomic-pathologic descriptions of craniocervical junction abnormalities were reported in the early part of the 19th century (43,99). Although these autopsy examinations stimulated clinical interest, confirmation of the diagnosis was lacking until death (48,49). With the advent of roentgenographic studies in the early part of the 20th century, craniocervical abnormalities, as well as trauma to this region, took new meaning. However, it was only after Chamberlain's classic radiographic study of basilar invagination that lesions at and around the craniocervical junction emerged from the realm of anatomic and pathologic curiosity to the practical clinical field of neuroscience (19). Postmortem reports were replaced by clinical and radiographic studies of abnormalities in this region.

Recent advances in neurodiagnostic imaging and microsurgical instrumentation have increased our surgical armamentarium. Up until the early 1970s, anteriorly placed lesions at the craniocervical border were approached via a posterior decompression and at times an associated fusion. The morbidity and mortality for such ventrally situated lesions were extremely high (9,26, 38,52,143). A physiologic approach to operative treatment that was based on an understanding of craniocervical dynamics, the stability of the craniocervical junc-

tion, and the site of encroachment was adopted by the author at the University of Iowa Hospitals and Clinics in 1977 (Fig. 1) (99). Since then, 2,100 patients with craniocervical abnormalities have been evaluated by the author and 821 underwent treatment on the Neurosurgical Service at the University of Iowa Hospitals and Clinics (Fig. 2) (102). The pathology of these abnormalities is extensive. A thorough knowledge of the bony anatomy, embryology, and biomechanics at the craniocervical junction is necessary to understand the etiology of abnormalities in this area, and thus their treatment.

DIAGNOSIS OF CRANIOCERVICAL JUNCTION ABNORMALITIES

The symptoms and signs of craniocervical junction abnormalities stem from the osseous changes; brainstem, cervical cord, and cerebellar dysfunction; abnormal cerebrospinal fluid dynamics; and changes that occur in the vertebral basilar vascular tree (9,22,27, 29,44,65,81,88,98,101,106,111,139). Perhaps the most interesting feature of this region's pathology is its diverse presentation (6,50,69,75,81). Compromise of the cervicomedullary junction results in a multiplicity of symptoms and signs, which may be indicated by brainstem and cervical myelopathy, cranial nerve and cervical root dysfunction, and alterations of the vascular supply to these structures (36,37,105,135,138). The symptoms

A. H. Menezes, M.D.: Professor and Vice Chairman, Division of Neurosurgery, University of Iowa Hospitals and Clinics, Iowa City, Iowa, 52242.

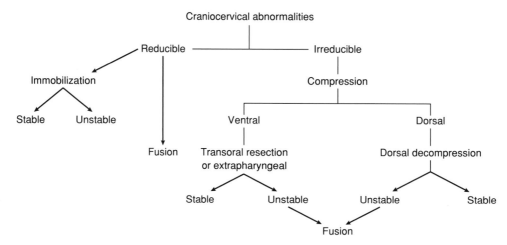

FIG. 1. Treatment of craniocervical abnormalities.

may be insidious and present as a puzzling clinical condition with false localizing signs, or may be precipitated by minor trauma. In a significant number of patients, there is rapid neurologic deterioration, which can be followed by sudden death (27,116,141).

Method of Approach

The factors (Fig. 1) influencing specific treatment are as follows (99,103):

1. Reducibility—whether the bony abnormality can be "reduced" to normal position to relieve compression of the cervicomedullary junction. This also implies restoration of anatomic relationships of the craniospinal axis.
2. The etiology of the lesion—whether bony or soft tissue. Vascular abnormalities, syrinx, Chiari malformations, and tumors are in this category.
3. The presence of ossification centers and epiphyseal growth plates in certain congenital lesions—e.g., fetal

warfarin syndrome, Klippel-Feil syndrome, and Goldenhar's syndrome.
4. The mechanics of compression and the direction of encroachment.

The primary treatment for reducible craniocervical lesions is stabilization, whereas surgical decompression is performed in patients with irreducible pathology. When irreducible lesions are encountered, the decompression is performed in the manner in which encroachment occurs. If a ventral encroachment is present, a transoral-transpalatal-pharyngeal decompression or other appropriate ventral procedure is done; in the case of dorsal compression, a posterior decompression is mandated. If instability exists after either situation, posterior fixation is required (Fig. 2).

Neuroradiologic Investigations

The factors influencing specific treatment are determined by plain radiographs; pleuridirectional tomogra-

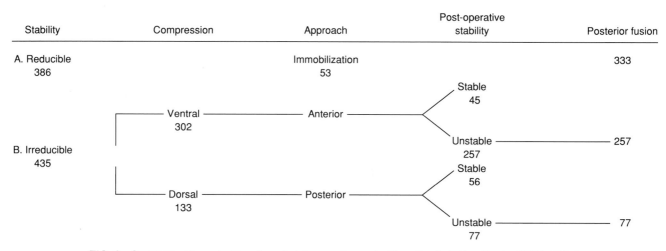

FIG. 2. Summary of surgical treatment at the craniocervical junction in 821 patients (1977–1994).

phy with associated dynamic studies, including the flexed and extended positions; computed tomography (CT) of the craniocervical area, including cerebrospinal fluid enhancement with Lohexol; and magnetic resonance imaging (MRI) (59,93,102,133,141). All of these techniques are important and provide complementary information about the craniocervical junction and the presence of incidental and pathologic changes in the normal and abnormal relationships (Fig. 3).

With the advent of MRI, there has been a gradual trend toward making it the only diagnostic procedure, apart from plain radiographs of the craniocervical border (18,82,102,133,150). However, MRI does not completely visualize osseous pathology and is unable to delineate the true extent of congenital and developmental lesions in this area (122). Imaging of the craniocervical junction should start with an outline of the bony pathology with tomography. This is best served with CT with thin-section frontal and lateral reconstructions from facet to facet (96). In addition, dynamic imaging in the flexed and extended position must be obtained with pleuridirectional tomography and to assess the results of cervical traction. This cannot be done with CT. The combination of CT and pleuridirectional tomography defines the bony pathology and acts as a preoperative assessment of stability in the anteroposterior, lateral, and vertical dimensions. MRI follows in the axial, sagittal, and coronal planes. Dynamic views of the flexed and extended positions are obtained in the mid-sagittal as well as parasagittal planes. Cervical traction with an MRI-compatible halo is subsequently used to determine the

stability of the lesion (Fig. 4). In selected patients, CT myelotomography is essential for identifying and locating the abnormality in relation to the subarachnoid space as well as its proximity to the vascular structures. At times, vertebral angiography is necessary to locate abnormal vessels and to see the effects of head rotation in the flexed and extended positions if this is part of the symptomatology.

In the case of tumors around the craniocervical region, it is imperative that diagnostic imaging be carried out using CT as well as gadolinium-enhanced images on MRI (102). In selected individuals, preoperative angiography is useful in understanding the dynamics of collateral circulation as well as tumor vascularity. Temporary balloon occlusion is a means of assessing the tolerance to vascular occlusion of the carotid or vertebral circulation before surgery (20). This is useful information before embarking on an operative procedure and at times may permit total resection of a difficult lesion by preoperative balloon occlusion of the major vessels encased in tumor. A precise definition and depiction of tumor extent and its relationship to the vital structures of the brainstem, cervical cord, cranial nerves, and the vascular structures require a complementary multi-modality approach (16,88,102,130,131).

APPROACHES TO THE CRANIOCERVICAL JUNCTION

The aims of treatment of osseous pathology certainly differ from those for neoplastic disease, for which com-

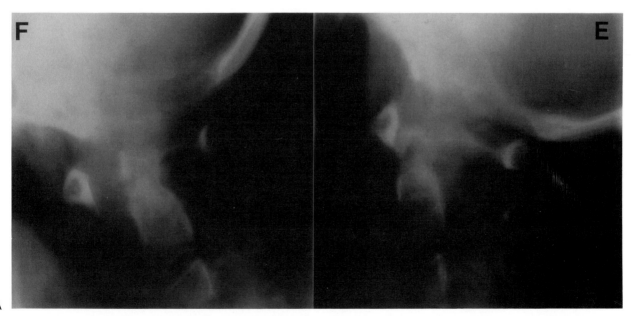

FIG. 3. A: Case D.M. Midline pleuridirectional tomograms of the craniocervical junction (CCJ) in the flexed (left) and extended (right) positions. This 42-year-old rheumatoid patient was known to have a reducible atlantoaxial luxation for several years. Recent loss of arm and hand function prompted further evaluation.

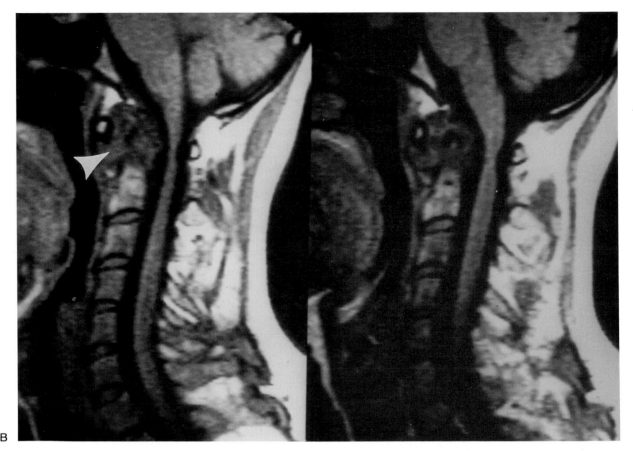

B

FIG. 3. (*Continued.*) **B:** Case D.M. Mid-sagittal T1-weighted MRIs of the craniocervical junction revealed a large mass (arrowhead) enveloping the entire odontoid process with ventral cervicomedullary (CM) neural compression.

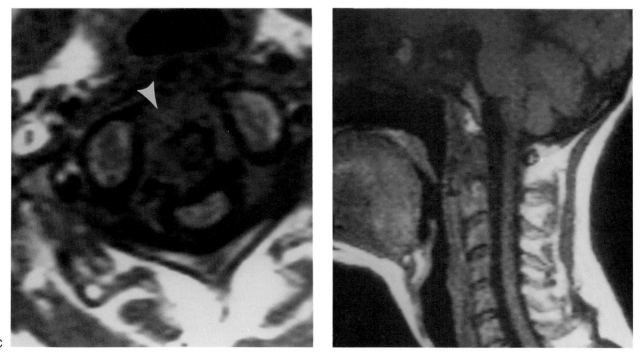

C

D

FIG. 3. (*Continued.*) **C:** Case D.M. Axial T1-weighted MRI at the craniocervical junction outlines pannus (arrowhead) surrounding the odontoid process with ventral cervicomedullary junction compression. **D:** Case D.M. Mid-sagittal T1-weighted MRI in halo traction, 6 days after transoral operation for cervicomedullary compression. Note the odontoid and pannus resection and the normal neural structures.

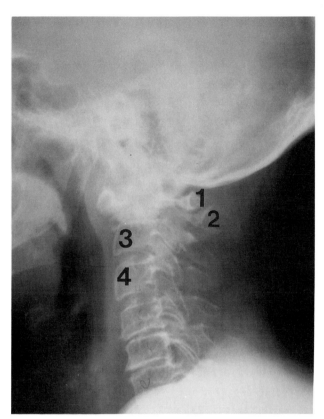 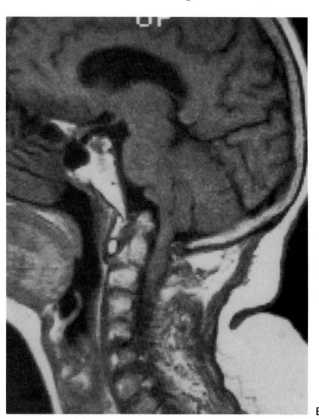

A   B

FIG. 4. A: Case M.T. Lateral skull and cervical radiographs in a 67-year-old patient with long-standing rheumatoid arthritis. There is "cranial settling." The anterior atlantal arch has telescoped down to the C2–C3 interspace, while the dorsal C1 arch is within the spinal canal. **B:** Case M.T. Mid-sagittal T1-weighted MRI of the craniocervical junction. The odontoid has migrated into the ventral aspect of the posterior fossa, compressing the medulla oblongata.

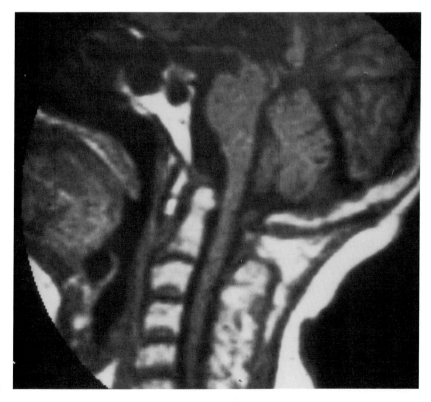

C

FIG. 4. *(Continued.)* **C:** Case M.T. Mid-sagittal T1-weighted MRI in halo traction at 8 lb. There is marked reduction in the odontoid invagination into the medulla.

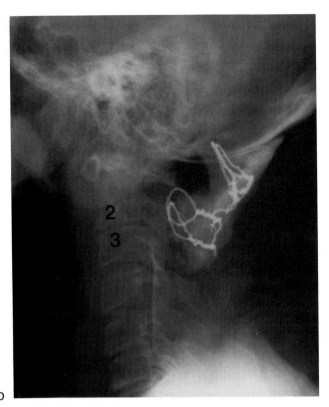

D

FIG. 4. (*Continued.*) **D:** Case M.T. Lateral cervical spine radiograph made 1 week after C1 posterior decompression and dorsal occipitocervical fusion with rib graft, wire, and methyl methacrylate. Note the reduction of the cranial settling.

plete excision is a goal. Likewise, degenerative disease differs from congenital and developmental abnormalities. The ability to work through the orodigestive tract in the ventral and ventrolateral aspects of the craniocervical junction has made direct access to this region easy and relatively safe. However, this avenue of approach itself carries potential risks to the cranial nerves, the vertebral and carotid systems, and the eustachian tubes. Primary lesions of the clivus and ventral aspect of the craniocervical junction tend to expand into the prevertebral space, with the only limitations being the temporal fossae and the expansion into the pterygopalatine and the sphenomaxillary regions. Thus, lateral approaches that allow entrance into this space give a better chance for resection (34,41,42,45,57,73,78,90,130).

Several surgical limitations and considerations must be given attention in designing an approach to the craniocervical junction. These include violation of the orodigestive tract, the need to cross the midline, the ability to look around the corner, and the limitations of the narrow circumference ringed by the carotid and the vertebral basilar systems as well as the mobile joints. Thus, stability and cosmesis also come into play.

The surgical approaches to the craniocervical junction are divided into the ventral approaches, the lateral, and the

dorsal approaches (2,4,7,11,17,28,30,31,71,73,78,80,83, 85,88,90,117–119). Each of these has further subdivisions, as listed in Table 1. The advantages, limitations, and indications for each approach are tabulated (Table 2), and the extent of exposure is illustrated (Fig. 5).

A variety of techniques for fusion in the craniocervical region have been described. Selecting the appropriate level to include in the fusion is often a point of controversy. In general, all levels demonstrating instability must be spanned in the fusion construct. Certain exceptions exist, such as inclusion of the occiput in patients with unstable dystopic os odontoideum and rheumatoid cranial settling.

Occipitocervical and atlantoaxial arthrodesis are generally performed by a posterior approach. Anterior approaches and fusions have been described less frequently. The difficulties inherent in fusing this crucial region led to the development of a number of techniques and innovations in both the approach and the instrumentation used, as shown in Table 3. As with any fusion, long-term stability is dependent upon osseous integration. The goal of instrumentation is to provide immediate stability until bony fusion is obtained. Ultimately, repetitive stress will result in fatigue and failure of the fusion construct if bony fusion cannot be achieved.

Transoral-Transpalatal-Pharyngeal Approach

The transoral-transpalatal-pharyngeal approach to the craniocervical region provides safe, effective, and rapid exposure to the median 4 cm of the craniocervical junction from the mid-clivus to the C3 vertebral body (Fig. 6) (2,12,13,17,24,33,34,38,56,60–62,66,

TABLE 1. *Surgical approaches to the craniocervical junction*

I. Ventral
   A. Midline
      Transoropharyngeal
      Transpalatal-transseptal
      Lateral rhinotomy
      Transbasal
      LeForte I with maxillary "down fracture"
      Median labiomandibular glossotomy
   B. Ventrolateral
      Transcervical extrapharyngeal
      Infratemporal preauricular
II. Lateral
   Lateral transcervical with translocation of vertebral
      artery and occipital condyle resection
   Postauricular infratemporal fossa transpetrosal
III. Dorsal
   Posterolateral decompression with vertebral artery
      translocation and condylar resection
   Midline posterior fossa and upper cervical
      decompression
   Fusions—occipitocervical; atlantoaxial

TABLE 2. *Surgical approaches to the foramen magnum and upper cervical spinal canal*

Approach	Indications	Extent of exposure	Advantages	Disadvantages	Complications
Transsphenoethmoidal	Extradural clivus and sella pathology	Ventral clivus and opposite side of transethmoid route	Short midline approach	Limited to midline and opposite side. Foramen magnum not reached.	Injury to cavernous sinus and optic nerves
Transfacial LeForte I drop-down maxillotomy	Angiofibromas, fibrous dysplasia, extradural chordoma	Paranasal sinuses, clivus, and anterior skull base	Wide anterior base exposure. Can be combined with transoral.	Poor dural coverage if arachnoid violated. Needs miniplate fixation.	Needs tracheostomy. Dural coverage poor.
Transoral transpalatopharyngeal	Extradural lower clivus and C1–C2 pathology	30-mm width of lower clivus, C1–C2 and C3 vertebrae	Procedure done in extension. May be combined with transpalatal and mandibulotomy.	Pterygoid plates limit lateral extension as well as hypoglossal nerves and eustachian tube and vertebral artery.	CSF leakage, retropharyngeal abscess, instability requiring occipitocervical fusion
Lateral extrapharyngeal	Chordoma, metastasis, some bony malformations and fusions	Clivus to petrous apex and down to C2 if the facial nerve is released in parotid	No oropharyngeal contamination. Ventral CVJ fusion possible.	May cause central nervous system IX, X, and XII palsies. Difficulty swallowing. Narrow field.	Limited exposure, lower cranial nerve dysfunction
Median mandibulotomy with glossotomy	Extradural pathology including oropharyngeal malignancy	Wide exposure if combined with palatal split clivus to C4	May be combined with all ventral procedures.	May lose a central incisor; tracheostomy, miniplate fixation.	Same as transoral. Mandibular infection, malocclusion, tracheostomy.
Far lateral "transcondylar"	Meningioma, neurinoma, chordoma	Lower clivus and jugular bulb to C3 and below	No oropharyngeal contamination. Good vertebral artery control. May be combined with posterior fossa and infratemporal procedures.	Sigmoid and venous sinuses	CSF leakage, vascular injury, potential instability
Infratemporal fossa approaches	Intradural tumors of clivus, middle and posterior fossa, and skull base	Petrous bone, upper clivus, foramen magnum	No brainstem or cerebellar retraction. Good control of carotid artery. Good muscle pedicle flaps possible.	Needs combined approaches to access lower clivus. Sacrifice of condyle of mandible and eustachian tube.	Problems chewing, hearing loss, facial palsy
Posterolateral "lateral cerebellar"	Extradural and intradural pathology of CVJ	90° to 120° arc from lateral condyles to past midline	No brainstem retraction with good vertebral artery control. Fusion possible.	Limited by sigmoid sinus, basilar artery, and occipitocervical joints	CSF collection, vascular injury
Posterior midline decompression and upper cervical laminectomies	Dorsal and lateral tumors, bony decompression of foramen magnum	Covers 120° of dorsal foramen magnum	Can easily be combined with fusions	Not indicated for ventral and lateral lesions	Very few disadvantages if indicated

CSF, cerebrospinal fluid; CVJ, craniovertebral junction.

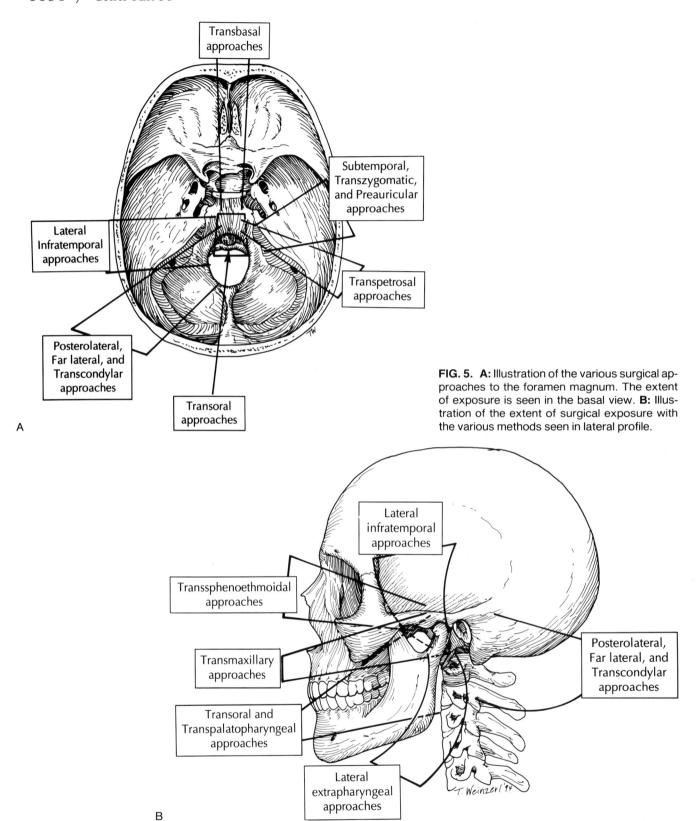

FIG. 5. A: Illustration of the various surgical approaches to the foramen magnum. The extent of exposure is seen in the basal view. **B:** Illustration of the extent of surgical exposure with the various methods seen in lateral profile.

TABLE 3. *Techniques for craniocervical arthrodesis*

I. Occipitocervical fusion
  A. Posterior
      Bone, wire, acrylic fusion
      Plate and screw or wire fusion
      Contoured loop instrumentation
      Plate and transarticular C1–C2 screw
  B. Anterior
      Post-odontoidectomy bone baffle
      Anterolateral extrapharyngeal
II. Atlantoaxial fusion
  A. Posterior
      Bone, wire, acrylic
      Interlaminar clamps
      Plate fixation
      Transarticular screw fixation
  B. Anterior
      Odontoid screw fixation
      Facet screw fixation
      Anterolateral extrapharyngeal

76,86,94,107,115,129,148). Further inferior access may be gained by a median labiomandibular glossotomy (4,30,58,68,78,79,90,110). Rostral extension of the exposure may be provided by limited resection of the caudal hard palate or by a sublabial LeForte I maxillary osteotomy with maxillary "down fracture" (5,72,89,127,140). An alternate operation is a lateral rhinotomy combined with the transoral-transpalatal-pharyngeal approach (88,123).

The main indication for a transoral procedure is irreducible ventral compression on the cervicomedullary junction due to osseous pathology, neoplasm, or inflammatory lesions (97,102). Bony tumors and chordomas have been approached in this manner. Meningiomas and schwannomas, which are primary intradural lesions, are best approached by the dorsal route, as they reside within the subarachnoid space. However, should this not be possible, a ventral operative approach may be essential (12,24,102). Similarly, midline vertebral basilar artery aneurysms have been clipped via this route with exposure through the clivus when no other route would suffice (34,61,62,66,86). Even though there appears to be host immunity to the oropharyngeal flora, the main indication for an anterior transoral midline operative procedure is an extradural lesion. It is important to bear in mind that even though lesions may appear to be irreducible, stabilization of cervical traction is essential during the ventral transoral procedure.

Preoperative Assessment

The nutritional status of symptomatic patients must be evaluated. In some individuals, a high caloric intake may be achieved only by nasogastric feedings or intravenous hyperalimentation. This is an important part of the preoperative and perioperative management because

oral intake is not permitted during the first week after operation.

In circumstances such as rheumatoid arthritis affecting the temporomandibular joint, the ability to open the mouth may be limited. It is important to obtain a working distance of 2.5 to 3 cm between the upper and lower incisor teeth. If this is not possible, an alternative route may be sought. If not, a median mandibular split with midline glossotomy becomes essential to the transoral operation.

Preoperative oropharyngeal cultures are obtained 3 days before a surgical procedure. No antibiotics are given unless pathologic flora are present. Should the lower cranial nerves be compromised, it is imperative that preoperative assessment of the swallowing mechanism and respiratory function be made. This may determine whether a tracheostomy will be needed at the time of the transoral procedure.

Operative Procedure

The patient is transported to the operating theater on a fracture bed with skeletal traction applied via an MRI-compatible halo at 7–8 lb. Topical and regional block

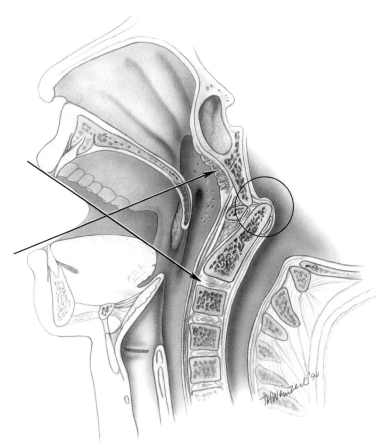

FIG. 6. Illustration of the extent of exposure (between arrows) via the transoral-transpalatal route to the craniocervical junction.

anesthesia facilitates an awake fiberoptic oral endotracheal intubation. The awake patient is then examined to ensure that no change in neurologic status has occurred during positioning. A nasotracheal intubation should be avoided as this tends to disrupt the integrity of the high nasopharyngeal mucosa, which is the avenue for approach to the craniocervical region. The patient is then positioned supine with the head resting in a Mayfield horseshoe head holder. Traction is maintained during the operation with mild extension of the neck. Once it is established that no neurologic deficit has occurred, general endotracheal and intravenous anesthesia is accomplished. In young or uncooperative patients, general anesthesia is performed while traction is maintained and a cervical collar is in place. Fiberoptic intubation is then made through a vent in the mask.

Tracheostomy is performed only when the operative procedure involves the craniocervical junction and structures rostral to it. In situations in which there is brainstem compromise, a tracheostomy is performed after the intubation. Following the intubation or tracheostomy, a gauze packing is placed to occlude the laryngopharynx and to prevent secretions and blood from draining into the stomach.

A modified Dingman self-retaining mouth retractor secures the armored endotracheal tube and allows exposure of the oral cavity as well as the pharynx. In operative procedures involving the clivus and foramen magnum, it is essential to split the soft palate to give the necessary exposure. The operating microscope provides magnification and a concentrated light source. The oral cavity is cleansed with 10% povidone-iodine and hydrogen peroxide and rinsed with saline. A midline incision is made in the soft palate extending from the hard palate to the base of the uvula and deviating to one side (Fig. 7). Stay sutures are applied to the incised soft palate, retracting the palate flaps to either side to expose the high posterior nasopharynx down to the C3 vertebral level. The posterior pharyngeal wall is anesthetized with topical 2.5% cocaine, and the median raphe is infiltrated with 0.5% Xylocaine® with 1:200,000 epinephrine. The midline posterior pharynx is now incised (Fig. 8A). The posterior pharyngeal flap is then retracted to either side with stay sutures, exposing the clivus down to the upper border of C3. The prevertebral fascia and longus colli muscles are dissected free of the osseous and ligamentous attachments to expose the axis and the atlas vertebra, as well as the caudal clivus. The ligaments are now swept away to expose the midline anterior arch of the atlas from one lateral mass to the other, the caudal clivus and the axis body, and the base of the dens.

Lateral exposure is limited to 2 cm to either side of the midline to preserve the integrity of the eustachian tube orifice and prevent injury to the hypoglossal nerves and the vertebral arteries.

The anterior arch of the atlas is removed with a high-speed drill, as is the caudal clivus (Fig. 8B). The soft tissue ventral to the odontoid process is now resected with rongeurs. Removal of the odontoid process is carried out in a rostral-caudal dimension using a high-speed drill with a Diamond burr (Fig. 8C). Chronic instability is indicated by pannus and must be resected (Fig. 8D). Division of the odontoid process at its base and downward traction have been advocated by some, yet these endanger the patient and are fraught with difficulty. This is especially so if pannus is tough and the odontoid has now

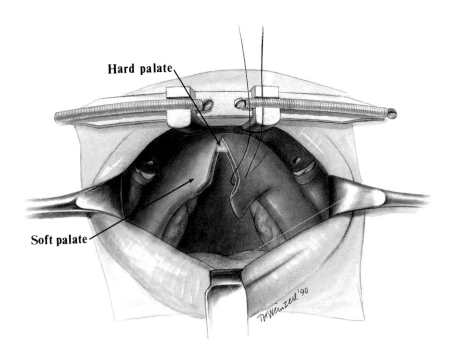

Hard palate

Soft palate

FIG. 7. Illustration of operative procedure. The mouth retractor is in position and the soft-palate incision is made.

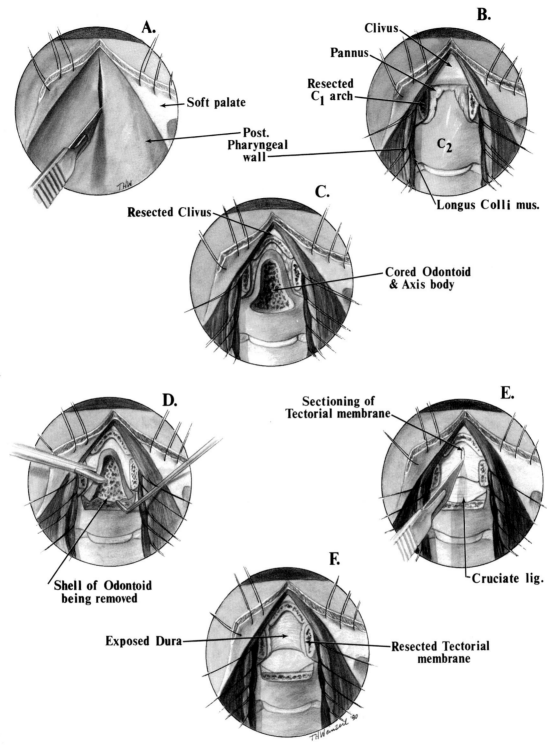

FIG. 8. Views through the operating microscope. **A:** Incision of the posterior pharyngeal wall. **B:** Resection of the anterior atlas arch and caudal clivus brings the invaginated odontoid process into relief. **C:** The odontoid is cored out. **D:** The odontoid shell is being removed. **E:** The tectorial membrane is incised. **F:** Dural decompression.

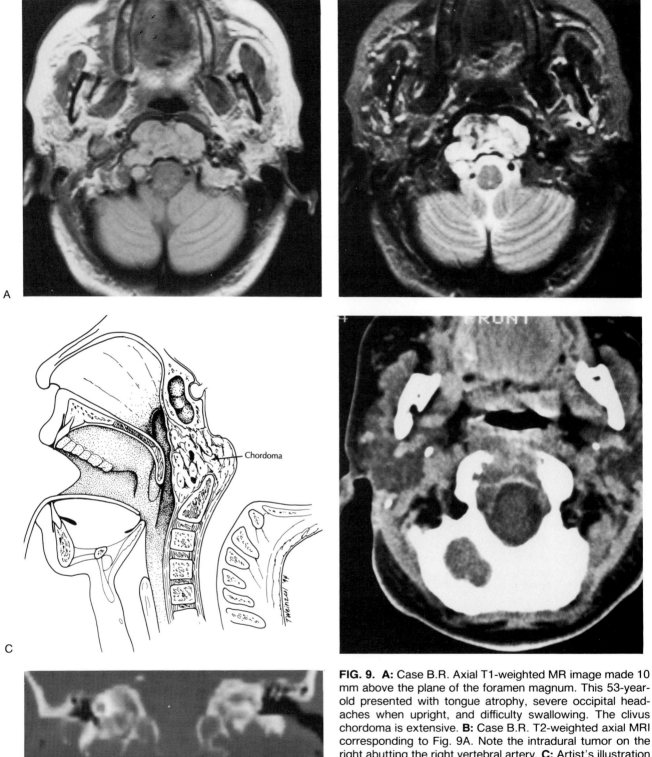

Chordoma

FIG. 9. A: Case B.R. Axial T1-weighted MR image made 10 mm above the plane of the foramen magnum. This 53-year-old presented with tongue atrophy, severe occipital headaches when upright, and difficulty swallowing. The clivus chordoma is extensive. **B:** Case B.R. T2-weighted axial MRI corresponding to Fig. 9A. Note the intradural tumor on the right abutting the right vertebral artery. **C:** Artist's illustration of the chordoma destroying the clivus and atlas. The majority of the tumor is extradural. **D:** Case B.R. Axial CT with intravenous Renografin contrast enhancement through the plane of the occipital condyles. The chordoma has eroded the clivus and medial aspect of the occipital condyles. **E:** Case B.R. Coronal reformatted CT images of the craniocervical region through the plane of the odontoid process. The chordoma has eroded the occipital condyles bilaterally.

achieved a subarachnoid location. After removal of the tectorial membrane (Fig. 8E), the surgeon is assured of adequate bony decompression by the pulsatile dura protruding into the decompression site (Fig. 8F). It is wise to leave the transverse portion of the cruciate ligament intact in children because it lends to partial stability of the atlas.

This author has used median nerve evoked responses during the operation to record brainstem latencies (134,146,147). Change in this parameter requires judicious handling of tissues and minimizing compression of the neural structures. However, this is felt to have little value to the clinical course during the operation. Its use would instead be appropriate during the commencement of anesthetic maneuvers and in the process of turning the patient.

If a tumor such as a chordoma is encountered, direct visualization of its extent is possible (Fig. 9). Piecemeal removal is necessary without undue traction in the case of dural penetration of the tumor. In situations in which an intradural lesion is encountered, a midline incision of the ventral dura must be made, starting inferiorly and proceeding upward. Resection of an intradural lesion requires relieving the cerebrospinal fluid turgidity by having previously placed a lumbosubarachnoid drain. The dura is opened in a midline fashion, extending up as high as necessary into the ventral posterior fossa. A cruciate dural incision is made by converting the vertical incision to a cruciform one below the foramen magnum, thus avoiding the circular sinus. Once the intradural operation is completed, it is essential to bring the dural leaves together in a closure as watertight as possible. If the dura has been violated, it is important to harvest external oblique aponeurosis for fascia to be laid against the dural closure. This must be reinforced with a fat pad before closure of the operative wound.

The longus colli muscles are approximated in the midline, with subsequent anatomic closure of the posterior pharyngeal musculature and the posterior pharyngeal mucosa. Each of these layers is approximated with interrupted sutures of polyglycolic acid.

If the opening into the clivus is large, a pharyngeal pack is used for compression at the high nasopharynx, with traction tubes brought out through the nostrils. In any case, a soft nasogastric feeding tube in inserted via the nose and passed into the stomach. This allows early feeding in the postoperative phase.

Closure of the soft palate is done by bringing the nasal mucosa together with interrupted sutures. The muscularis and oral mucous membrane of the soft palate are approximated with interrupted vertical mattress sutures of similar strength. In situations in which surgery is necessary through the clivus, or in patients with a foreshortened clivus and platybasia, the hard palate is exposed and the posterior 7 to 10 mm is resected (Fig. 10). This allows high nasopharyngeal exposure without splitting the mandible or doing a median glossotomy. The patient is maintained in 5 to 7 lb of skeletal traction after surgery if gross instability was evident. Otherwise, a Philadelphia collar suffices until fusion is made. Intravenous hyperalimentation is continued for 6 days, and no oral intake is permitted. Nasogastric tube feedings may be initiated on

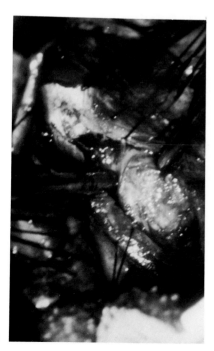

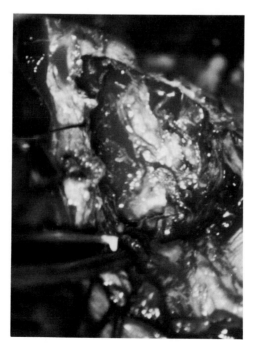

FIG. 10. A: Case B.R. Intraoperative photograph through the microscope during transpalatopharyngeal exposure of the clivus chordoma (arrow). **B:** Case B.R. The clivus chordoma is resected. The vascular ventral dura of the posterior fossa is seen.

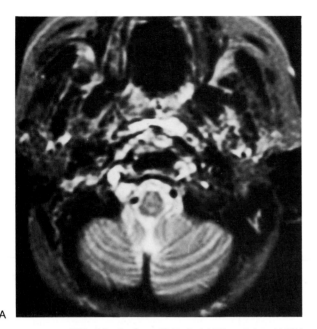
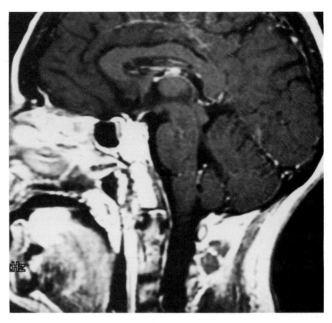

A   B

FIG. 11. A: Case B.R. Axial T2-weighted MR image made 6 days after transpalatopharyngeal resection of the clivus chordoma. There is residual intradural right lateral gutter tumor against the vertebral artery. A fat and fascial graft fills the clivus void. **B:** Case B.R. Mid-sagittal T1-weighted gadolinium-enhanced MRI of the craniocervical junction. A fascial fat pad occupies the lower half of the clivus.

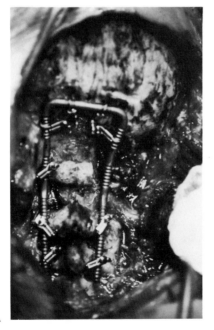
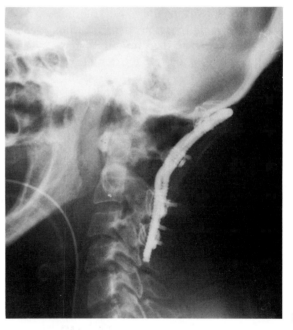

A   B

FIG. 12. A: Case B.R. Operative photograph after a right posterolateral transcondylar resection of the remaining tumor in the right occipital lateral gutter (white arrow). The titanium custom-contoured threaded loop has been affixed to the dorsal occiput–C1-C2-C3 regions with titanium cables and supplemented with bone grafts. **B:** Case B.R. Postoperative lateral cervical radiograph reveals the dorsal occipitocervical instrumentation and fusion.

TABLE 4. *Pathology encountered using the transoral-transpalatopharyngeal approach to the craniocervical junction (1977–1994; author's series)*

Primary basilar invagination and congenital anomalies	143
Rheumatoid "irreducible cranial settling"	62
Dystopic os odontoideum	19
Basilar invagination after malunion O-C1-C2 dislocation	13
Unfused C2 fracture	8
Granulation masses	8
Pseudogout	6
Osteoblastoma	1
Plasmacytoma	4
Clivus chordoma	23
Chondroma—clivus-C1	1
Miscellaneous (inflammatory ileitis, psoriasis, Goldenhar's syndrome, fetal warfarin, osteogenesis imperfecta, metastasis)	14
Total	302

the day after surgery. This is followed by clear liquids and subsequently full liquids by mouth until a regular diet is resumed 15 to 18 days later.

If the dura was opened, intravenous antibiotics (cefotaxime, Flagyl®, and methicillin) and spinal drainage are maintained for 10 days after the operation. The tracheostomy is discontinued only if a stabilization procedure is not required. If no tracheostomy was performed, the armored endotracheal tube is left in place for the first 48 hours to counteract any lingual or pharyngeal swelling.

Postoperative Evaluation

The postoperative stability is evaluated with pleuridirectional lateral tomography 1 week after the transoral operation. This is done in the flexed and extended positions and without and with traction to assess vertical stability. An offset at the lateral occipito-atlantal articulation or vertical displacement of the craniospinal axis is indicative of instability. MRI is performed at this time to assess decompression and the extent of tumor resection (Fig. 11). Should instability exist at the craniocervical junction, occipitocervical fixation must be done. Of the author's series of 302 patients who underwent ventral decompression, 257 required dorsal fixation procedures (Fig. 12).

Neurologic improvement was seen in all of the author's patients who underwent a transoral operation. The youngest patient was 4 years old and the oldest 82. Table 4 outlines the pathology encountered during this operation. Patients who were ventilator dependent after previous primary posterior fossa decompression from a dorsal route had resolution of their neurologic symptoms and signs (Fig. 13). More important, patients with a Chiari malformation and basilar invagination who underwent primary ventral decompression had resolution of their symptoms (97). In addition, the syrinx, if present, showed objective regression on MRI.

Intradural pathology was encountered in 6 children and 32 adults (Fig. 14). This was handled in the manner described previously. In the author's own series, there were no episodes of meningitis after the transoral procedure. However, *Haemophilus influenzae* meningitis oc-

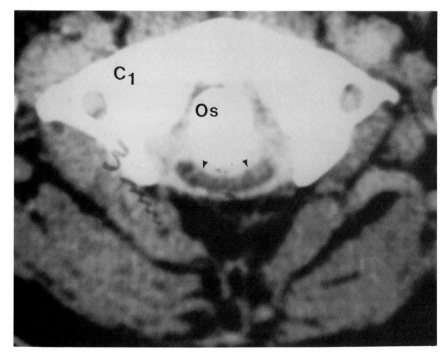

A

FIG. 13. A: Case D.P. Axial CT myelogram at the C1 level. This 23-year-old quadriparetic male worsened neurologically after dorsal C1–C3 laminectomies for os odontoideum with spinal cord compression. The ventrally located os odontoideum still causes cord compression despite the posterior decompression.

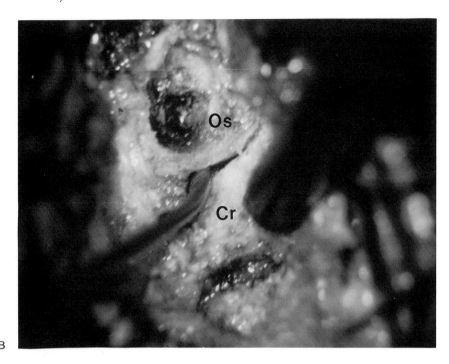

B

FIG. 13. (*Continued.*) **B:** Case D.P. View through the operating microscope during removal of the dystopic os odontoideum (Os) via the transoral route. The cruciate (Cr) ligament is below the os fragment and is incompetent.

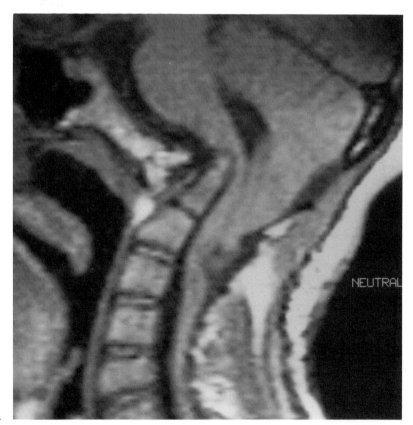

A

FIG. 14. A: Case M.T. Mid-sagittal T1-weighted MR image at the craniocervical junction. This 24-year-old male had previously undergone posterior fossa and upper cervical decompression for Chiari malformation. He had difficulty swallowing, sleep apnea, and inability to walk. There is severe odontoid invagination into the ventral aspect of the medulla, atlas assimilation, and Chiari malformation.

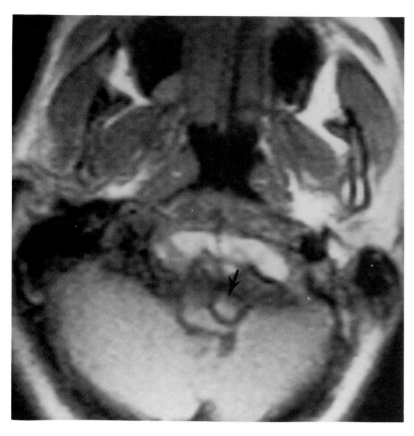

B

FIG. 14. (*Continued.*) **B:** Case M.T. Axial T1-weighted MRI made 15 mm above the foramen magnum. The odontoid process (arrow) is intradural in location, abutting the fourth ventricle. This was successfully excised via the transoral route.

curred recently in an individual 4 weeks after having undergone a transoral procedure and a subsequent dorsal occipitocervical fixation. A lumboperitoneal shunt has never been required. No septomucoperiosteal flap or pharyngeal flap has been needed for closure of the posterior pharyngeal wall or the dura. A pharyngeal wound dehiscence was seen in two individuals; this responded to intravenous hyperalimentation and antibiotics. The lack of infections or complications associated with this operation leads one to believe that there is host immunity to the existing flora within the oral cavity. Two individuals died. One expired 4 weeks after radical resection of a clivus chordoma that had expanded during radiation treatment elsewhere. The tumor had been excised via a ventral palatopharyngeal route and dorsolateral decompression with resection of the tumor and fusion. The cause of death was vertebral artery blowout between C1 and C2, 3 weeks later. In another individual, a cerebellar abscess was encountered 6 months after he had undergone a transoral procedure.

Unfortunately, the morbidity and mortality attached to the earlier reported series by Fang and Ong (38) are still cited as reasons to avoid the transoral operation. The present-day results speak for themselves.

Transcervical Extrapharyngeal Approach

The anterior retropharyngeal approach to the upper cervical spine has been described by several authors

(28,83,84,92,95,136,145). This approach provides anterior access to the neural elements from the clivus to the third cervical vertebra without entrance into the oral cavity and allows ventral fusion procedures (28,92,145). This author has used a modification of this procedure for exposure from the clivus to the lower cervical spine (102).

The awake patient undergoes fiberoptic intubation via a nasal endotracheal route. The oral cavity is kept free of any tubes. The same precautions are taken regarding intubation and anesthesia as with the transoral route.

The patient is positioned supine with the head maintained in traction resting on a padded headrest. It is turned slightly to the patient's left for a right-handed operating surgeon. The cervical incision starts behind the ear, proceeds over the mastoid process, and extends 1.5 cm below the angle of the mandible toward the midline above the hyoid bone (Fig. 15A). An inferior extension of this converts the transverse incision into a "T." This is done at the level of the omohyoid muscle and is brought down over the sternomastoid. The extent of the vertical limb of the incision depends on the amount of cervical spine that must be exposed. Subcutaneous dissection allows mobilization in the subplatysmal plane of the superficial fascia. The inferior division of the facial nerve is identified. The superficial draining veins into the jugular vein are dissected free and ligated before their entrance into the common facial vein or the jugular vein. The superficial branches of the facial nerve are protected by

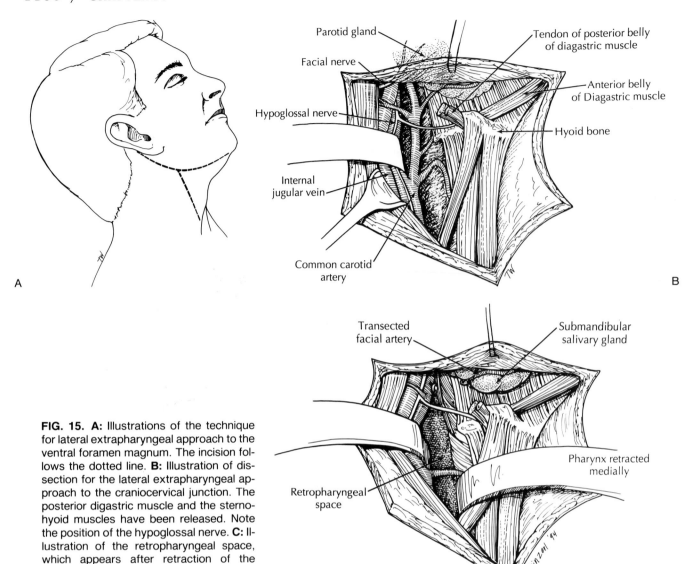

Parotid gland

Facial nerve

Hypoglossal nerve

Internal
jugular vein

Common carotid
artery

Tendon of posterior belly
of diagastric muscle

Anterior belly
of Diagastric muscle

Hyoid bone

A

B

Transected
facial artery

Retropharyngeal
space

Submandibular
salivary gland

Pharynx retracted
medially

C

FIG. 15. A: Illustrations of the technique for lateral extrapharyngeal approach to the ventral foramen magnum. The incision follows the dotted line. **B:** Illustration of dissection for the lateral extrapharyngeal approach to the craniocervical junction. The posterior digastric muscle and the sternohyoid muscles have been released. Note the position of the hypoglossal nerve. **C:** Illustration of the retropharyngeal space, which appears after retraction of the carotid sheath and the cervical strap muscles.

staying deep to this plane. The deep fascia at the anterior border of the sternomastoid is incised, allowing visualization of the carotid sheath. Dissection is made anterior to the carotid sheath (Fig. 15B). The submandibular salivary gland may be elevated. However, resection of the submandibular salivary gland has no consequences if its duct is sutured properly to prevent a salivary fistula. The nodes in the carotid and the digastric triangle are removed. The posterior belly of the digastric is traced to its tendon, where it is transected and transfixed with a suture for subsequent reapproximation. The stylohyoid muscle is divided to allow medial retraction of the laryngopharynx. Care is taken to identify the hypoglossal nerve as it swings between the internal and the external carotid arteries at the greater cornu of the hyoid bone. The hypoglossal nerve is then mobilized superiorly, taking care to preserve the descendens hypoglossi. The ret-

ropharyngeal space is achieved with blunt dissection (Fig. 15C). At this point, it is important to mention that veins crossing over into the jugular have to be sectioned. The prevertebral fascia is incised in a vertical manner to expose the longus colli muscles. These are retracted from their medial origins to expose the anterior arch of the atlas. Care must be taken in retraction to prevent injury to the hypoglossal nerve as it emerges from the condylar foramen. Orientation to the midline must be maintained at all times. The osseous ligamentous structures are swept away so that the caudal clivus and the upper cervical vertebra can be visualized in their anterior aspect.

Anterior decompression is accomplished using a high-speed drill, and the procedure is carried out as described for the transoral operation. Once decompression has been accomplished, fusion may be done using a tricorticate iliac crest graft or a fibular strut interposed between the caudal clivus and the inferior aspect of the axis vertebra. Closure of the cervical wound is first accomplished by approximating the longus colli muscles in the midline with 2-0 polyglycolic acid sutures. The digastric tendon is approximated with 3-0 Neurolon® sutures. The deep fascia of the anterior border of the sternomastoid is approximated, as is the platysma. Skin approximation is done in a standard fashion. No drains are used.

The author has used this procedure infrequently because of the high risk of hypoglossal nerve injury and difficulty in visualizing deep medial structures at the true craniocervical border. However, this approach is ideal for extradural lesions at the axis and subaxial level. Postoperative care includes placement in a halo vest by the third or fourth day; this is maintained until the fusion is documented. Anterior fusion was described by McAfee et al. as "conferring compressive stability only" (92), and the patient should be kept in skull traction until stabilization is achieved if the pathologic process has made the spine unstable. This approach requires a fair degree of dissection of the carotid sheath and structures of the carotid bifurcation. It is mandatory that the carotid system be scanned for changes such as fibromuscular hyperplasia before embarking on such a procedure, as intraoperative stroke with embolization is a rare possibility.

Posterolateral, Far Lateral, and Transcondylar Approach

This approach has been labeled the "extreme lateral," the "transcondylar," the "lateral suboccipital," the "transjugular," and the "dorsolateral suboccipital condylar" approach (1,11,46,47,63,119,131,142). Although the technique used in each of these approaches varies slightly, they all represent an attempt to expose the lower clivus, foramen magnum, craniovertebral junction, and the upper cervical spine without retracting the cerebellum or spinal cord (102). This is accomplished by performing an extensive posterior and lateral bony resection, which includes the lateral rim of the foramen magnum and the posterior aspect of the occipital condyle. Depending on the pathology, the posterior arch of the atlas vertebra as well as the posterior aspect of the foramen transversarium and the lateral atlantal masses may be resected. If one is approaching lesions that are solely within the upper cervical canal, resection of the occipital condyle is unnecessary. The advantages of the far lateral approach are control of the extracranial and intracranial vertebral body, the ability to work in front of the brainstem and cervical cord, and the ability to carry out a fusion construct.

The indications for a posterolateral approach are intradural neoplasms located entirely anterior to the brainstem and cervical cord, and aneurysms to the vertebral artery and the proximal basilar trunk. Extradural lesions

of the clivus and the upper cervical canal may be approached by this exposure. This route combined with the posterior retrosigmoid or presigmoid approach provides control of both intradural and extradural tumors that involve the jugular foramen and the upper cervical region (102).

Operative Technique

This procedure has been performed in the lateral, sitting, and the modified decubitus or park bench position. The author prefers the prone position with the head turned slightly to the side of the exposure and fixed in a multipinned headrest secured to the operating table so as to allow rotation of the table intraoperatively. The sitting position is an excellent one but is fraught with the danger of air emboli. It requires the skills of a competent neuroanesthesiologist and placement of a right atrial and pulmonary artery catheter, as well as Doppler monitoring of the heart for air embolism and respirating gases.

A lateral position allows the cerebellum to fall away from the side of the operative field, and tilting of the head upward provides venous drainage without the concern of air emboli.

The incisions have varied. The author prefers an inverted "U"-shaped skin incision or an inverted hockey stick incision that starts at the mastoid process and proceeds beneath the superior nuchal line to come down the midline (Fig. 16A). The advantage of this is that a cuff of nuchal fascia and muscle inferior to the insertion of this can be left for closure. This prevents cerebrospinal fluid leakage. The paraspinal muscles are split along the spinous process, and the dissection is carried out laterally to the side of the lesion. The paraspinal muscles are retracted with weights and fishhooks. A self-retaining retractor should never be used because of the bulk of cervical musculature that protrudes into the wound, obscuring vision. Care is taken in dissecting free the lateral mass of C1 because of the possibility of injury to the vertebral artery (especially in older individuals), and the venous plexus is spared. The ipsilateral occipital bone is removed to include the condylar fossa, the posterior rim of the occipital condyle, and the dorsolateral rim of the foramen magnum (Fig. 16B). The posterior arch of the atlas including the transverse process and the lamina of C2 may be exposed as necessary. The exposure of bone should include the sigmoid and transverse sinuses to the jugular bulb. A craniectomy may be necessary to expand the exposure. The vertebral artery is elevated from the sulcus arteriosus and dissected free from the transverse foramen of the atlas to the penetration of the occipital-atlantal membrane. Lateral exposure into the posterior fossa as well as the upper cervical spine is obtained only by transposition of the vertebral artery. This requires exposure and section of the second cranial nerve and ex-

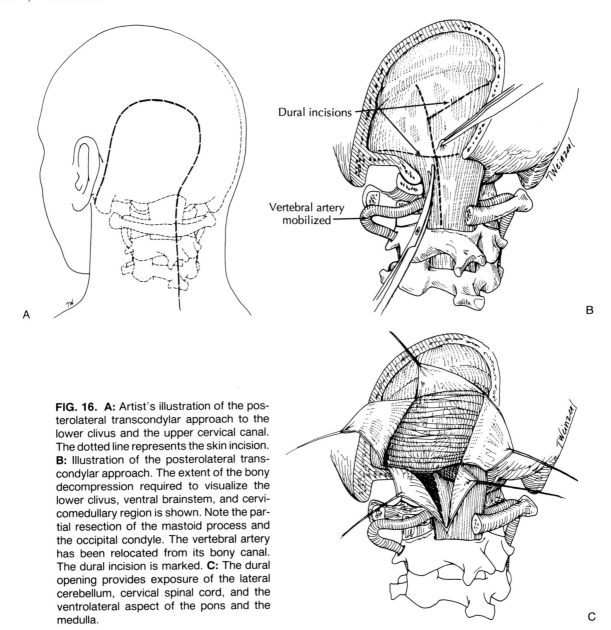

FIG. 16. A: Artist's illustration of the posterolateral transcondylar approach to the lower clivus and the upper cervical canal. The dotted line represents the skin incision. **B:** Illustration of the posterolateral transcondylar approach. The extent of the bony decompression required to visualize the lower clivus, ventral brainstem, and cervicomedullary region is shown. Note the partial resection of the mastoid process and the occipital condyle. The vertebral artery has been relocated from its bony canal. The dural incision is marked. **C:** The dural opening provides exposure of the lateral cerebellum, cervical spinal cord, and the ventrolateral aspect of the pons and the medulla.

tension of the subperiosteal dissection into the foramen transversarium. The foramen transversarium of the atlas is removed from its dorsal aspect of the vertebral artery, unroofed, and dissected down the axis vertebra. The extreme lateral resection of bone into the condylar process and, at times, the medial aspect of the occipital condyle is the key to being able to approach the front of the brainstem and cervical spinal cord without retraction.

Once craniectomy is completed, the capsule of the atlantal-occipital joint is coagulated, and the posteromedial aspect of the occipital condyle and the lateral mass of the atlas are removed. Dissection into the anterior portion of the occipital condyle must be avoided to prevent injury to the hypoglossal canal.

When a dumbbell neurilemoma is encountered, the neural foramen of the involved level is exposed by drilling the adjacent bone superiorly and inferiorly. The intradural extent of the neurilemoma determines the level at which the facetectomy must be performed.

A curvilinear dural incision extends from the sigmoid sinus to the lateral cervical exposure (Fig. 16C). This incision runs medial to the vertebral artery. Several secondary incisions are made perpendicular to the primary incision to allow retraction and intracranial and interspinal exposure.

The operating microscope is essential for magnification and a concentrated light source. The intradural vertebral artery is immediately encountered. The dentate ligament is now sectioned, and the cervicomedullary junction is rotated upward and away from a ventrally placed lesion. In rare circumstances, dorsal rootlets of C1 and at times C2 may need to be sacrificed. In the case of clivus meningiomas, the involved clival dura may be resected close to the entrance of the lower cranial nerve into the parietal dura (Fig. 17).

The specific pathology encountered is now treated, and hemostasis must be exact. The mastoid air cells are carefully waxed, and a fat pad may be necessary. Meticulous dural closure is essential. This may require supplementation with a fascial graft. Paraspinal muscle closure is anatomically done in layers. Should there be concern for cerebrospinal fluid leakage despite this, a lumbosub-arachnoid drain may be necessary for drainage in the early postoperative period.

In circumstances in which only the medial aspect of one occipital condyle has been resected, instability does not occur. However, if a significant portion of the lateral mass of C1 and facetectomy is made at C2, preoperative instability will result, and a fusion must be created on the opposite side. This can also be done on the same side, spanning the operative defect and going to one vertebral level below (100). Instrumentation used may consist of a contoured threaded Steinmann loop or a bent-angled plate (Fig. 12B). This may be secured to the occiput as

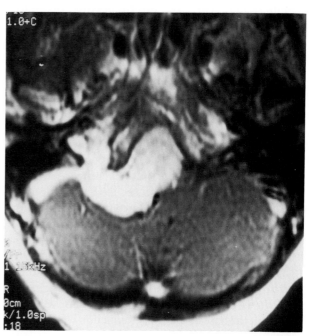

FIG. 17. A: Case P.S. Gadolinium-enhanced axial MRI through the plane of the jugular foramen. Note the lower clival and cerebellopontine angle meningioma. This extended in front of the cervical cord to the C2 level. The individual presented quadriparetic with lower cranial nerve palsies. B: Case P.S. Intraoperative view during posterolateral (left) approach to the foramen magnum. The vertebral artery (*white arrow*) is exposed, as is the lateral C1 posterior arch. C: Case P.S. Operative photograph reveals left posterior fossa craniectomy with removal of the posterior arch of C1 and the posterior aspect of the bony foramen transversarium. There is a relocated vertebral artery (*white arrow*). The lower point is against the medial aspect of the occipital condyle. D: Case P.S. Operative photograph through the microscope. The meningioma is both dorsal and ventral to the dentate ligaments. The spinal accessory nerve is dorsally displaced.

A

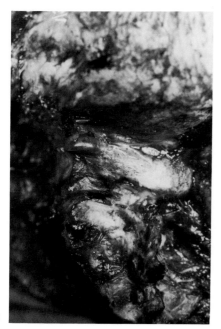
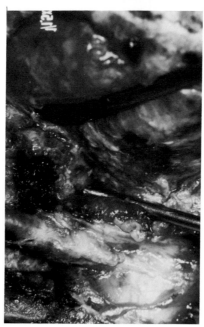
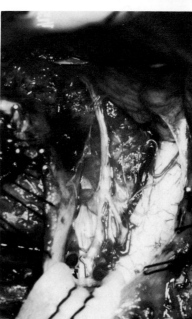

B,C

D

well as the upper cervical spine where possible, and at times may be supplemented with the use of lateral mass pedicular screw fixation from the axis to the atlas vertebra.

Complications

The far lateral transcondylar approach as described by Sen and Sekhar (131) has been fraught with severe complications due to vertebral artery injury as well as cerebrospinal fluid leakage. In the series by George et al. (47), 3 of 14 patients died. One succumbed from massive air embolization in the sitting position. Lower cranial nerve palsies have been described with excision of foramen magnum tumors. However, this results from dissection of the tumor from the cranial nerve itself and is not due to the operative exposure. The true posterolateral exposure described here has few if any complications.

Posterior Fusion for Reducible Lesions

The majority of the author's patients required skeletal traction for a few days to achieve realignment of the craniocervical junction (104). This occurred in 80% of patients with cranial settling, thus obviating the need for an anterior decompressive procedure in addition. In other reducible lesions such as Down syndrome, traction was initiated at 7 lb and followed by graded increases to a maximum of 15 to 18 lb (100). The author has been unsuccessful in realigning the craniocervical junction by cervical traction in those patients with rheumatoid arthritis in whom the odontoid process had invaginated more than 20 mm in the foramen magnum or who had a fracture at the base of the dens. Reduction was not possible in those individuals with complete separation of the anterior and posterior arches of the atlas and basilar invagination. Granulation tissue at the sites of instability fixes the odontoid process to the atlas-clivus junction. This was especially true in patients with atlas assimilation who were older than 16 years.

Dorsal Occipitocervical Fusion
(21,39,51,53,54,59,77,100,112,114,144)

Skeletal traction is maintained via a halo ring throughout the maneuvers of anesthesia induction. An awake fiberoptic oral or nasal endotracheal intubation is made. After this, the patient is placed prone on the operating table; traction is maintained and the face and the halo ring rest on a padded Mayfield-Kees horseshoe headrest. The head and neck are placed in the position that showed the least neural compromise on preoperative studies (Fig. 18). The chest is elevated on laminectomy rolls or a Wilson frame. The neurologic status is assessed and a lateral radiograph documents the optimal position for reduction, which is guided by the preoperative dynamic studies. After radiographic studies have been performed and the position adjusted, general anesthesia ensues. Cervical traction is maintained over a pulley bar so as to allow dynamic changes during the operation. A fixed head position with the pinned headrest or the halo vest allows changes in alignment between the prone and supine positions as well as during the operation. This is obviated by the use of a constantly moving mobile traction device that adapts to the patient's position.

The posterior scalp and cervical regions are prepared, as is the area for harvesting donor bone; namely, the posterior inferior rib cage or the iliac crest. Starting 12 hours

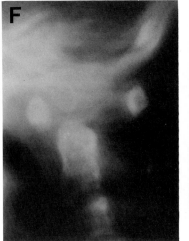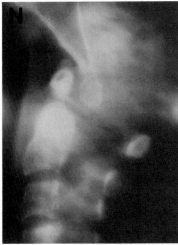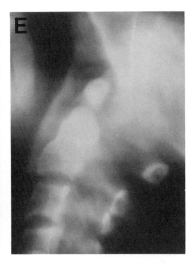

FIG. 18. A: Case V.D. Composite of midline polytomograms of the craniocervical junction in the flexed (F), neutral (N), and extension (E) positions. This 15-year-old gymnast suffered sudden hemiparesis on the parallel bars. There is craniocervical instability secondary to a dystopic os odontoideum.

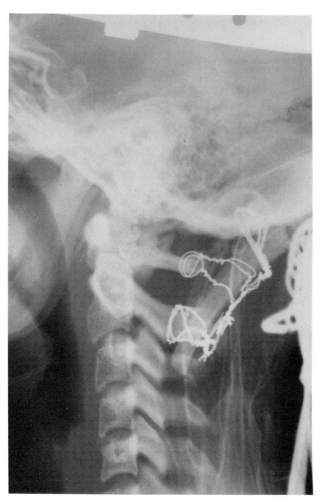

FIG. 18. (*Continued.*) **B:** Case V.D. Plain lateral cervical x-ray made in halo vest immobilization 1 week after C1 decompression and occipitocervical fusion.

foramen magnum is excised using Kerrison punch rongeurs, and bone is preserved for use in the construct. A craniectomy is done to excise the posterior rim of the foramen magnum and ascends 1.5 cm (Fig. 19). It is essential to remove the exoccipital bony ridge to facilitate passage of soft cable from a laterally placed trephine toward the midline. Trephines are made 2.5 cm to either side of the midline and 2 cm above the foramen magnum. Epidural braided no. 22 wire or soft cables are passed from the occipital trephine opening to the midline craniectomy. Similarly, braided wire or cables are passed beneath the lamina of the axis vertebra individually. An unbraided no. 20 wire is used, or no. 2 silk is passed beneath the lamina of C1 because this prevents the saw-like action from cutting the posterior arch of the atlas, which is often thin. The donor bone is harvested from the rib or ilium. The author has consistently used full-thickness rib that was removed close to the head of the rib to provide the contour and approximation between the occiput and the dorsal surface of the atlas and axis vertebrae. Decortication of the spinous processes and laminae is essential at the recipient site and at the occiput. The donor bone is secured to the occiput, atlas, and axis vertebrae by passing the wire through the graft to anchor it into position. Matchstick slivers of bone are then packed into the remaining crevices at the donor-recipient side. In situations such as Chiari malformation with basilar invagination and craniocervical instability, or in dorsally approached tumors that require a simultaneous fusion, the technique of occipitocervical fusion is modified as in Fig. 20. The atlantoaxial purchase is lateral.

Atlantoaxial Fusion (3,14,15,32,40,97,113,114,120,128,132,149)

Dorsal atlantoaxial arthrodesis is carried out in the same manner except that the grafts do not extend to the occiput (Fig. 21). A modified Gallie fusion can be made in older individuals in whom a satisfactory tricorticate bone graft can be removed from the iliac crest to be fashioned to fit between the undersurface of the dorsal arch of C1 and the superior aspect of the posterior arch of C2, with a notch being made for the spinous process. This is then maintained in position by placement of Gallie-type wiring that goes underneath the lamina of C1 and then hooks underneath the spinous process of C2 (Fig. 22A). The anterior portions of the wiring then pass around the wedge graft to be tied behind it and to anchor it into position (Fig. 22B).

The patient is maintained in a Philadelphia collar for 3 to 4 days after surgery before immobilization in a halo vest. Immobilization is required for 3 months for atlantoaxial arthrodesis and for 5 to 6 months for occipito-atlantoaxial arthrodesis (74). In the latter circumstance,

before the procedure and continuing for 48 hours afterward, 1 g of intravenous cephalothin-sodium (Keflin®) is administered every 6 hours.

A midline incision from the external occipital protuberance to the spinous process of the fifth cervical vertebra is made. A subperiosteal exposure is obtained of the squamous-occipital bone and the posterior arches of the upper three cervical vertebrae using sharp dissection. If gross instability is present, a towel clip is passed through the spinous process of the axis for stabilization. This is also done to the posterior arch of the atlas when muscle dissection is performed. Stabilization of the operative exposure can be obtained by placing the D'Errico or Miskimon retractors at a 90° angle to each other. This placement stretches and fixes the bone-muscle relationship so as to prevent motion of the occipitocervical and atlantoaxial joints. In those patients with occipito-atlantoaxial instability, the fusion must include the occiput as well as the atlas and axis vertebrae. The posterior rim of the

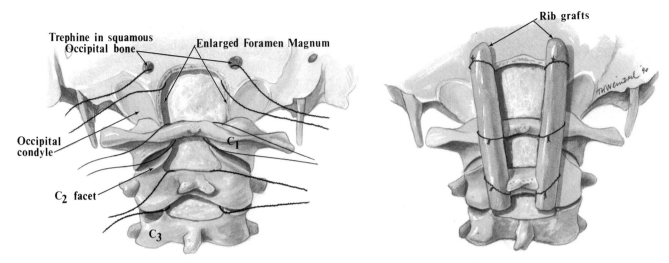

Trephine in squamous Occipital bone

Enlarged Foramen Magnum

Occipital condyle

C₁

C₂ facet

C₃

Rib grafts

FIG. 19. Illustration of the dorsal occipitocervical fusion technique.

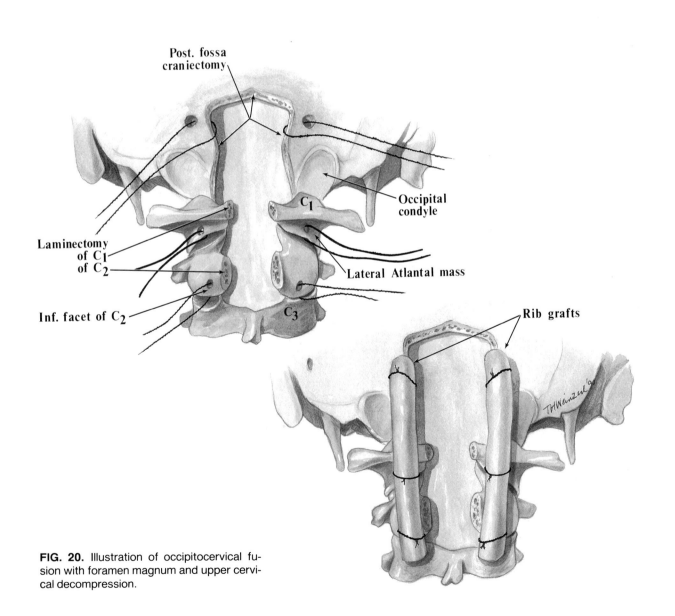

Post. fossa craniectomy

Occipital condyle

C₁

Laminectomy of C₁ of C₂

Lateral Atlantal mass

Inf. facet of C₂

C₃

Rib grafts

FIG. 20. Illustration of occipitocervical fusion with foramen magnum and upper cervical decompression.

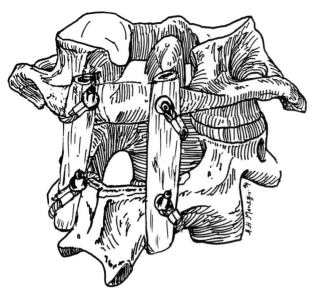

FIG. 21. Illustration of dorsal interlaminar atlantoaxial fusion.

shorter immobilization may result in nonunion, union in an abnormal position, or, in those patients with Down syndrome, additional cranial settling with subsequent increased neurologic deficit.

In severely disabled patients such as those with rheumatoid arthritis, immediate internal stabilization can be obtained by supplementing the bone fusion construct with methyl methacrylate and wire fixation (21,35, 91,104,137). In this situation, the wires anchoring the bone grafts are preserved for a length of 2 cm. These are then converted into hooks to act as pegs for the ongoing acrylic onlay. Methyl methacrylate is fashioned in a

horseshoe-shaped manner, with the horizontal connecting limb being molded to the occiput and the vertical stripes cascading over the bone grafts, enveloping the wire pegs but staying free of the lateral surface of bone. This allows muscle to approximate over the bone construct, thus providing vascularization (Fig. 4D).

Dorsal Occipito-Atlantoaxial Instrumentation

Several instrumentation procedures have been introduced into the armamentarium for atlantoaxial and occipitocervical fusion. These include clamps (25,54, 67,108,109,124), screws (8,10,55,125), rods, and contoured loops (23,64,70,87,121,126). The success of any fusion construct is ultimately dependent on achieving a solid bony fusion. This must be obtained before stress fatigue, hence there is always a race to achieve osseous integration before construct fatigue. For this reason, postoperative immobilization is mandatory. The placement of instrumentation serves only for the immediate postoperative period until osseous fusion has occurred. Clamp devices that approximate the atlas to the axis or in the Gallie-type fusion will only worsen a situation such as cranial settling in the rheumatoid patient. The ideal atlantoaxial arthrodesis should maintain spacing, prevent rotation, and accommodate flexion and compressive forces.

Custom contoured loop instrumentation spanning the occiput and upper cervical spine has achieved much popularity recently. The advent of titanium instrumentation with titanium cables allows postoperative MRI and has improved the management of patients with rheumatoid arthritis as well as tumors.

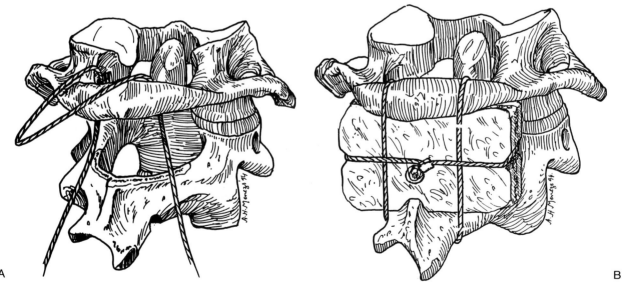

A   B

FIG. 22. A: Illustration of braided wire-cable placement for modified (Gallie) fusion. **B:** Illustration of dorsal atlantoaxial arthrodesis with a fitted wedge bone graft in place.

RESULTS

In no circumstance in the author's experience has there been an increase in the neurologic deficit. The rate of nonunion in more than 660 craniocervical arthrodeses was less than 2%. This is attributed to the design of the fusion construct, the extent of immobilization, and the removal of the anterior compressive pathology of the craniocervical junction before posterior fixation. There were two wound infections in 17 years.

SUMMARY

The choice of surgical approaches to the craniocervical junction requires precise definition and depiction of the pathology, as well as its relationship to the vital neural structures within. Surgical limitations and considerations include violation of the orodigestive tract, the need to cross the midline, the ability to look around a corner, and the limitations of the narrow circumference of the craniocervical junction ringed by the vertebrobasilar and carotid systems and the mobile joints. Thus, cosmesis and stability must be considered. The surgical approaches to this region have been divided into the ventral, lateral, and dorsal approaches. Ideally, the surgeon must be capable of combining a decompression and resection with fusion, should this be necessary.

REFERENCES

1. Anson JA, Spetzler RF (1993): Endarterectomy of the intradural vertebral artery via the far lateral approach. *Neurosurgery* 33: 804–811.
2. Apuzzo MLJ, Weiss MH, Heiden J (1978): Transoral exposure of the atlanto-axial region. *Neurosurgery* 3:201–207.
3. Aprin H, Wharf R (1988): Stabilization of atlantoaxial instability. *Orthopedics* 11:1687–1693.
4. Arbit E, Patterson RH Jr (1981): Combined transoral and median labiomandibular glossotomy approach to the upper cervical spine. *Neurosurgery* 8:672–674.
5. Archer DJ, Young S, Uttley D (1987): Basilar aneurysms: A new transclival approach via maxillotomy. *J Neurosurg* 67:54–58.
6. Aring CE (1981): Lesions about the junction of medulla and spinal cord (editorial). *JAMA* 229:1879.
7. Aryanpur J, Hurko O, Francomano C, et al. (1990): Craniocervical decompression for cervicomedullary compression in pediatric patients with achondroplasia. *J Neurosurg* 73:375.
8. Barbour JR (1971): Screw fixation and fractures of the odontoid process. *S Aust Chir* 5:20–24.
9. Barucha EP, Dastur HM (1964): Craniovertebral anomalies. *Brain* 87:469–480.
10. Benzel EC, Kesterson L (1989): An implant clamp for atlanto-axial fusion. *J Neurol Neurosurg Psychiatry* 52:291–292.
11. Bertalanffy H, Seeger W (1991): The dorsolateral, suboccipital, transcondylar approach to the lower clivus and anterior portion of the craniocervical junction. *Neurosurgery* 29:815–821.
12. Bonkowski JA, Gibson RD, Snape L (1990): Foramen magnum meningioma: Transoral resection with a bone baffle to prevent CSF leakage. Case report. *J Neurosurg* 72:493–496.
13. Bonney G (1970): Stabilization of the upper cervical spine by the transpharyngeal route. *Proc R Soc Med* 63:896–897.
14. Brattstrom H, Granholm L (1976): Atlanto-axial fusion in rheu-

matoid arthritis. A new method of fixation with wire and bone cement. *Acta Orthop Scand* 47:619–628.
15. Brooks AL, Jenkins EB (1978): Atlanto-axial arthrodesis by the wedge compression method. *J Bone Joint Surg [Am]* 60:279–284.
16. Bundschuh C, Modic MT, Kearney F, Morris R, Deal C (1988): Rheumatoid arthritis of the cervical spine. Surface-coil MR imaging. *AJR* 151:181–187.
17. Cannoni M (1978): La voi trans-orale dans l'abord des lesions de la region du clivus. *J Fr Otorhinolaryngol* 27:81–85.
18. Chaljule A, Van Fleet R, Geinito FC Jr, et al. (1992): MR imaging of clival and paraclival lesions. *AJR* 159:1069–1074.
19. Chamberlain WE (1939): Basilar impression (platybasia): A bizarre developmental anomaly of occipital bone and upper cervical spine with striking and misleading neurological manifestations. *Yale J Biol Med* 11:487–496.
20. Choi IS, Berenstein A (1988): Surgical neuroangiography of the spine and spinal cord. *Radiol Clin North Am* 26:1131–1141.
21. Clark CR, Goetz DD, Menezes AH (1989): Arthrodesis of the cervical spine in rheumatoid arthritis. *J Bone Joint Surg [Am]* 71: 381–392.
22. Cohen L, Macrae D (1962): Tumors in the region of the foramen magnum. *J Neurosurg* 19:462–469.
23. Crockard HA, Pozo JL, Ransford AO, Stevens JM, Kendall BE, Essigman WK (1986): Transoral decompression and posterior fusion for rheumatoid atlanto-axial subluxation. *J Bone Joint Surg [Br]* 68:350–356.
24. Crockard HA, Bradford R (1985): Transoral transclival removal of a schwannoma anterior to the craniocervical junction. *J Neurosurg* 62:293–295.
25. Cybulski GR, Stone JL, Crowell RM, et al. (1988): Use of Halifax interlaminar clamps for posterior C1-C2 arthrodesis. *Neurosurgery* 22:429–431.
26. Dastur DK, Wadia NH, DeSai AD, et al. (1965): Medullospinal compression due to atlanto-axial dislocation and sudden hematomyelia during decompression. *Brain* 88:897–924.
27. Davis FW Jr, Markley HE (1951): Rheumatoid arthritis with death from medullary compression. *Ann Intern Med* 35:451–454.
28. DeAndrade JR, MacNab I (1969): Anterior occipito-cervical fusion using an extra-pharyngeal exposure. *J Bone Joint Surg [Am]* 51:1621–1626.
29. Delamarter RB, Dodge L, Bohlman HH, Gambetti PL (1988): Postmortem neuropathologic analysis of eleven patients with paralysis secondary to rheumatoid arthritis of the cervical spine. *Orthop Trans* 12:54.
30. Delgado TE, Garrido E, Harwick RD (1981): Labiomandibular, transoral approach to chordomas in the clivus and upper cervical spine. *Neurosurgery* 8:675–679.
31. Derome PJ (1977): The transbasal approach to tumors invading the base of the skull. In: Schmidek HH, Sweet WH, eds. *Current techniques in neurosurgery.* New York: Grune and Stratton, pp. 223–245.
32. Dickman CA, Sonntag VK, Papadopoulos SM, et al. (1991): The interspinous method of posterior atlantoaxial arthrodesis. *J Neurosurg* 74:190–198.
33. DiLorenzo N, Palatinsky E, Bardella L, et al. (1987): Benign osteoblastoma of the clivus removed by a transoral approach: Case report. *Neurosurgery* 20:52–55.
34. Drake CG (1981): Progress in cerebrovascular disease. Management of cerebral aneurysm. *Stroke* 12:273–283.
35. Eismont FJ, Bohlman HH (1981): Posterior methylmethacrylate fixation for cervical trauma. *Spine* 6:347–353.
36. El-Khoury GY, Tozzi JE, Clark CR, et al. (1985): Massive calcium pyrophosphate crystal deposition at the craniovertebral junction. *Am J Radiol* 145:777–778.
37. Elsberg CA, Strauss I (1929): Tumors of the spinal cord which project into the posterior cranial fossa. *Arch Neurol Psychiatry* 21: 261–273.
38. Fang HSY, Ong GB (1962): Direct anterior approach to the upper cervical spine. *J Bone Joint Surg [Am]* 44:1588–1604.
39. Fielding JW, Griffin PP (1974): Os odontoideum. An acquired lesion. *J Bone Joint Surg [Am]* 56:187–190.
40. Fielding WJ, Hawkins RJ, Ratzan SA (1976): Spine fusion for atlantoaxial instability. *J Bone Joint Surg [Am]* 58:400–407.
41. Fisch U, Matton D (1988): Infratemporal fossa approach. In:

Fisch U, Matton D, eds. *Microsurgery of the skull base.* New York: Thieme, pp. 136–281.

42. Fisch U, Pillsbury HC (1979): Infratemporal fossa approach to lesions in the temporal bone and base of the skull. *Arch Otolaryngol* 105:99–107.

43. Foerster O (1927): *Die Leitungsbahnen des Schmerzgefuhls und die chiruurgische Behandlung der Schmerzzustaude.* Berlin: Urban and Schwarzenberg, p. 266.

44. Fremion AS, Garg BP, Kalsbeck J (1984): Apnea as the sole manifestation of cord compression in achondroplasia. *J Pediatr* 104:398–401.

45. Gates GA (1988): The lateral facial approach to the nasopharynx and infratemporal fossa. *Otolaryngol Head Neck Surg* 99:321–325.

46. George B, Atallah A, Laurian C, et al. (1989): Cervical osteochondroma (C2 level) with vertebral artery occlusion and second cervical nerve root irritation. *Surg Neurol* 31:459–464.

47. George B, Dematons C, Cophignon J (1988): Lateral approach to the anterior portion of the foramen magnum. Application to surgical removal of 14 benign tumors: Technical note. *Surg Neurol* 29:484–490.

48. Giacomini C (1886): Sull' esistenza dell' "os odontoideum" nell' uomo. *Gior Accad Med Torino* 49:24–28.

49. Gladstone J, Erickson-Powell W (1914–1915): Manifestation of occipital vertebra and fusion of atlas with occipital bone. *J Anat Physiol* 49:190–199.

50. Goffin J, Wilms G, Plets C, et al. (1992): Synovial cyst at the C1-C2 junction. *Neurosurgery* 30:914–916.

51. Grantham SA, Dick HM, Thompson RC Jr, et al. (1969): Occipito-cervical arthrodesis. Indications, technique and results. *Clin Orthop* 65:118–129.

52. Greenberg AD, Scoville WB, Davey LM (1968): Trans-oral decompression of the atlantoaxial dislocation due to odontoid hypoplasia. Report of two cases. *J Neurosurg* 28:266–269.

53. Grob D, Dvorak J, Gschwen N, et al. (1990): Posterior occipito-cervical fusion in rheumatoid arthritis. *Arch Orthop Trauma Surg* 110:38–44.

54. Grob D, Dvorak J, Panjabi M, et al. (1991): Posterior occipito-cervical fusion. A preliminary report of a new technique. *Spine* 16(3S):917–924.

55. Grob D, Jeanneret B, Aebi M, Markwalder TM (1991): Atlantoaxial fusion with transarticular screw fixation. *J Bone Joint Surg [Br]* 972–976.

56. Hadley MN, Spetzler RF, Sonntag VK (1989): The transoral approach to the superior cervical spine. A review of 53 cases of extradural cervicomedullary compression. *J Neurosurg* 71:16–23.

57. Hakuba A, Nishimura S, Jang BJ (1988): A combined retroauricular and preauricular transpetrosal-transtentorial approach to clivus meningiomas. *Surg Neurol* 30:108–116.

58. Hall JE, Denis F, Murray J (1977): Exposure of the upper cervical spine for spinal decompression by a mandible and tongue-splitting approach. *J Bone Joint Surg [Am]* 59:121–123.

59. Hamblen DL (1967): Occipitocervical fusion. Indications, technique and results. *J Bone Joint Surg [Br]* 49:33–45.

60. Harkey HL, Crockard HA, Stevens JM, et al. (1990): The operative management of basilar impression in osteogenesis imperfecta. *Neurosurgery* 27:782.

61. Hashi K, Hakuba A, Ikuno H, et al. (1976): A midline vertebral artery aneurysm operated via transoral transclival approach. *Nishinkei Geka-Neurol Surg [Japan]* 4:183–189.

62. Hayakawa T, Kamikawa K, Ohnishi T, Yoshimine T (1981): Prevention of postoperative complications after a transoral transclival approach to basilar aneurysms. *J Neurosurg* 54:699–703.

63. Heros RC (1986): Lateral suboccipital approach for vertebral and vertebrobasilar artery lesions. *J Neurosurg* 64:559–562.

64. Heywood AW, Learmonth ID, Thomas M (1988): Internal fixation for occipito-cervical fusion. *J Bone Joint Surg [Br]* 70:708–711.

65. Hirata Y, Matsukado Y, Kaku M (1985): Syringomyelia associated with a foramen magnum meningioma. *Surg Neurol* 23:291–294.

66. Hitchcock E, Cowie R (1983): Transoral-transclival clipping of a midline vertebral artery aneurysm. *J Neurol Neurosurg Psychiatry* 46:446–448.

67. Holness RO, Huestis WS, Howes WJ, et al. (1984): Posterior stabilization with an interlaminar clamp in cervical injuries: Technical note and long term experience with the method. *Neurosurgery* 14:318–322.

68. Honma A, Murota K, Shiba R, et al. (1989): Mandible and tongue splitting approach for giant cell tumor of axis. *Spine* 14:1204–1210.

69. Howe JR, Taren JA (1973): Foramen magnum tumors. Pitfalls in diagnosis. *JAMA* 225:1061–1066.

70. Itoh T, Tsuji H, Katoh Y, Yonezawa T, Kitagawa H (1988): Occipito-cervical fusion reinforced by Luque's segmental spinal instrumentation for rheumatoid disease. *Spine* 13:1234–1238.

71. Jackson IT (1986): Craniofacial osteotomies to facilitate skull base tumor resection. *Br J Plast Surg* 39:153–160.

72. James D, Crockard HA (1991): Surgical access to the base of skull and upper cervical spine by extended maxillotomy. *Neurosurgery* 29:411–416.

73. Janecka IP, Sen CN, Sekhar LN, et al. (1990): Facial translocation: A new approach to the cranial base. *Otolaryngol Head Neck Surg* 103:413–419.

74. Johnson RM, Hart DL, Simmons EF, et al. (1977): Cervical orthoses. A study comparing their effectiveness in restricting cervical motion in normal subjects. *J Bone Joint Surg [Am]* 59:332–339.

75. Julieu J, Riemens V, Vithal CI, et al. (1978): Cervical cord compression by solitary osteochondroma of the atlas. *J Neurol Neurosurg Psychiatry* 41:479–481.

76. Kennedy DW, Papel ID, Holliday M (1986): Transpalatal approach to the skull base. *Ear Nose Throat J* 65:48–53.

77. Kransdorf MJ, Wehrle PA, Moser RP Jr (1988): Atlanto-axial subluxation in Reiter's syndrome. *Spine* 13:12–14.

78. Krespi YP, Har-El G (1988): Surgery of the clivus and anterior cervical spine. *Arch Otolaryngol Head Neck Surg* 114:73–78.

79. Krespi YP, Sisson GA (1984): Transmandibular exposure of skull base. *Am J Surg* 148:534–538.

80. Lalwani AK, Kaplan MJ, Gutin PH (1992): The transsphenoethmoid approach to the sphenoid sinus and clivus. *Neurosurgery* 31:1008–1014.

81. Leach RE, Goldstein HH, Younger D (1967): Osteomyelitis of the odontoid process. *J Bone Joint Surg [Am]* 49:369–374.

82. Lee BCP, Deck MDF, Kneeland JB, et al. (1985): MR imaging of the craniocervical junction. *AJNR* 6:209–213.

83. Lesoin F, Jomin M, Pellerin P, Pruvo JP, Carini S, Servato R (1986): Transclival transcervical approach to the upper cervical spine and clivus. *Acta Neurochir (Wien)* 80:100–104.

84. Lesoin F, Pellerin P, Thomas CE 3rd, et al. (1984): Acrylic reconstruction of an arthritic cervical spine using the transcervical-trans-clival approach. *Surg Neurol* 22:329–334.

85. Levy ML, Chen TC, Weiss MH (1991): Monostotic fibrous dysplasia of the clivus. Case report. *J Neurosurg* 75:800–803.

86. Litvak J, Sumners TC, Barron JL, Fisher LS (1981): A successful approach to vertebrobasilar aneurysms. Technical note. *J Neurosurg* 55:491–494.

87. MacKenzie AI, Uttley D, Marsh HT, et al. (1990): Craniocervical stabilization using Luque/Hartshill rectangles. *Neurosurgery* 26:32–36.

88. Malis LI (1985): Surgical resection of tumors of the skull base. In: Wilkins RH, Rengachary SS, eds. *Neurosurgery.* New York: McGraw-Hill, pp. 1010–1021.

89. Maloney F, Worthington P (1984): The origin of the LeForte I maxillary osteotomy: Cheever's operation. *J Oral Surg* 39:731–734.

90. Martin H, Tollefsen RH, Gerold FP (1961): Median labiomandibular glossotomy. Trotter's median (anterior) translingual pharyngotomy. *Am J Surg* 102:753–759.

91. McAfee PC, Bohlman HH, Ducker T (1986): Failure of stabilization of the spine with methyl methacrylate. *J Bone Joint Surg [Am]* 68:1145–1157.

92. McAfee PC, Bohlman HH, Riley LH, Robinson RA, Southwick WO, Nachlas NE (1987): The anterior retropharyngeal approach to the upper part of the cervical spine. *J Bone Joint Surg [Am]* 69:1371–1373.

93. Menezes AH (1988): Os odontoideum—Pathogenesis, dynamics

and management. In Marlin AE, ed. *Concepts in pediatric neurosurgery,* Vol. 8. Switzerland: Karger, pp. 133–145.

94. Menezes AH (1990): Transoral approach to the clivus and upper cervical spine. In: Wilkins R, Rengachary S, eds. *Neurosurgery update.* New York: McGraw-Hill, pp. 306–313.

95. Menezes AH (1991): Anterior approaches to the craniocervical junction. In: *Clinical neurosurgery: Proceedings of the Congress of Neurological Surgeons.* New York: Williams and Wilkins, pp. 756–769.

96. Menezes AH (1991): Surgical approaches to the craniocervical junction. In: Frymoyer J, ed. *The adult spine: Principles and practice,* Vol. 2. New York: Raven Press, pp. 967–986.

97. Menezes AH (1992): Complications of surgery at the craniovertebral junction—Avoidance and management. *Ped Neurosurg* 17:254.

98. Menezes AH (1992): Normal and abnormal development of the craniocervical junction. In: Hoff JT, Crockard HA, Hayward R, eds. *Neurosurgery—The scientific basis of clinical practice,* 2nd ed. London: Blackwell Scientific Publishers, pp. 63–83.

99. Menezes AH, Graf CJ, Hibri N (1980): Abnormalities of the craniovertebral junction with cervicomedullary compression. *Child's Brain* 7:15–30.

100. Menezes AH, Ryken TC (1994): Instrumentation of the craniocervical region. In: Benzel E, ed. *Spinal instrumentation.* Park Ridge: American Association of Neurological Surgeons, pp. 47–62.

101. Menezes AH, Smoker WRK, Dyste GN (1990): Syringomyelia, Chiari malformations and hydromyelia. In: Youmans J, ed. *Neurological surgery,* 3rd ed. Philadelphia: W.B. Saunders, pp. 1421–1459.

102. Menezes AH, Traynelis VC, Gantz BJ (1994): Surgical approaches to the craniovertebral junction. In: Loftus CM, Traynelis VC, eds. *Clinical neurosurgery,* Vol 41, Congress of Neurological Surgeons. Baltimore: Williams and Wilkins, pp. 187–203.

103. Menezes AH, VanGilder JC (1988): Transoral-transpharyngeal approach to the anterior craniocervical junction. 10-year experience with 72 patients. *J Neurosurg* 69:895–903.

104. Menezes AH, VanGilder JC, Clark CR, El-Khoury G (1985): Odontoid upward migration in rheumatoid arthritis. An analysis of 45 patients with "cranial settling." *J Neurosurg* 63:500–509.

105. Michie I, Clark M (1968): Neurological syndromes associated with cervical and craniocervical anomalies. *Arch Neurol* 18:241–247.

106. Mikulowski P, Wollheim FA, Rotmil P, et al. (1975): Sudden death in rheumatoid arthritis with atlanto-axial dislocation. *Acta Med Scand* 198:445–451.

107. Miller E, Crockard HA (1987): Transoral transclival removal of anteriorly placed meningiomas at the foramen magnum. *Neurosurgery* 20:966–968.

108. Mills KL, Scotland TR, Wardlaw D, et al. (1988): An implant clamp for atlanto-axial fusion. *J Neurol Neurosurg Psychiatry* 51:450–451.

109. Mitsui H (1984): A new operation for atlanto-axial arthrodesis. *J Bone Joint Surg [Br]* 66:422–425.

110. Moore LJ, Schwartz HC (1985): Median labiomandibular glossotomy for access to the cervical spine. *J Oral Maxillofacial Surg* 43:909–912.

111. Muhonen M, Menezes AH, Sawin P, et al. (1992): Scoliosis in pediatric Chiari malformations without myelodysplasia. *J Neurosurg* 77:69.

112. Newman P, Sweetman R (1969): Occipito-cervical fusion: An operative technique and its indications. *J Bone Joint Surg [Br]* 51:423–431.

113. Osenbach RK, Youngblood LA, Menezes AH (1990): Atlantoaxial instability secondary to solitary eosinophilic granuloma of C2 in a 12-year-old girl. *J Spinal Disord* 3:408–412.

114. Papadopoulos SM, Dickman CA, Sonntag VK (1991): Atlantoaxial stabilization in rheumatoid arthritis. *J Neurosurg* 74:1–7.

115. Pasztor E, Vajda J, Piffko P, Horvath M, Gador I (1984): Transoral surgery for craniocervical space-occupying processes. *J Neurosurg* 60:276–281.

116. Pauli RM, Gilbert EF (1986): Upper cervical cord compression

117. Pech A, Cannoni M, Magnan J, et al. (1974): The transoral approach in otoneurosurgery. *Ann Otolaryngol Chir Cervicofac* 91:281–292.

118. Price JC (1986): The midfacial degloving approach to the central skull base. *Ear Nose Throat J* 65:46–48.

119. Pritz MG (1991): Evaluation and treatment of intradural tumors located anterior to the cervicomedullary junction by a lateral suboccipital approach. *Acta Neurochir* 113:74–81.

120. Ranawat CS, O'Leary P, Pellicci P, Tsairis P, Marchisello P, Dorr L (1979): Cervical spine fusion in rheumatoid arthritis. *J Bone Joint Surg [Am]* 61:1003–1010.

121. Ransford AO, Crockard HA, Pozo JL, Thomas NP, Nelson IW (1986): Craniocervical instability treated by contoured loop fixation. *J Bone Joint Surg [Br]* 68:173–177.

122. Robertson WD (1991): Magnetic resonance imaging of the skull base. *Can Assoc Radiol J* 42:210–215.

123. Robin PE, Powell DJ (1981): Treatment of carcinoma of the nasal cavity and paranasal sinuses. *Clin Otolaryngol* 6:401–414.

124. Roosen K, Trauschel A, Grote W (1982): Posterior atlanto-axial fusion. A new compression clamp for laminar osteosynthesis. *Arch Orthop Trauma Surg* 100:27–31.

125. Roy-Camille R, Mazel C (1992): Stabilization of the cervical spine with posterior plates and screws. In: Camins MB, O'Leary PF, ed. *Disorders of the cervical spine.* Baltimore: Williams and Wilkins, pp. 577–591.

126. Sakou T, Kawaida H, Morizono Y, et al. (1989): Occipito-atlantoaxial fusion utilizing a rectangular rod. *Clin Orthop* 239:136–144.

127. Sandor GK, Charles DA, Lawson VG, et al. (1990): Transoral approach to the nasopharynx and clivus using the LeForte I osteotomy with midpalatal split. *Int J Oral Maxillofac Surg* 19:352–355.

128. Santavirta S, Sandelin J, Slatis P (1985): Posterior atlanto-axial subluxation in rheumatoid arthritis. *Acta Orthop Scand* 56:298–301.

129. Seifert V, Laszig R (1991): Transoral transpalatal removal of a giant premesencephalic clivus chordoma. *Acta Neurochir (Wien)* 112:141–146.

130. Sekhar LN, Schramm VL Jr, Jones NF (1987): Subtemporal preauricular infratemporal fossa approach to large lateral and posterior cranial base neoplasms. *J Neurosurg* 67:488–499.

131. Sen CN, Sekhar LN (1990): An extreme lateral approach to intradural lesions of the cervical spine and foramen magnum. *Neurosurgery* 27:197–206.

132. Sherk HH (1978): Atlantoaxial instability and acquired basilar invagination in rheumatoid arthritis. *Orthop Clin North Am* 9:1053–1063.

133. Smoker WR, Keyes WD, Dunn VD, Menezes AH (1986): MRI versus conventional radiologic examinations in the evaluation of the craniovertebral and cervicomedullary junction. *Radiographics* 6:953–994.

134. Sollazzo D, Bruni P (1985): Brainstem auditory evoked potential (BAEP) abnormalities in subjects with craniovertebral malformations. *Ital J Neurol Sci* 6:185–189.

135. Spillane JD, Pallis C, Jones AM (1957): Developmental abnormalities in the region of the foramen magnum. *Brain* 80:11–48.

136. Stevenson GC, Stoney RJ, Perkins RK, Adams JE (1966): A transcervical transclival approach to the ventral surface of the brain stem for removal of a clivus chordoma. *J Neurosurg* 24:544–551.

137. Taitsman JP, Saha S (1977): Tensile strength of wire-reinforced bone cement and twisted stainless steel wire. *J Bone Joint Surg [Am]* 59:419–425.

138. Taylor AR, Chakravorty BC (1964): Clinical syndromes associated with basilar impression. *Arch Neurol* 10:475–484.

139. Taylor AR, Byrnes DP (1974): Foramen magnum and high cervical cord compression. *Brain* 97:473–480.

140. Uttley D, Moore A, Archer DJ (1989): Surgical management of midline skull base tumors: A new approach. *J Neurosurg* 71:705–710.

141. VanGilder JC, Menezes AH, Dolan K (1987): *Craniovertebral*

as a cause of death in osteogenesis imperfecta type II. *J Pediatr* 108:579.

junction abnormalities. Mount Kisco, New York: Futura Publishing Company, pp. 1–255.

142. Vera CL, Kempe LA, Powers JM (1980): Plasmacytoma of the clivus presenting with an unusual combination of symptoms. *J Neurosurg* 52:857–861.

143. Wadia NH (1967): Myelopathy complicating congenital atlantoaxial dislocation (a study of 28 cases). *Brain* 90:449–474.

144. Wertheim SB, Bohlman HH (1987): Occipitocervical fusion. Indications, technique, and long-term results in thirteen patients. *J Bone Joint Surg [Am]* 69:833–836.

145. Whitesides TE Jr, McDonald AP (1978): Lateral retropharyngeal approach to the upper cervical spine. *Orthop Clin North Am* 9: 1115–1127.

146. Yamada T, Ishida T, Kudo Y, et al. (1986): Clinical correlates of abnormal P14 in median SEP's. *Neurology* 36:765–771.

147. Yamada T, Machida M, Tippin J (1985): Somatosensory evoked potentials. In: Owen JH, Davis H, eds. *Evoked potential testing: clinical testing.* New York: Grune & Stratton, pp. 109–158.

148. Yamaura A, Makino H, Isobe K, Takashima T, Nakamura T, Takemiya S (1979): Repair of cerebrospinal fluid fistula following transoral transclival approach to a basilar aneurysm. Technical note. *J Neurosurg* 50:834–838.

149. Zoma A, Sturrock RD, Fisher WD, Freeman PA, Hamblen DL (1987): Surgical stabilisation of the rheumatoid cervical spine. A review of indications and results. *J Bone Joint Surg [Br]* 69:8–12.

150. Zygmunt S, Saveland H, Brattstrom H, et al. (1988): Reduction of rheumatoid periodontoid pannus following posterior occipitocervical fusion visualized by magnetic resonance imaging. *Br J Neurosurg* 2:315–320.

The Adult Spine: Principles and Practice,
2nd edition, J.W. Frymoyer, Editor-in-Chief.
Lippincott-Raven Publishers, Philadelphia © 1997.

CHAPTER 56

Anterior and Posterior Surgical Approaches to the Cervical Spine

Thomas S. Whitecloud III and Lee A. Kelley

The surgical approaches to the cervical spine have been developed and modified by numerous surgeons. Generally, these make use of natural anatomical planes and are relatively bloodless and relatively safe if the surgeon has a thorough knowledge of surgical anatomy of the region. This chapter describes the approaches to the anterior spine from C3 to C7, the anterior approach to C1 and C2, three different types of anterior retropharyngeal approaches to the upper cervical spine, and the standard posterior approaches to the upper cervical and lower cervical spine.

ANTERIOR APPROACHES

Skin Landmarks and Fascial Planes

The skin on the anterior portion of the neck is highly mobile, thin, and highly vascular. In the lower portion of

  T. S. Whitecloud III, M.D.: Professor and Chairman: Department of Orthopaedic Surgery, Tulane University School of Medicine, New Orleans, Louisiana 70112.
  L. A. Kelley, M.D.: Peachtree Road, NE, Atlanta, Georgia 30309.

the neck, the anterior skin creases run transversely, and then course obliquely in the more cephalad portion near the mandible. Skin incisions should be placed in these skin creases so that the surgical wound heals with minimal cosmetic compromise. Relatively small horizontal incisions on the anterior portions of the neck are possible for one- and two-level anterior fusions because retraction of the mobile skin affords excellent exposure through these relatively small incisions. Various palpable landmarks may be a clue to identifying vertebral levels about the anterior aspect of the neck. The arch of the atlas is generally located at the level of the hard palate. The C1-C2 interspace is generally at the level of the angle of the mandible, while the lower border of the mandible is generally at the level of C2-C3. The hyoid bone correlates to the level of C3, and the upper border of the thyroid cartilage generally correlates to the level of C4-C5. The cricoid cartilage is usually at the level of the C6 vertebral body, and this may be confirmed by palpation of the carotid tubercle (Chassaignac's tubercle), which is the tubercle on the anterior transverse process of the C6 vertebral body. Despite the anatomic landmarks, a lateral roentgenogram of the neck prior to incision can help ensure accurate placement of the skin incision. The skin incision should be placed in relation to the patient's shoulder as visualized on the lateral roentgenogram of the neck (Fig. 1).

Just beneath the skin is the superficial fascia, which contains the platysma muscles anteriorly. The platysma muscles are paired muscles of variable development that extend from the lower border of the mandible to the superficial fascia over the chest. The mediolateral extent of the muscles is generally from midline to the lateral border of the sternocleidomastoid muscle. These are innervated by the cervical branch of the facial nerve (cranial nerve VII). These muscles are pierced by the anterior cutaneous nerves as these course to innervate the skin. The muscle fibers of the platysma may be transected in the transverse plane during the course of an approach or may be split longitudinally in line with their fibers. These are usually closed as a separate layer at the conclusion of an anterior approach to the cervical spine.

Just deep to the superficial fascia lies the first layer of the deep cervical fascia. Within this layer are the four nerve trunks of the cutaneous nerves of the neck, which emanate from the posterior border of the sternocleidomastoid muscle near its midpoint. The most superior of these nerves is the lesser occipital nerve, which is derived from the second cervical nerve root and courses to the posterior aspect of the neck to supply the skin over the lateral occipital region. The great auricular nerve arises from the second and third cervical roots and may be seen to emanate just caudal to the lesser occipital nerve. This nerve crosses superficial to the sternomastoid and is parallel to the external jugular vein, supplying the area over the parotid gland and some of the skin about the ear. The

anterior cervical cutaneous nerve arises from the second and third roots as well. It crosses superficial to the sternocleidomastoid muscle and supplies the region of skin about the hyoid bone. The fourth nerve is the supraclavicular nerve, which arises from the third and fourth cervical roots and divides into three main branches that supply the skin about the clavicle and anterior trapezius muscle. Injury to any of these nerves in the course of an anterior or lateral approach to the neck will result in areas of cutaneous sensory deficit. However, in the standard anterior approach using short transverse incisions in the anterior cervical triangle, only the terminal branches of these sensory nerves are generally encountered. When longitudinal incisions in the anterior triangle are used or transverse incisions posterior to the sternocleidomastoid muscle are used, the larger nerve trunks are vulnerable and may result in larger areas of cutaneous sensory deficit should they be transected (Fig. 2).

Deep to the superficial fascia and platysma muscles, the anterior and posterior triangles, divided by the large sternocleidomastoid muscle, are encountered. The anterior and posterior cervical triangles are then subdivided by the digastric and omohyoid muscles into smaller triangles, which are named for their local anatomic features (digastric, carotid, or subclavian triangles). These are useful in anatomic description of various approaches; however, the most common anterior approach is entirely within the anterior cervical triangle (Fig. 3).

The fascial layers of the neck were described by Grodinsky and Holyoke (7) and have proven to be very useful as guides to dissection throughout the neck (Fig. 4). In performing the anterior approach, detailed knowledge of these fascial planes is essential to avoid injury to the contiguous viscera and neurovascular structures in the neck. The cervical fascia is divided into one superficial and four deep layers. The superficial fascia, as previously mentioned, is that portion of the fascia that contains the platysma muscle in its deeper portion. This layer of fascia is noted to surround the entire neck at the level of the subcutaneous tissue. Deep to the superficial fascia lies the superficial layer of the deep cervical fascia, the first of the four components of the deep cervical fascia. It surrounds the neck and encloses the sternocleidomastoid and trapezius muscles. The next three layers of deep fascia are considered to be the middle layers of the deep fascia. The first of these layers encloses the strap muscles and the omohyoid muscle in the anterior cervical region, then extends laterally to the scapula. The deepest component of the middle layer is the visceral fascia, which surrounds the larynx, trachea, esophagus, and thyroid. The recurrent laryngeal nerve is also enclosed within the visceral fascia. Care should be taken to avoid entering this fascial plane so that the enclosed structures as mentioned above will not be injured. The fourth portion of the deep fascia is the alar fascia, which spreads like wings (hence its name) behind the esophagus and surrounds

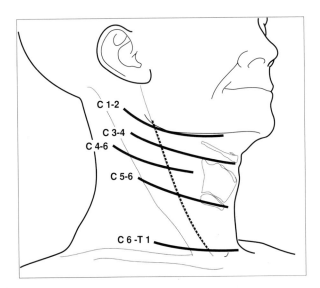

FIG. 1. Placement of skin incision for various levels in the cervical spine. Note that transverse incisions course from midline to the medial border of the sternocleidomastoid muscle. The oblique incision for multiple-level exposure courses along the medial border of the sternocleidomastoid muscle.

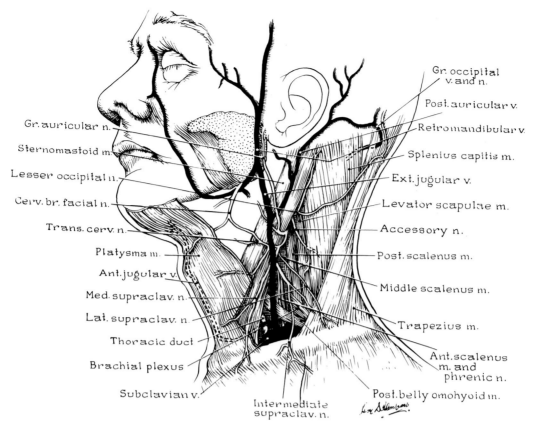

Gr. occipital
v. and n.

Post. auricular v.

Retromandibular v.

Splenius capitis m.

Ext. jugular v.

Levator scapulae m.

Accessory n.

Post. scalenus m.

Middle scalenus m.

Trapezius m.

Ant. scalenus
m. and
phrenic n.

Post. belly omohyoid m.

Gr. auricular n.

Sternomastoid m.

Lesser occipital n.

Cerv. br. facial n.

Trans. cerv. n.

Platysma m.

Ant. jugular v.

Med. supraclav. n.

Lat. supraclav. n.

Thoracic duct

Brachial plexus

Subclavian v.

Intermediate
supraclav. n.

FIG. 2. Cutaneous nerves of the neck in relation to the sternocleidomastoid muscle. Short transverse incisions will usually encounter small terminal branches of these nerves, but large trunks may be encountered with oblique or longitudinal incisions.

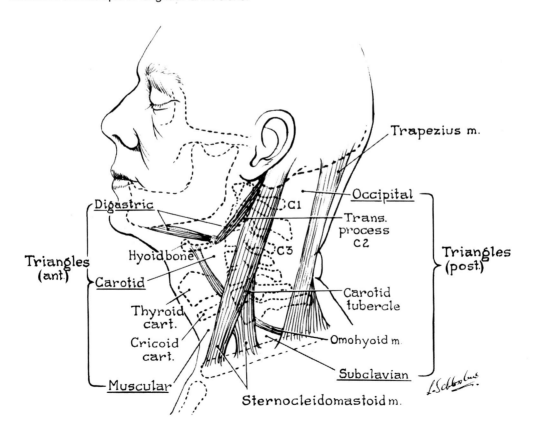

Trapezius m.

Occipital

Trans.
process
C2

Triangles
(post.)

Carotid
tubercle

Omohyoid m.

Subclavian

Digastric

C1

C3

Triangles
(ant.)

Hyoid bone

Carotid

Thyroid
cart.

Cricoid
cart.

Muscular

Sternocleidomastoid m.

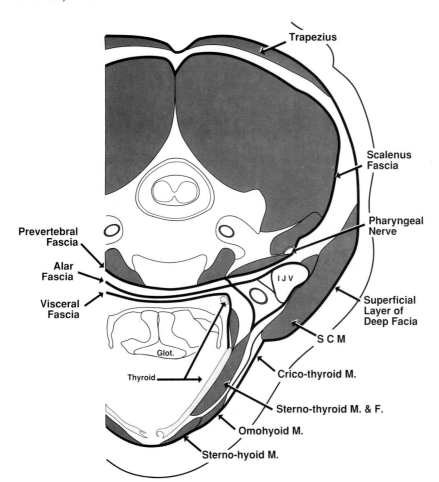

Trapezius

Scalenus
Fascia

Pharyngeal
Nerve

Prevertebral
Fascia

Alar
Fascia

Visceral
Fascia

IJV

Superficial
Layer of
Deep Facia

SCM

Crico-thyroid M.

Glot.

Thyroid

Sterno-thyroid M. & F.

Omohyoid M.

Sterno-hyoid M.

FIG. 4. Cross-section of the fascial compartments of the neck at the level of the thyroid cartilage.

the carotid sheath structures laterally. The deepest layer of fascia in the neck is the prevertebral fascia, which surrounds the vertebral bodies in the paraspinous muscles. Also enclosed in this layer are the phrenic nerve and the scalene muscles. It is noted to be continuous with the lumbodorsal fascia in its caudal-most extent. The prevertebral fascia and alar fascia are both considered portions of the deepest layer of the deep fascia. The alar fascia is noted to blend with the prevertebral fascia at the level of the transverse processes, but generally it does not have connections with the prevertebral fascia in the midportions of the neck. When performing a standard anteromedial approach to the cervical spine, the fascial layers are transected as follows: The superficial fascia is transected in conjunction with the platysma muscle; the superficial layer of the deep fascia is transected sharply at the medial border of the sternocleidomastoid muscle; the middle layer of the deep fascia is transected just anterior to the anterior border of the carotid artery, generally by finger dissection; and the alar fascia and prevertebral fascia are transected sharply directly in the midline to obtain access to the vertebral bodies and discs of the anterior cervical spine (Fig. 5).

Anteromedial Approach to the Vertebral Bodies and Intervertebral Discs from C3 Through C7

This approach has been previously described by Robinson and Southwick (14,16), and Riley (13) and is the standard approach to the anterior cervical spine from C3 through C7. This approach allows the discs between C2 and C3 and between C7 and T1, and all intervening discs, to be exposed in a relatively easy manner.

There has been considerable discussion about whether the approach is more advantageous on the right or left side of the midline. The rationale for approaching on the left side of the midline is that the recurrent laryngeal nerve ascends in the neck on the left side between the trachea and the esophagus, having branched off from its parent nerve, the vagus, at the level of the arch of the aorta. The right recurrent laryngeal nerve travels alongside the trachea in the neck after passing beneath the right subclavian artery. In the lower part of the neck, the right recurrent laryngeal nerve is vulnerable to damage as it crosses from the subclavian artery to the tracheoesophageal groove. Its course in relation to the groove is more variable on the right than on the left and, therefore,

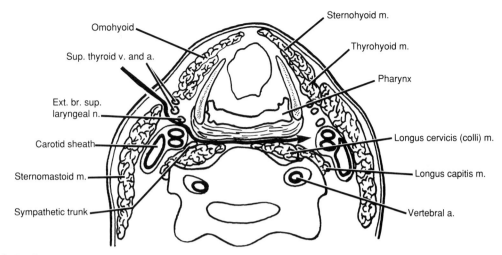

FIG. 5. Order of transection of cervical fascial layers in the anteromedial approach to C3-C7.

the right recurrent laryngeal nerve is slightly more vulnerable to injury than the left. The approach from the left side has the possibility of injuring the thoracic duct, which enters the jugular vein–subclavian vein junction at the base of the neck on the left. However, many surgeons prefer to perform the incision and approach to the right of the midline if they are right-handed, believing that this facilitates both orientation and technical performance in the procedure. Still others feel that the incision should be made on the side of the predominant pathology. However, because generous exposure of the anterior cervical spine can be obtained from either side, the surgical approaches should be done on the side that is most comfortable to the surgeon.

The operation may be performed through a transverse or longitudinal skin incision. In general, the transverse skin incision is sufficient to expose three consecutive vertebral bodies and two consecutive intervertebral discs. If more than two intervertebral discs must be exposed and a prolonged segment of the cervical spine needs to be accessed, such as would be needed in multiple vertebrectomy and strut grafting, then an oblique incision should be made paralleling the anterior border of the sternocleidomastoid muscle. A transverse skin incision should extend to the midline and be centered over the anterior border of the sternocleidomastoid muscle overlying the segment of the spine to be exposed (Fig. 6). Generally, the fifth, sixth, and seventh cervical segments should be approached through a transverse incision placed two to three fingerbreadths superior to the clavicle; and the third, fourth, and fifth cervical segments should be approached through a transverse skin incision placed three to four fingerbreadths superior to the clavicle. As previously mentioned, a lateral roentgenogram made prior to the initiation of the incision will help ensure proper placement of the incision. A longitudinal or oblique in-

cision should be made overlying the medial border of the sternocleidomastoid muscle and may extend from the tip of the mastoid process to the suprasternal notch if this degree of exposure is necessary.

Once the skin incision is made, the platysma muscle is sharply incised at the level of the lateral limb of the transverse incision or at the caudal limb of the longitudinal or oblique incision. It may then be bluntly separated from the underlying structures by passing an instrument deep to the muscle. This is important to prevent inadvertent incision of the underlying structures, which would include the sternocleidomastoid muscle at the lateral-most extent of the transverse incision or at the caudal extent of an oblique incision. On the medial aspect of the incision, the thyroid gland may be vulnerable to injury during the course of transecting the platysma muscle. The anterior border of the sternocleidomastoid muscle is clearly identified once the platysma muscle has been transected. The fascia investing the sternocleidomastoid muscle should be sharply incised at the medial border of the sternocleidomastoid muscle so that it may be retracted laterally. The middle layer of the cervical fascia is now well demonstrated, and the omohyoid muscle will be seen to cross the field in the midportion of the neck, generally just above the level of the sixth cervical vertebral body. This muscle may be mobilized and retracted inferiorly or superiorly, or divided and retracted to provide adequate exposure. The external jugular vein may be encountered deep to the sternocleidomastoid muscle, and both the external jugular vein and the anterior jugular vein may require division and ligation if these interfere with adequate exposure.

It is in the layer of the middle portion of the deep cervical fascia that the vessels and nerves coursing from lateral to medial are generally located. Palpation beneath the sternocleidomastoid muscle for the carotid pulse will

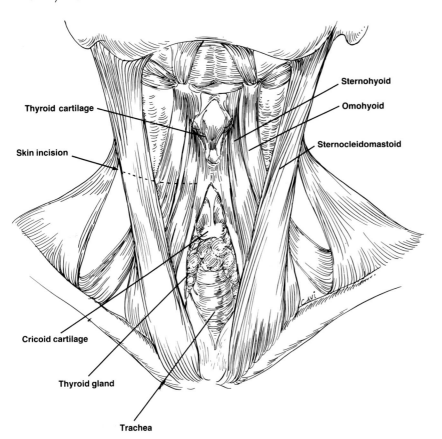

Thyroid cartilage

Skin incision

Cricoid cartilage

Thyroid gland

Trachea

Sternohyoid

Omohyoid

Sternocleidomastoid

FIG. 6. Transverse and longitudinal incision in relation to underlying muscles of the neck. The head should be placed in neutral position prior to making a transverse incision. We prefer to make both types of incisions on the right side.

identify the contents of the carotid sheath. The sterno-cleidomastoid muscle and the carotid sheath should be retracted together laterally, and the middle cervical fascia should be transected by finger dissection during the course of the lateral retraction of these structures. The following structures should be identified in the middle layer of the deep cervical fascia. The digastric muscle, hypoglossal nerve, and glossopharyngeal nerve are found in the superior-most portion of this exposure. These should be retracted superiorly. The superior thyroid artery and vein and the superior laryngeal nerve are the next structures encountered inferiorly. These should be identified and retracted as necessary. The middle thyroid vein courses from lateral to medial below the thyroid vessels and may be transected and ligated if necessary. The inferior thyroid vein and artery are the inferior-most vascular structures during this approach and may be retracted inferiorly or superiorly, according to the level being exposed.

Once the deep layer of the middle cervical fascia is traversed by blunt dissection and the appropriate structures are retracted, palpation of the anterior surface of the cervical spine is usually possible. At this point, the viscera and the midline should be inspected. The esophagus may be seen just posterior to the trachea, and more superiorly, it lies posterior to the larynx. The esophagus is often thin and ribbonlike and should be retracted with care to

avoid perforation. A blunt retractor such as a Cloward retractor is ideal for medial retraction of the esophagus, trachea, and thyroid gland (Fig. 7).

The prevertebral fascia may then be incised longitudinally in the midline of the neck and retracted to either side. This fascia must be incised as close to the midline of the cervical spine as possible to avoid injury to the other structures in the neck (Fig. 8). It has been emphasized that one must not mistake the palpable anterior tubercles of the transverse processes for the vertebral bodies. Otherwise, an incision that was intended to be made through the prevertebral fascia in the midline of the cervical spine may be made instead through the longus colli muscle, which lies immediately lateral to the midline of the cervical spine. This can result in possible damage to the cervical sympathetic chain or to the vertebral artery that lies deep in the longus colli muscle and may also result in excessive bleeding. Once the prevertebral fascia is incised in the midline, the longus colli muscles may be sharply elevated from the intervertebral disc and the vertebral bodies. They are then retracted laterally to allow more complete exposure to the entire segment of the vertebral bodies and intervertebral disc. Before elevating the longus colli muscle, its medial edge should be coagulated. This will prevent unnecessary bleeding. At this point, there should be adequate exposure of the vertebral bodies and disc spaces for performing a variety of proce-

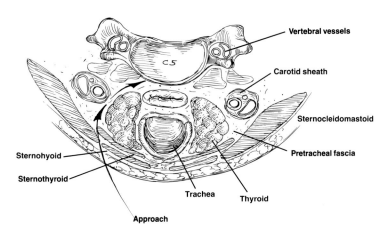

FIG. 7. The midline musculovisceral column may be bluntly retracted medially as a unit. The lateral structures include the sternocleidomastoid muscle and the contents of the carotid sheath.

dures, including discectomy, corpectomy, biopsy, or fusion.

Consequences of Injury to the Neurovascular Structures During the Anterior Approach

The vertebral artery is at risk for injury during the anterior approach. This can occur during excision of a cervical disc when the dissection is carried posterolateral to the joints of Luschka. The vertebral arteries pass through the transverse foramen at each cervical level from C6 cephalad to C1. Once the vertebral artery reaches the first cervical vertebra, it curves posteriorly immediately over the lateral masses between C1 and C2 and then follows a groove in the posterior arch of the atlas to pass into the foramen magnum. The vulnerability of these vessels at this location will be discussed in the next section on the posterior approaches. At each level, the cervical nerve root passes directly behind the vertebral artery. Thus, the roots are also in jeopardy if the vertebral artery is tied blindly when surgical injury occurs. If the artery is injured and bleeding cannot be controlled by tamponade, it must be exposed in the region of the transverse fora-

men and controlled proximally and distally prior to ligation. In young individuals, it is usually safe to ligate one vertebral artery, but this may result in cerebral or cerebellar ischemia in older individuals. This is due to one vertebral artery being compromised by spurring about the foramen and also may be due to traumatic disruption or occlusion of one vertebral vessel. In these circumstances, surgical compromise of the contralateral vessel results in significant ischemia.

Injury to neural structures during the approach can include damage to the cervical sympathetic chain, which is a deep structure located near the longus colli muscles. The sympathetic chain lies deep in a reflection of the carotid sheath along the anterior surface of the lateral masses and prevertebral muscles. It extends from the second cervical vertebra downward and exhibits three ganglionic enlargements: the superior ganglion in front of the second and third cervical vertebrae, the middle ganglion in front of the sixth cervical vertebra, and the inferior ganglion, frequently fused with the first thoracic ganglion just below the seventh cervical vertebra, called the stellate ganglion. Injury to the cervical sympathetic chain can result in a Horner's syndrome.

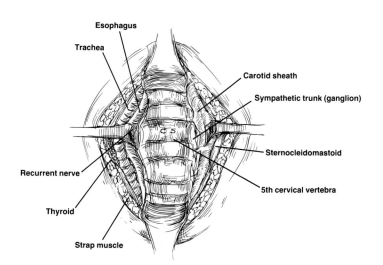

FIG. 8. Once the prevertebral fascia is visualized by appropriate retracting of medial and lateral structures, it should be incised as close to the midline as possible to minimize damage to contiguous structures.

Other nervous structures vulnerable to injury include the pharyngeal and superior laryngeal branches of the vagus nerve, which run deep to the carotid and superior thyroid arteries. These supply the tracheal muscles of the back of the pharynx and sensory innervation to the larynx and the cricothyroid. These are generally retracted with the viscera, and since they run in a longitudinal oblique course, they are not damaged as part of usual exposures.

The recurrent laryngeal nerve arises from the vagus at the level of the subclavian artery on the right, it recurs below the subclavian artery, and then it ascends between the trachea and esophagus, protected by the visceral fascia. The left recurrent laryngeal nerve arises at the level of the aortic arch and passes around the arch to ascend in a similar manner as on the right. Retraction may cause temporary paralysis of the recurrent laryngeal nerve during the anterior approach, but this is less likely to happen with a left-sided approach because the recurrent laryngeal nerve is more frequently located in the tracheoesophageal groove on the left than on the right. The

nerve gives branches to all muscles of the larynx except the cricothyroid. It communicates with the internal laryngeal nerve and supplies sensory filaments to the mucous membrane of the larynx below the level of the vocal cords. It also carries afferent fibers from the stretch receptors in the larynx. Injury to both recurrent laryngeal nerves causes the vocal folds to be motionless in the same position they are normally found in tranquil respiration. When only one recurrent laryngeal nerve is injured, the vocal fold of the same side is motionless. The function in the fold of the opposite side will allow phonation to be possible, but the voice will be altered and weak in timbre. Injury to the superior laryngeal nerve will result in anesthesia of the mucous membrane in the upper part of the larynx so that foreign bodies can readily enter the cavity. Because the nerve supplies the cricoid thyroid, the vocal folds cannot be made tense and the voice is deep and hoarse (21) (Fig. 9).

There is a less commonly known motor nerve injury which is encountered in the course of dissections of the neck. This involves a branch of the facial nerve known

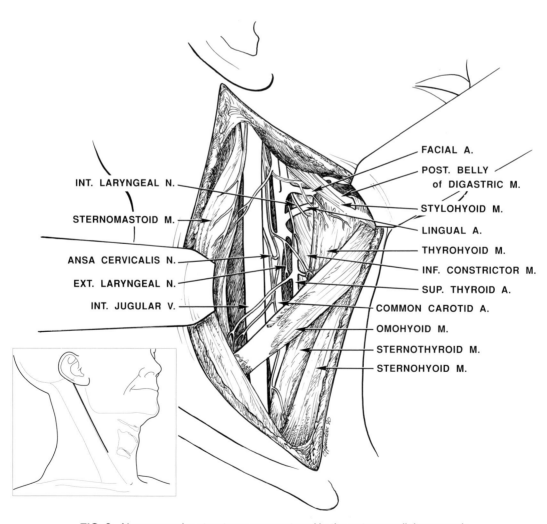

INT. LARYNGEAL N.
STERNOMASTOID M.
ANSA CERVICALIS N.
EXT. LARYNGEAL N.
INT. JUGULAR V.

FACIAL A.
POST. BELLY of DIGASTRIC M.
STYLOHYOID M.
LINGUAL A.
THYROHYOID M.
INF. CONSTRICTOR M.
SUP. THYROID A.
COMMON CAROTID A.
OMOHYOID M.
STERNOTHYROID M.
STERNOHYOID M.

FIG. 9. Neurovascular structures encountered in the anteromedial approach.

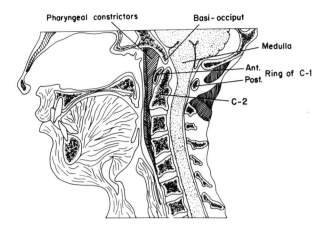

FIG. 10. Relationship of C1 ring and C2 body to the posterior pharynx. Note the relationship of the hard and soft palates to the atlantoaxial junction.

as the marginal mandibular nerve. This nerve is a branch of the facial nerve that originates within the parotid gland along with the cervical branches of the facial nerve. The marginal mandibular branch of the facial nerve exits the parenchyma of the parotid gland along the anterior inferior aspect of the gland and then runs deep to the platysma muscle. It then follows a looping course extending in a general downward arch along the posterior aspect of the inferior border of the mandible, then courses superiorly above the inferior border of the mandible, and then crosses the facial artery to innervate the depressors of the lower lip. These muscles include the depressor anguli oris, the depressor labii inferioris, the risorius (which is a portion of the orbicularis oris), and the mentalis. There is also a portion of the anterior platysma which is innervated by the marginal mandibular nerve. This nerve may be injured during the course of retraction when the upper cervical spine in the C2-C3 and perhaps C3-C4 area is being approached. Paralysis of the marginal mandibular nerve causes an inability to move the lower lip downward and laterally and an inability to evert the vermillion border of the lip. The deformity that is diagnostic of injury to the marginal mandibular nerve involves an inability to bring the lower lip downward and laterally during the course of a full dental smile. This results in a deformity which involves elevation of the palsied lower lip with an apparent drooping of the normal side. These almost always represent neurapraxic injuries and observation is indicated for a period of 6 weeks to 6 months as the majority of these will recover in time.

Anterior Approach to C1 and C2

This approach is attributed to Crowe and Johnson by Robinson and Southwick (14,16). However, Riley (13) attributes this approach to Fang and Ong (6). Histori-

cally, this approach has been used primarily for drainage of retropharyngeal abscesses and biopsy of the anterior arch of the first cervical vertebra and the body of the second cervical vertebra. A midline longitudinal incision is carried through the pharyngeal membrane and fascial planes directly to the mass or to the bone. The mid pharynx is usually avascular, and the small number of vessels that are cut may be ligated with absorbable sutures. Partial closure with interrupted gut sutures is usually used. When used to drain abscesses, this incision should not be closed. The transoral approaches have the obvious limitations of being small exposures with small spaces in which to work. However, with the use of the operating microscope, it is possible to perform such procedures as odontoid resection transorally. There is a reported high rate of infection using these exposures. For more extensive work in the upper cervical spine, alternative exposures should be considered (Figs. 10,11).

Anterior Retropharyngeal Approaches to the Upper Cervical Spine

Three retropharyngeal approaches to the upper cervical spine have been used as alternatives to transpharyngeal approaches. These include approaches described by De Andrade and Macnab (3) as well as the approach described by Riley (13), which requires anterior dislocation of the mandible on the side of the approach along with resection of the submaxillary gland with an extensive dissection of the anatomic structures in this area. Both of these approaches are medial to the carotid sheath. The lateral retropharyngeal approach to the upper cervical spine, as described by Whitesides et al. (19,20), is a modification of Henry's (9) approach to the vertebral artery and is carried anterior to the reflected sternocleidomastoid but posterior to the carotid sheath. The approach can then be extended medially into the retropharyngeal space, exposing all the vertebral bodies of C1 through C7.

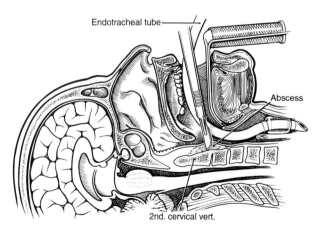

FIG. 11. Transoral pharyngeal approach for drainage of retropharyngeal abscess.

The retropharyngeal approaches may be used for treatment of a variety of problems in the cervical spine in which the upper cervical spine exposure is required. These include os odontoideum, fracture, non-union or mal-union, and postlaminectomy deformity. These may also be undertaken for purposes of stabilization in problems relating to inflammatory and collagen diseases, such as rheumatoid arthritis, ankylosing spondylitis, scleroderma, and lupus erythematosus. Biopsy and treatment of tumor in the upper cervical spine are common reasons for utilizing this approach. Although infection may be treated by this approach, the transoral retropharyngeal approach may be used more commonly to approach the upper cervical spine in this situation.

Lateral Retropharyngeal Approach to the Upper Cervical Spine

Whitesides et al. originally described the use of this approach for an anterior cervical fusion in a patient with neurofibromatosis who required extensive anterior fusion for a recurrent deformity (19,20). It may be performed with the neck in halo traction in slight extension and rotation to the contralateral side to be approached if possible. However, neither rotation nor extension is required to successfully approach the anterior cervical spine by this method. Because of potential respiratory problems from swelling after extensive retropharyngeal dissection, elective tracheostomy may be performed prior to commencing the procedure. If this is not anticipated, then nasotracheal intubation may be carried out in order to allow the mandible to be unobstructed during the course of the procedure. It is helpful to prep the ipsilateral ear inside and out and sew the earlobe anteriorly to the cheek in order to facilitate the exposure of the sternocleidomastoid insertion through the posterior limb of the hockey-stick incision. The hockey-stick incision is the initial horizontal portion of the incision, which begins just posterior to the tip of the mastoid process and is carried across the tip of the mastoid process anteriorly until the anterior border of the sternocleidomastoid muscle is reached, and then the incision is turned inferiorly in an oblique fashion along the anterior border of the sternocleidomastoid muscle (Fig. 12). Once the skin is incised, the greater auricular nerve should be identified and may be retracted cephalad. However, if retraction is not possible and this structure impedes further exposure, it may be divided and ligated, resulting in a minor sensory deficit in the distribution of the terminal portion of the greater auricular nerve. At this point, the platysma muscle is divided along the oblique portion of the incision just anterior to the sternocleidomastoid muscle, and the deep fascia along the medial border of the sternocleidomastoid muscle is divided sharply (Fig. 13). The interval between the sternocleidomastoid muscle and the

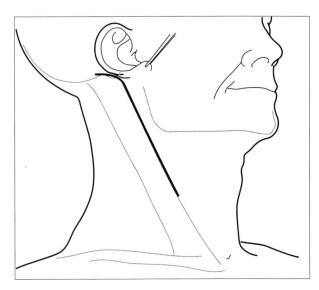

FIG. 12. Incision for lateral retropharyngeal approach (Whitesides technique).

contents of the carotid sheath may then be developed by finger dissection in the cephalad portion of the wound. If only the upper portion of the cervical spine need be approached, the sternocleidomastoid muscle may be retracted posterolaterally and the carotid sheath contents retracted anteromedially and the dissection continued in this interval. However, if the sternocleidomastoid muscle is well developed, or if exposure of both the upper and lower cervical spine is required for the procedure, the sternocleidomastoid muscle will be divided at its insertion along the mastoid process. Prior to dividing the sternocleidomastoid muscle at its insertion, the entrance of the spinal accessory nerve into the sternocleidomastoid muscle should be visualized. The spinal accessory nerve generally enters the sternocleidomastoid muscle 2 to 3 cm caudal to the tip of the mastoid process. Care should be exercised in retraction of the sternocleidomastoid muscle posterolaterally after the division of its insertion so that excessive traction is not placed on the spinal accessory nerve. It may be necessary to dissect the spinal accessory nerve from the jugular vein in the direction toward the jugular foramen in order to effect safe lateral retraction with the sternocleidomastoid muscle. After reflection of the sternocleidomastoid muscle, the interval just posterior to the carotid sheath contents is developed by finger dissection, and the prominent transverse process of C1 is palpated. It should be noted that if the patient's head is turned toward the contralateral side of the body, then the transverse process of C1 will be rotated away from the transverse process of C2.

Henry's original description of this approach involved access to the vertebral artery for ligation (9). A portion of the vertebral artery extending between the transverse foramen of C2 and the transverse foramen of C1 was a cephalad extent of Henry's second stage of the vertebral

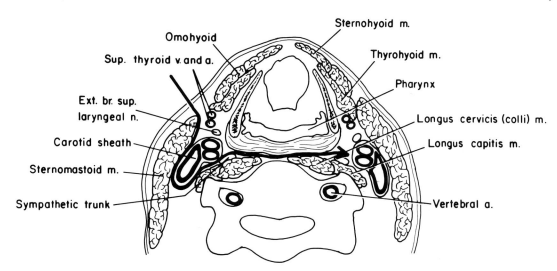

FIG. 13. Plane of dissection in lateral retropharyngeal approach is anterior to the sternocleidomastoid muscle and posterior to the carotid sheath.

artery, and since there is a relatively larger interval between the C2 transverse foramen and the C1 transverse foramen compared to the other contiguous transverse foramina of the cervical spine, this site is accessible for ligation of the vertebral artery (Figs. 14,15).

As the dissection is carried medially from the transverse processes of the upper cervical vertebral bodies, the sagittal fascial band, which binds the midline viscera to the prevertebral fascia (the fibers of Charpey), may be divided in order that the anterior musculovisceral column may be retracted anteromedially; thus the retropharyngeal space is entered with the prevertebral fascia being visible along the anterior cervical vertebral bodies and the longus colli and longus capitus muscles evident in the more anterolateral aspect of these vertebral bodies. Sharp transection of the prevertebral fascia may be performed after coagulation of the edges of the muscle fibers in the area. Subperiosteal dissection may then be performed to expose the anterior cervical vertebral bodies and their intervening disc spaces. The anterior cervical muscles down to the level of the upper thoracic region may be removed during the course of this anterior subperiosteal exposure if such exposure is required.

This approach may be used for simultaneous exposure of the right and left lateral C1-C2 articulations for procedures such as screw fixation, as described by Barbour (1), du Toit (4), and Simmons and du Toit (15). Other uses for this exposure include vertebrectomy and incision of the odontoid, biopsy of lesions in all areas of the anterior cervical spine, fusion of C1 to T1, and exposure of a small amount of the basiocciput for fusion to that area when necessary. Once the procedure is concluded, the sternocleidomastoid muscle may be reapproximated to its origin at the mastoid tip using absorbable suture, and a drain should be allowed to remain deep within the

wound. The platysma is closed using absorbable suture and the skin approximated with a subcutaneous stitch. External immobilization with a halo vest may be required for certain types of fusion in this area.

Complications associated with the approach have included facial nerve palsy, which may be secondary to retraction on the digastric muscle and subsequent injury to the seventh cranial nerve. Also, there is potential to injure the spinal accessory nerve, which would denervate the sternocleidomastoid muscle. Obviously, it is important to positively identify the jugular vein in the course of dissecting posterior to the contents of the carotid sheath so that this structure may not be injured during the course of this dissection. Infection rate has been acceptably low, especially as compared to the transoral approach. In Whitesides' series, a 2.5% incidence of infection was reported (20). In general, this approach offers a safe, effective means of exposing both the upper cervical spine and the combined upper and lower cervical spine.

Anteromedial Retropharyngeal Approach to the Upper Cervical Spine and Basiocciput

This approach was described by De Andrade and Macnab in order to gain access to the basiocciput in order to accomplish occipitocervical fusion (3). As described, it is a cranial extension of the approach popularized by Smith and Robinson and Bailey and Badgley. It involves extending the oblique incision just along the medial border of the sternocleidomastoid muscle as used in the anteromedial approach cephalad to the angle of the mandible. The platysma muscle and deep cervical fascia are divided sharply, and the lower cervical spine is approached by the same dissection used in the anteromedial approach. The branches of the external carotid artery,

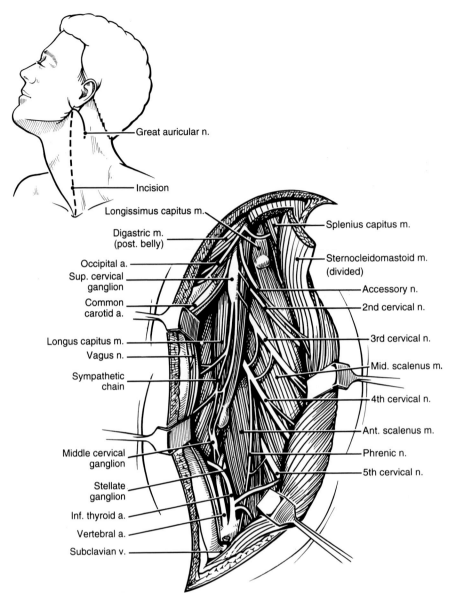

FIG. 14. Nerves and vessels in retropharyngeal approach.

which prevent access to the retropharyngeal space in the upper cervical spine, are divided and ligated to facilitate this portion of the exposure. These include the superior thyroid, lingual, and facial arteries. The other structures that hinder access to the retropharyngeal space in the upper cervical and craniocervical junction are the digastric muscle and hypoglossal nerve, which are retracted during the course of the procedure, and the pharyngeal and laryngeal branches of the vagus nerve, which are also retracted during the course of the procedure. The traction on the pharyngeal and laryngeal branches of the vagus nerve may result in temporary or permanent hoarseness and other problems related to the timbre of the voice (Fig. 16).

Anteromedial Retropharyngeal Approach to the Upper Cervical Spine (Riley's Technique)

This technique (13) is essentially an alternative means of extending the standard anteromedial approach cephalad to the C1-C2 vertebral bodies. The two major differences involve the use of a modified Shoebringer incision and the excision of the submaxillary gland and anterior dislocation of the temporomandibular joint to improve access to the upper cervical spine. The incision is begun in the submandibular area, just inferior to the edge of the mandible, and carried posteriorly in a horizontal fashion to the angle of the mandible. The incision is then carried inferiorly in an oblique fashion, just at the

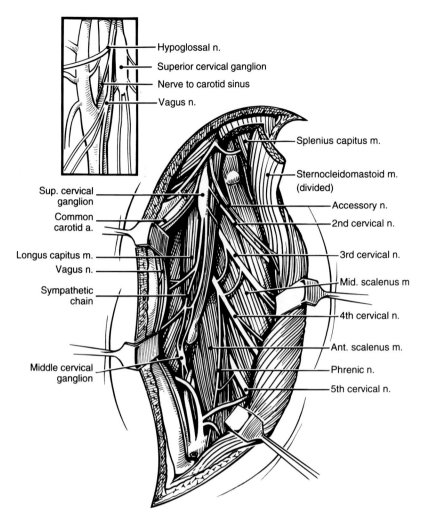

Hypoglossal n.
Superior cervical ganglion
Nerve to carotid sinus
Vagus n.

Sup. cervical ganglion
Common carotid a.
Longus capitus m.
Vagus n.
Sympathetic chain
Middle cervical ganglion

Splenius capitus m.
Sternocleidomastoid m. (divided)
Accessory n.
2nd cervical n.
3rd cervical n.
Mid. scalenus m
4th cervical n.
Ant. scalenus m.
Phrenic n.
5th cervical n.

FIG. 15. Cervical sympathetic chain demonstrated.

posterior edge of the sternocleidomastoid muscle. At the lower third of the sternocleidomastoid muscle, the incision is then gently curved anteriorly and inferiorly to cross the clavicle and terminate near the suprasternal space (Figs. 17,18). The deeper part of the incision involves transecting the subcutaneous tissue and platysma muscle in the same line as the incision and then retracting skin, subcutaneous tissue, and platysma as a single flap medially exposing the underlying sternocleidomastoid muscle at the lateral border of the dissection and the musculovisceral column medially. Superiorly the mandible and submaxillary fascia will be visible. At this point the mandibular branch of the facial nerve should be identified just inferior to the angle of the mandible and should be protected throughout the course of the dissection. The sternocleidomastoid muscle is then freed along its medial and lateral borders and retracted laterally. The omohyoid muscle is divided in its portion, which lies just deep to the sternocleidomastoid muscle, and then retracted superiorly and inferiorly. The blunt dissection through the middle layer of the cervical fascia is then carried medially to the carotid sheath toward the preverte-

bral fascia. The medial musculovisceral column may then be retracted medially and the contents of the carotid sheath retracted laterally with the sternocleidomastoid muscle. This will provide access to the vertebral bodies from the C2-C3 disc space to the C7-T1 disc space.

The superior development of the dissection to access C1 and C2 involves identifying the superior thyroid artery, which crosses the field horizontally from lateral to medial as it exits the external carotid artery *en route* to the thyroid gland. The superior thyroid artery may be divided and ligated in order to proceed superiorly to the superior laryngeal neurovascular bundle and the hypoglossal nerve. Both of these structures should be identified and protected during the course of the superior dissection. The stylohyoid muscle and digastric muscle are then identified, divided, and retracted. As the larynx and pharynx are retracted medially and the external carotid artery laterally, the floor of the submaxillary triangle will then be visualized. This may be retracted superiorly in order to visualize the base of the skull and anterior arch of C1. At this point, the exposure may be improved by excising the submaxillary gland and by manual anterior

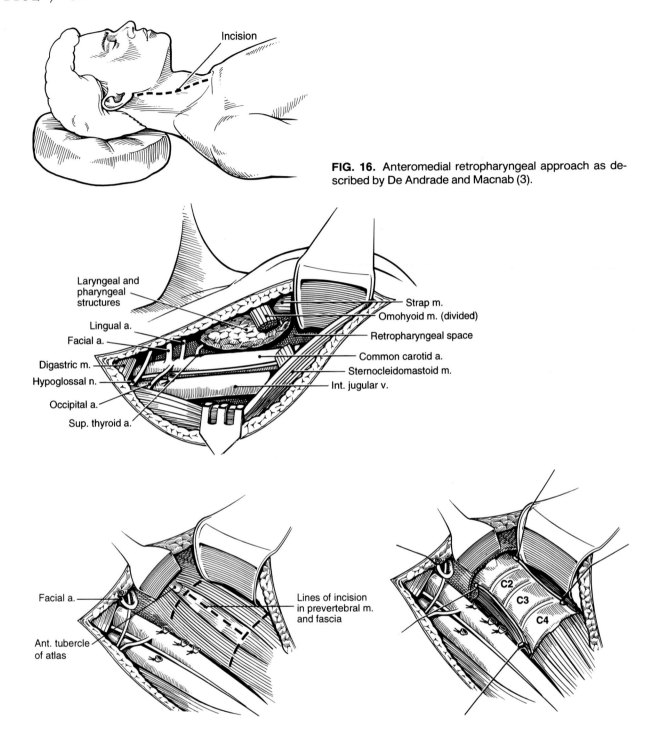

FIG. 16. Anteromedial retropharyngeal approach as described by De Andrade and Macnab (3).

dislocation of the temporomandibular joint (Fig. 19). The mandible may then be rotated out of the field of dissection, which improves the superior retraction of the floor of the submaxillary triangle to expose the base of the skull and the entire anterior aspect of C1. This allows adequate access to C1-C2, and the vertebral arteries are visualized in the course of this approach and may be controlled as necessary. Subperiosteal dissection of the longus colli muscle in a lateral direction will expose the transverse processes and the vertebral artery. Closure

may be accomplished by relocating the dislocated temporomandibular joint and repairing the digastric and stylohyoid tendons. A suction drain should be placed deep within the wound and the platysma muscle reapproximated throughout the course of the incision. A subcuticular absorbable suture is used for closure of the skin (Fig. 20).

The disadvantages of this approach involve not only the need to excise the submaxillary gland and the potential problems with dislocation of the temporomandibu-

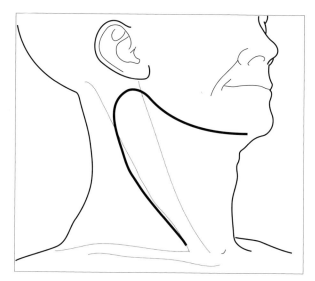

FIG. 17. Neck incision in Riley's anteromedial retropharyngeal approach.

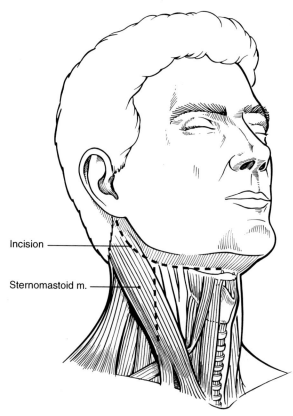

FIG. 18. Modified Shoebringer incision, which may be used in Riley's retropharyngeal approach to the upper cervical spine.

lar joint, but also the same risk as in the approach described by De Andrade and Macnab (3). The hypoglossal nerve and superior laryngeal nerve remain vulnerable to injury during this procedure, because they must be retracted as work is performed through this interval.

Supraclavicular Approach to the Lower Cervical Spine

This approach was also described by Riley as a means of accessing the lower cervical spine through an anterolateral approach (13). It provides excellent access to the transverse processes, pedicles, and vertebral artery.

A transverse incision is placed one fingerbreadth above the clavicle extending from the midline of the neck to just beyond the posterior border of the sternocleidomastoid muscle (Fig. 21). Transection of the platysma muscle is then performed in line with the skin incision,

and the medial and lateral borders of the sternocleidomastoid muscle are defined by blunt and sharp dissection. The sternocleidomastoid muscle should then be separated from its underlying structures by blunt dissection, and the anterior jugular vein and external jugular vein identified and ligated if necessary. The sternocleidomastoid muscle is then divided by incising it from its lateral border to its medial border, taking special care to

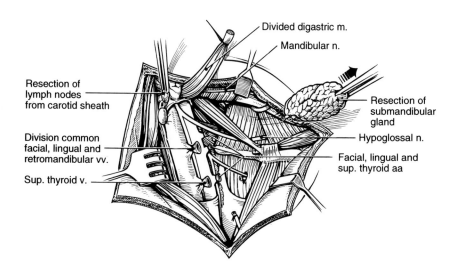

FIG. 19. Excision of submaxillary gland to improve exposure.

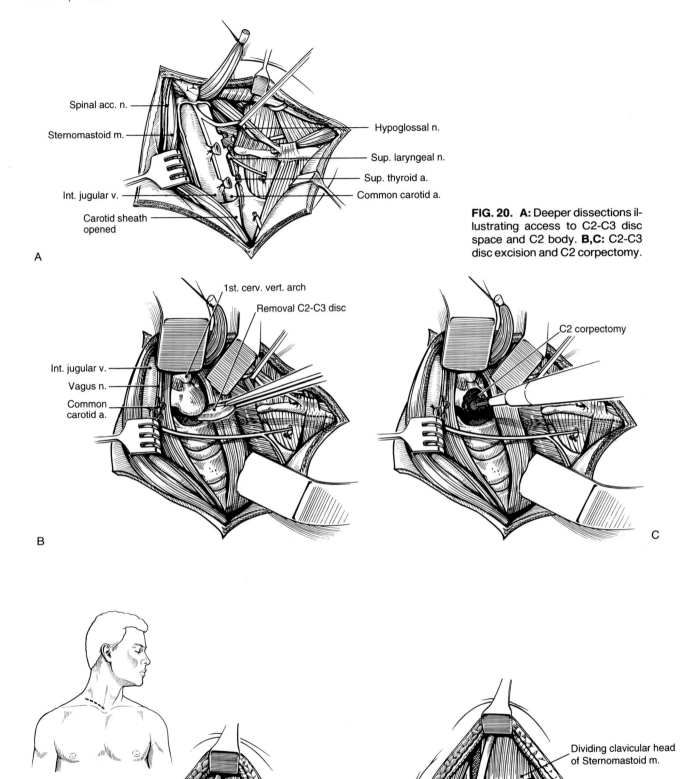

FIG. 20. A: Deeper dissections illustrating access to C2-C3 disc space and C2 body. **B,C:** C2-C3 disc excision and C2 corpectomy.

A

Spinal acc. n.

Sternomastoid m.

Int. jugular v.

Carotid sheath opened

Hypoglossal n.

Sup. laryngeal n.

Sup. thyroid a.

Common carotid a.

B

1st. cerv. vert. arch

Removal C2-C3 disc

Int. jugular v.

Vagus n.

Common carotid a.

C

C2 corpectomy

FIG. 21. Incision for supraclavicular approach.

External jugular v.

Med. supraclavicular n.

Clavicular head of Sternomastoid m. lobe divided

Platysma m.

Sternal head of Sternomastoid m.

Dividing clavicular head of Sternomastoid m.

avoid the internal jugular vein. The muscle is then re-tracted superiorly and inferiorly to access the area of the middle cervical fascia. The omohyoid and sternohyoid muscles should then be visualized. The middle cervical fascia is bluntly dissected lateral to the carotid sheath in order to access the surface of the anterior scalene muscle (Fig. 22). The omohyoid muscle may be divided and re-tracted in a fashion similar to the sternocleidomastoid muscle to improve access to this area. The phrenic nerve should be identified lying on the surface of the anterior scalene muscle. It crosses from lateral to medial in its superior to inferior course. The phrenic nerve may be retracted medially after it is gently freed from the surface of the anterior scalene muscle. The cords of the brachial plexus will be noted to emerge from beneath the lateral border of the anterior scalene muscle, and these should be visualized and protected throughout the course of the dissection. The anterior scalene muscle is then sharply divided approximately 1 inch inferior to the side of the desired exposure. The entire superior portion of the mus-cle may be excised; however, it should be noted that the slips of origin of the anterior scalene muscle emanate from the anterior tubercles of the cervical transverse pro-cesses, so the vertebral arteries are vulnerable to injury as they pass between the bony foramen and the transverse processes of the cervical vertebrae as these slips are being resected (Fig. 23). The standard approach involves lat-eral retraction of the carotid sheath; however, if possible, the internal jugular vein and carotid sheath may be re-tracted medially. Also, the anterior scalene muscle may be retracted laterally rather than resected if possible. The close relationship of the anterior scalene muscle to the parietal pleura should be noted. The deep surface of the anterior scalene muscle is covered by a continuation of the prevertebral fascia known as Sibson's fascia, and the deep surface of Sibson's fascia is formed by the apex of the parietal pleura and lung. Care should be taken not to violate this fascial plane, as this would involve entering the thoracic cavity. Sibson's fascia may then be followed medially toward the transverse processes of the cervical

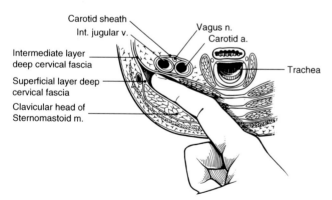

FIG. 22. Transection of clavicular head of sternocleidomas-toid muscle and plane of dissection.

vertebrae, where it may be incised and bluntly retracted inferiorly (Fig. 24). The recurrent laryngeal nerve should be retracted medially with the carotid sheath and the me-dial musculovisceral column. The prevertebral fascia may then be sharply transected in the midline, and subp-eriosteal dissection of the fascial attachment and longus colli muscle may then be performed. The dissection may then be carried superiorly to expose vertebral bodies up to the C2-C3 disc space. If the transverse processes, ped-icles, or neural foramina are to be exposed, then the lon-gus colli muscle may be reflected medially (Fig. 25).

As previously mentioned, a left-sided approach places the thoracic duct vulnerable to injury. During the course of this approach, if it is performed from the left side, the thoracic duct should be carefully sought at its junction with the internal jugular–subclavian vein complex. If in-jury to this structure is noted during the course of the dissection, it may be tied proximally and distally to pre-vent formation of a chylothorax. The other poten-tial complications involve pneumothorax as previously mentioned and injury to the cervical sympathetic chain as it ascends along the longus colli muscle.

Modified Anterior Approach to the Cervicothoracic Junction

This approach has been described by Kurz et al. (10) to obtain exposure of the cervicothoracic juncture. It will provide exposure from C3 to T4 for a resection of tumor and correction of kyphosis in this area. It can also be used for upper thoracic disc herniations to be approached an-teriorly in a patient with a short neck. This is actually a modification of a combined cervicothoracic approach described by Micheli and Hood (12). In the approach de-scribed by Kurz (10), the medial clavicle is excised and used as a strut graft, which gives a further advantage of harvesting a strut graft from the same operative site as the approach. Advantages of this approach include direct visualization of the anterior structures extending from C3 to T4, hemostatic access to the great vessels, a cervi-cothoracic approach that does not involve a transtho-racic approach, and, as already mentioned, the strut graft obtained from the operative site.

This approach is performed with the patient in supine position and a rolled towel between the scapulae. The neck is slightly extended and rotated toward the right. The neck and anterior thoracic area are prepped and draped sterilely. An angled incision is made in the skin overlying the anterior aspect of the left side of the neck. The vertical limb extends distally just past the manubri-osternal junction. The transverse limb is approximately 1 inch proximal and parallel to the left clavicle and ex-tends laterally to the lateral border of the left sternoclei-domastoid muscle. The incision extends through the skin and subcutaneous tissue and then the platysma

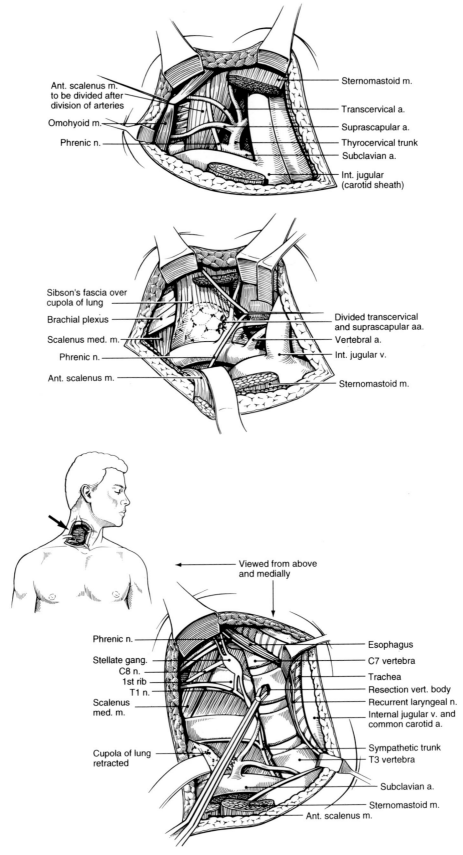

FIG. 23. Deeper dissection in supraclavicular approach.

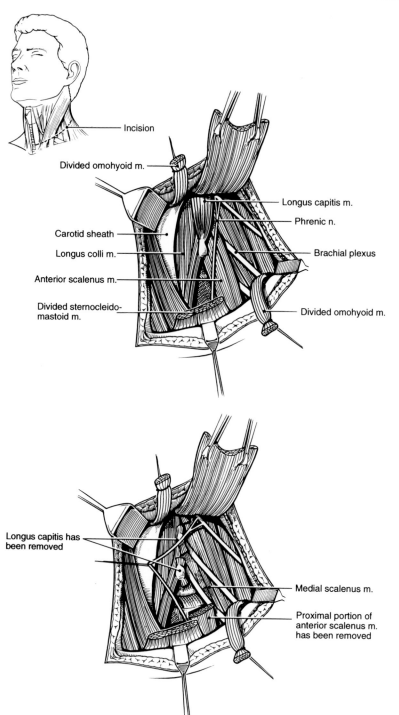

Incision

Divided omohyoid m.

Longus capitis m.

Phrenic n.

Carotid sheath

Longus colli m.

Brachial plexus

Anterior scalenus m.

Divided sternocleido-
mastoid m.

Divided omohyoid m.

FIG. 24. Exposure of transverse process by retraction of divided sternocleidomastoid muscle and resection of the cephalad portion of anterior scalene muscle.

Longus capitis has
been removed

Medial scalenus m.

Proximal portion of
anterior scalenus m.
has been removed

muscle is incised over the same length as the skin incision. Superficial anterior veins are ligated. The larger veins such as internal and external jugular veins are preserved and retracted. The medial supraclavicular nerve is retracted as well. The manubrial and cervical heads of the sternocleidomastoid muscle are elevated off of their distal attachments and retracted laterally and proximally. The strap muscles are severed just below the level of the clavicle and elevated in the proximal and medial

directions. The left half of the manubrium and the medial third of the clavicle are subperiosteally stripped. The clavicle is then cut at the junction of its medial and middle thirds with a Gigli saw. Great care must be utilized to avoid injuring the subclavian vein, which is just posterior and inferior to the clavicle. Once the medial third of the clavicle is sharply dissected from the manubrium, it is preserved for use as a strut graft. The inferior thyroid vein may be ligated if this prevents further retraction. In

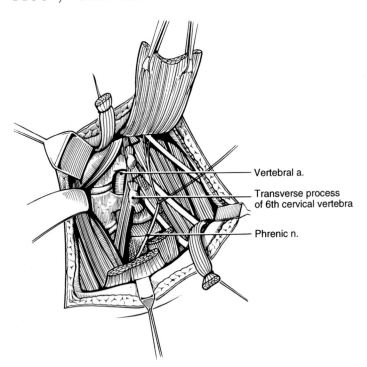

Vertebral a.

Transverse process
of 6th cervical vertebra

Phrenic n.

FIG. 25. Reflection of longus colli muscle improves access to vertebral bodies, neural foramina, and vertebral artery.

the proximal portion of the wound, a plane is dissected between the carotid sheath and the lateral edge of the trachea and esophagus. The recurrent laryngeal nerve is identified between the esophagus and trachea and should be retracted with the medial musculovisceral structures. Richardson retractors are placed medially and laterally and the prevertebral fascia is identified. At this point, incision and subperiosteal dissection of the prevertebral fascia will allow visualization of the T1, T2, and T3 vertebral bodies. Corpectomy may be performed, if necessary, and the medial clavicle head is fashioned into an appropriate-size strut graft and placed between intact vertebral bodies. Once the procedure is concluded, a deep drain is generally placed. Strap muscles are reapproximated and the sternocleidomastoid muscle is sutured to the clavicular periosteum. Closure of the subcutaneous tissues and skin is performed in the standard fashion. If a brace is to be used, it is placed prior to removal from the operating table.

In the original description of this approach, four patients with cervicothoracic tumors underwent this type of reconstruction with successful outcomes.

Direct Anterior Approach to the Upper Cervical Spine

This approach was described by Fang and Ong in order to gain access to the first four cervical vertebrae and their intervertebral discs, including the atlantoaxial and atlanto-occipital joints (6). The transthyrohyoid approach involves making a transverse incision along the uppermost crease of the neck at a level between the hyoid

bone and thyroid cartilage and extending it laterally to the level of the carotid sheath. The platysma muscle is then transected in line with the transverse incision. The sternohyoid muscles are in the next layer, and these are isolated near their attachment to the hyoid bone and sharply divided, which exposes the underlying thyrohyoid muscles. This next layer of muscle may also be delineated and divided near its attachment to the hyoid bone. The thyrohyoid membrane then comes into view. This structure is detached from the lower edge of the hyoid bone from the greater cornu on either side, with care to avoid cutting the epiglottis, which lies immediately deep to this structure. The most important structures exposed during the course of this dissection are the internal laryngeal nerves and the superior laryngeal arteries at their entrance on either side of the thyrohyoid membrane. The mucous membrane lining the valleculae is then exposed and the pharynx is entered by cutting through it. Retraction of the hyoid bone and epiglottis with a self-retaining retractor exposes the posterior pharyngeal wall, which lies immediately superficial to the second, third, and fourth cervical vertebral bodies. A midline incision may then be made straight down to bone in order to expose these vertebral levels. The soft tissues are then dissected by subperiosteal dissection laterally on either side of the midline, and long sutures may be used to maintain the retraction of these flaps. If care is taken to perform electrocautery along the edges of these subperiosteal flaps prior to raising them, there will be little bleeding during the course of the dissection. Once the procedure is completed, the posterior pharyngeal walls may be closed in three layers using O-chromic catgut. The thyrohyoid

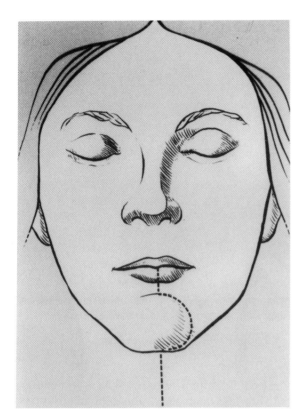

FIG. 26. Incision for mandibular–tongue–pharynx splitting approach to upper cervical spine.

all of the approaches that violate the pharynx have a high incidence of postoperative infection.

If wider exposure is necessary, this may be achieved through the anterolateral open-mouth approach. The mandibular–tongue–pharynx splitting approach offers direct anterior wide exposure of the cervical vertebral bodies from the clivus to C6. This was described by Stauffer and has been used successfully by him for a variety of procedures in this area (2). A vertical incision is made from the center of the lower lip and carried inferiorly to the prominence of the chin, where the incision turns posteroinferiorly to the posterior aspect of the chin (Fig. 26). The mucous membrane is then divided longitudinally and the mandible is pre-drilled to facilitate closure. The mandible is then cut in a step-cut fashion to facilitate accurate approximation of the bone during the closure (Fig. 27). The tongue is divided longitudinally through its central raphe, and the two portions of the mandible and the tongue are each retracted laterally away from midline, exposing the posterior structures of the epiglottis and palate. Palpation through the posterior pharyngeal wall will allow location of the bony prominences of the C1-C2 vertebral bodies (Fig. 28). A longitudinal incision then transects the posterior pharyngeal wall and mucosa in the midline; this incision may be carried down through the periosteum to the bone of the upper cervical segments. Subperiosteal dissection may then be performed after electrocoagulating the edges of the flaps and raising a subperiosteal flap to the lateral aspect on either side (Fig. 29). Extending this exposure cephalad allows exposure to the level of the clivus. The inferior extent of the exposure may go down to C6. Closure is then performed by reapproximating the tongue with absorbable sutures and repairing the mandible through the

membrane may be reattached and the thyrohyoid and sternohyoid muscles repaired to their tendinous attachments at the hyoid bone. A drain is placed at this level, and the platysma muscle and skin are sutured as separate layers to complete the closure. As previously mentioned,

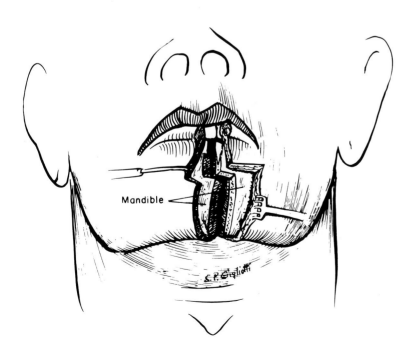

FIG. 27. Step-cut the mandible to facilitate closure.

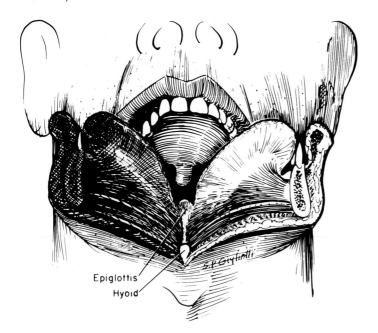

FIG. 28. The tongue is split down its central raphe exposing the epiglottis and palate.

Epiglottis

Hyoid

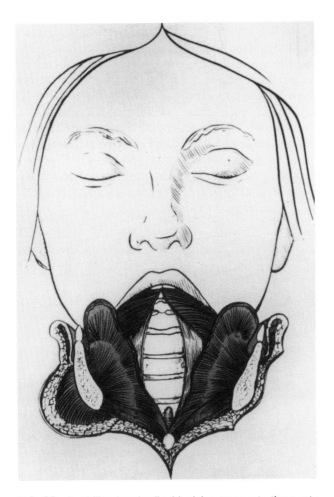

FIG. 29. A midline longitudinal incision transects the posterior pharyngeal wall and mucosa exposing the upper cervical segments.

pre-drilled holes with wire suture. The skin should be repaired with fine interrupted nonabsorbable sutures for optimal cosmesis.

Postoperatively, a halo jacket will usually be required for immobilization, as this will supplant any orthosis that would place pressure on the underside of the mandible. The halo jacket will also facilitate the patient's respiration through tracheostomy, which will have been performed prior to the commencement of the procedure. Stauffer (2) has reported a minimal postoperative morbidity, which he feels is acceptable when compared with the safety of the improved exposure of the upper cervical spine and neural canal.

POSTERIOR APPROACHES

Posterior Approach to C1-C2

The posterior approach to C1-C2 is used for fusions involving both the C1-C2 articulations and the occipitocervical articulations. The exposure may be extended cephalad to include the occiput and caudad to include the lower cervical spine.

The patient is prone on the operating table, and the head may be supported with either a headrest or self-retaining head fixation device that is attached to the table. The standard incision for a C1-C2 posterior fusion involves a midline incision from the caudal aspect of the occiput to the C3 spinous process. This is carried through the skin with a scalpel blade, and deeper dissection may be carried out with either a scalpel blade or electrocautery. The midline avascular structure, the median raphe

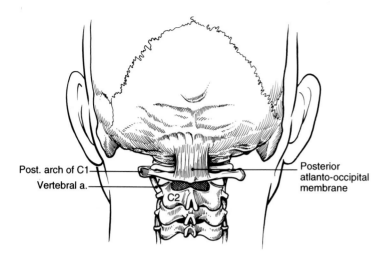

FIG. 30. The relationship between the C1 ring, C2 posterior elements, atlanto-occipital membrane, and the vertebral artery.

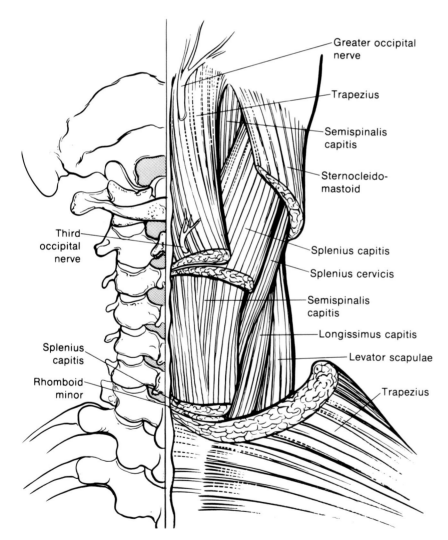

FIG. 31. Posterior cervical muscles: superficial layer.

or the ligamentum nuchae, follows a tortuous course; this generally prevents dissection in a straight line from posterior to anterior if this plane is to be followed. Care should be taken to remain within this raphe, as straying into the paraspinous muscle masses will cause unnecessary bleeding. The dissection may be carried down to the occiput in the cephalad extent into the spinous processes in the caudal portion of the exposure. In children, exposure of unnecessary levels should be avoided in order to avoid spontaneous fusion at levels adjacent to those necessary for the procedure. The ligamentous attachments to C2 are most prominent in this area, and dissection may begin at the C2 spinous process using either electrocautery or a subperiosteal elevator. The dissection then proceeds from the C2 spinous process out to the lamina of C2 in a lateral direction. The dissection will often be carried caudal to the C2 level in order to provide adequate exposure. The exposure of the C2 and C3 laminae should extend to the medial one third of the facet joint at the base of the laminae, but it should not extend beyond the facet joints during the course of the lateral exposure. The occiput may be subperiosteally exposed in a similar fashion. The intervening area will contain the ring of C1, which may be very deep with respect to C2. The posterior tubercle of C1 is usually palpable in

the midline, and subperiosteal dissection using a small subperiosteal elevator may proceed from the posterior tubercle of C1 laterally.

Care must be taken during the course of this dissection to avoid excessive pressure on the C1 ring, as it may be thin and easily fractured. Slipping off of the C1 ring in a cephalad direction during the course of subperiosteal dissection may cause penetration of the atlanto-occipital membrane and injury to the underlying structures. In the case of atlantoaxial instability, direct pressure of the C1 ring against the dura may leave the dura vulnerable to injury during the course of dissection. The dura may be penetrated on both the superior and inferior edges of the ring of C1, so care must be taken during the course of this portion of the dissection, and the pathology involved must be taken into account during the course of this dissection as well.

The lateral extent of exposure at C1 is approximately 1.5 cm. The lateral landmark at the ring of C1 is the second cervical ganglion, which lies approximately 1.5 cm on the lamina of C1 in the area of the groove for the vertebral artery. The medial aspect of the groove for the vertebral artery must be carefully identified, as this is found on the superior border of the C1 ring. The vertebral vein is usually visualized first and noted by its bluish

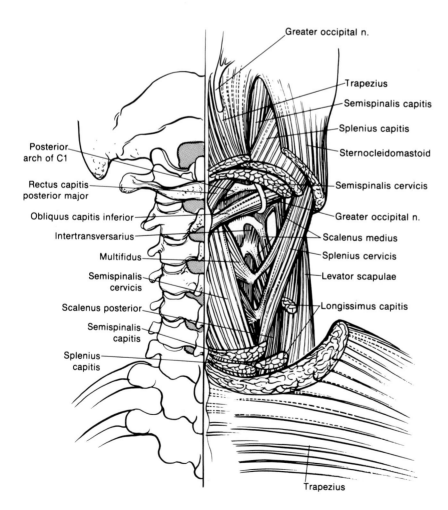

FIG. 32. Posterior cervical muscles: deeper layer.

color. Care must be taken in this area to avoid damage to the vertebral artery as it courses from the slightly posteriorly placed foramen transversarium of C1 in a posterior medial direction to enter the foramen magnum just above the ring of C1. The vertebral artery and vein, then, are vulnerable not only in the groove at C1, but also as the artery passes from the foramen transversarium of C2 to the foramen transversarium of C1, where it is in close lateral and posterior proximity to the joint (Fig. 30). The vertebral vein will be encountered first as the dissection is carried from medial to lateral along the lamina. Penetration of the atlanto-occipital membrane just off the superior border of the ring of C1, more medial than the usually safe 1.5-cm margin from the midline, may also result in damage to the vertebral artery. It is therefore imperative that these relationships be known in exposure of the C1, C2, and occipital portions of the upper cervical spine. Self-retaining retractors are useful in maintaining retraction of the cervical paraspinous muscles during procedures in the upper and lower cervical spine. If a more lateral approach to the C1-C2 facet joint is desired, the vertebral artery between the C1 and C2 articulation must be identified. It should be noted that in rotatory dislocations of the C1-C2 articulation, the artery is stretched tightly across the joint on the side that C1 is anterior to C2 and is easily damaged.

It should be noted that the position of the head is important during all posterior cervical spine procedures, and the head is generally held in as close to neutral alignment as possible. Flexion will often aid in the exposure by bringing the occiput away from the C1-C2 articulations in a cephalad direction. However, the pathology being treated must be considered, in that flexion of the occiput may not be possible in order to retain reduction of the C1-C2 articulation. The ultimate position of the cervical spine must be evaluated with a lateral x-ray prior to commencing any surgical incision. This should be assessed for both position of the neck with respect to the procedure to be performed and radiographic accessibility to the areas undergoing surgery, so that evaluation of the procedure may be performed radiographically during the course of the procedure.

Posterior Exposure of the Lower Cervical Spine

In exposure of the lower cervical spine, the prominent C7 spinous process should be palpated to determine the level and length of the midline posterior cervical incision. Once again, it is important to remain within the ligamentum nuchae during the course of the procedure to keep bleeding from the paraspinous muscles to a minimum. Once the skin and subcutaneous tissues are tran-

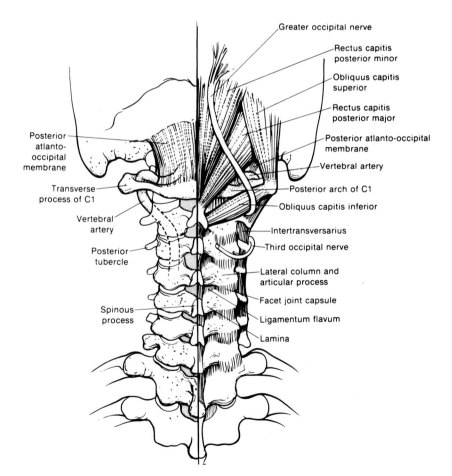

FIG. 33. Muscle attachments of upper cervical spine.

sected with a scalpel blade, the trapezius fascia is incised and retraction of the muscle mass on the side of the lesion is then performed. Subperiosteal dissection of the cervical paraspinous muscles can then be performed. These muscles include the splenius, the semispinalis capita, the lower semispinalis cervicis, and the multifidus. Dissection of these muscles may be performed using Bovie electrocautery, which is the method preferred by some. If not indicated, the extensor muscular insertions at C2 should not be removed, to preserve both function and stability. Exposure of the laminae in the lower cervical spine is therefore performed with relative impunity and may be carried laterally to expose the medial two thirds of the zygapophyseal joints. Dissection beyond the zygapophyseal joints may result in denervation of the paraspinous muscles; this may also make the vertebral artery vulnerable to injury, should the dissection be carried beyond the joint and slightly anterior to the crossing of the vertebral artery between the foramen transversarium of two adjacent bodies (Fig. 31).

Just as in exposure of the upper cervical spine, a lateral roentgenogram taken prior to commencing the surgical prep is of paramount importance (Figs. 32,33).

REFERENCES

1. Barbour JR (1971): Screw fixation in fractures of the odontoid process. *S Aust Clin* 5:20–24.
2. The Cervical Spine Research Society, Editorial Committee (1989): *The cervical spine*, 2nd ed. Philadelphia: JB Lippincott, pp. 805–807.
3. De Andrade JR, Macnab I (1969): Anterior occipito-cervical fusion using an extra-pharyngeal exposure. *J Bone Joint Surg [Am]* 51:1621–1626.
4. Du Toit G (1976): Lateral atlantoaxial arthrodesis. A screw fixation technique. *S Afr J Surg* 14:9–12.
5. Ellenbogen, R (1979): Pseudoparalysis of the mandibular branch of the facial nerve after platysmal face-lift operation. *Plast Reconstr Surg* 63:364–369.
6. Fang HSY, Ong GB (1962): Direct anterior approach to the upper cervical spine. *J Bone Joint Surg [Am]* 49:1588–1604.
7. Grodinsky M, Holyoke EA (1938): Fascial and fascial spaces of the head, neck and adjacent regions. *Am J Anat* 63:367.
8. Hall JE, Denis F, Murray J (1977): Exposure of the upper cervical spine for spinal decompression by a mandible and tongue-splitting approach. *J Bone Joint Surg [Am]* 59:121–123.
9. Henry AK (1973): *Extensile exposure.* New York: Churchill Livingston.
10. Kurz LT, Pursel SE, Herkowitz HN, et al. (1991): Modified anterior approach to the cervicothoracic junction. *Spine* 16(10 Suppl): S542–S547.
11. Liebman EP, Webster RC, Gaul JR, Griffin T (1988): The marginal mandibular nerve in rhytidectomy and liposuction surgery. *Arch Otolaryngol Head Neck Surg* 114:179–181.
12. Micheli LJ, Hood RW (1983): Anterior exposure of the cervicothoracic spine using a combined cervical and thoracic approach. *J Bone Joint Surg* 65A:992–997.
13. Riley LH Jr (1973): Surgical approaches to the anterior structures of the cervical spine. *Clin Orthop* 91:16–20.
14. Robinson RA, Southwick WO (1978): Surgical approaches to the cervical spine. *AAOS Instr Course Lect* 17:299–330.
15. Simmons EH, du Toit G (1978): Lateral atlantoaxial arthrodesis. *Orthop Clin North Am* 9(4):1101–1113.
16. Southwick WO, Robinson RA (1976): Surgical approaches to the vertebral bodies in the cervical and lumbar regions. *J Bone Joint Surg [Am]* 39:631–644.
17. Watkins RG (1983): *Surgical approaches to the spine.* New York: Springer-Verlag.
18. Whitecloud TS, LaRocca H (1976): Fibular strut graft in reconstructive surgery of the cervical spine. *Spine* 1(1):33–43.
19. Whitesides TE Jr, Kelly RP (1966): Lateral approaches to the upper cervical spine for anterior fusion. *South Med J* 59:879–883.
20. Whitesides TE Jr, McDonald AP (1978): Lateral retropharyngeal approach to the upper cervical spine. *Orthop Clin North Am* 9(4): 1115–1127.
21. Williams PL, Warwick R, eds. (1980): *Gray's anatomy*, 36th ed. Philadelphia: WB Saunders.

The Adult Spine: Principles and Practice,
2nd edition, J.W. Frymoyer, Editor-in-Chief.
Lippincott-Raven Publishers, Philadelphia © 1997.

CHAPTER **57**

Congenital Anomalies of the Cervical Spine

Mark R. Brinker, Steven H. Weeden, and Thomas S. Whitecloud III

Congenital anomalies of the cervical spine are uncommon conditions that arise from abnormal fetal development (55,137). Most individuals with these conditions are asymptomatic or have only a minimal restriction of neck motion. These anomalies may present as an incidental finding of little functional significance or as gross failures of development that may be incompatible with life. Abnormal development can occur during any of the complicated stages of vertebral column growth and in association with other congenital anomalies. Several of these osseous defects present in adulthood and are unrecognized in the child. The physician must be aware of these abnormalities and the possible associated anomalies of other major organ systems, as early recognition and treatment of these abnormalities may prevent serious neural deficits and prevent further cervical deformity.

The diagnosis of congenital anomalies of the cervical spine begins with a history and physical examination. Typically, the symptoms and findings are due to neural compression. The diagnostic assessment can be difficult

in a child and requires a variety of radiographic views. The interpretation of radiographs is complicated by the dynamic process of bony growth in the developing child. The evaluation of a patient with a congenital cervical spine defect must also include a total body examination in a search for associated congenital abnormalities. Recognition and prompt management are essential for the prevention of possible neurologic or vascular complications.

UPPER CERVICAL SPINE

Basilar Impression

Basilar impression is the most common congenital anomaly affecting the atlanto-occipital region (106). It may result from failure of formation/fusion of the occipital somites, or it may be secondary to a disease process of bone. A deformity of the bony structures in the area of the foramen magnum results in a basilar impression and an upward bulging of the floor of the skull. In this condition, the floor of the skull appears to be indented by the cervical spine. The tip of the odontoid process is cephalad to its normal position and may even protrude into the opening of the foramen magnum, potentially resulting in compression of the brain stem. This compression may present with neurologic damage, circulatory obstruction, or impaired cerebrospinal fluid flow.

There are two types of basilar impression. Primary (or congenital) basilar impression is the result of occipital

  M. R. Brinker, M.D.: Clinical Associate Professor, Department of Orthopaedic Surgery, Tulane University School of Medicine; and Texas Orthopedic Hospital, Houston, Texas 77030.
  S. H. Weeden, M.D.: Scott and White Memorial Hospital, Texas A&M University Health Science Center, College of Medicine, Temple, Texas 76508.
  T. S. Whitecloud III, M.D.:Professor and Chairman, Department of Orthopaedic Surgery, Tulane University School of Medicine, New Orleans, Louisiana 70112.

hypoplasia and may be associated with other vertebral defects. The associated vertebral defects that occur with a primary basilar impression include atlanto-occipital fusion, a bifid posterior arch of the atlas, odontoid abnormalities, and the Klippel-Feil syndrome (19,57,72). Although a defect of embryologic or fetal development, most patients do not present with primary basilar impression until adulthood. Secondary (or acquired) basilar impression is usually attributed to softening of the osseous structures comprising the base of the skull. Secondary basilar impression is a disease of adulthood, often associated with systemic diseases such as Paget's disease, rickets, osteoporosis, renal osteodystrophy, rheumatoid arthritis, neurofibromatosis, and ankylosing spondylitis (11,18,19,27,58). One report describes a unique case in which basilar impression and numerous other midline fusion abnormalities occurred after intrauterine exposure to phenytoin (77).

Presentation

Most patients with congenital basilar impression do not develop symptoms until the second or third decade of life (16). The signs and symptoms of this abnormality are usually secondary to neurologic or vascular impingement at the level of the foramen magnum. Long-tract symptoms including motor weakness, spasticity, and sensory defects are frequent and variable. One may also observe lower cranial nerve involvement, cerebellar ataxia, and bizarre respiratory patterns (129). A downbeat nystagmus is another common symptom. In addition, transient ischemia to the brain secondary to vertebral artery occlusion can present with altered states of consciousness or confusion (129). DeBarros et al. (16) have noted a high incidence of basilar impression in a particular population found in northeast Brazil and have reported that paresthesias and weakness of all four extremities are the most common symptoms. He also noted that a headache in the distribution of the greater occipital nerve may be another common complaint (16). Several other conditions may present with signs and symptoms similar to those of basilar impression. These conditions include polymyositis, posterior fossa tumors, multiple sclerosis, amyotrophic lateral sclerosis, and syringomyelia.

Several authors have observed that hydrocephalus and vertebral artery anomalies may be associated with basilar impression (16,81,137). Increased intracranial pressure with resultant hydrocephalus may result from posterior encroachment on the aqueduct of Sylvius. Vertebral artery anomalies or vertebral artery compression as the vessels pass through the foramen magnum may result in symptoms of vertebral artery insufficiency (5,81). The symptoms of vascular compromise demand immediate attention and accurate management.

Radiographic Evaluation

The radiographic evaluation of basilar impression is difficult; however, numerous radiologic measurements have been described. Chamberlain's line (13), McGregor's line (81), McRae's line (84,85), and Fischgold-Metzger's (33) line have been used in the evaluation of suspected basilar impression. Chamberlain felt that any projection of the odontoid process and body of C1 above a line connecting the posterior border of the foramen magnum and dorsal edge of the hard palate (Chamberlain's line; Fig. 1) on the lateral radiograph constituted basilar impression. McGregor's line (Fig. 1) connects the superior surface of the posterior edge of the hard palate to the most caudal point of the occipital curve of the skull. McGregor's line is one of the preferred methods for screening because the line can easily be defined in all age groups (58). To detect basilar impression, the odontoid tip is measured in relation to McGregor's line. A distance of 4.5 mm above this line is within the upper limit of normal (81). McRae's line (Fig. 1) defines the opening of the foramen magnum. McRae has suggested that when the odontoid tip lies below the opening of the foramen magnum, the patient is likely to be asymptomatic (84).

Fischgold and Metzger (33) described a line to be used in the assessment of basilar impression that connects the two digastric grooves on an anteroposterior laminograph. These authors felt that McGregor's line and Chamberlain's line could possibly be distorted by anatomic changes other than those involving the base of the skull, such as an abnormally long or short odontoid process, a highly arched palate, or abnormal facial bone structure. In patients with basilar impression, the distance from the digastric line to a line that crosses the center of the atlanto-occipital joint is reduced to less than the normal distance of 10 mm.

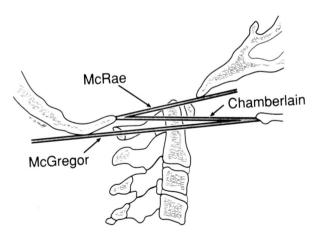

FIG. 1. The three lines used in the diagnosis and evaluation of basilar impression. See text for explanation. Adapted with permission from ref. 55.

With the advent of computed tomography (CT) and magnetic resonance imaging (MRI), the anatomic relationships of the cervico-occipital junction are now viewed in much greater detail (69,79). Although the McGregor's and McRae's lateral reference lines are still important for preliminary screening, CT reconstructions and MRI are invaluable in further delineating abnormal bony and neural tissues.

There are a variety of other imaging measurements described for the evaluation of a suspected basilar impression. Decker et al. (17) have reported that the tip of the odontoid lies between 10 mm above and 3 mm below the bimastoid line in normal individuals. Bull et al. (9) described an angle formed by the intersection of a line along the plane of the hard palate and a line along the plane of C1. This angle (Fig. 2) normally is not greater than 13°, although hard palate abnormalities or excessive flexion or extension about the neck can lead to angle variation (4,58). Additionally, there is a height index described by Klaus (65) for use in the assessment of basilar impression assessment. Klaus measured the height of a line from the tip of the odontoid process perpendicular to a line connecting the tuberculum sellae to the most superior aspect of the internal occipital protuberance. Although the normal range varies widely, a Klaus height index of 30 to 36 mm is suggestive of basilar impression (65).

Treatment

Symptomatic basilar impression requires surgical decompression. Interestingly, it is possible to have a severe basilar impression on radiographic evaluation without any neurologic symptoms. Therefore, the treatment of basilar impression is dictated by neurologic symptomatology and not the radiographic findings. The symp-

toms that occur secondary to anterior impingement from a hypermobile odontoid process are best treated with stabilization of the occipital cervical junction in extension (57). If one is unable to reduce the odontoid process, anterior excision of the odontoid followed by surgical stabilization in extension may be considered. Posterior impingement is reduced by suboccipital craniectomy and decompression of the posterior arch of the atlas. Decompression of C2 may also be of therapeutic value. Opening the dura mater to look for constrictive posterior dural and arachnoid bands with subsequent lysis has also been recommended (16). The proper management of basilar impression often requires the combined efforts of the orthopedic surgeon, the neurosurgeon, the neurologist, and the radiologist.

Atlanto-Occipital Fusion

Atlanto-occipital fusion is a congenital condition in which a partial or a complete bony union between C1 and the base of the skull is present. Common findings include fusion between the anterior aspect of the atlas and the rim of the foramen magnum, posterior displacement of the odontoid process, and an abnormal size of the odontoid process. Occipitalization of the atlas, occipito-cervical synostosis, and atlas assimilation are terms that have been used to describe this defect. The Klippel-Feil syndrome, basilar impression, condylar hypoplasia, and occipital vertebrae are frequently associated with atlanto-occipital fusion (121). Atlanto-occipital fusion in conjunction with other malformations may have significant adverse neurologic consequences.

Presentation

Most patients with atlanto-occipital fusion display abnormal neck features, which include a short broad neck, a low hairline, torticollis, a high scapula, and restricted neck motion (6,57,86,121). Other associated defects include dwarfism, a funnel chest, jaw abnormalities, cleft palate, cervical ribs, external ear deformities, hypospadias, and urinary tract anomalies (6,86,121).

Neurologic complications are rare in childhood and do not usually appear until the fourth or fifth decade of life. Similar to basilar impression, the signs and symptoms of atlanto-occipital fusion are related to bony impingement on neural tissues. The symptoms typically occur in a slow, unrelenting manner. In atlanto-occipital fusion, an odontoid process of abnormal size, position, or mobility is often the cause of symptoms (6,86,135). McRae (84) has suggested that when the odontoid process lies below the foramen magnum, the patient will usually be asymptomatic. However, if the tip of the odontoid process is in a position superior to McRae's line and is angled posteriorly, impingement of anterior

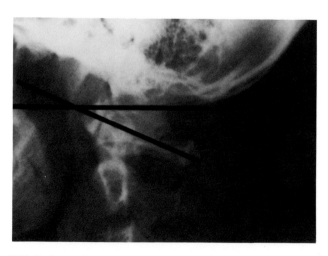

FIG. 2. Lateral radiograph demonstrating the construction of Bull's angle, the intersection of a line along the plane of the hard palate with a line along the plane of C1. From ref. 137.

neurologic structures with subsequent symptoms is likely. Patients with atlanto-occipital fusion may display pyramidal tract signs including muscle wasting, weakness, spasticity, abnormal reflexes, and ataxia (6,86). Less frequently, this defect may compress the cranial nerves and result in the development of dysphagia, diplopia, and tinnitus. In a minority of patients the posterior columns are involved. A loss of proprioception and vibration sense may develop as the posterior margin of the foramen magnum or a dural band impinges on the spinal cord. Vertical and horizontal nystagmus are not uncommon and should alert the physician to the possibility of tonsilar herniation.

Similar to a basilar impression, progressive ligament laxity (which occurs with aging) has been implicated as an etiology for the late onset of symptoms in atlanto-occipital fusion. Several authors have suggested that repeated neck extension and flexion leads to progressive ligamentous laxity about the odontoid process (6,86,135). In addition, the aging neurologic structures may become less tolerant of episodic compression by the odontoid process. The aging sclerotic vertebral vasculature may also become less compliant and thus more susceptible to extrinsic compression from occipitalization of the atlas.

Radiographic Evaluation

The standard radiographs of the atlanto-occipital articulation can be difficult to interpret. To visualize pathology of the atlanto-occipital articulation it may be necessary to use CT, myelography, or MRI. Imaging of affected individuals frequently displays the anterior arch of C1 to be displaced in the posterior direction, C1 assimilation into the occiput, and an associated hypoplastic posterior arch. Radiographic evaluation should also define the shape, length, and orientation of the odontoid process. McRae (84,86) noted that a neurologic deficit would likely be present if the distance from the posterior aspect of the odontoid process to either the posterior arch of the atlas or to the posterior lip of the foramen magnum (whichever is closer) is less than 19 mm on a lateral radiograph. McRae has suggested that approximately 60% of the patients with occipitalization of the atlas will have greater than 3 mm of displacement of the odontoid process with respect to the anterior arch of C1 (84–86).

A thorough radiographic search for associated anomalies of atlanto-occipital fusion should be performed. Gehle and von Torklus (134) have noted that atlanto-axial instability develops in approximately 50% of patients with atlanto-occipital fusion. A dysmorphic and posteriorly displaced odontoid process may also occur in association with occipitalization of the atlas. Additionally, a congenital fusion of C2 and C3, basilar impression, occipital vertebrae, and condylar hypoplasia may also be present in this population of patients. The evalu-

ation should also attempt to rule out herniation. Radiographic findings that are highly suggestive of herniation include blockage of myelographic material at the level of the foramen magnum (86) and vertebral angiography demonstrating a posterior inferior cerebellar artery in the cervical canal.

Treatment

The initial non-operative treatment of symptomatic atlanto-occipital fusion consists of immobilization of the affected area. Non-operative measures should be attempted first because surgical intervention is associated with a high mortality rate (84,135). A reduction of the odontoid process is obtained via skeletal traction before operative intervention. Symptomatic, posterior displacement with severe anterior compression of the spinal cord or brain stem requires upper cervical laminectomy and a suboccipital craniectomy. The results of posterior surgical decompression range from complete remission to extreme neurologic deficits and death (6).

Atlanto-Axial Instability

Atlanto-axial instability often presents secondary to trauma or, less commonly, as a congenital abnormality (43). The integrity of the odontoid process, the transverse ligament of C1, and the alar ligaments provide stability for the atlanto-axial joint. When these structures are abnormal or absent, instability may arise. Instability may present secondary to a reduction in size of the spinal canal, with subsequent impingement of the spinal cord or brain stem. Numerous conditions are associated with atlanto-axial instability. The associated conditions include Down syndrome (Fig. 3), congenital scoliosis, osteogenesis imperfecta, neurofibromatosis, Morquio's syndrome, Larsen's syndrome, and a short or webbed neck. The presence of atlanto-axial instability in Down syndrome patients is estimated to be between 10% and 40% (104).

Approximately one half of all rotational motion in the cervical spine occurs between C1 and C2. Extension between the atlas and the axis is normally limited to approximately 10° and flexion is limited to 5°. In conjunction with rotational motion, the atlas and axis tend to shift laterally with respect to one another (2). Because this joint is so mobile, it is consequently the least stable articulation of the cervical spine. The lack of stability of the atlanto-axial joint is accentuated by being surrounded by the atlanto-occipital and C2-C3 joints, which are relatively immobile.

Presentation

A patient with atlanto-axial instability may present with cardiopulmonary arrest, motor weakness, vertigo,

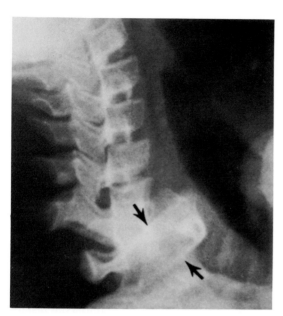

FIG. 3. Radiograph of an 11-year-old child with Down syndrome and gross atlanto-axial instability (*arrows*). Adapted from ref. 55.

neck pain, torticollis, quadriplegia, and even projectile vomiting (43,82). The symptoms typically manifest in adulthood and are likely the combination of ligament laxity and increasing rigidity in the aging neural structures (57). The symptoms of atlanto-axial instability are commonly inconsistent and transient. In a patient with deficient ligaments and an intact odontoid process, the spinal cord is at risk of becoming compressed when the neck is flexed. When anterior impingement occurs, the signs and symptoms include muscle weakness, muscle atrophy, hyper-reflexia, ataxia, and spasticity (58). If cerebellar herniation occurs, one may observe nystagmus and ataxia. Glannestras et al. (45) have described symptoms of dizziness, syncope, and seizures with compromised blood flow.

The clinical manifestations of atlanto-occipital instability resulting in dislocation in patients with anomalies of the odontoid process were divided into three groups by Nagashima (94): (a) acute (traumatic), (b) delayed (traumatic), and (c) chronic (nontraumatic). In the acute type, dislocation and immediate death may occur if bony displacement is great and severe damage to the cervical cord or vertebral arteries occurs (94). Symptoms in the delayed (traumatic) type may occur months to years following the inciting trauma. In the chronic type (with no history of trauma), symptoms may progress to permanent cervical myelopathy (94).

Radiographic Evaluation

The stability of the atlanto-axial joint may be assessed via a lateral radiograph. The atlanto-dens interval (ADI)

is the distance between the posterior edge of the anterior arch of the atlas and the anterior portion of the odontoid process (Fig. 4). This interval is useful in assessing the space available for the cord (SAC). The internal span of the ring of the atlas on the lateral radiograph (anterior/posterior span) of an adult measures approximately 30 mm (29,47). Steel (125) has suggested that the odontoid and spinal cord each occupy 10 mm of the 30 mm ring, and that there is a 10 mm area of "free space" available for displacement.

The normal ADI in adults is less than 3 mm (58). Even a small increase in the ADI, with the neck held in the neutral position, is suggestive of disruption of the transverse ligament. Fielding et al. (30) have suggested that an ADI of 3 to 5 mm implicates disruption of the transverse ligament. An ADI of 5 to 10 mm suggests additional ligamentous damage, and an ADI of 10 mm or more represents disruption of all ligaments. Fielding et al. (30) have recommended flexion-extension radiographs in all suspected cases of atlanto-axial instability where there are no signs of spinal cord involvement. Flexion and extension of the cervical spine should be performed by the patient alone. Changes in the ADI and SAC with flexion-extension are important in assessing the degree and direction of displacement.

The ADI is of little value in evaluating patients with anomalies of the odontoid process. In this patient population, measurement of the SAC is of greater clinical value. The SAC represents the distance from the posterior ring of the atlas to the posterior aspect of the odontoid process or posterior aspect of C2 (whichever value is less). In the patient with atlanto-axial instability and a freely mobile odontoid process (as in os odontoideum), flexion and extension result in a reduction of the SAC with no change in the ADI (137).

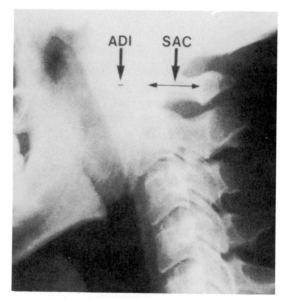

FIG. 4. Lateral radiograph of the cervical spine displaying the SAC and the ADI. From ref. 137.

McRae (84) studied the relationship between neurologic involvement and SAC and suggested that a measurement of less than 19 mm was always accompanied by symptomatology. Greenberg (47) suggested that in the adult cervical spine, cord compression always occurs if the anterior/posterior diameter behind the odontoid process is 14 mm or less, and never occurs if the diameter is 18 mm or more. More recently, Spierings and Braakman (120) have reported that 13 mm or less of SAC is associated with neurologic sequelae. Fielding et al. (29) have suggested that anterior displacement of the atlas on the axis is less dangerous in the patient with an abnormal odontoid process, which may be carried forward with the atlas.

The normal ADI interval in children is believed to be less than 4 mm (30,71). Locke et al. (71) studied the lateral radiographs of 200 normal pediatric patients and reported no cases of ADI greater than 4 mm. The authors recommended radiographs be performed in the neutral position and cautioned that an ADI greater than 4 mm was suggestive of atlanto-axial subluxation. Normal values for the SAC in children vary with age (58,71). The diameter of the SAC on the lateral radiograph is greatest at the atlas and progressively narrows to C5.

Myelography is of value in defining areas of spinal cord impingement in atlanto-axial instability. Several authors have recommended the use of gas or water-soluble contrast rather than oil contrast (40,84,100,107). A CT scan in conjunction with myelography may be useful in evaluating the SAC (40,107). If available, MRI in flexion and extension is a useful diagnostic test. In addition, Marijke et al. (76) have stated that radiographic imaging in children with Down syndrome is one of the best methods to detect atlanto-axial instability and is superior to physical examination for generalized ligament laxity.

Treatment

The treatment of atlanto-axial instability is based on the extent of instability, the etiology, and the patient's activity level (30,57). Fielding et al. (30) have stated that "even when there is minimal instability, trivial trauma superimposed on an already weakened and compromised structure can be catastrophic." In contrast, Cremers et al. (14) have reported that there is no reason radiographically to screen children with Down syndrome for atlanto-axial instability before they engage in athletic activity. Cremers and colleagues have also suggested that a physician need not inhibit these children from playing certain sports (14).

The indications for surgical arthrodesis in atlanto-axial instability as outlined by Fielding et al. (30) include central nervous system involvement, persistent cervical signs and symptoms, and an ADI (atlanto-axial distance in cases of odontoid pathology) greater than 5 mm. In older patients and in patients with rheumatoid arthritis in whom surgery is contraindicated or associated with a high complication rate, temporary immobilization of the neck may be a more practical treatment (30). Fielding et al. (30) do not employ the use of preoperative traction in asymptomatic patients with less than 7 mm of displacement. These authors described the importance of proper orientation of the atlas on the axis at the time of spinal arthrodesis. Axial CT views are extremely useful for evaluating the architecture of the lateral mass of C1 and the facets of C2. The normal anatomic relationship between C1 and C2 should be restored before surgical arthrodesis. The exception to this principle would be a deformity that is not correctable with traction or one with severe neurologic deficit. Standard arthrodesis of the Gallie or Brooks type is performed with or without the use of sublaminar wires. Sagher et al. (114) have described the use of autologous occipital bone for posterior atlanto-axial arthrodesis in surgical repair of atlanto-axial instability. Sagher and colleagues described the advantages of occipital bone harvest for atlanto-axial instability repair: ease of harvest, lack of postoperative discomfort from iliac bone retrieval, and suitability of occipital bone for fusion. In addition, Marcotte et al. (75) described the use of posterior atlanto-axial facet screw fixation for immediate multidirectional rigid fixation of C1-C2 in this population of patients. The use of facet screw fixation circumvents the need for rigid external orthosis and is particularly useful in the treatment of pseudoarthrosis (75).

Malformation of the Odontoid Process

Several congenital anomalies of the odontoid process have been described in the literature (36,37,45,48,51, 61,64,66,94,136,141). Malformations of the dens include aplasia, hypoplasia, duplication, condylicus tertius, os terminale, and os odontoideum. Odontoid aplasia is an extremely rare anomaly. Odontoid hypoplasia, a relatively common anomaly, appears as a short, stubby peg of odontoid. In odontoid hypoplasia it is not uncommon to find an associated os odontoideum. Os odontoideum is the most common anomaly of the odontoid. An os odontoideum appears as a radiolucent oval or round ossicle with a smooth dense border of bone. If the ossicle is located where the odontoid tip normally would be, it is said to be orthotopic; if the ossicle is located near the base of the occiput in the region of the foramen magnum, it is termed dystopic (137). The condylicus tertius syndrome occurs when an abnormally large odontoid process articulates with a third occipital condyle on the anterior rim of the foramen magnum. In condylicus tertius, brain stem compression may occur with narrowing of the foramen magnum. A patient may be asymptomatic or suffer debilitating neurologic sequelae.

The frequency of anomalies of the odontoid process is uncertain. Fielding et al. (31) have suggested that an odontoid process abnormality is often discovered on radiographic evaluation following head or neck trauma or after the spontaneous onset of symptoms. The early recognition of odontoid process anomalies is essential as they may result in atlanto-axial instability with subsequent neurologic involvement and possible death. Wolin (141), in 1963, reported an average age of diagnosis of 30 years in his series of patients with os odontoideum. In contrast, Fielding et al. (31) reported an average age at diagnosis of 18.9 years in their 1980 report. With the index of suspicion increasing, odontoid lesions are now being more commonly recognized. Additionally, malformations of the dens are more common in individuals with Klippel-Feil syndrome, Down syndrome, and certain skeletal and spondyloepiphyseal dysplasias (8,12, 15,28,32,53,70,78,116,120,135).

Presentation

A patient with a congenital malformation of the odontoid process may appear with no symptoms, local neck symptoms (pain, torticollis, headache), transitory episodes of paresis after minor trauma, myelopathies, or ischemia secondary to vertebral artery compression or death (31,126,135). The neurologic symptoms arise as a result of displacement of the atlas on the axis with spinal cord compression. In patients who are asymptomatic or who have minimal symptoms of local neck pain only, the prognosis is excellent (31,117). However, patients with symptoms that gradually worsen or display increasing neurologic signs have a poor prognosis and may be expected to deteriorate without treatment (31). In addition to spinal cord compression and frank neurologic symptoms, patients may display multiple congenital anomalies along with the odontoid process defect. Weakness and ataxia are also not uncommon findings and the insult may involve anterior and/or posterior neural structures (57). Additionally, patients may present with signs and symptoms of cerebral and brain stem ischemia, mental deterioration, syncope, vertigo, visual disturbances, and seizures (71,113,117). These confusing symptoms may result in a delayed and even an incorrect diagnosis. Trauma is frequently associated with the onset of symptoms and radiographic examination of the trauma patient may reveal an abnormal odontoid process.

Radiographic Evaluation

An odontoid process anomaly may frequently be seen on standard radiographs of involved individuals. The open-mouth (anteroposterior) and lateral, flexion, and extension studies and CT reconstructions aid in the visualization of the lesion along with the presence or absence of associated atlanto-axial instability. In os odontoideum, the radiographic evaluation reveals a radiolucent gap between the body of the axis and the dens (Fig. 5). Hensinger et al. (56) have suggested that displacement greater than 3 mm indicates the presence of odontoid process pathology. The extent of displacement is evaluated by measuring the anteroposterior distance between the posterior aspect of the body of C2 and the posterior aspect of the anterior arch of C1. In addition, the SAC distance should be measured and documented. The radiolucent gap of an os odontoideum may be mistaken for the normal epiphyseal line in children under 5 years of age. In patients younger than 5 years, radiographic evidence of motion between the odontoid process and the body of C2 is highly suggestive of os odontoideum (56).

The radiographic appearance of os odontoideum should not be confused with a traumatic non-union of the odontoid process. The radiolucent gap in traumatic non-union is typically narrow with an irregular border. In contrast, in os odontoideum the gap appears wide, with smooth margins. The lesion of os odontoideum typically appears to extend above the level of the superior facets of C2 and the free ossicle is oval in shape with a uniform rounded off cortex (55,56,88). In aplasia of the odontoid process, the odontoid is typically absent on the open-mouth (odontoid) view, and a depression may be seen between the superior articular facets (57). A short osseous remnant of the odontoid process is observed in odontoid hypoplasia. It is not uncommon for congenital anomalies of the odontoid process to be detected as an

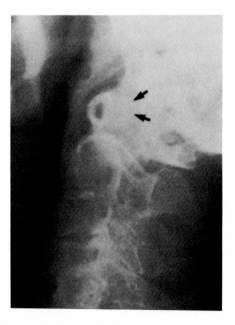

FIG. 5. Lateral radiograph displaying anos odontoideum. *Arrows* indicate an oval free ossicle in the orthrotopic position. From ref. 137.

incidental finding in a patient who has radiographs taken following trauma.

Treatment

In patients with odontoid process abnormalities, the major concern is that minor trauma superimposed on an already weakened structure may be catastrophic. There is no consensus of opinion as to the preferred treatment of the asymptomatic patient or once symptomatic now asymptomatic patient with anomalies of the dens. Several authors (38,44,88,117) have suggested that surgery is associated with a significant risk of mortality and increasing neurologic deficit. Therefore, surgical intervention is recommended only in those patients with progressive or recurrent neurologic symptoms. All other patients are treated with conservative measures, including instructions to avoid activities associated with head or neck trauma.

Reduction of the atlanto-axial joint should be obtained via careful positioning of the patient or by skeletal traction before surgery. Hensinger and MacEwen (57) have recommended that the patient remain in a reduced position for 1 to 2 weeks before operative intervention to allow a complete return of neurologic function. Early surgical reduction before adequate stabilization is not recommended because of the high rate of morbidity and mortality (38). Fielding et al. (30) have recommended surgical stabilization via a posterior cervical fusion of C1-C2 with wire fixation and iliac crest bone graft. A posterior approach is sufficient for atlanto-axial arthrodesis in atlanto-axial instability secondary to congenital anomalies of the odontoid process. During the surgical correction, care must be taken to expose only the bony elements to be fused. Postoperatively, a halo cast or a vest is preferred (123) and is usually left on the patient for about 6 weeks. This is followed by the use of a brace for an additional 6-week period.

Congenital Anomalies of the Ring of the Atlas and Axis

Malformations of the atlantal ring are not uncommon and often are detected on radiographs obtained for other purposes (73). In normal development, ossification of C1 begins during the seventh week of gestation (73), and at birth the anterior arch is cartilaginous. The anterior arch of the atlas normally fuses to the lateral masses by 6 to 8 years of age. In contrast, the posterior arches fuse during the third or fourth year of age (41,132). Congenital defects of the ring of the axis and atlas are caused by failure of fusion of the synchondroses of the developing cervical vertebrae. Chigira et al. (12) have reported that hypoplastic development is another common etiology of anomalies of C1. Defects of the anterior arch of the atlas are extremely rare (41,42,73,132). Geipel (42) reported a

0.1% incidence of clefts in the anterior arch of the atlas in 2,749 post mortem specimens, and found no cases of anterior arch aplasia. Although defects of the posterior arch of the atlas are extremely rare, they occur at least four times as often as those of the anterior arch (41,73). Congenital defects of the posterior elements of the axis are far more rare than those of the atlas (91,137). It is not uncommon for partial or complete absence of the posterior arch of C1 to occur along with a failure in closure of the anterior arch (Fig. 6). Defects in the posterior arch of C1 range from a midline cleft to partial or complete arch absence (unilateral or bilateral) (135).

The first large study to review the congenital defects of the ring of C1 was reported by Dubouset (23). The author described several patients in whom he was able to document the absence of a facet of C1. As the patients aged, they progressed to severe torticollis, usually in early childhood. The deformity is flexible initially, but as the child grows the torticollis becomes severe and eventually becomes fixed.

Congenital defects in the ring of the atlas and axis may be asymptomatic or may present with neurologic symptoms secondary to atlanto-axial instability. Congenital anomalies in the ring of the atlas and axis are often detected on x-ray following minor trauma to the head and neck, with or without the presence of symptoms. In the patient with an arch defect, malrotation and instability between C1 and C2 is not an uncommon finding. Radiographs of the cervical spine, which include oblique views, are helpful in demonstrating arch defects. Lateral radiographs often show soft tissue swelling anterior to C1 with congenital absence of a portion of the posterior arch (56) (Fig. 7). A CT image reconstruction may be useful in delineating the location and extent of bony defects. Careful radiographic evaluation is also useful in differentiating an arch fracture from a congenital defect. It is important to screen a patient for the presence of other possible associated occipito-atlanto-axial defects during the radiographic evaluation.

The treatment of patients with anomalies of C1 and C2 depends on the amount of instability present and the severity of the neurologic symptoms. When nonsurgical treatment is the chosen therapy, careful follow-up evaluation is mandatory.

Congenital spondylolisthesis in the upper cervical spine is rare (7,25,130). The failure of fusion between the neural arch and the centrum of the axis manifests as bilateral defects. These defects are usually not associated with atlanto-axial instability, but they have been associated with aplasia of the odontoid process (34,62,130). Bilateral fusion defects may allow for forward displacement of the vertebral body and spinal cord compression (26,50,58). Spondylolisthesis of the axis is similar to the hangman's fracture, and treatment therefore includes stabilization at the C2-C3 articulation with or without a posterior arthrodesis from C1 to C3 (63). When severe

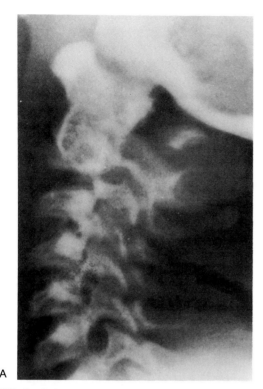
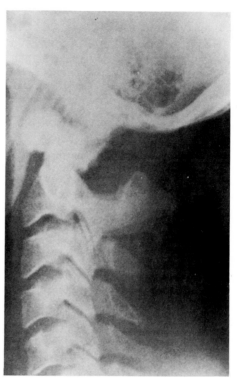

A

B

FIG. 6. A: Lateral radiograph of an asymptomatic patient with failure of fusion of the neural arches of the atlas. **B:** Lateral radiograph of a 34-year-old white man who presented with a complaint of diffuse back pain for 1 week. Radiograph reveals complete absence of the posterior arch of C1. From ref. 137.

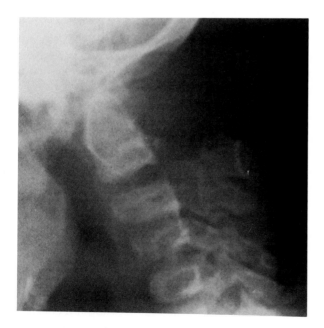

FIG. 7. Lateral radiograph of the cervical spine (in extension) that displays absence of the posterior arch of C1, failure of fusion of the posterior arch of C2, and fusion of the posterior elements of C2 and C3. From ref. 137.

neurologic compromise evolves, both an anterior and a posterior arthrodesis with stabilization are warranted. CT of patients with suspected congenital spondylolisthesis is usually sufficient to make a confident diagnosis in questionable cases (130).

LOWER CERVICAL SPINE

Osseous malformations of the lower cervical spine have been extensively reviewed in the literature (1,7,10,26,46,74). Cervical spine differentiation proceeds from the mesenchymal phase to that of chondrification and subsequent ossification. A disruption during any of these phases can lead to anomalous growth. When a pathologic process disrupts the normal bony development, the physical proximity of various other developing structures may result in a number of systems being involved. It is of no surprise that malformations of the central nervous system can coexist with congenital bony anomalies of the cervical spine (98). The etiology of bony anomalies in the lower cervical spine is likely multifactorial. Genetic (115), vascular (3), maternal substance abuse (77,131), and failure of differentiation (68) are several of the possible causative factors. The existence of an osseous malformation of the lower cervical spine is an important indicator of possible associated systemic malformation (7,25,130).

Klippel-Feil Syndrome and Associated Abnormalities

In 1912, Klippel and Feil (67) described their findings in a 46-year-old man who had recently died. The post mortem evaluation of this patient revealed complete fusion of the cervical vertebrae. The authors described several notable characteristics, including a low posterior hairline, restriction of neck motion, and an obvious short neck (67). These features constitute the classic triad of the condition now described as the Klippel-Feil syndrome. The anatomic and clinical expressions of this syndrome vary widely, ranging from mild deformity to severe disability.

Gray and associates (46) noted that only 53% of patients with Klippel-Feil syndrome display the classic clinical triad. The associated occult abnormalities may be more detrimental to the patient's general well-being than the obvious deformities of the neck (Table 1). Hen-

---

TABLE 1. *Associated anomalies in the Klippel-Feil syndrome[a]*

Musculoskeletal
Scoliosis
Torticollis
Pterygium colli (webbed neck)
Sprengel's anomaly
Cervical ribs and other costal abnormalities
Syndactyly
Hypoplastic thumbs
Supernumerary digits

Central nervous system
Spinal cord compression (anterior/posterior)
Facial nerve palsies
Deafness

Urinary system
Doubling of the collecting system
Agenesis of the kidney (unilateral > bilateral)
Horseshoe kidney
Tubular ectasia
Renal ectopia
Hydronephrosis

Reproductive system
Absence of the vagina
Agenesis of the ovaries

Cardiovascular system
Ventricular septal defect
Patent ductus arteriosus
Coarctation of the aorta
Atrial septal defect

[a] Adapted with permission from ref. 127.

---

singer et al. (57) noted the high incidence of related congenital defects and emphasized the importance of thoroughly evaluating all patients with Klippel-Feil syndrome. Most of these patients are asymptomatic or display only mild restriction of neck motion. Usually the symptoms attributed to the cervical spine occur in the adult and are due to areas of hypermobile articulations. The symptoms may also be related to degenerative changes. The relatively favorable prognosis of these cervical bony lesions is overshadowed by the poor prognosis related to the unrecognized associated anomalies.

Presentation

Along with the classic triad of physical findings in Klippel-Feil syndrome, the associated bony malformations include lordosis, torticollis, scoliosis, kyphosis, hemivertebrae, cervical fusion, and other musculoskeletal deformities. Patients with Klipppel-Feil syndrome may also develop congenital duplication of the mandibular rami and may present with an abnormal bony mass in the mandibular ramus region (22).

The symptoms associated with Klippel-Feil syndrome originate at the open segments of the fused cervical vertebrae, where the remaining free articulations may become compensatorily hypermobile. This hypermobility can lead to frank instability, caused either by trauma or early degenerative changes with a delayed onset of symptoms. The most consistent finding is limited neck motion (46). Flexion and extension are usually better preserved than rotational or lateral bending. If fusion of the cervical spine is present at only one or two vertebral levels, the patient may not be aware of the anomaly and may be surprised when radiographs reveal the deformity. In addition, patients may have weakness, paresthesias, and pain in the arms and lower limbs, which are often secondary to the musculoskeletal deformities.

Facial asymmetry is often seen in association with torticollis in this syndrome. However, less than 20% of patients with Klippel-Feil syndrome have an obvious facial asymmetry, webbing of the neck (pterygium colli), or torticollis (54,57). If torticollis is present, it is commonly the result of either sustained contracture of the sterno-cleidomastoid muscle or bony abnormalities. A cervical lordosis and pterygium colli are two other associated abnormalities. Pterygium colli consists of webbing of the skin on the lateral side of the neck and usually occurs bilaterally (35). Pterygium colli may be an innocent finding accompanying cervical bony defects or a secondary finding in patients with Turner's syndrome. Turner's syndrome may be present with or without a coexisting Klippel-Feil syndrome. Cubitus valgus and the presence of streaked gonads suggest the possibility of Turner's syndrome. Cervical lordosis is often associated with iniencephaly and demands immediate evaluation.

Iniencephaly is a rare craniocervical deformity characterized by marked, fixed retroflexion of the head and a short, immobile neck (93).

Sprengel's deformity is another frequently associated anomaly in Klippel-Feil syndrome. The relationship between these two conditions is best explained by the clear understanding of the embryology of the scapula. The scapula develops at 3 weeks' gestation from the mesodermal tissue high in the neck at the level of the third and fourth cervical vertebrae. In the eighth week of development the scapula descends to its normal thoracic position. It is the abnormal descent or nondescent of the scapula that results in an obvious scapular deformity. It is not surprising that this deformity occurs in patients with Klippel-Feil syndrome. Scapular descent occurs at the eighth week of development, the same time that the lesions of Klippel-Feil syndrome are believed to occur (46).

Congenital elevation (failure of descent) of the scapula can be varied in degrees of severity. Elevation of the affected shoulder with an omovertebral bone extending from the cervical spine to the scapula are detected on an anteroposterior radiograph of many affected individuals (Fig. 8). In Sprengel's deformity, a small palpable scapula with an abnormal neck contour and limited abduction of the shoulder on the affected side are observed clinically.

Scoliosis occurs in approximately 60% of patients and is considered the most frequently associated skeletal deformity in Klippel-Feil syndrome (31,80). Scoliosis is often associated with a hemi-vertebrae at C7 and T1 vertebral levels. The commonly seen cervicothoracic curve may cause severe physical deformity and even paraplegia (139,140). For this reason, most patients with scoliosis require treatment and continued evaluation. If compensatory curves above and below the cervicothoracic curve do not develop, an obvious loss of eye position and head tilt are present. The high incidence of scoliosis in patients with Klippel-Feil syndrome necessitates the radiographic evaluation of the complete spine. A progressive scoliosis of the thoracic spine may also seriously compromise pulmonary function (57).

The structural and mechanical abnormalities present in Klippel-Feil syndrome place the cervical spinal cord at risk. The fusion of cervical osseous segments reduces the ability of the cervical spine to compensate for the excessive forces that occur during neck movement. Spinal stenosis is also observed in many patients with Klippel-Feil syndrome and increases the risk of symptomatic spinal cord compression (103). The presence of congenital stenosis and synostosis of the cervical vertebral column can be clearly visualized on plain film radiographs—the narrow sagittal width of the vertebral body at the level of the obliterated disk is unmistakable.

Compression neuropathy of the nerve roots and myelopathy due to spinal stenosis associated with Klippel-Feil syndrome was reported by Prusick et al. (103). These patients are particularly prone to develop neurologic symptoms following even minor trauma (101–103). Symptoms may arise from mechanical irritation of the joint, allowing compression or irritation of the spinal cord, and are generally localized to the head, upper extremity, and neck (87,102). An osteophytic spur (87) causing foramina stenosis is another frequent cause of symptoms. Symptoms of spinal cord involvement range from mild spasticity, hyper-reflexia, muscular weakness, and sudden complete quadriplegia. Osteoarthritis and other degenerative changes have been known to occur in adults with Klippel-Feil syndrome.

Urologic and cardiac anomalies have also been associated with the original syndrome described by Klippel and Feil (46,57,80,102). Common urinary tract abnormalities include agenesis of the kidney, hydronephrosis, tubular ectasia, horseshoe kidney, renal ectopia, and a doubling of the collecting system (24,57,89,99,105). The most common urologic anomaly is unilateral renal agenesis. Renal dysgenesis with obvious abnormal renal function is rare, but it does occur 40 times more frequently than in the general population (89). The young patient with abnormal renal function is usually asymptomatic. Therefore, serial renal function testing is recommended. An ultrasound evaluation of the renal system is an essential noninvasive tool in evaluating the Klippel-Feil patient (57). Intravenous pyelography is another useful clinical tool.

Greene et al. (49) described the MURCS association: an association of mullerian duct aplasia, renal agenesis, and cervical and thoracic spine dysplasias. The authors described these structures' intimate spacial relationship during development and how a disruption of growth

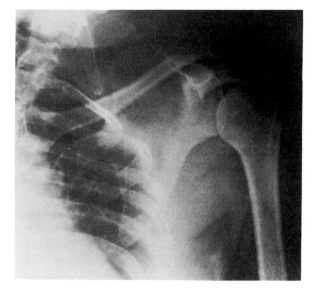

FIG. 8. Sprengel's deformity with omovertebral bone extending from the cervical spine to the scapula.

would alter all three structures (mullarian duct, renal collecting system, and spine) and their subsequent development.

Morrison et al. (92) noted that patients with Klippel-Feil syndrome have a greater risk of congenital heart defects (4.2% of cases). A ventricular septal defect is the most common associated cardiovascular anomaly. The Klippel-Feil population of patients may also have an associated patent ductus arteriosus, an atrial septal defect, dextrocardia, and anomalies of the pulmonary veins (95). When the cardiovascular system is involved, symptoms may include cyanosis, digital clubbing, and dyspnea on exertion (92,95). Noncardiogenic respiratory symptoms may also exist in Klippel-Feil syndrome. Rosen et al. (112) reported two children with severe sleep-disordered breathing associated with Klippel-Feil syndrome. In both patients, minor cervical vertebral anomalies were associated with major hindbrain aberrations (112).

McLay and Maran (83) described the findings of deafness and other anomalies in the Klippel-Feil patient. The literature reports numerous ear deformities, facial malformations, and deafness in association with this syndrome (22,83,96,124). The structures involved include the outer ear, the ossicles, the semicircular canals, the mandible, maxilla, and the hyoid bone. Deafness is often described as a sensorineural impairment. Less often, malformations of the middle ear ossicles result in a conductive hearing impairment that is amenable to operative correction. An absence of the auditory canal and microtia are less common defects. It is recommended that the Klippel-Feil patient undergo audiometric testing when otologic defects are suspected.

Klippel-Feil syndrome and mirror motion was first described by Bauman (2). Mirror motions (synkinesia) involve the involuntary paired movements of the limbs. Bauman (2) found mirror motions to occur in four of six patients with Klippel-Feil syndrome. Synkinesia may suggest the presence of significant central nervous system defects and malformations of the spinal cord along with central lesions of the corpus callosum. Fortunately, this condition tends to resolve with age. Occupational therapy and confirmation of synkinesia with an electromyogram may assist in the treatment of this disorder.

There are numerous reports that describe the various deformities in patients with iniencephaly (90,93,118, 119,138). In this disorder, congenital deformities include cervical synostosis, a fixed retroflexion of the head, severe lordosis, and varying degrees of incomplete posterior cervical spine closure. In severe cases, the deformities associated with iniencephaly are too debilitating to permit survival and the patient rarely lives into adult life. Patients who do survive to adulthood usually are severely handicapped by the fixed hyperextension of the neck (Fig. 9). The bony defect in iniencephaly permits the cerebellum and medulla to occupy the space outside,

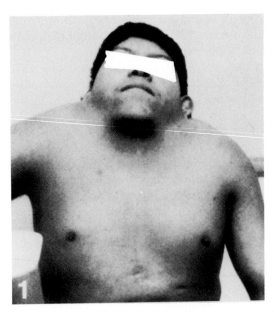

FIG. 9. A 17-year-old patient with iniencephaly. Severe fixed retroflexion of the head is present. From ref. 93, with permission.

below, and behind the cranium (118). Consequently, the severity of iniencephaly and its associated deformities have led to the development of prenatal diagnostic techniques (90). In the less severe forms, the deformity is correctable (39). In patients suspected of having iniencephaly, Munden et al. (93) have described the use of three-dimensional CT imaging to identify and estimate the severity of anomalies before surgery.

Radiologic Evaluation

The numerous imaging techniques now available have significantly enhanced our understanding of the congenital bony changes first described by Klippel and Feil (67). The initial radiographic evaluation of the Klippel-Feil patient should include an anteroposterior, and anteroposterior open-mouth, and lateral extension and flexion views of the cervical spine. In the severely involved patient, radiographic evaluation is often difficult, as fixed bony deformities may hamper proper positioning of patients. When the proper radiographic images are obtained, the clinician can define the pattern of congenital fusion, determine the amount of instability at the atlanto-axial joint, demonstrate a coexisting occipitalization of C1, and clearly visualize the area above and below the defect(s).

The radiographic hallmark of Klippel-Feil syndrome is fusion of the cervical vertebrae at one or multiple vertebral levels (Fig. 10). The lateral radiograph displays obliteration of the disc spaces. The fused vertebral bodies appear to be smaller in width than the normal vertebrae above and below the defect. This appearance, as viewed

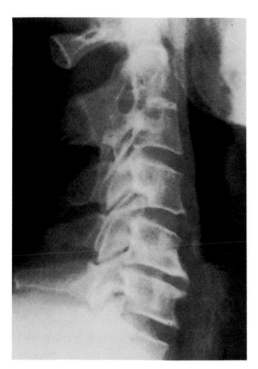

FIG. 10. Lateral radiograph of the cervical spine showing C2-C3 fusion.

on the lateral radiograph, has been described as having a "wasp-waist" (20). The flexion and extension laminagraphic views help to provide the information needed to assess stability. In the evaluation of infants, the radiograph may appear normal until the vertebrae are sufficiently ossified to define clearly the congenital bony changes. The spinal canal is usually of normal width; however, if an enlarged canal is detected, syringomyelia, Arnold-Chiari malformation, and hydromyelia must be excluded (21).

In older patients, lateral flexion and extension radiographs are essential in diagnosing and monitoring intersegmental vertebral instability. Historically, precise positioning of the head and neck is provided by the images of cineradiography. Cineradiography is a dynamic technique that allows one to evaluate axial rotation, lateral bending, and flexion-extension while being able to avoid the confusion of malrotation. The CT scan may be used to evaluate a patient for the presence of brain stem anomalies, spinal cord anomalies, spinal stenosis, and bone deformities about the occipitocervical junction. An MRI is not indicated initially in the Klippel-Feil individual, but it may be a useful tool in further defining anatomic defects. The ability of MRI to display bony and soft tissue defects has replaced the need for cineradiography. The use of CT and MRI in acquired and congenital abnormalities of the cervical spine and cord in the Klippel-Feil patient was evaluated by Ulmer and colleagues (133). Ulmer et al. (133) determined that spon-

dylosis or disk herniations were the most common radiologic abnormalities (observed in 42% of cases). Moreover, Ulmer et al. (133) reported that in most patients, spondylitic changes were seen widely distributed throughout the lower cervical vertebral column.

Pizzutillo et al. (101) have described a radiographic classification for Klippel-Feil syndrome. The authors discuss three high-risk patterns of cervical spine motion. The first pattern (Pattern 1) involves a fusion of C2 and C3 with atlanto-occipital fusion. As the patient with Pattern 1 ages, the odontoid process may become hypermobile and eventually compress the brain stem and spinal cord. Therefore, the risk of neurologic symptoms is not evident until adulthood. With the second pattern (Pattern 2), there is a long bony fusion in association with an abnormal occipitocervical junction. In the Pattern 2 patient, the forces of flexion-extension and rotation are concentrated about an abnormal odontoid process or a poorly developed atlantal ring. In the third pattern (Pattern 3), there is a single open interspace between two fused segments. If hypermobility is present in a Pattern 3 patient, frank instability or degenerative osteoarthritis may develop (46,87,102). Pizzutillo et al. (101) noted that the patients who had an upper segment instability were more likely to be children or adolescents and frequently suffered from neurologic symptoms at a younger age. In contrast, a low segment hypermobility was more common in the adult. The authors also described the presence of degenerative changes in most affected adults. The low segment pattern is stable throughout early life and the symptoms typically result after many years. In a more recent report, Pizzutillo et al. (102) reported that a statistically significant difference of increased motion per open interspace in the upper cervical segment was noted in individuals with Klippel-Feil syndrome when compared to controls. Moreover, the total motion of the lower cervical spine was significantly decreased in the Klippel-Feil population. Pizzutillo et al. (102) observed that individuals with hypermobility of the upper cervical spine are at an increased risk for neurologic sequelae, whereas those with lower cervical spine anomalies are predisposed to degenerative disease.

Treatment

The treatment of the Klippel-Feil patient is confined primarily to the area of associated conditions; however, several treatment modalities are available for the cervical spine abnormalities. A patient with minimal Klippel-Feil syndrome involvement can be expected to lead a normal life with only minor restrictions or symptoms.

Immediately after birth and continuing throughout the growth period, passive range-of-motion exercises are recommended. This improves the long-term chances for normal range of motion. At present, the treatment options for the cervical spine bony anomalies are limited. All patients with cervical synostosis should be advised to avoid high-risk motions that stress the cervical spine. The cervical defects in the Klippel-Feil patient are less capable of withstanding traumatic insults, and minor trauma may result in severe neurologic damage. The use of traction, a cervical collar, and analgesics are recommended for the treatment of symptomatic degenerative osteoarthritis. Before an operative intervention in a patient with neurologic symptoms is undertaken, it is recommended that a thorough examination be performed to determine the site of neurologic involvement. Attempts should be made to reduce any displaced bony architecture (via traction) before surgical stabilization. Surgical efforts are directed toward the improvement of both function as well as cosmetic appearance.

A torticollis secondary to contracture of the sternocleidomastoid muscle may be corrected by surgery. A fixed torticollis posturing may also respond favorably to long-term bracing followed by physical therapy. An associated cervical congenital scoliosis will commonly respond to a halo cast in combination with a posterior cervical fusion. A brace is used in cases of a worsening scoliosis deformity in a younger patient. Serial assessment with repeated radiographic studies is imperative to assess adequately the effectiveness of a cervicothoracic orthosis. If an operative intervention is considered, a preoperative CT scan is obtained to determine if any associated anomalies are located in the area to be surgically fused. A posterior arthrodesis extending to the uppermost level of the cervicothoracic curve with an autologous iliac bone graft is performed in severe cases of bony maldevelopment. The patient's head alignment should be maintained by an orthosis or a plaster jacket.

Sprengel's deformity may be corrected surgically. In Sprengel's deformity, the high scapula may be restored to its normal anatomic position, thereby increasing the apparent length of the neck. The symptoms of nerve root irritation, especially if mild, may frequently be relieved by traction or immobilization. If the neurologic symptoms are resistant to conservative measures, a decompression of the nerve root is frequently required.

As a general rule, the use of cosmetic surgery in the Klippel-Feil patient should be approached with caution because of the inherent high risks of neurologic compromise and limited possible gains.

Cervical Ribs

In the developing fetus the limb bud may occasionally be located abnormally high. A high limb bud may receive its major developmental contribution from the cervical vertebrae rather than the thoracic vertebrae with which it is normally associated. This situation favors the development of a larger rib element at the seventh cervi-

cal vertebral level. This abnormal costal element is called a cervical rib (Fig. 11). A cervical rib ranges in size from a nonsignificant osseous growth to a fully formed rib. The cervical rib occurs in approximately 1% of the population and of these, up to 80% are bilateral (111). Although most cervical ribs are considered to result from anomalous growth, Rogers et al. (109) described a dose-related increase in cervical ribs at the seventh cervical vertebral level after animals were exposed to methanol.

A patient with a cervical rib is frequently asymptomatic; however, cervical ribs at the C7 vertebral level may result in thoracic outlet syndrome (111). During the evaluation of this patient population, one must attempt to differentiate the cervical rib from the presence of other congenital osseous defects previously described. Compression and irritation of the brachial plexus or the surrounding vascular structures requires immediate evaluation and treatment. Resnick (108) noted that 15% of patients with Klippel-Feil syndrome may have accessory cervical ribs, and most patients with the costal anomaly are women. Another report describes the association of Marfan's syndrome and a symptomatic cervical rib.

Whereas a large proportion of patients with a cervical rib are asymptomatic, some are aware of the osseous anomaly but suffer no functional impairment. A small proportion of patients present with thoracic outlet syndrome. If the thoracic outlet syndrome is present, the symptoms usually result from either neurologic or vascular involvement. The most common symptom of the thoracic outlet syndrome is pain in the distribution of the median or ulnar nerve or pain about the shoulder joint and neck (128). The pain is usually continuous and includes paresthesia, hyperesthesia, and anesthesia after

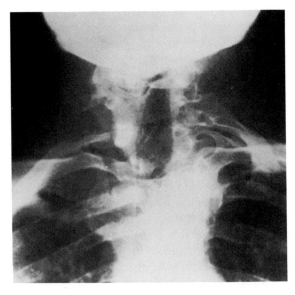

FIG. 11. Anteroposterior radiograph that displays multiple malformations of the cervical spine and cervical ribs.

strenuous upper limb exertion. The findings suggestive of vascular compression include a history of neck pain, pain in the upper limbs, or signs of vascular occlusion. An arteriogram of the affected side may reveal arterial stenosis as the subclavian artery passes superior or inferior to the cervical rib. During the physical examination the physician may occasionally palpate the cervical rib at the base of the neck. The examiner may also be able to reproduce the symptoms with the use of the Adson's test. The Adson's test is positive when a diminution of the radial pulse is detected after turning the head toward the affected side while the arm is placed in either a backward and downward direction or in hyperabduction (60). A minority of patients display symptoms after minor trauma to the involved area. In addition, persistent pruritus, located on the flexor aspect of the elbow and proximal forearm, may be suggestive of a cervical rib (110).

The treatment of a cervical rib usually involves conservative measures and patient education. If symptoms are present one may recommend several ameliorating measures. The use of exercises designed to lessen the compressive effect of the bony defect and anti-inflammatory medications have been shown to relieve the symptoms in a significant number of patients with thoracic outlet syndrome (52,119). The recommended exercises include proper posture while walking or running and active range-of-motion neck maneuvers. Occasionally, one may elect to brace the shoulders to alleviate the symptoms. The surgical removal of a cervical rib is necessary if symptoms do not respond to conservative measures or when significant neurologic or vascular compromise is observed. Operative intervention is rarely indicated because most of these patients remain asymptomatic throughout life.

Meningomyelocele

Spina bifida (meningomyelocele) in the cervical vertebral column is an extremely rare condition. In patients with meningomyelocele, it is not uncommon to find multiple congenital cervical anomalies, including vertebral artery anomalies, hemangiomas, dermoid tumors, frontonasal dysplasia, and congenital deafness (28,97). In meningomyelocele, the principle defect is the arrested development of the laminae. The developing neural structures are abnormal and there is myelodysplasia of the spinal cord. Cervical meningomyeloceles are frequently covered with full-thickness skin at the base and a tough, opaque, squamous epithelium at the dome (97). In contrast, thoracolumbar and lumbosacral meningomyelocele sacs are usually covered by thin arachnoid, not infrequently torn at birth. Unlike lower vertebral meningomyeloceles, cervical meningomyeloceles virtually never leak cerebrospinal fluid. When present, a neurologic deficit typically occurs caudal to the level of the

lesion. During the evaluation of cervical meningomyelocele and before surgical intervention, an evaluation for associated anomalies should be undertaken.

Treatment

The treatment and rehabilitation of patients with meningomyelocele is a long, complicated processes. The operative treatment of the primary defect in cervical meningomyelocele usually does not fall into the realm of the orthopedic surgeon. The neurosurgeon and orthopedic surgeon should work in concert to correct the underlying defect(s). Pang and Dias (97) recommend that initial surgical treatment should include a two-level laminectomy, intradural exploration, and, if present, excision of any tethering bands or septa. The care of each patient is individualized and centered around the extent of neural involvement and the presence of associated anomalies.

REFERENCES

1. Avery LW (1936): The Klippel-Feil syndrome: a pathological report. *Arch Neurol Psychiatry* 36:1068–1076.
2. Bauman GI (1932): Absence of the cervical spine: Klippel-Feil syndrome. *JAMA* 98:129–136.
3. Baurinck ON, Weaver DD (1983): Subclavian artery supply disruption sequence: hypothesis of a vascular etiology for Poland, Klippel-Feil syndrome, and mullerian anomalies. *Am J Med Genetics* 23:903–918.
4. Bergenhoff W (1958): Uber die messtechnische beurteilung der basilaren impression im rontgenbild. *Zentralbl Neurochir* 18:149–162.
5. Bernini FP, Elefante R, Smaltino F, Tedeschi G (1969): Angiographic study on the vertebral artery in cases of deformities of the occipitocervical joint. *Am J Roentgenol Radium Ther Nucl Med* 107:526–529.
6. Bharucha EP, Dastur HM (1964): Caraniovertebral anomalies (a report of 40 cases). *Brain* 87:469–480.
7. Black KS, Gorey MT, Seideman B, Scuderi DM, Cinnamon J, Hyman RA (1991): Congenital spondylolisthesis of the 6th cervical vertebrae: CT findings. *J Comput Tomogr* 15:335–337.
8. Blaw ME, Langer LO (1969): Spinal cord compression in morquio-brailsford's disease. *J Pediatr* 74:593–600.
9. Bull JWD, Nixon WLB, Pratt RTC (1955): Radiological criteria and familial occurence of primary basilar impression. *Brain* 229–247.
10. Cattel HS, Fitzer DL (1965): Pseudosubluxation and other normal variations in the cervical spine in children. *J Bone Joint Surg [Am]* 47:1295–1309.
11. Chakrabarti AK, Johnson SC, Samantray SK, Reddy ER (1974): Osteomalacia, myopathy and basilar impression. *J Neurol Sci* 23:227–235.
12. Chigira M, Kaneko K, Mashio K, Watanabe H (1994): Congenital hypoplasia of the arch of the atlas with abnormal segmentation of the cervical spine. *Arch Orthop Trauma Surg* 113:110–112.
13. Chamberlain WE (1939): Basilar impression (platybasia)—a bizarre developmental anomaly of the occipital bone and upper cervical spine with striking and misleading neurologic manifestations. *Yale J Biol Med* 11:487–486.
14. Cremers MJG, Bol E, Roos F, Gijn JV (1993): Risk of sports activities in children with Down's syndrome and atlantoaxial instability. *Lancet* 342:511–514.
15. Curtis BH, Blank S, Fisher RL (1968): Atlanto-axial dislocation in Down's syndrome. Report of two patients requiring surgical correction. *JAMA* 3205:464–465.

16. DeBarros MC, Farias W, Ata'ide L, Lins S (1968): Basilar impression and Arnold-Chiari malformation: A study of 66 cases. *J Neurol Neurosurg Psychiatry* 1:596–605.

17. Decker K, Fischgold H, Haker H, Metzger J (1956): Entwicklungsstorungen am atlanto-okzipitalen ubergang. *Fortschr Geb Rontgenstr* 84:47–57.

18. Dirheimer Y, Babin E (1971): Basilar impression and hereditary fragility of the bones. *Neuroradiology* 3:41–43.

19. Dolan KD (1977): Cervicobasilar relationships. *Radiol Clin North Am* 15:155–166.

20. Dolan KD (1977): Developmental abnormalities of the cervical spine below the axis. *Radiol Clin North Am* 15:167–175.

21. Dolan KD (1977): Expanding lesions of the cervical spinal canal. *Radiol Clin North Am* 15:203–214.

22. Douglas PS, Moos KF, Hislop WS (1992): Abnormal bone masses in Klippel-Feil syndrome. *Br J Oral Maxillofac Surg* 30:382–386.

23. Dubouset J (1986): Torticollis in children caused by congenital anomalies of the atlas. *J Bone Joint Surg [Am]* 68:178–188.

24. Duncan PA (1977): Embryologic pathogenesis of renal agenesis associated with cervical vertebral anomalies (Klippel-Feil phenotype). *Birth Defects* 13:91–101.

25. Durbin FC (1956): Spondylolisthesis of the cervical spine. *J Bone Joint Surg [Br]* 38:734–735.

26. Edwards MG, Wesolowski D, Benson MT, Wang AA (1991): Computed tomography of congenital spondylolisthesis of the sixth cervical vertebra. *Clin Imag* 15:191–195.

27. Epstein BS, Epstein JA (1969): The association of cerebellar tonsillar herniation with basilar impression incident to Paget's disease. *Am J Roentgenol Radium Ther Nucl Med* 107:535–542.

28. Erbengi A, Oge HK (1994): Congenital malformation of the craniovertebral junction: classification and surgical treatment. *Acta Neurochir* 127:180–185.

29. Fielding JW, Cochran GVB, Lawsing JF, Hohl M (1974): Tears of the transverse ligament of the atlas. A clinical and biomechanical study. *J Bone Joint Surg [Am]* 56:1683–1691.

30. Fielding JW, Hawkins RJ, Ratzan SA (1976): Spine fusion for atlanto-axial instability. *J Bone Joint Surg [Am]* 58:400–407.

31. Fielding JW, Hensinger RN, Hawkins RJ (1980): Os odontoideum. *J Bone Joint Surg [Am]* 62:376–383.

32. Finerman GA, Sakai D, Weingarten S (1976): Atlanto-axial dislocation with spinal cord compression in a mongoloid child. A case report. *J Bone Joint Surg [Am]* 58:408–409.

33. Fischgold H, Metzger J (1952): Etude radiotomographique de l'impression basilaire. *Rev Rhum Mal Osteoartic* 19:261–266.

34. Forsberg AA, Martinez S (1990): Cervical spondylolysis, imaging finding in 12 patients. *Am J Roentgenol Radium Ther Nucl Med* 154:751–755.

35. Frawley JM (1925): Congenital webbing. *Am J Dis Child* 29:799–809.

36. Fromm GH, Pitner SE (1963): Late progressive quadriparesis due to odontoid agenesis. *Arch Neurol* 9:291–296.

37. Frymoyer JW, Ducker TB, Hadler NM, Kostuik JP, Weinstein JN, Whitecloud TS III, eds. (1991): *The adult spine: principles and practice,* vol 2. New York: Raven Press, pp. 1017–1035.

38. Garber JN (1964): Abnormalities of the atlas and axis vertebrae: congenital and traumatic. *J Bone Joint Surg [Am]* 47:1782–1791.

39. Gartman JJ, Melin TE, Lawrence WT, Powers SK (1991): Deformity correction and long-term survival in an infant with iniencephaly. *J Neurosurg* 75:126–130.

40. Gechr RB, Rothman SLG, Kien EL (1978): The role of computed tomography in the evaluation of upper cervical spine pathology. *Comput Tomogr* 2:79–97.

41. Gehweiler JA, Daffner RH, Roberts L (1983): Malformation of the atlas vertebra simulating the Jefferson fracture. *Am J Roentgenol* 140:1083–1086.

42. Geipil P (1955): Zur kenntnis der spaltbidungen das atlas und epistropheus. Teil IV. *Zantralbl Allg Pathol* 94:19–84

43. Georgopoulos G, Pizzutillo PD, Lee MS (1987): Occipito-atlantal instability in children. A report of five cases and review of the literature. *J Bone Joint Surg [Am]* 69:429–436.

44. Gillman E (1959): Congenital absence of the odontoid process of the axis: report of a case. *J Bone Joint Surg [Am]* 41:345–348.

45. Glannestras NJ, Mayfield FH, Provencio FP, Maurer J (1964): Congenital absence of the odontoid process. A case report. *J Bone Joint Surg [Am]* 46:839–843.

46. Gray SW, Romaine CB, Pascoe DJ (1965): Congenital fusion of the cervical vertebrae. *Surg Gyneco Obstet* 118:373–385.

47. Greenberg AD (1968): Atlanto-axial dislocations. *Brain* 91:655–684.

48. Greenberg AD, Scoville WB, Davey LM (1968): Transoral decompression of atlanto-axial dislocation due to odontoid hypoplasia. Report of two cases. *J Neurosurg* 28:266–269.

49. Greene RA, Bloch MJ, Huff DS, Iozzo RV (1986): MURCS association with additional anomalies. *Hum Pathol* 17:88–91.

50. Guillane J, Roulleau J, Fardou H, Trail J, Manelfe C (1976): Congenital spondylolysis of cervical vertebrae with spondylolisthesis. *Neuroradiology* 11:159–168.

51. Gwinn JL, Smith JL (1962): Acquired and congenital absence of the odontoid process. *Am J Roentgenol* 88:424–431.

52. Haggart GE (1948): Value of conservative management in cervico-brachial pain. *JAMA* 137:508–512.

53. Harley EH, Collins MD (1994): Neurologic sequelae secondary to atlantoaxial instability in down syndrome. *Arch Otolaryngol Head Neck Surg* 120:159–165.

54. Hensinger RN (1986): Osseous anomalies of the craniovertebral junction. *Spine* 11:323–333.

55. Hensinger RN (1991) Congenital anomalies of the cervical spine. *Clin Orthop* 264:16–38.

56. Hensinger RN, Fielding JW, Hawkins RJ (1978): Congenital anomalies of the odontoid process. *Orthop Clin North Am* 9:901–912.

57. Hensinger RN, MacEwen GD (1982): Congenital anomalies of the spine. In: Rothman RH, Simone FA, eds. *The spine,* 2nd ed. Philadelphia: WB Saunders Company, pp. 188–216.

58. Hinck VC, Hopkins CE, Savara BS (1961): Diagnostic criteria of basilar impression. *Radiology* 76:572–585.

59. Hinck VC, Hopkins CE, Savara BS (1962): Sagittal diameter of the cervical spinal canal in children. *Radiology* 79:97–108.

60. Hoppenfeld S (1976): *Physical examination of the spine and extremities.* Norwalk: Appleton-Century-Crofts, p. 127.

61. Ivie, J (1946): Congenital absence of the odontoid process. Report of a case. *Radiology* 46:268–269.

62. Jeffreys TE (1980): *Disorders of the cervical spine.* London: Butterworths pp. 35–37.

63. Kane RJ, O'Connor AF, Morrison AW (1982): Primary basilar impression. An aetiological factor in Meniere's disease. *J Laryngol Otol* 96:931–936.

64. Karlen A (1962): Congenital hypoplasia of the odontoid process. *J Bone Joint Surg [Am]* 44:567–570.

65. Klaus E (1957): Roatgendiagnostik der platybasic und basilaren impression. Weitere Enfahrungen mit einer never untersuchungsmetnode. *Fortschr Geb Rontgenstr* 86:460–469.

66. Kline DG (1966): Atlanto-axial dislocation simulating a head injury: hypoplasia of the odontoid. Case report. *J Neurosurg* 24:1013–1016.

67. Klippel M, Feil AL (1912): Anomalie de la colonne vertebrale par absence dis vertebrae cervicales. *Bull Soc Arthrop* 65:101–109.

68. Kosher RA (1976): Inhibition of "spontaneous", notochord induced, and collagen induced in vitro somite chondrogenesis by cyclic AMP derivatives and theophylline. *Dev Biol* 53:265–276.

69. Kulkarni MV, Williams JC, Yeakley JW, et al. (1987): Magnetic resonance imaging in the diagnosis of the cranio-cervical manifestations of the mucopolysaccharidoses. *Mag Reson Imag* 5:317–323.

70. Lipson SJ (1977): Dysplasia of the odontoid process in morquio's syndrome causing quadriparesis. *J Bone Joint Surg [Am]* 59:340–344.

71. Locke GR, Gardner JI, Van Epps EF (1966): Atlas-dens interval (ADI) in children: a survey based on 200 normal cervical spines. *Am J Roentgenol Radium Ther Nucl Med* 97:135–140.

72. Luyendij KW, Marticoli B, Thomeer R (1978): Basilar impression in an achondroplastic dwarf. Causative role in tetraparesis. *Acta Neurochir* 41:243–25.

73. Mace SE, Holiday R (1986): Congenital absence of the C-1 vertebral arch. *Am J Emerg Med* 4:326–329.

74. MacEwen GD, Winter RB, Hardy JH (1972): Evaluation of kid-

ney anomalies in congenital scoliosis. *J Bone Joint Surg [Am]* 54:1451–1454.

75. Marcotte P, Dickman CA, Sonntag VKH, Karahalios DG, Drabier J (1993): Posterior atlantoaxial facet screw fixation. *J Neurosurg* 79:234–237.

76. Marijke JG, Cremers MD, Beifer HJM (1993): No relation between general laxity and atlantoaxial instability in children with down syndrome. *J Pediatr Orthop* 13:318–321.

77. Marks P, Mills B, West L (1994): Basilar invagination and midline skeletal abnormalities due to in utero exposure to phenytoin. *Br J Neurosurg* 8:365–368.

78. Martel W, Tishler JM (1966): Observations on the spine in mongoloidism. *Am J Roentgenol Radium Ther Nucl Med* 97:630–638.

79. McAfee PC, Bohlman HH, Han JS, Salvagno RT (1986): Comparison of nuclear magnetic resonance imaging and computed tomography in the diagnosis of upper cervical spinal cord compression. *Spine* 11:295–304.

80. McElfresh E, Winter R (1973): Klippel-Feil syndrome. *Minn Med* 56:353–357.

81. McGregor M (1948): The significance of certain measurements of the skull in the diagnosis of basilar impression. *Br J Radiol* 21:171–176.

82. McKeever FM (1968): Atlanto-axial instability. *Surg Clin North Am* 48:1375–1390.

83. McLay K, Maran AG (1969): Deafness and the Klippel-Feil syndrome. *J Laryngol Otol* 83:175–184.

84. McRae DL (1953): Bony abnormalities in the region of the foramen magnum: correction of the anatomic and neurologic findings. *Acta Radiol* 40:335–342.

85. McRae DL (1960): The significance of abnormalities of the cervical spine. *Am J Roentgenol Radium Ther Nucl Med* 84:3–11.

86. McRae DL, Barnum AS (1953): Occipitalization of the atlas. *Am J Roentgenol* 70:23–46.

87. Michie I, Clark M (1968): Neurological syndromes associated with cervical and craniocervical anomalies. *Arch Neurol* 18:241–247.

88. Minderhoud JM, Braakman R, Pening L (1969): Os odontoideum. clinical, radiological, and therapeutic aspects. *J Neurol Sci* 8:521–544.

89. Moore WB, Matthews TJ, Rabinowitz R (1975): Genitourinary anomalies associated with Klippel-Feil syndrome. *J Bone Joint Surg [Am]* 57:355–357.

90. Morey I (1986): Prenatal diagnosis and pathoanatomy of iniencephaly. *Clin Genet* 30:81–86.

91. Morizono Y, Sakou T, Machara T (1987): Congenital defect of posterior elements of the axis. *Clin Orthop* 216:120–123.

92. Morrison SG, Perry LW, Scott LP III (1968): Congenital brevicollis (Klippel-Feil syndrome) and cardiovascular anomalies. *Am J Dis Child* 115:614–620.

93. Munden MM, Macpherson RI, Cure J (1993): Iniencephaly:3D-computed tomography imaging. *Pediatr Radiol* 23:572.

94. Nagashima C (1970): Atlanto-axial dislocation due to agenesis of the os odontoideum or odontoid. *J Neurosurg* 33:270–280.

95. Nora JJ (1961): Klippel-Feil syndrome with congenital heart disease. *Am J Dis Child* 102:110–117.

96. Palant DI, Carter BL (1972): Klippel-Feil syndrome and deafness. A study with polytomography. *Am J Dis Child* 123:218–221.

97. Pang D, Dias MS (1993): Cervical myelomeningoceles. *Neurosurgery* 33:363–373.

98. Payne EE (1957): The cervical spine: An anatomic-pathological study of 70 specimens using a special technique with particular reference to the problem of cervical spondylosis. *Brain* 80:571–596.

99. Perez HJ, Tella BP, Herrera ML, Rodriquez VJ (1970): Klippel-Feil syndrome associated with horseshoe kidney and brown and white spots. *Rev Clin Esp* 119:263–275.

100. Perovic MN, Kopits SE, Thompson RC (1973): Radiologic evaluation of the spinal canal in congenital atlanto-axial dislocations. *Radiology* 109:713–716.

101. Pizzutillo PD, Woods MW, Nicholson L (1987): Risk factors in the Klippel-Feil syndrome. *Ortho Trans* 11:473–482.

102. Pizzutillo PD, Woods M, Nicholson L, MacEwen GD (1994): Risk factors in Klippel-Feil syndrome. *Spine* 19:2110–2116.

103. Prusick VR, Samberg LC, Wesolowski DP (1985): Klippel-Feil syndrome associated with spinal stenosis. A case report. *J Bone Joint Surg [Am]* 67:161–164.

104. Pueschel SM, Scola FH (1987): Atlantoaxial instability in individuals with down syndrome: epidemiologic, radiographic, and clinical studies. *Pediatrics* 80:555–560.

105. Ramsey J, Bliznak J (1971): Klippel-Feil syndrome with renal agenesis and other anomalies. *Am J Roentgenol Radium Ther Nucl Med* 113:460–463.

106. Raynor RB (1989): Congenital malformations of the base of the skull: the arnold chiari malformation. In: *The cervical spine*, 2nd ed. Philadelphia: JB Lippincott, pp. 226–235.

107. Resjo IM, Harwood-Nash DC, Fitz CR, Chuang S (1979): Normal cord in infants and children examined with computed tomographic metrizamide myelography. *Radiology* 130:691–696.

108. Resnick D (1988): Additional congenital or heritable anomalies and syndromes. In: Resnick D, Niwayama eds. *Diagnosis of bone and joint disorders.* Philadelphia: Saunders pp.124–145

109. Rogers JM, Mole ML, Chernoff N, et al. (1993): The developmental toxicity of inhaled methanol in the CD-1 mouse, with quantitative dose-response modeling for estimation of benchmark doses. *Tetrology* 47:175–188.

110. Rongioletti F (1992): Pruritus as presenting sign of cervical rib. *Lancet* 339:55.

111. Roos D (1976): Congenital anomalies associated with thoracic outlet syndrome: anatomy, symptoms. *Am J Surg* 132:771–784.

112. Rosen CL, Novotny EJ, D'Andrea LA, Petty EM (1993): Klippel-Feil sequence and sleep-disordered breathing in two children. *Am Rev Respir Dis* 147:202–204.

113. Rowland LP, Shapiro JH, Jacobson HG (1958): Neurological syndromes associated with congenital absence of the odontoid process. *Arch Neurol Psychiatry* 80:286–291.

114. Sagher O, Malik JM, Lee JH, Shaffrey CI, Shaffrey ME, Szabo TA, Jane JA (1993): Fusion with occipital bone for atlantoaxial instability. *Neurosurgery* 33:926–928.

115. Schapera J (1987): Autosomal dominant inheritance of cervical ribs. *Clin Genet* 31:386–388.

116. Schiff DC, Parke WW (1973): The arterial blood supply of the odontoid process. *J Bone Joint Surg [Am]* 55:1450–1456.

117. Shapiro R, Youngberg AS, Rothman SL (1973): The differential diagnosis of traumatic lesions of the occipio-atlanto-axial segment. *Radiol Clin North Am* 11:505–526.

118. Sherk HH, Shut L (1976): Correction of neck deformities in iniencephaly. *Jefferson Orthop J* 5:51–55.

119. Sherk HH, Shut L, Chung, S (1974): Iniencephalic deformity of the cervical spine with Klippel-Feil anomalies and congenital elevation of the scapula: report of three cases. *J Bone Joint Surg [Am]* 56:1254–1259.

120. Spierings EL, Braakman R (1982): The management of os odontoideum: analysis of 37 cases. *J Bone Joint Surg [Br]* 64:422–428.

121. Spillane K, Nagendran K, Pedoe DST (1993): Marfan's syndrome in association with cervical rib syndrome. *Muscle Nerve* 16:979.

122. Spillane JD, Pallis C, Jones AM (1957): Developmental abnormalities in the region of the foramen magnum. *Brain* 80:11–48.

123. Stabler CL, Eismont FJ, Brown MD, Green BA, Malinin TI (1985): Failure of posterior cervical fusions using cadaveric bone graft in children. *J Bone Joint Surg [Am]* 67:371–375.

124. Stark EW, Borton TE (1972): Hearing loss and the Klippel-Feil syndrome. *Am J Dis Child* 123:233–235.

125. Steel HH (1968): Anatomical and mechanical considerations of the atlanto-axial articulations. *J Bone Joint Surg [Am]* 50:1481–1482.

126. Stratford J (1957): Myelopathy caused by atlanto-axial dislocation. *J Neurosurg* 14:97–104.

127. Tachdjian MO, ed. (1990): *Pediatric Orthopaedics,* 2nd ed. Philadelphia: WB Saunders, p. 129.

128. Takagi K, Yamage M, Morisawa K, Kitagawa T (1987): Management of thoracic outlet syndrome. *Arch Orthop Trauma Surg* 106:78–81.

129. Taylor AR, Chakravorty BC (1964): Clinical syndromes associated with basilar impression. *Arch Neurol* 10:475–484.

130. Tokgozoglu AM, Alpaslan AM (1994): Congenital spondylolisthesis in the upper spinal column. Management of two cases. *Spine* 19:99–102.

131. Tredwell SJ, Smith DF, Macleod PJ, Wood BJ (1982): Cervical spine anomalies in fetal alcohol syndrome. *Spine* 7:331–334.

132. Truex RC, Johnson CH (1978): Congenital anomalies of the upper cervical spine. *Orthop Clin North Am* 9:891–900.

133. Ulmer JL, Elster AD, Ginsberg LE, Williams DW (1993): Klippel-Feil syndrome: CT and MR of acquired and congenital abnormalities of cervical spine and cord. *J Comput Assist Tomogr* 17:215–224.

134. von Torklus D, Gehle W (1972): *The upper cervical spine.* New York: Grune & Stratton, pp.254–279.

135. Wadia NH (1967): Myelopathy complicating congenital atlanto-axial dislocation. (A study of 28 cases). *Brain* 90:449–472.

136. Weiler HG (1942): Congenital absence of odontoid process of the axis with atlantoaxial dislocation. *J Bone Joint Surg* 24:161–165.

137. Whitecloud TS III, Brinker MR (1992): Congenital anomalies of the base of the skull and the atlanto-axial joint. In: Camins MB, O'Leary PF, eds. *Disorders of the cervical spine.* Baltimore: Williams and Wilkins, pp. 199–211.

138. Wilson WG, Randall ME, Babler WJ (1985): Palatal anteversion as part of the iniencephaly malformation sequence. *J Craniofac Genet Dev Biol* 5:5–10.

139. Winter RB, Moe JH, Lonstein JE (1984): The incidence of Klippel-Feil syndrome in patients with congenital scoliosis and kyphosis. *Spine* 9:363–366.

140. Winter RB, Moe JH, Wang JF (1973): Congenital kyphosis. Its natural history and treatment as observed in a study of one-hundred and thirty patients. *J Bone Joint Surg [Am]* 55:223–256.

141. Wolin DG (1963): The os odontoideum. Separate odontoid process. *J Bone Joint Surg [Am]* 45:1459–1471.

The Adult Spine: Principles and Practice,
2nd edition, J.W. Frymoyer, Editor-in-Chief.
Lippincott-Raven Publishers, Philadelphia © 1997.

CHAPTER 58

Diagnosis and Treatment of Congenital Neurologic Abnormalities Affecting the Cervical Spine

Francis W. Gamache, Jr.

There are congenital neurologic abnormalities that may affect the structure or function of the cervical spine, and the one that concerns the clinician most often is Arnold-Chiari malformation with or without syringomyelia. The higher bony deformities are all discussed in other chapters. In those diseases, there are abnormalities found on neurologic examination and a characteristic radiographic appearance. This chapter is intended to provide a practical update of the more common disorders of the nervous system.

DIAGNOSIS

Clinical (Neurologic) Examination

Unfortunately, there are no neurologic findings on examination that are pathognomonic for a congenital spinal cord disorder. The clinician must integrate the information from the patient's history and physical examination with the findings obtained from diagnostic testing. Table 1 provides a simplified summary of neurologic findings that may be helpful in localizing the level

F. W. Gamache, Jr., M.D.: Associate Professor, Department of Surgery, The New York Hospital—Cornell Medical Center, New York, New York, 10021.

of the problem affecting the cervical spine. The C1 and C2 nerve roots usually have no disc component ventral to them. All the remaining cervical roots are susceptible to encroachment by disc herniation or degenerative changes. Disc herniations most frequently occur at C7, followed by C6 and then C8 (58). Multilevel disc herniation is distinctly uncommon in the neck, and compression of roots by degenerative (spondylitic) disease is two to three times as frequent as disc compression (58). While the clinician is faced frequently with the common problems of disc herniation and degenerative disease of the neck, these facts must be kept in mind when patients present in a fashion involving multiple levels or in a manner in which spondylosis is an unlikely explanation for the patient's problem. Pain in the area of the back of the head has been attributed to the greater occipital nerve and referred to as "occipital neuralgia." Operations directed at relieving this condition with occipital neurectomy generally have not been successful. On the other hand, unilateral painful arthrosis of the atlantoaxial joint may present with ipsilateral suboccipital pain and point tenderness over the area of the abnormality, with limited motion of the neck. This condition is frequently relieved by a small amount of local anesthetic applied to the posterior aspect of the atlantoaxial joint.

Cervical roots 5, 6, 7, and 8 as well as the first thoracic

TABLE 1. *Summary of neurologic findings*

Root	Area of sensation affected	Major muscle affected	Comments
C1	Usually no sensory component	Nuchal	Not susceptible to disc encroachment
C2	Face bordering trigeminal skin zone to "high collar" area	Nuchal/strap	
C3-C4	Side of neck to corner of shoulder, clavicle-shoulder	Diaphragm/nuchal strap, rhomboids	Single root lesion, generally causes no significant motor loss
C5	Biceps, radial arm	Supraspinatus, infraspinatus, deltoid, biceps	Decrease of biceps reflex, pain may mimic angina
C6	Thumb, index finger	Extensor carpi rad brachioradialis	Decrease of biceps/brachioradialis reflexes
C7	Index, middle finger	Triceps, latissimus dorsi, pectoralis maj, ext. carpi ulnaris, ext. digitorum	Decrease in triceps reflex
C8	Fourth, fifth fingers	Wrist/finger flexors, intrinsic hand muscles	

root supply the arm and hand via the anterior primary divisions of the spinal nerves and brachial plexus. The paraspinal muscles are innervated by the posterior divisions of these spinal nerves. Irritation of any of these lower cervical roots produces pain in the base of the neck, scapular region, and shoulder (2). Thus, the precise level of involvement usually may not be determined simply by noting the distribution of pain, muscle tenderness, or neck position. Of note, lesions involving the T1 root may produce weakness of intrinsic hand muscles as well as ptosis, miosis, or anhydrosis.

Neurophysiologic Testing

Electromyography/nerve conduction velocity (EMG/NCV) testing may help confirm findings identified on a neurologic examination. Abnormalities in these tests frequently require days (NCV) or weeks (EMG) of neurologic dysfunction before the test patterns become frankly abnormal. Many weeks must pass after an offending lesion is removed before the EMG pattern may return to normal. Similarly, in senior citizens who routinely harbor degenerative changes in the neck, mild baseline abnormalities in EMG/NCV should be anticipated. Particularly in these patients or patients with an old injury, another pathologic process beginning in the cervical spine will make interpretation of EMG/NCV findings difficult. As a result, changes in the EMG/NCV frequently are not pathognomonic.

Routine somatosensory evoked potentials (SSEP) may not be able to localize a neurologic problem to the cervical spinal cord. At times it is difficult electrophysiologically to pinpoint the level of dysfunction to the brachial plexus, cervical spinal cord, or medulla. Emerson and Pedley (22) have suggested the use of additional recording electrodes and recording points to delineate cervical cord pathology. A normal SSEP response does not rule out anterior spinal cord pathology. In fact, in more than 1,000 patients undergoing spinal surgery at this institution, where SSEP studies were employed, five alarms were triggered suggesting neurologic dysfunction. All alarms were found to be the result of technical errors involving electrode malfunction. One patient did awaken with weakness in a lower extremity despite fully normal SSEP tracings throughout surgery. Motor evoked responses as well as magnetic evoked responses remain largely experimental procedures for preoperative or intraoperative diagnosis of spinal cord dysfunction (personal communication, Dr. Michael Rubin, Director, Neurophysiology Laboratory).

Radiographic Evaluation

Plain films of the spine are still quite useful in providing information regarding basic anatomic abnormalities involving the cervical spine, such as spina bifida, malformed vertebrae, fused vertebrae (a single unit or in blocks), and malalignment. Anteroposterior, lateral, and oblique films provide basic information about structure but not about motion of the spine (9). For that reason, voluntary gentle flexion-extension views are frequently useful, particularly in the case of congenital abnormalities that may cause hypermobility or instability, such as Klippel-Feil syndrome, Down syndrome, or neurofibromatosis, which may cause abnormal motion segments in the cervical spine.

Computed tomography (CT) of the cervical spine with or without myelography has been the radiographic cornerstone for the diagnosis and evaluation of bony malformations, meningoceles, or parenchymal spinal cord pathology. In the case of cavitary lesions of the cervical spine, myelography with CT frequently is necessary (66).

Magnetic resonance imaging (MRI) is especially useful in the diagnosis of abnormalities of the nervous system at the skull base and cervical spine. However, this diagnostic modality is frequently not available on an emergency basis and is still not available to all clinicians on demand. Where available, MR scanning has replaced myelography and CT in many instances. Because cerebrospinal fluid (CSF) appears bright on T2-weighted images, T2 views are especially useful for documenting spinal cord compression. T1-weighted images provide better morphologic detail about the cord, helping to provide useful pathoanatomic information such as cyst formation. Many radiologists believe that good-quality MRI scans in combination with plain films make CT and/or myelography unnecessary. The exception to this rule, however, would be the evaluation of syringomyelia or neurofibromatosis with an associated curvature (i.e., scoliosis), for which MR images are deformed. In this situation, myelography with post-myelography CT through individual segments of the cervical scoliosis provides useful information. Perhaps through better resolution of MRI in the future, myelogram/CT may be unnecessary. Where issues of instability are concerned, MR images taken in rapid sequence with the patient flexing or extending the neck ("dynamic MRI") provide extremely useful information. However, the diameter of the MRI unit limits the amount of flexion-extension.

Surgical Exploration

A clear diagnosis of a problem may not always rest with simply ascertaining the presence of an abnormality on the above-mentioned radiographic studies. Occasionally, tumor is suggested in the spinal canal based on a vague abnormality identified on one or more imaging techniques. In these instances, surgical exploration may become necessary to confirm or refute the diagnosis. In some cases, tumor may have been suspected but not found at surgical exploration; the cause of the imaging abnormality is speculative, although contrast enhancement of multiple sclerosis plaques may be one cause of "misinterpreted tumor." On the other hand, overinterpretation of an MRI finding may lead to unnecessary surgical exploration (i.e., negative exploration for a lesion that did not exist). One is thus cautioned about proceeding with surgical procedures based on minimal radiographic documentation of such lesions. Although MRI is extremely useful, the meaning of some findings remains to be elucidated. It is frequently useful to have other confirmatory imaging information and compelling clinical reasons before proceeding with a surgical exploration. However, in certain and undoubtedly rare circumstances, the ultimate diagnostic test may have to rest in such an exploratory approach.

DISEASES

Syringomyelia

Syringomyelia is a condition defined by the presence of a fluid-filled cavity within the substance of the spinal cord. The condition may develop from traumatic injury

to the spinal cord, may be related to tumor in the spinal cord, or may follow arachnoiditis. Most commonly the condition is associated with congenital malformations such as meningomyelocele or Chiari malformation, or may develop idiopathically. In Chapter 57, the four types of Arnold-Chiari malformation are presented. An uncertain number of nontraumatic syringes appear to communicate with the fourth ventricle, especially those associated with the various Chiari malformations. In the case of post-traumatic syrinx, the cavity within the spinal cord usually does not communicate with the fourth ventricle. Because of the variety of anatomic locations in which syringes begin within the spinal cord, as well as the variation with time and anatomic direction in which they grow, patients may present with a variety of complaints or neurologic symptoms. Classic teaching has been that because of the central location of the cavitation within the spinal cord, commonly in the cervical area, the lesion interrupts ascending pain and temperature pathways from each side of the body. A resultant loss of pain and temperature sensibility in a segmental distribution in the upper extremities thus follows, whereas proprioception and simple touch are usually spared. As the disease progresses and extends to the anterior gray horns of the spinal cord, weakness and atrophy of muscles innervated by the involved anterior horns will be demonstrated. A pattern of muscle wasting in the upper extremities, with capelike sensory loss in the upper extremities as well, has been considered diagnostic of syringomyelia.

Presently, with the widespread use of MR scanning of the head and neck, the classic findings are no longer being reported by clinicians because the diagnosis is made earlier. Motor and sensory symptoms remain frequent (6,80), but pain is a common complaint early in the disease in many patients (6,37,38,47). The mean age at presentation is approximately 32 years, with patients complaining of diffuse pain rather than a radicular pain.

On neurologic examination, the combination of pain and sensory dysfunction in a syringomyelic pattern has been found in approximately 50% to 80% of patients (7,10,13,38,47,51,72,79). An associated scoliosis is often present early in the disease and is frequently centered in the upper thoracic spine (13,37). It is not unusual for sensory and motor findings to develop after the observation of the scoliosis.

Plain film examination of the cervical spine should always be obtained. Historically, further radiologic evaluation has involved myelography with delayed CT scanning performed approximately 12 to 24 hours after myelography (3,66). Today, MRI has generally become the neurodiagnostic imaging study of choice. In those individuals with scoliotic curves, for which an MR image may be deformed, myelography with delayed CT remains the standard for neuroradiographic evaluation.

Multiple surgical procedures have been advocated for the treatment of syringomyelia. These procedures in-

clude posterior fossa decompression by suboccipital craniectomy, with cervical laminectomy as necessary and
some form of duraplasty. The advantages of large, medium, or small duraplasty reconstruction continue to be
debated (41,61,71). The decision to perform additional
procedures in the posterior fossa such as tonsillectomy,
fourth ventricular shunting, or other diversionary
procedures remains controversial (7,13,25,31,48,67).
Laminectomy and myelotomy remain other primary
procedures used for the treatment of these lesions. Percutaneous aspiration of the syrinx has been found to provide temporary relief in nearly 40% of cases, although the
explanation for this phenomenon remains unclear (67).

Various shunting procedures of the syrinx itself—
syringosubarachnoid (SS) shunt, syringopleural shunt,
and syringoperitoneal (SP) shunt—have also gained favor recently (45,46,64,77). However, a critical review of
drainage procedures for syrinx cavities has caused them
to be discouraged by some (74). Indirect shunting of the
syrinx by means of ventricular shunting (VS) was introduced in 1969 by Benini and Krayenbuhl (10). This has
not gained widespread favor, however, and the follow-up
reported in 1974 was generally very brief (43).

In patients with hindbrain malformation, primary
shunting of the syrinx has been considered by some to be
contraindicated because of the possibility of precipitating additional hindbrain herniation. Wisoff (80), however, did not find this to be a problem when using syringopleural shunts as the primary procedure in dysraphic
children presenting with hydromyelia. Tator et al. (77)
had the same experience and recently commented that
"drainage of the syrinx should be the primary surgical
procedure."

The natural history of untreated syringomyelia remains unclear (7,11,47). This is probably due to the generally short period of follow-up for patients with this diagnosis. One series with excellent long-term follow-up is
that of Boman and Iivanainen (12); they reported on 55
patients, some of whom were followed for 40 years. Just
under half of those patients were stable with regard to
their disease for up to 10 years. On the other hand, more
than half of the patients had gradual progression of
symptoms over a period of 2 to 45 years. Of the 55 patients, 43 had changes in the anatomy of the spine, such
as scoliosis (12). Thus, length of follow-up contributes
substantially to the clinical definition of the neurologic
implications of syringomyelia (1). Brief follow-up may
falsely suggest arrest of syringomyelia (6).

Probably because of the variation in follow-up, one
may find various surgical series treating hydromyelia
with Chiari malformations with rates of improvement or
stabilization ranging from 10% to 90% (7,25,31,47,
48,51,67,72,77).

It is interesting that patients may remain remarkably
intact neurologically despite considerable distortion of
the spinal cord observed on CT or MRI scanning. Per-

haps earlier diagnosis and treatment may lead to more
satisfactory results. Nevertheless, in view of the variations in the natural history, anatomy, treatment, and follow-up periods reported to date, very few firm conclusions regarding syringomyelia may be drawn. Generally,
no single surgical procedure predictably remedies syringomyelia for the long term. This was suggested by me in
1990 (29) and by other authors recently (74). Frequently,
multiple procedures are required. Direct treatment of the
syrinx cavity makes intuitive sense, particularly for those
syringes that do not communicate with the fourth ventricle. Because a syrinx cavity may be septated, complete
drainage may require attention to more than one area of
the lesion.

To complete the frustrating nature of the problem,
even when the syrinx cavity may be totally drained, not
all of the patient's symptoms necessarily clear, and sometimes may progress. The ultimate treatment for syringomyelia thus remains to be defined. Recent reviews may
be consulted for additional updated information regarding the pathophysiology and neurologic and surgical aspects of syringomyelia (29,55,61). The reported cases of
Oldfield et al. (61) are too few (seven) and too recent
(1994) to allow any long-term observations. The present
author has experienced mixed results (as with other techniques) using the procedure redescribed by Oldfield et al.
of post-fossa and cervical decompression (61).

Klippel-Feil Syndrome

Klippel-Feil syndrome refers to patients with congenital fusion of cervical vertebrae. It is a bony anomaly,
as discussed in Chapter 57, that may be associated with
neurologic problems (5,39,40,42,50). In this syndrome,
the bony problem may include two segments or the entire cervical spine.

The neurologic symptoms are generally localized to
the head, neck, and arms as a result of irritation or impingement of the cervical nerve roots (34). With time,
the neural foramina become compromised by osteophytes. This may be compounded by instability of the
motion segment because of repetitive trauma over time.
Findings range from cervical radiculopathy with mild
spasticity in the lower extremities, to hyporeflexia and
frank myelopathy with muscular weakness in the upper
extremities and gross spasticity in the lower extremities
secondary to spinal cord and root compression.

Patients with a mild degree of fusion of the cervical
spine should be expected to lead a normal life (5). On the
other hand, those patients with severely involved spines
have a better prognosis if early preventive measures are
taken to avoid the complications resulting from undue
stress or compression of the nervous system. The role of
prophylactic surgical stabilization in the asymptomatic
patient remains controversial. In a small percentage of

patients, however, when instability is documented, reduction of misalignment and surgical stabilization are appropriate. Either the anterior or posterior approach to treat myelopathy, outlined in Chapters 64 and 65, may be appropriate.

Surgical intervention, however, may be dangerous if other associated abnormalities of the brainstem and spinal cord have not been considered during the patient's work-up. This involves a team effort of neurologists, neurosurgeons, and orthopaedists working together (68).

Medical treatment for the hidden and often unrecognized associated anomalies, including scoliosis, renal abnormalities, cardiac abnormalities, and hearing problems, may provide more benefit to the patient than preoccupation with the cervical fusion itself (4,27, 52,56,57,60,62).

Congenital Atlantoaxial Instability

This problem is discussed in Chapter 55. However, the bony anomalies can be associated with other anomalies. Congenital scoliosis, Down syndrome, bone dysplasias, osteogenesis imperfecta, and neurofibromatosis are all capable of producing important degrees of atlantoaxial instability. In Down syndrome, approximately 20% of patients have been found to have laxity of the transverse atlantal ligament (TAL) (49,76). These patients appear to have attenuation or rupture of the transverse ligament with reduction of the space available to the spinal cord. As long as the alar ligaments remain intact, they may limit movement of the odontoid process and help to prevent spinal cord compression. With time and chronic stress, however, the alar ligaments may become incompetent, and cord compression then develops. Similar findings occur in neurofibromatosis and the other disorders listed above.

Patients may present neurologically with a puzzling clinical picture characterized by intermittent pain, numbness, and weakness in the arms or legs. Should the medulla be indented by the odontoid, the patient may present with cranial nerve palsies and/or respiratory difficulties. If the vertebral arteries are compressed, a clinical picture of syncope may develop.

Whereas the normal space seen on the lateral roentgenogram between the anterior aspect of the dens and the posterior aspect of the anterior ring of the atlas (ADI) is usually no more than 3 mm in the adult, patients with chronic atlantoaxial instability (AAI) (e.g., congenital anomalies, rheumatoid arthritis, Down syndrome, neurofibromatosis) may present with a larger ADI. Because of these conditions, the odontoid is frequently found to be hypermobile, particularly in flexion. Surprisingly, however, few patients are symptomatic (18). This is because the more important space for the spinal cord is the space available between the posterior aspect of the odontoid and the posterior arch of the atlas. Because this distance may change with flexion or extension, flexion-extension views should be performed routinely in a gentle manner on each patient suspected of having AAI. For those patients with formation of abnormal bone, CT may be useful. With the advent of MRI scanning, radiolucent soft-tissue masses posterior to the odontoid, such as those occurring in rheumatoid arthritis, may be well imaged and help to explain what otherwise might be neurologic dysfunction in a seemingly adequate-size canal. Anatomic studies by McRae (53) and Greenberg (35) revealed that spinal cord compression invariably occurs when this distance is 14 mm or less. When soft-tissue masses may exist and MRI scanning is not available, myelography with post-myelography CT may be extremely useful in further identifying intracanalicular anatomy.

The role of prophylactic surgical stabilization in patients with documented congenital AAI is reviewed in Chapter 55. If marked instability is demonstrated or the patient is frankly symptomatic neurologically, there is general agreement that surgical fusion (posterior) of C1 and C2 is appropriate and sufficient. Because respiratory dysfunction occurs more frequently in these patients than anticipated (33,44), pulmonary function testing preoperatively is well advised. In addition, attention should be addressed to compromise of lower cranial nerve function, as preoperative tracheostomy may also be necessary. Before surgical intervention, reduction of the atlantoaxial malalignment is best achieved by traction (26,30). Operative reduction without preoperative realignment has been associated with increased morbidity and mortality (75,78). The patient should be left in the reduced position preoperatively until improvement or stabilization of the neurologic condition has been observed. Should no neurologic improvement appear, additional neurologic work-up may be necessary. For those cases in which an abnormality in C1 may also be associated with TAL abnormality, an occiput-to-C2 stabilization may be necessary.

Scoliosis is a well-recognized feature of von Recklinghausen's neurofibromatosis, occurring in approximately one-quarter of such patients. Whereas the spine deformity in neurofibromatosis may lead to the neurologic problems described above, the scoliotic deformity infrequently involves the cervical spine. As a result, a more detailed description of neurofibromatosis and scoliosis will be found in Chapter 73.

Chiari Malformation

The eponym *Arnold-Chiari* historically is incorrect, because it was Cleland in 1883 (17) who first described and illustrated downward displacement of the cerebellum as well as deformity of the medulla. Chiari acknowledged Cleland's work and further described these lesions in 1891 (15) and 1895 (16). Arnold's contribution consisted of a later case report of an infant with multiple abnormalities, including a "ribbon-like" herniation of cerebellar tissue into the midcervical spine (2). Arnold did not provide details regarding the nature of the cerebellar tissue or any associated brainstem abnormalities. Colleagues of Arnold proposed that the term *Arnold-Chiari malformation* be used to designate the cerebellar herniation with brainstem deformity, disregarding Cleland's original work (73). Thus, the term was commonly used and became implanted in medical terminology despite attempts to rename the entity the Cleland-Chiari malformation. The individual subtypes are reviewed in detail in Chapter 55.

Abnormalities of the skull and cervical spine associated with a Chiari malformation are common. The Chiari malformation, though congenital, may remain silent and be discovered accidentally during routine CT or MRI studies of the cranial cervical junction performed for evaluation of other problems. In a review by Garcin and Oeconomos (32), 60% of their cases were documented between the second and third decades of life. The delay in the appearance of neurologic dysfunction may reflect slow, progressive restructuring of the foramen magnum. Perhaps progressive ligamentous distraction develops with resultant AAI. A water hammer effect of CSF on posterior fossa structures also may be important when free egress of CSF from the fourth ventricle is not possible, as with Chiari anatomy.

Seemingly minor trauma may be responsible for bringing a Chiari malformation to medical attention, as relatively unimportant flexion injuries to the neck may bring out AAI. When hydrocephalus is present, the evidence of increased intracranial pressure or symptoms of normal-pressure hydrocephalus prompt the diagnosis of Chiari malformation. In the case of compression of the cerebellum and medulla, patients may present with dizziness, vertigo, nystagmus, and/or ataxia. Tonsillar herniation may be manifest at times by the simple nonspecific complaint of neck pain, though this diagnosis should be reached after eliminating other obvious causes of neck pain. If high cervical spinal cord compression is the primary problem, patients may present with spastic quadriparesis, proprioceptive abnormalities, and perhaps weakness and paresthesias greater in the upper extremities than in the lower extremities. Cranial nerve palsies may present as compromise in gagging, coughing, or swallowing. Many times, however, the symptoms are rather vague and the diagnosis is difficult to make until imaging studies prompt the diagnosis.

The advent of MRI has made arteriography and myelography generally unnecessary. MRI nicely demonstrates hindbrain abnormalities as well as those of the cervical spinal cord (Figs. 1, 2, and 3). Bony abnormalities, however, remain better demonstrated with plain skull and cervical spine films, augmented by CT where necessary. In view of the association of syringomyelia with a Chiari malformation, MRI also satisfactorily describes the anatomy of the syrinx without the need for myelography and post-myelography CT. A CT or MR

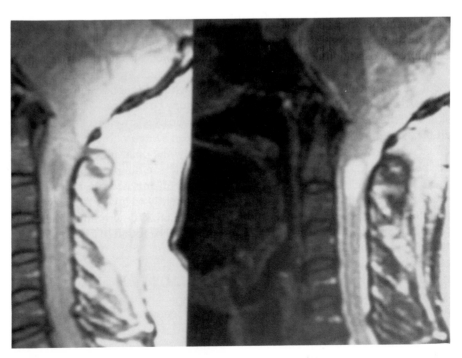

FIG. 1. Sagittal MRI demonstrating Chiari malformation with cerebellar tonsil displacement through the foramen magnum down to C1-C2 and associated C2-C3 cord syrinx.

33. Grantham SA, Dick HM, Thompson RC Jr, et al. (1969): Occipitocervical arthrodesis. Indication, technic and results. *Clin Orthop* 65:118–129.

34. Gray SW, Romaine CB, Skandalakis JE (1964): Congenital fusion of the cervical vertebrae. *Surg Gynecol Obstet* 118:373–385.

35. Greenberg AD (1968): Atlanto-axial dislocations. *Brain* 91:655–684.

36. Gunderson CH, Greenspan RH, Glaser GH, Lubs HA (1967): Klippel-Feil syndrome: Genetic and clinical reevaluation of cervical fusion. *Medicine* 46:491–512.

37. Hall PV, Holden RW, Matthews TJ (1981): Syringomyelia. *Contemp Neurosurg* 3:1–6.

38. Hankinson J (1978): The surgical treatment of syringomyelia. In: Krayenbuhl H, ed. *Advances and technical standards in neurosurgery,* Vol. 5. New York: Springer-Verlag, pp. 127–151.

39. Hensinger RN, Lang JE, MacEwen GD (1974): Klippel-Feil syndrome: A constellation of associated anomalies. *J Bone Joint Surg* [*Am*] 56:1246–1253.

40. Hensinger RN, MacEwen GD (1982): Congenital anomalies of the spine. In: Rothman RH, Simeone FA, eds. *The spine.* Philadelphia: W.B. Saunders, pp. 188–315.

41. Isu T, Sasaki H, Takamura H, et al. (1993): Foramen magnum decompression with removal of the outer layer of the dura as treatment for syringomyelia occurring with Chiari I malformation. *Neurosurgery* 33:845–850.

42. Jalladeau J (1936): *Malformations congenitales associees au syndrome de Klippel-Feil.* Theses de Paris, University of Paris, Paris.

43. Krayenbuhl H (1974): Evaluation of the different surgical approaches in the treatment of syringomyelia. *Clin Neurol Neurosurg* 2:110–128.

44. Krieger AJ, Rosomoff HL, Kuperman AS, et al. (1969): Occult respiratory dysfunction in a craniovertebral anomaly. *J Neurosurg* 31:15–20.

45. Laha RK, Malik HG, Langille RA (1975): Post-traumatic syringomyelia. *Surg Neurol* 4:519–522.

46. Lesoin F, Petit H, Thomas CE III, et al. (1986): Use of the syringoperitoneal shunt in the treatment of syringomyelia. *Surg Neurol* 25:131–136.

47. Levy WJ, Mason L, Hahn JF (1983): Chiari malformation presenting in adults: A surgical experience in 127 cases. *Neurosurgery* 12:377–390.

48. Logue V, Edwards MR (1981): Syringomyelia and its surgical treatment. An analysis of 75 patients. *J Neurol Neurosurg Psychiatry* 44:273–284.

49. Martel W, Tishler JM (1966): Observations on the spine in mongoloidism. *AJR* 97:630–638.

50. McElfresh E, Winter R (1973): Klippel-Feil syndrome. *Minn Med* 56:353–357.

51. McIlroy WJ, Richardson JC (1965): Syringomyelia: A clinical review of 75 cases. *Can Med Assoc J* 93:731–734.

52. McLay K, Maran AG (1969): Deafness and the Klippel-Feil syndrome. *J Laryngol Otol* 83:175–184.

53. McRae DL (1953): Bony abnormalities in the region of the foramen magnum: Correlation of the anatomic and neurologic findings. *Acta Radiol* 40:335–355.

54. Milhorat T (1972): *Hydrocephalus and the cerebrospinal fluid.* Baltimore: Williams and Wilkins.

55. Milhorat TH, Nobandegani F, Mille JI, Rao C (1993): Non communicating syringomyelia following occlusion of central canal in rats. Experimental model and histological findings. *J Neurosurg* 78:274–279.

56. Moore WB, Matthews TJ, Rabinowitz R (1975): Genitourinary anomalies associated with Klippel-Feil syndrome. *J Bone Joint Surg* [*Am*] 57:355–357.

57. Morrison SG, Perry LW, Scott LP 3d (1968): Congenital brevicollis (Klippel-Feil syndrome) and cardiovascular anomalies. *Am J Dis Child* 115:614–620.

58. Murphey F, Simmons JC, Brunson B (1973): Chapter 2. Ruptured cervical discs, 1939–1972. *Clin Neurosurg* 20:9–17.

59. Naik DR (1970): Cervical spinal canal in normal infants. *Clin Radiol* 21:323–326.

60. Nora JJ, Cohen M, Maxwell GM (1961): Klippel-Feil syndrome with congenital heart disease. *Am J Dis Child* 102:858–864.

61. Oldfield EH, Mruaszko K, Shawker TH, Patronas NJ (1994): Pathophysiology of syringomyelia associated with Chiari I malformation of the cerebellar tonsils. *J Neurosurg* 80:3–15.

62. Palant DI, Carter BL (1972): Klippel-Feil syndrome and deafness. A study with polytomography. *Am J Dis Child* 123:218–221.

63. Pang D, Dias MS (1993): Cervical myelomeningoceles. *Neurosurgery* 33:363–373.

64. Paul KS, Lye RH, Strang FA, et al. (1983): Arnold-Chiari malformation. Review of 71 cases. *J Neurosurg* 58:183–187.

65. Phillips TW, Kindt GW (1981): Syringoperitoneal shunt for syringomyelia: A preliminary report. *Surg Neurol* 16:462–466.

66. Resjo IM, Harwood-Nash DC, Fitz CR, et al. (1979): Computed tomographic metrizamide myelography in syringohydromyelia. *Radiology* 131:405–407.

67. Rhoton AL Jr (1976): Microsurgery of Arnold-Chiari malformation in adults with and without hydromyelia. *J Neurosurg* 45:473–483.

68. Rothman R, Simeone F, eds. (1982): *The spine.* Philadelphia: W.B. Saunders, pp. 216–233.

69. Rozen MJ (1977): Pathophysiology and spinal deformity in myelomeningocele. In: McLaurin RL, ed. *Myelomeningocele.* New York: Grune & Stratton, pp. 565–579.

70. Russell DS, Donald C (1935): The mechanism of internal hydrocephalus in spina bifida. *Brain* 58:203–215.

71. Sahuguillo J, Rubio E, Poca MA, et al. (1994): Posterior fossa reconstruction: A surgical technique for the treatment of Chiari I malformation and Chiari I/syringomyelia complex—Preliminary results and magnetic resonance imaging. *Neurosurgery* 35:874–885.

72. Schlesinger EB, Antunes JL, Michelsen WJ, et al. (1981): Hydromyelia: Clinical presentation and comparison of modalities of treatment. *Neurosurgery* 9:356–365.

73. Schwalbe E, Gredig M (1907): Uber Entwicklungs-storungen des kleinhirns, hirnstamms und halsmarks bei spina bifida (Arnoldsche und Chiarische missbildung). *Beitr Pathol Anat* 40:132–194.

74. Sgouros S, Williams B (1995): A critical appraisal of drainage in syringomyelia. *J Neurosurg* 82:1–10.

75. Sinh G, Pandya SK (1968): Treatment of congenital atlanto-axial dislocations. *Proc Aust Assoc Neurol* 5:507–514.

76. Spitzer R, Rabinowitch JY, Wybar KC (1961): A study of the abnormalities of the skull, teeth and lenses in mongolism. *Can Med Assoc J* 84:567–572.

77. Tator CH, Meguro K, Rowed DW (1982): Favorable results with syringosubarachnoid shunts for treatment of syringomyelia. *J Neurosurg* 56:517–523.

78. Wadia NH (1967): Myelopathy complicating congenital atlantoaxial dislocation (a study of 28 cases). *Brain* 90:449–472.

79. West RJ, Williams B (1980): Radiographic studies of the ventricles in syringomyelia. *Neuroradiology* 20:5–16.

80. Wisoff JH (1988): Hydromyelia: A critical review. *Childs Nerv Syst* 4:1–8.

Traumatic Disorders
of the Cervical Spine

The Adult Spine: Principles and Practice,
2nd edition, J.W. Frymoyer, Editor-in-Chief.
Lippincott-Raven Publishers, Philadelphia © 1997.

CHAPTER **59**

Cervical Acceleration Injuries: Diagnosis, Treatment, and Long-Term Outcome

Henry LaRocca, James C. Butler, and Thomas S. Whitecloud III

SCOPE OF THE PROBLEM

Acceleration injury of the neck is the term preferred by these authors to define that cluster of clinical symptoms following the application of a propulsive force to the head and neck complex in which tissue damage occurs directly as a result of that propulsion. This definition distinguishes acceleration injury from contact injury, in which an object impacting the head or neck (a swinging beam or the bottom of a pool) imparts a compressive or transitory force that creates internal loading to failure. The acceleration injury is variously called neck sprain, neck strain, whiplash, or soft-tissue neck injury, all of which share the inference of tissue stretching. Contact injuries, on the other hand, encompass a spectrum of fracture(s) and dislocation(s) of the vertebral column itself. The diagnostic and therapeutic approaches to the management of the effects of these two mechanisms of injury are substantially different. Moreover, although acceleration injuries are common, they appear to have received less attention than contact injuries, which are conceptually more simple.

During the past 40 years, a wide variety of clinical

H. LaRocca, M.D. (*deceased*): Clinical Professor of Orthopaedic Surgery, Tulane University School of Medicine, New Orleans, Louisiana 70112.

J. C. Butler, M.D., Associate Professor; T. S. Whitecloud III, M.D., Professor and Chairman: Department of Orthopaedic Surgery, Tulane University School of Medicine, New Orleans, Louisiana 70112.

problems associated with acceleration injury have been identified (Table 1). The first description of acceleration injuries to the neck was that of Gay and Abbott in 1953 (13). They identified a clinical syndrome produced generally by rear-end motor vehicle collisions, in which oscillations of the head and neck into flexion and extension result in a variety of pathologic states. In 1955, Severy et al. (39) described a precise experimental study of the rear-end collision that correlated mechanical events with medical phenomena. Their work established that there was a significantly forceful deflection and acceleration of the head and upper torso upon impact when the head and neck projected above the seat of the automobile models in use at that time. Their observation and those of others led to a proposition that neck injuries due to rear-end collisions could be minimized by restraining the head and neck with altered seat design, an eminently reasonable and even obvious conclusion. Regrettably, as recently as 1987, despite contemporary automobile seat designs, Deans et al. (11) reported that 62% of 137 patients attending a hospital after a motor vehicle accident suffered pain in the neck at some time following the accident; five had continuous pain 1 year later. In fact, during the last few decades, there has been a growing number of acceleration injuries as a result of motor vehicle accidents. In 1971, the National Safety Council estimated that there were approximately 4 million rear-end collisions in the United States alone, resulting in as many as 1 million reported injuries per year (8,30). McNabb (20–23) has estimated that cervical injury occurs in 20% of all accidents involving rear-end collisions.

TABLE 1. *Clinical problems arising from acceleration injury*

Spinal symptoms
1. Diffuse neck pain with nonradicular radiation and normal radiographs
2. Diffuse neck pain with or without radicular symptoms, and with radiographic evidence of pre-existing cervical spondylosis of varying extent
3. Cervical radiculopathy
4. Cervical myelopathy
5. Lumbar pain syndromes, including herniated nucleus pulposus

Central nervous system
1. Cerebral concussion
2. The Barre syndrome (sympathetic dysfunction)
3. Multiple cranial nerve dysfunction
4. Chronic headache (including migraine)
5. Cognitive impairment

Psychiatric symptoms
1. Mood and personality change
2. Sleep disturbance
3. Psychoneurotic reaction
4. Depression
5. "Litigation neurosis"

Other
1. Temporomandibular joint derangement
2. Esophageal laceration with or without mediastinitis

CLINICAL ISSUES

Many treating clinicians fail to regard cervical sprains/whiplash syndrome as a legitimate injury, but experimental and clinical evidence leaves little doubt that the majority of these patients have a physiologic cause for their symptoms. The clinical picture of whiplash is dominated by neck, head, and upper thoracic pain, often associated with a variety of poorly explained and sometimes bizarre symptoms such as dizziness, altered vision, and tinnitus. The symptom complex is frequently complicated by various psychosocial factors including anger, anxiety, depression, and pending litigation. Table 2 summarizes potential presenting symptoms seen in the cervical sprain syndrome.

In their 1953 report, Gay and Abbott (13) noted that about 15% of vehicular accidents that resulted in death, injury, or property damage were caused by a rear-end collision. A basic paradox existed in that seemingly inconsequential trauma resulted in a clinical problem of extraordinarily long duration. Ninety percent of these patients ascribed the onset of symptoms to a rear-end collision. The victim had typically been seated in a stationary vehicle which was struck from the rear by another traveling at a low velocity. Unlike the demographics of other types of trauma, 70% of the victims were women instead of men, and their occupations tended to have low physical demands. There were no heavy laborers in the cohort, and the typical victim was a housewife, skilled laborer, manager, clerk, or professional. The age distribution was between 30 and 50 years. None had re-

ceived a direct blow to the head or neck. Presenting symptoms included neck pain and limited neck motion with spasm, accompanied by tenderness of the cervical musculature. Pain was accentuated by motion. The physical examination often revealed paracervical spasm and tenderness extending into the interscapular region and into the shoulder girdles. The neurologic examination was generally normal. The authors noted that the patient "showed hypertonicity of the neuromuscular system and general nervous symptoms" (13).

In addition to this general set of complaints, Gay and Abbott (13) described five different clinical presentations: (a) cervical radiculitis, (b) cerebral concussion, (c) intervertebral disc herniation, (d) psychoneurotic reactions, and (e) low back pain. Radiographic examination demonstrated no abnormality in half of the 50 patients; the remainder showed some manifestations of degenerative disease. Approximately half of these patients required temporary hospitalization, and the response to treatment was slow, leading the authors to conclude that the whiplash injury was a chronic condition often associated with some form of psychoneurotic reaction.

In 1980, Balla (3) reported on the "late whiplash syndrome," defining it as a collection of symptoms and disabilities seen more than 6 months after a neck injury from a motor vehicle accident. Of the 300 patients they analyzed, symptoms persisted in 88% for more than 1 year after the injury and in 64% for more than 2 years afterward. Balla noted that there was no real difference in the symptoms of patients seen at 6 months or 2 years after injury. Women outnumbered men by nearly 2 to 1; the majority were in the age range of 21 to 50 years. Nerve root pain was reported in only 14 patients (5%), a clear sensory disturbance in an anatomic distribution was observed in only 13 (4%), and only 2 (0.7%) had a reflex loss. The complex of headache, neck pain, and stiffness was present in nearly all patients, and at some stage after injury, almost 40% complained of arm pain. A high proportion of patients also complained of anxiety, irritability, depression, and sleep disturbance. Correlation of plain-film radiologic changes with symptoms was

TABLE 2. *Potential presenting symptoms in acceleration injury*

Neck and shoulder pain
Headache
Arm pain/paresthesias/weakness
Dysphasia
Visual symptoms
Dizziness/vertigo
Tinnitus
Low back pain
Temporomandibular joint symptoms
Depression
Anxiety

poor. Thirty-nine percent of the cases exhibited mild degenerative changes, whereas the remainder were considered normal. Balla's data confirmed the observation of Gay and Abbott (13) that the occupations of the victims of late whiplash syndrome were less physically demanding types of employment. Balla concluded that the late whiplash syndrome was the result of an interaction between physical, psychosocial, and sociological factors combining to produce the symptom complex.

Norris and Watt (31) addressed the issue of prognosis of neck injuries resulting from rear-end collisions. They noted that there had been no simple method of estimating prognosis at or soon after the injury because of the heterogeneous and miscellaneous nature of the published reports. They attempted to establish a simple prognostic classification system that might be of utility in estimating future disability and likelihood of litigation. A group of 61 patients was evaluated, and each was placed into one of three subgroups based upon the symptoms and signs at the time of initial presentation. The maximum time elapsing between the injury and initial evaluation was 7 days. Group 1 patients complained of symptoms but had no abnormality on physical examination. Group 2 patients had symptoms accompanied by the clinical findings of a reduced range of cervical spine motion but no neurologic abnormality. Group 3 patients had symptoms, reduced range of motion, and evidence of objective neurologic deficits. Patient gender and age distribution were the same in each group. Approximately 20% of the patients in each of the three groups reported a delayed onset of symptoms up to 48 hours after the collision. The overwhelming majority of patients in the three groups were seated in stationary vehicles at the time of impact. After following these patients over an average interval of 19 months, the authors were unable to establish any definite trends for recovery in each of the groups. On the other hand, the groupings of patients did prove to have merit. Those with more objective signs had a poor prognosis, with greater time off from work accompanied by persistence of symptoms grave enough to affect recreation. Legal claims were also greater in group 3, suggesting that litigation is more dependent upon the severity of injury than upon some neurotic tendency, based on the fact that the patients were all classified within 7 days of injury before any legal action had been taken. Persistent headache was more likely to be associated with filing legal claims than was residual neck pain. Group 1 patients improved after the settlement of the claim or were no worse. However, in group 3, only two of ten patients were improved following settlement. These findings suggested to Norris and Watt that litigation itself has little influence on symptoms, and persons with milder syndromes are less likely to file a claim. Those with more serious injuries (group 3) all filed claims, but most failed to show any improvement after settlement. Finally, the authors suggested that pre-

existing radiographic evidence of degenerative changes in the cervical spine, however slight, did alter the prognosis adversely. Further, radiographic evidence of abnormal curves in the cervical spine, such as loss of lordosis, was more common in patients who reported a poor outcome.

Deans et al. (11) attempted to learn the true prevalence of pain in the neck after motor vehicle accidents. They studied 137 patients between 1 and 2 years after they had presented to a hospital because of a motor vehicle accident. Eighty-five patients (62%) complained of pain in the neck after their accident. In 36 patients (26%), the pain persisted longer than 1 year, and five patients (3.7%) had severe and continuous pain. Only 10 of the 137 patients (7%) had experienced pain in the neck before the accident. Most accident victims (77%) experienced the onset of pain within 12 hours of injury, whereas 7% reported that more than 48 hours elapsed before symptom onset. Regarding the direction of impact, the data confirmed that pain in the neck occurs after impact from any direction but was disproportionately more frequent after rear-end collision. Impact from behind was associated with pain almost twice as frequently as were front-end collisions.

The most common syndrome arising after acceleration injury is the complex of neck, interscapular, and arm pain associated with occipital headache. Frank disc herniation may occur but is rare (Fig. 1). However, other types of neurologic syndromes have been reported and merit mention. Rosa et al. (34) described a case report of multiple cranial nerve palsies due to hyperextension injury of the neck in a patient without other evidence of central nervous system injury. The patients in their case report showed signs of a unilateral injury to the sixth cranial nerve as well as bilateral injury to the lower cranial nerves from 9 through 12. These palsies were thought to be the result of severe stretching occurring with hyperextension of the neck. Scher (37) has emphasized that hyperextension trauma to the neck in the elderly may give arise to a central cord syndrome as a result of indirect cervical spine trauma to a neck with pre-existing advanced spondylosis.

Internal derangement of the temporomandibular joint was encountered in 25 patients reported by Weinberg and Lapointe in 1987 (41). They proposed that the shear stress applied to the intra-articular discs resulted in loss of synchronization of the disc and the mandibular condyle, which progressed to the classic syndrome of internal derangement of the temporomandibular joint with clicking and pain. This displacement is considered to be produced by hyperextension of the neck in which the mandible moves posteriorly less quickly than the cranium, resulting in downward and forward displacement of the disc-condyle complex relative to the cranial base. Stretching and tearing of the posterior attachment and synovial tissues along with loosening or tearing of the at-

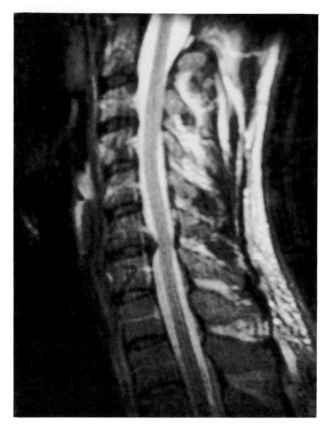

FIG. 1. Magnetic resonance scan of the cervical spine after acceleration injury, demonstrating frank herniation of the disc at L7.

tachment to the condylar poles occurs after hyperextension, reactive flexion occurs in the head and neck, and the attachment tissues are crushed between the mandibular condyle and glenoid fossa of the temporal bone. After injury, muscle spasm may produce additional displacement of the disc and perpetuate the temporomandibular joint syndrome.

Frankel (12) reported that 15 of 40 patients with acceleration injuries had signs and symptoms consistent with damage to the area of the temporomandibular joint. Frankel's theory was that direct injury to the temporomandibular joint could be caused by sequential extension and flexion of the head accompanied by simultaneous jaw movement, resulting in shear stresses and tearing of the retrodiscal posterior attachment tissues. One theory of indirect injury suggests that whiplash-induced myospasm leads to abnormal jaw posturing and muscle parafunctional activity, which result in eventual disc-condyle uncoordination and internal derangement (36).

A graver injury that can be produced by hyperextension of the neck is perforation of the esophagus (40). This condition may lead to cervical sepsis and descending mediastinitis (35). Presumably, the perforation results from impingement of the esophagus against a degenerative anterior cervical osteophyte.

Among the most challenging features of acceleration injury of the neck is the Barre syndrome (6). In this constellation, there are complaints of suboccipital headache, vertigo, tinnitus, intermittent aphonia and hoarseness, fatigue, temperature changes, and dysesthesia of the hands and forearms provoked by emotion, temperature, humidity, or noise. Craniofacial complaints can also occur, associated with pain, numbness, nausea, vomiting, and even diarrhea. Objective neurologic findings are generally absent, although there may be an absent corneal reflex. These symptoms are generally considered to be the result of hypertonia of the sympathetic nervous system. This may arise from stretch injury and hemorrhage within the sympathetic ganglia or from irritation of the ventral nerve roots from C5 to T1, all of which contain sympathetic fibers. Various arterial structures including the carotid plexus, external carotid artery, and the external maxillary, lingual, occipital, postarticular, superficial temporal, and internal maxillary arteries could be induced into vasospasm, giving rise to the bizarre symptom complexes described. Sympathetic blocks and surgical sympathectomies have occasionally resulted in relief of the Barre syndrome, thus leading some credence to the sympathetic hypertonia theory.

Headache is a prominent symptom in whiplash injury. In a retrospective study of 5,000 patients, Balla (3) reported that 25% of the patients had continuous disability 2 years after the trauma, with most experiencing headaches. Indeed, up to 80% of patients with cervical acceleration injury report complaints of headache within 2 months after injury (24). The acceptance of headaches as a potentially disabling symptom following minor trauma to the neck has gradually won acceptance in the medical community (25).

Only a few studies on the cognitive functions of whiplash patients have been performed (5,38). A recent report by Rajanov et al. (33) described the occurrence of cognitive deficits in patients who suffered acceleration injury of the neck. Fifty-one such patients underwent clinical and psychometric examination, which included formal testing of self-estimated cognitive impairment as well as auditory and visual information processing. Their results suggested the existence of two different syndromes. The first, termed "cervicoencephalic syndrome," was characterized by headache, fatigue, dizziness, poor concentration, disturbed accommodation, and impaired adaptation to light intensity. The second, termed "lower cervical spine syndrome," had the added features of neck and arm pain. In the cervicoencephalic syndrome, there was demonstrated abnormality of auditory information processing, whereas visual information processing was reduced to an equal degree in both syndromes. The authors assumed that there is reduced processing of work memory as a result of acceleration injury, which they consider may be responsible for more global cognitive problems as well as secondary neurotic reaction.

Considering all of the foregoing, acceleration injury of the neck presents multiple diagnostic and therapeutic challenges. Symptoms vary from brief discomfort in the neck all the way to both sympathetic and central nervous system dysfunction. Psychological and sociological factors play important contributing roles in many cases. The clinician is best advised not to prejudge and categorize victims of acceleration injury but instead to approach each one with an informed awareness of the possibilities at hand.

EXPERIMENTAL STUDIES

Much of the information needed to understand what happens in vehicular collisions to produce acceleration injury has long been available. Severy et al. conducted studies of such collisions and described their experimental results as long ago as 1955 (39). Their work deserves far greater currency than it has received. These authors produced controlled rear-end collisions and measured the forces and deflection that resulted using accelerometers and motion picture technique. Human volunteers participated in some of the runs, and anthropomorphic models were used in the others. A front car was placed in a stationary position and was impacted from the rear by a second car moving at low speeds of approximately 10 miles per hour. In this model, the impact imparted energy to the stationary vehicle, causing it to accelerate forward. These forces were applied to the seat on which the unrestrained subject was sitting. The subject's torso and shoulders accelerated with the seat, but because the head was not supported by the seat, there was a delay in its acceleration owing to its translational and rotational anuria, as it was propelled from below its center of rotation. Hence, the magnitude of acceleration of the head was greater than the peak acceleration of the car because the delayed reaction resulted in a shorter time to overcome the differential velocity between the head and car.

These findings reported by Severy et al. (39) can be further verified by the experimental work of White and Ponjabi (43) and are illustrated in Fig. 2. Enormous forces were applied to the head and neck complex even though this was a low-speed impact. For example, Severy et al. recorded typical head accelerations of 11 times gravity, resulting in the application of traction forces in excess of 100 lb to the head-neck complex. These data demonstrate conclusively that a low-speed rear-end collision is capable of applying seriously damaging forces to the head and neck, especially in anterior neck structures.

Animal experimentation has been conducted to investigate the pathology that results from the application of such forces. McNab (20) performed experiments in which monkeys were exposed to gravitational forces, re-

sulting in hyperextension strain. Dissection demonstrated a variety of pathologic lesions, ranging from tears of the sternocleidomastoid muscles to ruptures of the longissimus colli muscles with associated retropharyngeal hematoma, all consistent with destructive elongation of these anterior structures from the excessive excursion of the neck into extension. Also observed were esophageal injury and disruption of the cervical sympathetic plexus. In some animals there was disruption of the anterior longitudinal ligament and, most important, avulsion of the upper surface of the intervertebral disc from the intervertebral body above. Hence, a pathoanatomic basis for cervical intervertebral disc injury from hyperextension strain was established that is different from classic disc herniation. When avulsion of the disc from the bone deprives it of its normal nutritional pathway, disc degeneration is a likely outcome. That such pathologies occur in humans was established by Harris et al. (16), who operated upon a patient with intractable symptoms following a whiplash injury. They found separation of the C6-C7 disc from bone with an inspissated fragment of end-plate cartilage located within degenerated disc tissue.

Wickstrom et al. (44–47) conducted a variety of studies of whiplash injury in hares and primates that help clarify the etiology of protracted symptomatology. These exhaustively detailed experiments yielded a profusion of data. The Belgium hare used in initial experiments was found not to be the most appropriate animal for comparison with humans, because of the extreme flexibility of its neck and the proportionately lighter weight of its head in contrast to that of humans. A more appropriate subject for comparison proved to be the monkey, and a number of experiments were undertaken. An inventory of the tissue injury produced in primates included brain damage in 32%, spinal cord damage in 5%, and nerve root damage in 0.7%. Ligamentous injury concentrated between C4 and C7 was noted in 11% and intervertebral disc damage in 2.3% of the animals. Other pathologic changes included retropharyngeal hemorrhage, laryngeal hyperemia, and hemorrhage beneath the posterior longitudinal ligament or within the paraspinous muscles. The skeletal injuries observed often involved apophyseal joint damage not apparent on x-ray examination. Studies in which experimental animals and cadavers have been subject to whiplash motion have demonstrated that cervical zygapophyseal joint injuries are among the most common and consistent lesions produced (2,7,22). Postmortem studies of victims of motor vehicle accidents have shown that zygapophyseal joint injuries are common, being present in 86% of the necks examined (18).

Complementing all of these experimental studies is the report of Hohl (17), who reviewed 146 patients at a mean of 7 years after acceleration injury. None of the victims had evidence of pre-existing degenerative changes on an

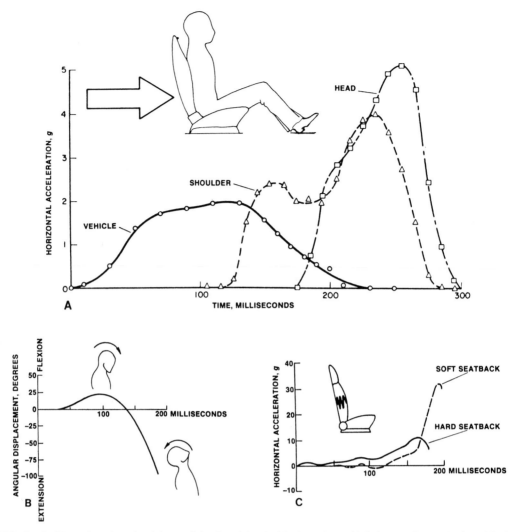

FIG. 2. A: Note that the shoulder and the head lag behind as the vehicle is accelerated when hit, but they catch up and within 0.3 seconds they reach accelerations 2 to 2.5 times the maximum vehicle acceleration. (Based on results from Severy DM, Mathewson JH, Bechtol CD (1955): Controlled automobile related engineering and mechanical phenomena. Medical aspects of traffic accidents. *Proceedings of Montreal Conference,* p. 152.) **B:** The head first goes into flexion and then into hyperextension within the first 0.2 seconds. **C:** The horizontal acceleration of the head for two different stiffnesses of the seat back. The harder seat back has a lower acceleration and therefore is associated with less injurious loading. (**B** and **C** based on results from McKenzie JA, Williams JF (1971): The dynamic behavior of the head and cervical spine during whiplash. *J Biomech* 4:477.)

acute phase radiographic examination, but at follow-up 39% demonstrated such changes, a prevalence more than six times greater than the expected 6% for this age group. More detailed statistical analysis revealed that 60% of those with more severe injury had evidence of degenerative change. Increased severity was defined as those individuals who (a) were rendered unconscious by the injury, (b) demonstrated restricted motion at one level on dynamic lateral roentgenograms, or (c) were required to wear a collar for symptom control for 3 months or longer after injury. The prognostic significance of radiologic abnormalities after acceleration injury was analyzed in a group of 73 patients by Miles et al. (29). Radiographs were evaluated for specific changes, and the clinical condition at 2 years after injury was then assessed. Patients who had degenerative changes at initial presentation were significantly more likely to have persisting problems at follow-up, whereas those with angular deformities had a better prognosis regarding symptom persistence at 2 years. The authors found no late effect related to the presence of prevertebral soft-tissue swelling in the absence of bony injury.

Because cervical sprain hyperextension injuries often show minimal radiographic abnormalities, Davis et al. (10) studied whether magnetic resonance imaging (MRI) could be used to define the nature and severity of hyperextension cervical injuries and to relate the findings to reported pathologic and radiographic features. Fourteen patients, nine with acceleration hyperextension whiplash injuries and five injured by direct frontal head trauma, underwent MRI within 4 months of injury. Five of seven patients with anterior spinal column injuries showed characteristic separation of the disc from the vertebral end plate, lesions still evident as late as 9 months after injury. These lesions, anterior longitudinal ligament injuries, anterior annular tears, and occult anterior vertebral end-plate fractures usually occurred at multiple levels except when there was pre-existing degenerative disc narrowing that had reduced spine mobility. Seven patients had acute cervical disc herniations causing cord impingement. The authors admitted that the role and timing of MR imaging in the absence of neurologic signs are difficult to establish, but they concluded that many of the lesions produced by hyperextension can be shown only with MRI. They also acknowledged that the patients included in their study probably represent those with a greater severity of injury, and this is a small minority of all patients sustaining this type of trauma. These data indicate that the intervertebral disc injury found in the various laboratory experiments is probably a significant and frequent component of the human acceleration injury as well. If so, this helps explain why the clinical course is often protracted. Thus, based on experimental, postmortem, clinical, and radiologic studies, the more common structural lesions due to acceleration injuries of the cervical spine can be summarized (Fig. 3).

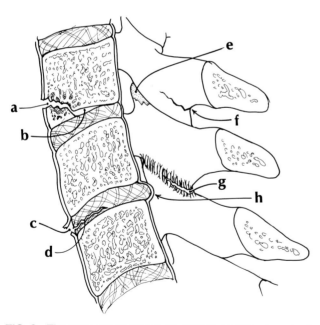

FIG. 3. The more common structural lesions following acceleration injury to the cervical spine include (*a*) vertebral end plate fracture, (*b*) separation of the disc from the vertebral end plate, (*c*) tear of the anterior longitudinal ligament, (*d*) tear of the annulus fibrosus, (*e*) fracture of the articular surface of the zygapophyseal joint, (*f*) articular pillar fracture, (*g*) rupture or tear of the zygapophyseal joint capsule, (*h*) posterior disc herniation.

EFFECTS OF LITIGATION

There has been much speculation and disagreement in both the scientific and medical communities with respect to the effects of litigation and compensation on symptomatic recovery from whiplash injury. Interest in the relationship between compensable injury, persistent pain, and treatment outcome has been long-standing and controversial (27,28).

Only a few prospective studies have evaluated the long-term outcome of cervical sprain and whiplash injuries following motor vehicle accidents. Norris and Watt (31) evaluated patients after cervical injury caused by rear-end collisions. As discussed in the preceding section on clinical issues, the maximum time elapsed between injury and evaluation was 7 days, and these patients were arbitrarily assigned into three different groups depending on whether any abnormality was demonstrated on physical examination, as opposed to a limitation of motion and/or objective neurologic deficit. Claims of personal injury were filed by 56% of the patients in group 1, 67% in group 2, and 100% in group 3. In their long-term follow-up surveillance, there was no statistical difference among the groups regarding improvement of symptoms after settlement. In other words, symptomatic improvement (not necessarily resolution) after litigation occurred in only 39% of the subjects overall. Unfortunately, Norris and Watt did not compare these subjects with non-litigants to determine whether the rate of improvement was higher than would be expected with the passage of time.

In another prospective study, Maimaris et al. (24) followed 120 consecutive patients seen in an emergency room after sustaining a cervical strain injury. Of the 102 patients able to be evaluated 18 to 30 months after injury, 66% were symptom-free but 34% still reported residual symptoms. Approximately half of the patients who were still experiencing symptoms had already settled their legal claims. Therefore, it is clear that settlement of litigation did not predictably resolve these patients' symptoms. The conclusion to be drawn from these prospective studies is that there is no apparent relationship between legal settlement and resolution of symptoms.

Various retrospective studies have also been published. McNab (23) reviewed 145 patients 2 or more years after settlement of litigation and found that 121 were still having symptoms, which in a majority were "a continuing nuisance rather than a significant disability." In a group of 266 patients, 45% continued to have symptoms after settlement of claims. Gotten (15) evaluated patients who had sustained a cervical neck strain or whiplash injury and attempted to determine their symptoms related to the status of their legal claim. Of 100 patients who were located and interviewed, 46 reported some continued discomfort or residual symptoms, and

12 of these patients had continued difficulty even after settlement of their legal claim. Numerous other retrospective studies in the literature all refute the contention that settlement of litigation leads to resolution of whiplash and cervical strain-related symptoms (14,17,32). Thus, it can be concluded that settlement of litigation is not necessarily associated with resolution of symptomatology in a significant percentage of patients involved in a cervical strain injury.

Few studies have examined the effects of litigation or compensation on the outcome and treatment for acceleration injuries. Weiss et al. (42) found little evidence that litigation hampered treatment response for patients with such injuries. Similarly, Abbott et al. (1) concluded that litigation appeared to have little effect upon the therapeutic outcome of patients sustaining cervical strain injuries.

Litigation following acceleration injury is so common that it may even be considered part of the syndrome, and most authors have accepted it as a fact of life. We believe that the litigant often has serious injury even if there are psychosocial factors at play, and medical evaluation and treatment should not be denied. The physician is the only professional who can establish the facts and the extent of the physical injury. The psychologist-consultant can be useful in establishing the degree to which psychological factors are affecting the clinical problem. Furthermore, contemporary imaging pathology lends credence to the presence of demonstrated tissue injury in those with severe injuries and suggests that the natural course of whiplash injuries may be more serious than previously assumed. In prospective studies, after patients have sustained acceleration injuries, residual symptoms may be seen for extended periods in up to 66% of patients (31). In conclusion, these studies indicate that between 14% and 42% of patients with whiplash injuries develop significant, chronic neck pain and that approximately 10% will have constant, severe pain for an indefinite period. These studies also suggest that the vast majority of individuals recover within the first 3 months after injury, with the rate of recovery then slowing over the next 2 years.

MANAGEMENT

Precise, detailed history elicitation is the essential beginning of management for any victim of an acceleration injury, for it provides the best measure of the magnitude of the force to which the head-neck complex has been exposed. The greater the magnitude, the more ominous is the prognosis. Physical examination also can provide prognostic information, as established so well by Norris and Watt (31). Radiographic study is imperative, including flexion and extension laterals (48). Most errors lead-

ing to missed or delayed diagnosis of cervical spine injuries are caused by either failure to obtain a technically adequate three-view cervical spine series (anteroposterior, lateral, and open-mouth odontoid views) or simply misinterpretation of roentgenograms (9). Should there be straightening of the normal cervical lordotic curve, acute cervical reversal on dynamic study, or pre-existing degenerative changes, again the prognosis is less favorable for early recovery (17). Which therapeutic modalities are appropriate in a given case is determined by the severity of the problem (19). The customary conservative measures include the use of cervical collars, physical therapy, and anti-inflammatory, muscle relaxant, and analgesic medications. Although treatment is generally administered on an outpatient basis, those patients with intense symptoms may require a brief hospitalization. The role of epidural injection of a narcotic and steroid has not been evaluated systematically, but based on anecdotal experience, it may be reasonably considered to interrupt the "pain-spasm" cycle. The application of mobilization principles of sports medicine has been reported to show promise in the treatment of acceleration injuries (26). Diagnostic and therapeutic blocks may be considered when conservative treatments fail, although the efficacy is not established. These sometimes include trigger point injections and cervical nerve and facet joint blocks. A recent report by Barnsley et al. (4) compared the efficacy of a depot injection of a corticosteroid preparation with the efficacy of an injection of anesthetic agent in patients with painful cervical zygapophyseal joint. The hypothesis tested was that a depot corticosteroid preparation injected into a painful joint would relieve the pain for a longer period than would an injection of a local anesthetic agent. The results of the study, however, demonstrated that less than half of the patients reported relief of pain for more than 1 week, and fewer than one in five patients reported relief for more than 1 month regardless of the treatment received. The authors concluded that intra-articular injection of betamethasone was not effective in treating painful zygapophyseal joint after a whiplash injury.

Surgery is reserved for the more severe and intractable cases and only when there is clear and unequivocal evidence of a remedial lesion. Definite and certainly progressive neurologic deficits may demand early decompression. Disc avulsion injuries with attendant disc degeneration may require disc excision and fusion if they persist in provoking intolerable symptoms for 6 to 12 months despite acceptable conservative therapy.

Based on the total diversity of available data, we conclude that acceleration injuries of the neck do produce a symptom complex that has a basis in anatomic dysfunction. Although litigation is frequently involved, the patient should not be denied appropriate care and diagnostic evaluation.

ACKNOWLEDGMENT. The authors acknowledge the late Henry LaRocca, M.D., for his contributions to their education in spinal surgery and to their understanding of spinal diseases.

REFERENCES

1. Abbott P, Rounsfell B, Fraser R, Goss A (1990): Intractable neck pain. *Clin J Pain* 6:26–31.
2. Abel MS (1958): Moderately severe whiplash injuries of the cervical spine and their roentgenologic diagnosis. *Clin Orthop* 12:189–208.
3. Balla JI (1980): The late whiplash syndrome. *Aust N Z J Surg* 50:610–614.
4. Barnsley L, Lord S, Wallis B, Bogduk N (1994): Lack of effect of intraarticular corticosteroids for chronic pain in the cervical zygapophyseal joints. *N Engl J Med* 330:1047–1050.
5. Berstad JR, Baerum B, Lochen EA, Mogstad TE, Sjaastad O (1975): Whiplash: Chronic organic brain syndrome without hydrocephalus ex vacuo. *Acta Neurol Scand* 51:268–284.
6. Bland JH (1987): *Disorders of the cervical spine.* Philadelphia: W.B. Saunders, pp. 224–225.
7. Bogduk N (1986): The anatomy and pathophysiology of whiplash. *Clin Biomech* 1:92–101.
8. Croft AC (1988): Biomechanics. In: Foreman SM, Croft AC, eds. *Whiplash injuries: The cervical acceleration deceleration syndrome.* Baltimore: Williams & Wilkins, p. 1072.
9. Davis JW, Phreaner DV, Hoyt DB, Mackersie RC (1993): The etiology of missed cervical spine injuries. *J Trauma* 34:342–346.
10. Davis SJ, Terisi LM, Bradley WG Jr, Ziemba MA, Bloze AE (1991): Cervical spine hyperextension injuries: M R findings. *Radiology* 180:245–251.
11. Deans GT, Magalliard JN, Kerr M, Rutherford WH (1987): Neck sprain—A major cause of disability following car accidents. *Injury* 18:10–12.
12. Frankel VA (1969): Temporomandibular joint pain syndrome following deceleration injury to the cervical spine. *Bull Hosp Jt Dis* 26:47.
13. Gay JR, Abbott KH (1953): Common whiplash injuries of the neck. *JAMA* 152:1698–1704.
14. Gore DP, Sepic SB, Gardner GM, Murray MP (1987): Neck pain: A long-term follow-up of 205 patients. *Spine* 12:1–5.
15. Gotten N (1956): Survey of 100 cases of whiplash injury after settlement of litigation. *JAMA* 162:865–867.
16. Harris WH, Hamblen DL, Ojemann RE (1968): Traumatic disruption of cervical intervertebral disc from hyperextension injury. *Clin Orthop* 60:163–167.
17. Hohl M (1974): Soft tissue injuries of the neck in automobile accidents. *J Bone Joint Surg* 56:1675–1682.
18. Jonsson H Jr, Bring G, Rauschning W, Sahlstedt B (1991): Hidden cervical spine injuries in traffic accident victims with skull fractures. *J Spinal Disord* 4:251–263.
19. LaRocca H (1978): Acceleration injuries of the neck. *Clin Neurosurg* 25:209–217.
20. MacNab I (1964): Acceleration injuries of the cervical spine. *J Bone Joint Surg* 46A:1797–1799.
21. MacNab I (1969): Acceleration extension injuries of the cervical spine. *AAOS symposium of the spine.* St. Louis: C.V. Mosby, pp. 10–17.
22. MacNab I (1971): The "whiplash syndrome." *Orthop Clin North Am* 2:389–403.
23. MacNab I (1982): Acceleration extension injuries of the cervical spine. In: Rothman RH, Simeon FA, eds. *The spine,* 2nd ed. Philadelphia: W.B. Saunders, pp. 647–660.
24. Maimaris C, Barnes MR, Allen MJ (1988): "Whiplash injuries" of the neck: A retrospective study. *Injury* 18:393–396.
25. Mandel S (1989): Minor head injury may not be "minor." *Postgrad Med* 85:213–225.
26. Mealy K, Brennan H, Fenelon GC (1986): Early mobilization of acute whiplash injuries. *BMJ* 292:656–657.
27. Mendelson G (1982): Not "cured by a verdict." *Med J Aust* 2:132–134.
28. Mendelson G (1992): Compensation and chronic pain. *Pain* 48:121–123.
29. Miles KA, Maimaris C, Finlay D, Barnes MR (1988): The incidence and prognostic significance of radiological abnormalities in soft tissue injuries to the cervical spine. *Skeletal Radiol* 17:493–496.
30. National Safety Council (1971): *Accident facts.* Chicago: National Safety Council, p. 47.
31. Norris SH, Watt I (1983): The prognosis of neck injuries resulting from rear-end vehicle collisions. *J Bone Joint Surg* [Br] 65:608–611.
32. Packard RC (1992): Posttraumatic headache: Permanency and relationship to legal settlement. *Headache* 32:496–500.
33. Radanov BP, Dvorak J, Valach L (1992): Cognitive deficits in patients after soft tissue injury of the cervical spine. *Spine* 17:2;127–131.
34. Rosa L, Carol M, Bellegarrigue R, Ducker TB (1984): Multiple cranial nerve palsies due to a hyperextension injury to the cervical spine. *J Neurosurg* 61:172–173.
35. Rotstein OD, Rhame FS, Molina E, Simmons RL (1986): Mediastinitis after whiplash injury. *Can J Surg* 29:54–56.
36. Towe NL, Killey HC (1968): *Fractures of the facial skeleton,* 2nd ed. Edinburgh: Churchill Livingstone, p. 144.
37. Scher AT (1983): Hyperextension trauma in the elderly: An easily overlooked spinal injury. *J Trauma* 23:1066–1068.
38. Schwartz DP, Barth JT, Dane JR, et al. (1987): Cognitive deficits in chronic pain patients with and without head/neck injury: Development of a brief screening battery. *Clin J Pain* 3:94–101.
39. Severy DM, Mathewson JH, Bechtol CO (1955): Controlled automobile rear-end collisions; an investigation of related engineering and medical phenomena. *Can Serv Med J* 11:727–759.
40. Stringer WL, Kelly DL Jr, Johnston FR, Holliday RH (1980): Hyperextension injury of the cervical spine with esophageal perforation. *J Neurosurg* 53:541–543.
41. Weinberg S, Lapointe H (1987): Cervical extension flexion injury (whiplash) and internal derangement of the temporomandibular joint. *J Oral Maxillofac Surg* 45:653–656.
42. Weiss HD, Stern BJ, Goldberg J (1991): Post-traumatic migraine: Chronic migraine precipitated by minor head or neck trauma. *Headache* 31:451–456.
43. White AA, Panjabi MM (1978): *Biomechanics of the spine.* Philadelphia: J.B. Lippincott, pp. 153–158.
44. Wickstrom JK, LaRocca H (1975): Management of patients with cervical spine and head injuries from acceleration forces. In: Ahstrom JP Jr, ed. *Current practice in orthopaedic surgery.* St. Louis: C.V. Mosby, pp. 83–98.
45. Wickstrom JK, Martinez J, Rodriguez RP (1967): Cervical sprain syndrome, experimental acceleration injuries of the head and neck. In: *Proceedings of the symposium on the prevention of highway injury.* Ann Arbor: The University of Michigan Press, pp. 182–187.
46. Wickstrom JK, Martinez JL, Rodriguez RP, Haines DM (1970): Hyperextension and hyperflexion injuries to the head and neck of primates. In: Gurdjian ES, Thomas LM, eds. *Neckache and backache.* Springfield, Illinois: CC Thomas, pp. 108–117.
47. Wickstrom JK, Rodriguez RP, Martinez JL (1968): Experimental production of acceleration injuries of the head and neck. In: *Accident pathology.* Washington, DC: U.S. Government Printing Office, pp. 185–189.
48. Winston KR (1987): Whiplash and its relationship to migraine. *Headache* 27:452–457.

The Adult Spine: Principles and Practice,
2nd edition, J.W. Frymoyer, Editor-in-Chief.
Lippincott-Raven Publishers, Philadelphia © 1997.

CHAPTER **60**

Cervical Spine Trauma

Jens R. Chapman and Paul A. Anderson

Injuries to the cervical spine present a diagnostic and therapeutic challenge to treating physicians. Two percent to 4.6% of patients presenting with blunt trauma are reported to have cervical spine injuries (52,68,90, 107,141,150,218). Timely diagnosis and institution of treatment avoid the deleterious effects of missed injuries. Understanding the injury at hand and implementing established treatment algorithms should optimize recovery of a functional, stable, pain-free cervical spine, while optimizing chances for recovery of neurological injury. Advances in diagnostic modalities and recent developments in the surgical instrumentation of unstable cervical spines allows for improved care of patients with cervical injuries.

  J. R. Chapman, M.D.: Assistant Professor; Chief, Orthopaedic Spine Service, Department of Orthopaedic Surgery, Harborview Medical Center, University of Washington School of Medicine, Seattle, Washington, 98104.
  P. A. Anderson, M.D.: Clinical Associate Professor, Department of Orthopaedic Surgery, University of Washington School of Medicine; and Orthopaedics International, Seattle, Washington, 98104.

RESUSCITATION AND EMERGENT MEASURES

Patient Retrieval

Successful treatment starts with appropriate retrieval of the injured patient. The trauma algorithm emphasizing establishment of airway, breathing, and circulation should be implemented. Strict immobilization during extraction and transportation prevents secondary injury. The cervical spine should be immobilized with a cervical collar or sandbags, with the patient secured on a rigid backboard. Extraction and endotracheal intubation can be performed while an assistant applies gentle manual traction. Transfers should be accomplished under strict spine precautions utilizing trained personnel and performing log-rolling if necessary. The injury history and an initial assessment of mental status, neurological function, and region of pain should be obtained and recorded by the emergency personnel on the scene. Intravenous access and nasal oxygen should be established in patients with suspected spinal cord injury. Expedient transport to a medical center staffed and equipped to handle trauma without delay should be arranged. In cases of pediatric spine injuries, the use of a standard backboard may lead to kyphosis of the cervical spine because of the relatively larger skull size (220). Use of a modified backboard with a recess for the occipital cranium has been suggested for these patients. Implementation of comprehensive spine precautions is particularly important in patients with altered mental status, facial or head trauma, or multiple injuries. Such patients should be assumed to have serious spine injuries until proven otherwise.

Emergency Room Assessment

Upon arrival at an emergency department, comprehensive reassessment of the patient following the standard ABC principles as suggested by the Advanced Trauma Life Support system is done (9). All patients with high-energy injury mechanisms or with altered mental status should have a lateral cervical spine radiograph, as well as an anteroposterior (AP) chest and an AP pelvis x-ray exam. An attempt is made to visualize the lower cervical spine by pulling the patient's arms caudally. A systematic physical examination should be performed, inspecting the head and neck region for obvious injuries. Using the log-rolling technique for turning, inspection, and palpation of the posterior aspect of the patient should be performed from the occiput to the coccyx. Particular emphasis should be placed on focal tenderness, interspinous gaps, and areas of bruising or ecchymosis. Neurological examination should follow the standards established by the American Spinal Injury Association (ASIA) (10) (Fig. 1). Motor strength of key myotomes of all extremities is recorded using the six-scale manual-resistance method. Systematic sensory evaluation of the key dermatomes of the trunk and extremities should utilize light touch, pinprick, and proprioception. Deep tendon reflexes and assessment for pathological reflexes are recorded.

In examining patients with suspected spinal cord injury, particular emphasis should be placed on anal sphincter tone, perianal sensation, and presence of a bulbocavernosus reflex. Detection of sacral sparing indicates presence of an incomplete spinal cord injury. In patients who are unable to comply with a formal neurological examination, assessment of spontaneous muscle tone, deep tendon reflexes, and sphincter tone should be completed. It is crucial to chart all findings of the neuro-logical examination systematically to facilitate communication and later comparisons.

Upon completion of the initial evaluation and resuscitation of a traumatized patient, the radiographic workup of the spine is completed. Radiographic evaluation of a patient with a cervical injury is detailed later in this chapter.

Emergent Treatment

Patients with spinal cord injuries or severely displaced spine fractures require normalization of vital signs and maintenance of adequate oxygenation and hematocrit. Emergent intervention measures are aimed at realigning a displaced spinal column, protecting the spinal column from further injury, and instituting appropriate pharmacological intervention. If traumatic malalignment of the cervical spine is detected on initial radiographs, the application of cranial traction using Gardner-Wells tongs is recommended (41,44,144,224), provided the patient has no skull fracture. An initial weight of about 5 to 10 pounds is applied and the effect is assessed by repeat neurological examinations and cross-table lateral radiographs.

In neurologically intact patients with facet dislocations, consideration may be given to obtaining an MRI study prior to reduction, to rule out a large herniated intervertebral disc (75). In neurologically compromised patients, achieving reduction of the deformity prior to obtaining additional imaging studies is preferred. The reduction sequence of a traumatic cervical spine deformity should follow principles of cervical traction as described by White et al. (224) (Table 1). Following successful reduction and realignment of the cervical spine, the traction weight is reduced to about 20 pounds and the neck is secured with a cervical collar. If closed reduction attempts fail, manipulation has been recommended. We recommend obtaining an expedient computed tomography (CT) scan of the injury zone and prefer open reduction and internal fixation to the more uncontrolled closed manipulation efforts (41,44,55). Following assessment of the entire spine, patients should be removed from the backboard, using precautions to protect the spine and prevent early soft tissue breakdown.

Methylprednisolone should be administered in spinal cord injury patients who present within 8 hours of injury (39) to decrease swelling and prevent propagation of secondary injury.

Indications for emergent surgical intervention are

FIG. 1. American Spine Injury Association (ASIA) Spinal Cord Injury Assessment Form. (Reproduced with permission from the American Spine Injury Association: Standards for Neurological and Functional Classification of Spinal Cord Injury, revised. Chicago: American Spine Injury Association, 1992.)

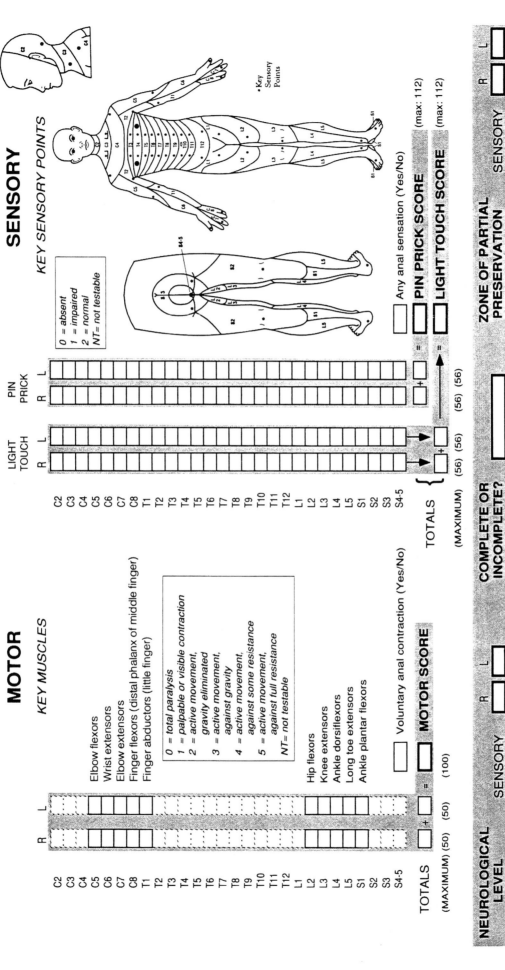

STANDARD NEUROLOGICAL CLASSIFICATION OF SPINAL CORD INJURY

MOTOR

KEY MUSCLES

C2
C3
C4
C5 — Elbow flexors
C6 — Wrist extensors
C7 — Elbow extensors
C8 — Finger flexors (distal phalanx of middle finger)
T1 — Finger abductors (little finger)
T2
T3
T4
T5
T6
T7
T8
T9
T10
T11
T12
L1
L2 — Hip flexors
L3 — Knee extensors
L4 — Ankle dorsiflexors
L5 — Long toe extensors
S1 — Ankle plantar flexors
S2
S3
S4-5

0 = total paralysis
1 = palpable or visible contraction
2 = active movement, gravity eliminated
3 = active movement, against gravity
4 = active movement, against some resistance
5 = active movement, against full resistance
NT = not testable

R L

TOTALS + = (50) (50)

(MAXIMUM) (100)

Voluntary anal contraction (Yes/No)

MOTOR SCORE

SENSORY

KEY SENSORY POINTS

0 = absent
1 = impaired
2 = normal
NT = not testable

• Key Sensory Points

LIGHT TOUCH   PIN PRICK

R L   R L

C2
C3
C4
C5
C6
C7
C8
T1
T2
T3
T4
T5
T6
T7
T8
T9
T10
T11
T12
L1
L2
L3
L4
L5
S1
S2
S3
S4-5

TOTALS + = + =
(56) (56) (56) (56)

(MAXIMUM)

Any anal sensation (Yes/No)

PIN PRICK SCORE (max: 112)

LIGHT TOUCH SCORE (max: 112)

NEUROLOGICAL LEVEL
The most caudal segment with normal function

R L
SENSORY
MOTOR

COMPLETE OR INCOMPLETE?
Incomplete = presence of any sensory or motor function in lowest sacral segment

ZONE OF PARTIAL PRESERVATION
Partially innervated segments

R L
SENSORY
MOTOR

Version 4d
GHC 1992

This form may be copied freely but should not be altered without permission from the American Spinal Injury Association

TABLE 1. *Stretch test*

1. It is recommended that the test be done under the supervision of an orthopedic surgeon.
2. Traction is applied by secure skeletal fixation or a head halter. If the latter is used, a small portion of gauze sponge between the molars improves comfort.
3. A roller is placed under the patient's head.
4. Place the film as close as possible to the patient's neck. The tube distance is 183 cm.
5. Take an initial lateral x-ray.
6. Add weight up to 12 kg. (If initial weight was 12 kg, omit this step.)
7. Increase traction by 5 kg increments. Take lateral film and measure it as before.
8. Continue by repeating step 7 until either one third of body weight or 30 kg is reached.
9. After each additional weight application, the patient is checked for any change in neurologic status. The test is is stopped and considered positive should this occur or if there is any abnormal separation of the anterior or posterior elements of the vertebrae. There should be at least 5 minutes between incremental weight applications; this will allow for the developing of the film, necessary neurologic checks, and "creep" of the viscoelastic structures involved.

From ref. 224.

open spine fractures or dislocations, inability to realign the spinal canal by closed means in the presence of neurological deficit, and neurological deterioration in the presence of documented compression of neural structures.

RADIOGRAPHIC ASSESSMENT OF THE CERVICAL SPINE

Standard Radiographs

Plain radiographs remain the best initial imaging study of the cervical spine (52,68,186). Lateral radiographs should be obtained early in the care of a traumatized patient (150). A lateral cervical spine radiograph should visualize the base of the cranium to the upper vertebral endplate of T1 (149). In order to facilitate visualization of the caudal cervical spine, both arms should be pulled in the distal direction when obtaining the lateral radiograph. If the desired view cannot be obtained with this technique, a Swimmer's view should be performed (186). Failure to visualize the cervicothoracic junction with these techniques necessitates a CT scan with reconstructions, or a magnetic resonance imaging (MRI) scan (110) (Fig. 2). In addition to alignment, fractures, or bony abnormalities, attention should be directed toward assessing the prevertebral soft tissue shadow for undue enlargement, widening of the posterior interspinous distance, and vertebral endplate or facet joint discongruity. Similarly, disc space widening of 1.5 times or more com-

pared to adjacent levels is suggestive of trauma (224). Digitally enhanced radiographic imaging may allow for enhancement of bony details in large patients.

The AP view is cranially limited by the mandible; the C3 vertebral body can be visualized to about T2. An open-mouth odontoid view is essential for radiographic visualization of the occiput-to-C2 region in the AP plane. In patients with multiple injuries or oromaxillofacial trauma, open-mouth odontoid views may be impractical, and AP tomography of C1-C2 or a CT scan should be substituted. Trauma oblique radiographs or pillar views may be helpful in delineating subtle facet injuries, and they allow for assessment of patency of the neuroforamina. In patients with obvious bony or ligamentous injury, or with incomplete or unclear visualization of the cervical spine on plain radiographs, further imaging studies such as CT or MRI are warranted (110,149).

Dynamic Radiographs

In patients with persistent neck pain, and normal neurological examination and plain radiographs, immobilization in a cervical collar should continue. Upright lateral radiograph may be helpful. Flexion–extension radiographs are able to detect disco-ligamentous instability in patients with otherwise normal radiographs. Some authors have suggested the use of these studies in the emergency room, and others have recently described video fluoroscopy-aided flexion–extension manipulation in intubated unconscious patients (67,68,224). We strongly caution against the use of these dynamic techniques in the acute postinjury phase. Neck pain and nuchal rigidity may limit the flexion and extension effort, thus limiting the validity of the study. Complications such as vertebral subluxation and acute neurological deterioration have been described as a result of flexion–extension radiographs obtained in the early postinjury setting (47,56). Flexion–extension radiographs are contraindicated in patients with altered mental status, obvious head and neck injuries, or neurological injury (31). Flexion–extension films in patients with a history of cervical trauma should be supervised by a physician. Normal plain radiographs are mandated prior to obtaining the dynamic motion study. The flexion–extension excursion should be voluntary, and patients should be instructed to stop their effort if pain or neurological symptoms are experienced.

In patients with injury mechanism for significant neck trauma, we recommend obtaining a flexion–extension radiograph after 1 or 2 weeks if plain upright radiographs are normal and the patient remains neurologically normal upon return visit (55). Patients with altered mental status or severe neck pain are not good candidates for flexion–extension radiographs, because they are either

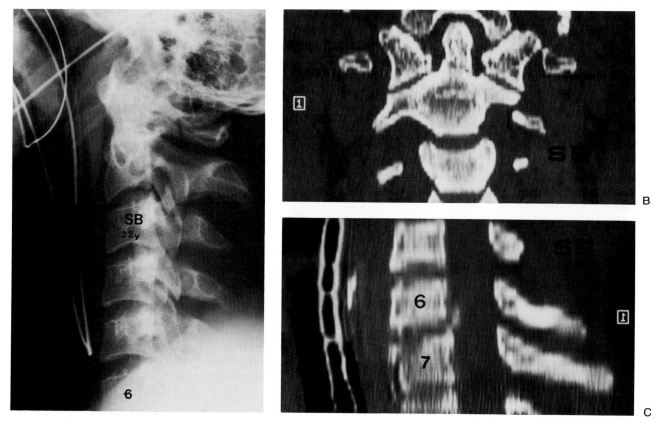

FIG. 2. A: The lateral cervical spine radiograph of a 22-year-old man injured in a 70-foot fall demonstrates a posterior arch fracture of C1, but it fails to demonstrate the C7 segment despite use of the shoulder pull-down technique. **B:** CT coronal reformatted view of the upper cervical spine demonstrates a type II odontoid fracture and allows for assessment of the integrity of the occipitocervical junction. **C:** CT sagittal reformatting of the cervicothoracic junction reveals an unstable C7 burst fracture. Inability to adequately visualize a segment of the cervical spine in a traumatized patient on plain radiographs should prompt further study of the region with CT or MRI.

unable to perform a meaningful excursion of neck motion or they lack protective pain inhibition to prevent excessive motion. Alternate imaging modalities such as MRI screens or bone scans may be safer techniques for assessment of occult trauma in such patients. If doubt exists, the patient can remain immobilized in an extraction collar for a 1- to 2-week period after the injury, prior to returning for clinical and radiographic reevaluation. The role of video fluoroscopy has yet to be verified. We feel there is a significant danger of missing injuries, because this technique is operator dependent, and it may not allow for adequate visualization of the cervicothoracic junction.

Tomography

Conventional polytomography has been largely replaced by CT. Lateral polytomography is a very useful diagnostic tool, but it is limited because of the need for the patient to be in the lateral decubitus position. Sagittal and coronal reformations derived from CT obviate the need for these studies. Linear AP tomography available in the emergency room can allow for rapid visualization of the upper cervical spine. This enables early assessment of the anatomic correlation of occiput and C1 to C2 during the initial trauma work-up, without transferring the patient to another imaging facility.

Bone Scan

The main role of the bone scan in spine trauma is focused on identification of occult trauma, non-union of fusions, and skeletal infection. In adult and pediatric trauma patients, some authors have suggested the use of technetium bone scans for detection of occult fractures as early as 48 hours after injury (23,125). Except for unusual cases, the combination of serial physical examinations and plain radiographs, supplemented by additional imaging studies such as CT and MRI, should adequately assess the cervical spine.

Computed Tomography

Prior to the advent of CT, 33% to 66% of cervical spine injuries were missed during the initial evaluation (33,52,68,90,141,190). CT can be performed rapidly with a patient safely positioned in a supine position. Also, the patient can remain in cervical traction while undergoing scanning. Indications for CT are evidence or suspicion of fracture or dislocation based on plain x-rays, or an inability to visualize any part of the cervical spine. CT can also help assess the age of the bony injury. Because spinal CT images are obtained in the axial plane in 3-mm increments, injuries limited to the axial plane can be missed. Slanting the gantry angle, reformatting the sagittal and coronal views, or using fine-cut CTs (1.5-mm cut) can avoid this problem (Fig. 2).

Magnetic Resonance Imaging

MRI allows for visualization of the spinal cord and cerebrospinal fluid, intervertebral discs (75), and some ligamentous structures (213). Traumatic effects such as hemorrhage, swelling, or edema in the soft tissues can be identified with proper MRI technique (119). The application of MRI allows for prognostic assessment of the final outcome of motor function (97,193). Indications for MRI include patients with incomplete neurological deficits, worsening neurological status, or neurological deficits above the level of skeletal injury (97,110,119). In certain injuries, presence of a soft tissue mass compromising neural elements, such as disc herniation or epi-

dural hematoma, should be ruled out prior to treatment (Fig. 3). Ligamentous tears or facet capsule disruptions can be visualized from fat-suppression techniques (213).

SPINAL CORD INJURY

The first few hours after spinal cord injury may have a significant impact on a patient's neurological recovery and possibility for functional improvement. Patients presenting with acute spinal cord injury therefore should be evaluated promptly to allow for early treatment. It is important that the evaluating physician understand the pathophysiology of spinal cord injury to address abnormal processes and create an environment conducive to maximum neurological recovery.

Pathophysiology of Spinal Cord Injury

Anatomically, the gray central aspect of the spinal cord consists of neural cell bodies, whereas the myelinated, ascending and descending axons are positioned in the peripheral white matter. Spinal cord injury can be differentiated into primary and secondary trauma. Primary injury is incurred at the time of injury as a result of compressive and distractive forces. Spinal cord transection is rare. In animal experiments, the severity of neurological injury and extent of histological damage was found to be proportionate to the kinetic energy imparted to the spinal cord (18,76). In Rhesus monkeys, irreversible neurological damages were found after subjecting the spinal cord to a 500 g/cm force; however, reversible

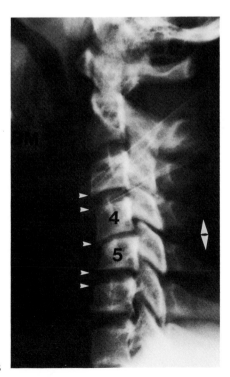 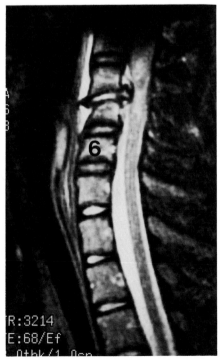

FIG. 3. A: This 16-year-old boy presented with a C5 level complete spinal cord injury. This lateral cervical spine radiograph shows loss of disc space height at the C4-C5 segment. *Large arrows* indicate interspinous widening. **B:** In patients with unexplained neurological deficits, an MRI should be obtained. The MRI demonstrates an extruded C4-C5 disc compressing the spinal cord.

A,B

neurological deficits were found after 300 g/cm force application (76). In an *in vitro* study, Chang et al. (53) found no correlation of residual spinal deformity to transient neural canal compression or vertebral displacement that occurred at the time of injury.

Following a traumatic event, there is immediate disruption of transmission of electric signals as a result of disruption of cell membranes, leading to potassium leakage and impaired blood flow to the cord. An expanding area of neuronal necrosis and axonal separation can be found over the first days after an injury. The gray matter is initially more severely affected by early posttraumatic changes than the myelinated white matter (19,20,73, 76,229,231). Within 3 to 5 minutes, petechial hemorrhage is found in the gray matter. Central neural hemorrhage and glial and neural necrosis can be identified by 30 minutes. Swollen but intact axons are found within the white matter at that point. By 4 hours, extensive gray matter necrosis can be identified. In the white matter, increased axonal swelling and necrosis of oligodendroglia is found. After 8 hours, maximal axonal swelling is present, axonal necrosis has started, and vesicular degeneration of myelin is under way (20).

Important therapeutic consequences arise from the finding that progressive changes evolve after a spinal cord injury and that they affect myelinated structures less than gray matter. These progressive changes have been identified as secondary injury and are caused by continued mechanical cord compression, ischemia, biochemical events, and an inflammatory response (212,229,231). Biochemical factors causing progressive neural tissue destruction are initiated by failure of the calcium-dependent enzymes and membrane transport systems. Release of phospholipase A_2 occurs, which in turn leads to release of arachidonic acid. This substance, through direct and indirect mechanisms, leads to further decrease of local blood flow, platelet aggregation, and release of lysosomal enzymes and formation of peroxide free radicals. Disruption of the lipid-based cell membranes by hydrolytic enzymes and peroxidation are thought to be important contributors to the secondary injury following spinal injury (132,134). Current research is under way to interrupt lipid peroxidation in an attempt to limit the biochemical component of secondary injury. Through cellular necrosis, a local autoimmune response is triggered. At the level of injury, a local infiltration of phagocytes, macrophages, and plasmacytes leads to further neural cell destruction and prepares the setting for fibroblast invasion. This subsequent scarring permanently prevents neurological recovery by blocking neural tissue regeneration (132,212).

Classification of Neurological Injury

Spinal cord injuries are divided into complete or incomplete neurological injuries. In patients with complete injuries, the most caudal level with at least antigravity motor strength is used to describe the level of injury. Sensory preservation of light touch is classified using standard dermatomal chart (Fig. 1). Preservation of perianal sensation or voluntary sphincter contractility identifies an incomplete lesion (10). The neurological level of injury (NLI) is established and correlated to the skeletal level of injury (SLI). A divergence of the two levels should be investigated with MRI or CT myelography. Meticulous serial documentation of the neurological examination of spinal cord injury patients is important for patient care, prognostication of rehabilitation needs, and research. A variety of incomplete spinal cord injury patterns have been described (Fig. 4). The functional level of a spinal cord injury has been classified by Frankel (Table 2) (100).

Pharmacological Treatment of Spinal Cord Injury

Methylprednisolone succinate is a corticosteroid that decreases lipid peroxidation. Intravenous high dose administration of this drug has been shown to improve preservation of neuronal structures and to decrease lipid peroxidation in animal spinal cord injury studies (38,39,120). The efficacy of methylprednisolone administered in a high dose within 8 hours of injury has been confirmed by a randomized double-blind study in which the effects of placebo, naloxone, and methylprednisolone on spinal cord injury recovery was measured on 476 patients. The group treated with methylprednisolone had statistically significant improvement of motor and sensory scores compared to the other groups. However, the overall improvement of motor function was small (39). Effects of this protocol on injuries to the nerve roots and conus medullaris, or on penetrating trauma to the spinal cord, were not evaluated in this study. Currently, the administration of a methylprednisolone loading dose of 30 mg/kg followed by a 23-hour intravenous drip of 5.4 mg/kg is recommended for adult patients presenting within 8 hours of a spinal cord injury (39).

Triliazoid is an amino-steroid without glucosteroid action, that acts as a lipid peroxidase inhibitor, and it is currently being investigated in a national randomized, double-blind study (12). Gangliosides are undergoing investigation for their potential to induce neural cytogenesis and have a neurotrophic effect on spinal cord injury patients. Initial reports have demonstrated decreased cerebral edema and more expedient recovery in patients with close head injuries. Geisler et al. have reported improved recovery in spinal cord injury patients who received GM-1 ganglioside, compared to the group given a placebo (106). Unlike methylprednisolone, gangliosides can be administered effectively up to 3 days after injury. Although these initial results are encouraging, further studies are necessary to confirm the role of gangliosides in the treatment of spinal cord injury patients.

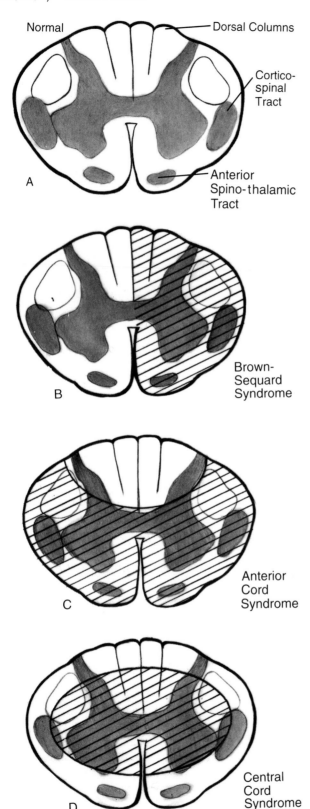

Normal — Dorsal Columns

Cortico-spinal Tract

A

Anterior Spino-thalamic Tract

B — Brown-Sequard Syndrome

C — Anterior Cord Syndrome

D — Central Cord Syndrome

FIG. 4. Incomplete spinal cord injury syndromes (10). *Anterior cord syndrome:* Neural function of the anterior two thirds of the spinal cord is disrupted. Proprioception and the sense of vibration and light touch are maintained; motor function and pain and temperature sensation are lost completely. *Central cord syndrome:* The central cord is injured, leading to

TABLE 2. *Frankel classification of spinal cord injury*

Frankel A	Complete loss of motor and sensory function below the level of injury
Frankel B	Preservation of some sensory function distal to the level of injury, but absent motor function
Frankel C	Motor function below level of injury retained but useless
Frankel D	Retained useful motor and sensory function below level of injury
Frankel E	Neurologically normal motor and sensory function

From ref. 100.

Mechanical Factors in Spinal Cord Injuries

Mechanical factors (instability of the injured segment, malalignment, and residual cord compression) continue to play an important role following the primary injury. Continued instability of an injured segment may lead to recurrent traumatization of neural tissue, thus exacerbating the neurological damage. In a primate study, Ducker et al. found immobilization to be the only therapeutic intervention that had a beneficial effect on neurological recovery, compared to a variety of pharmacological agents (79). Nursing techniques frequently used in spinal cord injury patients, such as log-rolling and use of a turning frame or a Roto-Rest bed, have been shown to cause significant fracture-site motion (89,100,154).

Breig (40,41) studied the anatomic effect of residual kyphosis and spinal cord compression in the human spine. He found that kyphosis created abnormal tension in the axonal tracts and led to displacement and narrowing of intramedullary vessels. Anterior spinal cord compression led to a lateral and posterior displacement of the anterior tracts. These effects were reversed with return to a physiological alignment (40,41,121). The physiological alignment of the cervical spine is one of lordosis. Kyphosis in this area, especially if focal in nature, can lead to compression of the cord against the posterior wall of the vertebral body (14).

Boehler recognized the detrimental role of extrinsic cord compression on spinal cord function and recovery. He advocated fracture reduction rather than laminectomy as an effective tool for spinal cord decompression

greater loss of neurological function in the arms than in the legs. Typically, the lower cervical roots are more affected than the upper roots. The lumbar and sacral tracts are spared because of the lamination of the fibers in the anterior spinothalamic and lateral corticospinal tracts, where the cervical fibers are more medial and the lumbosacral fibers more lateral. *Brown-Séquard syndrome:* Injury to one half of the cervical spinal cord can lead to ipsilateral loss of motor and dorsal column function, and loss of contralateral pain and temperature sensation.

(27). Several animal studies confirm a inverse relationship between duration of compression and recovery from spinal cord injury (33,70,71,74,212). In a canine spinal cord injury model, Delamarter et al. (70) found a statistically significant correlation between duration of spinal cord compression and recovery of somatosensory evoked potentials and neurological function. Delay of the decompression of 6 hours or more resulted in paraplegia, absence of bowel and bladder function, and severe histological changes. Bohlmann and Bolesta showed that delayed anterior decompression of the spinal cord up to 3 months after the injury was beneficial to neurological recovery in a dog model (34). In several clinical studies, meaningful neurological improvement could be gained in spinal cord injury patients with residual compression, with decompression and fusion up to a year following injury (14,32).

Timing of surgical intervention in cervical spinal cord injury remains controversial. Should closed reduction with traction succeed in realigning the spinal column and decompressing neural structures, definitive surgical stabilization can be deferred for several days (44,48,154). In a large multicenter study, Marshall found neurological deterioration in four patients with surgical treatment within 5 days from injury. He therefore recommended a 4- to 5-day delay prior to surgical intervention (154). Review of the data presented, however, demonstrates a higher incidence of neurological deterioration in the non-operatively treated group. The value of the study is limited, because it did not attempt to control for the type of surgery performed. In a comparison of 22 patients with cervical spinal cord injury who received surgical decompression and fusion within 4 days, and 21 patients who received surgery 5 days or later, no statistically significant differences in Frankel score recovery or motor score were found (42). However, 19% of patients in the delayed treatment group developed adult respiratory distress syndrome (ARDS) and required prolonged after care compared to 4% in the early treatment group. In thoracolumbar spinal cord injuries, Krengel et al. (140) and Edwards and Levine (84) have demonstrated improved neurological improvement in patients operated within 24 hours and within 10 hours from injury, respectively. Despite clear advantages of early decompression and stabilization in animal studies, well-controlled human studies on timing of surgical intervention are still missing.

Mortality from complete cervical spinal cord injury has been assessed to range from 23% to 60% after 1 year from injury (5,78,100), and 100% of patients over the age of 65 years expired (5). In contrast, a 4% mortality rate was found in patients with incomplete spinal cord injuries after 1 year (5).

Based on currently available data, timely reduction of deformity, atraumatic decompression of neurological tissue, and stabilization are indicated in patients with spinal cord injury (144). Pharmacological intervention may be able to increase the window of opportunity for intervention and maximize chances for recovery.

UPPER CERVICAL SPINE INJURIES

Occipitocervical Injuries

The occiput forms a functional unit with the C1 and C2 vertebrae. Any injury to any one of these elements should lead to a careful neurological examination and assessment of the bony and ligamentous structures of the upper cervical spine. A 90% incidence of injuries of the occiput to the C2 ring was found in a review of 382 fatal-motor-vehicle injury patients (66). Bucholz estimated a survival chance of 0.65% to 1% for patients with occipitocervical dissociations, based on a prospective morgue study (46). Improved patient recovery techniques and emergency services may have increased the survival chances of patients with serious occipitocranial injuries.

Occipital Condyle Fractures

Isolated occipital condyle fractures can be difficult to identify on standard plain radiographs. Asymmetry of the occipitocervical joints, increased prevertebral soft tissue space, or fragments around the foramen magnum on a CT of the head should lead the clinician to obtain a narrow-section CT with reformats in sagittal and coronal planes of the occipitocervical region. Until a better understanding of the injury is obtained, cranial traction should not be applied, to avoid overdistraction.

Occipital condyle fractures have been classified by Anderson and Montesano (17) (Fig. 5). Type I includes comminuted impaction fractures of the skull base, and these are usually expected to be stable. Type II fractures are shear-type injuries through the occipital condyles and may be unstable. Type III fractures are alar ligament avulsions that can be unstable (Fig. 6). The stability of these injuries ranges from actual dislocations to stable injuries.

Patients should be carefully examined for cranial nerve deficiencies, bulbar symptoms, and long tract signs. Stable bony injuries without joint-line asymmetry or neurological deficits can be treated with craniocervical orthoses. Predominately bony injuries with minimal displacement require reduction with cranial traction and application of a halo ring and vest. Ligamentous injuries and injuries with significant displacement are likely to be unstable and should be treated by open reduction, stable internal fixation, and fusion (17). Determination of stability of occipital condyle fractures can be difficult and necessitates close follow-up of patients undergoing conservative treatment.

Type I

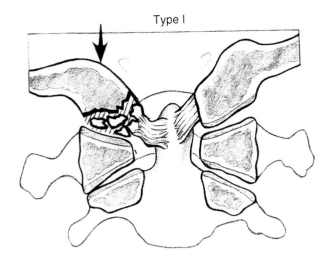

Type II

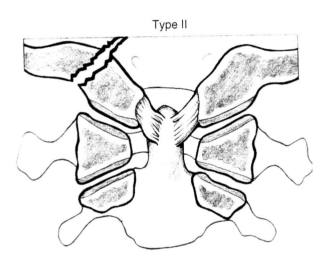

Type III

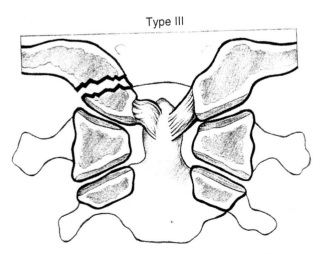

FIG. 5. Anderson and Montesano's (17) classification of occipital condyle fractures. Type I is an impaction fracture. Type 2 is a fracture of the occipital condyle involving the skull base. Type III is an avulsion fracture. This type III injury may represent occipitocervical instability.

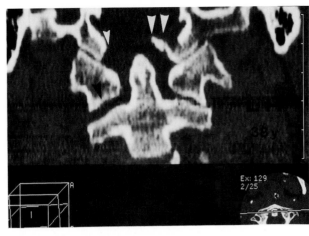

FIG. 6. The CT coronal reformation of the upper cervical spine reveals a type III occipital condyle fracture on the patient's left side (*large arrow*), and a type 2 avulsion injury on the right side (*small arrow*). Note the unilateral widening of the atlantoaxial joint indicating instability. The patient was successfully treated in a halo-vest.

Occipitocervical Dissociation

Diagnosis

Despite being severe injuries, occipitocervical dissociations often have delays in diagnosis (175). A high degree of clinical suspicion is necessary for the timely discovery of these injuries. Patients with craniofacial trauma, severe head injuries, occipital tenderness, or dysesthesia may have associated occipitocervical instability (159). Diagnostic difficulties arise from the unique anatomy of this region. In humans, the important structures are the alar ligaments and the tectorial membrane (82,222). Identification of ligament injuries can be accomplished indirectly by assessment of bony displacement and soft-tissue swelling, or more directly with specific MRI imaging techniques. Careful review of lateral cervical spine radiographs can allow for preliminary diagnosis. On horizontal beam, lateral beam radiographs obtained at a 40-inch target distance, congruency of the occipitocervical joints and prevertebral swelling are scrutinized. A variety of radiographic criteria have been suggested to assess the spatial relationship of the osseous structures of the occipitocervical junction (226). The basilar line has been described as a continuation of a line drawn from the posterior slope of the clivus to the posterior tip of the dens. The normal variability of the inclination angle of the clivus makes this an unreliable diagnostic tool for the identification of occipitocervical injuries. The *X-line* describes lines drawn from the posteroinferior axis body to the opisthion, from the tip of the basion to the midsection of the C2 spinolaminar line, and several other lines with reference to their intersection with the odontoid (145) (Fig. 6). Limited radiographic visualization of the opisthion and anatomic variability of the posterior spinolaminar dimension have limited the reliability of this test (124). *Powers' ratio* describes the quotient derived from the distance of the basion (A) to the anterior spinal laminar line of C1 (C), and the posterior aspect of the anterior arch of the atlas (B) to the opisthion (D) (Fig. 7). The test is considered positive if the ratio of AC to BD is less than 0.8. The test is limited to anterior atlantoaxial dissociations (175).

Recently, Harris and associates developed normal measurements of the occipitocervical junction based on the radiographs of 400 adults (123). The basion–dental interval (BDI) is established by measuring the distance from the caudad end of the basion to the rostral tip of the dens axis. In 95% of patients, this distance was less than 12 mm. A higher value is suggestive of for vertical atlanto-occipital displacement (Fig. 6). The basion–axial interval (BAI) is the distance between the posterior axial line and a parallel line drawn through the basion, and it should be between 0 and 12 mm. A larger value indicates

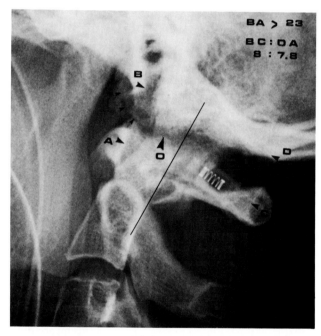

FIG. 7. This lateral cervical spine radiograph demonstrates an occipitocervical dissociation in this 22-year-old patient with respiratory-dependent quadriplegia. Note the anterior arch of the atlas (A), the basion (B), the posterior arch of the atlas (C), the opisthion (D), and the tip of the odontoid (O). Harris recommended extending a line along the posterior aspect of the axis body, the posterior axial line. The distance from the basion to the odontoid tip is the basion dens interval (BDI), which should measure 12 mm or less. In this patient, the BDI was 13 mm. The basion axis interval (BAI) is the distance from the basion to the posterior axial line and should measure less than 12 mm. In this patient, the BAI measured 20 mm. Powers' ratio is derived from the quotient of the length of AD divided by the length of BC, and it should be greater than 0.9. In this case, the quotient was 0.94, despite the patient having a atlanto-occipital dissociation. The patient was treated with occipitocervical fusion and recovered independent ambulatory function 6 months postoperatively.

the possibility of an anterior displacement, and a negative value should raise the suspicion of posterior displacement. In a comparison study, Harris et al. found a statistically significant lower sensitivity and specificity of the Powers' ratio and X-line measurement techniques compared with the BAI and the BDI (124).

A computed axial tomography (CAT) scan with 1.5-mm cuts and reformatted images in sagittal and frontal plane should be obtained if there is any clinical or radiographic concern for a craniocervical injury. MRI is helpful in identifying hematoma formation and ligamentous disruption. Significant injuries in this area may manifest as epidural or prevertebral hematomas. In cases of neurological deficits, additional insight may be gained from assessment of cord signal changes on MRI.

Classification

Traynelis et al. described anterior, posterior, vertical, and lateral dislocation patterns (214) (Fig. 8). Varying degrees of occipitocervical dissociation ranging from mild instability to complete craniocervical ligamentous separation exist. Provocative stability tests, such as traction or flexion–extension studies, are potentially life threatening and are therefore not recommended. Comprehensive assessment by imaging studies is recommended for determination of stability. If there is loss of the integrity of the alar ligaments and tectorial membrane, then the spine is highly unstable (82,222).

The occipitocervical region can be subject to a perplexing variety of neurological injury patterns. Cruciform paralysis (Bell's cruciate paralysis) is a rare incomplete spinal cord injury pattern uniquely associated with this region (72,142). It has been described as consisting of a varying degree of lower cranial nerve palsies and upper extremity weakness. To date, the exact neurophysiological basis of this disorder remains poorly understood. Because it shares some similarities with the central cord syndrome, clinical overlap or misdiagnosis may account for the rarity of diagnosis.

Treatment

Because of the ligamentous nature of the craniocervical junction, any injury leading to translational or vertical displacement should be considered unstable (82,222) (Fig. 9). Similarly, patients with neurological injury at the craniocervical junction should be carefully assessed for structural instability and are candidates for surgical stabilization. The application of longitudinal skeletal traction for the initial care of patients with craniocervical injuries is dangerous and usually not indicated (61). Immobilization with sandbags and cervical collar or application of a halo ring with vest is recommended. A congruous reduction with the head in neutral position can

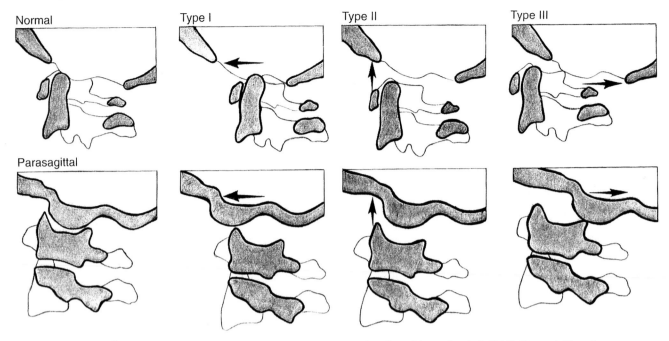

Normal   Type I   Type II   Type III

Parasagittal

FIG. 8. Classification of occipitocervical instabilities modified from Traynelis et al. (214). Normal. Type I-anterior. Type II vertical. Type III posterior.

be obtained by careful positioning of the head relative to the thorax (177). Attention should be directed to avoid any form of traction effect of the halo fixateur. Both upright and recumbent films should reflect continued anatomic reduction. In cases of craniocervical instability, posterior occiput to C2 instrumentation and fusion is recommended. Several fusion and instrumentation techniques have been described (177,187,192,206,223). Simple wiring techniques and the use of a preformed metallic rectangle affixed with sublaminar wire are effective but require stabilization in a halo fixateur (177). Recently, the use of small fragment plates bridging the occiput to the upper cervical spine has been reported (187,192,206). Successful fusion was achieved in all patients without loss of reduction and without neurological complications.

Injuries of the Atlas and C1-C2 Motion Segment

The atlas is a ring-like structure that acts as a washer between the occipital condyles and the lateral masses of the axis. The C1 lateral masses are wedge-like in cross section and connected by anterior and posterior arches. A strong ligamentous structure, the transverse ligament, connects the anterior portion of the left to right lateral masses, thus providing additional stability to the bony ring (82). Ten percent of cervical spine fractures involve the atlas. Other spine fractures, most commonly of the axis, are present in about 50% of cases (80,81,118, 143,147). Injury of the atlas should prompt careful review for additional spine or head injuries. Because of the

larger canal space, neurological injuries as a result of an isolated fracture of the atlas are rare (143).

Diagnosis

Most injuries of the C1 segment can be readily identified by plain radiographs (13). Standard radiographs of the C1 ring include the open-mouth odontoid view and a lateral cervical spine radiograph. The open-mouth odontoid view should show the lateral margins of both lateral masses and should demonstrate the odontoid to be equidistant to the lateral masses. In patients with significant craniofacial trauma, an open-mouth odontoid view frequently cannot be obtained. In such patients, tomography allows for rapid evaluation of the spatial relationship of the C1 lateral masses to the occipital condyles and axis. Spreading of the lateral masses of the occipital condyles over the lateral masses of the axis indicates a Jefferson type fracture. If the combined spread is more than 6.9 mm, then the transverse ligament is ruptured and stability of the C1-C2 junction is impaired (81,83,129). Because of x-ray magnification on open mouth odontoid views, transverse ligament insufficiency is suspected when the lateral mass overhang exceeds 8.1 mm on radiographs (129).

Plain lateral radiographs should be interpreted for any bony discontinuity, and for the relationship of the atlas to the dens axis. The distance between the posterior cortex of the anterior ring of C1 and the anterior cortex of the dens should be less than 3 mm in adults and 5 mm

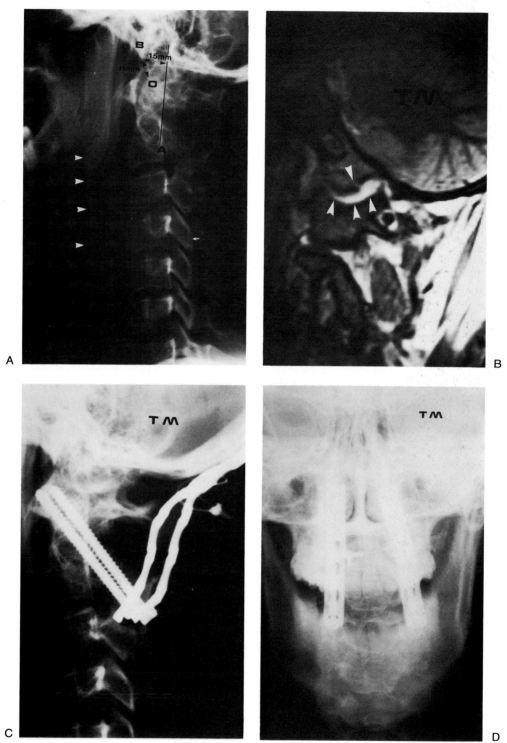

FIG. 9. A: Lateral cervical spine radiograph of a neurologically intact, 22-year-old woman involved in a high-speed motor vehicle crash demonstrates prevertebral soft-tissue swelling (*arrows*) and anterior subluxation of the occipital condyles on the lateral masses of the atlas. The BDI measures 11 mm and the BAI (B–O) measures 15 mm. **B:** Increased signal intensity of the occipitocervical and atlantoaxial joints on T2-weighted MR images correlates with severe ligamentous injuries of the cervicocranial junction. *Arrows* indicate anterior and vertical subluxation of the occipital condyles on the atlas. **C:** The lateral flexion C-spine radiograph taken 3 months postoperatively demonstrates solid occipitocervical fusion achieved with titanium reconstruction plates and atlantoaxial transarticular screw fixation with cortico-cancellous iliac crest bone graft. The patient remained neurologically normal and is pain free. **D:** Antero-posterior radiograph demonstrating occipitocervical plating.

in children (80,81,83). Occult instability of the C1-C2 junction can be identified on flexion–extension radiographs. Presence of prevertebral swelling is an important diagnostic finding for the presence of significant occult cervical spine trauma. In such patients, we recommend obtaining a CT scan or, preferably, an MRI scan. CT scans of the of the occiput to C2 should be obtained in case of any identified or suspected fractures of the atlas. Because the atlas is a thin bony structure, it is important to have CT cuts of 1.5-mm thickness with the gantry angle placed collinear with the axial plane of the atlas.

Classification

Atlas fractures usually reflect the injury mechanism incurred. Classification is based on the location of the fracture and its stability (116,118,143) (Fig. 10).

Anterior arch fractures. These injuries usually are result of a hyperextension mechanism and are classified as minimally displaced, comminuted, and unstable. Severity of fracture ranges from avulsions of the longus colli muscle to extension injuries that can leave the atlantodens joint unstable. As in all injuries of the occiput–C2 unit, possible atlanto-occipital instability has to be considered. Low-weight-traction lateral radiographs can be obtained to rule out significant ligamentous disruption of this segment. Unstable injuries are usually a displaced blowout of the anterior arch where the dens axis protrudes into the anterior arch. Similarly, significant ante-

rior arch comminution may reflect possible C1-C2 instability.

Lateral mass fractures. These injuries usually result from lateral loading mechanisms and can be easily missed on lateral radiographs. Decrease of lateral mass height or bony discontinuity on open-mouth odontoid views can be the only clues to an injury. CT scans may show an avulsion of the transverse ligament contralateral to the affected lateral mass. Identification of this injury pattern should raise concern regarding C1-C2 stability. Treatment of these injuries follows guidelines for bursting injuries of the atlas.

Posterior arch fractures. These fractures are caused by forced hyperextension together with axial loading, creating impaction of the occiput and the posterior arches of C1 and C2. These injuries may involve the greater and lesser occipital nerves, with the patient suffering severe occipital pain or numbness. Posterior arch fractures are usually stable and can be treated with a neck collar.

Burst fractures. Jefferson described the four-part burst fractures of C1 prior to the advent of CT scans (137) (Fig. 11). These fractures usually result from axial loading and can present as two-, three-, or four-part fractures. Because of the wedge-like cross section of the C1 lateral masses, these are pushed further lateral by increasing vertical force. Based on cadaver studies, the transverse ligament is likely torn or avulsed if the left- and right-sided C1 lateral masses overhang those of C2 by more than 6.9 mm (83). On lateral radiographs, transverse ligament insufficiency is present if the

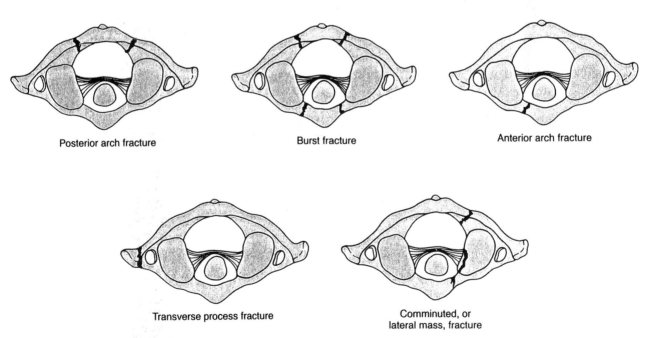

Posterior arch fracture   Burst fracture   Anterior arch fracture

Transverse process fracture   Comminuted, or lateral mass, fracture

FIG. 10. C1 ring injuries. [Reprinted with permission from Browner, Jupiter, Levine, Trafton (1992). In: Bruce D. Browner, et al, eds. *Skeletal trauma, fractures, dislocations, ligamentous injuries,* 1st ed. Chapter 27. Philadelphia: WB Saunders.]

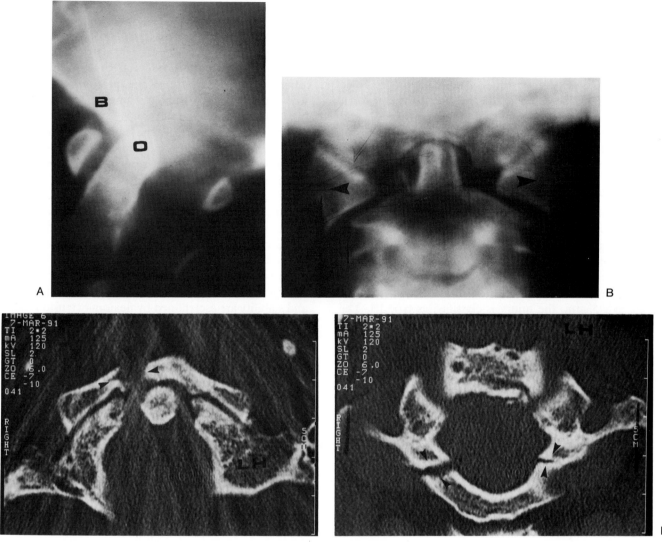

FIG. 11. A: Lateral tomography demonstrates cranial migration of the dens (O) to the foramen magnum (B) resulting from the unstable burst injury of the atlas and resultant loss of height of the C1 ring. An increased atlanto–dens interval of 5 mm is present. Following reduction with cranial traction, this 42-year-old patient was successfully treated with a halo vest. **B:** The open-mouth odontoid view demonstrates overhang of 6 mm on the left C1 lateral mass over the C2 lateral mass and 8 mm on the right. A combined lateral mass overhang of more than 6.9 mm is suggestive of an unstable axis fracture with transverse ligament disruption. **C:** Axial CT demonstrates a displaced three-part atlas fracture with avulsion of the transverse ligament. The anterior arch fracture is seen on this CT scan (*arrow*). **D:** The posterior arch fractures are visualized on this CT scan (*arrows*).

atlanto–dens interval is greater than 3 mm, or if the lateral mass overhang exceeds 8.1 mm (83,129).

Atlantoaxial Instability

Classification

There are three general patterns of atlantoaxial instability: flexion–extension, distraction, and rotatory (80, 81,83,162). These patterns may exist singly or in combination. They may also be associated with fractures of the

craniocervical junction. The transverse ligament is the primary checkrein against atlantoaxial AP translation. If the atlanto–dens interval increases beyond 7 mm, the spinal cord is endangered from compression of the dens into the medulla oblongata anteriorly and posterior impingement from the C2 lamina (83). Vertical displacement of the atlas on the axis is identified by widening of the C1-C2 facet joint (see Fig. 6). The tip of the dens axis lies within the arch of C1 or even caudad to it (162). The underlying pathology is disruption of the alar ligament and tectorial membrane (80,82). This condition is inherently unstable and is similarly treated as an atlanto-occipital dissociation.

Traumatic rotatory displacement of the atlas on the axis can range from a subtle subluxation to actual dislocation of the facet joints (81,86). Open-mouth odontoid radiographs will demonstrate the odontoid process to be eccentrically located between the lateral masses. Measurement of any shift between the anterior ring of C1 and the C2 is an important predictor of stability. A fine-cut CT scan with reformatting is important to demonstrate the extent of displacement. Fielding and Hawkins suggested a four-part classification (95) (Fig. 12). Type I is a simple rotatory displacement with an intact transverse ligament, the odontoid acting as a pivot. These injuries are a stable subluxation. Type II injuries are characterized by an anterior displacement of C1 on C2 of 3 to 5 mm, with one lateral mass serving as a pivot, and a deficient transverse ligament. Type II injuries are potentially unstable subluxations. If the forward displacement of C1 exceeds 5 mm, the injury is classified as type III. The lateral masses are either severely subluxed or actually dislocated, leaving the C1-C2 junction destabilized. Type IV injuries are present in case of posterior displacement of C1 on C2. This injury is usually associated with a fractured or deficient dens axis and is highly unstable.

Spinal cord injuries associated with these injuries are rare (146). The most common neurological injuries are dysesthesia resulting from injury to the C2 nerve roots. Vertebral artery occlusion or injury is a devastating but rare occurrence in patients with displaced rotatory C1-C2 injuries. Following expedient and cautious reduction of rotatory C1-C2 with traction, careful clinical reevaluation of cerebral and spinal cord function should be undertaken. If any changes in mental status or cranial nerve function are found, additional investigations with transcranial Doppler, MRI angiography, or vertebral arteriography should be obtained to rule out vascular damage.

Treatment

Treatment decisions are based on proper diagnosis and classification of injury. Initial treatment is aimed at protecting the spinal cord from further damage, reducing any deformities, decompressing compromised neural tissue, and stabilizing unstable segments until healing of the spinal column has occurred.

Fractures of the atlas. Because approximately 50% of atlas fractures are associated with other spine fractures, the definitive treatment decision has to be made after thorough evaluation of the entire spine (146,147). In general, nondisplaced, minimally displaced, or avulsion fractures are stable and can be treated with a simple orthotic device. Upright lateral radiographs are helpful in identifying an occult unstable ligamentous injury early. Stable burst and lateral mass fractures of C1 usually require a cervicothoracic orthosis such as a Minerva brace. After a 2- to 3-month period of immobilization, healing and stability are ascertained by flexion–extension radiographs. In patients with concomitant severe maxillofacial trauma, braces are not appropriate. In these cases, a halo ring and vest are recommended. Potentially unstable atlas injuries are comminuted anterior arch "blowout" fractures, injuries associated with transverse ligament insufficiency, and vertically or rotationally displaced C1-C2 segment injuries (146). Patients with such injuries are reduced with tong traction or a halo vest. If satisfactory reduction of the C1 ring cannot be maintained with a patient in a halo vest, return to continuous traction is recommended.

C1-C2 subluxation or dislocation. Greater than 3 mm of atlas–dens interval indicates transverse ligament insufficiency. Healing of such purely ligamentous injury in the adult is unlikely, and therefore posterior C1-C2 fusion is recommended (83). Vertically disrupted C1-C2 segments are highly unstable and indicate disruption of

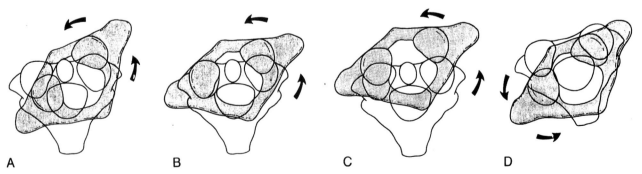

FIG. 12. Fielding's classification of rotary subluxation. (Reprinted with permission from Browner, Jupiter, Levine, Trafton (1992). In: Bruce D. Browner, et al., ed. *Skeletal trauma, fractures, dislocations, ligamentous injuries,* 1st ed. Chapter 27. Philadelphia: WB Saunders.] **A:** Type I, rotation about the dens without anterior translation. **B:** Type II, rotation about one lateral mass with anterior translation of 3 to 5 mm. **C:** Type III, rotation about one lateral mass with anterior translation greater than 5mm. **D:** Type IV, posterior displacement of C1 on C2.

alar and apical ligaments. Traction in these cases is dangerous. These patient should be treated with posterior occiput to C2 fusion. In patients with rotatory subluxation or dislocation, the treatment decisions are influenced by the time to discovery (95). Acute deformities can be reduced with cranial traction and evaluated by follow-up radiographs. Type III and type IV injuries are likely to be unstable because of transverse ligament disruption, and they may require open reduction and C1-C2 fusion in cases of lateral mass dislocations (95). In patients with an unstable C1-C2 segment without atlas fracture, posterior fusion using wire techniques, transarticular facet screws, and occipitocervical fusion are options (157). The wiring technique described by Gallie (101) has the advantage of not requiring sublaminar C2 wire passage, but it lacks the stiffness of the Brooks wire technique (43,112). The Gallie technique requires an inherently stable C1-C2 motion segment and presence of a structurally sound C2 posterior spinous process. If applied for trauma, it is preferable that both of these fusion techniques be supplemented externally with a halo vest.

The use of Halifax clamps has been proposed as an alternative to wiring techniques at C1-C2 (65,131,208). Although *in vitro* biomechanical testing has shown these devices to offer stiffness similar to a Brooks fixation construct (60,112,122), these devices offer no clinical advantage, in our opinion, and are accompanied by unacceptably high complication rates (131). In patients with a fractured C1 ring and an unstable C1-C2 segment, wiring techniques cannot stabilize the C1-C2 motion segment adequately. In such cases, transarticular facet screws or occipitocervical fusion have been recommended (157). *In vitro* stability of the C1-C2 fused motion segment is by far stiffest using two Magerl transarticular screws (112). However, anatomic reduction of the C1 lateral masses on the C2 lateral masses is a prerequisite for attempting this technique. Surgeons who are not familiar with this technique can consider occipitocervical fusion with plates or wire fixation techniques.

Complications

Most fractures of the atlas appear to heal uneventfully (146). Failure to maintain reduction of an unstable atlas fracture can lead to translational or vertical displacement of the occiput towards the C2 segment. Such loss of reduction imperils the medulla oblongata and requires surgical intervention. Patients with late deformity frequently present with myelopathy. Closed reduction of the deformity with skeletal traction should be undertaken. If reduction can be obtained, a C1-C2 fusion with transarticular facet screws can be considered. If closed reduction attempts fail, occipitocervical fusion combined with a C1 laminectomy may be indicated. Nonunions of C1-C2 fusion attempts have an incidence of

4% to 10% (43,116,146). Revision of non-unions requires adequate preoperative preparation with imaging studies and rigid internal fixation with autologous bone graft. If technically possible, transarticular facet screws are the preferable form of internal fixation. Alternatively, an occipitocervical fusion may be performed. Occipital neuralgia is a rare complication following atlantoaxial trauma (146). It is associated with posterior arch fractures and iatrogenic injury during fusion procedures. Treatment options, should conservative treatment fail, are decompression or ligation of the affected C2 nerve or C1-C2 fusion. Vertebral artery injuries may elude early clinical detection. In order to minimize any compression or undue tension on the arteries, early reduction of the C1 and C2 segments should be accomplished. In cases of intimal damage, anticoagulant treatment has been recommended (146).

Fractures of the Axis

Fractures of the Dens

Diagnosis

Odontoid fractures are 15% of all spine fractures, and they are the most frequent spine fractures in patients below 8 years and above 70 years of age (2,28,29). Most commonly, these injuries are a result of high-energy injury mechanisms involving a flexion or extension moment. In elderly patients, a simple fall on the head may cause this fracture. Ninety-four percent of odontoid fractures can be diagnosed with open-mouth anteroposterior and lateral standard radiographs (58,87). Difficulties in diagnosis may arise in pediatric patients and with initially nondisplaced fractures at the junction of the odontoid process to the base. Fractures may also be difficult to identify in the osteopenic skeletons of geriatric patients (173,188).

A transverse synchondrosis lies below the base of the odontoid process within the body of C2. This synchondrosis usually closes radiographically by age 7 (96). In an adult, an injury to this synchondrosis would represent a type III fracture of the Anderson D'Alonzo classification system (13). Similarly, nondisplaced fractures at the base of the odontoid may enter the medial eminence of the lateral mass and may be difficult to identify. Polytomography is an effective imaging device to assess this area for nondisplaced fractures. Axial CT scans may miss odontoid fractures if the fracture plane lies in the plane of the gantry. Sagittal and coronal image reformatting may minimize this problem. Motion artifacts during image acquisition may cause an artifact that can be mistaken for a dens fracture on reformatted images. To date, the efficacy of CT scans in the diagnosis of odontoid fractures has not been established.

Classification

Classification of odontoid fractures is important because of therapeutic and prognostic implications. Anderson and D'Alonzo (13) have described three fracture types (Fig. 13):

Type I fractures are rare oblique avulsions in the tip of the dens. They result from tension of alar ligaments. The importance of a type I fracture is that it may be associated with an atlanto-occipital dissociation.

Type II fractures are the most common odontoid fractures. They are located in the narrowest region at the waist of the process in the area caudad to the area covered by the transverse ligament and above the body of the axis. These fractures are likely to be unstable. Hadley

has suggested subclassifying comminuted fractures of the base of the odontoid as type IIa, because of their inherent instability (116,117). Further differentiation into the type of displacement may be helpful because of treatment implications. Displacement can be expressed as angulatory deformity and anterior, posterior, or vertical translation (195). Anterior and posterior translation can be affected by change of the head position. Vertically distracted dens fractures are inherently unstable (58). The incidence of neurological injuries associated with odontoid fractures ranges between 5% and 10% (58,117, 173,188,195).

Type III fractures are located in the body of the axis and usually have a well-vascularized broad cancellous fracture surface area. Fracture displacement is expressed

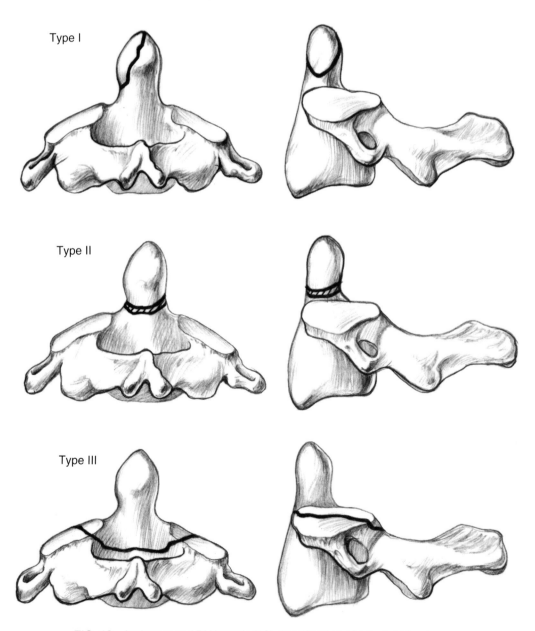

Type I

Type II

Type III

FIG. 13. Anderson and D'Alonzo's (13) classification of odontoid fractures.

in degrees of angulation and fracture distraction. Fracture stability is dependent on the initial displacement. In the series of Clark and White (58), 58% of type III fractures were displaced. A 20% incidence of neurological injuries was found for this injury type. Displacement exceeding 5 mm and angulation exceeding 10° was associated with an increased risk of non- or malunion in their series.

Treatment

Type I fractures. Prior to treatment of a type I fracture, the stability of the atlanto-occipital joint has to be determined. If an atlanto-occipital dissociation has been identified, a craniocervical fusion should be performed. Isolated type I fractures are stable injuries and can be treated with a rigid collar until radiographic union has been achieved. Following radiographic fracture union, stability should be verified by flexion–extension radiographs.

Type II fractures. Treatment protocols for this injury type remain controversial. All type II fractures are unstable. Non-operative treatment includes closed reduction and immobilization for 10 to 12 weeks in a halo vest (148,200). Skeletal traction should be applied with caution, because vertical displacement can readily occur. For closed treatment to succeed, it is imperative to achieve and maintain an anatomic reduction in the AP and lateral planes. The maximum acceptable displacement in both planes is 20% in order to maintain a surface contact of 64% (5,126,194). Any visible fracture gap is unacceptable toward the goal of fracture union (5,198).

Close serial radiographic monitoring for 2 to 5 months is required in order to verify adequate healing progress. Healing of these fractures may be difficult to ascertain. It is recommended that flexion–extension radiographs be obtained when healing appears accomplished (58). Repeat tomography or CT scans may be necessary in some patients. Although the closed treatment of choice for type II fractures is a halo, this may not be possible or advisable for a variety of reasons (148,200). In such circumstances, nondisplaced fractures can be treated in a brace such as a Minerva brace, but union is less likely to occur. Displaced fractures should be considered for internal fixation or primary C1-C2 fusions. Type II fractures have been associated with non-union rates of 4% to 32%. Risk factors for non-union include failure to institute treatment, and fractures with significant initial translational or angulatory displacement. Patient factors such as age above 60 years, delay of seeking medical help, and smoking have been associated with an increased risk for non-union (2,5,13,36,54,58,93,148,196,200,207).

In a multicenter study of 106 type II dens fractures, Clark and White (58) found posterior cervical C1-C2 fusions to lead to successful stability in 96% of patients,

compared with 66% treated with halo (Fig. 14). However, there were more complications in the surgically treated group. Statistically significant risk factors for non-union were more than 5 mm displacement, more than 9° of angulation, or a combination of these deformities. Although patients with age above 40 had more non- and malunions, the differences were not statistically significant (58). In the presence of such risk factors, or if a halo ring cannot be used, surgical treatment should be considered. Two options exist: closed reduction and anterior internal fixation of the dens with screws, or posterior C1-C2 fusion with instrumentation. Integrity of the atlas and concomitant trauma influences the surgical decision making considerably.

Internal fixation of the dens with cannulated small fragment screws has been reported to be successful in patients with fractures less than 3 weeks old (2,29,36, 54,92,93,160,191) (Fig.15). The theoretical advantages of direct screw fixation of the odontoid are preservation of the C1-C2 motion segment and avoidance of bone grafting. Further, this technique does not require the atlas to be intact. The successful placement of dens screws requires clear visualization of the dens on C-arm in two planes, and adequate closed reduction with anterior access to the body of C2 (29). A small dens, presence of a delayed union or non-union, comminution of the base of C-2, and very osteoporotic bone are relative contraindications (92). Studies have suggested the use of either one or two screws. A single screw was shown to offer sufficient stiffness in an *in vitro* comparison of one- and two-screw fixation techniques (191). A two-screw construct is expected to improve rotational control of the dens fragment. In clinical comparisons to posterior C1-C2 fusions, healing rates of the odontoid fracture fixation were similar, but with higher complication rates (2,92, 135,160). The role of anterior screw fixation of type II odontoid fractures remains to be established.

Posterior fusion techniques utilize autologous bone graft and wire constructs, clamps, or supplemental transarticular facet screws. Healing rates of primary C1-C2 fusion and delayed procedures for dens non-unions are similar. Transarticular facet screws have the advantage of achieving the highest C1-C2 stiffness of all constructs (112,113,151). With this technique, a supplemental halo is usually not required postoperatively. This is the preferred technique should a C1 or C2 ring fracture or laminectomy be present. The technique has the disadvantage of being more demanding and requiring intraoperative fluoroscopy. Congruous lateral mass reduction of C1 on C2 remains a prerequisite of this technique. Misdirection during drilling or screw placement may risk vertebral artery injury (122,153). In a series of 14 patients, Jeanneret and Magerl achieved union in all patients and had one instance of screw misplacement (135) (Fig. 16). Further studies will be necessary to assess the clinical success of this technique.

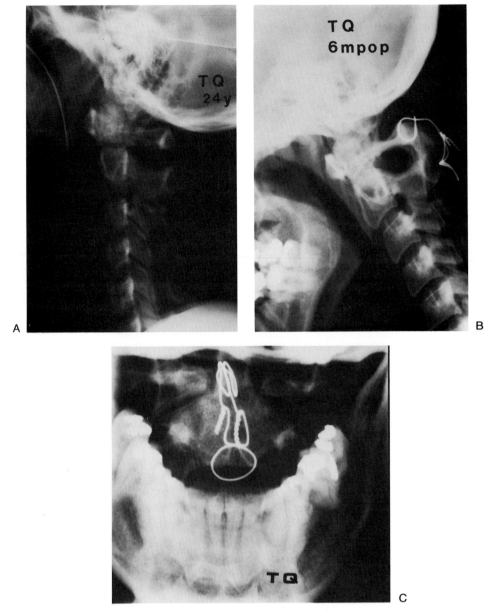

FIG. 14. A: This type II odontoid fracture in a 24-year-old woman failed to unite despite a 4-month treatment in a halo vest. The lateral cervical spine radiograph demonstrates an established non-union at the base of the odontoid. **B:** Successful fusion was achieved using the Gallie technique. The lateral view demonstrates remodeling of the posterior bone graft and healing of the fracture 6 months postoperatively. **C:** The AP view demonstrates correct wire placement.

Posterior C1-C2 fusion techniques using wire constructs or clamps require an intact C1 and C2 ring. In concomitant C1 ring fractures and dens fractures, it has been suggested that healing of the atlas should occur prior to commencing with a posterior C1-C2 fusion (58,195). This approach, however, may necessitate halo immobilization for 5 to 6 months. Healing rates for primary C1-C2 fusions have been reported as 96% (58). The use of compression clamps between the posterior elements of C1-C2 has been recommended by some (65,208). Disadvantages are the need for sublaminar

hook placement at both vertebral levels, lack of rotational control of a single clamp, loosening from cyclical loading, and need for axial stability of the two vertebral segments. Complication rates of 31% have been reported using this device (208). We do not recommend this device for the care of traumatic conditions of the upper cervical spine.

Type III fractures. Unstable type III dens fractures have an increased risk of non- or malunion. Closed treatment of displaced type III fractures should consist of a halo, with an attempt at anatomic realignment (58,

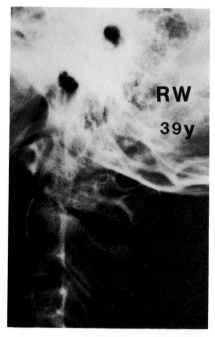

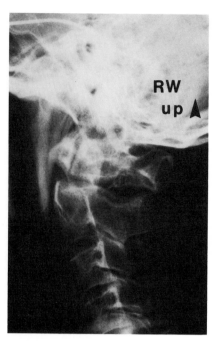

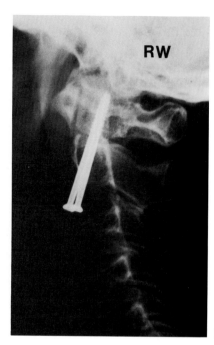

A

B,C

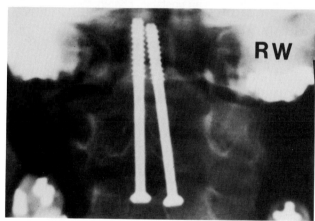

D

FIG. 15. A: The lateral radiograph taken in a recumbent position demonstrates a well-reduced type II odontoid fracture in this 42-year-old man. B: An upright view taken in the halo vest shows posterior translation of the dens. Despite several repeat reduction attempts carried out in the upright position, a stable reduction could not be maintained. C: Surgical stabilization of the odontoid in anatomically reduced position was carried out with two 3.5-mm cannulated screws, as seen on the postoperative lateral radiographs. D: Postoperative AP radiograph. Note slight convergence of the odontoid screws.

148,195,207). In patients with displacement in excess of 5 mm and angulation greater than 10°, consideration for surgical stabilization becomes relevant, because non-union rates between 22% and 40% have been described (58,196). Anterior dens screw fixation is not recommended for type III fractures unless they are of a "shallow" type (2,29,160). Posterior fusion techniques are more commonly applicable for fractures that require surgical stabilization.

Complications

Spinal cord injury as a result of a dens axis fracture are rare. Under normal circumstances, the spinal cord has ample space in the spinal canal formed by the C1 and C2 segments (146). Steels's rule of thirds approximates the distribution of components of the upper cervical spine on a lateral radiograph. The bony anterior column, the

spinal cord, and the dural sac with cerebrospinal fluid occupy one third each. Clark and White described a 13% incidence of spinal cord injuries for type II fractures and a 6% occurrence in type III fractures (58).

Spinal cord injuries can vary in severity from complete injuries with absence of respiratory impulse to incomplete injuries such as cruciform paralysis as described by Bell (25). Radiculopathies may present as greater occipital neuralgia or involve lower cervical roots and occur in 5% to 12% of patients with types II and III fractures (58).

Non-unions of type I dens fractures are rare and may in part explain the os odontoideum. Treatment outlines for a non-union of a type I dens fracture are similar to those for an os odontoideum. Making a decision between operative and non-operative treatment is guided by the age and activity level of the patient, and by evidence of instability on flexion–extension radiographs or MRI. Type II odontoid non-unions have been reported to range from 10% to 67% with non-operative treatment

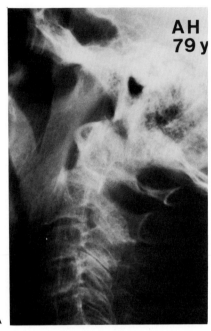
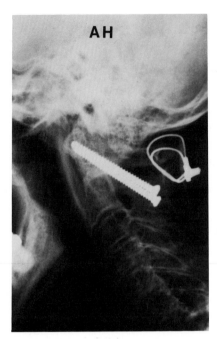
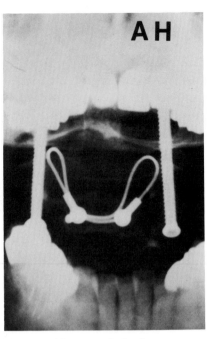

A   B,C

FIG. 16. A: This 76-year-old neurologically intact woman presented with an unstable, posteriorly displaced, type II odontoid fracture. Because of the age of the patient and initial fracture displacement, surgical stabilization of the C1-C2 segment was performed. **B:** Atlantoaxial fusion was achieved with transarticular facet screws, using the technique described by Magerl and Seemann (151), and iliac crest bone graft. The screws angle properly toward the midpoint of the anterior atlantal arch. **C:** Postoperative open-mouth view.

and 100% in missed, nontreated dens fractures (29, 58,92,135,196). A dens non-union has been described as a failure of achieving a stable union between the dens and the body of the axis by 4 months (196). Treatment of an established non-union should be performed with a posterior C1-C2 fusion technique as described previously. Anterior screw fixation of the dens is controversial and is not recommended.

Fractures of the Ring of C2

Diagnosis

Fractures of the C2 neural arch most frequently involve the pars interarticularis (146). Less common are fractures of the body, or isolated lateral mass fractures. These injuries are rare and therefore no formal classification system has been established. The most common injury is a fracture of the neural arch between the superior and inferior articular processes (86). This injury type has been described as the *Hangman's fracture*, implying an extension–distraction injury mechanism (99). The far more common mechanism is secondary to axial load, with extension or flexion mechanism from vehicular trauma or falls, and it is more appropriately termed *traumatic spondylolisthesis* (146). Lateral cervical spine ra-

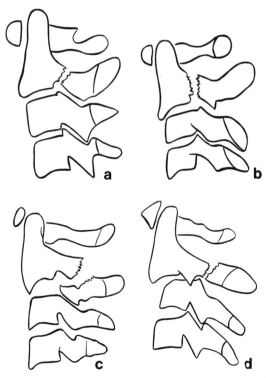

FIG. 17. Levine classification of traumatic spondylolisthesis of the axis. **a**, Type I. **b**, Type II. **c**, Type IIa. **d**, Type III.

diographs usually identify this injury as a disruption of the neural arch of the axis. More subtle signs of a fracture of the axis are angulation or translation across the C2-C3 intervertebral disc, posterior displacement of the C2 posterior spinal lamina, and prevertebral soft-tissue swelling. Traction may exhibit instability of the C2-C3 segment and therefore should be applied cautiously, starting with low weights and increasing them incrementally as required, after serial clinical and radiographic examinations (146). Lateral tomography or CT is helpful for the understanding of the injury, in particular when rotatory displacement is present. CT reformatting is helpful in identifying displacements of facet joints.

Classification

The most widely accepted classification for traumatic spondylolisthesis is Levine's modification of Effendi's system (86,146), based on lateral cervical spine radiographs (Fig. 17).

Type I injuries include all nondisplaced fractures, fractures with less than 3 mm displacement, and those with no malangulation. These injuries are expected to be stable.

Type II fractures have more than 3-mm anterior translation and angulation. The injury mechanism is postulated to be a sequence of extension axial loading followed by flexion. These injuries are potentially unstable (Fig. 17). The neural canal is widened in this injury, and neurological injury is accordingly rare. A subgroup, type IIa, is a flexion–distraction type of injury with less translation but more angulatory deformity. The angulatory deformity of these injuries increases with traction.

Type III injuries demonstrate severe angular and translational deformity and associated unilateral or bilateral C2-C3 facet dislocation. This type of injury is

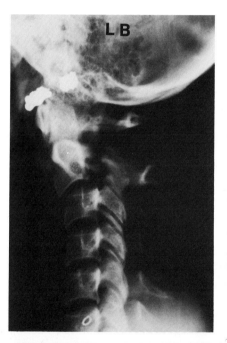

A

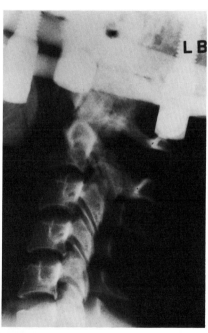

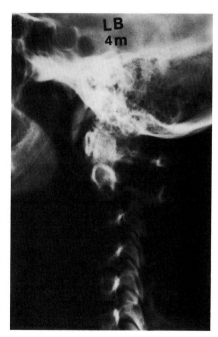

C,D

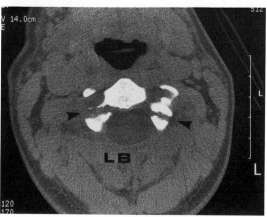

B

FIG. 18. A: The lateral cervical spine radiograph of this 36-year-old woman demonstrates a type II traumatic spondylolisthesis of the axis. **B:** The fracture of both pars interarticulares of the axis is demonstrated on this axial CT scan. **C:** Closed reduction and fracture realignment was achieved with a halo vest. **D:** Successful fracture healing could be verified on flexion–extension radiographs 3 months after injury. Despite residual displacement of C2-C3, the patient remained neurologically intact and pain free.

most frequently associated with neurological injuries. The injury is usually the result of a flexion–compression mechanism.

Treatment

Fractures of the vertebral body or lateral masses of C2 are rare. The treatment principles for those injuries are very similar to those applicable to the lower cervical spine. A type I traumatic spondylolisthesis is considered stable and can be treated with a cervical collar for 12 weeks. Reduction of the deformity of a type II fracture requires a halo for definitive treatment. Levine recommends temporary traction for more severely displaced fractures for a 3-week period prior to immobilization with a halo (146) (Fig. 18). Type IIa injuries are described as increasing in kyphotic angulation with traction. In order to avoid this deformity, Levine recommended immediate halo reduction and immobilization (146). Instability may result from C2-C3 discoligamentous disruption when it fails to heal with bone ankylosis (99). In such patients, we recommend a late anterior C2-C3 fusion with anterior plate fixation. A posterior instrumentation and fusion, if desired, will require a C1-C3 arthrodesis and therefore sacrifices an additional motion segment (99). The type III injury with unilateral or bilateral C2-C3 facet dislocations is unreducible by closed techniques (146). An open posterior reduction with stabilization is required. Surgical stabilization from the posterior may include placement of bilateral lag screws into the C2 body, stabilizing the pars fracture in conjunction with a C2-C3 wire or plate fixation.

LOWER CERVICAL SPINE INJURIES

Diagnosis

Plain radiographs of the lower cervical spine should be interpreted for obvious fracture lines, malalignment, and soft-tissue swelling. Missed injuries predominately affect the upper cervical spine or the region from C6 to T1. Therefore, visualization of the cervicothoracic junction is important (31,56,94,141,178). Loss of facet parallelism, facet overlap, and widening of the interspinous process distance between adjacent vertebrae may indicate ligamentous injury in the lower cervical spine.

Determination of stability is based on clinical assessment and radiographic parameters. The criteria established by White et al. (224) have become a standard for determination of stability of the lower cervical spine (Table 3). The radiographic parameters for instability are based on a straight lateral radiograph taken at a tube–plate distance of 183 cm. Although some authors recommend flexion–extension radiographs to assess stability, we do not recommend this test because of the possibility of incurring neurological injury. Trauma oblique radio-

TABLE 3. *Checklist for the diagnosis of clinical instability in the lower cervical spine*

Element	Point value
Anterior element destroyed or unable to function	2
Posterior element destroyed or unable to function	2
Relative sagittal plane translation > 3.5 mm	2
Relative sagittal plane rotation > 11°	2
Positive stretch test	2
Medullary (cord) damage	2
Root damage	1
Abnormal disc narrowing	1
Dangerous loading anticipated	1

Total point value of 5 or more indicates instability.

graphs are useful to assess neuroforamina and details of facet joints. Because of positional requirements, standard column radiographs are unsafe for traumatized patients. CT is best suited to evaluate the lower cervical spine comprehensively and should be obtained in traumatized patients with suspicion of radiographic abnormalities on plain radiographs.

Classification

Classification of cervical injuries should include evaluation of the osteoligamentous injury as well as the neurological injury. Currently, no accepted system combines both of these entities. Neurological injuries are classified as intact, complete, or incomplete. Several syndromes of incomplete spinal cord injuries have been described. Anterior, central, Brown-Séquard and posterior cord injuries are typical cord injuries. Many patients have isolated root injuries that are easily overlooked. The neurological level of injury is the level with at least antigravity motor function (10).

Classification systems of skeletal injury are based on morphology, mechanisms of injury, or combinations of the two. Critical in the application of the classification systems is the stability of an injury (170). Bohlman introduced a classification system that combines anatomic and mechanistic terms. Anterior element fractures are differentiated into avulsion fractures, fractures through the disc space, and compression fractures of the vertebral body. Posterior element injuries involve spinous process fractures, lamina fractures, unilateral and bilateral facet dislocations, or fracture dislocations and perched facets. Fractures involving the lateral mass constitute a separate subgroup (155). The Orthopaedic Trauma Association has accepted a modified form of this system for its comprehensive skeletal classification (108,170) (Table 4). After a review of force vectors on the C- Spine and resulting injuries Ducker described a "resultant force clock" identifying injury mechanisms and correlating injuries (155).

Allen and Ferguson have suggested a more complex but comprehensive classification system based on six

TABLE 4. *Cervical spine trauma classification, from the Orthopaedic Trauma Association*

51 Upper cervical spine

51 A1	Occipital cervical dislocation
A1.1	Anterior
A1.2	Vertical
A1.3	Posterior
51 A2	Cervical spine, occipital condyle
A 2.1	Type 1
A 2.2	Type 2
A 2.3	Type 3
51 A3	Atlas
A 3.1	Jefferson
A 3.2	Lateral mass
A 3.3	Posterior arch
A 3.4	Anterior arch
51 B1	Cervical spine, transverse ligament
B 1.1	Rupture, mid substance
B 1.2	Rupture avulsion
51 B2	Cervical spine, dens fracture
B 2.1	Type 1
B 2.2	Type 2
B 2.2.2	Type 2a
B 2.3	Type 3
51 C	Cervical spine, traumatic spondylolisthesis of the axis
C 1	Type 1
C 2	Type 2
C 2.2	Type 2a
C 3	Type 3

52 Lower cervical spine

A 1.1	Spinous process fracture
A 1.2	Extension avulsion or teardrop
A 1.3	Lateral mass fracture without subluxation
A 1.4	Isolated lamina fracture
A 1.5	Ligamentous strain
52 B 1.1	Facet injury
B 1.1.1	Perched unilateral
B 1.1.2	Perched bilateral
52 B 2.2.1	Facet dislocation
B 2.2.1	Without fracture, unilateral
B 2.2.2	Without fracture, bilateral
B 3.3.1	With displacement, unilateral
B 3.3.2	With displacement, bilateral
52 C	Severe injuries
C 1.1	Flexion teardrop
C 1.2	Severe ligamentous injury
C 3.1	Compression fracture
C 3.2	Burst fracture

From ref. 170.

different mechanisms of injuries grouped into separate phylogenies (Fig. 19). The individual injury severity is reflected as a stage within each of these six phylogenies, indicating a increasing severity of injury (6).

Distractive flexion. In this group of injuries, a forward flexion moment is coupled with a disruption of posterior elements. Because of the posterior ligamentous disruption, all of these injuries are at risk for instability and have a high rate of failure with non-operative treatment. Stage I injuries present disruption of posterior ligaments with subluxation. Stage II lesions are unilateral facet dislocations and stage III lesions are bilateral facet dislocations. Stage IV lesions are distractive lesions creating a "floating" vertebra with complete body displacement.

Vertical compression. In general, these fractures involve mostly bone and have little posterior ligamentous disruption. Stage I injuries afflict only the superior or inferior endplate. In contradistinction to distractive flexion injuries, stage I vertical compression fractures have no posterior ligament disruption. Stage II lesions have fractures of both superior and inferior endplates. Stage III lesions show centrifugal bursting of vertebral body fragments.

Compressive flexion. This phylogeny has five stages. Stage I has blunting of the anterior superior caused by impression of the more superior vertebral body. In stage II, the vertebral body is wedged. Stage III fractures have an oblique fracture from the ventral vertebral body to the inferior endplate. Stage IV lesions have subluxation of the posterior vertebral wall not exceeding 3 mm. In stage V fractures, the subluxation exceeds 5 mm. The facet joints in this subgroup are subluxed as well, indicating joint disruption. Stage I and II are usually stable injuries requiring bracing. Stages III and IV require close supervision to avoid undue collapse of the vertebral body. Stage V injuries are highly unstable and incompletely reduce with traction.

Compressive extension. This phylogeny also has five subgroups. Depending on the forces exerted, increasing comminution of the posterior elements and increasing separation of anterior vertebral bodies results. Stages I and II have either unilateral or bilateral posterior element fractures and are usually stable. In stages III through V, comminution of the lamina and lateral masses occurs with vertebral or disc space separation. Instability of the cervical spine has to be anticipated in case of disruption of anterior, middle, and posterior ligaments.

Distractive extension. Two subgroups are identified in this phylogeny, reflecting the severity of displacement. In contrast to compressive extension injuries, lesions in this group do not entail fractures of the posterior elements. They occur infrequently and are the opposite of distractive flexion injuries.

Lateral flexion. These injuries are rare and are classified in one of two subgroups. Increasing comminution and displacement is reflected in a higher grouping.

The classification system proposed by Allen and Ferguson necessitates intricate knowledge of the multiple subgroups (6). It is limited because it does not specifically address the osseous and ligamentous structures injured, and it is confusing because of its multiple subgroups.

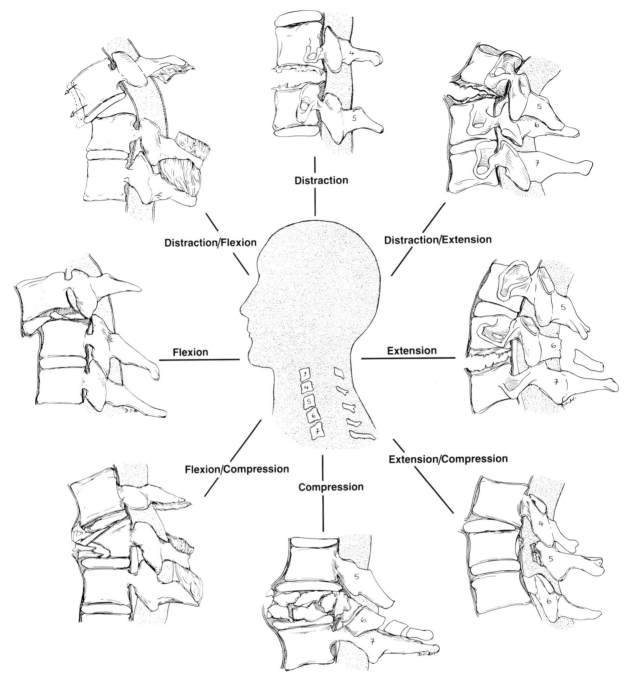

FIG. 19. Mechanistic classification of lower cervical spine injury mechanisms as modified from Allen et al. (6).

We recommend the use of a comprehensive classification system that covers all areas of the cervical spine and is easily reproducible. The system proposed by the Orthopaedic Trauma Association currently fulfills this requirement best (170) (Table 4).

Ligamentous Stability

Based on cadaveric studies and clinical experience, White et al. recommended a checklist that attempts to quantify clinical stability of the lower cervical spine (224). A specific point value is assigned to location of injuries, sagittal plane translation, sagittal plane rotation, abnormal disc diastasis during a stretch test, cord or root injury, preexistent disc disease, and likelihood of noncompliance (Table 3).

In patients with potential ligamentous instability, the application of a stretch test helps identify such lesions more safely than the more uncontrolled flexion–extension radiograph obtained in an emergent setting.

This test should be performed under physician supervision in an awake patient only. Longitudinal traction is applied with a 5 to 10 pound initial weight. Lateral cervical spine radiographs and repeat neurological examinations are performed with incremental weight increases not exceeding one third of the body weight. The stretch test is considered positive at any point at which a disc space or facet joint widens by more than 1.7 mm or angulates more than 7.5° (see Fig. 20). The point values of the various categories are then summated, and if the values are more than 5, the spine is probably clinically unstable.

Treatment

Treatment decisions require complete clinical and radiographic assessment of the patient. Determination of stability using an accepted classification system is a prerequisite prior to embarking on treatment. Any neurological injury is generally classified as unstable.

Minor lower cervical spine fractures. Isolated anterior longitudinal ligament avulsions, nondisplaced laminae or lateral mass fractures, and spinous process fractures are examples of minor lower cervical spine fractures. Provided there is no translational or angulatory deformity, these isolated injuries usually are stable and heal with immobilization in a rigid neck collar or cervicothoracic orthosis over 2 to 3 months. Upright radiographs in the brace should be obtained to verify proper alignment. Flexion–extension radiographs are obtained at the end of healing to verify adequate healing.

Ligamentous injuries. The severity of ligament injuries of the cervical spine is variable and ranges from minor sprains to complete disruptions (Figs. 20,21). Determination of stability is assessed with plain radiographs, stretch tests, or flexion–extension radiographs. Recently, MRI with fat-suppression technique has been described as diagnostic of acute ligamentous injuries in the cervical spine (213). Minor ligament injuries without instability are immobilized in a rigid orthosis for 2 months and re-

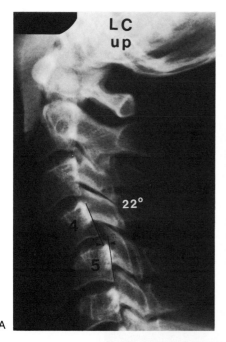
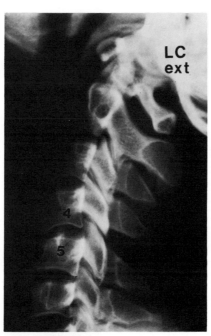
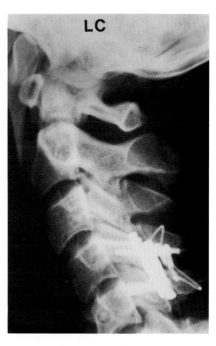

A

C,D

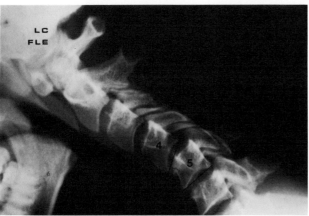

B

FIG. 20. A: This 24-year-old neurologically intact man presented with persistent neck pain 4 months following a motorcycle accident. The neutral upright lateral radiograph shows a focal kyphosis at C4-C5 measuring 22°, with 3 mm anterior translation. Interspinous widening is present between C4 and C5. **B:** Flexion radiographs showing increased kyphosis to 35° at C4-C5. **C:** Kyphosis corrects to 19° with full extension. Sagittal translation of 4 mm was found on the flexion lateral radiograph (B), but it was reduced in extension. **D:** Anatomic reduction and stable fusion were achieved with a posterior cervical fusion using lateral mass plates, interspinous cable fixation, and iliac crest bone graft. The patient has remained pain free.

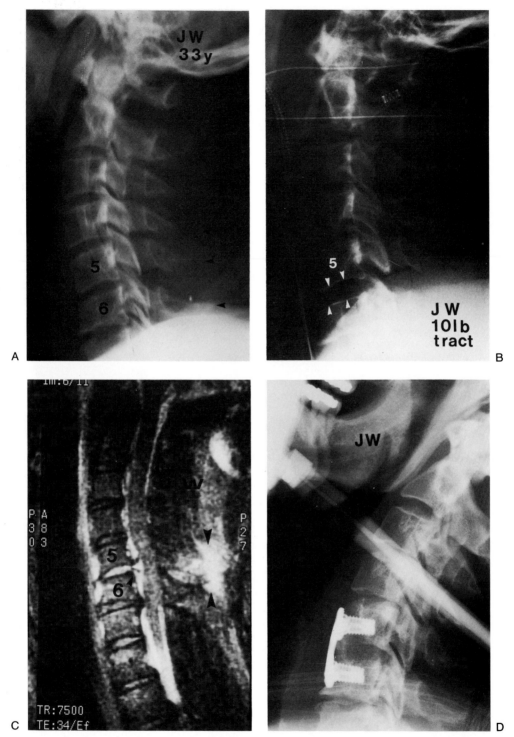

FIG. 21. A: The lateral cervical spine radiograph of a 33-year-old man involved in a rollover motor vehicle crash demonstrates interspinous widening at C5-C6. The patient presented with a C5 complete quadriplegia and three extremity open, long-bone fractures. *Arrows* indicate interspinous widening. Note the narrowed C5-C6 disc space. **B:** Cranial traction of 10 pounds demonstrates abnormal intervertebral widening, exceeding by 1.5 times the disc space of adjacent levels. This is indicative of total ligamentous disruption between C5 and C6. **C:** An emergently obtained a T2, fat-suppressed MRI demonstrates a large extruded disc fragment compressing the spinal cord at the C5-C6 level (*small arrow*). High-intensity signal is present in the nuchal ligaments confirming ligamentous disruption (*large arrows*). **D:** Following emergent anterior discectomy and intervertebral bone grafting, an anterior cervical locking plate was used for stabilization. The patient became independently ambulatory with bilateral ankle–foot orthoses by 6 months after injury.

assessed radiographically. Persistent pain and localized tenderness are an indication for late posterior cervical fusion (224). Radiographically more significant unstable ligamentous injuries have increased interspinous distance, loss of facet parallelism, and localized kyphosis. Ligament injuries in the cervical spine usually heal under scar formation in elongation and lead to poor functional recovery. Therefore, posterior cervical fusion is recommended for patients with documented ligamentous instability (45,224).

Unilateral facet dislocations. The goal of treatment is anatomic realignment of the injured segments using skeletal traction under physician supervision. Successful outcome requires maintenance of anatomic alignment of the spine, regardless of treatment (24,26,48,57,198). Initial treatment consists of closed reduction with skeletal tong traction. Patients with a pure unilateral facet dislocation that has been reduced successfully may be treated non-operatively in a halo vest (57). Serial radiographic evaluation should be carried out to assess for loss of reduction. Loss of anatomic joint alignment should be addressed by surgical stabilization (203). Unilateral facet dislocations associated with fractures of an articular process are usually easy to reduce, but they frequently redisplace with non-operative treatment (26,57). We recommend surgical stabilization with lateral mass plates or oblique wires (Fig. 22). Patients with unilateral facet dislocations frequently have radiculopathies. These patients should be assessed by CT myelography or MRI to evaluate foraminal patency (75,119,152,203). If foraminal stenosis is present, a foraminotomy and stabilization with lateral mass plates is recommended.

Bilateral facet dislocations. These injuries are highly unstable and are frequently associated with neurological injury (15,24,63,184). Timely reduction of the injury deformity is recommended to minimize deleterious pres-

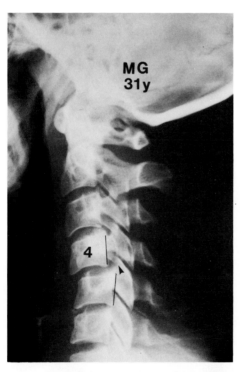

A

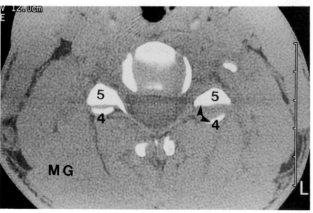

B

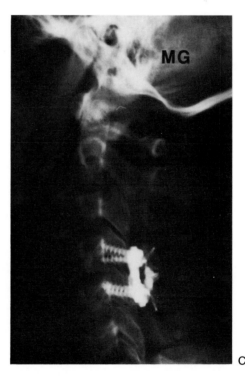

C

FIG. 22. A: This lateral cervical spine radiograph of a neurologically intact 24-year-old man demonstrates a 25% vertebral body translation resulting from a unilateral facet dislocation. Anatomic reduction was achieved with skeletal traction. **B:** Postreduction CT shows residual left facet joint diastasis. **C:** Posterior cervical fusion was carried out with iliac crest bone graft and posterior lateral mass plates following interspinous cable fixation.

sure on neural structures (Fig. 23). The protocol described by White et al. should be followed for the reduction sequence (224). Extrusion of the intervertebral disc following closed reduction has been described in 15% to 42% of patients with these injuries (88,176,180). In neurologically intact patients, imaging with MRI or CT myelography prior to reduction can influence treatment decisions (75). In patients with a large extruded disc fragment, anterior discectomy and fusion with bone graft and instrumentation can minimize the risk of neurological injury (88,176,180,181).

Delaying reduction to perform imaging is of little benefit to the patient with spinal cord injury. Reduction of the dislocation should take precedence over initial imaging, but the reduction should be followed by an imaging study to assess the status of the intervertebral disc. Definitive treatment decision are then made, based on the need for neurological decompression and stabilization (55). Non-operative treatment has been associated with loss of reduction in up to 48% of patients treated with halo vests (15,24). In patients with bilateral facet dislocations without significant disc herniation, closed reduction followed by posterior fusion and instrumentation is recommended (31,88,198) (Fig. 23). If a large disc herniation is identified, anterior discectomy and fusion with instrumentation is preferable (176,181) (Fig. 21).

Although *in vitro* studies have demonstrated significantly greater stiffness of posterior instrumentation compared with anterior plates, clinical outcome studies have not shown statistically significant differences (42,211).

Burst fractures. Burst fractures in the cervical spine result from axial and flexion loading forces and are frequently associated with neurological injury (31). Radiographic findings include retropulsion of vertebral body fragments into the spinal canal and posterior element disruptions such as lamina or spinous process fractures. Realignment of the spinal column with skeletal traction can achieve indirect spinal canal decompression if the posterior longitudinal ligament is intact. Overdistraction can occur if the posterior interspinous ligament is insufficient or if the applied weight exceed 70% of body weight (224). Non-operative treatment is indicated if canal decompression can be achieved and alignment maintained in a halo vest. Surgical stabilization is preferable in patients with neurological deficits and in those in whom there was failure to achieve a satisfactory reduction by closed means (Fig. 24). For single-level burst fractures, a vertebral corpectomy with strut grafting and anterior instrumentation can restore alignment and achieve canal decompression. In patients with multilevel fractures, closed reduction and posterior cervical fusion with lateral mass plates is preferable (16). Late decom-

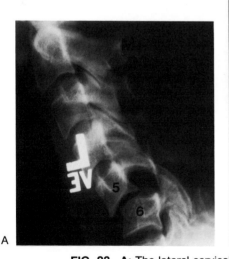
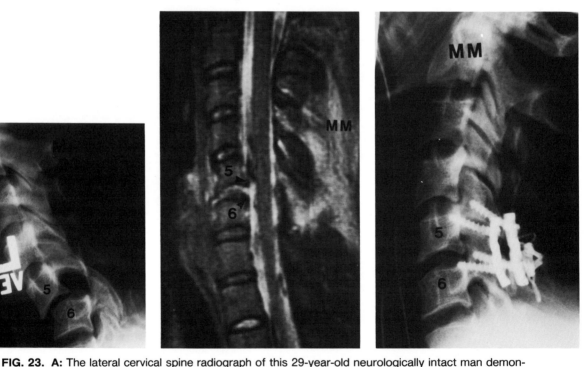

A

B,C

FIG. 23. A: The lateral cervical spine radiograph of this 29-year-old neurologically intact man demonstrates a bilateral C5-C6 facet dislocation. Sequentially increasing traction applied with Gardener-Wells tongs succeeded in injury reduction at 105 pounds. The patient remained neurologically intact following reduction. **B:** Postreduction MRI does not reveal a traumatic disc herniation, but it does demonstrate torn posterior longitudinal and nuchal ligaments. **C:** Posterior cervical fusion of the injured segment was carried out with lateral mass plates, interspinous cable fixation, and iliac crest bone graft.

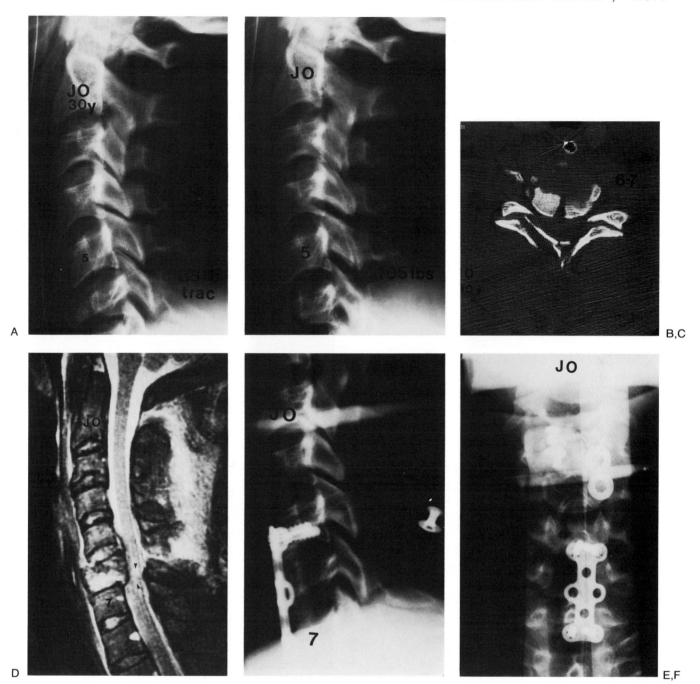

FIG. 24. A: This unfortunate 30-year-old presented with C5 complete tetraplegia following a fall. The lateral radiograph demonstrates the collapsed C6 vertebral body and interspinous widening between C5 and C6. **B:** Skeletal traction of 65 pounds succeeded in indirect fracture reduction via ligamentotaxis. **C:** This axial CT scan demonstrates an unstable C6 burst fracture with comminution of the vertebral body and posterior elements. **D:** MRI shows displacement of fragments of the vertebral body against the spinal cord. High-intensity signal in the cord substance represents edema or acute hemorrhage (*arrows*). **E:** Lateral radiographs following C6 cervical corpectomy. Reconstruction with autologous iliac crest and stabilization with an anterior cervical locking plate were carried out. Despite complete spinal cord decompression, the patient failed to make any neurological recovery. **F:** Postoperative AP radiograph.

pression and fusion has been recommended for patients with residual neurological deficits and persistent cord compression (14,32).

Extension injuries. Extension injuries frequently afflict elderly patients who have preexistent spinal column abnormalities such as ankylosing spondylitis or severe cervical spondylosis. In the presence of a narrowed canal, neurological injuries such as central or anterior cord syndromes can occur following hyperextension without obvious fracture (31,199) (Fig. 25). The spinal cord is pinched between anterior osteophytes and the buckling posterior ligamentum flavum. Initial treatment consists of reduction of the deformity by application of skeletal traction, with the patient's head in a neutral position. Extension of the neck is avoided. Definitive treatment decisions are based on posterior element injuries and neurological status of the patient. Single-level inju-

ries without posterior element comminution usually are stable and can be treated with a hard collar after traction for several days. Extensive posterior impaction injuries are unstable and should be treated with anterior fusion and instrumentation (Fig. 26). In patients with neurological injuries, surgical decompression and stabilization may allow a more predictable neurological recovery. Surgical stabilization is also the recommended treatment for patients with displaced fractures in ankylosing spondylitis or diffuse idiopathic skeletal hyperostosis.

Complications

Delay in diagnosis of an injury to the cervical spine can lead to serious sequelae. It is estimated that injuries in 3% to 25% of patients are missed, and of these, one

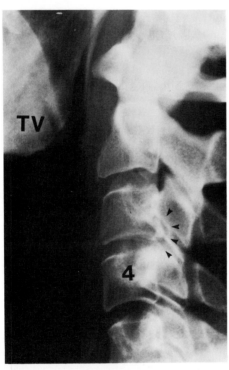

A

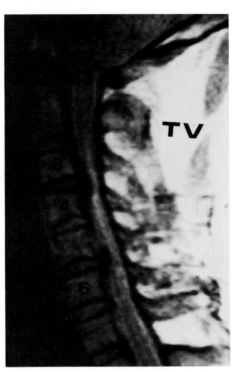

B

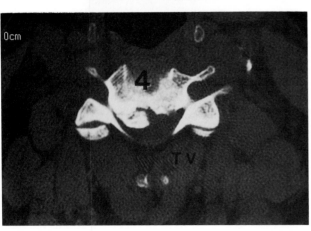

C

FIG. 25. A: The lateral cervical spine radiograph demonstrates an avulsion of the C3 inferior endplate in this 44-year-old man injured with a hyperextension mechanism during a bicycle accident. The patient presented with C3 complete tetraplegia. Large osteophytes (*arrows*) can be seen on the lateral radiographs at C3-C4 and C5-C6. **B:** The sagittal MRI shows presence of cervical spondylosis at C3-C4 and C5-C6 with discoligamentous injury of the C3-C4 motion segment. Severe spinal stenosis is present. **C:** A noncontrast axial computed tomogram of the C3-C4 disc space shows a large osteophyte emanating from the right uncovertebral joint of C4. In the presence of severe spinal stenosis and anterior osteophytes, even minor hyperextension trauma can lead to severe neurological injury. To maximize chances for neurological recovery, a C4 and C5 corpectomy, autologous iliac crest strutgraft reconstruction, and anterior plating from C3 to C6 was carried out.

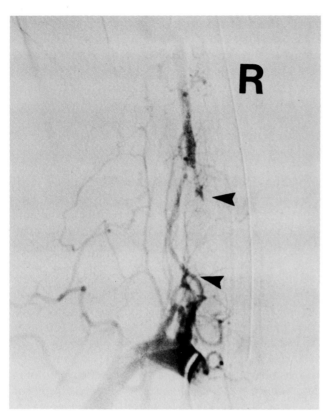

FIG. 26. Vertebral angiography of a 42-year-old man with C7 radiculopathy and mental status changes. Plain radiographs demonstrated a 25% subluxation of C6 on C7. Mental status changes, including confusion and imbalance, were noted 5 days after injury. CT showed fractures of the transverse processes of C6 and C7 and bilateral facet fracture dislocation. MR angiography was suggestive of bilateral vertebral artery injuries. Selective angiography was ordered because of the unexplained mental status change. Bilateral vertebral artery injuries with obstruction of flow were found (right side shown). Both vertebral arteries reconstitute through retropharyngeal collaterals. Bilateral cerebellar infarcts were found on MRI and CT as result of embolization emanating from the vertebral artery injuries. The patient was successfully treated with anterior cervical discectomy, anterior interbody fusion, and instrumentation C6 on C7.

third develop neurological sequelae. Failure to obtain a standard radiograph is the most common cause of missed injuries (31,52,68,90,107,149,150,178,186,190). Clinical suspicion and skilled image interpretation are necessary first steps to avoid these potentially serious complications. Cervical spine fractures are associated with injuries to other organ systems in 5% to 61% of patients (90,150,190,218). In polytraumatized patients, a full radiographic work-up of the spine is sometimes not possible. In such patients, spine precautions should be maintained until appropriate imaging studies have been obtained and have received expert review.

Vertebral artery injuries as a result of fractures and dislocations of the lower cervical spine have been estimated to occur in 0.9% to 46% of patients. In a prospective study using vertebral angiography, 9 of 12 patients with bilateral facet dislocations had vertebral artery occlusion (111,227). Bony obstruction of the foramen transversarium had a statistically significant association with disruption of flow of the vertebral artery. A possible association of occlusion of a single vertebral artery and neurological deficits is presently unknown. Routine vascular studies for determination of vascular injury are not recommended. In patients presenting with cervical spine trauma, with altered mental status and without identifiable head injury, normal vertebral artery flow should be verified (227).

Iatrogenic injuries to the vertebral artery have been described in case reports (111). If feasible, repair of the artery and local hemostasis, followed by angiography-guided embolization, have been recommended. Awareness of the location of the vertebral artery during the surgical care of the injured spine is important.

Neurological complications from reduction of cervical spine dislocations have been reported with an incidence of less than 1% (75,88,144,152,180,181). In a retrospective study of the National Spinal Injuries Center, no correlation to age, sex, mechanism of injury, or level or type of dislocation was found. Mechanical factors, such as a small spinal canal size, were found to be likely causes (152).

Disc herniation into the spinal canal is also a possible cause of postreduction neurological deterioration and has been associated with bilateral facet dislocations (31,88,176,180,181,198). In neurologically intact patients, a prereduction MRI or CT myelogram can assess the intervertebral disc and spinal canal space.

Late effects of cervical fusions include pain and degenerative changes rostral or caudal to fused segments. In a review of 61 patients examined at an average of 8 years after posterior fusion for cervical spine trauma, moderate or severe degenerative changes were found in 9%. The motion segment caudad to the fused segment was significantly more frequently affected by instability or degenerative changes than the cranial one. Pain and degenerative changes were significantly associated with kyphosis of 20° or more. It can be hoped that maintenance of physiological spine alignment with rigid internal fixation will decrease these adverse effects (138).

NON-OPERATIVE TREATMENT TECHNIQUES

Orthotic Devices

Orthotic devices are applied with the goal of supplying comforting support and motion restriction to an injured neck. Neck collars are made with materials of varying stiffness, ranging from foam to rigid plastic or metal. They may cover the neck area alone (category 1 devices), extend via head band to the patient's cranium (category

2 devices), or attach to the trunk via vest (category 3 devices) (21). The effectiveness of neck collars is limited by neck size and by the need for mandibular and shoulder girdle contact area for support. If the goal of treatment is immobilization, soft neck collars are generally ineffective. In biomechanical studies 70% to 75% of normal flexion–extension was possible in a soft neck collar, 78% to 82% of rotation, and 87% to 92% of lateral tilt (77,139). More rigid devices, such as a Philadelphia collar, allowed 26% to 29% of flexion–extension, 44% to 51% of rotation, and 66% to 71% of lateral bending. Rigid plastic collars, such as the Miami J or Stifneck devices, allow 15% to 37% of original flexion–extension, 37% to 49% of lateral tilt, and 24% to 35% of rotation to take place.

Cervicothoracic braces appeared to limit spine motion most effectively. Flexion–extension was limited to 13% of normal, rotation to 18%, and lateral bending to 50% (77). Category 2 devices, such as the SOMI brace, were found to mostly limit motion of the upper cervical spine, whereas cervicothoracic braces (category 3) were most effective between the fifth cervical and first thoracic vertebrae (139). Craniofacial pressures and comfort of different cervical orthoses were compared in a study on volunteers. The Philadelphia collar created occipital pressures in excess of capillary closing pressure with the volunteers in a supine position. The Miami J and Newport collars were best tolerated and were well below capillary closing pressures on all contact points. A single piece collar (Stifneck) exceeded capillary closing pressures on most contact points (174). These measurements are important in the long-term immobilization of patients with altered mental status. Compliance with brace wear may also be affected by pressure points. Particular care to the soft tissues of patients with altered mental status or frail integument who receive external immobilization is necessary to avoid decubital ulcers.

Cervical orthoses in general have limited potential for immobilization. Their main role is to provide supportive immobilization for postoperative needs or for stable injuries. If orthotic devices alone are used in the treatment of fractures, supine and upright plain radiographs should be obtained to rule out malalignment. Unstable osteoligamentous injuries of the cervical spine are not adequately treated by external orthoses alone.

Cranial Traction

A variety of devices are available to facilitate safe manipulation of the cervical spine. A head halter device can apply limited traction with a padded chin and occipital strap. This has a limited application in the care of the majority of spine fractures and can be tolerated only for a limited time period.

When reduction or stabilization of a patient with injured unstable cervical spine is required, cranial tong traction or a halo ring is used. Prior to application of any cranial traction device, the presence of a skull fracture has to be ruled out. Clinical evaluation, lateral skull radiographs, or a head CT scan should be obtained in all patients with head injuries.

Cranial tong traction originated from a modification of femoral traction by Crutchfield in 1933 (64). The requirements for skeletal traction are ease of application, ability to withstand substantial loads, and the avoidance of penetration of the inner skull table. Gardner-Wells tongs, introduced in 1973, fulfill these needs and are the device most commonly used for cervical spine trauma (21). One of the skull pins is a spring-loaded tension meter designed to prevent skull penetration. Both pins are directed at an upward angle to maximize pull-out strength. The pins are inserted under local anesthesia approximately one finger-breadth above the external auditory meatus, below the greater diameter of the skull. Locking nuts are secured against the tongs to minimize the risk of inadvertent pin twisting. The width of the tongs prevents rolling the patient on the side and serves as a visible warning signal of the patient's neck injury status. Since MRI is a frequently required diagnostic tool, graphite tongs with titanium pins are now preferred. If patients with unstable cervical spines require prolonged traction, the pins should be retightened after 24 hours (21,102). Patients who require prolonged traction are placed on a Roto-Rest bed to prevent skin breakdown and improve pulmonary function. Initial traction weights should reflect the level and type of injury and the patient's body weight. A lateral radiograph should be obtained after application of the initial low weight to check for overdistraction. Aside from skull fractures, cranial traction is contraindicated in patients with occipitocervical dissociations and purely distractive spine injuries. In these cases, a halo vest is recommended.

Halo Orthoses

Halo devices consist of a cranial ring and a trunk vest. The halo concept was introduced as an external immobilization device for polio patients in 1959 by Perry and Nickel (21). The cranial rings are of either closed or open design and are manufactured of stainless steel or graphite composites. The halo ring is secured with a minimum of four pins to the skull. Proper pin and ring placement is crucial to avoid complications (37). Presence of a skull fracture has to be ruled out. The ring is applied under local anesthesia, with the head shaven and disinfected in the area of pin application. Incisions are unnecessary (21,102). The ring should be below the skull equator to prevent ring pullout, and it should have about 1 cm clearance to the skin. The anterior pins should be placed above the lateral half of the eyebrows with the patient holding the eyes shut. The ring should be 1 cm or less from the eyebrows and ears. Pins are tightened by securing opposing pins synchronously to avoid ring displacement. Using a torque screw driver, the pins are initially tightened to 6 inch-pounds in adults. Retightening to 6 or 8 inch-pounds should be performed at least once (21,37,102).

Biomechanical tests have demonstrated that the stability of a halo assembly depends on the fit of the vest to the patient's torso (15,103,158). Most commercially available vests are assembled from an anterior and posterior shell. In one study, motion of the cervical spine was reduced to 4% of its original flexion–extension, 1% of original rotation, and 4% of original lateral bending (184). Anderson et al. (15) studied fracture site motion between supine and upright positions in patients treated with halo vests. In 77% of patients, fracture site motion of greater than 3° or 1 mm translation was found (see Fig. 15). Loss of reduction was encountered in 46% of patients (15,225). Halo vests do not necessarily prevent a "snaking" motion with flexion at one level and extension at an adjacent level (201).

Because most vertebral fractures require at least 2 months for healing, durability of the halo vest becomes an issue. In a series of 179 patients, pin-related problems were very common. Loosening was found in 36% of patients, pin site infections in 20%, severe pin discomfort in 18%, and disfiguring scars in 9% of patients. Other complications include pressure sores in 11% and dural penetration in 1% of patients (102). While the halo vest is the most rigid form of external immobilization device, its clinical usefulness is somewhat limited (45,158, 184,200,201,225). Successful treatment requires application with attention to detail and close follow-up (37). Radiographs made after application should include supine and upright comparison lateral radiographs to rule out unacceptable instability (15). There should be close clinical follow-up of pin tracts. In elderly individuals and patients with quadriplegia, these devices may be associated with skin breakdown, aspiration, and pulmonary complications (45,184,201,225).

ANTERIOR SURGERY

Indications

Anterior surgery for cervical spine injuries was introduced by Smith and Robinson in 1953 (205) and was popularized by Cloward (59) and Bohlman (31). This technique consists of a direct approach to the spine and allows for decompression of the ventral surface of the spinal cord. Indications for anterior procedures are unstable cervical burst fractures with incomplete reduction, and other injuries with residual ventral spinal cord im-

pingement. The importance of removing any anterior mechanical obstruction of the spinal cord in patients with cord injury was demonstrated by Bohlmann (14,32,35). Neurological improvement was found in 72% of patients with incomplete quadriplegia. Sixty-one percent of patients in this group regained the ability to ambulate (32). Sixty percent of patients with complete quadriplegia had improved upper extremity motor strength after anterior decompression and stabilization. Outcome was significantly improved in patients who received the anterior cervical decompression and fusion within 12 months. Only one patient of the 110 in the series deteriorated neurologically (14). In patients with unstable cervical burst fractures, restoration of the anterior vertebral column with a strutgraft and anterior instrumentation improves the biomechanical stability compared to posterior procedures or non-operative treatment (30).

Technique of Anterior Decompression and Fusion

Positioning of the patient is performed on a horseshoe headrest with traction extension or with Mayfield tongs. The shoulder girdle is slightly elevated with a rolled-up towel. Both arms are padded and tucked along the sides of the patient. The shoulders are gently pulled caudally by tape to facilitate intraoperative radiographic visualization. The anterolateral approach described by Robinson usually allows for exposure of the base of C2 to the T2-T3 disc space (182,183). With the retropharyngeal modification described by McAfee, exposure of the C2 vertebra is possible (155). A longitudinal neck incision along the medial border of the sternocleidomastoid muscle is suggested if more than three vertebral bodies need to be exposed. In order to minimize risk of iatrogenic injury to the recurrent laryngeal nerve, we recommend a left-sided approach. McAfee has recommended a right-sided incision for the retropharyngeal approach (155). Prior to making an incision, a sterile needle is placed on the operative field to determine the best level of the incision on a lateral radiograph. The incision should be centered on the injured segment to facilitate exposure. The skin incision of a standard Smith Robinson approach is transverse from the medial border of the sternocleidomastoid muscle to the midline (182,205). The platysma is transected with electrocautery. The interval between the sternohyoid muscles medially and the sternocleidomastoid muscle laterally is identified, and the superficial layer of the deep cervical fascia is incised. The medial border of the sternocleidomastoid muscle is now released to improve the exposure of the deeper layers. The posterior fascial envelope of the sternocleidomastoid connects to the sternothyroid muscle as the middle layer of the deep cervical fascia. After palpation of the carotid pulse, the artery is gently displaced laterally with a retractor.

The trachea and esophagus are displaced medially as a unit, using a blunt retractor. The deep layer of the deep cervical fascia is the prevertebral fascia. After visualization of this structure, it is incised sharply, allowing for inspection of the longus colli muscle. This muscle is incised along the midline and reflected laterally to both sides, together with the anterior longitudinal ligament. Iatrogenic injury to the cervical sympathetic chain is avoided by limiting the lateral dissection to the uncovertebral joints. Radiographic documentation of the level of surgical exposure is obtained with placement of a double-bent spinal needle into a disc space. The final step of the exposure is placement of self-retaining transverse and longitudinal retractors with the blades anchored under the reflected longus colli.

Depending on the clinical needs of the patient, a discectomy or corpectomy is performed. The annulus is sharply separated from the endplates and disc material is removed with cervical curettes and pituitary rongeurs. The depth of the vertebral body is best gauged by carefully completing the discectomy until the posterior longitudinal ligament is exposed. Laterally, the discectomies are carried out to the uncovertebral joints. Discectomies can be facilitated by use of endplate or vertebral body spreaders. In corpectomies, removal of the cranial and caudal disc helps the surgeon determine the depth of the vertebral body. The corpectomy is performed by removal of loose fragments using rongeurs and a high speed burr. Iatrogenic injury to the vertebral artery is avoided by limiting the lateral decompression to the level of the uncovertebral joints. Completion of the decompression is achieved when the posterior longitudinal ligament bulges forward. Removal of the posterior longitudinal ligament can be associated with significant epidural blood loss and is usually not necessary. However, displaced disc fragments can perforate the epidural space and may require removal of the posterior longitudinal ligament. The decompression phase is completed upon achieving adequate homeostasis.

The reconstruction of the spinal column is preferably accomplished with an autologous tricortical iliac bone graft. A variety of grafting techniques have been described. The endplates adjoining the corpectomy are cleared of cartilage with curettes. The endplates are then flattened with a burr to allow for flush seating of the bone graft ends. Smith and Robinson recommended creating a central recess into the cranial and caudal endplates. A tricortical iliac bone graft is then cut to fit the defect length (205). The graft is then trimmed in width to allow for 1 to 2 mm of space on the lateral sides. This permits drainage of a possible epidural hematoma. It is crucial to establish the depth of the vertebral body defect correctly. The graft depth should be several millimeters less in order to avoid iatrogenic cord impingement during graft insertion (98). If the technique of Smith and Robinson is used, small pegs are created on either end of the graft.

These pegs serve as anchor points in the vertebral body recesses created previously (182,205). A variation of this technique has been described as a reversed Smith Robinson graft. The modification consists of the cortical part of the tricortical iliac crest graft placed towards the spinal canal. Improved graft fixation has been attributed to this technique (155).

With the advent of safe anterior instrumentation techniques, we have abandoned the Smith Robinson technique and now place a graft flush against the flattened endplates of the adjacent vertebrae. Gentle distraction is exerted during the graft insertion. Upon graft placement, traction is removed and a lateral radiograph is obtained. Quality of the decompression, alignment of the spinal column, and graft placement are then judged. If a corpectomy of more than two levels is carried out, autologous crest graft becomes impractical. In such circumstances, a fibula auto- or allograft is a suitable alternate graft. Fibula grafts have significant biomechanical advantages over the iliac crest, but they may have decreased bony healing (228). Bone graft substitutes are being studied for their application in anterior interbody fusions (202). Currently, the use of these substitutes is not established in applications for trauma patients.

Anterior Instrumentation

Biomechanics

The procedure of anterior decompression and fusion decreases spinal stability through loss of longitudinal ligaments and intervertebral discs (98,209). With traumatically disrupted posterior elements or laminectomy, anterior grafts require rigid external immobilization or stable internal fixation (216). Neurological complications following anterior decompression and fusion alone have been reported by Flynn (98), Stauffer and Kelly (209), and others (29). Graft fragmentation and collapse of the strutgraft into the adjacent vertebral bodies can lead to malunion with cervical kyphosis. Maintenance of cervical lordosis appears to be related to satisfactory patient outcome. Kyphosis of 20° or more was associated with severe neck pain in a long-term outcome assessment (138). A 64% incidence of loss of reduction and graft displacement of anterior decompressions and strutgrafts without instrumentation has been demonstrated in several studies (4,30,61,98,121,209,216). In order to improve stability after anterior fusion, a posterior cervical procedure as a second stage surgery has been advocated (209,216). This has the advantage of excellent biomechanical stability, but it does necessitate a separate surgical intervention.

Anterior instrumentation has been developed to provide an immediately stable environment for graft healing in a single procedure. Several implant systems are available. The first generation anterior procedure used stainless steel plates with standard bone screws that required bicortical purchase. The Caspar plate was created with slotted screw holes to allow for some graft collapse during healing (51). The Orozco H-plate used conventional AO/ASIF (American Society of Internal Fixation) inventory (169). Because the screws of both systems have no purchase within the plate, the posterior cortex needs to be engaged with the screw tip in order to prevent screw loosening and loss of screw–plate alignment (189).

In vitro biomechanical comparison of first generation anterior plates to posterior instrumentation techniques demonstrated anterior plates to be superior in extension loading. In flexion, these devices had only 25% to 50% of the stiffness of posterior implants. Caspar plates were found to become progressively unstable during cyclical loading (1,60,215).

Because of the lack of biomechanical stiffness and the dangers inherent to placement of bicortical bone screws, a second generation of anterior plate systems has been introduced (161). These plating systems are manufactured from titanium and have a rigid screw–plate interface. They rely on unicortical cancellous bone fixation. The AO/ASIF system uses a hollow screw with an expansion head to lock the screw into the plate (163). The Orion plate by Danek uses an interference screw to lock the vertebral body screws to the plate. *In vitro* comparison of second generation to first generation plates revealed significantly higher load to failure and increased fatigue strength (1,115). Published union rates are similar for noninstrumented and instrumented anterior fusions in trauma. Noninstrumented anterior fusion after corpectomy or discectomy has resulted in published union rates of 36% to 98% (31,98,209,210). First generation AO/ASIF plates had 92% to 100% fusion rates (3,22,30,49,51,69,104,169,179). Complication rates of up to 36%, primarily related to hardware, have been reported (22,98,216). Second generation plates have been available for a limited time only. Published fusion rates are 100% to date (22,163,210). We compared the outcomes of spinal cord injury patients randomized to either anterior fusion and instrumentation with AO/ASIF locking plates, or posterior fusion with lateral mass plates. There was no statistically significant difference in neurological recovery, healing of fusions, or pain. We found a 10% non-union rate in the anterior group, and there were no non-unions in the posterior group (42).

Technique

The first generation plates offer few advantages and have increased risks, and we do not recommend their use. The second generation devices are titanium, which allows repeat imaging with an MRI scan. The screws are intended for unicortical purchase only. They are locked into the plate by means of expanding head screws [AO/ASIF-CSLP (cervical spine-locking plate)], interference screws (Orion, Danek), or locking nuts (Spinetek). Screws are usually available in 14-mm lengths, but they should be checked on preoperative CT or MRI. After decompression and placement of the strutgraft, the traction is released. Any anterior osteophytes or overhangs are planed down with a burr. A lateral radiograph is taken with an appropriately sized plate placed anteriorly on the spine. This allows for assessment of plate position and size. Ideally, the plate holes are located at approximately the mid body level (22). The plates may be contoured to reproduce cervical lordosis. The screws require drilling with a set-depth 3.0 drill and 4.0- or 4.35-mm tapping if needed. Penetration into adjacent disc spaces will adversely affect screw purchase and should be avoided. While the plate is held in position, the screw heads are inserted until they are flush with the plate surface. Prior to placement of locking screws, a repeat radiograph should be taken to confirm proper screw placement. The hardware placement is completed by placement of locking screws. Layered wound closure of the platysma and skin is performed. Postoperative immobilization is achieved with a rigid collar or class 3 orthosis for 2 to 3 months. Fusion is checked with flexion–extension radiographs.

Complications

Complications of anterior cervical decompressions and fusions are most commonly reported after surgical intervention for degenerative conditions. Risks of the anterior surgical approach include dysphagia, esophageal or pharyngeal perforation, and laryngeal nerve injury (98,167). We recommend a left-sided approach because of the unpredictable course of the recurrent laryngeal nerve on the right side (22,55). Myelopathic deterioration as a result of anterior cervical spine surgery was estimated to have an occurrence of 0.1% in a large retrospective questionnaire. Possible causes for this occurrence are direct surgical dissection trauma, cord impingement with an epidural hematoma or graft displacement, or spinal column malalignment (98). Another possible cause, change in cord perfusion, has been hypothesized but not documented. Published non-union rates of anterior fusions are widely divergent, possibly reflecting author bias.

Graft displacements have been reported in 50% to 68% of unstable spine fractures that received anterior interbody fusions or corpectomies with strutgrafts without internal fixation. Three contributing factors were identified: (a) failure to identify posterior instability, (b) insufficient anterior strut-grafting technique, and (c) inadequate postoperative external immobilization (98,209, 216). With exacting surgical technique and halo vest application, successful fusion rates as high as 98% have been described (31). Because these results were not widely reproducible in all centers, alternatives such as posterior fusions have been suggested (216).

Anterior instrumentation offers the chance to achieve the goal of adequate stabilization without a second surgery. In recent studies, the more extensive surgical exposure necessary for plate placement into adjacent vertebrae has not been accompanied by higher complication rates (22). Wound infections, neurological injuries, and esophageal injuries appear to have incidences similar to grafting procedures alone (167). Graft displacement and malunions appear to be consistently much lower than with noninstrumented anterior fusions. The incidence of hardware failure ranges from 0% to 8% (22). In our review of patients with anterior stabilization of cervical spinal cord injuries, we found an incidence of 5% anterior hardware failure in unstable three-column spine injuries. There were no significant differences in the fusion and hardware failure rates when anterior and posterior implants were compared. Loss of fixation can be found as toggle loosening around screw threads or as screw backout. Exacting drilling and screw placement technique in bone is important. Not all hardware failures reflect delayed or non-union of the anterior fusion. Discovery of hardware failure should, however, raise the level of suspicion for such a complication and lead to a further work-up. Loose hardware or plates and screws that have pulled loose should be treated by hardware removal in order to prevent esophageal erosion (22,167). Non-unions of anterior fusions without significant hardware displacement can be treated with posterior cervical fusion.

Dens Screw Fixation

Indications

Type II dens fractures have been associated with a high rate of non-union, despite halo vest treatment (13,58, 105,195,196). For closed treatment to succeed, a nearly anatomic fracture reduction must be maintained (126,198). If unacceptable displacement of the odontoid is encountered, anterior internal fixation of the fracture can be considered. The advantage of this technique is possible preservation of the C1-C2 motion segment. Fracture extension into the base of the axis, fractures of the tip of the dens, or patients with osteoporosis are contraindications for internal fixation (2). Treatment of delayed unions or non-unions of the odontoid with anterior fixation have been attempted but are controversial (29,54,92,165,191). Prior to screw placement, closed reduction of the odontoid must be achieved. Fluoroscopic imaging of the dens must be performed in two planes to avoid iatrogenic injury (160) (see Fig. 15). Non-union has been reported in 12% of patients with screw fixation

of type II dens fractures. The overall complication rate was reported as 28%. The authors of one study attributed these results in part to poor patient selection (3,29,160). These complication rates are, however, similar to some studies of posterior C1-C2 fusions. To date, anterior fixation of the odontoid remains under evaluation in major spine centers and has not become routine treatment for odontoid fractures.

Technique

The intubated patient is positioned supine on a radiolucent operating table. The patient's head is secured with Mayfield head tongs. A radiolucent bite block is placed into the opened mouth of the patient to allow for an open-mouth odontoid view. Closed reduction of the fracture is then performed under image intensification in two planes. The technique of anterior internal fixation of the odontoid should be continued only if the odontoid can be clearly imaged in both planes and can be anatomically reduced. We found the use of two C-arms placed at right angle projections to one another to be helpful.

A left-sided Smith Robinson approach is made over the C4-C5 or C5-C6 disc space. Upon identification of the longus colli muscle, the dissection is carried cranially. At the C2-C3 disc space, the longus colli muscle is split in midline and reflected laterally. A radiolucent mandibular retractor is secured into the base of C2. Two 1.1-mm-threaded guidewires are then inserted into the odontoid in slightly convergent fashion. After confirming pin length, overdrilling of the axis body is performed. A self-tapping cannulated screw is then inserted over the guide wire. The goal is to engage the posterior cortex of the odontoid tip with the terminal screw thread. We prefer placement of two screws because of the decreased likelihood of spinning the odontoid during single screw insertion. The dimensions of the odontoid should be preoperatively measured on the fine-cut CT scan of the region. If a small dens size precludes placement of two screws, single screws have been reported to provide adequate stability (126,191).

POSTERIOR SURGERY

Posterior Approach

Indications

The posterior approach to the cervical spine usually is direct and extensile. If indicated, a posterior decompression, such as a foraminotomy and laminectomy, can be performed in conjunction with a fusion. Posterior instrumentation and fusion can restore the posterior tension side of the cervical spine and maintain a physiological alignment. Indications for posterior surgery include decompression of posterior neural impingement and treatment for disrupted posterior elements that result in instability of the cervical spine. The posterior approach allows for open reduction and stabilization of ligamentous and facet fracture dislocations. New techniques such as posterior plating have increased the biomechanical stability of complex lower cervical spine injuries.

Technique

Intubation of the awake patient is accomplished by the nasotracheal route with fiberoptic guidance. During turning of the patient into a prone position, cranial traction is maintained and proper spine precautions are observed. Prone positioning with the patient awake allows for direct monitoring of neurological changes. Intraoperative electrodiagnostic monitoring is recommended for patients requiring manipulation of the spinal column (160). A Stryker or other turning frame is used for the posterior surgery of the unstable spine. In patients with significant spinal deformity, such as ankylosing spondylitis, a Stryker frame cannot be used safely. Awake prone positioning on a cushioned chest buildup with the head secured in Mayfield tongs is preferable. The arms are padded and tucked to the side. The shoulders are padded to minimize pressure on the brachial plexus. Gentle, caudally directed traction on the shoulders with tape can allow for improved intraoperative radiographic visualization of the lower cervical spine. A lateral radiograph should be taken immediately after positioning of the patient. Corrections in alignment and traction are made preoperatively, prior to draping. A midline approach limited to the area to be fused is made in order to avoid inadvertent extension of the fusion. The intact interspinous ligaments and facet capsules are preserved in order to minimize the risk of destabilization of levels adjacent to a fusion. The surgeon should be fully aware of any posterior element injuries and should perform the subperiosteal exposure with care in anticipation of exposed neural tissue and without any downward pressure on fractured segments. The level is identified radiographically. Laterally, the exposure is carried to the far edge of the lateral masses (16).

Decompression

Indications

Posterior cervical approaches allow for decompression of the spinal canal and foramina. A laminectomy is indicated for depressed laminar fractures causing cord compression and removal of an epidural hematoma. *In vitro* studies have shown that laminectomies do not have any decompressive effect on anterior spinal cord compression (7). Moreover, cervical laminectomies without con-

comitant fusion have been associated with increased deformity and loss of neurological function (50,204).

If a cervical laminectomy is indicated, the affected segments should be arthrodesed with facet bone grafting and instrumentation. We have found lateral mass plates to be effective means of internal fixation in such cases. Facet fractures and fracture dislocations can lead to nerve root impingement. The nerve root obstruction may persist despite reduction of the deformity. A postreduction CT myelography or MRI should be scrutinized for foraminal obstruction. If present, a posterior foraminotomy can be performed at the time of posterior fusion. We recommend segmental instrumentation of affected levels to avoid deformity and pain.

Technique of Posterior Decompression

After exposure of the identified levels, a foraminotomy is performed by elevating the lateral insertion of the ligamentum flavum and the facet capsule with a cervical curette. A limited laminotomy is performed with 1- to 2-mm Kerrison rongeurs. An air-powered small burr is used to resect the medial half of the caudad inferior articular process. Similarly, the medial half of the superior articular process is then removed. The exposure of the posterior aspect of the neuroforamen is then completed with small cervical curettes and Kerrison rongeurs. With small flat dissectors, loose fragments around the nerve root and spinal cord are elevated and removed. The decompression is completed if a small blunt probe can be passed laterally into the foramen without difficulty. Foraminotomies in the injured cervical spine are less difficult if performed before loose bone fragments have become adherent to the dura. Laminectomies are inefficient for the decompression of ventral spinal cord compression (7,50,204). This procedure is recommended for depressed lamina fragments and the evacuation of epidural hematoma. Depressed lamina fragments require particular care during the exposure. After exposure of the superior and inferior margins of the lamina, the ligamentum flavum insertion is removed sharply. Any downward pressure on the depressed segment is avoided. Elevation of the depressed segment can be accomplished with small, angled cervical curettes. Remaining jagged fracture ends should be smoothed with Kerrison rongeurs. An epidural hematoma can be a rare cause of posttraumatic spinal cord compression. The decompression technique depends on identification of the extent of the mass lesion and its severity. A fresh hematoma can be removed with a simple laminotomy at one or two levels without removal of the midline structures. A consolidated hematoma will require complete laminectomy to the extent of the lesion. After laminectomy in trauma patients, we routinely perform a posterior fusion (16).

Posterior Wire Fixation

Indications

Interspinous wire techniques have been the most commonly performed cervical spine stabilization techniques. Rogers (185) described the long-term results of 37 patients with spinal cord injury treated with interspinous wire fixation. He found a 95% success rate and one loss of reduction with unsatisfactory result. Posterior interspinous wires are able to increase stiffness in flexion by 110% compared to an intact spine (60,211). Satisfactory results can be achieved with interspinous wires in facet dislocations and ligamentous disruptions. Fractures of posterior elements and the presence of a laminectomy may make interspinous fixation of the injured vertebral levels with this technique impractical. Extending the fusion construct to adjacent vertebrae with intact posterior elements is required. Interspinous wires are less effective biomechanically if extended over multiple segments. Rotationally unstable cervical injuries, such as fracture dislocation treated with interspinous wires, have been accompanied by loss of reduction (221).

Several modifications of the standard interspinous wire fixation have been described. Bohlmann and McAfee reported 100% union rates in two series totaling 172 patients using the triple wire technique (156,221). Although the addition of the triple wire technique has been shown to add rotational stability to the cervical spine (156), the limitations associated with interspinous wire fixation remain the same despite this modification. Facet wiring techniques that gain bone purchase in the inferior articular process have been described by Robinson and Southwick (183). Edwards et al. (85) modified this technique by passing a wire from the inferior articular process to the next caudad spinous process. They reported successful union in 26 of 27 patients treated with the "oblique wire" technique for unilateral facet dislocations with rotational instability. Although facet wire techniques can be used in patients with deficient laminae, they are difficult to perform, they achieve limited biomechanical stability, and tey do not provide rotational or axial control in complex instability patterns. Because of the absence of biomechanical advantages and the potential for iatrogenic neurological injury, sublaminar wire fixation in the lower cervical spine is not recommended. McAfee et al. demonstrated no increase in stiffness when they compared sublaminar and simple interspinous wires (156). In trauma patients, the neural tissue may be swollen and therefore sublaminar wires may cause impingement of the spinal cord (155).

Technique of Wire Fixation for the Subaxial Spine

Interspinous wire. After exposure, the facet joints of the level to be arthrodesed are decorticated with a small curette or burr. Care is taken to not remove any bone from the lateral masses. Autologous cancellous bone is fit into the posterior half of the facet joint. A 3-mm burr hole is made at the base of the spinous processes and widened with a Lewen clamp. A titanium cable or 20-gauge wire is then passed through the hole and looped around the spinous process. The same process is repeated for the next level and the wires are then tightened (see Fig. 12, Chapter 54 on page 1134). Hyperextension or posterior translation of the instrumented vertebrae can occur during wire tightening. In such cases a small corticocancellous H-shaped bone graft can be placed between the spinous processes prior to tightening of the wires. An intraoperative lateral radiograph is obtained after wire insertion, to assess the quality of reduction. The lamina is decorticated and covered with iliac crest bone graft.

Bohlmann triple wire. In order to increase rotational stability, Bohlmann suggested the triple wire technique (156). After completion of a standard interspinous wire construct as described, one 22-gauge wire is passed through the superior spinous process, and another through the inferior. Two corticocancellous grafts are then sized to cover the superior and inferior spinous processes with their cancellous surfaces. Each of the 22-gauge wires is then passed through two small perforations made in the grafts, and the wires are tightened, compressing the strutgrafts against the spinous processes and laminae (see Fig. 13, Chapter 54 on page 1134).

Facet wire. Facet wires require a 3-mm hole to be drilled from the center of the lateral mass downward into the facet joint (183). While gently distracting the facet joint, a 22-gauge wire is passed through the hole into the facet joint and pulled out with a small grasper. This wire can then be tightened to another facet wire on the same side (see Fig. 15, Chapter 54 on page 1137). Some authors have recommended passing the facet wires through perforations of a corticocancellous bone graft to facilitate fusion and to minimize the risk of the wire breaking out. Edwards et al. recommend passing the facet wire of the cranial vertebra around the spinous process of the next caudad level (85). With this modification, the facet joint at the caudad level of the fusion remains intact and the cranial level is pulled towards the midline. An interspinous wire and bone graft are added. Postoperative immobilization depends on the instability and strength of fixation and ranges from a hard collar to a halo vest.

Posterior cervical clamps. Several clamps for posterior cervical fusions have been introduced. The Halifax clamp consists of two curved metallic hooks designed for sublaminar or facet joint insertion, which are connected by a threaded rod. Stabilization is achieved by compressing the two clamps against one another (208). Biomechanically, the Halifax clamp offers no increase in flexion, extension, or torsional stiffness compared to interspinous wire fixation (211). Holness et al. reported good results with this device (131). There are several conceptual disadvantages: (a) because posterior spine elements are compressed to achieve stabilization, the device is not applicable in the presence of lamina or lateral mass fractures; (b) multilevel fixation is not possible; (c) rotationally unstable spine injuries are poorly stabilized; and (d) we have observed loss of reduction and dangerous translation secondary to compression of the Halifax clamp. Clamps necessitate instrumentation into the adjacent motion segments at both ends of the construct, and they require sublaminar hardware placement with associated increased risk of neurological injury. We therefore do not recommend the use of this device in the lower cervical spine.

Posterior Cervical Plate Fixation

Indications

Posterior plate fixation of the cervical spine offers the possibility of immediate stability with limited levels of fusion, even in the presence of deficient posterior elements. Screw purchase for plate fixation of the lower cervical spine has been described for lateral masses and pedicles (11,16,114,136,171,187). However, close proximity of the spinal cord, nerve roots, and vertebral artery requires precision of screw placement to avoid iatrogenic injuries. Improved stiffness of a cervical spine instrumented with posterior plate fixation should be weighed against the risk of serious neurological or vascular damage (109).

Three different techniques of screw placement into lateral masses have been described. Roy-Camille et al. (187) first described the technique of posterior lateral mass plating. They recommended placing a screw starting in the center of a lateral mass, with a lateral trajectory of 15°. Fusion was achieved with plates without facet arthrodesis. Roy-Camille et al. reported good or excellent result in 85% of 221 patients. Using a similar technique, Nazarian and Louis (166) and Cooper (63) reported successful results in 41 of 42 patients. Jeanneret et al. (136) recommended lateral mass screw placement with cranial inclination of 25°. By using this screw direction, the length of screws used could be increased from an average of 14 mm with the Roy-Camille technique to 20 mm with the Magerl technique (136). The Magerl technique was found to significantly improve stiffness compared to the Roy-Camille technique (160). In a cadaver study, Heller et al. (127) found that 92% of the screws placed using the Roy-Camille technique had posed no danger to neurovascular structures, compared to 42% in specimens instrumented with the technique of Magerl. The technique of Roy-Camille was found to penetrate the facet joint caudal to the instrumented lateral mass more frequently than the technique of Magerl.

In conjunction with his suggestions for screw place-

ment, Magerl also introduced the Hook plate (136). This device combines sublaminar purchase of a cranially pointing hook at a lower vertebral level with lateral mass screw fixation in the next higher level. Biomechanically, this device offers the highest stiffness of all cervical spine implant systems (114). Jeanneret et al. reported 51 successful fusions using the hook plate and screw placement of Magerl (136).

Anderson further modified the technique of Magerl by suggesting a starting point of lateral mass screws 1 mm medial to the posterior center of the lateral mass with 30° to 40° angulation and 10% to 25% lateral angulation (11,16). All 30 patients prospectively followed after treatment with posterior cervical reconstruction plates healed anatomically. In one patient, subtle loss of reduction was found. No iatrogenic neurovascular injuries resulting from posterior lateral mass fixation were found in this series. Heller et al. found a 0.6% incidence of iatrogenic nerve root injury and a 0.2% incidence of fact joint violation in 654 lateral mass screws. Other complications included 0.3% broken screws, 1.3% broken plates, 0.2% screw avulsion, and screw loosening in 1.1% of screws (128). The authors identified technical difficulties in obtaining purchase in the C7 segment because of the narrow dimensions of its lateral mass and the increased likelihood of an iatrogenic nerve root injury. Present indications for posterior cervical plating versus interspinous wire fixation include patients with laminectomy, deficient or fractured posterior elements, and multilevel instability. In rotationally unstable cervical spines, lateral mass plates have been shown to offer superior stiffness compared to all other instrumentation techniques (60,91,109,211,215) (Figs. 22,23). Displaced lateral mass fractures or bilateral facet fracture dislocations are prone to displace with posterior wire fixation alone, and they are preferably treated with lateral mass plates.

Technique of Lateral Mass Plate Fixation

The posterior approach was described previously in this chapter. The important landmarks of the posterior cervical spine are the lateral masses. The posterior surface of the lateral masses forms a square, superiorly and inferiorly limited by the facet joints (16). The lateral margin is the far edge of the facet, and the medial margin is at the valley marking the junction of the lamina to the lateral mass. The center of the most cranial lateral mass is then determined. Roy-Camille et al. recommended directing a drill perpendicular to the cervical spine axis with 10° to 15° lateral direction (187). Jeanneret et al. recommended a 25° to 30° cranial angulation of the screws starting in the center of the lateral mass (136). Anderson et al. recommended a starting point 1 mm medial to the center, with screw direction similar to that of Magerl (16) (see Fig. 19, Chapter 54 on page 1140). Drilling is performed free-handed with a 2-mm Kirschner wire. An adjustable drill guide prevents plunging. After initial drilling depth of 12 to 14 mm, this length is increased by 2-mm increments until the far cortex is reached. Blunt probing of the drill hole is performed after each drill step to avoid lateral mass penetration. Bicortical screw purchase is associated with increased stiffness of fixation compared to unicortical screws. It is, however, potentially dangerous and therefore not recommended routinely (109,127).

After placement of the most cranial and most caudal drill hole, a posterior plate with the best match for screw hole spacing is selected. The Axis system (Danek) has plate hole spaces of 11, 13, and 15 mm, with double space holes. The posterior cervical reconstruction plates (Synthes) have plate hole spaces of 12 and 8 mm. After plate contouring and facet arthrodesis, the plate is secured with the cranial- and caudal-most screws. Intercalary screws are then placed as needed, following the previously described method. Cancellous bone graft is placed in the facet joints and along the decorticated spinous processes and laminae of the levels to be fused.

At the C2 level, the lateral masses are small and offer insufficient space for safe screw placement (11). Screw placement in this level can be obtained by following the pedicle alignment. A cranial angulation of 25° to 40° with medial direction of 10° to 15° degrees is recommended (11). Visualization of the medial margin of the C2 pedicle helps in accurate screw direction. An intraoperative lateral radiograph of the cervical spine is taken to confirm satisfactory hardware placement.

Posterior C1-C2 Fusion with Wire

The two basic wire fixation techniques have been described by Gallie (101) and Brooks and Jenkins (43). Several modifications exist for each technique. Contraindications to atlantoaxial wire fixation are posterior translation and fractures of the atlas. The surgical exposure for both techniques consists of posterior midline exposure of the base of the occiput, the lamina of the atlas, the axis, and the upper half of the C3 posterior elements. Dangers specific to the surgical approach are the vertebral artery and the C2 nerve. The vertebral artery lies lateral to the C1-C2 facet joint and courses adjacent to the superior rim of the C1 lamina into the cranium. Exposure of the C1 lamina exceeding 1.5 cm from the midline risks injury to the vertebral artery. The C2 nerve root emerges posterior to the C1-C2 facet joint encased by multiple epidural veins. In order to avoid injury to this structure, dissection from the C2 isthmus cranially is helpful. The C2 nerve root is cranially retracted to allow for exposure of the C1-C2 facet joint (151). Facet joint exposure is performed if a facet arthrodesis is required, or for placement of C2-C1 facet arthrodesis

screws. Sublaminar wire passage in patients with displaced vertebral segments is potentially hazardous to the spinal cord and dura and should be carefully weighed preoperatively.

The Gallie technique requires sublaminar C1 wire passage, which is secured to the spinous process of C2. Twenty-gauge wires are tightened over a corticocancellous iliac crest graft (43) (see Fig. 6, Chapter 54 on page 1126). Sublaminar wire passage under C1 usually is safe because of the more copious space available for the cord. The atlanto-occipital and atlantoaxial membranes are released from the cranial and caudal side of the C1 lamina 1.5 to 2 cm lateral to the midline. Using small cervical curettes or probes, a continuous passageway under the C1 lamina is created. Using a low-profile suture passer, a #2 suture is passed under the C1 lamina. This suture is threaded through a looped 18- or 20-gauge stainless steel wire, which in turn is pulled under the C1 lamina in a cranial direction. The wire loop end is then placed over the base of the C2 spinous process. Sectioning of the C2-C3 interspinous ligament is necessary to seat the wire appropriately. The laminae of atlas and axis are decorticated. A corticocancellous graft of 3 × 4 cm is now trimmed to congruously fit the C1 lamina and closely straddle the C2 spinous process and lamina. Small notches are created on both sides of the graft to control placement of the free end of the wire. The free ends of the wires are then crossed over the graft and tightened (see Fig. 14). Intraoperative lateral radiographs are then checked to evaluate reduction.

Brooks and Jenkins described placement of a pair of sublaminar wires under C1 and C2 (43). The advantage of this method compared to the Gallie technique is increased biomechanical stability and preservation of the C2-C3 interspinous ligament (112). The inherent disadvantage of the technique is the placement of sublaminar wires at the C2 segment. The surgical exposure is identical to that of the technique described for a Gallie procedure. In addition, a C2-C3 laminotomy is created and a sublaminar passage under the axis is established. Sutures are passed separately for the left and right sides under the axis and atlas, respectively. A looped 18- or 20-gauge wire is then passed from cranial to caudal on the left- and right-sided laminae of the atlas and axis. Two corticocancellous grafts are contoured on their cancellous surfaces to achieve maximum contact to the laminae of the axis and atlas. The wires are then tightened over two corticocancellous iliac crest grafts (see Fig. 7, Chapter 54 on page 1127). Postoperative immobilization with a Minerva brace or halo vest is recommended.

Transarticular C1-C2 Facet Arthrodesis

Transarticular C1-C2 facet screws have been recommended as a method of fixation for an unstable atlantoaxial segment (113,135,151,153). In the presence of deficient laminae in the C1-C2 region, transarticular screws are able to provide stability, provided a reduction of the atlas on the axis can be obtained. Preoperative evaluation of the quality of reduction is mandatory, preferably with a CT scan with reformatting. This procedure should be considered only if a congruous reduction of the C1 lateral mass onto the C2 joint can be obtained (135).

The patient is positioned prone, with the head secured with a halo ring or Mayfield tongs. It is important to flex the head, under fluoroscopic control, far enough to maintain reduction, yet allow for appropriate space for drilling. A posterior midline exposure from the occiput to the C3 segment is performed. The C1-C2 facet joints are dissected and the posterior third joint cartilage is removed with a small cervical curette. The medial wall of the isthmus of the axis is dissected with a small blunt probe. A starting point for the screws is created in the inferior articular process of C2 at the junction of the medial to center third of the facet joint with a 3-mm burr (see Fig. 8, Chapter 54 on page 1127). A 2.5-mm terminally threaded guide wire is then inserted through a small stab wound, paraspinously through the trapezius muscle at about the level of C7-T1, and directed into the starting point. This guide wire is then advanced, under lateral C-arm guidance, in a 45° to 60° angle of vertical inclination. The guide wire is aimed to stay just lateral to the medial wall of the isthmus of the axis. Intra-articular passage of the guide wire can be visualized by direct inspection of the joint. The anterior cortex of the anterior arch of the atlas is engaged but not penetrated with the wire (see Fig. 16). After the left- and right-sided wires have been inserted, the wire insertion depth is measured and the near cortex of the drill hole is tapped. Screws of 3.5- or 4.0-mm diameter with lengths between 40 and 50 mm are used. Each screw should engage the anterior cortex of the anterior arch of the atlas. Prior to screw insertion, an appropriately dimensioned wafer of cancellous bone is inserted into the facet joint. A small-fragment, cannulated screw set with self-tapping screws can make the exchange of the initial drill to screw easier. However, deflection of small guidewires may pose a challenging problem. The procedure is completed by performing a midline fusion using a corticocancellous bone graft and a Gallie wire technique. In some patients, reduction can be enhanced by use of posterior C1-C2 wires.

Occipitocervical Fusion

Several techniques for occipitocervical fusion have been described (177,187,206,223). We recommend occipitocervical fusion with cervical reconstruction plates (see Fig. 9). Preoperative skeletal traction is helpful in patients with basicervical invagination or malalignment.

In patients with atlanto-occipital dissociation, a halo vest is preferable to maintain reduction of the deformity.

With the patient positioned prone using Mayfield tongs or a halo, the reduction of the occipitocervical junction is carefully evaluated. Congruous reduction of the occipitocervical facet joints in a neutral position is important to achieve a physiological cervical spine alignment. A posterior midline exposure is carried out from the inion to the C3 segment. Further caudal exposure may be required in some conditions. After carrying out a C1-C2 facet arthrodesis, a cervical reconstruction plate is contoured to extend from the level of the inion to the lateral mass of C2 or C3. If possible, a C1-C2 transarticular facet screw is drilled. If not feasible, a C2 pedicle screw site is prepared. The cervical reconstruction plate is then contoured to fit the occipitocervical junction, and it is then secured to the prepared C2 segment by placement of a 3.5-mm C2 pedicle or a transarticular C1-C2 screw (see Fig. 4, Chapter 54 on page 1124). The plate is then affixed to the occiput by drilling both cortices of the skull base, arduously avoiding any plunging. After tapping, a 8- to 10-mm, 3.5-mm cortical screw is placed. Drilling above the level of the inion is contraindicated, to avoid injury to the transverse sinus. Because the skull base around the area of the foramen magnum is too thin to allow for safe screw placement, we do not recommend screw placement in this region. Usually three screws can be placed into the occiput on either side. A plate spacing of 4 to 6 cm is maintained between both plates for placement of a corticocancellous bone graft. The graft is shaped to match the occiput and C2 vertebrae closely. A slot is placed at the caudal end of the graft to straddle the C2 spinous process. This "clothespin" graft is secured with wires or cables that are looped around the plates at their cranial and cervical ends or through two small burr holes placed into the skull base. For an occipitocervical fusion without subaxial instability, the caudal instrumentation ends at C2. Caudal extension can be achieved with longer plates if required. Postoperatively, patients are immobilized in a Minerva brace or halo vest.

Fusion across the Cervicothoracic Junction

Cervicothoracic injuries are rare and frequently missed on initial patient survey (31,56,94). Closed reduction of cervicothoracic dislocations is difficult, as is nonoperative treatment, because of inability to provide adequate external immobilization (94). The cervicothoracic junction also poses considerable challenges to posterior instrumentation because of anatomic and biomechanic factors. Treatment choices include placement of sublaminar wires or rods with hooks. These devices are anchored within the neural canal in an area where the spinal cord is in close contact to the spinal canal. Posterior plate fixation of the cervicothoracic junction offers the

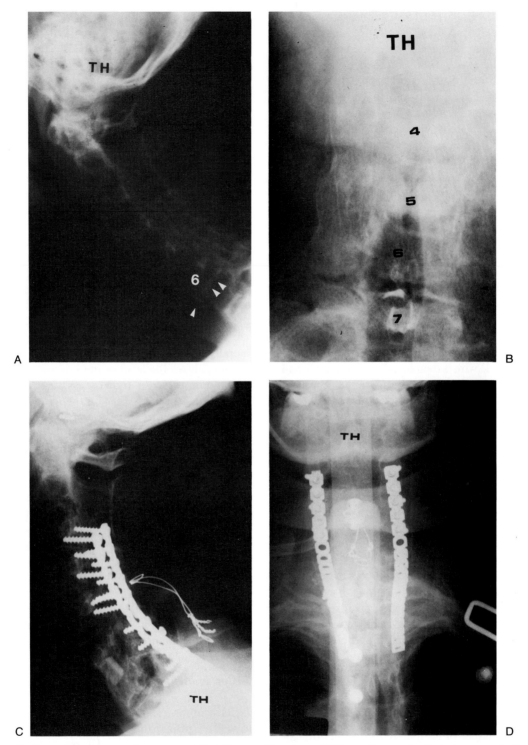

FIG. 27. **A:** The lateral radiographs of this 75-year-old patient with long history of ankylosing spondylitis shows an unstable C6-C7 shear fracture. The patient was neurologically intact. **B:** AP radiograph indicating that the fracture extends through both lateral masses. **C:** Postoperative lateral radiographs following posterior cervicothoracic plate fixation. An anterior interbody fusion was carried out because a 15° correction of cervical kyphosis had been achieved from the posterior approach. The patient remained neurologically intact and healed uneventfully. **D:** Postoperative AP radiograph. Screws were placed in the cervical spine and into the pedicles of the thoracic spine and C7.

possibility of crossing this region without intrusion into the spinal canal. Knowledge of the relationship of the pedicles of the upper thoracic spine to the posterior elements of these vertebrae is important to avoid iatrogenic injuries of neural or vascular structures (11,56).

The patient is positioned prone. Limited intraoperative radiographic visualization is possible with both arms tucked to the patient's sides. Midline subperiosteal exposure of the posterior cervicothoracic junction is performed (56). The facet capsules of C7-T1 and those levels caudally that require fusion are exposed. The medial and lateral margins of the superior articular processes are identified. The starting point for screw placement is 1 mm inferior to the articular ridge below the facet joint, and 1 mm lateral to the center of the superior articular process. Drilling is performed with a 2-mm K-wire with adjustable depth guide in a 10° medial and 15° caudal direction. Blunt probing of the drill hole is checked to identify any perforation of the pedicle. A final depth of 22 to 24 mm provides adequate screw purchase in the upper thoracic spine. All drillholes of the upper thoracic spine are then marked with a K-wire. Drilling of the most cranial cervical level to be instrumented is then performed as described previously. If the surgeon desires to verify screw placement, direct inspection of the medial wall of the upper thoracic spine pedicles is possible with a small laminotomy. After decortication, cancellous bone graft is placed into the facet joints and into the lateral gutter. Particular attention is directed toward decorticating and grafting the C7-T1 junction. A cervical reconstruction plate with hole intervals to match the upper thoracic spine is then selected and contoured. Screws (3.5 or 4 mm) are then placed sequentially from the cervical spine to the thoracic spine (Fig. 27). Final tightening of the screws is deferred until all screws have been deployed. Intraoperative radiographs to assure alignment and hardware placement are then obtained. Postoperative immobilization with a Minerva brace is recommended for 2 to 3 months.

SPECIAL CONDITIONS

Gunshot Wounds to the Cervical Spine

Efforts at decreasing spinal cord injuries from motor vehicle accidents have been successful, but gunshot injuries to the spinal cord have increased (219); penetrating injuries by guns have become the third largest cause of spinal cord injuries (133). In urban areas, low velocity gunshot wounds are among the leading causes for spinal cord injury. Gunshot wounds to the cervical spine are life-threatening injuries and have a higher mortality rate than injuries to the trunk (230). The proximity of trachea, esophagus, carotid, and vertebral arteries can pre-

sent the treating physician with complex life-threatening injury constellations necessitating urgent intervention.

Surgical intervention for the treatment of spinal cord or spinal column injuries has received limited attention. Although instability after low velocity gunshot wounds to the cervical spine was thought to be rare, it is found in 25% of patients (219). Surgical stabilization was recommended for patients showing instability according to the criteria established by White et al. (133,217,224). No neurological improvement occurred with surgical stabilization (133). The removal of bullets from the cervical spinal canal has remained controversial (Fig. 28).

High velocity gunshot wounds to the neck are usually fatal. If the patient survives, there is usually a high degree of soft tissue and bone destruction that requires surgical debridement. Stability of the spinal column may also be impaired by these projectiles.

The treatment of patients who have sustained low velocity gunshot injuries to the spine remains controversial. Advantages of bullet removal include decreased incidences of vertebral osteomyelitis, meningitis, and lead toxicity, and possibly improved neurological recovery. However, complications of surgical intervention may outweigh the incidence of complications resulting from retained bullets. The presence of a bullet within the spinal canal may affect neurological recovery. In a small series, Waters and Adkins (219) found improved neurological recovery in patients with incomplete cervical spinal cord injury who had the bullet removed, compared to patients who did not. No differences were found in patients with complete neurological injuries. In the thoracic spinal cord, no differences in neurological recovery were found in patients who underwent bullet removal, compared to those who did not. Patients with spinal cord injury below T12 made more recovery with bullet removal than those with the bullet left in the spinal canal; the difference was statistically significant (211). To date, there are no definitive recommendations regarding spinal cord decompression and surgical intervention.

Spinal Cord Injury without Radiographic Abnormalities

Children with immature spinal column may suffer spinal cord injuries without radiographic abnormalities, termed SCIWORA (172). Increased elasticity of the fibrocartilaginous tissues in the pediatric age group may lead to temporary subluxation of the spinal column, thus exposing the spinal cord to compressive or distractive forces without accompanying obvious radiographic abnormalities (197,220). Motor vehicle accidents and falls are the most common causes of SCIWORA in children 6 months to 16 years old. In a study by Pang and Wilberger (172), 54% of patients developed delayed neurological deficits, between 30 minutes and 4 days from injury. All

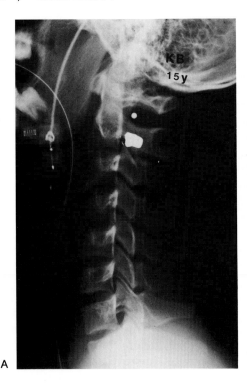

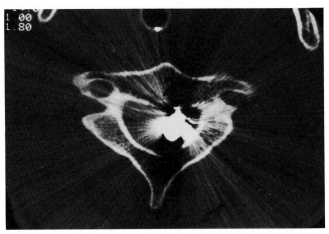

FIG. 28. A: This lateral cervical spine radiograph demonstrates a metallic foreign body posterior to the axis in this 15 year-old-victim of a gunshot wound. The patient presented with immediate complete C2 quadriplegia. **B:** Axial CT confirmed the presence of a bullet fragment within the spinal canal. The bullet was removed via C2 laminectomy 4 days after the injury. The dura was found to be intact at the time of surgery. The patient recovered to a Frankel D status 8 months after surgery.

of these patients had temporary initial neurological deficits and did not receive further diagnostic work-up. In patients less than 8 years old, an increased incidence of upper cervical spinal cord injuries was found, compared to children older than 8 years (172). Hypermobility of the C2-C3 and C4-C5 segments is a possible cause for this finding (197).

We recommend expedient MRI evaluation of traumatized patients with neurological deficits when no obvious skeletal injury is seen on plain radiographs or CT scan. Occult fractures, ligamentous injury, disc herniation, epidural bleeding, or cord signal changes are possible findings in patients with SCIWORA. Congenital abnormalities of the cervical spinal column or cord should be ruled out. A patient presenting with SCIWORA should be treated just as any patient presenting with spinal cord injury. External immobilization is recommended for a minimum of 4 weeks (172,220) in patients without any instability or spinal cord compression. Flexion radiographs are recommended at the conclusion of the immobilization period to ensure stability. Patients with cord compression or instability should be considered for expedient surgical decompression and surgical stabilization. Pang and Wilberger (172) found the neurological outcome of pediatric patients with SCIWORA to be closely related to the severity of the initial neurological presentation, regardless of age. Because of the high incidence of delayed onset of spinal cord injury in children, these authors recommended thorough work-up of children with history of head or neck injury and any form of neurological symptoms.

Fractures in Ankylosing Spondylitis

Patients with ankylosing spondylitis are at increased risk for spine fractures because of the lack of mobility of the spinal column (62). As a result of deformity and the associated difficulty in visualizing the entire spine on plain radiographs, fractures in patients with ankylosing spondylitis can be easily missed. In ankylosing spondilitis patients, fractures occur most frequently in the cervicothoracic junction and the midthoracic spine (164). Fractures in an ankylosed spine are inherently unstable and frequently are of a shear pattern. Because of the fracture instability, calcification of the ligamentum flavum, and risk of propagating epidural hematoma, neurological compromise is common (164). Non-operative treatment is hampered by difficulty in maintaining reduction with external means and a high percentage of complications. Early surgical stabilization allows mobilization with simple collar or brace (164). Awake, fiberoptically guided intubation and awake positioning are important in these patients, who frequently present with severe deformities. Turning tables, such as Stryker frames, may cause uncontrolled hyperextension and therefore are usually not suitable for patients with severe kyphotic deformities of the spine.

In patients with an ankylosed spine, instrumentation is subjected to considerable forces from the long lever arm of the ankylosed segments cranial and caudal to the fracture. It is therefore helpful to extend a posterior instrumentation several levels beyond the fracture. In selected patients, a partial correction of a preoperatively present kyphotic deformity is possible through the fracture site. Intraoperative electrodiagnostic monitoring or the Stagnara wake-up test should be performed if such attempts are made (168). For patients with cervical fractures in the presence of ankylosing spondylitis, we recommend posterior stabilization with lateral mass plates (Fig. 28). Anterior strut grafting and plate fixation should be added if an anterior defect remains after posterior instrumentation. Postoperatively, the spine is immobilized with a Minerva brace for 2 to 3 months.

CONCLUSIONS

The goals of treatment of spinal injury patients are to protect the cord from further neurological injury, to reduce fractures and dislocations, to stabilize the injured segment, and to provide a stable, painless spine for the long term. Fulfillment of these goals requires a high index of suspicion for cervical injury, meticulous evaluation, and complete radiological imaging. Newer imaging techniques can clearly document both neural and skeletal pathology. Early treatment, both by pharmacological agents and by addressing abnormal adverse mechanical factors, may lead to improved recovery. The choice of treatment is dictated by fracture type and resultant stability, the presence of residual neural compression, and the neurological status of the patient. Both anterior and posterior approaches, when performed for appropriate indications and by the correct technique, can result in successful outcomes.

REFERENCES

1. Abitbol JJ, Zdeblick T, Kunz D, McCabe R, Cooke M (1992): *A biomechanical analysis of modern anterior and posterior cervical stabilization techniques.* Presented at the Cervical Spine Research Society, Palm Desert, CA.
2. Aebi M, Etter C, Coscia M (1989): Fracture of the odontoid process. Treatment with anterior screw fixation. *Spine* 14:1965–1070.
3. Aebi M, Mohler J, Zaech GA, Morscher E (1986): Indication, surgical technique, and results of 100 surgically treated fractures and fracture-dislocations of the cervical spine. *Clin Orthop* 203:244–257.
4. Aebi M, Zuber K, Marchesi D (1991): Treatment of cervical spine injuries with anterior plating: indications, techniques, and results. *Spine* 16:538–545.
5. Alander DH, Andreychik DA, Stauffer S (1994): Early outcome in cervical spinal cord injured patients older than 50 years of age. *Spine* 19:2299–2301.
6. Allen BL, Ferguson RL, Lehmann TR, O'Brien RP (1982): A mechanistic classification of closed, indirect fractures and dislocations of the lower cervical spine. *Spine* 7:1–27.
7. Allen BL, Tencer AF, Ferguson RL (1987): The biomechanics of decompressive laminectomy. *Spine* 12:803–808.
8. Althoff B, Goldie IF (1977): The arterial supply of the odontoid process of the axis. *Acta Orthop Scand* 48:622–629.
9. American College of Surgeons (1992): *Advanced trauma life support manual.* Chicago, American College of Surgeons.
10. American Spinal Injury Association and International Medical Society of Paraplegia (1992): *Standard for neurologic and func-

11. tional classification of spinal cord injury,* revised. American Spinal Injury Association, Atlanta, GA.
11. An HS, Gordin R, Renner K (1991): Anatomic considerations for plate-screw fixation of the cervical spine. *Spine* 16:548–551.
12. Anderson DK, Braughler JM, Hall ED, Waters TR, McCaall JM, Means ED (1988): Effects of treatment with U-74006F on neurologic outcome following experimental spinal cord injury. *J Neurosurg* 69:562–567.
13. Anderson LD, D'Alonzo RT (1974): Fractures of the odontoid process of the axis. *J Bone Joint Surg* 56(A):1663–1674.
14. Anderson PA, Bohlmann HH (1992): Anterior decompression and arthrodesis in patients with traumatic, complete motor cervical spinal cord injury: long term neurological recovery in 52 patients. Part II. *J Bone Joint Surg* 74A:683–692.
15. Anderson PA, Budorick TE, Easton KB, Henley MB, Salciccioli GG (1991): Failure of Halo vest to prevent in vivo motion in patients with injured cervical spines. *Spine* 16:S501–505.
16. Anderson PA, Henley MB, Grady MS, Montesano PX, Winn HR (1991): Posterior cervical arthrodesis with AO reconstruction plates and bone graft. *Spine* 16:72–79.
17. Anderson PA, Montesano PX (1988): Morphology and treatment of occipital condyle fractures. *Spine* 13:731–736.
18. Assenmacher DR, Ducker TB (1971): Experimental traumatic paraplegia. *J Bone Joint Surg* 53(A):671–680.
19. Balentine JD (1978): Pathology of experimental spinal cord injury: I. The necrotic lesion as a function of a vascular injury. *Lab Invest* 39:236–253.
20. Balentine JD (1978): Pathology of experimental spinal cord trauma: II. Ultrastructure of axons and myelin. *Lab Invest* 39:254–266.
21. Barr Jr JS, Krag MH, Pierce DS (1989): Cranial traction and the Halo orthosis. *The cervical spine,* 2nd ed. Philadelphia: Lippincott, 1989;239–311.
22. Bassett T, Zdeblick TA (1994): Complications of cervical spine instrumentation. *Tech Orthop* 9:18–17.
23. Batillas J, Vasilas A, Pizzi WF, Gokcebay T (1981): Bone scanning in the detection of occult fractures. *J Trauma* 21:564–569.
24. Beatson TR (1963): Fractures and dislocations of the cervical spine. *J Bone Joint Surg* 45(B):21–35.
25. Bell HS (1970): Paralysis of both arms from the injury of the upper portion of the pyramidal decussation: "Cruciate paralysis." *J Neurosurg* 33:376–380.
26. Beyer CA, Cabanela ME, Bergquist TH (1992): Unilateral facet dislocations and fracture-dislocations of the cervical spine. *Orthopedics* 15:311–315.
27. Boehler J (1935): *The treatment of fractures,* 4th ed. Baltimore: W Wood.
28. Boehler J (1965): Fractures of the odontoid process. *J Trauma* 5:386–391.
29. Boehler J (1982): Anterior stabilization for acute fractures and nonunions of the dens. *J Bone Joint Surg* 64(A):18–27.
30. Boehler J, Gaudernak T (1980): Anterior plate stabilization for fracture-dislocations of the lower cervical spine. *J Trauma* 20:203–205.
31. Bohlmann HH (1979): Acute fractures and dislocations of the cervical spine. An analysis of three-hundred hospitalized patients and review of the literature. *J Bone Joint Surg* 61(A):1119–1142.
32. Bohlmann HH, Anderson PA (1992): Part I: Anterior decompression and arthrodesis of the cervical spine. Long term motor improvement. Part I: Improvement in incomplete traumatic quadriparesis. *J Bone Joint Surg* 74A:671–682.
33. Bohlmann HH, Bahniuk E, Raskulinecz G, Field G (1979): Mechanical factors affecting recovery from incomplete spinal cord injury: a preliminary report. *Johns Hopkins Med J* 145:115–125.
34. Bohlmann HH, Bolesta M (1992): *Experimental conus medullaris compression.* Read at the annual meeting of the American Academy of Orthopaedic Surgeons March 7–12, Anaheim Calif.
35. Bohlmann HH, Kirkpatrick JS, Delamarter RB, Leventhal M (1994): Anterior decompression for late pain and paralysis after fractures of the thoracolumbar spine. *Clin Orthop* 300:24–29.
36. Borne GM, Bedou GL, Pinaudeau M, Cristino G, Hussein A (1988): Odontoid process fracture osteosynthesis with a direct screw fixation technique in nine consecutive cases. *J Neurosurg* 68:223–226.

37. Botte MJ, Garfin SR, Byrne TP, Woo SLY, Nickel VL (1989): The Halo skeletal fixator. *Clin Orthop* 239:12–18.

38. Bracken MB, Collins WF, Freeman DF, Shepard MJ, Wagner FW, et al. (1984): Efficacy of methylprednisolone in acute spinal cord injury. *JAMA* 251:45–51.

39. Bracken MB, Shephard MJ, Collins WF, et al. (1990): A randomized controlled trial of methylprednisolone in acute spinal cord injury: results of the Second National Acute Spinal Cord Injury study. *N Engl J Med* 322:1405–1411.

40. Breig A (1972): The therapeutic possibilities of surgical bioengineering in incomplete spinal cord lesions. *Paraplegia* 9:173–182.

41. Breig A, El-Nadi F (1966): Biomechanics of the cervical spinal cord. Relief of contact pressure on and overstretching of the spinal cord. *Acta Radiol Diagn* 4:602–604.

42. Brodke DS, Anderson PA, Newell D, Grady MS, Harthan B, Chapman JR (1995): Anterior versus posterior stabilization of cervical spine fractures in spinal cord injured patients. Presented at the 23rd annual meeting of the Cervical Spine Research Society Nov 30–Dec 2, Sante Fe, New Mexico.

43. Brooks AL, Jenkins EW (1978): Atlanto-axial arthrodesis by the wedge compression method. *J Bone Joint Surg* 60(A):279–284.

44. Brunette DS, Rockswold GL (1987): Neurological recovery following rapid spinal realignment for complete cervical spinal cord injury. *J Trauma* 27:445–447.

45. Bucci MN, Dauser RC, Maynard FA, Hoff JT (1988): Management of posttraumatic cervical spine instability: operative fusion versus halo vest immobilization: analysis of 49 cases. *J Trauma* 28:1001–1006.

46. Bucholz RW, Burkhead WZ (1979): The pathologic anatomy of fatal atlanto-occipital dislocations. *J Bone Joint Surg* 61(A):248–249.

47. Budorick TE, Anderson PA, Rivara FP, Cohen W (1991): Flexion-distraction fracture of the cervical spine. A case report. *J Bone Joint Surg* 73(A):1097–1100.

48. Burke DC, Berryman D (1972): The place of closed manipulation in the management of flexion-rotation dislocations of the cervical spine. *J Bone Joint Surg* 53(B):165–182.

49. Cabanela ME, Ebersold MJ (1988): Anterior plate stabilization for bursting teardrop fractures of the cervical spine. *Spine* 13:888–891.

50. Capen DA, Nelson RW, Zigler JE (1987): Decompressive laminectomy in cervical spine trauma: a review of early and late complications. *Contemp Orthop* 17:21–29.

51. Caspar W, Barbier DD, Klara PM (1989): Anterior cervical fusion and Caspar plate stabilization for cervical trauma. *Neurosurgery* 25:491–502.

52. Chan RNW, Ainscow D, Sikorski JM (1980): Diagnostic failures in the multiple injured. *J Trauma* 20:684–687.

53. Chang DG, Tencer AF, Ching RP, Treece B, Senft D, Anderson PA (1994): Geometric changes in the cervical spine during impact. *Spine* 18:973–980.

54. Chang KW, Liu YW, Cheng PG, Chang L, Suen KL, Chung WL, Chen UL, Liang PL (1994): One Herbert double-threaded compression screw fixation of displaced type II odontoid fractures. *J Spinal Disord* 7:62–69.

55. Chapman JR, Anderson PA (1991): Internal fixation techniques for the treatment of lower cervical spine injuries. *J Int Orthop Trauma* 1(4):205–219.

56. Chapman JR, Anderson PA (1994): Posterior plate fixation of the cervicothoracic junction. *Tech Orthop* 9:80–85.

57. Cheshire DJE (1969): The stability of the cervical spine following the conservative treatment of fractures and fracture dislocations. *Paraplegia* 7:193–203.

58. Clark CR, White AA (1985): Fractures of the dens. A multicenter study. *J Bone Joint Surg* 67(A):1340–1348.

59. Cloward RB (1960): Treatment of acute fractures and fracture dislocations of the cervical spine by vertebral-body fusion. *J Neurosurg* 18:201–209.

60. Coe JD, Warden KE, Sutterlin CE, McAfee PC (1989): Biomechanical evaluation of cervical spinal stabilization methods in human cadaveric model. *Spine* 14:1122–1130.

61. Cone W, Nicholoson JT (1937): The treatment of fracture-dislocations of the cervical vertebrae by skeletal traction and fusion. *J Bone Joint Surg* 19(A):584–587.

62. Cooper C, Carbone L, Michet CJ, Atkinson EJ, O'Fallon WM, Melton LJ (1994): Fracture risk in patients with ankylosing spondylitis: a population based study. *J Rheumatol* 21:1877–1882.

63. Cooper PR, Cohen A, Rosiello A, Koslow M (1988): Posterior stabilization of cervical spine fractures and subluxations using plates and screws. *J Neurosurg* 23:300–306.

64. Crutchfield WG (1957): Further observations on the treatment of fracture dislocations of the cervical spine with skeletal traction. *Surg Gynecol Obstet* 63:513–517.

65. Cybulski GR, Stone JL, Crowell RM, et al. (1988): Use of Halifax interlaminar clamps for posterior C1-2 arthrodesis. *Neurosurgery* 22:429–431.

66. Davis D, Bohlmann HH, Walker AE, Fisher R, Robinson R (1971): The pathologic findings in fatal cranio-spinal injuries. *J Neurosurg* 34:603–613.

67. Davis JW, Parks SN, Detlefs, Williams GG, Williams JL, Smith RW (1995): *Clearing the cervical spine in obtunded patients: the use of dynamic fluoroscopy.* Presented at the 25th annual meeting of the Western Trauma Association, Big Sky, Montana, March 1.

68. Davis JW, Phreaner DL, Hoyt DB, Mackersie RC (1993): The etiology of missed cervical spine injuries. *J Trauma* 34:342–345.

69. de Oliveira J (1987): Anterior plate fixation of traumatic lesions of the lower cervical spine. *Spine* 12:324–329.

70. Delamarter RB, Sherman J, Carr JB (1995): Pathophysiology of spinal cord injury. Recovery after immediate and delayed decompression. *J Bone Joint Surg* 77(A):1042–1049.

71. Delamarter RB, Sherman JE, Carr JB (1991): Cauda equina syndrome: neurologic recovery following immediate, early, or late decompression. *Spine* 16:1022–1029.

72. Dickman CA, Hadley MN, Pappas CTE, Sonntag VKH, Geisler FH (1990): Cruciate paralysis of injuries to the cervicomedullary junction. *J Neurosurg* 73:850–858.

73. Dohrmann GJ, Wagner FC, Bucy PC (1972): Transitory traumatic paraplegia: electron microscopy of early alterations in myelinated nerve fibers. *J Neurosurg* 36:407–415.

74. Dolan EJ, Tator CH, Endrenyi L (1980): The value of decompression for acute spinal cord compression injury. *J Neurosurg* 53:749–755.

75. Doran SE, Papadopoulos SM, Ducker TB, Lillehei KO (1993): Magnetic resonance image documentation of coexistent traumatic locked facets of the cervical spine and disc herniation. *J Neurosurg* 79:341–345.

76. Ducker T, Kindt G, Kempe L (1971): Pathological findings in acute spinal cord trauma. *J Neurosurg* 35:700–708.

77. Ducker TB (1990): *Restriction of cervical motion by cervical collars.* Scientific exhibit; 58th annual meeting. American Association of Neurological Surgeons. April 28-May 3, Nashville, TN.

78. Ducker TB (1990): Treatment of spinal cord injuries. *N Engl J Med* 322:1459–1461.

79. Ducker TB, Saleman M, Daniell HB (1978): Experimental spinal cord trauma, part III: therapeutic effect of immobilization and pharmacologic agents. *Surg Neurol* 10:71–76.

80. Dvorak J, Hayek J, Zehnder R (1987): CT functional diagnostics of the rotatory instability of the upper cervical spine. Part 2. An evaluation on healthy adults and patients with suspected instability. *Spine* 12:726–731.

81. Dvorak J, Panjabi M, Gerber M, Wichman W (1987): CT functional diagnostics of the rotatory instability of the upper cervical spin. Part 1: An experimental study on cadavers. *Spine* 12:197–205.

82. Dvorak J, Panjabi MD (1987): Functional anatomy of the alar ligaments. *Spine* 12:183–186.

83. Dvorak J, Schneider E, Saldinger P, Rahn B (1988): Biomechanics of the cervicocranial region: the alar and transverse ligaments. *J Orthop* 6:452–461.

84. Edwards CC, Levine AM (1986): Early rod-sleeve stabilization of the injured thoracic and lumbar spine. *Orthop Clin North Am* 17:121–145.

85. Edwards CC, Matz SO, Levine AM (1986): The oblique wiring technique for rotational injuries of the cervical spine. *Orthop Trans* 10:455.

86. Effendi B, Roy D, Cornish B, Dussault RG, Laurin CA (1981): Fractures of the ring of the axis. A classification based on the analysis of 131 cases. *J Bone Joint Surg* 63(B):319–327.

87. Ehara S, El-Khoury GY, Clark CR (1992): Radiologic evaluation of dens fractures. Role of plain radiography and tomography. *Spine* 17:475–479.

88. Eismont FJ, Aruna MJ, Green BA (1991): Extrusion of an intervertebral disc associated with traumatic subluxation or dislocation of cervical facets. *J Bone Joint Surg* 73(A):1555–1560.

89. Eismont FJ, Green BA, McGuire E (1988): Comprison of stability provided to the unstable spine using the Kinetic Therapy Table and the Stryker Frame. *Neurosurgery* 22:842–845.

90. Enderson BL, Reath DB, Meadors J, Dallas W, DeBoo JB, Maull KI (1990): The tertiary trauma survey: a prospective study of missed injury. *J Trauma* 30:666–669.

91. Errico T, Uhl R, Cooper P, Casar R, McHenry T (1992): Pull-out strength comparison of two methods of orienting screw insertion in the lateral masses of the bovine cervical spine. *J Spinal Disord* 5:459–469.

92. Esses SI, Bednar DA (1991): Screw fixation of odontoid fractures and nonunions. *Spine* 16:S483–485.

93. Etter C, Coscia M, Jaberg H, Aebi M (1991): Direct anterior screw fixation of dens fractures with a cannulated screw system. *Spine* 16:S25–32.

94. Evans DK (1983): Dislocations at the cervicothoracic junction. *J Bone Joint Surg* 65(B)124–127.

95. Fielding JW, Hawkins RJ (1977): Atlanto-axial rotatory fixation. *J Bone Joint Surg* 59(A):37–44.

96. Fielding JW, Hensinger R, Hawkins RJ (1980): Os odontoideum. *J Bone Joint Surg* 62(A):376–383.

97. Flanders AE, Schaefer DM, Doan HT, Mishkin MM, Gonzalez CF, Northrop BE (1990): Acute cervical spine trauma: correlation of MR imaging findings with degree of neurologic deficit. *Radiology* 177:25–33.

98. Flynn TB (1982): Neurologic complications of anterior cervical interbody fusion. *Spine* 7:536–539.

99. Francis WR, Fielding JW, Hawkins RJ, Pepin J, Hensinger R (1981): Traumatic spondylolisthesis of the axis. *J Bone Joint Surg* 63(B):313–318.

100. Frankel H, Hancock DO, Hyslop G (1969): The value of postural reduction in the initial management of closed injuries of the spine with paraplegia and tetraplegia: I. *Paraplegia* 7:179–192.

101. Gallie WE (1939): Fractures and dislocations of the cervical spine. *Am J Surg* 46:494–499.

102. Garfin SR, Botte MJ, Waters RL, Nickel VL (1986): Complications in the use of the Halo fixation device. *J Bone Joint Surg* 68(A):320–325.

103. Garfin SR, Shackford SR, Marshall LF, Drummon JC (1989): Care of the multiply injured patient with cervical spine injury. *Clin Orthop* 239:19–29.

104. Gassman J, Seligson D (1983): The anterior cervical plate. *Spine* 8:700–707.

105. Geisler FH, Cheng C, Poka A, Brumback R (1989): Anterior screw fixation of posteriorly displaced type II odontoid fractures. *Neurosurgery* 25:30–38.

106. Geisler FH, Dorsey FC, Coleman WP (1991): Recovery of motor function after spinal cord injury: a randomized, placebo-controlled trial with GM-1 ganglioside: *N Engl J Med* 324:1829–1838.

107. Gerrelts BD, Petersen EU, Mabry J, Petersen SR (1991): Delayed diagnosis of cervical spine injuries. *J Trauma* 31:1622–1626.

108. Gertzbein SD (1992): Classification of thoracic and lumbar fractures. In: Gertzbein SD, ed. *Fractures of the thoracic and lumbar spine.* Baltimore: Williams & Wilkins, pp.25–57.

109. Gill K, Paschal S, Corin J, Ashman R, Bucholz RW (1988): Posterior plating of the cervical spine, a biomechanical comparison of different posterior fusion techniques. *Spine* 13:813–816.

110. Goldberg AL, Rothfus WE, Deeb ZL, Daffner RH, Lupetin AR, Wilberger JE, Prostko ER (1988): The impact of magnetic resonance on the diagnostic evaluation of acute cervicothoracic spinal trauma. *Skeletal Radiol* 17:89–95.

111. Golfinos JF, Dickman CA, Zabranski JM, Sonntag VKS, Spetzler RF (1994): Repair of vertebral artery injury during anterior cervical decompression. *Spine* 19:2552–2556.

112. Grob D, Crisco JJ, Panjabi M, Wang P, Dvorak J (1992): Biomechanical evaluation of four different posterior atlantoaxial fixation techniques. *Spine* 17:480–490.

113. Grob D, Jeanneret B, Aebi M, Markwalder TM (1991): Atlanto-axial fusion with transarticular screw fusion. *J Bone Joint Surg* 73(B):972–976.

114. Grob D, Magerl F (1987): Dorsal spondylodesis of the cervical spine using a hooked plate. *Orthopade* 16:55–61.

115. Grubb MR, Currier BL, Bonin V, Grabowski JJ, Chao EYS (1994): *Biomechanical evaluation of the anterior spine stabilization in a porcine model. Ortho Trans* 18:338.

116. Hadley MN, Browner CB, Sonntag VKH (1985): A comprehensive review of management and treatment in 107 cases. *Neurosurgery* 17:281–289.

117. Hadley MN, Browner CM, Liu SS, Sonntag VKH (1988): New subtype of acute odontoid fracture (type IIa). *Neurosurgery* 22:67–71.

118. Hadley MN, Dickman CA, Browner CM, Sonntag VKM (1988): Acute traumatic atlas fractures: management and long term outcome. *Neurosurgery* 23:31–35.

119. Hall AJ, Wagle VG, Raycroft J, Goldman RL, Butler AR (1993): Magnetic resonance imaging in cervical spine trauma. *J Trauma* 34:21–26.

120. Hall ED (1988): Effects of the 21-aminosteroid U74006F on post-traumatic spinal cord ischemia in cats. *J Neurosurg* 68:462–465.

121. Hamilton A, Webb JK (1994): The role of anterior surgery for vertebral fractures with and without cord compression. *Clin Orthop* 300:79–89.

122. Hanson PB, Montesano PX, Sharkey N, Rauschning W (1991): Anatomic and biomechanical assessment of transarticular screw fixation for atlanto-axial instability. *Spine* 16:1141–1145.

123. Harris JH, Carson GC, Wagner LK (1994): Radiologic diagnosis of traumatic occipitovertebral dissociation: 1. Normal occipito-vertebral relationships on lateral radiographs of supine subjects. *Am J Radiol* 162:881–886.

124. Harris JH, Carson GC, Wagner LK, Kerr N (1994): Radiologic diagnosis of traumatic occipitocervical dissociation: 2. Comparison of three methods of detecting occipitocervical relationships on lateral radiographs of supine subjects. *Am J Radiol* 162:887–892.

125. Heinrich SD, Gallagher D, Harris, Nadell JM (1994): Undiagnosed fractures in severely injured children and young adults. Identification with technetium imaging. *J Bone Joint Surg* 76(A):561–572.

126. Heller JG, Alson D, Schaffler MB, Garfin SR (1992): Quantitative internal dens morphology. *Spine* 17:861–866.

127. Heller JG, Carlson GD, Abitbol JJ, Garfin SG (1991): Anatomic comparison of the Roy-Camille and Magerl techniques for screw placement in the lower cervical spine. *Spine* 16:S552–557.

128. Heller JG, Silcox DH, Sutterlin CE (1995): Complications of posterior cervical plating. *Spine* 20:2442–2448.

129. Heller JG, Viroslav S, Hudson T (1993): Jefferson fractures: the role of magnification artifact in assessing transverse ligament integrity. *J Spinal Disord* 6:392–396.

130. Hochberg MC (1990): Ankylosing spondylitis. *Semin Spine Surg* 2:86–94.

131. Holness RO, Huestis WS, Howes WJ, Langille RA (1984): Posterior stabilization with an interlaminar clamp in cervical injuries: technical note and review of the long term experience with the model. *Neurosurgery* 14:318–322.

132. Ikata T, Iwasa K, Morimoto K, Tonai T, Tasoka Y (1989): Clinical considerations and biochemical basis of prognosis of spinal cord injury. *Spine* 14:1096–1101.

133. Isiklar ZU, LindsayP.W (1995): Cervical spine instability following low velocity civilian gunshot wounds to the cervical spine. *Orthop Trans* 19:183.

134. Janssen L, Hansebout RR (1989): Pathogenesis of spinal cord injury and newer treatments: a review. *Spine* 14:23–32.

135. Jeanneret B, Magerl F (1992): Primary posterior fusion C1/2 in odontoid fractures: indications, technique, and results of transarticular screw fixation. *J Spinal Disord* 5:464–475.

136. Jeanneret B, Magerl F, Haterward E (1991): Posterior stabilization of the cervical spine with hook plates. *Spine* 16:56–63.

137. Jefferson G (1927): Fractures of the first cervical vertebra. *Br Med J* 2:153–157.

138. Jenkins LA, Capen DA, Zigler JE, Nelson RW, Nagelberg S

(1994): Cervical spine fusions for trauma. A long-term radiographic and clinical evaluation. *Orthop Rev* Suppl:13–19.

139. Johnson RM, Hart DL, Simmons EF, Ramsby GR, Southwick WO (1977): Cervical orthoses. *J Bone Joint Surg* 59(A):332–339.

140. Krengel WF, Anderson PA, Henley MB (1993): Early stabilization and decompression for incomplete paraplegia due to a thoracic level spinal cord injury. *Spine* 18:2080–2087.

141. Laasonen EM, Kivioja A (1991): Delayed diagnosis of extremity injuries in patients with multiple injuries. *J Trauma* 31:257–260.

142. Ladouceur D, Veilleux M, Levessque RY (1991): Cruciate paralysis secondary to C1 on C2 fracture-dislocation. *Spine* 17:1383–1385.

143. Landells CD, Van Peteghem PK (1988): Fractures of the atlas: classification, treatment and morbidity. *Spine* 13:450–452.

144. Lee AS, MacLean JCB, Newton DA (1994): Rapid traction for reduction of cervical spine dislocations. *J Bone Joint Surg* 76(B):352–356.

145. Lee C, Woodring JH, Golstein SJ, Daniel TL, Young AB, Tibbs PA (1987): Evaluation of traumatic atlano-occipital dislocations. *Am J Neuroradiol* 8:19–26.

146. Levine AM, Edwards CC (1989): Traumatic lesions of the atlantoaxial complex. *Clin Orthop* 239:53–68.

147. Levine AM, Edwards CC (1991): Fractures of the atlas. *J Bone Joint Surg* 73(A):680–691.

148. Lind B, Nordall A, Sihlbom H (1987): Odontoid fracture treated with Halo-vest. *Spine* 12:173–177.

149. MacDonald RL, Schwartz ML, Mirich D, Sharkey PW, Nelson WR (1990): Diagnosis of cervical spine injury in motor vehicle crash victims: how many X-rays are enough? *J Trauma* 30:392–397.

150. Mackersie RC, Shackford SR, Garfin SR, Hoyt DB (1991): Major skeletal injuries in the obtunded blunt trauma patient: a case for routine radiologic survey. *J Trauma* 28:1450–1453.

151. Magerl F, Seemann PS (1987): Stable posterior fusion of the atlas and axis by transarticular screw fixation. In: Kehr P, Weidner PA, eds. *Cervical spine*, 1st ed. New York: Springer-Verlag pp.322–327.

152. Mahale YJ, Silver JR, Henderson NJ (1993): Neurological complications of the reduction of cervical spine dislocations. *J Bone Joint Surg* 73(B):403–409.

153. Marcotte P, Dickman CA, Sonntag VKH, Karahalios DG, Drabier J (1993): Posterior atlantoaxial facet screw fixation. *J Neurosurg* 79:234–237.

154. Marshall LF, Knowlton S, Garfin SR, Klauber MR, Eisenberg HM, Kopaniky D, Miner ME, Tabbador KT, Clifton GL (1987): Deterioration following spinal cord injury. A multicenter study. *J Neurosurg* 66:400–404.

155. McAfee P (1991): Cervical spine trauma. In: Frymoyer J, ed. *The adult spine.* New York: Raven Press; pp.1063–1107.

156. McAfee PC, Bohlman HH, Wilson WL (1985): The triple wire technique for stabilization of acute cervical fracture dislocations: a biomechanical analysis. *Orthop Trans* 9:142.

157. McGuire RA, Harkey HL (1995): Primary treatment of unstable Jefferson's fractures. *J Spinal Disord* 8:233–236.

158. Mirza S, Moquin R, Anderson PA, Steinman J, Tencer A, Varnau D (1994): Stabilizing properties of the Halo-vest. *Orthop Trans* 18:697–698.

159. Montane I, Eismont FJ, Green BA (1991): Traumatic occipitoatlantal dislocation. *Spine* 16:112–116.

160. Montesano PX, Anderson PA, Schlehr F, Thalgott JG, Lowrey G (1991): Odontoid fractures treated by anterior odontoid screw fixation. *Spine* 16:S33–37.

161. Montesano PX, Juach EC, Anderson PA, Benson DR, Hanson PB (1991): Biomechanics of cervical spine internal fixation. *Spine* 16:10–16.

162. Monu J, Bohrer SP, Howard G (1987): Some upper cervical spine norms. *Spine* 12:515–519.

163. Morscher E, Sutter F, Jennis M, Olerud S (1986): Die vordere Verplattung der Halswirbelsaeule mit dem Hohlschraubenplattensystem. *Chirurg* 57:702–707.

164. Murray GC, Persellin RH (1981): Cervical fracture complicating ankylosing spondylitis: a report of eight cases and review of the literature. *Am J Med* 70:1033–1041.

165. Nakanishi T, Sasaki T, Tokita N, Hirabayashi K (1982): Internal fixation of the odontoid fracture. *Orthop Trans* 6:176.

166. Nazarian SM, Louis RP (1991): Posterior internal fixation with screw pates in traumatic lesions of the cervical spine. *Spine* 16:S64–S71.

167. Newhouse KE, Lindsey RW, Clark CR, Lieponis J, Murphy MJ (1989): Esophageal perforation following anterior cervical spine surgery. *Spine* 14:1051–1053.

168. Nuwer MR, Dawson, Carlson LG, Kanim LEA, Sherman JE (1995): Somatosensory evoked potential spinl cord monitoring reduces neurologic deficits after scoliosis surgery: results of a large multicenter survey. *Electroencephalogr Clin Neurophysiol* 96:6–11.

169. Orozco Delclos R, Llovet Tapies J (1971): Osteosintesis en las lesiones traumaticas y degenerativas de la columna vertebral. *Rev Traumatol Cirurjia Rehabil* 1:45–52.

170. Orthopaedic Trauma Association (1996): Comprehensive classification of fractures. *J Orthop Trauma* (in press).

171. Pait TG, McAllister PV, Kaufmann HH (1995): Quadrant anatomy of the articular pillars (lateral cervical mass) of the cervical spine. *J Neurosurg* 82:1011–1014.

172. Pang D, Wilberger JE (1982): Spinal cord injury without radiographic abnormalities in children. *J Neurosurg* 57:114–129.

173. Pepin JW, Bourne RB, Hawkins RJ (1985): Odontoid fractures with special reference to the elderly patient. *Clin Orthop* 193:178–183.

174. Plaisier B, Gabram SGA, Schwartz, RJ, Jacobs LM (1940): Prospective evaluation of craniofacial pressure in four different cervical orthoses. *J Trauma* 37:714–720.

175. Powers B, Miller MD, Kramer RS, Martinez S, Gehweiler JA (1979): Traumatic anterior atlanto-occipital dislocation. *J Neurosurg* 4:12–17.

176. Pratt ES, Green DA, Spengler DM (1990): Herniated intervertebral discs associated with unstable spinal injuries. *Spine* 15:662–666.

177. Ransford AO, Crackard HA, Pozo JL, Thomas NP, Nelson IW (1986): Craniocervical instability treated by contoured loop fixation. *J Bone Joint Surg* 68(B):173–176.

178. Reid DC, Henderson R, Saboe L, Miller JDR (1987): Etiology and clinical course of missed spine fractures. *J Trauma* 27:980–986.

179. Ripa DR, Kowall MG, Meyer PR, Rusin JJ (1991): Series of ninety-two traumatic cervical spine injuries stabilized with anterior ASIF plate fixation technique. *Spine* 16:S46–55.

180. Rizzolo SJ, Piazza MR, Cotler JM, Balderston RA, Schaefer D, Flanders A (1991): Intervertebral disc injury complicating cervical spine trauma. *Spine* 16:S187–189.

181. Robertson PA, Ryan MD (1992): Neurologic deterioration after reduction of cervical subluxation: mechanical compression by disc tissue. *J Bone Joint Surg* 74(B):224–227.

182. Robinson RA, Smith GW (1953): Anterolateral disc removal and interbody fusion for cervical disc syndrome. *Johns Hopkins Hosp Bull* 96:223–224.

183. Robinson RA, Southwick WO (1960): Indications and techniques for early stabilization of the neck in some fracture dislocations of the cervical spine. *South Med J* 53:565–579.

184. Rockswold GL, Bergmann T, Ford SE (1990): Halo immobilization and surgical fusion: relative indications and effectiveness in the treatment of 140 cervical spine injuries. *J Trauma* 30:893–898.

185. Rogers WA (1957): Fractures and dislocations of the cervical spine: end-result study. *J Bone Joint Surg* 39:341–376.

186. Ross SE, Schwab CW, David ET, Delong WG, Born CT (1987): Clearing the cervical spine: initial radiologic evaluation. *J Trauma* 27:1055–1060.

187. Roy-Camille R, Saillant G, Mazel C (1989): Internal fixation of the unstable cervical spine by a posterior osteosynthesis with plates and screws. In: *The cervical spine*, 2nd ed. Philadelphia: JB Lippincott 1989; pp390–403.

188. Ryan MD, Taylor TKF (1993): Odontoid fractures in the elderly. *J Spinal Dis* 6:397–401.

189. Ryken TC, Goel VK, Clausen JD, Traynelis C (1995): Assessment of unicortical and bicortical fixation in a quasistatic cadav-

eric model. Role of bone mineral density and screw torque. *Spine* 20:1861–1867.

190. Saboe LA, Reid DC, Davis LA, Warren SA, Grace MG (1991): Spine trauma and associated injuries. *J Trauma* 31:43–48.

191. Sasso R, Doherty BJ, Crawford MJ, Heggeness MH (1993): Biomechanics of odontoid fracture fixation: comparison of one and two screw techniques. *Spine* 18:1950–1953.

192. Sasso RC, Jeanneret B, Fischer K, Magerl F (1994): Occipitocervical fusion with posterior plate and screw insertion. A long term follow-up study. *Spine* 19:2364–2368.

193. Schaefer DM, Flanders AE, Osterhol JL, Northrup BE (1992): Prognostic significance of magnetic resonance imaging in the acute phase of cervical spinal cord injury. *J Neurosurg* 76:218–223.

194. Schaffler MB, Alson MD, Heller JG, Garfin SR (1992): Morphology of the dens: a quantitative study. *Spine* 17:738–743.

195. Schatzker J, Rorabeck CH, Waddell JP (1971): Fractures of the dens (odontoid process). *J Bone Joint Surg* 53(B):392–405.

196. Schatzker J, Rorabeck CH, Waddell JP (1975): Non-union of the odontoid process. *Clin Orthop* 108:127–137.

197. Scher AT (1976): Cervical spinal cord injury without evidence of fracture or dislocation. An assessment of the radiological features. *S Afr Med J* 50:962–965.

198. Schiff DC, Parke WW (1973): The arterial blood supply of the odontoid process. *J Bone Joint Surg* 55(A):1950–1956.

199. Schneider RC, Crosby EC, Russo RH, Gosh HH 1972 Traumatic spinal cord syndromes and their management. *Clin Neurosurg* 20:424.

200. Schweigel JFL (1987): Management of the fractured odontoid with Halo-thoracic bracing. *Spine* 12:838–839.

201. Sears W, Fazl M (1990): Prediction of stability of cervical fractures managed in the Halo vest and indications for surgical intervention. *J Neurosurg* 72:426–432.

202. Senter HJ, Kortyna R, Kemp WR (1989): Anterior cervical discectomy with hydroxyl apatite fusion. *Neurosurgery* 25:39–42.

203. Shapiro SA (1993): Management of unilateral locked facet of the cervical spine. *Neurosurgery* 33:832–837.

204. Sim FH, Svien HJ, Bickel WH, Janes JM (1974): Swan neck following extensive laminectomy. A review of 21 cases. *J Bone Joint Surg* 56(A):564–580.

205. Smith GW, Robinson RA (1958): The treatment of certain cervical spine disorders by anterior removal of the intervertebral disc and interbody fusion. *J Bone Joint Surg* 40(A):607–623.

206. Smith MD, Anderson PA (1994): Occipital cervical fusion. *Tech Orthop* 9:37–42.

207. Southwick WO (1980): Management of fracture of the dens (odontoid process). *J Bone Joint Surg* 62(A):482=n486.

208. Statham P, O'Sullivan M, Russell T (1993): The Halifax interlaminar clamp for posterior cervical fusion: initial experience in the United Kingdom. *Neurosurgery* 32:396–399.

209. Stauffer ES, Kelly EG (1977): Fracture-dislocation of the cervical spine: instability and recurrent deformity following treatment by anterior interbody fusion. *J Bone Joint Surg* 59(A):45–48.

210. Suh PB, Kostuik JP, Esses SI (1990): Anterior cervical plate fixation with the titanium hollow screw plate system. A preliminary report. *Spine* 15:1079–1081.

211. Sutterlin III CE, McAfee PC, Warden KE, Rey RM, Farey ID (1988): A biomechanical evaluation of cervical spinal stabiliza-tion of cervical spinal stabilization methods in a bovine model. *Spine* 13:795–802.

212. Tator CH, Fehlings MH (1991): Review of the secondary injury theory of acute spinal cord trauma with emphasis on vascular mechanisms. *J Neurosurg* 75:15–26.

213. Tien RD (1992): Fat-suppression MR Imaging in neuroradiology: technique and clinical application. *Am J Radiol* 158:369–379.

214. Traynelis VC, Marano GD, Dunker RO, Kaufman HH (1986): Traumatic atlantooccipital dislocation: case report. *J Neurosurg* 65:863–870.

215. Ulrich C, Woersdorfer O, Kalff R, Claes L, Wilke HJ (1991): Biomechanics of fixation systems to the cervical spine. *Spine* 16:54–59.

216. Van Peteghem PK, Schweigel JF (1979): The fractured cervical spine rendered unstable by anterior cervical fusion. *J Trauma* 19:110–114.

217. Velmahos G, Demetriades D (1994): Gunshot wounds of the spine: should retained bullets be removed to prevent infection? *Ann R Coll Surg Engl* 76:85–87.

218. Ward WG, Nunley JA (1991): Occult orthopaedic trauma in the multiply injured patient. *J Orthop Trauma* 5:308–312.

219. Waters RL, Adkins RH (1991): The effects of removal of bullet fragments retained in the spinal canal: a collaborative study to the National Spinal Cord Injury Model Systems. *Spine* 16:934–939.

220. Webb JK, Broughton RBK, McSweeney T (1976): Hidden flexion injury of the cervical spine. *J Bone Joint Surg* 58(B):322–327.

221. Weiland DJ, McAfee PC (1991): Posterior cervical fusion with triple wire strut graft technique: one hundred consecutive patients. *J Spinal Disord* 4:15–21.

222. Werne S (1957): Studies in spontaneous atlas dislocation. *Acta Orthop Scand Suppl* 32:1–140.

223. Wertheim SB, Bohlmann HH (1987): Occipitocervical fusion. Indications, technique, and long-term results in thirteen patients. *J Bone Joint Surg* 69(A):833–836.

224. White AA, Southwick WO, Panjabi MM (1976): Clinical instability of the lower cervical spine. A review of past and current concepts. *Spine* 1:15–27.

225. Whitehill R, Richman JA, Glaser JA (1986): Failure of immobilization of the cervical spine by the halo vest. A report of 5 cases. *J Bone Joint Surg* 68(A):326–332.

226. Wholey MH, Bruwer AJ, Hillier LB (1958): The lateral roentgenogram of the neck (with comments on the atlanto-odontoid-basion relationship). *Radiology* 71:350–353.

227. Willis BK, Greiner F, Orrison WW, Benzel EC (1994): The incidence of vertebral artery injury after midcervical spine fracture or subluxation. *Neurosurgery* 34:435–442.

228. Wittenberg RH, Moeller J, Shea M, White AA, Hayes WC (1990): Compressive strength of autologous and allogenous bone grafts for thoracolumbar and cervical spine fusion. *Spine* 16:1073–1078.

229. Yashon D (1978): Pathogenesis of spinal cord injury. *Orthop Clin North Am* 9:247–261.

230. Yoshida GM, Garland D, Waters RL (1995): Gunshot wounds to the spine. *Orthop Clin North Am* 26:107–116.

231. Young W (1993): Secondary injury mechanisms in acute spinal cord injury. *J Emerg Med* 11:13–22.

The Adult Spine: Principles and Practice,
2nd edition, J.W. Frymoyer, Editor-in-Chief.
Lippincott-Raven Publishers, Philadelphia © 1997.

CHAPTER 61

Late Complications of Cervical Fractures and Dislocations and Their Management

Michael J. Bolesta and Henry H. Bohlman

Tremendous progress has been made over the past decade to improve the care of trauma victims. Highly skilled emergency medical technicians stabilize the seriously injured and rapidly transport them to designated trauma centers. Once there, experienced personnel thoroughly evaluate, stabilize, reevaluate, and manage problems systematically. Refined protocols help identify all important injuries, but as Bohlman and others have pointed out, cervical injuries often occur in association with other injuries, which can divert attention away from the neck (13,15,62). Despite the progress made, every spine surgeon still faces a number of problems after the acute phase. Early identification and appropriate management of cervical injuries under the best of circumstances will still be plagued by some late complications. These include instability, persistent neural compression, progressive loss of neurologic function, and a miscellaneous group of infections and failures of previous stabilizations.

M. J. Bolesta, M.D.: Assistant Professor of Orthopaedic Surgery, University of Texas Southwestern Medical Center, Dallas, Texas, 75235-8883.
H. H. Bohlman, M.D.: Professor and Vice Chairman of Orthopaedics, Case Western Reserve University, University Hospitals of Cleveland, Cleveland, Ohio, 44106.

INSTABILITY WITH PAIN OR DEFORMITY

Etiology

White and Panjabi (76) defined instability as a loss of the ability of the spine under physiologic loads to maintain relationships between vertebrae in such a way that there is neither damage nor subsequent irritation to the spinal cord or nerve roots and there is no development of incapacitating deformity or pain due to structural changes. In broad terms, stability is dependent on the integrity of the bones, joints, joint capsules, and ligaments of the spine. Trauma can render the cervical spine unstable by disrupting any or all of these components. The cervical musculature can splint the spine acutely, but cannot substitute for osteoligamentous integrity.

Bohlman (13) has documented that the torn posterior ligament complex in flexion injuries may not heal even after long rigid immobilization (Fig. 1). White and Panjabi (76) consider the atlanto-occipital joint to be relatively unstable, and injuries are usually fatal. Most are produced by a blow to the head.

Atlantoaxial stability depends on the integrity of the lateral joint capsules and, more important, on the transverse portion of the cruciate ligament, although

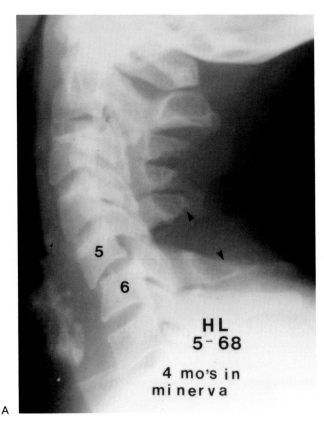 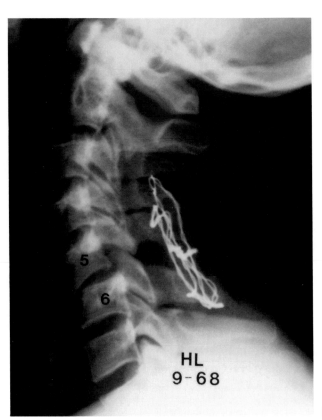

FIG. 1. A middle-aged man with C5-C6 subluxation treated in a Minerva jacket for 4 months. **A:** Lateral radiograph after 4 months of immobilization, showing persistent subluxation. **B:** Solid fusion after open reduction and internal fixation.

there are many secondary support structures. The transverse ligament may be ruptured with flexion or in association with a severe C1 burst injury (Jefferson fracture). Complete dislocation can occur with minor trauma in Down syndrome (51). Depending on the amount of anterior stability, the late presentation is with cervical occipital pain, usually without a neurologic deficit. Approximately 12% of atlantoaxial injuries, treated operatively and nonoperatively, will produce chronic pain; some investigators have postulated a demyelinating process, as several of these patients describe Lhermitte's phenomenon (36). A torticollis deformity is seen with rotary subluxation, which can occur with or without significant trauma.

Traumatic spondylolisthesis of the axis, or the hangman's fracture, occurs through the pedicles of the axis and may be associated with disruption of the C2-C3 disc and ligament complex. In the Maryland series of 52 patients, early conversion of traction to halo vest was associated with significant residual deformity, which also correlated with their classification scheme (53). In a larger series of 123 cases, no correlation was found between nonunion and time of bed rest, displacement, or angulation (40). Those patients were divided into three treatment groups: traction for 4 to 12 weeks, traction for

3 days to 3 weeks, or an orthosis alone. Regardless of the treatment method, only seven required an operation: six for nonunion and one for a painful kyphosis at C3-C4 after C2 healed.

Denis popularized the three-column concept of the thoracolumbar spine (31,32) and related this to stability. Cybulski et al. (28) applied this model to the subaxial cervical spine. Not surprisingly, patients with involvement of all three columns were very unstable, and simple posterior wiring failed. Their criteria for three-column damage are retrolisthesis and angulation of the superior vertebra on the subjacent one, or disruption of the posterior interspinous ligaments sufficient to allow facet subluxation or dislocation in conjunction with a "shear" dislocation of one vertebra on another. They recommended combined anterior and posterior fusion for three-column injuries. Although more complex, a mechanistic classification was proposed by Allen et al. (1).

Experimentally, White et al. (74) sequentially divided the soft tissue in cadaveric cervical spines from anterior to posterior or posterior to anterior trauma, eventually producing instability. The extent of this damage, as well as its location, will influence the timing of presentation. Severe trauma with neurologic deficit is unlikely to present late, unless there is an associated head injury or other multiple injuries that obscure the cervical fracture-dislocation. More subtle injuries will take time to manifest themselves, usually as persistent pain or deformity (48). The most common deformity is kyphosis secondary to flexion and axial loading injuries. This deformity can produce pain, probably secondary to muscle spasms as the patient attempts to maintain head position (54), or neural compression even without paralysis. There can be a rotary deformity in addition to the kyphosis with a unilateral facet injury. Such deformity can be reduced closed in the early period, but reduction may be lost, even with halo fixation (77).

Evaluation

A detailed history will cover details of the accident, catalog all associated injuries, and review the management to date. This will provide valuable information about the mechanism of injury by also documenting sites of head or facial injury. Physical examination will localize the portion of the cervical spine involved and document clinical deformity and loss of motion. A thorough neurologic examination is essential.

Plain radiographs provide information about the location of injury and the presence of malalignment or deformity. As in the acute situation, it is essential to visualize the body of C7 and ideally T1, which may require the use of arm traction or the swimmer's view. Oblique films should be obtained to evaluate the facet joints. The odontoid view provides information not present on the standard anteroposterior (AP) film. With rotary subluxation or dislocation, there is asymmetry between the dens and the lateral masses of the atlas as well as the atlantoaxial joint (Fig. 2). Goddard et al. (43) classified these findings into two types. In Type I, which occurs in children and adults, the C1-C2 joints are fixed in partial rotation but are not dislocated. On the AP view, the anteriorly rotated lateral mass of C1 appears to be widened, closer to the odontoid, and slightly elevated. In Type II, one inferior facet of C1 is anteriorly dislocated and locked, which they believe occurs only in children. On the AP view, again, the anteriorly rotated mass of C1 appears widened, but seems further from the odontoid and tilted downward (43). When there is concern about the atlanto-occipital joint, a lateral view of the skull may give better detail of this region than the standard lateral of the cervical spine, and comparison should be made with films obtained at the time of injury when possible.

Abnormalities at the atlanto-occipital level prompt further diagnostic studies and may require stabilization. At the atlantoaxial level, the interval between the posterior cortex of the anterior arch of C1 and the dens should not exceed 3 mm in adults and 5 mm in children. Of even greater importance is the distance between the dens and the posterior arch of C1, which in adults should nor-

mally measure 22 to 24 mm. Boden et al. (11) determined 14 mm to be the critical value for the posterior atlantodental interval in rheumatoid patients; stabilization was recommended for values of 14 mm or less, regardless of neurologic status. Extrapolation to the trauma patient is probably reasonable. Voluntary flexion/extension lateral radiographs are helpful in this evaluation of late instability in the subaxial spine. By White and Panjabi's criteria (74,76), greater than 3.5 mm of vertebral body translation or more than 11° rotation denotes instability. A complete facet dislocation, either unilaterally or bilaterally, should be considered acutely unstable because of disruption of the facet capsules and ligaments.

Plain tomography is a valuable technique to define bony anatomy, particularly in the upper cervical spine as well as the lower cervical spine posterior elements.

Myelography, combined with computed tomography (CT), is used to assess the neural elements in patients with paralysis. The two will identify associated disc herniation and posterior element fractures not readily appreciated on plain films. Water-soluble dye inserted at the atlantoaxial level is well tolerated, and the technology is readily available. Magnetic resonance imaging (MRI) provides direct sagittal imaging, demonstrates the cord directly, and is noninvasive. Bondurant et al. (18) and others found prognostic information in cord images shortly after injury (66). Later, MRI is the modality of choice for diagnosing syringomyelia. The resolution of MRI for osseous structures is inferior to that of CT. Dynamic studies are possible and can be quite useful in demonstrating neural compression in certain positions (58).

Treatment

The patient who survives a traumatic dislocation of the atlanto-occipital joint requires occipitocervical fusion for stability. Wertheim and Bohlman described a technique of posterior arthrodesis (73). A midline incision is used (Fig. 3A). A burr creates a ridge at the external occipital protuberance, preserving the inner table. Twenty-two-gauge wire is passed through this, looped, and passed through the hole again. A sublaminar wire is passed at C1. A spinous process wire is placed at C2 (Fig. 3B). Large corticocancellous grafts are harvested through a separate incision (Fig. 3C) and secured by the wires (Fig. 3D). Additional cancellous bone is packed between the grafts and interstices between the grafts and underlying bone (Fig. 3E). Depending on the surgeon's assessment of preoperative instability, the patient is immobilized for 8 to 12 weeks in either a halo or two-poster orthosis.

More recently, Smith et al. (67) described a plating method that is useful in situations when midline decompression is necessary or when the arthrodesis must ex-

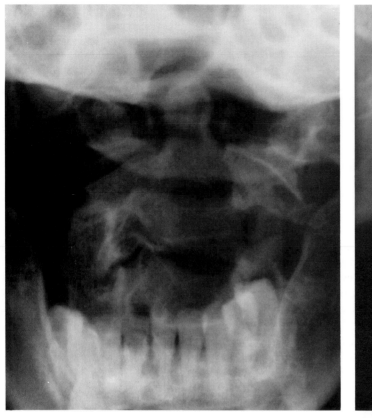

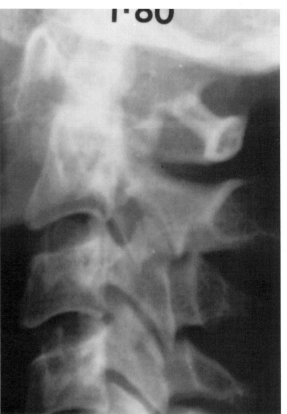

FIG. 2. A young woman with post-traumatic torticollis. **A:** AP odontoid view demonstrating offset between the lateral mass of the atlas and the superior facet of the axis. **B:** The lateral view reveals rotation of C1 as well as a fracture of the atlas. **C:** Lateral view showing a posterior atlantoaxial arthrodesis without reduction. Clinically, there was resolution of the torticollis and pain.

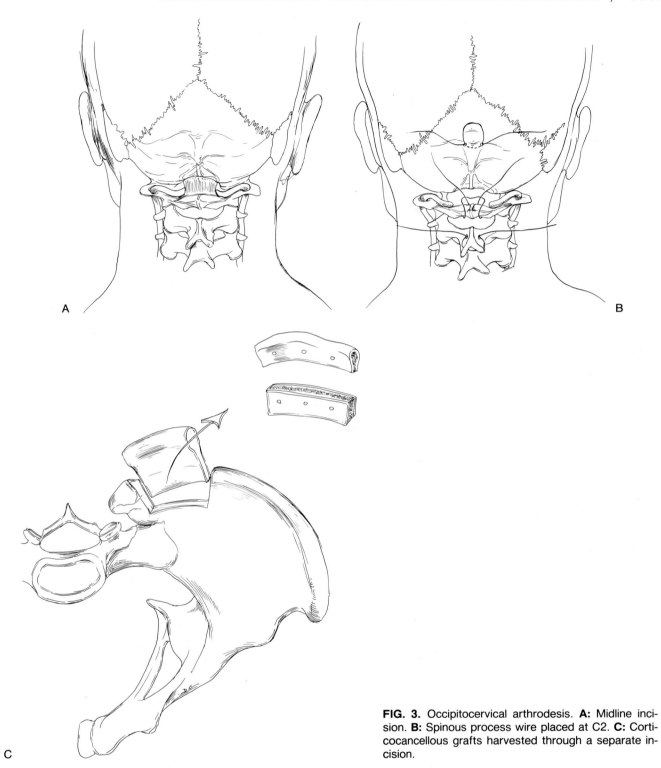

FIG. 3. Occipitocervical arthrodesis. **A:** Midline incision. **B:** Spinous process wire placed at C2. **C:** Corticocancellous grafts harvested through a separate incision.

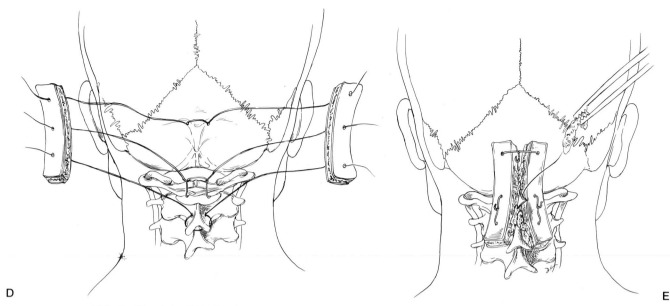

D

E

FIG. 3. (*Continued*.) **D:** Corticocancellous graft secured by wires. **E:** Additional cancellous bone.

tend over multiple subaxial segments. This is an extension of the technique developed for the lower cervical spine (3).

Kahanovitz et al. (50) described an unusual case in which the atlas dislocated and became fixed intracranially. This was missed because of significant intracranial trauma, which masked the dislocation. When recognized late, it was stable and did not require treatment. For late atlantoaxial instability secondary to a torn transverse ligament or Type II odontoid fracture, posterior arthrodesis is the standard treatment (Fig. 4). A variety of techniques may be used, depending on the surgeon's preference. A modification of the Gallie technique is to place a sublaminar wire at C1 (Fig. 5A). A second wire is placed through and around the spinous process of C2. The cortical cancellous grafts are harvested, and holes are placed to accommodate the wires (Fig. 5B). Grafts are firmly secured by the wires, and cancellous bone is placed between the grafts and the bone (Fig. 5C). This technique is technically less demanding than the Brooks fusion, does not require a C2 sublaminar wire, and provides excellent, immediate stability and a high fusion rate. Posterior wiring and fusion are also effective in children and adolescents (68).

In the Brooks technique, wire or braided wire is passed beneath the arch of C1 and the lamina of C2. This is done bilaterally. A corticocancellous bone graft is placed between the arch of the atlas and the lamina of the axis and secured by the wire, which is tied posteriorly.

Although there have been trials of anterior screw fixation of dens fractures (5), this technique has not been applied to established nonunions. Halifax clamps obviate the need to pass sublaminar wires at C1, but the bulky clamps do reduce the area available for fusion, and the

published follow-up has been short (29). Yablon et al. (79) reported the use of a Harrington compression rod and hooks for fixation after open reduction of a C4-C5 dislocation; this was complicated by migration of one rod into the cerebellum noted 4 years after surgery (79). Bohler (12) described combined anterior and posterior fusion for dens nonunions in 13 patients.

In the unusual event that there is a congenitally absent posterior arch of the atlas with atlantoaxial instability, there are three options. First, screw fixation of the atlantoaxial facet joints may be performed through an anterior extraoral approach (44,59). A 2.5-cm screw is inserted through the lateral mass of C1 into the body of C2. With the head in neutral rotation, the drill is directed in the line from the mastoid process to the tip of the transverse process of C1. Because of the angle used, bilateral anterolateral exposure is required. Alternatively, facet screws may be placed via a posterior exposure. A longer incision than usual is made, which allows for far lateral exposure. If this technique fails or if the atlanto-occipital joint is diseased, or if these two approaches are too extensive for the patient, a posterior occipital cervical arthrodesis can be performed as described above.

If the preoperative evaluation reveals cervical cord compression by the posterior arch of C1 that is fixed and cannot be reduced, then simple atlantoaxial arthrodesis is contraindicated because there is not enough room to pass a sublaminar C1 wire (14). The arch of C1 is therefore resected, and an occipital cervical arthrodesis is performed. If the compression is anterior, as with a dens malunion, posterior arthrodesis may be followed with anterior resection of the odontoid. The transoral approach has been described (4,37,55,65), as have several extraoral dissections (59). The latter have the distinct ad-

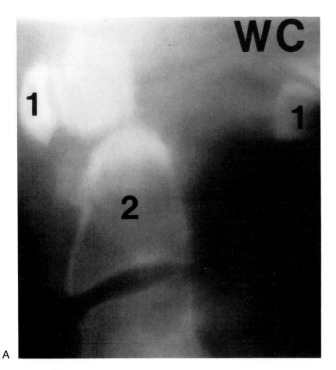

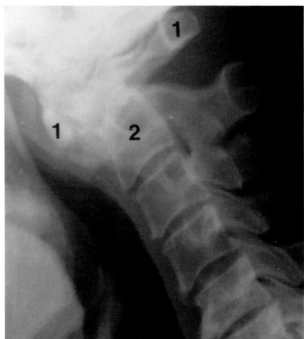

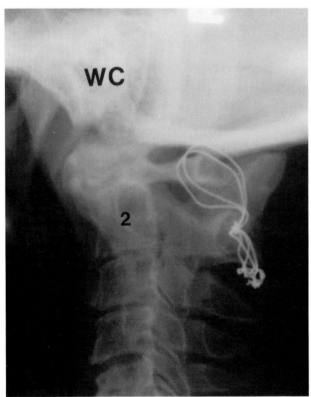

FIG. 4. A 61-year-old polytrauma victim with a dens fracture treated in a halo. Nonunion was recognized, but surgical stabilization was delayed because of cardiac instability after anesthesia induction. The patient was later fused successfully. He was free of symptoms until dying from pneumonia 15 months later. **A:** Lateral tomogram demonstrating the nonunion. **B:** Anterior atlantoaxial instability with flexion. **C:** Healed posterior atlantoaxial arthrodesis.

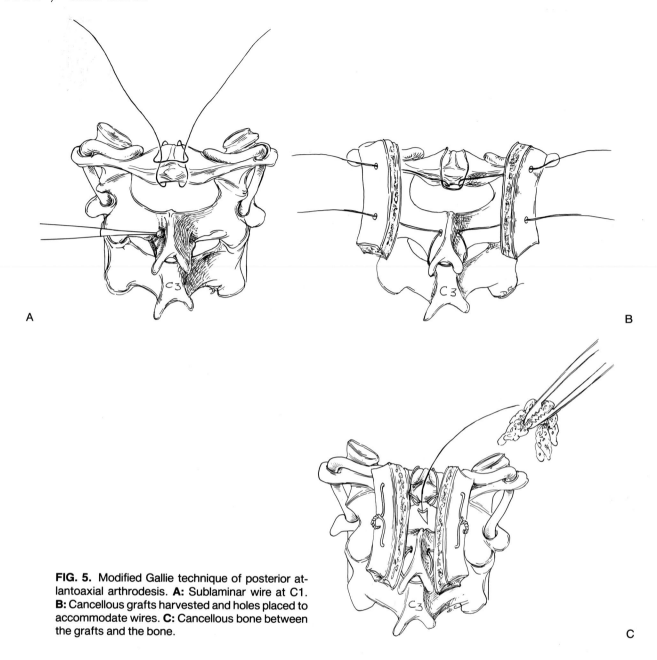

A

B

C

FIG. 5. Modified Gallie technique of posterior atlantoaxial arthrodesis. **A:** Sublaminar wire at C1. **B:** Cancellous grafts harvested and holes placed to accommodate wires. **C:** Cancellous bone between the grafts and the bone.

vantage of being less disfiguring and carrying a lower risk of infection and death. Nonetheless, the transoral approach remains popular.

In a series of 123 cases of traumatic spondylolisthesis of the axis, one patient developed a painful C3-C4 kyphosis below a healed C2 fracture. This responded to a C2-C4 posterior cervical fusion (40).

Pain and instability without kyphotic deformity in the subaxial spine are treated with posterior arthrodesis using a triple-wire technique. After exposure through a midline incision, a 20-gauge tethering wire is placed through and around the spinous processes and tied to itself, providing immediate stability (Fig. 6A). Twenty-two-gauge wires are passed through and around the spinous processes (Fig. 6B) and are used to secure cortico-

cancellous grafts (Fig. 6C). Six to eight weeks in a two-poster orthosis is generally sufficient to assure a solid fusion.

Some surgeons advocate polymethylmethacrylate as a substitute for or adjuvant to bone graft in selected patients (27,61). In the absence of bone graft, such constructs are experimentally inferior (78). McAfee et al. (57) reported 24 cases of severe complications in patients treated with methylmethacrylate stabilization, including loss of fixation, increased neurologic deficit, and deep infection.

Roy-Camille has developed an alternative fixation with plates applied to the articular processes (33,46,64). Experience is accumulating in this country (3,6). The advantages include fixation in the presence of posterior el-

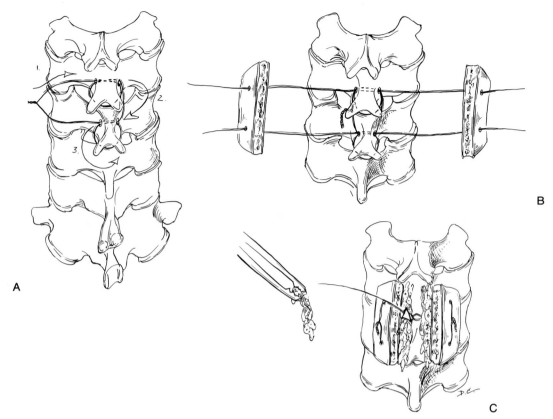

FIG. 6. Triple-wire technique of posterior cervical arthrodesis. A 20-gauge tethering wire **(A)** provides immediate stability, and 22-gauge wires are passed through and around the spinous processes **(B)** to secure corticocancellous grafts **(C).**

ement fractures, fixation in the absence of lamina, improved rotational stability, and possibly reduced need for external support. Disadvantages are increased cost and potential injury to the nerve roots and vertebral artery.

Another alternative for posterior instability is anterior cervical discectomy and fusion (63), but experimentally this has proven biomechanically inferior to posterior fixation (69). Bucci et al. (24) have advocated nonoperative management of cervical instability with halo fixation, but eight (40%) of their patients so treated had persistent symptoms; five of them underwent delayed surgery, and two of these five had worsening of neurologic symptoms before the operation.

When there is significant late fixed kyphosis of the lower cervical spine, an anterior approach is used. Corpectomies are performed followed by a strut fusion. Up to two bodies can be spanned by iliac crest, but longer fusions require the use of fibula. Intraoperative traction helps provide correction and intraoperative stability. Some investigators are using anterior plates to fix the graft, but follow-up is short (21) and this fixation is unstable in flexion. We routinely use intraoperative evoked potential monitoring. Depending on the status of the posterior column, posterior arthrodesis may also be indicated if there is an associated torn ligament complex

(80). This also affects the postoperative immobilization required. Depending on neurologic function, the patient may be maintained in traction or stabilized with a posterior arthrodesis and early mobilization in a halo (45).

In patients with ankylosing spondylitis, the fracture deformity may be corrected through the fracture with halo traction, but careful neurologic monitoring is necessary with slow gradual correction to avoid overdistraction and retrolisthesis. These fractures may be quite unstable; displacement and neurologic injury are often delayed relative to the fracture (23).

PERSISTENT NEURAL COMPRESSION

Etiology

Unless obscured by other injuries, major neurologic deficit is generally apparent at the time of the injury. Most of the damage probably occurs at the initial impact. This was recently corroborated in an elegant burst fracture model by Chang et al. (26). The more severe loss of canal length and area during injury could not be correlated to the recoil position post-trauma. The physician has no control over this, but can address residual canal

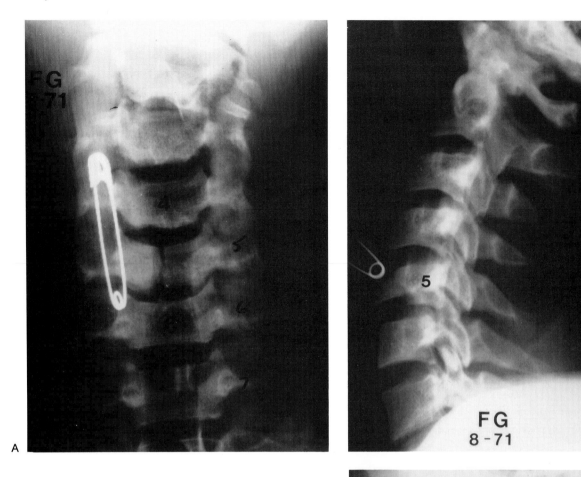

A

B

C

FIG. 7. A 20-year-old man with developmental stenosis who developed an anterior cord syndrome after a C5 fracture. He enjoyed complete recovery after an anterior fusion. Four years later, he again injured his neck and again developed anterior cord syndrome secondary to a C3-C4 herniated disc above his fusion. After anterior discectomy and fusion, he recovered completely. AP **(A)** and lateral **(B)** radiographs of the original C5 compression fracture. One year later **(C)**, there was healing of the anterior graft from C4 to C6. Note the marked narrowing of the cervical canal.

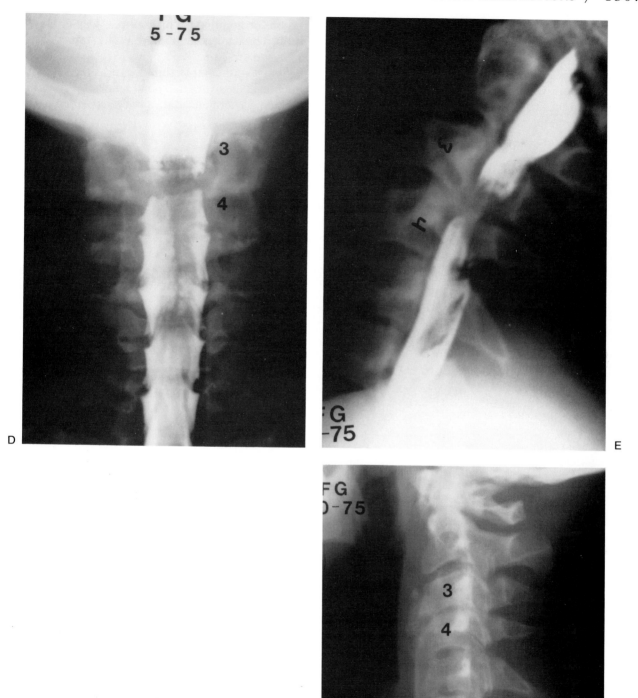

FIG. 7. (*Continued.*) AP **(D)** and lateral **(E)** myelograms revealing C3-C4 disc herniation. Lateral radiograph **(F)** after C3-C4 discectomy and fusion.

compromise as indicated. When the compression is milder, the deficit may be more subtle; in some cases, pain is the only manifestation of neural compression. Therefore, a careful preoperative assessment, as described previously, is essential. In other cases, the neural compression occurs later with secondary deformity, mal-

union, or nonunion. For example, Day et al. (30) described basilar invagination resulting from an untreated Jefferson's fracture.

Spinal cord compression occurs as the result of a reduction in the size of the spinal canal for various reasons, including a herniated disc, a fractured vertebra, or dislo-

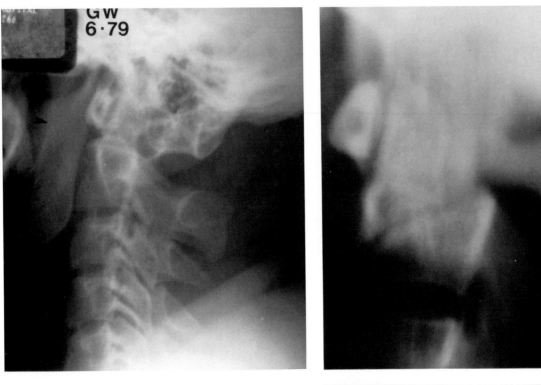

FIG. 8. Man with an unrecognized nondisplaced dens fracture who went on to unstable nonunion and myelopathy. **A:** Lateral radiograph from the time of injury. Note the soft-tissue swelling anterior to the upper cervical spine. **B:** Lateral tomogram revealing a displaced nonunion. **C:** Lateral radiograph after posterior atlantoaxial arthrodesis. The patient's myelopathy improved significantly.

cation. In a developmentally narrow spinal canal, a bulging disc without herniation can produce cord compression. Eismont et al. (35) were able to correlate the severity of neurologic deficit to the size of the spinal canal (Fig. 7). Instability also can produce cord compression (Fig. 8).

Anterior nerve root compression may result from a lateral disc herniation (Fig. 9), whereas fractures of the pedicles or fracture-dislocations of the facets may compromise the spinal nerves posteriorly.

Anterior spinal cord decompression facilitates recovery from incomplete nerve root or spinal cord injury,

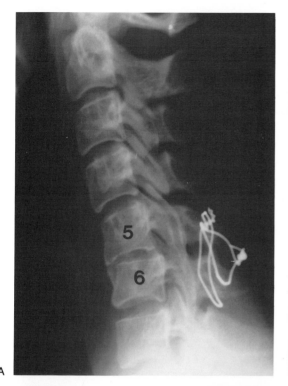

A

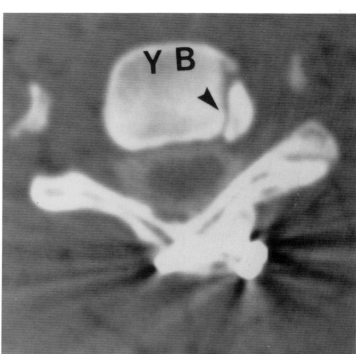

B

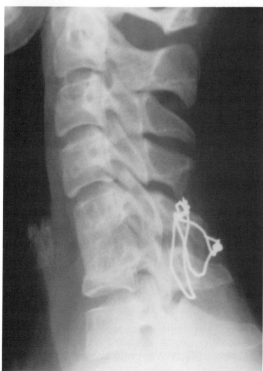

C

FIG. 9. Young woman who sustained a C5-C6 fracture-subluxation, treated with posterior cervical fusion. One year later, she presented with hypesthesia and weakness in the C6 distribution. **A:** Lateral radiograph 1 year after injury reveals a healed posterior fusion with mild residual C5-C6 subluxation. **B:** CT with contrast demonstrates unilateral root compression at the level of the uncovertebral joint. **C:** Lateral radiograph after anterior discectomy and fusion at C5-C6. The patient experienced complete resolution of radiculopathy.

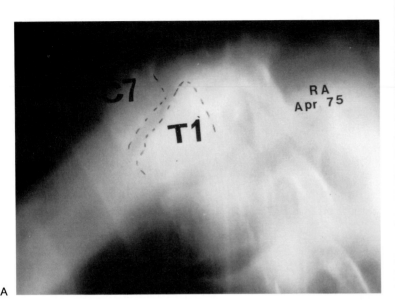

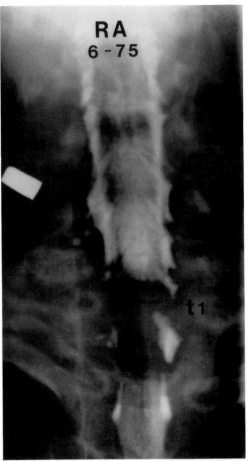

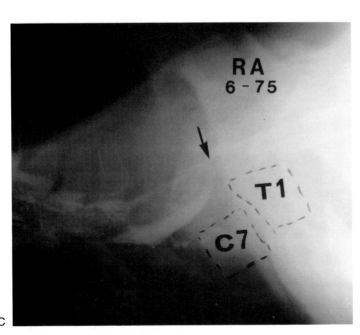

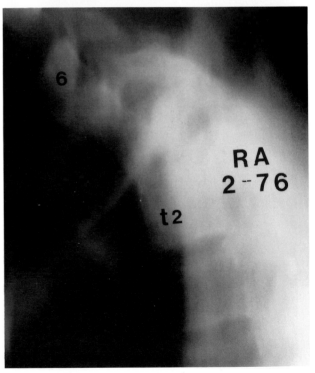

FIG. 10. Man with C7-T1 fracture-dislocation and anterior cord syndrome treated with laminectomy without reduction. He did not improve and was left with a kyphotic deformity. **A:** Lateral tomogram demonstrating a C7-T1 dislocation and a healed compression fracture of T1. AP **(B)** and lateral **(C)** myelograms revealing high-grade block at this level. **D:** Lateral tomogram after anterior corpectomy and strut grafting with iliac crest. The patient regained significant motor function.

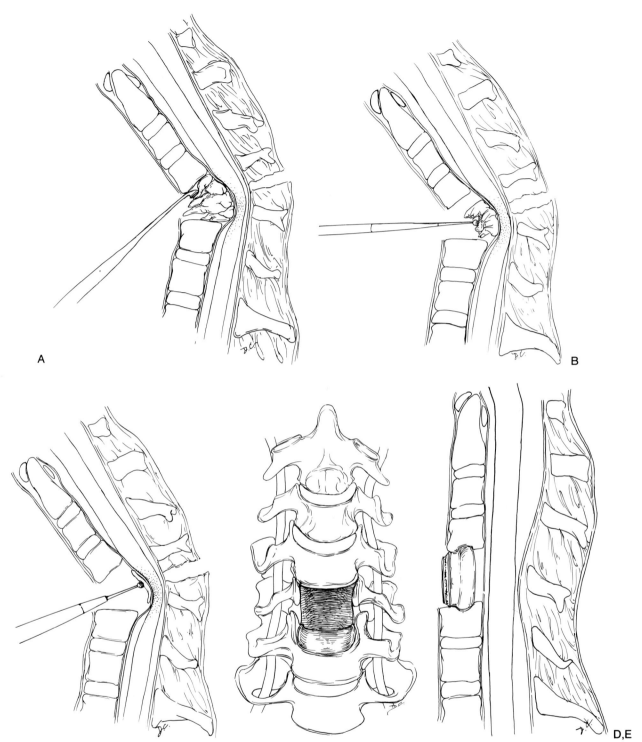

FIG. 11. Anterior corpectomy and strut arthrodesis. **A:** Discectomies rostral and caudal to each involved body. **B:** Rongeurs or burrs remove the central portion of the body. **C:** Diamond burr removes the posterior cortex of the body. **D:** Concavities in the remaining rostral and caudal vertebral bodies. **E:** Strut fashioned from iliac crest.

which has been demonstrated experimentally and clinically (2,13,16,17,56). In the patient with complete spinal cord injury, there is currently no way to restore distal cord function; however, root function may recover, with decompression resulting in significant improvement in the activities of daily living (2,8,9). Late unreduced dislocations should be treated operatively.

Evaluation

Evaluation is very similar to that described for instability. Myelography with CT, MRI, and plain tomograms help the surgeon localize and characterize the nature of the root or cord compression (58). This should be correlated with the patient's symptoms and any neurologic deficit. It is also essential to identify any coexisting instability.

Treatment

In a patient with a healed malunion of an odontoid or axis body fracture and anterior cord compression with myelopathy, an anterior approach is indicated, which may be transoral (10,55) or, as we prefer, by the retropharyngeal approach with arthrodesis (59). In a patient presenting late with root compression from an unreduced facet subluxation, dislocation, or fracture, a posterior approach is used to remove partially the superior articular process with a power burr, which will facilitate a foraminotomy and reduction, followed by posterior arthrodesis. An unusual case of nerve compression was reported by Cartwright et al. (25), in which a synovial cyst developed below anterior C5-C6 and posterior C2-C3 fusions for trauma, which was treated by resection.

Traumatic disc herniations are safely and reliably treated by anterior cervical discectomy and fusion (Fig. 7), and biomechanical studies have established the Robinson technique to be superior to other anterior constructs (75). An anterior approach should be used for all central and lateral disc herniations. Tamura (70) has described the associated cranial symptoms with C4 root compression after trauma, postulating sympathetic involvement. These 40 patients had headaches, vertigo, tinnitus, or ocular problems. They responded well to discectomy and fusion. Eismont et al. (34) pointed out the potentially catastrophic association of disc herniation with facet dislocations. Most of their seven patients had significant deficits. Probst and Karli (60) found a 50% incidence of disc herniation in those patients approached ventrally. The true incidence and significance of these combined lesions are unknown at this time.

When there is malunion of a vertebral body burst fracture with compression of the spinal cord or in the presence of a kyphotic deformity, corpectomies are necessary (Fig. 10). An anterior approach is again used. Discecto-

mies are performed rostral and caudal to each involved body (Fig. 11A). Rongeurs or burrs are used to remove the central portion of the body (Fig. 11B). Lateral cortices are preserved to avoid damage to the vertebral arteries. Enough disc is removed proximally and distally to identify the posterior longitudinal ligament. The posterior cortex of the body is removed with a diamond burr (Fig. 11C). Concavities are created in the remaining rostral and caudal vertebral bodies (Fig. 11D). A strut is fashioned from iliac crest or fibula, depending on the number of vertebral bodies resected. One or two corpectomies can be spanned with iliac crest (Fig. 11E); more than that require a fibula because of the curvature of the crest. The patient is maintained postoperatively for 6 to 12 weeks in an orthosis or halo, depending on the integrity of the posterior column. A posterior arthrodesis, using the triple-wire technique described above, may be necessary if there has been extensive damage to the posterior column. Lateral mass plating and facet fusion are employed if a laminectomy had been performed earlier.

PROGRESSIVE LOSS OF NEURAL FUNCTION

Etiology

Multiple studies have demonstrated the potential for neural recovery after decompression following cervical injury (2,8,9,13,16,17,56). This can occur even with delayed decompression. However, chronic persistent compression can result in irreversible neurologic dysfunction. Anderson and Bohlman reported worse results after decompression more than 12 months after incomplete and 18 months after complete cervical cord injuries (2,16). The exact mechanism for this is unknown, but may be due to chronic ischemia caused by stretching and occlusion of capillaries and small intrinsic vessels. Pressure itself may be a factor. Late deterioration may be a manifestation of the aging nervous system.

Post-traumatic cysts of the spinal cord, one type of syringomyelia, may present with pain or progression of a previously static neurologic deficit. The mechanism by which these cysts develop is unknown. They may result from liquefaction of necrotic cord, absorption of hematoma, or increased pressure within the central canal and may be found from months to years after trauma.

Evaluation

Assessment in the case of chronic compression has been described, and is best accomplished with myelography, CT, and MRI.

MRI is clearly the best modality for evaluating intrinsic cord pathology such as a post-traumatic cyst (19,20,42,49) by providing direct sagittal and transverse images (Fig. 12). It is noninvasive and can be repeated

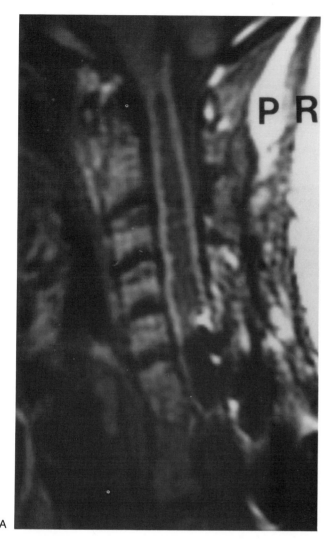

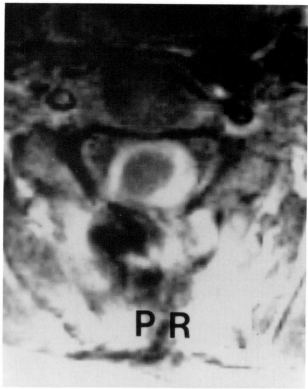

FIG. 12. Man with long-standing complete quadriplegia at the C7 level, treated with anterior decompression and fusion. He developed new pain and ascending weakness. Sagittal **(A)** and transverse **(B)** MRI demonstrate a large posttraumatic cyst, which extends proximally within the cord. He experienced significant recovery with myelotomy and drainage.

serially, which is useful when these cysts are small and when the correlation with clinical symptoms is equivocal. Worsening symptoms and ascending paralysis with a documented increase in size should prompt drainage of the cyst. In addition, MRI is ideal in evaluating the success of a shunt in decompressing the spinal cord.

If MRI is unavailable, delayed CT after the administration of intrathecal contrast may be used. Because this is an invasive procedure, it cannot be repeated as easily as MRI. Furthermore, timing of the scan is critical; it is easier to underestimate the size of a cyst or miss it entirely using this technique.

Another less common neurologic manifestation of cord injury is reflex sympathetic dystrophy. Wainapel (72) described two people with sympathetic dystrophy associated with central cord syndrome.

Treatment

The surgical treatment of persistent neural compression is detailed above. Large post-traumatic cysts and those documented as increasing in size should be drained by a posterior exposure; microscopic myelotomy is performed and a tube is placed to shunt the cyst cavity into the subarachnoid space. Smaller cysts may be followed clinically with serial MRI studies (see Chapter 28).

OTHER COMPLICATIONS

Infection

Although rare, the esophagus can be injured at the time of initial insult (7,52,71). Patients sustaining cervical fractures and dislocations often have other injuries, so there is often a lag between the time of injury and resumption of oral feedings. Contamination of the neck can occur secondary to a ruptured esophagus. Cervical and often mediastinal abscesses will generally present with sepsis. However, unsuspected abscesses have been encountered at the time of tracheostomy. A high index of suspicion is necessary to make the diagnosis. Esophagoscopy may not be possible because of the cervical injury. Contrast studies with a barium swallow followed by CT usually confirm the diagnosis. Adequate drainage and antibiotics are essential for successful management of this potentially lethal complication.

Instability at Another Level

Careful initial evaluation and management will minimize this rare complication. When another more subtle level presents after treatment of a different cervical lesion, the same principles are used as described above. Decompression and/or arthrodesis are performed as indicated.

Nonunion and Malunion

Nonunion of odontoid fractures may be painful, with or without instability. These require posterior atlantoax-

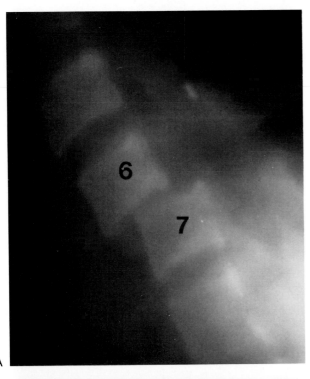

A

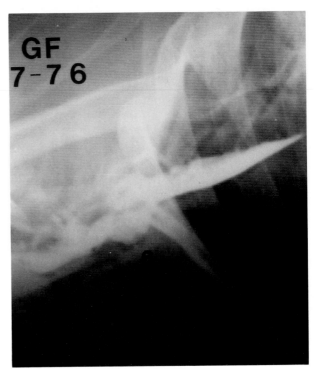

B

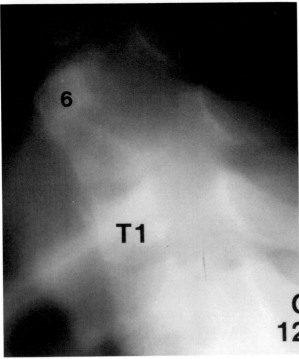

C

FIG. 13. Man with a C6-C7 dislocation that was never reduced. **A:** Lateral radiograph demonstrating a 50% translation of C6 on C7 consistent with bilateral facet dislocation. **B:** Lateral myelogram revealing cord compression at the level of the dislocation. **C:** Lateral tomogram after C7 corpectomy and C6-T1 anterior strut graft with iliac crest.

ial arthrodesis. Os odontoideum likely represents disruption of the vasculature about the dens, secondary to a remote fracture altering odontoid growth, and results in late instability requiring arthrodesis (39,47).

Traumatic spondylolisthesis of the axis, or hangman's fracture, can usually be treated with traction and a halo. Of the 123 patients of Francis et al. (40), 5.5% went on to nonunion. This type of instability can be treated by anterior C2-C3 or posterior C1-C3 arthrodesis. In addition, that series included one posterior C2-C4 arthrodesis for a painful kyphosis at C3-C4 after the axis healed.

Malunion in the lower cervical spine can lead to loss of motion, pain, and perhaps neurologic deficit. Radiologic evaluation will define the pathology. Based on this, the appropriate fusion or decompression can be performed (Fig. 13).

Finally, nonunion of a previous attempt at cervical fusion may be diagnosed by flexion/extension plain films and tomography. Myelography, CT, and MRI should be used if there is suspicion of persistent neural compression. If present, this should be addressed at the time of revision fusion. The surgeon may wish to consider posterior fusion for a failed anterior fusion (22,38). The location of the persistent recurrent neural compression will usually dictate the operative approach required, though Farey et al. (38) recommended a posterior approach for failed anterior surgery, using foraminotomy to decompress the involved nerve roots. Fuji et al. (41) recommended wiring without graft if stability can be obtained, if the nonunion is hypervascular, and if there is not excessive delay between the initial and revision procedures.

REFERENCES

1. Allen BL Jr, Ferguson RL, Lehmann TR, O'Brien RP (1982): A mechanistic classification of closed, indirect fractures and dislocations of the lower cervical spine. *Spine* 7:1–27.
2. Anderson PA, Bohlman HH (1992): Anterior decompression and arthrodesis of the cervical spine: Long-term motor improvement. Part II—Improvement in complete traumatic quadriplegia. *J Bone Joint Surg* [Am] 74A:683–692.
3. Anderson PA, Henley MB, Grady MS, Montesano PX, Winn HR (1991): Posterior cervical arthrodesis with AO reconstruction plates and bone graft. *Spine* 16:S72–S79.
4. Ashraf J, Crockard HA (1990): Transoral fusion for high cervical fractures. *J Bone Joint Surg* [Br] 72B:76–79.
5. Barbour JR (1971): Screw fixation in fracture of the odontoid process. *South Aust Clin* 5:20.
6. Barquet A, Pereyra D (1988): An unusual extension injury to the cervical spine: A case report. *J Bone Joint Surg* [Am] 70-A:1393–1395.
7. Benoit BG, Russell NA, Cole CW, Clark AJ, McIntyre RW (1983): Meningitis secondary to retropharyngeal abscess. Report of a case occurring in association with cervical spine fracture. *Spine* 8:438–439.
8. Benzel EC, Larson SJ (1986): Recovery of nerve root function after complete quadriplegia from cervical spine fractures. *Neurosurgery* 19:809–812.
9. Benzel EC, Larson SJ (1987): Functional recovery after decompressive spine operation for cervical spine fractures. *Neurosurgery* 20:742–746.
10. Blazier CJ, Hadley MN, Spetzler RF (1986): The transoral surgical approach to craniovertebral pathology. *J Neurosci Nurs* 18:57–62.
11. Boden SD, Dodge LD, Bohlman HH, Rechtine GR (1993): Rheumatoid arthritis of the cervical spine. A long-term analysis with predictors of paralysis and recovery. *J Bone Joint Surg* [Am] 75A:1282–1297.
12. Bohler J (1982): An approach to non-union of fractures. *Surg Annu* 14:299–315.
13. Bohlman HH (1979): Acute fractures and dislocations of the cervical spine. An analysis of three hundred hospitalized patients and review of the literature. *J Bone Joint Surg* [Am] 61:1119–1142.
14. Bohlman HH (1985): Surgical management of cervical spine fractures and dislocations. *Instr Course Lect* 34:163–187.
15. Bohlman HH (1986): Complications of treatment of fractures and dislocations of the cervical spine. In: Epps CH Jr, ed. *Complications in orthopaedic surgery*, 2nd ed. Philadelphia: J.B. Lippincott, pp. 897–918.
16. Bohlman HH, Anderson PA (1992): Anterior decompression and arthrodesis of the cervical spine: Long-term motor improvement. Part 1—Improvement in incomplete traumatic quadriparesis. *J Bone Joint Surg* [Am] 74A:671–682.
17. Bohlman HH, Bahniuk E, Raskulinecz G, Field G (1979): Mechanical factors affecting recovery from incomplete cervical spinal cord injury: A preliminary report. *Johns Hopkins Med J* 145:115–125.
18. Bondurant JF, Cotler HB, Kulkarni MV, McArdle CB, Harris JH Jr (1990): Acute spinal cord injury. A study using physical examination and magnetic resonance imaging. *Spine* 15:161–168.
19. Bosley TM, Cohen DA, Schatz NJ, Zimmerman RA, Bilaniuk LT, Savino PJ, Sergott RS (1985): Comparison of metrizamide computed tomography and magnetic resonance imaging in the evaluation of lesions at the cervicomedullary junction. *Neurology* 35:485–492.
20. Bradway JK, Kavanagh BF, Houser OW (1986): Post-traumatic spinal cord cyst: A case report. *J Bone Joint Surg* [Am] 68A:932–933.
21. Bremer AM, Nguyen TQ (1983): Internal metal plate fixation combined with anterior interbody fusion in cases of cervical spine injury. *Neurosurgery* 12:649–653.
22. Brodsky AE, Khalil MA, Sassard WR, Newman BP (1992): Repair of symptomatic pseudarthrosis of anterior cervical fusion. *Spine* 17:1137–1143.
23. Broom MJ, Raycroft JF (1988): Complications of fractures of the cervical spine in ankylosing spondylitis. *Spine* 13:763–766.
24. Bucci MN, Dauser RC, Maynard FA, Hoff JT (1988): Management of post-traumatic cervical spine instability: Operative fusion versus halo vest immobilization. Analysis of 49 cases. *J Trauma* 28:1001–1006.
25. Cartwright MJ, Nehls DG, Carrion CA, Spetzler RF (1985): Synovial cyst of a cervical facet joint: Case report. *Neurosurgery* 16:850–852.
26. Chang DG, Tencer AF, Ching RP, Treece B, Senft D, Anderson PA (1994): Geometric changes in the cervical spinal canal during impact. *Spine* 19:973–980.
27. Clark CR, Keggi KJ, Panjabi MM (1984): Methylmethacrylate stabilization of the cervical spine. *J Bone Joint Surg* [Am] 66A:40–46.
28. Cybulski GR, Douglas RA, Meyer PR Jr, Rovin RA (1992): Complications in three-column cervical spine injuries requiring anterior-posterior stabilization. *Spine* 17:253–256.
29. Cybulski GR, Stone JL, Crowell RM, Rifai MH, Gandhi Y, Glick R (1988): Use of Halifax interlaminar clamps for posterior C1-C2 arthrodesis. *Neurosurgery* 22:429–431.
30. Day GL, Jacoby CG, Dolan KD (1979): Basilar invagination resulting from untreated Jefferson's fracture. *AJR* 133:529–531.
31. Denis F (1983): The three column spine and its significance in the classification of acute thoracolumbar spinal injuries. *Spine* 8:813–831.
32. Denis F (1984): Spinal instability as defined by the three-column spine concept in acute spinal trauma. *Clin Orthop* 189:65–76.
33. Domenella G, Berlanda P, Bassi G (1982): Posterior-approach osteosynthesis of the lower cervical spine by the Roy-Camille technique: Indications and first results. *Ital J Orthop Traumatol* 8:235–244.
34. Eismont FJ, Arena MJ, Green BA (1991): Extrusion of an inter-

vertebral disc associated with traumatic subluxation or dislocation of cervical facets. Case report. *J Bone Joint Surg* [Am] 73:1555–1560.

35. Eismont FJ, Clifford S, Goldberg M, Green B (1984): Cervical sagittal spinal canal size in spine injury. *Spine* 9:663–666.

36. Ersmark H, Kalen R (1987): Injuries of the atlas and axis: A follow-up study of 85 axis and 10 atlas fractures. *Clin Orthop* 217:257–260.

37. Fang HSY, Ong GB (1962): Direct anterior approach to the upper cervical spine. *J Bone Joint Surg* [Am] 44A:1588–1604.

38. Farey ID, McAfee PC, Davis RF, Long DM (1990): Pseudarthrosis of the cervical spine after anterior arthrodesis. Treatment by posterior nerve-root decompression, stabilization, and arthrodesis. *J Bone Joint Surg* [Am] 72A:1171–1177.

39. Fielding JW, Hensinger RN, Hawkins RJ (1980): Os odontoideum. *J Bone Joint Surg* [Am] 62A:376–383.

40. Francis WR, Fielding JW, Hawkins RJ, Pepin J, Hensinger R (1981): Traumatic spondylolisthesis of the axis. *J Bone Joint Surg* [Br] 63B:313–318.

41. Fuji T, Yonenobu K, Fujiwara K, Yamashita K, Ono K, Okada K (1986): Interspinous wiring without bone grafting for nonunion or delayed union following anterior spinal fusion of the cervical spine. *Spine* 11:982–987.

42. Gabriel KR, Crawford AH (1988): Identification of acute posttraumatic spinal cord cysts by magnetic resonance imaging: A case report and review of the literature. *J Pediatr Orthop* 8:710–714.

43. Goddard NJ, Stabler J, Albert JS (1990): Atlanto-axial rotatory fixation and fracture of the clavicle. *J Bone Joint Surg* [Br] 72B:72–75.

44. Henry AK (1957): *Extensile exposure,* 2nd ed. Edinburgh: Churchill Livingstone, pp. 58–72.

45. Hershman EB, Bercik RJ, Allen SC, Fielding JW (1985): Correction of chin-on-chest deformity in ankylosing spondylitis through a fracture site: A case report. *Clin Orthop* 201:201–204.

46. Honnart F, Patel A, Fumo P (1982): Fractures of cervical spine with neurological lesion treated by reduction and fixation with plates. *Ann Acad Med Singapore* 11:186–193.

47. Hukuda S, Ota H, Okabe N, Tazima K (1980): Traumatic atlanto-axial dislocation causing os odontoideum in infants. *Spine* 5:207–210.

48. Johnson JL, Cannon D (1982): Nonoperative treatment of the acute tear-drop fracture of the cervical spine. *Clin Orthop* 168:108–112.

49. Jourdan P, Pharaboz C, Ducolombier A, Pemod P, Desgeorges M (1987): Early syringomyelia following benign cervical injury: Contribution of postoperative MRI. *Neurochirurgie* 33:57–61.

50. Kahanovitz N, Mehringer MC, Johanson PH (1981): Intracranial entrapment of the atlas complicating an untreated fracture of the posterior arch of the atlas: A case report. *J Bone Joint Surg* [Am] 63A:831–832.

51. Kobori M, Takahashi H, Mikawa Y (1986): Atlanto-axial dislocation in Down's syndrome: Report of two cases requiring surgical correction. *Spine* 11:195–200.

52. Krespi YP, Grossman BG, Berktold RE, Sisson GA (1985): Mediastinitis and neck abscess following cervical spinal fracture. *Am J Otolaryngol* 6:29–31.

53. Levine AM, Edwards CC (1985): The management of traumatic spondylolisthesis of the axis. *J Bone Joint Surg* [Am] 67A:217–226.

54. Levine AM, Edwards CC (1986): Complications in the treatment of acute spinal injury. *Orthop Clin North Am* 17:183–203.

55. Louis R (1992): Anterior surgery of the upper cervical spine. *Chir Organi Mov* 77:75–80.

56. Maiman DJ, Barolat G, Larson SJ (1986): Management of bilateral locked facets of the cervical spine. *Neurosurgery* 18:542–547.

57. McAfee PC, Bohlman HH, Ducker T, Eismont FJ (1986): Failure of stabilization of the spine with methylmethacrylate. A retrospective analysis of twenty-four cases. *J Bone Joint Surg* [Am] 68A:1145–1157.

58. McAfee PC, Bohlman HH, Han JS, Salvagno RT (1986): Comparison of nuclear magnetic resonance imaging and computed tomog-

raphy in the diagnosis of upper cervical spinal cord compression. *Spine* 11:295–304.

59. McAfee PC, Bohlman HH, Riley LH, Robinson RA, Southwick WO, Nachlas NE (1987): The anterior retropharyngeal approach to the upper part of the cervical spine. *J Bone Joint Surg* [Am] 69A:1371–1383.

60. Probst C, Karli HU (1989): Traumatic dislocations/dislocation fractures of the cervical spine. Neurosurgical experiences in 42 surgical patients. *Aktuel Traumatol* 19:47–56.

61. Raco A, Di-Lorenzo N, Delfini R, Ciappetta P, Cantore G (1993): The acrylic-wire option in cervical spine fixation. A retrospective study. *Acta Neurochir* 120:53–58.

62. Reiss SJ, Raque GH Jr, Shields CB, Garretson HD (1986): Cervical spine fractures with major associated trauma. *Neurosurgery* 18:327–330.

63. Rifkinson-Mann S, Mormino J, Sachdev VP (1986): Subacute cervical spine instability. *Spine Neurol* 26:413–416.

64. Roy-Camille R, Saillant G, Mazel C (1989): Internal fixation of the unstable cervical spine by a posterior osteosynthesis with plates and screws. In: Sherk HH, ed. *The Cervical Spine Research Society: The cervical spine,* 2nd ed. Philadelphia: J.B. Lippincott, pp. 390–403.

65. Sakou T, Morizono Y, Morimoto N (1984): Transoral atlantoaxial anterior decompression and fusion. *Clin Orthop* 187:134–138.

66. Schweighofer F, Ranner G, Passler JM, Wildburger R, Hofer HP (1992): The value of magnetic resonance tomography in diagnosis and follow-up of cervical spine injuries. *Unfallchirurgie* 95:599–602.

67. Smith MD, Anderson P, Grady MS (1993): Occipitocervical arthrodesis using contoured plate fixation. An early report on a versatile fixation technique. *Spine* 18:1984–1990.

68. Smith MD, Phillips WA, Hensinger RN (1991): Fusion of the upper cervical spine in children and adolescents. An analysis of 17 patients. *Spine* 16:695–701.

69. Sutterlin CE III, McAfee PC, Warden KE, Rey RM Jr, Farey ID (1988): A biomechanical evaluation of cervical spinal stabilization methods in a bovine model: Static and cyclical loading. *Spine* 13:795–802.

70. Tamura T (1989): Cranial symptoms after cervical injury. *J Bone Joint Surg* [Br] 71B:283–287.

71. Tomaszek DE, Rosner MJ (1984): Occult esophageal perforation associated with cervical spine fracture. *Neurosurgery* 14:492–494.

72. Wainapel SF (1984): Reflex sympathetic dystrophy following traumatic myelopathy. *Pain* 18:345–349.

73. Wertheim SB, Bohlman HH (1987): Occipitocervical fusion. Indications, technique, and long-term results in thirteen patients. *J Bone Joint Surg* [Am] 69A:833–836.

74. White AA III, Johnson RM, Panjabi MM, Southwick WO (1975): Biomechanical analysis of clinical stability in the cervical spine. *Clin Orthop* 109:85–96.

75. White AA, Jupiter J, Southwick WO, Panjabi MM (1973): An experimental study of the immediate load bearing capacity of three surgical constructions for anterior spine fusions. *Clin Orthop* 91:21–28.

76. White AA III, Panjabi MM (1990): The problem of clinical instability in the human spine: A systematic approach. In: White AA III et al., eds. *Clinical biomechanics of the spine,* 2nd ed. Philadelphia: JB Lippincott, pp. 277–378.

77. Whitehill R, Richman JA, Glaser JA (1986): Failure of immobilization of the cervical spine by the halo vest. A report of five cases. *J Bone Joint Surg* [Am] 68A:326–332.

78. Whitehill R, Stowers SF, Fechner RE, Ruch WW, Drucker S, Gibson LR, McKeman DJ, Widmeyer JH (1987): Posterior cervical fusions using cerclage wires, methylmethacrylate cement and autogenous bone graft. An experimental study of a canine model. *Spine* 12:12–22.

79. Yablon IG, Cowan S, Mortara R (1993): The migration of a Harrington rod after cervical fusion. *Spine* 18:356–358.

80. Zdeblick TA, Bohlman HH (1989): Cervical kyphosis and myelopathy: Treatment by anterior corpectomy and strut-grafting. *J Bone Joint Surg* [Am] 71A:170–182.

The Adult Spine: Principles and Practice,
2nd edition, J.W. Frymoyer, Editor-in-Chief.
Lippincott-Raven Publishers, Philadelphia © 1997.

CHAPTER 62

Posttraumatic Syringomyelia

Thomas A. Zdeblick and Thomas B. Ducker

Improvement in emergency medical services as well as increased awareness of spine injuries in the trauma patient have led to an increase in the survival of the patient with an injured spinal cord. Neurologic deficit is primarily a result of the initial traumatic event. Neurologic worsening in the acute phase after injury, has been thought to be due to either spinal cord edema or hemorrhage. However, untoward management events may also play a role in acute worsening (21).

Increasing neurologic deficit in the chronic phase following spinal cord injury may also occur. Spine instability with progressive deformity may lead to increasing neurologic deficit. However, the most common cause of delayed neurologic loss, such as late ascending neurologic loss, is the development of a posttraumatic syringomyelia.

OVERVIEW

Syringomyelia was first described in 1827 by Ollivier, who felt that the spinal cord was distended by fluid from within (42). In 1871, Hallopeau described a cystic lesion of the spinal cord at autopsy in a patient who had suffered a spinal cord injury (12). In 1915, Holmes noted oval or cylindrical cavities in spinal cord specimens from patients with spinal gunshots wounds (13). It was Free-

man in 1953 who was the first to equate "ascending spinal paralysis" in the posttraumatic patient with syringomyelia (8).

The development of a progressive neurologic deficit extending to previously uninvolved segments months or years after a spinal cord injury, and due to a syrinx, is uncommon. The incidence of posttraumatic syringomyelia has been estimated to be between 0.3% and 2.3% of spinal cord injuries (29,41). In a large series, Barnett found that 1.8% of spinal cord–injured patients developed a symptomatic syrinx, compared to the incidence of idiopathic syringomyelia of 0.01% (4). Rossier et al. noted an overall incidence of 3.2% in 951 patients with spinal cord injury. With complete tetraplegia, 8% developed syringomyelia (28). Most authors state that thoracic and lumbar lesions are more common than cervical lesions (10,42). As we use MRI more and more, the true incidence of this problem is probably higher than previously stated.

SYMPTOMS

The presentation of a posttraumatic syrinx may be quite subtle. The classic sign is the presence of severe pain unrelieved by analgesics, an ascending disassociated sensory loss, or progression of an incomplete lesion. Pain is the most commonly reported symptom, and numerous authors have stressed the importance of pain that increases with coughing, straining, or sneezing (17,31, 33,36,37). Occasionally, radicular pain is present, although axial pain is more common. Dissociate sensory loss describes a state in which the patient has objective loss of sensation to pain and temperature but preserva-

T. A. Zdeblick, M.D.: Associate Professor, Division of Orthopaedic Surgery, University of Wisconsin Hospital, Madison, Wisconsin 53792.

T. B. Ducker, M.D.: Professor, Department of Neurological Surgery, The Johns Hopkins University School of Medicine, Baltimore, Maryland 21205.

tion of touch sensation (5,17,33). This sensory loss may increase distal to the injury or, more commonly, ascend to previously unimpaired levels.

Signs of muscle wasting or lower extremity spasticity are also found, although less commonly. In incomplete lesions, progression of the motor paralysis may occur. In thoracic or lumbar level injuries, signs of cranial nerve involvement may occur rarely with syringomyelia (36). In cervical level injuries that develop a syrinx, up to 25% will have bulbar signs (33). A much less common finding, and quite rare at presentation, is the presence of a neuropathic joint (16,26). Charcot joints, particularly of the upper extremity, may result from syringomyelia. Rarely, an increase in urinary dysfunction may herald the onset of a syrinx (34).

The onset of symptoms from a posttraumatic syrinx is often quite delayed from the time of injury. Delays from 6 months to 16 years have been reported (4,21,31). Typically, a syrinx will develop several years after the injury. Several studies have shown that syringomyelia presents earlier in patients with complete spinal cord lesions than in those with incomplete lesions. Lyons et al. (20) and Barnett et al. (4) demonstrated an average delay of approximately 4 years in patients with complete lesions, compared to 9 years in patients with incomplete spinal cord injury.

PATHOPHYSIOLOGY

The pathophysiology of posttraumatic syringomyelia is not completely understood. The etiology of spinal cord cavitation is probably multifactorial. Most syrinxes form in the gray matter between the dorsal horns and the posterior columns (41). Autopsy examination has shown that the cavity forms in the partially damaged level of the cord, adjacent to an area of complete injury (7). Williams et al. feel that the intramedullary hematoma, which forms at the time of injury, liquefies (41). This eventually leads to a cystic degeneration within the cord. Kao et al. favor the theory that trauma leads to neural disruption and the formation of myelin microcysts (14). These microcysts then coalesce into an intramedullary cavity. Other possible causes for syrinx formation include vascular lesions remote from the injury, micro-infarcts, and arachnoiditis causing local scarring and cord tethering (35).

The mechanisms for extension of the cavity are better understood. The "slosh" mechanism of Williams et al. states that the hydrodynamic dissection of the spinal cord is caused by rapid movement of fluid within the cavity in response to pressure changes in the subarachnoid cerebrospinal fluid (CSF) space (42). This compression of the CSF space may result from pressure changes in the epidural venous plexus or direct changes due to coughing, sneezing, or straining. Syrinx fluid may accumulate due to continued cord necrosis, transudation of proteinaceous fluid, direct passage of fluid via diffusion through the cord, or "sucking" of fluid through the cisternae during pressure changes (9).

DIAGNOSIS

Confirmation of a syrinx by radiologic means is currently undergoing change. In the past, demonstration of an enlarged cord at the level of injury by air or Pantopaque contrast myelography was considered presumptive evidence of a syrinx. Water-soluble myelography increased the visualization of the cord, and delayed-contrast computed tomography (CT) scanning further refined the definition of the syrinx (10,25,33). Contrasted CT is particularly helpful in following the postoperative course of a syrinx. Endomyelography, in which water-soluble dye is injected within the cavity itself, is quite good at outlining the extent of a syrinx (33). This technique, however, may miss the multicentric cord cavitation.

Rarely, nonradiologic means are helpful in delineating a syrinx. Radioisotope ventriculography has been found to be useful (11). Electrodiagnostic studies will demonstrate normal nerve conduction velocities. Electromyography shows an increase in polyphasic spikes with an increase in motor unit action potential duration (5). Percutaneous ultrasound has not proven effective in the initial diagnosis of a syrinx. However, some believe that intraoperative ultrasound is beneficial in delineating the exact location of the syrinx, while others have felt that postlaminectomy, postdrainage ultrasound is helpful in following syrinx size (2,22).

The best current method to diagnose posttraumatic syringomyelia is magnetic resonance imaging (MRI). This test is noninvasive and provides excellent visualization of the spinal cord and the craniovertebral junction. It has been shown to be as accurate as contrasted CT scanning in making the diagnosis (15,24). The low density intramedullary signal on T1 imaging, or a bright signal on T2 imaging, is evidence of a syrinx. MRI, however, has some drawbacks. In patients with spinal instrumentation, it is technically less helpful. False positives have been seen with MRI scanning: the low density signal of myelomalacia is indistinguishable from that of an intramedullary cyst (24). The use of gadolinium contrast enhances the ability of MRI to delineate small tumors from cystic cavities (18,23,27,38,40). Examples of posttraumatic syrinx are shown in Chapter 34 and in Figure 1.

TREATMENT

The treatment of posttraumatic syrinx should be surgical. The natural history of an untreated syrinx is progressive. Vernon et al. followed 40 symptomatic patients

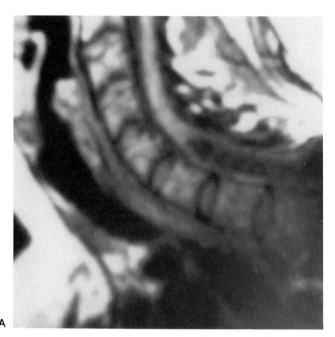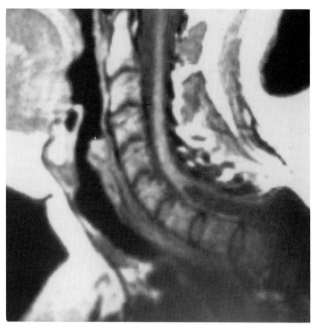

A

B

FIG. 1. A,B: Eight years after having a high thoracic fracture, the patient developed a progressive syrinx going up into the spinal cord, causing numbness and weakness in the hands.

non-operatively and found that all progressed and demonstrated an increase in severity and an ascending level of pain and sensory loss (37). Rarely, spontaneous collapse of a syrinx has been reported.

In 1892, Abbe and Coley first demonstrated the feasibility of syringostomy performed at autopsy (1). Freeman and Wright, in a series of experiments with cats and dogs, found that spinal cord trauma led to intramedullary cavities, and they proceeded to drain these cavities (8). In 1959, Freeman performed the first syringostomy in humans (31). Other early surgeons treated syringomyelia in patients with complete lesion by cord transection, allowing drainage of the syrinx. However, in both simple syringostomy and cord transection, the problem of resealing the opening leading to recurrent syrinx occurred (17,31). Percutaneous drainage has been attempted but has not led to long-term success (19).

Shunting procedures have the benefit of being minimally invasive and of keeping an open channel for decompression of the cavity. Both syringoperitoneal (SP) shunts and syringosubarachnoid shunts have been popularized (3,32,33). Suzuki et al. demonstrated that 22 of 29 patients treated with an SP shunt improved (32). Tator and Briceno felt that SP shunting led to a higher complication rate and treated 40 patients with syringosubarachnoid shunting (33). They had good to excellent results in 29 of 40 patients, with 10 of the 14 posttraumatic patients making an excellent recovery. Vernon et al. demonstrated that pain or motor recovery can be expected in about 50% of patients treated with shunting, that sensory symptoms improve in 33%, and that the

procedure failed to halt the progression of symptoms in 10% of patients (37). Pillay et al. noted that 3 of 6 patients with posttraumatic syrinx benefit from SP shunting (23).

The procedure of choice is either the syringosubarachnoid shunt or the syringopleural shunt. When possible, the operation is performed with somatosensory evoked potential monitoring to assess cord function during surgery. Following laminectomy and durotomy, intraoperative ultrasonography is often helpful in locating the cystic cavity. A posterior midline myelotomy is then performed and, in most cases, the scarring should be dissected so that the spinal cord lies relaxed and one is confident that good CSF flow is possible. The operating microscope is helpful in taking down arachnoid adhesions. Some surgeons first perform needle aspiration for localization. A small Silastic catheter is then placed in the cavity, extended to the subarachnoid or pleural space, and sewn to the dura. Others prefer to have the catheter enter at the dorsal root entry zone. The dura is then closed. Postoperative monitoring of the syrinx is then performed by physical exam, MRI, or contrasted CT scan.

CONCLUSION

The occurrence of posttraumatic syringomyelia is rare and its diagnosis may be difficult. However, once found. surgical treatment can lead to improvement in the majority of cases. Dissecting adjacent scar to promote normal CSF dynamics locally, and drainage of the cyst (syrinx) to reduce an abnormal intramedullary pressure, constitute the two goals of operative care.

REFERENCES

1. Abbe R, Coley WB (1892): Syringomyelia, operation, exploration of cord; withdrawal of fluid. Exhibition of patient. *J Nerv Ment Dis* 9:512–520.
2. Aschoff A, Albert F, Mende U, St. Kunze: Intra-operative sonography in syringomyelia—technique, results, limitation. In: Donauer E. *100 years of syrinx surgery,* 176–177.
3. Barbaro MN, Wilson CB, Gutin PH, Edwards MS (1984): Surgical treatment of syringomyelia. Favorable results with syringoperitoneal shunting. *J Neurosurg* 61:531–538.
4. Barnett HJ, Jousse AT, Morley TP, Lougheed WM (1971): Post-traumatic syringomyelia. *Paraplegia* 9:33–37.
5. Benedetto MD, Rossier AB (1977): Electrodiagnosis in post-traumatic syringomyelia. *Paraplegia* 14:286–295.
6. Birbamer G, Buchberger W, Felber S, Posch A, Russegger L (1993): Spontaneous collapse of post-traumatic syringomyelia: serial magnetic resonance imaging. *Eur Neurol* 33:378–381.
7. Foo D, Bignami A, Rossier AB (1989): A case of post-traumatic syringomyelia. Neuropathological findings after one year of cystic drainage. *Paraplegia* 27:63–69.
8. Freeman LW, Wright TW (1953): Experimental observations of concussion and contusion of the spinal cord. *Ann Surg* 137:433–443.
9. Gardner WJ (1965): Hydrodynamic mechanism of syringomyelia: its relationship to myelocele. *J Neurol Psychiatry* 28:247–259.
10. Griffiths ER, McCormick CC (1981): Post-traumatic syringomyelia (cystic myelopathy). *Paraplegia* 19:81–88.
11. Hall PV, Kalsbeck E, Wellman HN, Campbell RL, Lewis S (1976): Radioisotope evaluation of experimental hydrosyringomyelia. *J Neurosurg* 45:181–187.
12. Hallopeau FM (1871): Sur une faite de sclerose diffuse de la substance grise et strophie musculaire. *Gaz Med de Paris* 25:183.
13. Holmes G (1915): The Goulstonian lectures on spinal injuries of warfare. *Br Med J* 2:769–774.
14. Kao CC, Chang LW, Bloodworth JM Jr (1977): The mechanism of spinal cord cavitation following spinal cord transaction. *J Neurosurg* 46:745–756.
15. Kokmen E, Marsh WR, Baker HL (1985): Magnetic resonance imaging in syringomyelia. *Neurosurgery* 17:267–270.
16. Kolawole T, Banna M, Hawass N, Khan F, Rahman N (1987): Neuropathic arthropathy as a complication of post-traumatic syringomyelia. *Br J Radiol* 60:702–704.
17. Laha RK, Malik HG, Langille RA (1975): Post-traumatic syringomyelia. *Surg Neurol* 4:519–522.
18. Lee BC, Zimmerman RD, Manning JJ, Deck MDF (1985): MR imaging of syringomyelia and hydromyelia. *Am J Radiol* 144:1149–1156.
19. Levy R, Rosenblatt S, Russell E (1991): Percutaneous drainage and serial magnetic resonance imaging in the diagnosis of symptomatic post-traumatic syringomyelia: a case report and review of the literature. *Neurosurgery* 29(3):429–434.
20. Lyons BM, Brown DJ, Calvert JM, Woodward JM, Wriedt CHR (1987): The diagnosis and management of post-traumatic syringomyelia. *Paraplegia* 25:340–350.
21. Marshall LF, Knowlton S, Garfin SR, et al. (1987): Deterioration following spinal cord injury: a multicenter study. *J Neurosurg* 66:400–404.
22. Mende U, Aschoff A, Wannenmacher M: Technique and limitations of percutaneous sonography in the evaluation of the contents of the spinal canal. In: Donnauer E. *100 years of syrinx surgery,* 172–173.
23. Pillay PK, Awad LA, Little JR, Hahn JF (1988): Surgical management of syringomyelia: a five year experience in the era of magnetic resonance imaging. *Acta Neuro* 43:13–16.
24. Pojunas & Williams AL, Daniels DI, Haughton VM (1984): Syringomyelia and hydromyelia: magnetic resonance evaluation. *Radiology* 153:679–683.
25. Quencer RM, Green BA, Eismont FJ (1983): Post-traumatic spinal cord cysts: clinical features and characterization with metrizamide computed tomography. *Radiology* 146:415–423.
26. Rhoades CE, Neff JR, Renagachary SS, et al. (1983): Diagnosis of post-traumatic syringohydromyelia presenting as neuropathic joints: report of two cases and review of the literature. *Clin Orthop* 180:182–187.
27. Roosen N, Dahlhaus P, Lumenta CB, Lins E, Stork W, Gahlen D, Bock WJ (1988): Magnetic resonance (MR) imaging in the management of primary and secondary syringomyelic cavities and of other cystic lesions of the spinal cord. *Acta Neurol [Scand]* 43:13–16.
28. Rossier AB, Foo D, Shillito J, Dyro FM (1985): Post-traumatic cervical syringomyelia. *Brain* 108:439–461.
29. Rossier AB, Foo D, Shillito J, et al. (1981): Progressive late post-traumatic syringomyelia. *Paraplegia* 19:96–97.
30. Santoro A, Delfini R, Innocenzi G, Di Biasi C, Trasimeni G, Gualdi G (1993): Spontaneous drainage of syringomyelia. *J Neurosurg* 79:132–134.
31. Shannon N, Symon L, Logue V, Cull D, Kang J, Kendall B (1981): Clinical features, investigation and treatment of post-traumatic syringomyelia. *J Neurol Neurosurg Psychiatry* 44:35.
32. Suzuki M, Davis C, Symon L, Gentili F (1985): Syringoperitoneal shunt for treatment of cord cavitation. *J Neurol Neurosurg Psychiatry* 48:620–627.
33. Tator CH, Briceno C (1988): Treatment of syringomyelia with a syringosubarachnoid shunt. *Can J Neurol Sci* 15:48–57.
34. Umbach I, Heilporn A (1988): Evolution of post-traumatic cervical syringomyelia: case report. *Paraplegia* 25:56–61.
35. Umbach I, Heilporn A (1991): Review article: post-spinal cord injury syringomyelia. *Paraplegia* 29:219–221.
36. Vernon JD, Silver JR, Ohry A (1982): Post-traumatic syringomyelia. *Paraplegia* 20:339–364.
37. Vernon JD, Silver JR, Symon L (1983): Post-traumatic syringomyelia: the results of surgery. *Paraplegia* 21:37–46.
38. Williams AL, Haughton VM, Pojunas KW, Daniels DL, Kilgore DP (1987): Differentiation of intramedullary neoplasms and cysts by MR. *Am J Radiol* 149:159–164.
39. Williams B (1990): Post-traumatic syringomyelia, an update. *Paraplegia* 28:296–313.
40. Williams B (1990): Syringomyelia. *Neurosurg Clin N Am* 1(3):653–685.
41. Williams B, Terry AF, Jones F, McSweeney T (1981): Syringomyelia as a sequel to traumatic paraplegia. *Paraplegia* 19:67–80.
42. Williams B, Weller RO (1973): Syringomyelia produced by intramedullary fluid injection in dogs. *J Neurol Neurosurg Psychiatry* 36:467–477.

Degenerative Conditions
of the Cervical Spine

The Adult Spine: Principles and Practice,
2nd edition, J.W. Frymoyer, Editor-in-Chief.
Lippincott-Raven Publishers, Philadelphia © 1997.

CHAPTER 63

Differential Diagnosis and Nonoperative Management

Charles R. Clark

Degenerative conditions of the cervical spine are common. In a survey of 10,000 adults in Norway, 34% of respondents complained of neck pain within the past year and approximately 14% complained of neck pain lasting greater than 6 months (17). Schmorl and Junghann (155) reported that 90% of males older than age 50 and 90% of females over 60 had radiographic evidence of degeneration. Chronic cervical degeneration is the most common cause of progressive spinal cord and nerve root deterioration (37). *Cervical spondylosis* is the term used to describe degeneration of the cervical spine. It is a generalized disease process that initiates in the intervertebral disc. It involves degenerative changes in the disc, osteophytosis of the vertebral bodies, hypertrophy of the facets and laminar arches, and ligamentous and segmental instability (104). Normal aging contributes to the pathophysiologic changes (35). The condition progresses with age and often develops at multiple interspaces (91). Because the natural history of cervical spondylosis is associated with the aging process, senescent and pathologic

processes may be morphologically indistinguishable (104). Cervical spondylitic myelopathy is the most serious consequence of cervical intervertebral disc degeneration, especially when associated with a narrow cervical vertebral canal (107).

This chapter focuses on cervical spondylosis, including spondylitic radiculopathy as well as spondylitic myelopathy. It is important to differentiate between these conditions. Many authors in the past have failed to do so, which may affect the interpretation of their findings. In addition to describing the clinical diagnosis of cervical spondylosis, this chapter highlights the differential diagnosis of degenerative conditions. This encompasses intrinsic cervical conditions including inflammatory, neoplastic, infectious, and miscellaneous afflictions, as well as extrinsic disorders affecting the upper extremity, which often pose problems in differential diagnosis. The last section of this chapter deals with principles of treatment. Although nonoperative approaches will be the main emphasis, operative management is discussed briefly to put it in its proper perspective in the overall management of patients with cervical degenerative disease.

C. R. Clark, M.D.: Professor, Orthopaedic Surgery, University of Iowa College of Medicine, Iowa City, Iowa, 52242.

CERVICAL SPONDYLOSIS

Cervical spondylosis can be divided into three primary groups of clinical manifestations. The first group of patients present primarily with neck pain without a true radicular or myelopathic component. These patients complain of intrinsic neck pain as well as pain that is referred locally. Internal disc derangement is included in this group. The second group of patients includes those who have radicular complaints, that is, signs and symptoms primarily in the distribution of a nerve root. Multiple nerve roots may be involved. The last group of patients are those with myelopathy secondary to spondylosis. Patients may have combinations of these three types of involvement or may progress from intrinsic neck pain to radiculopathy and then on to frank myelopathy. Progression may be insidious and not readily apparent to the patient or examiner.

The introduction notes the importance of differentiating cervical spondylitic radiculopathy from myelopathy. This is important not only in the clinical management of patients, but also when reviewing the medical literature. In general, the results of management of cervical spondylitic radiculopathy tend to be more favorable than those described for the treatment of myelopathy. If this distinction is not made and all patients are grouped together, the operative outcome may be biased, with the inclusion of a large group of one of these two types of patients. In addition to these two conditions, it is important to differentiate cervical spondylosis from intrinsic degeneration of the central nervous system (37). Epstein et al. (53) have pointed out the importance of recognizing patients with motor neuron disease, particularly amyotrophic lateral sclerosis (ALS), as well as multiple sclerosis (MS). Indeed, such intrinsic conditions may coexist with cervical spondylosis.

An understanding of the natural history of cervical spondylosis helps to put treatment into its proper perspective. Gore et al. (66) reported a 10-year follow-up of patients with neck pain. They found that after this interval, 79% of patients had a decrease in their neck pain and 43% of patients actually had no pain. Thirty-two percent, however, had residual moderate or severe pain. The authors concluded that patients with the most severe involvement appeared not to have improved. They also found that a large number of patients did not respond to nonoperative treatment. Patients presenting with neck pain alone should be approached with reluctance regarding operative intervention, as intermittent flare-ups with subsidence and ultimate overall improvement can be expected in most cases (86).

Myelopathy may result from cervical spondylosis (183) and is the most serious consequence of intervertebral disc degeneration (107). Spondylitic myelopathy is the most common cervical cord disorder during and af-

ter middle age (38). Patients with this myelopathy often have very long periods without the development of new or worsening signs or symptoms.

The early operative results for the treatment of cervical spondylitic myelopathy described by Northfield (129) and Campbell and Phillips did not notably differ from the natural history of the condition, and therefore Lees and Turner (102) concluded that nonoperative management should be the rule. The natural history of 114 patients treated nonoperatively revealed that 36% actually improved, whereas 64% showed no increase in symptoms and only 26% of patients worsened. Therefore, there is some evidence to justify a nonoperative approach to this group of patients (18,102,131,150). Operative management may be particularly effective in selected patients, and this will be discussed later; however, the natural history of this condition is a prerequisite for developing a rational plan for treatment.

Crandall and Batzdorf (37) described five categories of cervical spondylitic myelopathy based on the predominant neurologic findings (in order of decreasing frequency):

1. Transverse lesion syndrome (corticospinal and spinothalamic tracts and posterior columns are involved).
2. Motor syndrome (primarily corticospinal or anterior horn cell involvement).
3. Central cord syndrome (motor and sensory involvement of the upper extremities greater than the lower extremities).
4. Brown-Sequard syndrome (unilateral cord lesion with ipsilateral corticospinal tract involvement and contralateral anesthesia below the level of the lesion).
5. Brachialgia and cord syndrome (predominant upper limb pain and some associated long tract involvement).

This classification has been described in many subsequent papers and appears to be clinically useful, particularly when comparing the results of various treatment modalities.

Pathophysiology

The pathophysiology of cervical spondylosis is multifactorial, including anatomic, genetic, biomechanical, and electrophysiologic factors. Anatomic factors include the blood supply (with the potential for ischemia) and the bony architecture (with the potential for compression). The blood supply of the spinal cord per se as well as the dimensions of the spinal canal are additional important anatomic factors. Parke (136) described in detail the blood supply of the spinal cord, which consists of three major longitudinal arteries: a large ventral (anterior) spinal artery and two dorsolateral arteries that are fed by medullary vessels of segmental origin. The location of the anterior spinal artery makes it vulnerable to direct compression by osteophytes and degenerative disc material. In addition, medullary feeder vessels may be compressed as they traverse along the neuroforamina to the midventral surface of the cord (30,136).

A study involving matched lateral cervical spine radiographs of 23 pairs of twins showed that the degenerative changes in the cervical spines of twins follow a very similar pattern. The suggestion was made that the shape of the individual vertebrae is of considerable importance in the development of the changes that are found with aging, and that this similarity in shape explains the familial pattern of spondylosis (134).

Canal size must also be considered. Narrowing of the spinal canal may either be congenital/developmental or acquired. The former groups include such conditions as Klippel-Feil syndrome, achondroplasia, spinal bifida, spondylolisthesis, isolated congenital anomalies, and congenital narrowing (15,24,176). Acquired conditions include degenerative disease (cervical spondylosis), rheumatoid arthritis, ankylosing spondylitis, inflammation, and tumors (15). Congenitally narrow canals per se are usually asymptomatic; however, the spinal cord may be more vulnerable to additional encroachment (176). Further compromise may occur from protrusion of disc material, subluxation of the vertebra (139), buckling of the ligamentum flavum, and development of osteophytes (7,30). Compression of the cord and interference with the blood supply and subsequent ischemia may result.

Several parameters have been used to describe canal size. These include the sagittal diameter of the canal as well as the cross-sectional area. The developmental sagittal diameter of the cord is measured at the midlevel of the vertebral body and represents the baseline midsagittal size of the canal before degenerative change. The spondylitic sagittal diameter is measured at the level of the intervertebral disc. This latter measurement takes into consideration the effects of osteophytes (50). Measurements involving ratios have been developed that are useful because they eliminate the effect of image magnification present on plain radiographs. Pavlov's ratio compares the relationship between the sagittal diameter of the spinal canal to the vertebral body (169). Plain radiographs are typically used to determine canal size, and measurements are discussed further in the section on clinical diagnosis. Computed tomography (CT) scan is useful to quantitate the cross-sectional area of the spinal canal as well as the spinal cord. Magnetic resonance imaging (MRI) provides perhaps the best appraisal of canal size because in addition to determining the area, it details characteristics of the spinal cord as well as the degree of encroachment of anterior and posterior defects on the subarachnoid spine and neural structures (116). Batzdorf and Batzdorff (8) felt that spinal curvature is an addi-

tional important anatomic factor. However, they found no clear correlation between the severity of myelopathy and the degree of sagittal curvature. Severe myelopathy was present in patients with straight, lordotic, as well as hyperlordotic spines; however, neck pain was most severe in patients with reversed cervical curvature, and the degree of curvature seemed to correlate with postoperative results. Patients with normal curvature showed the greatest improvement in symptomatology after treatment. One should bear in mind that sagittal alignment of the cervical spine is dependent to some degree on contraction of the neck musculature, and straight alignment or reversal of cervical lordosis may occur in patients having cervical muscle strain. The geometry of the spinal canal is an important factor in the selection of patients when operative intervention is considered.

Static and dynamic factors place abnormal stresses and strains on the spinal canal and, potentially, the spinal cord. Panjabi and White described the biomechanics of the spine in cervical spondylitic myelopathy. Static factors include those previously mentioned such as a small canal, osteophytes, disc herniation, hypertrophy of the ligamentum flavum, and apophyseal joint deformation. Dynamic factors include normal and abnormal motion, normal and abnormal loads applied, and the mechanical properties of the spinal cord and spinal column (30,135,180). Good and Mikkelsen (64) identified a correlation between discogenic spondylosis and motion (normal, hypomobility, hypermobility, paradoxic motion) found in the sagittal planes of the intervertebral motion units of the lower cervical spine. Intervertebral motion units that had discogenic spondylosis had a greater likelihood of exhibiting motion abnormalities, and all types of motion seem to be dependent on its severity. Hypomobility became predominant overall as moderate and severe discogenic spondylosis was found (64).

Bohlman and Emery (14) reported that electrophysiologic changes occur in the pathophysiology of this condition. They noted alterations of evoked potentials as the disease progresses. Intrinsic changes occur within the spinal cord. These include blockage of axoplasmic flow, distortion of cord tissue, and stretching of intrinsic transverse terminations of the spinal artery. These authors found tissue destruction with demyelination of white matter in severe cases, and concluded that the pathologic findings appear to correlate with clinical severity (4,30).

Spondylosis may involve the entire vertebral column, but tends to be more pronounced in the cervical and lumbar regions where mobility is greatest. It is important to keep this in mind because patients may have multiple levels of involvement. In a retrospective clinical review of 214 patients treated for symptomatic spinal spondylosis, Edwards and LaRocca (51) found that 28 (13%)

had symptoms relative to both the cervical and lumbar spine. Further, in this group of patients with combined disease of the cervical and lumbar spine, 18 of the 28 (64%) had spinal canal diameters below the accepted average values.

Pain may result from stimulation of the intrinsic nerves in the cervical spine. McLain (121) has demonstrated mechanoreceptors in human cervical facet joints. The presence of mechanoreceptive and nociceptive nerve endings in cervical facet capsules proves that these tissues are monitored by the central nervous system and implies that neural input from the facet is important in proprioception and pain sensation in the cervical spine.

Cervical Spondylitic Radiculopathy

Cervical spondylosis may result in radicular pain (i.e., pain in the distribution of a nerve root). This may be the result of a herniation of nuclear material through the annulus fibrosis (soft disc) (Fig. 1) or encroachment on the neural foramina by osteophytes (hard disc). The most mobile segments of the spine are the most frequently involved levels in cervical degeneration (44). The C5-C6 interspace is the most commonly involved, followed by C6-C7 and C4-C5 (22).

The anteromedial wall of the neuroforamen is formed by the uncovertebral joint, and the posterolateral wall is formed by the apophyseal or facet joint. Osteophytes involving either of these articulations may compress the neuroforamina, resulting in radicular pain. Soft-disc herniation actually is a spectrum of entities ranging from tears of the annulus fibrosis with mild bulging of nuclear material to frank herniation with sequestration. The most common location of a soft-disc herniation is posterolateral; however, herniation may also occur anteriorly or posteriorly (central herniation). Posterior herniations may produce myelopathy and will be discussed later. Anterior herniations may cause extrinsic compression of the esophagus. In addition, anterior osteophytes along the anterior surface of the vertebral bodies may compress the esophagus.

Dysphagia may result from anterior soft- or hard-disc encroachment upon the esophagus (59). Bony protuberances into the hypopharynx or esophagus may be accompanied by soft-tissue inflammation, resulting in increased symptoms (95). Dysphagia due to organic, anatomic narrowing of the gut lumen must be differentiated from muscular or neuromuscular disorders. Typically, such anatomic dysphagia is worse for solid foods than for liquids, and there is no difficulty in expelling food from the pharynx to the hypopharynx (95). The di-

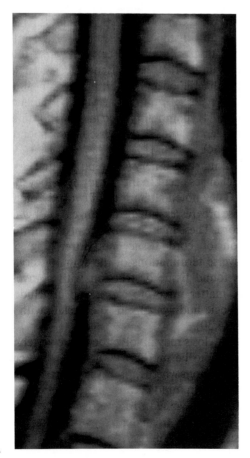

A

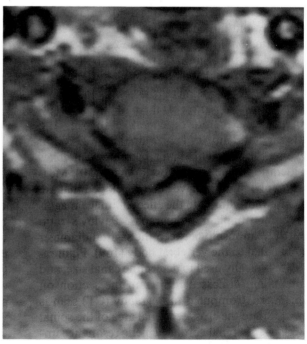

B

FIG. 1. MR images from a 35-year-old patient with an acute soft-disc herniation at C6-C7. **A:** Sagittal image demonstrating the herniation with cord compression. **B:** Transverse image.

agnosis is confirmed by having the patient ingest barium-impregnated solids and obtaining lateral radiographs. Hyperostosis of the cervical spine is common but is only rarely a cause of dysphagia (80). The initial treatment of this condition is conservative, as dysphagia may be magnified by local edema; in some cases, treatment with nonsteroidal anti-inflammatory agents or steroids may be useful. All other conditions causing dysphagia should be excluded before operating on the sespurs (175). Long-term follow-up is necessary to determine the validity of operative excision of osteophytes in the treatment of this condition (80).

Radicular and myelopathic syndromes are produced by nerve root and spinal cord compression, respectively. Intrinsic neck pain is less clearly understood. The patterns of local and referred pain syndromes may be mediated by the synovertebral nerves or the medial branches of the posterior rami (75). Internal disc derangement may produce local and referred symptoms in the neck and is included in this section; typically, however, it does not produce radicular pain. Whitecloud and Seago (182) reported 34 patients who underwent cervical arthrodesis because of a positive discogram. Reproduction of the patient's symptoms at the time of disc space injection was used to determine the involved levels. The authors reported 70% good or excellent results using their technique. They cautioned, however, that the cervical discogram should be considered only after a complete diagnostic work-up including myelography, CT scan, and/or MRI, and following a prolonged period of an unsuccessful nonoperative management. They reported positive operative results in approximately two thirds of patients when the pain pattern is reproduced by the disc space injection and specific guidelines are followed (30,182).

Cervical Spondylitic Myelopathy

Myelopathy may occur secondary to cervical spondylosis, particularly in patients older than 55 years (27). Typical neurologic findings include lower motor neuron and reflex changes at the level of the lesion and upper motor neuron involvement below. The gait abnormality

TABLE 1. *Nurick's classification of disability in spondylitic myelopathy*

Grade 0	Root signs and symptoms No evidence of cord involvement
Grade I	Signs of cord involvement Normal gait
Grade II	Mild gait improvement Able to be employed
Grade III	Gait abnormality prevents employment
Grade IV	Able to ambulate only with assistance
Grade V	Chair bound or bedridden

With permission from ref. 130.

TABLE 2. *The assessment scale proposed by the Japanese Orthopaedic Association*

I. Motor dysfunction of the upper extremity
   Score
   0 = Unable to feed oneself
   1 = Unable to handle chopsticks, able to eat with a spoon
   2 = Handle chopsticks with much difficulty
   3 = Handle chopsticks with slight difficulty
   4 = None
II. Motor dysfunction of the lower extremity
   Score
   0 = Unable to work
   1 = Walk on flat floor with walking aid
   2 = Up and/or down stairs with handrail
   3 = Lack of stability and smooth reciprocation
   4 = None
III. Sensory deficit
   A. The upper extremity
      Score
      0 = Severe sensory loss or pain
      1 = Mild sensory loss
      2 = None
   B. The lower extremity, same as A
   C. The trunk, same as A
IV. Sphincter dysfunction
   Score
   0 = Unable to void
   1 = Marked difficulty in micturition (retention, strangury)
   2 = Difficulty in micturition (pollakiuria, hesitation)
   3 = None

With permission from ref. 78.

is often the most common clinical concern of the patient, and Nurick classified cervical spondylitic myelopathy largely on the basis of gait (Table 1) (130,131,181).

As in cervical spondylosis without myelopathy, myelopathy may coexist with lumbar spinal stenosis. A study by Laroche et al. (99) revealed that 19 patients with cervical and lumbar canal stenosis also had advanced ankylosing spinal hyperostosis.

Patients with early myelopathy may present with a clinical picture mimicking bilateral carpal tunnel syndrome (57). Careful diagnostic evaluation including a detailed neurologic examination with imaging studies should establish the proper diagnosis. Electromyography with nerve conduction velocities may be necessary to exclude carpal tunnel syndrome.

The Japanese Orthopaedic Association (JOA) (78) has devised an objective assessment scale to quantitate the degree of involvement secondary to spondylitic myelopathy. The scale involves four categories: motor dysfunction of the upper extremity, motor dysfunction of the lower extremity, sensory deficit, and sphincter dysfunction (Table 2). The maximum number of points is 17 (normal). Hirabayashi et al. described a formula, based on the JOA score, to assess the recovery rate after operative intervention in patients with myelopathy secondary to ossification of the posterior longitudinal ligament (Table 3) (27,78). This formula has also been used to quan-

TABLE 3. *Recovery rate after surgery*

1. Maximum gain = maximum score − preoperative score
2. Maximum rate of recovery (%) =
$$\frac{\text{maximum score} - \text{preoperative score}}{17 \text{ (full score)} - \text{preoperative score}} \times 100$$
3. Final gain = final score − preoperative score
4. Final rate of recovery (%) =
$$\frac{\text{final score} - \text{preoperative score}}{17 \text{ (full score)} - \text{preoperative score}} \times 100$$

With permission from refs. 27 and 78.

titate recovery in patients with cervical spondylitic myelopathy.

Premature cervical spondylosis may occur secondary to movement disorders such as torticollis and athetosis. Cervical radiculopathy as well as myelopathy may be superimposed on a chronic dystonia. Cervical myelopathy or radiculopathy should be suspected in any patient with a chronic movement disorder of the head, neck, or arm, who presents with decreased neurologic function (143). Involuntary movement disorders may be present in patients with cerebral palsy, and myelopathy may be superimposed on the underlying pathology (81,112). Such patients may benefit from operative intervention if their neurologic status deteriorates. Abnormalities in the cervical spine resulting in myelopathy may occur in patients with Down syndrome. Typically there is upper cervical involvement secondary to instability; however, patients with Down syndrome and degeneration of the lower cervical spine may develop myelopathy, as reported in two patients (133). Patients with such chronic, static underlying conditions should be evaluated for the possibility of a superimposed myelopathy if their condition deteriorates. Patients with cervical spondylosis may be more prone to myelopathy after sustaining an injury, even a rather minor fall (60). Most patients with cord injury sustain obvious bony and/or ligamentous damage commensurate with their neurologic function. Regenbogen et al. (146) found that in approximately 30% of the patients in their series who were older and had cervical spondylosis and spinal cord injuries, there was no obvious bony abnormality, and approximately 20% of patients had only minimal evidence of damage on radiographs. Therefore, the radiographs may be seemingly unremarkable in patients who sustain major injury, including cord damage. The narrowing of the canal secondary to degenerative change may make the cord more susceptible to damage (146).

CLINICAL DIAGNOSIS

History and Physical Findings

Symptoms referable to cervical degenerative disease can be divided into three categories: neck pain, radicular symptoms, and myelopathic symptoms. An individual patient may manifest findings from one, two, or all three of these areas. The neck pain referable from cervical degenerative disease tends to be posterior, located in the paraspinous muscular region. Associated with this, patients may have occipital headaches as well as interscapular pain. The pain may be exacerbated by neck motion as well as use of the arms in the over-the-shoulder position. Patients also tend to complain of neck stiffness with pain at the extremes of motion. The pain may be lessened or relieved by immobilization of the neck with a cervical orthosis.

Radicular symptoms secondary to cervical degenerative disease are characterized by proximal pain and distal paresthesias. In general, the symptoms are referable to an individual nerve root. However, there is overlap between the dermatomes innervated by a particular nerve, and it is rare to have findings strictly isolated to the distribution of a single dermatome. The upper extremity is primarily supplied by the C5 through C8 and T1 nerve roots. The sensory dermatomes of these roots follow a relatively simple pattern. If one thinks of the upper extremity with the arm positioned in the anatomic position (i.e., the palms supinated), the sensory dermatomes follow a circular pattern. The C5 dermatome provides sensation to the lateral arm. The C6 dermatome provides sensation to the lateral forearm, including the thumb. The C7 dermatome includes the middle portion of the hand and middle finger. The C8 dermatome provides sensation to the medial forearm, and the T1 dermatome provides sensation to the medial arm. There is also overlap of the innervation to the muscles in the upper extremity, and this is also true of the reflexes. A helpful way to remember the nerve supply of the upper-extremity muscles is to think of the primary joint(s) innervated by a particular root. The C5 root involves the shoulder (deltoid muscle—shoulder abduction). The C6 root primarily supplies the elbow flexors (biceps and brachialis muscles) and the wrist extensors (extensor carpi radialis longus and brevis and extensor carpi ulnaris muscles). The C7 root is basically the antagonist of the C6 root (elbow extension—triceps muscle, wrist flexion—flexor carpi radialis and flexor carpi ulnaris muscles), with the addition of finger extension at the metacarpal phalangeal (MP) joints. The C8 and T1 roots primarily supply the hand intrinsic muscles, with the C8 roots primarily responsible for flexion at the MP joints and the T1 roots supplying the abductors and adductors of the fingers.

The reflex innervation is as follows: The biceps reflex is mediated by C5 and C6; the brachioradialis is primarily mediated by C6; the triceps is primarily mediated by C7.

The cervical nerve roots exist above the corresponding vertebral body. For example, the C5 root exists above the C5 vertebral body. Therefore, a disc rupture of the C4-C5 intervertebral disc will usually compress the C5 root. Because the C8 root comes out above the T1 body, the relationship of the nerve root to the disc space is different below the cervical-thoracic junction.

As previously noted, patients with cervical radiculopathy have a predominance of proximal pain and distal paresthesias. Therefore, a patient with cervical degeneration at C5-C6 with compression of the C6 root tends to have pain in the lateral arm, with paresthesias in the lateral forearm down into the thumb. In addition, the patient may have weakness of the elbow flexors and wrist extensors with hyporeflexia of the biceps and/or brachioradialis reflexes.

The onset of symptoms with cervical radiculopathy secondary to a hard disc or degenerative disease is insidious in many cases. However, a patient often will ascribe the onset to a specific incident such as lifting, a vigorous recreational activity, or a household work project. Patients who present with the abrupt onset of symptoms may have a soft-disc rupture superimposed upon their cervical degenerative disease.

Patients with a ruptured cervical disc may have relief of pain with arm abduction. This maneuver is similar to relieving tension in the nerve by bending the knee during Laseque's maneuver. Such relief, however, is uncommon in patients with cervical radiculopathy secondary to spondylosis (10).

Myelopathy secondary to cervical spondylosis typically has an insidious onset, developing gradually over a long period (Fig. 2) (37,183). The most common clinical pattern involves short periods of worsening followed by long intervals of relative stability (102). The sudden onset of myelopathy may occasionally develop in the presence of cervical spondylosis. Severe hyperextension injuries, acute superimposed soft-disc herniation, or torsion dystonia may cause an acute myelopathy (3,12,83,107). When the onset is acute and there is rapid deterioration, a vascular etiology should also be considered (177). It is important to rule out motor neuron disease when considering the diagnosis of myelopathy secondary to spondylosis. Conditions such as MS and particularly ALS must be excluded (53). (Further discussion of the differential diagnosis of cervical myelopathy is presented later in this chapter.)

A deep, aching pain and burning sensation is clinical evidence of spinal cord involvement (55). Patients often complain of loss of hand dexterity. Many will have painful dysesthesias and difficulty writing. Diffuse nonspe-

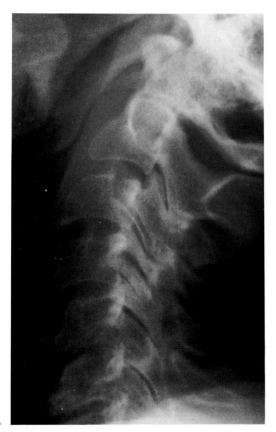
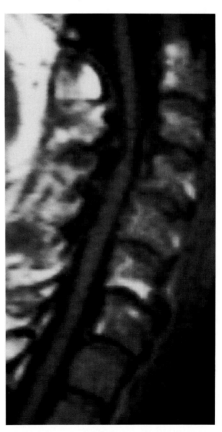

FIG. 2. Diagnostic images of a 72-year-old patient who presented with myelopathy. The patient had a gradual onset over a period of several years. She had a broad-based unsteady gait. **A:** Lateral radiograph demonstrating multilevel cervical spondylosis. **B:** Sagittal MR image demonstrating cord compression at multiple levels.

cific weakness may be present. Patients also complain of difficulty walking and often lose their balance. The typical walking pattern is a broad-based gait. Bladder incontinence may also be present (27,161).

Patients with cervical spondylitic myelopathy tend to exhibit myelopathic findings more commonly than root symptoms, and motor and reflex changes more commonly than sensory changes. Analgesia is more common than anesthesia, which is more common than proprioceptive loss (108).

The typical motor findings are lower motor neuron involvement at the level of the lesion and upper motor neuron manifestations below the level. This includes the lower levels of the upper extremities as well as the lower extremities. Upper-extremity involvement tends to be unilateral, whereas the lower extremities are typically affected bilaterally (27). Sensory findings are often variable because compression of sensory pathways occurs at several levels. Typically, sensory findings occur at a level below the area of compression, touch sensation is often preserved, and pain and temperature may be diminished as well as proprioception and vibratory sense (27). Cervical spondylosis is the most common cause of loss of position and vibratory sense (174). Reflex changes usually follow the pattern of motor involvement, that is, lower motor neuron findings (hyporeflexia) at the level of involvement and upper motor neuron findings (hyperreflexia) below. A positive Hoffmann and/or Babinski sign may be present, indicating an upper motor neuron lesion. Denno and Meadows (41) have described a dynamic Hoffmann's sign, which they found useful in the early diagnosis of cervical spondylitic myelopathy. The Hoffmann's sign was checked in neutral (static) and during multiple active full flexion to extension movements (dynamic), as tolerated by the patient. A positive dynamic Hoffmann's sign was consistent with a narrow diameter of the cervical canal and aided clinically in making the diagnosis of early cervical spondylitic myelopathy or congenital cervical narrowing (41).

As noted previously, Crandall and Batzdorf (37) described five categories of presentation (transverse, motor, central, Brown-Sequard, and brachial cord). This classification is useful when categorizing the clinical presentation of a patient with myelopathy. It may also relate to the prognosis of treatment. Jabbari et al. (88) described a rapidly progressive myelopathy of the Brown-Sequard type even in younger individuals, which was often a presenting clinical feature of cervical spondylosis.

Ebara et al. (48) have described a condition known as "myelopathy hand," characterized by muscle wasting. The main clinical features were localized wasting and weakness of the extrinsic and intrinsic muscles of the hand, not accompanied by either sensory loss or spastic quadriparesis. The authors recommended that attention be paid to the narrow anteroposterior canal diameter of the cervical spine (less than 13 mm), multisegmental spondylosis at C5-C6 and C6-C7, and reduced transactional area of the cord at the C7, C8, or T1 levels.

High cervical spondylosis (C3-C5) may present with a distinctive clinical syndrome of "numb, clumsy hands" and stereoanesthesia of the hands (63). Such higher lesions cause a different syndrome compared with the more common lower lesions. This syndrome is characterized by paresthesia and proprioceptive loss in the hands, with minimal sensory changes in the legs. Relative sparing of primary sensory modalities and motor and bladder function are other features. This is similar to the central cord syndrome of Crandall and Batzdorf (37). The clinical picture of lower cervical involvement (C5-C8) typically includes spasticity as well as proprioceptive loss in the legs (52,63,68,109,118).

Physical findings include a positive Spurling's maneuver (present in 25% of patients) (37). Oblique extension with compression of the head and neck produces cervical root compression, resulting in pain. Lhermitte's sign is a shock-like sensation in the trunk or limbs following quick extension or flexion of the neck. This sign is present in approximately 25% of patients with myelopathy secondary to cervical spondylosis (37). Spasticity is almost invariably present in these patients.

Imaging and Laboratory Investigation

Imaging modalities play a major role in the diagnosis and management of patients with cervical spondylitic myelopathy. It is important, however, that diagnostic studies be correlated with the patient's history and clinical findings, particularly before considering therapeutic intervention. Modic et al. (125) have outlined the advantages and disadvantages of the various studies used to image degenerative disease of the cervical spine. Plain x-rays are rapid and provide an inexpensive screen of osseous pathology; however, they are unable to visualize directly encroachment or compression of the neural structures. Noting the relationship of various portions of the vertebrae on a plain lateral radiograph may suggest the presence of stenosis. If the base of the spinous process is immediately adjacent to the dorsal aspect of the articular process, stenosis may be present. Hayashi et al. (72) reported that cervical spondylitic radiculopathy is likely to develop when the superior articular process is anterior to the posterior margin of the vertebral body. Plain radiographs provide an inexpensive initial means of evaluating the degenerative cervical spine if viewed within the context of the patient's history and physical examination (144). However, Heller et al. (74) questioned the value of routine radiographic examinations of the cervical spine. They suggested that radiographs should be performed only when there is a clinical suspicion of malignancy or infection, after trauma, or when operative intervention may be indicated. They believe that there is little point in taking radiographs of the neck to diagnose cervical spondylosis.

Water-soluble nonionic contrast myelography is able to image the entire cervical region except in cases of high-grade stenosis. However, it is invasive and lacks diagnostic specificity. CT with intrathecal contrast provides excellent differential between bone and soft-tissue lesions, directly demonstrates canal size and foraminal narrowing, is minimally operator dependent, and can visualize abnormalities distal to severe narrowing or blockage (5,33,39,47,96,125,127,156). CT myelography may indicate the degree of uncovertebral and facet joint involvement, indentation of the fecal sac, encroachment of the nerve root in the neural foramen, and the degree of spinal stenosis (16). MRI provides excellent, noninvasive evaluation of the spinal cord, other neural structures, and soft tissues. This operator-dependent study primarily reflects the physiology of the imaged area rather than the anatomy per se. Modic et al. (125) feel that MRI might now be the appropriate first test to evaluate the cervical spine in a patient with signs or symptoms referable to degenerative disease when therapeutic intervention is considered. MRI is ideally suited to exclude intramedullary lesions of the central nervous system (116). The additional information provided by this study may compensate for its additional cost. It is important to understand, however, that MRI may be positive in asymptomatic individuals with degenerative disease. Modic et al. (125) have shown that disc protrusions are present in 20% of patients aged 45 to 55 years and in 57% of patients older than 64. In addition, spinal cord impingement may be present in 16% of patients less than age 64 and in 26% of patients older than 64.

Several dimensions of the spine have clinical importance. These include the sagittal diameter of the spinal canal, the cross-sectional area of the canal, the mobility of the spinal cord, and spinal curvature (8). The sagittal diameter is most commonly assessed on a plain radiograph. Measurements determined on lateral radiographs should be obtained on radiographs with a focus-grid distance of 72 inches (151). Normally, the spinal canal is oval shaped in the midcervical region and there is a sagittal diameter of 17 mm (186). The cervical cord diameter varies little from C1 to C7 and averages 10 mm (151). The diameter of the spinal canal increases with flexion and decreases with extension. The spinal cord moves rostrally as much as 3 mm at C7 during flexion and extension and results in angulation of the nerve roots at their foramina (19).

Okada et al. (132) reported that the transverse area of the spinal cord on T1-weighted MR images at the level of maximum compression was closely correlated with the severity of myelopathy, duration of disease, and recovery rate as determined by the JOA score. Nagata et al. (126) found T1-weighted MRI accurate in diagnosing compressive myelopathy, deciding the level of disease focus,

and assessing operative results. The value of the signal intensity on MRI has been debated. Mehalic et al. (123) evaluated 19 patients before and after operation. They found increased signal intensity within the spinal cord in T2-weighted images at the point of maximum compression and felt that this carried prognostic significance. Yone et al. (187), in a study of pre- and postoperative patients with cervical myelopathy, found that the presence or absence of areas of high signal intensity did not correlate with the severity of myelopathy or operative recovery in the group of patients with ossification of the posterior longitudinal ligament and in the group with cervical spondylitic myelopathy. Koyanagi et al. (94) evaluated the transverse area and the so-called flattening ratio of the spinal cord on CT-myelograms. In cervical spondylitic myelopathy and ossification of the posterior longitudinal ligament, the transverse area of the spinal cord and duration of symptoms could be used to predict recovery after operation. In cervical disc disease, however, recovery was good regardless of the transverse area and the duration of symptoms.

The role of a narrow cervical spinal canal in relation to clinical syndromes was investigated by Edwards and LaRocca (50). They described several measurements (Fig. 3). The developmental segmental sagittal diameter

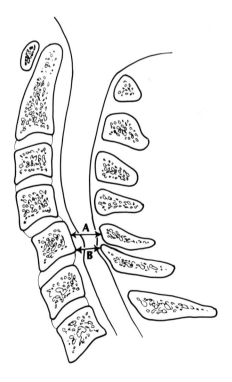

Spondylosis Index = A - B

FIG. 3. Schematic diagram depicting the developmental segmental sagittal diameter (DSSD) (label A) and the spondylitic segmental sagittal diameter (SSSD) (label B). The spondylosis index (SI) is the difference between the DSSD and SSSD (see text for details). With permission from ref. 50.

(DSSD) is determined at the level of the pedicle. A perpendicular line is drawn to the posterior margin of the spinal canal, as determined by the most anterior bony landmark for the segment. A second perpendicular line is drawn at the level of the disc, indicating the spondylitic segmental sagittal diameter (SSSD). The difference between these two measurements is the spondylosis index (SI), which represents the amount of narrowing due to the disease process (21,50,51). Edwards and LaRocca stated that the ultimate importance of the developmentally narrow canal will depend on the amount of reserve space within the canal and the rate of progression of the disease (50). They used midcervical (C4-C6) diameters as predictors. Patients with developmental diameters of 10 to 13 mm and spondylitic narrowing of 2 to 4 mm per segment were in the premyelopathic group. Patients with diameters greater than 13 mm were less prone to develop myelopathy, however, and tended to have symptomatic cervical spondylosis. Patients with greater than 17-mm diameters tolerated spondylosis without notable symptoms. The authors found that, using a measurement of 17 mm as the normal cutoff between wide and narrow as determined by Wolf et al. (186), patients with a narrow canal tolerated a spondylosis index of 2.1 mm per segment, compared with an index of 3.3 mm per segment for patients with a wide canal.

One concern about making absolute measurements on plain radiographs is the variability of magnification. Torg et al. (168) described a ratio method (Pavlov's ratio) that eliminates this variable (Fig. 4). Their method involves determining the sagittal diameter of the spinal canal from the midpoint of the posterior aspect of the vertebral body to the nearest point on the corresponding spinolaminar line. This ratio compares the sagittal diameter of the spinal canal with the anteroposterior width of the vertebral body measured through the midpoint of the body. Furthermore, these authors investigated neurapraxia of the cervical spinal cord with transient quadriplegia in athletes and found that the control group of normal individuals had a Pavlov's ratio of 1 or greater. They found statistically significant spinal stenosis (p < 0.0001) in patients with cord neurapraxia compared with controls. This group had a ratio of less than 0.8. They found, however, no evidence that the occurrence of neurapraxia of the spinal cord predisposed to permanent injury (168).

Patients with a stenotic spinal canal are usually asymptomatic (176). However, they are more vulnerable to encroaching lesions such as herniated discs, protruding or bulging of the annulus fibrosis, osteophytes, and/or infolding of the ligamentum flavum.

Besides canal diameter, sagittal spinal alignment should be evaluated on lateral plain radiographs. As previously noted, Batzdorf and Batzdorff (8) found that neck pain was most severe in patients with a reversal of the cervical curve. Further, they believed that the degree

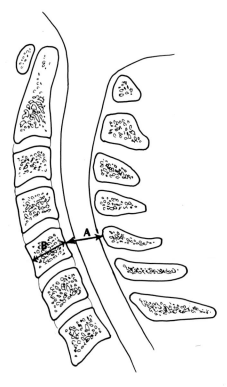

Pavlov's Ratio = A / B

FIG. 4. Schematic diagram depicting the measurements made on a plain lateral radiograph to determine Pavlov's ratio. Pavlov's ratio = A/B (see text for details). With permission from ref. 168.

of spinal curvature correlated with postoperative outcome. Patients with normal curvature showed the greatest improvement in signs and symptoms after operation. Spinal geometry should be considered in patient selection for operation (8). The rationale for laminectomy includes dorsal migration of the spinal cord into the space developed by the removal of the ligamentum flavum and laminae (2,157). Posterior decompression allows the cord to migrate dorsally, thereby decreasing the axial tension and improving vascular perfusion of the cord (54). If a patient has a major kyphotic deformity, the majority of compression may be anterior to the cord. Such a deformity is a relative contraindication to a posterior approach (29).

Dynamic MR images obtained in hyperflexion, neutral, and hyperextension positions are useful in the diagnosis of cord compression in patients with spinal stenosis and myelopathy (56). In addition, these studies are useful to determine the relief of cord compression after operative intervention.

Controversy surrounds the use of cervical discography as a diagnostic test. Conner and Darden (36) reported a relatively high complication rate of 15% (4 of 31 patients) with this procedure and felt that diagnostic cervical discography did not provide the degree of clinical predictive value necessary to justify its potential risks and complications. Cervical discography appears to be most reliable when a patient's signs and symptoms are repeatedly reproduced with a noxious stimulus and diminished with an analgesic agent.

Electrodiagnostic studies play a limited but increasingly important role in the evaluation of cervical spondylitic myelopathy and hold great promise for the future. Nerve conduction velocities, cervical somatosensory evoked potentials (SEPs), and concentric needle electromyography (EMG) are useful tests for distinguishing cervical root lesion and peripheral entrapment neuropathy (92). EMG may be less sensitive than SEPs in detecting cervical root lesions (100). The greatest role for EMG is the differentiation of radicular disease from peripheral involvement. In many cases, nerve conduction velocities can rule out a peripheral nerve compression that may mimic cervical radiculopathy and/or myelopathy. Electrodiagnostic changes preferably in combination with mixed nerve SEP testing may be important in evaluating cases of early cervical myelopathy (141). Restuccia et al. (147) evaluated SEPs in the diagnosis of cervical spondylitic myelopathy. These authors studied median, ulnar, radial, and common perineal nerve evoked potentials. They found common perineal nerve SEP abnormalities in all patients, but these were of no value in identifying the cervical spine as a site of the lesion. Leblhuber et al. (100) evaluated the diagnostic value of different electrophysiologic tests in cervical disc prolapse. They found abnormal EMGs in 67% of patients and abnormal dermatomal SEPs in 85%. Restuccia et al. (148) evaluated SEPs in patients with cervical spondylitic myelopathy and found that the subclinical abnormalities of the spine N13 potential probably resulted from reduced blood supply due to compression of the anterior spinal artery in patients with cervical spondylitic myelopathy.

Transcranial magnetic stimulation of the motor cortex may be useful to measure conduction within the central motor pathways of patients with cervical spondylosis or disc herniation. Maertens de Noordhout et al. found that muscle action potentials (MAPs) due to cortical stimulation were abnormal in 84% of patients with, and in 22% of those without, radiologic signs of cervical cord compression. Jaskolski et al. (89) reported that magnetic stimulation provides objective confirmation of upper motor neuron involvement and may provide some measure of its degree, but it does not appear to be superior to clinical methods of diagnosing its presence. DiLazzaro et al. (42) felt that owing to their high degree of sensitivity, central motor conduction studies may have considerable value in the functional assessment of central motor pathways in cervical spondylitic myelopathy. Tang and Ren (167) concluded that noninvasive and painless magnetic transcranial stimulation of the motor pathways is useful in the assessment and management of patients with cervical spondylitic myelopathy and is better than electrical

stimulation. Direct stimulation of the motor tracts may be of value in functional assessment of the motor pathways in cervical spondylosis (1). However, this is an invasive procedure. Certainly the use of evoked potentials, particularly the motor evoked potential, is an evolving technology at present and holds promise for the future. Currently, evoked potentials are primarily used investigationally to monitor the status of patients intraoperatively. Pre- and postoperative studies are being done to assess the changes occurring after operative intervention and to compare the changes in potentials with the clinical findings. Jaskolsio et al. (90) reported notable improvement in motor conduction times in patients with myelopathy who improved clinically, but they felt that preoperative motor conduction times provided no clear predictive information. Heiskari et al. (73) found that SEP abnormalities are common in cervical radiculopathy and particularly in cervical myelopathy, and seem to be quite persistent postoperatively despite clinical improvement, especially in the form of pain relief. As the technology becomes more refined, it will undoubtedly play a more prominent role in the management of patients with cervical spondylitic myelopathy.

Voiding dysfunction may occur as a result of cervical spondylitic myelopathy. Hattori et al. (70) evaluated 37 patients with cervical spondylitic myelopathy and found that 30 (81%) had voiding symptoms. Urodynamic studies revealed abnormalities in a number of these patients. Urodynamic investigations seem to provide additional information regarding the severity of the disease (165).

DIFFERENTIAL DIAGNOSIS

This section highlights the major clinical conditions that should be considered in the differential diagnosis of patients presenting with symptoms referable to the neck. It includes two major subheadings: intrinsic and extrinsic conditions. Intrinsic cervical conditions include inflammatory, neoplastic, infectious, and miscellaneous disease processes. Extrinsic conditions include degenerative, inflammatory, neoplastic, infectious, and miscellaneous conditions of the upper extremity that may have a clinical presentation similar to that of degenerative disease of the cervical spine and must be considered in the differential diagnosis. This section discusses these various disorders, pointing out clinical features that differentiate these conditions from manifestations of cervical spondylosis. One must keep in mind that many of these conditions may coexist with cervical spondylosis.

Intrinsic Cervical Conditions

Inflammation: Rheumatoid Arthritis

Rheumatoid arthritis frequently affects the cervical spine, and the majority of patients with this disease have cervical involvement. The pathophysiology of cervical involvement is similar to that in the peripheral joints. The primary disease process involves the synovium with resultant destruction of bone, cartilage, and ligaments. This may produce marked instability of the cervical spine with neurologic compromise. There are three common patterns of involvement: atlantoaxial subluxation (C1-C2), cranial settling (also known as atlantoaxial or occipitoatlantoaxial impaction), and subaxial subluxation (25). Any or all of these conditions may coexist in the same patient. Atlantoaxial subluxation results from loss of integrity of the transverse, alar, and/or apical ligaments and is present in 19% to 71% of patients (34,45,113,117,159,163). Instability is determined on lateral flexion and extension radiographs (Figs. 5 and 6). When the anterior atlantodental interval (ADI) is greater than 3 mm, integrity of the transverse atlantoaxial ligament is jeopardized and instability may be present. When the ADI is greater than 10 to 12 mm, all of the supporting ligaments of the atlantoaxial complex are disrupted, and the segment is grossly unstable (58). The posterior atlantodental interval (PADI) is the area between

the posterior aspect of the dens and the anterior portion of the posterior arch of the ring of C1, and represents the space available for the cord. When this interval measures less than 13 mm on a plain lateral radiograph, the extra space available for the cord is either minimal or no longer present, and cord compression may be present or imminent. Some patients may stabilize in the subluxed position; therefore, instability is considered present when mobility is demonstrated on flexion and extension radiographs. Cranial settling results from destruction of the occipitoatlantal and atlantoaxial joints with the dens protruding through the foramen magnum, providing the potential for brainstem compression. This condition is present in 5% to 32% of patients with rheumatoid arthritis (45,117,140,145). Several parameters based on plain radiographs are used to determine and quantitate the degree of cranial settling (Fig. 7). The McGregor line (McG) is drawn from the posterior edge of the hard palate to the most inferior portion of the occiput. Normally the tip of the odontoid process should not protrude more than 4.5 mm above this line (76). The method of Redlund-Johnell involves determining the distance from

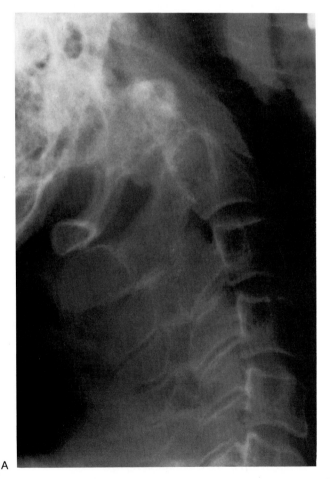

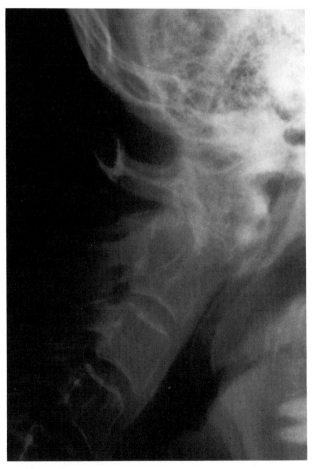

A   B

FIG. 5. Lateral flexion and extension radiographs from a rheumatoid patient with severe atlantoaxial subluxation. **A:** Extension view demonstrating reduction of the subluxation. **B:** Flexion view demonstrating significant mobile atlantoaxial subluxation.

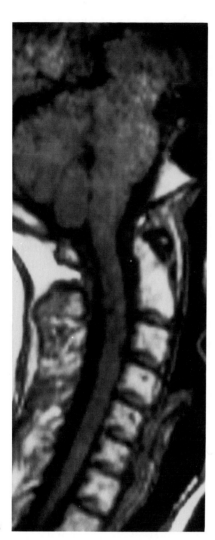
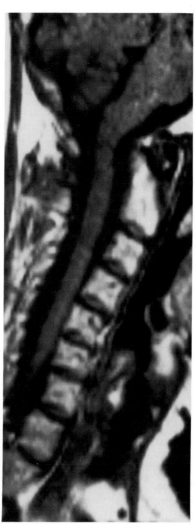

A,B

FIG. 6. Dynamic MR images of the rheumatoid patient in Fig. 5 with atlantoaxial subluxation. **A:** Extension image (C1-C2 reduced). **B:** Cervicomedullary junction.

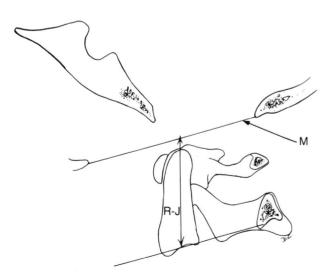

FIG. 7. Schematic diagram depicting McGregor's line (M) and the measurement of Redlund-Johnell (see text for details). With permission from ref. 31.

the base of C2 to McGregor's line. Normally this distance is greater than 17 mm. Cranial settling is considered present when this interval is less than 15 mm in males and 13 mm in females (28). The simplest way to screen quickly for the possibility of cranial settling is to note the relationship of the anterior arch of C1 to C2. This parameter is known as the station of the atlas and was described by Clark et al. (28) (Fig. 8). The station of the atlas is determined by dividing the axis into thirds along its sagittal plane. Normally the anterior arch of C1 is adjacent to the tip of the dens (station 1). As cranial settling progresses, the anterior arch of C1 may be adjacent to the base of the dens (station 2). In cases of severe cranial settling, the anterior arch of the atlas may be adjacent to the body of the axis (station 3) or even lower (28). The advantage of this parameter is that a determination can be made with relative ease on plain radiographs. Subaxial (below C2) subluxation may be present in 10% to 20% of patients (6,124,158). This condition

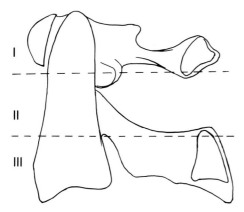

FIG. 8. Schematic diagram depicting the station of the atlas (see text for details). With permission from ref. 28.

may be present at one or several levels and results from synovitis of the apophyseal as well as uncovertebral joints, with resulting ligamentous and capsular laxity.

The clinical presentation of patients with rheumatoid involvement of the cervical spine is varied. Patients may complain of neck pain, but many are asymptomatic. Such patients have multiple joint involvement and frequently suffer from chronic disease. Therefore, they may present with relatively few cervical complaints. Symptoms result from tissue inflammation, neurologic dysfunction, and/or vertebral artery insufficiency. Synovitis and mechanical instability may result in referred pain into the intrascapular area, chest, shoulder, and/or upper extremity. Neurologic dysfunction is present in 7% to 34% of patients and may include the brainstem, spinal cord, and/or nerve roots (34,140,163). Cranial settling may include impingement of the dens on the lower cranial nerves as well as the cardiorespiratory center and pyramidal tracts. Atlantoaxial subluxation may cause cord compression with spasticity, pathologic reflexes, and urinary retention or incontinence. Vertebral artery insufficiency is perhaps the least common mode of presentation. Such patients may present with dysequilibrium, tinnitus, vertigo, visual disturbances, diplopia, dysphagia, and nystagmus (105).

The treatment of rheumatoid arthritis is somewhat controversial and beyond the scope of this chapter. However, because of the likelihood of progressive instability, posterior arthrodesis should be considered when there is radiographic evidence of major instability and cord compression demonstrated on neuroradiographic studies. This may be necessary even in the absence of pain or neurologic deficit (28).

Neoplastic Conditions

Primary cervical neoplasms are rare and account for approximately 1% of patients with primary bone tumors (161). Spinal lesions in older patients are most frequently malignant; spinal lesions in children and adolescents are usually benign (179). Benign primary cervical neoplasms include hemangioma, osteochondroma, osteoid osteoma, osteoblastoma, and giant cell tumor of bone. Malignant primary cervical neoplasms are less common than the benign tumors and include chordoma, multiple myeloma, osteosarcoma, and chondrosarcoma.

The spine is a common site for skeletal metastases regardless of the primary tumor (157). Approximately 75% of vertebral metastases originate from carcinoma of the breast, prostate, kidney, or thyroid, or from lymphoma or myeloma (69).

The clinical presentation of patients with neoplastic disease includes localized pain in the area of involvement. Neck pain tends to be the most common presenting symptom (13). The pain tends to be unremitting. It is often more intense at night, at rest, or during times of inactivity. It may be associated with headaches and upper-extremity pain. Neurologic abnormalities frequently develop in patients with primary cervical neoplastic disease. Radicular pain is common and the spinal cord level is usually discrete (4).

Intrinsic spinal cord tumors are extremely rare. Only a small percentage of primary central nervous system tumors are intraspinal. These tumors are classified as extradural, intradural-extramedullary, and intramedullary. Extradural tumors account for approximately 22% of primary spinal cord tumors. The rest are intradural. Approximately 71% of these are extramedullary, with the most common tumors being meningiomas and schwannomas. The remaining 29% are intramedullary tumors, and these include ependymomas and astrocytomas (106). The clinical presentation of spinal cord tumors includes nocturnal and rest pain. The pain may be local as well as referred and is often localized to a discrete neurologic level. Intradural-extramedullary lesions may produce asymptomatic myelopathic deficits. Extramedullary lesions produce radicular sensory and motor loss. Bladder dysfunction may also be present with these tumors (106).

Infections

Spinal sepsis constitutes only a small portion of all cases of skeletal infection due to pyogenic organisms (164). Of these, approximately 3% to 4% occur in the cervical spine (63). This condition generally occurs in children and the elderly, as well as in medically compromised patients (62,82,103). Spread to the epidural space occurs in up to one third of patients. Antecedent infection can be identified in only a minority of patients.

The clinical presentation includes tenderness, guarding, and limited spine motion. Pain is increased with axial compression or percussion of the spinous process of the involved vertebrae. Radiculopathy or myelopathy may be present if structural instability or epidural extension exists.

Although the spine is the most common site of tuberculous skeletal involvement, only approximately 3% to 5% of cases of spondylitis involve the cervical spine (46,115). Neurologic deficit may result from direct pressure of granulation tissue, abscess formation, extruded necrotic bone or disc material, or spinal instability. The clinical findings include progressive pain and neck stiffness. Pain may be referred to the shoulders, upper extremities, or occiput. When myelopathy is present, there tends to be lower motor neuron findings at the level of infection and upper motor neuron findings distal to the level (84).

Miscellaneous Differential Conditions

Cervical spondylosis is a relatively common cause of myelopathy, and the clinical presentation may mimic several types of neurologic disease, including MS and ALS. Cervical spondylosis with myelopathy is one of the most frequently unrecognized and misdiagnosed, yet treatable, conditions affecting the nervous system (142). Distinguishing between cervical spondylitic myelopathy and ALS can be difficult. Careful neurologic examination with attention to clinical details, muscle biopsy in some patients, and routine EMG will usually lead to the proper diagnosis (101).

MS is often considered "the great imitator" in neurologic disease (137). MS has a prevalence of approximately 30 to 80 per 100,000 people in the northern United States and southern Canada (120). Because of the ubiquitous nature of this condition, it should be considered in the differential diagnosis of patients presenting with cervical myelopathy. The average age at onset is approximately 32 years (137). In the younger patient, the clinical course tends to be one of remission and relapse; however, an older patient often has a chronically progressive course.

The clinical presentation involves acute loss of central vision in 16% to 30% of patients, with slightly greater than 10% of patients complaining of diplopia. Incoordination, fatigability, dysarthria, dysphasia, urinary tract dysfunction, and acute loss of sensory and/or motor function in the upper or lower extremities may be present. Up to one third of patients may have a positive Lhermitte's sign. Patients typically have reduced vibratory and position sense, and approximately 30% exhibit absent deep tendon reflexes. Muscular atrophy is an infrequent finding (137).

The diagnosis of MS is confirmed by a combination of clinical, neuroimmunologic, electrophysiologic, and/or neuroradiologic findings. The evaluation of a patient with known MS who develops new signs of cervical spinal cord dysfunction should include spinal neural im-

aging studies because cervical spondylosis and MS may coexist (20). Sometimes the etiology of a myelopathy is not obvious. Marti-Fabregas et al. (114) reviewed a series of 72 patients in whom the etiology of myelopathy was not apparent. The most frequent diagnosis was either definite or probable MS. MRI was of great value in detecting asymptomatic brain lesions.

Ossification of the posterior longitudinal ligament (OPLL) is a common cause of myelopathy in Oriental populations. However, this condition is being recognized more frequently in non-Asian populations (119). The diagnosis is suspected on a clinical basis and frequently the ossification is easily seen on plain lateral radiographs; however, neuroradiographic studies may be required to confirm the diagnosis and determine the extent of cord compression. Patients who present with hyperextension/hyperflexion injuries of the cervical spine (the so-called "whiplash syndrome") will often present with neck and shoulder pain. These patients should be considered in the differential diagnosis. However, the history of preceding trauma often confirms the diagnosis. A hyperextension or hyperflexion injury may also aggravate a preexisting cervical spondylosis. This subject is discussed in greater depth in the Chapter 59 on the cervical sprain syndrome.

Apical lung or Pancoast tumors must be considered in the differential diagnosis of patients presenting with neck and upper extremity pain as well as neurologic symptoms. These lesions constitute approximately 5% of all bronchogenic tumors and arise in the apical parietal pleura (160). The tumor may invade the stellate ganglia of the sympathetic chain as well as elements of the brachial plexus, resulting in Horner's syndrome as well as upper-extremity symptoms. Early diagnosis is essential to successful management. About 60% of cases are operatively resectable, with a 5-year survival of approximately 31% and a 15-year survival of approximately 22% (138). The clinical presentation includes local pain in the area of the scapula and shoulder. Pain may radiate into the ulnar distribution of the upper extremity. Wasting of hand intrinsic muscles and Horner's syndrome may be present. Radiographs may reveal thickening of the apical pleura, destruction of the first to third ribs, and erosions of the vertebral bodies (160). The tumor may be seen on an AP radiograph of the cervical spine if the lung fields are carefully scrutinized on this view (Fig. 9).

Syringomyelia may result from a congenital or developmental disorder or may be post-traumatic in origin. Generally, there is combined sensory and motor dysfunction (154). Patients typically present with paresthesias or dysesthetic pain, producing a prickling or tingling sensation (184). Sensory loss is present in 90% of patients. Pain is present in only 20% and may be radicular and simulate nerve root compression. Thermal and pain modalities are affected more than proprioception and light touch. Motor weakness is present in the majority of

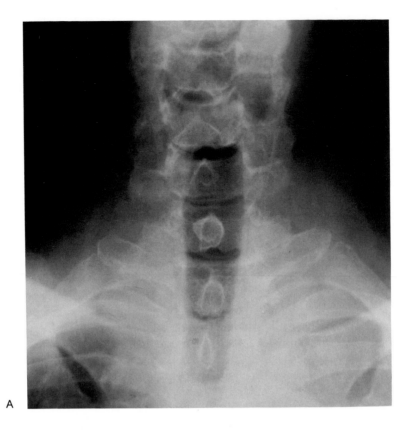

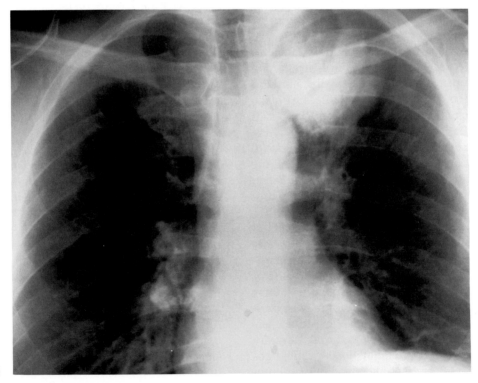

FIG. 9. Middle-aged patient with Pancoast tumor of the left upper lobe of the lung. The patient presented with neck and radicular pain in the C8-T1 distribution. He had Horner's syndrome. **A:** AP cervical radiograph suggesting a fullness in the apex of the left lung. **B:** Posteroanterior chest radiograph depicting the lesion at the apex of the left lung.

patients. The characteristic cerebrospinal fluid findings include low protein (154).

Extrinsic Conditions: Upper Extremity

Shoulder

Extrinsic shoulder problems are perhaps the most common conditions that must be differentiated from cervical pathology. Indeed, conditions in both areas may coexist, but typically one condition precedes the onset of the other. Primary cervical conditions that refer pain to the shoulder include cervical spondylosis with foraminal encroachment, acute soft-disc herniation with nerve root compression and radicular pain, post-traumatic degeneration with foraminal compromise, and miscellaneous cervical conditions including tumors (71). Referred pain to the shoulder from the cervical spine can initiate the process of tendinitis in the shoulder with a resultant "frozen shoulder." The keys in differentiating cervical from shoulder conditions are the history and physical examination. Clinically, patients with cervical spine disorders complain of neck pain and headaches. Pain is typically at the top of the shoulder, may be increased at night, and is often relieved with the use of a cervical orthosis. Pain secondary to shoulder impingement or rotator cuff problems is located predominantly over the deltoid insertion and is not relieved by a cervical orthosis (71).

When evaluating shoulder conditions, it is helpful to separate those that limit passive glenohumeral motion from those that do not. Therefore, physical examination is essential to determine a specific diagnosis. Conditions that typically do not limit passive shoulder motion will be discussed first.

Rotator cuff tendinitis results from impingement of the rotator cuff between the acromion and the humeral head. The coracoacromial ligament is also important in the pathophysiology of this condition. Neer (128) identified three stages of impingement. Stage 1 consists of edema and hemorrhage of the rotator cuff. Stage 2 involves tendinitis, fibrosis, and calcification of the supraspinatus tendon; in addition there is thickening and fibrosis of the subacromial bursa. In stage 3, rotator cuff tendinitis occurs with partial or complete rupture of the rotator cuff. The clinical presentation consists of an aching or gnawing pain in the deltoid region. Pain is often worse at night and exacerbated with overhead work. Abduction and external rotation against resistance increase the symptoms. Impingement may be reproduced by forward elevation of the humerus against resistance. With a torn rotator cuff, there is loss of active motion, particularly in abduction or external rotation.

Bicipital tendinitis may develop secondary to inflammation of the rotator cuff. Typically, patients complain of shoulder pain in the region of the bicipital groove. Increased symptoms result from resistance to forward flexion of the shoulder with the elbow in extension and the forearm supinated.

Calcific tendinitis of the rotator cuff occurs most frequently in the supraspinatus tendon. Calcification is a different pathologic process than impingement (122, 172). Symptoms result from rupture of calcium deposits into the subacromial bursa producing an acute, extremely painful, crystal-induced bursitis. The clinical findings are characterized by an atraumatic, acute onset of pain in the region of the greater tuberosity. Diagnosis is confirmed by a positive radiograph.

Another important group of disorders that do not typically limit passive glenohumeral range of motion includes acromioclavicular (AC) joint problems. Such patients complain of pain in the region of the AC joint. Symptoms may be aggravated by adducting the affected upper extremity or extreme glenohumeral abduction.

Several intrinsic shoulder conditions limit full passive glenohumeral motion. Adhesive capsulitis generally results from immobilization for a painful condition such as rotator cuff inflammation, glenohumeral arthritis, pulmonary disease, or myocardial infarction. Clinically, patients typically present with poorly localized intense pain about the shoulder. Pain may also be referred to the deltoid insertion. The earliest motion that is lost is external rotation. Disuse atrophy of the shoulder is often present.

Glenohumeral arthritis also tends to limit passive glenohumeral motion. Both inflammatory and degenerative disorders produce painful limitation of motion and a weakness of the shoulder girdle; crepitation is frequently present. The range of motion is limited because of capsulitis. Radiographic findings are characteristic and confirm the diagnosis.

Pyogenic arthritis of the glenohumeral joint must also be considered in the differential diagnosis. Clinically, patients present with pain, swelling, and limitation of shoulder motion. Systemic manifestations are infrequent. The only abnormalities may be a mild elevation of temperature and leukocyte count.

Many extrinsic disorders result in referred pain to the shoulder region. Symptoms may result from irritation of the phrenic nerve. Such patients typically present with pain in the supraclavicular or trapezial regions or at the superior angle of the scapula. Disorders that may produce diaphragmatic irritation include pneumonia, pulmonary infarct, hepatobiliary disease, and subphrenic abscess.

Brachial plexitis is an inflammatory process of uncertain etiology. It may be viral in origin. The majority of patients have involvement of the upper portion of the plexus. Approximately one third of patients recover from symptoms in 1 year, and 90% recover in 3 years (171). Recovery is generally more rapid with lesions of the proximal plexus. Patients who have recurrent or prolonged pain and no sign of motor recovery after 3 months have a poor prognosis. The clinical presentation consists of acute onset of pain and tenderness in the region of the shoulder. Pain is maximal at the time of onset in three-fourths of cases. The pain may be sharp, stabbing, throbbing, or achy in character. Pain may radiate into the scapula or the upper extremity (43). Muscle weakness develops within the first 2 weeks of onset in approximately 70% of patients (171). The most frequent muscles involved include the deltoid, supraspinatus, infraspinatus, serratus anterior, biceps, and triceps (43).

Compressive Neuropathies

The suprascapular nerve originates from the first branch of the brachial plexus and is derived from the C5-C6 roots. Entrapment occurs at the suprascapular notch and produces atrophy of the supraspinatus and infraspinatus muscles. Patients typically exhibit weakness of glenohumeral external rotation and abduction.

The thoracic outlet syndrome may be the result of congenital, developmental, or post-traumatic abnormalities of osseous or soft-tissue structures. Approximately 30% of cases are due to osseous abnormalities including first-rib or clavicular fractures, cervical ribs, or osteochondromas of the clavicles (40). Approximately 70% are due to soft-tissue problems, including involvement of the scalenus anticus, scalenus medius, and pectoralis minor I muscles, and/or fibrous bands. Functional factors play an important role, such as overuse, poor posture, and trauma. Clinical findings include pain in the neck, shoulder, or upper extremity. Paresthesias or weakness may be present. Less commonly there is vascular involvement. Provocative tests include adduction/external rotation, costoclavicular, and hyperabduction tests. Pulse obliteration with the arm and/or head in various positions (Adson's test) is a normal finding in the majority of asymptomatic people and has no relation to the etiology or presence of symptoms (152). Therefore, it is not useful in diagnosing this condition. Patients with upper plexus involvement typically have tenderness with palpation in the region of the C5-C6 roots. Tilting of the head to the opposite side is painful. Patients may have weakness of the biceps, triceps, and wrist. In addition, they may have hypesthesia in the radial nerve distribution. Patients with lower plexus involvement tend to have tenderness in the supraclavicular area and along the course of the ulnar nerve, and weakness of hand grip and interosseous muscles (153).

The median nerve may be compressed at several sites along its anatomic course, producing various neuropathies. Anatomic sites include the supracondylar process, Lacertus fibrosis, pronator teres, arch of the flexor digitorum superficialis, and the carpal tunnel. Carpal tunnel syndrome is the most common entrapment neuropathy of the upper extremity. Patients typically present with pain and paresthesias in the median nerve distribution of the hand. The pain tends to be worse at night and with use of the hand. Clinical examination may include a positive Tinel's sign, a positive Phalen's sign, thenar atrophy, and weakness with altered sensibility in the median nerve distribution of the hand. It is not unusual to find an increased prevalence of cervical arthritis and diabetes in patients with carpal tunnel syndrome. The phenomenon of the "double-crush" syndrome has been suggested as an explanation of this association (173).

The ulnar nerve is typically compressed at two sites: the cubital tunnel and Guyon's canal. Symptoms include aching pain in the medial side of the proximal forearm and paresthesias within the ulnar nerve distribution. Sensory changes include the area supplied by the dorsal cutaneous branch of the ulnar nerve. Weakness of the intrinsic muscles of the hand may also be present.

Shoulder Hand Syndrome

This condition is a type of reflex sympathetic dystrophy (RSD). Typically it results from trauma to the shoulder or upper extremity or from pain due to a visceral lesion such as a stroke or myocardial infarction (98). The pathogenesis includes a "vicious cycle" of pain, immobility, edema, tissue reaction, and vasospasm leading to a stiff, nonfunctional dystrophic extremity (97). Clinically, patients often present with adhesive capsulitis of the shoulder with pain, swelling, and limitation of motion. With time, pain and swelling develop particularly over the dorsum of the hand. Characteristic atrophy of the skin with irreversible flexion deformities of the fingers develop later in the disease process. The diagnosis is typically made on a clinical basis; however, nuclear diagnostic studies may be useful to confirm this condition. A diffusely positive late image on a three-phase bone scan, with all areas showing increased activity, is considered diagnostic of RSD, with both sensitivity and specificity greater than 95% (110).

PRINCIPLES OF TREATMENT

The treatment of a patient with cervical spondylosis should begin with the obvious: a careful clinical history and physical examination. This should be followed by an appropriate diagnostic evaluation to establish an accurate diagnosis. These factors are essential in the successful management of patients with spondylosis; however, they may be easily overlooked.

When considering management of patients with cervical spondylosis, it is important to categorize patients according to the predominance of the signs and symptoms. Patients should be divided into three primary groups: neck pain alone, radiculopathy, and myelopathy. The role of operative management of patients with neck pain alone is controversial and very limited. Certainly there is a role for nonoperative management of patients with radiculopathy and/or myelopathy, and the vast majority of patients are treated in this manner.

Several factors are very important when planning treatment. First, the severity of neurologic involvement must be considered. Second, the rate of progression is important. Patients with a rapidly progressive neurologic deficit may be identified for prompt operative management provided a vascular etiology is ruled out. Duration of symptoms should also be considered. Several studies suggest that patients with cervical spondylitic radiculopathy and/or myelopathy have the best prognosis after operation when symptoms have been of relatively short duration (11,12,29,49,85).

Relative contraindications to operative management include a long history of nonprogressive symptoms (29,49). Patients with profound neurologic deficit may not respond well to operative management. In addition, other disorders of the nervous system may coexist with cervical spondylosis and portend a poorer prognosis from operative management (49). The differential diagnosis must be considered to rule out other disorders that may have a similar clinical presentation. ALS and MS may mimic spondylitic myelopathy (29). In addition, patients with associated cerebrovascular disease, multiple strokes, or low-pressure hydrocephalus may present in a similar manner (27,29,54).

Patients with spinal cord atrophy or myelomalacia on imaging studies may not be good candidates for operative intervention. MRI is particularly helpful in this regard (9,32).

The overall medical status of the patient must be considered when developing a treatment plan. Severe cardiac disease, diabetes melitis, poorly controlled hypertension, as well as various psychological disorders may be contraindications to operative intervention.

The cornerstone of successful nonoperative management of patients with cervical spondylosis is accurate diagnosis. Many patients can be adequately managed with nonsteroidal anti-inflammatory medication, the short-term use of a cervical orthosis, and judicious physical therapy modalities. Physical therapy tends to be most effective when used during acute exacerbations of symptoms. Such treatments include transcutaneous electrical nerve stimulation, ultrasound, neuroprobe, and cervical traction. A double-blind, controlled study of manipulation in patients with chronic neck pain by Sloop et al. (162) failed to show a significant difference between manipulation and control groups. These authors concluded that the value of a single manipulation of the cervical spine has not been established for this condition. Manipulation of the cervical spine may be dangerous in patients with cervical spondylitic myelopathy and is usually contraindicated (170).

One of the most important components of nonoperative treatment is the longitudinal follow-up of patients, including a careful neurologic examination to rule out the development or progression of neurologic signs and symptoms. Because this disease process tends to be slowly progressive, it is important to document the neurologic status of patients at regular intervals to monitor for any insidious change.

Therapeutic injections may have a role in the treatment of patients with cervical spondylosis. Injections should be used judiciously and tend to work best when symptoms are acute. Trigger point and facet injections may provide prompt improvement of symptomatology. Cervical epidural steroid injections (CESI) may have a role in the nonoperative management of patients with cervical pain with or without radicular symptoms. Wilson et al. (185) reported a series of 100 patients who underwent 235 CESIs. Patients in this study had had no previous cervical spine procedures. Complications consisted of a dural puncture rate of 1 in 50 patients. These investigators found that CESI was most effective in patients with radicular pain and signs. CESI supports the pathophysiology of root inflammation as a source of radicular pain.

Pain treatment centers may play an important role in the nonoperative management of patients, particularly those with symptoms of long duration. In addition to traditional treatment modalities including therapeutic injections, many centers use specialized techniques including behavioral modification, biofeedback, acupuncture, and acupressure in the management of such patients. If neck pain becomes chronic, the accompanying psychosocial dysfunction should be addressed through behavioral modification techniques, particularly in such a multidisciplinary setting (166). Patients in long-term treatment for chronic pain should be evaluated periodically to verify the underlying diagnosis and to rule out occult neurologic progression.

Chemonucleolysis has been reported as a treatment option for a herniated cervical disc (149). This treatment, however, is extremely controversial, and certainly the experience in the lumbar spine has been associated with important neurologic risk, including transverse myelitis. A recent review of 38 patients undergoing cervical chemonucleolysis reported good to excellent results in 83% of the cases (149). However, the group of patients who respond best to this type of management are those who respond very effectively to standard treatment modalities, that is, patients with radicular signs and symptoms who have failed nonoperative treatment and have positive neuroradiologic studies that correspond to the clinical signs and symptoms. Contraindications to this procedure include the previous use of chymopapain, cord involvement, cervical spine instability, and isolated neck pain (149). Because of the relative lack of well-controlled studies, one must view this treatment modality for cervical spondylosis with major skepticism at the present time.

Cervical discography may play a role in the management of patients with cervical spondylosis. In general, discography is reserved for those cases in which the diagnosis cannot be established by more traditional methods (65). Indeed, the cervical discogram should be considered last as a diagnostic technique following myelography, CT scan, and/or MRI (30). Diagnostic cervical disc injection may be used to determine symptomatic levels in patients with internal disc derangement. Cervical arthrodesis should be considered only when prolonged treatment fails. As previously mentioned, positive operative results have been reported in approximately two thirds of patients when the pain pattern is reproduced by the injection (182).

It is beyond the scope of this chapter to discuss the operative management of patients with cervical spondylosis. However, it is important to understand the advantages and disadvantages of operative intervention in order to put nonoperative treatment in its proper perspective. There are two basic approaches to the cervical spine: anterior and posterior. Anterior procedures primarily include intervertebral disc excision with or without arthrodesis and vertebrectomy. The major posterior procedures include laminectomy and laminoplasty. Patients with single-level disease and radicular findings may respond adequately to anterior intervertebral disc

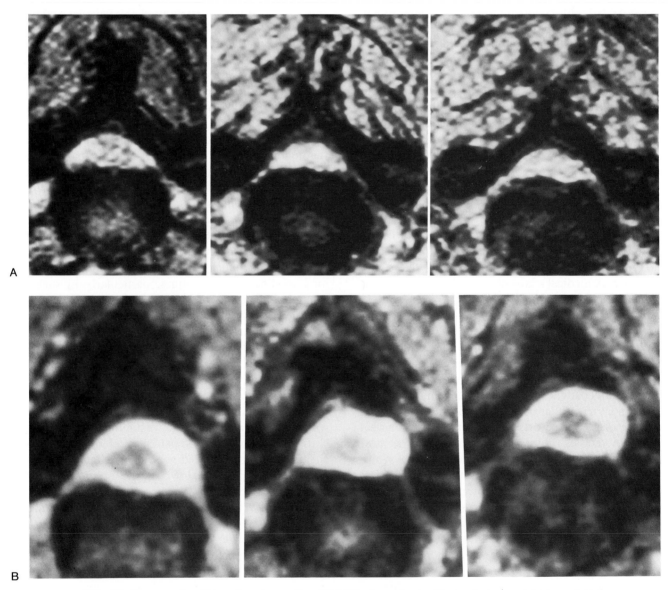

FIG. 10. Preoperative **(A)** and postoperative **(B)** MRI of a patient with cervical spondylosis and early myelopathy who underwent a cervical laminoplasty. The left image in each sequence is C4/C5, the middle image is C5/C6, and the right image is C6/C7. Note the marked increase in space available for the cord after laminaplasty.

excision. Such patients may also respond to posterior laminotomy/laminectomy, with excision of disc material and/or osteophytes encroaching upon the neuroforamen. The number of levels involved may be important in deciding the approach to a patient with cervical spondylitic myelopathy. In general, patients with fewer than two or three levels of involvement may be judiciously managed by an anterior procedure. Patients with greater than three to four levels involved may be best managed by a posterior approach. Certainly there are many different ways to manage myelopathy secondary to cervical spondylosis. Often the procedure that the treating physician is most comfortable with produces the best result. However, it is very important to individualize the operative treatment plan based on the characteristics of the patient as well as the neuroradiographic findings. Therefore, the spine surgeon should be skilled in multiple approaches. The following general principles apply. Patients with central cord compression may be managed most directly with an anterior approach. The most direct approach to a specific anatomic lesion is often the most effective. Cervical kyphosis may be a contraindication to posterior procedures, particularly laminectomy, as adequate decompression may not be obtained and the cord is not allowed to migrate dorsally because of the sagittal plane deformity. A study involving postoperative MRI confirmed that posterior migration of the spinal cord after laminectomy may be inadequate to clear osteophytes in patients with straight or reversed curvatures of the cervical spine (8).

Cervical laminoplasty is playing an increasingly important role in the management of patients with cervical spondylosis (Fig. 10). Yonenobu et al. (188) reviewed a series of patients with cervical spondylitic myelopathy treated operatively and followed for a minimum of 2 years, and concluded that laminoplasty was the treatment of choice for multisegmental cervical spondylitic myelopathy. The Japanese have had a long and successful experience with the use of this procedure in patients with myelopathy secondary to ossification of the posterior longitudinal ligament as well as spondylosis (77,79,93). Laminoplasty has the advantages of maintaining the osseous protection of the spinal cord as well as potentially retaining stability (93). The development of a late swan-neck deformity has been a concern in patients undergoing multilevel laminectomies (38). This may be a particular problem in younger patients with more mobile spines, but is less of a concern in older patients with relatively immobile spines.

Patients treated operatively must be followed up because progression of the underlying disease may occur. Goto et al. (67) found a disturbing prevalence of progressive myelopathy 10 years after operation. These authors noted newly developed intervertebral disc herniation and progression of spondylosis associated with spinal malalignment in both the cephalic and caudal directions,

and reported that MRI was useful in identifying many of the causes.

In summary, many patients with cervical spondylosis can be effectively managed nonoperatively, and in most cases operative intervention is not considered until the patient has undergone an adequate trial of nonoperative management. Certainly, the duration as well as severity of neurologic signs and symptoms are important considerations in this regard. Accurate diagnosis and careful patient selection are essential to the successful management of this condition.

ACKNOWLEDGMENT

The author wishes to acknowledge the assistance of William A. Roberts, M.D., who provided important input for the section on differential diagnosis.

REFERENCES

1. Abbruzzese G, DallAgata D, Morena M, Simonetti S, Spadavecchia L, Severi P, Andrioli GC, Favale E (1988): Electrical stimulation of the motor tracts in cervical spondylosis. *J Neurol Neurosurg Psychiatry* 51:796–802.
2. Aboulker J, Metzger J, David M, Engel P, Balliret J (1965): Les myelopathies cervicals d'origine rachidienne. *Neurochirurgie* 11:87–198.
3. Angelini L, Broggi G, Nardocci N, Savoiardo M (1982): Subacute cervical myelopathy in a child with cerebral palsy. Secondary to torsion dystonia? *Childs Brain* 9:354–357.
4. Austin GM (1960): The significance and nature of pain in tumors of the spinal cord. *Surg Forum* 10:782–785.
5. Badami JP, Norman D, Bardaro NM, Cann CE, Weinstein PR, Sobel DF (1985): Metrizamide CT myelography in cervical myelopathy and radiculopathy: Correlation with conventional myelography and surgical findings. *AJR* 144:675–680.
6. Ball J, Sharp J (1971): Rheumatoid arthritis of the cervical spine. In: Hill AGS, ed. *Modern trends in rheumatology*, Vol. 2. London: Butterworth, p. 117.
7. Barnes MP, Saunders M (1984): The effect of cervical mobility on the natural history of cervical spondylitic myelopathy. *J Neurol Neursurg Psychiatry* 47:17–20.
8. Batzdorf U, Batzdorff A (1988): Analysis of cervical spine curvature in patients with cervical spondylosis. *Neurosurgery* 22:827–836.
9. Batzdorf U, Flannigan BD (1991): Surgical decompressive procedures for cervical spondylitic myelopathy. A study using magnetic resonance imaging. *Spine* 16:123–127.
10. Beatty RM, Fowleer FD, Hanson EJ Jr (1987): The abducted arm as a sign of ruptured cervical disc. *Neurosurgery* 21:731–732.
11. Bernard TN Jr, Whitecloud TS (1987): Cervical spondylitic myelopathy and myeloradiculopathy. Anterior decompression and stabilization with autogenous fibula strut graft. *Clin Orthop* 221:149–160.
12. Bertalanffy H, Eggert HR (1988): Clinical long-term results of anterior discectomy without fusion for treatment of cervical radiculopathy and myelopathy. A follow-up of 164 cases. *Acta Neurochir (Wein)* 90:127–135.
13. Bohlman HH, Sachs BL, Carter JR, Riley L, Robinson RA (1986): Primary neoplasms of the cervical spine. *J Bone Joint Surg [Am]* 68:483–494.
14. Bohlman HH, Emery SE (1988): The pathophysiology of cervical spondylosis and myelopathy. *Spine* 13:843–846.
15. Boni M, Denaro V (1982): The cervical stenosis syndrome with a review of 83 patients treated by operation. *Int Orthop* 6:185–195.
16. Boot DA, Khan RH, Sellar RJ, Hughes SP, Kirkpatrick AE

(1987): Computed tomogram myelopathy in cervical spondylosis. *Int Orthop* 11:249–254.

17. Bovim G, Schrader H, Sand S (1991): Neck pain in the general
population. *Spine* 19:1307–1309.

18. Bradshaw P (1957): Some aspects of cervical spondylosis. *Q J Med* 26:177–208.

19. Breig A, Turnbull I, Hassler O (1966): Effects of mechanical
stresses on the spinal cord in cervical spondylosis: A study on
fresh cadaver material. *J Neurosurg* 25:45–56.

20. Burgerman R, Rigamonti D, Randle JM, Fishman P, Panitch HS,
Johnson KP (1992): The association of cervical spondylosis and
multiple sclerosis. *Surg Neurol* 38:265–270.

21. Burrows EH (1963): The sagittal diameter of the spinal canal in
cervical spondylosis. *Clin Radiol* 14:77–86.

22. Buszek MC, Szymke TE, Honet JC, Raikes JA, Gass HH,
Leuchter W, Bendix SA (1983): Hemidiaphragmatic paralysis:
An unusual complication of cervical spondylosis. *Arch Phys Med Rehabil* 64:601–603.

23. Campbell AM, Phillips DG (1960): Cervical disk lesions with
neurological disorder. Differential diagnosis, treatment, and prognosis. *BMJ* 2:481–485.

24. Chozick BS, Knuckey NW, Epstein MH (1993): Congenital
anomaly of the second cervical vertebra predisposing to progressive cervical myelopathy. *Spine* 18:339–342.

25. Clark CR (1984): Cervical spine involvement in rheumatoid arthritis. A primer for the practitioner. *Iowa Med* 74:57–62.

26. Clark CR (1987): Surgical treatment of bone destruction in the
cervical spine. *Semin Orthop* 2:84–93.

27. Clark CR (1988): Cervical spondylitic myelopathy: History and
physical findings. *Spine* 13:847–849.

28. Clark CR, Goetz DD, Menezes AH (1989): Arthrodesis of the
cervical spine in rheumatoid arthritis. *J Bone Joint Surg [Am]* 71:
381–392.

29. Clark CR (1989): Indications and surgical management of cervical myelopathy. *Semin Spine Surg* 1:254–261.

30. Clark CR (1990): The cervical spine. Pediatric and reconstructive
aspects. In: Pos R, ed. *Orthopaedic knowledge update*,
3rd ed. Park Ridge, Illinois: American Academy of Orthopaedic
Surgeons, pp. 379–394.

31. Clark CR (1993): Rheumatoid arthritis. Surgical considerations.
In: Rothman RH, Simeone FA, eds. *The spine*, 3rd ed. Philadelphia: W.B. Saunders.

32. Clifton AG, Stevens JM, Whitear P, Kendall BE (1990): Identifiable causes for poor outcome in surgery for cervical spondylosis.
Post-operative computed myelography and MR imaging. *Neuroradiology* 32:450–455.

33. Coin CG, Coin JT (1981): Computed tomography of cervical disc
disease. Technical consideration with representative case reports.
J Comput Assist Tomogr 5:275–280.

34. Conlon PW, Isdale IC, Rose BS (1966): Rheumatoid arthritis of
the cervical spine. An analysis of 333 cases. *Ann Rheum Dis* 25:
120–126.

35. Connell MD, Wiesel SW (1992): Natural history and pathogenesis of cervical disk disease. *Orthop Clin North Am* 23:369–380.

36. Connor PM, Darden BV (1993): Cervical discography complications and clinical efficacy. *Spine* 18:2035–2038.

37. Crandall PH, Batzdorf U (1966): Cervical spondylitic myelopathy. *J Neurosurg* 25:57–66.

38. Crandall PH, Gregorius FK (1977): Long-term follow-up of surgical treatment of cervical spondylitic myelopathy. *Spine* 2:139–
146.

39. Daniels DL, Grogan JP, Johansen JG, Meyer GA, Williams AL,
Haughton VM (1984): Cervical radiculopathy. Computed tomography and myelography compared. *Radiology* 151:109–113.

40. Daskalakis MK (1983): Thoracic outlet compression syndrome:
Current concepts and surgical experience. *Int Surg* 68:337–344.

41. Denno JJ, Meadows GR (1991): Early diagnosis of cervical spondylitic myelopathy. A useful clinical sign. *Spine* 16:1353–1355.

42. Di Lazzaro V, Restuccia D, Colosimo C, Tonali P (1992): The
contribution of magnetic stimulation of the motor cortex to the
diagnosis of cervical spondylitic myelopathy. Correlation of central motor conduction to distal and proximal upper limb muscles
with clinical and MRI findings. *Electroencephalogr Clin Neurophysiol* 85:311–320.

43. Dillin L, Hoaglund FT, Schenck M (1985): Brachial neuritis. *J
Bone Joint Surg [Am]* 67:878–883.

44. Di Lorenzo N, Fortuna A (1987): High cervical (C2-C3) spondylogenic myelopathy treated by transoral approach. Case report. *J
Neurosurg Sci* 31:71–74.

45. Dirheimer Y (1977): *The craniovertebral region in chronic inflammatory rheumatic disease.* Berlin: Springer-Verlag.

46. Dobson J (1951): Tuberculosis of the spine. An analysis of the
results of conservative treatment and of the factors influencing
the prognosis. *J Bone Joint Surg [Br]* 33:517–531.

47. Dublin AB, McGahan JP, Reid MH (1983): The value of computed tomographic metrizamide myelography in the neuroradiological evaluation of the spine. *Radiology* 146:79–86.

48. Ebara S, Yonenobu K, Fujiwara K, Yamashita K, Ono K (1988):
Myelopathy hand characterized by muscle wasting. A different
type of myelopathy hand in patients with cervical spondylosis.
Spine 13:785–791.

49. Editorial (1984): Management of cervical spondylitic myelopathy. *Lancet* 1:1058.

50. Edwards WC, LaRocca H (1983): The developmental segmental
sagittal diameter of the cervical spine canal in patients with cervical spondylosis. *Spine* 8:20–27.

51. Edwards WC, LaRocca H (1985): The developmental segmental
sagittal diameter in combined cervical and lumbar spondylosis.
Spine 10:42–49.

52. Ehni G (1982): Extradural spinal cord and nerve root compression from benign lesions of the cervical area. In: Youmans JR, ed.
Neurological surgery, Vol. 4. Philadelphia: W.B. Saunders, pp.
2574–2612.

53. Epstein JA, Janin Y, Carras R, Lavine LS (1982): A comparative
study of the treatment of cervical spondylitic myeloradiculopathy. Experience with 50 cases treated by means of extensive laminectomy, foraminotomy, and excision of osteophytes during the
past 10 years. *Acta Neurochir (Wein)* 61:89–104.

54. Epstein JA (1985): Management of cervical spinal stenosis, spondylosis and myeloradiculopathy. In: Tindall GT, ed. *Contemporary neurosurgery*, Vol. 7. Baltimore: Williams and Wilkins, pp.
1–6.

55. Epstein NE, Epstein JA, Carras R, Murphy VS, Hyman RA
(1984): Coexisting cervical and lumbar spinal stenosis. Diagnosis
and management. *Neurosurgery* 15:489–496.

56. Epstein NE, Hyman RA, Epstein JA, Rosenthal AD (1988): Dynamic MRI scanning of the cervical spine. *Spine* 13:937–938.

57. Epstein NE, Epstein JA, Carras R (1989): Coexisting cervical
spondylitic myelopathy and bilateral carpal tunnel syndromes. *J
Spinal Disord* 2:36–42.

58. Fielding JW, Cochran Gvan B, Lawsing JF 3rd, Holh M (1974):
Tears of the transverse ligament of the atlas. A clinical and biomechanical study. *J Bone Joint Surg [Am]* 56:1683–1691.

59. Flynn JM (1991): Anterior cervical osteophytes causing dysphagia. *Bol Asoc Med P R* 83:47–53.

60. Foo D (1986): Spinal cord injury in forty-four patients with cervical spondylosis. *Paraplegia* 24:301–306.

61. Forsythe M, Rothman RH (1978): New concepts in the diagnosis
and treatment of infections of the cervical spine. *Orthop Clin
North Am* 9:1039–1051.

62. Garcia A Jr, Grantham SA (1960): Hematogenous pyogenic vertebral osteomyelitis. *J Bone Joint Surg [Am]* 42:429–436.

63. Good DC, Couch Jr, Wacaser L (1984): Numb, clumsy hands
and high cervical spondylosis. *Surg Neurol* 22:285–291.

64. Good CJ, Mikkelsen GB (1992): Intersegmental sagittal motion
in the lower cervical spine and discogenic spondylosis: A preliminary study. *J Manipulative Physiol Ther* 15:556–564.

65. Gore DR, Sepic SB (1984): Anterior cervical fusion for degenerated or protruded discs. A review of one hundred forty-six patients. *Spine* 9:667–671.

66. Gore DR, Sepic SB, Gardner GM, Murray MP (1987): Neck pain.
A long-term follow-up of 205 patients. *Spine* 12:1–5.

67. Goto S, Mochizuki M, Watanabe T, Hiramatu K, Tanno T, Kitahara H, Moriya H (1993): Long-term follow-up study of anterior surgery for cervical spondylitic myelopathy with special reference to the magnetic resonance imaging findings in 52 cases.
Clin Orthop 291:142–153.

68. Gregorius FK, Estrin T, Crandall PH (1976): Cervical spondylitic

radiculopathy and myelopathy. A long-term follow-up study. *Arch Neurol* 33:618–625.

69. Harrington KD (1986): Metastatic disease of the spine. *J Bone Joint Surg [Am]* 68:1110–1115.

70. Hattori T, Sakakibara R, Yasuda K, Murayama N, Hirayama K (1990): Micturitional disturbance in cervical spondylitic myelopathy. *J Spinal Disord* 3:16–18.

71. Hawkins RJ (1985): Cervical spine and the shoulder. *Instr Course Lect* 34:191–195.

72. Hayashi K, Tabuchi K, Yabuki T, Kurokawa T, Seki H (1977): The position of the superior articular process of the cervical spine. Its relationship to cervical spondylitic radiculopathy. *Radiology* 124:501–503.

73. Heiskari M, Siivola J, Heikkinen ER (1986): Somatosensory evoked potentials in evaluation of decompressive surgery of cervical spondylosis and herniated disc. *Ann Clin Res* 47(18 Suppl):107–113.

74. Heller CA, Stanley P, Lewis-Jones B, Heller RF (1983): Value of x-ray examinations of the cervical spine. *BMJ* 287:1276–1278.

75. Heller JG (1992): The syndromes of degenerative cervical disease. *Orthop Clin North Am* 23:381–394.

76. Hensinger RN (1984): Cervical spine: Pediatric. In: Asher MA, ed. *Orthopedic knowledge update,* 1st ed. Park Ridge, Illinois: American Academy of Orthopaedic Surgery, p. 191.

77. Herkowitz HN (1989): The surgical management of cervical spondylitic radiculopathy and myelopathy. *Clin Orthop* 239:94–108.

78. Hirabayashi K, Miyakawa J, Satomi K, Maruyama T, Wakano K (1981): Operative results and postoperative progression of ossification among patients with ossification of cervical posterior longitudinal ligament. *Spine* 6:354–364.

79. Hirabayashi K, Satomi K (1988): Operative procedure and results of expensive open-door laminoplasty. *Spine* 13:870–876.

80. Hirano H, Suzuki H, Sakakibara T, Higuchi Y, Inove K, Suzuki Y (1982): Dysphagia due to hypertrophic cervical osteophytes. *Clin Orthop* 167:168–172.

81. Hirose G, Kadoya S (1984): Cervical spondylitic radiculomyelopathy in patients with athetoid-dystonic cerebral palsy: Clinical evaluation and surgical treatment. *J Neurol Neurosurg Psychiatry* 47:775–780.

82. Holzman RS, Bishko F (1971): Osteomyelitis in heroin addicts. *Ann Intern Med* 75:693–696.

83. Hoff JT, Wilson CB (1877): The pathophysiology of cervical spondylitic radiculopathy and myelopathy. *Clin Neurosurg* 24:474–487.

84. Hsu LCS, Yau ACMC (1983): Infections: Tuberculosis. In: Bailey RW, ed. *The cervical spine,* 1st ed. Philadelphia: J.B. Lippincott, pp. 336–355.

85. Hukuda S, Mochizuki T, Okata M, Shichikawa K, Shimomura Y (1985): Operations for cervical spondylitic myelopathy. A comparison of the results of anterior and posterior procedures. *J Bone Joint Surg [Br]* 67:609–615.

86. Hunt WE (1980): Cervical spondylosis: Natural history and rare indications for surgical decompression. *Clin Neurosurg* 27:466–480.

87. Iansek R, Heywood J, Karnaghan J, Balla JI (1987): Cervical spondylosis and headaches. *Clin Exp Neurol* 23:175–178.

88. Jabbari B, Pierce JF, Boston S, Echols DM (1977): Brown-Sequard syndrome and cervical spondylosis. *J Neurosurg* 47:556–560.

89. Jaskolski DJ, Jarratt JA, Jakubowski J (1989): Clinical evaluation of magnetic stimulation in cervical spondylosis. *Br J Neurosurg* 3:541–548.

90. Jaskolski DJ, Laing RJ, Jarratt JA, Jukubowski J (1990): Pre and postoperative motor conduction times, measured using magnetic stimulation, in patients with cervical spondylosis. *Br J Neurosurg* 4:187–192.

91. Kadoya S, Nakamura T, Kwak R, Hirose G (1985): Anterior osteophytectomy for cervical spondylitic myelopathy in developmentally narrow canal. *J Neursosurg* 63:845–850.

92. Khan MR, McInnes A, Hughes SP (1989): Electrophysiological studies in cervical spondylosis. *J Spinal Disord* 2:163–169.

93. Kimura I, Oh-Hama M, Shingu H (1984): Cervical myelopathy treated by canal-expansive laminaplasty. Computed tomographic and myelographic findings. *J Bone Joint Surg [Am]* 66:914–920.

94. Koyanagi T, Hirabayashi K, Satomi K, Toyama Y, Fujimura Y (1993): Predictability of operative results of cervical compression myelopathy based on preoperative computed tomographic myelography. *Spine* 18:1958–1963.

95. Lambert JR, Tepperman PS, Jimenez J, Newman A (1081): Cervical spine disease and dysphagia. Four new cases and a review of the literature. *Am J Gastroenterol* 76:35–40.

96. Landman JA, Hoffman JC Jr, Braum IF, Barrow DL (1984): Value of computed tomographic myelography in the recognition of cervical herniated disk. *AJNR* 5:391–394.

97. Lankford LL, Thompson JE (1977): Reflex sympathetic dystrophy, upper and lower extremity: Diagnosis and management. *Instr Course Lect* 26:163–178.

98. Lankford LL (1983): Reflex sympathetic dystrophy. In: Evarts CM, ed. *Surgery of the musculoskeletal system.* New York: Churchill Livingstone, pp. 145–201.

99. Laroche M, Moulinier L, Ariet J, Arrue P, Rousseau H, Cantagrel A, Mazieres B (1992): Lumbar and cervical stenosis. Frequency of the association, role of the ankylosing hyperostosis. *Clin Rheumatol* 11:533–535.

100. Lebhluber F, Reisecker F, Boehm-Jurkovic H, Witzmann A, Diesenhammer E (1988): Diagnostic value of different electrophysiologic tests in cervical disk prolapse. *Neurology* 38:1879–1881.

101. Lee KS, Kelly DL Jr (1987): Amyotrophic lateral sclerosis and severe cervical spondylitic myelopathy in a patient with a posterior fossa arachnoid cyst: Diagnostic dilemma. *South Med J* 80:1580–1583.

102. Lees F, Turner JW (1963): Natural history and prognosis of cervical spondylosis. *BMJ* 2:1607–1610.

103. Leonard A, Comty CM, Shapiro FL, et al. (1973): Osteomyelitis in hemodialysis patients. *Ann Intern Med* 78:651–658.

104. Lestini WF, Wiesel SW (1989): The pathogenesis of cervical spondylosis. *Clin Orthop* 239:69–93.

105. Lipson SJ (1984): Rheumatoid arthritis of the cervical spine. *Clin Orthop* 182:143–149.

106. Long DM (1983): Cervical cord tumors. In: Bailey RW, ed. *The cervical spine,* 1st ed. Philadelphia: J.B. Lippincott, pp. 323–335.

107. Lunsford LD, Bissonette DJ, Zorub DS (1980): Anterior surgery for cervical disc disease. Part 2: Treatment of cervical spondylitic myelopathy in 32 cases. *J Neurosurg* 53:12–19.

108. MacFadyen DJ (1984): Posterior column dysfunction in cervical spondylitic myelopathy. *Can J Neurol Sci* 11:365–370.

109. Macnab I (1975): Cervical spondylosis. *Clin Orthop* 109:69–77.

110. Mackinnon SE, Holder LE (1984): The use of three-phase radionuclide bone scanning in the diagnosis of reflex sympathetic dystrophy. *J Hand Surg [Am]* 9:556–563.

111. Maertens-de-Noordhout A, Remacle JM, Pepin JL, Born JD, Delwaide PJ (1991): Magnetic stimulation of the motor cortex in cervical spondylosis. *Neurology* 41:75–80.

112. el-Mallakh RS, Rao K, Barwick M (1989): Cervical myelopathy secondary to movement disorders: Case report. *Neurosurgery* 24:902–905.

113. Martel W (1961): The occipito-atlanto-axial joints in rheumatoid arthritis and ankylosing spondylitis. *AJR* 86:223–240.

114. Marti-Fabregas J, Martinez JM, Illa I, Escartin A (1989): Myelopathy of unknown etiology. A clinical follow-up and MRI study of 57 cases. *Acta Neurol Scand* 80:455–460.

115. Martin NS (1970): Tuberculosis of the spine: A study of the results of treatment during the last twenty-five years. *J Bone Joint Surg [Br]* 52:613–628.

116. Masaryk TJ, Modic MT, Geisinger MA, Standefer J, Hardy RW, Boumphrey F, Duchesneau PM (1986): Cervical myelopathy: A compression of magnetic resonance and myelography. *J Comput Assist Tomogr* 10:184–194.

117. Mathews JA (1969): Atlanto-axial subluxation in rheumatoid arthritis. *Ann Rheum Dis* 28:260–266.

118. Mayfield FH (1979): Cervical spondylitic radiculopathy and myelopathy. *Adv Neurol* 22:307–321.

119. McAfee PC, Regan JJ, Bohlman HH (1987): Cervical cord compression from ossification of the posterior longitudinal ligament in non-Orientals. *J Bone Joint Surg [Br]* 69:569–575.

120. McFarlin DE, McFarland HF (1982): Multiple sclerosis (second of two parts). *N Engl J Med* 107:1246–1251.

121. McLain RF (1994): Mechanoreceptor endings in human cervical facet joints. *Spine* 19:495–501.

122. McLaughlin HL (1962): Rupture of the rotator cuff. *J Bone Joint Surg [Am]* 44:979–983.

123. Mehalic TF, Pezzuti RT, Applebaum BI (1990): Magnetic resonance imaging and cervical spondylitic myelopathy. *Neurosurgery* 26:217–217.

124. Meikle JA, Wilkinson M: Rheumatoid involvement of the cervical spine. *Ann Rheum Dis* 30:154–161.

125. Modic MT, Ross JS, Masaryk TJ (1989): Imaging of degenerative disease of the cervical spine. *Clin Orthop* 239:109–120.

126. Nagata K, Kiyonaga K, Ohashi T, Sagara M, Miyazaki S, Inoue A (1990): Clinical value of magnetic resonance imaging for cervical myelopathy. *Spine* 15:1088–1096.

127. Nakagawa H, Okumura T, Sugiyama T, Iwata K (1983): Discrepancy between metrizamide CT and myelography in diagnosis of cervical disk protrusions. *AJNR* 6:604–606.

128. Neer CS 2nd (1983): Impingement lesions. *Clin Orthop* 173:70–77.

129. Northfield DW (1955): Diagnosis and treatment of myelopathy due to cervical spondylosis. *BMJ* 2:1474–1477.

130. Nurick S (1972): The pathogenesis of the spinal cord disorder associated with cervical spondylosis. *Brain* 95:87–100.

131. Nurick S (1972): The natural history and the results of surgical treatment of the spinal cord disorder associated with cervical spondylosis. *Brain* 95:101–108.

132. Okada Y, Ikata T, Yamada T, Sak R, Katoh S (1993): Magnetic resonance imaging study the results of surgery for cervical compression myelopathy. *Spine* 18:2024–2029.

133. Olive PM, Whitecloud TS, Bennett JT (1988): Lower cervical spondylosis and myelopathy in adults with Down syndrome. *Spine* 13:781–784.

134. Palmer PE, Stadalnick R, Arnon S (1984): The genetic factor in cervical spondylosis. *Skeletal Radiol* 11:178–182.

135. Panjabi M, White A 3rd (1988): Biomechanics of nonacute cervical spinal cord trauma. *Spine* 13:838–842.

136. Parke WW (1988): Correlative anatomy of cervical spondylitic myelopathy. *Spine* 13:831–837.

137. Paty DW, Poser C (1984): Clinical symptoms and signs of multiple sclerosis. In: Poser CM, ed. *The diagnosis of multiple sclerosis*. New York: Thieme-Stratton, pp. 27–43.

138. Paulson DL (1975): Carcinomas in the superior pulmonary sulcus. *J Thorac Cardiovasc Surg* 70:1095–1104.

139. Payne EE (1959): The cervical spine and spondylosis. *Neurochirurgia* 1:178–196.

140. Pellicci PM, Ranawat CS, Tsairis P, Bryan WJ: A prospective study of the progression of rheumatoid arthritis of the cervical spine. *J Bone Joint Surg [Am]* 63:342–350.

141. Perlik SJ, Fisher MA (1987): Somatosensory evoked response evaluation of cervical spondylitic myelopathy. *Muscle Nerve* 10:481–489.

142. Peterson DI, Dayes LA (1977): Myelopathy associated with cervical spondylosis: A frequently unrecognized disease. *J Fam Pract* 4:233–236.

143. Polk JL, Maragos VA, Nicholas JJ (1992): Cervical spondylitic myeloradiculopathy in dystonia. *Arch Phys Med Rehabil* 73:389–392.

144. Rahim KA, Stambough JL (1992): Radiographic evaluation of the degenerative cervical spine. *Orthop Clin North Am* 23:395–403.

145. Rasker JJ, Cosh JA (1978): Radiological study of cervical spine and hand in patients with rheumatoid arthritis of 15 years' duration: An assessment of the effect of corticosteroid treatment. *Ann Rheum Dis* 37:529–535.

146. Regenbogen VS, Rogers LF, Atlas SW, Kim KS (1986): Cervical spinal cord injuries in patients with cervical spondylosis. *AJR* 146:277–284.

147. Restuccia D, Di-Lazzaro V, Lo-Monaco M, Evoli A, Valeriani M, Tonali P (1992): Somatosensory evoked potentials in the diagnosis of cervical spondylitic myelopathy. *Electromyogr Clin Neurophysiol* 32:389–395.

148. Restuccia D, Di-Lazzaro V, Valeriani M, Tonali P, Mauguiere F (1992): Segmental dysfunction of the cervical cord revealed by abnormalities of the spinal N13 potential in cervical spondylitic myelopathy. [Published erratum appears in *Neurology* 1992 Aug; 42:1614–1615.] *Neurology* 42:1054–1063.

149. Richaud J, Lazorthes Y, Verdie JC, Bonafe A (1988): Chemonucleolysis for herniated cervical disc. *Acta Neurochir (Wein)* 91:116–119.

150. Roberts AH (1966): Myelopathy due to cervical spondylosis treated by collar immobilization. *Neurology* 16:951–954.

151. Robinson RA, Afeiche N, Dunn EJ, Northrop BE (1977): Cervical spondylitic myelopathy: Etiology and treatment concepts. *Spine* 2:89.

152. Roos DB (1976): Congenital anomalies associated with thoracic outlet syndrome: Anatomy, symptoms, diagnosis and treatment. *Am J Surg* 132:771–778.

153. Roos DB (1982): The place for scalenectomy and first-rib resection in thoracic outlet syndrome. *Surgery* 92:1077–1085.

154. Schlesinger ED, Antunes JL, Michelsen WJ, Louis KM (1981): Hydromyelia: Clinical presentation and compression of modalities of treatment. *Neurosurgery* 9:356–365.

155. Schmorl G, Junghann S (1932): *Die gesunde and kranke wirbel saule in Rontgenbild*. Leipzig.

156. Scotti G, Scialfa G, Pieralli S, Boccardi E, Valsecchi F, Tonon C (1983): Myelopathy and radiculopathy due to cervical spondylosis. Myelographic-CT correlations. *AJNR* 4:601–603.

157. Scoville WB (1961): Cervical spondylosis treated by bilateral facetectomy and laminectomy. *J Neurosurg* 18:423–428.

158. Sharp J, Purser DW, Lawrence JS (1958): Rheumatoid arthritis of the cervical spine in the adult. *Ann Rheum Dis* 17:303–313.

159. Sharp J, Purser DW (1961): Spontaneous atlanto-axial dislocation in ankylosing spondylitis and rheumatoid arthritis. *Ann Rheum Dis* 20:47–77.

160. Shaw RR (1984): Pancoast's tumor. *Ann Thorac Surg* 37:343–345.

161. Simeone FA, Rothman RH (1982): Cervical disc disease. In: Rothman RH, Simeone FA, eds. *The spine*. Philadelphia: W.B. Saunders, pp. 440–476.

162. Sloop PR, Smith DS, Goldenberg E, Dore C (1982): Manipulation for chronic neck pain. A double-blind controlled study. *Spine* 7:532–535.

163. Stevens JC, Cartlidge NE, Saunders M, Appleby A, Hall M, Shaw DA (1971): Atlanto-axial subluxation and cervical myelopathy in rheumatoid arthritis. *Q J Med* 40:391–408.

164. Stone DB, Bonfiglio M (1963): Pyogenic vertebral osteomyelitis. A diagnostic pitfall for the internist. *Arch Intern Med* 112:491–500.

165. Tammela TL, Heiskari MJ, Lukkarinen OA (1992): Voiding dysfunction and urodynamic findings in patients with cervical spondylitic spinal stenosis compared with severity of the disease. *Br J Urol* 70:144–148.

166. Tan JC, Nordin M (1992): Role of physical therapy in the treatment of cervical disk disease. *Orthop Clin North Am* 23:435–449.

167. Tang XF, Ren ZY (1991): Magnetic transcranial motor and somatosensory evoked potentials in cervical spondylitic myelopathy. *Clin Med J (Engl)* 104:409–415.

168. Torg JS, Pavlov H, Genuario SE, Sennett B, Wisneski RJ, Robie BH, Jahre C (1986): Neurapraxia of the cervical spinal cord with transient quadriplegia. *J Bone Joint Surg [Am]* 68:1354–1370.

169. Torg JS (1989): Pavlov's ratio: Determining cervical spinal stenosis on routine lateral roentgenograms. *Contemp Orthop* 18:153–160.

170. Toto BJ (1986): Cervical spondylitic myelopathy: A case report. *J Manipulative Physiol Ther* 9:43–46.

171. Tsairis P, Dyck PJ, Mulder DW (1972): Natural history of brachial plexus neuropathy. *Arch Neurol* 27:109–117.

172. Uhthoff HK, Sarkar K, Gomez J (1977): Calcifying tendinitis: A new concept of its pathophysiology. In: Abstracts XV. *Int Congress Rheum;* p. 106.

173. Upton AR, McComas AJ (1973): The double crush in nerve entrapment syndromes. *Lancet* 2:359–362.

174. Valergakis FE (1976): Cervical spondylosis: Most common cause of position and vibratory sense loss. *Geriatrics* 31:51–56.

175. Van-Wellen P, Klaes R, De-Boeck H (1989): Hypertrophic cervi-

cal osteophytes presenting with pharyngeal symptoms. *Acta Orthop Belg* 55:599–603.

176. Veidlinger OF, Colwill JC, Smyth HS, Turner D (1981): Cervical myelopathy and its relationship to cervical stenosis. *Spine* 6:550–552.

177. Verbiest H (1973): The management of cervical spondylosis. *Clin Neurosurg* 20:262–294.

178. Weidner A, Immenkamp M (1981): The operative management of extradural tumors of the cervical spine. *Orthop Trans* 5:116.

179. Weinstein JN, McLain RF (1987): Primary tumors of the spine. *Spine* 12:843–851.

180. White AA 3rd, Panjabi MM (1988): Biomechanical considerations in the surgical management of cervical spondylitic myelopathy. *Spine* 13:856–860.

181. Whitecloud TS (1983): Management of the radiculopathy and myelopathy by the anterior approach. In: Bailey R, ed. *The cervical spine*. Philadelphia: J.B. Lippincott, pp. 411–424.

182. Whitecloud TS 3rd, Seago RA (1987): Cervical discogenic syndrome: Results of operative intervention in patients with positive discography. *Spine* 12:313–316.

183. Wilberger JE Jr, Chedid MK (1988): Acute cervical spondylitic myelopathy. *Neurosurgery* 22:145–146.

184. Williams B (1979): Orthopaedic features in the presentation of syringomyelia. *J Bone Joint Surg [Br]* 61:314–323.

185. Wilson SP, Iacobo C, Rocco AG, Ferrante FM, Lipson SJ (1989): *Cervical epidural steroid injection (CESI): Clinical classification as predictor of therapeutic outcome.* Read before the annual meeting of the Cervical Spine Research Society, New Orleans.

186. Wolf BS, Khiinani M, Malis LI (1956): The sagittal diameter of the bony cervical spinal canal and its significance in cervical spondylosis. *J Mt Sinai Hosp* 23:283–292.

187. Yone K, Sakou T, Yanase M, Ijiri K (1992): Preoperative and postoperative magnetic resonance image evaluation of the spinal cord in cervical myelopathy. *Spine* 17(10 Suppl):S388–S392.

188. Yonenobu K, Hosono N, Iwasaki M, Asano M, Ono K (1992): Laminoplasty versus subtotal corpectomy. A comparative study of results in multisegmental cervical spondylitic myelopathy. *Spine* 17:1281–1284.

The Adult Spine: Principles and Practice,
2nd edition, J.W. Frymoyer, Editor-in-Chief.
Lippincott-Raven Publishers, Philadelphia © 1997.

CHAPTER **64**

Thoracic Outlet Syndrome

James N. Campbell

Physicians who see patients with pain or neurological problems in the neck and upper extremities encounter patients with so-called thoracic outlet syndrome (TOS). TOS refers to a group of disorders characterized by compression of the structures that pass between the neck and chest. Indeed, patients with cervical spondylosis may present with symptoms similar to those of TOS. In this chapter, the etiology, diagnosis, and treatment of these disorders will be considered.

The term *thoracic outlet syndrome* is inaccurate (12): the true thoracic outlet is at the level of the diaphragm. The syndromes discussed herein actually occur in the thoracic inlet. The thoracic inlet provides passage for the subclavian artery, the subclavian vein, and the brachial plexus. Accordingly, three clinical syndromes may occur in patients with compressive lesions in this region: arterial obstruction, venous obstruction, and brachial plexus compression. Compression of the brachial plexus is by far the most common form of TOS.

ANATOMY

The thoracic inlet (10) is formed rostrally by the scalenic triangle. This triangle is formed by the first thoracic rib below and the anterior and middle scalene muscles in

front and behind, respectively, as shown in Figure 1. The scalene muscles arise from the anterior tubercle of the transverse process of cervical vertebrae and insert on the first thoracic rib. A key anatomic relationship is the passage of the subclavian vein in front of the anterior scalene muscle, and the passage of the subclavian artery posterior and lateral to the scalene muscle. After going through the scalenic triangle, the neurovascular bundle passes through the costoclavicular space bordered by the clavicle, the subclavian muscle superiorly, and the first thoracic rib below.

Cervical ribs are often discussed in the context of TOS, but their role in producing symptoms is far from clear. In patients with intrinsic muscle wasting of the hands attributable to brachial plexus compression, cervical ribs are common. Otherwise, the presence of cervical ribs is not particularly helpful diagnostically. Occasionally, it is possible to palpate the cervical rib in the supraclavicular fossa. If this area is tender, it may be inferred that the cervical rib plays some role in the symptoms.

Congenital bands are thought by many to play an important role in the production of TOS (14). Many varieties have been described and attempts have been made to classify them. For example, bands have been described that arise anomalously from the cervical vertebrae and course across the brachial plexus to insert on the first thoracic rib. A band may course on the inside of the first rib and compress and elevate the T1 root. Bands may also be associated with Sibson's fascia.

Patients with TOS are often women with long necks

J. N. Campbell, M.D.: Professor, Department of Neurosurgery, Johns Hopkins University School of Medicine, Baltimore, Maryland, 21287-7509.

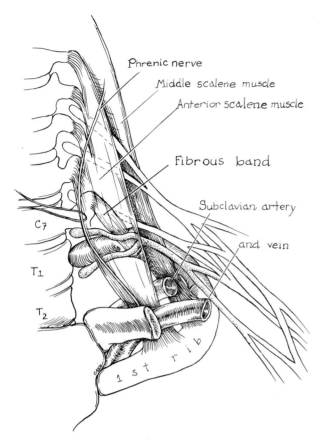

FIG. 1. The relationship of vascular and normal structures in the scalenic triangle. An anomalous fibrous band is seen compressing the C7, C8, and T1 roots.

and sloping shoulders. The ability to see the T2 vertebra on a standard lateral cervical spine x-ray is common in these patients. An anatomic explanation for this is that the first thoracic rib is high relative to the plexus and vessels, which are therefore compressed as they pass over the rib.

Anomalies undoubtedly play an important role in TOS. However, the onset of symptoms often occurs immediately after a traumatic event (11). Although trauma should be considered a contributing cause, it may not by itself be sufficient to cause TOS. Most likely, TOS is caused by a combination of a congenital anomaly and a precipitating traumatic event (7).

COMPRESSION OF THE BRACHIAL PLEXUS

Entrapment neuropathy of the brachial plexus is the most common form of TOS (1). Just as with carpal tunnel syndrome (CTS) and various spinal disorders, some patients present with pain but little or no neurological deficit, whereas others present with an impressive degree of neurological deficit but little or no pain (6). The ele-

ments of the plexus most commonly affected in TOS are the C8 and T1 roots and the lower trunk. The signs and symptoms thus relate to these structures.

Differential Diagnosis of Intrinsic Muscle Weakness in the Hand

Intrinsic weakness with thenar involvement means that there is involvement of muscles innervated by both median and ulnar nerves. There are two clinically useful intrinsic muscle to test. The first dorsal interosseus muscle, which abducts the index finger, is innervated by the ulnar nerve and is easily visualized on the dorsum of the hand between the index finger and the thumb. The abductor pollicis brevis muscle, which abducts the thumb in a direction perpendicular to the plane of the palm, is innervated by the median nerve and is easily visualized in the thenar eminence.

The differential diagnosis for intrinsic hand weakness includes (a) an intramedullary lesion of the spinal cord (e.g., syringomyelia), (b) a lower plexus lesion, (c) a dual lesion of the ulnar and median nerves, and (d) TOS. Diminished reflexes and a dissociated sensory loss point to an intramedullary lesion, in particular when there are bilateral findings. Nerve conduction studies will typically distinguish entrapment neuropathies of the median and ulnar nerves from TOS. The sensory nerve action potential helps distinguish plexus lesions from spinal root and spinal cord lesions. With nerve root lesions (e.g., foraminal lesions from disc herniations) and spinal cord lesions, the involvement of sensory fibers is proximal to the dorsal root ganglion, and thus the sensory nerve action potential is unaffected. However, with plexus lesions, the sensory fibers are affected distal to the dorsal root ganglion, so the sensory nerve action potential is reduced.

Cervical ribs are often present in TOS in cases where there is intrinsic muscle weakness. However, cervical ribs are frequently present in patients who do not have TOS.

Malignant lesions should always be considered in patients who present with TOS symptoms. All patients suspected of having TOS should be inspected for the presence of Horner's syndrome, which may be the harbinger of a tumor at the apex of the lung with compromise of the brachial plexus (Pancoast syndrome). Brachial plexus metastases from breast carcinoma can result in TOS; there may be a palpable mass in the axilla.

There is a rare form of muscular atrophy that occurs typically in the juvenile years that involves the intrinsic muscles of the hand. There is rapid progression of weakness for two or three years, then slower progression in the years that follow. The cause is unknown. Absence of sensory involvement and pain distinguishes this syndrome from thoracic outlet syndrome (15).

Patients with TOS most commonly present with the complaint of pain but without clear signs of weakness. Quite often in these patients, the neurological examination is normal. Patients often ascribe the onset of symptoms to a particular event such as an auto accident, a fall, or a blow to the shoulder. Other patients have a more insidious onset of symptoms and may relate them to particular job-related routine tasks. A teacher may indicate that symptoms are brought on by writing on the blackboard. A cellist may ascribe symptoms to holding the left arm in an abducted position. A painter may ascribe symptoms to painting a ceiling.

Symptoms include pain in the region of the supraclavicular fossa, upper arm, and hand, particularly in the ulnar distribution. Pain is worsened by arm abduction in the majority of cases. There are four signs, some or all of which may be present in this form of TOS:

1. Distinct tenderness in the supraclavicular fossa.
2. Tinel's sign in the supraclavicular fossa. Tapping this area with the head turned to the contralateral direction evokes tingling paresthesias in the hand.
3. Tingling paresthesias in the hand with downward tugging on the arm.
4. Tingling paresthesias in the hand with abduction of the arm to a position above the head.

When all of these signs are present, the patient quite likely has TOS. In the majority of cases, however, the patient presents with only some aspects of the syndrome. The key, therefore, is to consider what other conditions may have similar presentations. Before CTS was appreciated as a common entrapment neuropathy, TOS was cited as the cause of the finger numbness and hand weakness that was probably due to carpal tunnel syndrome. The advent of nerve conduction studies and knowledge of the features of CTS makes it unlikely that CTS will continue to be confused with TOS.

Ulnar neuropathy may also be confused with TOS, because lower plexus lesions (C8 and T1 root lesions) and ulnar neuropathy give rise to sensory symptoms on the ulnar aspect of the hand. Positive nerve conduction studies, absence of involvement of the abductor pollicis brevis, Tinel's sign at the elbow, and clear sensory changes on the ulnar (as opposed to the radial) aspect of the ring finger, all serve to help distinguish the two disorders.

It is more difficult to distinguish cervical spondylosis from TOS. A patient with a disc herniation in the cervical spine may present with symptoms that closely mimic TOS. Even a disc herniation at C4-C5 may lead to pain and sensory symptoms in an ulnar distribution. The following findings are helpful:

1. Patients with cervical spondylosis, but not with TOS, have pain with hyperextension of the neck.
2. Patients with cervical spondylosis may have tenderness in the region of the trapezius, whereas patients with TOS tend to have more tenderness in the supraclavicular fossa.
3. Arm abduction usually does not lead to paresthesias in the hand in patients with cervical spondylosis.
4. A positive Tinel's sign in the supraclavicular fossa is highly specific for TOS.
5. Patients with cervical spondylosis may have tenderness over the spinous processes, unlike those with TOS.
6. Patients with TOS are much more likely to complain of anterior chest pain and pain radiating to the angle of the jaw.

Another word of caution is in order. It is "neater" if patients have only one diagnosis that accounts for their symptoms. However, patients with TOS frequently have more than one diagnosis. For example, ulnar nerve entrapments at the elbow and radial tunnel syndrome appear to coexist with TOS in some patients.

ANCILLARY TESTS

Plain x-rays are helpful to examine the cervicothoracic junction for cervical ribs. Recently, magnetic resonance imaging (MRI) of the thoracic inlet has been used to look for distortion in the course of the plexus and vessels; the MRI scan has been cited to be both moderately sensitive and specific for TOS (9). Electromyogram studies are useful whenever muscle atrophy is suspected. Nerve conduction studies probably do not contribute to the diagnosis, except when there are clear neurological signs.

VASCULAR COMPRESSION SYNDROMES

Subclavian artery compression and subclavian vein compression represent additional types of TOS. In most series, these cases account for less than 10% of all cases.

Patients with arterial compression present with symptoms and signs of loss of blood supply to the arm and hand with arm abduction maneuvers. Pain and tingling paresthesias referred to the hand in a vague distribution may occur when the arm is abducted and externally rotated at the shoulder. Less commonly, patients may develop poststenotic dilatation and aneurysmal formation. Some of these patients present with distal thromboembolic complications. There may or may not be an associated cervical rib.

Another group of patients present with signs and symptoms of subclavian vein compromise (also referred to as Pajet–von Schrötter syndrome). These patients complain of hand swelling, bluish discoloration of the hand, and arm pain after exertion or maneuvers that require shoulder abduction. At the time of presentation, patients may have frank thrombosis of the subclavian vein. Because vigorous activity may induce the thrombosis, this entity is also known as effort thrombosis (17,18).

Diagnosis of the vascular compression syndromes depends on clinical suspicion and arteriography or venography, as appropriate. Ultrasound studies also have a major role in diagnosis (2).

TREATMENT

The treatment alternatives include physical therapy, surgery, and doing nothing at all. Many patients with mild symptoms need to learn what they can and cannot do, and to modify their life styles accordingly. Data demonstrating that physical therapy is effective are scant (19). Enthusiasm for surgery should be balanced with estimates of surgical risk. Major morbidity from transaxillary approaches ranges from less than 1% to between 15% and 20% (16,20), probably depending on the experience and skill of the surgeon.

The history of surgical approaches is worth reviewing briefly. Even in the earliest accounts of TOS, attention was directed to the role of ribs in the compression. In 1861, Coote (4) reported resection of a cervical rib from a young girl with arterial and plexus compression. Removal of the first thoracic rib to relieve neurovascular compression was reported by Murphy in 1910 via a supraclavicular approach (8). Resection of the first rib from this approach is hazardous, however, and this treatment of TOS was abandoned until 1962, when Clagett (3) introduced first-rib resection through a posterior thoracotomy approach. Clagett maintained that the first rib was the key structure in TOS, because it was the one structure common to both the scalenic triangle and the costoclavicular space. The posterior approach requires considerable muscle dissection; Falconer and Li (5) suggested first-rib resection via the anterior supraclavicular approach.

Roos (13) reported on the transaxillary approach for removal of the first thoracic rib. This approach has been widely used since then and has led to a surge in the number of operations for thoracic outlet syndrome.

Another alternative is the supraclavicular approach with neurolysis of the brachial plexus (16). The first thoracic rib may be resected from this vantage point, but the approach is difficult.

Because there have been no prospective studies of the various surgical approaches, it cannot be said which affords the best results. If the surgery is for venous or arterial disease, there seems to be general satisfaction with transaxillary first-rib resection (combined with resection of the cervical rib, if present) as a first choice. For brachial plexus compression, both the supraclavicular and transaxillary approaches have been advocated, and some patients appear to require both.

Resection of the First Rib from the Transaxillary Approach

There is no easy way to remove the first thoracic rib. The postthoracotomy approach requires a large incision and considerable muscle dissection. The supraclavicular approach puts the vessels and the brachial plexus between the surgeon and the rib. Retraction of the plexus could lead to inadvertent nerve injury.

The transaxillary approach for first-rib resection is my preference. This operation requires considerable skill, particularly in the region of the first thoracic root. Although this operation has been associated with a high morbidity rate, there are techniques and precautions that allow it to be performed quite safely.

The use of a headlight is important, and loupe magnification is helpful. The patient is placed under general anesthesia *without muscle paralysis*. Absence of muscle paralysis provides greater safety with dissection in the area of important nerves (e.g., the long thoracic nerve). A small amount of padding is placed beneath the shoulder (Fig. 2). The arm is abducted 135° and further rotated anteriorly 45°. The arm is suspended with a 3- to 5-pound weight attached in pulley fashion. A curved incision (approximately 7 cm) is made at the caudal portion of the axilla at the point the skin comes away from the chest wall. Dissection is done bluntly down to the chest wall, then upwards to the level of the first rib. The first rib is distinctive as a broad, flat structure. The intercostobrachial nerve can usually be dissected free and protected as it emerges from the second intercostal space. The initial dissection of the rib is done bluntly with the fingers. Two narrow Deaver retractors are used to hold the soft tissues away from the first rib. The intercostal muscles are taken down with cautery at the caudal edge of the rib. The pleura is separated from the rib. The axillary artery and vein and the plexus are appreciated as they drape over the rib. The right-angle retractor is placed around the anterior scalene muscle as it inserts on the first rib between the subclavian artery and vein. Once isolated, the muscle is divided. The middle scalene muscle is similarly taken down. Other soft-tissue attachments to the rib are taken down with a periosteal elevator and cautery.

Some surgeons then insert a rib cutter to remove the rib anteriorly and posteriorly. I prefer to remove the rib with rongeurs in piecemeal fashion. The Lexel double-action rongeurs are suitable for this purpose. The rib is removed posteriorly to within 2 cm of the transverse process. The T1 nerve root arises from the foramen just below the insertion of the rib on the transverse process, and

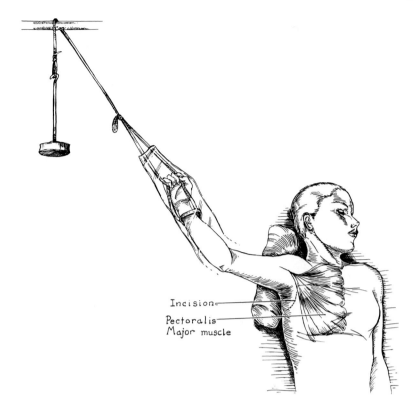

Incision

Pectoralis
Major muscle

FIG. 2. The patient is positioned for a right trans-axillary resection of the first thoracic rib.

then it joins the C8 root and both then course over the rib at the lower trunk. The lower trunk and T1 root must be free of all compression. All sharp spicules of bone are carefully removed. The lower plexus should now be free of any compression. The resection is carried anteriorly until the subclavian vein is free of any contact with the first rib. If the pleura is torn, a $\frac{1}{8}$-inch Hemovac drain is inserted, followed by a subcuticular closure. If a hole in the lung is created, a chest tube is needed, but this complication is rare.

It is often difficult for the surgeon to know intraoperatively whether the plexus or the vessels are indeed compressed. One thing to look for is a fibrous band that courses posteriorly and superiorly from the top of the first rib. One can imagine that such a structure would compress any structures draped over the first rib. Cervical ribs constitute a variant of this form of compression. The cervical rib is essentially an extension of the transverse process of the C7 vertebra. The cervical rib or a fibrous extension of it typically inserts on the rib in such a way that the lower plexus is compressed. The cervical rib is excised with bony rongeurs as part of the transaxillary approach.

Neurolysis of the Brachial Plexus via the Supraclavicular Approach

General anesthesia without muscle paralysis is used. An incision of about 6 cm is made parallel to the clavicle (Fig. 3). The platysma is opened, and often the lateral third of the sternocleidomastoid muscle is divided. The omohyoid muscle is divided as the scalene fat pad is mobilized to reveal the upper trunk of the plexus (Fig. 4). The anterior scalene muscle is encountered, along with the phrenic nerve, which courses along the axis of the muscle fibers in its position on top of the scalene muscle. A neurolysis of the phrenic nerve is performed and the nerve is mobilized in this manner away from the muscle. The anterior scalene muscle is then severed. The middle trunk comes into view. The middle and lower trunks of the plexus lie in a position inferoposterior to the upper trunk. A neurolysis of the middle trunk is performed, followed by a neurolysis of the lower trunk. Vessel loops are placed around the middle trunk (the C7 root) and around the C8 and T1 roots. The T1 root emerges from the anterior side of the posterior aspect of the first rib. Several different anomalies may be observed. Any fibrous bands that arise from the apex of the pleura or the first rib should be taken down (Fig. 5). On occasion, an arterial compression is observed from branches of the subclavian artery. Ligation and division of such branches may be necessary. A high arching subclavian artery may be seen, and mobilization of the artery may be useful to fully decompress the plexus. Dissection down to the first rib and apex of the lung can be done either between the lower and middle trunk, or alternatively between the middle and upper trunk. Resection of an anomalous cervical rib is quite easy with this approach. Some surgeons perform resection of the first thoracic rib with this ap-

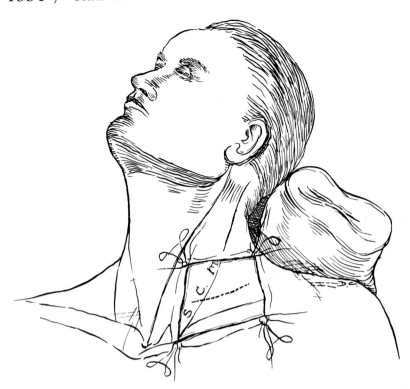

FIG. 3. The incision used for the supraclavicular approach to the brachial plexus.

proach, but the traction of the plexus that may be necessary to perform an adequate first-rib resection is worrisome.

If the patient does not achieve satisfactory benefit from either the supraclavicular or transaxillary approach, then the alternative operation is done. If neither operation works, it is well to consider whether the first rib was adequately removed posteriorly.

The success of surgery varies with the patient's presentation. If the patient fulfills only some of the diagnostic criteria and pain is the chief complaint, the success rate may be only about 50%. Even with adequate decompression, some patients may continue to have annoying symptoms. First rib resection is generally successful for vascular compression. Patients with profound intrinsic

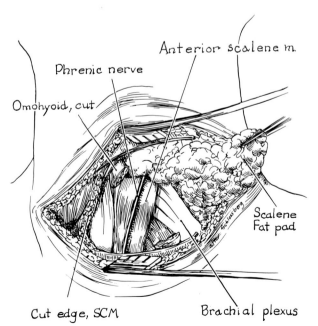

FIG. 4. Early stage of dissection in the supraclavicular approach to the brachial plexus.

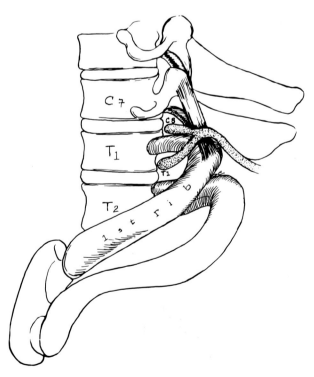

FIG. 5. Close-up of an anomalous band that compresses the lower plexus.

hand weakness are not likely to have much recovery of strength. However, pain is generally relieved by surgery.

CONCLUSION

TOS represents a spectrum of compression disorders with involvement of the subclavian artery or vein, or the brachial plexus. Patients may present with signs of arterial insufficiency in the arm, signs of subclavian vein thrombosis, or signs and symptoms of brachial plexus involvement. Brachial plexus compression is the most common form of the disorder. Pain is the most common feature, but patients may present with painless loss of intrinsic hand muscle function as well. Exacerbation of symptoms with maneuvers that tug downward on the shoulder, or that involve abduction of the shoulder, is common in TOS. Unfortunately, patients with other disorders may present similarly. Tinel's sign in the supraclavicular fossa is probably more specific for TOS than other signs. Surgery is reserved for patients who present with vascular compromise, neurological loss, or persistent pain unresponsive to conservative measures. The transaxillary resection of the first thoracic rib is preferred for the vascular variants of the disease. Transaxillary first-rib resection or supraclavicular neurolysis of the brachial plexus (or both) may be done for the cases of brachial plexus compression.

REFERENCES

1. Campbell JN, Naff NJ, Dellon AL (1991): Thoracic outlet syndrome. Neurosurgical perspective. *Neurosurg Clin North Am* 2: 227–233.
2. Chengelis KL, Glover JL, Bendick P, Ellwood R, et al. (1994): The use of intravascular ultrasound in the management of thoracic outlet syndrome. *Am Surg* 60:592–596.
3. Clagett OT (1962): Presidential address. Research and prosearch. *J Thoracic Cardiovasc Surg* 44:153–166.
4. Coote H (1861): Exostosis of the left transverse process of the seventh cervical vertebra surrounded by blood vessels and nerves: successful removal. *Lancet* 1:360.
5. Falconer MA, Li FWP (1962): Resection of the first rib in costoclavicular compression of the brachial plexus. *Lancet* 1:59–63.
6. Gilliatt RW (1984): Thoracic outlet syndromes. In: Dyck PJ, Thomas PK, Lambert EH, et al., eds. *Peripheral neurology.* Philadelphia, WB Saunders, p. 1409.
7. Makhoul RG, Machleder HI (1992): Developmental anomalies at the thoracic outlet: an analysis of 200 consecutive cases. *J Vasc Surg* 16:534–542.
8. Murphy T (1910): Brachial neuritis caused by pressure of first rib. *Aust Med J* 15:582.
9. Panegyres PK, Moore N, Gibson R, Rushworth G, Donaghy M (1993): Thoracic outlet syndromes and magnetic resonance imaging. *Brain* 116:823–841.
10. Pang D, Wessel B (1988): Thoracic outlet syndrome. *Neurosurgery* 22:105.
11. Razi DM, Wassel HD (1993): Traffic accident induced thoracic outlet syndrome: decompression without rib resection, correction of associated recurrent thoracic aneurysm. *Int Surg* 78:25–27.
12. Robb CG, Standeven A (1958): Arterial occlusion complicating thoracic outlet compression syndrome. *Br Med J* 2:709.
13. Roos DB (1966): Transaxillary approach for first rib resection to relieve thoracic outlet syndrome. *Ann Surg* 163:354.
14. Roos DB (1976): Congenital anomalies associated with thoracic outlet syndrome. *Am J Surg* 132:771.
15. Sobue I, Saito N, Iida M, Ando K (1978): Juvenile type of distal and segmental muscular atrophy of upper extremities. *Ann Neurol* 3:429–432.
16. Swenson WM, Vigesaa RE, Heib RE, et al. (1986): Thoracic outlet syndrome: the supraclavicular approach to first-rib resection. *Surg Rounds* 9:73.
17. Thompson RW, Schneider PA, Nelken NA, Skioldebrand CG, Stoney RJ (1992): Circumferential venolysis and paraclavicular thoracic outlet decompression for effort thrombosis of the subclavian vein. *J Vasc Surg* 16:723–732.
18. Urschel HC Jr, Razzuk MA (1991): Improved management of the Paget-Schroetter syndrome secondary to thoracic outlet compression. *Ann Thorac Surg* 52:1217–1221.
19. Walsh MT (1994): Therapist management of thoracic outlet syndrome. *J Hand Ther* 7:131–144.
20. Wilbourn AJ, Porter JM (1988): Thoracic outlet syndrome. In: Weiner MA, ed. *Spine: State of the art reviews.* Philadelphia: Hanley and Belfus, p. 597–626.

The Adult Spine: Principles and Practice,
2nd edition, J.W. Frymoyer, Editor-in-Chief.
Lippincott-Raven Publishers, Philadelphia © 1997.

CHAPTER 65

Cervical Spondylosis and Disc Herniation: The Anterior Approach

Thomas S. Whitecloud III and Joseph G. Werner, Jr.

Degenerative disease of the cervical spine can produce a variety of clinical signs and symptoms, most of which are amenable to nonoperative management. There are instances, however, when pain or neurologic dysfunction is best managed by operative intervention. Depending on where pressure is exerted on neural structures, radiculopathy, myelopathy, or a combination of both may be produced (130). These symptoms may not be produced by the same etiologic factors, although the resultant neurologic lesion is the same. A soft-disc herniation can produce an acute medullary or radicular symptom complex; progressive disc deterioration without a frank herniation may lead to the formation of posterior and posterolateral osteophytes, with resultant similar compression on neurologic structures. Disc degeneration without any frank neurologic deficits may result in a condition known as a discogenic syndrome, which is characterized by chronic neck, shoulder, and interscapular pain and is frequently associated with occipital headaches (36,142,184). Failure of nonoperative management for any of these symptom complexes may require the treating physician to consider operative intervention. The timing of such surgery may have important pragmatic implications. It is now recognized that early

surgical intervention, especially in cases of cervical spondylitic myelopathy, will generally result in a better clinical outcome (5,6,11,62,73,82,90,93,108,115,127,136, 154,187).

Historically, the routine surgical approach for symptoms produced by cervical spondylosis was posterior. As early as 1928, Stookey (163) noted difficulty in removing "chondromas" by the posterior transdural route. During the past 40 years, it became recognized that the primary problem with this approach was the technical difficulty encountered in attempting to expose and remove compressive structures that lie primarily anterior to the spinal cord and nerve roots. The need for easier access to anterior compressive structures led to development of the anterior surgical approach to the cervical spine. This approach was developed and popularized in the early 1950s. Bailey and Badgley performed an anterior cervical stabilization procedure in 1952 for a patient suffering from a lytic lesion of the fourth and fifth cervical vertebrae. The first published report of their technique of an onlay strut graft appeared in 1960 (8) (Fig. 1). This was recommended for use in destructive lesions of the vertebral column and in fracture dislocations. In 1955, Robinson and Smith (143) described an operative technique for stabilizing a pathologic cervical segment using a horseshoe-shaped graft (Fig. 2). Cloward, with no knowledge of the work done by others, first published his technique of anterior disc excision and direct removal of compressive structures in 1958 (35) (Fig. 3). Dereymaeker and Mulier, in 1956 (51), had developed a tech-

   T. S. Whitecloud III, M.D.: Professor and Chairman, Department of Orthopaedic Surgery, Tulane University School of Medicine, New Orleans, Louisiana, 70112.
   J. G. Werner, Jr., M.D.: Orthopaedic Surgeon, Browne & Reichard, PSC, Suite 1000, Baptist East Office Park, Louisville, Kentucky 40207.

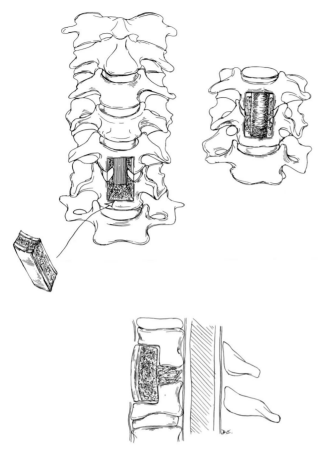

FIG. 1. A Bailey-Badgley-type arthrodesis in which only a portion of the disc is removed, the posterior disc space is filled with cancellous bone, and an on-lay graft is inserted. No attempt is made to remove compressive structures.

nique similar to that of Smith and Robinson. It is interesting that these various techniques were reported to result in good or excellent results in the majority of patients.

The primary difference between the Cloward procedure and that of Robinson and Smith is not the configuration of graft constructs. The Cloward technique emphasizes direct visualization and removal of compressive structures (35,37,38), whereas Robinson and Smith felt that the removal of these offending structures was not necessary and that posterior and posterolateral osteophytes will be resorbed once stabilization has been achieved (143,144).

Numerous refinements have been made in the anterior approach to the cervical spine for the treatment of cervical radiculopathy, myelopathy, or myeloradiculopathy. There are variations in configurations of bone graft (7,10,19,20,40,71,156), as well as variations in the source of graft material (27,39,43,66,73,83,151,152, 166). Use of operative magnification allows better visualization of neural structures so that compressive lesions can be easily seen and removed (9,18,58,60,86,94,99, 104,107,109,148,159).

SURGICAL TECHNIQUE

The anterior approach to the cervical spine is relatively safe, technically easy, and relatively bloodless, and uses natural anatomic planes. The approach is essentially the same for any type of operative procedure to be performed on the anterior cervical spine. Anatomic details of the surgical approach have been well described (158).

Preoperative broad-spectrum antibiotics are administered and maintained for 24 hours. Cefazolin is used routinely; vancomycin may be substituted in penicillin-allergic patients. Dexamethasone should be administered at this time and given for 24 hours. Somatosensory evoked potential monitoring should be considered when vertebrectomy or radical decompression is anticipated (61).

Positioning of the patient for the surgical approach is critical. The patient is supine on the operating table with a head halter or skeletal traction in place. Traction helps to stabilize the spine in a neutral position. Distraction of

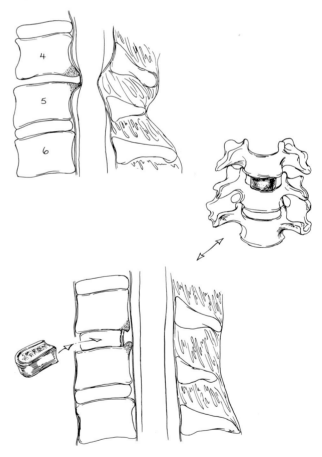

FIG. 2. An anterior disc excision followed by insertion of a cortical cancellous horseshoe-shaped Robinson-Smith bone graft. No attempt is made to remove posterior or posterolateral compressive structures. The cortical portion of the graft is inserted anteriorly in the original description of this procedure.

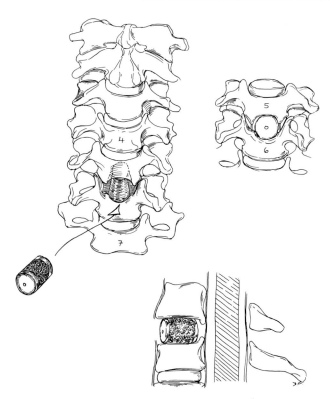

FIG. 3. The Cloward technique of insertion of a dowel of bone into the prepared disc space and vertebral bodies. Neural structures are decompressed directly posteriorly to the posterior longitudinal ligament, which may be removed at the discretion of the surgeon. With this graft configuration, care must be taken to insert the bone graft so that both cortical ends of the graft are within the disc space, otherwise there is a tendency for graft collapse or extrusion.

the disc space can be obtained by adding more weight at the time of graft insertion, or a vertebral body spreader can be used. A distraction system with pins inserted into the vertebral bodies above and below the disk space to be grafted is yet another method of obtaining distraction. It is not necessary to elevate one side of the pelvis to harvest an iliac crest graft if one is to be used. Operative draping must be done so that the cervical spine can be easily evaluated radiographically.

Although anatomic landmarks are present that will help guide the surgeon to the pathologic interspace, a lateral roentgenogram taken before making the skin incision can help assure an accurate approach to the appropriate level. The incision can then be placed in relationship to the shoulders as they appear on the roentgenogram. The approach to the cervical spine can be made from either the right or the left side, although most right-handed surgeons prefer to work from the right side. Generally, only one or two discs will be removed at the time of the operative procedure, and this can be adequately accomplished through a transverse skin incision. However, if three or more levels are involved, it is easier to place the skin incision obliquely along the border of

the sternocleidomastoid. Generally, we harvest bone graft material before making the neck incision.

Once the anterior aspect of the cervical spine has been exposed, it is mandatory to obtain a roentgenogram identifying the proper disc level. Proper illumination is necessary at the time of disc removal and can be obtained from a fiberoptic light source or an operating microscope. Magnification loupes or an operating microscope allow better visualization for removal of compressive structures.

Retractors, either self-retaining or hand-held, are placed to maintain exposure of the involved level. Care is taken to avoid prolonged retraction pressure on vital structures, especially the esophagus.

The anterior longitudinal ligament and anterior annulus are excised parallel to the vertebral end plate. Discectomy is performed using pituitary rongeurs and microcurettes. Interbody spreaders or pin distraction is used to enhance disk space exposure. Cartilage end plates are removed while maintaining cortical contact with the subchondral bone at all times. This prevents inadvertent dissection outside the disk space. Dissection is continued in this fashion back to the posterior longitudinal ligament. Removal of posterior structures and details of graft types and insertion are discussed below.

GRAFT CONFIGURATIONS FOR ANTERIOR CERVICAL FUSIONS

The pioneers of the anterior approach to the cervical spine for the treatment of a variety of pathologic conditions are considered to be Bailey and Badgley (8), Robinson and Smith (143), and Cloward (35). Based on biomechanical studies, White and Hirsch (178) concluded that the horseshoe-shaped graft of Robinson and Smith resists compressive forces better than the other graft configurations. Although their grafts are of different configurations, all of these authors believe that stabilization is necessary following disc excision to achieve the best possible clinical result. As stated, Cloward emphasized the direct visualization and removal of compressive structures at the time of surgical intervention. Robinson and Smith did not recommend removal of compressive structures; but if desired, it is possible to remove compressive structures with the Robinson-Smith technique, especially with use of the operating microscope. The original technique of Bailey and Badgley simply stabilizes the involved segment and does not require complete disc removal.

The individual surgeon must decide whether direct removal of compressive structures enhances the overall clinical result. However, it does appear that the risk of spinal cord injury at the time of surgery increases if there is a direct attempt to remove compressive structures or resect the posterior longitudinal ligament (9,16,61,75, 111,125,142,165,186).

Robinson and Smith were the first to describe a technique of anterior cervical fusion done for symptoms of cervical disc degeneration (143). They postulated that disc degeneration led to osteophyte formation, disc narrowing, subluxation, instability of one cervical vertebra on another, or disc protrusion. Their technique of interbody fusion restores disc height and, by stopping excessive motion, theoretically allows resorption of posterior and posterolateral osteophytes (Fig. 4). Their method of graft insertion consists of removing the pathologic disc or discs at the appropriate interspace. In their early description, they recommended removal of cartilaginous end plates and subchondral bone at the top and bottom of the disc space to be fused. Subsequently, Robinson and Smith recommended that the subchondral bone be left in place. No attempt is made to remove any compressive structures. The prepared disc space is then measured, and a horseshoe-shaped graft obtained from the iliac crest is inserted and countersunk. The graft is inserted so that its cancellous portion is directed posteriorly.

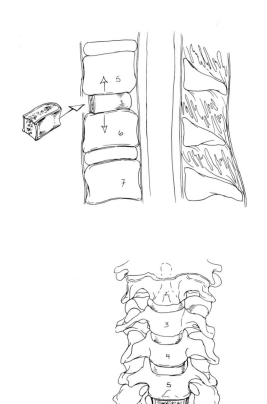

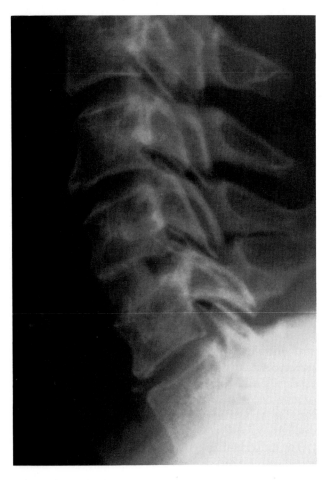

FIG. 4. Postoperative roentgenogram after anterior disc excision and fusion at C5-C6. No attempt was made to remove the posterior or posterolateral osteophytes. In this instance, the Robinson-Smith graft has been reversed. The patient had an excellent clinical result.

FIG. 5. A variation of the Robinson-Smith graft technique in which the graft is reversed so that the cortical portion is posterior. This ensures placement of a maximum amount of cortical bone within the disc space to resist compressive forces and extrusion. The graft does not have to be inserted in line with the posterior aspect of the vertebral bodies. The arthrodesis rate using this technique is somewhat higher than that reported in the literature for the original description of bone graft insertion.

Technical difficulties, such as collapse, extrusion, or nonunion (6,42,49,68,140,144,179,185), which occurred on occasion with this type of graft, led to a modification described by Bloom and Raney (14). The graft is prepared in a similar fashion, but the cortical portion is inserted directly posteriorly (Fig. 5). This assures placement of the maximum amount of cortical bone within the disc space and allows better maintenance of disc height. Whitecloud and Levet (183) reported a clinical series using this modification, with a lower pseudarthrosis rate than found in series in which the original technique was used (Fig. 6). Brodke and Zdeblick (25) also reported similar results in a group of 51 patients.

Cloward's technique of interbody fusion consists of drilling a round hole in the region of the intervertebral disc and inserting a pre-fit dowel of bone (35). He modified instrumentation previously designed for posterior lumbar interbody fusion. A drill is used with a guard that permits drilling of the intervertebral disc space and adja-

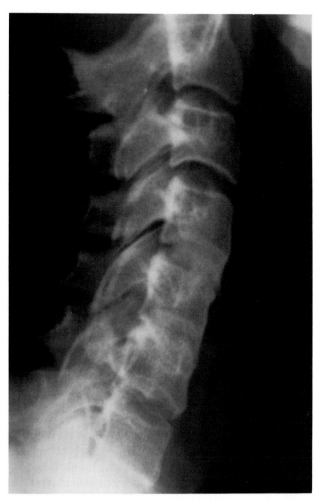

FIG. 6. Lateral roentgenogram of two-level cervical spondylosis treated by the modified Robinson-Smith technique.

cent vertebra to any desired depth. The drill and guard are removed several times to check their location. Drilling is continued downward until the bone at the bottom of the hole is entirely cortical in nature. This remaining cortical bone is then removed with curettes and rongeurs to expose the posterior longitudinal ligament. With care, the direct removal of posterior and posterolateral osteophytes or a soft disc is then possible. Once decompression has been carried out, a pre-cut dowel of bone obtained from the iliac crest is then tapped into place. It should be slightly shorter than the depth of the drill hole. The dowel of bone is cancellous in its midportion, with cortical bone at both ends. Cloward recommends the use of allograft where possible (39). One of the difficulties with use of a dowel of bone is that care must be taken to place it exactly in the prepared hole, otherwise there is a tendency for graft extrusion or collapse. If this occurs, a kyphotic deformity may develop (105). Because of this, Cloward subsequently modified multiple-level fusions so that a Robinson-Smith type of graft may be inserted at

one disc space, with a dowel of bone at an adjacent space (40). He also uses large blocks of bone when one or more vertebral bodies needs to be replaced.

The original technique of Bailey and Badgley required the preparation of a trough in the anterior aspect of the vertebral body approximately one-half inch in width and three-sixteenths of an inch in depth (8). The trough is cut into the full vertical height of the vertebra, and the discs are cleaned with a rongeur to a depth of approximately one-half inch. The cartilaginous end plates of the inferior and superior aspects of the vertebral bodies to be fused are removed. A cortical cancellous graft from the iliac crest is shaped to fit into the prepared trough. Chips of cancellous bone are packed into the cleaned disc spaces, and the cortical cancellous graft is mortised into the trough. If possible, sutures placed through the prevertebral fascia are tied over the graft, helping to maintain it in its correct position.

Besides these original three techniques regarding graft constructs, other graft configurations have been developed. They include the keystone graft of Simmons and subsequent modification by Gore (20,71,156). With the advent of subtotal vertebrectomy for thorough removal of all compressive structures that may be contributing to compression of the spinal cord in patients with cervical spondylitic myelopathy, other surgeons have developed and described different graft configurations and techniques for insertion that will span multiple cervical segments (7,10,15,19,66,73,160,192). These grafts are either cortical cancellous bone obtained from the iliac crest or cortical bone generally obtained from the fibula.

There have been numerous reports in the literature on the clinical results and the rate of fusion in patients undergoing anterior disc excision and interbody fusion. As would be expected, the reported pseudarthrosis rates vary (6,17,20,25,38,42,49,72,144,156,164,179,185). There is no doubt that there is increased risk of pseudarthrosis if more than one level is fused (17,25,42,179). This is not true, however, if one long piece of cortical cancellous graft or cortical bone is used to span multiple segments (10,19,48,192). The presence of a pseudarthrosis does not necessarily compromise the clinical result (49), although the surgeon's goal is to stabilize the involved pathologic spinal segment.

RESULTS OF ANTERIOR DISC EXCISION AND FUSION

Because of different preoperative criteria and length of follow-up, it is not possible to compare critically the numerous reports that have appeared in the literature describing the clinical results of anterior disc excision and interbody fusion (17,20,25,33,42,49,52,72,76,79,101,140, 144,156,164,179,185,194). Table 1 is a list of selected series from the literature that have used Odom's criteria

TABLE 1. *Clinical results of anterior disc excision and fusion*

Reference	No. of cases	Good, excellent (%)	Fair (%)	Poor (%)
Robinson (144)	55	73	22	5
Stuck (164)	151	73	21	6
Connolly (42)	63	54	24	22
Dohn (52)	210	51	29	20
Williams (185)	60	63	15	22
Riley (140)	93	71	18	10
Simmons (156)	68	81	15	22
Jacobs (101)	62	82	13	5
DePalma (49)	229	63	29	8
White (179)	65	67	22	11
Green (76)	33	97	1	0
Chirls (33)	467	92	6	2
Gore (72)	133	96	2	2
Brodke (25)	51	92	6	2
Grossman (79)	42	88	7	5
Totals	1,782	76.2	15.3	8.2

or a modification thereof for evaluation of postoperative clinical results (129). These criteria are listed in Table 2. Patients in the excellent, good, or fair category have benefited from surgical intervention. In the series presented in Table 1, Stuck (164), Dohn (52), and Chirls (33) used a Cloward technique, whereas the Robinson-Smith technique was used by all the other authors except for Simmons and Gore, who reported on their keystone type of arthrodesis. Brodke and Zdeblick (25) reversed a Robinson-Smith graft and removed bony end plates down to bleeding cancellous bone. Grossman et al. (79) reported on allograft fibula as a graft material.

Other large series, which cannot be listed in Table 1 because results were not reported by Odom's criteria, include that of Mosdal (123). In 1984, he reported on the results of 740 patients undergoing anterior disc excision with interbody fusion by the Cloward technique. For those patients having primarily radicular symptoms, 19% were totally pain-free and 62% had partial relief of their preoperative symptoms. These would correspond to good or excellent results if they had been judged by Odom's criteria. Eighty-three percent of these patients had heterologous graft material used (Kiel surgibone). Kyphotic angulation was noted in 12% of patients and was found to be more prevalent when more than one level was fused. This did not seem to compromise the surgical result.

In 1992, Bosacco et al. (20) reported on 202 patients in whom 87% of results were good or excellent by Odom's criteria. Average follow-up was 6.8 years. A unique interlocking autograft configuration was thought to contribute to the low pseudarthrosis rate of 6.5%.

In 1993, Bohlman et al. (17) published a 6-year average follow-up of 122 patients who underwent anterior

cervical discectomy and fusion at 195 segments. The results showed that 171 of 195 segments fused, for an overall pseudarthrosis rate of 13%, higher than in most reports. Pseudarthrosis was found in 11% of single-level fusions, 27% of two- and three-level fusions, and in the one four-level fusion. Clinical results were encouraging: 108 of 122 patients had no functional impairment and were able to resume work and daily activities. Thirty-seven had residual neck pain; six had residual arm pain. Sixteen of 24 patients with pseudarthrosis were symptomatic, but only four required revision. A statistically significant association between the presence of pseudarthrosis and postoperative neck or arm pain was found.

It has been noted by several authors that the results of surgery on patients involved in litigation are not statistically different from those on patients who are not in a litigious situation (17,25,179,184). Furthermore, White et al. (179) pointed out that there is no difference in results in patients with an abnormal psychological profile.

There is no question that the best surgical results can be anticipated from those patients who present with a monoradiculopathy and a duration of symptoms of less than 1 year (5,6,17,62,72,93,107). Multilevel disease requiring surgery at more than one level usually does not provide an excellent result, especially as regards the relief of neck pain. It must be remembered that cervical disc degeneration is a progressive disease, and a recurrence or progression of symptoms should not be unanticipated (29). The large series of Mosdal, in which follow-up of 13 years has been possible, shows a deterioration of his 81% good or excellent results to 71% on longer follow-up (123).

The series presented here did not directly address the question of cervical spondylitic myelopathy. Several of the authors included a few patients in this diagnostic category and generally found the results to be much poorer than those for patients with radiculopathy only (52,108,123,154,179). Again, it must be emphasized that early surgical intervention will allow the best results from anterior surgery for cervical spondylitic myelopathy (13,17,25,62,90,115,187).

Without question, anterior disc excision followed by stabilization with any variety of graft configuration should result in satisfaction of both patient and surgeon

TABLE 2. *Odom's criteria*

Excellent:	All pre-operative symptoms relieved; abnormal findings improved
Good:	Minimal persistence of pre-operative symptoms; abnormal findings unchanged or improved
Fair:	Definite relief of some pre-operative symptoms; other symptoms unchanged or slightly improved
Poor:	Symptoms and signs unchanged or exacerbated

most of the time. The literature review indicates that approximately 90% of patients undergoing this procedure derive benefit from it, and 70% can be anticipated to have a good or excellent result. It is not possible to ascertain whether compressive structures should be removed at the time of disc excision, as comparable results are found in those patients in whom the diseased cervical segment is simply immobilized by fusion. Each individual surgeon must decide whether direct neural decompression provides more benefit to each individual patient.

ANTERIOR DISC EXCISION WITHOUT FUSION

In addition to the controversy that has developed between surgeons who favor direct removal of compressive structures and those who favor simple stabilization of the involved segment after disc removal, another has developed between surgeons who do not insert a graft after disc removal and those who do (Fig. 7). Clinical results of those who recommend fusion and those who do not are very similar; that is, 90% of patients undergoing disc excision without fusion will derive benefit from the procedure (9,11,13,18,47,54,69,80,86,92,94,99,104,107,109, 120,125,141,145,154,173,186).

In 1960, Hirsch first described partial anterior excision of a cervical disc without an accompanying interbody fusion (92). His operative technique consisted of incising the anterior annulus and curetting the disc. No attempt was made to remove the cartilaginous end plates, posterior annulus, osteophytes, or posterior longitudinal ligament. Twenty-nine of 35 patients (83%) undergoing this procedure had a good or excellent clinical result. All patients achieved a fibrous or bony union at the area of disc excision. Subsequent series demonstrated a bony union in 70% to 100% of cases (9,11,13,18,47,54,69,80,86, 92,94,99,104,109,120,125,141,145,173,186). Hirsch was unable to explain why this procedure would eliminate the patients' symptoms.

Murphy and Gado reported on a similar operation in a group of 26 patients undergoing anterior disc excision for a lateral cervical disc syndrome (125). Twenty-four of their patients, or 92%, had a good clinical result. Follow-up radiographic evaluation in 20 patients showed that 72% had fused when discectomy alone was performed at a single level. Even in those patients who did not have a complete fusion, dynamic roentgenograms demonstrated apparent increased stability at the operative site, as measured by reduced motion. It is interesting that half of their patients demonstrated some degree of resorption of posterior and posterolateral osteophytes at 12 months. This compares favorably with reported series of anterior cervical discectomy with interbody fusion, in which approximately half the patients

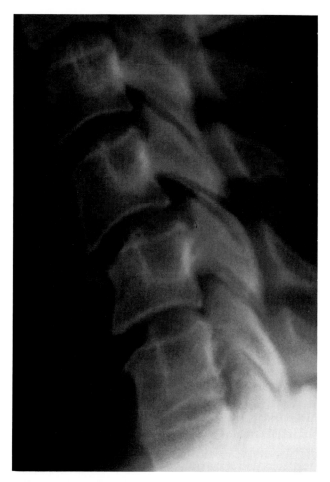

FIG. 7. Lateral radiograph of a patient after anterior disc excision without fusion at C6-C7. Spontaneous arthrodesis has occurred. The patient has had an excellent result from surgery performed for soft-disc herniation with radiculopathy.

studied demonstrated posterior osteophyte remodeling (17,72,144).

Although these surgical results were satisfactory, subsequent reported series emphasized the need for a much more radical decompression of neural structures (11,13,18,54,94,99,107,109,115,119,120,173). Most authors who prefer an anterior disc excision without fusion feel that the primary goal in obtaining relief of clinical symptoms is the removal of compressive structures to relieve the pressure on the cervical nerve root and/or the spinal cord (54,99,116,120,125,141,173). Numerous series emphasize the importance of removing posterior and posterolateral osteophytes in association with bilateral foraminotomies to prevent root compression by narrowing of the intervertebral space, which occurs after radical discectomy (11,13,18,54,56,94,99,107,109, 115,120,125,141,161,173). A controversy exists regarding resection of the posterior longitudinal ligament. Some authors find that it is unnecessary and dangerous to resect the ligament (7,9,75,125,141,142,186), whereas others feel that it is an essential part of the procedure to visualize the roots and dura to be sure the decompression is adequate (11,13,86,99,109,113,120,159,173,176).

Use of the operating microscope has made the radical decompression procedures, which now seem to be favored, technically feasible. One of the first reported series of a more radical excision was by Robertson in 1973 (141). He compared 53 patients who had undergone anterior disc excision and fusion with 40 patients who had not. He could find no difference in the clinical results, but felt that a simple discectomy avoided the morbidity of bone grafting, and thus he preferred this technique. He recommended thorough curettage of all disc material, including the cartilaginous end plates. The operating microscope was used to allow inspection for a hole in the posterior annulus through which a disc fragment could have migrated, and also for removal of posterior annulus and posterior longitudinal ligament if necessary. Clinically, 16 patients with radiculopathy had an excellent result, and 80% of the patients with a painful disc syndrome were markedly improved. A slightly different technique using the operating microscope was reported by Hankinson and Wilson in 1975 (86). They emphasized preserving columns of disc material on both sides of the disc space, recommending a central opening of no more than 10 mm. Using the operating microscope and an air drill with an angled adapter, a portion of the superior intervertebral body is removed, thus allowing more vertical exposure in the central portion of the disc. Posterior and posterolateral osteophytes are then removed under direct vision. If possible, the posterior longitudinal ligament is generally opened. This series reported on the clinical results in 51 patients. In 26 of these, disc removal was performed at multiple levels, and three had four discs removed at the time of surgery. Instability did not develop in any of these patients, possibly because of preservation of lateral column disc material and the minimal removal of anterior bone. Their results were similar to those of others, with 84% of their patients showing good or excellent results.

A more radical surgical procedure was described by Martins in 1976 (120). His operative technique consisted of radical discectomy with foraminotomy. The entire disc is removed along with cartilaginous end plates. In addition, the posterior aspect of the superior and inferior vertebral bodies is removed to facilitate exposure of the posterior longitudinal ligament. The ligament is excised and removed along with any posterior osteophytes. At the end of the procedure, the dura and nerve roots are checked visually to be certain they are free of any encroachment. Ninety-two percent of the patients undergoing surgery fell in the good or excellent category. This series of patients was compared with another group who underwent Cloward interbody fusion. The results were similar, with both groups having 92% good or excellent results. Comparing these results, Martins raised the question of why a fusion should even be done.

Dunsker also reported a small series in which two similar groups of patients either were fused or underwent a radical disc excision without fusion (54). He felt that grafting should be considered if a large amount of bone was removed from the posterior aspect of the vertebral bodies to visualize and decompress the neural structures. Again, the results in these patients undergoing either a radical disc excision or excision and fusion were quite similar, most falling in the good or excellent category. Martins also recommended grafting with the dowel technique in cases of advanced spondylosis requiring surgery at multiple levels (120).

Several large series have appeared in the literature that emphasize the value of radical disc excision and removal of all compressive structures to relieve pressure on the cervical nerve roots and/or the spinal cord (11,13, 18,54,94,99,107,109,115,119,120,125,141,173). Use of the operating microscope allows relatively safe neural decompression. A detailed description of the generally accepted technique with the microscope is given by Seeger (148) (Fig. 8).

Bertalanffy and Eggert (13) performed anterior microsurgical discectomy at one or more cervical segments without interbody fusion in 251 cases between 1976 and 1983. They were able to follow 164 cases between 1 and

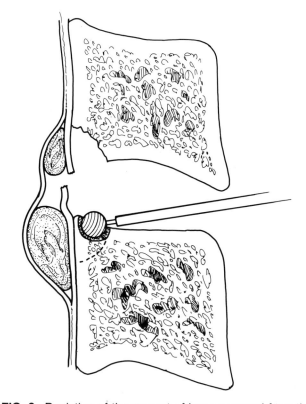

FIG. 8. Depiction of the amount of bone removed from the posterior superior and posterior inferior aspects of the vertebral body for removal of a soft-disc herniation in which a fusion will not be done. This is the technique described by Seeger and is performed using an operating microscope.

8 years. Diagnostic categories included 109 patients with radiculopathy and 55 patients with myelopathy. As expected, the best results were found in patients with radicular symptoms; 82% had good or excellent long-term results. Fifty-five percent of those patients with myelopathy had good or excellent long-term benefit from surgery. These authors felt that their results clearly demonstrated that anterior cervical disc excision is an effective treatment of cervical myelopathy. This stands in contrast to other reports (117,123,127,128,153,187).

Another series by Lesoin et al. analyzed the results of 1,000 surgical procedures done for radicular myelopathy over a 20-year period (115). Eight hundred cases were performed by an anterior incision and 200 were posterior. The investigators were able to analyze the surgical results in 700 of these patients, and although the specific numbers treated by the various techniques are not possible to ascertain, they felt that 66% of the patients achieved excellent or good results. This large series allowed these authors to state that they prefer the radical discectomy to discectomy followed by a Cloward bone graft.

Laus et al., in 1992, reported on 57 cases in which they found no difference in good/excellent results between microscopic (84%) and macroscopic (80%) decompression (113). They did observe that those treated microscopically had a more rapid regression of pain. Furthermore, they found no difference in outcome in patients who had discectomies with fusion versus discectomies alone. On this basis, they recommended microdiscectomy without fusion. Similarly, Klaiber et al. (107) treated 196 patients with anterior microdiscectomy without fusion and found good or excellent results in 66% of patients at 2 years.

It is obvious from the literature reviewed that radical decompression anteriorly without bone grafting is an accepted modality for the treatment of cervical radiculopathy, myelopathy, or myeloradiculopathy, which will be discussed later in this chapter.

Critical evaluation of the series available in the literature reveals that the results of disc excision without fusion are comparable to those in which an interbody fusion is performed. Obviously, the elimination of the donor site from the operative procedure decreases operative morbidity. Although generally minor in nature, complications from the donor site have been reported in approximately 20% of patients undergoing autologous grafting (180). Lunsford et al. (116) compared a series of 334 patients in which some had undergone fusion and some had not, and stated that the postoperative complications were much more frequent and hospital stays were longer in those patients undergoing fusion.

Despite these reports, restoration of disc height and stabilization of the pathologic cervical segment with bone graft is a much more commonly used surgical technique.

ANTERIOR SURGERY FOR CERVICAL SPONDYLITIC MYELOPATHY

The most serious consequence of degenerative disease of the cervical spine is cervical spondylitic myelopathy (Fig. 9). This condition is obviously different from cervical spondylosis causing a radiculopathy. Myelopathy is due to direct compression on the spinal cord itself, as opposed to nerve root compression only. It is the most common disease of the spinal cord developing during and after middle age (22,45), but must be differentiated from other diseases affecting the spinal cord such as amyotrophic lateral sclerosis or multiple sclerosis (30,57,146).

The pathophysiology of cervical spondylitic myelopathy is due to factors causing a reduction in the volume of the spinal canal (131,167,168). These can be both static and dynamic mechanical factors, and are frequently associated with vascular compromise (169). Anatomic factors that lead to reduction in the volume of the spinal canal include hypertrophy of the posterior arch, thickening of the ligamentum flavum, dural hypertrophy, tethering of the spinal cord by dentate ligaments, compression of radicular vessels by foraminal osteophytes, compression of the spinal cord by anterior osteophytes, ossification of the posterior longitudinal ligaments, and ossification of the ligamentum flavum (1–3,34,55,58–60,67,108,112,126,128,131,132,134,162,167–169,175). Experimental studies have indicated that both compression and ischemia contribute to myelopathy (70,78,98,188). These are additive factors, producing more symptoms in combination than when acting singly (70). Dynamic compression, which has been described by various authors, further reduces the functional diameter of the osseous canal (1,81,135,168). This occurs with motion, as flexion stretches the cord across ventral spurs and extension may cause retrolisthesis of a vertebral body or in-buckling of the ligamentum flavum (24,138).

The clinical presentation of this disease is highly variable. The most common presenting symptoms are upper-extremity weakness associated with a gait disturbance. Other findings can include spasticity, muscle atrophy, intrinsic bladder dystrophy, and, on occasion, radicular pain. In the most severe cases, posterior column dysfunction is noted. This is an ominous prognostic sign that indicates permanent spinal cord damage and is a poor prognostic sign as regards a patient's response to surgical intervention (16).

The natural history of cervical spondylitic myelopathy is one of intermittent progression with long periods in which the disease is static, followed by periods of exacerbation (57). Only a small group of patients will ever show a rapidly deteriorating disability. Few deaths are directly attributed to cervical spondylitic myelopathy (77). The episodic nature of this disease process has been documented by Lees and Turner (114) and by Clark and

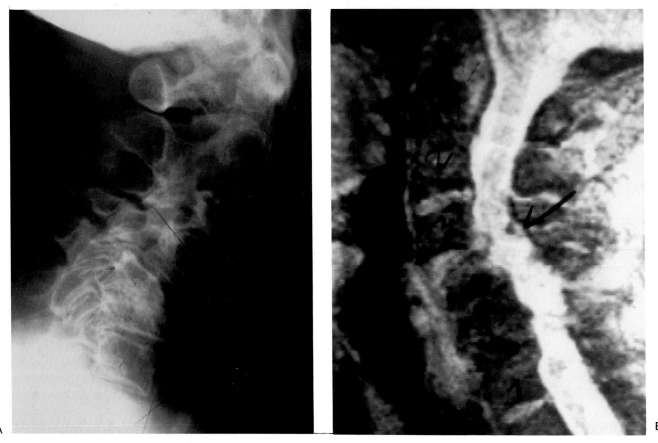

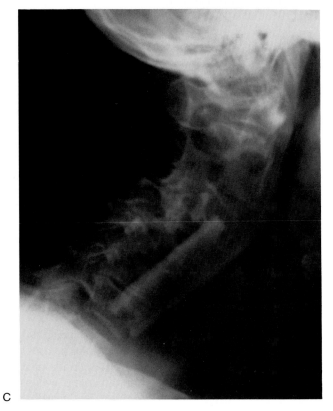

FIG. 9. Radiograph **(A)** and MRI **(B)** of a patient with severe cervical spondylosis with a secondary kyphotic deformity and herniation of the C3-C4 cervical disc. The patient manifested signs and symptoms of cervical spondylitic myelopathy. **C:** Surgery consisted of subtotal vertebrectomy of C4 and excision of herniated cervical disc at C3-C4, and anterior stabilization with a fibular allograft from C3-C7.

Robinson (34). These authors felt that there was no prognostic sign that would identify those patients who would deteriorate rapidly.

Lees and Turner also pointed out that the long-term follow-up results of posterior surgery for cervical spondylitic myelopathy showed no significant difference between those treated operatively and those treated nonoperatively (114). Delayed loss of neurologic function after laminectomy as well as the hazards of perioperative neurologic deficit are well recognized and estimated to occur 19% to 53% of the time (23,34,45,77,82,136,172).

These relatively poor results from posterior procedures led to the use of the anterior approach for operative intervention in patients suffering from this disease process (10,16,19,41,42,45,46,48,50,52,58–60,73,81,84, 85,87,100,108,124,136,147,150,189,190,192,195). However, the type of anterior procedure to be performed on patients with cervical spondylitic myelopathy has not been delineated. Favorable surgical outcome has been reported in patients undergoing simple disc excision without fusion (4,11,13,54,80,99,102,107,115,119,130,149) and also in patients undergoing disc excision plus radical decompression followed by stabilization procedures (10,19,41,42,45,46,50,52,58–60,73,81,84,85,87, 100,124,136,147,150,189,190,192,195). It has been noted that early operative intervention will provide the best clinical results (5,6,11,13,58,60,62,72,81,90,93,108,115,136, 154,187).

Some of the early series reporting on clinical results of anterior disc excision and fusion included patients who had cervical spondylitic myelopathy. In Dohn's large series, 39 of his 210 patients were in this diagnostic category (52). Overall, he noted that the results were poorest in this group of patients. White et al. also reported an overall poor result in patients with this disease process (179). In Connolly's series, two-thirds of the patients with this diagnosis had good or excellent results from anterior disc excision and stabilization (42). Aronson et al. (5,6) had three patients with cervical spondylitic myelopathy from soft-disc herniations, and all were treated successfully by the anterior approach. They found that the duration of symptoms in these patients with soft-disc herniations was short and represented a disease process somewhat different from that of patients with long-standing deficits.

One of the earliest reports dealing only with the results of anterior disc excision and fusion for cervical spondylitic myelopathy was published in 1966 by Crandall and Batzdorf (45). They had 21 patients treated by the Cloward technique, and noted a 71% improvement after surgery. In 1969, Guidetti and Fortuna reported 45 patients undergoing a similar operative procedure; 82% had results in the very good, good, or fair category (81). They did note that two patients were made worse by surgery, and one continued to deteriorate after surgery. Phillips reported a 74% improvement rate after Cloward

procedures performed in 65 patients (136). He felt that the results of anterior surgery were markedly superior to those of laminectomy or conservative management.

Crandall and Gregorius compared the results of laminectomy with those of anterior decompression followed by a Cloward fusion in 33 patients (46). Twelve of the 18 patients undergoing laminectomy deteriorated, whereas only 5 of the 15 patients lost function after decompression and fusion. In 1977, Bohlman reported on 17 patients who required ambulatory aids before surgery who were treated by simple stabilization of the involved segment (16). Fifteen patients became independent ambulators after surgery.

Although simple stabilization of the pathologic segment was shown by Bohlman (16) to be beneficial, most series now recommend both decompression and stabilization of the involved spinal segments. This may be done at the disc level only (42,45,46,50,52,81,84,85,87,100, 107,124,136,147,150,189,190,192,195) or in combination with a partial vertebrectomy (7,10,19,84,85,87,108, 189,190).

Another series with long-term follow-up was reported by Irvine and Strachan in 1987 (100). Forty-six patients were evaluated at a mean of 10 years post-surgery, and it was found that 36 patients (78%) remained improved, 6 remained unchanged (13%), and 4 (9%) showed progression of the disease. It should be noted that these patients underwent surgery only at one or two levels.

One of the few series in which the Smith-Robinson technique was used exclusively was published by Zhang et al. in 1983 (195). A total of 121 patients were presented; the average number of discs removed and fused per patient was 2.9. They reported a 91% improvement after surgery and a 73% rate of patients' being able to return to their former activities.

Another series reporting the results of patients undergoing decompression and Cloward fusion for one- or two-level disease has been published by Moussa et al. (124). Among 125 patients, 70% were improved by surgery and 30% were able to return to their former employment. The average follow-up was 2.3 years.

Surgery in the before-mentioned series was for disease at one or two levels. Use of the Cloward or the Smith-Robinson technique is difficult over multiple segments, and the pseudarthrosis rate is higher. For this reason, various techniques of partial vertebrectomy with decompression followed by stabilization with a variety of graft configurations have been described (10,19,84,85,87, 189,190) (Fig. 10). Techniques for vertebral body resection and decompression were initially described for the treatment of trauma (15,160).

All the techniques developed for grafting after vertebral body resection have in common the use of purely cortical or cortical cancellous bone, which is fashioned in such a way as to be locked into the vertebral bodies above and below the area of resection. The purely corti-

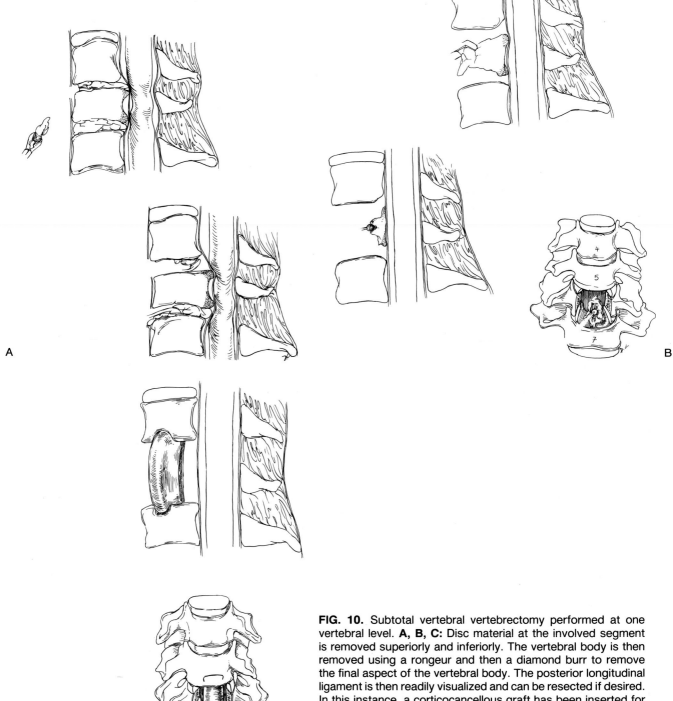

FIG. 10. Subtotal vertebral vertebrectomy performed at one vertebral level. **A, B, C:** Disc material at the involved segment is removed superiorly and inferiorly. The vertebral body is then removed using a rongeur and then a diamond burr to remove the final aspect of the vertebral body. The posterior longitudinal ligament is then readily visualized and can be resected if desired. In this instance, a corticocancellous graft has been inserted for vertebral body replacement. It is recommended that if more than two vertebral bodies are removed, a purely cortical graft be inserted, which resists compressive forces better than a corticocancellous graft.

cal bone used for graft material is usually obtained from the fibula or tibia, whereas the cortical cancellous graft material is generally obtained from the iliac crest. The grafts are usually inserted over at least two disc spaces. The published rates of fusion vary, with some reports approaching 100% (48,60,64).

Several series have been reported in which multilevel subtotal vertebrectomy with resection of all compressive structures has been performed. Senegas and Guerin (150) reported such a technique in 1975 (Fig. 11). Boni et al. (19) reported on 39 cases in which the central portion of three or more vertebral bodies was removed, followed by stabilization with a cortical cancellous graft. Fifty-three percent of patients were reported as having good results, with moderate improvement shown in 39%. Boni et al. initially removed the disc and the portion of the vertebral body using a Cloward drill (Fig. 12). Graft material was obtained from the iliac crest. Sakou et al. (147) reported on a similar procedure in 22 patients suffering from ossification of the posterior longitudinal ligament. Results were considered excellent in 2, good in 16, and fair in 4. Hanai et al. reported on a series of 15 patients undergoing subtotal vertebrectomy and fusion using iliac crest graft (84). This series again was in patients with ossification of the posterior longitudinal ligament.

Shireffs and Reeves (154) reported 40 consecutive cases of central corpectomy and grafting, with a cure rate of 57%. Kojima et al. reported good results with vertebrectomy and fusion for patients with cervical spondylosis and ossification of the posterior longitudinal ligament (108).

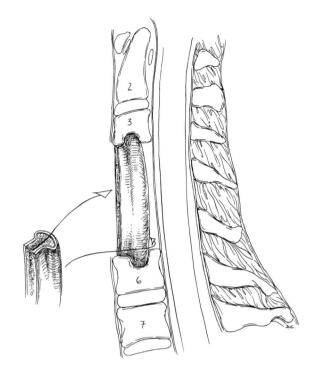

FIG. 12. Corticocancellous graft locked into place after two-level vertebral body resection.

A somewhat different method of vertebral body resection and grafting has been reported by Bernard and Whitecloud (10,182) (Fig. 13). In their operative technique, discs in the involved area are removed first, as would be done in performing a Smith-Robinson procedure. The intervening vertebral bodies are then removed using a dental burr and rongeurs. The midportion of the vertebral body is removed down to the posterior longitudinal ligament. Compressive structures in the region of the disc itself are then removed using curettes and rongeurs. Decompression is thus carried out from a region of minimal compression toward the region of maximum compression. After decompression, the superior and inferior vertebral bodies are undercut in such a way as to retain the anterior portion of the vertebra (Fig. 14). The posterior extension of a previously notched fibula can then be locked into place. In the initial reported series of 21 patients, 19 benefited from surgical intervention. Autologous fibula was used in this series, but subsequently has been changed to fibular allograft (Fig. 15). With either type of graft, the fusion rate approaches 100%.

Zdeblick and Bohlman (192) reported on eight patients with cervical spondylitic myelopathy treated with a similar procedure, but varied the method of insertion of the graft (Fig. 16). Aswasthi and Voorhies described a technical modification of strut graft stabilization (7).

Yonenobu et al. compared three surgical procedures for multisegment cervical spondylitic myelopathy in 95 patients (189). From the 21 patients undergoing subtotal

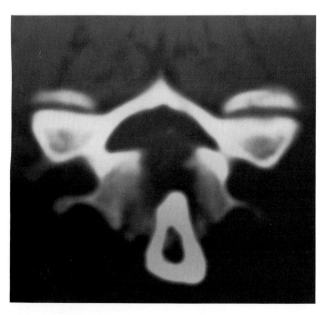

FIG. 11. Postoperative CT scan of partial vertebrectomy done for removal of compressive structures causing cervical spondylitic myelopathy.

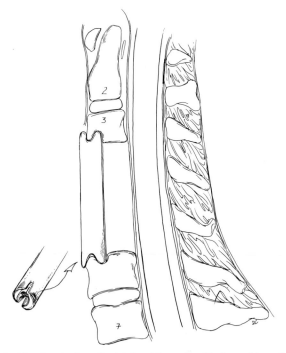

FIG. 13. Cortical graft obtained from the fibula and inserted so that it is notched into place. This graft is inserted with traction applied to the cervical spine. The neck does not have to be extended for insertion. This graft configuration helps prevent migration of the graft posteriorly into the area of the neural canal either at the time of insertion or in the postoperative period.

vertebrectomy and fusion, he felt that the results were superior to the other techniques of laminectomy and anterior fusion alone. He did state that if there is involvement of more than four segments, a posterior procedure should be carried out.

Epstein has made numerous contributions to the recent literature on ossification of the posterior longitudinal ligament (58–60). In her series of 43 patients, the 20 patients with the most severe neurologic deficits underwent anterior corpectomy and strut grafting (60). Ten patients with intermediate deficits underwent laminectomy. The remainder of the patients who had the least severe deficits were treated with discectomies alone. The most severely affected patients who underwent anterior surgery had the best outcomes, as judged by improvement on the Ranawat grading system (137). She emphasized the use of operative microscopy, the necessity of an adequately wide decompression, and the routine use of somatosensory evoked potentials (58–61).

Not all reports of anterior decompression and stabilization have been optimistic. Galera and Tovi noted only a 39% improvement in 33 patients undergoing a Cloward procedure (68). They felt that there was a definite tendency toward deterioration with prolonged follow-up. Likewise, Lunsford et al. (117) noted only 50% improvement in patients who had undergone anterior cer-

vical surgery who were followed for 1 to 7 years. Fifty percent of the patients were not improved or deteriorated despite operative intervention. In this series, various types of anterior procedures were performed, none showing any better results than another. The authors did not feel that surgical intervention results were any better than nonoperative management. Roland questioned whether surgical results offered improvement over the natural history of cervical spondylitic myelopathy (146). In his review, he emphasized the need for a multicenter trial using standardized treatment procedures and methods of outcome assessment.

Some patients have been managed successfully by disc excision alone. Bertalanffy and Eggert (13) performed radical disc excision in 105 patients having medullary or radiculomyelopathy signs and symptoms. The best results in this group of patients were in those who had a soft-disc herniation causing medullary symptoms. Overall, 55% of patients with myelopathy had an excellent or good long-term result. Bollati et al. (18) performed a similar radical decompression in ten patients having

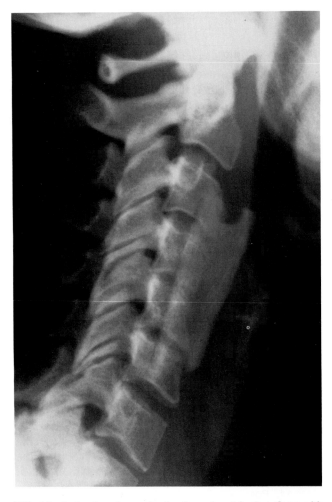

FIG. 14. Lateral radiograph of a three-level fusion done with fibula allograft. Three months have elapsed since surgery.

myelopathy and reported that eight were in the excellent or good category. In Wilson and Campbell's series (186), nine patients with myelopathy had one excellent, five good, two satisfactory, and one poor result. Klaiber et al. reported good to excellent results in two-thirds of 64 patients treated with microdiscectomy alone (107).

It is quite difficult to compare directly the various series that appear in the literature regarding results of anterior cervical surgery for cervical spondylitic myelopathy. Most results are evaluated according to Nurick's six grades of disability, which are based on the degree of difficulty in walking (127). Despite the numerous series that indicate anterior surgery should benefit the patient, in approximately 70% to 80% of cases, there are still no clear criteria as to when or how surgery should be performed. A short duration of symptoms before operative intervention does appear to give a better chance of a favorable surgical result. Patients younger than 70 with less severe myelopathy have been noted to fare better postoperatively (154).

Just as there is no clear indication when surgery should

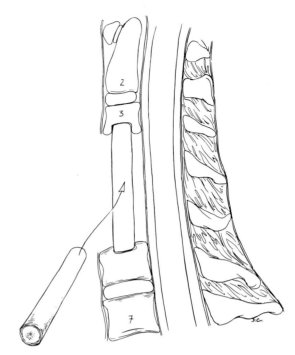

FIG. 16. Entire piece of fibula may be inserted following multiple-level subtotal vertebrectomies. For this graft to be inserted, the neck must be extended. This cannot be done safely unless any compressive structures have been totally removed. Care must be taken at the time of graft insertion not to impact the graft into the spinal canal.

be considered, it has not been conclusively shown whether the anterior approach is better than the posterior one (181). Epstein's reports aside, quite favorable results have been published on the different varieties of laminoplasties developed primarily for the treatment of ossification of the posterior longitudinal ligament (91,97, 106,153,174). The answer to when and how to operate for a cervical spondylitic myelopathy cannot be obtained until controlled prospective series have been initiated and completed.

INTERNAL FIXATION IN CERVICAL SPONDYLOSIS

Internal fixation techniques developed by the AO group have been adapted to the cervical spine. Orozco and Houet, in 1971, described the application of small fragment plates for rigid fixation after cervical fusion for traumatic and degenerative conditions (133). Most early reports described anterior plating of unstable cervical fracture-dislocations. Ricciardi and Whitecloud (139) reviewed the results and complications of AO plating in 630 patients. Hardware failure was reported in 13 patients, with only one pseudarthrosis.

In 1989, Caspar et al. described their technique and instrumentation and the results in 60 patients with un-

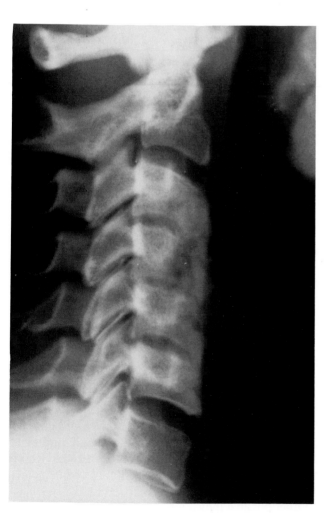

FIG. 15. Roentgenogram of cervical spine fused using allograft, 4 years after surgery.

stable cervical spines (31). All patients had fusion without external stabilization. They reported no neurologic or vascular complications. Five patients required reoperation, including one technically inadequate graft and plating, two cases of persistent instability after plating, one deep infection, and one hardware loosening. In the article, they noted using plate osteosynthesis in 128 patients with myelopathy or radiculopathy, but did not report the results from these patients. Similar results and complications from Caspar's plating and trauma indications are reported elsewhere in this volume and in the literature (139).

Inherent in the AO and Caspar techniques is the necessity of bicortical bone screw penetration. Herein lies the fearful potential for catastrophic neurologic injury. In 1986, Morscher et al. (122) developed a titanium screw locking plate (TSLP), which does not require penetration of the posterior vertebral cortex for adequate fixation. Early hardware failures were attributable to a fenestrated screw design, which has subsequently been modified (95). Kostuik et al. reported on TSLP use in 42 patients undergoing anterior decompression and fusion, 25 of whom were operated on for spondylitic conditions (110). They reported a 100% fusion rate and seven minor

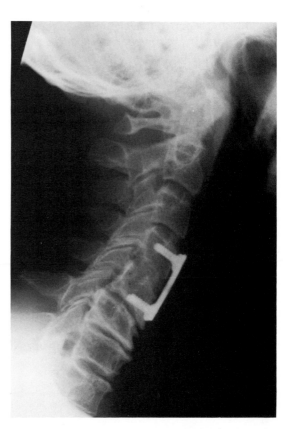

FIG. 18. Maintained position and early evidence of fusion at 9 months' follow-up. Functional improvement was noted postoperatively.

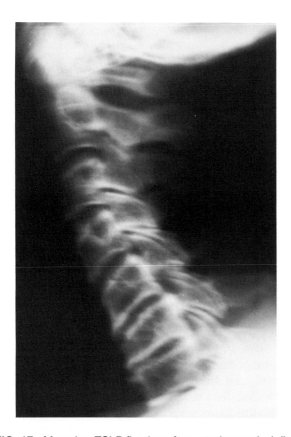

FIG. 17. Morscher TSLP fixation after anterior cervical discectomy and fusion. The patient is a 35-year-old spastic quadriplegic with C-4,5 radiculopathy. Conservative measures had been exhausted. Because of athetoid movements, postoperative immobilization would not have been tolerated.

hardware-related problems, for which one patient required subsequent removal of plate and screws. No major complications or deep infections were noted. Based on these results, they recommended consideration of anterior TSLP plating for patients requiring multilevel cervical arthrodesis.

Two cases of esophageal perforation after screw loosening have been reported (157). Animal studies show no increase in the fusion rate versus uninstrumented segments (193). Regional vascularity may be compromised by plate and screw application (193). Clinical reports, however, show an increased fusion rate when screws and plates are employed (31,95,110,133,139).

Potentially disastrous neurologic complications have not been reported. The risk of spinal cord injuries should be lessened with the Morscher screw design (122). This theoretic risk must be weighed against the satisfactory rate of fusion and clinical outcomes reported with current uninstrumented methods. At this time, anterior plating in spondylitic patients should remain limited to those in whom excess instability is proven and in whom postoperative external immobilization would be poorly tolerated (Figs. 17 and 18).

Other possible indications for internal fixation in degenerative disease are for revision of pseudarthrosis when kyphosis must be corrected, and for stabilization below a previous fusion. Obviously, the cost/benefit ratio and potential complications of internal fixation must be considered before internal fixation is routinely used in cervical degenerative disease.

COMPLICATIONS OF ANTERIOR CERVICAL SURGERY

The anterior approach to the cervical spine is relatively easy and uses natural anatomic planes. The results of surgery are generally satisfactory to both the patient and the surgeon in approximately 90% of procedures. This is true whether or not an interbody fusion is done. As with any surgical procedure, there are inherent risks related to the surgical approach. This is due to the diversity of anatomic structures encountered as the anterior portion of the cervical spine is exposed. Once exposure has been achieved, disc excision, with or without removal of compressive structures, has a potential for injury to the spinal cord or cervical nerve roots (12,65,74,111,165). If the pathologic segment is stabilized after disc removal, bone graft and donor-site problems can be encountered (8,37,42,49,140,144,171,180). The spinal surgeon must be aware of these potential complications, their incidence according to the literature, and how to prevent them. Only then can the surgeon intelligently discuss with the patient the risks and benefits of a surgical procedure which, in most cases, is elective in nature.

In the surgical exposure of the anterior cervical spine, there are a number of soft-tissue structures that must be recognized, avoided, and/or retracted. Virtually any of the anatomic structures encountered are susceptible to injury, and such injuries have been reported.

The necessity for retraction of the pharynx, trachea, and esophagus across the midline for disc exposure renders these structures susceptible to injury. In most circumstances, injury is caused by penetration by the sharp blades of a retractor (37,170). These structures should be carefully retracted, and if self-retaining retractors are used, their blades should be carefully placed under the edge of the longus colli muscles. Retractor blades should not be sharp. Prolonged retraction against the *in situ* tracheal tube can lead to the common complication of temporary dysphagia and hoarseness (121,177). This can be eliminated by not applying constant pressure against the trachea and by using dexamethasone in the perioperative period (180).

Vocal cord paralysis can occur with injury to the recurrent laryngeal or vagus nerve (28,88). It is unlikely that these structures are divided directly during the exposure; more than likely it is again caused by prolonged pressure against the trachea. Fortunately, most of these injuries are transient. Heeneman (88) reported on 85 cases evaluated after anterior cervical surgery and found that 11% had postoperative voice changes, with three permanent vocal cord paralyses. Anatomically, the recurrent laryngeal nerve is less likely to be injured when approached from the left side of the neck because of its longer course and more protective position in the trachea-esophageal groove (158).

Another complication that can occur as the disc and vertebral bodies are approached is an injury to the sympathetic chain (170,171). This can be avoided if care is taken not to dissect lateral to the longus colli muscles and to avoid improper retractor placement. Most of these injuries are transient in nature and of little clinical consequence.

Vascular injuries to the carotid artery or jugular vein are fortunately rare, but have been reported (115,136). Again, the most common cause of injury is penetration by a sharp retractor. Prolonged, forceful retraction against the carotid artery can lead to cerebral ischemia.

Direct injury to the vertebral artery is, again, a rare complication and almost invariably occurs from direct injury by an instrument (44). Direct exposure is necessary at the foramen transversarium to control the resultant hemorrhage.

Use of a drain inserted down to the anterior portion of the cervical spine generally prevents accumulation of a postoperative hematoma (180). This is a potentially serious problem if unrecognized in the early postoperative course. Tew and Mayfield (171) have recommended that a cervical collar not be applied in the operating room so that the postoperative dressing can be inspected easily. This recommendation was made after one of their patients had a respiratory arrest due to tracheal compression secondary to hematoma accumulation. Fortunately, the incidence of postoperative wound infection of the cervical spine is less than 1% (170). This is probably due to the vascularity of the area. There is an increased risk of infection at the donor site if a graft has been harvested. Proper draping of the donor site, proper placement of the incision, use of a drain, and obtaining the graft and closing the wound before beginning the approach to the cervical spine can decrease this problem (180).

Many surgeons who prefer anterior disc excision without fusion have been led to this preference because of the complications that occur at the donor site and with the grafts themselves once inserted (8,37,42,140,144,171, 180). The use of any type of graft configuration can result in partial graft extrusion, frank dislodgment, or graft collapse. Partial graft extrusion is of little consequence and usually does not require any treatment. Complete graft extrusion, however, especially when multiple levels have been stabilized, obviously requires replacement of the graft (182). Another potential complication encountered with the use of grafts at individual interspaces is the occurrence of avascular necrosis of the remaining vertebral body (123). This is more prone to occur using the Cloward technique at two adjacent levels. Cloward has reported on alternating graft configurations at adjacent levels to help avoid this problem (40). When avascular necrosis or graft collapse occurs, an anterior kyphotic deformity may result (96,105). This, again, can be avoided by use of a cortical strut graft over multiple levels or by alternating the types of grafts inserted.

The pseudarthrosis rate using different varieties of graft techniques varies from zero to as high as 26% (6,42,49,64,72,140,144,156,164,179,185). Pseudarthrosis is frequently asymptomatic and may not merit revision (144). Bohlman et al., however, reported a statistically significant correlation between pseudarthrosis after anterior cervical discectomy and fusion and postoperative pain (17). Farey et al. (63) reported good results and a 100% fusion rate of symptomatic anterior pseudarthrosis using posterior decompression and arthrodesis with a triple-wire technique. Brodsky et al. (26) treated 34 patients with symptomatic pseudarthrosis of anterior cervical fusions. Anterior repair was performed in 17 patients, with a 76% fusion rate. Of 17 patients treated posteriorly with triple wiring and arthrodesis, 94% fused. Excellent/good results were reported in 59% versus 94%, respectively. Based on these results, posterior fusion was recommended for repair of anterior cervical pseudarthrosis.

The donor site is a source of a number of complications. These are generally minor and can consist of persistent drainage, hematoma formation, superficial or deep wound infection (which has been addressed previously), hernia through the area of bone removal, injury to the lateral femoral nerve, and chronic bone-site pain. A review of 1,244 cases from various series reported a complication rate of 20% at the donor site, whereas there was only a 0.2% complication rate occurring from the neck incision (180).

Use of other materials to obtain fusion obviously eliminates donor-site problems and is another strategy preferred by some. Reports have appeared in the literature of Kiel bone grafts, hydroxyapatite, or polymethylmethacrylate (43,83,151,152,166). Titanium and carbon fiber cages have been introduced to be used in combination with cancellous autograft bone (155). The frequency of donor-site complications has enhanced the appeal of allograft bone for interbody and multilevel strut grafts. Fusion rates approaching 100% have been reported for allograft fibular struts (147,182,191). Ferneyhough et al. (64) presented the results from a retrospective study of 126 consecutive multilevel discectomies and vertebrectomies for cervical spondylosis using autograft or allograft fibular strut. They found a pseudarthrosis rate of 27% with autograft and 41% with allograft. Zdeblick found autogenous graft superior to allograft in anterior cervical discectomy and fusion in goats (193). In a separate article, he discussed the follow-up of 87 patients undergoing Robinson-Smith anterior cervical fusions (194). At 1 year, pseudarthroses were noted in 8% of pa-

tients with autograft and 22% of patients with allograft. Nonunion in one-level procedures, however, was 5% in each group. In addition, he found that relief of neck and arm pain was similar in both groups. Grossman et al. (79) found a 92% union rate using freeze-dried fibular allografts in anterior cervical discectomy and fusion. Good or excellent results were reported in 88%. Allograft bone appears to be an effective graft substitute for autogenous bone. The increased incidence of radiographic nonunion may be offset by the lack of graft donor-site complications and excellent report of clinical outcomes.

Although disc excision without fusion obviously eliminates donor-site and graft complications, there are definite complications that can occur when disc excision alone is performed. One major problem is a transient exacerbation of cervical pain after disc removal. Most series report a 15% to 20% prevalence (12,80,94). One series had a 60% occurrence; for that reason the author elected to abandon the procedure (103). Wilson and Campbell consider postoperative neck pain as directly proportionate to the extent of vertebral spreading at the time of disc removal (186).

Another reported complication of this procedure is a radiculopathy occurring on the extremity opposite to what was present preoperatively. This is thought to be due to inadequate anterior foraminotomy performed bilaterally (12,69,86,99,116). Several series have reported an increased angular deformity occurring at the site of disc excision (12,125,171). This is generally of no consequence, but on occasion is significant enough to require bone grafting (12,125). This is more likely to occur when multiple levels are operated on, especially if radical disc excision is carried out (12,171).

Although there are successful reports of treating myelopathy with anterior disc excision alone, several reports indicate a definite increased risk of worsening of symptoms (12,69), especially in elderly patients with multilevel disease or in patients with congenital stenosis.

By far the most devastating complication of anterior cervical surgery is injury to the spinal cord or nerve root. The exact incidence of this serious complication is not known; there are, however, a few mentioned in most large series. Flynn (65) has published the most ambitious attempt to determine the magnitude of neurologic problems after anterior cervical surgery. Members of the American Association of Neurological Surgeons were polled, and 52% responded. An analysis of the responses showed a 0.38% incidence of neurologic complications. A radiculopathy was reported in 158 cases and a myelopathy in 129. There were 70 cases in which a myelopathy resulted in which detailed evaluation could be made. Fifty-three of these were immediate and 17 were delayed. Surgical re-exploration did not make much difference in recovery.

The Cervical Spine Research Society has obtained further information regarding the incidence of complications in cervical spine surgery (74). This organization is composed primarily of orthopaedists and neurosurgeons. Five years' experience of this group has been obtained and published. In 3,894 reported anterior procedures, the incidence of neurologic complication has ranged from a low of 0.265% in 1983 and 1984 to a high of 0.91% in the period between 1985 and 1986. These large retrospective series indicate that the risk of spinal cord injury in anterior cervical surgery is probably less than 1%.

There remains speculation as to what causes cord injuries at the time of the surgical procedure. Some undoubtedly are due to intraoperative trauma caused by actual impaction of the bone graft (136) or the use of instrumentation within the spinal canal (37,111). A postoperative epidural hematoma has been implicated in other cases (165,176). The vascular supply of the cord can be damaged at the time of surgery (111).

It must be remembered that mechanical factors such as manipulation of the neck during intubation or hyperextension of the neck in an anesthetized patient can cause in-buckling of the ligamentum flavum and annulus fibrosus and thus cause a cord injury (24,56,165). Some authors have recommended testing the tolerance of neck motion before surgery and making certain that it is not exceeded during the intubation procedure (165,170).

Radical neural decompression with removal of all compressive structures and the posterior longitudinal ligament remains controversial. There have been reported cases of the extensive dissection required for removal of these structures resulting in an increased incidence of epidural bleeding (176). It is apparent that adequate visualization using accessory illuminative sources and operative magnification is necessary for safe removal of compressive structures. Also, epidural bleeding must be thoroughly controlled. A bone graft of any configuration must be properly shaped and inserted without excessive force. Obviously, care must be taken not to impact the bone graft into the neural canal.

Intraoperative monitoring of neurologic function is another strategy and may alert the surgeon to mechanical or vascular causes of neurologic compromise. Epstein reported an evaluation of somatosensory evoked potential monitoring in 100 patients undergoing cervical spine surgery (161). Using historic controls, she found a reduced incidence of neurologic injury from 4% to 6.9% in unmonitored patients versus 0.7% in patients monitored with somatosensory evoked potentials.

Sugar (165) has made several recommendations regarding what to do if an increased neurologic deficit is noted postoperatively. Certainly each case must be treated individually, but general guidelines are useful. Make certain that the blood pressure is maintained at proper levels. Intravenous corticosteroids are now shown to be of limited benefit in traumatic injury to the spinal cord in humans (21). Methylprednisolone should be administered intravenously using the protocol described by Bracken et al. (21). Prompt administration within 8 hours of injury is imperative for maximal effectiveness. A lateral roentgenogram of the neck should be made to visualize placement of the graft carefully. An anesthetist should be notified that surgery may have to be performed as soon as possible, especially if the graft is obviously within the canal. This could be done under local anesthesia to avoid manipulation of the already compromised cord.

If there is no evidence of direct compression of the cord by the bone graft, diagnostic studies such as myelography, computed tomography (CT), or magnetic resonance imaging (MRI) can be obtained to evaluate for the presence of a compressive lesion. Further anterior or posterior decompression can be considered. Consultation should be sought. It must be remembered that an etiologic factor for deterioration in neurologic function after anterior surgery is often not found, and the cause is never known.

Although their occurrence is rare, a number of serious complications can result from anterior cervical spine surgery. Because this operative procedure is relatively easy, there is a tendency to underestimate the seriousness of these potential problems. The spinal surgeon must know how to discuss these potential problems intelligently with the patient before embarking on any type of anterior cervical procedure. Certainly, the surgeon also must know how to deal with them if any are encountered.

REFERENCES

1. Adams CBT, Logue V (1971): Studies in cervical spondylitic myelopathy: I. Movement of the cervical roots, dura and cord, and their relation to the course of the extrathecal roots. *Brain* 94:557–568.
2. Adams CBT, Logue V (1971): Studies in cervical spondylitic myelopathy: II. The movement and contour of the spine in relation to the neural complications of cervical spondylosis. *Brain* 94: 569–586.
3. Adams CBT, Logue V (1971): Studies in cervical spondylitic myelopathy: III. Some functional effects of operations for cervical spondylitic myelopathy. *Brain* 94:587–594.
4. Arnasson O, Carlsson CA, Pellettieri L (1987): Surgical and conservative treatment of cervical spondylitic radiculopathy and myelopathy. *Acta Neurochir (Wien)* 84:48–53.
5. Aronson NI (1973): The management of soft cervical disc protrusions using the Smith-Robinson approach. *Clin Neurosurg* 20: 253–258.
6. Aronson N, Filtzer DL, Bagan M (1968): Anterior cervical fusion by the Smith-Robinson approach. *J Neurosurg* 29:397–404.
7. Aswasthi D, Voorhies R (1992): Anterior cervical vertebrectomy and interbody fusion. *J Neurosurg* 76:159–163.
8. Bailey RW, Badgley CE (1960): Stabilization of the cervical spine by anterior fusion. *J Bone Joint Surg* [Am] 42:565–594.
9. Benini A, Krayenbuhl H, Bruderl R (1982): Anterior cervical discectomy without fusion. Microsurgical technique. *Acta Neurochir (Wien)* 61:105–110.
10. Bernard TN Jr, Whitecloud TS III (1987): Cervical spondylitic myelopathy and myeloradiculopathy: Anterior decompression

and stabilization with autogenous fibula strut graft. *Clin Orthop* 221:149–160.

11. Bertalanffy H, Eggert H-R (1988): Clinical long-term results of anterior discectomy without fusion for treatment of cervical radiculopathy and myelopathy: A follow-up of 164 cases. *Acta Neurochir (Wien)* 90:127–135.

12. Bertalanffy H, Eggert H-R (1989): Complications of anterior cervical discectomy without fusion in 450 consecutive patients. *Acta Neurochir (Wien)* 99:41–50.

13. Bertalanffy H, Eggert H-R (1990): Anterior discectomy without fusion for treatment of cervical degenerative disc disease. Twelve years' experience based on 450 consecutive cases. In: Louis R, Weidner A, eds. *Cervical spine II. Marseille 1988.* New York: Springer-Verlag, pp. 208–215.

14. Bloom MH, Raney FL Jr (1981): Anterior fusion of the cervical spine: A technical note. *J Bone Joint Surg* [Am] 63:842.

15. Bohlman HH (1972): Pathology and current treatment for cervical spine injuries. *AAOS Instructional Course Lectures,* Vol. 21. St. Louis: C.V. Mosby, pp. 108–115.

16. Bohlman HH (1977): Cervical spondylosis with moderate to severe myelopathy: A report of 17 cases treated by Robinson anterior cervical discectomy and fusion. *Spine* 2:151–162.

17. Bohlman HH, Emery SE, Goodfellow DB, Jones PK (1993): Robinson anterior cervical discectomy and arthrodesis for cervical radiculopathy. *J Bone Joint Surg [Am]* 75:1298–1307.

18. Bollati A, Galli G, Gandolfini M, Marini G, Gatta G (1983): Microsurgical anterior cervical disk removal without interbody fusion. *Surg Neurol* 19:329–333.

19. Boni M, Cherubino P, Benazzo F (1984): Multiple subtotal somatectomy: Technique and evaluation of a series of thirty-nine cases. *Spine* 9:358–362.

20. Bosacco DN, Berman AT, Levenberg RJ, Bosacco SJ (1992): Surgical results in anterior cervical discectomy and fusion using a counter sunk interlocking autogenous iliac bone graft. *Orthopedics* 15:923–925.

21. Bracken MB, Shepherd MF, Collins WF, et al. (1990): A randomized controlled trial of methylprednisolone or naloxone in the treatment of acute spinal cord injury: Results of the second national acute spinal cord injury study. *N Engl J Med* 322:1405–1411.

22. Brain R (1954): Spondylosis: The known and the unknown. *Lancet* 1:687–693.

23. Brain WR, Northfield D, Wilkerson M (1952): The neurological manifestations of cervical spondylosis. *Brain* 75:187–225.

24. Breig A, Turnbull I, Hassler O (1966): Effects of mechanical stresses on the spinal cord in cervical spondylosis. *J Neurosurg* 25:45–56.

25. Brodke DS, Zdeblick TA (1992): Modified Smith-Robinson procedure for anterior cervical discectomy and fusion. *Spine* 17(10Suppl):S427–430.

26. Brodsky AE, Khalil MA, Sassard WR, et al. (1992): Repair of symptomatic pseudarthrosis of anterior cervical fusion: Posterior versus anterior repair. *Spine* 17(10Suppl):1137–1143.

27. Brown MD, Malinin TI, Davis PB (1976): A roentgenographic evaluation of frozen allografts versus autografts in anterior cervical spine fusions. *Clin Orthop* 119:231–236.

28. Bulgar RF, Rejowski JE, Beatty RA (1985): Vocal cord paralysis associated with anterior cervical fusion: Considerations for prevention and treatment. *J Neurosurg* 62:657–661.

29. Busch G (1978): Anterior fusion for cervical spondylosis. *J Neurol* 219:117–126.

30. Campbell A, Phillips D (1960): Cervical disc lesion with neurological disorder. Differential diagnosis, treatment, and progression. *BMJ* 2:481–485.

31. Caspar W, Dragos DB, Klara PM (1989): Anterior cervical fusion and Caspar plate stabilization for cervical trauma. *Neurosurgery* 25:491–502.

32. Chapman MW, Younger EM (1989): Morbidity of bone graft donor sites. *J Orthop Trauma* 3:192–195.

33. Chirls M (1978): Retrospective study of cervical spondylosis treated by anterior interbody fusion (in 505 patients performed by the Cloward technique). *Bull Hosp Joint Dis* 39:74–82.

34. Clark E, Robinson PK (1956): Cervical myelopathy: A complication of cervical spondylosis. *Brain* 79:483–510.

35. Cloward RB (1958): The anterior approach for removal of ruptured cervical disks. *J Neurosurg* 15:602–617.

36. Cloward RB (1959): Cervical discography contribution to the etiology and mechanism of neck, shoulder and arm pain. *Ann Surg* 150:1052.

37. Cloward RB (1962): New method of diagnosis and treatment of cervical disc disease. *Clin Neurosurg* 8:93–132.

38. Cloward RB (1963): Lesions of the intervertebral disks and their treatment by interbody fusion methods. *Clin Orthop* 27:51–77.

39. Cloward RB (1980): Gas-sterilized cadaver bone grafts for spinal fusion operations: A simplified bone bank. *Spine* 5:4–10.

40. Cloward RB (1988): The anterior surgical approach to the cervical spine: The Cloward procedure: Past, present and future. *Spine* 13:823–827.

41. Concha S, McQueen J (1977): Anterior cervical fusions for spondylitic myelopathy: A preliminary report. *Spine* 2:147–150.

42. Connolly ES, Seymore RJ, Adams JE (1965): Clinical evaluation of anterior cervical fusion for degenerative cervical disc. *J Neurosurg* 23:431–437.

43. Cook SD, Dalton JE, Tan EH, Tejeiro WV, Young MJ, Whitecloud TS (1994): In vivo evaluation of anterior cervical fusions with hydroxyapatite graft material. *Spine* 19:1856–1866.

44. Cosgrove GR, Theron J (1987): Vertebral arteriovenous fistula following anterior cervical spine surgery. Report of two cases. *J Neurosurg* 66:297–299.

45. Crandall PH, Batzdorf U (1966): Cervical spondylitic myelopathy. *J Neurosurg* 25:57–66.

46. Crandall PH, Gregorius FK (1977): Long-term follow-up of surgical treatment of cervical spondylitic myelopathy. *Spine* 2:139–146.

47. Cuatico W (1981): Anterior cervical discectomy without interbody fusion: An analysis of 81 cases. *Acta Neurochir (Wien)* 57:269–274.

48. Cummins B (1991): The treatment of spondylitic cervical myelopathy by multiple subtotal vertebrectomy and fusion. *Br J Neurosurg* 5:249–255.

49. DePalma AF, Rothman RH, Lewinneck RE, Canale S (1972): Anterior interbody fusion for severe cervical disc degeneration. *Surg Gynecol Obstet* 134:755–758.

50. Dereymaeker A, Ghosez J-P, Henkes R (1963): Le traitement chirurgical de la discopathie cervicale. Resultats comparés de l'abord posterieur (laminectomie) et de l'abord ventral (fusion corporeale) dans une cinquantaine de cas personels. *Neurochirurgie* 9:13–20.

51. Dereymaeker A, Mulier J (1956): Nouvelle cure neurochirurgicale des discopathies cervicales. *Neurochirurgie* 2:233–234.

52. Dohn DF (1966): Anterior interbody fusion for treatment of cervical disk condition. *JAMA* 197:897–900.

53. Doi K, Kawa S, Sumiura S, Sakai K (1988): Anterior cervical fusion using the free vascularized fibular graft. *Spine* 13:1239–1244.

54. Dunsker SB (1977): Anterior cervical discectomy with and without fusion. *Clin Neurosurg* 24:516–521.

55. Epstein J, Carras R, Epstein B, Levine L (1970): Myelopathy in cervical spondylosis with vertebral subluxation and hyperlordosis. *J Neurosurg* 32:421–426.

56. Epstein JA, Carras R, Levine LS, Epstein BS (1969): The importance of removing osteophytes as part of the surgical treatment of myeloradiculopathy in cervical spondylosis. *J Neurosurg* 30:219–226.

57. Epstein JA, Janin Y, Carras R, Levine LS (1982): A comparative study of the treatment of cervical spondylitic myeloradiculopathy: Experience with 50 cases treated by means of extensive laminectomy, foraminotomy, and excision of osteophytes during the past 10 years. *Acta Neurochir (Wien)* 61:89–104.

58. Epstein NE (1993): The surgical management of ossification of the posterior longitudinal ligament in 51 patients. *J Spinal Disord* 6:432–455.

59. Epstein NE (1994): Ossification of the posterior longitudinal ligament in evolution in 12 patients. *Spine* 19:673–681.

60. Epstein NE (1994): The surgical management of ossification of the posterior longitudinal ligament in 43 North Americans. *Spine* 19:664–672.

61. Epstein NE, Danto J, Nardi D (1993): Evaluation of intraopera-

tive somatosensory-evoked potential monitoring during 100 cervical operations. *Spine* 18:737–747.

62. Eriksen EF, Buhl M, Fode K, et al. (1984): Treatment of cervical disc disease using Cloward's technique. The prognostic value of clinical preoperative data in 1,106 patients. *Acta Neurochir (Wien)* 70:181–197.

63. Farey ID, McAfee PC, Davis RF, Long DM (1990): Pseudarthrosis of the cervical spine after anterior arthrodesis: Treatment by posterior nerve-root decompression, stabilization, and arthrodesis. *J Bone Joint Surg [Am]* 72(8):1171–1177.

64. Ferneyhough JC, White JI, Larocca H (1991): Fusion rates in multilevel cervical spondylosis comparing allograft fibula with autograft fibula in 126 patients. *Spine* 16:S561–564.

65. Flynn TB (1982): Neurologic complications of anterior cervical fusion. *Spine* 7:536–539.

66. Freidberg SR, Gomley GJ, Pfeifer BA, Mybels RL (1989): Vascularized fibular graft to replace resected cervical vertebral bodies. *J Neurosurg* 71:283–286.

67. Frykholm R (1951): Cervical nerve root compression resulting from the disk degeneration and nerve root sleeve fibrosis: A clinical investigation. *Acta Chir Scand Suppl* 160:1–149.

68. Galera GR, Tovi D (1968): Anterior disc excision with interbody fusion in cervical spondylitic myelopathy and rhizopathy. *J Neurosurg* 28:305–310.

69. Giombini S, Solero CL (1980): Consideration on 100 anterior cervical discectomies without fusion. In: Grote W, Brook M, Clar HE, Klinger M, Nau HE, eds. *Advances in neurosurgery*, Vol. 8. Berlin: Springer-Verlag, pp. 302–307.

70. Gooding MR, Wilson CB, Hoff JT (1975): Experimental cervical myelopathy: Effects of ischemia and compression of the canine cervical spinal cord. *J Neurosurg* 43:9–17.

71. Gore DR (1984): Technique of cervical interbody fusion. *Clin Orthop* 188:191–195.

72. Gore DR, Sepic SB (1984): Anterior cervical fusion for degenerated or protruded discs: A review of one hundred forty-six patients. *Spine* 9:667–671.

73. Goto S, Mochizuki M, Kita T, et al. (1993): Anterior surgery in four consecutive technical phases for cervical spondylitic myelopathy. *Spine* 18:1968–1973.

74. Graham J (1989): Complication of cervical spine surgery. In: *The cervical spine*, 2nd ed. The Cervical Spine Research Society. Philadelphia: J.B. Lippincott, pp. 831–837.

75. Granata F, Taglialatela G, Graziussi G, Avella F (1981): Management of cervical disc protrusions by anterior discectomy without fusion. *J Neurosurg Sci* 25:231–234.

76. Green PWB (1977): Anterior cervical fusion: A review of thirty-three patients with cervical disc degeneration. *J Bone Joint Surg [Br]* 59:236–240.

77. Gregorius F, Estrin T, Crandall P (1976): Cervical spondylitic radiculopathy and myelopathy. A long-term follow-up study. *Arch Neurol* 33:618–625.

78. Griffiths IR (1972): Some aspects of the pathology and pathogenesis of the myelopathy caused by disc protrusions in the dog. *J Neurol Neurosurg Psychiatry* 35:403–413.

79. Grossman W, Peppelmam WC, Baum JA, Kraus DR (1992): The use of freeze-dried fibular allograft in anterior cervical fusion. *Spine* 17:565–569.

80. Guarnaschelli JJ, Dzenitis AJ (1982): Anterior cervical discectomy without fusion: Comparison study and follow-up. In: Brock M, ed. *Modern neurosurgery I*. New York: Springer-Verlag, pp. 284–291.

81. Guidetti B, Fortuna A (1969): Long-term results of surgical treatment of myelopathy due to cervical spondylosis. *J Neurosurg* 30:714–721.

82. Haft H, Shenkin HA (1963): Surgical end results of cervical ridge and disk problems. *JAMA* 186:312–315.

83. Hamby WB, Glaser HT (1959): Replacement of spinal intervertebral discs with locally polymerizing methylmethacrylate. Experimental study of effects upon tissue and report of a small clinical series. *J Neurosurg* 16:311–313.

84. Hanai K, Fujiyoshi F, Kamei K (1986): Subtotal vertebrectomy and spinal fusion for cervical spondylitic myelopathy. *Spine* 11:310–315.

85. Hanai K, Inouye Y, Kawai K, Tago K, Itoh Y (1982): Anterior

decompression for myelopathy resulting from ossification of the posterior longitudinal ligament. *J Bone Joint Surg [Br]* 64:561–564.

86. Hankinson HL, Wilson CB (1975): Use of the operating microscope in anterior cervical discectomy with fusion. *J Neurosurg* 43:452–456.

87. Harsh GR IV, Sypert GW, Weinstein PR, Ross DA, Wilson CB (1987): Cervical spine stenosis secondary to ossification of the posterior longitudinal ligament. *J Neurosurg* 67:349–357.

88. Heeneman H (1973): Vocal cord paralysis following approaches to anterior cervical spine. *Laryngoscope* 83:17–21.

89. Herkowitz HN, Kurz LT, Overholt DP (1990): Surgical management of cervical soft disc herniation: A comparison between the anterior and posterior approach. *Spine* 15:1026–1030.

90. Hicks D, Whitecloud T, LaRocca SH (1980): Cervical spondylitic myelopathy: Results of anterior decompression and stabilization. *Orthop Trans* 4:44.

91. Hirabayashi K, Watanabe K, Wakano K, Suzuki N, Satomi K, Ishii Y (1983): Expansive open-door laminoplasty for cervical spinal stenotic myelopathy. *Spine* 8:693–699.

92. Hirsch C (1960): Cervical disc rupture: Diagnosis and therapy. *Acta Orthop Scand* 30:172–186.

93. Hirsch C, Wickbon I, Lidstrom A, et al. (1964): Cervical disc resection. A follow-up of myelographic and surgical procedure. *J Bone Joint Surg [Am]* 46:1811–1821.

94. Hoff JT, Wilson CB (1979): Microsurgical approach to the anterior cervical spine and spinal cord. *Clin Neurosurg* 26:513–528.

95. Hollowel JP, Reinarts J, Pintar FA, et al. (1994): Failure of Synthes anterior cervical fixation device by fracture of the Morscher screws: A biomechanical study. *J Spinal Disord* 7:120–125.

96. *Horwitz NH, Rizzoli HV (1967): Postoperative complications in neurosurgical practice: Recognition, prevention, and management. Baltimore: Williams and Wilkins.*

97. Hukuda S, Mochizuki T, Ogata M, Shichikawa K, Shimomura Y (1985): Operations for cervical spondylitic myelopathy. *J Bone Joint Surg [Br]* 67:609–615.

98. Hukuda S, Wilson C (1972): Experimental cervical myelopathy: Effects of compression and ischemia on the canine cervical cord. *J Neurosurg* 37:631–652.

99. Husag L, Probst C (1984): Microsurgical anterior approach to cervical discs. Review of 60 consecutive cases of discectomy without fusion. *Acta Neurochir (Wein)* 73:229–242.

100. Irvine GB, Strachan WE (1987): The long-term results of localised anterior cervical decompression and fusion in spondylitic myelopathy. *Paraplegia* 25:18–22.

101. Jacobs B, Krueger EG, Leivy DM (1970): Cervical spondylosis with radiculopathy: Results of anterior discectomy and interbody fusion. *JAMA* 211:2135–2140.

102. Jomin M, Lesoin F, Lozes G, Thomas CE III, Rousseaux M, Clarisse J (1986): Herniated cervical discs. Analysis of a series of 230 cases. *Acta Neurochir (Wien)* 79:107–113.

103. Kadoya S, Kwak R, Hirose G, Yamamoto T (1982): Cervical spondylitic myelopathy treated by a microsurgical anterior approach with or without interbody fusion. In: Brock M, ed. *Modern neurosurgery I*. Berlin: Springer-Verlag, pp. 292–297.

104. Kadoya S, Nakamura T, Kwak R (1984): A microsurgical anterior osteophytectomy for cervical spondylitic myelopathy. *Spine* 9:437–441.

105. Keblish PA, Keggi KJ (1967): Mechanical problems of the dowel graft in anterior cervical fusion. *J Bone Joint Surg [Am]* 49:198–199.

106. Kimura I, Oh-Hama M, Shingu Y (1984): Cervical myelopathy treated by canal-expansive laminaplasty. *J Bone Joint Surg [Am]* 66:914–920.

107. Klaiber RD, vonAmmon K, Sarioglu AC (1992): Anterior microsurgical approach for degenerative cervical disc disease. *Acta Neurochir (Wien)* 114:36–42.

108. Kojima T, Waga S, Kubo N, et al. (1989): Anterior cervical vertebrectomy and interbody fusion for multilevel spondylosis and ossification of the posterior longitudinal ligament. *Neurosurgery* 24:864–872.

109. Kosary IZ, Braham H, Shacked I, Shacked R (1976): Microsur-

gery in anterior approach to cervical discs. *Surg Neurol* 6:275–277.

110. Kostuik JP, Connolly PJ, Esses SI, Suh P (1993): Anterior cervical plate fixation with the titanium hollow screw plate system. *Spine* 18:1273–1278.

111. Kraus DR, Stauffer ES (1975): Spinal cord injury as a complication of elective anterior cervical fusion. *Clin Orthop* 112:130–141.

112. Kubota M, Babe I, Sumida T (1981): Myelopathy due to ossification of the ligamentum flavum of the cervical spine: A report of two cases. *Spine* 6:553–559.

113. Laus M, Pignatti G, Alfonso C, et al. (1992): Anterior surgery for the treatment of soft cervical disc herniation. *Chir Organi Mov* 77:101–108.

114. Lees F, Turner JWA (1963): Natural history and prognosis of cervical spondylosis. *BMJ* 2:1607–1610.

115. Lesoin F, Bouasakao N, Clarisse J, Rousseaux M, Jomin M (1985): Results of surgical treatment of radiculomyelopathy caused by cervical arthrosis based on 1,000 operations. *Surg Neurol* 23:350–355.

116. Lunsford LD, Bissonette DJ, Jannetta PJ, Sheptak PE, Zorub DS (1980): Anterior surgery for cervical disc disease. Part 1: Treatment of lateral cervical disc herniation in 253 cases. *J Neurosurg* 53:1–11.

117. Lunsford LD, Bissonette DJ, Zorub DS (1980): Anterior surgery for cervical disk disease: Treatment of cervical spondylitic myelopathy in thirty-two cases. *J Neurosurg* 53:12–19.

118. McAfee PC, Bohlman HM, Wilson WL (1985): The triple wire fixation technique for stabilization of acute cervical fracture-dislocations: A biomechanical analysis. *Orthop Trans* 9:142.

119. Mann KS, Khosla VK, Gulati DR (1984): Cervical spondylitic myelopathy treated by single-stage multilevel anterior decompression: A prospective study. *J Neurosurg* 60:81–87.

120. Martins AN (1976): Anterior cervical discectomy with and without interbody bone graft. *J Neurosurg* 44:290–295.

121. Mayfield F (1966): Cervical spondylosis: A comparison of the anterior and posterior approaches. *Clin Neurosurg* 13:181–188.

122. Morscher F, Sutter F, Jennis M, et al. (1986): Die vordere Verplattung der Halswirbelsäule mit dem Holschrauben-plattensystem. *Chirurg* 57:702–707.

123. Mosdal C (1984): Cervical osteochondrosis and disc herniation. Eighteen years' use of interbody fusion by Cloward's technique in 755 cases. *Acta Neurochir (Wien)* 70:207–255.

124. Moussa AH, Nitta M, Symon L (1983): The results of anterior cervical fusion in cervical spondylosis: Review of 125 cases. *Acta Neurochir (Wien)* 68:277–288.

125. Murphy MG, Gado M (1972): Anterior cervical discectomy without interbody bone graft. *J Neurosurg* 37:71–74.

126. Nugent GR (1959): Clinicopathologic correlations in cervical spondylosis. *Neurology* 9:273–281.

127. Nurick S (1972): The natural history and the results of surgical treatment of the spinal cord disorder associated with cervical spondylosis. *Brain* 95:101–108.

128. Nurick S (1972): The pathogenesis of the spinal cord disorder associated with cervical spondylosis. *Brain* 95:87–100.

129. Odom GL, Finney W, Woodhall B (1958): Cervical disk lesions. *JAMA* 166:23–28.

130. O'Laire SA, Thomas DGT (1983): Spinal cord compression due to prolapse of cervical intervertebral disc (herniation of nucleus pulposus): Treatment in 26 cases by discectomy without interbody bone graft. *J Neurosurg* 59:847–853.

131. Olsson SE (1958): The dynamic factor in spinal cord compression: A study on dogs with special reference to cervical disc protrusion. *J Neurosurg* 15:308–321.

132. Ono K, Ota H, Tada K, Hamada H, Takaoka K (1977): Ossified posterior longitudinal ligament. *Spine* 2:126–138.

133. Orozco DR, Houet J (1971): Osteosynthesis en los lesiones traumáticos y degenerativos de la columna vertebral. *Rec Traumatol Ciruj Rehabil* 1:45–52.

134. Payne EE, Spillane JD (1957): The cervical spine. An anatomico-pathological study of 70 specimens (using a special technique) with particular reference to the problem of cervical spondylosis. *Brain* 80:571–576.

135. Penning L, Van der Zwaag P (1966): Biomechanical aspects of spondylitic myelopathy. *Acta Radiol* 5:1090–1103.

136. Phillips DG (1973): Surgical treatment of myelopathy with cervical spondylosis. *J Neurol Neurosurg Psychiatry* 36:879–884.

137. Ranawat CS, O'Leary P, Pellicci P, Tsairis P, Marchisello P, Dorr L (1979): Cervical fusion in rheumatoid arthritis. *J Bone Joint Surg* 61A:1003–1010.

138. Reid JD (1960): Effects of flexion-extension movements of the head and spine upon the spinal cord and nerve roots. *J Neurol Neurosurg Psychiatry* 23:214–221.

139. Ricciardi JE, Whitecloud TS (1995): Complications of cervical spine fixation. In: *Seminars in spine surgery.* [In press].

140. Riley LH Jr, Robinson RA, Johnson KA, et al. (1969): The results of anterior interbody fusion of the cervical spine: Review of ninety-three consecutive cases. *J Neurosurg* 30:127–133.

141. Robertson JT (1973): Anterior removal of cervical disc without fusion. *Clin Neurosurg* 20:259–261.

142. Robertson JT (1978): Anterior operations for herniated cervical disc and for myelopathy. *Clin Neurosurg* 25:245–250.

143. Robinson RA, Smith GW (1955): Anterolateral cervical disc removal and interbody fusion for cervical disc syndrome. *Bull Johns Hopkins Hosp* 96:223–224.

144. Robinson RA, Walker AE, Ferlic DC, et al. (1962): The results of an anterior interbody fusion of the cervical spine. *J Bone Joint Surg [Am]* 44:1579–1586.

145. Rosenorn J, Hansen EB, Rosenorn M-A (1983): Anterior cervical discectomy with and without fusion: A prospective study. *J Neurosurg* 59:252–255.

146. Rowland LP (1992): Surgical treatment of cervical spondylitic myelopathy: Time for a controlled trial. *Neurology* 42:5–13.

147. Sakou T, Miyazaki A, Tomimura K, Maehara T, Frost HM (1979): Ossification of the posterior longitudinal ligament of the cervical spine: Subtotal vertebrectomy as a treatment. *Clin Orthop* 140:58–65.

148. Seeger W (1982): *Microsurgery of the spinal cord and surrounding structures.* New York: Springer-Verlag.

149. Selladurai BM (1992): Cervical myelopathy due to nuclear herniations in young adults: Clinical and radiological profile, results of microdiscectomy without interbody fusion. *J Neurol Neurosurg Psychiatry* 55(7):604–608.

150. Senegas J, Guerin J (1975): Technique de decompression medullaire anterieure dans les stenoses canalaires estendues. *Rev Chir Orthop* 61:219–223.

151. Senter HJ, Kortyna R, Kemp WR (1989): Anterior cervical fusion with hydroxylapatite fusion. *Neurosurgery* 25:39–42.

152. Shima T, Keller JT, Alvirn MM, Mayfield FH, Dunsker SB (1979): Anterior cervical discectomy and interbody fusion: An experimental study using a synthetic tricalcium phosphate. *J Neurosurg* 51:533–538.

153. Shinomiya K, Okamoto A, Kamikozuru M, et al. (1993): An analysis of failures in primary cervical anterior spinal cord decompression and fusion. *J Spinal Disord* 6:277–288.

154. Shireffs TG, Reeves AG (1991): Central corpectomy for cervical spondylitic myelopathy: A consecutive series with long-term follow-up evaluation. *J Neurosurg* 74:163–170.

155. Shono Y, McAfee PC, Cunningham BW, Brantigan JW (1993): A biomechanical analysis of decompression and reconstruction methods in the cervical spine. Emphasis on a carbon-fiber-composite cage. *J Bone Joint Surg* 75:1674–1684.

156. Simmons EH, Bhalla SK (1969): Anterior cervical discectomy and fusion: A clinical and biomechanical study with eight year follow-up. *J Bone Joint Surg [Br]* 51:225–237.

157. Smith MD, Bolesta MJ (1992): Esophageal perforation after anterior cervical plate fixation: A report of two cases. *J Spinal Disord* 5:357–361.

158. Southwick WO, Robinson RA (1957): Surgical approaches to the vertebral bodies in the cervical and lumbar regions. *J Bone Joint Surg [Am]* 39:631–644.

159. Spetzler RF, Roski RA, Selman WR (1982): The microscope in anterior cervical spine surgery. *Clin Orthop* 168:17–23.

160. Stauffer ES, Kaufer H (1975): Fractures and dislocations of the spine. In: Rockwood CA, Green DP, eds. *Fractures.* Philadelphia: J.B. Lippincott, pp. 851–853.

161. Stevens JM, Clifton AG, Whiten P (1993): Appearance of posterior osteophytes after sound anterior interbody fusion in the cer-

vical spine: A high definition computed myelographic study. *Neuroradiology* 35:227–228.

162. Stoltmann H, Blackwood W (1964): The rule of the ligamenta flava in the pathogenesis of myelopathy in cervical spondylosis. *Brain* 87:45–50.

163. Stookey B (1928): Compression of the spinal cord due to ventral extradural cervical chondromas: Diagnosis and surgical treatment. *Arch Neurol Psychiatry* 20:275–291.

164. Stuck RM (1963): Anterior cervical disc excision and fusion: Report of two hundred consecutive cases. *Rocky Mount Med J* 60: 25–30.

165. Sugar O (1981): Spinal cord malfunction after anterior cervical discectomy. *Surg Neurol* 15:4–8.

166. Taheri ZE, Gueramy M (1972): Experience with calf bone in cervical interbody spinal fusion. *J Neurosurg* 36:67–71.

167. Tarlov IM, Klinger H (1954): Spinal cord compression studies: II. Time limits for recovery after acute compression in dogs. *Arch Neurol Psychiatry* 71:271–290.

168. Tarlov IM, Klinger H, Vitale S (1953): Spinal cord compression studies: I. Experimental techniques to produce acute and gradual compression. *Arch Neurol Psychiatry* 70:813–819.

169. Taylor AR (1953): Mechanism and treatment of spinal-cord disorders associated with cervical spondylosis. *Lancet* 1:717–723.

170. Tew JM Jr, Mayfield FH (1975): Complications of surgery of the anterior cervical spine. *Clin Neurol* 23:424–434.

171. Tew JM, Mayfield FH (1981): Surgery of the anterior cervical spine: Prevention of complications. In: Dunsker SB, ed. *Cervical spondylosis.* New York: Raven Press, pp. 191–208.

172. Tezuka A, Yamada K, Ikata T (1976): Surgical results of cervical spondylitic radiculo-myelopathy observed more than five years. *Tokushima J Exp Med* 23:9–18.

173. de Tribolet N, Zander E (1981): Anterior discectomy without fusion for the treatment of ruptured cervical discs. *J Neurosurg Sci* 25:217–222.

174. Tsuji H (1982): Laminoplasty for patients with compressive myelopathy due to so-called spinal canal stenosis in cervical and thoracic regions. *Spine* 7:28–34.

175. Tsuyama N (1981): The ossification of the posterior longitudinal ligament of the spine (OPLL). *J Jpn Orthop Assoc* 55:425–440.

176. U HS, Wilson CB (1978): Postoperative epidural hematoma as a complication of anterior cervical discectomy. *J Neurosurg* 49: 288–291.

177. Verbiest H, Paz Y, Geuse HD (1966): Anterolateral surgery for cervical spondylosis in cases of myelopathy or nerve root compression. *J Neurosurg* 25:611–622.

178. White AA III, Hirsch C (1971): An experimental study of the immediate load bearing capacity of some commonly used iliac grafts. *Acta Orthop Scand* 42:482–490.

179. White AA III, Southwick WO, DePonte RJ, Gainor SW, Hardy R (1973): Relief of pain by anterior cervical spine fusion for spondylosis: A report of sixty-five cases. *J Bone Joint Surg* [Am] 55: 525–534.

180. Whitecloud TS III (1978): Complication of anterior cervical fusion. In: *American Academy of Orthopaedic Surgeons: Instructional course lectures,* Vol. 27. St. Louis: C.V. Mosby, pp. 223–227.

181. Whitecloud TS III (1988): Anterior surgery for cervical spondylitic myelopathy: Smith-Robinson, Cloward and vertebrectomy. *Spine* 13:861–863.

182. Whitecloud TS III, LaRocca SH (1976): Fibular strut graft in reconstructive surgery of the cervical spine. *Spine* 1:33–43.

183. Whitecloud TS III, Levet B (1993): Smith-Robinson graft reversal. In: Whitecloud TS, Dunsker SB, eds. *Anterior cervical spine surgery.* New York: Raven Press, pp. 39–42.

184. Whitecloud TS III, Seago RA (1987): Cervical discogenic syndrome: Results of operative intervention in patients with positive discography. *Spine* 12:313–315.

185. Williams JL, Allen MD Jr, Harkess JW (1968): Late results of cervical discectomy and interbody fusion: Some factors influencing the results. *J Bone Joint Surg* [Am] 50:277–286.

186. Wilson DH, Campbell DD (1977): Anterior cervical discectomy without bone graft: Report of seventy-one cases. *J Neurosurg* 47: 551–555.

187. Wohlert L, Buhl M, Eriksen EF, et al. (1984): Treatment of cervical disc disease using Cloward's technique. III. Evaluation of cervical spondylitic myelopathy in 138 cases. *Acta Neurochir (Wien)* 71:121–131.

188. Wolf BS, Khilnani M, Malis L (1956): The sagittal diameter of the bony cervical spinal canal and its significance in cervical spondylosis. *J Mount Sinai Hosp* 23:283–292.

189. Yonenobu K, Fuji T, Ono K, Okada K, Yamamoto T, Harada N (1985): Choice of surgical treatment for multisegmental cervical spondylitic myelopathy. *Spine* 10:710–716.

190. Yonenobu K, Hosono N, Iwasaki M, et al. (1992): Laminoplasty versus subtotal corpectomy: A comparative study of results in multisegmental cervical spondylitic myelopathy. *Spine* 17:1281–1284.

191. Young WF, Rosenwassen RH (1993): An early comparative analysis of the use of fibular allograft versus autologous iliac crest graft for interbody fusion after anterior cervical discectomy. *Spine* 18: 1123–1124.

192. Zdeblick TA, Bohlman HH (1989): Myelopathy, cervical kyphosis and treatment by anterior corpectomy and strut grafting. *J Bone Joint Surg* [Am] 71:170–182.

193. Zdeblick TA, Cooke ME, Wilson D, et al. (1993): Anterior cervical discectomy, fusion and plating: A comparative animal study. *Spine* 18:1974–1983.

194. Zdeblick TA, Ducker TB (1991): The use of freeze-dried allograft bone for anterior cervical fusions. *Spine* 16:726–729.

195. Zhang ZH, Yin H, Yang K, Zhang T, Dong F, Dang G, Lou SQ, Cai Q (1983): Anterior intervertebral disc excision and bone grafting in cervical spondylitic myelopathy. *Spine* 8:16–19.

The Adult Spine: Principles and Practice,
2nd edition, J.W. Frymoyer, Editor-in-Chief.
Lippincott-Raven Publishers, Philadelphia © 1997.

CHAPTER 66

Cervical Radiculopathies and Myelopathies: Posterior Approaches

Thomas B. Ducker and Seth M. Zeidman

When spinal surgery developed at the turn of the century, the neurologist made an anatomic diagnosis and advised the surgeon where to make the incision. An extendible midline incision over the spinous processes enabled progressive exposure of segments until the pathology was found. In the early 1920s, the conditions of nerve root pain (sciatica) and myelopathy became better appreciated and differentiated. Specific root syndromes were identified in the 1940s, and by the 1950s the posterior decompression keyhole surgical procedure for removal of a lateral ruptured cervical intervertebral disc and/or osteophytes had been described (59,62,63). By the 1960s, neurosurgeons and orthopedists could treat various radicular syndromes resulting from disc rupture (45). Myelopathies due to cervical spondylitic stenosis, either acquired or congenital, were reported (6), and

their treatment via the posterior approach was well defined (1,11,18,42). Utilization of an anterior approach to the cervical spine began in the late 1950s, and debate on which route was preferable began (10,42,61). The debate regarding the posterior versus the anterior procedure continues to the present day. Posterior procedures are not only acceptable but may be preferable for certain patients with cervical spondylosis. Physicians utilizing the posterior approach to the exclusion of an anterior procedure and vice versa are not providing optimal care, because each patient's case must be individualized.

The posterior approach has certain advantages over the anterior route. The midline structures and musculature can be rapidly and safely divided without endangering major vessels or nerves, the esophagus, or the trachea. Careful muscle reapproximation, utilizing multiple layers, yields an acceptable cosmetic result. The posterior exposure carries minimal potential for producing instability or malalignment, providing the integrity of the facet joints and capsules is preserved. Multilevel stenosis can easily be decompressed from the posterior approach with good visualization over several segments and full appreciation of the extent of decompression. Furthermore, the entire cervical spine can be easily treated because there is access to lesions as high as C1 and as low as T1.

    T. B. Ducker, M.D.: Professor of Neurosurgery, Department of Neurosurgery, The Johns Hopkins University School of Medicine, Baltimore, Maryland, 21205.
    S. M. Zeidman, M.D.: Clinical Instructor, The Johns Hopkins University School of Medicine, Baltimore, Maryland; Assistant Professor, Departments of Surgery and Critical Care Medicine, The Uniformed Services University of the Health Sciences, and Staff Neurosurgeon, Division of Neurosurgery, Department of Surgery, Walter Reed Army Medical Center, Washington, D.C., 20307.

The posterior exposure is not ideal for all patients, however. Clear cut pathology at one or two disc levels anteriorly, and/or focal instability at a single interspace, is an indication for an anterior procedure, which can be safely and rapidly performed with minimal morbidity or mortality. When preoperative diagnostic images reveal the predominant pathology to be anterior, posterior operations are not as successful. In particular, anterior compression with cervical kyphosis is a clear indication for anterior decompression and fusion. Multilevel laminectomies in children can produce instability and result in a postlaminectomy kyphotic deformity. Appreciation of each patient's complaints and analysis of imaging studies will allow selection of an appropriate procedure.

CLINICAL ASSESSMENT

Before undertaking surgical therapy for radiculopathy or myelopathy, sequential evaluations should be performed and a treatment using non-operative modalities attempted. The interval between visits varies widely. A patient with an acute problem, such as severe pain or progressive neurological loss, requires rapid performance of definitive diagnostic studies with early re-evaluation to allow expeditious treatment. A patient with chronic and/or recurrent pain, with minimal associated weakness, requires re-evaluation on a weekly or monthly basis, permitting full appreciation of the neurological syndrome. Accurate neurological diagnosis is essential to appropriately treat radiculopathies and myelopathies. Posterior operations rely on specific identification and decompression of the involved nerve root(s) and/or spinal cord. Although axial cervical pain with referred pain can occasionally be relieved with anterior cervical fusion, this is rarely the case posteriorly. Clinical identification of the involved neural structure facilitates radiologic confirmation of the lesion.

Plain cervical spine radiographs, often with flexion and extension views to evaluate stability, are the essential first step in the radiologic diagnostic evaluation. The more bony abnormalities identified on plain films, the more likely a computed tomographic (CT) scan will permit definitive diagnosis. The CT is an excellent study in many older patients. Radiographs without noteworthy bony pathology should focus attention on a soft tissue lesion, and magnetic resonance imaging (MRI) is the next indicated study. Unfortunately, some patients have an osteophyte at one level and a soft disc herniation at the next, and isolated use of MRI or CT may not fully define the pathological abnormality. If CT and MRI do not provide a diagnosis, and a neurological syndrome is strongly suspected, other, more invasive, studies may be required. Depending on the index of suspicion and the seriousness of pathology, one can choose an enhanced CT scan or a myelogram followed by selected CT images

at levels of involvement (i.e., a CT myelogram). At the same time, the cerebrospinal fluid should be fully evaluated. Finally, there are those patients in whom the clinical symptoms and signs are not straightforward. In these patients, intracranial pathology needs to be excluded by MRI of the brain. Some patients have multiple pathological processes, such as a myelopathy accompanied by multiple sclerosis (MS). Improved diagnostic techniques increase the probability of accurate diagnosis.

Concurrent disease influences the outcome of care of the patient with myelopathies and radiculopathies. The metabolic disease with the most wide-ranging adverse influence is diabetes. Particularly in the older patient, vascular, heart, and pulmonary disease may preclude operative treatment. Finally, neurological disorders (such as MS and amyotrophic lateral sclerosis) always make diagnosis challenging. Each spinal surgeon has his own rare case wherein standard surgery failed to relieve the patient of his problem and the extremely rare diagnosis was made later. An example is a patient succumbing to Shy-Drager syndrome (severe dysautonomia and concurrent myelopathy). Repeat assessments generally permit identification of each patient's neurological syndrome.

INFORMED CONSENT AND ANTICIPATED RESULTS

The natural histories of untreated radiculopathies and myelopathies are quite different. Radiculopathies, even when severe, tend to improve even though there may be persistent weakness and pain. A devastating outcome from an untreated radiculopathy is rare. Therefore, decisions regarding surgical treatment should consider the quality of the patient's life more than any other single factor. With radiculopathies, persistent pain or weakness often interferes with activities despite adequate medical treatment including anti-inflammatory drugs.

The natural history of untreated myelopathies, on the other hand, is a different matter. Two thirds of patients will have progression of their myelopathy, with numbness and clumsiness of the hands and weakness in the legs, and over a period of years they may become confined to a wheelchair or a bed. When operative intervention is delayed until the late stages of the disease, irreversible harm will have been done to the cord, and substantial recovery is unlikely. Myelopathy complicated by ossification of the posterior longitudinal ligament is common in the Orient and rare in the Western hemisphere. It carries the same ominous prognosis as spondylitic myelopathy. The description of end-stage myelopathy with spinal cord scarring and gliosis is well documented.

When operative intervention is planned, and anticipated results are being explained to the patient to obtain an informed consent, it is necessary to discuss both general information about operative care and specific details about the patient's disorder. General broad statements addressing the risks of anesthesia and drug reactions are appropriate, but these complications are rare. A general statement about infection should be included. The infection rate in spinal procedures typically is 1% to 2% and appears to be even less when 24 hours of antibiotic coverage is provided (12,30,31,56,57,60). Although the consequences of infection need to be outlined, a reassuring statement to the effect that most surgical infections can be successfully treated with antibiotics can be added. Thrombophlebitis in the lower extremities, or thrombophlebotic phenomenon, can occur and is more common in older patients, especially when the operation is protracted. Again, this occurs in less than 1 patient per 100. In our experience, use of the intermittent pressure device or sequential compression stockings on the lower extremities intraoperatively and immediately postoperatively has reduced the incidence of lower extremity venous thrombosis to almost zero. Postoperative urinary tract infections still occur, and if a man has preexisting prostatism or a woman has a history of recurrent urinary tract infection, it is a greater risk. Specific problems related to the surgery itself include iatrogenic spinal instability and spinal cord or nerve root injury. Treating radiculopathies with intervertebral disc removal, foraminal decompression, or reduction of an osteophytic spur will impair neurological function in the specific nerve root in 2% to 3% of cases. In treating radiculopathies, damage to the spinal cord is rare but does occur in 1 out of 200 to 300 cases. Systemic disease, such as longstanding insulin-dependent diabetes mellitus, increases the risk of neurological injury. Such patients may have diabetic end-artery disease, and manipulation of the root can lead to a central ischemic episode in the spinal cord itself. Spinal instability after laminoforaminotomies is extremely rare, providing careful attention is paid to facet integrity. In summary, 90% to 97% of patients undergoing posterior cervical surgery for radiculopathies have a satisfactory outcome (17,22,33,44,46,50,59,62,63). Our success rate has been 97%. A total of 172 patients (93 men and 79 women) were operated on for cervical radiculopathy. The majority of patients had pathology at C5-C6 and C6-C7. The average age of patients undergoing posterior cervical laminoforaminotomy for radiculopathy was 49 years. Sixty patients (35%) required a posterolateral discectomy for herniated disc fragments. Patients operated on for herniated discs were younger (mean age, 43 years) than those without discectomy. A group of 68 patients (40%) who were somewhat older (mean age, 55 years) were operated on at multiple levels. Multiple-level foraminotomies were carried out to relieve the patients of more diffuse symptoms in the upper extremities.

Relief of radicular pain was obtained in 167 patients (97%) who had laminoforaminotomies. In 77% of patients, evaluation was at follow-up 2 or more years after the procedure, and it was after 1 year for the remaining 23%. Failure to relieve radicular pain was noted in five patients (3%), four of whom had operations at multiple levels. Improvement in motor weakness, back to baseline function, was achieved in 36 of the 39 patients (93%) with preoperative motor deficits who underwent laminoforaminotomies with discectomy. The 68 patients who underwent multiple-level laminoforaminotomies presented initially with pain and weakness, and they obtained significant relief of their pain with minimal relief of their weakness. Four of these patients (5.8%) received substantial relief of their preoperative motor deficits. The overwhelming majority of patients undergoing laminoforaminotomy with discectomy or single-level laminoforaminotomies had improvement in preoperative sensory abnormalities. In contrast, the degree of improvement in sensory deficits was not as great in patients who underwent multiple-level laminoforaminotomies. The only significant morbidity was a central cord syndrome in one diabetic patient, which resolved in part within a few months with some residual deficit.

These outcome numbers exceed the number reported in general cervical spine or lumbar spine operations, and the radiculopathic patients clearly responded better than the myelopathic patients. Outcome assessments by independent third person reviews are not so optimistic. The latest Cervical Spine Research Society data, not yet published, probably tell more accurately what happens in cervical spine operations. When there is an independent third-party interview before an operation and at 6 months and 1 year, the number of good results is less. When one studies all patients who have had similar operations, and outcome is graded on a scale by a person not in the doctor's office, over 70% of the patients are truly improved. Improvement in cervical radiculopathy is best determined by pain reduction. It should be noted that many lumbar spine outcome studies show similar numbers. Although the single-root cervical decompressive procedure with a posterior approach is one of the best operations on the spine, a true outcome number for this operation varies from over 70% to over 90%, with 80% being probably the fairest figure.

Compared to the treatment of radiculopathies, operative decompression for myelopathy is much more hazardous. If it were not for the grave prognosis without decompression, surgeons would be hesitant to do these procedures. In providing informed consent for these patients, the evidence indicates that two thirds of the patients will continue to deteriorate without surgery (5,6,39,49,55). However, a well-executed decompressive laminectomy with limited foraminotomies as needed will lead to partial or complete improvement in the patient's clinical condition in over 77% of patients (2,8,16,20,43). How aggressive the surgeon is in removing osteophytes in and around the foramen depends on preference and skills, but certainly the experience reported by Epstein et al. (20) indicates that foraminotomy may further enhance recovery after the surgical procedure. Use of dural grafts, with or without dentate ligament sectioning, does not improve the patient's chances of a favorable outcome (2,11,26,28,29,43,50,52,66). The major goal is adequate posterior decompressive laminectomy, and this is usually all that is required (8,11,16,17,23).

COMPARISON OF SURGICAL RESULTS AFTER ANTERIOR AND POSTERIOR DECOMPRESSION

In Table 1, the posterior and anterior approaches are compared by adding together several large series. In many of these series, the patients treated with posterior procedures were older and had a more severe cord deficit (8,17). Yet, the results of treatment are comparable. These data support both anterior and posterior operative approaches, but they also indirectly support the concept that individualizing each case to select the most appropriate decompressive procedure is the responsibility of the surgeon (6,8,11,17,22,28,42,53,67,69). However, it also must be recognized that not all patients do well. Older patients with severe myelopathy, who are unable to ambulate, run a risk of dying from the procedure. As previously noted, these patients are more prone to cardiovascular and thromboembolic complications. The percent of patients actually worse following a decompressive laminectomy varies from 3% to 10% [in our experience, it is 4% to 5% (8)]. We have recently reviewed our experience with 300 patients operated on via either an anterior or a posterior approach. One hundred twenty-two patients underwent an anterior procedure, 165 a posterior procedure, and 13 a combined procedure. Of those patients undergoing anterior surgery, 72 (59%) had a single-level procedure, 47 (39%) a two-level procedure, and 3 patients (2%) a three-level discectomy and fusion. Of those patients undergoing a posterior decompressive procedure, 135 (72%) had decompressive procedures alone, and 30 of the patients (18%) un-

derwent a laminectomy and fusion. In the 1970s, decompressive laminectomies were generally confined to three or four levels, but, in the 1980s, five-level procedures were performed in nearly every patient.

The two groups of patients (anterior and posterior approaches) differed in several ways. Patients operated on by a posterior approach were older (mean age, 60 years) and worse neurologically (average preoperative clinical grade, 3.2). Patients undergoing anterior procedures were younger (mean age, 47 years) with an average preoperative clinical grade of 2.4. The average postoperative grade was 0.8 for patients operated on by the anterior route and 1.5 for patients decompressed from the posterior route. Eighty-five percent of the patients undergoing an anterior procedure improved, compared to 77% for posterior procedures, with the *amount* of improvement being equivalent between the two groups (1.6 versus 1.7 Nurick grade). Overall, the results were comparable.

KYPHOSIS

The contour of the cervical spine should be carefully assessed preoperatively. With a lordotic or straight curve and myelopathy, a laminectomy over several segments allows posterior cord migration, relieving anterior impingement. However, a kyphotic curve places the spinal cord under tension over the angular deformity. Laminectomy will be ineffective in relieving cord impingement and may further destabilize the spine, increasing kyphosis (4,8,27,28,42,67,69). Coexistence of myelopathy and cervical kyphosis is a clear indication for anterior decompression and fusion.

OSSIFICATION OF POSTERIOR LONGITUDINAL LIGAMENTS

Myelopathy associated with ossification of the posterior longitudinal ligament (OPLL) is a serious problem (13). Ossification of the posterior longitudinal ligament can take on many configurations; for example, there may be protrusions into the canal, and they may be square-shaped, mushroom-like, or Hill types (see Fig. 15) (3,13,25,35,37,47,48). When bony compression impinges on the anterior spinal artery complex, ischemic spinal cord injury may result. Surgical results for OPLL do not have the 70% good results for myelopathy associated with degeneration; even the Japanese can only improve 60% of these patients (34,35,38). The OPLL continues to progress and impinge upon the spinal cord even after operative intervention in 25% to 80% of patients (37). Fusion with laminoplasties retards the transverse and longitudinal growth of the OPLL. Standard decompressive procedure is less commonly carried out on this particular subgroup of patients. This subgroup of patients, which exceeds 10% in some series, has a higher

TABLE 1. *Comparing anterior and posterior decompressive procedures in cervical myelopathy patients. Numbers reflect summations of several large series*

Approach	Patients	Improved	Unimproved
Anterior	434	73%	27%
Posterior	685	71%	29%

References for this table are available in the articles by Epstein (16) and Carol and Ducker (8). Additional references concerning the anterior approach are in Chapter 69 by Whitecloud (this volume) and in references 27, 43, 67, 68, and 69.

There is no randomized comparative series. In most comparative evaluations, the patients having the posterior decompressive procedures were older, had disease at many levels, and presented with worse neurological deficits (8).

probability of being neurologically worse after the decompression.

PREOPERATIVE PLANNING AND ADJUNCTS TO SURGERY

Anesthesia: Positioning and Monitoring

Patient positioning should reflect the surgeon's and anesthesiologist's preference. The prone position causes engorgement of adjacent veins and tissues, which impairs visualization and could compromise the decompression. Although the sitting position produces less venous engorgement and drains fluid and blood away from the surgical field, there is a risk of air emboli and cardiovascular instability. Unfortunately, if an adverse problem develops with either position, there are self-styled experts who travel the country claiming the physician or anesthesiologist made the wrong choice. Either the prone or sitting position is acceptable for the treatment of radiculopathies and myelopathies. For a variety of reasons, surgeons tend to use the sitting position for the radicular nerve root decompressions and the prone position for myelopathy. In treating radiculopathies, bony resection is unilateral and quite limited, and the operation is swiftly carried out. It is in those positions that we consistently work in front of the nerve root to remove a herniated disc or osteophyte. Good visualization of the nerve root without engorgement of fluid or blood is important. In our experience of over 500 cases, we have not had serious air emboli leading to cardiovascular instability or alteration in the end-tidal PCO_2. While the Doppler has detected air on a few occasions, this has never been of clinical consequence. Our experience parallels that of Henderson et al. (33). Although the prone position is more common for myelopathy, the experience of Epstein et al. (18,20) clearly shows that patients properly positioned and hydrated can have these procedures carried out in the sitting position as well. If the patient has a severe myelopathy that leads to altered sympathetic tone causing low blood pressure and compromised spinal cord perfusion, the prone position may be safer. A more complete analysis of over 500 cases by Matjasko et al. is available for review (41).

Holding the patient's head during operative intervention of the cervical spine is usually done by the three-pin Mayfield head holders. In some of the patients who have severe myelopathies, traction can afford some minor pain relief prior to operative intervention. In those patients who have had an acute traumatic event, utilization of traction in the hospital bed with the head and shoulders elevated 10° to 20° helps. The 15 to 20 pounds of traction opens up the joints, decompressing the collapsed ligaments. In patients with significant myelopathy, skeletal tong traction with 15 to 20 pounds during

the operation is recommended (8). Traction can be done with an operative wedge or a Stryker frame, or it can be carried out with standard operating room equipment with horseshoe head apparatus and a traction attachment. Gardner-Wells tongs facilitate the rotation from supine to prone without unusual positioning. Traction is most commonly used in myelopathy patients undergoing decompression.

Intubation techniques depend on the patient's diagnosis. If the patient has a supple neck and radiculopathy, a standard intubation technique is safe. When the endotracheal tube is in position, primary extension is at the occipital C1-C2 area, with flexion occurring in the lower cervical areas, where the pathology commonly occurs. In patients with early myelopathy who have a good cervical range of motion, transient extension to place the endotracheal tube rarely causes a problem. However, in patients with severe myelopathies and stenosis involving C3-C4 or higher, most anesthesiologists and surgeons prefer an awake fiberoptic-assisted intubation under local anesthesia. These patients are more likely to be operated on in a Stryker frame and with traction. Once properly intubated, the patient can be placed under general anesthesia, maintained or placed in traction, and turned safely without significant risks. In some instances, patient positioning prior to administration of general anesthesia is preferable after awake intubation.

Intravascular volume, controlled by peripheral and central venous lines, is assessed on an individual basis. If the sitting position is used, it is wise to keep the patient well hydrated unless there is a specific cardiovascular contraindication. Certain centers advocate central line placement in all these patients. One rationale for a central line is aspiration of air from the right atrium in the event of air embolism. Based on our experience, we have been unimpressed with the ability to remove air through these lines. In fact, suction applied to a central line may further compromise cardiac output. Using the central line as a measure of central blood volume is of more value (19,41) and justified in an unstable patient.

With limited laminoforaminotomies for root decompression, adequate hydration, Doppler monitoring for air embolism, and careful monitoring of vital signs and end-tidal PCO_2 are all that is required. End-tidal PCO_2 monitoring will also alert the anesthesiologist to kinks in the endotracheal tube. Placing a central line in all of these patients is unnecessary and may lead to complications (33). In our experience treating radiculopathies with one- or two-level laminoforaminotomies, we have had more difficulty with pneumothoraces from line placement (three patients) than serious air emboli (no patients). Doppler will detect air in roughly 3% of patients, but the vital signs, end-tidal PCO_2, and other indicators do not change and the volume of air must be minimal (41). Consequently, for simple unilateral laminoforaminotomies, we place a central venous or pulmonary wedge pressure line in less than half of our patients, and the decision is left to the anesthesiologist.

If the patient to be treated has a myelopathy, especially if it is an elderly patient taking antihypertensive medications, monitoring to include central venous pressure and/or pulmonary arterial wedge pressures may be necessary. Central lines are often helpful in the prone patient. These patients have an abnormal sympathetic nervous system due to cervical spinal cord compression. The central fibers of the reticulospinal system are damaged along with the motor and sensory fibers. With an unstable sympathetic system, and if there is an unstable cardiac condition, these patients may be more difficult to manage in either position. If one elects to use the sitting position in this group of patients, proper hydration and monitoring are warranted (41). Furthermore, in these patients treated in the sitting position, the importance of Doppler monitoring cannot be overemphasized. When air is heard, even though it may not alter the vascular dynamics, the source of the air should be identified and the vessel coagulated with a bipolar cautery. If it is inaccessible, temporarily packing the wound with wet sponge for a minute or two will often stop this air influx permanently. Doppler monitoring should be utilized by the surgeon as a warning to find the source of any open vessel. Once the air is heard, the next important monitor is the end-tidal PCO_2. If there is significant air, the end-tidal PCO_2 will fall and blood pressure and cardiac output may be diminished. If this occurs, the wound must be packed with wet sponges until hemodynamic stability is regained.

Evoked Potentials

Somatosensory evoked potential monitoring of the spinal cord during operations for myelopathy is now commonplace (14). Evoked potential monitoring is not needed for treating radiculopathies, but it is helpful for certain myelopathy patients. By utilizing certain anesthetic agents, an evoked potential not present on routine study can be augmented, allowing recording throughout the surgical procedure (4). Most evoked potential monitoring techniques measure the sensory systems through the posterior columns. This is a valuable tool with posterior cervical operations and decompression, although there are limitations. Many anesthetic agents depress the response, making interpretation difficult. Moreover, patients with severe myelopathy may have impaired evoked potentials preoperatively, which makes intraoperatively assessment impossible. Information from evoked potentials alters the care in only 3% of patients (9). Patient position is often modified because of evoked potentials. We have found that having the patient in a neutral, slightly flexed position yields the strongest potentials. Hyperflexion or hyperextension is detrimental

to the evoked potentials and to the cord. Hypotension is definitely detrimental to the evoked potentials. Any pressure applied to the spinal cord during the surgical procedure will alter the potential (9).

Intraoperative Radiography

No matter how trivial or unnecessary it may seem, a single localizing intraoperative x-ray should be utilized. This film helps the surgeon confine dissection to the pathological area, and it prevents exploration of a nerve root that does not require inspection. It also is a means of defense in a litigious society that may accuse the surgeon of not carrying out the procedure properly.

Antibiotics and Steroids

Use of perioperative antibiotics and steroids remains controversial. Our early research shows that steroids are more helpful when administered prior to spinal cord injury than when administered afterwards (15). There is a definite place for this medication, even though it is limited (7,8,32). It is common for surgeons to give the patient 4 to 6 mg of dexamethasone, or an equivalent dose of methylprednisolone, 2 hours before the procedure and intraoperatively, and two or three doses every 6 hours after the surgical procedure. Twenty-four-hour coverage is all that is needed. Utilizing the medication for longer periods, while advocated by some, seems unnecessary (8,17). Conversely, the short time use of steroids appears beneficial experimentally and clinically (7,32).

Perioperative antibiotics appear to be beneficial (12,30,31,40,56,57,60,64). Haines (30) reviewed and summarized the more than 100 articles on this subject and recommends that an antibiotic be given in the perioperative period. The major intraoperative infectious organism is *Staphylococcus*. Consequently, a newer penicillin or one of the cephalosporins is acceptable. If the patient is allergic to penicillin, then either no drug or an entirely different family of medications such as vancomycin would be needed.

OPERATIVE TECHNIQUE

Laminotomy and Laminoforaminotomy

Exposure of the lamina and the foramen to decompress the nerve root for a radiculopathy can be from either a straight posterior incision or a posterior lateral incision. The former is the traditional approach (17,22,33,46,53,59,63), whereas the latter has been developed more recently and is quite effective (Fig. 1) (44). The pure posterior approach takes down the muscle attachments

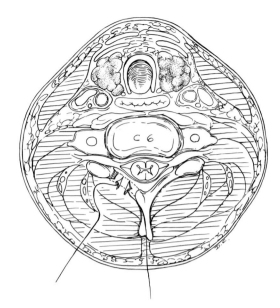

FIG. 1. The most common posterior approach to the cervical spine for radiculopathy is midline posterior, but the postero-lateral approach is equally acceptable. Both approaches to the nerve root allow adequate views of any pathology.

off the midline and the spinous processes in order to expose the lamina and facets. The posterolateral approach is more of a muscle-splitting procedure, but, again, the muscles are taken off part of the lamina and facet area. The older posterior procedure was developed, in part, in the 1940s, and it was clearly described in the 1950s (50,59,62,63). The "keyhole" foraminotomy became common in the 1950s and the early 1960s (21,46,58) (Fig. 2). The incision has to be long enough for the instruments to be placed in the operative hole without obliterating the surgeon's view. With good exposure of the lamina and two thirds of the facet, a single blade re-

tractor is all that is required to hold the muscles laterally. Although we have had special instruments made for this common procedure, commercially available retractors accomplish the same task. If the neck is hyperflexed, the muscles and adjacent tendons are extremely tight, making it difficult to retract the muscles laterally. If the neck is only slightly flexed, the retraction is easily achieved without a great deal of strain on the tissues. If the neck is extended, it is harder to get into the interlaminar space to accomplish the exposure for decompression. Neck position is a factor in both the sitting and prone positions.

A localizing x-ray is commonly employed at the dissecting stage of exposure. An instrument such as a small dissector probe is placed into the apophyseal joint at the level that has been exposed, and the intraoperative film will confirm that the correct interlaminar space has been reached (Fig. 3). The marker will point to the vertebral body slightly above the joint space itself. Others prefer to mark a spinous process or an intraspinous process area for the film. All of these techniques are acceptable and provide intraoperative confirmation, at the time of initial exposure, that the bony removal is at the correct level. Because the incisions are not long and the exposures are limited, it is difficult to count, with certainty, the various spinous processes to be confident of proper exposure without an intraoperative film.

Studying both the lateral and AP plain x-rays, with identification of the last bifid spine, whether C5 or C6, aids in creating the proper limited exposure. If a straight

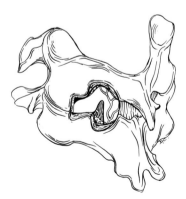

FIG. 2. For three decades, "keyhole" laminoforaminotomies have provided good exposure to the nerve root and the lateral dura. Only a very small portion of the ligamentum flavum needs to be removed. Although tiny cotton pledgets can be placed laterally to compress epidural veins, there are occasions when posterior epidural veins need to be coagulated. The dura covering the spinal cord is not retracted for this laterally extruded disc.

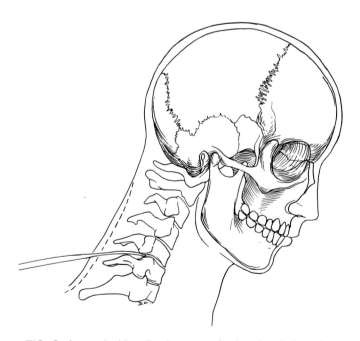

FIG. 3. In cervical hemilaminectomy for herniated disc, the incisions now are shorter, making it difficult to identify the vertebral level with certainty. Therefore, an intraoperative localizing film is necessary. Placing a probe at the laminoforaminotomy site or in the facet joint makes the identification of the decompressive level absolutely accurate.

posterior exposure is used, one side of a bifid spine may be excised without any loss of mobility or stability, in order to achieve a better visualization of the lamina and facet areas. Removing that small part of the spinous process may also facilitate the placing of retractors to hold the muscle laterally. Bony removal is initiated in the intervertebral joint area. This can be safely done without introducing any instruments into the canal or onto the nerve root. The same bone can be taken away quickly with a high speed drill. Either the drill or rongeur forceps can be used to reduce the bulk of the bone superiorly, even in the facet area. In patients who have a lateral disc rupture without canal stenosis, small rongeurs and the very small angled Kerrison punches can be safely used. However, in patients who have any canal compromise and severe bony stenosis, high speed drills work better in thinning down the bone. In either case, the roof of the foramen or spinal root canal can be further decompressed with angled 2-0 and 3-0 curettes. This can be carried out by undercutting one third or one half of the facet area and the joint. The majority of the posterior apophyseal joint is maintained, and spinal instability is rarely

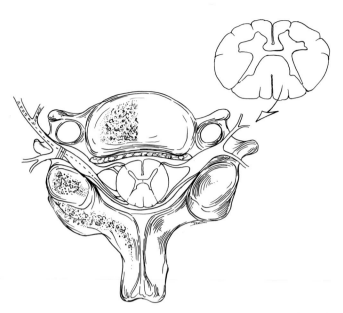

FIG. 5. The normal cross-sectional anatomy at C5-C6 illustrates the relation of the roots to the spinal cord itself. Gentle retraction of the roots in the axilla of the dura sleeve results in very little pressure on the cord.

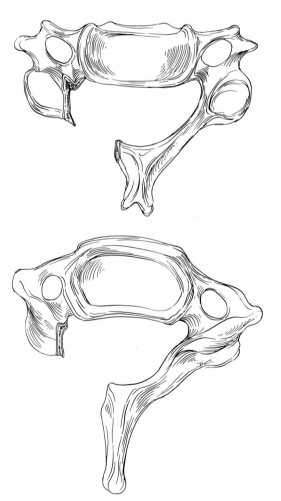

FIG. 4. In removing the bone posteriorly for radiculopathy, only one third of the facet itself needs to be removed, and this will not cause any instability.

an issue (53,54,70). Spinal instability does not occur when surgery is performed posteriorly for radiculopathy (Fig. 4).

When focal instability develops at one level, it is usually associated with neurofibroma tumor surgery in which much of the facet anatomy was destroyed prior to surgery and changed further with the operative exposure required to rid the patient of the tumor. If the bony removal is carried out properly, the lateral aspects of the dura sac can readily be visualized by removing only the lateral one third of the remaining ligamentum flavum and soft tissues. The nerve root as it exits from the dura sac should be visualized above and below, although most of the visualization is clearly inferiorly. The anatomy is usually clearly identified by gently sweeping aside any remaining small epidural fat present, by bipolar coagulation of any obvious veins, and by removing fibrous tissue over the posterior aspect of the nerve root itself. In the majority (90%) of clinical situations, the decompression of a cervical nerve root and the dura sac can be accomplished through this limited exposure. By taking a small dissector, the plane between the nerve root and the dura sac can be developed well up into the axilla of that junction of the dura (Fig. 5). The nerve root can be gently mobilized superiorly and then retracted without fear of significant damage, especially when the foraminotomy has been carried out so that the nerve root is free (Fig. 6). Again, any veins that are a problem can be treated with bipolar coagulation at that time, or a small micropledget or a cutdown pledget may be placed inferiorly if there is any oozing. Hemostatic cellulose material is rarely needed but can be placed epidural and laterally if required.

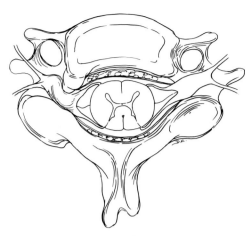

FIG. 6. Soft disc herniation in radiculopathy is lateral and beneath the nerve root. In some cases, it can be pulled from beneath the nerve root, and in others it remains beneath a thinned layer of posterior longitudinal ligament.

By holding the nerve root axilla superiorly, a small, blunt, micro–nerve hook may then be passed beneath the nerve root and the dura, and with a 360-degree sweeping motion, removal of any herniated disc fragments that have traversed the posterior longitudinal ligament can be safely accomplished (Fig. 7). The 90-degree nerve root hook sizes recommended are 2 mm, 3 mm, and, on very rare occasions, 4 mm. If the posterior longitudinal ligament is deformed over a disc or spur, it will be apparent at this stage of the operation, and the actual pathology can be appreciated with the smaller and shorter nerve hook. To remove a disc fragment that is still beneath the ligament, or to reduce an osteophyte in the same area, the posterolateral aspect of the posterior and longitudinal ligament needs to be incised. This is done with a pointed No. 11 knife, while one hand carefully holds the nerve root superiorly and the dura sac slightly medially. The cut into the posterior longitudinal ligament should extend directly behind the small dissector, which is holding the nerve root superiorly and slightly medially, and it should be made inferiorly and laterally (Fig. 8). In this fashion, the movement of the knife is always away from the spinal cord and the nerve root sleeve itself. If there is any bleeding at this time, bipolar coagulation can be utilized. If a soft disc is the diagnosis as proven by the preoperative study (such as MRI), the right-angled small nerve hooks or dissectors can again be introduced, and with a sweeping motion the herniated disc fragment will commonly present itself. Removing the disc fragment is easily done with toothed forceps (Fig. 9). Rarely are larger pituitary forceps needed. If there are herniated disc fragments, it is important to try to mobilize them so that they present away from the spinal cord and nerve root into the small opening made in the posterior and longitudinal ligament. By repeated sweeping motions, the sizeable disc fragments can be removed. One must remember that a large cervical disc would be very small for the lumbar area. Rarely, if ever, is a single huge disc fragment removed. In the two cases in which this was done, it was regretted: in one case it was definitely associated with a transient worsening

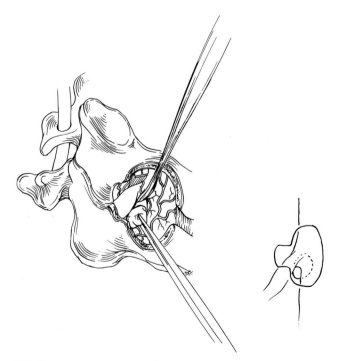

FIG. 7. In nearly all cases, the nerve root can be lifted safely. A micro–nerve hook will mobilize the disc. Long, small, toothed forceps can then remove a free fragment of disc.

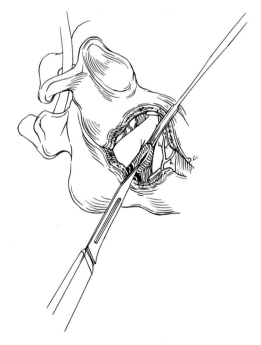

FIG. 8. In some cases, the disc herniation is beneath the posterior longitudinal ligament, so the ligament needs to be cut open. The incision is down and lateral away from the cord and roots.

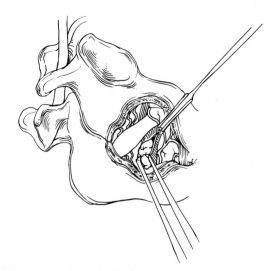

FIG. 9. Once there is an opening in the posterior longitudinal ligament, the micro–nerve hook can free the herniated fragments. Then, the herniated disc can be removed with the forceps.

of a patient's neurological signs and symptoms, and in the other case a transient central cord symptom developed. Fortunately, these neurological problems entirely cleared.

If, on opening the posterior longitudinal ligament, the problem beneath the nerve root is an obvious osteophyte (Fig. 10), this can easily be reduced with a small reverse-angled curette, utilizing a motion that again is both inferiorly and slightly laterally coming away from the cord and root (Fig. 11). These techniques have been available since the 1960s (17,19,46). If there is not a single bony spur or hump, a carefully executed laminoforaminotomy with decompression posteriorly will achieve relief of the patient's symptoms. This type of bony stenosis

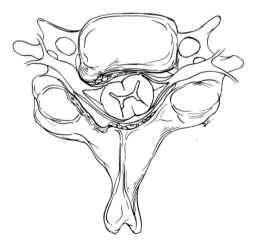

FIG. 10. Diffuse foraminal stenosis will respond to posterior decompression. In the drawing, the bone posterior to the root has been removed. In many cases, the foraminotomy is all that is required, but in some cases, the osteophyte from the uncinate process distorts the nerve root.

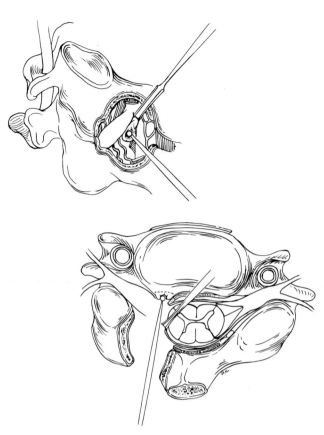

FIG. 11. When there is focal distortion of the nerve root due to osteophyte, removal of that bony prominence assures decompression. The posterior longitudinal ligament in front of the root needs to be incised, with bipolar coagulation. Either a small reverse-angled curette or a 2-mm diamond burr is needed to remove that bone.

can be identified on preoperative CT scan and is often a reflection of facet hypertrophy more than any anterior spurring. It is also in this group of patients that the clinical syndrome between two adjacent roots makes it difficult to identify a single root as the cause of the patient's symptoms. Consequently, it is in this group of patients that a two-level foraminotomy is carried out to relieve the patients of the diffuse symptoms in the upper extremity that could be either a C6 or C7 root syndrome (Fig. 12). In these cases, the pain extends down into the arm, is often worse with traction, is unrelenting, and is present for a long period of time. There is some triceps weakness and the sensory loss is more diffuse and rarely dermatomal. When the patient has this diffuse foraminal or nerve root canal stenosis due to facet disease and the apophyseal joint needs to be undercut some 50%, the straight posterior approach is better because over 50% of the posterior aspect of that joint can be maintained in the surgical procedure. If one is removing a simple lateral disc herniation or a very focal osteophytic posterior spurring coming off aspects of the uncovertebral joint, the posterolateral approach is equally good and, on occasion, superior. Control of bleeding is often easily

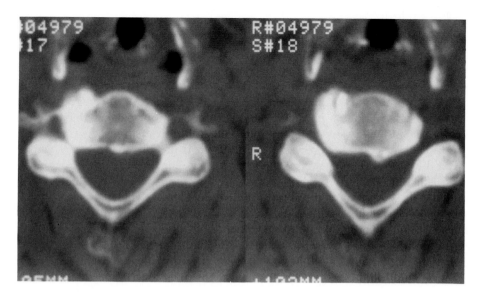

FIG. 12. A high-quality plain CT often will confirm the level of diffuse foraminal stenosis. In a few cases, the stenosis will be at two levels. Posterior laminoforaminotomies are quick, safe, and effective in these cases.

achieved with bipolar coagulation or temporary placement of micropaddies. If that fails, using hemostatic cellulose agents with small pledgets will achieve the hemostasis needed. Placing large pledgets is contraindicated. If one simply waits with a small pledget, the bleeding will stop. If there is a minor ooze at the end of the procedure, a small drain may be placed and removed in 12 to 24 hours. Postoperative hematomas for the laminotomies and the laminoforaminotomies are extremely rare.

Closure of even the simpler laminoforaminotomies needs to be carefully done. If the posterolateral exposure was chosen, the incision is mere muscle splitting, and simply by removing the retractors, the wound appears to close almost on its own. The outer two layers of fascia need to be closed with 1-0 polyglactin suture, a subcutaneous layer can be closed with 3-0 polyglactin, and the skin may be closed with either a small subcuticular nylon suture or staples. Patients prefer the former for comfort and cosmetic reasons. If the straight posterior exposure was chosen, four layers of polyglactin suture are needed. The deep muscles next to the spinous processes should be closed. Then the heavy fascial layer needs to be closed in two layers, getting the inferior aspect and then the superior aspect with different rows of sutures. The second fascial layer includes much of the ligamentum nuchal layer, especially in the inferior aspect of the cervical area. Even the deep subcutaneous tissue should be closed with inverted polyglactin to prevent spreading of the wound. The subcutaneous layer can then be closed with 3-0 polyglactin and the skin closed with either a small subcuticular nylon, a nonlocking running nylon, or staples. All of these lead to good cosmetic results. The most important aspect of closure of posterior cervical wounds is to prevent any separation of the muscles that can lead to an unsightly indentation or cavitation.

If immediately after the operative procedure the patient is worse neurologically, either at the root or cord level, it is the surgeon's responsibility to become aware of this problem in the recovery room, and not to leave the hospital until it is certain that the patient's arms and legs are functioning as well as they did preoperatively. If there is any problem, an immediate lateral cervical spine x-ray is indicated to check for alignment. After that, the patient needs a contrast diagnostic study. In the past, a full myelogram was utilized. More recently, an intrathecal enhanced CT scan with good visualization of the operative area will suffice to rule out any retained disc fragments or hematoma. If the myelogram and CT scan show no compression at the operative area, the patient should be treated as if there is a vascular spinal cord injury, which includes maintenance of good blood volume, adequate profusion pressure, and maintenance of normal blood pressure. If there is any suspicion of spinal instability, either traction or a firm cervical collar should be applied. If there is any contrast blockage or compression documented on the CT diagnostic study, such as hematoma, the patient should be taken back to the operating room within a few hours, for a wider decompressive laminectomy and removal of any residual pathology. The wound should be closed meticulously, and a small suction drainage catheter should be placed at the base of the wound to prevent reoccurrence of the same problem. In closure after a cervical laminectomy or a complicated laminotomy, utilization of a small suction catheter at the base of the wound is recommended. If the surgery went well and there is only a minor ooze, these catheters can be removed in 24 hours. If there is any persistent drainage, removal of such catheters after 48 hours is equally acceptable.

Postoperative Care

Postoperative care after a laminotomy for pathology on a nerve root should include encouraging the patient to be up and active as soon as possible; this includes bathroom privileges the day of the operation. For comfort, a soft cervical collar can be utilized; however, the majority of patients prefer to have no collar. For the first 18 to 24 hours after the procedure, antibiotic and steroid coverage can reduce the incidence of wound infection and nerve root swelling and pain, respectively. If steroids are used for 12 to 24 hours, it is wise to warn patients that at 48 hours after surgery they will be considerably stiffer than they were the day immediately after the operation. By 24 to 48 hours, all drains, medicines such as intravenous fluids, steroids, and antibiotics should be stopped and patients should be fully ambulatory so that they can be sent home. The skin closure, be it a 4-0 or 5-0 nylon suture or staples, should be removed 7 to 10 days after the procedure. The better the closure of the subcutaneous layer, the less separation there will be of the skin itself.

Patients need to be encouraged to maintain good posture in holding their head erect. We discourage neck motion in the early postoperative period because it leads to fibrosis and tearing on the deep fascial suture line. In the neck, exercises are not needed at any time to increase muscle strength or range of motion. It is more important to constantly emphasize that the patient have good posture and maintain proper curvature of the spine. We also instruct the patients not to read or study in a position that results in marked flexion of the neck. Commonly, patients having a one- or a two–nerve root decompression on one side are back to work within 2 to 3 weeks. Few patients are unable to work more than 1 month. Heavy laborers may miss 6 weeks of work, because the large muscles attaching to the scapula and the upper part of the shoulder girdle posteriorly need to be well healed before they can do extremely heavy shoveling, pulling, etc. Even those patients returning to professional contact sports have resumed all of their activities by the end of 8 weeks. Spinal instability, as previously mentioned, is such a rare problem that follow-up x-rays are probably unnecessary.

Laminectomy for Myelopathy

A standard decompressive laminectomy in the cervical area over several segments now can be safely carried out in the majority of patients. The reported rate of serious neurological deterioration with such procedures is now in the range of 2% to 3% (8), although there are reports of a higher incidence (27,49). The patient in whom such a problem occurs usually already has a severe neurological myelopathy, accompanying cardiovascular disease, and, not infrequently, a poor nutritional status. In that subgroup of patients, the risks are considerable, but there is really no alternative therapy.

The exposure for cervical decompressive laminectomy has to be sufficient for good visualization. This is certainly not microscopic surgery. The skin should be marked before draping, for the midline may be elusive once all the drapes are placed. For most cervical decompressive laminectomies for spinal stenosis, the spinous processes in the laminae from C3 through C7 inclusive must be removed. For this, the incision has to begin over the C2 spinous process and extend over the C7 spinous process. Once the skin is incised, skin bleeders can be controlled using cautery. The muscle dissection is in the midline, using self-retaining retractors to pull the tissues laterally to reduce the cautery dissection. If one uses self-retaining retractors, constantly moving them deeper and deeper, the amount of tissue that is cauterized or burned is kept to a minimum. Bleeders are quickly identified. Dissection can be carried out in the midline more accurately right down to the spinous processes on the back of C2 so that one can feel the bifid spines of C3, C4, and C5, and then the more straight nonbifid spines of either C6 or C7. The C6 spinous process may or may not be bifid. With good identification of the spinous processes, the muscles can be detached around the end of the spinous processes. If the bifid parts are in the way of good exposure of the lamina, they can be removed at this initial exposure. If at all possible, the muscles arising from the superior aspect of C2 should be kept intact if C2 is not to be removed, because the major extensors of the neck insert here.

Once the muscles are detached from the ends of the spinous process, the muscles can easily be stripped subperiosteally from the lamina. Operative exposure is aided by turning the cautery down to a lower electrical intensity when placing the retractors deeper and deeper. The retractors can then be placed well down the lateral to the C7 lamina and well lateral to the C3 and C4 lamina, with retraction in between if necessary. Throughout this part of the exposure, the blood loss should be less than 50 cc. With good visualization of all of the spinous processes, the lamina, and at least half of the facet area, the full laminectomy can begin. This is done by removing the spinous processes, typically from caudal to cephalad.

After the spinous processes are off, one can judge the position of the hidden spinal canal more accurately. Removing the lamina is done either with large bony rongeur forceps or with a high speed drill. If bony rongeurs are utilized, they have to be kept parallel to the spinal canal and at no time should the lip of the instrument enter the canal. Standard Kerrison punches should not be used in the initial part of the laminectomy. The spinal canal is often compromised in these cases; we have observed diameters down to 5 mm. The tighter the stenosis, obviously, the more caution is used in removing the bone. Placing a 3 mm Kerrison punch beneath the lamina obviously can compromise the canal very severely. In any canal below 14 mm in AP central diameter, there

giving a large dose with a longer interval of time between doses. The new patient control devices for intravenous narcotics for the first 24 to 48 hours are equally effective. Pain medication may include an injection at night, with the patient on the oral synthetic codeine–acetaminophen combination drugs by the second postoperative night. Bracing and collars are only rarely used. However, if a fusion is required with the laminectomy, obviously the patient will have to be immobilized. Finally, when patients are out of the recovery area, placing them in a slight jack-knife position with the head of the bed up about 20° will promote venous drainage from the operative area and may minimize some of the swelling. For those patients who do not have a significant myelopathy and do not require canes or crutches for ambulation, discharge on the 3rd or 4th day is common. In those patients with a marked gait disturbance, up to a week of hospitalization is required. Many of these patients also require physical therapy in order to improve their strength and ambulation. Patients who have severe neurological deficit with a very spastic myelopathy may require transfer to a rehabilitation center.

Soft Central Disc Herniation

Soft central disc herniations should not be removed posteriorly. Now that we have modern CT scans and MRIs, these problems can be identified prior to operative intervention. In the past, before diagnostic studies could completely outline the pathology, the disc was mobilized and removed. In two thirds of such cases, the patients had a satisfactory outcome; however, removing a soft disc posteriorly when it is placed central and anterior can be associated with a transient neurological deterioration (27). Now that surgical procedures have been developed for removing soft discs anteriorly with a cervical discectomy, decompression, and fusion, this is the recommended surgical approach (10,42,61,69). This is true even if it means closing a patient posteriorly, turning him or her over, and proceeding with the anterior decompression, when a soft central disc is identified during posterior decompression.

Recently, the Mayo Clinic neurosurgical service treated some of these patients with a transdural exposure to remove such disks under direct exposure. While this is an accepted technique, a direct anterior removal is preferred in the majority of cases.

Laminoplasty

Laminoplasty has been found to be of benefit in those patients with OPLL (Fig. 15) (3). It is our Japanese colleagues who have championed this procedure (34,35, 37,38,47,48,51,65). In the Japanese Public Health study (37), longitudinal and transverse growth of OPLL in

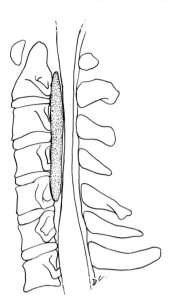

FIG. 15. In many cases of OPLL, the pathology is as high as C2 and, therefore, the decompression needs to include even C1.

asymptomatic patients was found to be 24% and 11%, respectively, over 5 years. This means that nearly one quarter of the patients in a 5-year period have longitudinal extension of the OPLL by the natural course of the disease. Once a laminectomy is done, this longitudinal extension may increase to 85% to 90% of patients (35). If a laminectomy is converted back to a laminoplasty so that there are some posterior elements, this extension is reduced to 34%. If a solid spinal fusion is achieved anteriorly, it is further reduced to 20%, or approximately equal to the natural course of the disease if left untreated. Data of this kind have led to the laminoplasty, especially in the patient who is young and has OPLL. There are five common ways to carry out laminoplasty (Fig. 16) (35), two of which require bone grafts. Currently, it is difficult to say which is the most effective technique. Our experience is limited, but we have found the open-door hemilateral technique utilizing a bone graft to be effective. In over half of these cases, the spinous process itself has been used as the bone graft to fill in the lamina on the side where the opening is achieved. In other cases, the graft is from the ilium. Banked bone can also be safely used.

To carry out a laminoplasty, a high speed drill is essential. The basic exposure is the same as the laminectomy with a fusion. With good visualization of the lamina and spinous process, the spinous process is cut away, with one bone cut so that it can be used as a bone graft. Then the high speed drill is used to thin the bone down to a single cortical layer posterolateral to the spinal cord on both sides. On the side to be opened, a very small angled curette can be used to crack through the remaining thin bone. The bone can then be opened gently. A small hole can be made into the lamina with the 1 mm drill. Then,

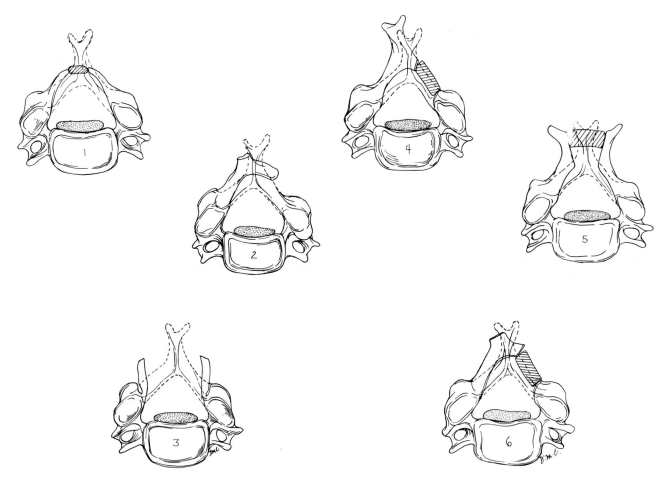

FIG. 16. There are at least six different ways to do cervical laminoplasty: (*1*) Hattori, (*2*) Hirabayashi, (*3*) Iwaski, (*4*) Itoh and Matsuzaki, (*5*) Kurokawa, and (*6*) Ducker. Hirabayashi's review (ref. 35) provides the data for this operation, which is considerably more common in Japan.

2-0 nylon suture can be passed through the hole and to the graft, affixing the graft to the lateral aspect of interfacet area (see illustration 6 in Fig. 16). We do not use wire for bone fixation in these cases; the grafts are commonly incorporated quickly. The closure of the wound is slightly different from that in the standard laminectomy. The muscles next to the laminoplasty are not closed. Instead of the four-layer closure, a three-layer closure of the fascia is all that is required. The placement of a small suction drainage should be on the bony side away from the graft.

The results in terms of stopping the progression of myelopathy in OPLL are not as good as the success rates after treating degenerative cervical spondylitic stenotic myelopathy. Instead of 70% of the patients improving, good results are around 60% (34,36,37). Practically speaking, half of the patients should remain improved over an extended period. Older patients, patients with superimposed trauma, and patients who have a kyphotic spinal curvature do poorly. Unfortunately, there are no alternative treatments that offer better results. The anterior procedure has major limitations in this disease.

Posterior Cervical Fusion for Degenerative Disease

Posterior spinal fusion is an appropriate operative procedure for patients who have recurrent osteophytes and/or failed anterior cervical discectomy and fusion with continued pain and deformity. If a radiculopathy is the major symptom, the standard lateral laminoforaminotomy, as previously described, is chosen.

After decompressive laminoforaminotomies, some fusion technique is indicated to stabilize the spine and prevent progression of radicular disease. The three most commonly used procedures in our practice include: local bone fusion with spine process and laminar morcellized bone, posterior plating in conjunction with local bone, and triple wire fusion using Songer cables and iliac strip grafts (Figs. 17,18).

Front and Back

In selected cases, approximately 3% to 4%, front and back decompression and fusion is performed in one op-

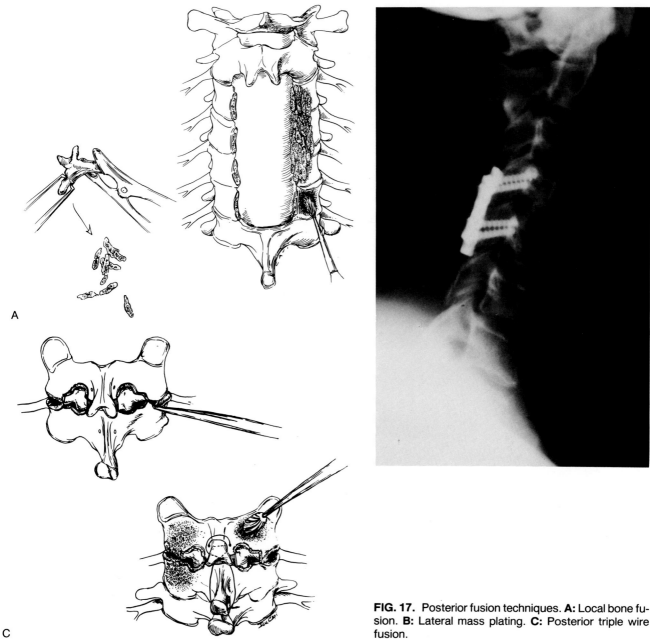

FIG. 17. Posterior fusion techniques. **A:** Local bone fusion. **B:** Lateral mass plating. **C:** Posterior triple wire fusion.

eration. This is indicated in cervical stenosis patients with central disc herniation in front, or in patients with a central disc with highly accelerated myelopathy (Fig. 19). Initial performance of either the front or back procedure and subsequent salvage with the other does not do as well.

Failed Anterior Cervical Fusion

Between 4% and 12% of anterior cervical fusions will progress to a non-union. Approximately half of these patients remain symptomatic with neck and arm pain. With myelopathy and continued canal compromise, re-peat anterior decompression and fusion can be successful. This requires a partial or hemicorpectomy above and below the disc space to safely remove the posterior osteophyte ridge. A tall tricortical bone graft can then be used (70). In the non-union of an anterior cervical fusion, where neck and arm pain or neck pain alone persists, we prefer a posterior approach. As previously described, a keyhole foraminotomy is performed for decompression of the symptomatic nerve root. A limited decompression is done on the asymptomatic side. This is followed by posterior interspinous process wiring and bone grafting at the non-union level. With a solid posterior fusion, the anterior non-union often will consolidate (24).

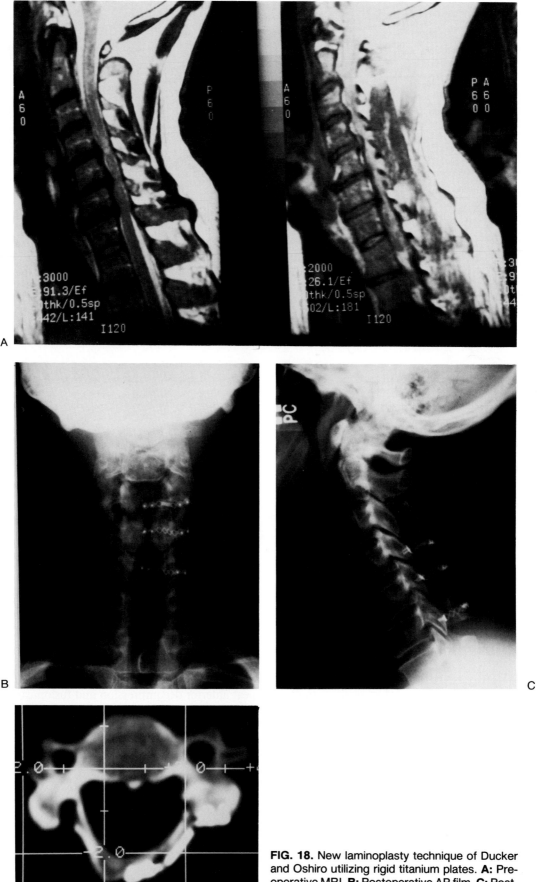

FIG. 18. New laminoplasty technique of Ducker and Oshiro utilizing rigid titanium plates. **A:** Preoperative MRI. **B:** Postoperative AP film. **C:** Postoperative lateral film. **D:** Postoperative CT scan.

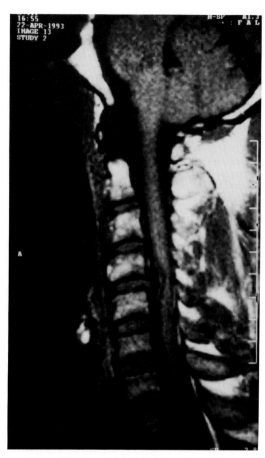

FIG. 19. Preoperative studies (MRI) in a patient who had both an acute disc herniation and congenital spinal stenosis. In 4 weeks, this patient progressed to a grade V (Nurick) paralysis.

REFERENCES

1. Aboulker J, Metzger J, David M, Engel P, Ballivet J (1965): Les myelopathies cervicales d'origine rachidienne. *Neurochirurgie* 11: 87.
2. Allen KL (1968): Cervical spondylosis with accompanying myelopathy: its alleviation by removal of the bony spur. *S Afr J Surg* 6:5.
3. Bakay L, Cares HL, Smith RJ (1970): Ossification in the region of the posterior longitudinal ligament as a cause of cervical myelopathy. *J Neurol Neurosurg Psychiatr* 33:263.
4. Batzdorf U, Batzdorf A (1988): Analysis of cervical spine curvature in patients with cervical spondylosis. *Neurosurgery* 5:827–836.
5. Bradshaw P (1957): Some aspects of cervical spondylosis. *Q J Med* 26:177.
6. Brain WR, Wilkinson JL (1967): *Cervical spondylosis and other disorders of the spine.* Philadelphia: WB Saunders.
7. Braughler JM, Hall ED (1985): Current application of "high-dose" steroid therapy for CNS injury. *J Neurosurg* 62:806–810.
8. Carol MP, Ducker TB (1988): Cervical spondylotic myelopathies: surgical treatment. *J Spinal Disord* 1:59–65.
9. Cassidy J, Ducker TB (1990): Clinical correlations of intraoperative evoked potential monitoring in spinal cord disorders. In: *Spinal cord monitoring and electrodiagnosis.* Heidelberg: Springer-Verlag.
10. Cloward RB (1952): Treatment of ruptured intervertebral discs: observations on their formation and treatment. *Am J Surg* 84:151.
11. Crandall PH, Barzdorf I (1966): Cervical spondylotic myelopathy. *J Neurosurg* 25:57.
12. Dempsey R, Rapp RP, Young B, et al. (1988): Prophylactic parenteral antibiotics in clean neurosurgical procedures: a review. *J Neurosurg* 69:52–57.
13. Dietemann JL, Dirheimer Y, et al. (1985): Ossification of the posterior longitudinal ligament (Japanese disease): a radiological study in 12 cases. *J Neuroradiol* 12:212.
14. Ducker TB, Brown RH (1988): *Neurophysiology and standards of spinal cord monitoring.* New York: Springer-Verlag.
15. Ducker TB, Hamit HF (1969): Experimental treatments of acute spinal cord injury. *J Neurosurg* 6:693–697.
16. Epstein JE, Carras R, Lavine LS, Epstein BS (1969): The importance of removing osteophytes as part of the surgical treatment of myeloradiculopathy in cervical spondylosis. *J Neurosurg* 30:219.
17. Epstein JA, Epstein NE (1989): The surgical management of cervical spinal stenosis, spondylosis, and myeloradiculopathy by means of the posterior approach. In: Sherk HH, et al., eds. *The cervical spine,* 2nd ed. Philadelphia: JB Lippincott, pp. 625–643 .
18. Epstein JA, Epstein BS, Lavine LS (1963): Cervical spondylotic myelopathy: the syndrome of the narrowed canal treated by laminectomy, foraminotomy, and the removal of osteophytes. *Arch Neurol* 8:307.
19. Epstein JA, Epstein BS, Lavine LS, et al. (1978): Clinical monoradiculopathy caused by arthrotic hypertrophy. *J Neurosurg* 49:387.
20. Epstein JA, Janin Y, Carras R, Lavine LS (1982): A comparative study of the treatment of cervical spondylotic myeloradiculopathy: experience with 50 cases treated by means of extensive laminectomy, foraminotomy and excision of osteophytes during the past 10 years. *Acta Neurochir (Wein)* 61:89–104.
21. Epstein JA, Lavine LS, Aronson HA, et al. (1965): Cervical spondylotic radiculopathy. *Clin Orthop* 40:113–122.
22. Fager CA (1976): Management of cervical disc lesions and spondylosis by posterior approaches. *Clin Neurosurg* 24:488.
23. Fager CAL (1973): Results of adequate posterior decompression in the relief of spondylotic cervical myelopathy. *J Neurosurg* 38:6–84.
24. Farey ID, McAfee PC, Davis RF, Long DM (1990): Posterior foraminectomies, stabilization, and fusion for failed anterior cervical fusion. *J Bone Joint Surg* 72A:1171–1177.
25. Firooznia H, Rafii M, et al. (1984): Computed tomography of calcification and ossification of posterior longitudinal ligament of the spine. *J Comput Assist Tomogr* 8:317.
26. Gorter K (1976): Influence of laminectomy on the course of cervical myelopathy. *Acta Neurochir (Wein)* 33:265.
27. Gregorius FK, Estrin T, Crandall PR (1976): Cervical spondylotic radiculopathy and myelopathy. A long term follow-up study. *Arch Neurol* 33:618–625.
28. Guidetti B, Fortuna A (1969): Long term results of surgical treatment of myelopathy due to cervical spondylosis. *J Neurosurg* 30: 714–721.
29. Haft H, Shenkin HA (1963): Surgical end results of cervical ridge and disc problems. *JAMA* 186:312.
30. Haines SF (1980): Systemic antibiotic prophylaxis in neurological surgery. *Neurosurgery* 6:355–361.
31. Haines SJ (1985): Prophylactic antibiotics. In: Wilkins RH, Rengachary SS, eds. *Neurosurgery,* vol. 1. New York: McGraw-Hill, 448–452.
32. Hall ED, Wolf MS, Braughler MJ (1984): Effects of a single large dose of methylprednisolone sodium succinate on experimental post-traumatic spinal cord ischemia. *J Neurosurg* 61:124–130.
33. Henderson CA (1983): Posterolateral foraminotomy as exclusive operative technique for cervical radiculopathy: a review of 846 consecutively operated cases. *Neurosurgery* 13:504–512.
34. Hirabayashi K, Miyakawa J, Satomi K, et al. (1981): Operative results and postoperative progression of ossification among patients with cervical posterior longitudinal ligament. *Spine* 6:354–364.
35. Hirabayashi K, Satomi K, Sasaki T (1989): Ossification of the posterior longitudinal ligament in the cervical spine. In: Sherk HH, et al., eds. *The cervical spine,* 2nd ed. Philadelphia: JB Lippincott, pp. 678–691.
36. Hirabayashi K, Watanabe K, Wakano K, et al. (1983): Expansive open-door laminoplasty for cervical spinal stenotic myelopathy. *Spine* 8:693.
37. Japanese Ministry of Public Health and Welfare (1981-1985): Investigation committee reports on OPLL. Tokyo.

38. Kojima T, et al. (1989): Anterior cervical vertebrectomy and interbody fusion for multi-level spondylosis and ossification of the posterior longitudinal ligament. *Neurosurgery* 6:864–872.
39. Lees F, Aldren Turner JS (1963): Natural history and prognosis of cervical spondylosis. *Br Med J [Clin Res]* 2:1607–1610.
40. Malis LI (1979): Prevention of neurosurgical infection by intraoperative antibiotics. *Neurosurgery* 5:339–343.
41. Matjasko J, Petrozza P, Cohen M, Steinberg P (1985): Anesthesia and surgery in the seated position: analysis of 554 cases. *Neurosurgery* 17:695.
42. Mayfield FH (1965): Cervical spondylosis: a comparison of the anterior and posterior approaches. *Clin Neurosurg* 13:181.
43. McPherson RW, Ducker TB (1988): Augmentation of somatosensory evoked potential waves in patients with cervical spinal stenosis. In: Ducker TB, Brown RH, eds. *Neurophysiology and standards of spinal cord monitoring.* New York: Springer-Verlag, pp. 168–176.
44. Miller C, Hunt W (1985): Management of cervical reticulopathy. *Clin Neurosurg* 33:485–502.
45. Mollman HD, Haines SJ (1986): Risk factors for postoperative neurosurgical wound infection. A case-control study. *J Neurosurg* 64:902–906.
46. Murphey F, Simmons J (1966): Ruptured cervical discs. *Am J Surg* 32:83–88.
47. Nagashima C (1972): Cervical myelopathy due to ossification of the posterior longitudinal ligament. *J Neurosurg* 37:653–660.
48. Nakanishi T, Mannen T, Toyokura Y, et al. (1974): Symptomatic ossification of the cervical spine. *Neurology* 24:1139–1140.
49. Nurick S (1972): The natural history and the results of surgical treatment of the spinal cord disorder associated with cervical spondylosis. *Brain* 9(S):101.
50. Odom GL, Finney W, Woodhall B (1958): Cervical disk lesions. *JAMA* 166:23–28.
51. Ono K, Ota H, Tada K, Yamamoto T (1977): Cervical myelopathy secondary to multiple spondylotic protrusions. *Spine* 2:218.
52. Piepgras DG (1977): Posterior decompression for myelopathy due to cervical spondylosis: laminectomy alone vs laminectomy with dentate ligament section. *Clin Neurosurg* 24:508–515.
53. Raynor RB (1983): Anterior or posterior approach to the cervical spine: an anatomical and radiographic evaluation and comparison. *Neurosurgery* 12:7.
54. Raynor RB, Pugh J, Shapiro I (1985): Cervical facetectomy and its effect on spine strength. *J Neurosurg* 63:278–282.
55. Roberts AH (1966): Myelopathy due to cervical spondylosis treated by collar immobilization. *Neurology* 16:951–954.
56. Savitz MH, Katz SS (1981): Rationale for prophylactic antibiotics in neurosurgery. *Neurosurgery* 9:142–144.
57. Savitz MH, Katz SS (1986): Prevention of primary wound infection in neurosurgical patients: A 10-year study. *Neurosurgery* 18: 685–688.
58. Scoville WB (1961): Cervical spondylosis treated by bilateral facetectomy and laminectomy. *J Neurosurg* 18:423–428.
59. Scoville WB, Whitcomb BB, McLaurin RL (1951): The cervical ruptured disc: report of 115 operative cases. *Trans Am Neurol Assoc* 76:222–224.
60. Shapiro M, Wald U, Simchen E, et al. (1986): Randomized clinical trial of intra-operative antimicrobial prophylaxis of infection after neurosurgical procedures. *J Hosp Infect* 8:283–295.
61. Smith GW, Robinson RA (1955): Anterior lateral cervical disc removal and interbody fusion for cervical disc syndrome. *Bull Johns Hopkins Hosp* 96:223.
62. Spurling RG, Scoville WB (1955): Lateral rupture of the cervical intervertebral discs: a common cause of shoulder and arm pain. *Surg Gynecol Obstet* 78:350.
63. Spurling RB, Segerberg LH (1953): Lateral intervertebral disc lesions in the lower cervical region. *JAMA* 151:354.
64. Tenney JH, Valahov D, Salcman M, Ducker TB (1985): Wide variation in risk of wound infection following clean neurosurgery: implications for perioperative antibiotic prophylaxis. *J Neurosurg* 62: 243–247.
65. Tsuji H (1982): Laminoplasty for patients with compressive myelopathy due to so-called spinal canal stenosis in cervical and thoracic regions. *Spine* 7:28–34.
66. Thomalski G, Wilk von K, Lammert E (1972): Zur chirurgischen behandlung der cervicales myelopathie. *Nervenarzt* 43:520–524.
67. Veidlinger OF, Coleill JC, Smyth HS, Turner D (1981): Cervical myelopathy and its relationship to cervical stenosis. *Spine* 6:550–552.
68. Verbiest H (1973): The management of cervical spondylosis. *Clin Neurosurg* 20:262.
69. Verbiest H, Paz Y, Geuse HD (1966): Anterolateral surgery for cervical spondylosis in cases of myelopathy or nerve root compression. *J Neurosurg* 25:611.
70. Zdeblick T, Bohlman HH (1989): Cervical kyphosis and myelopathy. Treatment by anterior corpectomy and strut-grafting. *J Bone Joint Surg* 71(A):170–182.
71. Zdeblick T, Zou D, Warden KE (in press): Cervical stability after foraminotomy. A biomechanical in-vitro analysis. *J Bone Joint Surg [AM]* 1992;74(1):22–27.
72. Zeidman SM, Ducker TB (1993): Posterior cervical laminoforaminotomy for radiculopathy: review of 172 cases. *Neurosurgery* 33(3):356–363.
73. Zeidman SM, Ducker TB. Cervical spondylotic myelopathy: determination of the appropriate operative approach. Review of 300 cases. *Neurosurgery (in press)*.

The Adult Spine: Principles and Practice,
2nd edition, J.W. Frymoyer, Editor-in-Chief.
Lippincott-Raven Publishers, Philadelphia © 1997.

CHAPTER **67**

Complex Cervical Myelopathies

Ulrich Batzdorf

Cervical spondylotic myelopathy is defined as a neurologic disorder generally manifested in its severe (complex) form by a spastic gait, sometimes spastic hands with atrophy and sensory impairment, sphincter disturbances, and related underlying spondylosis of the cervical spine. These symptoms may exist in every different combination and proportion. Although there is often some degree of associated neck stiffness, severe neck pain is not usually part of the syndrome.

PATHOPHYSIOLOGY

Two major schools of thought exist with respect to the basic mechanisms responsible for the myelopathic clinical features and the often profound changes seen in autopsy specimens of the cervical cord.

U. Batzdorf, M.D.: Professor, Department of Surgery/Neurosurgery, University of California, Los Angeles, School of Medicine, Los Angeles, California 90095-6901.

Mechanical

The classical concept is that spondylotic myelopathy is the result of spinal cord compression, focal or extending over several segments, with osteophytes or a combination of osteophytes and degenerated disc constituting the compressive material (18). The varying mechanisms by which osteophyte growth or disc degeneration might be produced are discussed below in the section on etiologies. Even this very elementary concept must, however, be qualified. While it is inherent in the postulated mechanism that the osteophyte or degenerated disc is hard, it is also known that the spinal cord can tolerate quite extensive compression by osteophyte or disc, as judged by magnetic resonance (MR) scans for example, without any clinical manifestations of myelopathy (27).

The development of significant myelopathy seems to depend on the interaction of at least three factors: (a) degree of cord compression; (b) the period of time (i.e., rate) over which these compressive changes have taken place; and (c) the constancy or intermittency of the compressive force. Thus, the spinal cord notoriously will tolerate extensive compression if the narrowing of the canal develops very slowly, that is, over a period of many years. Relatively constant compression also seems to be better tolerated by the spinal cord than frequent repetitive compressive forces, such as might be seen in the patient with a hypermobile spine segment. Intermittent subluxation at a motion segment, or several adjacent motion segments, as is sometimes seen, seems to resemble repeated episodes of sub-acute trauma rather than chronic compression. However, as discussed below, once the spinal cord is compressed, though asymptomatically, it sometimes takes very little additional compression (such as might result from a seemingly trivial fall) to produce sudden and severe neurologic deterioration. Changes in viscoelastic properties of the degenerated cord may also play a role (24), particularly as they might relate to the known normal stretching of the spinal cord with physiologic motion of the spine (4).

Vascular

A vascular mechanism for the development of spinal cord changes and the associated myelopathic symptoms and signs has been postulated for many years (26). The close resemblance of the clinical syndrome of anterior spinal artery occlusion to that seen in many patients with severe cervical myelopathy led to the belief that the rough anterior osteophytes rub against the spinal cord and produce focal areas of ischemia or hypoperfusion. Some have also shown that fibrosis of the root sleeve due to foraminal compression can involve the delicate accompanying radicular vessels which contribute to spinal cord perfusion.

The strongest argument against the vascular theory has always been the slow clinical progression in most instances of myelopathy due to spondylosis, whereas a vascular occlusive mechanism would be expected to present more abruptly.

Combination of Mechanical and Vascular

The possibility that mechanical and vascular factors may work in combination to produce myelopathic changes must be considered. A compressed cord will tolerate diminished perfusion poorly; a marginally vascularized cord will tolerate compression equally poorly. One must further consider the added injury to the cord that might come about from temporarily reduced perfusion on a systemic basis, similar to that postulated in the secondary insult concept considered responsible for some of the more severe effects of a head injury (6).

ETIOLOGIES

A number of different etiologies of cervical myelopathy must be considered. All may cause cord injury by either compression, vascular changes, or a combination thereof, as discussed above and in Chapters 64 and 65.

Acute Disc Herniation

A significant disc herniation, particularly if central, can result in acute myelopathy.

Spondylosis

Typically, spondylosis consists of protrusion and calcification of the annulus fibrosus due to intrinsic degenerative changes of the intervertebral disc, which involve loss of water and changes in collagen, resulting in loss of disc height with some spreading effect, i.e., increase in disc diameter. Not infrequently, this process occurs at several levels simultaneously.

While normal aging processes result in these changes in many patients, chronic repetitive disc trauma such as produced by certain occupations (for example, hod carriers) or even a single episode of severe disc injury, can accelerate these degenerative changes. Ligamentous changes following a spine injury conceivably could also favor the late development of disc and intervertebral joint degeneration.

A sequence of related changes may follow degenerative disc pathology (9):

1. bony overgrowth at the annulus margin to form an osteophytic ridge;
2. facet joint stress leading to joint narrowing, cartilage degeneration, and osteoarthritic spurs originating from the joint margin;
3. hypermobility of the spine or segments thereof, including subluxation of vertebrae with secondary stretching of the supporting ligaments of the spine (8,10);
4. loss of disc height leading to telescoping of the cervical spine with shingling of cervical vertebrae and contraction of the ligamentum flavum which, in its contracted state, is thicker;
5. spontaneous fusion due to bridging osteophytes.

Loss in Height of Vertebrae and Postural Changes

Vertebral compression may occur as an aftermath to the vertical component of spine trauma, or as a consequence of osteoporosis, or from other less clearly understood mechanisms such as impairment of bone vascularity.

When these forces are applied in an uneven manner, they will result in a change in the shape of the vertebral body. Most commonly this is in the form of wedging, the result of the anterior vertebral body being compressed more than the posterior margin. This may then result in an alteration of the curvature of the spine from its lordotic curve. Secondary ligamentous stretching may then occur and ultimately a combination of soft tissue, bony, and cartilaginous changes may make the deformity irreversible.

Postural changes of the cervical spine probably can also result from primary ligamentous problems, i.e., ligamentous weakness or stretching, such as might occur following a flexion injury (10). Finally, severe kyphotic deformities of the upper thoracic spine, such as are sometimes seen in the elderly, may generate a compensatory lordotic deformity of the cervical area as a result of the patient's need to look forward (Fig. 1).

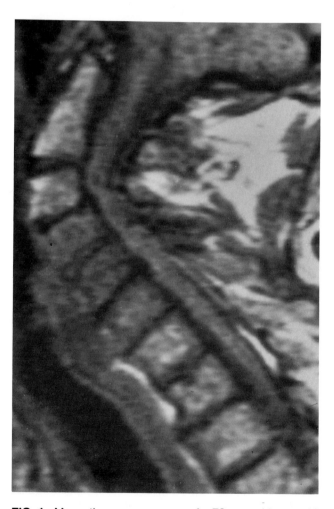

FIG. 1. Magnetic resonance scan of a 79-year-old man with hyperlordotic deformity resulting in cord compression at the C3 and C4 levels. Patient was treated with a C1 to C5 laminectomy.

Degenerative Changes Superimposed on Previous Acute Trauma

As noted above, the normal processes of aging of the intervertebral disc may be given a premature start or accelerated by the internal disruption of a disc following an acute injury.

Degenerative Changes Superimposed on Congenital Abnormalities of the Cervical Spine

Three categories are important. They are (a) the congenitally narrow spinal canal (Fig. 2); (b) Klippel-Feil deformities; and (c) craniocervical junction abnormalities. These entities are discussed in Chapters 57, 58, 64, and 65. Whereas Klippel-Feil and craniocervical junction abnormalities tend to be immediately recognizable on plain radiographs, the congenitally narrow canal may be less obvious. Complete overlapping of the facet joints on the laminae in a lateral cervical radiograph is strongly suggestive of a congenitally narrow canal. A thin-slice CT scan in the axial projection would provide the best confirmation of short pedicles.

The significance of a congenitally narrow canal in the context of cervical myelopathy is that a relatively small osteophyte or disc protrusion can result in spinal cord compression and myelopathy when the "tolerance" for the cord is marginal at the outset. This is exemplified to the extreme in achondroplastics.

Klippel-Feil deformities, characterized by block vertebrae, may show evidence of accelerated degenerative change at the first mobile segment above and below the block vertebra; presumably motion, which is normally distributed over many segments, is greater at the remaining mobile segment when a block vertebra is present. Craniocervical junction abnormalities can cause myelopathy by a number of different mechanisms, including displacement of the cord by a nonunited odontoid, basilar invagination, and congenital anomalies of the atlantoaxial joint (19).

Idiopathic Ossification of the Posterior Longitudinal Ligament

The cause of this condition is poorly understood. Calcified thickening of the posterior longitudinal ligament may be focal or spread over several spinal segments. Incorporation of the dura into the calcified or ossified ligament has been described and obviously creates management problems.

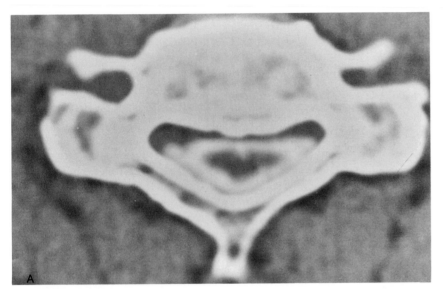

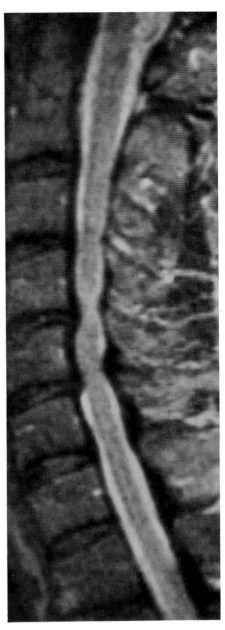

FIG. 2. Computed tomographic scan of the cervical spine in a 58-year-old patient following intrathecal injection of Omnipaque. **A:** The spinal canal is very narrow in the anterior-posterior dimension due to unusually short pedicles. **B:** Multiple levels of cord compression are evident in the sagittal scan of the same patient. Even small disc protrusions or osteophytes like these can cause myelopathy in a patient with a congenitally narrow canal; treated by laminectomy.

CLINICAL DIAGNOSIS

Symptoms

In a comprehensive analysis (11), gait abnormalities, together with lower extremity weakness, sensory symptoms, and sphincter disturbances were noted in over 60% of patients with cervical myelopathy (Fig. 3). Signs on examination (Fig. 4) reflected a similar pattern, with upper and lower extremity spasticity and lower extremity weakness being most common. Upper extremity weakness was almost as common, with atrophy present in the proximal or distal portion of the limb in many patients. Shoulder, arm, forearm, or hand pain often signal the coexistence of radiculopathy.

Differential Diagnosis

The differential diagnosis should include a consideration of vascular malformations of the cord, syringomyelia, and cord tumors. These conditions should be readily differentiated by magnetic resonance imaging. More difficult might be the differential diagnosis of amyotrophic lateral sclerosis, particularly in the elderly patient who also has some spondylotic changes of the cervical spine. The major point in the differential diagnosis of this condition, as well as multiple sclerosis, is the presence of findings, clinical or by imaging, above the spinal level. Sub-acute combined degeneration and even early stages of extrapyramidal disorder may mimic cervical spondylotic myelopathy.

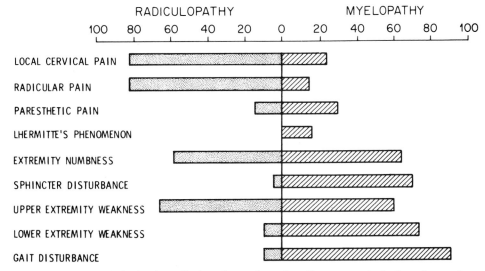

FIG. 3. Symptoms at admission in radiculopathy and myelopathy groups, including all symptoms in all patients. From Gregorius et al. (11) with permission.

Confirmatory Tests

The diagnosis of cervical spondylotic myelopathy is today often made by an initial magnetic resonance scan, the appeal of this study being its noninvasive nature, its capacity to generate both sagittal and axial images, and the ability to exclude almost immediately several other conditions such as tumor or syringomyelia. This diagnostic technique does, however, have some limitations quite aside from those relating to the technical features of the particular scanner. MR scans are, for the most part, static and do not reflect abnormalities that may be seen in positions of flexion or extension, but occasionally such studies can be requested. Gliosis due to chronic

cord compression is sometimes recognizable on MR scans and may correlate with a fixed myelopathic picture (25). Actual cord compression is best recognized in the sagittal MR image. MR scans are, however, not ideal for visualization of bony abnormalities, and such features as congenital narrowing of the canal or certain craniocervical abnormalities may not be immediately apparent. For this reason, it is best to obtain plain films of the cervical spine, as well as flexion and extension views (22). The latter are particularly helpful in assessing abnormal motion of the cervical spine.

Computed tomography (CT) scans, especially when obtained in conjunction with a myelogram using water-soluble contrast material, provide an excellent means of

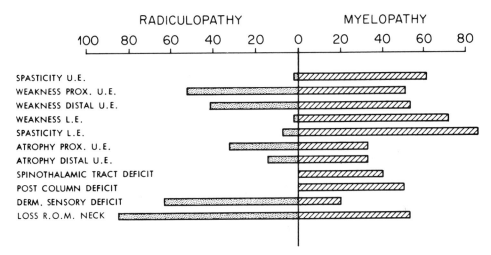

FIG. 4. Physical findings at admission in radiculopathy and myelopathy groups, including all signs in all patients. UE, upper extremity; PROX, proximal part; LE, lower extremity; DERM, dermatoma; ROM, range of motion. From Gregorius et al. (11) with permission.

assessing the patient with spondylotic myelopathy. CT scans show bony abnormalities very clearly, and with contrast will demonstrate deformation or compression of the cord, especially on axial views. The same limitations of a static examination do, however, apply. When performed with intrathecal contrast, this study is invasive, although very few complications have been encountered with currently used contrast agents.

PRINCIPLES OF TREATMENT

Nonsurgical Treatment

Medical therapy can be instituted to help relieve some symptoms of cervical myelopathy, notably spasticity. Carefully titrated doses of baclofen seem to be effective for some patients. Sometimes spasticity may generate pain in spastic muscle groups, and medical therapy in conjunction with physical medicine may be very helpful.

In patients in whom hypermobility of the cervical spine can be demonstrated, external stabilization will help to protect the cord from additional trauma. Only rarely would such immobilization be expected to achieve any clinical improvement, but it may be a useful interim measure while plans for definitive therapy await completion.

Surgical Considerations

The preoperative evaluation of patients with complex spondylotic cervical myelopathy should take the following into consideration:

1. hypermobility or instability of the cervical spine;
2. abnormal curvature of the cervical spine;
3. number of vertebral levels involved in the spondylotic process;
4. presence of congenital canal narrowing or other congenital anomalies;
5. evaluation of relative degrees of anterior spinal pathology (e.g., osteophytes, discs) versus posterior spinal pathology (e.g., ligamentous hypertrophy, shingling);
6. a history of previous cervical spine surgery or of recent ligamentous injury with its implications for spine mobility and stability.

As a general rule, the surgeon must be cognizant of potential long-term effects of arthrodesis, both on neck mobility and on adjacent interspaces. Surgery should be planned to sacrifice no more motion segments than absolutely necessary. This may sometimes be accomplished by judicious staged combination of anterior arthrodesis and foraminotomies at different spinal levels, a strategy which may preserve one motion segment. In addition, the patient's general condition should be taken

into account, particularly the presence of osteopenia if some form of arthrodesis is under consideration as part of the surgical management. Maintenance of the patient's blood pressure during surgery is particularly important.

Hypermobility or Instability

Subluxation of the cervical spine at one or more segments, in the presence of myelopathy, requires that stabilization be part of the operative management. Hypermobility implies disc degeneration and ligamentous stretching, including the capsular ligaments of the intervertebral joints. In the author's experience, stabilization and anterior decompression is best performed by an anterior cervical disc excision and interbody fusion. External immobilization is essential postoperatively until complete fusion has been achieved, as evidenced by serial cervical spine radiographs. Both the Cloward dowel construct (5) and the tricortical wafer-type bone graft (23), as discussed in Chapters 64 and 65, are acceptable techniques for achieving stability in these cases.

When multiple levels of disc protrusion or osteophyte formation require decompression, vertebrectomy and fusion, as opposed to several individual interspace decompressions and fusions, has also been advocated (16). In situations in which two adjacent interspaces are involved, the author has found partial vertebrectomy and placement of a single graft spanning both interspaces mechanically stable and very satisfactory (3). There is a role for anterior plating in conjunction with bone grafts spanning two or more interspaces and in situations of unusual instability, including patients who had a prior laminectomy. In selected situations, anterior plating has also been used to restore lordosis to the cervical spine. Some surgeons prefer to accomplish decompression and stabilization from a posterior approach using lateral mass plating techniques and bone graft as discussed in Chapter 68. In severe cases of subluxation and instability, preoperative tractions may be helpful in improving vertebral alignment. Halo immobilization as well as surgical stabilization may be necessary to maintain the alignment, at least until surgical fixation has been accomplished.

Abnormal Curvature

Kyphosis, straightening, and hyperlordosis of the cervical spine may all be seen in conjunction with spondylotic myelopathy, whereas in other patients the normal curvature is preserved (1) (Fig. 5). These alterations in curvature must be taken into consideration during preoperative surgical planning.

When the cervical spine is straightened or kyphotic, anterior osteophyte removal and decompression of the cord is indicated; laminectomy cannot be expected to ac-

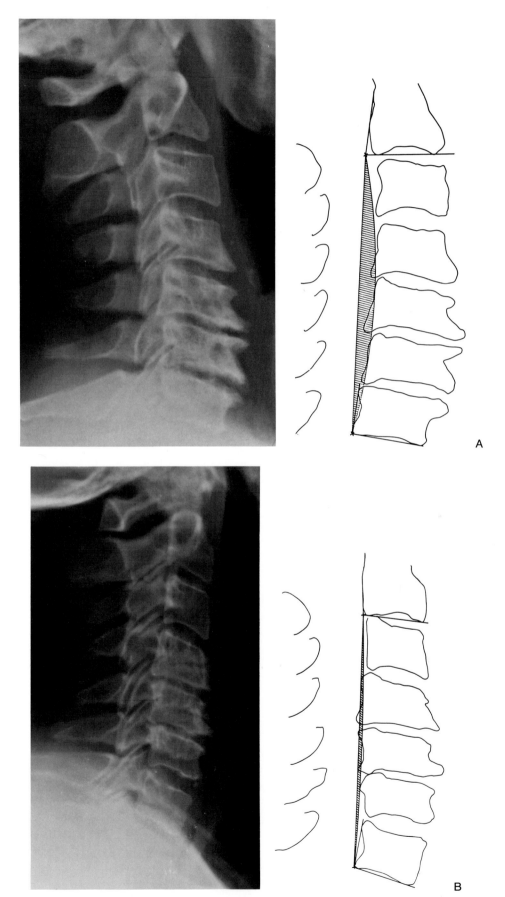

FIG. 5. A–D. Spondylosis may give rise to varying deformities of the spine, often in conjunction with narrowing of the spinal canal. **A:** Normal cervical curvature. **B:** Straightened cervical spine.

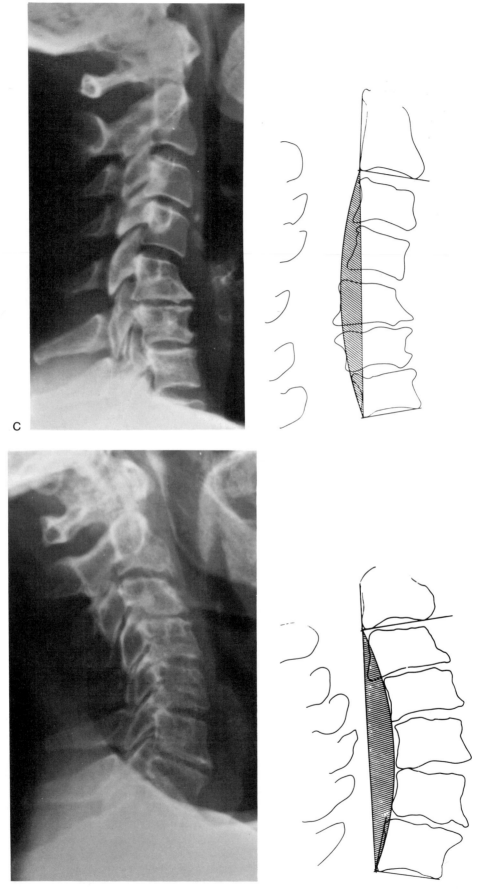

FIG. 5. *(Continued.)* **C:** Kyphotic spine. **D:** Hyperlordotic spine. The shaded area represents the area under the arc, constructed from C2 to C7, and quantifies the degree of deformity. From Batzdorf et al. (1) with permission.

complish adequate canal decompression of a kyphotic spine. When the spine is straightened but not angulated, laminectomy may be considered, particularly if the consideration of spine geometry includes removal of the C2 and C1 laminae, as well as the mid- and lower cervical vertebrae (extended laminectomy). A postoperative MR scan should be obtained and any osteophytes still compromising the cord should be removed by the anterior approach as a staged, secondary procedure (2) (Fig. 6).

In the patient with a normally preserved lordosis, anterior osteophyte removal with interbody fusion or posterior laminectomy can be considered. In general, if three or more vertebral levels are involved, this author prefers laminectomy to multiple arthrodeses, because of the somewhat greater risk of nonunion and the more significant reduction in spine mobility when fusion occurs. Multiple level vertebrectomies with fusion have, however, been performed (16). The same option mentioned

previously, of dealing with a remaining compressive osteophyte by the anterior approach if this is indicated on the basis of a postoperative MR scan, should be considered. The resulting decrease in mobility would probably still be less than with a multiple-level arthrodesis. When one or two levels of anterior compression are the basis of the patient's myelopathy, the anterior approach of osteophyte and disc removal with arthrodesis is the preferred approach.

Decompressive laminectomy covering multiple levels is also the indicated procedure for patients with myelopathy and a congenitally narrow spinal canal. In patients in whom the normal lordotic cervical curvature is preserved, cord disengagement from the osteophytes can usually be achieved without removing the C1 and C2 laminae. The normally wider canal diameter at these two levels is a well-recognized anatomic feature. Section of the dentate ligament (15) and dural grafting (7) are no longer carried out by this author as part of a standard decompressive laminectomy.

Hyperlordosis of the spine may pose a difficult management problem. A laminectomy covering many levels, even the commonly performed C3 to C7 laminectomy covering the most frequently involved levels, may result in such extensive posterior migration of the cord that excessive angulation or tension can be applied to several nerve roots. The accompanying radicular vessels may also be compromised. An anterior procedure will often do little to eliminate the factors causing cord compression in such patients. A judiciously planned, limited laminectomy, with geometrical considerations in mind, is the preferred approach.

Laminoplasty, described in Chapter 65, may be useful in these patients by preventing excessive dorsal migration of the dura and spinal cord.

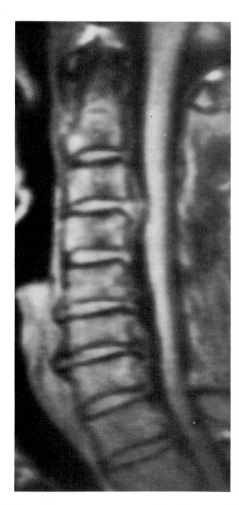

FIG. 6. Magnetic resonance scan of a 48-year-old patient who underwent a C2–C7 laminectomy. The scan shows that the cervical spine is straightened and the cord is not disengaged from a large osteophyte at C3–C4. Some cord atrophy is also evident.

"S" Curves and Postlaminectomy Deformities

Kyphosis and hyperlordosis may coexist and this gives rise to an S-shaped deformity of the spine, causing greater instability and management problems. Both S-type deformities and reversed S-type deformities have been described in patients following cervical laminectomy (14). The S-type has a kyphosis in the lower cervical level and increased lordosis in the upper cervical region; the reversed S-type has an increased lordosis in the lower cervical segment, and kyphosis in the upper cervical area, the more typical "swan" deformity. Such deformities can also exist preoperatively as a result of the multifactorial degenerative changes of spondylosis (Fig. 7). These patients may require both anterior decompression (for the kyphotic deformity) and posterior decompression (at the hyperlordotic levels) at one operation. The potential role of upper cervical muscle and ligamentous injury at the time of surgery is cited as playing a

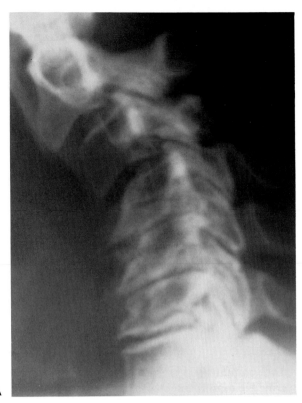
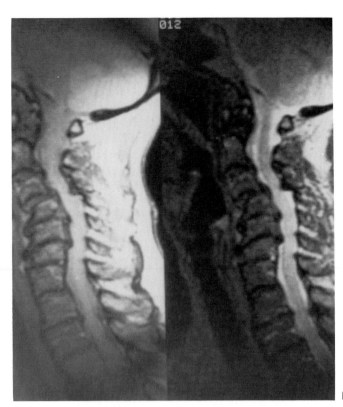

A   B

FIG. 7. Radiograph (**A**) and magnetic resonance scan (**B**) of a male patient with a kyphotic deformity at C4–C6 and hyperlordosis of C2–C4 with instability at the C2–C3 and C3–C4 levels, an "S-type" deformity. He was managed by upper cervical laminectomy and anterior decompression and fusion below (with permission from Dr. Thomas B. Ducker).

role in the postoperative deformities. It is tempting to speculate that relatively minor ligamentous injuries may set the stage for later spontaneous cervical spine deformities that occur in spondylosis (10).

The foregoing should make it clear that detailed decision making is necessary preoperatively, based on considerations particular to the patient, rather than on a preexisting formula. The potential delayed hazards of laminectomy, particularly if the facet joints are injured, have been analyzed in detail and are discussed below (14).

Congenital Canal Narrowing and Other Anomalies

Laminectomy has already been mentioned as the preferred technique for decompressing the cord in the patient with a congenitally narrow canal. Klippel-Feil deformities tend to be associated with degenerative disc changes at the first mobile segment above and below the block vertebra. Anterior osteophyte and disc excision with arthrodesis is generally the preferred surgical approach, even with the recognition of diminished cervical mobility, but in specific limited situations laminectomy may be preferable. Craniocervical junction abnormalities may be very complex. If there is evidence of odontoid impingement on the spinal cord that cannot be re-

lieved by realignment in gradual traction, odontoid resection must be considered (20). When the cord compression can be relieved with realignment, posterior fusion should be performed. This would usually be limited to a C1–C2 arthrodesis, although occasionally the occiput must be included in the fusion. High cervical laminectomy and foramen magnum decompression may be indicated in certain specific instances of high cervical cord compression (1).

Ossification of the Posterior Longitudinal Ligament (OPLL)

OPLL can result in severe myelopathy (Fig. 8). Recent experience (12,16) has favored extensive anterior resections at multiple levels, stabilization being accomplished by fibular strut graft or iliac crest. Depending on the particular spine alignment, some patients with OPLL may also be managed by laminectomy, with or without fusion, or by laminoplasty. The laminoplasty techniques are described in Chapter 65.

Delayed Sequelae of Surgical Management

Late changes, not properly called complications, may develop after either anterior or posterior cervical proce-

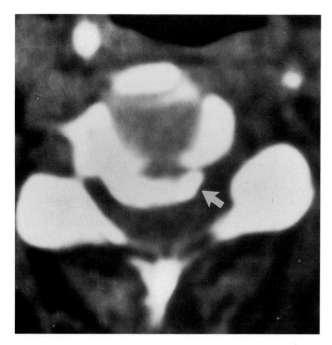

FIG. 8. Computed tomographic scan of a 63-year-old patient with OPLL. The densely calcified ligament (*arrow*) occupies more than a third of the anterior-posterior dimension of the spinal canal.

dures for myelopathy, and such changes may result in secondary deterioration of the patient's condition. Secondary deformity of the cervical spine after extensive laminectomy has been well described and was studied extensively (14). Concerns over spinal instability, delayed deformities, dural compression by epidural scar formation, and lack of bony protection of the cervical cord led to the development of a modified laminectomy technique (21). Suspension laminotomy, a form of laminoplasty described by Ohmori et al. (21), preserves the posterior arches as one unit by using an air drill to divide the laminae on each side. The resulting laminar flap is then suspended from the preserved nuchal and supraspinous ligaments and anchored to several of the facets. Bone grafts may be interposed to maintain the position of the laminar flap. A lower incidence of spinal deformity and dural constriction is reported for this procedure (14) compared to conventional laminectomy. This author has had no personal experience with the technique. The importance of preserving the integrity of the facet joints in performing a laminectomy is well recognized. The development of a laminectomy membrane has also been described extensively (17), although its role in producing recurrent cervical cord compression is not clear.

Late changes may also follow anterior cervical disc excision and interbody fusion. The technical problems of early graft absorption and nonunion are well recognized. The use of properly prepared bank bone in place of autologous bone is particularly justified in the osteopenic patient. Excessive late bone formation at the site of an anterior interbody fusion (autologous bone graft) can result in recurrent cord compression. Such problems should be helped by laminectomy.

Combined Anterior and Posterior Surgical Procedures

Reference has already been made to the occasional patient with multilevel spondylotic disease (or congenital canal stenosis) for whom staged posterior and anterior decompressive procedures would appear to be the most appropriate form of therapy. For example, a patient with three levels of spondylotic cord, or cord and nerve root, compression may fare better with a laminectomy that might decompress two of three affected levels completely, followed by an anterior procedure at the remaining level. The alternative, a three-level anterior decompression and fusion, would eliminate three cervical motion segments, with its attendant disadvantages. Such combined operations can be performed as staged procedures at a suitable time interval or, in appropriate circumstances as reported by Ducker, on the same day. Anterior or posterior plating must be considered in such situations because significant instability may exist when combined procedures are performed simultaneously.

Staged procedures can also be considered for patients who develop nerve root symptoms at an interspace level adjacent to a previous anterior fusion, a problem encountered in several patients by the author. In this situation a foraminotomy with nerve root decompression has proved very helpful.

Anterior spine decompression and fixation also is the general approach to patients who develop myelopathy as a result of a postlaminectomy kyphotic deformity of the spine. As reported by Herman and Sonntag (13), these patients very often present with both radicular and myelopathic symptoms, including nerve root pain, in addition to neck instability. Complete anatomic reduction of the spine is often not possible in these patients, even with preoperative traction. Anterior decompression, usually by corpectomy, with bone fusion and plate fixation, is the treatment of choice. The authors report improvement in 55% of their patients, cure in 10%, a clinically stable course in 30%, and late progression in 5% of their patients. The inherent problem of creating a long, solidly fused segment of the cervical spine appears unavoidable at present.

Anterior versus Posterior Surgical Approach: An Epilogue

The details of surgical decompressive procedures by the anterior and posterior approaches are covered in Chapters 64 and 65. Each has its advocates. Careful preoperative analysis is essential, and the special considerations that affect decision making have been detailed in this chapter. It is of greatest importance that the surgeon be prepared to employ either approach, or a combination of staged procedures, in the management of any patient with spondylotic myelopathy.

REFERENCES

1. Batzdorf U, Batzdorff A (1988): Analysis of cervical spine curvature in patients with cervical spondylosis. *Neurosurgery* 22:827–836.
2. Batzdorf U, Flannigan B (1991): Evaluation of the efficacy of surgical decompressive procedures for cervical spondylotic myelopathy: a study utilizing magnetic resonance imaging. *Spine* 16:123–127.
3. Batzdorf U, Johnson JP (1993): A new technique for cervical fusion without instrumentation (abstract). *Joint Section on Disorders of the Spine and Peripheral Nerves*.
4. Breig A (1978): *Adverse mechanical tension in the central nervous system.* Stockholm: Almquist & Wiksell International.
5. Cloward RB (1958): The anterior approach for removal of ruptured cervical disks. *J Neurosurg* 15:602–617.
6. Cooper PR (1985): Delayed brain injury: secondary insults. In: Becker DP, Povlishock JT, eds. *Central nervous system trauma status report.* Bethesda: National Institutes of Health, pp. 217–228.
7. Crandall PH, Batzdorf U (1966): Cervical spondylotic myelopathy. *J Neurosurg* 25:57–66.
8. Epstein JA, Carras R, Epstein BS, et al. (1970): Myelopathy in cervical spondylosis with vertebral subluxation and hyperlordosis. *J Neurosurg* 32:421–426.
9. Epstein JA, Davidoff LM (1951): Chronic hypertrophic spondylosis of the cervical spine with compression of the spinal cord and nerve roots. *Surg Gynecol Obstet* 93:27–38.
10. Green JD, Harle TS, Harris JH Jr (1981): Anterior subluxation of the cervical spine: hyperflexion sprain. *AJNR* 2:243–250.
11. Gregorius FK, Estrin T, Crandall PH (1976): Cervical spondylotic radiculopathy and myelopathy. *Arch Neurol* 33:618–625.
12. Harsh GR IV, Sypert GW, Weinstein PR, et al (1987): Cervical spine stenosis secondary to ossification of the posterior longitudinal ligament. *J Neurosurg* 67:349–357.
13. Herman JM, Sonntag VKH (1994): Cervical corpectomy and plate fixation for postlaminectomy kyphosis. *J Neurosurg* 80:963–970.
14. Ishida Y, Suzuki K, Ohmori K, et al. (1989): Critical analysis of extensive cervical laminectomy. *Neurosurgery* 24:215–222.
15. Kahn EA (1947): The role of the dentate ligaments in spinal cord compression and the syndrome of lateral sclerosis. *J Neurosurg* 4:191–199.
16. Kojima T, Waga S, Kubo Y, et al. (1989): Anterior cervical vertebrectomy and interbody fusion for multi-level spondylosis and ossification of the posterior longitudinal ligament. *Neurosurgery* 24:864–872.
17. LaRocca H, Macnab I (1974): The laminectomy membrane: studies in its evolution, characteristics, effects and prophylaxis in dogs. *J Bone Joint Surg* [Br] 56:545–550.
18. Mair WGP, Druckman R (1953): The pathology of spinal cord lesions and their relation to the clinical features in protrusion of cervical intervertebral discs. *Brain* 76:70–91.
19. McRae DL (1960): The significance of abnormalities of the cervical spine. *Am J Roentgenol Radium Ther* 84:3–25.
20. Menezes AH, VanGilder JC, Graf CJ, et al. (1980): Craniocervical abnormalities: a comprehensive surgical approach. *J Neurosurg* 53:444–455.
21. Ohmori K, Ishida Y, Suzuki K (1987): Suspension laminotomy: a new surgical technique for compression myelopathy. *Neurosurgery* 21:950–957.
22. Payne EE, Spillane JD (1957): The cervical spine: an anatomico-pathological study of 70 specimens (using a special technique) with particular reference to the problem of cervical spondylosis. *Brain* 80:571–596.
23. Robinson RA, Smith GW (1955): Antero-lateral cervical disc removal and interbody fusion for cervical disc syndrome. *Bull Johns Hopkins Hosp* 96:223–224.
24. Stevens JM, O'Driscoll DM, Yu YL, et al. (1987): Some dynamic factors in compressive deformity of the cervical spinal cord. *Neuroradiol* 29:136–142.
25. Takahashi M, Sakamoto Y, Miyawaki M, et al. (1987): Increased MR signal intensity secondary to chronic cervical cord compression. *Neuroradiol* 29:550–556.
26. Taylor AR (1964): Vascular factors in the myelopathy associated with cervical spondylosis. *Neurology* 14:62–68.
27. Teresi LM, Lufkin RB, Reicher MA, et al. (1987): Asymptomatic degenerative disk disease and spondylosis of the cervical spine: MR imaging. *Radiology* 164:83–88.

The Adult Spine: Principles and Practice,
2nd edition, J.W. Frymoyer, Editor-in-Chief.
Lippincott-Raven Publishers, Philadelphia © 1997.

CHAPTER **68**

Postlaminectomy Instability of the Cervical Spine

Etiology and Stabilization Technique

John G. Heller and D. Hal Silcox III

The choice of an anterior or a posterior approach to the cervical spine should be based on a thorough understanding of the lesion, its natural history, and the relevant pathomechanics. Despite its waxing and waning in popularity over the years, the posterior approach provides convenient, extensile, and appropriate access for certain disorders of the cervical spine and spinal cord. However, adequate exposure requires detachment of the extensor muscle groups and ligaments, as well as violation of the posterior column, which has implications for spinal stability. This chapter explores the variables influencing cervical stability and the spectrum of techniques for managing postoperative cervical instabilities.

The posterior column is defined as the osteoligamentous complex dorsal to the posterior longitudinal ligament (77). This complex includes the laminae, facet joints, and spinous processes, as well as the supraspinous and interspinous ligaments, ligamentum flavum, and facet capsules. *In vitro* biomechanical testing has dem-

onstrated the importance of these structures to cervical stability (35,55,65,77,78). The lateral masses actively participate in force transmission. In vertical compression, the anterior column transmits only 36% of the applied load, while each pillar of facets transmits 32% of the total applied load (54). Flexion–extension testing has demonstrated that stability requires that at least one of the posterior column elements must be intact, in addition to all of the anterior column (77).

Considerable controversy exists over the relative incidence of instability following posterior cervical procedures (Fig. 1). Review of the published literature over the last four decades makes it apparent that controversy has arisen from heterogeneity in patient populations, pathological processes, and surgical procedures. An all-encompassing reference to postlaminectomy instability is too nebulous. The importance of age, preoperative cervical alignment, disease type, number and location of laminae excised, and degree of facet violation must be specified (40).

The occurrence of postlaminectomy deformity in children is well recognized, with the highest incidence occurring in the cervical spine (6,8,12,43,73,81,82). In reviewing 89 children who underwent cervical laminectomy, Bell et al. found a 37% incidence of kyphosis and a 15% incidence of hyperlordosis (8). When laminectomy was

J. G. Heller, M.D.: Associate Professor, Department of Orthopaedic Surgery, Emory University School of Medicine, Decatur, Georgia 30033.

D. Hal Silcox III: Assistant Professor, Department of Orthopaedic Surgery, Emory University School of Medicine, Decatur, Georgia, 30033.

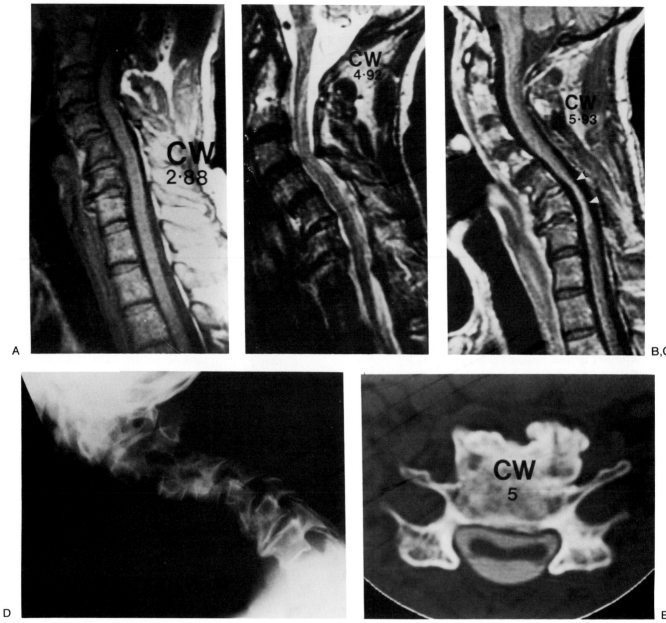

FIG. 1. Postlaminectomy cervical kyphosis. **A:** T1-weighted sagittal MRI of the cervical spine showing anterolisthesis C4-C5, herniated nucleus pulposus C5-C6, and cervical spondylosis C6-C7 prior to treatment. **B:** Follow-up T2-weighted sagittal MRI showing cervical stenosis at C3-C4 and development of cervical kyphosis. **C:** T1-weighted sagittal MRI after C3-C7 laminectomy, with findings of myelomalacia (*arrowheads*) and continued cervical kyphosis. **D:** Standing lateral radiograph of the cervical spine showing severe cervical kyphosis. **E:** Postmyelogram CT of the cervical spine showing flattening of the cervical spinal cord and absence of posterior elements.

F 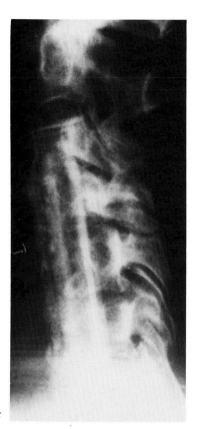 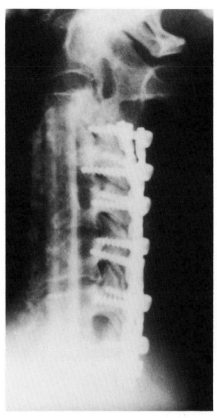 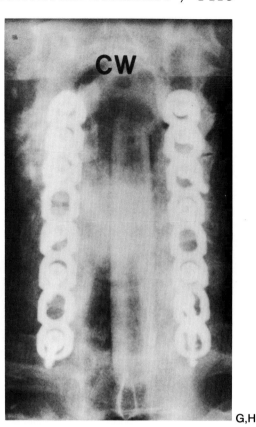 G,H

FIG. 1. (Continued.) F: Lateral radiograph of cervical spine after anterior C4-C7 corpectomies with fibular strut graft. Cervical kyphosis has been corrected. G: Lateral radiograph of cervical spine showing placement of posterior cervical lateral mass plates. H: AP radiograph of cervical spine showing lateral mass plates and C3-T1 fibular strut graft.

combined with suboccipital decompression, Aronson et al. found instability in 95% of operated children (6). Yasouka et al. noted that postoperative kyphosis will develop in children without preexisting deformity or facet violation (Fig. 2). They felt that the evolution of kyphosis and vertebral wedging was a reflection of altered static and dynamic stabilization amplified through their influence on spinal growth and development (81,82). As an alternative approach, Raimondi and co-workers have performed multilevel *en bloc* excision of laminae with reconstruction of the posterior arch, thereby avoiding the risk of kyphosis and the need for fusion (57).

In adults with normal cervical alignment and no preoperative instability, laminar excision alone usually is not associated with a significant incidence of postoperative instability or kyphosis (5). However, finite element analysis (65) suggests that removal of one or more spinous processes and/or ligaments (ligamentum flavum, interspinous ligaments) transfers tensile forces to the facet joints, whereas they normally experience compressive loads (54). The presence of preoperative kyphosis or instability will enhance the probability of progressive deformity or instability (Fig. 1) (39,47,67). Because of disproportionately poor results from laminectomies in patients with spondylotic myelopathy and cervical malalignment, Miyazaki et al. began to include posterolateral fusion in all such cases. They reported improved results with this approach and emphasized the tendency for malalignment to progress when fusion was not performed. In spite of attempted fusion, 50% of their patients developed either new deformity or worsening of preexisting malalignment (48). These results are all the more compelling because their operative technique was a laminoplasty variant in which the majority of the ligamentum flavum was preserved and no facetectomy was performed. Yonenobu et al. (83), in comparing laminoplasty to subtotal corpectomy for cervical spondylotic myelopathy, found 10% of their laminoplasty patients developed kyphosis and 5% developed anterolisthesis of greater than 3 mm despite not performing facetectomies.

The contribution of facetectomy to postoperative instability must be emphasized (45,85). Scoville's assertion that partial or complete facetectomy engendered no risk of instability (66) has been proven false. Fager often performed laminectomy from C1 to T1 without significant postoperative instability; however, he carefully distinguished between laminectomy alone and laminectomy combined with facetectomy (21,22). More recent biome-

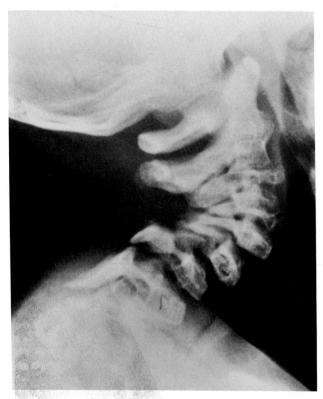

FIG. 2. Cervical kyphosis in a skeletally immature patient after laminectomies at C4, C5, and C6 for arteriovenous malformation.

chanical work by Nowinski et al. (53), which compared multilevel laminectomy and laminoplasty of the cervical spine, found kyphosis was induced by as little as 25% facetectomy. Thus, they felt that multilevel cervical laminectomies deserved serious consideration for prophylactic fusion. The authors further stated that laminoplasty appeared to obviate the need for such prophylactic fusions.

Several other authors have expounded on the problems associated with partial facetectomy in addition to cervical laminectomy (83,53,85). Epstein underscored the importance of the facet's contribution to stability as he emphasized that not more than one quarter to one third of the facet should be removed in foraminal decompression (19). Laboratory data support these clinical deductions. Munechika demonstrated the relative contribution of facets and laminae to spinal stability in monkeys. Laminectomy alone was not associated with deformity when fewer than five laminae were removed; however, a gibbus developed when laminectomy was combined with resection of even one facet joint (50).

Raynor et al. have shown that bilateral facetectomy of greater than 50% significantly reduces resistance to loads in shear (59). His group has also demonstrated alterations in coupled cervical motions secondary to facetectomy that might predispose motion segments to injury or degeneration (58). White et al. demonstrated with flexion loads that clinical instability in horizontal translation is significantly greater following facetectomy (77). Cusick et al. examined the influence of complete facetectomy on cervical stability in compression–flexion loading (16). They noted 32% and 53% reductions in strength with unilateral and bilateral facetectomies, respectively. Zdeblick et al. studied the effect of progressive facetectomy (85) and facet capsule resection (84) on cervical stability. This work is particularly important in that human specimens were tested in axial load, flexion, extension, and torque. Each test was performed on the intact specimen and then repeated after 25%, 50%, 75%, and complete C5-C6 bilateral facetectomy. Facetectomy of greater than 50% caused a statistically significant loss of stability in flexion and torsion (85) (Fig. 3). Similarly, in the study of facet capsule resection, specimens were studied intact and after 25%, 50%, 75%, and 100% C5-C6 bilateral capsule resection. As with facetectomy, 50% capsule resection caused a significant loss of stability.

It had been assumed that the cervical muscle groups contribute little to clinical stability (77). Perry and Nickel demonstrated that severe paracervical muscle pa-

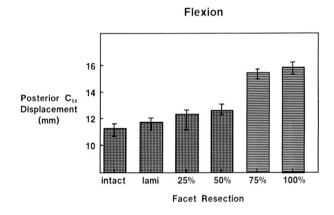

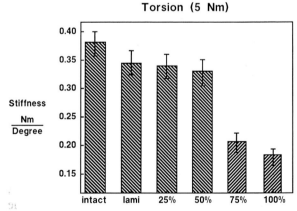

FIG. 3. The effect of progressive facetectomy on cervical spine stability. **A:** In flexion testing, a significant increase in posterior displacement occurs when more than 50% facetectomy is performed. **B:** Likewise, torsion stiffness decreases significantly with more than 50% facetectomy (courtesy Dr. Thomas A. Zdeblick).

ralysis did not necessarily lead to significant instability as long as the bony and ligamentous structures remained intact (56). However, Nolan and Sherk have questioned the validity of these observations. Based on their cadaveric dissections and biomechanical modeling, they reasoned that the semispinalis cervicis and semispinalis capitis groups are primarily responsible for head and neck extension. Because of this presumed dynamic role in stabilizing the head and neck, they recommend preserving the insertion of these muscle groups into the arch of C2 and the occiput whenever possible (52). In an *in vitro* study, Saito et al. (65) found that as the gravitational center of the head shifts forward after posterior laminectomy, kyphosis of the cervical spine is more likely to occur. The tendency towards kyphosis may be potentiated further by denervation or fibrosis of the extensor muscles following posterior procedures. Epstein advocates similar restraint in posterior cervical exposures (19).

In summary, there are many determinants of clinical stability that must be kept in mind during posterior cervical surgery. The extent of soft-tissue stripping is presumed to have potential influence on postoperative stability. Clinical and laboratory data have demonstrated the adverse consequences of excessive facet resection. Preexisting segmental instability or deformity amplify any adverse influence of laminectomy or facetectomy in the adult. Children represent a distinct high-risk subgroup because of their remaining growth potential and relative ligamentous laxity. The judgment to recommend addition of a stabilization procedure at the time of posterior cervical surgery must be based on a thorough understanding of these variables.

POSTERIOR CERVICAL FUSION TECHNIQUES

Subaxial Cervical Fusion

Operative Preparation

For most posterior cervical procedures in which fusion is anticipated, the patient should be positioned prone or in some degree of reverse Trendelenburg position. The sitting position does not allow access to the iliac crests for bone graft harvest. The head and neck are held in appropriate alignment by Mayfield cranial tongs, a halo ring, or Gardner-Wells tongs with a horseshoe headrest. If a halo vest will be used postoperatively, the ring should be applied before positioning the patient, because this gives optimal control of the head and neck and minimizes postoperative manipulation. Adapters are available to rigidly fix most halo rings to the operating table.

With the patient appropriately positioned, lateral radiographs or fluoroscopic images are used to confirm proper positioning. Generous fields should be prepped

for both the primary surgical site and the intended graft donor site. The surgeon must anticipate the need to significantly extend the exposure if required by intraoperative findings. Both iliac crests should be prepped for access in case of inadequate graft from one side or graft fracture.

On-lay Fusion Technique

The fundamental subaxial fusion technique is illustrated in Figure 4. The principles of an on-lay fusion are critical in that they are the cornerstone on which all other techniques build. Without meticulous attention to detail, results will be compromised. The levels to be fused are determined by the variables discussed above. Meticulous subperiosteal exposure proceeds laterally to the edge of the lateral masses, but only over the levels of intended fusion: the facet capsules of unfused segments must not be disturbed. Decortication of the exposed bone surfaces and dorsal articular surfaces is performed with a high-speed burr. Cancellous and corticocancellous strips of iliac autograft are then placed over the decorticated areas. In the presence of a laminectomy, care should be taken not to displace the grafts when closing the wound. Both the cervical and iliac wounds are drained appropriately. A halo vest is recommended postoperatively in most circumstances because the technique does not provide immediate stability.

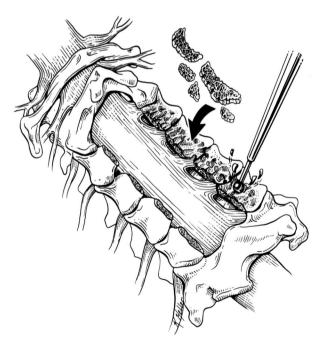

FIG. 4. On-lay fusion technique from C3 to C6. The facet capsules at C2-C3 and C6-C7 must be left intact. A high-speed burr is used to decorticate the lateral masses. Cancellous autograph is then placed over the decorticated surfaces. Care is taken during closure to avoid graft displacement medially.

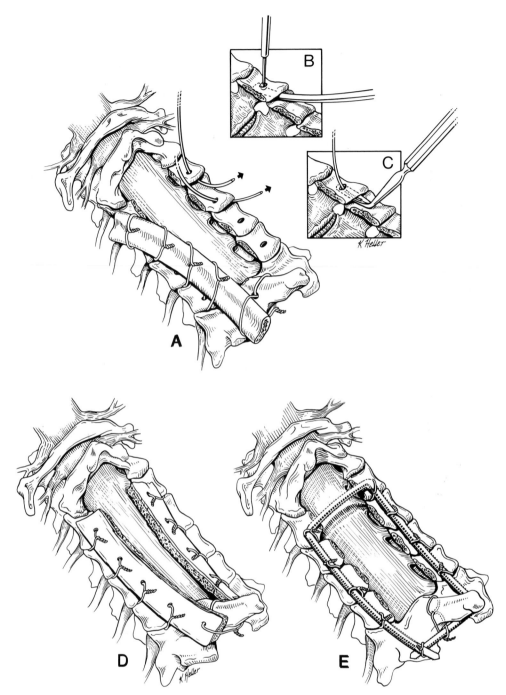

FIG. 5. A–J: Southwick fusion technique. **A:** The facet wiring construct illustrated with a rib graft. Note that the subjacent intact level is included in the fusion. **B:** A high-speed burr is used to drill a hole in each lateral mass. The Freer elevator defines the depth and orientation of each hole and protects against overdrilling. **C:** Passage of each wire is facilitated by an angled dural guide. **D:** A variation of Southwick's original construct in which the wires are passed through drill holes in an iliac strut graft rather than around it. Supplemental cancellous graft is added lateral to each strut. **E:** Metallic implants may be used to enhance segmental stability, especially when bone grafts are mechanically deficient or in the event of malignancy. In this case, a threaded Steinmann pin has been fashioned into a contoured rectangular implant.

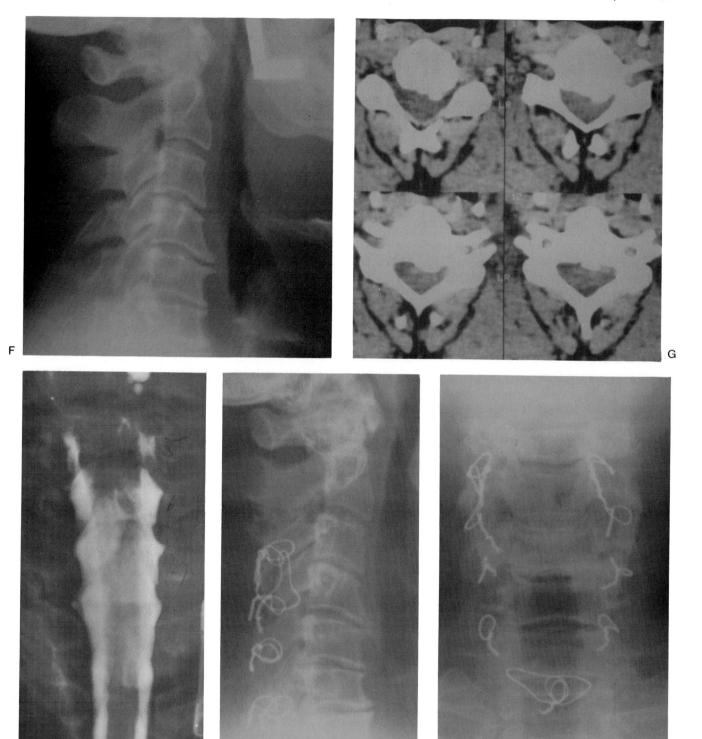

FIG. 5. (*Continued.*) **F:** Lateral cervical spine x-ray in a 52-year-old man showing marked degenerative changes and very early kyphotic reversal of the normal spinal curvature. **G:** Axial cuts in the CT scan at several levels show diffuse spinal stenosis with multiple osteophytic ridging. **H:** Myelogram in the same patient demonstrates spinal cord compression and blockage from C5-C6 up to C3-C4, with three levels involved and the osteophytes extending not only behind the discs, but behind the vertebral bodies as well. **I:** Postoperative film of the same patient after decompressive cervical laminectomy. In addition, posterolateral facet wiring fusion was done in order to immobilize the spine completely, stop the arthritic changes, and prevent further kyphotic deformity. **J:** AP spine x-ray of the same patient shows the wire placement (see Figs. 5B,C). The patient has a long, segmental decompression as well as a stable fusion. The patient did extremely well with complete clearing of his myelopathy and radiculopathy complaints.

Facet Wiring Technique

The Southwick facet wiring technique provides some immediate internal stability in the absence of spinous processes or laminae (11,26,60) (Fig. 5). Figure 5A demonstrates the construct utilizing a rib graft. Southwick preferred iliac crest to rib (11), but he secured his grafts as seen in Figure 5A. Figure 5D illustrates a modified iliac technique, which may increase the strength of the construct. Cancellous graft chips are then placed laterally between the strut grafts and the cervical musculature. The strength of the Southwick technique, and indeed its weakness, has always been the quality of the host bone, both in the graft and at the wire–facet interface (26). Proper positioning of the drill hole will maximize the latter. Graft strength may be poor in the elderly and in patients with connective tissue disease, steroid use, or long-standing spinal cord injuries. When autogenous graft strength is poor, purchase may be enhanced by using segmental fixation to a contoured rectangle fashioned from a threaded Steinmann pin, a stainless steel rod (25) (Fig. 5E), or a Luque rectangle. Bone graft is then applied to all exposed decorticated surfaces, as in the on-lay grafting procedure. Alternatively, if one wishes to avoid metallic implants, allograft bone struts can be used in association with autogenous cancellous bone. In any of the above constructs, postoperative immobilization is recommended (11).

Lateral Mass Plating

As an alternative to wiring, posterior cervical fixation with lateral mass screws and plates was introduced by Roy-Camille and Saillant (62) (Fig. 6). Clinical experience with posterior cervical plating has been encouraging. Reported fusion rates are good, but the studies are all relatively short in follow-up and some are wanting in the evaluation of results and complications (4,23,28, 38,42,51,63,69). A variety of screw insertion techniques have been proposed. Each shares the goal of obtaining screw purchase in the lateral articular mass. Biomechanical studies have documented the efficacy of these constructs compared to standard wiring configurations (14,20,49,72). In most testing modes, posterior plates are equivalent or superior to anterior plates in stabilizing cervical motion segments (14,49,72,75).

In the presence of intact posterior arches and spinous processes, wiring techniques are simple, cost effective, and mechanically sound (16,49,61,71,72,75). However, when the posterior arches are surgically removed or fractured, the wiring techniques may be less applicable. Lateral mass plating restricts fusion to the destabilized or injured segments only, whereas transspinous wiring generally requires extension to one level above and one level below the laminectomized segments (71). Southwick recommended fusing to the first intact level below the decompression (11).

If posterior plating is biomechanically equivalent to the best-known wiring techniques and is able to spare additional fusion levels, why has it not replaced wiring? The procedures are technically demanding with greater inherent risks. In an attempt to define these risks, Heller et al. (30) performed a cadaveric study to compare two competing methods of screw insertion. Figure 7 illustrates the differences between the Roy-Camille and Magerl screw techniques. Each method avoids the central zone ventral to the articular mass through which the exit-

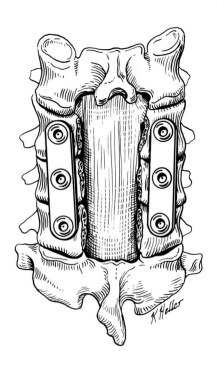

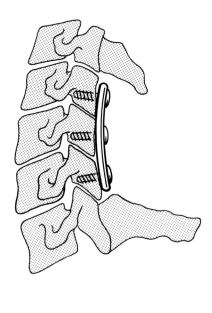

FIG. 6. Roy-Camille plates used for stabilization and fusion from C4 to C6 after laminectomy. Decortication and bone grafting are recommended.

Magerl

Roy – Camille

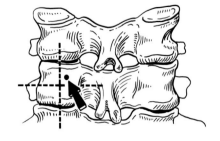
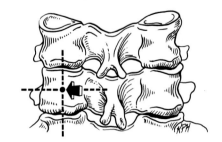

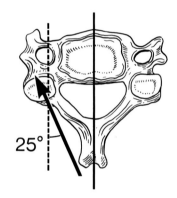
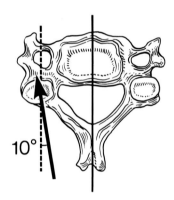

25°   10°

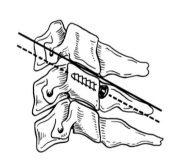
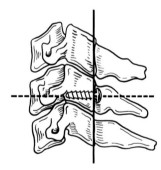

FIG. 7. Comparison of the Magerl and Roy-Camille techniques for lateral mass screw insertion. Magerl's starting point is 2 to 3 mm medial and cephalad to the intersection of lines bisecting the exposed lateral mass. Roy-Camille's starting point is at the intersection of these lines. Magerl then angles the drill 25° laterally and parallel to the surface of the superior articular process. Roy-Camille screws are angled 10° laterally and perpendicular to the posterior vertebral cortex.

ing nerve root traverses. The study demonstrated a learning curve, in that the accuracy of insertion tended to improve with increasing operator familiarity with the procedure and the relevant cervical anatomy. This learning curve was independent of the operators' years of experience with spinal surgery. Heller et al. did not find a statistically significant difference in the rate of nerve root injury between the Roy-Camille and Magerl techniques (2% and 6%, respectively). However, the trajectory of a given screw placed a nerve root "at risk" for injury in 33% of the Magerl screws but only 6% of the Roy-Camille screws. In such a circumstance, injury could have occurred with insertion of too long a screw or past-pointing with a drill (Fig. 8). An et al. have recommended a modified screw trajectory that puts the nerve root and facet at the least apparent risk (2). Thirty-four percent of Roy-Camille screws violated their associated facet joint, whereas no Magerl screw did so (30).

As early reports of posterior cervical plating surface, the complications attributable to these procedures are being defined. Unfortunately, many of these early reports did not elaborate on complications, failing to report on them or their absence (Table 1). Fehlings et al. (23) addressed follow-up and complications associated with lateral mass screw application, but their work was limited in that it evaluated instrumentation of only one or two motion segments (23). A more representative study of the complications associated with posterior cervical plating was reported by Heller et al. (32). They described their results for 78 patients with complex reconstructive procedures averaging 8.4 lateral mass screws per case. Clinically observed complications were compared to the theoretical risks previously reported by Heller et al. (30). They found that nerve root injuries and facet violations occurred much less frequently than predicted (Table 2). There were no spinal cord or vertebral

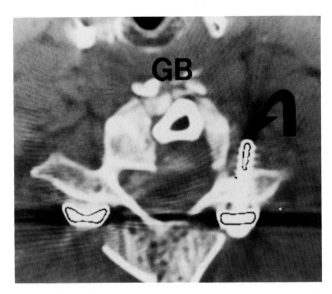

FIG. 8. CT scan of the cervical spine after lateral mass plating. The *arrow* points to the lateral mass screw, which was too long, causing nerve root impingement. This screw was subsequently exchanged for a shorter screw.

artery injuries as predicted in the cadaveric study. Some observed complications, such as an anterior horn cell infarct, implant failure, loss of reduction, wound infection, adjacent segment degeneration, and pseudarthrosis could not have been predicted in the cadaveric study.

A troublesome complication of posterior cervical plating is screw loosening or avulsion that at times causes a loss of reduction. In vitro biomechanical testing has demonstrated variability in lateral mass screw purchase, with a tendency to be weakest at the upper and lower ends of the cervical spine (31). In looking for better ways to purchase the cervical vertebrae, investigators have reported on cervical transpedicular screw fixation. Anatomic studies of the cervical spine have found the lateral masses of C2 and C7 relatively deficient for screw fixation. An et al. (2) described the anatomic dimensions of the pedicles of C2, C7, T1, and T2, and they found these pedicles to be suitable for screw fixation. Work by Xu et al. (80) and Tominaga et al. (74) has further defined the anatomic suitability of the C2 pedicle for screw fixation. In testing the difference in pull-out resistance of cervical lateral masses to that of cervical pedicle screws, Jones and Heller (38) found the strength of pedicle fixation in C2-C7 was significantly greater than lateral masses during uniaxial pull-out. Despite the enhanced purchase of cervical pedicle screws, the clinical feasibility of utilizing the C3 through C6 pedicles is unlikely because of their small size, steep angulation from the midline, and proximity to unforgiving structures. Anatomic and early clinical studies by Jeanneret et al. (37) reported no significant complications, but the number of samples and patients was small. Abumi et al. (1) reported their results with cervical pedicle screw fixation in 13 patients with injuries to the lower cervical spine. They reported no neurovascular injuries due to screw insertion, no implant failures, and no pseudarthroses, although they were not specific about the follow-up time interval.

While cervical pedicle screw fixation appears to be an attractive means of purchasing the cervical spine, the clinical efficacy of this type of fixation remains unknown. Presently, we do not advocate the use of cervical pedicle screws in the mid cervical spine (C3 to C6), but pedicle fixation of C2 and C7, as well as across the cervicothoracic junction to T1 or T2, may be necessary to achieve optimal fixation.

A variety of other plating techniques are available. Figure 9 demonstrates the use of Magerl's hook plate. When the interspinous bone block is properly seated, this technique is biomechanically equivalent to other posterior

TABLE 1. *Compilation of reported complications with the use of lateral mass screws and posterior cervical plates*

Study (ref.)	Heller (32)	Fehlings (23)	Grob (28)	Smith (70)	Levine (43)	Roy-Camille (64)	Jeanneret (38)	Anderson (4)
Number of patients	78	44	33	14	24	197	51	30
Number of screws	654	210						
Nerve Injury	4	0		0	6			0
Iatrogenic foraminal stenosis	2							
Spinal cord injury	2[a]			0				0
Vertebral injury	0	0		0				0
Facet penetration	1							2
Screw loosening	6	8		4				3
Screw avulsion	1	2						
Screw breakage	1							0
Plate breakage	1							0
Adjacent segment degeneration	3		2					
Fusion extension	0							3
Lost reduction	2	3			4	33		0
Pseudarthrosis	1	3	2	0	0			
Infection	1	2		0	3			1

From Heller et al., ref. 32.
[a] Injuries not due to screw placement.

TABLE 2. *Complications encountered with lateral mass screw placement*

Type of complication	Observed cases (%)	Predicted[30]
Directly attributable to screw insertion		
Nerve root injury[a]	4 (0.6)	(≤3.6)
Facet violation[a]	1 (0.2)	(≤3.6)
Vertebral artery injury[a]	0 (0)	(0)
Spinal cord injury[a]	0 (0)	(0)
Neurologic deficit due to other causes		
Spinal cord injury	2 (2.6)	(0)
Iatrogenic stenosis	2 (2.6)	NA
Implant failure		
Broken screw[a]	2 (0.3)	NA
Broken plate	1 (1.3)	NA
Screw avulsion[a]	1 (0.2)	NA
Screw loosening[a]	7 (1.1)	NA
Lost reduction	2 (2.6)	NA
Miscellaneous		
Infection	1 (1.3)	NA
Adjacent segment degeneration	3 (3.8)	NA
Pseudarthrosis[b]	1 (1.4)	NA

[a] From Heller et al., ref. 32. Percentages based on the number of screws (N = 654). All other percentages are based on the number of patients (N = 78).

[b] The denominator for this rate was N = 71, because 3/74 intended fusions could not be reliably assessed prior to patients' deaths.

NA, not available.

cervical plates (72,75). However, this technique has a relative disadvantage: each plate must grasp a portion of an intact lamina at the caudal end of the fusion. Furthermore, it is generally limited to one or two motion segments. The Halifax clamp, which has fallen in popularity

in recent years, (34) also requires an intact lamina above and below the laminectomy level. Despite some authors' claims to the contrary, autogenous graft is always employed with a Halifax clamp. It should be placed over the exposed decorticated surfaces of the lateral masses.

The key to safe insertion of lateral mass screws is a thorough grasp of cervical anatomy and osteology (30). The surgeon should be aware that posterior landmarks are distorted by degenerative disease. Osteophytes should be excised to reveal the true boundaries of the lateral masses. An image intensifier will increase the margin of safety. Pointed, self-tapping screws may increase the risks of nerve root injury unnecessarily and are biomechanically less sound. Therefore, smooth-tipped 3.5-mm cortical screws should be inserted after tapping the drill hole when concerned about host bone quality or purchase strength. Screw purchase should be bicortical (41) as 3.2-mm and larger screws with bicortical purchase have been found to be biomechanically superior (31). As always, care must be taken not to penetrate beyond the ventral cortex of the lateral mass. In some instances, a long, multihole plate is needed for fixation of multiple cervical levels. In these cases, the most superior and most inferior lateral mass screws can be inserted according to conventional landmarks, but the intermediate screws may be difficult to place because the plate restricts the surgeon from achieving the desired starting point on the lateral mass. An et al. (2) implied that the importance is not necessarily the starting point on the lateral mass, but rather the end point of the drill bit and screw. Consequently, the interval screws can be applied by utilizing a fluoroscopic C-arm for a lateral view of the cervical spine, aiming the drill bit towards the root of the transverse process, and directing the drill bit in an appropriate lateral direction.

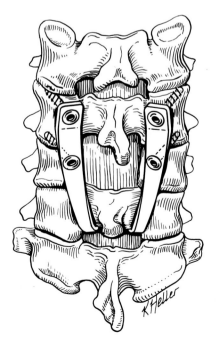

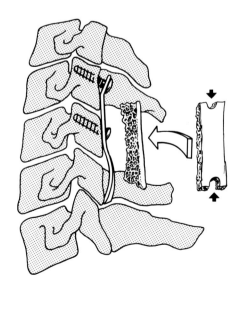

FIG. 9. Magerl's hook plate used for stabilization and fusion from C4 to C6 after C5 laminectomy. A corticocancellous bone block is contoured and fitted into notches in the spinous processes of C4 and C6. The graft blocks overreduction of the facets and increases the construct's stiffness. Cancellous graft is added lateral to the plates.

In circumstances in which the superior articular process of one level is deficient as a result of fracture or excision, other fusion methods can be adapted to maintain anatomic alignment. The use of a "tile plate" is illustrated in Figure 10. This angled plate serves as a prosthetic replacement for the absent superior articular process (63,64). Alternatively, if a subjacent spinous process is present, an oblique wiring technique may be used to supplement the construct of choice (10,16,18,71). Also important to the safe insertion of lateral mass screws is the use of spinal cord monitoring. Care must be taken to ensure that all nerve roots are monitored through the appropriate peripheral nerves at the levels at which lateral mass screws are to be inserted. Heller et al. (32) reported a case of a false-negative somatosensory evoked potentials while inducing a C8 root injury with an excessively long C7 screw. In this case, the median nerve had been monitored but the ulnar nerve was not.

The type of brace to be used after cervical plating must be individualized. In general, these constructs provide immediate stiffness similar to that of the intact spine. Sutterlin et al. demonstrated that these constructs endure short-term fatigue testing. However, they rightly observed that healing of a fusion occurs over months (72), and the properties of screw–plate constructs during such an interval cannot be determined from short-term biomechanical studies (79).

In deciding about postoperative support, it is critical to remember that the quality and duration of fixation depends on the host's bone. Relatively deficient bone requires greater protection until there is radiographic evidence of healing.

Cervicocranial Fusion

Atlantoaxial Fusion

Instability of the atlanto-occipital and atlantoaxial joints can present a difficult problem. With an intact C1 posterior arch, any number of techniques may be used to perform atlantoaxial (71) or occipitocervical fusion (76). When a laminectomy of C1 is required, possibly in combination with a suboccipital decompression, other techniques may be considered. Atlantoaxial fusion must be performed with posterior transarticular screws as described by Magerl (27,44) (Fig. 11). The transarticular screw technique has been found to be superior to Gallie wiring, Brooks Jenkins wiring, and Halifax clamp fixation in biomechanical testing in flexion–extension, rotation, and lateral bend (29). Although 51 consecutive cases have been reported without significant complications (27), Magerl cautioned that this procedure is exacting. The entrance point and trajectory of the screws are critical and difficult to achieve. Intraoperative fluoroscopy is essential. Deviation medially can injure the spinal cord, and lateral deviation threatens the vertebral artery. Failure to angle the screws sufficiently cephalad will compromise purchase in the C1 articular mass; too steep an angle risks injury to the atlanto-occipital joints. Furthermore, examination of a large number of C2 specimens has demonstrated that the size and location of the vertebral arteries within the lateral masses of C2 are quite variable. On occasion, a vertebral artery and its associated venous plexus may fill an entire lateral mass (74,80). Because of these potential problems, careful analysis of thin section computed tomography (CT) scans with appropriate re-formations should identify these high-risk variants. We are aware of only one incident of vertebral artery laceration that was controlled by local measures, without adverse neurological sequelae (3). Magerl does not recommend postoperative immobilization when this technique is used to augment a conventional fusion (27). However, in the absence of a C1 posterior arch, bracing or a halo is probably advisable.

In the absence of a C1 posterior arch there is another alternative to occipitocervical fusion, the Barbour anterior atlantoaxial screw fixation technique (7). The procedure requires bilateral lateral approaches to the upper cervical spine with the application of bilateral transartic-

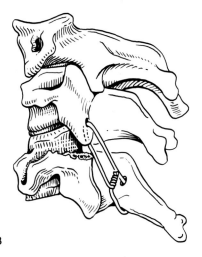
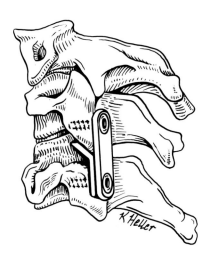

A,B

FIG. 10. Stabilization techniques in the presence of a fractured or resected superior articular process. Rotational and translational stability can be increased by using (**A**) an oblique facet wiring technique or (**B**) a "tile plate" in conjunction with a screw-plate construct.

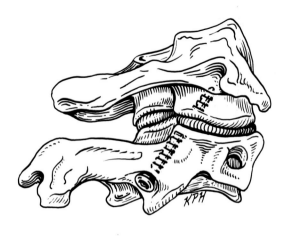

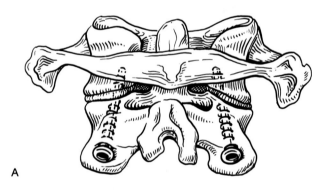

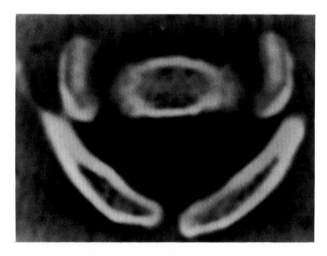

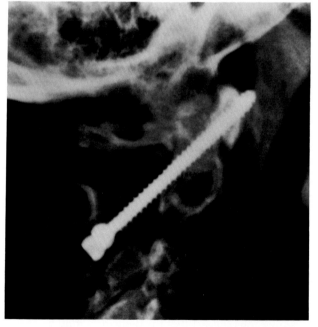

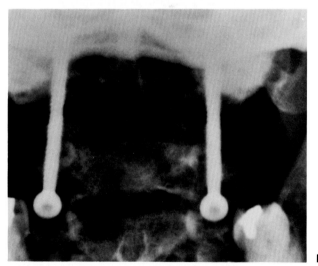

A

B

C

D

FIG. 11. A: Magerl's C1-C2 transarticular screw technique. **B:** CT scan of the cervical spine showing the posterior arches at C1 that failed to form fully. This malformation precludes the use of sublaminar wire techniques for C1-C2 fusion in this rheumatoid arthritic patient with C1-C2 instability. **C:** Postoperative lateral radiograph of the cervical spine showing placement of transarticular screws at C1-C2. **D:** AP open-mouth odontoid radiograph showing transarticular screws at C1-C2.

ular screws. Besides the obvious advantage of preserving atlanto-occipital motion, this procedure allows the surgeon to avoid the previously violated posterior anatomy and place new graft under compression in a highly vascular bed.

Occipitocervical Wiring

Occipitocervical fusion can be made more difficult and less predictable after C1 laminectomy or suboccipital decompression. The diminished bone surface available for fusion is a theoretical concern. Again, standard techniques may be readily adapted to this situation. Figure 12 illustrates the technique of Wertheim and Bohlman (76) (see Chapter 65), except that the C1 sublaminar wire is conspicuously absent. A high-speed burr is used to create a trough on either side of the inion process. The troughs are then connected by undermining the outer cortex with a burr and angled curettes. Care should be taken to preserve the full thickness of the cortical bone. Transspinous holes are prepared in C2 and as many other spinous processes as deemed appropriate. Either 18- or 20-gauge wires or braided cables are then passed twice through each hole to increase their pull-out strength (70). The hazards of passing transspinous wires are well defined (13). Care should be taken in choosing the location of the burr holes and in the passage of the wires. Bone grafts are harvested from the outer table of the iliac crest. Two stout corticocancellous struts are required in addition to a generous amount of cancellous bone. If the patient's iliac bone is unsuitably weak, consideration should be given to using allograft iliac struts supplemented by cancellous autograft. The cancellous bone is used to fill the voids ventral to the strut grafts. In these instances, halo immobilization is required for 3 to 6 months. Alternatively, internal fixation may be added to the standard occipitocervical fusion to avoid halo immobilization (36). Figure 13 illustrates the use of a contoured threaded Steinmann pin to provide additional stability.

Occipitocervical Plating

Posterior occipitocervical plating (Fig. 14) affords rigid internal fixation (28,64,69) and is growing in popularity. Grob et al. (28) and Smith et al. (69) report fusion rates of 94% and 100%, respectively, using posterior plating techniques for occipitocervical fusion. In both of these studies, postoperative immobilization involved the use of a soft or semirigid cervical collar: no halo immobilization was used. No significant complications occurred in these studies, but Grob et al. (28) reported subjacent segment degeneration in two patients that required further surgery.

Methylmethacrylate

The indications for methylmethacrylate stabilization techniques in the cervical spine are well defined (17,46). Such constructs are considered for instabilities secondary to malignancy when life expectancy is less than 1 year. Methylmethacrylate serves well as an anterior load-bearing column, but posterior arthrodesis is frequently recommended for additional stability and durability (17,46). Methylmethacrylate is a grouting material; it does not induce fusion. Adverse biological effects, such as local immune response suppression and infection rates higher than implants, have been associated with methylmethacrylate. In total joint replacement, the cement may be associated with a synovial-like membrane sometimes associated with osteolysis and implant failure. It is for these reasons that we do not recommend the use of methylmethacrylate as a choice for cervical spine fixation posteriorly.

ALTERNATIVES TO THE POSTERIOR APPROACH

The first portion of this chapter has dealt with the recognition of patients at risk for postlaminectomy kyphosis (PLK) and the surgical options available at the time of decompression to stabilize and fuse the cervical spine from a posterior approach. Certainly it is easier to manage such problems by preventing their occurrence. However, patients will be encountered who have developed PLK, possibly in association with other iatrogenic instabilities that require surgical management. Formulating an optimal surgical strategy for such patients requires consideration of anterior procedures as alternatives or adjunctive measures to posterior procedures. Recommendations for surgical management of any particular patient require an analysis of the patient's spinal alignment, its degree of passive malalignment, its degree of passive correctability, and any associated neurological compression.

Passively Correctable Kyphosis

Patients with PLK, with or without associated neurological compression, may have a passively correctable alignment. If flexion–extension radiographs or traction radiographs suggest that the deformity may be passively correctable, then a period of preoperative skeletal traction should be undertaken to see what degree of correction will be achieved. If suitable alignment can be restored, then one has the option of proceeding with the direct anterior reconstruction and stabilization. For patients without neurological compromise, multilevel anterior fusion must be achieved. Multiple levels of ante-

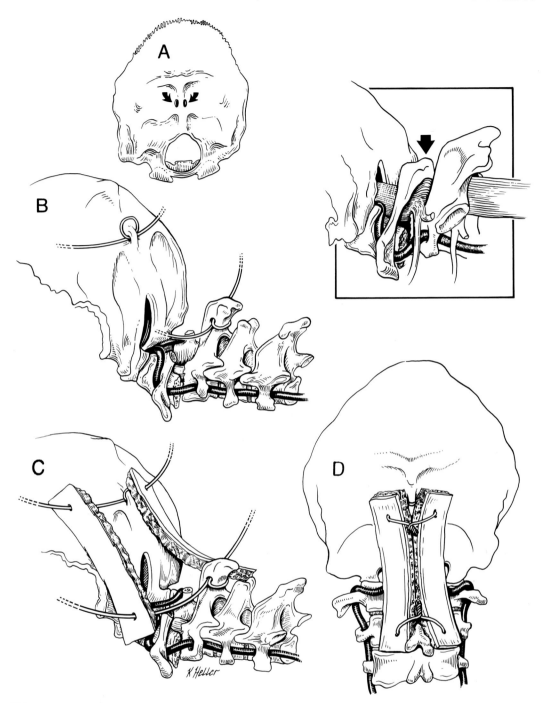

FIG. 12. Occipitocervical fusion technique to stabilize the cervicocranium after C1 laminectomy or sub-occipital decompression. The example is cord compression due to irreducible atlantoaxial subluxation requiring C1 laminectomy (*inset*). **A:** Burr holes on either side of the inion process are connected to provide purchase of the skull by wire. **B:** Transspinous drill holes are made at the appropriate levels. Double looped wires are then passed at each level. **C:** The exposed bone surfaces are decorticated before wiring contoured iliac struts in place. Cancellous graft is used to fill any voids between the struts and the underlying recipient surfaces. **D:** Posterior view of an occiput to C2 construct.

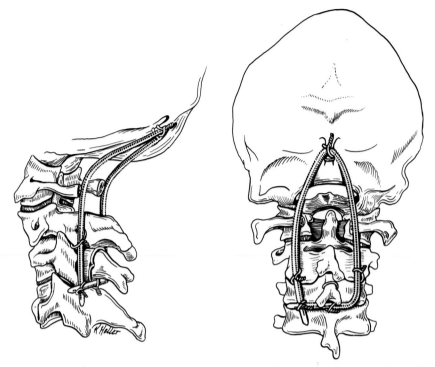

FIG. 13. A contoured threaded Steinmann pin can be wired in place to impart greater immediate stability when autogenous struts are mechanically inadequate. Bone grafting is still performed as in Fig. 12.

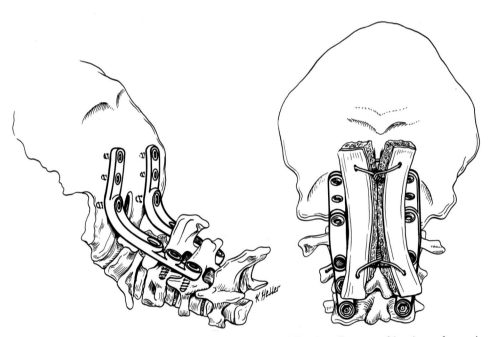

FIG. 14. Roy-Camille occipitocervical plates for rigid internal fixation. Bone grafting is performed as in Fig. 12.

rior interbody fusions with tricortical iliac autografts may be attempted. However, non-union rates tend to be lower if a single fibular autograft strut is utilized (9). The channel cut through the intercalary vertebral bodies must be deep enough and wide enough to accommodate the strut such that it is well seated at both ends. The local cancellous bone from these intervening subtotal corpectomies should be saved, morcelized, and applied to the lateral and end portions of the autograft strut (Fig. 15).

When neurological compromise remains after passive correction of a kyphosis, then decompression must be achieved in association with the reconstruction. Most commonly, corpectomies will be appropriate to ensure adequate decompression. Reconstruction and strut graft should proceed as described above. Local cancellous bone should be saved and utilized because of its enhanced osteogenic potential. We tend to favor the use of iliac crest autograft struts in cases of reconstructions spanning two to three disc spaces. Fibular autograft struts are ideally suited to anterior reconstructions spanning three or more intervertebral disc spaces. The use of allograft struts carries a higher risk of non-union (24). If a surgeon chooses to employ these struts, supplementation with local cancellous graft becomes a greater imperative.

Anterior reconstruction for PLK has an inherently higher non-union risk than such reconstructions done for pathology in the absence of a laminectomy. Accordingly, adjunctive immobilization, whether external or

internal, may be of relatively greater importance in these patients. If supplemental internal fixation is not employed, then halo-vest immobilization is highly recommended. Whether internal fixation obviates the need for a halo or yields net lower non-union rates is unclear. The indications for and contribution of anterior cervical plating requires further study. The first anterior cervical plate systems required bicortical purchase in the vertebral body, placing the spinal cord and nerve roots at potential risk for injury. Fortunately, new systems are available that do not require purchase of the posterior cortex. It remains to be seen whether these constrained plate screw unicortical devices provide adequate fixation for anterior reconstruction in the setting of PLK. Herman and Sonntag (33) reported on 20 patients with PLK treated with anterior corpectomy and plate fixation. All 20 patients had anterior cervical plates applied over an average of 3.8 levels. The authors reported a 100% union rate but did not specify how union was determined. Their patients had a mean residual kyphosis of 16%. A few patients were additionally immobilized using a halo vest. Curtin and Heller (15) compared the fusion results obtained using a halo versus anterior cervical plating versus posterior cervical plating in stabilizing multilevel (more than three levels) cervical corpectomies with strut fusions. They found that three of seven cases utilizing anterior cervical plates were judged to be non-unions on flexion–extension lateral radiographs. Although this study was small, it suggests that the question of efficacy of anterior plating is still unanswered. Interestingly, 100% of the patients who were treated with anterior corpectomy and posterior plate stabilization were judged to be solidly fused (Fig. 16).

As an alternative to anterior reconstruction and plating, consideration can be given to anterior reconstruction followed by posterior segmental instrumentation and fusion. Biomechanical data suggest that such posterior fixation is inherently more stable than anterior fixation. This approach requires considerably longer anesthesia time as well as the inherent difficulty of repeat dissection following cervical laminectomy. Nonetheless, this more aggressive strategy may be well indicated in patients who are considered to be at high risk for non-union. Patients with a compromised healing potential, poor bone quality, malnutrition, steroid-dependent illnesses, or particularly long anterior segmental reconstructions may profit from this more aggressive strategy.

Rigid Postlaminectomy Kyphosis

Rigid PLK present a far more challenging problem. One must first determine whether deformity alone is the problem or whether there is associated symptomatic neurological compression. If deformity is the sole issue, then it must be determined whether the treatment objec-

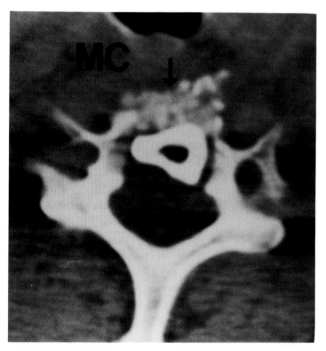

FIG. 15. CT scan of the cervical spine after anterior corpectomy with fibular strut graft reconstruction. The fibular strut graft is augmented with morcelized cancellous bone from the vertebral bodies placed over the fibular strut graft (*arrow*).

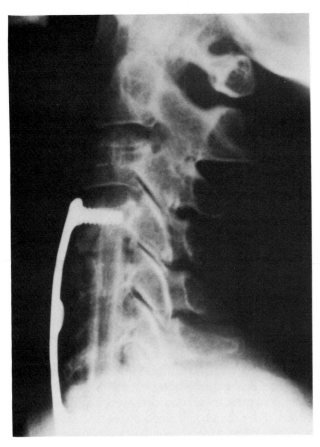

FIG. 16. Lateral radiograph of the cervical spine after anterior corpectomies of C5-C6 with fibular strut graft reconstruction and anterior cervical plate placement from C4 to C7.

tive is to simply stabilize the deformity or to correct it. Arresting a progressive kyphosis in the absence of neurological compromise is a matter of achieving arthrodesis over the involved segments. Any one of a number of the anterior and posterior strategies described above will suffice. More commonly, such PLK cases come to medical attention because of either unacceptable deformity or associated neurological compression. As the neurological compromise is anterior, then some component of the surgical strategy will involve anterior decompression. Once again, whether decompression alone with reconstruction is appropriate or whether to pursue restoration of normal alignment is a matter of the degree of malalignment and physician judgment. The most challenging circumstance arises when multisegmental decompression and realignment are to be achieved for a rigid PLK.

When cases of PLK do not passively correct with flexion–extension views or traction, one must determine why they are rigid. It is possible that the posterior facet joints have ankylosed. In such cases, correction cannot be achieved until the ankylosed posterior elements have been released. In this case, the first stage would usually require multiple posterior osteotomies prior to an anterior procedure that releases the tethering of the anterior column in the process of the decompression. The deformity may then be corrected and the second-stage anterior procedure may be employed to achieve reconstruction and stabilization. The factors influencing the judgment to use supplemental internal fixation with or without halo immobilization are as noted above.

In the event that the posterior facet joints are not ankylosed, the surgeon may wish to proceed directly to anterior decompression, intraoperative reduction of deformity, and reconstruction. Under such circumstances, the procedure begins with complete discectomy procedures over the involved segments so that the lateral extreme of the uncovertebral joints is fully defined. As much of the anterior and lateral annulus as possible must be resected. Unlike deformity surgery in the lumbar and thoracic spine, circumferential resection of the annulus is probably ill advised in the cervical spine. The proximity of the vertebral arteries and their surrounding venous plexus are problematic in releasing the posterolateral portions of the cervical annulus. In either case, if these discectomies and releases are performed at the beginning of the procedure, then proper orientation to the midline is achieved and maintained for the purposes of decompression. Also, intraoperative skull-tong traction and/or the use of an intraoperative vertebral interbody distraction device can facilitate stretching of the residual annulus and optimization of cervical alignment. Once the spinal cord and nerve roots are decompressed, reconstruction proceeds according to the same options noted above. When decompression is not necessary, the posterior cortical walls of the vertebral bodies are usually preserved to facilitate additional surface for union between the graft and host vertebra. Local cancellous bone is saved and used to supplement or to promote more rapid healing of the strut. The decision to use supplemental anterior plating and/or a second-stage posterior fusion procedure must be individualized.

When neurological compression occurs in the presence of a mild but evolving PLK, intervention should be undertaken to relieve the compression, but correction of the deformity may not be necessary. This circumstance most commonly arises in cervical spondylosis initially treated with a laminectomy. If the evolution of kyphosis is appreciated early enough, then anterior decompression and fusion with one-stage reconstruction is the treatment of choice (Fig. 17). Reduction of kyphosis becomes a secondary goal in such procedures, as the reduction is a substantial intraoperative risk necessary to correct a minor deformity and probably unwarranted.

Occasionally, more complicated circumstances may arise wherein a patient has been arthrodesed in kyphosis and is experiencing progressive deformity and/or neurological symptoms (Fig. 18). In such circumstances, it may be excessively hazardous to try to osteotomize

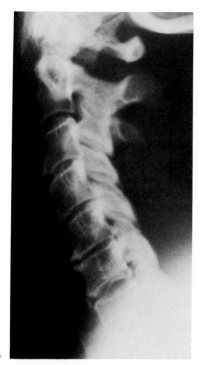

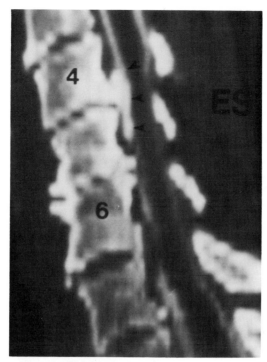

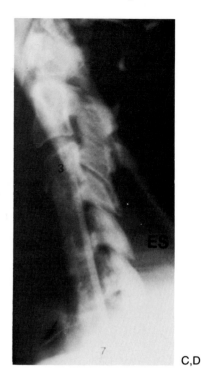

A

C,D

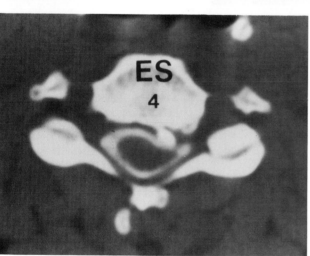

B

FIG. 17. Lateral radiograph of the cervical spine after laminectomy of C4, C5, and C6 with relative kyphosis. This patient persisted in having myelopathic symptoms after posterior decompression. **B:** Postmyelogram CT of the cervical spine shows ossification of the posterior longitudinal ligament displacing the spinal cord. **C:** Sagittal reconstructions of the postmyelogram CT scan of the cervical spine showing ossification of the posterior longitudinal ligament at the C4-C5 level with continued cervical stenosis from C4 to C7. **D:** Lateral radiograph of the cervical spine after anterior cervical corpectomies of C4, C5, and C6 with fibular strut graft reconstruction.

multiple previously fused levels. This is particularly the case if the arthrodesis has been done both anteriorly and posteriorly by the previous surgeons. In such cases, one may wish to compromise by performing a realigning osteotomy at an appropriate segment below the deformity. The magnitude of the correction obtained with the osteotomy should be sufficient to restore spinal balance, with an attempt to achieve alignment so that the spinal cord is no longer draped over the kyphosis. Cervicothoracic osteotomies are similar in concept to those done for ankylosing spondylitis; unfortunately one cannot count on fracture through the disc space anteriorly as is commonly done with a single-stage posterior osteotomy in ankylosing spondylitis. Therefore, the first stage requires anterior discectomy at the intended level of the osteotomy. A generous amount of cancellous autograft should be placed into and around the site of the discectomy so that a suitable amount of bone graft is present once the osteotomy and realignment are done from behind. The second-stage procedure is as described by Simmons (68) for cervicothoracic osteotomy. The planned resection of the posterior elements should be based on degrees of correction desired and must remove enough of the posterior elements so that iatrogenic foraminal stenosis and dorsal cord compression are not created as the osteotomy is extended to the desired position. Simmons recommended varied halo-cast or halo-vest immobilization of ankylosing spondylitics following such osteotomies (68).

We support rigid posterior internal fixation spanning at least two to three levels above and below the osteotomy. Fluoroscopically assisted pedicle screw insertion is recommended in the upper thoracic spine. Fixation in

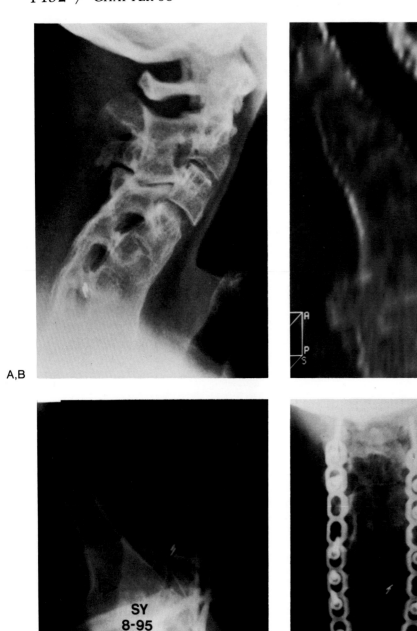

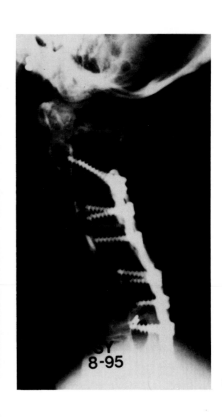

A,B

C

D,E

FIG. 18. A: Standing lateral radiograph of the cervical spine showing postlaminectomy cervical kyphosis with solid arthrodesis at C2-C3 and C4-C7, with pseudarthrosis at C3-C4. **B:** Sagittal reconstruction of a CT scan of the cervical spine postoperatively. The *arrow* points to morcelized cancellous bone placed in the anterior cervical discectomy site of C7-T1. Note the lordosis created at the C7-T1 segment due to the closing wedge osteotomy posteriorly at C7-T1. **C:** Follow-up lateral radiograph showing posterior cervical plates and lateral mass screws. **D:** Swimmer's view lateral of the cervical spine showing pedicle screws in T1-T3. *Open arrow* points to the healed C7-T1 discectomy/fusion site. *Closed arrows* point to the anterior aspect of the cervical and thoracic spine. **E:** Follow up AP radiograph showing posterior cervical plate fixation.

the cervical spine generally requires multiple lateral mass screws. The decision as to what kind of supplemental external immobilization to use must be a matter of judgment, taking into account patient compliance, healing potential, stability of the internal fixation, and bone quality. At a minimum, a cervicothoracic orthosis with a long thoracic extension should be used. If there is any concern that this would be insufficient, then halo-vest immobilization is recommended.

CONCLUSION

PLK may be one of the most challenging problems in spine surgical management. Obviously, prevention of the deformity is the optimal strategy for physician and patient alike. For those patients with multiple risk factors for evolution of PLK, stabilization at the time of their laminectomy is recommended. Any of the posterior techniques described above may be suitable in a particular circumstance. The choice of technique should be based on the evaluation of the patient's local anatomy and surgeon experience and comfort with the various options. In the event that PLK has evolved and requires treatment, management strategies must be based on an appreciation of the presence or absence of neurological compromise, the passive correctability or the deformity, local anatomic considerations, and the patient's healing potential. Such problems are technically demanding and warrant care by surgeons highly experienced in these matters. Patients and their family members should be counselled appropriately with regard to the inherent risks of the treatment.

REFERENCES

1. Abumi K, Itoh H, Taneichi H, Kaneda K (1994): Transpedicular screw fixation for traumatic lesions of the middle and lower cervical spine: description of the techniques and preliminary report. *J Spinal Dis* 7:19–28.
2. An HS, Gordin R, Renner K (1991): Anatomic considerations for plate–screw fixation of the cervical spine. *Spine* 16:S548–S551.
3. Anderson PA (1995). [*Unpublished.*]
4. Anderson PA, Henley MB, Grady MS, Montesano PX, Winn HR (1991): Posterior cervical arthrodesis with AO reconstruction plates and bone graft. *Spine* 16(S):72–79.
5. Aronson DD, Filtzer DK, Bagan M (1968): Anterior cervical fusion by the Smith-Robinson approach. *J Neurosurg* 29:397–404.
6. Aronson DD, Kahn RJ, Canady A (1989): *Cervical spine instability following suboccipital decompression and cervical laminectomy for Arnold-Chiari syndrome (abstr).* Presented at the 56th annual meeting of the American Academy of Orthopaedic Surgeons, Las Vegas.
7. Barbour JR (1971): Screw fixation in fracture of the odontoid process. *S Aust Clin* 5:20–24.
8. Bell DF, Walker JL, O'Connor G, Tibshirani R (1994): Spinal deformity after multiple-level cervical laminectomy in children. *Spine* 4:406–411.
9. Bernard TN, Whitecloud TS (1987): Cervical Spondylotic myelopathy and myeloradiculopathy. *Clin Orthop* 221:149–164.
10. Branch CL, Kelly DL, Davis CH, McWhorter JM (1989): Fixation of fractures of the lower cervical spine using methylmethacrylate

11. Callahan RA, Johnson RM, Margolis RN, Keggi KJ, Albright JA, Southwick WO (1977): Cervical facet fusion for control of instability following laminectomy. *J Bone Joint Surg* 59:991–1002.
12. Cattell HS, Clark GL (1977): Cervical kyphosis and instability following multiple laminectomies in children. *J Bone Joint Surg* 59:991–1002.
13. Coe JD, Simpson MB (1989): *Potential neurological hazards with interspinous wiring in the cervical spine (abstr).* Presented at the 17th annual meeting of the Cervical Spine Research Society, New Orleans.
14. Coe JD, Warden KE, Sutterlin CE, McAfee PC (1989): Biomechanical evaluation of cervical spinal stabilization methods in a human cadaveric model. *Spine* 14:1123–1131.
15. Curtin S, Heller JG (1995): (*unpublished*).
16. Cusick JF, Yoganandan N, Pintar F, Myklebust J, Hussain H (1988): Biomechanics of cervical spine facetectomy and fixation techniques. *Spine* 13:808–812.
17. Dunn EJ (1977): The role of methylmethacrylate in the stabilization and replacement of tumors of the cervical spine: a project of the Cervical Spine Research Society. *Spine* 2:15–24.
18. Edwards EC, Matz SO, Levins A (1985): The oblique wiring technique for ratational injuries of the cervical spine. *Trans Orthop* 9:142.
19. Epstein JA (1988): The surgical management of cervical spinal stenosis, spondylosis, and myeloradiculopathy by means of the posterior approach. *Spine* 13:864–869.
20. Errico T, Uhl R, Cooper P, Casar R, McHenry T (1992): Pullout strength comparison of two methods of orienting screw insertion in the lateral masses of the bovine cervical spine. *J Spinal Dis* 4:459–463.
21. Fager CA (1973): Results of adequate posterior decompression in the relief of spondylotic cervical myelopathy. *J Neurosurg* 38:684–692.
22. Fager CA (1977): Management of cervicaldisc lesions and spondylosis by posterior approaches. *Clin Neurosurg* 24:488–507.
23. Fehlings MG, Cooper PR, Errico TJ (1994): Posterior plates in the management of cervical instability: long-term results in 44 patients. *J Neurosurg* 81:341–349.
24. Fernyhough JC, White JI, Larocca H (1991): Fusion rates in multilevel cervical spondylosis comparing allograft fibula with autograft fibula in 126 patients. *Spine* 16:S561–S564.
25. Garfin SR, Moore MR, Marshall LF (1988): A modified technique for cervical facet fusion. *Clin Orthop* 230:149–153.
26. Goel VK, Clark CR, Harris KG, Kim YE, Schulte MR (1989): Evaluation of effectiveness of a facet wiring technique: an in vitro biomechanical investigation. *Ann Biomed Eng* 17:115–126.
27. Greenfield GQ Jr, Jeanneret B, Magerl F (1989): *Transarticular screw fixation for atlanto-axial instability (abstr).* Presented at the 56th annual meeting of the American Academy of Orthopaedic Surgeons, Las Vegas.
28. Grob D, Dvorak J, Panjabi MM, Antinnes JA (1994): The role of plate and screw fixation in occipitocervical fusion in rheumatoid arthritis. *Spine* 19:2545–2551.
29. Hanson PB, Montesano PX, Sharkey NA, Rauschning W (1991): Anatomic and biomechanical assessment of transpedicular screw fixation for atlantoaxial instability. *Spine* 16:1141–1145.
30. Heller JG, Carlson GD, Abitbol JJ, Garfin SR (1991): Anatomic comparison of the Roy-Camille and Magerl techniques for screw placement in the lower cervical spine. *Spine* 16(S):552–557.
31. Heller JG, Estes B (1996): *Cervical lateral mass screws: biomechanical study of variables affecting pull-out strength. J Bone Joint Surg* [*in press*]
32. Heller JG, Silcox DH III, Sutterlin CE (1995): Complications of posterior cervical plating. *Spine* 20(22):2442–2448.
33. Herman JM, Sonntag VKH (1994): Cervical corpectomy and plate fixation for postlaminectomy kyphosis. *J Neurosurg* 80:963–970.
34. Holness RO, Huestis WS, Howes WJ, Langille RA (1984): Posterior stabilization with an interlaminar clamp in cervical injuries: technical note and review of the long term experience with the method. *Neurosurgery* 14:318–322.
35. Huelke DF, Nusholtz GS (1986): Cervical biomechanics: a review of the literature. *J Orthop Res* 4:232–245.

and wire: technique and results in 99 patients. *Neurosurgery* 25:503–513.

36. Itoh TI, Tsuji H, Katoh Y, Yonezaw AT, Kitagawa H (1988): Occipito-cervical fusion reinforced by Luque's segmental spinal instrumentation for rheumatoid arthritis. *Spine* 13:1234–1238.

37. Jeanneret B, Gebhard JS, Magerl F (1994): Transpedicular screw fixation of articular mass fracture-separation: results of an anatomical study and operative techinque. *J Spinal Dis* 7:222–229.

38. Jeanneret B, Magerl F, Ward EH, Ward J-CH (1991): Posterior stabilization of the cervical spine with hook plates. *Spine* 16:S56–S63.

38a. Jones L, Heller JG, Silcox DH (1996): Cervical pedicle screws versus lateral mass screws: a biomechanical comparison and anatomic feasibility. Presented at the 63rd Annual Meeting of the American Academy of Orthopaedic Surgeons, Atlanta, Georgia, February 23.

39. Kamioka Y, Yamamoto H, Tani T, Ishida K, Sawamoto T (1989): Postoperative instability of cervical OPLL and cervical radiculopathy. *Spine* 14:1177–1183.

40. Katsumi Y, Honma T, Nakamura T (1989): Analysis of cervical instability resulting from laminectomies for removal of spinal cord tumor. *Spine* 14:1172–1176.

41. Krag MH (1990): Spinal Instrumentation: biomechanics of transpedicle spinal fixation. In: Weinstein JN, Wiesel SW, eds. *The lumbar spine*. Philadelphia: WB Saunders, pp. 916–940.

42. Levine AM, Mazel C, Roy-Camille R (1992): Management of fracture separations of the articular mass using posterior cervical plating. *Spine* 17:S447–S454.

43. Lonstein JE (1977): Post-laminectomy kyphosis. *Clin Orthop* 128:93–100.

44. Magerl F, Seemann P (1985): Stable posterior fusion of the atlas and axis by transarticular screw fixation. In: Kehr P, Weidner A, eds. *Cervical spine I*. New York: Springer-Verlag.

45. Mayfield FH (1965): Cervical spondylosis: a comparison of the anterior and posterior approaches. *Clin Neurosurg* 13:181–188.

46. McAfee PC, Bohlman HH, Ducker T (1986): Failure of stabilization of the spine with methylmethacrylate: a retrospective analysis of twenty four cases. *J Bone Joint Surg* 68(A):1145–1157.

47. Mikawa Y, Shikata J, Tamamuro T (1987): Spinal deformity and instability after multilevel cervical laminectomy. *Spine* 12:6–11.

48. Miyazaki K, Tada K, Matsuda Y, Oluno M, Yasuda T, Murakami H (1989): Posterior extensive simultaneous multisegment decompression with posterolateral fusion for cervical instability and kyphotic and/or S-shaped deformities. *Spine* 14:1159–1170.

49. Montesano PX, Juach EC, Anderson PA, Benson DR, Hanson PB (1991): Biomechanics of cervical spine internal fixation. *Spine* 16(S):11–16.

50. Munechika Y (1973): Influence of laminectomy on the stability of the spine: an experimental study with special reference to the extent of laminectomy and the resection of the intervertebral joint. *J Jap Orthop Assn* 47:111–125.

51. Nazarian SM, Louis RP (1991): Posterior internal fixation with screw plates in traumatic lesions of the cervical spine. *Spine* 16:S64–S71.

52. Nolan JP, Sherk HH (1988): Biomechanical evaluation of the extensor musculature of the cervical spine. *Spine* 13:9–11.

53. Nowinski GP, Visarious H, Nolte LP, Herkowitz HN (1993): A biomechanical comparison of cervical laminaplasty and cervical laminectomy with progressive facetectomy. *Spine* 18:1995–2004.

54. Pal GP, Sherk HH (1988): The vertical stability of the cervical spine. *Spine* 13:447–449.

55. Panjabi MM, Summer DJ, Pelker RR, Videman T, Friedlaender GE (1986): Three-dimensional load-displacement curves due to forces on the cervical spine. *J Orthop Res* 4:151–152.

56. Perry J, Nickel VL (1959): Total cervical spine fusion for neck paralysis. *J Bone Joint Surg* 41:37–60.

57. Raimondi AJ, Gutierrez FA, Dirocco C (1976): Laminotomy and total reconstruction of the posterior spinal arch for spinal canal surgery in childhood. *J Neurosurg* 45:555–560.

58. Raynor RB, Moskovich R, Zidel P, Pugh J (1987): Alterations in primary and coupled neck motions after facetectomy. *Neurosurgery* 21:681–687.

59. Raynor RB, Pugh J, Shapiro I (1985): Cervical facetectomy and its effect on spine strength. *J Neurosurg* 63:278–282.

60. Robinson RA, Southwick WO (1960): Indication and techniques for early stabilization of the neck in some fracture dislocations of the cervical spine. *South Med J* 53:565–579.

61. Rogers WA (1957): Fractures and dislocations of the cervical spine. *J Bone Joint Surg* 39A:341–376.

62. Roy-Camille R, Saillant G (1972): Chirurgie du rachis cervical. *Nouv Presse Med* 1:2707–2709.

63. Roy-Camille R, Saillant G, Laville C, Benazet JP (1992): Treatment of lower cervical spinal injuries—C3 to C7. *Spine* 17(S):442–446.

64. Roy-Camille R, Saillant G, Mazel C (1989): Internal fixation of the unstable cervical spine by a posterior osteosynthesis with plates and screws. In: Sherk HH, Dunn EJ, Eismont FJ, et al., eds. *The cervical spine*. Philadelphia: JB Lippincott, pp. 390–403.

65. Saito T, Yamamuro T, Shikata J, Oka M, Tsutsumi S (1991): Analysis and prevention of spinal column deformity following cervical laminectomy. I. Pathogenetic analysis of postlaminectomy deformities. *Spine* 16:494–502.

66. Scoville WB (1961): Cervical spondylosis treated by bilateral factectomy and laminectomy. *J Neurosurg* 18:423–428.

67. Sim FH, Svien HJ, Bickel WH, Janes JM (1974): Swan-neck deformity following extensive cervical laminectomy: a review of twenty-one cases. *J Bone Joint Surg* 56A:564–580.

68. Simmons EH (1992): Ankylosing spondylitis: surgical considerations. In: Rothman RH, Simeone FA, eds. *The spine*. Philadelphia: WB Saunders, pp. 1447–1511.

69. Smith MD, Anderson P, Grady MS (1993): *Occipitocervical arthrodesis using contoured plate fixation: an early report on a versatile fixation technique (abstr)*. Spine Palm Desert, CA: 1984–1990.

70. Stambrough JL, Jauch EC, Norrgran CL (1989): *Posterior spinous process wiring in the cervical spine (Abstr)*. Presented at the 17th annual meeting of the Cervical Spine Research Society, New Orleans.

71. Stauffer ES (1988): Wiring techniques of the posterior cervical spine for the treatment of trauma. *Orthopaedics* 11:1543–1548.

72. Sutterlin CE, Mcafee PC, Warden KE, Rey RM, Farey ID (1988): A biomechanical evaluation of cervical spinal stabilization methods in a bovine model: static and cyclical loading. *Spine* 13:795–802.

73. Taddonio RF, King AG (1982): Atlantoaxial rotatory fixation after decompressive laminectomy: a case report. *Spine* 7:540–544.

74. Tominaga T, Dickman CA, Sonntag VKH, Coons S (1995): Comparative anatomy of the baboon and the human cervical spine. *Spine* 20:131–137.

75. Ulrich C, Woersdoerfer O, Claes L, Magerl F (1987): Comparative study of the stability of anterior and posterior cervical spine fixation procedures. *Arch Orthop Trauma Surg* 106:226–231.

76. Wertheim SB, Bohlman HH (1987): Occipitocervical fusion: indications, technique, and long-term results in thirteen patients. *J Bone Joint Surg* 69(A):833–836.

77. White AA, Johnson RM, Panjabi MM, Southwick WO (1988): Biomechanical analysis of clinical stability in the cervical spine. *Clin Orthop* 109:85–96.

78. White AA, Panjabi MM (1988): Biomechanical considerations in the surgical management of cervical spondylotic myelopathy. *Spine* 13:856–860.

79. Whitehall R, Barry JC (1985): The evolution of stability in cervical spinal constructs using either autogenous bone graft or methylmethacrylate cement. *Spine* 10:32–41.

80. Xu R, Nadaud MC, Ebraheim NA, Teasting RA (1995): Morphology of the second cervical vertebra and the posterior projection of the C2 pedicle. *Spine* 20:259–263.

81. Yasouka S, Peterson HA, Laws ER, MacCarty CS (1995): Pathogenesis and prophylaxis of postlaminectomy deformity of the spine after multiple level laminectomy: difference between children and adults. *Neurosurgery* 9:145–152.

82. Yasouka S, Peterson HA, MacCarty CS (1982): Incidence of spinal deformity after multilevel laminectomy in children and adults. *J Neurosurg* 57:441–445.

83. Yonenobu K, Hosono N, Iwasaki M, Asano M, Ono K (1992): Laminoplasty versus subtotal corpectomy: a comparative study of results in multisegmental cervical spondylotic myelopathy. *Spine* 17(11):1281–1284.

84. Zdeblick TA, Abitbol J-J, Kunz DN, McCabe RP, Garfin S (1993): Cervical stability after sequential capsule resection. *Spine* 18:2005–2008.

85. Zdeblick TA, Zou D, Warden KE, McCabe R, Kunz D, Vanderby R (1992): Cervical stability after foraminotomy: a biomechanical in vitro analysis. *J Bone Joint Surg* 74:22–27.

Subject Index

Subject Index

Note: Page numbers in *italics* refer to illustrations; page numbers followed by t refer to tables.

ISBN 0-7817-0329-8